CONVERSION TO SYSTEME INTERNATIONAL (SI) FOR COMMON SERUM CHEMISTRY DATA

Measurement	SI Unit	Common Unit	Common → SI*	SI → Common*
Albumin	g/L	g/dl	10.0	0.100
Bile acids	μmol/L	mg/L	2.55	0.392
Bilirubin	μmol/L	mg/dl	17.10	0.058
Calcium	mmol/L	mg/dl	0.250	4.00
Carbon dioxide content	mmol/L	mEq/L →ᵐ L	1.00	1.00
Cholesterol	mmol/L	mg/dl	0.026	38.7
Chloride	mmol/L	mEq/L	1.00	1.00
Creatinine	μmol/L	mg/dl	88.40	0.011
Creatinine clearance	ml/s	ml/min	0.017	60.0
Glucose	mmol/L	mg/dl	0.056	18.0
Inorganic phosphorus	nmol/L	mg/dl	0.323	3.10
Osmolality	nmol/kg	mOsm/kg	1.00	1.00
Potassium	mmol/L	mEq/L	1.00	1.00
Protein, total	g/L	g/dl	10.0	0.100
Sodium	mmol/L	mEq/L	1.00	1.00
Urea nitrogen	mmol/L	mg/dl	0.357	2.8

*Factor to multiply to convert from one unit to other.

CANINE *and* FELINE
ENDOCRINOLOGY
and REPRODUCTION

THIRD EDITION

CANINE *and* FELINE ENDOCRINOLOGY *and* REPRODUCTION

EDWARD C. FELDMAN, DVM
Diplomate, American College of Veterinary Internal Medicine
Professor, Department of Medicine and Epidemiology
School of Veterinary Medicine
University of California
Davis, California

RICHARD W. NELSON, DVM
Diplomate, American College of Veterinary Internal Medicine
Professor, Department of Medicine and Epidemiology
School of Veterinary Medicine
University of California
Davis, California

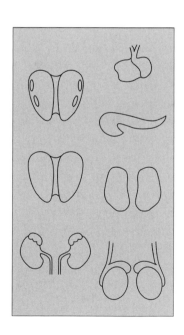

With 850 illustrations

SAUNDERS
An Imprint of Elsevier

SAUNDERS
An Imprint of Elsevier

11830 Westline Industrial Drive
St. Louis, Missouri 63146

CANINE AND FELINE ENDOCRINOLOGY AND REPRODUCTION, THIRD EDITION   0-7216-9315-6

NOTICE

Companion animal practice is an ever-changing field. Standard safety precautions must be followed, but as new research and clinical experience broaden our knowledge, changes in treatment and drug therapy may become necessary or appropriate. Readers are advised to check the most current product information provided by the manufacturer of each drug to be administered to verify the recommended dose, the method and duration of administration, and contraindications. It is the responsibility of the licensed prescriber, relying on experience and knowledge of the patient, to determine dosages and the best treatment for each individual patient. Neither the publisher nor the author assumes any liability for any injury and/or damage to persons or property arising from this publication.

Previous editions copyrighted 1996, 1987

Library of Congress Cataloging in Publication Data
Feldman, Edward C.; Nelson, Richard W.
  Canine and feline endocrinology and reproduction/Edward C. Feldman, Richard W.
    Nelson.—3rd ed.
      p.; cm.
  Includes bibliographical references and index.
  ISBN 0-7216-9315-6
      1. Dogs—Diseases. 2. Cats—Diseases. 3. Dogs—Endocrinology. 4. Cats—Endocrinology.
      5. Dogs—Reproduction. 6. Cats—Reproduction. I. Nelson, Richard W. (Richard William),
  1953-II. Title.
      [DNLM: 1. Dog Diseases. 2. Endocrine Diseases—veterinary. 3. Cat Diseases. 4. Genital
  Diseases, Female—veterinary. 5. Genital Diseases, Male—veterinary. SF 992.E53 F312c 2004]
  SF992.E53F45 2004
  636.7'08964—dc22
                                                                                    2003059096

Acquisitions Editor: Ray Kersey
Developmental Editor: Denise LeMelledo
Publishing Services Manager: Linda McKinley
Senior Project Manager: Jennifer Furey
Designer: Julia Dummitt

Printed in the United States of America.

Last digit is the print number: 9 8 7 6 5 4 3 2 1

DEDICATION

To
our colleagues and clients who have provided us
with cases and supported our work through the years.
Also, with special thanks to our residents, technicians, and students
who have helped perform much of our clinical research
and who refuse to allow us to stop searching for answers

ECF & RWN

To
Kay, Beth Ann, and Christopher

RWN

To
an appreciation for the knowledge that life, like the experience
of the long distance runner, is filled with "trials of miles and miles of trials."
During the initial years since publishing the second edition of this text,
the miles and trials were long uphill battles.
At such times, support and understanding can be a blessing. I dedicate this effort,
in part, to my daughters Rhonda and Shaina, who were not judgmental
and to my family: Bernie, Jack, Judy, Karen, Rebecca, and Mitchell
who were there when I needed them most. Also to my friends who helped level
the trail and make the trials tolerable:
Steve, Pat, Lori, Nancy, Jimmy, Mary, Peter, Thelma Lee, Dick, Kay,
Jennifer, Stefan,
Chuck, Terri, Eli, Meg, Jamie, Marie, & Aunt Anne....

Most importantly,
to Shawn Marie
with you the miles were shorter & they sloped gently downhill, the trials became
lenient. Thank you for providing the energy that allowed me to complete this task
and thank you for teaching me the meaning of beauty, sincerity, and compassion
I cherish you so.

ECF

PREFACE

The goal of the third edition of our textbook on canine and feline endocrinology and reproduction is similar to that of the first two editions: to provide veterinarians with a concise but complete source of information on pathophysiology, clinical signs, diagnosis, and treatment of endocrine, metabolic, and reproductive disorders in dogs and cats. The tremendous expansion of information on these diseases since the last edition prevented us from supplying the profession with an edition that represented "simple editing and minor revisions." This third edition is, once again, a complete revision of the last edition. We did maintain the format of the first two editions but with significant changes and additions that we believe will enhance the clinical usefulness of this resource.

After glancing at the table of contents, the reader will quickly notice that this textbook has been divided into endocrine and reproductive disorders. Two extremely important new chapters have been added to the endocrine section: one on Feline Hyperadrenocorticism, and the other on Feline Diabetes Mellitus. We have long been aware that cats are not small dogs. As our knowledge base regarding cats and their diseases expands, the need for specific information on pathophysiology, clinical signs, diagnosis, and treatment of feline disease becomes distinct and obvious.

This third edition again attempts to emphasize clinically relevant information. Virtually all other chapters have undergone extensive re-writing and updating of material, provision of new or updated tables, addition of new or updated figures and algorithms, and alterations to previously used algorithms that demonstrate our continuing evolution in understanding how to explain disease processes. This same approach was used in determining how to improve our diagnostic strategies while continuing to make them practical, cost-effective, and expedient. Finally, we continue to examine how veterinarians can better manage each endocrine or reproduction condition to achieve longer and healthier lives for the cats and dogs owned by our clients. Treatment recommendations were consistently developed with practicality, cost-effectiveness, and compassionate care in mind. We never want to underestimate the importance of the history, physical examination, and general clinical status of each canine or feline patient.

We hope this book will be of help to veterinary students, practitioners, interns, residents, breeders, and owners. The development of this textbook provided us with a challenging, informative, and laborious but rewarding task. We do not believe that final answers are provided for any subject. We do hope this textbook provides the reader with complete, current, applicable information on endocrine and reproductive disorders of dogs and cats. We do not claim that the information is presented completely without bias. Indeed, our extensive clinical experience creates bias, which we are convinced provides a positive and well established foundation to our recommendations on diagnostic and management strategies.

A book of this nature cannot be produced without the support of many people. Our families have endured another period where we spent nights, weekends, and spare time completing this dream of creating a useful resource for people we do not know, but with whom we share a common love of animals. We wish to offer a sincere thank you to the editorial and production staffs at Saunders and Elsevier and to JoAnn Adams, Allen Reinero, and the others at the University of California—Davis who helped in various ways to make the task easier and the product better.

EDWARD C. FELDMAN
RICHARD W. NELSON

CONTENTS

CANINE *and* FELINE ENDOCRINOLOGY *and* REPRODUCTION

THE PITUITARY GLAND

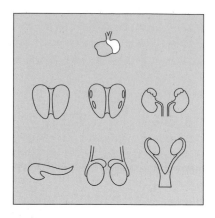

1

WATER METABOLISM AND DIABETES INSIPIDUS

Water consumption and urine production are controlled by complex interactions between plasma osmolality, fluid volume in the vascular compartment, the thirst center, the kidney, the pituitary gland, and the hypothalamus. Dysfunction in any of these areas results in the clinical signs of polyuria and polydipsia. Vasopressin (antidiuretic hormone [ADH]) plays a key role in the control of renal water resorption, urine production and concentration, and water balance. In the presence of vasopressin and dehydration, the average dog and cat can produce urine concentrated to or above 2300 mOsm/kg. In the absence of vasopressin or vasopressin action on the kidneys, the urine may be as dilute as 20 mOsm/kg.

Diabetes insipidus results from deficiencies in secretion of vasopressin or in its ability to interact normally with receptors located in the distal and collecting tubular cells of the kidney. The result of either disorder is impaired ability to conserve water and concentrate urine, with production of dilute urine and compensatory polydipsia. Because of the dramatic polyuria and polydipsia associated with diabetes mellitus and diabetes insipidus, the term *diabetes* was historically used for both conditions. However, the urine is tasteless (insipid) with diabetes insipidus because, unlike in diabetes mellitus (in which the urine is sweet from sugar), polyuria in diabetes insipidus is not the result of a glucose-induced osmotic diuresis.

PHYSIOLOGY OF WATER METABOLISM

OVERVIEW. Plasma osmolality and its principal determinant, the plasma sodium concentration, are normally maintained within remarkably narrow ranges. This stability is achieved largely by adjusting total body water to keep it in balance with the serum sodium concentration. Water balance is controlled by an integrated system that involves precise regulation of water intake via thirst mechanisms and control of water output via stimulation of vasopressin secretion (Fig. 1-1). The major sources of fluid loss from the dog and cat include urine, the respiratory tract, and feces. As long as free access to water is allowed, total body water in humans rarely varies by more than 1% to 2% (Aron et al, 2001). Some of the water necessary to maintain homeostasis is taken in with food; the majority is ingested as water.

The capacity of the kidney to produce concentrated urine plays an important part in maintenance of water balance. Animals eat a diet that produces osmotically active material ultimately excreted in urine, thus requiring water in which to be excreted. The more

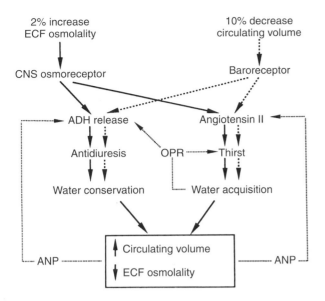

FIGURE 1–1. Schematic illustration of the primary mechanisms involved in maintenance of water balance. Solid lines indicate osmotically stimulated pathways, and dashed lines indicate volume stimulated pathways. The dotted lines indicate negative feedback pathways. *ANP,* atrial natriuretic peptide; *ADH,* antidiuretic hormone; *CNS,* central nervous system; *ECF,* extracellular fluid; *OPR,* oropharyngeal reflex. (From Reeves WB, Andreoli TE: The posterior pituitary and water metabolism. *In* Wilson JD, Foster DW (eds): Williams Textbook of Endocrinology, 8th ed. Philadelphia, WB Saunders, 1992, p 311.)

concentrated urine the kidney can produce, the less water is required to excrete those solutes.

Urine-concentrating mechanisms can reduce but not completely prevent loss of water into the urine. Even if an animal is maximally concentrating urine, obligatory fluid loss is still considerable. This situation is exacerbated in a warm environment, in which significant quantities of fluid may be lost via dissipation of heat through panting. Body fluid can be brought back to normal only through increasing water intake. Not surprisingly, the mechanisms involved in the control

of thirst and of vasopressin secretion have many similarities.

THE NEUROHYPOPHYSIS. The neurohypophysis consists of a set of hypothalamic nuclei (supraoptic and paraventricular) responsible for the synthesis of oxytocin and vasopressin; the axonal processes of these neurons, which form the supraopticohypophysial tract; and the termini of these neurons within the posterior lobe of the pituitary (Fig. 1-2; Reeves et al, 1998). The neurosecretory cells in the paraventricular and supraoptic nuclei secrete vasopressin or oxytocin in response to appropriate stimuli. The neurosecretory cells receive neurogenic input from various sensor elements, including low-pressure baroreceptors located in the heart and arterial circulation and two circumventricular organs, the subfornical organ and the organum vasculosum of the lamina terminalis. These organs lie outside the blood brain barrier and may be important for osmoreception and interaction with blood-borne hormones, such as angiotensin II.

VASOPRESSIN: BIOSYNTHESIS, TRANSPORT, AND METABOLISM. Vasopressin and oxytocin are nonapeptides composed of a six-membered disulfide ring and a three-membered tail on which the terminal carboxyl group is amidated (Fig. 1-3). Arginine vasopressin (AVP) is the antidiuretic hormone in all mammals except swine and other members of the suborder Suina, in which lysine vasopressin is synthesized (Reeves et al, 1998). Vasopressin differs from oxytocin in most mammals only in the substitution of phenylalanine for isoleucine in the ring and arginine for leucine in the tail. The ratio of antidiuretic to pressor effects of vasopressin is increased markedly by substituting D-arginine for L-arginine at position 8. This modification, as well as removal of the terminal amino group from cysteine, yields 1 deamino (8 D-arginine) vasopressin (DDAVP), a synthetic commercially available product (see Fig. 1-3). DDAVP is a clinically useful analogue with prolonged and enhanced antidiuretic activity that does not require injection to be effective.

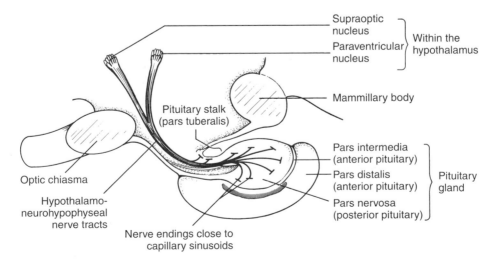

FIGURE 1–2. Schematic illustration of the relationship between the hormone synthesizing areas of the hypothalamus and the pituitary gland

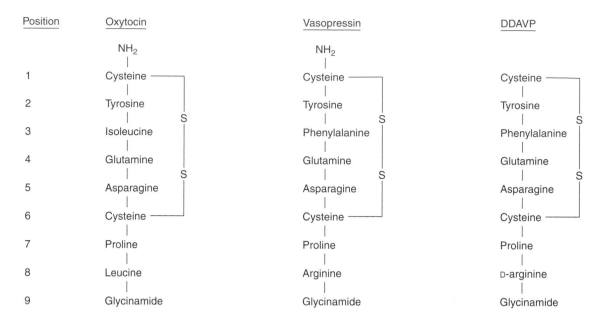

FIGURE 1–3. The chemical structures of oxytocin, vasopressin, and 1 deamino (8 D-arginine) vasopressin (DDAVP).

The production of vasopressin and oxytocin is associated with synthesis of specific binding proteins called *neurophysins*. One molecule of neurophysin I (estrogen-stimulated neurophysin) binds one molecule of oxytocin, and one molecule of neurophysin II (nicotine-stimulated neurophysin) binds one molecule of vasopressin (Reeves et al, 1998). The neurophysin peptide combination, often referred to as *neurosecretory material,* is transported along the axons of the hypothalamo-neurohypophyseal nerve tract and stored in granules in the nerve terminals located in the posterior pituitary gland (see Fig. 1-2). Release of vasopressin into the bloodstream occurs following electrical activation of the neurosecretory cells containing AVP. Secretion proceeds by a process of exocytosis, with release of vasopressin and neurophysin II into the bloodstream. In plasma, the neurophysin-vasopressin combination dissociates to release free vasopressin. Nearly all of the hormone in plasma exists in an unbound form, which because of its relatively low molecular weight, readily permeates peripheral and glomerular capillaries. Metabolic degradation of AVP appears to be mediated through binding of AVP to specific hormone receptors, with subsequent proteolytic cleavage of the peptide (Reeves et al, 1998). Renal excretion is the second method for elimination of circulating hormone and accounts for about one-fourth of total metabolic clearance.

ACTIONS OF VASOPRESSIN. ***Cellular Actions.*** AVP acts via tissue receptors classified as V_1 receptors in smooth muscle and V_2 receptors in renal epithelia (Reeves et al, 1998). Only the latter receptors activate adenylate cyclase. The antidiuretic action of AVP is mediated through V_2 cyclic AMP-dependent receptors, whereas its vasoconstrictive action is mediated through V_1 phosphatidylinositol dependent receptors.

Vasopressin stimulates V_1 and V_2 receptors, whereas the vasopressin analogue, desmopressin (DDAVP), which is commonly used for the treatment of central diabetes insipidus, has a strong affinity for V_2 receptors with minimal pressor (V_1) activity.

The major antidiuretic contribution of AVP is to increase the water permeability of terminal nephron segments or collecting ducts. The effects of AVP are mediated primarily by the intracellular second messenger cAMP (Fig. 1-4). AVP binds to the V_2 receptors of hormone-responsive epithelial cells and activates membrane-associated adenylate cyclase to catalyze cAMP generation from ATP. cAMP-dependent activation of the protein kinase system leads to an increase in the water permeability of the luminal membrane of the cell as a result of insertion of aquaporin-2 water channels into the apical membrane of the epithelial cell. Transmembrane water movement occurs through these water channels, rather than by diffusion across the lipid bilayer or through junctional complexes (Fig. 1-5; Kanno et al, 1995; Lee et al, 1997). In essence, AVP, working via cAMP and protein kinase, alters water transport in hormone-responsive epithelia by causing the microtubule-dependent insertion of specialized membrane units (aquaporin-2 water channels) into the apical plasma membranes of these cells. The increase in water permeability in these segments augments osmotic water flow from the tubular lumen into a hypertonic medullary interstitium, thus providing for maximal urine concentration during antidiuresis (Reeves et al, 1998).

The intracellular concentration of cAMP appears to be the primary factor regulating the cellular actions of AVP. Increased concentrations of cAMP result from either enhanced formation (i.e., stimulation of adenyl cyclase following the interaction of AVP with receptors)

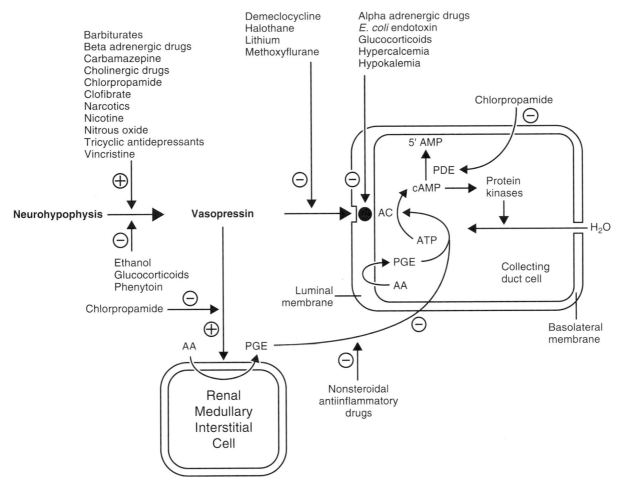

FIGURE 1–4. Effects of selected drugs and electrolytes on vasopressin release and action. *AA,* arachidonic acid; *AC,* adenyl cyclase; *PGE,* prostaglandin E; *ATP,* adenosine triphosphate; *cAMP,* cyclic adenosine monophosphate; *PDE,* phosphodiesterase; *5'AMP,* 5'-adenosine monophosphate. (From DeBartola SP: Disorders of sodium and water: Hypernatremia and hyponatremia. *In* DiBartola SP (ed): Fluid Therapy in Small Animal Practice, 2nd ed. Philadelphia, WB Saunders, 2000, p 52.)

or decreased catabolism. cAMP phosphodiesterase catalyzes the breakdown of cAMP to 5'AMP. Several drugs, hormones, and disease conditions change the renal tubular response to AVP by altering the interaction of AVP with its receptor, the activation of adenyl cyclase, or the catabolism of cAMP.

The collecting ducts convey urine from the distal tubule and collecting tubule to the renal pelvis. As the collecting ducts traverse the renal medulla, the urine within the ducts passes through regions of ever-increasing osmolality, up to a maximum of 2000 to 2500 mOsm/kg of water at the tip of the canine renal papilla. In the presence of vasopressin, collecting duct fluid moves into and equilibrates with this hyperosmotic environment until urine osmolality approaches that of medullary interstitial fluid. Vasa recta distribute absorbed water into the systemic circulation, maintaining the hypertonicity of the medullary interstitium. Vasopressin also increases the permeability of the papillary collecting duct epithelium to urea. Thus urine production is low in the presence of vasopressin and high in its absence.

Clinical Effect. The primary effect of AVP is to conserve body fluid by reducing the volume of urine production (Table 1-1). This antidiuretic action is achieved by promoting the reabsorption of solute free water in the distal and/or collecting tubules of the

TABLE 1–1   ACTIONS OF VASOPRESSIN

Target Organ	Action
Kidney	
Cortical and outer medullary collecting ducts	Enhances water permeability
Papillary collecting ducts	Enhances water and urea permeability
Thick ascending limb of the loop of Henle	Suppresses renin release
Juxtaglomerular cells	
Heart	Bradycardia
Arterioles	Constriction
Brain	Enhances passive avoidance behavior
Liver	Enhances glycogenolysis and fatty acid synthesis
Adenohypophysis (anterior pituitary)	Promotes ACTH secretion

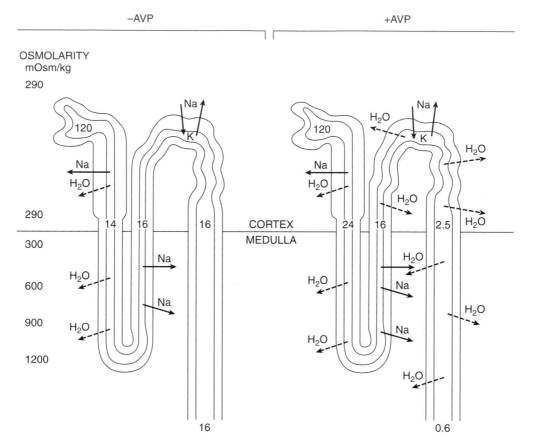

FIGURE 1–5. Schematic representation of the effect of vasopressin on the formation of urine by the human nephron. The osmotic pressure of tissue and tubular fluid is indicated by the density of the shading. The numbers within the lumen of the nephron indicate typical rates of flow in milliliters per minute. Arrows indicate reabsorption of sodium (Na) or water (H_2O) by active *(solid arrows)* or passive *(broken arrows)* processes. Note that vasopressin acts only on the distal nephron, where it increases the hydro-osmotic permeability of tubular membranes. The fluid that reaches this part of the nephron normally amounts to between 10% and 15% of the total filtrate and is hypotonic owing to selective reabsorption of sodium in the ascending limb of the loop of Henle. In the absence of vasopressin, the membranes of the distal nephron remain relatively impermeable to water, as well as to solute, and the fluid issuing from Henle's loop is excreted essentially unmodified as urine. With maximum vasopressin action, all but 5% to 10% of the water in this fluid is reabsorbed passively down the osmotic gradient that normally exists with the surrounding tissue. Remember that the concentration of the canine renal medullary interstitial fluid can be greater than 2500 mOsm/kg. (Reprinted with permission from Frohman LA, Krieger DT: *In* Felig P, et al (eds): Endocrinology and Metabolism. New York, McGraw Hill Book Co, 1981, p 258.)

kidney. In the absence of AVP, the membranes lining this portion of the nephron are uniquely resistant to the diffusion of both water and solutes. Hence the hypotonic filtrate formed in the more proximal portion of the nephron passes unmodified through the distal tubule and collecting duct. In this condition, referred to as *water diuresis*, urine osmolality is low and urine volume is great (see Fig. 1-5).

In the presence of AVP and normal renal receptor activity, the hydro-osmotic permeability of the distal and collecting tubules increases, allowing water to back-diffuse down the osmotic gradient that normally exists between tubular fluid and the isotonic or hypertonic milieu of the renal cortex and medulla. Because water is reabsorbed without solute, the urine that remains within the lumen of the nephron has an increased osmotic concentration, as well as a decreased rate of flow through the tubules. The amount of water

reabsorbed in the distal nephron depends on the plasma AVP concentration and the existence of a significant osmotic gradient in the renal interstitium. Vasopressin does not cause an active (i.e., energy-requiring) reabsorption of solute free water. It merely "opens the water channels" in the luminal membrane to allow water to flow in the direction of the higher osmolality (along the osmotic gradient). In the normal animal, the osmolality of the filtrate entering the distal tubule is low, whereas that of the renal interstitium is high, promoting reabsorption of water when the pores are open. Increasing the renal medullary interstitial osmolality increases the ability to reabsorb water and concentrate urine; thus desert rodents with extremely concentrated medullary interstitium can produce urine more concentrated than that of dogs and are remarkably capable of conserving fluid. Conversely, loss of the renal medullary hypertonicity may inhibit vasopressin's antidiuretic activity (see Fig. 1-5). Decreased medullary hypertonicity (or lack thereof) can result from various causes, such as chronic water diuresis or reduced medullary blood flow. However, because a majority of fluid flowing from the loop of Henle can still be reabsorbed isotonically in the distal convoluted tubule and proximal collecting duct, loss of the hypertonic medullary concentration gradient alone rarely results in marked polyuria (Robertson, 1981).

It should be noted that 85% to 90% of the fluid filtered by the glomerulus is reabsorbed isosmotically with sodium and glucose in the proximal portion of the nephron. Sodium is then selectively reabsorbed from the remaining fluid, making the fluid hypotonic as it reaches the distal nephron. An additional 90% of this remaining fluid can be reabsorbed under the influence of AVP (Robertson, 1981). However, if the oral intake of salt is high or if a poorly reabsorbed solute such as mannitol, urea, or glucose is present in the glomerular filtrate, fluid resorption from the proximal tubule is impaired. The resultant increase in fluid volume presented to the distal nephron may overwhelm its limited capacity to reabsorb water. As a consequence, urine osmolality decreases and volume increases, even in the presence of large amounts of vasopressin. This type of polyuria is referred to as *solute diuresis* to distinguish it from that due to a deficiency of vasopressin action (see Complications of the Modified Water Deprivation Test, page 29). Conversely, in clinical situations such as congestive heart failure, in which the proximal nephron reabsorbs increased amounts of filtrate, the capacity to excrete solute free water is greatly reduced, even in the absence of vasopressin.

The physiologic significance of other vasopressin actions, listed in Table 1-1, is less clear. It has been suggested that the pressor actions of vasopressin are somehow important in the maintenance of blood pressure during hypovolemia. Vasopressin also acts on the gastrointestinal tract and the central nervous system (CNS). The neurophysins have no recognized biologic action apart from complexing oxytocin and vasopressin in neurosecretory granules of the neurohypophysis.

THIRST CENTER. Consumption of water to preserve body fluid tonicity is governed by the sense of thirst, which in turn is regulated by many of the same factors that determine AVP release. The sensation of thirst is controlled by osmoreceptors located close to the AVP synthesizing cells in the hypothalamus. The specificities of the osmoregulation of thirst and of AVP release are similar (e.g., hypertonic NaCl stimulates both thirst and AVP release), whereas hypertonic urea or glucose stimulates neither (Reeves et al, 1998). In spite of the functional similarities of the osmoregulation of thirst and AVP secretion, electrophysiologic studies indicate that they are mediated by two distinct but adjacent osmoreceptors.

REGULATION OF THIRST AND VASOPRESSIN SECRETION. Changes in plasma osmolality and blood volume are the most important mechanisms controlling thirst and vasopressin secretion.

Plasma Osmolality. The most important stimulus for thirst and vasopressin secretion under physiologic

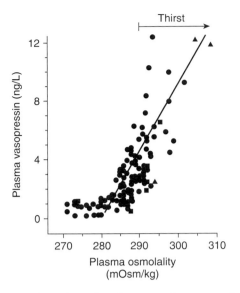

FIGURE 1–6. The relationship between plasma osmolality and plasma vasopressin level. (Adapted from Robertson GL, Berl T: Water metabolism. *In* Brenner BM, Rector FC Jr (eds): The Kidney, 3rd ed. Philadelphia, WB Saunders, 1986, p 385.)

conditions is plasma osmolality. At plasma osmolalities below a certain minimum or threshold value (approximately 280 mOsm/kg), plasma vasopressin is uniformly suppressed to low or undetectable levels. Above this point, plasma vasopressin and the sensation of thirst increase in direct proportion to increases in plasma osmolality (Fig. 1-6). The relationship among thirst, plasma AVP concentration, and plasma osmolality is quite sophisticated. Increases of as little as 1% in plasma osmolality result in stimulation of water intake and vasopressin secretion (Hammer et al, 1980).

The osmoreceptor is not equally sensitive to all plasma solutes. Sodium and its anions, which normally contribute more than 95% of the total osmotic pressure of plasma, are the most potent solutes known to stimulate thirst and vasopressin secretion. Certain sugars, such as mannitol and sucrose, are also effective when administered intravenously. Conversely, an increase in plasma osmolality due to urea or glucose causes little or no direct stimulation of vasopressin secretion. Precisely how and why the osmoreceptor discriminates so effectively between different kinds of plasma solutes are still unsettled. One theory involves the osmotic decrease in cellular water content (i.e., cellular dehydration) created by a given solute, which would depend on the permeability characteristics unique to the osmoreceptor cell membrane. Cellular dehydration occurs when extracellular fluid osmolality is increased by a solute that cannot penetrate cell membranes. This causes water to be withdrawn from cells in an effort to equilibrate the osmotic gradient that is formed. Cellular dehydration, in turn, provides the signal for secretion of vasopressin and consumption of water.

Studies indicate that an important role is also played by the blood-brain barrier, again suggesting unique permeability characteristics. Osmoreceptors appear to be situated in an area of the brain where the blood-brain barrier is deficient and are thus influenced by the composition of plasma rather than cerebrospinal fluid (Aron et al, 2001). Two circumventricular organs, the subfornical organ and the organum vasculosum of the lamina terminalis, lie outside the blood-brain barrier and are believed to be important for osmoreception, interaction with blood-borne hormones (e.g., angiotensin II), and regulation of AVP secretion by neurosecretory cells.

Blood Volume and Pressure. Thirst and AVP secretion may be stimulated by contraction of the extracellular fluid volume without a change in plasma osmolality. Such an extracellular fluid loss may occur secondary to hemorrhage, for example, and results in both increased fluid consumption and vasopressin secretion. Small decreases in volume have little effect on AVP secretion, but any reduction exceeding 10% of the extracellular fluid causes marked stimulation that not only conserves water but may also be important in maintaining blood pressure (Aron et al, 2001).

Volume-mediated release of AVP may occur as a consequence of stimuli arising from "volume receptors," or baroreceptors. Low pressure baroreceptors are located in the venous bed of the systemic circulation, the right side of the heart, and the left atrium, whereas high pressure baroreceptors are located within the systemic arterial system of the carotid sinus and aortic arch (Reeves et al, 1998). The electrical activity of the baroreceptor is related to the degree of stretch in the vessel wall. Increases in pressure and wall tension increase receptor firing rate, whereas decreases in blood pressure or blood volume decrease electrical activity. An inverse relationship exists between baroreceptor electrical activity and AVP secretion; that is, decreased electrical activity of the baroreceptor stimulates AVP secretion. The afferent pathways for the atrial and carotid bifurcation baroreceptors appear to be the vagus and glossopharyngeal nerves, respectively. Electrical activation of the thirst center and neurosecretory cells containing AVP is controlled by groups of neurons located in the anterior hypothalamus near, but distinct from, the supraoptic and paraventricular nuclei.

The renin angiotensin system also participates in the regulation of AVP release. In all animal species studied, angiotensin is an effective dipsogen (thirst stimulant). In addition, particularly in the presence of a raised plasma osmolality, angiotensin may stimulate AVP release by direct action on AVP producing neurons and by stimulating afferent pathways from other regions of the brain. Hypovolemia stimulates renin secretion, which promotes angiotensin formation. The relative roles of the direct baroreceptor input versus angiotensin mechanisms in the thirst response to extracellular dehydration have yet to be determined.

Interaction of Plasma Osmolality and Blood Volume. Normal day-to-day regulation of water balance involves interaction between osmotic and volume stimuli. In the case of vasopressin secretion, decreases in extracellular fluid volume sensitize the release of vasopressin to a given osmotic stimulus. Thus

for a given increase in plasma osmolality, the increase in plasma vasopressin concentration is greater in hypovolemic states than with normovolemia.

In dehydration, an increase in plasma osmolality results in withdrawal of fluid from cells. The reduction in total body water is shared equally between intracellular and extracellular fluid compartments. The increase in plasma osmolality and the reduction of extracellular fluid volume act synergistically to stimulate vasopressin release. In salt depletion, however, plasma vasopressin concentrations remain constant or are slightly increased despite a fall in plasma osmolality. Hypovolemia in this situation, as a result of osmotic movements of water from the extracellular into the intracellular fluid space, appears to provide the sensitizing influence.

Thirst mechanisms also involve interactions between extracellular fluid volume and osmolality. During periods of dehydration, increased plasma osmolality provides approximately 70% of the increased thirst drive, and the remaining 30% is due to hypovolemia. In salt depletion, the situation is less clear, but the normal drinking behavior or increased drinking observed in experimental animals has been attributed to the associated hypovolemia (Ramsay, 1983).

Miscellaneous Factors. A variety of nonosmotic and nonhemodynamic factors may also stimulate AVP secretion. With varying potency, these factors include nausea, hypoglycemia, the renin angiotensin system, and nonspecific stress caused by factors such as pain, emotion, and physical exercise. A large number of drugs and hormones have also been implicated in the alteration of vasopressin secretion. This list includes agents that either stimulate or inhibit AVP secretion, as well as substances that potentiate or inhibit the renal tubular response to AVP (Table 1-2; see Fig 1-4; Reeves et al, 1998).

SATIATION OF THIRST. Dehydrated animals have a remarkable capacity to consume the appropriate volume of water to repair a deficit. It has been demonstrated that dogs deprived of water for various periods of time drink just the volume of water needed to meet the deficit within 5 minutes. All animals have this capacity, although some species take longer to ingest the required amount of fluid. Satiation of thirst in dogs and cats requires restoration of normal plasma osmolality and blood volume, with correction of plasma osmolality playing the major role. In dogs with hypertonic volume depletion, restoration of osmolality in the carotid circulation without correcting osmolality outside the CNS caused a 70% decrease in drinking (Reeves et al, 1998). Restoration of blood volume in these dogs without ameliorating plasma hypertonicity reduced drinking by about 30%. Additional mechanisms may also play a minor role, including gastric distention and perhaps the participation of receptors in the liver. Similar inhibitory influences affect vasopressin secretion. Following voluntary rehydration in dehydrated animals, plasma vasopressin secretion returns to normal before redilution of the body fluids has been completed.

TABLE 1–2 DRUGS AND HORMONES REPORTED TO AFFECT VASOPRESSIN SECRETION OR ACTION

SECRETION

Stimulate AVP release	Inhibit AVP release
Acetylcholine	α-Adrenergic drugs
Anesthetic agents	Atrial natriuretic peptide
Angiotensin II	Glucocorticoids
Apomorphine	Haloperidol
β–Adrenergic drugs	Oxilorphan
Barbiturates	Phenytoin
Carbamazepine	Promethazine
Clofibrate	
Cyclophosphamide	
Histamine	
Insulin	
Metoclopramide	
Morphine and narcotic analogues	
Prostaglandin E_2	
Vincristine	

RENAL

Potentiate AVP action	Inhibit AVP action
Aspirin	α-Adrenergic drugs
Carbamazepine	Atrial natriuretic peptide
Chlorpropamide	Barbiturates
Nonsteroidal anti-inflammatory agents	Demeclocycline
Thiazides	Glucocorticoids
	Hypercalcemia
	Hypokalemia
	Methoxyflurane
	Prostaglandin E_2
	Protein kinase C
	Tetracyclines
	Vinca alkaloids

TABLE 1–3 DIFFERENTIAL DIAGNOSIS FOR POLYDIPSIA AND POLYURIA AND USEFUL DIAGNOSTIC TESTS

Disorder	Diagnostic Aids
Diabetes mellitus	Fasting blood glucose, urinalysis
Renal glycosuria	Fasting blood glucose, urinalysis
Chronic renal failure	BUN, creatinine, Ca:P, urinalysis
Postobstructive diuresis	History, monitoring urine output
Pyometra	History, CBC, abdominal radiography, abdominal ultrasonography
Escherichia coli & septicemia	Blood cultures
Hypercalcemia	Serum calcium
Hepatic insufficiency	Biochemistry panel, bile acids, ammonia tolerance test, abdominal radiography and ultrasonography
Hyperadrenocorticism	ACTH stimulation test, dexamethasone screening test, urine cortisol/creatinine ratio
Primary hyperaldosteronism	Serum sodium and potassium, blood pressure, abdominal ultrasonography, ACTH stimulation test (aldosterone)
Bacterial pyelonephritis	Urine culture, abdominal ultrasonography, excretory urography
Hypokalemia	Serum potassium
Hyponatremia	Serum sodium
Hypoadrenocorticism	Na:K, ACTH stimulation test
Hyperthyroidism	Serum thyroxine
Diabetes insipidus	Modified water deprivation test
Psychogenic polydipsia	Modified water deprivation test
Polycythemia	CBC
Acromegaly	Serum GH and IGF-I, CT scan
Paraneoplastic disorders	
Intestinal leiomyosarcoma	Abdominal ultrasonography, biopsy
Iatrogenic disorders	History
Very low protein diet	History

DIFFERENTIAL DIAGNOSES FOR POLYDIPSIA AND POLYURIA

Increased thirst (polydipsia) and urine production (polyuria) are common owner concerns in small animal veterinary practice. In dogs and cats, normal water intake varies from 20 to 70 ml/kg per day, and normal urine output varies between 20 and 45 ml/kg per day (Barsanti et al, 2000). Polydipsia and polyuria in the dog and cat have been defined as water consumption greater than 100 ml/kg/day and urine production greater than 50 ml/kg/day, respectively. It is possible, however, for individual dogs and cats to have abnormal thirst and urine production within the limits of these normal values. Polyuria and polydipsia usually exist concurrently, and determining the primary component of the syndrome is one of the initial diagnostic considerations when approaching the problem of polydipsia and polyuria (see page 13).

A variety of metabolic disturbances can cause polydipsia and polyuria (Table 1-3). These disorders can be classified, on the basis of underlying pathophysiology, into primary pituitary and nephrogenic diabetes insipidus; secondary nephrogenic diabetes insipidus resulting from interference with the normal interaction of AVP with renal tubular V_2 receptors, generation of intracellular cAMP, or renal tubular cell function, or from loss of the renal medullary interstitial concentration gradient; osmotic diuresis–induced polyuria and polydipsia; or interference with hypothalamic/pituitary secretion of AVP.

Osmotic diuresis

DIABETES MELLITUS. Diabetes mellitus is one of the most common endocrinopathies in the dog and cat. As glucose utilization diminishes as a result of relative or absolute insulin deficiencies, glucose accumulates in the blood. When the rising blood glucose concentration exceeds the renal tubular capacity for glucose reabsorption, glucose appears in the urine and acts as an osmotic diuretic, causing increased water loss into the urine. The water loss results in hypovolemia, which in turn stimulates increased water intake. Urinalysis and fasting blood glucose measurement are usually sufficient screening tests for diagnosing diabetes mellitus.

PRIMARY RENAL GLYCOSURIA. This uncommon disorder is seen primarily in the Basenji and Norwegian Elkhound. Primary renal glycosuria is a congenital renal tubular disorder resulting in an inability to reabsorb glucose from the ultrafiltrate in the nephron.

In some dogs and cats, renal glycosuria may also be a component of a Fanconi-like syndrome, in which phosphate, potassium, uric acid, amino acids, sodium, and/or bicarbonate may also be inadequately reabsorbed from the ultrafiltrate. As in diabetes mellitus, glucose appears in the urine and acts as an osmotic diuretic, causing polyuria and, in turn, polydipsia. Urinalysis and fasting blood glucose measurement are sufficient initial screening tests for this disorder.

CHRONIC RENAL FAILURE.   Chronic renal failure is a syndrome in which the number of functioning nephrons progressively decreases as a result of structural damage to the kidney, as occurs with chronic interstitial nephritis, medullary interstitial amyloidosis, and chronic pyelonephritis. A compensatory increase is seen in glomerular filtration rate (GFR) per surviving nephron, but the amount of fluid presented to the distal renal tubules is increased. Increased tubular flow rate causes less urea, sodium, and other substances to be reabsorbed. The result is an osmotic diuresis that is further complicated by a reduced renal medullary concentration gradient. These factors contribute to polyuria. The water loss results in hypovolemia, which causes compensatory polydipsia. Such animals may have increased blood urea nitrogen (BUN), creatinine, and inorganic phosphorus concentrations, as well as nonregenerative anemia and isosthenuric urine (urine specific gravity of 1.008 to 1.015).

POSTOBSTRUCTIVE DIURESIS.   Postobstructive diuresis may occur in any animal but is most common after urethral obstruction is relieved in male cats with feline lower urinary tract disease (i.e., feline urologic syndrome). These animals often have dramatic elevations in BUN, which results from the obstruction and creates a marked osmotic diuresis once the obstruction is relieved. Postobstructive diuresis is self-limiting. The veterinarian, however, must be aware of this problem and maintain the animal's hydration through aggressive fluid therapy, which can be slowly decreased over several days as the uremia clears and the osmotic diuresis declines.

Vasopressin (antidiuretic hormone) deficiency

Partial or complete lack of vasopressin production by the neurosecretory cells located in the supraoptic and paraventricular nuclei in the hypothalamus is called *central diabetes insipidus (CDI)*. This syndrome is discussed in subsequent sections (page 15).

Primary nephrogenic diabetes insipidus

A partial or complete lack of response of the renal tubule to the actions of AVP is called *nephrogenic diabetes insipidus* (NDI). Primary NDI results from a congenital defect involving the cellular mechanisms responsible for "opening the water channels" that allow water to be absorbed from the renal tubular ultrafiltrate. This syndrome is discussed in subsequent sections (page 17).

Acquired (secondary) nephrogenic diabetes insipidus

Several disorders may interfere with the normal interaction between AVP and its renal tubular receptors, affect renal tubular cell function, or decrease the hypertonic renal medullary interstitium, resulting in a loss of the normal osmotic gradient. Polyuria with a compensatory polydipsia results and can be quite severe. These disorders resemble primary NDI but are referred to as *acquired* or *secondary*, because AVP, AVP receptor sites, and postreceptor mechanisms responsible for water absorption are present.

PYOMETRA.   Bacterial endotoxins, especially those associated with *Escherichia coli*, can compete with AVP for its binding sites on the renal tubular membrane, causing a potentially reversible renal tubular insensitivity to AVP. The kidneys have an impaired ability to concentrate urine and conserve water, and polyuria with compensatory polydipsia develops. Pyometra is the most common infectious disorder associated with the development of polyuria and polydipsia, although it has also been reported with prostatic abscessation, pyelonephritis, and septicemia (Barsanti et al, 2000). Affected bitches and queens may produce extremely dilute urine, causing fluid depletion and compensatory polydipsia. Normal urine-concentrating ability usually returns within days of successfully eliminating pyometra. The diagnosis of secondary NDI is presumptive in any polyuric/polydipsic bitch or queen with pyometra.

HYPERCALCEMIA.   Increases in serum calcium concentration may inhibit binding of AVP to its receptor site, damage AVP receptors in the renal tubules, inactivate adenyl cyclase and interfere with the action of AVP at the renal tubular level (acquired NDI), or decrease transport of sodium and chloride into the renal medullary interstitium. Polydipsia and polyuria are common early signs of hypercalcemia, which is easily diagnosed with a serum biochemistry panel. Once hypercalcemia is identified, the clinician must undertake an often extensive diagnostic evaluation to determine its cause (see Chapter 16).

HEPATIC INSUFFICIENCY AND PORTOSYSTEMIC SHUNTS. Liver insufficiency and portosystemic shunts are recognized causes of polyuria and polydipsia. Many of the metabolic causes of polyuria and polydipsia (e.g., diabetes mellitus, hyperadrenocorticism, hypercalcemia) secondarily affect the liver, making it difficult to determine the role of the liver in causing polyuria and polydipsia. The exact cause of the polyuria is not known but may involve loss of medullary hypertonicity secondary to impaired urea nitrogen production or altered renal blood flow, increased GFR and renal volume, hypokalemia, impaired metabolism of cortisol, and primary polydipsia (Deppe et al, 1999). Urea nitrogen is a major constituent in the establishment and maintenance of the renal medullary concentration gradient. Without urea nitrogen the kidney loses the ability to concentrate urine, causing polyuria and compensatory polydipsia. Hepatic insufficiency and portosystemic shunts are usually suspected after evaluation of a complete blood count (CBC), serum biochemistry panel, urinalysis, and abdominal ultrasonography; these causes are confirmed with a liver function test (e.g., pre- and postprandial bile acids, ammonia tolerance test), specialized diagnostic imaging (e.g., positive contrast portogram, technetium scan) and histologic evaluation of an hepatic biopsy.

HYPERADRENOCORTICISM (CUSHING'S SYNDROME). Polyuria and polydipsia are common clinical signs of hyperadrenocorticism. Glucocorticoids inhibit AVP release by a direct effect within the hypothalamus and/or neurohypophysis (Papanek and Raff, 1994; Papanek et al, 1997). This inhibition of AVP release is characterized by both an increase in osmotic threshold and a decrease in the sensitivity of the AVP response to increasing osmolality (Biewenga et al, 1991). Hyperadrenocorticism also causes resistance to the effect of AVP in the kidney, possibly through interference with the action of AVP at the level of the renal collecting tubules or direct depression of renal tubular permeability to water. In a few patients, a deficiency in AVP may result from direct compression of neurosecretory cells by an enlarging pituitary tumor. Suspicion of hyperadrenocorticism is usually aroused after careful review of the history, physical examination, and results of CBC, serum biochemistry panel, and urinalysis. Confirmation requires appropriate pituitary adrenocortical function tests (see Chapter 6).

PRIMARY HYPERALDOSTERONISM. Polyuria and polydipsia have been reported in cats and dogs with primary hyperaldosteronism. The mechanism for polyuria and polydipsia is not clear, although mineralocorticoid-induced renal resistance to the actions of AVP and disturbed osmoregulation of AVP release has been documented in a dog with primary hyperaldosteronism (Rijnberk et al, 2001). Similar abnormalities have been identified in dogs with glucocorticoid excess, suggesting similar mechanisms of action for the polyuria and polydipsia in hyperaldosteronism and hyperadrenocorticism. The typical findings with primary hyperaldosteronism include weakness, severe hypokalemia, hypernatremia, systemic hypertension and adrenomegaly on abdominal ultrasound. Plasma aldosterone concentrations before and after ACTH administration are increased, and plasma renin activity is suppressed (see Chapter 6).

PYELONEPHRITIS. Infection and inflammation of the renal pelvis can destroy the countercurrent mechanism in the renal medulla, resulting in isosthenuria, polyuria, polydipsia, and eventually renal failure. Bacterial endotoxins, especially those associated with Escherichia coli, can also compete with AVP for its binding sites on the renal tubular membrane, causing a potentially reversible renal tubular insensitivity to AVP. A dog or cat with acute bacterial pyelonephritis may develop nonspecific systemic signs of lethargy, anorexia, and fever, and a neutrophilic leukocytosis may be identified on a CBC. Systemic signs are usually not present with chronic pyelonephritis. Pyelonephritis should also be suspected in a patient with recurring urinary tract infection. Urinalysis may reveal white blood cells and white blood cell casts, bacteria, and occasionally red blood cells. Culture of urine obtained by antepubic cystocentesis should be positive for bacterial growth. Abdominal ultrasonography and excretory urography may reveal abnormalities consistent with pyelonephritis (e.g., renal pelvis dilatation).

HYPOKALEMIA. Hypokalemia is believed to render the terminal portion of the nephron less responsive to AVP, possibly by suppressing the generation of intracellular cAMP in renal tubular cells. Hypokalemia may also affect the hypertonic medullary interstitial gradient by interfering with solute accumulation and may interfere with release of AVP from the pituitary. Polyuria and polydipsia are not common clinical signs of hypokalemia. The most common clinical signs are related to neuromuscular dysfunction of skeletal, cardiac, and smooth muscle (e.g., weakness, cervical ventriflexion). Hypokalemia usually develops secondary to another disorder (Table 1-4), many of which also cause polyuria and polydipsia.

HYPOADRENOCORTICISM (ADDISON'S DISEASE). Adrenocortical insufficiency results in impaired ability to concentrate urine (see Chapter 8). Despite normal kidney function and severe hypovolemia, most dogs with hypoadrenocorticism have a urine specific

TABLE 1–4 CAUSES OF HYPOKALEMIA IN THE DOG AND CAT

Transcellular Shifts (ECF to ICF)
Metabolic alkalosis
Diabetic ketoacidosis*
Hypokalemic periodic paralysis (Burmese cats)

Increased Loss
Gastrointestinal fluid loss*
Chronic renal failure, especially in cats*
Diet-induced hypokalemic nephropathy in cats
Distal (type I) renal tubular acidosis
Proximal (type II) renal tubular acidosis after sodium bicarbonate
    treatment
Postobstructive diuresis
Primary hyperaldosteronism
Secondary hyperaldosteronism*
    Liver insufficiency
    Congestive heart failure
    Nephrotic syndrome
Hyperthyroidism
Hypomagnesemia

Iatrogenic*
Potassium-free fluid administration (e.g., 0.9% NaCl)
Parenteral nutritional solutions
Insulin and glucose-containing fluid administration
Sodium bicarbonate therapy
Loop (e.g., furosemide) and thiazide diuretics
Low dietary intake

Pseudohypokalemia
Hyperlipidemia (dry reagent methods; flame photometry)
Hyperproteinemia (dry reagent methods; flame photometry)
Hyperglycemia (dry reagent methods)
Azotemia (dry reagent methods)

Modified from DiBartola SP and De Morais HA: Disorders of potassium: Hypokalemia and hyperkalemia. In, DiBartola SP, editor: *Fluid Therapy in Small Animal Practice*, ed 2, Philadelphia, 2000, WB Saunders, p. 93.
*Common cause.

gravity of less than 1.030. Mineralocorticoid deficiency results in chronic sodium wasting, renal medullary solute washout, and loss of the medullary hypertonic gradient. Adrenalectomy in rats also decreases AVP-stimulated activation of renal medullary adenylate cyclase, primarily because of impairment in the coupling between the AVP receptor complex and adenylate cyclase. Treatment with dexamethasone corrects the defect. Hypercalcemia occurs in some patients with hypoadrenocorticism and may also play a role in the generation of polyuria and polydipsia.

Polyuria and polydipsia typically develop early in the course of the disease and are quickly overshadowed by the more worrisome and obvious vomiting, diarrhea, anorexia, weakness, and depression seen in these patients. The polyuria of hypoadrenocorticism can be difficult to differentiate from primary renal failure unless specific tests of the pituitary adrenocortical axis (e.g., ACTH stimulation test) are performed. Initial suspicion for hypoadrenocorticism usually follows evaluation of serum electrolytes, although hyperkalemia and hyponatremia can also occur with renal insufficiency.

HYPERTHYROIDISM. Polyuria and polydipsia are common findings in cats and dogs with hyperthyroidism. The exact mechanism for the polyuria and polydipsia is not clear. Increased renal medullary blood flow may decrease medullary hypertonicity and impair water resorption from the distal portion of the nephron. Psychogenic polydipsia secondary to thyrotoxicosis and, in some patients, concurrent renal insufficiency may also contribute to the polyuria and polydipsia. The tentative diagnosis of hyperthyroidism is usually based on clinical signs, palpation of an enlarged thyroid lobe or lobes (i.e., goiter), and measurement of serum thyroxine (T_4) concentration.

ACROMEGALY. Excessive secretion of growth hormone (GH) in the adult dog or cat results in acromegaly (see Chapter 2). Acromegaly causes carbohydrate intolerance and the eventual development of overt diabetes mellitus. In most cats and dogs with acromegaly, the polyuria is assumed to be caused by an osmotic diuresis induced by glycosuria. Renal insufficiency from a diabetic or GH-induced glomerulonephropathy may also play a role (Peterson et al, 1990).

POLYCYTHEMIA. Polyuria and polydipsia may occur with polycythemia. Studies in 2 dogs with secondary polycythemia identified an increased osmotic threshold for AVP release, resulting in a delayed AVP response to increasing plasma osmolality (van Vonderen et al, 1997a). The authors attributed the abnormal AVP response to increased blood volume and hyperviscosity, which stimulate atrial natriuretic peptide (ANP) secretion and atrial and carotid bifurcation baroreceptors. ANP inhibits AVP release from the pituitary gland and the renal collecting duct's responsiveness to AVP (Dillingham and Anderson, 1986; Lee et al, 1987).

Primary and psychogenic polydipsia

Primary polydipsia is defined as a marked increase in water intake that cannot be explained as a compensatory mechanism for excessive fluid loss. In humans, primary polydipsia results from a defect in the thirst center or may be associated with mental illness (Reeves et al, 1998). Primary dysfunction of the thirst center resulting in compulsive water consumption has not been reported in the dog or cat, although an abnormal vasopressin response to hypertonic saline infusion has been reported in dogs with suspected primary polydipsia (van Vonderen et al, 1999). A psychogenic or behavioral basis for compulsive water consumption does occur in the dog but has not been reported in the cat. Psychogenic polydipsia may be induced by concurrent disease (e.g., hepatic insufficiency, hyperthyroidism) or may represent a learned behavior following a change in the pet's environment. Polyuria is compensatory to prevent overhydration. Psychogenic polydipsia is diagnosed by exclusion of other causes of polyuria and polydipsia and by demonstrating that the dog or cat can concentrate urine to a specific gravity in excess of 1.030 after water deprivation. This syndrome is discussed in more detail in subsequent sections (page 17).

Iatrogenic (drug-Induced) causes of polydipsia and polyuria

Several drugs have the potential to cause polyuria and polydipsia (Table 1-5). The most commonly encountered in small animal veterinary practice are glucocorticoids, diuretics, anticonvulsants (e.g., phenobarbital), synthetic levothyroxine, and salt supplementation. Drug-induced polyuria and polydipsia do not usually pose a diagnostic challenge. The polyuria and polydipsia should resolve following discontinuation of the drug. If polyuria and polydipsia persist, a concurrent disorder causing polyuria and polydipsia or renal medullary solute washout should be considered.

Renal medullary solute washout

Loss of renal medullary solutes, most notably sodium and urea, results in loss of medullary hypertonicity and impaired ability of the nephron to concentrate the ultrafiltrate. Renal medullary solute washout is usually

TABLE 1–5 DRUGS AND HORMONES CAUSING POLYURIA AND POLYDIPSIA IN DOGS AND CATS

Anticonvulsants*
Phenobarbital
Primidone
Dilantin
Glucocorticoids*
Diuretics*
Mannitol
Synthetic thyroid hormone supplements
Amphotericin B
Lithium
Methoxyflurane
Sodium bicarbonate
Salt supplementation*
Vitamin D (toxicity)

*Common cause

caused by one of the disorders previously described. It has also been associated with chronic diuretic therapy and abnormalities in circulation, such as hyperviscosity syndromes (polycythemia, hyperproteinemia), renal lymphatic obstruction (lymphosarcoma, lymphangiectasia), and systemic vasculitis (septicemia, systemic lupus erythematosus). Perhaps the most important clinical ramification of renal medullary solute washout is its potential to interfere with results of the modified water deprivation test (see page 32). Hypertonicity of the renal medulla is usually restored once the underlying cause of the polyuria and polydipsia is corrected.

DIAGNOSTIC APPROACH TO POLYURIA AND POLYDIPSIA

Depending on the cause, the cost and time expenditure for evaluating a dog or cat with polyuria and polydipsia may be brief and inexpensive (e.g., diabetes mellitus) or time-consuming and costly (e.g., partial CDI). Therefore, the clinician should be reasonably sure that polyuria and polydipsia exist, preferably based on a combination of history, multiple random urine specific gravity determinations, and if necessary, quantitation of water consumption over several days with the dog or cat in the home environment. The average daily volume of water consumed by a dog is usually less than 60 ml/kg of body weight, with an upper normal limit of 100 ml/kg of body weight. Similar values are used for cats, although most cats drink considerably less than these amounts. If an owner knows the volume of water the pet is consuming in an average 24-hour period and if that amount exceeds the upper limit of normal, a diagnostic evaluation to determine the cause is warranted. If 24-hour water intake is normal, pathologic polyuria and polydipsia are unlikely and another inciting factor (e.g., hot weather) should be sought, or misinterpretation of polyuria (e.g., dysuria instead of polyuria) should be considered. If the owner is certain that a change in the volume of water consumption or urination exists, even though water consumption is still in the normal range, a diagnostic evaluation may still be warranted.

Assessment of urine specific gravity may be helpful in identifying polyuria and polydipsia and may provide clues to the underlying diagnosis, especially if multiple urine specific gravities are evaluated (Table 1-6).

Urine specific gravity varies widely among healthy dogs and, in some dogs, can range from 1.006 to greater than 1.040 within a 24 hour period (van Vonderen et al, 1997b). Wide fluctuations in urine specific gravity have not been reported in healthy cats.

We prefer to have the owner collect several urine samples at different times of the day for 2 to 3 days, storing the urine samples in the refrigerator until they can be brought to the veterinary hospital for determination of urine specific gravity. Urine specific gravities measured from multiple urine samples that are consistently less than 1.030 (especially less than 1.020) support the presence of polyuria and polydipsia and the need for a diagnostic evaluation to determine the cause. Identification of one or more urine specific gravities greater than 1.030 supports normal urine concentrating ability and an intact, functioning pituitary vasopressin-renal tubular cell axis. Dogs and cats may still have polyuria and polydipsia despite identification of concentrated urine; possible differentials include disorders causing an osmotic diuresis (e.g., diabetes mellitus), psychogenic polydipsia and disorders in the regulation of AVP secretion (van Vonderen et al, 1999).

Many potential causes exist for the development of polyuria and polydipsia in dogs and cats (see Table 1-3), one of the least common being diabetes insipidus. An animal with a history of severe polydipsia and polyuria should be thoroughly evaluated for other causes of polydipsia and polyuria prior to performing specific diagnostic procedures for diabetes insipidus (Fig. 1-7). The array of differential diagnoses precludes premature or unsubstantiated formation of a diagnosis and treatment plan. It is necessary to establish a firm data base. Initial information allows inclusion or exclusion of the many common medical disorders associated with polyuria and polydipsia that are contrasted with the less common CDI, NDI, or psychogenic polydipsia.

Our diagnostic approach (see Fig. 1-7) to the animal with polyuria and polydipsia is initially to rule out the more common causes. Recommended initial diagnostic studies include a CBC, urinalysis with bacterial culture of urine obtained by antepubic cystocentesis, and a serum biochemistry profile that includes liver enzymes, BUN, calcium, phosphorus, sodium, potassium, cholesterol, blood glucose, total plasma protein, and plasma albumin. A serum thyroxine (T_4) concentration should be measured in older cats. Depending on the history and physical examination

TABLE 1-6 URINALYSIS RESULTS IN DOGS WITH SELECTED DISORDERS CAUSING POLYURIA AND POLYDIPSIA

Disorder	No. of Dogs	URINE SPECIFIC GRAVITY Mean	URINE SPECIFIC GRAVITY Range	Proteinuria	WBC (> 5/HPF)
Central diabetes insipidus	20	1.005	1.001–1.012	5%	0%
Psychogenic polydipsia	18	1.011	1.003–1.023	0%	0%
Hyperadrenocorticism	20	1.012	1.001–1.027	48%	0%
Renal insufficiency	20	1.011	1.008–1.016	90%	25%
Pyelonephritis	20	1.019	1.007–1.045	70%	75%

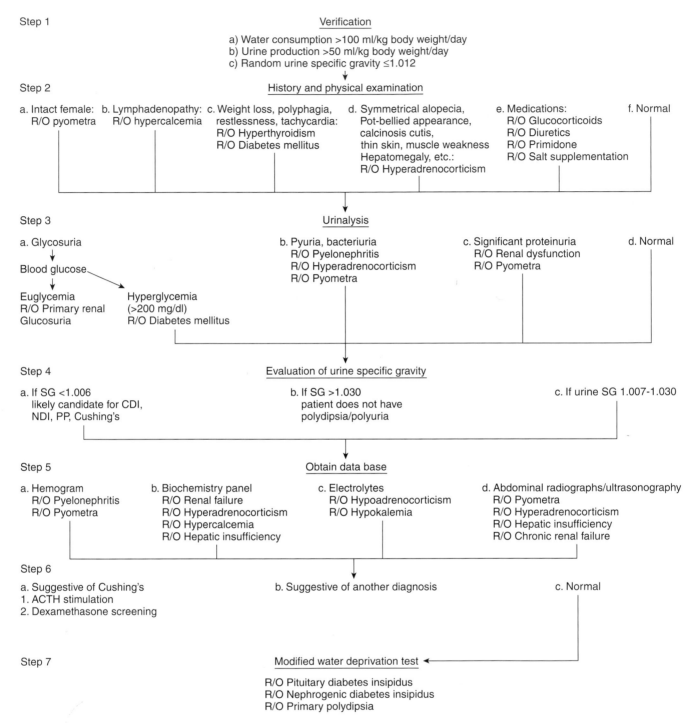

FIGURE 1–7. The diagnostic plan in a dog or cat with severe polydipsia and polyuria. *R/O,* rule out (a diagnosis); *CDI,* central diabetes insipidus; *NDI,* nephrogenic diabetes insipidus; *PP,* primary (psychogenic) polydipsia.

findings, abdominal ultrasonography may be warranted to evaluate liver, kidney, adrenal, or uterine size and to search for calcified adrenals in patients with suspected hyperadrenocorticism. Careful evaluation of the history, physical examination findings, and initial data base usually provides the diagnosis outright (e.g., diabetes mellitus, pyometra) or offers clues that allow the clinician to focus on the under-

lying cause (e.g., increased serum alkaline phosphatase and cholesterol in hyperadrenocorticism).

Occasionally, the physical examination and initial data base are normal in the dog or cat with polyuria and polydipsia. Viable possibilities in these dogs and cats include diabetes insipidus, psychogenic water consumption, unusual hyperadrenocorticism, renal insufficiency without azotemia, and possibly mild hepatic insufficiency. Hyperadrenocorticism, renal insufficiency, and hepatic insufficiency should be ruled out before performing tests to establish a diagnosis of diabetes insipidus or psychogenic polydipsia. Diagnostic tests to consider include tests of the pituitary adrenocortical axis, liver function tests (e.g., pre- and postprandial bile acids), urine protein:creatinine ratio, contrast imaging of the kidney. and if indicated, renal biopsy.

Careful evaluation of urine specific gravity and urine protein loss may provide clues to the underlying diagnosis (Table 1-6). For example, if the urine specific gravity measured on multiple urine samples is consistently in the isosthenuric range (1.008 to 1.015), renal insufficiency should be considered the primary differential diagnosis, especially if the BUN and serum creatinine concentration are high normal or increased (i.e., ≥25 mg/dl and ≥0.8 mg/dl, respectively) and proteinuria is present. Although isosthenuria is relatively common in dogs with hyperadrenocorticism, psychogenic water consumption, hepatic insufficiency, pyelonephritis, and partial central diabetes insipidus with concurrent water restriction, urine specific gravities tend to fluctuate above (hyperadrenocorticism, psychogenic water consumption, hepatic insufficiency, pyelonephritis) and below (hyperadrenocorticism, psychogenic water consumption, partial central diabetes insipidus) the isosthenuric range in these disorders. In contrast, if the urine specific gravity is consistently less than 1.006, renal insufficiency and pyelonephritis are ruled out and diabetes insipidus, psychogenic water consumption, and hyperadrenocorticism should be considered.

The diagnosis of diabetes insipidus and psychogenic water consumption should be based on results of the modified water deprivation test, measurement of plasma osmolality, and response to synthetic vasopressin therapy (see Confirming the Diagnosis of Diabetes Insipidus, page 21). Ideally, all realistic causes of secondary acquired NDI should be ruled out before performing tests (especially the modified water deprivation test) to diagnose diabetes insipidus and psychogenic polydipsia. The recommended initial laboratory studies not only ensure that the veterinarian is pursuing a correct diagnosis but also alert the clinician to any concomitant medical problems. A logical, systematic approach may appear cumbersome but avoids misdiagnosis. More important, problems may be avoided by not subjecting an animal to unnecessary, expensive, and potentially harmful procedures, should the presumptive diagnosis be incorrect.

ETIOLOGY OF DIABETES INSIPIDUS AND PRIMARY POLYDIPSIA

Vasopressin deficiency–central diabetes insipidus

DEFINITION. CDI is a polyuric syndrome that results from a lack of sufficient AVP to concentrate the urine for water conservation. This deficiency may be absolute or partial. An absolute deficiency of AVP causes persistent hyposthenuria and severe diuresis. Urine specific gravity in dogs and cats with complete lack of AVP usually remains hyposthenuric (≤1.006), even with severe dehydration. A partial deficiency of AVP, referred to as a *partial CDI*, also causes persistent hyposthenuria and a marked diuresis as long as the dog or cat has unlimited access to water. During periods of water restriction, however, dogs and cats with partial CDI can increase their urine specific gravity into the isosthenuric range (1.008 to 1.015) but cannot typically concentrate their urine above 1.015 to 1.020, even with severe dehydration. For any dog or cat with partial CDI, maximum urine-concentrating ability during dehydration is inversely related to the severity of the deficiency in AVP secretion; that is, the more severe the AVP deficiency, the less concentrated the urine specific gravity during dehydration.

PATHOPHYSIOLOGY. Destruction of the production sites for vasopressin—the supraoptic and paraventricular nuclei of the hypothalamus—and/or loss of the major ducts (axons) that carry AVP to the storage and release depots in the posterior pituitary (see Fig. 1-2) result in CDI. Permanent CDI requires an injury that is sufficiently high in the neurohypophyseal tract to cause bilateral neuronal degeneration in the supraoptic and paraventricular nuclei. Transection of the hypothalamic hypophyseal tract below the median eminence or removal of the posterior lobe of the pituitary usually causes transient (albeit severe) CDI and polyuria because sufficient hormone can be released from fibers ending in the median eminence and pituitary stalk to prevent occurrence of permanent diabetes insipidus (Fig. 1-8; Ramsay, 1983).

A triphasic response sufficient to cause diabetes insipidus has been reported following surgical damage to the hypothalamus of cats. Immediately following creation of the lesion, polydipsia and polyuria began and usually lasted 4 to 5 days. This was followed by a 6-day period of intense antidiuresis and then recurrence of permanent CDI. The first phase is believed to result from the acute damage that causes disruption in the ability to release stored AVP. The antidiuretic stage results from degeneration of hormone-laden tissue with release of excessive amounts of AVP into the circulation. This is supported by a lack of the usual diuretic response following administration of a water load during the second stage. If the posterior pituitary is also removed at the time of hypothalamic damage, the antidiuretic phase is not observed. With only minor damage to the hypothalamus, permanent CDI may not follow the second phase.

ETIOLOGY. CDI may result from any condition that damages the neurohypophyseal system. Recognized causes for CDI in the dog and cat are listed in Table 1-7. Idiopathic cases of CDI are the most common, appearing at any age in any breed in either gender. Necropsies performed in dogs and cats with idiopathic CDI fail to identify an underlying reason for the AVP deficiency.

Autoimmune hypothalamitis has been suggested as a possible cause of idiopathic CDI in humans (Salvi et al, 1988). Circulating AVP cell antibodies, which bind

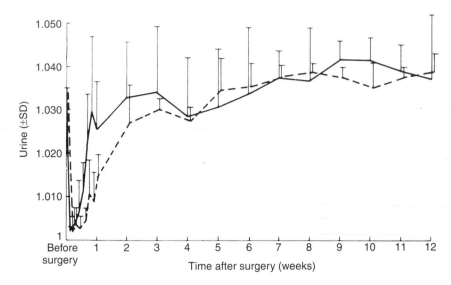

FIGURE 1–8. Mean urine specific gravity obtained before and for 3 months after hypophysectomy in four dogs treated with intraoperative polyionic fluids *(solid line)* and four dogs treated with intraoperative polyionic fluids and dexamethasone *(dashed line)*. (From Lantz GC, et al: Am J Vet Res 49:1134, 1988.)

TABLE 1–7 RECOGNIZED CAUSES OF CENTRAL DIABETES INSIPIDUS IN HUMANS, DOGS, AND CATS

Humans	Dogs/Cats
Acquired	
Idiopathic	Idiopathic
Traumatic	Traumatic
Neoplasia	Neoplasia
Craniopharyngioma	Craniopharyngioma
Germinoma	Chromophobe adenoma and
Meningioma	adenocarcinoma
Lymphoma	Metastases
Adenoma	Pituitary malformation
Metastases	Cysts
Granulomas	Inflammation
Infectious	
Viral	
Bacterial	
Vascular	
Sheehan's syndrome	
Aneurysms	
Autoimmune	
Familial (Autosomal Dominant)	**Familial (?)**

to cell membranes of hypothalamic preparations, have been identified in some humans with CDI (Scherbaum, 1987). AVP cell antibodies have been identified prior to the development of CDI, and titers of AVP cell antibodies decline eventually to negative values with increasing duration of the disease (Bhan and O'Brien, 1982; Scherbaum et al, 1986). These patients also show a significant association with other endocrine disorders (e.g., immune thyroiditis, Addison's disease), suggesting that, at least in some cases, polyendocrine autoimmunity may also involve the hypothalamus (see Chapter 3, page 91). A similar association between CDI and other endocrinopathies has not been identified

in dogs and cats, nor have studies examining a possible immune basis for CDI been reported.

The most common identifiable causes for CDI in dogs and cats are head trauma (accidental or neurosurgical), neoplasia, and hypothalamic/pituitary malformations (e.g., cystic structures). Head trauma may cause transient or permanent CDI, depending on the viability of the cells in the supraoptic and paraventricular nuclei. Trauma-induced transection of the pituitary stalk often results in transient CDI, usually lasting 1 to 3 weeks (see Fig. 1-8; Lantz et al, 1988; Authement et al, 1989). The duration of diabetes insipidus depends on the location of the transection of the hypophyseal stalk relative to the hypothalamus. Transection at more proximal levels, close to the median eminence, is associated with a longer time for hypothalamic axons to undergo regeneration and secretion of ADH. Trauma-induced CDI should be suspected when severe polydipsia and polyuria develop within 48 hours of head trauma or when hypernatremia, hyposthenuria and hypertonic dehydration develop in a traumatized dog or cat that is being treated with intravenous fluids rather than water ad libitum (see page 29).

Primary intracranial tumors associated with diabetes insipidus in dogs and cats include craniopharyngioma, pituitary chromophobe adenoma, and pituitary chromophobe adenocarcinoma (Fig. 1-9; Neer and Reavis, 1983; Goossens et al, 1995; Harb et al, 1996). Tumor metastases to the hypothalamus and pituitary can also cause CDI. In humans, metastatic tumors most often spread from the lung or breast (Reeves et al, 1998). Metastatic mammary carcinoma, lymphoma, malignant melanoma, and pancreatic carcinoma have been reported to cause CDI by their presence in the pituitary gland or hypothalamus in dogs (Capen and Martin, 1983; Davenport et al, 1986). Metastatic neoplasia as a cause for CDI has not yet been reported in the cat.

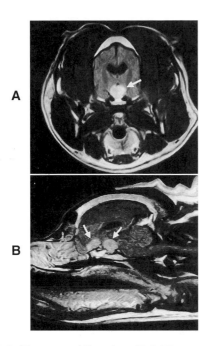

FIGURE 1–9. Transverse *(A)* and sagittal *(B)* magnetic resonance images of the pituitary region in a 12-year-old male Boxer with central diabetes insipidus, hypothyroidism, and neurologic signs. A mass is evident in the region of the pituitary gland, hypothalamus, and rostral floor of the calvarium *(arrows).*

A rare, hereditary form of CDI occurs in humans, is transmitted as an autosomal dominant trait, has equal occurrence in males and females, displays father-to-son transmission, and shows variable expression among affected individuals (Baylis and Robertson, 1981). This condition is believed to result from a degenerative disorder affecting the neurosecretory cells (Kaplowitz et al, 1982). Although CDI is well documented in kittens and puppies, hereditary CDI has not yet been documented. In one report, hereditary CDI was suggested in two sibling Afghan Hound pups that developed CDI at less than 4 months of age and were from a bitch suffering from polyuria and polydipsia "all her life" (Post et al, 1989). Necropsy of these puppies revealed vacuolated areas in the neurohypophysis and hypothalamohypophysial tracts of the median eminence of the tuber cinereum, findings that suggested hypomyelination or demyelination. We have also diagnosed CDI in a litter of five 8-week-old German Short-haired Pointers and three of five 7-week-old Schnauzers, suggesting possible familial CDI in these dogs.

Primary (familial) nephrogenic diabetes insipidus

DEFINITION. NDI is a polyuric disorder that results from impaired responsiveness of the nephron to the actions of AVP. Plasma AVP concentrations are normal or increased in animals with this disorder. NDI is classified as primary (familial) or secondary (acquired). Secondary or acquired NDI is common in dogs and cats and is discussed on page 10. Primary or familial NDI is a rare congenital disorder in dogs and cats;

polydipsia and polyuria typically become apparent by the time the dog or cat is 8 to 12 weeks of age.

ETIOLOGY. Two types of congenital or familial NDI have been identified in humans. X-linked NDI results from mutations in the AVPR2 gene that codes for the AVP antidiuretic (V_2) receptor. It is a rare recessive X-linked disease and occurs primarily in males (Fujiwara et al, 1995; van Lieburg et al, 1995). Autosomal recessive NDI is a non–X-linked form of NDI that results from mutations in the AQP2 gene that codes for the AVP-dependent water channel and results in a postreceptor (post-cAMP) defect (van Lieburg et al, 1994; Deen et al, 1994). X-linked NDI occurs more frequently than autosomal recessive NDI. For both disorders, clinical signs are apparent shortly after birth.

Only a few reports of congenital (primary) NDI in dogs have appeared in the veterinary literature (Breitschwerdt et al, 1981; Grunbaum et al, 1990; Grunbaum and Moritz, 1991). Primary NDI has not yet been reported in the cat. The cause of primary NDI in dogs and cats is unknown. Electron microscopic examination of the renal medulla in a Miniature Poodle with primary NDI revealed vacuoles in the cells of the Henle loops, blood vessels, and interstitium, but the significance of these lesions is not known. Necropsy failed to identify any lesions in the kidney of a German Shepherd with primary NDI.

Familial NDI has been reported in a family of Huskies, in which the female parent was diagnosed as a carrier of the NDI gene, and three of four male puppies in her litter had NDI (Grunbaum et al, 1990). Affected puppies possessed normal V_2 receptor numbers in the kidney inner medulla, but the receptors had a 10-fold lower binding affinity for AVP than in normal dogs (Luzius et al, 1992). Adenylate cyclase stimulation by AVP was similarly reduced in a dose response manner; however, stimulation of adenylate cyclase by non–AVP-mediated chemicals was comparable for normal and NDI-affected dogs, implying normal adenylate cyclase in the affected Huskies. The NDI-affected dogs also had antidiuretic responses to high doses of DDAVP, consistent with their possessing V_2 receptors of lower binding affinity.

Primary or psychogenic polydipsia

Primary polydipsia (compulsive water consumption) is a syndrome characterized by ingestion of water in excess of the capacity of the normal kidney to excrete it. In humans, primary polydipsia is one of several disorders categorized as hypotonic syndromes (Table 1-8). These conditions involve deranged water homeostasis, causing free water to be excreted at a rate not sufficient to maintain either normal serum sodium concentration or normal body fluid osmolality (Reeves et al, 1998). Hyponatremia is a hallmark finding with hypotonic syndromes, although the hyponatremia that occurs in humans with primary polydipsia is generally slight, with serum sodium concentrations generally in the range of 135 mEq/L.

TABLE 1–8   THE HYPOTONIC SYNDROMES DESCRIBED IN HUMANS

Excessive water ingestion
Decreased water excretion
  Decreased solute delivery to diluting segments of nephron
    Starvation
    Beer potomania
  AVP excess
    Syndrome of inappropriate antidiuretic hormone secretion
    Drug-induced AVP secretion
AVP excess with decreased distal solute delivery
    Congestive heart failure
    Cirrhosis of the liver
    Nephrotic syndrome
    Cortisol deficiency
    Hypothyroidism
    Diuretic use
  Renal failure

In humans, primary polydipsia is most commonly found in individuals with underlying psychiatric illness (Cronin, 1987; Victor et al, 1989) and rarely, in individuals with lesions involving the thirst center. The cause of the polydipsia in individuals with psychiatric illness is uncertain, and most patients have, in addition to polydipsia, some abnormality in water excretion, such as excessive AVP secretion (Goldman et al, 1988).

Primary polydipsia caused by a hypothalamic lesion affecting the thirst center has not been reported in the dog or cat. A psychogenic basis for compulsive water consumption occurs uncommonly in the dog and has not been reported in the cat. Affected animals are usually hyperactive dogs that are placed in exercise-restrictive environments. Some of these dogs have had significant changes to their environment, resulting in unusual stress. In some dogs, compulsive water consumption is a learned behavior to gain attention from the owner. Dogs with psychogenic water consumption can concentrate urine to greater than 1.030 during water deprivation (see page 29), although the latter may take hours because of concurrent renal medullary solute washout. Urine specific gravity may vary widely over time, and concentrated urine may be identified on random urine evaluation. Identification of concentrated urine implies hypothalamic AVP production, pituitary AVP secretion, and renal tubular responsiveness to AVP.

Abnormal AVP release in response to hypertonic saline stimulation was recently described in four dogs with suspected primary polydipsia (van Vonderen et al, 1999). All dogs presented for polyuria and polydipsia and had normal routine laboratory examinations except for hyposthenuria and concentrated urine during the water deprivation test. During serial measurements, urine osmolality spontaneously reached high concentrations (i.e., greater than 1000 mOsm/kg) in two dogs. During water deprivation, plasma AVP concentrations remained relatively low in all dogs. The AVP response to hypertonic saline infusion was abnormal in all dogs, with an increased threshold value in three dogs, an increased sensitivity in two dogs, and

an exaggerated response in one dog. These findings suggested a primary disturbance in the regulation of AVP secretion, although chronic overhydration may have caused down-regulation of AVP release in response to hypertonicity (Moses and Clayton, 1993). Subnormal AVP release during water deprivation and hypertonic stimulation has been documented in humans with primary polydipsia (Zerbe and Robertson, 1981); these individuals were subsequently classified as having partial diabetes insipidus. It is not clear whether the dogs described by van Vonderen et al (1999) represent a variant or early stage of partial diabetes insipidus. They were classified as having primary polydipsia based on their ability to concentrate urine to a specific gravity greater than 1.030, but the identified abnormalities suggest a problem with AVP release rather than the thirst center, per se.

CLINICAL FEATURES OF DIABETES INSIPIDUS AND PSYCHOGENIC POLYDIPSIA

Signalment

CENTRAL DIABETES INSIPIDUS. There is no apparent breed, gender, or age predilection for CDI (Fig. 1-10). Of 41 dogs diagnosed with CDI at our hospital, 23 different breeds were represented. The Boxer (five dogs), German Shepherd (four dogs), and Labrador Retriever (three dogs) were the breeds most commonly affected. The age at time of diagnosis in these 41 dogs ranged from 7 weeks to 14 years, with a median age of 5 years. Most dogs diagnosed with CDI were less than 2 years or greater than 6 years of age.

Seven cats with CDI have been reported in the literature (Burnie and Dunn, 1982; Winterbotham and Mason, 1983; Kraus, 1987; Brown et al, 1993; Pittari, 1996), and we have diagnosed an additional four cats at our hospital. Eight of these eleven were Domestic Short- or Long-haired, two were Persian, and one was an Abyssinian. Six of the cats were female or female/spayed, and five were male or male/castrated. The age at the time of diagnosis of CDI ranged from 8 weeks to 6 years, with a mean of 1.5 years.

PRIMARY NEPHROGENIC DIABETES INSIPIDUS. Primary NDI is rare in dogs and cats. To date, primary NDI has been reported in a 13-week-old male German Shepherd, an 18-month-old male Miniature Poodle, an 18-month-old female Boston Terrier, and a family of Huskies (Breitschwerdt et al, 1981; Grunbaum et al, 1990). We have also diagnosed NDI in a 5-month-old Norwegian Elkhound and a 1-year-old Boston Terrier. Both dogs had polyuria and polydipsia since acquired by their owners at 6 to 8 weeks of age. Primary NDI has not yet been reported in the cat.

PSYCHOGENIC POLYDIPSIA. Psychogenic polydipsia can be diagnosed in dogs of any age, either gender, and numerous breeds. Fifteen different breeds were represented in 18 dogs diagnosed with psychogenic polydipsia at our hospital. Eleven dogs were female or female/spayed, and the age at time of diagnosis ranged from 6 months to 11 years, with a mean and median

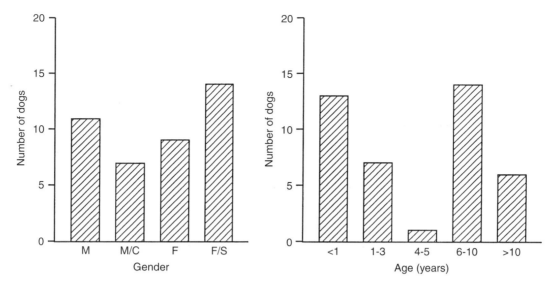

FIGURE 1–10. Gender and age distribution of 41 dogs diagnosed with central diabetes insipidus.

age of 4.5 and 4 years, respectively. Psychogenic polydipsia has not yet been reported in the cat.

Clinical signs

Polyuria and polydipsia are the hallmark clinical signs for diabetes insipidus and psychogenic polydipsia. Polyuria and polydipsia can be quite severe, as illustrated by two of our recent dogs with CDI that were observed to drink water while urinating in their cage. Polyuria and polydipsia have usually been present for 1 to 6 months before veterinary care is sought (Fig. 1-11). Many owners also report urinary incontinence, in part because of the frequency of urination and loss of normal "house broken" behavior and in part because of the inability to maintain continence because of the large volume of urine being produced, especially when the dog or cat is sleeping. Owners of cats with diabetes insipidus also complain about the increased frequency of changing the litter, which often needs to be done once or twice a day. An insatiable desire for water may result in the consumption of any liquid, including ice, snow, and urine. Occasionally, the afflicted pet's strong desire for water overrides its normal appetite (i.e., they would rather drink than eat), resulting in weight loss.

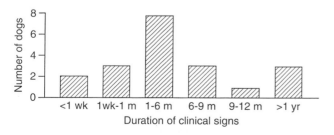

FIGURE 1–11. Duration of polyuria and polydipsia in 20 dogs with central diabetes insipidus before owners presented their pet to the veterinarian for examination.

Additional clinical signs depend, in part, on the underlying cause. Other historical abnormalities (e.g., vomiting, diarrhea, coughing) are usually not present in dogs or cats with congenital, idiopathic, or trauma-induced forms of diabetes insipidus. These pets are typically alert and playful and have normal exercise tolerance. However, dogs with acquired CDI secondary to a growing pituitary or hypothalamic neoplasm may develop additional signs related to the nervous system, including stupor, disorientation, anorexia, ataxia, seizures, and tremors (Harb et al, 1996). Neurologic signs may be present at the time CDI is diagnosed or, more typically, develop weeks to months after CDI is identified. In one study, 6 of 20 dogs with CDI developed neurologic signs from 2 weeks to 5 months (median, 1 month) after CDI was diagnosed (Harb et al, 1996). A tumor in the region of the hypothalamus and pituitary was identified by CT scan or necropsy in all six dogs. Neurologic signs may also develop secondary to hypertonic dehydration and severe hypernatremia (see page 29).

Physical examination

As with the history, the abnormalities found during the physical examination depend on the underlying cause. For most animals, the physical examination is unremarkable, although some dogs tend to be thin. Abnormalities of the cardiovascular, respiratory, gastrointestinal, and urogenital systems are usually absent. Animals with idiopathic or congenital diabetes insipidus are alert and active. Typically, as long as access to water is not restricted, hydration, mucous membrane color, and capillary refill time remain normal. The presence of neurologic abnormalities is variable in dogs and cats with trauma-induced CDI or neoplastic destruction of the hypothalamus and/or pituitary gland. Many of these animals have no perceptible neurologic alterations on physical examination. A few show mild to severe neurologic signs, including stupor, weakness, ataxia, circling, and proprioceptive deficits.

Clinical pathology abnormalities

COMPLETE BLOOD COUNT.   The CBC in dogs and cats with CDI or NDI is usually unremarkable. The white blood cell count and differential are normal, because these pets are not particularly susceptible to infection. The red blood cell count is normal or mildly increased. Polycythemia is not common and is the result of a mild, clinically imperceptible state of dehydration. Diabetes insipidus is a primary polyuric disorder with compensatory polydipsia, and affected dogs and cats are chronically, albeit mildly, fluid-depleted to stimulate the compensatory thirst response. Owners commonly tire of their pets' polyuria and polydipsia and begin restricting access to water, further exacerbating dehydration. Fluid depletion results in hemoconcentration with a mild increase in hematocrit, red blood cell count, and serum total protein concentration. The CBC in dogs with psychogenic polydipsia is rarely abnormal.

URINALYSIS.   Random urinalysis in dogs and cats with CDI, NDI, or psychogenic polydipsia typically reveals a urine specific gravity less than 1.006, with values of 1.001 and 1.002 occurring commonly (Fig. 1-12). The corresponding urine osmolality is usually less than 300 mOsm/kg. A urine specific gravity in the isosthenuric range (1.008 to 1.015) does not rule out diabetes insipidus (see Fig. 1-12) or psychogenic polydipsia (see Table 1-6), especially when the urine has been obtained after water is knowingly or inadvertently withheld (e.g., a long car ride and wait in the veterinary office). Dogs and cats with partial diabetes insipidus can concentrate their urine into the isosthenuric range if dehydrated. The remaining components of the urinalysis in these animals are usually normal.

Extremely dilute urine is not commonly seen in veterinary practice, being limited usually to animals with postobstructive diuresis, excessive intravenous fluid administration, diuretic use, or hyperadrenocorticism, as well as CDI, NDI, or psychogenic polydipsia. Numerous disorders can result in polydipsia and polyuria (see page 9). In our experience, most of those problems do not cause the severe polyuria suggested by remarkable depression in the specific gravity (<1.006). Although we have seen animals that were polyuric owing to hypercalcemia, hypokalemia, pyometra, pyelonephritis, and other disorders, the degree of urine dilution is less dramatic and typically in the 1.008 to 1.020 range. However, even mild disturbances in the ability to concentrate urine, resulting in urine specific gravities of 1.008 to 1.015, often alter behavior sufficiently to allow an owner to realize the change.

SERUM CHEMISTRIES.   The serum biochemistry panel is normal in most dogs and cats with diabetes insipidus and psychogenic polydipsia. The chronic and severe diuresis associated with CDI, NDI, and psychogenic polydipsia causes excessive loss of urea via the kidneys and may cause a subsequent reduction of BUN to levels of 5 to 10 mg/dl. In 20 of our dogs with CDI, 40% had a BUN less than 10 mg/dl at the time of initial presentation to our hospital. Inadequate access to water can cause severe dehydration and prerenal azotemia with hyposthenuria. Azotemia (BUN >30 mg/dl) and hypernatremia (>158 mEq/L) were identified in 15% of our dogs with CDI at the time of initial presentation to our hospital. These clinicopathologic abnormalities resolved after allowing the dogs access to water and initiating DDAVP therapy. Additional abnormalities identified occasionally on a serum biochemistry panel from dogs and cats with diabetes insipidus include a mild increase in serum alanine aminotransferase and alkaline phosphatase activities, as well as serum creatinine, cholesterol, and total protein concentrations.

SERUM ELECTROLYTES.   Serum electrolytes are usually normal in dogs and cats with diabetes insipidus and psychogenic polydipsia. Mild hyponatremia (140 to

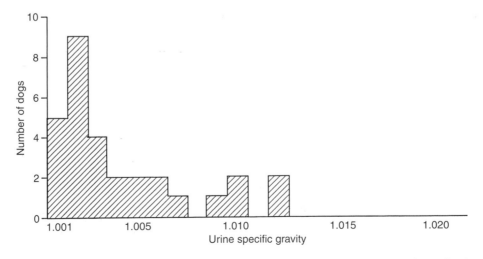

FIGURE 1–12. Urine specific gravity measured in 30 dogs with central diabetes insipidus at the time of initial presentation to the veterinarian.

144 mEq/L) and hypokalemia (3.8 to 4.0 mEq/L) have been identified in 20% of our dogs with CDI and psychogenic polydipsia. More important, severe hypernatremia (serum sodium, 159 to 165 mEq/L) and hyperkalemia (5.4 to 5.9 mEq/L) have been identified in 15% of our dogs with CDI, abnormalities presumably developing secondary to water restriction and dehydration. Rarely, hypertonic dehydration, severe hypernatremia, and neurologic signs may develop in a dog or cat with diabetes insipidus that is unable to drink (e.g., posttraumatic episode) or has restricted access to water (Reidarson et al, 1990). See Complications of the Modified Water Deprivation Test: Hypertonic Dehydration and Hypernatremia (page 29) for more information on this subject.

An intact renin angiotensin aldosterone axis succeeds in maintaining electrolyte homeostasis in most dogs and cats despite the remarkable urine output associated with CDI, NDI, and psychogenic polydipsia. Maintenance of fluid and electrolyte balance depends on functioning thirst and hunger centers in the hypothalamus. Water restriction can cause severe dehydration in a matter of hours. Because free water diuresis continues despite water restriction, vascular and systemic hyperosmolarity develops. Increases in serum sodium contribute significantly to this hyperosmolarity. Severe hypernatremia is associated with significant metabolic consequences and is a difficult therapeutic challenge. Water deprivation studies to confirm the diagnosis of diabetes insipidus are not without complications and require careful patient monitoring to avoid dangerous consequences (see Complications of the Modified Water Deprivation Test, page 29).

CONFIRMING THE DIAGNOSIS OF DIABETES INSIPIDUS

Several diagnostic approaches are used to confirm CDI, primary NDI, and primary (psychogenic) polydipsia. The modified water deprivation test (see below) is considered the best diagnostic test to differentiate between these three causes of polyuria and polydipsia. However, the test can be labor-intensive, time-consuming, and expensive, especially if urine and plasma osmolalities and plasma AVP concentrations are measured. Results of the test can also be confusing, especially with partial deficiency syndromes. Nevertheless, the modified water deprivation test is an excellent test to evaluate AVP secretion and renal tubular response to AVP and to identify psychogenic polydipsia by documenting an ability of the patient to concentrate urine to a specific gravity above 1.030 during water deprivation.

A simpler approach that is especially appealing in a busy practice is the measurement of random plasma osmolality to identify psychogenic polydipsia (see page 34), followed by evaluation of response to trial therapy with desmopressin (DDAVP) (see page 35). This approach requires that all other causes of polyuria and polydipsia except CDI, primary NDI, and psychogenic polydipsia be previously ruled out. Although random plasma osmolality measurement followed by trial DDAVP therapy is less time-consuming than the water deprivation test, the expense is often comparable, in part because of the expense of DDAVP. The modified water deprivation test may still need to be performed if nebulous results are obtained with this simpler approach.

MODIFIED WATER DEPRIVATION TEST

Principle of the Test

The modified water deprivation test is designed to determine whether endogenous AVP is released in response to dehydration and whether the kidneys respond to this stimulus. When the test is properly completed, one can differentiate CDI from NDI from psychogenic polydipsia. Occasionally the test also aids in separating these three disorders from hyperadrenocorticism. The modified water deprivation test serves no other purpose and is not meant to be a test of renal function. If the clinician successfully reduces the differential diagnoses in a polydipsic/polyuric dog or cat to CDI, NDI, or psychogenic polydipsia, the modified water deprivation test helps to complete the differentiation. Causes of secondary NDI, as well as other causes of polydipsia and polyuria, must be ruled out before accurate interpretation of the modified water deprivation test can be done. The following discussion assumes completion and review of the history, physical examination, and preliminary in-hospital screening tests as discussed on page 13 and focuses on the differences among CDI, NDI, and psychogenic polydipsia. In addition, canine hyperadrenocorticism is included because severe polydipsia and polyuria with dilute urine are frequent features of this relatively common endocrinopathy. The history, physical examination, and preliminary in-hospital routine testing, however, usually distinguish hyperadrenocorticism from CDI, NDI, and psychogenic polydipsia.

Contraindications to Performing the Test

The modified water deprivation test is not indicated to study the function of any organ system other than renal tubular response to AVP. This protocol is specifically contraindicated in patients suspected or known to have renal disease, those that are uremic owing to prerenal or primary renal disorders, and animals with suspected or obvious dehydration.

Terminology Used in Water Balance Studies

OSMOLALITY. Osmolality is continually a point of reference in discussions on polydipsia, polyuria, water balance, and water deprivation. The osmolal concentration of a substance in a fluid is measured by the degree to which the concentration depresses the freezing point: 1 mole/L of ideal solute depresses the freezing point 1.86° C. The number of milliosmoles per liter in a solution equals the freezing point depression divided by 0.00186. The osmolarity is the number of osmoles per liter of solution, such as plasma. The osmolality is the number of osmoles per kilogram of solvent. Therefore, osmolarity is affected by the volume of the various solutes in the solution and the temperature, whereas osmolality is not. Osmotically active substances in the body are dissolved in water and the density of water is 1. Therefore, osmolal concentrations can be expressed as osmoles per kilogram of water. In this discussion, osmolal (rather than osmolar) concentrations are considered, and osmolality is expressed in milliosmoles per kilogram (mOsm/kg).

The normal range for plasma osmolality is 280 to 310 mOsm/kg. It is important to note the relative contributions of the various plasma components to the total osmolal concentration of the plasma. Of the average 290 mOsm/kg, 270 are contributed by sodium and its accompanying anions, principally chloride and bicarbonate. Other cations and anions make a small contribution. Normal glucose concentrations make a small contribution of about 5 mOsm, because glucose does not dissociate and has a relatively large molecular weight of 180. The plasma proteins have a higher molecular weight than does glucose. Although present in large quantities, plasma proteins make an extremely small contribution to the plasma osmolality. The osmolal concentration of protein derivatives (other than electrolytes) is about 0.33 times that of BUN, or approximately 6 mOsm/kg. Because plasma is not an ideal solution, the osmolality of the plasma can be estimated from the following formula:

$$\frac{\text{Osmolality}}{\text{(mOsm/kg)}} = \frac{2(Na^+ + K^+)}{\text{(mEq/L)}} + \frac{0.05 \text{ (glucose)}}{\text{(mg/dl)}} + \frac{0.33 \text{ (BUN)}}{\text{(mg/dl)}}$$

This formula and others like it are useful in evaluating patients with fluid and electrolyte abnormalities, as well as assessing the contributions of the various components to normal plasma osmolality.

OSMOTIC PRESSURE. Osmotic pressure depends on the number rather than the type of particles in a solution. In effect, it is due to a reduction in the activity of the solvent particles in a solution. The activity of a substance is its effective concentration as evaluated by its behavior in solution. When a solute is dissolved in a solvent, the activity of the solvent molecules is decreased. A homogeneous solution of a single substance has an osmotic pressure, but this pressure can be expressed only when the solution is separated from a more dilute solution by a membrane permeable to the solvent but not to the solute. In this situation, solvent molecules diffuse from the area in which their activity is greater and the osmotic pressure is less (the dilute solution) to the area in which their activity is less and osmotic pressure is greater (the concentrated solution). Thus if a 10% aqueous solution of glucose is

placed in contact with distilled water across a membrane permeable to water but not to glucose, the volume of the glucose solution increases and its glucose concentration decreases as water molecules move into it from the water compartment.

TONICITY. All fluid compartments of the body are apparently in, or nearly in, osmotic equilibrium, except when there has been insufficient time for equilibration to occur following a sudden change in fluid composition. The term *tonicity* is used to describe the effective osmotic pressure of a solution relative to plasma. Solutions that have the same effective osmotic pressure as plasma are said to be isotonic, those with greater pressure are hypertonic, and those with lesser pressure are hypotonic. All solutions that are isosmotic with plasma would also be isotonic except that some solutes diffuse into cells and others are metabolized. Thus a 0.9% saline solution is isotonic because there is no net movement of the osmotically active particles in the solution into cells and the particles are not metabolized. However, urea diffuses rapidly into cells, so the effective osmotic pressure drops when cells are suspended in an aqueous solution that initially contains 290 mOsm/L of urea. Similarly, a 5% glucose solution is isotonic when initially infused intravenously; however, glucose is metabolized, so the net effect is that of infusing a hypotonic solution.

URINE SPECIFIC GRAVITY. It is much easier to place a drop of urine on a refractometer than to determine the osmolality of the urine. Therefore, specific gravity is still measured clinically as an index of urine concentration. The specific gravity of an ultrafiltrate of plasma is 1.010, whereas that of a maximally concentrated urine specimen is above 1.060. However, the specific gravity of a solution depends on the nature as well as the number of solute particles in it. For example, a subject excreting radiographic contrast medium may have a specific gravity of 1.040 to 1.050, with relatively low osmolality. The osmolality is more consistent and accurate than the specific gravity. Determination of specific gravity is a clinically useful tool in most situations, however, and is readily available and inexpensive. Prior to starting the modified water deprivation test, the clinician should check the accuracy of the refractometer by ensuring that a reading of 1.000 is obtained with distilled water (Barsanti et al, 2000).

Protocol (Table 1-9)

PREPARATION FOR THE TEST (PHASE I). The severity of renal medullary solute washout is a difficult variable to evaluate in an animal with severe polydipsia and polyuria; yet it may have an effect on test results. Theoretically, correction of renal medullary solute washout improves renal tubular concentrating ability and the accuracy of the modified water deprivation test in differentiating among CDI, NDI, and primary polydipsia. However, in animals with CDI, water restriction alone may not improve renal medullary solute washout; only after correction of polyuria and

TABLE 1–9   PROTOCOL FOR THE MODIFIED WATER DEPRIVATION TEST

Phase I. Preparation for the test
A. Determine total water intake per 24 hours based on unrestricted access to water
B. Three to five days prior to the test, gradually decrease total 24 hour water intake until the goal of 100 ml/kg/24 hours is attained or the animal becomes aggressive for water
C. Withhold food beginning 12 hours before the test

Phase II. Water deprivation
A. Prior to initiation
  1. Withdraw food and all water
  2. Empty bladder completely
  3. Obtain *exact* body weight
  4. Check urine osmolality/specific gravity
  5. Obtain serum osmolality
  6. Obtain BUN and serum electrolytes
  7. Check hydration and CNS status
B. During the test
  1. Completely empty bladder every 60–120 min
  2. Check *exact* body weight every 60 min
  3. Check urine osmolality/specific gravity at each interval
  4. Check hydration and CNS status at each interval
  5. Recheck BUN and serum electrolytes
  6. Recheck serum osmolality
C. End of Phase II
  1. If urine specific gravity exceeds 1.030
  2. When dog is clinically dehydrated or appears ill
  3. When dog has lost 3 to 5% body weight
    a. Obtain serum (plasma) for vasopressin concentration
    b. Empty bladder
    c. Check urine osmolality/specific gravity
    d. Check BUN and serum electrolytes
    e. Check serum osmolality

Phase III. Response to exogenous ADH
A. Administer aqueous vasopressin 2–5 U IM
B. Continue withholding food and water
C. Monitor patient
  1. Empty bladder every 30 min for 1–2 hours maximum
  2. Check urine osmolality/specific gravity
  3. Check serum osmolality
  4. Check BUN and serum electrolytes
  5. Check hydration and CNS status

Phase IV. End of test
A. Introduce small amounts of water (10–20 ml/kg) every 30 minutes for 2 hours
B. Monitor patient for vomiting, hydration status, CNS status
C. If patient is well 2 hours after ending test, return to ad lib water

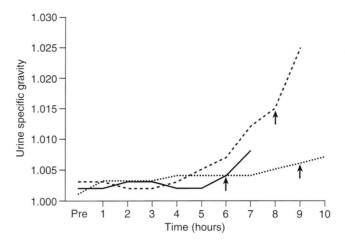

FIGURE 1–13. Results of the modified water deprivation test in a 1-year-old Persian cat with congenital central diabetes insipidus. *Solid line*, initial water deprivation test results. *Dotted line*, water deprivation test results after gradually restricting water consumption for 7 days prior to performing the test. *Dashed line*, water deprivation test results after gradual water restriction and twice daily injections of AVP for 7 days prior to performing the test. AVP injections were discontinued 24 hours prior to performing the test. ↑, 5% loss of body weight and aqueous AVP injection.

given at bedtime. No food is given within 12 hours of beginning the test or during the procedure.

BEGINNING THE TEST (PHASE IIA). The animal's bladder is catheterized and emptied; then an exact body weight is obtained just prior to initiating the test. Beginning at 8 or 9 a.m., water is completely withheld from the patient. Specific gravity and, if possible, osmolality should be determined on a pretest urine sample. Evaluation of plasma osmolality is also recommended but is not necessary for interpretation of test results. Periodic evaluation of BUN and serum sodium concentration, beginning at the start of the test, is helpful in identifying the development of uremia or hypernatremia. The onset of uremia or hypernatremia is a criterion for ending the test.

The water deprivation test should always be started at the beginning of the workday, because animals undergoing this test must be observed and evaluated frequently. Most dogs and cats with CDI or NDI dehydrate and lose 3 to 5% of their body weight (end point for the test) within 3 to 10 hours (Table 1-10). Withholding water and leaving the dog or cat with diabetes insipidus unattended for several hours or throughout the night may result in the development of severe complications and possibly death (see Complications of the Modified Water Deprivation Test, page 29). Frequent observation and proper methodology help avoid complications or severe dehydration.

DURING THE TEST (PHASE IIB). The urinary bladder must be completely emptied every 60 to 120 minutes. Dogs can either be catheterized initially with a Foley catheter sutured in place or be repeatedly catheterized. Some dogs urinate if taken for short walks. This decision is based on the size of the dog and the ease of the procedure. For cats, an indwelling bladder catheter is used. The specific gravity should be determined on

polydipsia with vasopressin therapy, in conjunction with water restriction, can the capacity of the renal tubule to concentrate urine be fully appreciated (Fig. 1-13). Nevertheless, we attempt to minimize the effects of severe medullary washout on the results of the modified water deprivation test, using progressive water restriction before initiating total water deprivation. The goal is to decrease 24-hour water intake to approximately 100 ml/kg the day prior to performing the water deprivation test. Total water intake per 24 hours should be determined by the owner and based on unrestricted access to water. Water restriction is begun once total 24-hour water intake has been quantified. The total 24-hour allotment of water is gradually decreased over 3 to 5 days until the goal of 100 ml/kg/24 hours is attained or the animal becomes aggressive for water. Each day's 24-hour allotment of water should be divided into six to eight aliquots with the last aliquot

TABLE 1–10   GUIDELINES FOR INTERPRETATION OF THE WATER DEPRIVATION TEST*

Disorder	URINE SPECIFIC GRAVITY			TIME TO 5% DEHYDRATION (HOURS)	
	Initially	5% Dehydration	Post-ADH	Mean	Range
Central DI					
Complete	<1.006	<1.006	<1.010	4	3-7
Partial	<1.006	1.008–1.020	<1.015	8	6-11
Primary nephrogenic DI	<1.006	<1.006	<1.006	5	3-9
Primary polydipsia	1.002–1.020	>1.030	NA	13	8-20

*Based on results from 20 dogs with central diabetes insipidus, 5 dogs with primary nephrogenic diabetes insipidus, and 18 dogs with primary (psychogenic) polydipsia.
DI = Diabetes insipidus; *NA* = not applicable.

each urine sample and an aliquot stored for osmolality determination, should it be desired at the end of the test. Most important, the dog or cat must be carefully weighed at least once an hour. Phase II ends when 3% to 5% of body weight has been lost or urine specific gravity exceeds 1.030. Additionally, the dog or cat should be assessed for clinical evidence of dehydration and changes in mentation or behavior. Periodic evaluation of BUN and serum sodium concentration should also be done. The test should be halted if the dog or cat becomes uremic, hypernatremic, or severely dehydrated or develops changes in mentation or behavior.

END OF PHASE II (PHASE IIC).   Maximal secretion of AVP and concentration of urine are achieved when an animal loses 3% to 5% of its body weight owing to urine loss of fluid with simultaneous water deprivation. The goal is to get as close to 5% loss of body weight as possible before ending phase II of the test. At that point the urinary bladder should be completely emptied, the urine checked for specific gravity and osmolality, and phase III of the water deprivation test initiated (see Table 1-9). A plasma vasopressin concentration obtained at this time is helpful in interpreting the test (see Plasma Vasopressin Determinations, page 33).

Normal dogs typically require more than 24 hours to lose 3% to 5% of body weight following water deprivation. In contrast, water deprivation usually causes 3% to 5% or greater loss of body weight within 3 to 10 hours if the animal has CDI or NDI (see Table 1-10). Dogs or cats with partial CDI or psychogenic polydipsia may require considerably longer than 10 hours to achieve 3% to 5% loss of body weight. The clinician should always be prepared to continue the water deprivation test into the late evening hours. If this is not possible and the dog or cat has not yet lost 3% to 5% body weight or attained a urine specific gravity greater than 1.030 by the end of the working hours, the dog or cat can be transferred to a veterinary hospital with overnight care so the test can be continued.

Alternatively, the study can be stopped and water offered, initially in small amounts to prevent over-zealous intake. The modified water deprivation test can then be repeated in a few days with the following adjustments in protocol: body weight is measured and water withheld beginning at midnight; the dog or cat is kept in a cage (or at home) for the remainder of the night, ideally with periodic visual assessment by individuals working at night (or by the owner if the patient is at home); the urinary bladder is completely emptied first thing in the morning and urine specific gravity and/or osmolality are measured; body weight is recorded; and phase II is continued as previously discussed. With this modification, the clinician is already 6 to 8 hours into phase II of the test at the beginning of the workday. Complete CDI and NDI must be ruled out before this modification to the modified water deprivation test is used; that is, the clinician must prove that the dog or cat requires at least 10 hours of water deprivation before 3% to 5% loss of body weight occurs. The modification described here should never be incorporated into the initial modified water deprivation test performed on the dog or cat.

Serial evaluation of body weight is a simple, inexpensive, reliable, and readily available method to determine the end point of phase II of the test. The goal is to exceed 3% (preferably, to reach close to 5%) loss of body weight during water deprivation. A 1% to 2% loss of weight due to dehydration may fail to maximally stimulate AVP secretion. False plateaus in urine osmolality and urine specific gravity have been observed with weight loss in the range of 2%, which can be misleading.

Other criteria have been used to determine whether and when maximal urinary concentration has been achieved through water deprivation. One method is recognition of a "plateau," or lack of increase, in urine osmolalities once 3% loss of body weight has occurred. This criterion is based on the knowledge that after the maximal renal response to water deprivation is achieved, the urine osmolality becomes relatively constant. This plateau in urine concentration is defined as a change in osmolality between three consecutive urine collection periods, 1 hour apart, of less than 5% or 30 mOsm/kg. Monitoring urine specific gravity in lieu of osmolality is less reliable than monitoring body weight, because false plateaus in urine specific gravity are common, even when 3% loss of body weight has occurred. Although the ability to ascertain a specific gravity is readily available, it is not sufficiently accurate to use as a criterion for ending phase II of the study, unless the urine specific gravity exceeds 1.030, which implies normal AVP secretion with renal responsiveness.

Monitoring skin turgidity and measuring the packed cell volume of blood have not proved to be reliable or consistent tools for recognizing dehydration. Measurement of total plasma protein concentration may be more reliable than the former two parameters, but monitoring cannot be considered as consistent or informative as body weight and patient observation. One important aid during phase II of the modified water deprivation test is the periodic check of the BUN and serum sodium concentration. Whenever the BUN rises above 30 mg/dl, the patient is azotemic and phase II should be ended. Azotemia developing during the modified water deprivation test has not been a problem in dogs and cats monitored as suggested above. However, assessment of BUN is simple and inexpensive. If azotemia is considered a possible sequela to water deprivation, it should be monitored or the water deprivation test should be postponed. Similarly, hypernatremia and increased plasma osmolality are potent stimulants of AVP secretion; when identified, these signs suggest that phase II of the water deprivation test be ended.

RESPONSE TO EXOGENOUS AVP (PHASE III). Phase II determines the effects of dehydration on endogenous AVP secretion and AVP action on the renal tubules. Phase III determines what effect, if any, exogenous AVP has on renal tubular ability to concentrate urine in the face of dehydration. This phase differentiates impaired AVP secretion from impaired renal tubular responsiveness to AVP.

After 3% to 5% or greater loss of body weight via water deprivation has occurred, aqueous vasopressin (Parke Davis, Morris Plains, NJ) is administered intramuscularly (IM) at a dose of 0.55 U/kg of body weight. The maximum dose in any dog or cat is 5 U. Water deprivation continues, and the bladder is emptied 30, 60, and 120 minutes following injection. Specific gravity and/or osmolality is determined on these urine samples. The test is now complete, and the dog or cat is offered small amounts of water over the next 2 hours. Ultimately, the animal is returned to free-choice water. The water is initially offered in small amounts to prevent overzealous intake, which could result in vomiting or water intoxication.

SUBCUTANEOUS (SC) AND INTRAVENOUS (IV) AVP ADMINISTRATION. The urine concentrating ability following subcutaneous administration of aqueous vasopressin is variable and not recommended. Results obtained after intravenous administration of AVP are reliable. Aqueous AVP, suggested for intravenous use, should be diluted in lactated Ringer's or 5% dextrose solution to attain 1 mU of AVP per milliliter of fluid solution. The patient then receives 10 ml of AVP containing intravenous fluids per kilogram of body weight (10 mU AVP/kg). This solution is administered slowly over 60 minutes, and urine samples are obtained at 0, 15, 30, 45, 60, 75, and 90 minutes. We have not had problems with intramuscular AVP administration and prefer this route of aqueous vasopressin administration. Either method of AVP administration, however, should provide the necessary information to differentiate CDI from NDI.

DESMOPRESSIN ACETATE (DDAVP) ADMINISTRATION. Desmopressin acetate is a synthetic analogue of vasopressin used for the treatment of CDI in dogs and cats (see page 37). DDAVP has been used in lieu of aqueous vasopressin during phase III of the water deprivation test, although appropriate timing of urine samples for assessment of urine osmolality and/or specific gravity has not been critically evaluated. The maximal effect of DDAVP, regardless of the route of administration, occurs from 2 to 8 hours after administration. Urine samples obtained every 1 to 2 hours for 8 hours and, if necessary, 12 and 24 hours after placement of 4 drops of DDAVP intranasal preparation in the conjunctival sac should be helpful in assessing renal response to vasopressin during phase III of the test. Alternatively, 10 to 20 µg of the parenteral or intranasal preparation of DDAVP can be administered intravenously or subcutaneously and urine specific gravity may be checked every 1 to 2 hours for 8 hours and, if necessary, at 12 and 24 hours (Barsanti et al, 2000). The intranasal preparation of DDAVP is not sterile, so the solution should be passed through a bacteriostatic filter before administration. Small amounts of water should be offered when a response to DDAVP is identified, hypernatremia or azotemia develops, or there is a change in hydration status or mental alertness of the animal.

Responses to the Modified Water Deprivation Test

NORMAL DOGS. Normal dogs dehydrate quite slowly (Fig. 1-14). The secretion of AVP in the normal dog results in exquisite conservation of fluid over long time periods. Random urine samples from normal dogs with free access to water reveal a specific gravity of 1.006 to greater than 1.040 and an osmolality of 160 to greater than 2500 mOsm/kg (van Vonderen et al, 1997b). In a report on laboratory dogs, the range of values was narrower and maximal urine concentration was achieved in 20 dogs after an average of approximately 40 hours of water deprivation. Maximal urine osmolality ranged from 1700 to 2700 mOsm/kg and specific gravity from 1.050 to 1.075. Urine concentration indices (specific gravity and osmolality) did not plateau after reaching maximal values. Most dogs reached a peak in urine concentration, followed by slight fluctuations below that value for the remaining period of water deprivation. No difference in testing parameters occurred between males and females. Although not specifically evaluated, similar findings are expected in the cat.

What happens if AVP is injected after maximal urine concentration is reached via water deprivation in normal dogs and cats? As expected, such animals are experiencing maximal endogenous AVP secretion, and

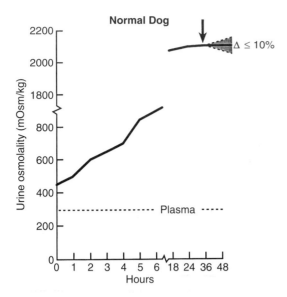

FIGURE 1–14. The effect of water deprivation on the urine osmolality of a normal dog. ↓ represents an injection of aqueous vasopressin, which alters urine osmolality 10% or less.

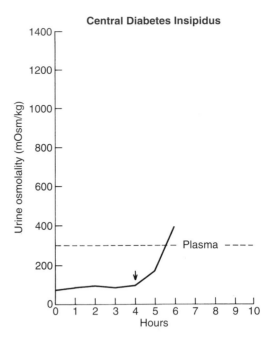

FIGURE 1–15. The effect of water deprivation on the urine osmolality of a dog with severe central diabetes insipidus (CDI). ↓ represents an injection of aqueous vasopressin administered after 5% or more body weight is lost, causing greater than 50% increase in urine osmolality. Note how quickly these dogs lose 5% of their body weight.

no further urine concentration can occur. Therefore, exogenous AVP should have little effect on urine concentration in these animals. After dehydration, changes in urine concentration of 10% or less of preinjection levels are not considered significant. Such lack of change is typical in dogs and cats with normal AVP secretion rates and renal responsiveness to AVP (see Fig. 1-14).

In a clinical setting, *normal* for the modified water deprivation test is defined as a urine osmolality significantly greater than plasma osmolality. Normal dogs and cats have urine that is typically greater than 1100 mOsm/kg and a urine specific gravity greater than 1.030 after dehydration. If urine osmolality and specific gravity exceed these values, pituitary AVP secretion, and renal responsiveness to AVP are considered intact and there is no need to evaluate renal responsiveness to exogenous AVP.

CDI. Dogs and cats with severe (complete) CDI cannot concentrate urine to levels greater than plasma osmolality (280 to 310 mOsm/kg), even with severe dehydration. In fact, the parameters of urine concentration change little, if any, with continuing water deprivation (Fig. 1-15). CDI may be subdivided into severe or partial deficiencies of AVP. The modified water deprivation test has been used to help differentiate between mild and severe forms of CDI. As previously described, mild states of dehydration, resulting in a 1% to 2% loss in body weight, cause sustained release of AVP in the normal subject. After maximal urine concentration occurs in the normal animal, it does not increase more than an additional 10% with the injection of aqueous vasopressin. If the administration of AVP to a dehydrated dog or cat causes a significant increase in the concentration of the urine, endogenous AVP production and/or secretion must be insufficient. In dogs and cats with severe AVP deficiency, the urine osmolalities do not reach

300 mOsm/kg with dehydration; however, the increase in osmolality after administration of vasopressin ranges from 50% to 600% greater than the preinjection level (Figs. 1-16 and 1-17).

Dogs and cats with partial AVP deficiencies can increase their urine osmolality above 300 mOsm/kg after dehydration, but they also experience a further 10% to 50% or greater increase in urine osmolality following administration of vasopressin (Fig. 1-18; see Fig. 1-17). Dehydration often increases plasma osmolality, which may become worrisome because of induction of cerebral damage (see page 29). Changes in urine specific gravity often behave in a manner similar to changes in urine osmolality (Fig. 1-19; see Table 1-10). However, in some dogs and cats, urine specific gravity is not as easy to interpret as is urine osmolality (Fig. 1-20).

Dogs and cats with either severe or partial CDI are brought to the veterinarian with similar owner concerns. These animals consume large quantities of water, are polyuric, and may appear incontinent to their owners. Some owners report the need to allow such dogs to go outside to urinate several times each night. It is often not until after completion of the modified water deprivation test that dogs and cats with partial CDI are distinguished from those with severe CDI. The differentiation is of interest academically but is also important clinically, because oral agents may be successfully used in the treatment of partial CDI, whereas synthetic AVP administration is necessary for treating severe CDI.

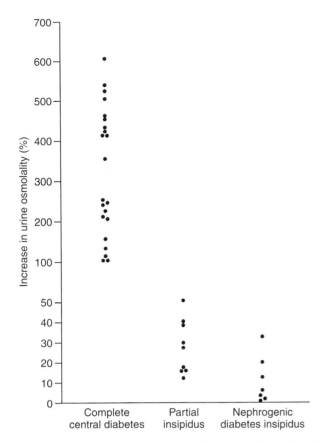

FIGURE 1–16. Increase in urine osmolality during phase III of the modified water deprivation test, that is, after IM administration of aqueous vasopressin, in 22 dogs with complete central diabetes insipidus, 9 dogs with partial central diabetes insipidus, and 7 dogs with primary nephrogenic diabetes insipidus. Note the marked increase in urine osmolality after vasopressin administration with complete central diabetes insipidus versus partial central or primary nephrogenic diabetes insipidus.

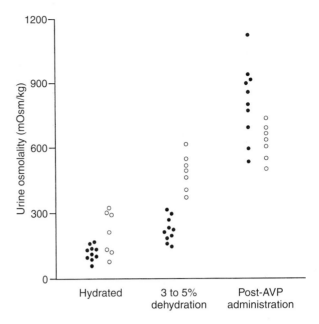

FIGURE 1–17. Urine osmolality in 10 dogs with complete central diabetes insipidus (solid circle) and 7 dogs with partial central diabetes insipidus (open circle) at the beginning (hydrated), end of phase II (3% to 5% dehydration), and end of phase III (post-AVP administration) of the modified water deprivation test. Note the relative failure of dogs with complete central diabetes insipidus to increase urine osmolality with dehydration and the marked increase in urine osmolality after aqueous vasopressin administration. The opposite occurred in the dogs with partial central diabetes insipidus.

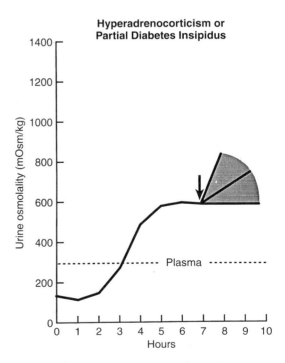

FIGURE 1–18. The effect of water deprivation on the urine osmolality of a dog afflicted with partial CDI or canine hyperadrenocorticism. ↓ represents an injection of aqueous vasopressin administered after 5% or more body weight is lost owing to fluid loss via the urine. The urine osmolality did increase, but subnormally, in response to dehydration. Vasopressin results in a further 10% to 50% increase in urine osmolality. Note that the dog with partial CDI takes longer to dehydrate than one with severe CDI (see Fig. 1-15).

NDI. Dogs, and presumably cats, afflicted with primary NDI cannot concentrate urine to levels greater than plasma osmolality (280 to 310 mOsm/kg), even after severe dehydration. As with CDI, the parameters of urine concentration change little, if any, with continuing water deprivation (Fig. 1-21; see Table 1-10). Unlike CDI, however, minimal to no increase in urine osmolality and urine specific gravity occurs after administration of vasopressin (see Fig. 1-16).

Similar to dogs with severe CDI, dogs with NDI dehydrate quickly without water (see Table 1-10). The only difference between NDI and severe CDI is the lack of response to an injection of vasopressin seen in NDI versus the dramatic increase in urine concentration seen in CDI after vasopressin injection. Spontaneous severe NDI appears to be a congenital disorder. Dogs with this condition have been young (see page 17). However, dogs and cats with acquired NDI are usually adults with a concurrent illness that interferes with AVP action at the renal tubular level (see page 10).

Acquired NDI patients are usually differentiated from those with CDI or spontaneous NDI after review

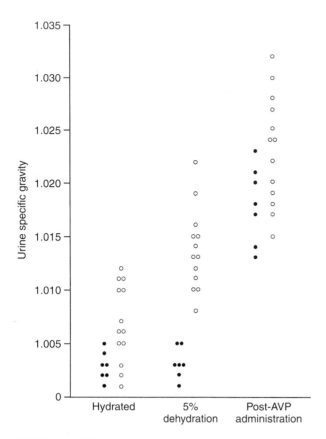

FIGURE 1–19. Urine specific gravity in 7 dogs with complete central diabetes insipidus *(solid circle)* and 13 dogs with partial central diabetes insipidus *(open circle)* at the beginning (hydrated), end of phase II (5% dehydration), and end of phase III (post-AVP administration) of the modified water deprivation test. Note the similarity of response between urine specific gravity and urine osmolality (see Fig. 1-17).

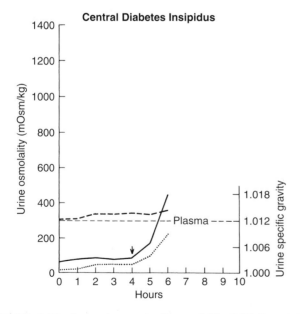

FIGURE 1–20. Same dog as in Figure 1-15. *Solid line,* urine osmolality; *dashed line,* increasing plasma osmolality caused by dehydrating a dog with CDI; *dotted line,* urine specific gravity, illustrating why it is a less precise and less obvious diagnostic marker with severe CDI (see Fig. 1-15).

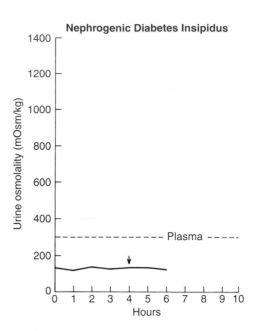

FIGURE 1–21. The effect of water deprivation on the urine osmolality of a dog afflicted with primary nephrogenic diabetes insipidus. Vasopressin is administered (↓) after 5% or more of body weight is lost (in this dog, after only 4 hours). Note the rapid loss of weight and the absence of any increase in urine concentration following 5% or more loss in body weight. The urine osmolality is not increased by vasopressin administration (<10% change).

of the history, physical examination, and routine clinical pathology. Therefore, dogs and cats with pyometra, pyelonephritis, hypercalcemia, hypokalemia, hyperadrenocorticism, diabetes mellitus, chronic renal failure, or renal glycosuria should be identified on screening studies, eliminating the need for the modified water deprivation test. Animals with acquired NDI respond to water deprivation and postdehydration AVP administration similarly to those with congenital spontaneous NDI (Breitschwerdt, 1981). Therefore, the modified water deprivation test fails to separate spontaneous/congenital from acquired/secondary NDI, just as the test fails to separate congenital from acquired CDI. This knowledge does not detract from the value of the study; rather, it lends strong support to the need for establishing a complete data base that may preclude the need for water deprivation.

Occasionally, preliminary testing on dogs or cats with acquired NDI does not reveal the underlying disorder. Such patients may undergo an unnecessary modified water deprivation test. Several disease states can be difficult to diagnose. These include pyelonephritis, in which the only clue may be sporadic bacteriuria; early renal failure, in which the BUN and creatinine are near the upper range of normal but isosthenuria is present; hyperadrenocorticism, if the only signs are polydipsia and polyuria, clinicopathologic abnormalities are not evident, and tests of the pituitary-adrenocortical axis are equivocal; and pyometra, in which the vaginal discharge is slight, the dog or cat keeps herself clean, the uterus is small, and the white blood count is normal. Each of these situations is uncommon but points out the potential indirect aid that a modified water deprivation test can provide. Any time a veterinarian establishes the diagnosis of NDI in a mature dog or cat, acquired disease must be considered likely (see page 10).

CANINE HYPERADRENOCORTICISM (CUSHING'S SYNDROME). Hyperadrenocorticism commonly causes severe polydipsia and polyuria. Occasionally, dogs have no other clinical signs and do not have the typical laboratory abnormalities associated with the disease. Results of the modified water deprivation test in dogs with hyperadrenocorticism are similar to results in dogs with partial CDI (see Fig. 1-18) and, sometimes, dogs with psychogenic polydipsia. Dogs with hyperadrenocorticism usually concentrate their urine above plasma osmolality after water deprivation. Subsequent injection of aqueous AVP may cause a further 10% to 50% increase in urine osmolality, results that resemble partial CDI. However, response in some dogs with hyperadrenocorticism resembles psychogenic polydipsia in that no increase occurs in urine osmolality after the injection of aqueous AVP. Thus the clinician should be able to distinguish between NDI, severe CDI, and hyperadrenocorticism using the modified water deprivation test. One may not always be able to distinguish between psychogenic polydipsia, partial CDI, and hyperadrenocorticism. However, the relative frequency of Cushing's syndrome in relation to CDI, NDI, and psychogenic polydipsia would make hyperadrenocorticism a strong possibility in any animal with equivocal test results, especially in an older dog.

PRIMARY OR PSYCHOGENIC POLYDIPSIA. Dogs, and presumably cats, with primary or psychogenic polydipsia have an intact hypothalamic pituitary renal axis for controlling fluid balance and variable severity of renal medullary solute washout. Because pituitary AVP secretion and renal tubular response to AVP are normal, these dogs can concentrate urine to an osmolality above that of plasma with complete water deprivation and, given enough time, can attain urine specific gravities in excess of 1.030. Depending on the severity of renal medullary solute washout, it may take 12 to 24 hours of water deprivation to attain concentrated urine. The previously described progressive water restriction procedure during the 72 hours preceding the water deprivation test aids in reestablishing the renal medullary concentration gradient in these dogs and shortens the time to attain concentrated urine. Phase III (response to aqueous AVP injection) is rarely needed in dogs with psychogenic polydipsia. If phase III is performed, injection of AVP in a dehydrated dog with psychogenic polydipsia causes little change (<10%) in urine osmolality (Fig. 1-22). This lack of change reflects the competent AVP secretory response of the posterior pituitary to dehydration and a response to AVP by the renal tubules.

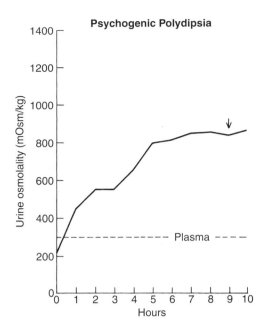

FIGURE 1–22. The effect of water deprivation on the urine osmolality of a dog afflicted with psychogenic polydipsia. Although these dogs are hormonally normal, the chronic diuresis may inhibit normal concentrating ability. ↓ represents an injection of aqueous vasopressin administered after 5% or more body weight is lost as a result of the unabated diuresis. The urine does show mild concentrating ability with dehydration, but less than 10% change in concentration following vasopressin administration.

Complications of the Modified Water Deprivation Test: Hypertonic Dehydration and Hypernatremia

An adult dog or cat is composed of 60% water. This water is subdivided into an intracellular compartment, which accounts for two-thirds of the total, and an extracellular compartment, which is one-third (Fig. 1-23). Movement of solutes that readily diffuse across all membranes (such as urea) is not accompanied by appreciable fluid shifts, because these solutes generate equal osmotic forces on either side of the cell membrane. Increased concentration of these solutes creates hyperosmolality in all fluid compartments because of a lack of water redistribution.

Solutes that are less permeable across cell membranes by virtue of molecular size, electrical charge, or active membrane pumps create an effective osmotic force. Intracellular solutes of this kind include potassium, phosphate, and protein. Sodium and its anions serve the same purpose in the extracellular fluid. Increased concentrations of such solutes in the extracellular fluid produce hyperosmolality and hypertonicity. The osmotic gradient that is formed results in movement of intracellular fluid into the extracellular space. Therefore, extracellular volume increases at the expense of cellular hydration. Alternatively, decreased concentrations of extracellular solutes produce a hyposmotic, hypotonic extracellular fluid that necessitates intracellular movement of water, causing both

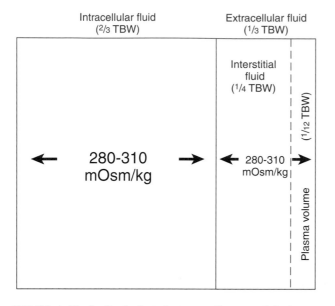

FIGURE 1–23. In the hydrated state, uniform total body water (TBW) distribution is maintained between the intracellular fluid and extracellular fluid compartments by osmotic forces (normal range, 280 to 310 mOsm/kg; average, 295 mOsm/kg) generated by solutes. (From Edwards DF, et al: JAVMA 182:973, 1983.)

hypovolemia and cellular overhydration (Edwards et al, 1983).

Three chemically distinct forms of dehydration (isotonic, hypotonic, and hypertonic) occur in veterinary practice. Isotonic dehydration is produced by proportional loss of water and electrolytes (solutes) (Fig. 1-24, A). Protracted vomiting and diarrhea are one cause of isotonic dehydration, in which water and electrolyte losses occur predominantly from the extracellular fluid compartment to the external environment. Serum sodium concentrations are generally normal, and clinical signs, such as skin turgidity/elasticity, are proportional to the degree of hypovolemia.

Hypotonic dehydration is produced by loss of electrolytes in excess of water, as is seen in hypoadrenocorticism. In this example, excessive sodium is lost in the urine and gastrointestinal tract, creating a hypotonic extracellular compartment that loses water to both the external environment and the intracellular space. Serum sodium values are generally low in this condition, prerenal azotemia is common, and these animals exhibit more obvious signs of hypovolemia than those with isotonic dehydration (see Fig. 1-24, B).

Hypertonic dehydration is produced by loss of water in excess of electrolytes and is the major concern after water deprivation in a dog or cat with CDI, NDI, or primary polydipsia and in dogs and cats with inadequate fluid intake following the onset of trauma-

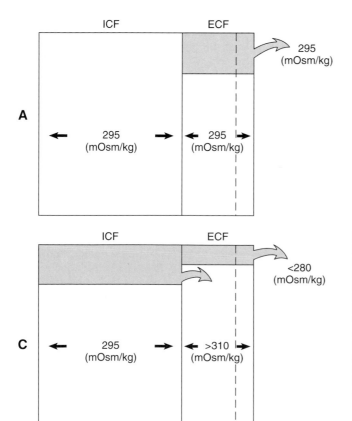

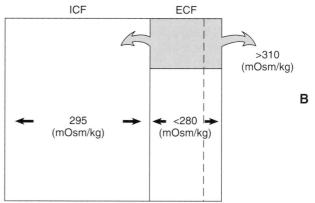

FIGURE 1–24. *A*, Isotonic dehydration results from extracellular fluid (ECF) loss of water and electrolytes isosmotic (295 mOsm/kg) to TBW. Because compartmental osmolality and tonicity remain unchanged (295 mOsm/kg), no major shift of intracellular fluid (ICF) occurs. *B*, Hypotonic dehydration results from ECF loss of water and electrolytes hyperosmotic (>310 mOsm/kg) to TBW. The ECF becomes hypo-osmolar and hypotonic (<280 mOsm/kg) to ICF. The intracellular movement of ECF reestablishes compartmental equilibrium at a lower osmotic pressure (<295 mOsm/kg) and minimizes fluid loss from the ICF space. *C*, Hypertonic dehydration results from ECF loss of water and electrolytes hyposmotic (<280 mOsm/kg) to TBW. The ECF becomes hyperosmolar and hypertonic (>310 mOsm/kg) and minimizes fluid loss from the ECF space. (From Edwards DF, et al: JAVMA 182:973, 1983.)

induced CDI (see Fig. 1-24, C). The hypertonic extracellular compartment preserves volume by dehydrating the intracellular compartment. The total water deficit is shared by fluid compartments in proportion to their normal content of water (Edwards et al, 1983). The cells, which contain two-thirds of the total body water, lose substantially more fluid than does the extracellular compartment. Plasma volume, constituting only one-twelfth of the total body water, is relatively well preserved under these circumstances. Thus hypertonic dehydration results in few of the expected signs of severe fluid depletion. Tachycardia, lack of skin turgidity/elasticity, decreased pulse pressure, and decreased vascular volume are not detected until severe dehydration is present. Weight loss is consistently seen much sooner and further emphasizes the importance of monitoring body weight during a water deprivation test.

Severe hypernatremia and hyposthenuria are classic markers for hypertonic dehydration in the dog or cat with CDI or NDI. Other causes of hypernatremia are not typically associated with hyposthenuria (Table 1-11). The predominant clinical signs associated with hypertonic dehydration result from CNS dysfunction. The initial critical signs include irritability, weakness, and ataxia; as the hypernatremia worsens, stupor progresses to coma and seizures. The progression and severity of these signs depend on the rate of onset, degree, and duration of hypernatremia. Sodium has limited access to brain cells and is slow to equilibrate with the cerebrospinal fluid (CSF). Rapidly developing severe hypernatremia results in a shift of water from the intracellular to the extracellular space and forces reduction in CSF volume as water crosses into the hyperosmotic fluid outside the CSF, causing shrinkage of the brain. Reduction in brain size leads to tearing of veins, subdural hemorrhage, and venous thrombosis. The brain synthesizes intracellular cerebral osmolar active substances (i.e., polyols) to compensate for the hyperosmolar extracellular fluid and to minimize the shift of fluid into the extracellular space. Osmolytes are produced in the brain beginning within 1 hour

after induction of persistent hyperosmolality of extracellular fluid (Pollock and Arieff, 1980).

The goal in treating hypernatremic, hypertonic dehydration is to restore the ECF volume to normal and correct water deficits at a fluid rate that avoids significant complications. Because the brain adjusts to hypertonicity by increasing the intracellular solute content via the accumulation of "idiogenic osmoles," the rapid repletion of body water with ECF dilution causes translocation of water into cells and can cause cerebral edema (Edwards et al, 1983; Reeves et al, 1998). If slower water repletion is undertaken brain cells lose the accumulated intracellular solutes and osmotic equilibration can occur without cell swelling.

The initial priority is to restore the extracellular fluid (ECF) volume to normal. The choice of fluid to be administered depends on whether circulatory collapse is present, the rate at which hypernatremia developed, and the magnitude of the hypernatremia. In patients with modest volume contraction (e.g., tachycardia, dry mucous membranes, slow skin turgor), fluid deficits should be corrected with 0.45% saline supplemented with an appropriate amount of potassium. With severe dehydration, 0.9% saline or plasma should be used to expand vascular volume. In replacing deficits, rapid administration of fluids is contraindicated unless there are signs of significant hypovolemia. Any fluid should be administered in a volume only large enough to correct hypovolemia. Worsening neurologic status or sudden onset of seizures during fluid therapy is generally indicative of cerebral edema and the need for hypertonic saline solution or mannitol therapy.

Once ECF deficits have been replaced, the intravascular compartment is stabilized, serum sodium concentration should be reevaluated and water deficits corrected if hypernatremia persists. An approximation of the water deficit in liters may be calculated using the formula:

$$0.6 \times \text{body weight (kg)} \times [1 - (\text{serum Na}^+_{desired} / \text{serum Na}^+_{present})]$$

Oral fluid administration is preferable to correct water deficits, with intravenous administration used when oral therapy is not possible. Half-strength (0.45%) saline solution with 2.5% dextrose or a 5% dextrose in water (D_5W) solution are used to correct the water deficit in hypernatremic animals. A 5% dextrose in water (D_5W) solution can be used to replenish body water in patients with acute onset of mild hypernatremia (<24 hours duration, serum sodium <165 mEq/L) in the absence of significant circulatory collapse, but the infusion rate must be less than the rate of glucose metabolism to avoid glycosuria and glucose-induced osmotic diuresis. Half-strength (0.45%) saline solution with 2.5% dextrose should be considered initially when severe hypernatremia (>170 mEq/L) is present, especially if it has developed gradually over more than a 24-hour period. D_5W solution can be substituted for 0.45% saline solution with 2.5% dextrose if the hypernatremia does not improve after 12 to

TABLE 1–11   CAUSES OF HYPERNATREMIA IN DOGS AND CATS

Water loss in excess of electrolytes
Central diabetes insipidus
Nephrogenic diabetes insipidus
Gastrointestinal fluid loss
Osmotic diuresis
  Renal failure
  Diabetes mellitus
  Mannitol
Heat stroke
Fever
Burns
Hypothalamic dysfunction (primary adipsia)
Excess sodium retention
Iatrogenic
  Salt ingestion
  Saline fluid therapy
  Sodium bicarbonate therapy
Primary hyperaldosteronism

24 hours of fluid therapy. The water deficit should be replaced slowly—approximately 50% in the first 24 hours and the remainder over the next 24 to 48 hours. Serum sodium concentrations should decline slowly, preferably at a rate less than 1 mEq/L/hour of fluid therapy. A gradual reduction in serum sodium concentration minimizes the fluid shift from the extracellular to the intracellular compartment, thereby minimizing neuronal cell swelling, cerebral edema, and intracranial pressure. Deterioration of CNS status after the initiation of fluid therapy suggests cerebral edema and the immediate need for a reduction in the rate of fluid administration. Frequent monitoring of serum electrolytes, with appropriate adjustments in the type of fluid and rate of fluid administration, is important in the successful management of hypernatremia. It is much simpler to avoid these complications by careful monitoring during water deprivation.

Misdiagnosis (Inaccuracies) Using the Modified Water Deprivation Test

The modified water deprivation test is an excellent study to differentiate severe NDI from severe CDI, but it may not differentiate partial CDI from primary poly-dipsia with complete certainty (Fig. 1-25). Difficulties in differentiating partial CDI from primary polydipsia may be explained by two associated changes in the renal response to AVP. First is the reduction in maximal concentrating capacity resulting from chronic polyuria itself (i.e., renal medullary solute washout), which is manifested as subnormal urine concentrations in the presence of excess levels of plasma vaso-pressin. Second, there appears to be an enhanced antidiuretic response to low levels of plasma AVP in patients with CDI; that is, these patients have a supersensitive response to the small amount of AVP they secrete endogenously (Block et al, 1981). The consequence of the enhanced antidiuretic effect is the amelioration of the urinary manifestations of partial AVP deficiency. Therefore, patients with partial CDI and those with primary polydipsia (that have not attained 3% to 5% loss of body weight) may respond to fluid deprivation with similar levels of urine concentration that cannot be increased further by injections of AVP (see Figs. 1-17 and 1-21). Thus neither the absolute level of urine osmolality achieved during fluid deprivation nor the percentage of increase evoked by exogenous AVP consistently permits a clear distinction between the two disorders (Zerbe and Robertson, 1981).

The modified water deprivation test may also occasionally misdiagnose human patients with NDI. This inconsistency arises because a small percentage of these patients are only partially resistant to the anti-diuretic effect of vasopressin and can concentrate their urine to some degree if the plasma levels of the hormone are quite high (Robertson and Scheidler, 1981). Because the standard diagnostic dose of aqueous AVP customarily produces marked hyper-vasopressinemia, patients with partial resistance may respond in this phase of the modified water deprivation test as though they had CDI (Zerbe and

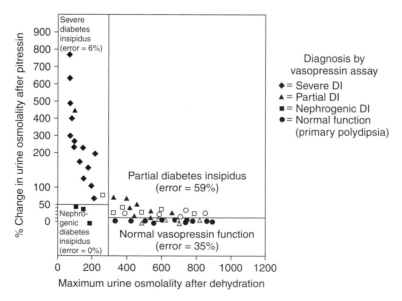

FIGURE 1–25. Relationship between maximum urine osmolality after dehydration and percentage of increase in urine osmolality after vasopressin administration in humans with central and nephrogenic diabetes insipidus (DI) and primary polydipsia. Note the overlap in results between patients with partial central diabetes insipidus and patients with normal vasopressin function (i.e., primary polydipsia). (From Robertson GL: The Endocrine Society 41st Postgraduate Annual Assembly Syllabus, New Orleans, October, 1989, p 25.)

Robertson, 1981). Partial resistance to the antidiuretic actions of vasopressin has been documented in Huskies with congenital NDI (Luzius et al, 1992), raising the possibility, albeit an uncommon one, that the modified water deprivation test could misdiagnose NDI in dogs too.

A number of humans have been incorrectly diagnosed as having primary (psychogenic) polydipsia. The diagnosis was initially based on results of a modified water deprivation test similar to that illustrated in Figure 1-22. However, sophisticated studies have revealed that some individuals have a metabolic explanation for such a test result. These patients have an abnormal "osmostat" (i.e., an abnormally elevated set point in their osmoreceptors for stimulating release of AVP). Therefore, at a relatively high plasma osmolality, which should cause release of AVP, these individuals remain "AVP free," polyuric, and thus polydipsic. Similarly, such patients may have a lower than normal set point for thirst (i.e., thirst may be stimulated at a plasma osmolality of 290 mOsm/kg when it should not be stimulated until the osmolality reaches 295 or 300 mOsm/kg). A similar phenomenon has been described in 4 dogs with suspected primary polydipsia, in which the AVP response to hypertonic saline infusion was abnormal and suggested a primary disturbance in the regulation of AVP secretion (van Vonderen et al, 1999).

Recognizing the potential misdiagnoses encountered in the modified water deprivation test does not eliminate its use. Rather, knowing the limitations of the test should allow veterinarians to interpret the results with a better degree of knowledge. The test has remained valuable in the dogs and cats we have studied. Incorporation of plasma vasopressin determinations into the test, as described in the following section, should improve the accuracy of the final diagnosis, as has been demonstrated in humans (Table 1-12; Zerbe and Robertson, 1981).

Plasma Vasopressin Determinations

The direct assay of plasma AVP substantially improves the accuracy of conventional tests used in the differential diagnosis of polyuria in humans (Zerbe and Robertson, 1981). The modified water deprivation test alone is consistently correct in establishing a diagnosis of severe CDI because direct measure of AVP concentrations does not alter the results of tests in which a patient did not concentrate urine during dehydration. However, inaccuracies may occur in differentiating patients with partial CDI from those with primary polydipsia and NDI; incorporating plasma AVP determinations into the modified water deprivation test helps differentiate these disorders.

Reports incorporating plasma AVP measurements into the modified water deprivation test are sporadic in the veterinary literature. Plasma AVP concentrations failed to increase after 5% loss of body weight by water deprivation in two dogs with congenital CDI compared with normal dogs (Post et al, 1989). Plasma AVP concentration was 3.3 and 3.7 pg/ml in these two dogs, versus a mean of 31.3 pg/ml in three healthy dogs after water deprivation. A similar deficiency in plasma AVP after water deprivation was identified in a cat with CDI (plasma AVP, 1.3 pg/ml versus a mean of 84.6 pg/ml in eight healthy cats) (Brown et al, 1993). Plasma AVP concentrations remained within or below the reference range (i.e., less than 7 pg/ml) during water deprivation in four dogs with suspected primary polydipsia that were subsequently identified with a disturbance in the regulation of AVP secretion (van Vonderen et al, 1999).

When measurement of plasma AVP is incorporated into the modified water deprivation test, plasma for AVP determination should be obtained after 3% to 5% loss of body weight is caused by water deprivation but before exogenous AVP is administered (i.e., at the end of phase II). Plasma for AVP determination can also be obtained prior to water deprivation, although this is not necessary. Although not widely available in commercial veterinary endocrine laboratories, plasma AVP assays are currently available at several medical and a few veterinary medical schools.

In humans, the plasma AVP value is interpreted in conjunction with the concurrent plasma and/or urine osmolality. When evaluating plasma AVP and plasma osmolality concurrently after dehydration, values from humans with severe or partial CDI fall below the normal range, whereas those from humans with NDI or primary polydipsia are almost always within or above the normal range (Fig. 1-26; Robertson, 1988). When plasma AVP and urine osmolality are evaluated after dehydration, values from humans with severe or partial CDI almost always fall within or above the

TABLE 1–12 RESULTS OF DIAGNOSTIC STUDIES IN DOGS WITH CDI, NDI, AND PSYCHOGENIC POLYDIPSIA

Test	CDI	NDI	Psychogenic Polydipsia
Random plasma osmolality	Normal or ↑	Normal or ↑	Normal or ↓
Random urine osmolality	↓	↓	↓
Urine osmolality after water deprivation (≥5% loss of body weight)	No change	No change	↑
Urine osmolality during hypertonic saline infusion	No change	No change	↑
Urine osmolality after vasopressin administration	↑	No change	No change or mild ↑
Plasma vasopressin after water deprivation (≥5% loss of body weight)	Low	Normal or high	Normal or high

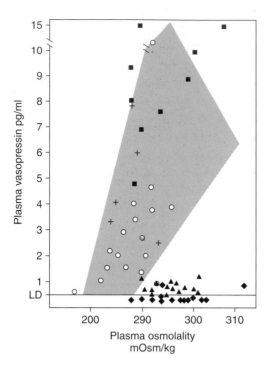

◆ = Severe diabetes inspidus
▲ = Partial diabetes inspidus
■ = Nephrogenic diabetes inspidus
○ = Primary polydipsia
+ = Normal subjects

FIGURE 1–26. Relationship of plasma AVP to plasma osmolality after dehydration in human beings with diabetes insipidus and primary polydipsia. Note that values from patients with central diabetes insipidus fall below the normal range *(shaded area),* whereas those from patients with nephrogenic diabetes insipidus and primary polydipsia are almost always within or above the normal range. (From Robertson GL: Posterior pituitary. *In* Felig P, et al (eds): Endocrinology and Metabolism, 2nd ed. New York, McGraw Hill, 1987, p 338.)

normal range, whereas those from humans with NDI fall uniformly below normal (Fig. 1-27). In most cases, the values from humans with primary polydipsia are normal, but a few may be subnormal, presumably as a consequence of renal medullary solute washout. Similar findings have yet to be reported in a large group of dogs and cats with primary polyuric and polydipsic disorders. Until more extensive studies have been completed, we interpret plasma AVP concentrations after dehydration as follows: patients with severe or partial CDI should have AVP deficiencies, and those with NDI or primary polydipsia should have normal or excessive concentrations of AVP in the face of dehydration and subnormal urine osmolality (see Table 1-12).

Approach If the Dog or Cat Is Brought into the Hospital Dehydrated

Occasionally, pets with severe polydipsia and polyuria appear clinically dehydrated or have developed hypernatremia before the modified water deprivation test can be undertaken. The most common cause for this dehydration is the owner's withholding of water in an attempt to reduce the likelihood of urination in the home. If the dehydrated dog or cat exhibits CNS symptoms, immediate fluid therapy should be initiated. However, if the pet is in no apparent distress, the bladder can be drained and the urine checked for specific gravity and osmolality. A serum sample can be obtained to assess the BUN, sodium, osmolality, and vasopressin concentrations. The clinician can then proceed with the next phase of the modified water deprivation test (Phase III; see Table 1-9) if the urine present in the bladder has a specific gravity of less than 1.030 (osmolality <1100 mOsm/kg) and the dog or cat is not uremic or hypernatremic. If the urine is more concentrated than 1.030 (1100 mOsm/kg), a normal pituitary-renal tubular concentrating axis probably exists. If the animal is truly polyuric/polydipsic, primary polydipsia and hyperadrenocorticism remain possible diagnoses. If the urine is dilute, response to exogenous vasopressin administration should help to establish the diagnosis.

RANDOM PLASMA OSMOLALITY AS A DIAGNOSTIC TOOL

In consideration of the pathophysiology resulting in CDI, NDI, or psychogenic polydipsia, the random sampling of plasma osmolality may be valuable. Dogs and cats with CDI and NDI have a primary polyuric disorder with secondary compensatory polydipsia; that is, they drink excessively because they urinate excessively. The stimulation for water intake in CDI and NDI is loss of free water through the kidneys, resulting in decreased blood volume and increased serum osmolality. Thus, patients with CDI and NDI should have high normal or high plasma osmolalities (Fig. 1-28). In contrast, dogs with primary or psychogenic polydipsia have a primary polydipsic disorder with secondary compensatory polyuria; that is, they urinate excessively because they drink excessively. In these dogs, uncontrollable fluid intake raises blood volume and decreases plasma osmolality, which in turn causes decreased secretion of AVP and a decreased renal medullary concentration gradient, resulting in large urine volumes. Dogs with psychogenic polydipsia, in theory, should have depressed plasma osmolalities.

It should be pointed out that the above discussion applies to the "classic" situation. Unfortunately, nature rarely provides us with "classic" patients. This is illustrated in a study of polyuric humans, in whom the serum osmolality varied from 281 to 298 mOsm/kg in CDI, 285 to 292 in NDI, and 275 to 291 in primary polydipsia (Zerbe and Robertson, 1981). In our series of dogs, as well as those reported in the literature, plasma osmolality varied from 281 to 339 mOsm/kg in CDI, 283 to 340 in NDI, and 274 to 304 in psychogenic polydipsia (see Fig. 1-28). Based on our experiences, a random plasma osmolality of less than 280 mOsm/kg obtained while the dog or cat has free access to water

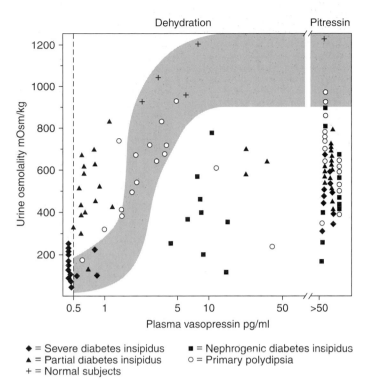

FIGURE 1–27. Relationship of urine osmolality to plasma vasopressin in human beings with diabetes insipidus and primary polydipsia. Note that values obtained during dehydration in humans with central diabetes insipidus almost always fall within or above the normal range, whereas those from patients with nephrogenic diabetes insipidus fall uniformly below normal. Values in most humans with primary polydipsia are normal, but a few may be subnormal, presumably as a consequence of washout of the medullary concentration gradient. (From Robertson GL: Posterior pituitary. *In* Felig P, et al (eds): Endocrinology and Metabolism, 2nd ed. New York, McGraw Hill, 1987, p 338.)

suggests primary or psychogenic polydipsia, whereas a plasma osmolality greater than 280 mOsm/kg is consistent with CDI, NDI, or psychogenic polydipsia.

RESPONSE TO DESMOPRESSIN [DDAVP] AS A DIAGNOSTIC ALTERNATIVE

A method of diagnosing CDI that is simpler, albeit less sophisticated, than the modified water deprivation test is evaluating the response of the dog or cat to DDAVP therapy. This should be considered only after the differential diagnostic list is narrowed to CDI, NDI, and primary (psychogenic) polydipsia. The owner should measure the patient's 24-hour water intake for 2 to 3 days before the test is begun, allowing free-choice water intake. The owner should also collect a urine sample at a given time each day to be checked for osmolality and specific gravity. After these initial 2 to 3 days, a half to a whole 0.1-mg or 0.2-mg DDAVP tablet is administered orally every 8 hours or 1 to 4 drops of DDAVP nasal spray is administered from an eye dropper into the conjunctival sac every 12 hours for 5 to 7 days (see page 37). Water intake should be monitored daily, and several urine samples obtained on the fifth to seventh day for evaluation of specific gravity and osmolality. A dramatic reduction in water intake and/or an increase in urine concentra-

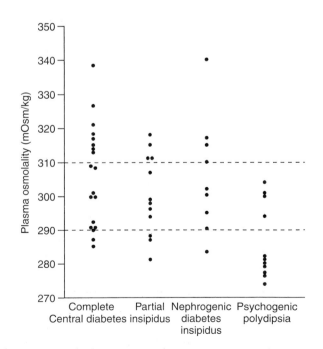

FIGURE 1–28. Random plasma osmolality in 19 dogs with complete central diabetes insipidus, 12 dogs with partial central diabetes insipidus, 9 dogs with primary nephrogenic diabetes insipidus, and 11 dogs with primary (psychogenic) polydipsia. Note the overlap in values between groups of dogs. *Dashed lines,* upper and lower limits for normal plasma osmolality.

tion (>50%) would provide strong evidence for CDI (see Table 1-12). Renal medullary solute washout often prevents a dog or cat with partial or severe CDI from forming highly concentrated urine in response to one or two administrations of DDAVP. The effect of DDAVP administration is, nonetheless, dramatic. If the effect is not dramatic, severe CDI should be eliminated from the differential diagnosis. Moderate response is consistent with partial CDI or hyperadrenocorticism.

Dogs with NDI are not helped by the administration of DDAVP, although a response may be observed with very large doses of DDAVP (Luzius et al, 1992). Those with primary polydipsia may exhibit a mild decline in urine output and water intake because the chronically low serum osmolality tends to depress AVP production. It is possible for a dog with primary polydipsia to have decreased urine output yet maintain abnormal water intake. Water intoxication is possible.

Dogs with hyperadrenocorticism may experience minimal to moderate increases in urine concentration and a reduction in urine output after administration of DDAVP. Dogs in the early stages of hyperadrenocorticism may be mistakenly diagnosed with CDI when the only clinical signs are polydipsia and polyuria, typical changes in initial blood work are not present, and tests of the pituitary-adrenocortical axis are ambiguous. An initial response to DDAVP treatment is observed, presumably because hyperadrenocorticism suppresses pituitary vasopressin secretion. With time, DDAVP treatment becomes ineffective as hyperadrenocorticism becomes more established. Reevaluation of routine blood work and tests of the pituitary-adrenocortical axis will usually reveal abnormalities consistent with hyperadrenocorticism—abnormalities which were not evident at the time of initial evaluation by the veterinarian.

SALINE INFUSION STUDY (HICKEY-HARE TEST)

The Hickey-Hare test assesses the pituitary and renal tubular ability to reduce urine volume in response to increasing plasma osmolality induced by the intravenous administration of hypertonic saline. Water is not allowed during saline infusion. Urine production per minute is determined by draining the bladder completely every 15 minutes during hypertonic saline administration and for an additional 15 minutes following completion of the infusion. A significant (>25%) reduction in urine flow rate is indicative of a normal pituitary-renal tubular concentrating axis. Dogs with psychogenic polydipsia should have reduced urine production rates, whereas those with CDI or NDI should not.

An alternative and more appealing approach uses measurement of plasma osmolality and AVP concentration in lieu of urine production during saline infusion. The AVP response to a progressive increase in plasma osmolality is evaluated by an intravenous

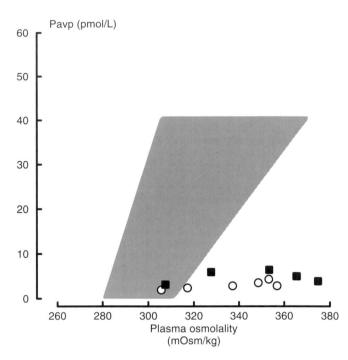

FIGURE 1–29. Relation of plasma vasopressin (Pavp) with plasma osmolality during hypertonic saline infusion in two dogs with central diabetes insipidus caused by pituitary tumor. The gray area represents the range in healthy dogs. (From Rijnberk A: Diabetes insipidus. *In* Ettinger SJ, Feldman EC (eds): Textbook of Veterinary Internal Medicine, 5th ed. Philadelphia, WB Saunders, 2000, p 1378.)

infusion of 20% saline for 2 hours at a rate of 0.03 ml/kg body weight per minute (Biewenga et al, 1987). Blood samples for plasma AVP and plasma osmolality are obtained at 20-minute intervals. The test requires very close monitoring of the animal and monitoring of plasma osmolality to avoid severe hyperosmolality. In a dog or cat with a normal hypothalamic pituitary renal axis, plasma AVP concentration should increase with increasing plasma osmolality. Dogs with CDI have decreased plasma AVP concentrations, compared with normal dogs (Fig. 1-29). Evaluating changes in plasma AVP concentration in relation to changes in plasma osmolality may also allow the clinician to identify disturbances in the regulation of AVP secretion (van Vonderen et al, 1999).

URINE-TO-PLASMA OSMOLALITY RATIOS

It has been suggested that the ratio of urine to plasma osmolality, after water deprivation–induced dehydration, may be used as a diagnostic tool. A ratio below 1.84 suggests severe CDI or NDI; 1.83 to 3.0 suggests partial CDI; and greater than 3.0 is normal or suggests primary polydipsia. In our experience, urine:plasma osmolality ratios have not been consistent and do not appear to be of real value in assessing animals with suspected primary polyuria or polydipsia disorders.

TREATMENT

Treatment options for controlling polydipsia and polyuria in dogs and cats with CDI, NDI, and primary (psychogenic) water consumption are outlined in Table 1-13 and discussed below. Evaluation of the hypothalamic and pituitary region of the brain using computed tomography or magnetic resonance imaging is indicated in dogs and cats diagnosed with acquired CDI and primary polydipsia (see Fig. 1-9). Radiation therapy should be considered if a mass lesion (i.e., tumor) is identified, especially if the mass is small and the dog or cat is healthy aside from polydipsia and polyuria (see Chapter 6).

Vasopressin analogues (used in CDI and partial CDI)

Historically, the standard therapy for CDI has been the parenteral administration of partially purified extracts of ADH prepared from bovine and porcine pituitaries (Pitressin Tannate in Oil; Parke Davis, Morris Plains, NJ). Pitressin Tannate in Oil was discontinued in the

TABLE 1–13   THERAPIES AVAILABLE FOR POLYDIPSIC/POLYURIC DOGS WITH CDI, NDI, OR PRIMARY (PSYCHOGENIC) POLYDIPSIA

A. Central diabetes insipidus (severe)
  1. DDAVP (desmopressin acetate)
    a. Effective
    b. Expensive
    c. May require drops in conjunctival sac if oral is ineffective
  2. LVP (lypressin [Diapid])
    a. Short duration of action; less potent than DDAVP
    b. Expensive
    c. Requires drops into nose or conjunctival sac
  3. No treatment–provide continuous source of water
B. Central diabetes insipidus (partial)
  1. DDAVP
  2. LVP
  3. Chlorpropamide
    a. 30–70% effective
    b. Inexpensive
    c. Pill form
    d. Takes 1–2 weeks to obtain effect of drug
    e. May cause hypoglycemia
  4. Clofibrate–untested in veterinary medicine
  5. Thiazides
    a. Mildly effective
    b. Inexpensive
    c. Pill form
    d. Should be used with low-sodium diet
  6. Low-sodium diet
  7. No treatment–provide continuous source of water
C. Nephrogenic diabetes insipidus
  1. Thiazides–as above
  2. Low sodium diet
  3. No treatment–provide continuous source of water
D. Primary (psychogenic) polydipsia
  1. Water restriction at times
  2. Water limitation
  3. Behavior modification
    a. Exercise
    b. Another pet
    c. Larger living environment

late 1980s following the successful development of vasopressin analogues for use in humans that could be administered by nasal spray or as eye drops. Aqueous Pitressin (Parke Davis, Morris Plains, NJ) is still manufactured but is not suitable for long term management of CDI. Its duration of action is only a few hours and therefore requires repeated injections; however, it is the ideal agent for the modified water deprivation test.

DDAVP (DESMOPRESSIN ACETATE; AVENTIS PHARMACEUTICALS, PARSIPPANY, NJ). A synthetic analogue of vasopressin, DDAVP (desmopressin; see Fig. 1-1) is approved for use in humans and is available for parenteral (DDAVP injection: 1- and 2-ml ampules containing 15 µg DDAVP/ml and 1- and 10-ml ampules containing 4 µg DDAVP/ml), intranasal (DDAVP nasal drops: 2.5- and 5.0-ml bottles containing 100 µg DDAVP/ml) and oral (DDAVP tablets: 0.1- and 0.2-mg DDAVP tablets) administration. DDAVP has strong antidiuretic (V2 receptor) activity with minimal vasopressor (V1 receptor) activity (Pliska, 1985). Several extrarenal actions of DDAVP have also been described: release of two coagulation factors (factor VIIIc and von Willebrand factor; Richardson and Robinson, 1985), a decrease in blood pressure and peripheral resistance, and an increase in plasma renin activity (Schwartz et al, 1985; Williams et al, 1986).

DDAVP has several advantages over the use of Pitressin Tannate in Oil. The synthetic alterations seen at positions 1 and 8 of the molecule double its antidiuretic potency, eliminate its pressor actions, and increase its resistance to metabolic degradation. DDAVP also appears to have greater affinity for the renal AVP (V2) receptor than does Pitressin Tannate in Oil (Schwartz-Porsche, 1980). The slow metabolic clearance, absorption through mucous membranes, stability in aqueous preparations, and lack of side effects make it an excellent drug for treating CDI.

The metabolism of DDAVP in humans follows a biexponential curve with first and second half-lives of 7.8 and 75.5 minutes, respectively. Similar findings are noted in experiments with normal dogs (Ferring, 1985) and in spontaneous canine cases of CDI. Additionally, blood chemistry studies and necropsies on treated dogs (Ferring) and clinical experience in dogs and cats with CDI (Kraus, 1987; Harb et al,1996) indicate that the drug is safe for use in dogs and cats. The intranasal DDAVP preparation is used most commonly for treating CDI in dogs and cats. In most humans with CDI, twice daily administration of 10 to 25 µg (0.2 ml of the 0.01% solution) by nasal insufflation affords complete relief of symptoms. Administration of medication to animals via the intranasal route is possible but not recommended. The DDAVP nasal preparation may be transferred to a sterile eye dropper bottle and drops placed in the conjunctival sac of the dog or cat. Although the solution is acidic, ocular irritation rarely occurs. One drop of DDAVP contains 1.5 to 4 µg of DDAVP, and one to four drops administered once or twice daily appear sufficient to control signs of CDI in most patients.

Recently, we have been using oral DDAVP tablets for treating CDI with good results. DDAVP is available as 0.1 and 0.2 mg tablets. Bioavailability of oral DDAVP is approximately 5% to 15% of the intranasal dose in humans. In humans, the initial dose is one-half of a 0.1-mg tablet twice a day and the dose is adjusted, as needed, to control clinical signs. The optimum therapeutic dose ranges from 0.1 to 0.8 mg a day given in two to three divided doses. Our initial oral DDAVP dose in dogs is 0.1 mg given three times a day. The dose is gradually increased to effect if unacceptable polyuria and polydipsia persists 1 week after initiating therapy. A decrease in frequency of administration to twice a day can be tried once clinical response is documented. To date, dogs have required 0.1 to 0.2 mg of DDAVP two to three times a day to control polyuria and polydipsia. We have not yet treated a cat with oral DDAVP.

DDAVP for parenteral (SC) administration can be used in lieu of eye drops or oral tablets. The initial parenteral dosage of DDAVP is 0.5 to 2 µg SC once or twice daily. Because of cost differences between parenteral and nasal preparations, the intranasal form of DDAVP, although not designed for parenteral use, has been given to dogs and cats by injection with no apparent adverse reactions (Nichols, 2000). However, the intranasal form of DDAVP is not sterile, so the solution should be passed through a bacteriostatic filter before administration.

The maximal effect of DDAVP, regardless of the route of administration, occurs from 2 to 8 hours after administration, and the duration of action varies from 8 to 24 hours. Larger doses of DDAVP appear to both increase its antidiuretic effects and prolong its duration of action; however, expense becomes a limiting factor. The medication may be administered exclusively in the evening as insurance against nocturia.

Ideally, the dog or cat should not be allowed free access to water immediately following each dose of DDAVP, especially if severe polydipsia and polyuria have redeveloped. Without such restriction, the pet may consume excessive amounts of water that cannot subsequently be excreted owing to the iatrogenic ADH effects of DDAVP on the renal tubules. Physiologically, inability to excrete free water causes a relative lowering of the extracellular fluid osmolality and subsequent cellular overhydration. The intracellular movement of water, especially within the brain, may lead to obvious disturbances, such as depression, increased salivation, vomiting, ataxia, muscle tremors, coma, and convulsions (Schwartz-Porsche, 1980). However, many of our owners have ignored this suggestion without harming their pets.

We have had excellent results in dogs and cats receiving daily medication for longer than 5 years. Owners of dogs and cats with CDI have reported that their pets become accustomed to receiving eye drops, mentioning eye or conjunctival irritation as an infrequent complication. If polyuria and polydipsia recur despite DDAVP therapy, several possibilities should be considered, including problems with owner compliance or administration technique, inadequate dose, outdated or inactivated DDAVP, or development of a concurrent disorder causing polyuria and polydipsia. Hyperadrenocorticism is the primary differential when polyuria and polydipsia recur despite DDAVP treatment in a dog with CDI.

DDAVP was effective in Husky puppies with familial NDI caused by a defect in V2 receptor binding affinity for AVP (Luzius et al, 1992). However, extremely high dosages (0.33 U/kg body weight intramuscularly three times a day) of DDAVP were required to obtain improvement in polyuria and polydipsia, dosages that most owners would consider cost-prohibitive. For practical purposes, DDAVP is considered ineffective in the treatment of NDI.

LVP (LYSINE-8-VASOPRESSIN). Another synthetic analogue is Diapid Nasal Spray (Novartis Pharmaceuticals, East Hanover, New Jersey). In humans, it is generally used only as an adjunct to other forms of therapy because the antidiuretic effect of each spray lasts only 2 to 6 hours. This drug's duration of activity, along with its mild antidiuretic action and its high cost, probably does not warrant its routine use in dogs or cats with CDI.

Oral agents (used in CDI, partial CDI, NDI, and primary polydipsia)

CHLORPROPAMIDE. Chlorpropamide (Diabinese; Pfizer Inc, New York, NY) is an oral sulfonylurea drug used for the treatment of hyperglycemia in humans (see Chapter 12). Largely by chance, chlorpropamide has also been found to be efficacious in treating humans with CDI and has been found to reduce urine output 30% to 70% in humans afflicted with partial CDI. This reduction is associated with a proportional rise in urine osmolality, correction of dehydration, and a reduction in fluid consumption similar to that observed with small doses of vasopressin (Robertson, 1981). The drug may also cause antidiuresis in normal humans or humans with primary polydipsia. For unknown reasons the effect in these latter situations is less pronounced than in humans with CDI.

The exact mechanism of the potentiating effect of chlorpropamide on the action of AVP in the kidney is not know. Chlorpropamide may enhance AVP stimulation of renal medullary cAMP by augmenting adenylate cyclase sensitivity to AVP or by inhibiting phosphodiesterase (Reeves et al, 1998). Inhibition of PGE_2 synthesis, thereby removing an antagonist of AVP, has also been proposed as a mechanism for chlorpropamide potentiation. Finally, chlorpropamide treatment may augment AVP dependent NaCl absorption by the medullary thick ascending loop of Henle, thereby increasing the driving force for water absorption in collecting ducts (Kusano et al, 1983). Like DDAVP, chlorpropamide is ineffective in treating patients with NDI. Other drugs of the sulfonylurea class do not have a significant antidiuretic effect in CDI and, in some humans, may actually be mildly diuretic.

The effectiveness of chlorpropamide in the treatment of canine CDI is a matter unresolved in the literature. As in humans, use of the drug in dogs requires the presence of some endogenous AVP. Some veterinarians have had little or no success using chlorpropamide, citing a reduction in urine volume of only 18% during 7 days of therapy (Schwartz-Porsche, 1980). Other veterinarians have claimed a 50% reduction in urine volume after 5 days of therapy. The drug has also had mixed results when used in cats with CDI (Kraus, 1987).

The inconsistent results of this therapeutic modality are most likely compatible with the presence of both severe and partial forms of CDI and the knowledge that severe forms do not respond whereas the partial forms may. Also, response may require several consecutive days of therapy. The optimal antidiuretic activity of chlorpropamide in humans is seen 3 to 10 days after beginning treatment. Finally, response may be dose-dependent. Doses of 250 to 750 mg chlorpropamide daily reduce polyuria in between 50% and 80% of humans with partial CDI (Reeves et al, 1998). An effective dosage of chlorpropamide for the treatment of partial CDI has not been determined in the dog or cat, although 10 to 40 mg/kg/day has been suggested (Hardy, 1982). The dose of chlorpropamide used in the unsuccessful study in dogs was 250 mg twice daily (Schwartz-Porsche, 1980) and was approximately 30 mg/kg/day in one cat that failed to respond (Kraus, 1987). The dosage was not mentioned in the dog study and was approximately 10 mg/kg/day in one cat in which chlorpropamide improved polyuria and polydipsia.

The primary adverse effect of chlorpropamide is hypoglycemia caused by chlorpropamide-induced insulin secretion. Regular feeding schedules should be adhered to if hypoglycemic problems are to be avoided. We have had little experience with chlorpropamide simply because our success with DDAVP has been excellent, and our owners have accepted the cost and difficulties encountered in treating their pets with this drug. If successful in a trial administration period, chlorpropamide may prove to be a valid alternative in treating partial CDI.

CLOFIBRATE. The hypolipidemic agent clofibrate may reduce the polydipsia and polyuria in humans with partial CDI but is ineffective in complete CDI and NDI. Clofibrate appears to work by directly stimulating the release of AVP from the hypothalamus. It is believed to be less effective than chlorpropamide. There are no reports of its use in dogs or cats.

CARBAMAZEPINE. The anticonvulsant carbamazepine may reduce polydipsia and polyuria in humans with partial CDI. Like clofibrate, carbamazepine is also ineffective in severe CDI and NDI. Carbamazepine's proposed mechanisms of action include direct stimulation of the release of AVP from the hypothalamus and increased sensitivity of the kidney to AVP (Gold et al, 1983). There are no reports of its use in dogs or cats.

THIAZIDES. The thiazide diuretics may reduce the polyuria in animals with diabetes insipidus (Breitschwerdt et al, 1981). This seemingly paradoxic effect is seen in NDI, as well as in CDI, suggesting that this therapeutic agent has a mode of action distinct from that of chlorpropamide or clofibrate. By inhibiting sodium reabsorption in the ascending limb of Henle's loop, the thiazides reduce total body sodium concentrations, thus contracting the extracellular fluid volume and increasing salt and water resorption in the proximal renal tubule. This results in lower sodium concentrations in the distal renal tubule and less osmotic effect to maintain tubular volume, resulting in a reduction in urine volume. The net effect in diabetes insipidus is to cause a slight rise in urine osmolality and a proportionate reduction in urine volume. Depending on sodium intake, polyuria can be reduced 30% to 50% in humans with NDI or CDI. Apart from occasional hypokalemia, significant side effects are rare. The thiazides reduce the ability to excrete a water load and, if given to a patient with primary polydipsia, may precipitate water intoxication (Robertson, 1981).

Chlorothiazides are recommended at a dose of 20 to 40 mg/kg twice daily, in concert with low-sodium diets. Periodic serum electrolyte determinations (every 2 to 3 months) should aid in avoiding iatrogenic problems.

SODIUM CHLORIDE (SALT) RESTRICTION. Restricting salt intake, as the sole therapy in diabetes insipidus, reduces urine output by increasing the volume of filtrate absorbed isosmotically in the proximal nephron. This simple therapy may be helpful in the treatment of both CDI and NDI. Salt content of commercial dog and cat foods is quite variable, ranging from 0.14 to 3.27 g/1000 kcal dietary metabolizable energy for dog foods and 0.3 to 4.0 g/1000 kcal dietary metabolizable energy for cat foods. Diets containing less than 0.6 g and 0.9 g/1000 kcal dietary metabolizable energy are considered low in sodium for dogs and cats, respectively (Table 1-14).

No treatment

Therapy for diabetes insipidus (CDI and NDI) and primary polydipsia is not mandatory as long as the dog or cat has unlimited access to water and is maintained in an environment where polyuria does not create problems. In most instances, untreated pets are outdoor animals. Some of our owners have elected not to treat their pets from the time the diagnosis is established. More commonly, owners have discontinued DDAVP treatment after 1 or 2 months of therapy, primarily because of the expense. Still others treat their pet with DDAVP periodically, when it is undesirable for the dog or cat to be exhibiting severe polyuria and polydipsia (e.g., relatives staying at the house). If an owner elects not to treat his or her pet, it is imperative that the dog or cat have access to a constant water supply because relatively short periods of water restriction can have catastrophic results (see Complications of Modified Water Deprivation Test, page 29).

TABLE 1–14 EXAMPLES OF CANINE AND FELINE DIETS THAT ARE SODIUM-RESTRICTED (NaCl < 0.6 g/1000 kcal ME) OR LOW IN SODIUM CONTENT (NaCl < 0.9 g/1000 kcal ME)

SODIUM RESTRICTED DIETS			
Canine Diet	Salt Content (g/1000 kcal ME)	Feline Diet	Salt Content (g/1000 kcal ME)
Hill's h/d (wet)	0.14 g	Purina NF (wet)	0.30 g
Hill's h/d (dry)	0.15 g	Waltham's low phosphorus and	
Purina CV	0.20 g	low protein	0.40 g
Purina GF	0.30 g	Hill's l/d (wet)	0.48 g
Hills k/d (wet)	0.38 g	Purina CV (wet)	0.50 g
Waltham low phosphorus and low protein	0.40 g	Purina NF (dry)	0.50 g
Purina NF	0.50 g	Hill's k/d (dry)	0.56 g
Hill's k/d (dry)	0.52 g	Purina UR (dry)	0.60 g
Eukanuba Maximum Calorie (wet)	0.55 g		
Eukanuba Restricted Calorie	0.55 g		

LOW SODIUM DIETS			
Hill's w/d (dry)	0.67 g	Hill's k/d (wet)	0.64 g
Science Diet Maintenance (dry)	0.70 g	Purina EN (wet)	0.70 g
Purina OM (dry)	0.70 g	Eukanuba Response LB (wet)	0.76 g
Waltham High Fiber	0.80 g	Hill's w/d (dry)	0.77 g
Eukanuba Maximum Calorie (dry)	0.84 g	Purina OM (dry)	0.80 g
		Purina DM (wet)	0.80 g
Purina EN	0.90 g	Eukanuba Restricted Calorie (dry)	0.82 g

Behavior modification (used in primary polydipsia)

WATER RESTRICTION. Gradually limiting water intake to amounts in the high normal range (60 to 80 ml/kg/24 hours) improves and may resolve polyuria and polydipsia in dogs with psychogenic polydipsia. In some dogs, rapid water restriction results in bizarre behavior, excessive barking, urine consumption, and dehydration. Therefore, we prefer to have the owner first calculate the dog's approximate water intake per 24 hours while free-choice water is allowed. This volume of water is then reduced by 10% per week until water volumes of 60 to 80 ml/kg/24 hours are reached. The total 24-hour volume of water should be divided into several aliquots, with the last aliquot given at bedtime. Oral salt (1 g/30 kg twice a day) and/or oral sodium bicarbonate (0.6 g/30 kg twice a day) may also be administered for 3 to 5 days, in order to reestablish the medullary concentration gradient. We have had excellent success with gradual water restriction and do not routinely use oral salt or sodium bicarbonate.

CHANGE IN ENVIRONMENT. Most dogs with psychogenic polydipsia respond to water restriction as described previously. In the nonresponsive patient, less scientific approaches may be attempted. These include (1) significant and routine daily exercise, such as running (jogging) with an owner or running behind a car or bicycle; (2) bringing a second pet into the home; (3) providing some distraction, such as a radio playing when the owners are not home; (4) moving the dog to an area with increased amount of contact with humans. If these techniques fail, placing the dog with a different family may be considered.

PROGNOSIS

Dogs and cats with idiopathic or congenital CDI usually become asymptomatic with appropriate therapy, and with proper care these animals have an excellent life expectancy. Unfortunately, many owners discontinue DDAVP therapy or elect euthanasia of their pet after a few months because of the expense of DDAVP. Without therapy, these animals often lead acceptable lives as long as water is constantly provided and they are housed in an environment that cannot be damaged by severe polyuria. However, the untreated animal is always at risk for developing life-threatening dehydration if water is withdrawn for longer than a few hours. Additionally, even mild illness that causes vomiting or reduces water intake can develop into one associated with severe dehydration. Thus, untreated dogs and cats carry a guarded prognosis.

In one study, long-term follow-up of 19 dogs with CDI found 7 of 19 dogs still alive a mean of 29 months (median, 30 months) from the time of diagnosis of CDI (Harb et al, 1996). Six of these seven dogs were 3 years of age or younger at the time CDI was diagnosed. Of the original 19 dogs, 12 had died within an average of 6 months (median, 2 months) after diagnosis of CDI. Three dogs died from unrelated or unknown causes, two dogs were euthanized shortly after the diagnosis of CDI was established, and seven dogs died or were euthanized because of development of neurologic disease. In these later seven dogs, neurologic signs developed 2 months (median, 1 month; range, 0.5 to 5 months) and the dogs were dead 3.3 months (median, 1.5 months; range, 1 to 7 months) after CDI was diagnosed (Harb et al, 1996). A mass in the region of the pituitary gland was identified by CT scan or at necropsy in six of the dogs in which these procedures were performed. The seven dogs that developed neurologic signs were older than 6 years of age.

Obviously, dogs with aggressive hypothalamic or pituitary problems, such as a growing tumor, have a grave prognosis. Treatment of tumors in the region of the hypothalamus and pituitary, using either irradiation (see Chapter 6) or chemotherapy (e.g., BCNU), can be tried; however, results are unpredictable. We have treated three dogs with CDI caused by a hypothalamic or pituitary mass. No obvious improvement in survival time was evident in two dogs with neurologic clinical signs at the time of radiation therapy. Polyuria and polydipsia resolved and DDAVP was discontinued in one dog with CDI and no neurologic clinical signs 2 months after completing radiation therapy (see Fig. 1-9); the dog is alive and asymptomatic for CDI 2 years after completing radiation treatment. Based on experience with pituitary macrotumors, successful response to radiation therapy is more likely when the tumor is small and before neurologic clinical signs develop. CT or MRI scan is warranted at the time of diagnosis of CDI, especially when CDI is acquired in an older dog or cat.

Because successful therapy in NDI is less than ideal, these dogs also have a guarded to poor prognosis. They are always more likely than other animals to have severe problems after contracting a mild illness. Owners must be made aware of the potential for development of severe dehydration in these pets. The prognosis with secondary NDI depends on the prognosis of the primary problem.

The prognosis in psychogenic polydipsia is usually excellent. Water restriction and some form of behavior modification help most of these animals to become asymptomatic, although relapses do occur.

SYNDROME OF INAPPROPRIATE VASOPRESSIN SECRETION: EXCESS VASOPRESSIN

A primary excess of AVP occurs in two clinical settings—in the syndrome of inappropriate antidiuretic hormone (SIADH) and as a consequence of drugs that enhance AVP release or action (see Table 1-2). In SIADH, sustained release of AVP occurs in the absence of either osmotic or nonosmotic stimuli (Reeves et al, 1998). In humans, SIADH has been observed in a variety of disorders, particularly pulmonary diseases, cranial disorders, and neoplastic disorders (Table 1-15). Vasopressin or a peptide having comparable biologic activity is produced by tumors. SIADH is rare in the dog and cat and has been reported in one dog with heartworm disease, one dog

TABLE 1–15 CONDITIONS ASSOCIATED WITH SIADH IN HUMANS*

Malignant Neoplasia
Carcinoma; bronchogenic, pancreatic, prostatic, bladder
Lymphoma and leukemia
Thymoma and mesothelioma

Central Nervous System Disorders
Trauma
Infection
Tumors
Porphyria

Pulmonary Disorders
Tuberculosis
Pneumonia

Drug-Induced
Clofibrate
Chlorpropamide
Thiazides
Vincristine
Cyclophosphamide
Others

Endocrine Diseases
Adrenal insufficiency
Hypothyroidism
Pituitary insufficiency

*Adapted from Ramsay DJ: Posterior pituitary gland. In Greenspan FS, Fosham PH (eds): Basic and Clinical Endocrinology. Los Altos, CA, Lange Medical Publications, 1983, p 120.

with an undifferentiated carcinoma, one dog with a tumor in the region of the hypothalamus, and was considered idiopathic in two dogs (Rijnberk et al, 1988; Houston et al, 1989).

As a result of sustained release of AVP or AVP-like substances, patients retain ingested water and become hyponatremic and modestly volume-expanded and generally gain body weight (Reeves et al, 1998). This volume expansion results in reduced rates of proximal tubular sodium absorption and, consequently, natriuresis. Increased levels of atrial natriuretic peptide also contribute to the natriuresis. Thus the diagnostic features that characterize this syndrome include hyponatremia, volume expansion without edema, hyposmolality of the plasma, osmolality of the urine greater than that appropriate for the concomitant osmolality of the plasma, and continued urinary excretion of sodium despite hyponatremia. A similar clinical picture can be produced experimentally by giving high doses of AVP to a normal subject who receives a normal to increased fluid intake. Water restriction results in the plasma osmolality and serum sodium concentrations returning to normal (Aron et al, 2001).

Four different patterns of plasma AVP secretion have been described in humans with SIADH, suggesting four patterns of osmoregulatory defects in this syndrome. The most common derangement (40%) is wide fluctuations of AVP levels independent of osmotic or nonosmotic control (Reeves et al, 1998). This erratic and irregular secretion of AVP can be associated with both malignant and nonmalignant disease. About one-third of humans with SIADH have a "reset osmostat"; their threshold for AVP secretion is abnormally low, but if sufficiently hyponatremic, these patients with SIADH can produce a maximally dilute urine. Approximately 20% of patients with SIADH exhibit the "AVP leak" pattern, namely, sustained AVP production below serum osmolality values of

278 mOsm/kg and normal release of AVP in response to osmotic stimuli. The least common are patients that have no detectable abnormality in AVP levels; they fail, for reasons not yet understood, to dilute urine maximally. Thus far, it has not been possible to correlate the pattern of AVP abnormality with the pathology of the syndrome. The threshold and sensitivity of vasopressin secretion were studied by infusion of hypertonic saline in two dogs with idiopathic SIADH (Rijnberk et al, 1988). One dog demonstrated a pattern of reset osmostat and the other, a pattern consistent with vasopressin leak.

Clinical signs are a result of water intoxication caused by hyponatremia and volume expansion and are primarily neurologic in origin as a consequence of brain swelling. The severity of clinical signs depends on the degree and duration of hyponatremia. In humans, clinical signs generally occur when the serum sodium concentration decreases to less than 120 mEq/L. Early signs include lethargy, inappetence, and weakness, which progress to muscle fasciculations, seizures, and coma as hyponatremia worsens.

The diagnosis of SIADH is made by excluding other causes of hyponatremia (see Table 8-11) and meeting the following criteria: hyponatremia with plasma hyposmolality; inappropriately high urine osmolality in the presence of plasma hyposmolality; normal renal and adrenal function; presence of natriuresis despite hyponatremia; no evidence of hypovolemia, ascites or edema; and correction of hyponatremia with fluid restriction (Reeves et al, 1998).

Treatment is directed toward alleviation of hyponatremia and elimination of the underlying disease. The goal of treatment directed at the hyponatremia is to correct body water osmolality and restore cell volume to normal by raising the ratio of sodium to water in extracellular fluid. The increase in extracellular fluid osmolality draws water from cells and therefore reduces their volume. The therapeutic approach depends on the severity of hyponatremia and the presence or absence of clinical signs. Patients with acute, severe hyponatremia (serum sodium concentration <120 mEq/L) and neurologic signs are treated with normal (0.9%) or hypertonic (3% to 5%) saline solutions and furosemide at levels that gradually increase the serum sodium concentration to 125 mEq/L or higher over 6 to 8 hours (Reeves et al, 1998). The diuretic induces urinary salt loss and reduces the risk of extracellular fluid volume expansion. Consequently, the combination of intravenously administered normal or hypertonic saline with a furosemide-induced diuresis of urine that is dilute compared with plasma provides an effective way of raising the serum sodium level in a volume-expanded patient with SIADH.

Rapid increase in serum sodium concentration to levels greater than 125 mEq/L is potentially dangerous and should be avoided. Because loss of brain solute represents one of the compensatory mechanisms for preserving brain cell volume during dilutional states, an increase in serum sodium concentration towards normal (greater than 140 mEq/L) is relatively hypertonic to brain cells that are partially depleted of solute as a result of hyponatremia (Sterns et al, 1989; Sterns et al, 1993). Consequently, raising the serum sodium concentration rapidly to greater than 125 mEq/L can cause CNS damage (Ayus et al, 1987; Sterns et al, 1994). The current recommendation for correcting severe hyponatremia in humans is to increase serum sodium concentration slowly at a rate of approximately 0.5 mEq/L per hour until the serum sodium concentration reaches 125 mEq/L. Once the serum sodium concentration is greater than 125 mEq/L, further correction of hyponatremia is accomplished by restricting water intake. Reduction of fluid intake to the point at which urinary and insensible losses induce a negative water balance leads to restoration of normal body fluid volume, reduction in urinary sodium excretion, and increased serum sodium concentration.

Alternative treatments in humans include demeclocycline and the nonapeptide AVP antagonist OPC-31260. Demeclocycline (Declomycin; Ledeerle Pharmaceutical, Pearl River, NY) is in the tetracycline family of antibiotics. Demeclocycline interferes with the renal tubular effects of AVP and reproducibly inhibits renal concentrating ability in humans with SIADH (Reeves et al, 1998). There are no reports on the use of demeclocycline for SIADH in dogs or cats. The nonapeptide selective AVP V2 receptor antagonist OPC-31260 (Otsuka Pharmaceutical Co., Tokyo, Japan) is effective in increasing free-water excretion in rats and humans with SIADH (Fujisawa et al, 1993; Ohnishi et al, 1993). Treatment of a dog with SIADH with OPC-31260 at a dose of 3 mg/kg orally every 12 hours resulted in a marked increase in free-water excretion and significant palliation of clinical signs with no discernible side effects detected over a 3-year treatment period (Fleeman et al, 2000).

HYPODIPSIC HYPERNATREMIA (ESSENTIAL HYPERNATREMIA)

Hypodipsic or essential hypernatremia is characterized by chronic hypernatremia in a setting of euvolemia, normal renal function, decreased thirst perception, and a normal renal response to exogenous AVP (Reeves et al, 1998). Despite elevations of serum sodium concentration and ECF osmolalities, affected patients exhibit hypodipsia and an inappropriately dilute urine for the corresponding plasma osmolality. The primary defect in human patients with essential hypernatremia appears to be an insensitivity of thirst centers and osmoreceptors to osmotic stimuli. Affected patients have a normal response of AVP release, measured either as a rise in urine osmolality or as an increase in plasma AVP levels, to baroreceptor stimulation following volume contraction.

Given the association of a diminished sensation of thirst and a diminished release of AVP in response to osmotic stimulation, it is likely that essential hypernatremia represents a more or less specific ablation of hypothalamic osmoreceptor function. In humans, essential hypernatremia has been reported in children as a congenital disease and in adults in association with CNS histiocytosis, pineal tumors, surgery for craniopharyngioma, head trauma, and vascular disturbances (e.g., ischemia, hemorrhage). Necropsy has been performed in five dogs with essential hypernatremia and revealed hypothalamic dysplasia in a 4.5-month-old Dalmatian (Bagley et al, 1993); hydrocephalus in an adult mixed-breed dog (DiBartola et al, 1994); astrogliosis and neuronal degeneration in the region of the hypothalamus and thalamus in a 7-month-old Miniature Schnauzer (Crawford et al, 1984); focal, severe meningoencephalitis in the hypothalamus in a 7-year-old Doberman Pinscher (Mackay and Curtis, 1999); and no identifiable lesions in the anterior, third cerebral ventricular area, hypothalamus or pituitary gland in a 5-month-old Great Dane (Hawks et al, 1991). Essential hypernatremia has also been described in a 14-month-old Miniature Schnauzer (Hoskins and Rothschmitt, 1984), but the dog was still alive at the time of the report. Essential hypernatremia was also reported in a 7-month-old Domestic Short-Haired cat in which hydrocephalus was identified with CT imaging (Dow et al, 1987).

All six dogs and the cat presented to the veterinarian with signs related to hypernatremia (i.e., lethargy, inappetence, weakness, neurologic signs). Consistent findings on physical examination and initial clinical pathology included dehydration, hypernatremia, hyperchloridemia, prerenal azotemia, and urine specific gravities greater than 1.030. Serum sodium concentrations ranged from 168 to 215 mEq/L; consequently, serum osmolalities were markedly increased. The dogs and cat were conscious and adipsic or hypodipsic despite severe hypernatremia and hyperosmolality, findings that strongly support the diagnosis of hypodipsic or essential hypernatremia. The diagnosis was confirmed in one dog by documenting lack of endogenous AVP secretion with worsening hyperosmolality induced by hypertonic saline infusion and marked AVP secretion in response to conjunctival administration of apomorphine (DiBartola et al, 1994).

Treatment is directed toward alleviation of the hypernatremia and, if possible, elimination of the underlying disease. Rapid correction of hypernatremia by administration of hypotonic fluids IV is not recommended, because hypernatremia typically has been developing for more than a week and intracellular osmoles have been produced within neurons in response to the increased osmolality of the extracellular fluid. Rapid reduction of plasma osmolality can result in an intracellular influx of water into neurons, thereby worsening neurologic signs (see Hypertonic Dehydration, page 29). Forced oral hydration is recommended in humans, but it does not consistently correct the hypernatremia. Addition of water to the food in excess of maintenance requirements and/or forced oral administration of water was beneficial in most, but not all, dogs and the cat

with essential hypernatremia. Chlorpropamide, a sulfonylurea drug that augments the antidiuretic effect of low levels of circulating AVP (see page 38), has been useful in restoring osmotic homeostasis in humans with essential hypernatremia (Reeves et al, 1998). Chlorpropamide, 33 mg/kg/day for 2 weeks, was ineffective in stimulating thirst or correcting hypernatremia in one dog (Crawford et al, 1984). Patients with neurologic signs induced by severe hypernatremia may require intensive fluid therapy to initially control the hypernatremia (see page 29).

REFERENCES

Aron DC, et al: Hypothalamus and pituitary. In Greenspan FS, Gardner DG (eds): Basic and Clinical Endocrinology. New York, McGraw Hill Co, 2001, p 100.

Authement JM, et al: Transient, traumatically induced, central diabetes insipidus in a dog. JAVMA 194:683, 1989.

Ayus JC, et al: Treatment of symptomatic hyponatremia and its relation to brain damage: A prospective study. N Engl J Med 317:1190, 1987.

Bagley RS, et al: Hypernatremia, adipsia, and diabetes insipidus in a dog with hypothalamic dysplasia. JAAHA 29:267, 1993.

Barsanti JA, et al: Diagnostic approach to polyuria and polydipsia. In Bonagura JD (ed): Current Veterinary Therapy XIII. Philadelphia, WB Saunders Co, 2000, p 831.

Baylis PH, Robertson GL: Vasopressin function in familial cranial diabetes insipidus. Postgrad Med J 57:36, 1981.

Bhan GL, O'Brien TD: Autoimmune endocrinopathy associated with diabetes insipidus. Postgrad Med J 58:165, 1982.

Biewenga WJ, et al: Vasopressin in polyuric syndromes in the dog. Front Horm Res 17:139, 1987.

Biewenga WJ, et al: Osmoregulation of systemic vasopressin release during long-term glucocorticoid excess: A study in dogs with hyperadrenocorticism. Acta Endocrinol 124:583, 1991.

Block LH, et al: Changes in tissue sensitivity to vasopressin in hereditary hypothalamic diabetes insipidus. Klin Wochenschr 59:831, 1981.

Breitschwerdt EB: Clinical abnormalities of urine concentration and dilution. Compend Cont Ed 3:413, 1981.

Breitschwerdt EB, et al: Nephrogenic diabetes insipidus in three dogs. JAVMA 179:235, 1981.

Brown BA, et al: Evaluation of the plasma vasopressin, plasma sodium, and urine osmolality response to water restriction in normal cats and a cat with diabetes insipidus [abstract]. J Vet Intern Med 7:113, 1993.

Burnie AG, Dunn JK: A case of central diabetes insipidus in the cat: Diagnosis and treatment. J Small Anim Pract 23:237, 1982.

Capen CC, Martin SL: Diseases of the pituitary gland. In Ettinger SJ (ed): Textbook of Veterinary Internal Medicine, 2nd ed. Philadelphia, WB Saunders Co, 1983, p 1523.

Crawford MA, et al: Hypernatremia and adipsia in a dog. JAVMA 184:818, 1984.

Cronin RE: Psychogenic polydipsia with hyponatremia: Report of eleven cases. Am J Kidney Dis 4:410, 1987.

Davenport DJ, et al: Diabetes insipidus associated with metastatic pancreatic carcinoma in a dog. JAVMA 189:204, 1986.

Deen PMT, et al: Requirement of human renal water channel aquaporin-2 for vasopressin-dependent concentration of urine. Science 264:92, 1994.

Deppe TA, et al: Glomerular filtration rate and renal volume in dogs with congenital portosystemic vascular anomalies before and after surgical ligation. J Vet Int Med 13:465, 1999.

DiBartola SP, et al: Hypodipsic hypernatremia in a dog with defective osmoregulation of antidiuretic hormone. JAVMA 204:922, 1994.

Dillingham MA, Anderson RJ: Inhibition of vasopressin action by atrial natriuretic factor. Science 231:1572, 1986.

Dow SW, et al: Hypodipsic hypernatremia and associated myopathy in a hydrocephalic cat with transient hypopituitarism. JAVMA 191:217, 1987.

Edwards DF, et al: Hypernatremic, hypertonic dehydration in the dog with diabetes insipidus and gastric dilatation volvulus. JAVMA 182:973, 1983.

Ferring AB: Product Information, DDAVP, Malmo, Sweden, 1985.

Fleeman LM, et al: Effects of an oral vasopressin receptor antagonist (OPC-31260) in a dog with syndrome of inappropriate secretion of antidiuretic hormone. Aust Vet J 78:825, 2000.

Fujisawa G, et al: Therapeutic efficacy of non-peptide ADH antagonist OPC-31260 in SIADH rats. Kidney Int 46:237, 1993.

Fujiwara TM, et al: Molecular biology of diabetes insipidus. Annu Rev Med 46:331, 1995.

Gold PW, et al: Carbamazepine diminishes the sensitivity of the plasma arginine vasopressin response to osmotic stimulation. J Clin Endocrinol Metab 57:952, 1983.

Goldman MB, et al: Mechanisms of altered water metabolism in psychotic patients with polydipsia and hyponatremia. N Engl J Med 318:397, 1988.

Goossens MMC, et al: Central diabetes insipidus in a dog with a pro-opiomelanocortin-producing pituitary tumor not causing hyperadreno-corticism. J Vet Int Med 9:361, 1995.

Grunbaum EG, Moritz A: Zur diagnostik des diabetes insipidus renalis beim hund. Tierarztliche Praxis 19:539, 1991.

Grunbaum EG, et al: Genetisch bedingter diabetes insipidus renalis beim hund. 35th Annual Meeting, Deutsche Veterinarmedizinische Gesellschaft DVG, Fachgeruppe Kleintierkrankheiten (ed. DVG), DVG, GieBen FRG, 1990, p 126.

Hammer M, et al: Relationship between plasma osmolality and plasma vasopressin in human subjects. Am J Physiol 238:E313, 1980.

Harb M, et al: Central diabetes insipidus: 20 dogs (1986-1995). J Am Vet Med Assoc 209:1884, 1996.

Hardy RM: Disorders of water metabolism. Vet Clin North Am [Small Anim Pract] 12:353, 1982.

Hawks D, et al: Essential hypernatremia in a young dog. J Small Anim Pract 32:420, 1991.

Hoskins JD, Rothschmitt J: Hypernatremic thirst deficiency in a dog. Vet Med 79:489, 1984.

Houston DM, et al: Syndrome of inappropriate antidiuretic hormone secretion in a dog. Can Vet J 30:423, 1989.

Kanno K, et al: Urinary excretion of aquaporin-2 in patients with diabetes insipidus. N Engl J Med 332:1575, 1995.

Kaplowitz PB, et al: Radioimmunoassay of vasopressin in familial central diabetes insipidus. J Pediatr 100:76, 1982.

Kraus KH: The use of desmopressin in diagnosis and treatment of diabetes insipidus in cats. Compend Cont Educ Small Anim Pract 9:752, 1987.

Kusano E, et al: Chlorpropamide action on renal concentrating mechanism in rats with hypothalamic diabetes insipidus. J Clin Invest 72:1298, 1983.

Lantz GC, et al: Transsphenoidal hypophysectomy in the clinically normal dog. Am J Vet Res 49:1134, 1988.

Lee J, et al: Atrial natriuretic factor inhibits vasopressin secretion in conscious sheep. Proc Soc Exp Biol Med 185:272, 1987.

Lee MD, et al: The aquaporin family of water channel proteins in clinical medicine. Medicine 76:141, 1997.

Luzius H, et al: A low affinity vasopressin V_2 receptor in inherited nephrogenic diabetes insipidus. J Receptor Res 12:351, 1992.

Mackay BM, Curtis N: Adipsia and hypernatremia in a dog with focal hypothalamic granulomatous meningoencephalitis. Aust Vet J 77:14, 1999.

Moses AM, Clayton B: Impairment of osmotically stimulated AVP release in patients with primary polydipsia. Am J Physiol 265: R1247, 1993.

Neer TM, Reavis DU: Craniopharyngioma and associated central diabetes insipidus and hypothyroidism in a dog. JAVMA 182:519, 1983.

Nichols R: Clinical use of the vasopressin analogue DDAVP for the diagnosis and treatment of diabetes insipidus. In Bonagura JD (ed): Current Veterinary Therapy XIII. Philadelphia, WB Saunders Co, 2000, p 325.

Ohnishi A, et al: Potent aquaretic agent: A novel nonpeptide selective vasopressin 2 antagonist (OPC-31260) in men. J Clin Invest 92:2653, 1993.

Papanek PE and Raff H: Chronic physiological increases in cortisol inhibit the vasopressin response to hypertonicity in conscious dogs. Am J Physiol 267:R1342, 1994.

Papanek PE, et al: Corticosterone inhibition of osmotically stimulated vasopressin from hypothalamic-neurohypophysial explants. Am J Physiol 272:R158, 1997.

Peterson ME, et al: Acromegaly in 14 cats. J Vet Intern Med 4:192, 1990.

Pittari JM: Central diabetes insipidus in a cat. Feline Pract 24:18, 1996.

Pliska V: Pharmacology of deamino-d-arginine vasopressin. In Czenichow P, Robinson AG (eds): Frontiers of Hormone Research. Vol 13. Diabetes Insipidus in Man. Basel, Switzerland, S. Karger, 1985, p 278.

Pollock AS, Arieff AI: Abnormalities of cell volume and their functional consequence. Am J Physiol 239:F195, 1980.

Post K, et al: Congenital central diabetes insipidus in two sibling Afghan Hound pups. JAVMA 194:1086, 1989.

Ramsay DJ: Posterior pituitary gland. In Greenspan FS, Forsham PH (eds): Basic and Clinical Endocrinology. Los Altos, CA, Lange Medical Publications, 1983, p 120.

Reeves WB, et al: The posterior pituitary and water metabolism. In Wilson JD, Foster DW, Kronenberg HM, Larsen PR (eds): Williams Textbook of Endocrinology, 9th ed. Philadelphia, WB Saunders Co, 1998, p 341.

Reidarson TH, et al: Extreme hypernatremia in a dog with central diabetes insipidus: A case report. JAAHA 26:89, 1990.

Richardson DW, Robinson AG: Desmopressin. Ann Intern Med 103:228, 1985.

Rijnberk A, et al: Inappropriate vasopressin secretion in two dogs. Acta Endocrinol 117;59, 1988.

Rijnberk A, et al: Aldosteronoma in a dog with polyuria as the leading symptom. Domest Anim Endocrinol 20:227, 2001.

Robertson GL: Diseases of the posterior pituitary. In Felig P, et al (eds): Endocrinology and Metabolism. New York, McGraw Hill Book Co, 1981, p 251.

Robertson GL: Differential diagnosis of polyuria. Ann Rev Med 39:425, 1988.

Robertson GL, Scheidler JA: A newly recognized variant of familial nephrogenic diabetes insipidus distinguished by partial resistance to vasopressin (type 2) [abstract]. Clin Res 29:555A, 1981.

Salvi M, et al: Role of autoantibodies in the pathogenesis and association of endocrine autoimmune disorders. Endocr Rev 9:450, 1988.

Scherbaum WA: Role of autoimmunity in hypothalamic disorders. Bailliere's Clin Immunol 1:237, 1987.

Scherbaum WA, et al: Autoimmune cranial diabetes insipidus: Its association with other endocrine diseases and with histiocytosis X. Clin Endocrinol 25:411, 1986.

Schwartz J, et al: Hemodynamic effects of neurohypophyseal peptides with antidiuretic activity in dogs. Am J Physiol 249:H1001, 1985.

Schwartz Porsche D: Diabetes insipidus. In Kirk RW (ed): Current Veterinary Therapy VII. Philadelphia, WB Saunders Co, 1980, p 1005.

Sterns RH, et al: Brain dehydration and neurologic deterioration after rapid correction of hyponatremia. Kidney Int 35:69, 1989.

Sterns RH, et al: Organic osmolytes in acute hyponatremia. Am J Physiol 264:F833, 1993.

Sterns RH, et al: Neurologic sequelae after treatment of severe hyponatremia: a multicenter perspective. J Am Soc Nephrol 4:1522, 1994.

van Lieburg AF, et al: Patients with autosomal nephrogenic diabetes insipidus homozygous for mutations in the aquaporin 2 water-channel gene. Am J Hum Genet 55:648,1994.

van Lieburg AF, et al: Clinical phenotype of nephrogenic diabetes insipidus in females heterozygous for a vasopressin type 2 receptor mutation. Hum Genet 96:70, 1995.

van Vonderen IK, et al: Polyuria and polydipsia and disturbed vasopressin release in two dogs with secondary polycythemia. J Vet Int Med 11: 300, 1997a.

van Vonderen IK, et al: Intra- and interindividual variation in urine osmolality and urine specific gravity in healthy pet dogs of various ages. J Vet Int Med 11: 30, 1997b.

van Vonderen IK, et al: Disturbed vasopressin release in four dogs with so-called primary polydipsia. J Vet Int Med 13: 419, 1999.

Victor W, et al: Failure of antipsychotic drug dose to explain abnormal diurnal weight gain among 129 chronically psychotic inpatients. Prog Neuropsychopharmacol Biol Psychiatry 13:709, 1989.

Williams TDM, et al: Hormonal and cardiovascular responses to DDAVP in man. Clin Endocrinol (Oxf) 24:89, 1986.

Winterbotham J, Mason KV: Congenital diabetes insipidus in a kitten. J Small Anim Pract 24:569, 1983.

Zerbe RL, Robertson GL: A comparison of plasma vasopressin measurements with a standard indirect test in the differential diagnosis of polyuria. N Engl J Med 305:1539, 1981.

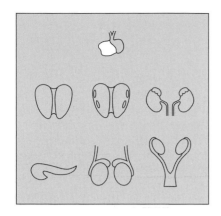

2

DISORDERS OF GROWTH HORMONE

BIOSYNTHESIS OF GROWTH HORMONE AND IGF-I

Growth hormone (GH; somatotropin) is a single-chain polypeptide with a molecular weight of approximately 22,000 daltons (Thorner et al, 1998). The amino acid sequence of canine GH has been elucidated and is identical to that of porcine GH (Mol and Rijnberk, 1997; Secchi et al, 2001). GH shares amino acid sequence homology with prolactin and placental lactogen, suggesting that these hormones evolved from a single ancestral gene. GH is synthesized and secreted by the somatotrophs of the anterior pituitary. GH's larger precursor peptide, PreGH, is also secreted but has no known physiologic significance (Aron et al, 2001). Secretion of GH occurs in a pulsatile ultradian fashion, with pulse intervals of 4 to 6 hours (French et al, 1987; Conzemius et al, 1998). In humans, plasma GH concentrations increase from birth onward, reach a maximum in late adolescence, and decline during adulthood. In contrast, in a study by Nap and colleagues (1993), mean plasma GH concentrations declined between 7 and 27 weeks of age (13.7 ± 2.2 versus 0.7 ± 0.4 µg/L, respectively) in Great Dane puppies. The pulsatile secretion pattern of GH also changes according to the phase of the estrus cycle in healthy bitches, with higher baseline GH secretion and less GH secreted in pulses during stages involving a high plasma progesterone concentration (Kooistra et al, 2000a). The pulse height of GH decreases with age in humans, cattle, and domestic fowl and is presumed to also decrease with age in other species, including dogs and cats (Mol and Rijnberk, 1997). High- and low-affinity GH-binding proteins (GHBPs) exist in plasma in humans and have been reported in dogs (Maxwell et al, 2000). GHBPs are believed to play a significant role in modulating the activity of growth hormone (Styne, 2001). The high-affinity GHBP is identical to the amino acid sequence of the extracellular domain of the GH receptor (Thorner et al, 1998). Protein-bound GH is metabolized differently, persists longer in plasma, and has a limited volume of distribution compared with monomeric GH, suggesting that protein binding may enhance the biologic activity of GH.

In the late 1950s researchers identified a "sulfation factor," which promoted growth and was controlled by GH, and a serum fraction, which had insulin-like activity that could not be abolished by antiinsulin antibodies. In the 1970s these factors were termed *somatomedins* (because they *mediate* the action of somatotropin) and *insulin-like growth factors*, respectively. Somatomedin C and insulin-like growth factor-I (IGF-I) were subsequently shown to be the same molecule. Most of the growth-promoting effects of GH are mediated by IGF-I. IGF-I has an approximately 50% homology of structure with proinsulin and insulin, and the IGF-I cell membrane receptor resembles the insulin receptor in its structure. IGF-I binds to insulin receptors and promotes glucose utilization, enhances tissue sensitivity to insulin, and decreases the blood glucose concentration. IGF-I is produced in most tissues and appears to be exported to neighboring cells to act upon them in a paracrine manner (Yakar et al, 1999; Styne, 2001). As such, serum IGF-I concentrations may not reflect the most significant actions of this growth factor. The liver is a major site of IGF-I synthesis, and much of the circulating IGF-I is believed to be derived from the liver. In humans, serum IGF-I concentrations vary in liver disease with the extent of liver destruction.

Secretion of IGF-I is under the direct control of GH. Serum IGF-I concentrations are low in GH deficiency and increased in acromegaly. The biologic effects of circulating IGF-I are modulated by several different IGF-binding proteins (IGFBPs), with IGFBP-3 being the most abundant in dogs and cats (Maxwell et al, 1998; Lewitt et al, 2000). In dogs, IGF-I binds primarily with IGFBP-3 and an acid-labile subunit (ALS) to form a ternary complex that does not cross the vascular endothelium, that prolongs the plasma half-life of IGF-I, and that functions as a storage pool for IGF-I (Maxwell et al, 2000). In one study, ALS concentrations were low in cats, compared with other species, and this limited the formation of IGFBP-3 ternary complexes (Lewitt et al, 2000). Interestingly, ALS concentrations were increased in diabetic cats, and the elevated levels, by promoting ternary complex formation, may have lead to the increase seen in serum IGF-I concentrations in the diabetic cats compared with healthy cats; this finding may have implications for the use of IGF-I as a diagnostic aid for feline acromegaly (see page 76).

IGFBP-1 is the only acute regulator of IGF-I bioavailability (Lee et al, 1997). The primary role of IGFBP-1 is the acute binding of IGF-I in the circulation; the greater the concentration of IGFBP-1, the lower the concentration of free IGF-I and vice versa. GH decreases IGFBP-1 concentrations in plasma. Results of in vitro and in vivo studies have shown that IGFBP-1 inhibits growth and differentiation stimulated by IGF-I and counteracts the insulin-like hypoglycemic activity of IGF-I (Ferry et al, 1999). Circulating IGF-I and its interaction with IGFBP-1 are believed to be important determinants of glucose homeostasis, providing an important link between nutrition and growth (Sandhu et al, 2002). For example, consumption of a meal stimulates ghrelin secretion, which stimulates GH secretion, which decreases IGFBP-1 and increases the amount of free IGF-I available for binding to insulin receptors and promoting glucose utilization. Insulin suppresses IGFBP-1, and studies have documented decreased IGFBP-1 levels in humans with obesity and type 2 diabetes mellitus; these findings suggest that measurement of IGFBP-1 may be useful as a marker for insulin resistance. Finally, some disease states increase the levels of IGFBP-1, which can have a deleterious effect on the diagnostic usefulness of IGF-I as a marker for GH excess. Renal failure and some solid tumors have been shown to increase the concentration of IGFBP-1 in humans, causing an increase in plasma total IGF-I concentrations by as much as 30% to 50%.

METABOLIC ACTIONS OF GROWTH HORMONE

GH is described as anabolic, lipolytic, and diabetogenic, concepts derived primarily from in vitro studies of isolated tissue and in vivo studies involving administration of pharmacologic amounts of GH. The primary function of growth hormone is promotion of linear growth (Conzemius et al, 1998). Most of the growth-promoting effects are mediated by IGF-I (Fig. 2-1). A dual-effector model of GH action has been proposed in which GH first stimulates prechondrocytes in the epiphyseal growth plate to undergo differentiation and stimulates the expression of IGF-I in hepatocytes and chondrocytes; IGF-I then acts as a mitogen to stimulate clonal growth of the differentiated cells (Isaksson et al, 1987; Scheven and Hamilton, 1991). In this way locally produced IGF-I, under GH regulation, contributes to the stimulatory effects of GH, particularly the enhancement of longitudinal growth.

Differences in adult body size of dog breeds is preceded by differences in GH release at a young age and not by differences in circulating IGF-I concentrations. In one study, young Great Danes and young Beagles both experienced a period of high GH release, but this period persisted much longer in Great Danes (Favier et al, 2001). There was no difference in circulating IGF-I concentrations between the two groups of young dogs. The authors speculate that the longer period of increased GH secretion in the Great Danes may have been caused by delayed maturation of the inhibitory influences of somatostatin on GH release. In contrast, during adulthood similar GH concentrations are found in the plasma of dog breeds of widely differing body sizes, but the serum IGF-I levels are quite different and positively correlated with body size (Eigenmann, 1987). Smaller breeds have lower concentrations of IGF-I than larger breeds. In one study, the mean IGF-I concentrations were 36 ± 27 ng/ml in Cocker Spaniels; 87 ± 33 ng/ml in Beagles; 117 ± 34 ng/ml in Keeshonds; and 280 ± 23 ng/ml in German Shepherd dogs (Eigenmann

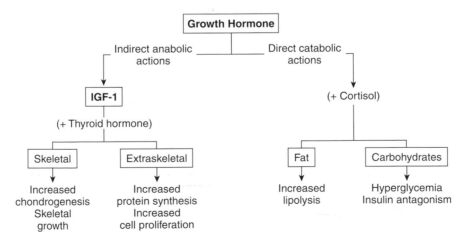

FIGURE 2–1. The anabolic and catabolic actions of growth hormone. (Modified from Underwood LE, Van Wyk JJ: *In* Wilson J, Foster D (eds): Williams Textbook of Endocrinology, 7th ed. Philadelphia, WB Saunders, 1985, p 155.)

et al, 1984b). In another study that compared IGF-I levels in different-sized dogs within the same breed (i.e., Toy, Miniature, and Standard Poodles), a linear correlation between body size and circulating IGF-I levels was established (Eigenmann et al, 1984a). All of these dogs secreted similar normal amounts of GH in response to provocative stimulation.

Another important anabolic action of GH is stimulation of protein synthesis, an action mediated by IGF-I (see Fig. 2-1). Cellular uptake of amino acids is enhanced; transcription and translation of mRNA is accelerated; and enzymatic steps necessary for protein synthesis are activated (Daughaday, 1985). DNA synthesis is stimulated in a variety of cell types, including fibroblasts, chondrocytes, muscle, and hematopoietic and hepatic tissue (Van Wyk et al, 1981). These actions result in the stimulation of cell proliferation or in cellular differentiation without obligatory proliferation. In all responding tissues, the production of cell products is characteristic of each target tissue.

GH tends to decrease protein catabolism by directly promoting lipolysis and enhancing the conversion of free fatty acids to acetyl coenzyme A (acetyl-CoA), from which energy is derived (see Fig. 2-1; Aron et al, 2001). GH also has a direct effect on carbohydrate metabolism. In excess, it decreases carbohydrate utilization and impairs glucose uptake into cells. GH-induced insulin resistance appears to be due to a post-receptor impairment in insulin action (Bratusch-Marrain et al, 1982; Rosenfeld et al, 1982). The net effect is promotion of hyperglycemia, carbohydrate intolerance, and, with sustained increases in plasma GH, the development of diabetes mellitus, which quickly becomes resistant to insulin treatment.

REGULATION OF GROWTH HORMONE SECRETION

In many domestic species, GH is secreted from the pituitary gland in a pulsatile manner that is under the dual regulation of hypothalamic GH-releasing hormone (GHRH; somatocrinin) and GH release–inhibiting factor (somatostatin) (Fig. 2-2). The two factors act in concert to precisely control GH secretion so as to maintain homeostasis in the growing body from fetal life through adolescence. These positive and negative regulating stimuli persist in adults as well.

GH-RELEASING HORMONE. GHRH stimulates both GH synthesis and secretion. GHRH causes a prompt increase in blood GH levels, followed by a rapid return of GH to basal concentrations (Thorner et al, 1983). The pulsatile increases in GH primarily reflect the pulsatile secretion of GHRH from the hypothalamus (Thorner et al, 1998). Sustained infusions of GHRH over several hours result in an initial rise and then a progressive decrease in plasma GH concentrations, suggesting that GHRH depends on pulsatile secretion for its physiologic effect (Reichlin, 1998). The effects of GHRH are almost completely specific for GH, although a minimal increase in plasma prolactin may also occur.

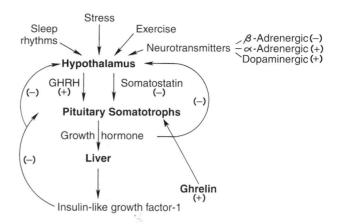

FIGURE 2–2. Proposed stimulatory and inhibitory influences involved in the regulation of growth hormone and insulin-like growth factor-I (IGF-I) secretion. (Modified from Reichlin S: *In* Wilson J, Foster D (eds): Williams Textbook of Endocrinology, 7th ed. Philadelphia, WB Saunders, 1985, p 492.)

SOMATOSTATIN. Somatostatin denotes a family of peptides, including somatostatin-14, which is a cyclic peptide containing 14 amino acids, and the N-terminal-extended somatostatin-28, which is a cyclic peptide containing 28 amino acids. Somatostatin-14 is identical with the terminal 14 amino acids of somatostatin-28. Somatostatin-14 is found predominately in the central nervous system (CNS), including the hypothalamus, and somatostatin-28 is found predominately in the gastrointestinal tract, including the pancreas (Reichlin, 1998). As a pituitary regulator, somatostatin is a potent inhibitor of GH secretion. Somatostatin secretion is increased by elevated levels of GH and IGF-I. Somatostatin appears to determine the timing and amplitude of GH pulses but has no effect on GH synthesis (Thorner et al, 1998). Somatostatin inhibits secretion of thyroid-stimulating hormone (TSH) and, under certain conditions, secretion of prolactin and adrenocorticotropic hormone (ACTH). It also has non-pituitary roles, including activity as a neuromodulator in the central and peripheral nervous systems and as a gut and pancreatic regulatory peptide (Table 2-1; Reichlin, 1998). Somatostatin blocks hormone release in many endocrine-secreting tumors, including insulinomas, glucagonomas, vasoactive intestinal polypeptide–secreting tumors (VIPomas), carcinoid tumors, and some gastrinomas (see Chapters 14 and 15). In humans, long-acting analogs of somatostatin have been used therapeutically in the management of GH excess and functioning neuroendocrine tumors (Reichlin, 1998).

STIMULI AFFECTING GH-REGULATING FACTORS. The influence of GHRH and somatostatin on GH secretion is tightly regulated by an integrated system of neural, metabolic, and hormonal factors, including GH itself (Tables 2-2 and 2-3) (Buonomo and Baile, 1990). Most of these stimuli exert their effects on GH secretion by influencing hypothalamic secretion of GHRH or somatostatin. The predominant influence of the hypothalamus on GH secretion is stimulatory, as evidenced by the fact that damage to the hypothalamic-pituitary

TABLE 2–1 BIOLOGIC ACTIONS OF SOMATOSTATIN OUTSIDE THE CENTRAL NERVOUS SYSTEM

Inhibition of Hormone Secretion	Inhibition of Gastrointestinal Actions
Pituitary gland	Gastric acid secretion
TSH, GH	Gastric emptying
Gastrointestinal tract	Pancreatic bicarbonate secretion
Gastrin	Pancreatic enzyme secretion
Secretin	Intestinal absorption
Gastrointestinal polypeptide	Gastrointestinal blood flow
Motilin	AVP-stimulated water transport
Enteroglucagon	Bile flow
VIP	
Pancreas	
Insulin	
Glucagon	
Somatostatin	
Genitourinary tract	
Renin	

Modified from Reichlin S: *In* Wilson JD, Foster DW, Kronenberg HM, Larsen PR (eds): Williams Textbook of Endocrinology, 9th ed. Philadelphia, WB Saunders Co, 1998, p 191.
TSH, thyrotropin; *GH,* growth hormone; *AVP,* arginine vasopressin; *VIP,* vasoactive intestinal polypeptide.

TABLE 2–2 FACTORS THAT STIMULATE GH SECRETION IN PRIMATES

Physiologic	Hormones and Neurotransmitters
Episodic, spontaneous	Insulin-induced hypoglycemia
Exercise (not dogs)	Amino acid infusions
Stress	(inconsistent in dogs)
Sleep	Peptide hormones
Postprandial	GHRH
Hyperaminoacidemia	Vasopressin
Hypoglycemia (relative)	Alpha-MSH
Fasting (hypoglycemia)	ACTH
	Glucagon
Pathologic	Low IGF-I
Acromegaly	Monoaminergic stimuli
Hypothyroidism (dogs not	Alpha-adrenergic agonists
primates)	Clonidine, epinephrine
Unregulated diabetes mellitus	Beta-adrenergic antagonists
Chronic renal failure	Propranolol
Hepatic cirrhosis	Dopamine agonists
Fasting, starvation	L-Dopa, bromocriptine
Protein depletion	Serotonin precursors
Ectopic GHRH production	Melatonin
Interleukins 1,2,6	Acetylcholine agonists
In acromegalics	Nonpeptide hormones
TRH	Estrogens
LHRH	Diethylstilbestrol
Glucose	Progesterone (dogs not
Arginine	primates)
	Potassium infusion

Modified from Reichlin S: *In* Wilson JD, Foster DW, Kronenberg HM, Larsen PR (eds): Williams Textbook of Endocrinology, 9th ed. Philadelphia, WB Saunders Co, 1998, p 210.

TABLE 2–3 FACTORS THAT INHIBIT GH SECRETION IN PRIMATES

Physiologic	Hormones and Neurotransmitters
Postprandial hyperglycemia	Somatostatin
(primates but not dogs)	Glucocorticoids
Increased free fatty acids	Progesterone (Primates but not
Serotonin antagonists	dogs)
Increased GH and IGF-I	High IGF-I
concentrations	Melatonin
Cyproheptadine	Alpha-adrenergic agonists
	Phentolamine
Pathologic	Beta-adrenergic antagonists
Hypothyroidism	Isoproterenol
(primates but not dogs)	Serotonin antagonists
Hyperthyroidism	Methysergide
Hyperadrenocorticism	Cyproheptadine
Obesity	Dopamine antagonists
In acromegalics	Phenothiazines
L-Dopa	Acetylcholine antagonists
Apomorphine	Theophylline
Phentolamine	Morphine
Bromocriptine	

Modified from Reichlin S: *In* Wilson JD, Foster DW, Kronenberg HM, Larsen PR (eds): Williams Textbook of Endocrinology, 9th ed. Philadelphia, WB Saunders Co, 1998, p 210.

gastric emptying and promote satiety. Ghrelin also stimulates GH secretion, which in turn increases IGF-I concentrations. IGF-I promotes glucose utilization by binding to insulin receptors in tissues. Growth hormone also decreases IGFBP-1 concentrations, resulting in increased free IGF-I concentrations. As mentioned previously, the primary role of IGFBP-1 is the binding of IGF-I, thereby decreasing the circulating concentration of IGF-I.

Differences in the effect of stimuli on GH secretion appear to exist between dogs and humans. For example, moderate exercise stimulates GH secretion in humans but apparently not in dogs. Arginine, a potent stimulant of GH secretion in humans, has given inconsistent results when administered to dogs. The GH response to insulin-induced hypoglycemia has also been inconsistent in dogs, with some investigators reporting a clear-cut elevation and others reporting only a sluggish response. Likewise, hyperglycemia resulting from a glucose infusion inhibits GH secretion in humans but has a minimal effect in dogs. Because of this species variability, it seems inappropriate to assume that factors that affect GH secretion in humans automatically have a similar effect in dogs.

The reader is referred to the first edition of *Canine and Feline Endocrinology and Reproduction* for more information on the metabolic actions of GH and the factors that regulate GH secretion.

CONGENITAL HYPOSOMATOTROPISM: PITUITARY DWARFISM

Etiology

Pituitary dwarfism results from a congenital deficiency of GH. GH deficiency may occur as an isolated deficiency or in combination with deficiencies in other

connection is followed by inhibition of both basal and induced GH release (Reichlin, 1998). One exception is ghrelin, a recently discovered hormone that is produced primarily in the stomach and to a lesser extent in the hypothalamus. Ghrelin is secreted after consumption of a meal; its primary actions are to decrease hormones of the anterior lobe of the pituitary gland (i.e., TSH, prolactin, ACTH, follicle-stimulating hormone [FSH], and luteinizing hormone [LH]). In dogs and probably cats, dwarfism is most commonly associated with pressure atrophy of the anterior lobe of the pituitary gland caused by cystic enlargement of the residual craniopharyngeal duct (i.e., Rathke's cleft) and with pituitary hypoplasia resulting from primary failure of differentiation of the craniopharyngeal ectoderm of Rathke's pouch into a normal anterior lobe.

PITUITARY CYST. Pituitary dwarfism may result from congenital cystic distention or persistence of the "intrasellar" portion of the craniopharyngeal duct (Rathke's pouch). The intrasellar portion is found within the sella turcica, the region of the skull "encasing" the pituitary. During embryonic development, the anterior pituitary (adenohypophysis) arises from Rathke's pouch, an evagination of the posterior wall of the pharynx. The portion of the pouch that comes in contact with the neurohypophysis differentiates into the pars intermedia of the anterior pituitary, and the anterior wall of the pouch differentiates into the pars distalis of the anterior pituitary. Lateral proliferations from the embryonic pouch extend around the infundibular stem to form the pars tuberalis (pituitary stalk). In the dog and cat, the distal and intermediate parts of the anterior pituitary are separated by the residual hypophyseal cleft, which is the residual lumen of Rathke's pouch. The stalk of Rathke's pouch is attenuated in the embryo to form the craniopharyngeal duct. This duct should disappear, although either or both ends of it commonly persist as vestiges in dogs. Persistence of the intrasellar portions of the duct is especially common in brachycephalic breeds. The degree of persistence and consequences varies. The remnants may become cystic; may be single or multiple, unilocular or multilocular; and frequently contain mucin produced by the epithelium that lines the cyst. The cysts are usually microscopic and clinically insignificant but sometimes are larger in volume than a normal pituitary gland (Fig. 2-3). Large cysts may cause pressure atrophy of pituitary cells.

Pituitary cysts are relatively common in the dog, yet dwarfism is rare. Also, dwarfism is most often encountered in the German Shepherd dog, and German Shepherd dwarfs have been identified with only a very small pituitary cyst. For these reasons, the theory that cystic distention of the craniopharyngeal duct is the primary cause of destruction of the adenohypophysis has been questioned. An alternative hypothesis suggests a primary failure in the differentiation of the adenohypophyseal cells into normal tropic hormone–secreting cells (Kooistra et al, 2000b).

PITUITARY HYPOPLASIA. The development of the anterior lobe of the pituitary gland is characterized by the expression of a series of homeodomain transcription factors, which are required for normal growth of the pituitary primordium (Treier et al, 1998; Watkins-Chow and Camper, 1998). After proliferation, different cell phenotypes arise in a distinct temporal fashion and undergo a highly selective determination and differentiation (Simmons et al, 1990; Voss and Rosenfeld,

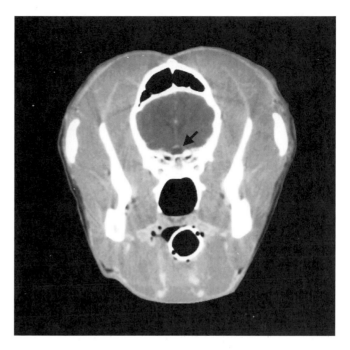

FIGURE 2–3. CT scan of the pituitary region of a small 2-year-old female spayed Great Dane presenting for diagnostic evaluation of pituitary function. A large radiolucent cyst is evident in the pituitary region (arrow).

1992). The corticotropic cell is the first distinct cell type that differentiates from the pituitary stem cell (Sheng et al, 1997). Ultimately, the mature pituitary anterior lobe is composed of five distinct endocrine cell types that are easily distinguished by the hormones they secrete. Any defect in the organogenesis of the pituitary gland may result in an isolated or combined pituitary hormone deficiency.

Pituitary dwarfism is encountered most often as a simple, autosomal recessive inherited abnormality in the German Shepherd dog (Kooistra et al, 2000b). Inherited pituitary dwarfism may be due to isolated GH deficiency or may be part of a combined anterior pituitary hormone deficiency syndrome. Concurrent deficiency in TSH and prolactin are most commonly identified in German Shepherd dwarfs; ACTH secretion is preserved (Fig. 2-4; Hamann et al, 1999; Kooistra et al, 2000b). Kooistra and colleagues (2000b) hypothesize that the disorder in German Shepherd dogs is caused by a mutation in a developmental transcription factor that precludes effective expansion of a pituitary stem cell after the differentiation of the corticotropic cells that produce ACTH. Mutations in the genes encoding for transcription factors Pit-1 or the Prophet of Pit-1 (Prop-1) cause combined pituitary anterior lobe hormone deficiencies in humans and mice (Pellegrini-Bouiller et al, 1996; Fofanova et al, 1998; Wu et al, 1998). Unfortunately, a mutation in the gene encoding transcription factors Pit-1 and Prop-1 was not identified in German Shepherd dwarfs, which indicates that another homeodomain gene is affected in dwarf German Shepherd dogs (Lantinga-van Leeuwen et al, 2000a and 2000b). Kooistra and colleagues (2000b)

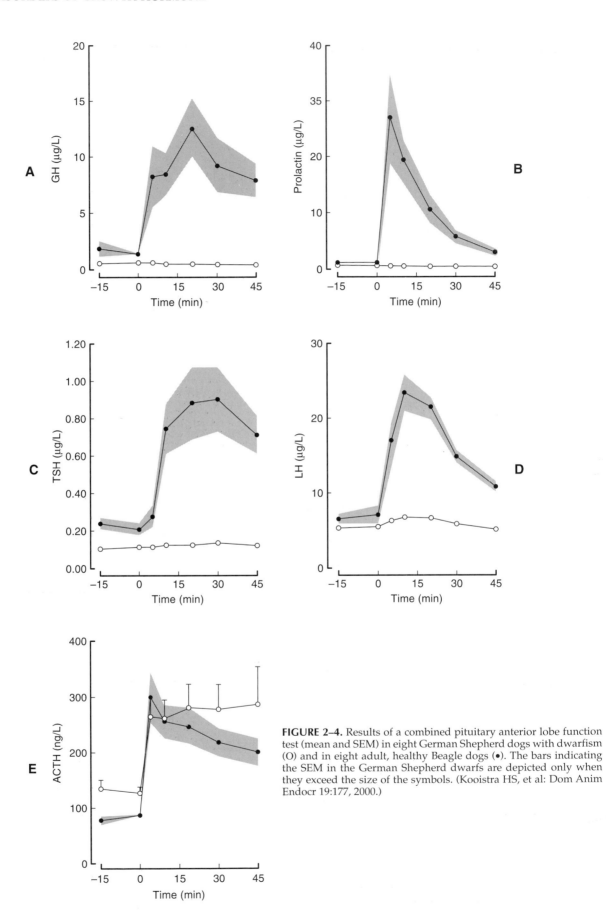

FIGURE 2–4. Results of a combined pituitary anterior lobe function test (mean and SEM) in eight German Shepherd dogs with dwarfism (O) and in eight adult, healthy Beagle dogs (•). The bars indicating the SEM in the German Shepherd dwarfs are depicted only when they exceed the size of the symbols. (Kooistra HS, et al: Dom Anim Endocr 19:177, 2000.)

speculate that the underlying defect may involve a mutation that precludes effective expansion of a pituitary stem cell. Because ACTH secretion remains intact, a combined pituitary hormone deficiency in German Shepherd dwarfs would most likely be caused by a mutation in a developmental transcription factor that precludes effective expansion of a pituitary stem cell after the differentiation of the corticotropic cells. Such a factor would be analogous to the pituitary transcription factors Pit-1 and Prop-1 but would act at an earlier stage of pituitary gland development (Kooistra et al, 2000b).

The cystic changes involving the pituitary gland in dogs with congenital GH deficiency may be the result of primary failure of differentiation of the anterior lobe of the pituitary gland rather than the cause of the GH deficiency. Undifferentiated adenohypophyseal cells may secrete osmotically active proteinaceous material into the craniopharyngeal duct (Eigenmann, 1983). Analysis of cystic fluid obtained from rats has shown that the osmotically active proteinaceous material could attract water and lead to cystic changes, which is compatible with the observation that the cysts enlarge with time (Benjamin, 1981; Kooistra et al, 1998).

GH INSENSITIVITY SYNDROMES. Pituitary dwarfism may develop from insensitivity to GH. The prototype of GH insensitivity is the syndrome of Laron-type dwarfism in human beings. Circulating levels of GH are increased in people with Laron-type dwarfism, but IGF-I levels are deficient. This disorder is due to inactivating mutations in the gene for the GH receptor, which results in absent or defective GH receptors and partial to complete GH insensitivity (Rosenfeld et al, 1994; Goddard et al, 1995). GH insensitivity can also result from an abnormality in the structure of GH (Takahashi et al, 1996), abnormalities of GH signal transduction (postreceptor defects), primary defects of synthesis of IGF-I, or lack of target tissue response to IGF-I (Lanes et al, 1980; Takahashi et al, 1996; Reiter and Rosenfeld, 1998).

Similar subcategories of dwarfism in dogs or cats have not yet been convincingly described. To date, all cases of pituitary dwarfism in the dog in which either GH or IGF-I concentrations were evaluated have revealed low to undetectable GH concentrations and low IGF-I concentrations. There has been no response of GH to stimulation tests (Rijnberk et al, 1993). Two dwarf German Shepherd dogs have been described with low IGF-I activity and histologically normal pituitary glands. Secondary GH deficiency (i.e., abnormal GH structure or nonresponsive target tissue) was proposed as the cause for the dwarfism, making the assumption that circulating GH levels were normal. Unfortunately, plasma GH concentrations were not evaluated to substantiate the claims. In another study in a German Shepherd dog, similar arguments were made for secondary GH deficiency as the cause of the dwarfism (Muller-Peddinghaus et al, 1980). In this study, basal GH concentrations rather than the GH secretory capacity of the pituitary were assessed. Unfortunately, basal GH concentrations in normal and hypopituitary dogs may be similar, rendering this parameter inadequate for assessing GH secretory capacity (Eigenmann and Eigenmann, 1981a).

Interestingly, two German Shepherd dogs have been described that had delayed growth, resulting in an initial stunted appearance, that eventually resolved by 1 year of age (Randolph et al, 1990). Both dogs had normal basal serum GH and IGF-I concentrations, normal GH secretory response to xylazine administration, and normal adrenal gland and thyroid gland function. These authors speculated that delayed growth was due to mild hypopituitarism or intermittent GH neurosecretory dysfunction. It seems logical that a spectrum of severity, from mild to severe, might exist with hypopituitarism and that the exhibited clinical signs would depend on the severity of impaired GH secretion.

Pathophysiology

The clinical manifestations of pituitary dwarfism result from the deficiency in GH (hyposomatotropism) and the secondary deficiency in circulating IGF-I (Eigenmann et al, 1984c). In the immature animal, hyposomatotropism impairs linear growth, resulting in the development of short stature. Dogs with combined anterior pituitary hormone deficiencies usually lack TSH and prolactin in addition to GH. Lack of TSH secretion may contribute to abnormal body maturation and growth (see Chapter 3). Normal physical development depends on the presence of normal plasma thyroid hormone concentrations, which act synergistically with GH and IGF-I to promote chondrogenesis. Lack of prolactin secretion would prevent mammary gland enlargement and lactation in the postpartum bitch. Dogs with combined anterior pituitary hormone deficiencies may have impaired secretion of gonadotropins (LH and FSH), resulting in hypogonadism and infertility. Studies in German Shepherd dwarfs suggest that corticotroph function and ACTH secretion are maintained in dogs with combined pituitary hormone deficiencies (Kooistra et al, 2000b). Secondary adrenal insufficiency does not occur in most dogs with combined anterior pituitary hormone deficiencies. Clinical manifestations resulting from deficiency of neurohypophyseal hormones (i.e., vasopressin, oxytocin) are not apparent in pituitary dwarfs. If the neurohypophysis were damaged, vasopressin secretion would continue directly from the hypothalamus, thereby preventing diabetes insipidus. Because of concurrent hypogonadism, any deficiency in oxytocin would be clinically insignificant.

Signalment

Pituitary dwarfism occurs primarily in the German Shepherd dog, although the condition has been described in other breeds, including the Weimaraner, Spitz, Toy Pinscher, and Carnelian Bear dog. Pituitary dwarfism has also been described in cats. A simple autosomal recessive mode of inheritance has been reported for the German Shepherd dog and the Carnelian Bear dog. In one study, plasma IGF-I concentrations were evaluated in a group of German Shepherd dwarfs and their relatives; interestingly, in the clinically unaffected relatives, IGF-I concentrations were intermediate between those of the normal dogs and those of the dwarfs, suggesting a gene-dosage effect (Willeberg et al 1975). This pattern would be expected if the unaffected relatives were heterozygous, expressing approximately 50% of the trait compared with the fully expressed homozygous dwarfs. Unfortunately, determinations of the basal GH concentrations and the responsiveness of the somatotrophs to provocative testing were not performed.

There does not appear to be a gender predilection for pituitary dwarfism. Affected animals begin to show clinical signs (i.e., lack of growth) around the second to third month of life; however, the age at which veterinary care is sought has been variable. Usually the animal is examined prior to 1 year of age for failure to grow or for dermatologic abnormalities.

Clinical signs

The most common clinical manifestations of pituitary dwarfism are a lack of growth (i.e., short stature), endocrine alopecia, and hyperpigmentation of the skin (Table 2-4). Affected animals are usually normal in size during the first 1 to 2 months of life, after which the rate of growth is slower than that of their littermates. By 3 to 4 months of age, affected dogs and cats are obviously "runts" of the litter and usually never attain full adult dimensions (Figs. 2-5 and 2-6). The initial normal growth is consistent with the concept that growth in early postnatal life in most animals and in humans proceeds for a certain period at a normal rate even in the absence of GH.

TABLE 2–4 CLINICAL SIGNS ASSOCIATED WITH PITUITARY DWARFISM

Musculoskeletal	Dermatologic
Stunted growth	Soft, woolly haircoat
Thin skeleton, immature facial features	Retention of lanugo hairs
	Lack of guard hairs
Square, chunky contour (adult)	Alopecia
Bone deformities	Bilaterally symmetrical
Delayed closure of growth plates	Trunk, neck, proximal extremities
Delayed dental eruption	Hyperpigmentation of skin
	Thin, fragile skin
Reproductive	Wrinkles
Testicular atrophy	Scales
Flaccid penile sheath	Comedones
Failure to cycle	Papules
	Pyoderma
	Seborrhea sicca
Other Signs	
Mental dullness	
Shrill, puppy-like bark	
Signs of secondary hypothyroidism	
Signs of secondary adrenal insufficiency	

Dwarfs with an isolated GH deficiency typically maintain a normal body contour and body proportions as they age (i.e., proportionate dwarfism), whereas dwarfs with combined anterior pituitary hormone deficiencies (most notably TSH) may acquire a square or chunky contour typically associated with congenital hypothyroidism (i.e., disproportionate dwarfism) (see Fig. 2-6) (see Chapter 3, page 104). Closure of the epiphyseal growth plates is usually delayed in pituitary dwarfs, and the fontanelles of the skull may remain open. Dental eruption may be delayed, but dentition is usually normal.

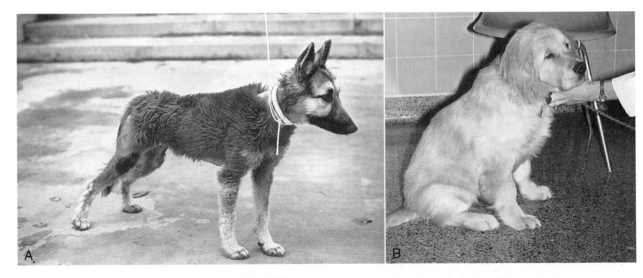

FIGURE 2–5. *A,* A 1.5-year-old female German Shepherd dog with pituitary dwarfism. This dog's size was similar to that of a 4-month-old German Shepherd puppy. *B,* An 11-month-old female Golden Retriever with pituitary dwarfism. This dog's size was similar to that of a 10-week-old Golden Retriever puppy. For both dogs, note the normal body contour, juvenile appearance, and retention of secondary hairs with concurrent lack of primary guard hairs.

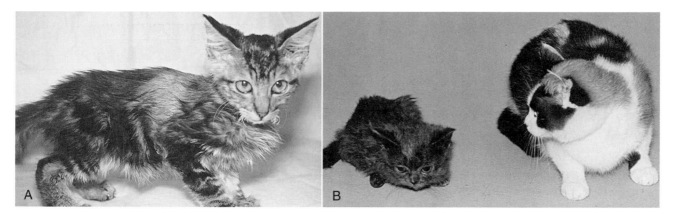

FIGURE 2–6. *A,* An 8-month-old male Domestic Short-Haired cat with pituitary dwarfism. This cat's size was similar to that of an 8-week-old kitten. Note the normal body contour and juvenile appearance. *B,* A 1-year-old Domestic Long-Haired cat with pituitary dwarfism. A cat of comparable age is present to illustrate the small size of the pituitary dwarf. Note the square, chunky contour of the head of the pituitary dwarf.

The most notable dermatologic sign is retention of the lanugo, or secondary, hairs, with concurrent lack of the primary, or guard, hairs. As a result, the hair coat in a dwarf is initially soft and woolly. The lanugo hairs are easily epilated, and bilateral symmetric alopecia gradually develops. Initially, hair loss is confined to areas of wear, such as the neck (collar) and postero-lateral aspects of the thighs (from sitting). Eventually the entire trunk, neck, and proximal limbs become alopecic, with primary hairs remaining only on the face and distal extremities.

The skin is initially normal but with time becomes progressively hyperpigmented (gray to brown to black), thin, wrinkled, and scaly. Comedones, papules, and secondary pyoderma frequently develop in the adult dwarf. Secondary bacterial infections of the skin and respiratory tract are common long-term complications.

Hypogonadism may also develop, although normal reproductive function has been reported in some pituitary dwarfs. In the male, testicular atrophy, azoospermia, and a flaccid penile sheath are typical; in the female, absence of estrus activity develops as a result of impaired secretion of pituitary gonadotropins. Most canine pituitary dwarfs retain a shrill, puppylike bark (Campbell, 1988). Most pituitary dwarfs remain alert and active when young. As they grow older, however, they may become progressively more listless, dull, and inactive. Inappetence may develop. These changes may reflect the various endocrine deficiencies associated with the condition or progressive expansion of a pituitary cyst or cysts.

Clinical pathology

The results of a complete blood count (CBC), biochemical panel, and urinalysis are usually normal in dogs and cats with pituitary dwarfism caused by isolated GH deficiency. A mild increase in renal parameters (urea nitrogen and creatinine) may develop secondary to maldevelopment of glomeruli or a functional decrease in the glomerular filtration rate (Feld and Hirschberg, 1996). Hypophosphatemia, hypoalbuminemia, and anemia have also been reported (Eigenmann, 1983). Additional clinicopathologic alterations may develop in pituitary dwarfs with combined anterior pituitary hormone deficiencies, primarily as a result of concurrent hypothyroidism (see Chapter 3).

Dermatohistopathology

The histopathologic alterations in the skin of dogs with hyposomatotropism are similar to those seen in many other endocrinopathies (Table 2-5). These skin alterations include varying degrees of orthokeratotic hyperkeratosis, follicular keratosis, follicular dilatation, follicular atrophy, telogenization of hair follicles, excessive trichilemmal keratinization, sebaceous gland atrophy, epidermal atrophy, epidermal melanosis, and dermal thinning (Scott et al, 2001). A highly suggestive finding of hyposomatotropism is the decreased amount and size of dermal elastin fibers. Elastin fibers are smaller, fragmented, and less numerous than normal. In dogs with concurrent secondary hypothyroidism, histopathologic findings may include vacuolated or hypertrophied arrector pili muscles.

Endocrinologic evaluation

BASAL GH CONCENTRATIONS. Reported normal basal GH concentrations range from 1.5 ± 1.2 ng/ml to 4.3 ± 1.1 ng/ml in dogs (Eigenmann, 1983) and 1.2 ± 1.0 ng/ml to 3.2 ± 0.7 ng/ml in cats (Eigenmann et al, 1984d; Peterson et al, 1990). Unfortunately, basal GH concentrations in dogs and cats with hyposomatotropism (both congenital and acquired) may also be in this range, which makes it difficult to document hyposecretion when relying solely on basal GH levels. Two dogs with congenital GH deficiencies did have consistently undetectable serum concentrations

TABLE 2–5 DERMATOHISTOPATHOLOGIC ALTERATIONS ASSOCIATED WITH ENDOCRINOPATHY-INDUCED ALOPECIA

Abnormality	Specific Endocrine Disorder
Nonspecific Abnormalities Supporting an Endocrinopathy	
Orthokeratotic hyperkeratosis	—
Follicular keratosis	—
Follicular dilatation	—
Follicular atrophy	—
Predominance of telogen hair follicles	—
Sebaceous gland atrophy	—
Epidermal atrophy	—
Epidermal melanosis	—
Thin dermis	—
Dermal collagen atrophy	—
Abnormalities Suggestive of Specific Endocrine Disorder	
Decreased amount and size of dermal elastin fibers	Hyposomatotropism
Excessive trichilemmal keratinization (flame follicles)	Growth hormone- and castration-responsive dermatosis
Vacuolated and/or hypertrophied arrector pilae muscles	Hypothyroidism
Increased dermal mucin content	Hypothyroidism
Thick dermis	Hypothyroidism
Comedones	Hyperadrenocorticism
Calcinosis cutis	Hyperadrenocorticism
Absence of arrector pili muscles	Hyperadrenocorticism

TABLE 2–6 GROWTH HORMONE STIMULATION TESTING PROTOCOLS

Test	Description and Results
Xylazine Stimulation Test*	
Protocol	100 µg/kg IV; plasma samples obtained before and at 15, 30, 45, and 60 minutes after administration of xylazine†
Normal results	Plasma GH, > 10 ng/ml 15 to 30 minutes after xylazine administration
Adverse reactions	Sedation (common), bradycardia, hypotension, collapse, shock, seizures
Clonidine Stimulation Test	
Protocol	10 µg/kg IV; plasma samples obtained before and at 15, 30, 45, and 60 minutes after administration of clonidine†
Normal results	Plasma GH, > 10 ng/ml 15 to 30 minutes after clonidine administration
Adverse reactions	Sedation (common), bradycardia, hypotension, collapse, aggressive behavior
GHRH Stimulation Test	
Protocol	1 µg/kg human GHRH IV; plasma samples before and at 10, 20, 30, 45, and 60 minutes after administration of GHRH
Normal results	Plasma GH, > 10 ng/ml 15 to 30 minutes after GHRH administration
Adverse reactions	None reported

* Currently preferred GH stimulation test.
† An abbreviated protocol in which plasma samples are obtained before and 20 and 30 minutes after stimulation can be done.
GH, Growth hormone; *GHRH,* growth hormone-releasing hormone.

TABLE 2–7 CONDITIONS THAT MAY AFFECT PITUITARY SOMATOTROPH RESPONSIVENESS TO GH STIMULATION TESTS IN HUMANS

Decreased Responsiveness	Increased Responsiveness
Old age	Poorly regulated diabetes mellitus
Delayed puberty	Malnutrition
Obesity	Renal failure
Hypothyroidism	Liver cirrhosis
Thyrotoxicosis	Metastatic carcinoma
Hyperadrenocorticism	Estrogen therapy
Stress	
Glucocorticoids	

Modified from Lazarus L: *In* Donald RA (ed): Endocrine Disorders: A Guide to Diagnosis. New York, Marcel Dekker, Inc, 1984, p 273.

(Rijnberk et al, 1993). Currently, assessment of random basal GH concentrations is inadequate for documentation of hyposomatotropism; assessment of GH secretory capacity after stimulation of the pituitary somatotrophs is recommended to establish the diagnosis.

GH STIMULATION TESTS. Several stimulation tests have been developed to evaluate the GH secretory capabilities of the pituitary. The most commonly used stimulation tests in the dog are the clonidine, xylazine, and GHRH stimulation tests and a combined pituitary anterior lobe function test using four releasing hormones: GHRH, thyrotropin-releasing hormone (TRH), gonadotropin-releasing hormone (GnRH), and corticotropin-releasing hormone (CRH) (Table 2-6). Use of these tests to assess GH secretion in cats has not yet been reported.

Interpretation of GH stimulation tests requires some knowledge of the conditions that may affect somatotroph responsiveness to various stimuli; this becomes especially important in the attempt to differentiate partial GH deficiency states from normal. A number of conditions may affect somatotroph responsiveness to stimuli in humans (Table 2-7) (Lazarus, 1984). Similar conditions have not been thoroughly evaluated in the dog, although hyperadrenocorticism, hypothyroidism, and some sex hormone imbalances may cause a reversible suppression of plasma GH concentrations (Peterson and Altszuler, 1981; Lothrop, 1988; Regnier and Garnier, 1995), and β-adrenergic antagonists potentiate the GH response to GHRH (Regnier et al, 1992).

Clonidine Stimulation Test. Clonidine is an α-adrenergic agonist that stimulates secretion of GHRH, which in turn stimulates secretion of GH. Injection of clonidine increases circulating GH and glucose concentrations and decreases plasma insulin concentrations in the dog (Hampshire and Altszuler, 1981). These effects are dose dependent. The use of clonidine to provoke GH secretion appears to be more reproducible and results in more dramatic changes in plasma GH concentrations than do the other stimulation tests. Currently, either the clonidine stimulation test or the GHRH stimulation test is preferred for diagnosing hyposomatotropism.

The dose of clonidine used in the test is somewhat variable and depends on the protocol established for the individual laboratory. An increase in GH may be seen at dosages as low as 3 µg/kg body weight given intravenously (Hampshire and Altszuler, 1981), although dosages of 10 µg/kg (Eigenmann, 1983), 16.5 µg/kg (Roth et al, 1980), and 30 µg/kg have been reported. The usual dosage is 10 µg/kg given intravenously. It should be kept in mind that larger dosages of clonidine (i.e., 16.5 and 30 µg/kg) produce a more pronounced and prolonged hyperglycemia but have a greater incidence of adverse reactions, including sedation, bradycardia, hypotension, collapse, and aggressive behavior (Lothrop, 1988; Eigenmann and Eigenmann, 1981a). Adverse reactions may last 15 to 60 minutes. If necessary, atropine can be used to reverse bradycardia, and the α-adrenergic antagonists phentolamine or yohimbine can be used to antagonize the hypotensive effects of clonidine (and xylazine). Plasma samples for GH determination should be obtained prior to clonidine administration and 15, 30, 45, 60, and 120 minutes after stimulation. GH is relatively stable for prolonged periods if frozen and maintained at -20° C.

In the normal dog, plasma GH concentrations should increase after clonidine administration, reaching peak concentrations 15 to 30 minutes after initiation of the test (Fig. 2-7) (Hampshire and Altszuler, 1981; Eigenmann, 1983). In healthy dogs, GH concentrations

TABLE 2–8 RESULTS OF A CLONIDINE STIMULATION TEST IN NINE ADULT DOGS WITH GH DEFICIENCY

| | GH (ng/ml) | | | | | |
Dog	0 Min	15 Min	30 Min	45 Min	60 Min	90 Min
1†	*	6.2	6.0	4.3	3.1	3.1
2†	*	5.8	2.0	0.5	*	*
3	*	*	2.0	0.5	*	*
4	*	0.5	*	*	*	*
5	*	*	*	*	*	*
6	*	*	*	*	*	*
7	*	*	*	*	*	*
8	*	0.8	1.0	0.9	0.9	*
9	*	*	*	*	*	*
Normal	1.5	29.6	44.4	16.5	10.3	6.0
±SEM	±0.1	±9.6	±13.9	±4.9	±2.9	±2.7

From Eigenmann JE, Patterson DF: JAAHA 20:741, 1984. Used with permission.
*Below detection limit (0.39 ng/ml)
†Dogs 1 and 2 are believed to have partial GH deficiency, while the remaining 7 dogs have complete GH deficiency. Clonidine, 10 µg/kg, was given IV at time 0.

should exceed 10 ng/ml after clonidine stimulation. The GH concentration should then decline rapidly toward basal levels. Pituitary dwarfs and dogs with adult-onset complete GH deficiency do not respond to clonidine (see Fig. 2-7). In these dogs, no increase in plasma GH concentrations follows clonidine administration. A partial GH deficiency may be suspected whenever subnormal results are obtained (Table 2-8) (Eigenmann and Patterson, 1984).

Evaluation of plasma glucose concentrations during clonidine-induced GH secretion may be helpful in evaluating somatotroph function. In the normal dog, plasma glucose concentrations increase after clonidine administration, an effect that is dose dependent (Hampshire and Altszuler, 1981). The peak increase in the plasma glucose concentration occurs approximately 90 minutes after clonidine administration. In contrast, no increase in plasma glucose occurs in hypophysectomized dogs or in dogs with hyposomatotropism (Eigenmann, 1981). The exact mechanism of the hyperglycemia is not known, although it seems likely to be a result of GH-induced insulin antagonism and decreased glucose uptake by cells.

Xylazine Stimulation Test. Xylazine is a sedative analgesic that is structurally related to clonidine. Injection of xylazine increases circulating GH concentrations in normal dogs (Hampshire and Altszuler, 1981). The use of xylazine to provoke GH secretion is a suitable test for hyposomatotropism. Plasma samples are obtained prior to and 15, 30, 45, 60, and 120 minutes after intravenous administration of xylazine at a dosage of 100 to 300 µg/kg. Although the higher dose is typically recommended to ensure maximal stimulation of GH secretion, profound sedation, hypotension, shock, and seizures (rarely) may develop at these higher dosages. The lower dose (i.e., 100 µg/kg) is an effective GH stimulant but does not appear to increase the blood glucose concentration (Hampshire and Altszuler, 1981). The incidence of adverse reactions (e.g.,

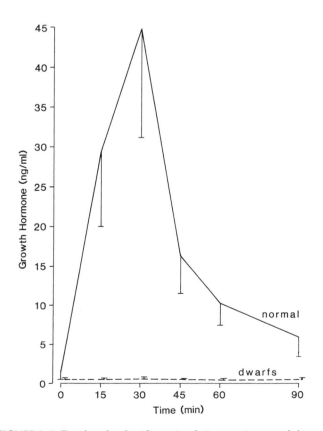

FIGURE 2–7. Results of a clonidine stimulation test in normal dogs and nine German Shepherd dogs with pituitary dwarfism. Clonidine, 10 µg/kg body weight, was given intravenously at time 0. (Eigenmann JE, et al: Acta Endocrinol 105:289, 1984.)

sedation, bradycardia, hypotension, collapse) is also lower at this lesser dose. Interpretation of this test is similar to that of the clonidine stimulation test. In one study, the normal mean-peak serum GH concentration was 43.5 ± 40.8 ng/ml at 15 minutes after xylazine administration (Schmeitzel and Lothrop, 1990).

Growth Hormone–Releasing Hormone Administration Test. The use of GHRH has been evaluated as a diagnostic test for canine congenital and adult-onset GH deficiency (Lothrop, 1986; Rijnberk et al, 1993; Kooistra et al, 2000b). Administration of human GHRH (1 µg/kg IV; Peninsula Laboratories, San Carlos, CA) results in a rapid increase in plasma GH, with peak concentrations occurring 10 to 30 minutes after GHRH administration (Fig. 2-8; Abribat et al, 1989; Meij et al, 1996). The mean ($\pm$ SE) plasma GH concentration was 14.7 ± 3.7 ng/ml at 10 minutes after GHRH administration (Meij et al, 1996). In eight German Shepherd dwarfs, basal GH concentrations were low and there was no increase in the plasma GH concentration after GHRH administration (see Fig. 2-4; Kooistra et al, 2000b). In six dogs with suspected adult-onset GH deficiency, basal GH concentrations were either low or within normal limits and there was no increase in GH after GHRH stimulation (Rijnberk et al, 1993). Adverse reactions were not observed after administration of GHRH. For the GHRH stimulation test, plasma samples for GH measurement should be obtained prior to and 5, 10, 20, 30, 45, and 60 minutes after intravenous administration of 1 µg of GHRH/kg body weight. Availability and cost are obvious disadvantages of GHRH.

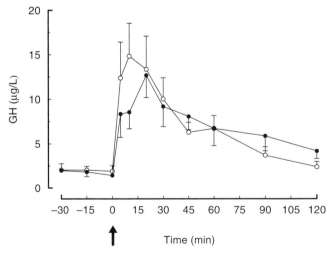

FIGURE 2–8. Plasma GH response (mean ± SE) in eight male Beagles after rapid (30 second) intravenous injection *(arrow)* of a combination of four hypothalamic releasing hormones (•) compared with single stimulation with 1 µg/kg GHRH (O). In the combined test, the releasing hormones were injected in the following order and doses: 1 µg of CRH/kg, 1 µg of GHRH/kg, 10 µg of GnRH/kg, and 10 µg of TRH/kg. The area under the curve (AUC) and the increment (peak basal level at 0 minutes) in the plasma GH concentration were not significantly different between combined and single stimulation tests. *CRH,* Corticotropin-releasing hormone; *GHRH,* growth hormone–releasing hormone; *GnRH,* gonadotropin-releasing hormone; *TRH,* thyrotropin releasing hormone. (Meij BP, et al: Dom Anim Endocr 13:161, 1996.)

Combined Anterior Pituitary Function Test. A combined anterior pituitary function test can be used to assess pituitary function in dogs that are suspected of having pituitary dysfunction or that have undergone hypophysectomy for Cushing's disease (see Chapter 6). The combined anterior pituitary function test consists of sequential, 30-second intravenous administrations of four hypothalamic releasing hormones in the following order and dosages: CRH, 1 µg/kg body weight; GHRH, 1 µg/kg; GnRH, 10 µg/kg; and TRH, 10 µg/kg (Meij et al, 1996). Plasma samples are collected prior to and 5, 10, 20, 30, 45, 60, 90, and 120 minutes after administration of the last releasing hormone for measurement of GH, ACTH, TSH, LH, FSH, and prolactin. In one study, the combined administration of these four hypothalamic releasing hormones caused no apparent inhibition or synergism with respect to the responses to GHRH, CRH, and TRH administered separately, but it did cause a 50% attenuation in the LH response compared with LH response to single GnRH administration (Meij et al, 1996). Adverse effects of the combined anterior pituitary function test include restlessness and nausea, which disappear shortly after administration of the releasing hormones. The combined anterior pituitary function test was used to document a combined deficiency of GH, TSH, and prolactin in 10 German Shepherd dwarfs (see Fig. 2-4; Hamann et al, 1999; Kooistra et al, 2000b). Availability and cost are obvious disadvantages of the combined anterior pituitary function test.

BASAL IGF-I CONCENTRATION. IGF-I concentrations are low in dogs with pituitary dwarfism. In one study involving nine German Shepherd dwarfs, the mean plasma IGF-I concentration in normal adults was 280 ± 23 ng/ml; in immature normal animals, 345 ± 50 ng/ml; and in the dwarf dogs, 11 ± 2 ng/ml (Eigenmann et al, 1984c). Low plasma IGF-I concentrations have also been documented in three additional studies involving nine pituitary dwarfs (Rijnberk et al, 1993; Kooistra et al, 1998; Kooistra et al, 2000b). These findings support the theory of GH control over plasma IGF-I concentrations (see Fig. 2-2) and imply the important role that IGF-I plays in the regulation of growth. Radioimmunoassays for measurement of IGF-I in humans have been validated in dogs (Randolph et al, 1990) and cats (Church et al, 1994) and are commercially available. Measurement of serum IGF-I concentrations by radioimmunoassay provides a way to gain further evidence of GH deficiency as the cause of poor growth in dogs and cats when measurement of GH is not available. However, interpretation of results in dogs must take into consideration the size of the breed (i.e., smaller breeds have lower normal IGF-I concentrations and larger breeds have higher normal concentrations) (Eigenmann et al, 1984b).

THYROID FUNCTION. Evaluation of thyroid gland function is imperative in any animal with suspected hyposomatotropism, because the clinical signs of hypothyroidism and hyposomatotropism are similar, making hypothyroidism an important differential diagnosis; also, TSH deficiency is the most common concurrent hormone deficiency in pituitary dwarfs with pituitary hypoplasia and combined hormonal deficiencies. In theory, the basal serum thyroxine, free thyroxine, and endogenous TSH concentrations should be low or undetectable in pituitary dwarfs with concurrent hypothyroidism. Unfortunately, an undetectable endogenous TSH concentration does not confirm pituitary TSH deficiency because the lower limit of the normal range using the TSH assay currently available extends below the sensitivity of the assay. In addition, low serum thyroxine or free thyroxine concentrations may be caused by extraneous factors affecting the thyroid gland function (e.g., euthyroid sick syndrome) rather than by pituitary TSH deficiency. The serum thyroxine concentration may also be within the reference range in a pituitary dwarf with impaired TSH secretion (Kooistra et al, 1998). For these reasons, evaluation of pituitary and thyroid gland function using thyrotropin-releasing hormone (TRH) stimulation testing is recommended (see Chapter 3, page 120). The results of TRH stimulation testing should be normal in dogs and cats with isolated GH deficiency. In dogs and cats with congenital hypothyroidism or pituitary dwarfism caused by combined anterior pituitary hormone deficiency, the baseline TSH, thyroxine, and free thyroxine concentrations should be low and there should be minimal to no increase in the concentrations of these hormones after administration of TRH (see Fig. 2-4). The reader is referred to Chapter 3 for more information on thyroid gland function tests.

ADRENOCORTICAL FUNCTION. Corticotroph function is usually normal in dogs with isolated GH deficiency and those with combined anterior pituitary hormone deficiencies (see Fig. 2-4). Evaluation of the pituitary-adrenocortical axis may be warranted in pituitary dwarfs that develop signs suggestive of cortisol deficiency (e.g., lethargy, inappetence, vomiting, weight loss). Evaluation of the baseline endogenous ACTH concentration and adrenocortical response to ACTH stimulation or, preferably, performance of a CRH stimulation test with measurement of plasma ACTH and cortisol concentrations should be done to confirm secondary hypoadrenocorticism. The reader is referred to Chapter 8 for more information on secondary hypoadrenocorticism.

Definitive and differential diagnosis

The signalment, history, and physical examination usually provide sufficient evidence to include pituitary dwarfism among the tentative diagnoses of short stature. Strong presumptive evidence can be obtained by ruling out other potential causes of small size (Table 2-9) after a thorough evaluation of the history and physical examination findings, as well as the results of routine laboratory studies (i.e., CBC, serum biochemistry panel, urinalysis, fecal examinations) and diagnostic imaging studies (Fig. 2-9). The most difficult differential diagnoses to rule out are cretinism, portovascular shunts, and hepatic microvascular dysplasia. A definitive diagnosis of hyposomatotropism should rely on

TABLE 2–9 SOME POTENTIAL CAUSES OF SMALL STATURE IN DOGS AND CATS

Endocrine	Nonendocrine
Hyposomatotropism	Malnutrition
Hypothyroidism	Gastrointestinal
Hyperadrenocorticism	Maldigestion
Hypoadrenocorticism	Pancreatic exocrine insufficiency
Diabetes mellitus	Malabsorption
	Heavy intestinal parasitism
	Hepatic
	Portosystemic vascular shunt
	Glycogen storage disease
	Renal disease
	Cardiovascular disease, anomalies
	Skeletal dysplasia; chondrodystrophy
	Mucopolysaccharidosis
	Hydrocephalus

an evaluation of somatotroph responsiveness to provocative testing. In most pituitary dwarfs, there is no increase in the plasma GH concentration after the administration of a GH secretagogue. A partial GH deficiency may be suspected whenever subnormal results are obtained. Baseline serum IGF-I concentrations should also be low to undetectable in dogs and cats with pituitary dwarfism.

Treatment

TREATMENT WITH GH. Therapy for pituitary dwarfism relies on the administration of GH. Unfortunately, an effective GH product is not readily available for use in dogs. Recombinant human GH is expensive and difficult to procure and may induce antibody formation, which can interfere with its effectiveness when administered to dogs (Van Herpen et al, 1994). Recombinant bovine GH is designed for use in cows and is not suitable for dilution to concentrations suitable for use in dogs. Porcine GH is immunologically similar to canine GH, but its availability is unpredictable (Ascacio-Martinez et al, 1994). If available, the recommended initial dose of porcine GH is 0.1 IU (0.05 mg)/kg given subcutaneously three times per week. Subsequent adjustments in the dosage and frequency of administration should be based on the clinical response and plasma IGF-I concentrations (Mandel et al, 1995; Kooistra et al, 1998). The goal of treatment is to have the plasma IGF-I concentrations increase to within the reference range; breed size should be considered when evaluating IGF-I test results. Interpretation of IGF-I results should take into consideration differences in the reference range. Hypersensitivity reactions (including angioedema), carbohydrate intolerance, and overt diabetes mellitus are the primary adverse reactions associated with GH injections. Frequent monitoring of the urine for glucose and of the blood for the development of hyperglycemia (blood glucose >150 mg/dl) is important, and GH therapy should be stopped if either develops. Failure to halt GH therapy can result in permanent insulin-dependent diabetes mellitus.

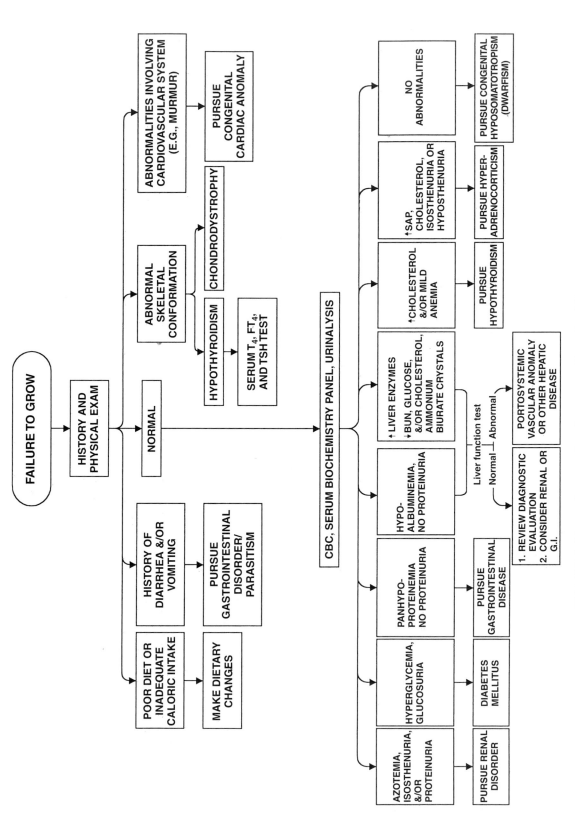

FIGURE 2–9. Diagnostic approach to the puppy or kitten that fails to grow.

Because of the synergistic influence of GH and thyroid hormone on growth processes, subnormal concentrations of thyroid hormone may diminish the effectiveness of GH therapy. For this reason, concurrent thyroid hormone supplementation should be provided for dogs and cats with suspected combined anterior pituitary hormone deficiencies and secondary hypothyroidism, as outlined in Chapter 3 (pages 136 and 148). Daily thyroid hormone supplementation should be continued for the rest of the animal's life.

TREATMENT WITH PROGESTINS. Prolonged treatment of dogs with progestins may cause GH hypersecretion, leading to acromegalic changes, carbohydrate intolerance, and diabetes mellitus (Eigenmann et al, 1983a). The progestin-stimulated plasma GH concentrations do not have a pulsatile secretion pattern, are not sensitive to stimulation with GHRH or clonidine, and are not inhibited by somatostatin (Watson et al, 1987; Selman et al, 1991). The progestin-stimulated increase in the plasma GH concentration does cause an increase in the plasma IGF-I concentration (Selman et al, 1994a). Subsequent studies identified foci of hyperplastic ductular epithelium of the mammary gland as the site of origin of GH production induced by progestins (Selman et al, 1994b). The expression of the gene encoding GH has been demonstrated in canine mammary gland tissue (Mol et al, 1995) and sequence analysis has revealed that the gene encoding GH in the mammary gland is identical to the pituitary GH gene (Mol et al, 1996). The locally produced GH and associated production of IGF undoubtedly participate in the cyclic development of the mammary gland in the bitch.

The progestin-stimulated increases in the plasma GH and IGF-I concentrations raise interesting possibilities for the use of progestins to treat pituitary dwarfism in dogs. Improvement in clinical signs has been reported in one male and one female German Shepherd dwarf treated with subcutaneous injections of medroxyprogesterone acetate (MPA) in doses of 2.5 to 5.0 mg/kg body weight, initially at 3-week intervals and subsequently at 6-week intervals (Kooistra et al, 1998). Dosage and interval adjustments were based on physical changes and the GH and IGF-I concentrations. Body size increased, and a complete adult hair coat developed in both dogs. Adverse reactions included pruritic pyoderma in both dogs, cystic endometrial hyperplasia with mucometra in the female dog, and signs of acromegaly in the male dog. Progestin-induced GH excess can also cause diabetes mellitus, necessitating periodic blood and urine glucose evaluations. Both dogs were alive and healthy 3 and 4 years after starting MPA treatment. In another study, increases in the serum IGF-I concentration and in body weight, as well as improvement in the hair coat, were identified in one male and one female German Shepherd dwarf after 9 weeks of proligestone treatment at a dosage of 10 mg/kg body weight given subcutaneously at 3-week intervals (Herrtage and Evans, 1998).

The usefulness of progestins for treating pituitary dwarfism in cats remains to be determined. The expression of the gene encoding GH has been demonstrated in feline mammary gland tissue that has undergone progestin-induced fibroadenomatous changes (Mol et al, 1995), suggesting that feline mammary gland tissue may be able to produce GH. However, Peterson (1987) found no significant rise in plasma GH concentrations in cats during 12 months of treatment with megestrol acetate, and Church and colleagues (1994) found no change in plasma IGF-I concentrations in cats treated with proligestone or megestrol acetate compared with cats treated with saline.

Response to therapy—prognosis

A beneficial response in the skin and hair coat usually occurs within 6 to 8 weeks of initiation of GH and thyroid hormone supplementation. The hair that grows back is predominantly lanugo, or secondary, hairs; growth of primary, or guard, hairs is variable and may occur sporadically over the body (Eigenmann, 1981). Growth is unpredictable and depends in part on the age of the animal and the status of the growth plates at the time GH or progestin treatment is initiated. The younger the animal, the more likely the growth plates are to still be open, and the more likely significant growth will take place. An increase in size will not occur or will be minimal if the growth plates have closed or are about to close at the time of the initial examination.

The long-term prognosis for pituitary dwarfism is guarded. In general, pituitary dwarfs have a shortened life expectancy. Pituitary dwarfs that are not treated typically die or are euthanized at an early age (typically less than 5 years of age). Death is usually a result of infections, degenerative diseases, or neurologic dysfunction, which develop as a consequence of chronic GH, IGF-I, and TSH deficiencies and continued enlargement of a pituitary cyst or cysts. The prognosis for dogs treated with GH or progestins is guarded and depends in part on maintaining normal IGF-I concentrations and avoiding complications associated with chronic or excessive progestin or GH administration (e.g., diabetes mellitus, pyometra, acromegaly).

ACQUIRED HYPOSOMATOTROPISM

Hyposomatotropism may develop in the adult dog or, less commonly, the adult cat as a result of destruction of the pituitary gland by inflammatory, traumatic, vascular, or neoplastic disorders; with suppression of somatotroph function caused by concurrent disease; or as an idiopathic disorder (Eigenmann et al, 1983b). Clinical manifestations of acquired hyposomatotropism are confined to the skin in the dog. Classic clinical signs are symmetric endocrine alopecia and hyperpigmentation. This syndrome has been termed *adult-onset, GH-responsive dermatosis*. Clinical manifestations of acquired hyposomatotropism have not been reported in the cat.

Deficiencies involving other pituitary hormones may also occur, depending on the etiology and extent of the destruction of the pituitary gland. Panhypopituitarism (i.e., a deficiency of all pituitary hormones) may ultimately develop. Clinical signs of hyposomatotropism may or may not be a predominant clinical feature. Clinical signs caused by concurrent deficiencies of vasopressin, ACTH, or TSH would be more obvious to owners than clinical signs caused by GH deficiency, whereas concurrent deficiencies in prolactin and the gonadotropins would be clinically silent and would go unnoticed by owners unless the affected animal was intact and intended for breeding. Depending on the etiology, clinical signs related to neurologic dysfunction may also be present (see Chapter 6).

In humans, suppressed secretion of GH may arise from many conditions, including obesity, hypothyroidism and hyperthyroidism, spontaneous hyperadrenocorticism, and exogenous glucocorticoids (Lazarus, 1984). In dogs, as in humans, excessive production of endogenous glucocorticoids (Cushing's syndrome) occurs secondary to either pituitary-dependent bilateral adrenocortical hyperplasia or adrenocortical neoplasia. Either syndrome can induce suppression of GH release, which is reversible with successful treatment of the primary illness (Peterson and Altszuler, 1981). Comparable suppression of GH secretion would also be expected after prolonged and/or excessive glucocorticoid administration. A similar reversible suppressive effect has been suggested with hypothyroidism in the dog (Lothrop, 1988). Although clinical signs related to GH deficiency are not usually evident with these disorders, recognition of potential suppressibility of somatotroph function must be considered when interpreting GH stimulation tests (see page 62).

ADULT-ONSET, GROWTH HORMONE–RESPONSIVE DERMATOSIS

Etiology

GH-responsive dermatosis is a poorly defined dermatologic disorder that affects adult dogs. GH-responsive dermatosis may represent an initially mild (partial?) but progressive form of congenital hyposomatotropism that is not severe enough to cause dwarfism but that in time results in dermatologic manifestations in young adult dogs. Alternatively, hyposomatotropism may be acquired after normal growth has occurred. Currently, the cause is unknown. Basal GH concentrations are low in these dogs and no increase in the plasma GH concentration occurs after stimulation of the somatotrophs, suggesting a problem with somatotroph function. Lack of necropsy data from dogs with GH-responsive dermatosis has hampered our understanding of this disorder. The necropsy results of three dogs with GH-responsive dermatosis revealed moderate atrophy of the pituitary gland in two dogs and no pituitary lesions in the other dog (Scott and Walton, 1986; Schmeitzel, 1990). It is not known whether the site of dysfunction in this disorder is the pituitary gland, the hypothalamus, or elsewhere. Given the strong breed predisposition for the disorder, genetics

undoubtedly plays a role, at least in some breeds. Gender may also play a role, given the predominance of this dermatosis in intact male dogs. One thing is certain: the lesion does not appear to be progressive or to involve other endocrine functions of the pituitary. Other pituitary tropic hormones are present and functional, as demonstrated by normal end-organ responsiveness to appropriate stimulation tests (e.g., ACTH and TSH stimulation). In addition, dogs with GH-responsive dermatosis have a good prognosis, as evidenced by the lack of necropsy cases after establishment of the diagnosis. This implies that only the pituitary-GH axis is affected in these animals.

In one study, 32 of 95 dogs evaluated for GH-responsive dermatosis had normal GH stimulation test results (Lothrop, 1988; Lothrop and Schmeitzel, 1990). Twenty-two (69%) of these 32 dogs were breeds with a documented predisposition for GH-responsive dermatosis (e.g., Chow Chow, Keeshond). In addition, basal IGF-I concentrations were normal, not low, in dogs with abnormal GH stimulation test results. Despite normal GH stimulation test results, some of these dogs responded to GH therapy. These findings suggest that true GH deficiency may not be present in some dogs with the syndrome of GH-responsive dermatosis (especially Chow Chows, Keeshonds, Pomeranians, and Samoyeds); that other, as yet poorly characterized causes of endocrine dermatosis exist that mimic GH-responsive dermatosis (see discussion on endocrine alopecia, page 62); and that dogs may respond to GH therapy without having hyposomatotropism. GH-responsive dermatosis may have multiple causes and may respond to other modes of therapy (e.g., castration, o,p'DDD therapy) in addition to GH administration.

Pathophysiology

Theoretically, clinical manifestations of GH-responsive dermatosis are due to hyposomatotropism; the other tropic cells of the pituitary are normal. Because hyposomatotropism occurs in the adult dog, signs related to impaired growth do not develop. Rather, the primary clinical manifestations are dermatologic, and they develop secondary to atrophy of the dermal and epidermal structures and retardation of hair growth. Clinical signs that mimic hyposomatotropism may also occur with gonadal-dependent or adrenal-dependent sex hormone imbalances (see page 64) (Schmeitzel and Lothrop, 1990). The results of GH stimulation tests may be normal or abnormal in these dogs, and in some of these dogs, hyposomatotropism may contribute to the clinical syndrome.

Signalment

Although GH-responsive dermatosis can occur in any dog, there seems to be a striking breed predilection for the Chow Chow, Pomeranian, Toy and Miniature Poodle, Keeshond, American Water Spaniel, and Samoyed (Parker and Scott, 1980; Eigenmann and

Patterson, 1984; Lothrop, 1988; Bell et al, 1993). We have also seen the condition in several Tibetan Terriers. Because the Chow Chow, Keeshond, Pomeranian, and Samoyed are overrepresented in the congenital adrenal hyperplasia–like syndrome (see page 66), any GH irregularity in these breeds may be either coincidental or a secondary problem. Most of the reported cases, as well as those seen by the authors, have been males, implying a possible gender predilection as well. Clinical signs usually develop in young animals (1 to 4 years of age), although the age for initial examination for related signs by the veterinarian may include dogs as old as 11 years of age.

Clinical signs

Hyposomatotropism in the mature dog primarily affects hair growth and skin pigmentation (Fig. 2-10). The onset of clinical signs usually occurs after 1 to 3 years of age. The disorder is characterized by bilaterally symmetric alopecia of the trunk, neck, pinnae, tail, and caudomedial thighs. Alopecia frequently begins in areas of friction or wear (e.g., around the neck in the vicinity of the collar). Initially there is gradual loss of guard (primary) hairs in affected areas, giving the hair coat a puppylike appearance. With time, undercoat (secondary) hairs are lost. Truncal primary hairs are then gradually lost, followed by secondary hairs. Complete truncal alopecia is uncommon. The head is not involved, and the legs are involved to a lesser degree than the trunk. Hair in affected areas is easily epilated, and the remaining hair coat is usually dry and lusterless. Hyperpigmentation develops in areas of alopecia. In chronic cases the skin becomes thin and hypotonic. These dogs are otherwise normal. Affected dogs have normal activity and appetite and would be

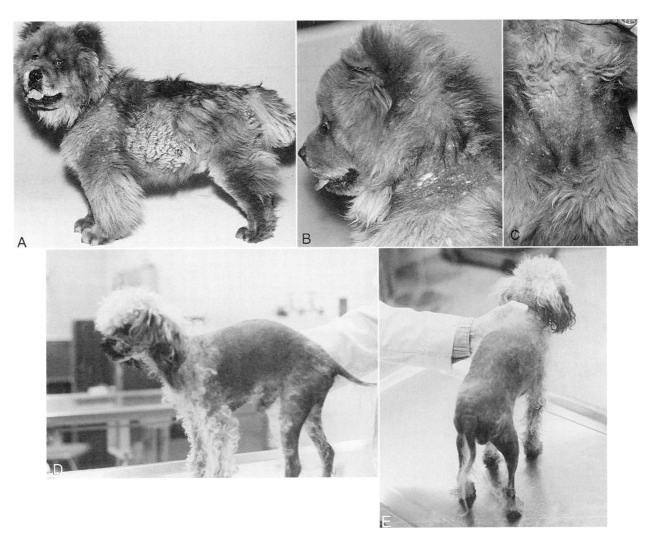

FIGURE 2–10. *A to C,* A 2-year-old male Chow Chow with adult-onset GH-responsive dermatosis. Note the symmetric alopecia and hyperpigmentation around the neck and the dry, lusterless quality of the remaining hair coat. Although not readily apparent from these pictures, alopecia was also developing on the trunk. The severity of alopecia on the neck was probably related to excessive epilation of hair caused by the dog's collar. *D* and *E,* A 5-year-old male Miniature Poodle with adult-onset, GH-responsive dermatosis. Note the symmetric alopecia and hyperpigmentation, which have spared the head and, to a lesser degree, the legs. (*A to C,* Courtesy D. Serra, Wyoming, RI.)

considered completely healthy by their owners were it not for the alopecia.

Clinical pathology

The results of routine clinicopathologic tests, including CBC, biochemistry panel, and urinalysis, are normal in the mature dog with GH-responsive dermatosis. These normal findings are helpful in distinguishing this disorder from hypothyroidism and hyperadrenocorticism, two important differential diagnoses. (The reader is referred to Chapters 3 and 6 for complete discussions of the abnormal clinicopathologic data associated with hypothyroidism and hyperadrenocorticism, respectively.)

Dermatohistopathology

Histologic assessment of a skin biopsy specimen may reveal nonspecific alterations found in endocrine skin diseases (see Table 2-4); a decrease in the amount and size of dermal elastin fibers; and flame follicles (Gross et al, 1992; Scott et al, 2001). Flame follicles are exaggerated forms of catagen follicles in which large spikes of fused keratin appear to protrude through the outer root sheath into the vitreous layer of the follicle. Flame follicles are seen with endocrine and developmental disorders, most notably GH-responsive dermatosis, castration-responsive dermatosis, postclipping alopecia, and the follicular dysplasia seen in Siberian Huskies. The tendency to form flame follicles may also be breed dependent; flame follicles may develop in dogs such as Chow Chows or Pomeranians as a result of other atrophic influences on the hair follicle (e.g., hyperestrogenism, hyperadrenocorticism). The epidermis and superficial follicular epithelium in dogs with GH-responsive dermatosis is of normal thickness, and epidermal hyperpigmentation usually is evident. Hair follicles are diffusely in hair growth cycle arrest, and the catagen stage predominates.

Endocrinologic evaluation

GROWTH HORMONE CONCENTRATIONS. Baseline GH concentrations are similar in normal dogs and dogs with GH-responsive dermatosis, making it difficult to document hyposecretion when relying solely on basal GH levels. Assessment of GH secretory capacity after stimulation of the pituitary somatotrophs using clonidine, GHRH, or xylazine is recommended to establish the diagnosis (see page 54). In the normal dog, the plasma GH concentration should exceed 10 ng/ml (it usually exceeds 30 ng/ml) 15 to 30 minutes after the administration of the secretagogue. Dogs with GH-responsive dermatosis should have undetectable plasma GH concentrations throughout the test, whereas the peak plasma GH concentration should remain less than 10 ng/ml in dogs with suspected partial GH deficiency syndrome (Bell et al, 1993). Hypothyroidism, hyperadrenocorticism, and sex hormone imbalances suppress pituitary GH secretion and should be ruled out before interpretation of GH stimulation tests (Lothrop, 1988; Schmeitzel and Lothrop, 1990; Rijnberk et al, 1993). Evaluation of plasma glucose concentrations during clonidine-induced stimulation of GH secretion may be helpful in the evaluation of somatotroph function, especially if a GH assay is not available (see page 54).

GROWTH HORMONE–RELEASING HORMONE TESTING. The use of GHRH has been evaluated as a diagnostic test for GH-responsive dermatosis (Lothrop, 1986; Rijnberk et al, 1993). Administration of human GHRH (1 µg/kg) to normal dogs results in an increase in the serum GH concentration within 5 minutes, with the peak GH concentration ranging from 10 to 60 ng/ml (Abribat et al, 1989; Meij et al, 1996). In six dogs with suspected adult-onset GH deficiency, basal GH concentrations were either low or within normal limits and there was no increase in GH after provocative stimulation with either GHRH or xylazine. The reader is referred to the section on GH stimulation tests (page 54) for more information on the GHRH stimulation test.

BASAL IGF-I CONCENTRATION. Although low basal IGF-I concentrations have been demonstrated in dogs with pituitary dwarfism (see page 56), basal IGF-I concentrations were normal in a small number of Chow Chows, Pomeranians, and Poodles with GH-responsive dermatosis (Lothrop, 1988; Rijnberk et al, 1993). The reason these dogs maintained normal IGF-I concentrations is not clear, although the clinical signs may have been the result of a disorder other than GH deficiency.

THYROID FUNCTION. Evaluation of thyroid gland function is indicated in any dog with suspected GH-responsive dermatosis, because hypothyroidism is an important differential diagnosis and a condition that may cause a reversible suppression of plasma GH concentrations (Lothrop, 1988). The reader is referred to Chapter 3 (page 111) for information on evaluating thyroid gland function.

ADRENOCORTICAL FUNCTION. Evaluation for hyperadrenocorticism is indicated in any dog with suspected GH-responsive dermatosis, because hyperadrenocorticism can cause endocrine alopecia without other clinical signs associated with the disease (e.g., polyuria, polydipsia, panting, weakness); also, hyperadrenocorticism and exogenously administered glucocorticoids may cause a reversible suppression of plasma GH concentrations (Peterson and Altszuler, 1981; Regnier and Garnier, 1995). An ACTH stimulation test can identify both iatrogenic and spontaneous hyperadrenocorticism and is recommended initially. The reader is referred to Chapter 6 (page 300) for information on diagnostic tests for hyperadrenocorticism.

Diagnostic approach to endocrine alopecia and establishing the diagnosis of GH-responsive dermatosis

Endocrine alopecia is a common clinical problem in dogs and to a lesser extent in cats. It is typically bilaterally symmetric, with the distribution pattern varying depending on the cause. Hairs are easily epilated, and the skin is often thin and hypotonic; hyperpigmentation is common. Other dermatologic lesions, such as scales, crusts, and papules, are absent. Seborrhea and pyoderma may develop, depending on the underlying cause.

The potential causes of endocrine alopecia are listed in Table 2-10. The history and physical examination findings frequently provide clues to the underlying cause, and the appropriate diagnostic tests can then be done to confirm the diagnosis. If the history and physical examination fail to provide insight into the cause, the clinician should sequentially rule out the causes of endocrine alopecia, beginning with the most likely one.

In dogs the most common causes of endocrine alopecia are hypothyroidism and glucocorticoid excess (iatrogenic or spontaneous). The diagnostic evaluation for endocrine alopecia should begin with a CBC, serum biochemistry panel, and urinalysis. If the results of initial blood work are not helpful (e.g., normal), definitive diagnostic tests for hypothyroidism (see Chapter 3) and hyperadrenocorticism (see Chapter 6) should be performed concurrently because of the suppressive effects of glucocorticoid excess on baseline thyroid hormone concentrations. Diagnosis becomes more difficult once hypothyroidism and hyperadrenocorticism

have been ruled out. GH-responsive dermatosis, gonadal-dependent sex hormone imbalance, and adrenal-dependent sex hormone imbalance then constitute the primary differential diagnoses. Unfortunately, differentiating between these conditions is difficult, partly because the clinical and histologic abnormalities affecting the skin are similar, and tests to establish a definitive diagnosis for most of these disorders are lacking. Follicular dysplasia can cause a similar clinical picture and should also be considered.

GH-responsive dermatosis has a characteristic signalment and a historical lack of clinical signs and physical findings other than endocrine alopecia and hyperpigmentation. GH-responsive dermatosis is diagnosed on the basis of the results of a GH stimulation test (see Table 2-6) and the dog's response to GH replacement therapy. Baseline GH concentrations are similar in normal dogs and dogs with GH-responsive dermatosis. The clonidine stimulation test is the most commonly used GH stimulation test. In normal dogs, the plasma GH concentration should exceed 10 ng/ml 15 to 30 minutes after administration of the secretagogue; it should remain less than 10 ng/ml (preferably undetectable) in dogs with suspected GH deficiency syndrome. Hypothyroidism, hyperadrenocorticism, and possibly sex hormone imbalances suppress pituitary GH secretion and should be ruled out before the

TABLE 2-10 DISORDERS CAUSING ENDOCRINE ALOPECIA

Disorder	Common Clinicopathologic Abnormalities	Diagnostic Tests
Hypothyroidism	Hypercholesterolemia, mild non-regenerative anemia	Baseline T_4, free T_4, cTSH measurement
Hyperadrenocorticism	Stress leukogram, increased SAP, hypercholesterolemia, hyposthenuria, urinay tract infection	ACTH-stimulation test, low-dose dexamethasone-suppression test, urine cortisol/creatinine ratio
Growth hormone deficiency–pituitary dwarfism	None	Signalment, physical findings, growth hormone response test
Growth hormone-responsive dermatosis-adult dog	None	Growth hormone response test, response to growth hormone supplementation
Castration-responsive dermatosis	None	Response to castration
Hyperestrogenism		
Functional Sertoli cell tumor-male dog	None (bone marrow depression uncommon)	Physical findings, histopathologic findings, plasma estrogen and inhibin concentration
Hyperestrogenism in intact female dog	None (bone marrow depression uncommon)	Abdominal ultrasonography, plasma estrogen concentration, response to ovariohysterectomy
Hypoestrogenism (?)		
Estrogen-responsive dermatosis of spayed female dogs	None	Response to estrogen therapy
Feline endocrine alopecia	See below	See below
Hypoandrogenism (?)		
Testosterone-responsive dermatosis-male dog	None	Response to testosterone therapy
Feline endocrine alopecia	None	Response to combined estrogen-testosterone or progestin therapy
Telogen defluxion (effluvium)	None	History of recent pregnancy or diestrus
Diabetes mellitus	Hyperglycemia, glycosuria	Blood and urine glucose measurement
Adrenal sex hormone dermatosis	None	Sex hormones and precursors before and after ACTH stimulation
Progestins	None	Blood progesterone and 17-OH-progesterone concentration

T_4, Tetraiodothyronine; *TSH*, thyroid-stimulating hormone; *SAP*, serum alkaline phosphatase; *ACTH*, adrenocorticotropic hormone.

results of GH stimulation tests are interpreted (Lothrop, 1988; Schmeitzel and Lothrop, 1990; Rijnberk et al, 1993). Unfortunately, the means to measure GH in the dog is severely limited. As such, a tentative diagnosis is made based on the signalment, the history and physical examination findings, an absence of clinico-pathologic alterations, the finding of appropriate dermatohistopathologic alterations on skin biopsy specimens, and the ruling out of more common causes of endocrine alopecia. If all of the findings support the existence of GH-responsive dermatosis, the animal's response to GH replacement therapy can be used to help establish the diagnosis.

Gonadal- or adrenal-dependent sex hormone imbalance (see the next section) should be suspected if the dog fails to show clinical improvement within 2 months of the initiation of GH therapy and if hypothyroidism and hyperadrenocorticism have been ruled out. Alternatively, if the history and physical examination suggest a sex hormone imbalance, appropriate diagnostic tests and, if indicated, treatment (e.g., castration, melatonin) can be pursued prior to initiation of GH therapy.

Disorders that resemble GH-responsive dermatosis

GONADAL-DEPENDENT SEX HORMONE IMBALANCE. Endocrine alopecia can result from an excess or deficiency of one of the sex hormones, most notably estrogens and androgens, or it may respond to treatment with one of the sex hormones (see Table 2-10). Dermatologic manifestations are similar for most sex hormone–induced or sex hormone–responsive dermatoses; they include endocrine alopecia that initially begins in the perineal, genital, and ventral abdominal regions and spreads cranially; dull, dry, easily epilated hair; failure of the hair coat to regrow after clipping; and variable presence of seborrhea and hyperpigmentation. Additional clinical findings depend on the underlying etiology. For example, in the male dog, additional clinical signs of hyperestrogenism may include gynecomastia, a pendulous prepuce, attraction of other male dogs, squatting to urinate, and unilateral testicular atrophy (contralateral to the testicular tumor); in the bitch, signs may include vulvar enlargement and persistent proestrus, estrus, or anestrus. Dermatologic signs of sex hormone–induced or sex hormone–responsive dermatosis can mimic those of GH-responsive dermatosis, creating a difficult diagnostic challenge for the veterinarian, especially when the alopecia occurs in a breed with a known predisposition for GH-responsive dermatosis (e.g., Pomeranians).

Diagnosis of sex hormone–induced or sex hormone–responsive dermatosis is based on the signalment, history, and physical examination findings; the results of routine biochemical and hormonal tests done to rule out other causes of endocrine alopecia; and the response to treatment. Histologic assessment of a skin biopsy specimen can be used to identify nonspecific endocrine-related alterations and to support the diagnosis of endocrine alopecia (see Table 2-5). There are no pathognomonic histologic changes for sex hormone–induced or sex hormone–responsive dermatoses. Identification of an increased plasma estrogen concentration would support the presence of a functional Sertoli cell tumor in the dog and hyperestrogenism in the bitch (assuming that the bitch is not in proestrus or early estrus). Abdominal ultrasonography may identify ovarian cysts or neoplasia in the bitch with hyperestrogenism. The diagnosis in animals with most of these disorders, however, ultimately depends on the animal's response to therapy (Table 2-11). Because of potentially serious adverse reactions to therapy, the more common causes of endocrine alopecia should always be ruled out before treatment is begun with one of the sex hormones (e.g., diethylstilbestrol, methyltestosterone). The hair coat should improve within 3 months of the start of therapy; if no improvement is seen within this time, another diagnosis should be considered.

ADRENAL-DEPENDENT SEX HORMONE IMBALANCE. Adrenal-dependent sex hormone imbalance may

TABLE 2–11   TREATMENT FOR SEX HORMONE–INDUCED OR SEX HORMONE–RESPONSIVE ENDOCRINE ALOPECIA

Disorder	Primary Treatment	Potential Adverse Reactions to Therapy
Sertoli cell neoplasia	Castration	None
Castration-responsive dermatosis	Castration	None
Hyperestrogenism in the intact female dog	Ovariohysterectomy	None
Estrogen-responsive dermatosis of spayed female dogs	Diethylstilbestrol, 0.1-1.0 mg PO q 24 hr 3 weeks per month; once responds, 0.1-1 mg 4-7 d	Aplastic anemia
Feline endocrine alopecia	Megestrol acetate, 2.5-5 mg/cat q 48 h until hair regrows; then 2.5-5 mg/cat q 7-14 d	Adrenocortical suppression, benign mammary hypertrophy, mammary neoplasia, pyometra (female cats); infertility (male cats), diabetes mellitus
Testosterone-responsive dermatosis	Methyltestosterone, 1 mg/kg (maximum 30 mg) PO q 48 h until hair regrows, then q 4-7 d	Aggression, hepatopathy
Telogen defluxion (effluvium)	None	None
Adrenal sex hormone	Growth hormone, castration, melatonin (see page 67), mitotane	Diabetes mellitus, hypoadrenocorticism

occur as a primary disorder or in association with hyperadrenocorticism. Sex hormones and their precursors may be increased in dogs with pituitary-dependent hyperadrenocorticism, but the predominant clinical signs in these dogs result from hypercortisolism (e.g., polyuria, polydipsia) (Frank et al, 2001). Sex hormones may also be increased in adrenal-dependent hyperadrenocorticism and may affect the dermatologic manifestations of the disease (e.g., alopecia of the flank, color change of the hair coat). Progesterone-secreting adrenocortical tumors have been described in cats (Boord and Griffin, 1999; Rossmeisl et al, 2000). Clinical features in affected cats mimic hyperadrenocorticism, presumably because progesterone acts as a glucocorticoid agonist. An increase in baseline and/or post-ACTH plasma 17-hydroxyprogesterone has also been documented in dogs with clinical manifestations of hyperadrenocorticism but normal plasma cortisol concentrations after administration of ACTH or dexamethasone (Ristic et al, 2001).

Congenital adrenal hyperplasia–like syndrome has clinical signs similar to those of GH-responsive dermatosis and has been identified in many breeds, especially the Pomeranian, Chow Chow, Keeshond, and Samoyed (Scott et al, 2001). Both genders are affected, but males are overrepresented. A partial deficiency of one of the adrenal enzymes—11-β-hydroxylase, 21-hydroxylase, or 3β-hydroxysteroid dehydrogenase—is believed to cause a partial deficiency of cortisol and aldosterone in affected dogs (Fig. 2-11) (Schmeitzel et al, 1995). A deficiency in cortisol and aldosterone in turn promotes pituitary ACTH secretion, the development of adrenocortical

hyperplasia, and an accumulation of precursor steroids proximal to the blocked steps in hormone synthesis. Elevations in progesterone and its precursors (e.g., 17-hydroxyprogesterone) are common in affected dogs. Progesterone can have antiandrogenic activity, and the alopecia may be attributable to local hypoandrogenism (Scott et al, 2001); regrowth of hair occurs in some affected dogs with methyltestosterone treatment (Lothrop and Schmeitzel, 1990).

Precursor steroids (i.e., 17-hydroxyprogesterone) may also be shunted into other metabolic pathways, particularly androgen biosynthesis, which ultimately results in increased concentrations of dehydroepiandrosterone and androstenedione (Frank et al, 2001). In one study that evaluated a group of Pomeranians with a suspected 21-hydroxylase deficiency, the mean serum 17-hydroxy-progesterone, dehydroepiandrosterone, and androstenedione concentrations were significantly increased compared with those of control dogs (Tables 2-12 and 2-13) (Schmeitzel and Lothrop, 1990). Interestingly, not all Pomeranians studied were clinically affected. It was proposed that affected Pomeranians have a "late" form of 21-hydroxylase deficiency that causes clinical signs to develop at the onset of puberty. Unaffected Pomeranians have a cryptic form of this enzyme deficiency, resulting in similar hormonal abnormalities, yet clinical signs are not manifested (Schmeitzel and Lothrop, 1990).

Skin biopsies from dogs with suspected congenital adrenal hyperplasia–like syndrome show the typical changes associated with endocrine alopecia (see Table 2-5) and may also show features of follicular dysplasia (Scott et al, 2001). Diagnosis requires evaluation of sex

TABLE 2–12 SERUM CONCENTRATIONS OF SEX HORMONES BEFORE AND AFTER ADRENOCORTICOTROPIN (ACTH) STIMULATION IN FEMALE CONTROL DOGS AND IN POMERANIANS AFFECTED AND UNAFFECTED BY GROWTH HORMONE–RESPONSIVE DERMATOSIS

Sex Hormone		Control Dogs ($n=9$)	Unaffected Pomeranians ($n=8$)	Affected Pomeranians ($n=3$)
Progesterone (ng/ml)	Before	0.4 (± 0.5)*	1.8 (± 1.2)†[a]	0.8 (± 0.5)‡
	After	1.4 (± 1.7)*	6.8 (± 1.4)†[a]	7.6§[a]
17-hydroxyprogesterone (ng/ml)	Before	0.4 (± 0.4)	1.3 (± 1.1)[a]	1.4 (± 1.1) ‖ [a]
	After	1.9 (± 1.1)	6.6 (± 2.8)[a]	18.9 (± 8.7) ‖ [b]
11-deoxycortisol (ng/ml)	Before	0.5 (± 0.1)	1.2 (± 0.6)[a]	2.0 (± 0.6) ‖ [a]
	After	5.6 (± 2.6)	7.0 (± 2.0)	13.5 (± 11.4) ‖
DHEAS (ng/ml)	Before	6.6 (± 2.0)	14.8 (± 7.8)[a]	15.8 (± 6.1) ‖ [a]
	After	8.4 (± 1.7)	20.4 (± 11.3)[a]	26.8 (± 14.8) ‖ [a]
Androstenedione (ng/ml)	Before	5.2 (± 6.4)	2.8 (± 1.4)	2.5 (± 0.7) ‖
	After	7.1 (± 12.8)	9.2 (± 5.1)	15.3 (± 5.9) ‖
Testosterone (ng/ml)	Before	0.1 (± 0.0)	0.0 (± 0.0)[a]	0.1 (± 0.2)
	After	0.1 (± 0.0)	0.0 (± 0.0)[a]	0.0 (± 0.0) ‖
17β-Estradiol (pg/ml)	Before	33.8 (± 21.2)	29.6 (± 19.8)	8.1 (± 10.5)[a]
	After	29.9 (± 16.1)	39.6 (± 21.7)	5.0 (± 7.1) ‖

From Schmeitzel LP, Lothrop CD Jr: Hormonal abnormalities in Pomeranians with normal coat and in Pomeranians with growth hormone-responsive dermatosis. JAVMA 197:1337, 1990.
*n = 8; 1 female had high progesterone concentration attributable to metestrus; results were omitted from statistical analysis.
†n = 5; 3 females had high progesterone concentration (metestrus); results were omitted from statistical analysis.
‡n = 2; 1 female had high progesterone concentration (metestrus); results were omitted from statistical analysis
§n = 1; 1 female not determined, 1 female had high progesterone concentration (metestrus); results were omitted from statistical analysis.
‖ n = 2; 1 female not determined.
Superscript letters denote significant ($P \le 0.05$) difference from value in control dogs[a] or from value in control dogs and unaffected Pomeranians.[b]
DHEAS, dehydroepiandrosterone sulfate.
Data are expressed as mean (± SD).

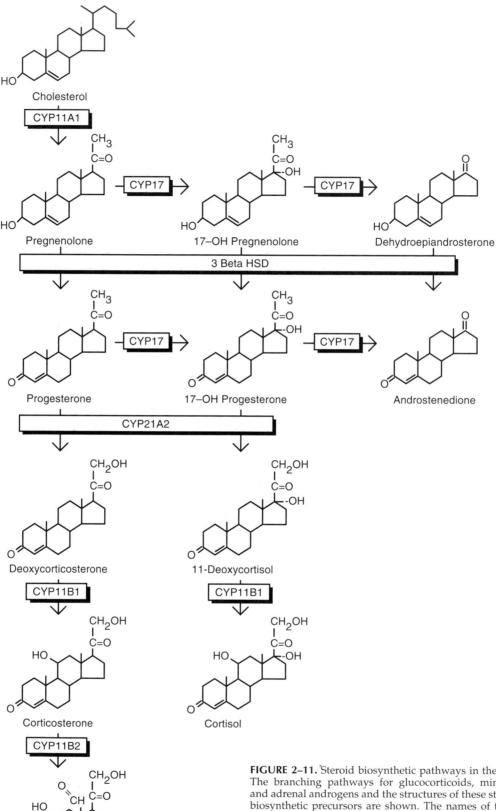

FIGURE 2–11. Steroid biosynthetic pathways in the adrenal cortex. The branching pathways for glucocorticoids, mineralocorticoids, and adrenal androgens and the structures of these steroids and their biosynthetic precursors are shown. The names of the biosynthetic enzymes are shown in the boxes. *CYP11A1*, Cholesterol side-chain cleavage enzyme; *CYP17*, 17α-hydroxylase; *3β-HSD*, 3β-hydroxysteroid dehydrogenase; *CYP21A2*, 21-hydroxylase; *CYP11B1*, 11β hydroxylase; *CYP11B2*, aldosterone synthase. (Modified from Orth DN and Kovacs WJ: *In* Wilson J, Foster D, Kronenberg H, Larsen P (eds): Williams Textbook of Endocrinology, 9th ed. Philadelphia, WB Saunders, 1998, p 523.)

TABLE 2–13 SERUM SEX HORMONE CONCENTRATIONS BEFORE AND AFTER ACTH STIMULATION IN MALE CONTROL DOGS AND MALE POMERANIANS AFFECTED AND UNAFFECTED BY GROWTH HORMONE–RESPONSIVE DERMATOSIS

Sex Hormone		Control Dogs (n=10)	Unaffected Pomeranians (n=4)	Affected Pomeranians (n=4)
Progesterone (ng/ml)	Before	0.4 (± 0.5)*	1.8 (± 1.7)†	0.4 (± 0.2)
	After	1.1 (± 1.2)	4.4 (± 1.1)*	2.7 (± 0.9)*
17-hydroxyprogesterone (ng/ml)	Before	0.3 (± 0.4)	1.2 (± 0.6)*	0.5 (± 0.2)
	After	1.4 (± 0.9)	3.2 (± 1.0)*	2.1 (± 1.0)
11-deoxycortisol (ng/ml)	Before	0.9 (± 1.0)	2.2 (± 2.1)	1.0 (± 0.3)
	After	4.7 (± 1.5)	6.8 (± 1.5)*	4.3 (± 1.8)
DHEAS (ng/ml)	Before	18.5 (± 11.5)	53.9 (± 34.0)*	33.3 (± 17.8)
	After	20.8 (± 10.9)	70.2 (± 24.7)*	34.7 (± 15.0)
Androstenedione (ng/ml)	Before	13.3 (± 24.1)	31.8 (± 24.1)	36.6 (± 30.0)*
	After	12.2 (± 6.7)	29.9 (± 18.4)*	33.0 (± 13.7)*
Testosterone (ng/ml)	Before	3.1 (± 4.2)	5.6 (± 4.6)	2.3 (± 3.6)
	After	2.6 (± 4.1)	2.6 (± 2.2)	1.0 (± 1.0)
17β-Estradiol (pg/ml)	Before	18.7 (± 14.6)	4.6 (± 5.3)	19.1 (± 4.7)
	After	15.6 (± 8.6)	9.4 (± 8.3)	17.2 (± 7.0)

From Schmeitzel LP, Lothrop CD Jr: Hormonal abnormalities in Pomeranians with normal coat and in Pomeranians with growth hormone-responsive dermatosis. JAVMA 197:1337, 1990.
*Significant (P ≤ 0.05) difference from value in control dogs.
†Significant (P ≤ 0.05) difference from value in unaffected Pomeranians.
Data are expressed as mean (± SD).
See Table 2–12 for key.

hormones and their precursors before and after ACTH administration. Treatment of congenital adrenal hyperplasia–like syndrome has included castration; methyltestosterone therapy (see Table 2-11); growth hormone therapy (see below); melatonin therapy (3 to 6 mg q12-24h for 6 weeks) (Ashley et al, 1999; Paradis, 2000); o,p'DDD therapy (induction dose, 15 to 25 mg/kg daily until post-ACTH plasma cortisol concentration is 2 to 5 μg/dl, then initiate maintenance therapy; see Chapter 6) (Rosenkrantz and Griffin, 1992; Schmeitzel et al, 1995); and observation. The drug o,p'DDD is reportedly the most effective therapy for congenital adrenal hyperplasia–like syndrome because of its ability to cause necrosis and atrophy of the zona fasciculata and the zona reticularis of the adrenal cortex (Schmeitzel at al, 1995). Dogs with congenital adrenal hyperplasia–like syndrome are healthy aside from the alopecia, and many owners elect not to treat the dog because of the expense and/or risk of complications associated with methyltestosterone, GH, or o,p'DDD treatment.

Treatment for GH-responsive dermatosis

Historically, treatment of GH-responsive dermatosis has involved the administration of GH. Unfortunately, an effective GH product is not readily available for use in dogs. Recombinant human GH is expensive and difficult to procure, and it may induce antibody formation, which can interfere with its effectiveness when administered to dogs. Recombinant bovine GH is designed for use in cows and is not suitable for dilution to concentrations acceptable in dogs. Porcine GH is immunologically similar to canine GH, but its availability is unpredictable. If porcine GH is available, the recommended dose is 0.1 IU (0.05 mg)/kg given subcutaneously three times per week for 4 to 6 weeks.

Hypersensitivity reactions (including angioedema), carbohydrate intolerance, and overt diabetes mellitus are the primary adverse reactions associated with GH injections. Frequent testing of the urine for glucose and of the blood for the development of hyperglycemia (blood glucose >150 mg/dl) should be performed, and GH therapy should be stopped if either develops. Regrowth of hair and thickening of the skin are measures used to assess the response to therapy. The hair coat should improve within 4 to 6 weeks of the start of therapy (Fig. 2-12). The hair that grows back consists primarily of lanugo, or secondary, hairs, with variable regrowth of primary, or guard, hairs. The duration of clinical remission in dogs with GH-responsive dermatosis that responds to GH treatment varies, but remission may last up to 3 years after therapy. A 1-week course of GH treatment should be given if dermatologic signs begin to recur.

Some dogs with suspected GH-responsive dermatosis fail to respond adequately to GH treatment (Fig. 2-13). Inactivated or outdated GH, an inappropriate treatment protocol, the development of GH antibodies, or misdiagnosis should be considered in these dogs. Alternative treatments that have been reported to be effective in some dogs with clinical manifestations suggestive of GH-responsive dermatosis include castration, melatonin therapy, and administration of o,p'DDD (see Disorders that Resemble GH-Responsive Dermatosis, page 64). Response to treatments other than GH casts doubt on the role of GH in the development of the clinical syndrome and emphasizes the difficulty in separating GH-responsive, sex hormone–induced, and sex hormone–responsive endocrine alopecia. Some dogs with suspected GH-responsive dermatosis that fail to respond to GH therapy may eventually undergo spontaneous resolution of the endocrine alopecia (Fig. 2-14).

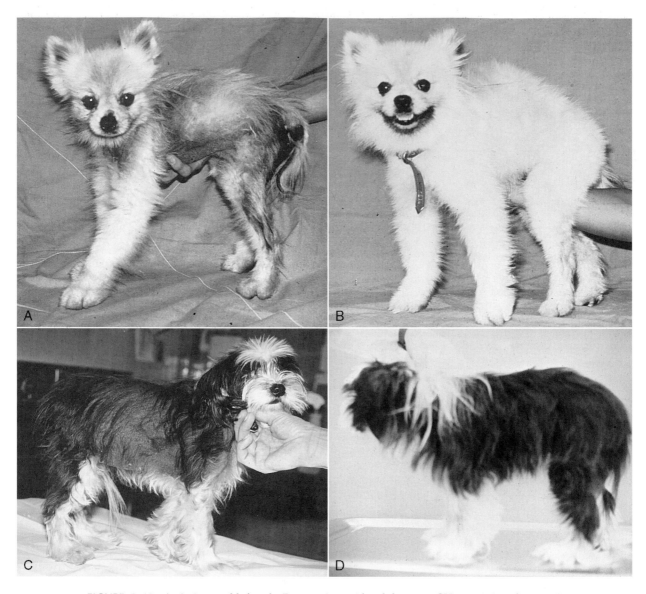

FIGURE 2–12. *A,* A 6-year-old female Pomeranian with adult-onset, GH-responsive dermatosis. *B,* Same dog as in *A* 3 months after initiation of exogenous porcine GH replacement therapy. *C,* A 3-year-old female spayed Tibetan Terrier with GH-responsive dermatosis. *D,* Same dog as in *C* 3 months after initiation of exogenous recombinant human GH replacement therapy.

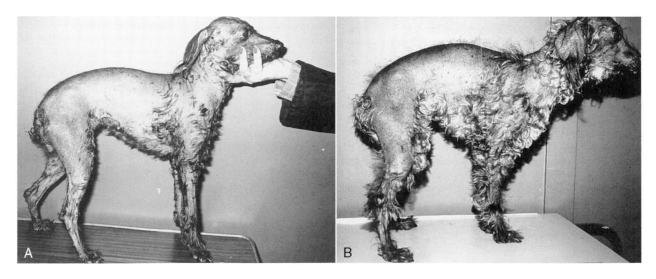

FIGURE 2–13. *A,* A 2-year-old female spayed Miniature Poodle with suspected adult-onset, GH-responsive dermatosis. *B,* Same dog as in *A* after two series of 10 injections of recombinant human growth hormone. (Courtesy of T. Olivery, Raleigh, NC.)

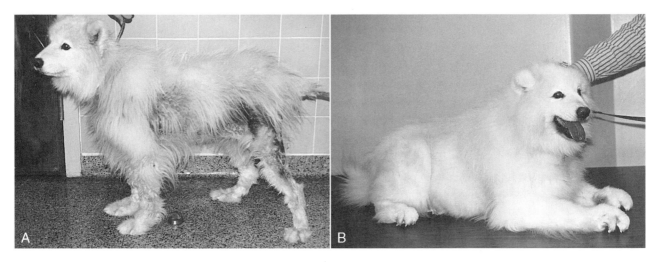

FIGURE 2–14. *A,* A 10-year-old female spayed Samoyed with endocrine alopecia of undetermined origin. Treatment with thyroid hormone, two series of injections of recombinant human GH, and sex hormones failed to improve the alopecia. *B,* Same dog as in *A* 6 months after all attempts at therapy had been discontinued.

Prognosis

The long-term prognosis is good, even in dogs not treated with GH. Most untreated dogs eventually lose most of their hair on the thorax and abdomen (the head and distal extremities are spared), and the skin turns black. The dogs are otherwise healthy.

FELINE ACROMEGALY

Etiology

PITUITARY NEOPLASIA. Chronic excessive secretion of GH in the adult cat results in acromegaly, a chronic disease characterized by overgrowth of connective tissue, bone, and viscera. In cats, the most common cause of acromegaly is a functional adenoma of the somatotropic cells of the pars distalis (Fig. 2-15; Peterson et al, 1990). In the overwhelming majority of cats, the pituitary tumor is easily visible with computed tomography (CT) or magnetic resonance imaging (MRI) at the time acromegaly is diagnosed. For most of these cats, the tumor is greater than 1 cm in diameter (i.e., macroadenoma) and extends dorsally into or compresses the hypothalamus and thalamus (Fig. 2-16). An obvious pituitary tumor may not be discernible with CT or MRI in acromegalic cats in the early stages of the disease but becomes identifiable with time and growth of the tumor (Fig. 2-17). GH secretion is increased by these tumors, and presumably feedback control of GH secretion is abnormal. In humans, secretion remains episodic; however, the number, duration, and amplitude of secretory episodes are increased, with the episodes occurring randomly through each 24-hour period (Thorner et al, 1998). The characteristic nocturnal surge is preserved, but the responses to suppression and stimulation testing are abnormal. Thus glucose suppressibility is lost, an abnormality that can be used as a diagnostic test for acromegaly.

PROGESTINS. Unlike with the dog, progesterone-induced acromegaly has not been documented in cats. The expression of the gene encoding GH has been demonstrated in feline mammary gland tissue that has undergone progestin-induced fibroadenomatous changes (Mol et al, 1995), which suggests that feline mammary gland tissue may be able to produce GH. However, Peterson (1987) found no significant rise in plasma GH concentrations in cats during 12 months of treatment with megestrol acetate, and Church and colleagues (1994) found no difference in plasma IGF-I concentrations between cats treated with proligestone or megestrol acetate and cats treated with saline.

MISCELLANEOUS ETIOLOGIES. In humans, excessive production of GHRH accounts for less than 1% of human acromegalic cases (Thorner et al, 1998). Excessive GHRH secretion has been documented with functional hypothalamic tumors, including hamartomas, choristomas, gliomas, and ganglioneuromas, and with peripheral tumors (see Fig. 2-15; Melmed, 1990; Thorner et al, 1998; Aron et al, 2001). Ectopic GHRH-secreting tumors include carcinoid tumors arising from the bronchus, gastrointestinal tract, and pancreas; pancreatic islet cell tumor; small cell carcinoma; adrenal adenoma; and pheochromocytoma. Acromegaly due to secretion of GH by an ectopic pancreatic islet cell tumor has also been described in a human (see Fig. 2-15; Melmed et al, 1985). Acromegaly caused by excessive GHRH or ectopic GH production has not yet been reported in the cat or dog. The potential for GH production by ductular epithelium of the mammary gland raises interesting possibilities for the development of acromegaly secondary to ectopic GH production by mammary gland adenocarcinoma in dogs and possibly cats (Selman et al, 1994b; Mol et al, 1995).

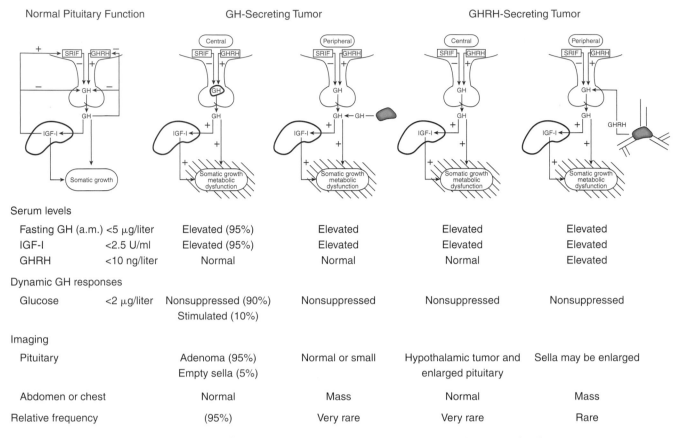

		Normal Pituitary Function	GH-Secreting Tumor		GHRH-Secreting Tumor	
Serum levels						
Fasting GH (a.m.)	<5 μg/liter	Elevated (95%)	Elevated	Elevated	Elevated	
IGF-I	<2.5 U/ml	Elevated (95%)	Elevated	Elevated	Elevated	
GHRH	<10 ng/liter	Normal	Normal	Normal	Elevated	
Dynamic GH responses						
Glucose	<2 μg/liter	Nonsuppressed (90%) Stimulated (10%)	Nonsuppressed	Nonsuppressed	Nonsuppressed	
Imaging						
Pituitary		Adenoma (95%) Empty sella (5%)	Normal or small	Hypothalamic tumor and enlarged pituitary	Sella may be enlarged	
Abdomen or chest		Normal	Mass	Normal	Mass	
Relative frequency		(95%)	Very rare	Very rare	Rare	

FIGURE 2–15. Pathophysiology and diagnosis of four types of acromegaly documented in humans. *GH,* Growth hormone; *GHRH,* growth hormone–releasing hormone; *IGF-I,* insulin-like growth factor-I; *SRIF,* somatostatin; +, stimulated secretion; -, suppressed secretion. (Melmed S: N Engl J Med 322:966, 1990.)

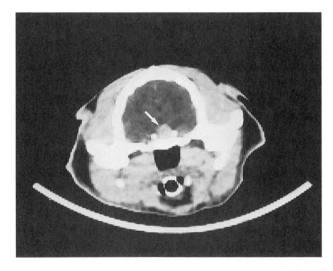

FIGURE 2–16. CT scan of the pituitary region of an 8-year-old male castrated cat with insulin-resistant diabetes mellitus and acromegaly. A mass is evident in the hypothalamic-pituitary region *(arrow).* This mass was visible without contrast enhancement.

Pathophysiology

Chronic GH hypersecretion has both catabolic and anabolic effects. The anabolic effects are caused by increased concentrations of IGF-I (Middleton et al, 1985; Abrams-Ogg et al, 1993). The growth-promoting effects of IGF-I result in proliferation of bone, cartilage, and soft tissues and in organomegaly. These anabolic effects are responsible for the classic clinical manifestations of acromegaly. The catabolic effects of GH are a direct result of the antiinsulin effects of GH on tissues. In excess, GH decreases carbohydrate utilization and impairs glucose uptake into cells. GH-induced insulin resistance appears to be due to a postreceptor impairment in insulin action (Rosenfeld et al, 1982; Bratusch-Marrain et al, 1982). The net effect is development of carbohydrate intolerance, hyperglycemia, and, with sustained increases in plasma GH, development of diabetes mellitus, which quickly becomes resistant to insulin treatment. Most but not all cats with acromegaly have diabetes mellitus at the time acromegaly is diagnosed, and most eventually develop severe insulin resistance. Twenty-two of 23 cats diagnosed with acromegaly at our hospital during the past decade had insulin-resistant diabetes mellitus at the time acromegaly was diagnosed.

Signalment

Acromegaly typically occurs in older male, Domestic Short-Haired or Long-Haired cats (Peterson et al, 1990). Twenty-two of 23 cats diagnosed with acromegaly at our hospital during the past decade were Domestic Short-Haired or Long-Haired cats, and one was

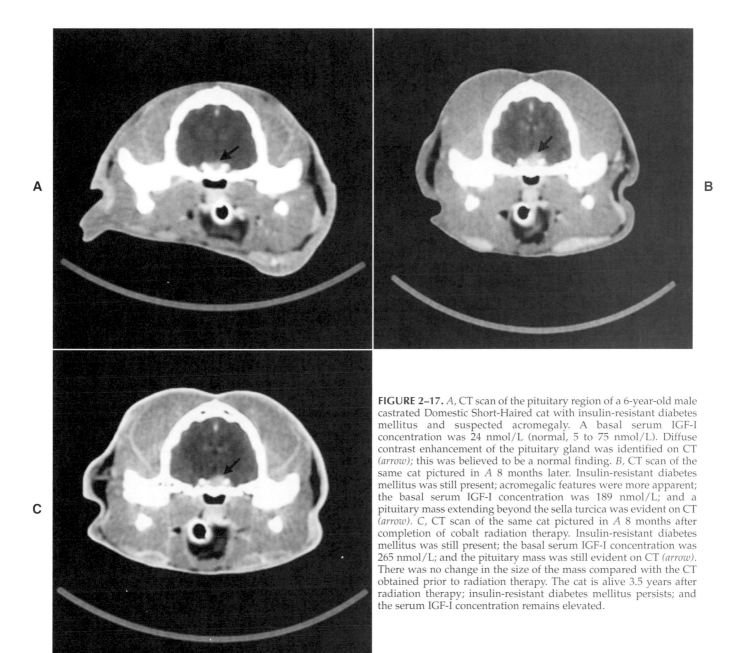

FIGURE 2–17. *A,* CT scan of the pituitary region of a 6-year-old male castrated Domestic Short-Haired cat with insulin-resistant diabetes mellitus and suspected acromegaly. A basal serum IGF-I concentration was 24 nmol/L (normal, 5 to 75 nmol/L). Diffuse contrast enhancement of the pituitary gland was identified on CT *(arrow)*; this was believed to be a normal finding. *B,* CT scan of the same cat pictured in *A* 8 months later. Insulin-resistant diabetes mellitus was still present; acromegalic features were more apparent; the basal serum IGF-I concentration was 189 nmol/L; and a pituitary mass extending beyond the sella turcica was evident on CT *(arrow)*. *C,* CT scan of the same cat pictured in *A* 8 months after completion of cobalt radiation therapy. Insulin-resistant diabetes mellitus was still present; the basal serum IGF-I concentration was 265 nmol/L; and the pituitary mass was still evident on CT *(arrow)*. There was no change in the size of the mass compared with the CT obtained prior to radiation therapy. The cat is alive 3.5 years after radiation therapy; insulin-resistant diabetes mellitus persists; and the serum IGF-I concentration remains elevated.

Siamese. Twenty cats were castrated males and three were spayed females. The average age at the time acromegaly was diagnosed was 10 years, with a median of 9 years and a range of 4 to 17 years.

Clinical signs

The clinical signs and physical examination findings result from the catabolic, diabetogenic effects of GH, the anabolic actions of IGF-I, and growth of the pituitary macroadenoma (Table 2-14). The earliest and most common clinical signs are polyuria (PU), polydipsia (PD), and polyphagia resulting from the concurrent diabetes mellitus (Table 2-15). Polyphagia may also develop as a direct result of hypersomatotropism, independent of the diabetes mellitus, and can

become quite intense. Weight loss varies and depends in part on whether the anabolic effects of IGF-I or the catabolic effects of insulin resistance and hyperglycemia predominate. Most acromegalic cats lose weight initially, but this is quickly followed by a period of stabilization and then a slow, progressive gain in body weight as the anabolic effects of IGF-I begin to dominate the clinical picture (see Table 2-15). Weight gain occurs despite severe insulin resistance. In most cats, the clinician considers acromegaly only after he or she realizes that insulin therapy has been ineffective in establishing glycemic control of the diabetic state. Insulin dosages in cats with acromegaly frequently exceed 2 U/kg body weight twice a day, with no apparent decline in the blood glucose concentration. The mean insulin dosage per injection in our

TABLE 2–14 CLINICAL SIGNS ASSOCIATED WITH ACROMEGALY IN DOGS AND CATS

Anabolic, IGF-I-Induced

Respiratory
  Inspiratory stridor
  Transient apnea
  Panting
  Exercise intolerance
  Fatigue
Dermatologic
  Myxedema
  Excessive skin folds
  Hypertrichosis
Conformational
  Increased size
  Increased soft tissue in
    oropharyngeal/laryngeal area
  Enlargement of:
    Abdomen
    Head
    Feet
    Viscera
  Broad face
  Prominent jowls
  Prognathia inferior
  Increased interdental space
  Rapid toenail growth
  Degenerative polyarthropathy

Catabolic, GH-Induced

Polyuria, polydipsia
Polyphagia

Iatrogenic

Progestins
Mammary nodules
Pyometra

Neoplasia-Induced

Lethargy, stupor
Adipsia
Anorexia
Temperature deregulation
Papilledema
Circling
Seizures
Pituitary dysfunction
  Hypogonadism
  Hypothyroidism
  Hypoadrenocorticism

IGF-I, Insulin-like growth factor-I.

TABLE 2-15 CLINICAL SIGNS AND PHYSICAL EXAMINATION FINDINGS IN 23 CATS WITH ACROMEGALY

Clinical Sign	Number of Cats (%)
Poorly-controlled diabetes mellitus	22 (96%)
Polyuria and polydipsia	19 (83%)*
Polyphagia	18 (78%)*
Increase in body weight	8 (35%)
Weight loss	2 (9%)
Lethargy	8 (35%)*
Increase in body size	3 (13%)*
Intermittent weakness (hypoglycemia)	2 (9%)
Respiratory distress, stridor	1 (4%)
Changes in behavior	1 (4%)

Physical Examination Findings	Number of Cats (%)
Large cat with big head, feet and abdomen	19 (83%)*
Prognathia inferior	8 (35%)*
Diabetic neuropathy	6 (26%)
Hepatomegaly	6 (26%)
Renomegaly	5 (22%)*
Poor, unkempt haircoat	5 (22%)
Heart murmur	4 (17%)*
Stridor	2 (9%)
Dull, stuporous	2 (9%)
Increased soft tissue-pharyngeal region	1 (5%)
Large tongue	1 (5%)
Increased interdental spacing	1 (5%)*
Degenerative arthropathy	1 (5%)

*Includes acromegalic cat without concurrent diabetes mellitus.

22 acromegalic cats with insulin-resistant diabetes mellitus was 2.2 U/kg body weight (median, 2.0 U/kg; range, 1.1 to 4.4 U/kg).

Clinical signs and physical examination findings related to the anabolic actions of excess GH secretion (see Table 2-14) may be evident at the time diabetes mellitus is diagnosed. More commonly, however, they become apparent several months after the diabetes has been diagnosed, often in conjunction with the realization that hyperglycemia is difficult to control with exogenous insulin therapy. Because of the insidious onset and slowly progressive nature of the anabolic clinical signs, owners often are not aware of the subtle changes in the appearance of their cat until the clinical signs are quite obvious. The most frequent anabolic changes identified by veterinarians are the presence of a big cat with a massive head and large abdomen (see Table 2-15; Fig. 2-18). The average body weight of our 23 acromegalic cats was 6.5 kg (range, 4.9 to 9.0 kg). Weight gain or stable body weight in a large cat with poorly regulated diabetes mellitus is an important diagnostic clue to acromegaly. Prognathia inferior is another important diagnostic clue and was identified in approximately one third of our acromegalic cats (Fig. 2-19). With time organomegaly develops, especially of the heart, kidney, liver, and adrenal gland. Renomegaly and hepatomegaly may be evident on physical examination. Diffuse thickening of soft tissues in the oropharyngeal region can lead to extrathoracic upper airway obstruction, respiratory distress, and stridor.

Cardiovascular abnormalities include systolic murmurs; gallop rhythms; radiographic evidence of cardiomegaly; echocardiographic evidence of hypertrophic cardiomyopathy, most notably septal and left ventricular wall hypertrophy; and, late in the course of the disease, signs of congestive heart failure (e.g., dyspnea, muffled heart sounds, ascites) (Peterson et al, 1990). Systemic hypertension is variably present and usually is identified in acromegalic cats with concurrent renal insufficiency. Myocardial histologic lesions include myofiber hypertrophy, multifocal myocytolysis, interstitial fibrosis, and intramural arteriosclerosis. The cause of cardiac disease is not clear, but it probably results from a direct effect of GH on protein synthesis and, if present, the effects of systemic hypertension (van den Heuvel et al, 1984).

Degenerative arthropathy was reported in 43% of 14 acromegalic cats (Peterson et al, 1990), although only half of these cats were symptomatic for joint disease. Affected joints included the shoulder, elbow, carpus, digits, stifle, and spine. Radiographic changes included periarticular periosteal reaction, osteophytes, soft tissue swelling, and collapse of the joint spaces in some cats. Pathologic findings included erosion and ulceration of articular cartilage with chondroid hyperplasia and fissure formation. Degenerative arthropathy was an infrequent finding in our acromegalic cats (see Table 2-15), which probably reflects diagnosis of the disease earlier in its development as our ability to recognize the disorder improves. The pathogenesis of acromegalic arthropathy is not completely

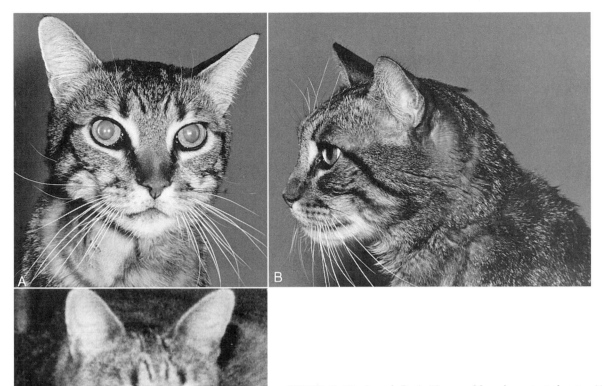

FIGURE 2–18. *A* and *B*, A 13-year-old male castrated cat with insulin-resistant diabetes mellitus and acromegaly. The owners had noticed a gradual increase in the size of the cat's head and feet. Note the broad face and mildly protruding mandible (prognathia inferior). *C*, Same cat as in *A* and *B* at 6 years of age, prior to the development of diabetes mellitus or acromegaly.

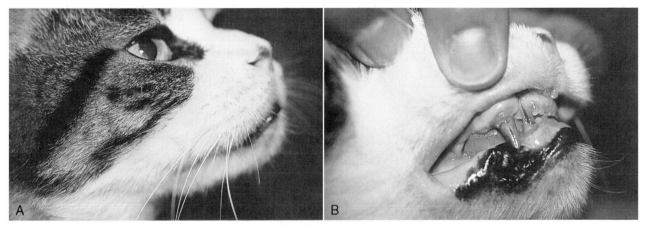

FIGURE 2–19. An 8-year-old male castrated Domestic Short-Haired cat with insulin-resistant diabetes mellitus and acromegaly. Note the prognathia inferior with displacement of the lower canine teeth. A CT scan of the pituitary region of this cat is shown in Fig. 2-16.

understood, but it is believed to be a noninflammatory condition in which cartilage hypertrophy and hyperplasia lead to the disruption of joint geometry and chondrocyte metabolism and ultimately to degenerative joint changes (Johanson et al, 1983).

Neurologic signs may develop as a result of pituitary tumor growth and the resultant invasion and compression of the hypothalamus and thalamus. Signs include stupor, somnolence, adipsia, anorexia, temperature deregulation, circling, seizures, and changes in behavior. Blindness is not common, because the optic chiasm is located anterior to the pituitary gland. Papilledema may be evident during an ophthalmic examination. Lethargy may develop as a result of pituitary tumor growth or, more commonly, as a result of poorly controlled diabetes mellitus and persistent severe hyperglycemia. Peripheral neuropathy, causing weakness, ataxia, and a plantigrade stance, as well as a poor hair coat from decreased grooming behavior, also develops as a result of poorly controlled diabetes mellitus. Other endocrine and metabolic abnormalities resulting from the compressive effects of the tumor on the pituitary are uncommon. The reader is referred to Chapter 6 for more information on pituitary macro-tumor syndrome.

Clinical pathology

Concurrent, poorly controlled diabetes mellitus is responsible for most of the abnormalities identified on a CBC, serum biochemical panel, and urinalysis, including hyperglycemia, glycosuria, hypercholesterolemia, and mild increase in alanine transaminase and alkaline phosphatase activities. Ketonuria is an infrequent finding. Mild erythrocytosis, persistent mild hyperphosphatemia without concurrent azotemia, and persistent hyperglobulinemia (total serum protein concentration of 8 to 10 mg/dl) with a normal pattern of distribution on protein electrophoretic studies may also be found (Peterson et al, 1990). Persistent hyper-

phosphatemia without concurrent azotemia is believed to be caused by GH-induced renal phosphate retention. The mild erythrocytosis found in some cats with acromegaly may also be caused by the anabolic effects of GH or IGF-I on the bone marrow. Renal failure is a potential sequela of acromegaly and, if present, is associated with azotemia, isosthenuria, and proteinuria. Progressive azotemia with clinical signs of renal failure developed in 7 of 14 acromegalic cats (Peterson et al, 1990). Kidneys were normal to enlarged, and mesangial thickening of the glomeruli was identified at necropsy. Glomerulonephropathy was the most probable cause of renal failure in these cats, and it may have developed secondary to poorly controlled diabetes mellitus and/or chronic GH excess.

Diagnostic imaging

CONVENTIONAL RADIOGRAPHY. Radiographic changes that have been identified in acromegalic cats include a diffuse increase of soft tissue in the oropharyngeal area; degenerative arthropathy of the shoulder, elbow, stifle, carpus and/or digits characterized by periarticular periosteal reaction and osteophytes with soft tissue swelling and collapse of the joint space; spondylosis deformans of the spine; enlargement of the mandible; and hyperostosis of the bony calvarium (Fig. 2-20) (Peterson et al, 1990). Thoracic radiographs may reveal mild to severe cardiomegaly and pulmonary edema or pleural effusion if congestive heart failure is present. Abdominal radiographs may reveal hepatomegaly and renomegaly. The presence and severity of radiographic changes depend on the duration of hypersomatotropism.

ABDOMINAL ULTRASOUND. Abdominal ultrasound results are often unremarkable in cats with acromegaly. Hepatomegaly is the most consistent abnormality identified but in most cats probably occurs secondary to diabetes mellitus–induced hepatic lipidosis (Table 2-16). Cats with long-standing acromegaly eventually

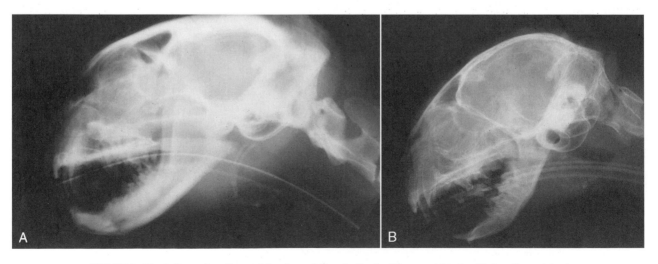

FIGURE 2–20. *A*, Lateral radiographic view of the skull of a 13-year-old cat with insulin-resistant diabetes mellitus and acromegaly. Note the hyperostosis of the bony calvarium. *B*, Lateral radiographic view of a normal cat skull.

TABLE 2-16   FINDINGS ON ABDOMINAL ULTRASOUND IN 17 CATS WITH ACROMEGALY

Ultrasound Finding	Number of Cats (%)
Hepatomegaly	9 (53%)
Renomegaly	5 (29%)
Dilation-renal pelvis	2 (12%)
Bilateral adrenomegaly	4 (24%)
Enlarged pancreas	3 (18%)
Splenomegaly	1 (6%)
Normal ultrasound	4 (24%)

develop renomegaly and adrenomegaly in addition to hepatomegaly. Identification of adrenomegaly in a cat with severe insulin-resistant diabetes mellitus is suggestive of but not confirmatory for hyperadrenocorticism; acromegaly should also be considered. Fortunately, in cats the remainder of the clinical presentation and clinicopathologic findings are different for acromegaly and for hyperadrenocorticism (see page 77).

COMPUTED TOMOGRAPHY/MAGNETIC RESONANCE IMAGING. CT and MRI play an important role in establishing the diagnosis of acromegaly in cats (see Definitive Diagnosis, page 77). Most cats have a visible pituitary tumor on CT or MRI at the time acromegaly is tentatively diagnosed (see Fig. 2-16). This finding, in conjunction with the clinical presentation and determinations of serum GH or IGF-I concentrations, helps establish the diagnosis. Intravenous administration of a contrast agent (iodinated contrast agent for CT; gadopentetate dimeglumine for MRI) is usually necessary to visualize the pituitary mass via CT or MRI. Failure to identify a pituitary mass on CT or MRI does not rule out acromegaly, especially if the disease is early in its development (see Fig. 2-17). The size and location of the tumor must be determined from the CT or MRI scan before radiation therapy is started; over the course of treatment, serial CT or MRI scans allow evaluation of tumor response to therapy (Fig. 2-21).

Hormonal evaluation

BASELINE GH CONCENTRATION. Baseline GH concentrations are variable and depend in part on the severity of the disease at the time GH is measured. Most acromegalic cats with severe insulin-resistant diabetes mellitus and physical examination abnormalities induced by the anabolic actions of IGF-I have baseline GH concentrations greater than 10 ng/ml and often greater than 25 ng/ml (normal concentration, less than 5 ng/ml). However, cats in the early stages of acromegaly (i.e., diabetes somewhat responsive to insulin, minimal anabolic changes on physical examination) may have baseline GH concentrations of 5 to 10 ng/ml. With time, baseline GH concentrations increase in these cats as insulin-resistance worsens and anabolic changes become more apparent.

In humans, GH is secreted episodically, in brief bursts. As such, a single, random serum GH concentration measurement may not be helpful for diagnosing or excluding acromegaly because a "normal" value may be a nadir level in an acromegalic patient; conversely, a "high" value may be a peak value in a normal individual (Thorner et al, 1998). Concurrent measurement of the serum IGF-I concentration (see below) or evaluation of the change in GH during an oral glucose tolerance test helps establish the diagnosis. In nonacromegalic humans, the serum GH concentration decreases to less than 1 ng/ml after ingestion of 50 to 100 g of glucose (Stewart et al, 1989). In human acromegalics, GH levels may decrease, increase, or show no change after glucose administration; however, GH

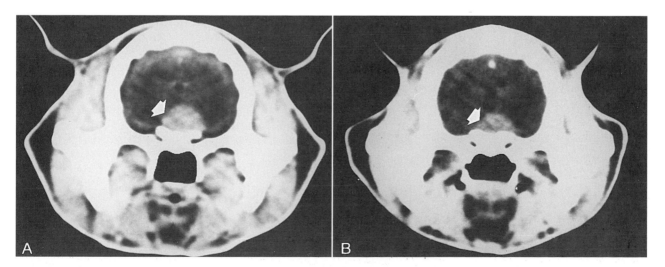

FIGURE 2–21. *A,* CT scan of the pituitary region of a 13-year-old male castrated cat with insulin-resistant diabetes mellitus and acromegaly (see Fig. 2-18). The concentration was 54 ng/ml (normal, less than 5 ng/ml). A mass is evident in the hypothalamic-pituitary region after intravenous administration of a positive contrast agent *(arrow). B,* CT scan of the same cat pictured in *A* 2 months after completion of cobalt radiation therapy. A basal GH concentration at this time was 7 ng/ml. Although pooling of the contrast agent is still evident in the hypothalamic-pituitary region *(arrow),* the mass had decreased in size by more than 50%.

levels should not decrease to less than 1 ng/ml. This lack of suppressibility confirms the diagnosis of acromegaly. Nonsuppressibility of basal GH levels after intravenous administration of glucose has been demonstrated in the acromegalic dog (see page 81) (Eigenmann and Venker-van Haagen, 1981). Similar studies have not been reported in cats. We do not assess the responsiveness of somatotrophs to glucose administration to establish the diagnosis of acromegaly in cats (see section on establishing the diagnosis, page 77).

BASELINE IGF-I CONCENTRATIONS. Measurement of the serum IGF-I concentration is considered the best screening test for acromegaly in humans. Serum IGF-I concentrations are considered to reflect overall GH secretion during the previous 24 hours. Because these concentrations vary minimally over 24 hours and correlate closely with the severity of clinical signs, they provide a reliable indicator of GH secretion (Thorner et al, 1998). IGF-I levels are increased in virtually all human patients with acromegaly. The role of IGF-I measurement as a screening test for GH excess in cats remains to be critically evaluated. Increased IGF-I concentrations have been found in acromegalic cats (Middleton et al, 1985; Abrams-Ogg et al, 1993), which suggests that IGF-I may be a useful diagnostic tool. However, the role of IGF-I measurement as a screen for GH excess was questioned in one study in which serum IGF-I concentrations were fourfold higher in eight randomly selected diabetic cats, compared with eight healthy cats (Lewitt et al, 2000). None of the diabetic cats were suspected to have acromegaly. In our experience, measurement of the serum IGF-I concentration has proven to be a useful screening test for GH excess when done in diabetic cats with insulin resistance (Fig. 2-22).

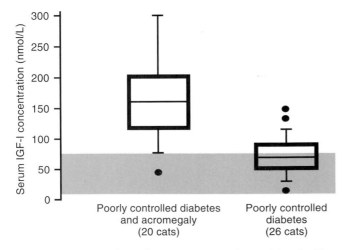

FIGURE 2–22. Box plots of serum concentrations of insulin-like growth factor-I (IGF-I) in 20 cats with poorly controlled diabetes caused by concurrent acromegaly and in 26 cats with poorly controlled diabetes caused by another disorder. For each box plot, T bars represent the main body of data, which in most instances is equal to the range. Each box represents interquartile range (25th to 75th percentile). The horizontal bar in each box is the median, and the solid circles represent outlying data points. (Modified from Nelson RW: *In* Nelson RW and Couto GC (eds): Small Animal Internal Medicine, 3rd ed. St. Louis, Mosby, 2003, p. 676.)

Measurement of serum IGF-I is available commercially (e.g., Diagnostic Endocrinology Laboratory, College of Veterinary Medicine, Michigan State University, East Lansing, Mich.). The reference range for the serum IGF-I concentration that is used by the Diagnostic Endocrinology Laboratory is 5 to 70 nmol/L; most cats with acromegaly have serum IGF-I concentrations greater than 100 nmol/L (see Fig. 2-22). Serum IGF-I values between 70 and 100 nmol/L are nondiagnostic; some nonacromegalic diabetic cats with insulin resistance have serum IGF-I values that fall in this range, and some acromegalic diabetic cats have serum IGF-I values that fall in the upper normal range in the early stages of the disease (see Fig. 2-17). Repeat measurements performed 3 to 6 months later usually demonstrate an increase in serum IGF-I if acromegaly is present. The increase in serum IGF-I typically coincides with the development and growth of the pituitary somatotropic adenoma. Because measurement of the serum GH concentration is not readily available commercially, we routinely use measurement of the serum IGF-I concentration as a screening test for acromegaly in cats. It is important always to interpret IGF-I results in conjunction with the history, physical examination findings, results of routine blood and urine tests, and severity of insulin resistance. A CT or MRI scan is recommended to confirm the existence of a pituitary macrotumor if the clinical picture supports acromegaly and if the serum IGF-I concentration is increased (see the section on establishing the diagnosis, page 77).

PANCREATIC β-CELL FUNCTION. The close association between diabetes mellitus, insulin resistance, and acromegaly and the recognition that insulin-requiring diabetes mellitus may resolve with treatment of acromegaly raises interesting questions concerning the status of pancreatic β-cell function in acromegalic cats. Baseline serum insulin concentrations are variable and depend in part on the duration and severity of hypersomatotropism, the severity of the pathology in the pancreatic islets, and the presence of glucose toxicity. Initially, the β-cells respond to GH-induced carbohydrate intolerance and insulin antagonism by increasing insulin secretion. Hyperinsulinemia represents an expected physiologic attempt to regulate blood glucose concentrations. Early in the development of hypersomatotropism, hyperinsulinemia keeps the blood glucose concentration in the normal range or mildly increased. Prolonged hypersomatotropism leads to worsening insulin resistance, hyperglycemia, and the eventual development of overt diabetes mellitus. In cats, hyperglycemia also suppresses β-cell function, a phenomenon referred to as *glucose toxicity* (see Chapter 12). The end result is acromegaly, insulin-resistant diabetes mellitus, and hypoinsulinemia. In theory, baseline serum insulin concentrations may be low, normal, or high in a cat with hypersomatotropism, depending on when in the progression of the disease the serum insulin concentration is measured. In reality, the serum insulin concentration is typically within or below the normal range (i.e., less than 10 μU/ml) at the time acromegaly is diagnosed; this finding suggests hypoinsulinemia in the face of often profound hyperglycemia. However, identification of a low serum insulin concentration in an acromegalic cat may or may not provide an accurate picture of the health of the β-cells and may or may not accurately predict the reversibility of the diabetic state if acromegaly is successfully treated. If islet pathology is severe and the population of β-cells is significantly reduced, insulin-requiring diabetes mellitus will be permanent. If islet pathology is minimal, if an adequate population of β-cells is present but their function is suppressed as a result of glucose toxicity, and if glucose toxicity resolves after treatment of acromegaly, the β-cells may regain function and overt diabetes mellitus may resolve.

THYROID FUNCTION. In humans, acromegaly-induced organomegaly may include enlargement of the thyroid gland and palpable thyroid nodules (Thorner et al, 1998). Adenomatous hyperplasia of the thyroid gland with normal serum thyroid hormone concentrations has also been documented in some cats with acromegaly (Peterson et al, 1990). Similar findings have not been reported in dogs. Basal thyroid hormone concentrations, when measured, are usually normal (Peterson et al, 1990). Low thyroid hormone concentrations would suggest the euthyroid sick syndrome (see Chapter 3, page 128). In theory, secondary hypothyroidism may develop late in the course of neoplasia-induced acromegaly, after normal pituitary tissue has been compressed by an expanding pituitary macrotumor, or with destruction of normal pituitary tissue by radiation treatment; however, these scenarios are uncommon. Increased thyroid hormone concentrations would suggest concurrent hyperthyroidism (see Chapter 4).

ADRENOCORTICAL FUNCTION. Hyperadrenocorticism and acromegaly are the primary differential diagnoses for severe insulin-resistant diabetes mellitus in cats (see below). Diagnostic tests to assess adrenocortical function are often performed in cats ultimately diagnosed with acromegaly. Mild to moderate multifocal nodular hyperplasia of the adrenal cortices has been documented in some cats with acromegaly (Peterson et al, 1990), and abdominal ultrasound may reveal mild bilateral adrenomegaly (maximum width of the adrenal gland, 0.5 to 1.0 cm); these findings are suggestive of pituitary-dependent hyperadrenocorticism. Urine cortisol/creatinine ratios may also be increased, presumably because of the effects of the poorly controlled diabetic state on baseline cortisol concentrations. Fortunately, acromegalic cats with insulin-resistant diabetes mellitus have a normal response to ACTH stimulation and dexamethasone suppression testing.

Definitive diagnosis

Acromegalic cats are usually brought to veterinarians for problems related to poorly controlled diabetes mellitus. Conformational alterations (see Table 2-15) are insidious in onset and often not noted by owners.

These alterations may be obvious to the veterinarian during the physical examination and, when present in conjunction with appropriate concurrent signs, are almost pathognomonic for acromegaly. Acromegaly is less likely to be suspected in the cat that lacks typical conformational alterations. For these animals, the diagnostic approach is aimed at ruling out more common causes of poor glycemic control (see Chapter 12, page 572). Acromegaly is usually not suspected until other causes of poor glycemic control have been ruled out or conformational alterations become apparent with the passage of time.

A definitive diagnosis of acromegaly requires documentation of an increased baseline serum GH concentration. The baseline GH concentration in cats with acromegaly typically exceeds 10 ng/ml (normal concentration, less than 5 ng/ml). Unfortunately, a commercial GH assay is not available for cats, and it may take months before results are obtained when blood samples are submitted to research laboratories. For most cats, the diagnosis is ultimately based on (1) identification of conformational alterations (e.g., increased body size, large head, prognathia inferior, organomegaly) in a cat with insulin-resistant diabetes mellitus; (2) a persistent increase rather than decrease in the body weight of a cat with poorly controlled diabetes mellitus; (3) an increase in the serum IGF-I concentration in an insulin-resistant cat with clinical manifestations consistent with acromegaly; and (4) documentation of a pituitary mass by CT or MRI scanning (see Fig. 2-16). In addition, hyperadrenocorticism must be ruled out before a tentative diagnosis of acromegaly can be made.

ACROMEGALY VERSUS HYPERADRENOCORTICISM. Hyperadrenocorticism and acromegaly are uncommon disorders that occur in older cats, Both of these disorders have a strong association with diabetes mellitus, can cause severe insulin resistance, and often give rise to a pituitary macrotumor (Elliot et al, 2000). Clinical signs related to poorly controlled diabetes mellitus are common in cats with hyperadrenocorticism and acromegaly. Additional clinical signs differ dramatically between these two disorders, and these differences form the basis for distinguishing between the two conditions. Hyperadrenocorticism is a debilitating disease that results in progressive weight loss, leading to cachexia and dermal and epidermal atrophy, which in turn lead to extremely fragile, thin, easily torn, and ulcerated skin (i.e., feline fragile skin syndrome). In contrast, conformational changes caused by the anabolic actions of chronic IGF-I secretion dominate the clinical picture in acromegaly, most notably an increase in body size, prognathia inferior, and weight gain despite poorly regulated diabetes mellitus. Feline fragile skin syndrome does not occur with acromegaly. For both disorders, most of the abnormalities identified on routine blood and urine tests are caused by the concurrent poorly controlled diabetes mellitus. Abdominal ultrasound scans may also reveal mild bilateral adrenomegaly with both disorders. Ultimately, differentiation of the two diseases is based on the results of tests of the pituitary-adrenocortical axis (see Chapter 7) and on the serum GH and/or IGF-I concentrations.

Treatment

The goals of treatment are to decrease the size and reverse the mass effects of the pituitary macrotumor, return GH secretion to normal, resolve insulin resistance and potentially revert to a non-insulin-requiring diabetic state, and preserve other anterior pituitary function. In humans, treatment options include surgical resection, pituitary radiation, and medical therapy with dopamine agonists or somatostatin analogs. Similar treatment options have been tried in acromegalic cats, but to date none has been consistently successful.

RADIATION THERAPY. Radiation therapy is currently considered the best treatment option for acromegaly in cats. Cobalt teletherapy involves administration of a total dose of 45 to 48 Gy in daily fractions 5 days a week for 3 to 4 weeks. The response to cobalt teletherapy is unpredictable and ranges from no response, to a partial decrease in pituitary tumor size or serum GH concentration (or both) and increased responsiveness to insulin, to a dramatic response characterized by significant shrinkage of the tumor, elimination of hypersomatotropism, resolution of insulin resistance and, in some cats, reversion to a subclinical diabetic state (Goossens et al, 1998) (see Fig. 2-17 and Fig. 2-23). Typically, tumor volume and the serum GH and IGF-I concentrations decrease and insulin responsiveness improves after cobalt teletherapy, although this improvement may take 6 months or longer after radiation treatment. In most treated cats that respond to radiation therapy, diabetes mellitus or insulin resistance (or both) recurs 12 to 24 months after treatment, although growth of the pituitary mass is often not evident on CT or MRI scans.

Ten acromegalic cats have undergone radiation treatment for pituitary macrotumors in our hospital during the past decade. Three cats developed problems with hypoglycemia within 6 months, and one of these cats died of severe hypoglycemic seizures 1 month after completing radiation therapy. Hypoglycemic

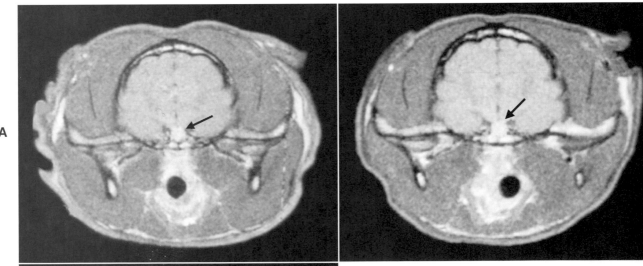

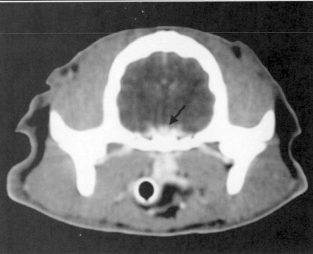

FIGURE 2–23. *A,* MRI scan of the pituitary region of a 4-year-old male castrated cat with insulin-resistant diabetes mellitus and acromegaly. A basal serum IGF-I concentration was 118 nmol/L (normal, 5 to 75 nmol/L). Diffuse contrast enhancement of the pituitary gland was identified on MRI *(arrow);* this was believed to be a normal finding. *B,* MRI scan of the same cat pictured in *A* 3 months later. Insulin-resistant diabetes mellitus was still present; the basal serum IGF-I concentration was greater than 153 nmol/L; and contrast enhancement of the pituitary gland was still evident on MRI *(arrow).* Measurement of the pituitary gland revealed a 0.1 by 0.2 cm increase in size compared with the gland's size measured 3 months earlier. *C,* CT scan of the same cat pictured in *A* 2.5 years after completion of cobalt radiation therapy. The insulin resistance resolved, and the need for insulin injections has fluctuated during the past 2 years. The basal serum IGF-I concentration was 100 nmol/L. Although pooling of the contrast agent was still evident in the pituitary region *(arrow),* the mass had decreased in size by approximately 70%.

seizures resulted from an insulin overdose caused by marked improvement in tissue responsiveness to insulin, not an increase in the insulin dosage. Insulin-requiring diabetes mellitus resolved in five cats 6 to 9 months after completion of radiation treatment. One of the five cats has had recurring transient diabetes mellitus for 2 years; two cats had recurrence of insulin-requiring diabetes mellitus 1 and 3 years later; and two cats have remained euglycemic for longer than 1 year after reversion to a non-insulin-requiring diabetic state.

Disadvantages of radiotherapy include limited availability, expense, the need for extended hospitalization, frequent anesthesia, and an unpredictable outcome. The most common complication after radiotherapy in our acromegalic cats was hypoglycemia resulting from resolution of insulin resistance. In human acromegalics, complications after radiation therapy include secondary hypothyroidism, secondary hypoadrenocorticism, and visual loss secondary to optic nerve damage (Thorner et al, 1998). Similar complications are possible in acromegalic cats, although we have not seen these problems in our acromegalic cats that have undergone radiotherapy. The reader is referred to Chapter 6 for more information on radiation therapy of pituitary tumors.

MEDICAL THERAPY.   An effective medical option for the treatment of feline acromegaly has not yet been reported. In humans, the dopamine agonist bromocriptine is effective in improving clinical signs and decreasing serum GH concentrations in 70% of treated patients (Thorner et al, 1998). The use of dopamine agonists for the treatment of acromegaly has not been reported in cats. Bromocriptine has been used for the treatment of canine hyperadrenocorticism with only marginal success (Drucker and Peterson, 1981) (see Chapter 6). Adverse reactions were common and included vomiting, anorexia, depression, and behavior changes.

Octreotide (Novartis Pharmaceuticals, East Hanover, NJ) is an 8-amino-acid cyclic peptide analog of somatostatin that suppresses GH release for up to 8 hours in healthy and acromegalic humans (Plewe et al, 1984; Davies et al, 1986). Approximately 90% of human acromegalics treated with octreotide have shown improvement in disease manifestations, a reduction in the serum GH and IGF-I concentrations, and, in approximately 30% of patients, a reduction in pituitary tumor size (Thorner et al, 1998). The therapeutic response to octreotide correlates directly with the density of somatostatin receptors in the adenoma (Reubi and Landolt, 1989). Unfortunately, octreotide has been unsuccessful in lowering the serum GH concentration or improving insulin sensitivity in acromegalic cats in which it has been used (Morrison et al, 1989; Peterson et al, 1990). Dosages have ranged from 10 to 200 µg given subcutaneously two to three times daily. The reason for this ineffectiveness in cats is not understood, especially because somatostatin is a peptide hormone that is highly conserved between species. It may be that GH-secreting somatotroph adenomas of cats lack the somatostatin receptors, the

receptors have abnormal binding affinity for the somatostatin analog, the treatment regiment is incorrect, or the duration of treatment has been inadequate to allow identification of a response.

Pegvisomant is a genetically engineered analog of human growth hormone that functions as a growth hormone–receptor antagonist (Fuh et al, 1992). In a 12-week, double-blind, placebo-controlled study, pegvisomant significantly ameliorated both the clinical and biochemical manifestations of acromegaly in 112 human acromegalics (Trainer et al, 2000). The drug was well tolerated, and the increase in serum GH concentrations during treatment was small, was not progressive, and was not associated with any evidence of tumor growth. Pegvisomant was subsequently shown to lower serum IGF-I concentrations to normal in approximately 90% of acromegalic humans during 1 year of treatment (van der Lely et al, 2001). The potential usefulness of pegvisomant for treatment of feline acromegaly remains to be determined.

SURGERY.   Transsphenoidal selective adenoma removal or hypophysectomy is the initial treatment of choice for acromegaly in humans. The surgical outcome depends on the size of the tumor and the expertise of the surgeon. Pituitary tumors less than 1 cm in diameter have the greatest possibility for a surgical cure; the presence of tumors greater than 1 cm in diameter, particularly with suprasellar extension or extension into the cavernous sinus, reduces the probability of a surgical cure (Thorner et al, 1998). Normal serum GH concentrations are attained postoperatively in approximately 60% of patients that undergo surgery, the best outcomes occurring with small tumors (Davis et al, 1993). Microsurgical transsphenoidal hypophysectomy has been shown to be effective for the treatment of feline pituitary-dependent hyperadrenocorticism (see Chapter 7) (Meij et al, 2001), but use of this specialized surgical technique for the treatment of feline acromegaly has not been reported. Successful use of transsphenoidal cryotherapy of a pituitary tumor has been described in a cat with acromegaly (Abrams-Ogg et al, 1993). Unfortunately, the role of surgical techniques in the treatment of feline acromegaly will remain limited for the foreseeable future because of the need for specialized surgical expertise and equipment.

Prognosis

The short-term and long-term prognoses for cats with tumor-induced acromegaly are guarded to good and poor, respectively. Survival time has ranged from 4 to 60 months (typically 1.5 to 3 years) from the time the diagnosis of acromegaly is established. The GH-secreting pituitary tumor usually grows slowly, and neurologic signs associated with an expanding tumor are uncommon until late in the disorder. Diabetes mellitus is very difficult to control, even with the administration of large doses of insulin (20 U or more per injection) given twice daily. Administration of large doses of insulin should be avoided. The severity of insulin resistance fluctuates unpredictably in cats with acromegaly, and severe, life-threatening hypoglycemia may suddenly develop after months of insulin resistance and blood glucose concentrations in excess of 400 mg/dl. Two of our untreated acromegalic cats died months after the diagnosis had been established because of hypoglycemic coma caused by a sudden and unexpected improvement in insulin sensitivity while the cats were receiving large amounts of insulin (i.e., 18 and 20 U per injection). To avoid severe hypoglycemia, insulin doses should not exceed 12 to 15 U per injection. Most cats with acromegaly eventually die or are euthanized because of the development of severe congestive heart failure, renal failure, respiratory distress, the neurologic signs of an expanding pituitary tumor, or coma caused by severe hypoglycemia.

CANINE ACROMEGALY

Etiology

PROGESTERONE. Progesterone-induced acromegaly is the most common type of acromegaly in the dog. Acromegaly may develop after prolonged administration of progestins, especially MPA, or during the diestrual phase of the estrous cycle in the intact older female dog (Eigenmann and Rijnberk, 1981; Eigenmann et al, 1983a). Hypersomatotropism does not appear to be common in the pregnant female dog in which elevated progesterone concentrations are also present. Progestin-stimulated plasma GH concentrations do not have a pulsatile secretion pattern, are not sensitive to stimulation with GHRH or clonidine, and are not inhibited by somatostatin (Watson et al, 1987; Selman et al, 1991). The progestin-stimulated increase in the plasma GH concentration does cause an increase in the plasma IGF-I concentration (Selman et al, 1994a). Subsequent studies identified foci of hyperplastic ductular epithelium of the mammary gland as the site of origin of GH production induced by progestins (Selman et al, 1994b). The expression of the gene encoding GH has been demonstrated in canine mammary gland tissue (Mol et al, 1995), and sequence analysis has revealed that the gene encoding GH in the mammary gland is identical to the pituitary GH gene (Mol et al, 1996). Stimulation of GH secretion by exogenous progestins appears to be dose related, with larger dosages producing higher basal GH concentrations (Scott and Concannon, 1983). Dosages of MPA ranging from 10 mg/kg every 3 weeks to as little as 50 mg/kg twice yearly have been shown to cause acromegaly (Eigenmann and Rijnberk, 1981; Eigenmann et al, 1983a). Estrogen priming amplifies MPA-induced GH overproduction in the ovariohysterectomized dog (Eigenmann and Eigenmann, 1981b). Estrogen priming has been shown to increase progesterone receptor concentrations in the brain, hypothalamus, and pituitary gland.

PITUITARY AND HYPOTHALAMIC NEOPLASIA. Acromegaly caused by a GH-secreting pituitary somatotropic adenoma is rare in the dog. Only one case has been reported in the literature involving a 9-year-old male Doberman Pinscher with severe insulin-resistant diabetes mellitus; acromegalic changes were not identified on physical examination. Although the serum GH and IGF-I concentrations were not measured, necropsy revealed a pituitary adenoma 0.5 cm in diameter, and immunohistochemical staining for GH showed a strong immunolabeling for GH within the cytoplasm of the tumor cells (van Keulen et al, 1996).

Hypersomatotropism has been reported in a young dog secondary to a hypothalamic astrocytoma (Nelson et al, 1981). The excessive secretion of GH suggested impaired secretion of somatostatin or increased secretion of GHRH in this dog. Interestingly, this animal was brought to a veterinarian because of signs consistent with the human diencephalon syndrome (i.e., alertness, polyphagia, severe weight loss), a syndrome potentially resulting from hypersomatotropism in infants.

Pathophysiology

See page 70.

Signalment

No apparent breed or age predilection exists for canine acromegaly. Almost all reported cases of spontaneously occurring disease have been seen in intact older female dogs because of the role progesterone plays in stimulating GH secretion. In one report of seven acromegalic female dogs, the mean age at the time of initial presentation to the veterinarian was 10 years, with a range of 8 to 11 years (Eigenmann and Venker-van Haagen, 1981). In the same study, the mean age was 7.7 years, with a range of 4 to 11 years, in 15 female dogs with progestin-induced acromegaly. These dogs had been receiving MPA (50 mg twice yearly) for an undisclosed period of time to prevent estrus.

Clinical signs

The anabolic IGF-I–induced clinical signs usually predominate in dogs with progestin-induced acromegaly, although carbohydrate intolerance and diabetes mellitus may develop (see Table 2-14). The length of time between initiation of progestin therapy and onset of clinical signs of acromegaly is variable and depends in part on the dosage and frequency of administration of the progesterone compound. In the dog, elevations in GH concentrations have been documented within 9 weeks of initiating MPA therapy (10 mg/kg body weight every 3 weeks) (Eigenmann and Rijnberk, 1981).

The most consistent clinical sign is inspiratory respiratory distress and stridor, which arise from an increase in the soft tissues in the orolingual, oropharyngeal, and orolaryngeal areas (Rijnberk, 2000). The resultant impairment in respiration results in exercise intolerance, fatigue, and frequent panting.

Cardiomyopathy may be a sequela of acromegaly and, if present, may also cause respiratory signs.

IGF-I–induced proliferation of bone and especially connective tissue results in an increase in body size, most frequently manifested as enlargement of the limbs, feet, head, and abdomen (Rijnberk, 2000). The face may become broad, with prominent jowls, a protruding mandible (prognathia inferior), and an increase in the interdental spaces. Degenerative arthropathies may develop in chronic cases, and enlargement of the viscera may be evident on palpation of the abdomen.

The skin becomes palpably thickened and develops excessive folds, especially about the head, neck, and distal extremities (Scott and Concannon, 1983). The dermal changes are a result of connective tissue proliferation and the accumulation of intercellular matrix. Dermal deposition of hyaluronates leads to interstitial edema (i.e., myxedema), causing the skin to feel puffy. Hypertrichosis and thick, hard claws may also develop (Scott et al, 2001).

Progestin-induced clinical signs may also develop, including mammary nodules or a vaginal discharge subsequent to development of an open cervix pyometra (Eigenmann and Venker-van Haagen, 1981). Clinical signs of a closed cervix pyometra may also develop (see Chapter 23).

Clinical pathology

See page 74.

Dermatohistopathology

Dermatohistopathologic findings in dogs with acromegaly include variable degrees of orthokeratotic hyperkeratosis, hypergranulosis, and dermal and epidermal hyperplasia (Scott and Concannon, 1983). Dermal hyperplasia is the most striking and characteristic feature, with an increased amount of collagen and increased numbers of fibroblasts giving the dermis a dense, compact, cellular, and often thickened appearance. Diffuse mucinous degeneration (myxedema) may also be present.

The primary histopathologic differential diagnosis for the cutaneous changes seen in canine acromegaly is hypothyroidism. Additional dermatohistopathologic findings suggestive of hypothyroidism include sebaceous gland atrophy, follicular keratosis and atrophy, a predominance of telogen hair follicles, and hypertrophied/vacuolated arrector pili muscles.

Diagnostic imaging

See page 74.

Hormonal evaluation

The serum GH and IGF-I concentrations are usually increased in dogs with progesterone-induced acromegaly. In one study, the serum GH concentration ranged from 11 to 1476 ng/ml in a group of dogs with spontaneous and progestin-induced disease (normal, less than 5 ng/ml) (Eigenmann and Venker-van Haagen, 1981). In another study, the mean (± SE) serum IGF-I concentrations were 679 ± 116 ng/ml and 280 ± 23 ng/ml in 20 acromegalic dogs and 13 normal German Shepherd dogs, respectively (Eigenmann et al, 1984b). Nonsuppressibility of basal GH levels after intravenous administration of glucose has also been demonstrated in the acromegalic dog and is further evidence for acromegaly (Eigenmann and Venker-van Haagen, 1981). Glucose (1 g/kg body weight, 50% solution) is given intravenously, and the GH concentration is measured before and 15, 30, 45, 60, and 90 minutes after glucose loading. Acromegalic dogs should show minimal to no decrease in serum GH concentrations after glucose administration, whereas GH concentrations should decrease well into the normal range in healthy dogs. The reader is referred to page 75 for more information on GH and IGF-I in acromegaly.

Although overt diabetes mellitus is not as common in dogs with progesterone-induced acromegaly as in cats with a GH-secreting pituitary tumor, the results of glucose tolerance testing in dogs with hypersomatotropism reveal glucose intolerance, hyperinsulinemia, and an abnormal insulin response to a glucose load (Eigenmann et al, 1983a). Increased baseline insulin concentrations may not increase further during the test, whereas more moderately elevated insulin concentrations may or may not increase after glucose administration. Glucose tolerance is extremely impaired in hypersomatotropism. In one study, the mean (± SE) glucose disappearance coefficient (K value) in 21 dogs with hypersomatotropism was 0.9 ± 0.1 (± SE), whereas it was 3.9 ± 0.2 in 20 healthy dogs (Eigenmann et al, 1983a). The reader is referred to Chapter 11 for details on performing the glucose tolerance test.

Baseline thyroid hormone concentrations, when measured, are usually normal but can be low in dogs with progesterone-induced acromegaly (Rijnberk et al, 1980; Eigenmann and Venker-van Haagen, 1981). Low thyroid hormone concentrations are presumably a result of the euthyroid sick syndrome (see Chapter 3, page 128) rather than primary hypothyroidism per se. The intrinsic glucocorticoid-like activity of exogenous progestins may suppress ACTH secretion, causing secondary adrenal insufficiency. As such, plasma cortisol concentrations may be low in dogs in which acromegaly is created by chronic administration of progestins (Concannon et al, 1980).

Definitive diagnosis

A tentative diagnosis of acromegaly in the dog is based on the presence of appropriate clinical signs and physical examination findings in an older, intact, cycling female or in a dog with a history of chronic progestin administration. The most common clinical manifestations are respiratory signs resulting from an increase in the soft tissues in the oropharyngeal area, an increase in body size (especially the skull and feet), prognathia inferior, an increase in the interdental spaces, and thickened, myxedematous skin thrown into excessive folds. A definitive diagnosis requires documentation of increased serum GH or IGF-I concentrations. Unfortunately, measurement of the GH concentration in dogs is not readily available commercially; the diagnosis, therefore, is usually based on appropriate clinical signs in conjunction with (1) identification of diestrus in an older female dog or (2) a history of chronic progestin administration.

Treatment

PROGESTERONE-INDUCED HYPERSOMATOTROPISM. Withdrawal of exogenous progestin therapy or ovariohysterectomy is the therapy of choice in female dogs with acromegaly arising from progesterone stimulation. In one study, serum GH concentrations returned to normal after ovariohysterectomy in 12 acromegalic female dogs (pretherapy the levels were 82.9 ± 35.9 ng/ml; posttherapy they were 2.8 ± 0.7 ng/ml) (Eigenmann and Venker-van Haagen, 1981). The anabolically induced clinical signs (e.g., increased soft tissue in the oropharyngeal region) are reversible after correction of the hypersomatotropism. Disappearance of the catabolic abnormalities, especially carbohydrate intolerance, depends on the functional status of the pancreatic β-cells. If an adequate population of functional β-cells is present at the time the source of progesterone is removed, as suggested by the presence of hyperinsulinemia, carbohydrate intolerance and hyperglycemia may be reversible after correction of the hypersomatotropism. If the population of functional β-cells is severely decreased, permanent diabetes mellitus can be anticipated.

PITUITARY NEOPLASIA. See page 78.

Prognosis

The prognosis for progesterone-induced hypersomatotropism is good. All of the clinical manifestations, except hypoinsulinemic diabetes mellitus, are potentially reversible after discontinuation of the exogenous progestin or ovariohysterectomy.

REFERENCES

Abrams-Ogg ACG, et al: Acromegaly in the cat: Diagnosis with magnetic resonance imaging and treatment by cryohypophysectomy. Can Vet J 34:682, 1993.

Abribat T, et al: Growth hormone response induced by synthetic human growth hormone releasing factor (1-44) in healthy dogs. J Vet Med 36:367, 1989.

Aron DC, et al: Hypothalamus and Pituitary. In Greenspan FS, Gardner DG (eds): Basic and Clinical Endocrinology, 6th ed. New York, Lange Medical Books/McGraw-Hill, 2001, p 100.

Ascacio-Martinez JA, et al: A dog growth hormone: cDNA codes for a mature protein identical to pig growth hormone. Gene 143:277, 1994.

Ashley PF, et al: Effect of oral melatonin administration on sex hormone, prolactin, and thyroid hormone concentrations in adult dogs. J Am Vet Med Assoc 215:1111, 1999.

Bell AG, et al: Growth hormone responsive dermatosis in three dogs. NZ Vet J 41:195, 1993.

Benjamin M: Cysts (large follicles) and colloid in pituitary glands. Gen Comp Endocrinol 45:425, 1981.

Boord M, Griffin C: Progesterone secreting adrenal mass in a cat with clinical signs of hyperadrenocorticism. J Am Vet Med Assoc 214:666, 1999.

Bratusch-Marrain PR, et al: The effect of growth hormone on glucose metabolism and insulin secretion in man. J Clin Endocrinol Metab 55:973, 1982.

Buonomo FC, Baile CA: The neurophysiological regulation of growth hormone secretion. Dom Anim Endocr 7:435, 1990.

Campbell K: Growth hormone–related disorders in dogs. Compend Cont Ed Sm Anim Pract 10:477, 1988.

Church DB, et al: Effects of proligestone and megestrol on plasma adrenocorticotrophic hormone, insulin and insulin-like growth factor-I concentrations in cats. Res Vet Sci 56:175, 1994.

Concannon P, et al: Growth hormone, prolactin, and cortisol in dogs developing mammary nodules and an acromegaly-like appearance during treatment with medroxyprogesterone acetate. Endocrinology 106:1173, 1980.

Conzemius MG, et al: Correlation between longitudinal bone growth, growth hormone, and insulin-like growth factor-I in prepubertal dogs. Am J Vet Res 59:1608, 1998.

Daughaday WH: The anterior pituitary. In Wilson JD, Foster DW (eds): Williams Textbook of Endocrinology. Philadelphia, WB Saunders, 1985, p 568.

Davies RR, et al: Effects of somatostatin analogue SMS 201-995 in normal man. Clin Endocrinol (Oxf) 24:665, 1986.

Davis DH, et al: Results of surgical treatment for growth hormone–secreting pituitary adenomas. J Neurosurg 79:70, 1993.

Drucker WD, Peterson ME: Advances in the diagnosis and management of canine Cushing's syndrome. Proceedings of the 31st Gaines Veterinary Symposium, Baton Rouge, La, 1981, p 17.

Eigenmann JE: Diagnosis and treatment of dwarfism in a German Shepherd dog. JAAHA 17:798, 1981.

Eigenmann JE: Diagnosis and treatment of pituitary dwarfism in dogs. Proceedings of the Sixth Kal Kan Symposium, Columbus, Ohio, 1983, p 107.

Eigenmann JE: Insulin-like growth factor-I in the dog. Front Horm Res 17:161, 1987.

Eigenmann JE, Eigenmann RY: Radioimmunoassay of canine growth hormone. Acta Endocrinol 98:514, 1981a.

Eigenmann JE, Eigenmann RY: Influence of medroxyprogesterone acetate (Provera) on plasma growth hormone levels and on carbohydrate metabolism. II. Studies in the ovariohysterectomized, oestradiol-primed bitch. Acta Endocrinol 98:603, 1981b.

Eigenmann JE, Patterson DF: Growth hormone deficiency in the mature dog. JAAHA 20:741, 1984.

Eigenmann JE, Rijnberk A: Influence of medroxyprogesterone acetate (Provera) on plasma growth hormone levels and on carbohydrate metabolism. I. Studies in the ovariohysterectomized bitch. Acta Endocrinol 98:599, 1981.

Eigenmann JE, Venker-van Haagen AJ: Progestagen-induced and spontaneous canine acromegaly due to reversible growth hormone overproduction: Clinical picture and pathogenesis. JAAHA 17:813, 1981.

Eigenmann JE, et al: Progesterone-controlled growth hormone overproduction and naturally occurring canine diabetes and acromegaly. Acta Endocrinol 104:167, 1983a.

Eigenmann JE, et al: Panhypopituitarism caused by a suprasellar tumor in a dog. JAAHA 19:377, 1983b.

Eigenmann JE, et al: Body size parallels insulin-like growth factor-I levels but not growth hormone secretory capacity. Acta Endocrinol (Copenh) 106:448, 1984a.

Eigenmann JE, et al: Insulin-like growth factor-I in the dog: A study in different dog breeds and in dogs with growth hormone elevation. Acta Endocrinol (Copenh) 105:294, 1984b.

Eigenmann JE, et al: Growth hormone and insulin-like growth factor-I in German Shepherd dwarf dogs. Acta Endocrinol (Copenh) 105:289, 1984c.

Eigenmann JE, et al: Elevated growth hormone levels and diabetes mellitus in a cat with acromegalic features. J Am Anim Hosp Assoc 20:747, 1984d.

Elliott DA, et al: Prevalence of pituitary tumors among diabetic cats with insulin resistance. J Am Vet Med Assoc 216:1765, 2000.

Favier RP, et al: Large body size in the dog is associated with transient GH excess at a young age. J Endocrinol 170:479, 2001.

Feld S, Hirschberg R: Growth hormone, the insulin-like growth factor system, and the kidney. Endocr Rev 17:423, 1996.

Ferry RJ, et al: Insulin-like growth factor binding proteins: new proteins, new function. Horm Res 51:34, 1999.

Fofanova O, et al: Compound heterozygous deletion of the PROP-1 gene in children with combined pituitary hormone deficiency. J Clin Endocrinol Metab 83:2601, 1998.

Frank LA, et al: Steroidogenic response of adrenal tissues after administration of ACTH to dogs with hypercortisolemia. J Am Vet Med Assoc 218:214, 2001.

French MB, et al: Secretory pattern of canine growth hormone. Am J Physiol 252:E268, 1987.

Fuh G, et al: Rational design of potent antagonists to the human growth hormone receptor. Science 256:1677, 1992.

Goddard AD, et al: Mutations of the growth hormone receptor in children with idiopathic short stature. N Engl J Med 333:1093, 1995.

Goossens MMC, et al: Cobalt 60 irradiation of pituitary gland tumors in three cats with acromegaly. J Am Vet Med Assoc 213:374, 1998.

Gross TL, et al: Veterinary Dermatopathology: A Macroscopic and Microscopic Evaluation of Canine and Feline Skin Disease. St Louis, Mosby–Year Book, 1992.

Hamann F, et al: Pituitary function and morphology in two German Shepherd dogs with congenital dwarfism. Vet Rec 144:644, 1999.

Hampshire J, Altszuler N: Clonidine or xylazine as provocative tests for growth hormone secretion in the dog. Am J Vet Res 42:1073, 1981.

Herrtage ME, Evans H: The effect of progestogen administration on insulin-like growth factor concentrations in two pituitary dwarfs. J Vet Int Med 12:212, 1998 (abstract).

Isaksson OGP, et al: Mechanism of the stimulatory effect of growth hormone on longitudinal bone growth. Endocr Rev 8:426, 1987.

Johanson NA, et al: Acromegalic arthropathy of the hip. Clin Orthop 173:130, 1983.

Kooistra HS, et al: Progestin-induced growth hormone (GH) production in the treatment of dogs with congenital GH deficiency. Dom Anim Endocr 15:93, 1998.

Kooistra HS, et al: Pulsatile secretion pattern of growth hormone during the luteal phase and mid-anoestrus in Beagle bitches. J Repro Fertil 199:217, 2000a.

Kooistra HS, et al: Confirmed pituitary hormone deficiency in German Shepherd dogs with dwarfism. Dom Anim Endo 19:177, 2000b.

Lanes R, et al: Dwarfism associated with normal serum growth hormone and increased bioassayable, receptorassayable, and immunoassayable somatomedin. J Clin Endocrinol Metab 50:485, 1980.

Lantinga-van Leeuwen IS, et al: Cloning, characterization, and physical mapping of the canine Prop 1 gene: exclusion as a candidate gene for combined pituitary hormone deficiency in German Shepherd dogs. Cytogenet Cell Genet 88:140, 2000a.

Lantinga-van Leeuwen IS, et al: Cloning of the canine gene encoding transcription factor Pit-1 and its exclusion as candidate gene in a canine model of pituitary dwarfism. Mamm Genome 11:31, 2000b.

Lazarus L: Growth hormone. In Donald RA (ed): Endocrine Disorders: A Guide to Diagnosis. New York, Marcel Dekker, 1984, p 273.

Lee PD, et al: Insulin-like growth factor binding protein-1: Recent findings and new directions. Proc Soc Exp Biol Med 216:319, 1997.

Lewitt MS, et al: Regulation of insulin-like growth factor binding protein-3 ternary complex in feline diabetes mellitus. J Endocrinol 166:21, 2000.

Lothrop CD: Growth hormone response to growth hormone–releasing factor in normal and suspected growth hormone–deficient dogs. Proceedings of the Fourth Annual Veterinary Medical Forum, Washington, DC, 1986, p 14.

Lothrop CD: Pathophysiology of growth hormone–responsive dermatosis. Compend Cont Educ Pract Vet 10:1346, 1988.

Lothrop CD, Schmeitzel LP: Growth hormone–responsive alopecia in dogs. Vet Med Rep 2:82, 1990.

Mandel S, et al: Changes in insulin-like growth factor-1 (IGF-1), IGF-binding protein-3, growth hormone (GH)–binding protein, erythrocyte IGF-1 receptors, and growth rate during GH treatment. J Clin Endocrinol Metab 80:190, 1995.

Maxwell A, et al: Nutritional modulation of canine insulin-like growth factors and their binding proteins. J Endocrinol 158:77, 1998.

Maxwell A, et al: Reduced serum insulin-like growth factor (IGF) and IGF-binding protein-3 concentrations in two Deerhounds with congenital portosystemic shunts. J Vet Intern Med 14:542, 2000.

Meij BP, et al: Assessment of a combined anterior pituitary function test in Beagle dogs: Rapid sequential intravenous administration of four hypothalamic releasing hormones. Dom Anim Endocr 13:161, 1996.

Meij BP, et al: Transsphenoidal hypophysectomy for treatment of pituitary-dependent hyperadrenocorticism in 7 cats. Vet Surg 30:72, 2001.

Melmed S: Acromegaly. N Engl J Med 322:966, 1990.

Melmed S, et al: Acromegaly due to secretion of growth hormone by an ectopic pancreatic islet cell tumor. N Engl J Med 312:9, 1985.

Middleton DJ, et al: Growth hormone–producing pituitary adenoma, elevated serum somatomedin C concentration and diabetes mellitus in a cat. Can Vet J 26:169, 1985.

Mol JA, Rijnberk A: Pituitary function. In Kaneko JJ, Harvey JW, Bruss MI (eds): Clinical Biochemistry of Domestic Animals. San Diego, Academic Press, 1997, p 517.

Mol JA, et al: Growth hormone mRNA in mammary gland tumors of dogs and cats. J Clin Invest 95:2028, 1995.

Mol JA, et al: New insights in the molecular mechanism of progestin-induced proliferation of mammary epithelium: Induction of the local biosynthesis of growth hormone (GH) in the mammary gland of dogs, cats and humans. J Steroid Biochem Molec Biol 57:67, 1996.

Morrison SA, et al: Hypersomatotropism and insulin-resistant diabetes mellitus in a cat. JAVMA 194:91, 1989.

Muller-Peddinghaus R, et al: Hypophysarer zwergwuchs beim deutschen schaferhund. Vet Pathol 17:406, 1980.

Nap RC, et al: Age-related plasma concentrations of growth hormone (GH) and insulin-like growth factor (IGF-I) in Great Dane pups fed different dietary levels of protein. Dom Anim Endocr 10:237, 1993.

Nelson RW, et al: Diencephalic syndrome secondary to intracranial astrocytoma in a dog. JAVMA 179:1004, 1981.

Paradis M: Melatonin therapy for canine alopecia. In Bonagura JD (ed): Kirk's Current Veterinary Therapy XIII. Philadelphia, WB Saunders, 2000, p 546.

Parker WM, Scott DW: Growth hormone–responsive alopecia in the mature dog: A discussion of 13 cases. JAAHA 16:824, 1980.

Pellegrini-Bouiller I, et al: A new mutation of the gene encoding the transcription factor Pit-1 is responsible for combined pituitary hormone deficiency. J Clin Endocrinol Metab 81:2790, 1996.

Peterson ME: Effects of megestrol acetate on glucose tolerance and growth hormone secretion in the cat. Res Vet Sci 42:354, 1987.

Peterson ME, Altszuler N: Suppression of growth hormone secretion in spontaneous canine hyperadrenocorticism and its reversal after treatment. Am J Vet Res 42:1881, 1981.

Peterson ME, et al: Acromegaly in 14 cats. J Vet Intern Med 4:192, 1990.

Plewe G, et al: Long-acting and selective suppression of growth hormone secretion by somatostatin analogue SMS 201-995 in acromegaly. Lancet 2:782, 1984.

Randolph JF, et al: Delayed growth in two German Shepherd dog littermates with normal serum concentrations of growth hormone, thyroxine, and cortisol. JAVMA 196:77, 1990.

Regnier A, Garnier F: Growth hormone responses to growth hormone–releasing hormone and clonidine in dogs with Cushing's syndrome. Res Vet Sci 58:169, 1995.

Regnier A, et al: Effect of propranolol on growth hormone response to GH-releasing hormone (GHRH 1-44) in the dog. Res Vet Sci 52:110, 1992.

Reichlin S: Neuroendocrinology. In Wilson JD, Foster DW, Kronenberg HM, Larsen PR (eds): Williams Textbook of Endocrinology, 9th ed. Philadelphia, WB Saunders, 1998, p 165.

Reiter EO, Rosenfeld RG: Normal and aberrant growth. In Wilson JD, Foster DW, Kronenberg HM, Larsen PR (eds): Williams Textbook of Endocrinology, 9th ed. Philadelphia, WB Saunders, 1998, p 1427.

Reubi JC, Landolt AM: The growth hormone responses to octreotide in acromegaly correlate with adenoma somatostatin receptor status. J Clin Endocrinol Metab 68:844, 1989.

Rijnberk A: Acromegaly. In Ettinger SJ, Feldman EC (eds): Textbook of Veterinary Internal Medicine, 5th ed. Philadelphia, WB Saunders, 2000, p 1370.

Rijnberk A, et al: Acromegaly associated with transient overproduction of growth hormone in a dog. JAVMA 177:534, 1980.

Rijnberk A, et al: Disturbed release of growth hormone in mature dogs: A comparison with congenital growth hormone deficiency. Vet Rec 133:542, 1993.

Ristic JME, et al: Plasma 17-hydroxyprogesterone concentrations in the diagnosis of canine hyperadrenocorticism. J Vet Int Med 15:298, 2001 (abstract).

Rosenfeld RG, et al: Both human pituitary growth hormone and recombinant DNA–derived human growth hormone cause insulin resistance at a postreceptor site. J Clin Endocrinol Metab 54:1033, 1982.

Rosenfeld RG, et al: Growth hormone (GH) insensitivity due to primary GH receptor deficiency. Endocr Rev 15:369, 1994.

Rosenkrantz WS, Griffin C: Lysodren therapy in suspect adrenal sex hormone dermatosis. Proceedings of the Second World Congress of Veterinary Dermatology, Montreal, Canada, May, 1992, p 121.

Rossmeisl JH, et al: Hyperadrenocorticism and hyperprogesteronemia in a cat with an adrenocortical adenocarcinoma. J Am Anim Hosp Assoc 36:512, 2000.

Roth JA, et al: Thymic abnormalities and growth hormone deficiency in dogs. Am J Vet Res 41:1256, 1980.

Sandhu MS, et al: Circulating concentrations of insulin-like growth factor-1 and development of glucose intolerance: a prospective observational study. Lancet 359:1740, 2002.

Scheven BAA, Hamilton NJ: Longitudinal bone growth in vitro: effects of insulin-like growth factor-I and growth hormone. Acta Endocrinol (Copenh) 124:602, 1991.

Schmeitzel LP: Sex hormone–related and growth hormone–related alopecias. Vet Clin North Am 20:1579, 1990.

Schmeitzel LP, Lothrop CD: Hormonal abnormalities in Pomeranians with normal coat and in Pomeranians with growth hormone–responsive dermatosis. JAVMA 197:1333, 1990.

Schmeitzel LP, et al: Congenital adrenal hyperplasia–like syndrome. In Bonagura JD (ed): Kirk's Current Veterinary Therapy XII. Philadelphia, WB Saunders, 1995, p 600.

Scott DW, Concannon PW: Gross and microscopic changes in the skin of dogs with progestagen-induced acromegaly and elevated growth hormone levels. JAAHA 19:523, 1983.

Scott DW, Walton DK: Hyposomatotropism in the mature dog: A discussion of 22 cases. JAAHA 22:467, 1986.

Scott DW, Miller WH, Griffin CE (eds): Muller & Kirk's Small Animal Dermatology, 6th ed. Philadelphia, WB Saunders, 2001, p 780.

Secchi C, et al: Amino acid modifications in canine, equine, and porcine pituitary growth hormones, identified by peptide-mass mapping. J Chromatography 757:237, 2001.

Selman PJ, et al: Progestins and growth hormone excess in the dog. Acta Endocrinol 125[suppl 1]:42, 1991.

Selman PJ, et al: Progestin treatment in the dog: I. Effects on growth hormone, IGF-1, and glucose homeostasis. Eur J Endocrinol 131:413, 1994a.

Selman PJ, et al: Progestin-induced growth hormone excess in the dog originates in the mammary gland. Endocrinology 134:287, 1994b.

Sheng HZ, et al: Multistep control of pituitary organogenesis. Science 278:1809, 1997.

Simmons DM, et al: Pituitary cell phenotypes involve cell-specific Pit-1 mRNA translation and synergistic interactions with other classes of transcription factors. Genes Dev 4:695, 1990.

Stewart PM, et al: Normal growth hormone response to the 75 g oral glucose tolerance test measured by immunoradiometric assay. Ann Clin Biochem 26:205, 1989.

Styne D: Growth. *In* Greenspan FS, Gardner DG (eds): Basic and Clinical Endocrinology, 6th ed. New York, Lange Medical Books/McGraw-Hill, 2001, p 163.

Takahashi Y, et al: Short stature caused by a mutant growth hormone. N Engl J Med 334:432, 1996.

Thorner MO, et al: Human pancreatic growth hormone–releasing factor selectively stimulates growth hormone secretion in man. Lancet 1:24, 1983.

Thorner MO, et al: The anterior pituitary. *In* Wilson JD, Foster DW, Kronenberg HM, Larsen PR (eds): Williams Textbook of Endocrinology, 9th ed. Philadelphia, WB Saunders, 1998, p 249.

Trainer PJ, et al: Treatment of acromegaly with the growth hormone receptor antagonist pegvisomant. N Engl J Med 342:1171, 2000.

Treier M, et al: Multistep signaling requirements for pituitary organogenesis in vivo. Genes Dev 12:1691, 1998.

van den Heuvel PACMB, et al: Myocardial involvement in acromegaly. Int J Cardiol 6:550, 1984.

van der Lely AJ, et al: Long-term treatment of acromegaly with pegvisomant, a growth hormone receptor antagonist. Lancet 358:1754, 2001.

Van Herpen H, et al: Production of antibodies to biosynthetic human growth hormone in the dog. Vet Rec 134:171, 1994.

van Keulen LJM, et al: Diabetes mellitus in a dog with a growth hormone–producing acidophilic adenoma of the adenohypophysis. Vet Pathol 33:451, 1996.

Van Wyk JJ, et al: Role of somatomedin in cellular proliferation. *In* Ritzen ER (ed): Biology of Normal Human Growth. New York, Raven Press, 1981, p 223.

Voss JW, Rosenfeld MG: Anterior pituitary development: short tales from dwarf mice. Cell 70:527, 1992.

Watkins-Chow DE, Camper SA: How many homeobox genes does it take to make a pituitary gland? Trends in Genetics 14:284, 1998.

Watson ADJ, et al: Effect of somatostatin analogue SMS 201-995 and antiprogestin agent RU486 in canine acromegaly. Front Horm Res 17:193, 1987.

Willeberg P, et al: Pituitary dwarfism in German Shepherd dogs: Studies on somatomedin activity. Nord Vet Med 27:448, 1975.

Wu W, et al: Mutations in Prop-1 cause familial combined pituitary hormone deficiency. Nature Genet 18:147, 1998.

Yakar S, et al: Normal growth and development in the absence of hepatic insulin-like growth factor-I. Proc Natl Acad Sci USA 96:7324, 1999.

THE THYROID GLAND

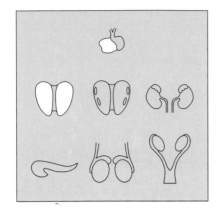

3

HYPOTHYROIDISM

PHYSIOLOGY OF THE THYROID GLAND

THYROID HORMONE SYNTHESIS. The basic functional unit of the thyroid gland is the follicle, a hollow sphere of cells surrounded by a basement membrane (Fig. 3-1). The wall of the follicle is a single layer of thyroid cells, which are cuboidal when quiescent and columnar when active. The follicular lumen contains colloid, a viscous gel that is primarily a store of thyroglobulin secreted by the thyroid cells. Thyroglobulin is a large glycoprotein dimer containing iodotyrosines that serve as precursors for thyroid hormone synthesis.

Adequate ingestion of iodide is a prerequisite for the normal synthesis of thyroid hormones by the thyroid. Iodide is actively transported from the extracellular fluid into the thyroid follicular cell, where it is rapidly oxidized by thyroid peroxidase into a reactive intermediate that is then incorporated into the tyrosine residues of acceptor proteins, primarily thyroglobulin (Greenspan, 2001). Iodinated tyrosine residues (monoiodotyrosine [MIT], diiodotyrosine [DIT]) in thyroglobulin combine to form iodothyronines—thyroxine and triiodothyronine (Fig. 3-2).

Thyroglobulin is stored extracellularly in the follicular lumen. As a prerequisite for thyroid hormone secretion into the blood, thyroglobulin must first reenter the thyroid cell and undergo proteolysis. Pseudopods from the apical cell surface extend into the colloid in the follicular lumen, and large colloid droplets enter the cytoplasm by endocytosis (Greenspan, 2001). Each colloid droplet is enclosed in a membrane derived from the apical cell border. Electron-dense lysosomes then fuse with the colloid droplets to produce phagolysosomes. These phagolysosomes migrate toward the basal aspect of the cell, during which time lysosomal proteases hydrolyze thyroglobulin. Thyroxine and, to a much lesser degree, triiodothyronine liberated from thyroglobulin by the proteolytic process pass from the phagolysosome into the blood, possibly by diffusion. Most of the liberated

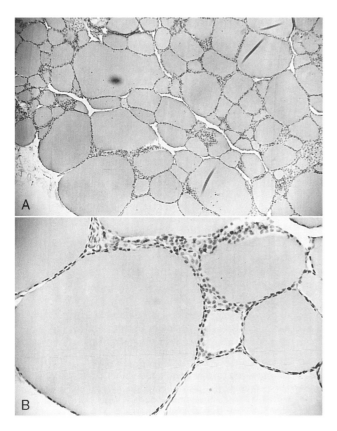

FIGURE 3–1. *A* and *B,* Histologic section of a thyroid gland from a healthy dog, illustrating variable-sized follicles, each lined by follicular epithelial cells and filled with an amorphous material, colloid. (*A,* H&E ×40; *B,* H&E ×160)

when the thyroid cells are damaged, such as occurs with lymphocytic thyroiditis.

REGULATION OF THYROID FUNCTION. Thyroid hormone synthesis and secretion are regulated by extrathyroidal (thyrotropin) and intrathyroidal (autoregulatory) mechanisms. Thyrotropin (TSH) is the major modulator of thyroid activity, the net result of which is increased thyroid hormone secretion (Fig. 3-3). TSH secretion by the pituitary is modulated by thyroid hormone in a negative feedback regulatory mechanism. At the pituitary, it is primarily 3,5,3'-triiodothyronine (T_3), produced locally by the monodeiodination of thyroxine (T_4), that inhibits TSH secretion (Greenspan, 2001). The "thermostat" setting of the thyroid hormone–TSH feedback loop is modulated by thyrotropin-releasing hormone (TRH) from the hypothalamus. Hypothalamic production and release of TRH are controlled by poorly understood neural pathways from higher brain centers.

The thyroid is able to regulate its uptake of iodide and thyroid hormone synthesis by intrathyroidal mechanisms independent of TSH. Examples of autoregulatory mechanisms include the Wolff-Chaikoff block (decrease in thyroglobulin iodination and thyroid hormone synthesis with increasing iodide intake), intrathyroidal alterations in thyroid sensitivity to TSH stimulation, and increased ratio of T_3 to T_4 secretion by the thyroid during periods of iodide insufficiency.

THYROID HORMONES IN PLASMA. Thyroid hormones in plasma are largely bound to protein, most notably thyroid hormone–binding globulin (TBG), thyroxine-binding prealbumin (TBPA), albumin, and certain plasma lipoproteins. Less than 1% of T_4 and T_3 circulate "free" in the unbound state. Free or unbound thyroid hormones enter cells, produce their biologic effects, and are in turn metabolized. Only the free hormone regulates the pituitary feedback mechanism. Protein-bound thyroid hormones serve as a large reservoir that

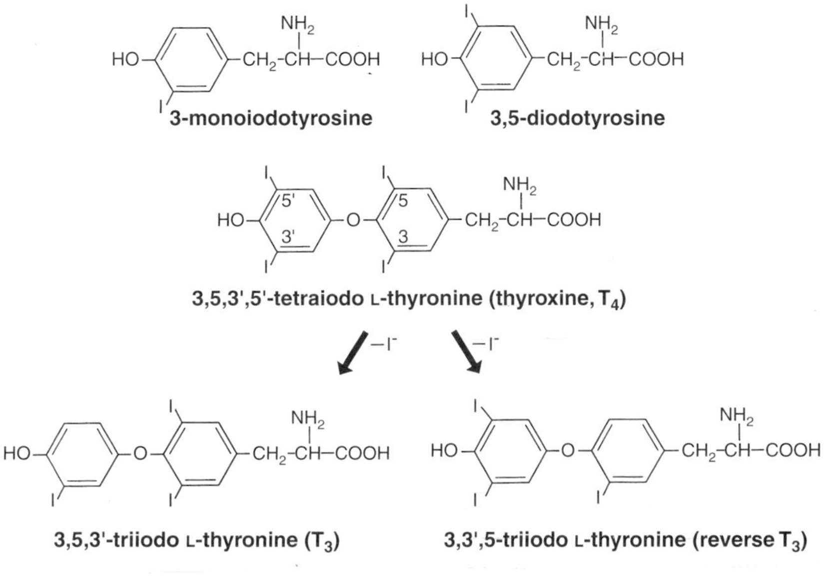

iodotyrosines (MIT, DIT) are deiodinated, thus releasing iodide, which can be reused for thyroglobulin iodination or can diffuse out into the circulation. A small quantity of intact thyroglobulin also enters the circulation. This leakage can be increased

3-monoiodotyrosine

3,5-diodotyrosine

3,5,3',5'-tetraiodo L-thyronine (thyroxine, T_4)

3,5,3'-triiodo L-thyronine (T_3)

3,3',5-triiodo L-thyronine (reverse T_3)

FIGURE 3–2. Structure of the thyroid hormones and their precursors.

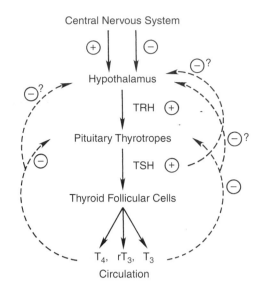

Central Nervous System

Hypothalamus

TRH $+$

Pituitary Thyrotropes

TSH $+$

Thyroid Follicular Cells

$T_4,$ $rT_3,$ T_3

Circulation

FIGURE 3–3. Schematic of the hypothalamic-pituitary-thyroid axis. *TRH,* Thyrotropin-releasing hormone; *TSH,* thyrotropin; $T_4,$ thyroxine; $T_3,$ 3,5,3′-triiodothyronine; $rT_3,$ reverse 3,3′,5′-triiodothyronine; +, stimulation; –, inhibition.

is slowly drawn upon as the free hormone dissociates from the binding proteins and enters the cells. Thyroid hormone secretion is precisely regulated to replenish the metabolized thyroid hormones.

THYROID HORMONE METABOLISM. Thyroxine is the major secretory product of the normal thyroid. The major pathway of T_4 metabolism is the progressive deiodination of the molecule. The initial deiodination of T_4 may occur in the outer ring, producing T_3, or in the inner ring, producing reverse T_3 (rT_3; Fig. 3-2). Because conversion of T_4 to T_3 represents a "step up" in biologic activity, whereas conversion of T_4 to rT_3 has the opposite effect, the conversion of T_4 to T_3 or rT_3 by outer or inner ring iodothyronine deiodinase is a pivotal regulatory step in determining thyroid hormone biologic activity. Less than 20% of total T_3 is produced in the thyroid, and the remaining 80% to 90% is derived from outer ring monodeiodination of T_4 in peripheral tissues. The tissues that concentrate the most thyroid hormone are liver, kidney, and muscle (Greenspan, 2001). Conjugation of thyroid hormone to soluble glucuronides and sulfates with subsequent excretion in the bile and urine represents another major metabolic pathway for thyroid hormone.

THYROID HORMONE ACTIONS. The thyroid hormones affect many metabolic processes, influencing the concentration and activity of numerous enzymes; the metabolism of substrates, vitamins, and minerals; the secretion and degradation rates of virtually all other hormones; and the response of their target tissues to them. Thyroid hormones are critically important in fetal development, particularly of the neural and skeletal systems. Thyroid hormones stimulate calorigenesis, protein and enzyme synthesis, and virtually all aspects of carbohydrate and lipid metabolism, including synthesis, mobilization, and degradation (Larsen et al, 1998). Furthermore, thyroid hormones have marked chronotropic and inotropic effects on the heart; are necessary for normal hypoxic and hypercapnic drive to the respiratory centers; stimulate erythropoiesis; and stimulate bone turnover, increasing both formation and resorption of bone (Greenspan, 2001). In essence, no tissue or organ system escapes the adverse effects of thyroid hormone excess or insufficiency.

CANINE HYPOTHYROIDISM

CLASSIFICATION

Structural or functional abnormalities of the thyroid gland can lead to deficient production of thyroid hormone. A convenient classification scheme is based on the location of the problem within the hypothalamic–pituitary–thyroid gland complex (Fig. 3-3). Primary hypothyroidism is the most common form of this disorder in the dog, resulting from problems within the thyroid gland. In the dog, destruction of the thyroid gland is the usual cause of primary hypothyroidism. Congenital defects in hormonogenesis have also been documented but are rare. Secondary hypothyroidism follows dysfunction within the pituitary thyrotropic cells, causing impaired secretion of TSH and a "secondary" deficiency in thyroid hormone synthesis. Secondary hypothyroidism, rare to uncommon in dogs, could follow destruction of pituitary thyrotrophs (e.g., pituitary neoplasia) or suppression of thyrotroph function by hormones or drugs (e.g., glucocorticoids). Tertiary hypothyroidism is defined as deficient TRH secretion by peptidergic neurons in the supraoptic and paraventricular nuclei of the hypothalamus. Tertiary hypothyroidism has not been reported in dogs and can be assumed to be extremely rare.

Disorders causing secondary or tertiary hypothyroidism would result in thyroid gland atrophy and no real "pathology." The thyroid gland remains potentially responsive to TSH or TRH administration, although the response may be absent or suppressed with chronic lack of stimulation from the pituitary gland. In contrast, progressive pathologic lesions within the thyroid are usually identifiable in dogs with

TABLE 3–1 POTENTIAL CAUSES OF HYPOTHYROIDISM IN THE DOG

Primary Hypothyroidism

Lymphocytic thyroiditis*
Idiopathic atrophy*
Follicular cell hyperplasia (dyshormonogenesis?)*
Neoplastic destruction*-
Iatrogenic*
    Surgical removal
    Antithyroid medications
    Radioactive iodine treatment

Secondary Hypothyroidism

Pituitary malformation*
Pituitary cyst
Pituitary hypoplasia
Pituitary destruction*
    Neoplasia
Pituitary thyrotroph cell suppression*
    Naturally acquired hyperadrenocorticism
    Euthyroid sick syndrome
Defective TSH molecule
Defective TSH-follicular cell receptor interaction
Iatrogenic*
    Drug therapy, most notably glucocorticoids
    Radiation therapy
    Hypophysectomy

Tertiary Hypothyroidism

Congenital hypothalamic malformation
Acquired destruction of hypothalamus
    Neoplasia
    Hemorrhage
    Abscess
    Granuloma
    Inflammation
Defective TRH molecule
Defective TRH-thyrotroph receptor interaction

Congenital Hypothyroidism

Thyroid gland dysgenesis (aplasia, hypoplasia, ectasia)*
Dyshormonogenesis: iodine organification defect*
Circulating thyroid hormone transport abnormalities
Ingestion of goitrogens
Deficient dietary iodine intake*

*Established etiology in the dog

primary disease. Thyroid responsiveness to TSH and TRH becomes severely impaired after significant primary disease. This failure of responsiveness of the thyroid gland to TSH or TRH has historically been used to diagnose the disorder.

ETIOLOGY

Primary Hypothyroidism

Primary hypothyroidism is the most common cause of naturally occurring thyroid failure in the adult dog, accounting for more than 95% of our hypothyroid cases. Two histologic forms of primary hypothyroidism predominate in the dog: lymphocytic thyroiditis and idiopathic atrophy (Table 3-1). The end result of both these forms is the same—progressive destruction of the thyroid gland and resultant deficiency of circulating thyroid hormones.

LYMPHOCYTIC THYROIDITIS. Lymphocytic thyroiditis is characterized histologically by a diffuse infiltration of lymphocytes, plasma cells, and macrophages within the thyroid gland, resulting in progressive destruction of follicles and secondary fibrosis (Gosselin et al, 1981a; Fig. 3-4). Neutrophils are usually not abundant and, when present, are associated with necrotic areas of the thyroid gland. Destruction of the thyroid gland is progressive, and clinical signs may not become evident until more than 75% of the gland is destroyed. Based on experiences following dogs with positive thyroglobulin autoantibody test results (see page 124), the onset of clinical signs and development of decreased serum thyroid hormone and increased serum TSH concentrations is usually a gradual process, often requiring 1 to 3 years to develop, suggesting that the destructive process is slow (Nachreiner et al, 2002). Graham et al (2001a) have proposed several stages in the development of lymphocytic thyroiditis in dogs, beginning with a subclinical stage characterized by positive thyroglobulin and thyroid hormone auto-antibody tests and minimal inflammation in the thyroid gland through progressively worsening inflammation and destruction of the thyroid gland and the eventual development of increased serum TSH and decreased serum thyroid hormone concentrations (Table 3-2). The terminal stages of destruction are characterized by few follicles and extensive adipose connective tissue replacement of atrophied parenchymal structures, with residual infiltrates of lymphocytes and plasma cells interspersed with nests of parafollicular cells and a few small follicles containing degenerating follicular cells and poorly staining colloid (Conaway et al, 1985b). Analysis of age distributions of dogs with laboratory test results (i.e., thyroglobulin antibody, T_4, and TSH) consistent with the different stages or classifications of lymphocytic thyroiditis suggest that the age of peak

TABLE 3–2 PROPOSED FUNCTIONAL STAGES OF LYMPHOCYTIC THYROIDITIS IN DOGS

Stage of Thyroiditis	Clinical Signs of Hypothyroidism	Serum T_4 and fT_4	Serum TSH	Serum Thyroglobulin Autoantibody
I-Subclinical thyroiditis	Not present	Normal	Normal	Positive
II-Subclinical hypothyroidism	Not present	Normal	Increased	Positive
III-Overt hypothyroidism	Present	Decreased	Increased	Positive
IV-Noninflammatory atrophic hypothyroidism	Present	Decreased	Increased	Negative

Adapted from Graham PA, et al: Lymphocytic thyroiditis. Vet Clin North Am 31:915, 2001.
T_4, thyroxine; fT_4, free thyroxine; TSH, thyrotropin.

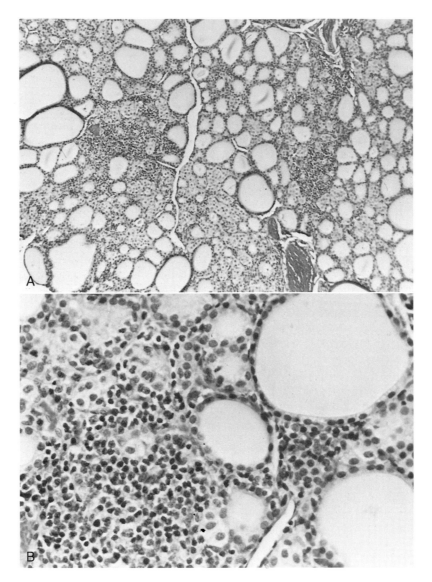

FIGURE 3–4. *A* and *B,* Histologic section of a thyroid gland from a dog with lymphocytic thyroiditis and hypothyroidism. Note the mononuclear cell infiltration, disruption of the normal architecture, and loss of colloid-containing follicles. (*A,* H&E ×63; *B,* H&E ×250)

prevalence progresses by 1 to 2 years through each of the classifications (Graham et al, 2001a). Studies also suggest that differences in progression rate or likelihood of progression may exist for different breeds of dogs.

Lymphocytic thyroiditis is an immune-mediated disorder. Involvement of humoral immune mechanisms is supported by these findings: increased incidence of circulating autoantibodies to thyroid antigens, including thyroglobulin, T_4, and T_3; identification by electron microscopy of thickened basement membranes containing electron-dense deposits, which are believed to be antigen-antibody complexes, in thyroid follicles; and the induction of lesions similar to lymphocytic thyroiditis in dogs following the intrathyroidal injection of thyroglobulin antibodies (Gosselin et al, 1980; 1981a; 1981b; 1981c; Gaschen et al, 1993). Antibody binding to the follicular cell, colloid, or thyroglobulin antigens is believed to activate the complement cascade,

antibody-dependent cell-mediated cytotoxicity, or both, causing follicular cell destruction. Identifiable thyroid antigens include the following: thyroglobulin, which is the main antigen in colloid and has the strongest correlation with the presence of lymphocytic thyroiditis; colloidal antigen (CA-2), a nonthyroglobulin, noniodine component of colloid; microsomal antigen and antinuclear substance antigen, located within the follicular cells; and cell-surface antigen (Gosselin et al, 1980; Vajner, 1997).

The cell-mediated immune system may also play an important, possibly primary, role in the development and perpetuation of lymphocytic thyroiditis. A defect in suppressor T cell function is suspected in this disorder. This would allow effector T lymphocytes to attack follicular cells and allow helper T cells to induce plasma cell differentiation, with subsequent production of thyroid antibodies (Strakosch et al, 1982).

The initiating factors involved in the development of lymphocytic thyroiditis are poorly understood. Genetics undoubtedly plays a major role, especially given the increased incidence of this disorder in certain breeds and in certain lines within a breed (see page 96). Lymphocytic thyroiditis is an inherited disorder in colony-raised Beagles, with a polygenic mode of inheritance, and was identified as an autosomal-recessive trait in a family of Borzoi dogs (Conaway et al, 1985a). An increased frequency of circulating thyroid hormone autoantibodies has also been found in certain breeds (Table 3-3; Nachreiner et al, 2002). Environmental risk factors have not been well defined in the dog. A link between infection and development of lymphocytic thyroiditis has been speculated but not proved (Penhale and Young, 1988). Infection-induced damage to the thyroid gland, causing release of antigens into the circulation and their subsequent exposure to the host's immune system, or antigenic mimicry of thyroid antigens by viral or bacterial agents could initiate the immune-mediated inflammatory process. Vaccine administration has also been hypothesized to be a contributing factor for development of lymphocytic thyroiditis (Smith, 1995; Allbritton, 1996). A recent study documented a significant increase in antibovine and anticanine thyroglobulin antibodies in research Beagles after repeated vaccinations beginning at 8 weeks of age (Scott-Moncrieff et al, 2002). A significant increase in anticanine thyroglobulin antibodies was also documented in adult pet dogs 2 weeks after vaccination. The clinical importance of this finding as it relates to development of lymphocytic thyroiditis is unknown. The study did not determine how long the thyroglobulin antibodies persisted, although antibody levels had decreased to prevaccination values by the time of the next vaccination in most research dogs. None of the dogs in the study, with the exception of three dogs believed to have developed spontaneous thyroiditis, developed evidence of thyroid dysfunction by 4.5 years of age. The authors speculated that the anti-thyroglobulin antibodies detected in their study was the result of contamination of the vaccine by bovine thyroglobulin. There is considerable sequence homology for thyroglobulin between species, and antibodies to thyroglobulin have some species cross-reactivity (Tomer, 1997).

LYMPHOCYTIC THYROIDITIS AND IMMUNOENDO-CRINOPATHY SYNDROMES (POLYGLANDULAR AUTOIMMUNE SYNDROMES). Because autoimmune mechanisms play an important role in the pathogenesis of lymphocytic thyroiditis, it is not surprising that lymphocytic thyroiditis may occur with other immune-mediated endocrine deficiency syndromes. In humans, two polyglandular autoimmune syndromes, type I and type II, predominate (Table 3-4). Polyglandular autoimmune syndrome type II (Schmidt's syndrome) is the most common of the immunoendocrinopathy syndromes in humans and is usually defined by the occurrence of primary adrenal insufficiency in combination with autoimmune thyroid disease, insulin-dependent diabetes mellitus, or both (Neufeld et al, 1981). Combinations of endocrine deficiency disorders (e.g., hypothyroidism and diabetes mellitus; Addison's disease and hypothyroidism) have been documented in dogs (Hargis et al, 1981; Haines and Penhale, 1985; Bowen et al, 1986; Ford et al, 1993; Kooistra et al, 1995; Greco, 2000), although occurrence is uncommon (Table 3-5). In a retrospective study of 225 dogs with hypoadrenocorticism, 4% of the dogs also had hypothyroidism, 0.5% had concurrent diabetes mellitus, and one dog had concurrent hypothyroidism, diabetes mellitus, and hypoparathyroidism (Peterson et al, 1996).

The initial lesion and precipitating events that result in these syndromes are unknown in dogs. Genetic predisposition to polyglandular autoimmune syndromes has been confirmed in humans (Eisenbarth and Jackson, 1992) and may play a role in the dog as well. Type II polyglandular autoimmune syndrome is the most common form in humans and is inherited as an autosomal dominant trait associated with human leukocyte antigens (HLA; Verge, 1998). Lymphocytic and plasmacytic destruction of affected endocrine glands is identified histologically, and circulating organ-specific autoantibodies are commonly present. Environmental factors combined with an HLA-associated genetic predisposition are thought to

TABLE 3–3 DOG BREEDS REPORTED TO HAVE AN INCREASED PREVALENCE OF THYROID HORMONE AUTOANTIBODIES

Breed	Odds Ratio*
Pointer	3.61
English Setter	3.44
English Pointer	3.31
Skye Terrier	3.04
German Wirehaired Pointer	2.72
Old English Sheepdog	2.65
Boxer	2.37
Maltese	2.25
Kuvasz	2.18
Petit Basset Friffon Vendeen	2.16
American Staffordshire Terrier	1.84
Beagle	1.79
American Pit Bull Terrier	1.78
Dalmatian	1.74
Giant Schnauzer	1.72
Rhodesian Ridgeback	1.72
Golden Retriever	1.70
Shetland Sheepdog	1.69
Chesapeake Bay Retriever	1.56
Siberian Husky	1.45
Brittany Spaniel	1.42
Borzoi	1.39
Australian Shepherd	1.28
Doberman Pinscher	1.24
Malamute	1.22
Cocker Spaniel	1.17
Mixed	1.05

From Nachreiner RF, et al: Prevalence of serum thyroid hormone autoantibodies in dogs with clinical signs of hypothyroidism. JAVMA 220:466, 2002.

*Odds of having serum thyroid hormone autoantibodies (THAA) among breeds with an increased risk of having THAA, compared with dogs of all other breeds.

TABLE 3–4 COMPONENT DISORDERS OF TYPE I AND TYPE II POLYENDOCRINE AUTOIMMUNE SYNDROMES

Type I (% Occurrence)	Type II (% Occurrence)
Adrenal insufficiency (100%)	Adrenal insufficiency (100%)
Hypoparathyroidism (76%)	Autoimmune thyroid disease (69%)
Mucocutaneous candidiasis (73%)	Insulin-dependent diabetes mellitus (52%)
Gonadal failure (17%)	Gonadal failure (4%)
Autoimmune thyroid disease (11%)	Diabetes insipidus (rare)
Insulin-dependent diabetes mellitus (4%)	Hypopituitarism (rare)

Miscellaneous Disorders

Alopecia (32%)	Vitiligo (5%)
Malabsorption (22%)	Pernicious anemia (1%)
Pernicious anemia (13%)	Alopecia (1%)
Chronic active hepatitis (13%)	Myasthenia gravis
Vitiligo (8%)	Collagen vascular disease
	Celiac disease

Data from Neufeld M, et al: Two types of autoimmune Addison's disease associated with different polyglandular autoimmune (PGA) syndromes. Medicine 60:355, 1981.

TABLE 3–5 NUMBER OF DOGS WITH VARIOUS ENDOCRINE DEFICIENCY SYNDROMES, SINGLY AND IN COMBINATIONS, SEEN AT OUR HOSPITAL BETWEEN 1990 AND 1994

Endocrine Disorder	Number of Dogs
Insulin-dependent diabetes mellitus	153
Primary hypothyroidism	124
Primary hypoadrenocorticism	72
Primary hypoparathyroidism	13
Diabetes mellitus and hypothyroidism	13
Diabetes mellitus and hypoadrenocorticism	9
Hypoadrenocorticism and hypothyroidism	3
Diabetes mellitus, hypoadrenocorticism, and hypothyroidism	2
Hypoparathyroidism and other endocrine deficiencies	0

trigger the destructive process. Both cell-mediated and humoral immunity appear to be involved in the destruction of target tissues. The most consistent abnormality is a functional defect leading to decreased suppressor T cell immunity. Lymphocytic and plasmacytic destruction of endocrine glands (e.g., lymphocytic thyroiditis, lymphocytic insulitis, lymphocytic adrenalitis) and circulating organ-specific autoantibodies (e.g., thyroglobulin autoantibodies, anti-islet cell antibodies, antiadrenal gland antibodies) have been identified in affected dogs (Haines and Penhale, 1985; Kooistra et al, 1995), findings that suggest etiopathogenic mechanisms in dogs similar to those that have been identified in human beings.

Immunoendocrinopathy syndromes should be suspected when multiple endocrine gland failure is identified in a dog. Hypoadrenocorticism, hypothyroidism, and to a lesser extent, diabetes mellitus, hypoparathyroidism, and primary gonadal failure are recognized combined endocrine deficiency syndromes. In most affected dogs, each endocrinopathy is manifested separately, with additional disorders following one by one after variable time periods (usually 3 to 18 months). Diagnosis and treatment are directed at each disorder as it becomes recognized, because it is not possible to reliably predict or prevent any of these problems. Furthermore, the clinician must consider the effects that one endocrine disorder may have on the tests used to diagnose another disorder (e.g., untreated diabetes mellitus suppresses circulating thyroid hormone concentrations) and the effects that treating one endocrine disorder may have on the treatment of concurrent endocrine disorders (e.g., initiation of thyroid supplementation may dramatically improve insulin sensitivity in a diabetic animal). Immunosuppressive drug therapy is not indicated in these syndromes and may actually create problems (e.g., insulin resistance or thyroid suppression with high-dose glucocorticoid therapy).

IDIOPATHIC ATROPHY. Idiopathic atrophy of the thyroid gland is characterized microscopically by loss of the thyroid parenchyma, which is replaced by adipose tissue (Fig. 3-5). An inflammatory infiltrate is lacking, even in areas in which small follicles or follicular remnants are present (Gosselin et al, 1981b) and tests for lymphocytic thyroiditis are negative. The parathyroid glands are rarely affected, and variable numbers of parafollicular cells remain.

The cause of idiopathic thyroid atrophy is not known. It has been suggested that idiopathic atrophy is a primary degenerative disorder involving individual follicular cells (Gosselin et al, 1981b). Degeneration of follicular cells is seen histologically early in the lesion, with their subsequent exfoliation into the colloid or the interfollicular spaces. Progressive reduction in the size of the follicles and replacement of the degenerating follicles with adipose tissue occur. This atrophy can be distinguished from the atrophy associated with decreased TSH secretion (i.e., secondary hypothyroidism), in which the follicles are lined by low cuboidal epithelial cells with no indication of degeneration.

Atrophy of the thyroid gland may also represent an end stage of lymphocytic thyroiditis. Evaluation of the morphologic changes involved in lymphocytic thyroiditis in a colony of related Borzoi dogs revealed initial degenerative thyroidal parenchymal changes, which progressed to progressively worsening inflammation, subsequent fibrosis, and an end stage of thyroid gland destruction, which manifested itself as an entity histologically similar to idiopathic follicular atrophy (Conaway et al, 1985b). However, residual inflammation was still evident histologically at the end stage of lymphocytic thyroiditis. In a recent study, the mean age at the time of diagnosis of hypothyroidism was older in dogs with suspected idiopathic atrophy, compared with dogs diagnosed with lymphocytic thyroiditis; a finding that supports the theory that idiopathic atrophy may be an end stage of lymphocytic thyroiditis (Graham et al, 2001a). Results for serum thyro-

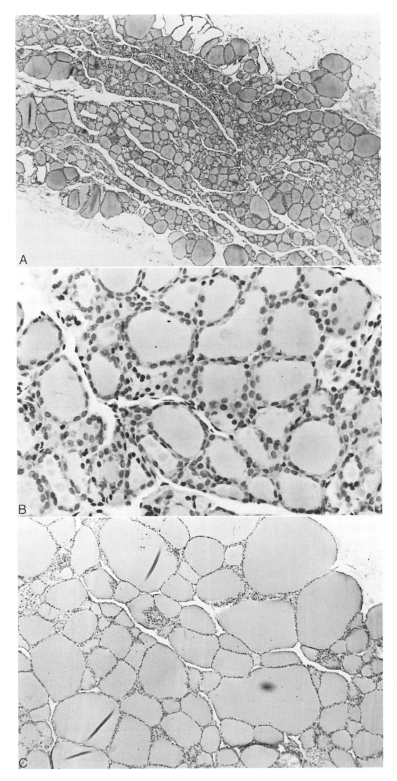

FIGURE 3–5. *A* and *B*, Histologic section of a thyroid gland from a dog with idiopathic atrophy of the thyroid gland and hypothyroidism. Note the small size of the gland (compare with *C*), decrease in follicular size and colloid content, and lack of a cellular infiltration (*A*, H&E ×40; *B*, H&E ×250). *C*, Histologic section of a normal thyroid gland at the same magnification as *A*. Note the increased size of the gland, the follicles, and the colloid content compared with the gland in A. (H&E ×40)

globulin and thyroid hormone autoantibody tests also progress from positive to negative with time in dogs with lymphocytic thyroiditis, suggesting that the inciting antigens for lymphocytic thyroiditis disappear with time. Although idiopathic atrophy may represent an end-stage form of autoimmune lymphocytic thyroiditis, the inability to demonstrate an inflammatory cell infiltrate, even when follicles are still present, on histopathologic examination of the thyroid gland in dogs diagnosed with idiopathic atrophy suggests that there may be more than one etiology for thyroid atrophy in the dog. Unlike for lymphocytic thyroiditis, there are no blood tests currently available that establish the diagnosis of idiopathic atrophy. Hence the diagnosis tends to be one of exclusion; that is, if the tests for lymphocytic thyroiditis are negative, the dog must have idiopathic atrophy. Until histologic evaluation of several thyroid gland biopsies obtained from the same dog over time has been done in a group of dogs in the early stages of naturally acquired lymphocytic thyroiditis, the relationship between lymphocytic thyroiditis and idiopathic atrophy of the thyroid gland will remain conjectural.

FOLLICULAR CELL HYPERPLASIA. Histologic evaluation of the thyroid gland in some dogs with hypothyroidism reveals small thyroid follicles that contain minimal amounts of colloid. Follicular cell hyperplasia is present, however. No appreciable inflammation is seen within the gland, and circulating antithyroglobulin antibody has been undetectable in a few dogs studied. The cause of these pathologic changes is not known, although the histologic changes resemble those found with iodine deficiency or in juvenile dogs and cats with defects in thyroid hormone biosynthesis (Chastain et al, 1983; Arnold et al, 1984). Iodine deficiency is extremely unlikely because these dogs have been fed nutritionally balanced, commercial dog foods. One possible explanation is impaired function of the follicular cells (e.g., dyshormonogenesis), resulting in a thyroid-deficient state. Follicular cell hyperplasia may develop secondary to the stimulatory effects of increased TSH secretion in response to thyroid hormone deficiency, assuming appropriate binding of TSH to its receptor occurs. It is interesting to note that ingestion of diets containing an excessive amount of iodine can cause significant impairment of thyroid function and hypothyroidism (Castillo et al, 2001). Excessive iodine intake inhibits iodide uptake and organification and thyroid hormone secretion by thyroid follicular cells, resulting in a compensatory increase in circulating TSH concentrations (Pisarev and Gartner, 2000).

NEOPLASTIC DESTRUCTION. Clinical signs of hypothyroidism may develop following destruction of more than 75% of the normal thyroid gland by an infiltrative tumor. Tumors may arise from the thyroid gland or from adjacent tissues, which then infiltrate the thyroid gland. Thyroid carcinoma and squamous cell carcinoma are the most common tumors causing extensive destruction of the thyroid gland.

In most dogs, thyroid tumors are hormonally inactive and do not secrete excessive amounts of thyroid hormone. As a result, clinical signs of hyperthyroidism are uncommon. In our hospital, 55% to 60% of dogs with thyroid neoplasia have normal serum thyroid hormone concentrations, 30% to 35% have low serum thyroid hormone concentrations and clinical signs supportive of hypothyroidism, and approximately 10% have increased serum thyroid hormone concentrations and signs supportive of hyperthyroidism (see Chapter 5).

Although most canine thyroid tumors have been considered "nonfunctioning," they may secrete inactive or altered forms of thyroid hormone. The altered hormone may not cause thyrotoxicosis and may not be detected by standard radioimmunoassay techniques. These products, however, may be capable of suppressing TSH secretion, in which case atrophy of the remaining normal thyroid tissue would result. This process was thought to have occurred in one dog described as having hypothyroidism and a follicular thyroid carcinoma involving only one lobe of the thyroid gland (Branam et al, 1982).

MISCELLANEOUS CAUSES. Primary hypothyroidism may result from the ingestion of toxic agents or antithyroid medications (e.g., propylthiouracil, methimazole) or following surgical removal of a thyroid tumor. Accessory thyroid tissue is common in dogs and may be found from the base of the tongue to the base of the heart. Therefore surgical removal of the thyroid gland rarely results in permanent hypothyroidism. Use of radioactive iodine (iodine-131) to treat hyperthyroidism may result in total ablation of the thyroid, especially if both thyroid lobes are affected and excessive doses are used (Meric et al, 1986).

SUMMARY. Although there are several potential causes (see Table 3-1), lymphocytic thyroiditis and idiopathic atrophy account for most of the clinical cases of primary hypothyroidism diagnosed in dogs. Both cause progressive loss of thyroid function as a result of either immune-mediated destruction (lymphocytic thyroiditis) or degeneration (idiopathic atrophy) of the thyroid. The result is a deficiency in thyroid hormone synthesis and secretion and development of clinical signs of hypothyroidism.

Secondary Hypothyroidism

Secondary hypothyroidism results from failure of pituitary thyrotrophs to develop (pituitary hypoplasia causing pituitary dwarfism) or dysfunction within the pituitary thyrotrophs causing impaired secretion of thyroid-stimulating hormone (TSH) and a "secondary" deficiency in thyroid hormone synthesis and secretion. Follicular atrophy gradually develops owing to the lack of TSH. Histologically, the follicles are distended with colloid and lined by low cuboidal epithelial cells. The colloid is uniformly dense, with little evidence of colloidal endocytosis (i.e., resorption vacuoles). Immunocyte infiltration and epithelial cell degeneration are absent.

Potential causes of secondary hypothyroidism include congenital malformations of the pituitary gland, pituitary destruction, and pituitary suppression. In the dog, secondary hypothyroidism caused by naturally acquired defects in pituitary thyrotroph function or destruction of pituitary thyrotrophs (e.g., pituitary neoplasia) is uncommon. In contrast, suppression of pituitary thyrotroph function by hormones or drugs (e.g., glucocorticoids, naturally occurring hyper-adrenocorticism) is quite common. Serum TSH concentrations should be decreased or undetectable with secondary hypothyroidism. Unfortunately, current assays used to measure endogenous TSH in dogs are unable to differentiate between normal and decreased concentrations (see page 118), making confirmation of secondary hypothyroidism difficult. Identification of an increased serum TSH concentration is consistent with primary hypothyroidism, and although one would expect the serum TSH concentration to be undetectable in a dog with secondary hypothyroidism, such a finding does not confirm the diagnosis.

PITUITARY MALFORMATION. Congenital abnormalities involving the pituitary gland have been recognized in many breeds but are reported most commonly in German Shepherd dogs. Cystic Rathke's pouch or hypoplasia of the anterior pituitary affecting the thyrotropic cells results in impaired secretion of TSH (Eigenmann, 1981; Hamann et al, 1999; Kooistra et al, 2000a). Because of the involvement of other anterior pituitary hormones, most notably growth hormone (GH), congenital defects affecting the anterior pituitary usually result in the development of dwarfism (see Chapter 2). If TSH but not GH secretion were affected, cretinism would develop (see page 104).

PITUITARY DESTRUCTION. Although uncommon, pituitary tumors may cause secondary hypothyroidism following destruction of thyrotrophs by an expanding, space-occupying mass. Neoplasia-induced pituitary destruction may create additional endocrinopathies, including hypocortisolism (secondary adrenal insufficiency), diabetes insipidus, reproductive dysfunction (i.e., irregular estrous cycles, failure to cycle, loss of libido, testicular atrophy, azoospermia), and pituitary dwarfism in immature animals. The owner's primary concern may depend, in part, on which endocrine system is most severely affected. The most common pituitary tumor affecting thyroid gland function in the dog is a functional corticotropic tumor causing pituitary-dependent hyperadrenocorticism. In these dogs, secondary hypothyroidism results from suppression of thyrotroph function (i.e., suppressed TSH secretion) rather than from destruction of thyrotrophs by the tumor.

PITUITARY THYROTROPH SUPPRESSION. Secondary hypothyroidism may develop following suppression of thyrotroph function by concurrent illness, drugs, hormones, or malnutrition (see Factors Affecting Thyroid Gland Function Tests, page 126). These are the most common causes of secondary hypothyroidism in the dog. From a clinical standpoint, perhaps the most important is the suppressive effect of glucocorticoids, either from exogenous administration or from naturally acquired hyperadrenocorticism. In a study of 102 dogs

with naturally acquired hyperadrenocorticism, randomly obtained basal serum T_4 and/or serum T_3 levels were decreased in 68% of the dogs (Ferguson and Peterson, 1986). The thyroid is usually subnormally responsive to TSH administration (see Chapter 6). Unlike the other causes, secondary hypothyroidism induced by suppression of thyrotroph function is potentially and usually reversible. Thyroid hormone supplementation is not required if the cause for the suppression can be identified and treated.

MISCELLANEOUS CAUSES. In humans, secondary hypothyroidism may also develop following production of a defective TSH molecule or impaired interaction between TSH and its receptor on follicular epithelial cells. These causes have not yet been reported in the dog. Secondary hypothyroidism can follow radiation therapy for expansile adrenocorticotrophic hormone (ACTH)–secreting pituitary tumors. Secondary hypothyroidism can also be caused by hypophysectomy (Lantz et al, 1988; Meij et al, 1998).

Tertiary Hypothyroidism

Tertiary hypothyroidism is defined as a deficiency in the secretion of thyrotropin-releasing hormone (TRH) by peptidergic neurons in the supraoptic and paraventricular nuclei of the hypothalamus. Lack of TRH secretion should cause a deficiency in TSH secretion and secondary follicular atrophy in the thyroid gland. Histologically, the thyroid gland would then resemble glands seen in dogs with secondary hypothyroidism. In humans, impaired secretion of TRH by the hypothalamus may result from a congenital defect, acquired destruction secondary to a mass lesion or hemorrhage, a defective TRH molecule, or defective TRH-thyrotroph receptor interaction (Larsen et al, 1998). Neurologic signs and additional pituitary dysfunction may be present, depending on the cause. In theory, differentiation between secondary and tertiary hypothyroidism would rely on changes in the serum TSH concentration after administration of TRH (see page 120). Tertiary hypothyroidism has not been reported in dogs and can be assumed to be rare.

Congenital Defects

The incidence of congenital hypothyroidism in the dog is not known. In a survey of 2642 dogs with hypothyroidism, 3.6% were less than 1 year of age (Milne and Hayes, 1981). It can be assumed that a percentage of these animals had congenital defects of the thyroid gland. Unfortunately, congenital hypothyroidism probably results in early death of most affected puppies, and the cause of death is inadvertently lumped into the broad diagnosis of "fading puppy syndrome." Thus most puppies with congenital hypothyroidism are not diagnosed or documented.

Congenital defects are divided into four categories in humans: thyroid dysgenesis, dyshormonogenesis, circulating thyroid hormone transport abnormalities, and metabolic defects following ingestion of goitrogens. Mutations in the TSH molecule that cause it to be ineffective as a thyroid stimulator or a defect in the TSH receptor that impairs the ability of the thyroid cell to respond to TSH have also been described in humans (Hayashizaki et al, 1990; Sunthornthepvarakul et al, 1994). In humans, the majority of congenital thyroid defects are due to thyroid dysgenesis (i.e., aplasia, hypoplasia, or ectasia; Larsen et al, 1998). Of the remaining categories, an inherited inability to organify iodide is the most common cause of congenital hypothyroidism in human infants. Only a few reports of canine congenital hypothyroidism have appeared in the literature. Documented causes of congenital primary hypothyroidism in the dog include deficient dietary iodine intake, dyshormonogenesis (i.e., iodine organification defect), and thyroid dysgenesis (Chastain et al, 1983; Greco et al, 1985). Secondary hypothyroidism resulting from an apparent deficiency of TSH has also been reported in a family of Giant Schnauzers (Greco et al, 1991) and a Boxer dog (Mooney and Anderson, 1993). Pedigree analysis suggested an autosomal recessive mode of inheritance in the family of Giant Schnauzers. Pituitary dwarfs with combined anterior pituitary hormone deficiencies usually lack TSH in addition to GH and prolactin (Hamann et al, 1999; Kooistra et al, 2000a; see Chapter 2). Lack of TSH secretion may contribute to abnormal body maturation and growth in pituitary dwarfs.

The development of an enlarged thyroid gland (i.e., goiter) depends on the etiology. If the hypothalamic-pituitary-thyroid gland axis is intact, appropriate binding of TSH occurs with its receptor, and the block in thyroid hormone production is within the thyroid gland itself (e.g., as occurs with an iodine organification defect), goiter will develop in response to increased serum TSH concentration. Treatment with levothyroxine sodium will cause a decrease in the serum TSH concentration, providing evidence for normal pituitary thyrotrophs. If the hypothalamic-pituitary-thyroid gland axis is not intact (e.g., as occurs with pituitary TSH deficiency), goiter will not develop. Serum TSH concentration is decreased, although current TSH assays used in dogs cannot detect low TSH concentrations (see page 118). If defects exist in the binding of TSH to its receptor, serum TSH concentration will be increased and goiter absent. TSH binding defects have not been documented in dogs.

An inability to convert T_4 to T_3 by peripheral tissues, presumably as a result of a deficiency in 5'-monodeiodinase, is often proposed to explain low serum T_3 but normal serum T_4 concentrations in some dogs. Unfortunately, conversion defects have not been documented in humans or dogs and are probably rare, if they exist at all. Seemingly, a deficiency in 5'-monodeiodinase would be incompatible with life and should cause fetal resorption, fetal abortion, or neonatal death (i.e., "fading puppy syndrome"). Low serum T_3 concentrations in conjunction with normal T_4 levels are quite common in euthyroid dogs because of

normal fluctuations in serum T_3 concentration, concurrent illness, and drug therapy (see page 115). Nondetectable serum T_3 concentrations can also occur in dogs with lymphocytic thyroiditis and T_3 autoantibodies in the circulation. Depending on the type of assay used to measure T_3 concentrations, T_3 autoantibodies may interfere with the assay and cause spuriously low results (see page 125).

Iodine Deficiency

Iodine deficiency is a rare cause of hypothyroidism in dogs because of the adequate amounts of iodine in commercial pet foods. The iodine requirement in the adult Beagle is 140 µg/day. In one study, decreased concentrations of serum T_4 and, to a lesser extent, serum T_3 did not occur until iodine intake was restricted to 20 to 50 µg/day. Clinical signs of hypothyroidism did not develop in these dogs. Free T_4 concentrations, determined by equilibrium dialysis, remained in the normal range regardless of the amount of dietary iodine restriction.

Two histologic changes were observed in the thyroids of dogs with iodine deficiency. In one group, thyroid follicles were small and contained minimal amounts of colloid. Follicular cell hyperplasia was present, and increased uptake and rapid release of radioiodine occurred. In the second group, thyroid follicles were larger and contained more colloid. Increased uptake but slower release of radioiodine occurred. TSH-secreting cells of the pituitary were enlarged and sparsely granulated, suggesting increased activity and secretion of TSH.

CLINICAL FEATURES OF PRIMARY HYPOTHYROIDISM IN THE ADULT DOG

Signalment

No single diagnostic test confirms the diagnosis of hypothyroidism in the dog. Therefore reports containing data regarding breed incidence and genetics for this disorder should always be examined critically, especially in terms of how the diagnosis of hypothyroidism was made. Evaluation for serum thyroglobulin and thyroid hormone autoantibodies provides insight into breeds that have an increased incidence of lymphocytic thyroiditis (Table 3-3) and may indicate a genetic role for the disorder in some of these breeds (Nachreiner et al, 2002). Local breed popularity can also influence a veterinarian's perception of which breeds are predisposed to developing hypothyroidism, a perception that may or may not be accurate. In our hospital, hypothyroidism is most commonly diagnosed in Doberman Pinschers, Golden Retrievers, Labrador Retrievers, and Cocker Spaniels (Table 3-6). Clinical signs usually develop during middle age (i.e., 2 to 6 years). Of 3206 dogs diagnosed with hypothyroidism, 32% were between 4 and 6 years of age,

TABLE 3–6 BREED DISTRIBUTION OF 130 DOGS WITH PRIMARY HYPOTHYROIDISM

Breed	Number (%) of Dogs
Golden Retriever	24 (18%)
Doberman Pinscher	22 (17%)
Labrador Retriever	8 (6%)
Cocker Spaniel	7 (5%)
German Shepard dog	7 (5%)
Mixed Breed	7 (5%
Dachshund	5 (4%)
Poodle	4 (3%)
Rottweiler	4 (3%)
Spaniels (Springer, King Charles)	4 (3%)
Akita	3 (2%)
Boxer	3 (2%)
Terriers (Fox, Scottish, Westie)	3 (2%)
Beagle	2 (2%)
Chesapeake Bay Retriever	2 (2%)
Chow Chow	2 (2%)
Maltese	2 (2%)
Mastiff	2 (2%)
Old English Sheepdog	2 (2%)
Samoyed	2 (2%)
Shetland Sheepdog	2 (2%)
13 breeds	< 1% each

and 22% each were between 2 and 3 years and 7 and 9 years of age (Milne and Hayes, 1981). Age of onset of symptomatic hypothyroidism may vary between breeds, presumably as a result of the underlying etiology and rate of progression of thyroid pathology. Individual variability also exists within a breed. In general, breeds at increased risk tend to develop clinical signs at an earlier age than other breeds (Milne and Hayes, 1981; Nesbitt et al, 1980; Muller et al, 1983). There is no apparent gender predisposition.

Clinical Signs

Thyroid hormone is needed for the normal cellular metabolic functions of the body. A deficiency in circulating thyroid hormone affects the metabolic function of almost all organ systems. As a result, clinical signs are quite variable and depend in part on the age of the dog at the time a deficiency in thyroid hormone develops (Table 3-7). Clinical signs may also differ between breeds. For example, different breeds appear to have markedly different hair cycles and follicular morphology, which may influence the clinical and histologic features of the disease (Credille et al, 2001). Similarly, dermatologic signs may predominate in some breeds, whereas neuromuscular signs may predominate in other breeds. Destruction of the thyroid gland tends to be a slow process, often taking more than a year from the time tests for lymphocytic thyroiditis are positive until tests of thyroid gland function become abnormal. Hence the onset of clinical signs is often gradual and subtle, and this can hamper the clinician's ability to establish the diagnosis. Important information regarding the existence of some clinical signs (e.g., metabolic signs) may not be evident

TABLE 3–7 CLINICAL MANIFESTATIONS OF HYPOTHYROIDISM IN THE ADULT DOG

Metabolic
Lethargy*
Mental dullness
Inactivity*
Weight gain*
Cold intolerance

Dermatologic
Endocrine alopecia*
Symmetric or asymmetrical
Areas of friction and pressure
"Rat tail"
Dry, brittle hair coat
Hyperpigmentation
Seborrhea sicca, oleosa, or
  dermatitis
Pyoderma
Otitis externa
Myxedema

Reproductive
Persistent anestrus
Weak or silent estrus
Prolonged estrual bleeding
Inappropriate galactorrhea or
  gynecomastia
Testicular atrophy (?)
Loss of libido (?)

Behavioral Abnormalities (?)

Neuromuscular
Weakness*
Knuckling
Ataxia
Circling
Vestibular signs
Facial nerve paralysis
Seizures
Laryngeal paralysis (?)

Ocular
Corneal lipid deposits
Corneal ulceration
Uveitis

Cardiovascular
Bradycardia
Cardiac arrhythmias

Gastrointestinal
Esophageal hypomotility (?)
Diarrhea
Constipation

Hematologic
Anemia*
Hyperlipidemia*
Coagulopathy

*Common

from the history simply because the clinical signs have been slow to develop, the owners have unconsciously adapted to the changes in their dog, and they do not recognize the problem. Only after the dog returns to normal following initiation of thyroid hormone supplementation does the owner have a reference point and can recognize that a problem existed.

In the adult dog, the most consistent clinical signs of hypothyroidism result from decreased cellular metabolism and the effects on the dog's mental status and activity (Table 3-8). Additional clinical signs typically involve the skin, neuromuscular system, or reproductive system. Other organ systems may be affected by thyroid hormone deficiency, but clinical signs related to these other systems are rarely the reason for presentation of the dog to the veterinarian.

GENERAL METABOLIC SIGNS. In our experience, most adult dogs with hypothyroidism have signs resulting from the effect of a generalized decrease in metabolic rate on mental status and activity. These signs include some degree of mental dullness, lethargy, exercise intolerance or unwillingness to exercise, and a propensity to gain weight without a corresponding increase in appetite or food intake. In one study, energy expenditure, as measured by indirect calorimetry, was approximately 15% lower in hypothyroid dogs, compared with healthy dogs, and energy expenditure returned to normal after initiating levothyroxine sodium treatment (Greco et at, 1998). Hypothyroid dogs have

TABLE 3–8 INCIDENCE OF CLINICAL SIGNS IN 100 ADULT DOGS WITH HYPOTHYROIDISM

Clinical Sign	Percent of Dogs
Gain in body weight	48%
Lethargy, mental "dullness"	35%
Dermatologic problems	
Hyperkeratosis	33%
Symmetric endocrine alopecia	25%
Thin hair coat	25%
Seborrhea	16%
Hyperpigmentation	15%
Otitis externa	13%
"Rat" tail	12%
Pyoderma	12%
Patchy endocrine alopecia	11%
Pruritus	9%
Myxedema of the face	8%
Neuromuscular problems	
Weakness, exercise intolerance	12%
Grand mal seizures	4%
Facial nerve paralysis	4%
Head tilt	3%
Dysphagia	3%
Laryngeal paralysis	3%
Reproductive problems	
Persistent anestrus	4%
Infertility (male)	1%
Goiter	1%
Corneal lipid deposits	1%
Nasal hemorrhage	1%
Asymptomatic; hyperlipidemia identified	4%

also been classified as "heat seekers" following development of an intolerance to cold. However, we have not found this to be historically useful information, because most dogs seem to be "heat seekers" at one time or another.

Metabolic signs are perhaps the most difficult for an owner to identify, in part, because of their gradual onset and subtle nature. The severity of these signs is also directly related to the duration of hypothyroidism. Thus metabolic signs may not be evident in the history and can be difficult to recognize during the physical examination, especially if the veterinarian is examining the dog for the first time. In one study involving 108 hypothyroid dogs, lethargy was observed in only 11%, and less than 10% had observable obesity or cold intolerance (Nesbitt et al, 1980). Most dogs with hypothyroidism, however, have improvement in activity and become more interactive with family members within 7 to 10 days of initiating thyroid hormone supplementation, regardless of the findings during the history and physical examination.

DERMATOLOGIC SIGNS. Alterations in the skin and hair coat are the most commonly observed abnormalities in dogs with hypothyroidism. Dermatologic changes can be quite varied and dependent on the breed of dog and severity and chronicity of the disease. The classic cutaneous sign of hypothyroidism is bilaterally symmetric, nonpruritic truncal alopecia. However, in a recent study evaluating the effect of induced hypothyroidism on the skin in Beagle dogs, none of the untreated hypothyroid dogs had a discernable

alopecia after 10 months of observation despite one-third fewer hair shafts than healthy Beagles (Credille et al, 2001). The most common finding was an inability of the hypothyroid dogs to regrow their hair after clipping. Hair failed to regrow because the overwhelming majority of hair follicles were in the telogen, or resting, phase of the hair cycle. The hair shafts in telogen follicles appear to be retained for long periods (months to years) without falling out. Retaining telogen hairs maintains the pelage, which explains why truncal alopecia does not usually develop in hypothyroid Beagle dogs. However, in contrast with the findings in healthy Beagles, lost telogen hairs were not replaced in hypothyroid Beagles, which explains how areas of alopecia could develop over pressure point regions and body sites exposed to friction. Presumably, dermatologic signs are different in other breeds of dogs because of different hair cycles and follicular morphology. The study by Credille et al illustrates why breed-specific studies on clinical manifestations and diagnostic testing for hypothyroidism are needed.

Thyroid hormone is necessary to initiate and maintain the anagen, or growing, phase of the hair cycle (Credille et al, 2001). With thyroid hormone deficiency, hair follicles prematurely enter the telogen phase of the hair cycle. Excessive shedding with lack of hair regrowth leads to alopecia. Decreases in cutaneous fatty acids and prostaglandin E_2 and sebaceous gland atrophy leads to hyperkeratosis, scales, and seborrhea sicca with a dry and lusterless haircoat (Campbell and Davis, 1990). In the early stages of hypothyroidism, hair loss is often asymmetric and develops over areas of excessive wear or pressure, such as the caudal thighs, ventral thorax, tail base, and tail (i.e., development of a "rat tail"; Fig. 3-6). As hypothyroidism becomes more severe or chronic, alopecia becomes more symmetric and truncal, eventually developing into the classic cutaneous finding of bilaterally symmetric, nonpruritic truncal alopecia that tends to spare the head and distal extremities (Fig. 3-7). Although nonpruritic endocrine alopecia is not pathognomonic for hypothyroidism (see page 62), when it is present in a dog with signs of altered cellular metabolism and no polyuria or polydipsia, hypothyroidism is certainly the most likely diagnosis.

Depending on the breed and the individual, hair may be easily epilated or may fail to shed out normally (e.g., Irish Setter), leading to hypertrichosis. In the short-coated breeds (e.g., Doberman Pinscher, Boxer), the hypertrichosis may produce a very dense "brush coat" usually involving focal areas over the head, extremities, or both (Rosychuk, 1998). In some dogs there is a loss of predominantly the undercoat, and the remaining primary hairs give the coat a coarse appearance. In others (e.g., arctic breeds), primary hairs are lost, giving the coat a "wooly" appearance. Some dogs develop thinning of the haircoat but not truncal alopecia (e.g., Beagles). In general, the head and distal extremities are spared with respect to development of alopecia in

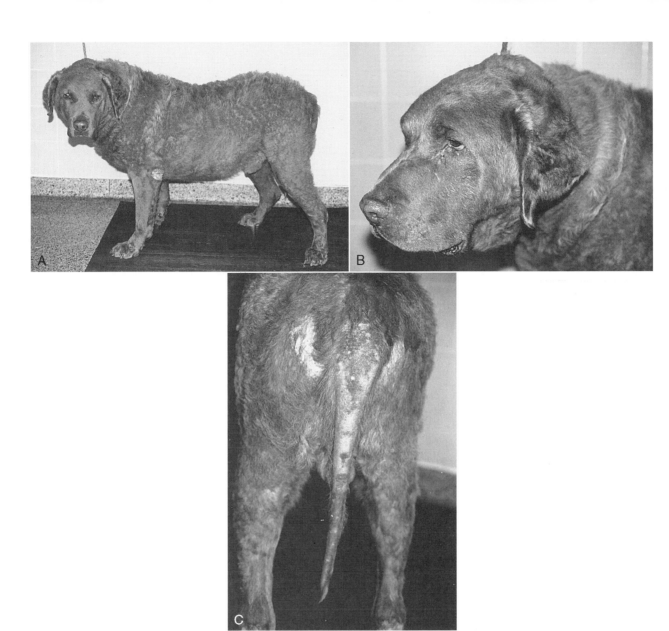

FIGURE 3–6. An 8-year-old male Chesapeake Bay Retriever with hypothyroidism. Note the poor hair coat, lethargic appearance, myxedema of the face with drooping of the eyelids *(A and B)*, and "rat" tail *(C)*.

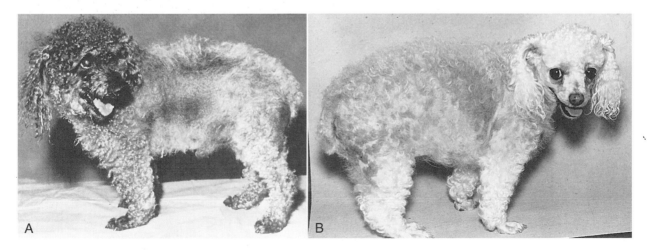

FIGURE 3–7. A 5-year-old male Miniature Poodle *(A)* and a 6-year-old spayed Miniature Poodle *(B)* with hypothyroidism and endocrine alopecia. Note the truncal alopecia and hyperpigmentation, which have spared the head and extremities, in both dogs.

dogs with hypothyroidism, although significant alopecia over the bridge of the nose (e.g., in Beagles), pinna of the ear (e.g., in Dachshunds), or lateral aspects of the distal extremities (e.g., in Newfoundlands) may develop (Rosychuk, 1998; Credille et al, 2001).

Hair regrowth is slow in part because the majority of hair follicles are in the telogen phase of the hair growth cycle. In dogs without obvious external manifestations of hypothyroidism, an initial suspicion is often raised when clipped hair fails to regrow, a sign also typical of hyperadrenocorticism and hyperestrogenism (i.e., Sertoli cell tumor).

Variable degrees of hyperpigmentation are common, especially in alopecic areas and areas of wear such as the axilla and inguinal regions (Fig. 3-8). Poor wound healing and easy bruisability may also be noted, but these are uncommon findings resulting from decreased fibroblast function, collagen synthesis, and protein metabolism. In severe cases of hypothyroidism, acid and neutral mucopolysaccharides and hyaluronic acid may accumulate in the dermis, bind water, and result in increased thickness of the skin. Referred to as *myxedema*, this skin thickening occurs predominantly in the forehead, eyelids, lips, and the distal extremities, resulting in rounding of the temporal region of the forehead, puffiness and increased thickness of facial skin folds, and in conjunction with dropping of the upper eyelids and lips, the development of a "tragic facial expression" (Fig. 3-6).

Dogs with hypothyroidism may develop superficial bacterial infections (folliculitis, superficial spreading pyoderma, impetigo) characterized by papules, pustules, epidermal collarettes, and/or focal areas of alopecia (Rosychuk, 1998). Bacterial infections are usually caused by *Staphylococcus intermedius* and are variably pruritic. Thyroid hormone has a direct enhancing effect on the immune response of lymphoid cells (Chen, 1980). Depletion of thyroid hormone suppresses humoral immune reactions, impairs T cell function, and reduces the number of circulating lymphocytes. These defects are reversible with administration of exogenous thyroid hormone supplementation; however, short-term penicillinase-resistant antibiotic administration and germicidal shampoos may be necessary initially to control the infectious process. Antibiotic therapy should be continued for 2 weeks beyond complete resolution of the infection to minimize the incidence of recurrence. Hypothyroidism may also predispose the dog to the development of adult onset demodicosis and chronic otitis externa (Duclos et al, 1994).

The skin changes associated with hypothyroidism are generally nonpruritic. If pruritis is noted, it is usually related to secondary bacterial and/or *Malassezia*

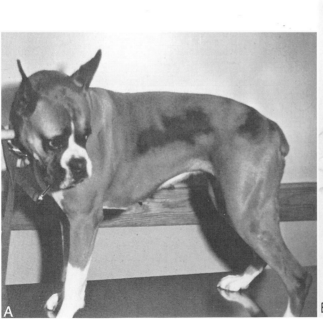

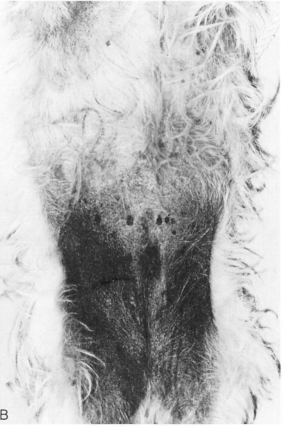

FIGURE 3–8. *A*, Truncal hyperpigmentation in a 4-year-old female spayed Boxer with hypothyroidism. *B*, Severe hyperpigmentation involving the inguinal region in a 6-year-old spayed mixed-breed dog with hypothyroidism.

infection, demodicosis, seborrheic changes (very dry or very oily skin), or concurrent pruritic diseases such as atopy or flea bite hypersensitivity (Rosychuk, 1998). Initial presentation of the dog for a pruritic skin disease does not rule out underlying hypothyroidism. However, interpretation of tests of thyroid gland function must be done with the realization that concurrent skin disease may suppress thyroid gland function test results (see page 128).

NEUROMUSCULAR SIGNS. Neurologic signs may be the predominant problem in some dogs with hypothyroidism. Hypothyroidism-induced segmental demyelination and axonopathy may cause signs referable to the central or peripheral nervous system (Bichsel et al, 1988). Central nervous system signs may also develop following mucopolysaccharide accumulation in the perineurium and endoneurium, cerebral atherosclerosis, or severe hyperlipidemia (Swanson et al, 1981; Liu et al, 1986). Central nervous system signs are uncommon and include seizures, ataxia, and circling. These signs are often present in conjunction with vestibular signs (e.g., head tilt, positional vestibular strabismus) or facial nerve paralysis. Clinical signs caused by peripheral neuropathies are more common and include facial nerve paralysis, weakness, and knuckling or dragging the feet with excessive wear of the dorsal part of the toenail (Jaggy et al, 1994). Muscle wasting may also be evident, although myalgia is not common. Thyroxine-responsive unilateral forelimb lameness has also been described in dogs with normal neurologic examinations but electromyography findings suggestive of generalized neuromyopathy (Budsberg et al, 1993). The relationship between hypothyroidism and laryngeal paralysis or esophageal hypomotility remains controversial, in part, because it is difficult to prove a cause and effect relationship between these disorders and because treatment of hypothyroidism usually does not improve the clinical signs caused by laryngeal paralysis or esophageal hypomotility.

Diagnostic tests of the neuromuscular system in dogs with hypothyroidism should reveal hyporeflexic tendon reflexes; slow nerve conduction velocities; and prolonged insertional activity, fibrillation potentials, and positive sharp waves on electromyography (Braund et al, 1981; Swanson et al, 1981; Indrieri et al, 1987; Budsberg et al, 1993; Jaggy et al, 1994). The most common histopathologic abnormality identified in muscle biopsies is type II myofiber atrophy, a hallmark of denervation atrophy. This histology is also found in muscle from hypothyroid humans with neuropathy (Braund et al, 1981; Indrieri et al, 1987). Additional histopathologic findings may include type I myofiber atrophy with a periodic acid–Schiff (PAS)-positive material in the fibers, hypertrophy of type I and type II myofibers, nemaline rods, and lack of inflammation (Jaggy et al, 1994; Delauche et al, 1998). Lymphocytic plasmacytic myositis has also been described (Muller et al, 1983).

Hypothyroidism is often not recognized as a potential cause of neuromuscular problems. However, routine blood tests are commonly evaluated in dogs with neurologic signs. Hypercholesterolemia and hyperlipidemia (i.e., hypertriglyceridemia) are common in dogs with hypothyroidism and should serve as a marker for possible thyroid dysfunction in dogs presented with neurologic signs.

REPRODUCTIVE SIGNS. Historically, hypothyroidism was believed to cause lack of libido, testicular atrophy, and oligospermia to azoospermia in male dogs. However, work by Johnson et al (1999) in Beagles failed to document any deleterious effect of experimentally induced hypothyroidism on any aspect of male reproductive function. Although other classic clinical signs and clinicopathologic abnormalities of hypothyroidism developed in dogs studied, libido, testicular size, and the total sperm count per ejaculate remained normal. These findings suggest that hypothyroidism may, at best, be an uncommon cause of reproductive dysfunction in male dogs, assuming the Beagle is representative of other dog breeds. However, reproductive dysfunction may not be a typical manifestation of hypothyroidism in Beagles, the duration of the study (2 years) may have been too short to allow reproductive abnormalities to develop, or the induced model used in the study may not be representative of what happens when Beagles develop hypothyroidism from lymphocytic thyroiditis, which is the most common form of hypothyroidism in that breed. It is also possible that lymphocytic thyroiditis and lymphocytic orchitis occur concurrently. In our experience, hypothyroidism is an uncommon cause of infertility in male dogs. However, it remains a possible explanation and should be considered when other causes for infertility cannot be identified, especially if decreased libido is part of the clinical picture (see Chapter 31).

Although thyroid hormone is believed to be necessary for normal follicle-stimulating hormone (FSH) and luteinizing hormone (LH) secretion, an association between hypothyroidism and infertility in the female dog has not been well documented in the veterinary literature. One study failed to identify an association between poor reproductive performance and hypothyroidism in Greyhounds (Beale et al, 1992). In our clinical experience, hypothyroidism can cause prolonged interestrus intervals and failure to cycle in the female dog, although these are uncommon clinical manifestations of the disease. Additional reproductive abnormalities that have been reported in the veterinary literature include weak or silent estrous cycles, prolonged estrual bleeding (which may be caused by acquired problems in the coagulation system), and inappropriate galactorrhea and gynecomastia. The latter is believed to develop following thyroid hormone deficiency–induced increase in TRH secretion, which in turn stimulates prolactin secretion (Chastain and Schmidt, 1980; Cortese et al, 1997).

In women, maternal thyroid hormone is important in maintaining pregnancy. Although many pregnancies are successfully carried to term in women with hypothyroidism, abortion may result from impaired progesterone production due to the diminished trophic and stimulatory effect of thyroid hormone on chorion and corpus luteum function (Maruo et al, 1992). A similar association between hypothyroidism and fetal resorption, abortion, and stillbirth has been suggested in the female dog, although no published documentation of this association is available. Evaluation of thyroid gland function is a recommended component of evaluating a female dog with persistent fetal resorption, fetal abortion, or stillbirth problems. However, in our experience, tests of thyroid gland function are almost always normal in these animals. Maternal hypothyroidism has also been suggested to cause the birth of weak puppies that die shortly after birth.

CARDIOVASCULAR SIGNS. Clinical signs related to dysfunction of the cardiovascular system are not common. Abnormalities identified on physical examination may include bradycardia and a weak apex beat. Atrial fibrillation has been suggested to be associated with hypothyroidism in dogs (Gerritsen et al, 1996), but this appears to be rare based on findings in other studies (Panciera, 2001). More commonly, functional abnormalities are identified on electrocardiography or echocardiography in dogs exhibiting the more common clinical signs of hypothyroidism. Electrocardiographic abnormalities include sinus bradycardia, decreased amplitude of the P and R waves, inversion of the T waves, and first-degree and second-degree atrioventricular block (Panciera, 1994; Panciera, 2001). Echocardiographic abnormalities include increased left ventricular end systolic diameter, prolonged pre-ejection period, and decreases in left ventricular posterior wall thickness during systole, percentage change in left ventricular posterior wall from diastole to systole, interventricular wall thickness during systole and diastole, aortic diameter, velocity of circumferential fiber shortening, and fractional shortening (Miller et al, 1984; Panciera, 1994). Many of the hemodynamic effects of hypothyroidism appear to be attributable to direct effects of hypothyroidism on the myocardium, which include decreased cardiac muscle myosin ATPase activity, decreased sarcoplasmic reticulum calcium-ATPase activity, decreased calcium channel activity, decreased sodium-potassium ATPase activity, and reduced β-adrenergic receptors in the myocardium (Bilezikian and Loeb, 1983; Haber and Loeb, 1988; Hawthorn et al, 1988; Dowell et al, 1994). Alterations in the circulatory system may also contribute to the decrease in cardiac output present in hypothyroidism, including increased systemic vascular resistance, decreased vascular volume, and atherosclerosis (Klein, 1990; Hess et al, 2002). It is not known which of these alterations contribute to the myocardial abnormalities identified in dogs with hypothyroidism. Fortunately, the decrease in cardiac contractility is usually mild and asymptomatic in dogs with hypothyroidism but may become relevant during a surgical procedure requiring prolonged anesthesia and aggressive fluid therapy. Cardiac abnormalities are usually reversible with thyroid hormone supplementation although it may take months of supplementation to restore normal cardiovascular function (Panciera, 1994).

It is important to emphasize that although hypothyroidism can induce echocardiographic changes, thyroid hormone deficiency alone rarely causes heart failure. Heart failure associated with primary hypothyroidism is considered to represent an exacerbation of intrinsic cardiac disease by the superimposed hemodynamic effects of thyroid hormone deficiency. Both cardiomyopathy and hypothyroidism are common problems in Doberman Pinschers, and Calvert et al speculated on a possible cause-and-effect relationship between these two disorders in 1982. However, subsequent studies failed to identify any relationship between hypothyroidism and cardiomyopathy in Doberman Pinschers (Lumsden et al, 1993; Calvert et al, 1998). Although low baseline serum thyroid hormone concentrations occur in dogs with idiopathic dilated cardiomyopathy and heart failure, the thyroid gland in most of these dogs is responsive to TSH, suggesting the euthyroid sick syndrome (see page 120).

Administration of thyroid hormone supplements to dogs with heart failure and low serum thyroid hormone concentrations remains controversial in part because there are no published reports documenting the benefits or complications of such treatment in dogs. Upregulation of thyroid hormone receptor β_1 and β_2 messenger RNA has been documented in the myocardium of dogs with dilated cardiomyopathy and chronic valvular disease, and appears to be a secondary effect of heart failure and alterations in thyroid hormone metabolism (Shahrara et al, 1999). These findings suggest that levothyroxine sodium treatment may improve cardiac performance in dogs with heart failure. Short-term administration of levothyroxine sodium has been shown to improve cardiac and exercise performance in humans with chronic heart failure and to decrease the concentration of thyroid hormone receptor β messenger RNA in the myocardium in vitro (Morkin et al, 1993; Drvota et al, 1995; Moruzzi et al, 1996). Administering thyroid hormone to a dog in heart failure should be done cautiously because of the potential increase in basal metabolic rate and demand for oxygen delivery to tissues caused by treatment (Greco et al, 1998). Until studies prove otherwise, we do not recommend thyroid hormone supplementation for dogs in heart failure that have low baseline thyroid hormone concentrations unless a strong suspicion exists for concurrent hypothyroidism.

OCULAR SIGNS. Ocular signs are rare and probably develop secondary to hyperlipidemia. Corneal lipid deposits (i.e., arcus lipoides corneae) have been described in a group of hypothyroid Alsatians with concomitant hyperlipidemia. Corneal ulceration, uveitis, lipid effusion into the aqueous humor, secondary glaucoma, keratoconjunctivitis sicca, and Horner's syndrome have also been associated with thyroid deficiency (Kern and Riis, 1980; Gosselin et al, 1981b; Peruccio, 1982; Kern et al, 1989).

GASTROINTESTINAL SIGNS. Clinical signs related to the gastrointestinal system have been described but are not common in hypothyroid dogs. Constipation may occur, presumably as a result of alterations in electrical control activity and smooth muscle contractile responses in the gastrointestinal tract. Diarrhea has also been reported with hypothyroidism, although a cause-and-effect relationship has not been established and some of these dogs may have the euthyroid sick syndrome rather than hypothyroidism.

Generalized megaesophagus has been identified in some dogs with hypothyroidism, and some investigators have theorized that megaesophagus is caused by hypothyroidism, presumably as a result of hypothyroid-induced neuropathy or myopathy (Jaggy et al, 1994). Unfortunately, no published reports document a cause-and-effect relationship between hypothyroidism and megaesophagus, and one recent study failed to identify an association between hypothyroidism and acquired megaesophagus in dogs (Gaynor et al, 1997). As with cardiomyopathy, a low baseline thyroid hormone concentration in a dog with generalized megaesophagus more often represents the euthyroid sick syndrome than hypothyroidism. The thyroid gland in most of these dogs is responsive to TSH, megaesophagus persists despite thyroid hormone supplementation, and treatment has minimal to no effect on clinical signs (Panciera, 1994; Jaggy et al, 1994).

Myasthenia gravis has been identified in dogs with hypothyroidism (Dewey et al, 1995) and is a well-recognized cause of acquired megaesophagus in the dog. In human beings, there is a link between autoimmune thyroiditis and acquired myasthenia gravis, and myasthenia gravis is a recognized component of type II polyendocrine autoimmune syndrome (see Table 3-4) Presumably a common abnormality in immune function allows development of autoimmunity to the thyroid gland and acetylcholine receptors. Myasthenia gravis was documented in only 1 of 162 dogs with hypothyroidism reviewed by Panciera (2001), implying that hypothyroidism is rarely associated with myasthenia gravis. A causal relation between hypothyroidism and myasthenia gravis remains to be established.

COAGULOPATHY SIGNS. In humans, hypothyroidism may cause any of several abnormalities in the coagulation system, including a reduction in circulating factors VIII and IX, a reduction in factor VIII–related antigen (von Willebrand factor), reduced platelet adhesiveness, and increased capillary fragility (Hymes et al, 1981; Rogers et al, 1982; Dalton et al, 1987). These abnormalities are believed to be caused by decreased protein synthesis in the hypothyroid state and account for the easy bruising observed in some humans with hypothyroidism. Clinically significant bleeding, however, is rare.

A similar reduction in factor VIII–related antigen has been reported in dogs with hypothyroidism (Avgeris et al, 1990), but subsequent studies suggest that hypothyroidism does not induce acquired von Willebrand disease or significant defects in primary hemostasis (Panciera and Johnson, 1994; Panciera and Johnson, 1996). Dogs with subclinical von Willebrand disease may become clinical if hypothyroidism develops. In our experience, however, it is rare for hypothyroid dogs to be presented with clinical signs

related to a bleeding disorder. Evaluation of the coagulation cascade or factor VIII–related antigen is not recommended in dogs with untreated hypothyroidism unless concurrent bleeding problems are present. In contrast, evaluation of thyroid gland function may be indicated in dogs with newly diagnosed von Villebrand disease to rule out hypothyroidism as a contributing factor for the disease. However, when reliance is placed on baseline thyroid hormone concentrations to diagnose hypothyroidism, the clinician must interpret test results critically because of the potential influence of the euthyroid sick syndrome (see page 128).

The effect of thyroid hormone treatment on circulating factor VIII–related antigen is controversial. One study identified an increase in the circulating concentration of factor VIII–related antigen in hypothyroid dogs after initiating levothyroxine sodium treatment (Avgeris et al, 1990), whereas subsequent studies documented a decrease in the concentration of factor VIII–related antigen in dogs with experimental hypothyroidism (Panciera and Johnson, 1996) and euthyroid dogs with von Willebrand disease (Johnstone et al, 1993) after initiating treatment. Thyroid hormone's mechanism of action for increasing the circulating concentration of factor VIII and factor VIII–related antigen is not known but may be related to a generalized increase in protein synthesis. Currently, thyroid hormone supplementation in the euthyroid dog with von Willebrand disease is not recommended.

ALTERATIONS IN BEHAVIOR. In humans, central nervous system function is extremely sensitive to thyroid hormones. Neurologic and psychiatric symptoms are prominent both in hyper- and hypothyroidism. Typical features of hypothyroidism include slowing of all cerebral functions, memory loss, and somnolence; some humans may develop psychosis. Symptoms are usually reversed with levothyroxine sodium treatment (Joffe, 1990; Szabadi, 1991; Monzani et al, 1993). In a study evaluating dogs with polyglandular endocrine disorders, it was postulated that hypothyroidism was associated with canine aberrant behavior, including aggression, submissiveness, shyness, fearfulness, excitability, passivity, irritability, moodiness, and unstable temperament (Dodds, 1995). To date, most reports on alterations in behavior and hypothyroidism have been verbal, anecdotal, and at best, based on apparent improvement in behavior following initiation of thyroid hormone treatment. In one clinical report, aggression may have improved following initiation of levothyroxine sodium treatment in two dogs diagnosed with hypothyroidism (Dodman et al, 1995). An inverse relationship between development of aggression and serotonin activity in the central nervous system has been documented in several species including dogs. Serotonin turnover and sympathetic activity in the CNS are increased in rats made hypothyroid following surgical thyroidectomy; dopamine receptor sensitivity is affected by thyroid hormone in rats; and thyroid hormone potentiates the activity of tricyclic antidepressants in humans suffering from certain types of depression (Crocker and Cameron, 1988; Extein and Gold, 1988; Henley et al, 1991). These studies suggest that thyroid hormone may have an influence on the serotonin-dopamine pathway in the CNS, regardless of the functional status of the thyroid gland. The benefits, if any, for using thyroid hormone to treat behavioral disorders such as aggression in dogs remain to be clarified.

MYXEDEMA COMA. Myxedema coma is a rare syndrome of severe hypothyroidism characterized by profound weakness, hypothermia, bradycardia, and a diminished level of consciousness, which can rapidly progress to stupor and then coma (Chastain et al, 1982; Kelly and Hill, 1984; Henik and Dixon, 2000). Common client complaints include mental dullness, depression, unresponsiveness, and weakness, in addition to the more typical dermatologic signs of hypothyroidism. Physical findings include profound weakness; hypothermia; nonpitting edema of the skin, face, and jowls (i.e., myxedema); bradycardia; hypotension; and hypoventilation. Myxedema results from the accumulation of acid and neutral mucopolysaccharides and hyaluronic acid in the dermis, which bind water and result in increased thickness of the skin. Laboratory findings may include hypoxemia, hypercarbia, hyponatremia, and hypoglycemia in addition to the typical findings of hyperlipidemia, hypercholesterolemia, and nonregenerative anemia. Serum thyroid hormone concentrations are usually extremely low or undetectable; serum TSH concentration is variable but typically increased.

Mortality is high with this disorder, primarily because of lack of recognition. Correctly identifying myxedema of the face and jowls (see Fig. 3-6) is the key to recognizing this syndrome. Early recognition and aggressive therapy are critical to survival. Consequently, the diagnosis should be made clinically, and therapy should be initiated without waiting for results of serum thyroid hormone concentrations.

Treatment consists of thyroid hormone administration and attempts to correct the associated physiologic disturbances, most notably the hypothermia, hypovolemia, electrolyte disturbances, and hypoventilation. Because of the sluggish circulation and severe hypometabolism, absorption of therapeutic agents from the gut or from subcutaneous or intramuscular sites is unpredictable. Thyroid hormone should be administered intravenously, if possible. Levothyroxine sodium (Synthroid; Knoll Pharmaceuticals, Mount Olive, NJ) for parenteral administration is commercially available. The recommended initial dosage is 5 μg/kg every 12 hours (Peterson and Ferguson, 1989). A 50% to 75% reduction in the dosage should be considered if preexisting cardiac disease or failure is present (Henik and Dixon, 2000). Oral administration of levothyroxine sodium can also be administered every 12 hours to provide sustained delivery of T_4. Appropriate supportive care should also be initiated, including intravenous sodium-containing fluids with dextrose supplementation; slow, passive rewarming with blankets; and assisted ventilation, if needed. Clinical improvement is usually seen within 24 hours. Once the dog has stabilized, reliance on oral thyroid hormone treatment can be started (see page 136).

CLINICAL FEATURES OF CONGENITAL HYPOTHYROIDISM: CRETINISM

Severe hypothyroidism in puppies is termed *cretinism*. As the age of onset increases, the clinical appearance of cretinism merges imperceptibly with that of adult hypothyroidism. Normal physical development depends on the presence of normal plasma thyroid hormone concentrations, which act synergistically with GH and insulin-like growth factor-I (IGF-I) to promote chondrogenesis. Retardation of growth and impaired mental development are the hallmarks of cretinism (Table 3-9). Abnormalities usually become obvious to owners by the time affected dogs are 12 weeks of age. Dogs with cretinism appear disproportionate, with large, broad heads; thick, protruding tongues; wide/square trunks; and short limbs (Fig. 3-9). This is in contrast to the proportionate dwarfism caused by GH deficiency (see Fig. 2-5). Delayed epiphyseal appearance and retarded epiphyseal growth with reduced long bone growth cause the disproportionate dwarf stature of congenital hypothyroidism (Saunders and Jezyk, 1991).

Cretins are mentally dull and lethargic and lack the typical playfulness seen in normal puppies. The soft, fluffy "puppy hair coat" usually persists, and diffuse truncal thinning of the hair develops, which may progress to complete alopecia. Seborrhea may be obvious. Additional clinical signs may include inappetence, constipation, delayed dental eruption, and goiter. The presence of goiter is variable and dependent on the underlying etiology (see page 95).

Abnormalities detected on neuromuscular examination may include mental dullness, weakness, hyporeflexia, joint laxity, spasticity, and muscle tremors. Lack of conscious proprioceptive positioning, exaggerated spinal reflexes, and diffuse hyperesthesia have also been reported (Greco et al, 1985).

Differential diagnoses for failure to grow include endocrine (e.g., dwarfism) and nonendocrine causes (see Table 2-9 and Fig. 2-9). See page 48 for more information on pituitary dwarfism.

TABLE 3–9 CLINICAL SIGNS ASSOCIATED WITH CRETINISM

Dwarfism	Gait abnormalities
Short, broad skull	Delayed dental eruption
Shortened mandible	Alopecia
Enlarged cranium	"Puppy" hair coat
Shortened limbs	Dry hair
Kyphosis	Thick skin
Mental dullness	Lethargy
Constipation	Dyspnea
Inappetence	Goiter

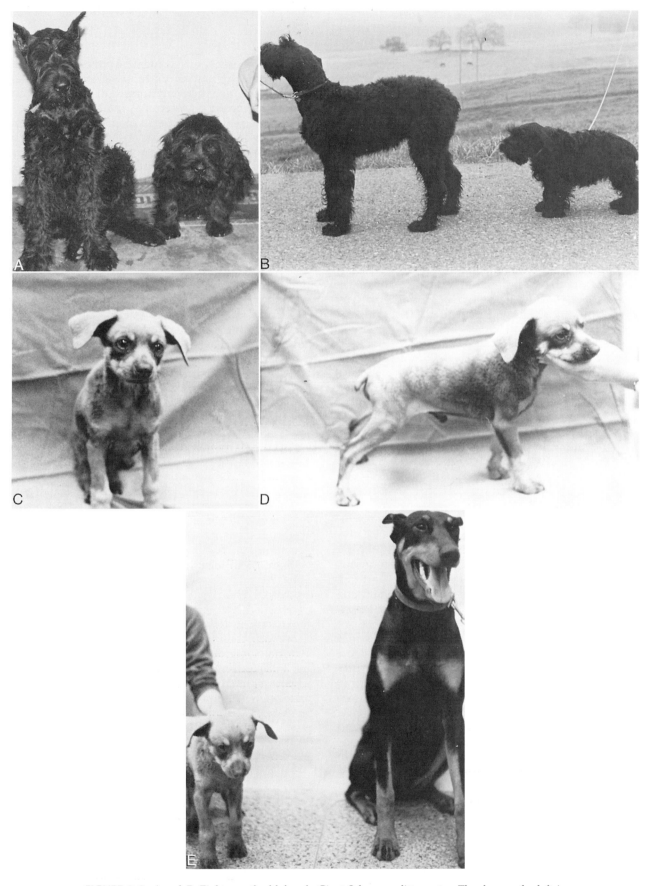

FIGURE 3–9. *A* and *B*, Eight-month-old female Giant Schnauzer littermates. The dog on the left is normal, whereas the smaller dog on the right has congenital hypothyroidism (cretinism). Note the small stature, disproportionate body size, large broad head, wide square trunk, and short limbs in the cretin. *C* and *D*, A 3-year-old male Doberman Pinscher with congenital hypothyroidism. Note the small stature, juvenile appearance, and retention of a soft, fluffy puppy hair coat. *E*, Same dog as in *C* and *D*, shown next to his female littermate.

CLINICAL FEATURES OF SECONDARY HYPOTHYROIDISM

The array of clinical signs is similar for primary and secondary hypothyroidism in the adult and juvenile dog. However, these signs may be minor compared with other, more dominant clinical signs produced by the underlying cause. In most adult dogs, acquired secondary hypothyroidism is caused by a pituitary tumor. The predominant clinical signs depend on the hormonal activity of the tumor and the amount of compression/destruction occurring to surrounding structures. Clinical signs of hypoadrenocorticism or hyperadrenocorticism, diabetes insipidus, or hypothalamic/thalamic dysfunction (i.e., lethargy, stupor, anorexia, adipsia, loss of temperature regulation) usually predominate. Subtle changes associated with hypothyroidism, GH deficiency, or reproductive dysfunction are less likely to be observed by an owner.

CLINICOPATHOLOGIC ABNORMALITIES OF HYPOTHYROIDISM

Well-recognized laboratory abnormalities are associated with hypothyroidism, the severity of which usually correlates with the severity and chronicity of the hypothyroid state. Many of these alterations are nonspecific and may be associated with many other diseases in the dog. Their presence, however, adds supportive evidence for a diagnosis of hypothyroidism in an animal with appropriate clinical signs.

COMPLETE BLOOD COUNT. The classic alteration on a complete blood count (CBC) is a normocytic, normochromic, nonregenerative anemia (packed cell volume [PCV], 28% to 36%). The total red blood cell count, hemoglobin, and PCV are all decreased. A nonregenerative anemia is identified in less than 50% of our hypothyroid dogs. Although the cause is not known, studies in the rat, dog, and human implicate a decrease in plasma erythropoietin concentration and subsequent lack of bone marrow stimulation; erythrocyte survival time is not affected by hypothyroidism. Decreased erythroid progenitor response to erythropoietin and a direct effect of thyroid hormone on early hemopoietic pluripotent stem cells may also contribute to the anemia of hypothyroidism (Green and Ng, 1988; Sainteny et al, 1990). Decreased oxygen consumption by peripheral tissues, a direct reducing effect on plasma erythropoietin, and an increase in 2,3-diphosphoglycerate concentrations in red blood cells (which increases O_2 release in peripheral tissues) are all associated with thyroid deficiency. These factors decrease the demand for red blood cell production. Hypothyroidism in humans has been associated with diminished bone marrow activity, reduced serum iron and iron-binding capacity, normal bone marrow iron stores, decreased plasma iron and red blood cell turnover rates, and decreased total red blood cell volumes.

The absorption of dietary iron by the gastrointestinal tract is also impaired in thyroid deficiency states. As a result, an iron deficiency anemia (i.e., hypochromic, microcytic) has been seen in as many as 15% of hypothyroid humans. Macrocytic megaloblastic anemia is also occasionally encountered in hypothyroid humans, developing secondary to impaired folic acid/vitamin B_{12} metabolism. Similar anemias have been reported in thyroid-deficient dogs but are uncommon (Muller et al, 1983).

Evaluation of red blood cell morphology may reveal increased concentrations of leptocytes (target cells). These cells are believed to develop from increased erythrocyte membrane cholesterol loading, a direct result of the concomitant hypercholesterolemia associated with thyroid deficiency.

The white blood cell count is variable. The presence of a leukocytosis is usually associated with infection, such as a concomitant pyoderma. Platelet counts are normal to increased, and platelet size is normal to decreased (Sullivan et al, 1993).

SERUM BIOCHEMISTRY PANEL. The classic abnormality seen on a screening biochemistry panel is fasting hypercholesterolemia, which is present in more than 75% of our hypothyroid dogs. Fasting hyperlipidemia and hypertriglyceridemia are also common. Thyroid hormones stimulate virtually all aspects of lipid metabolism, including synthesis, mobilization, and degradation (Larsen et al, 1998). Both the synthesis and degradation of lipids are depressed in hypothyroidism, with degradation affected more than synthesis. The net effect is an accumulation of plasma lipids in hypothyroidism and the potential for development of atherosclerosis (Hess et al, 2002).

Lipoprotein electrophoretic evaluation of plasma from 26 hypothyroid dogs revealed three general groups of findings: (1) normal plasma lipid concentrations and lipoprotein electrophoresis; (2) hypercholesterolemia with increased intensity of the alpha$_2$-lipoprotein band; and (3) hypercholesterolemia and hypertriglyceridemia with prominent pre-beta, beta, and alpha$_2$-lipoprotein bands (Rogers et al, 1975). Hyperlipidemia and altered lipoprotein electrophoretic patterns returned nearly to normal following supplementation with thyroid hormone. A more recent study used a combined ultracentrifugation and precipitation technique to quantify plasma lipoprotein concentrations in 10 dogs with hypothyroidism (Barrie et al, 1993). The plasma concentrations of cholesterol, very–low-density lipoprotein (VLDL) cholesterol, low-density lipoprotein (LDL) cholesterol, and high-density lipoprotein (HDL) cholesterol were significantly higher, compared with healthy dogs. Thyroid hormone deficiency-induced decrease in hepatic LDL receptor activity and reduced activities of lipoprotein lipase and hepatic lipase were proposed as the underlying mechanisms responsible for the lipoprotein cholesterol abnormalities identified in hypothyroid dogs (Valdermarsson et al, 1983).

Fasting hypercholesterolemia and hypertriglyceridemia can be associated with several other

TABLE 3–10   CAUSES OF HYPERLIPIDEMIA IN THE DOG AND CAT

Postprandial hyperlipidemia
Secondary hyperlipidemia
  Hypothyroidism
  Hyperadrenocorticism
  Diabetes mellitus
  Pancreatitis
  Cholestasis
  Hepatic insufficiency
  Nephrotic syndrome
  Protein-losing enteropathy
Primary hyperlipidemia
  Idiopathic hyperlipoproteinemia (Miniature Schnauzer)
  Idiopathic hyperchylomicronemia (cat)
  Lipoprotein lipase deficiency (cat)
  Idiopathic hypercholesterolemia
Drug-induced hyperlipidemia
  Glucocorticoids
  Megesterol acetate (cat)

disorders (Table 3-10) and thus are not pathognomonic for hypothyroidism. However, their presence in a dog with appropriate clinical signs is strong supportive evidence for hypothyroidism.

Occasionally, hypothyroid dogs may have a mild to moderate increase in serum lactate dehydrogenase, aspartate aminotransferase, alanine transaminase, and alkaline phosphatase activities. These increases are believed to be due to an associated myopathy or hepatic lipidosis. However, these increased activities are extremely inconsistent and may not be directly related to the hypothyroid state.

Mild hypercalcemia may be found in some dogs with congenital hypothyroidism. This alteration has been documented in hypothyroid children secondary to increased intestinal absorption and decreased urinary excretion of calcium.

An elevation in plasma creatine kinase (CK) is well recognized in hypothyroid humans and has been reported in dogs, although its incidence is controversial (Chastain and Schmidt, 1980; Braund et al, 1981; Muller et al, 1983). In humans, there is an inverse relationship between CK activity and thyroid function. Intuitively, an increase in CK activity could be expected to correspond with the development of hypothyroid myopathy. Dogs with histologically confirmed hypothyroid myopathy, however, may not have abnormal CK activity and vice versa (Braund et al, 1981). Therefore CK activity may also be a reflection of alterations in catabolic and anabolic processes within muscle or of alterations in the sarcolemmal membrane permeability, allowing release of the enzyme from muscle, in addition to a reflection of degenerative changes involving the type II muscle fibers.

URINALYSIS.   Results of urine evaluation are usually normal in dogs with hypothyroidism. In dogs with lymphocytic thyroiditis, immune-complex glomerulonephritis may result in proteinuria. Polyuria, hyposthenuria, and urinary tract infections are not typical of hypothyroidism.

NONTHYROID HORMONE CONCENTRATIONS.   Hypothyroidism can affect the secretion of nonthyroidal hormones from other endocrine glands, most notably the pituitary gland. In humans, dogs, and rats, hypothyroidism can result in a suppressed plasma growth hormone (GH) response to provocative stimuli (see page 54) (Froelich and Meserve, 1982; Greco et al, 1985). Despite suppressed GH secretion, GH treatment alone fails to promote statural growth in dwarf, hypothyroid children. Adequate thyroid hormone replacement, however, normalizes impaired GH secretion and leads to rapid "catch-up" skeletal growth in these individuals.

Thyroid hormone deficiency–induced increase in TRH secretion can stimulate prolactin secretion, resulting in hyperprolactinemia and, in some female dogs, inappropriate lactation (Chastain and Schmidt, 1980; Cortese et al, 1997). Thyroid hormone is also necessary for normal LH and FSH secretion. Pituitary LH and FSH secretion is suppressed in humans with hypothyroidism, resulting in diminished libido, ovulation failure, and oligospermia (Larsen et al, 1998). The metabolism of androgens and estrogens is also altered in hypothyroidism.

Finally, hypothyroidism may be a component of immunoendocrinopathy syndromes (polyglandular autoimmune syndromes; see page 91). Affected dogs may also have insulin-dependent diabetes mellitus, hypoadrenocorticism, hypoparathyroidism, or gonadal failure, with corresponding deficiencies in circulating hormone concentrations.

DERMATOHISTOPATHOLOGIC FINDINGS IN HYPOTHYROIDISM

The value of skin biopsies as part of the diagnostic evaluation for hypothyroidism is controversial. Pathologic changes in the skin have a finite number of clinical manifestations. Because of this, different problems can cause similar gross dermatologic alterations. Hypothyroidism is not an exception. Skin biopsies are often performed in dogs with suspected endocrine alopecia in which the typical screening diagnostic tests (including baseline thyroid hormone concentrations) have failed to identify the cause. For most dogs, findings on skin biopsy reveal nondiagnostic changes consistent with an endocrinopathy but fail to identify the underlying endocrine disorder (Table 3-11; Gross et al, 1992; Scott et al, 2001). Histopathologic findings highly suggestive of hypothyroidism may be identified and include vacuolated, hypertrophied arrector pili muscles, increased dermal mucin, and a thick dermis. The presence of "hypothyroid-specific" histopathologic alterations is an indication for further evaluation of thyroid gland function. Approximately 50% of biopsy specimens from dogs with hypothyroidism have variable degrees of inflammation, reflecting the common occurrence of secondary seborrhea, bacterial pyoderma, or both (Scott et al, 2001).

TABLE 3–11 DERMATOHISTOPATHOLOGIC ALTERATIONS ASSOCIATED WITH ENDOCRINOPATHY-INDUCED ALOPECIA IN THE DOG

Nonspecific Abnormalities Supporting an Endocrinopathy

Orthokeratotic hyperkeratosis
Follicular keratosis
Follicular dilatation
Follicular atrophy
Predominance of telogen hair follicles
Sebaceous gland atrophy
Epidermal atrophy
Epidermal melanosis
Thin dermis
Dermal collagen atrophy

Abnormalities Supportive of Hypothyroidism

Vacuolated arrector pilae muscles
Hypertrophied arrector pilae muscles
Increased dermal mucin content
Thick dermis

RADIOGRAPHY, ULTRASONOGRAPHY, AND NUCLEAR IMAGING

CONVENTIONAL RADIOGRAPHY. Conventional radiography is not a routine procedure for evaluation of canine hypothyroidism. Cervical radiography is ineffective in determining the status of the thyroid gland. If hypothyroidism develops following destruction of the thyroid gland by an invasive tumor, however, thoracic radiographs should be obtained to help rule out metastatic disease.

Bone surveys from dogs with congenital hypothyroidism are abnormal. Radiographic abnormalities include delayed epiphyseal ossification (Fig. 3-10); epiphyseal dysgenesis (i.e., irregularly formed, fragmented, or stippled epiphyseal centers), most common in the humeral, femoral, and proximal tibial condyles; short broad skulls; shortened vertebral bodies; and delayed maturation (Greco et al, 1991; Saunders and Jezyk, 1991; Mooney and Anderson,

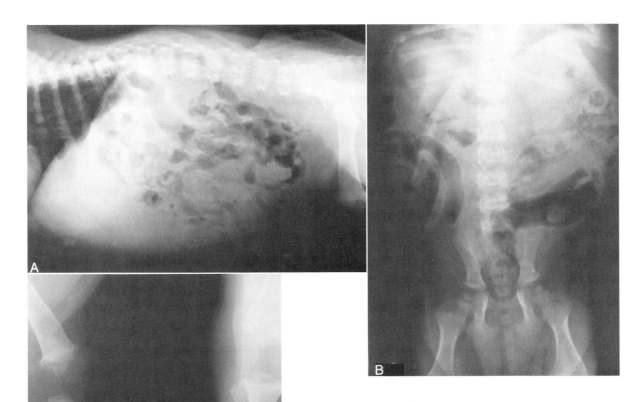

FIGURE 3–10. *A* and *B*, Lateral and ventrodorsal radiographs of the spine of a dog with congenital hypothyroidism. Note the shortened vertebral bodies with scalloped ventral borders and only partially calcified vertebral endplates. *C*, Lateral and anteroposterior radiograph of the tibia and fibula of a dog with congenital hypothyroidism, illustrating epiphyseal dysplasia and poor calcification of the bones.

1993). Ventral borders of vertebral bodies may be scalloped, suggesting lack of normal longitudinal growth (Fig. 3-10). Overall length of the diaphyses of long bones is reduced, and carpal and tarsal bones appear to have retarded ossification. Valgus deformities are common. Accelerated epiphyseal ossification occurs during thyroid hormone supplementation, but degenerative joint changes may develop despite thyroid hormone supplementation (Saunders and Jezyk, 1991). Owners should be informed of the arthritis invariably associated with this degenerative joint disease. Radiographic changes similar to congenital hypothyroidism have been reported in multiple epiphyseal dysplasia in Beagles and a Miniature Poodle (Saunders and Jezyk, 1991) and in dogs with pituitary dwarfism (see Chapter 2).

ULTRASONOGRAPHY. The thyroid gland can be identified and its size, shape, and echogenicity determined using real-time ultrasonography in dogs. Ultrasonography is a commonly employed diagnostic aid in dogs with suspected neoplastic thyroid masses, especially for guidance in performing needle biopsy (see Chapter 5). Ultrasound may also prove to be a diagnostic aid for differentiating between hypothyroidism and the euthyroid sick syndrome. Intuitively, lymphocytic thyroiditis and idiopathic atrophy should cause a decrease in the size and alterations in the shape and echogenicity of the thyroid lobe, compared with a normal thyroid lobe. Differences in thyroid lobe size and echogenicity were recently identified in hypothyroid versus healthy Golden Retrievers using ultrasonography (Brömel et al, 2001). The thyroid lobe in healthy Golden Retrievers was usually fusiform and triangular to oval in shape on longitudinal and transverse views, respectively (Fig. 3-11). Both thyroid lobes had a homogeneous echogenic pattern and were hyperechoic to isoechoic, compared with the echogenicity of the surrounding musculature. Similar findings were identified in Golden Retrievers with the euthyroid sick syndrome. Although differences in shape were not identified, there was a significant reduction in size and volume of the thyroid lobe in hypothyroid versus healthy and euthyroid sick Golden Retrievers. In addition, the echogenicity of the thyroid lobe in hypothyroid Golden Retrievers tended to be isoechoic to hypoechoic with hyperechoic foci and the echogenic pattern often differed between thyroid lobes in the same dog. Although the diagnostic value of ultrasound remains to be determined, these preliminary findings suggest that ultrasound evaluation of the thyroid lobe may be helpful in differentiating hypothyroidism from the euthyroid sick syndrome in dogs with nondiagnostic thyroid hormone test results. Unfortunately, a direct correlation between size of the dog breed and size and volume of the normal thyroid gland may exist; the smaller the size of the dog breed, the smaller the size and volume of the normal thyroid lobe (Brömel et al, 2002). Presumably, reference ranges for thyroid lobe size and volume will have to be established for each

breed before ultrasound can be used to confirm a decrease in thyroid lobe size and volume in dogs with suspected hypothyroidism.

NUCLEAR IMAGING. Thyroid scans using radioactive pertechnetate (see Chapter 4) may be clinically useful in evaluating the size, shape, and location of thyroid tissue. Although not recommended to evaluate function, pertechnetate scans may aid in differentiating between hypothyroidism, euthyroidism, and the euthyroid sick syndrome. The normal thyroid lobes appear as two uniformly dense, symmetric ovals in the midcervical area (Fig. 3-12). These ovals are slightly smaller than the salivary glands, which also concentrate pertechnetate. A 1:1 ratio normally exists between size and density because of pertechnetate uptake in the parotid salivary gland and uptake in normal thyroid glands. Adult dogs with primary hypothyroidism typically have low or nondetectable accumulation of pertechnetate by the thyroid gland, and the thyroid gland may also appear smaller than normal if pertechnetate does concentrate within the gland (Fig. 3-12). Similar results are found in puppies with congenital hypothyroidism caused by thyroid dysgenesis and dogs with secondary hypothyroidism (Kintzer and Peterson, 1991; Greco et al, 1991). In contrast, puppies with congenital hypothyroidism caused by iodination defects have normal to enlarged thyroid lobes and normal to increased pertechnetate accumulation. Dogs with nonthyroidal illness or drug-induced lowering of baseline serum thyroid hormone concentrations that is not secondary to suppression of pituitary TSH secretion should have normal or increased accumulation of pertechnetate (Hall et al, 1993). The latter suggests increased physiologic iodide trapping by the thyroid gland.

TESTS OF THYROID GLAND FUNCTION

Overview

Function of the thyroid gland is typically assessed by measuring baseline serum thyroid hormone concentrations or evaluating the responsiveness of the thyroid gland to provocative stimulation (e.g., TRH stimulation test). Several tests to assess thyroid gland function are available, including those that measure thyroxine (T_4), free T_4 (fT_4), 3,5,3'-triiodothyronine (T_3), free T_3 (fT_3), 3,3',5'-triiodothyronine (reverse T_3 [rT_3]), and endogenous thyrotropin (TSH) concentration. T_4 accounts for most of the thyroid hormone secreted by the thyroid gland, with only small quantities of T_3 and minor amounts of rT_3 released. Once secreted into the circulation, more than 99% of T_4 is bound to plasma proteins (see page 87). The unbound, or free, T_4 is biologically active, exerts negative feedback inhibition on pituitary TSH secretion (see Fig. 3-3), and is capable of entering cells throughout the body (Fig. 3-13). Protein-bound T_4 acts as a reservoir and buffer to maintain a steady concentration of free hormone in the plasma, despite rapid alterations in the delivery of

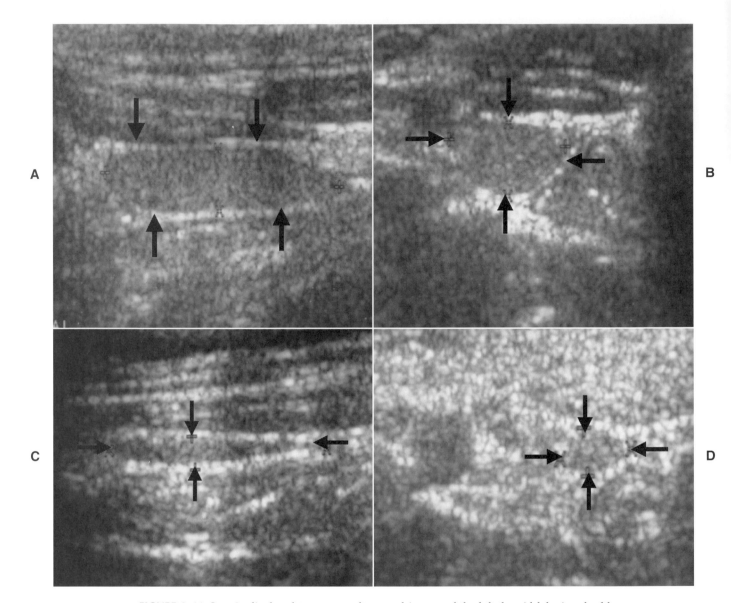

FIGURE 3–11. Longitudinal and transverse ultrasound images of the left thyroid lobe in a healthy Golden Retriever dog *(A and B)* and a Golden Retriever dog with hypothyroidism *(C and D)*. Note the smaller size of the thyroid lobe in the dog with hypothyroidism, compared with the healthy dog. The maximum length, width, and height of the thyroid lobe measured 24.8 mm, 7.9 mm, and 4.6 mm in the healthy dog and 20.2 mm, 4.1 mm, and 2.8 mm in the hypothyroid dog.

thyroid hormone to tissues. Serum T_4 concentrations generated by commercial endocrine laboratories represent the sum of the protein-bound and free levels circulating in the blood, unless fT_4 concentration is specifically requested.

As previously discussed, free thyroid hormone concentrations are biologically active and capable of entering cells throughout the body. Within the cell, fT_4 is deiodinated to form either T_3 or rT_3, depending on the metabolic demands of the tissues at that particular time. T_3 is preferentially produced during normal metabolic states, whereas rT_3, which is biologically inactive, appears to be produced during periods of illness, starvation, or excessive endogenous catabolism. Intracellular T_3 binds to receptors on the mitochondria, nucleus, and plasma membrane and exerts

its physiologic effects. T_3 is believed to be the primary hormone that induces physiologic effects, because of its greater biologic activity and volume of distribution compared with those of T_4, the preferential deiodination of T_4 to T_3 within the cell, and the presence of specific intracellular receptors for T_3 (Werner, 1982).

All serum T_4, both protein-bound and free, comes from the thyroid gland. Therefore tests that measure the serum total and free T_4 concentrations, in conjunction with the serum TSH concentration, are currently recommended for the assessment of thyroid gland function in dogs suspected of having hypothyroidism. In contrast, most T_3 and rT_3 is formed through the deiodination of T_4 in extrathyroidal sites, most notably the liver, kidney, and muscle. Serum T_3

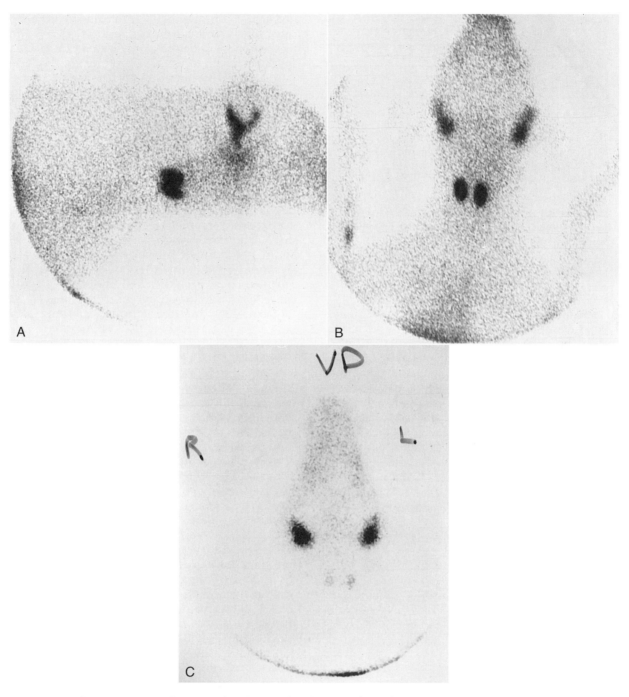

FIGURE 3–12. *A* and *B,* Lateral and ventrodorsal views of a sodium pertechnetate nuclear scan performed in a normal dog. The normal thyroid lobes appear as two uniformly dense symmetric spots in the cervical region. The parotid salivary glands are also visible. *C,* Ventrodorsal view of a sodium pertechnetate nuclear scan performed in a dog with primary hypothyroidism. Uptake of sodium pertechnetate is normal by the parotid salivary glands, which are readily visible, but is markedly reduced by the thyroid lobes, which are barely visible.

concentration is a poor gauge of thyroid gland function because of its predominant location within cells and the minimal amount secreted by the thyroid gland in comparison with the amount of T_4 secreted. Thus measurement of serum T_3, fT_3, and rT_3 concentration is not routinely recommended for the assessment of thyroid gland function in dogs.

Baseline Serum Total Thyroxine Concentration

ASSAY TECHNIQUE. Baseline serum total T_4 concentration is the sum of both protein-bound and free hormone circulating in the blood. Clinical chemistry laboratories currently use either a radioimmunoassay (RIA) technique or enzyme immunoassay for measuring

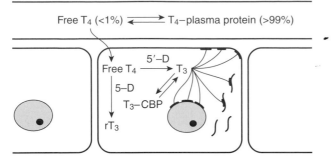

Blood vessel

$$\text{Free } T_4 (<1\%) \rightleftharpoons T_4\text{--plasma protein } (>99\%)$$

FIGURE 3–13. Schematic of intracellular metabolism of free T_4 to either T_3 or reverse T_3 by 5'- or 5-monodeiodinase, respectively. Intracellular T_3 formed from monodeiodination of free T_4 can interact with T_3 receptors on the cell membrane, mitochondria, or nucleus of the cell and stimulate the physiologic actions of thyroid hormone or bind to cytoplasmic binding proteins (CBP). The latter forms an intracellular storage pool for T_3.

T_4 concentrations in the blood. The RIA technique incorporating radiolableled hormone is considered the gold standard for measurement of serum T_4 concentration and is the generally accepted reference method. RIAs are competitive assays in which known quantities of iodine-125–labeled thyroid hormone and a specific amount of patient serum are mixed in a test tube containing antithyroid hormone antibody (Fig. 3-14). The radioactive thyroid hormone and the thyroid

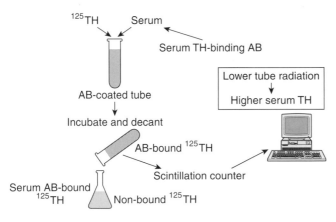

FIGURE 3–14. Schematic illustration of how antithyroid hormone antibodies may cause spuriously increased thyroid hormone values for a radioimmunoassay using a single-step, antibody-coated tube separation system. Patient serum and radiolabeled thyroid hormone (which comes with the assay) are added to a test tube coated with antithyroid hormone antibody. Thyroid hormone in serum competes with radiolabeled thyroid hormone for antibody-binding sites in the tube. After incubation, the liquid in the tube is decanted, the radioactivity of the tube is measured in a scintillation counter, and the serum thyroid hormone concentration is determined based on the tube radioactivity. An inverse relationship exists between tube radioactivity and serum thyroid hormone concentration. If antithyroid hormone binding antibodies are present in the patient's serum, these antibodies compete with the antibodies attached to the tube for serum thyroid hormone and radiolabeled thyroid hormone. Because serum thyroid hormone antibodies are not attached to the tube, they are decanted along with any radiolabeled thyroid hormone that has bound to them. This causes a falsely low radioactivity of the tube and a corresponding spuriously high serum thyroid hormone value. *TH*, thyroid hormone; *AB*, antibody.

hormone in the animal's serum compete for binding to the antithyroid hormone antibody. Following an incubation period, the antibody-bound radiolabeled thyroid hormone is separated from the unbound radiolabeled thyroid hormone, the radioactivity of the tube is counted, and the thyroid hormone concentration is extrapolated from a standard curve. Most laboratories use a single-phase separation system with the antithyroid hormone antibody bound to the test tube. For these systems, separation involves merely decanting the liquid contents from the tube and placing the tube in the scintillation counter. An inverse correlation exists between the amount of radioactivity measured and the concentration of thyroid hormone in the serum sample. The greater the concentration of thyroid hormone in the animal's serum, the less the binding of iodine-125–labeled thyroid hormone to the antibody and the lower the radioactivity of the tube. The opposite occurs when the thyroid hormone concentration in the animal's serum is decreased.

The normal range for serum T_4 concentration varies between laboratories because of differences in commercial RIA kits used, laboratory technique, and expertise. For most laboratories, the serum T_4 concentration in healthy dogs ranges between 1.0 and 3.5 µg/dl. The lower limit of the normal range varies between laboratories, depending on whether the laboratory wants greater specificity or sensitivity for the test (see Interpretation, below).

Most RIAs for measurement of serum thyroid hormones are actually produced for use in humans. These assays work in dogs because of good cross-reactivity of thyroid hormone between species. Baseline serum T_4 concentrations tend to be lower in healthy dogs than in humans (1.0 to 3.5 versus 4.0 to 10.0 µg/dl, respectively). Hence the RIA technique must be sensitive enough to detect T_4 concentrations less than 1.0 µg/dl to accurately differentiate hypothyroidism from euthyroidism in dogs. Some RIA kits accurately measure serum T_4 concentrations only as low as 2.0 to 5.0 µg/dl, values that are too high for assessment of canine thyroid dysfunction. The clinician must know the sensitivity of the assay (i.e., the lowest concentration the assay can reliably detect) being used, especially if the assays are completed in a human-oriented endocrine laboratory.

ENZYME IMMUNOASSAYS. A homogeneous enzyme-linked immunoassay (ELISA) (CEDIA Total T_4 Assay; Boehringer Mannheim Corp, Indianapolis, IN) for measurement of serum T_4 in humans was recently adapted for use in dogs and cats (Horney et al, 1999). This method uses recombinant fragments of *E. coli* β-galactosidase, which are inactive separately but combine spontaneously to form active enzyme. Thyroxine is covalently coupled to one of the fragments so that monoclonal antibody to T_4 blocks enzyme formation. Serum T_4 competes for antibody binding and thus allows formation of active enzyme. The amount of active enzyme formed is directly proportional to the concentration of T_4 in the patient's serum and is measured through hydrolysis of the reaction substrate 0-nitrophenyl-β-D-galactopyranoside.

Method comparison studies gave close agreement between RIA and ELISA results when the ELISA was evaluated on the Hitachi 911 automated analyzer (Boehringer Mannheim Corp, Indianapolis, IN), with correlation coefficients of 0.88 and 0.97 for canine and feline samples, respectively (Horney et al, 1999). The ELISA method was not sensitive to interference from hemolysis or moderate to high elevations in triglyceride (5 to 10 g/L) and was less sensitive than the RIA method to interference from T_4 autoantibodies, presumably because the RIA system used a polyclonal antibody, whereas the ELISA method used a mouse monoclonal antibody less susceptible to interference by cross-reactivity. The ELISA is a precise and accurate method for determination of T_4 concentration in canine and feline serum, can be adapted to automated photometric analyzers used routinely in veterinary clinical chemistry laboratories, and can be performed in conjunction with routine clinical chemistry tests, thereby providing an effective alternative to RIA.

Point-of-care ELISAs for measuring serum T_4 in dogs and cats are also available. The advantage of an in-house test is that it is economical, quick, easy to perform, and allows the clinician to make recommendations the same day the animal is evaluated. Evaluations of an in-house ELISA (Snap T_4 test kit and VetTest Snap Reader; IDEXX Laboratories Inc, Westbrooke, ME) for quantitative measurement of serum T_4 concentration in dogs and cats have been conflicting. In one study, substantial discrepancies between the in-house ELISA and RIA results for T_4 concentrations were detected (Lurye et al, 2002). In dogs, the in-house ELISA overestimated and underestimated the serum T_4 concentration obtained with RIA, and interpretation of the ELISA results from 62% of 50 samples would have lead to inappropriate clinical decisions. In cats, the in-house ELISA consistently overestimated the serum T_4 concentration obtained with RIA, and interpretation of the ELISA results from 50% of 50 samples would have lead to inappropriate clinical decisions. In contrast, another study found a good correlation between the in-house ELISA and RIA in feline (r=0.90) and canine (r=0.91) blood samples (Peterson et al, 2003). The overall accuracy of the in-house ELISA was considered excellent and results from the in-house ELISA would have lead to a different clinical decision compared with results from the RIA in only 5 of 105 samples. Because differences in point-of-care ELISA test results exist between veterinary hospitals, accuracy of any point-of-care ELISA should always be documented by the hospital in which it is used, preferably by comparing ELISA and RIA results from the same blood samples.

STABILITY AND FACTORS INTERFERING WITH MEASUREMENT. Thyroxine is a relatively stable hormone that enhances the chance of receiving accurate results when blood samples must be mailed to commercial laboratories. Blood T_4 is resistant to degradation by contact with cells in blood, long-term storage following centrifugation, hemolysis, or repeated thawing and freezing (Reimers et al, 1982). In addition, serum may be stored in plastic tubes for 8 days at room temperature and for 5 days at 37° C without affecting the concentration of T_4 (Behrend et al, 1998). This is also true for heparinized plasma and ethylenediamine-tetra-acetic acid (EDTA) plasma samples. However, storage of serum or plasma at 37° C in glass can cause a significant increase in serum T_4 concentration, compared with storage at –20° C (Behrend et al, 1998). Although T_4 is stable, whenever possible, serum samples should be frozen and stored in plastic tubes and sent to the laboratory on cold packs.

Many physiologic and pharmacologic factors affect the pituitary-thyroid axis and interfere with the accuracy of baseline serum T_4 concentration in differentiating hypothyroidism from euthyroidism (see Factors Affecting Thyroid Gland Function Tests, page 126). However, the only factor that interferes with the ability of the RIA to measure T_4 is anti-T_4 antibodies in the serum sample. Antithyroid hormone antibodies may develop in dogs with lymphocytic thyroiditis and cause spuriously increased or decreased serum T_4 values (Thacker et al, 1992). The effect of antithyroid hormone antibodies on the serum T_4 value depends on the type of assay being used by the laboratory (see page 125). Hyperlipidemia does not interfere with RIA measurement of T_4 in serum (Lee et al, 1991).

INTERPRETATION OF RESULTS. Measurement of the serum T_4 concentration can be used as the initial test for hypothyroidism or be part of a thyroid panel containing T_4, fT_4, TSH, and an antibody test for lymphocytic thyroiditis (Table 3-12). Theoretically, the interpretation of baseline serum T_4 concentration should be straightforward; that is, dogs with hypothyroidism should have low values compared with healthy dogs. Unfortunately, the range of serum T_4 concentration overlaps between hypothyroid dogs and healthy dogs, and this overlap becomes more evident in euthyroid dogs with concurrent illness. In one study, the range of serum T_4 concentration in 62 healthy dogs was 1.0 to 3.3 µg/dl and in 51 hypothyroid dogs was undetectable to 1.5 µg/dl (Nelson et al, 1991). The amount of residual thyroid gland function at the time the sample is obtained, the suppressive effects of extraneous factors on serum thyroid hormone concentrations, and the presence of circulating antithyroid hormone antibodies all affect the sensitivity and specificity of serum T_4 concentration in diagnosing hypothyroidism.

This overlap between euthyroidism and hypothyroidism creates a dilemma when a laboratory tries to establish its normal range for serum T_4 concentration. If the laboratory keeps the lower limit of the normal serum T_4 range high (e.g., 1.5 µg/dl), sensitivity of the test is sacrificed for specificity. That is, the number of hypothyroid dogs misdiagnosed as euthyroid is minimized, but the number of euthyroid dogs misdiagnosed as hypothyroid is increased, leading to inappropriate thyroid replacement treatment of euthyroid dogs. Alternatively, by decreasing the lower limit of the normal serum T_4 range (e.g., 0.8 µg/dl), specificity is sacrificed for sensitivity. The number of euthyroid dogs misdiagnosed as hypothyroid is minimized, but the number of hypothyroid dogs misdiagnosed as euthyroid increases, potentially creating diagnostic confusion.

TABLE 3–12   DIAGNOSTIC RECOMMENDATIONS FOR EVALUATING THYROID GLAND FUNCTION IN THE DOG

1. The decision to assess thyroid gland function should be based on results of the history, physical examination, and results of routine bloodwork (CBC, serum biochemistry panel, urinalysis)
2. Initial single screening tests include baseline serum T_4 and baseline serum free T_4 measured by equilibrium dialysis (MED).
   a. Treatment is indicated if the serum T_4 or free T_4 concentration is low and the initial evaluation of the dog strongly supports the diagnosis of hypothyroidism.
   b. Treatment is not indicated if the serum T_4 or free T_4 concentration is normal and the initial evaluation of the dog does not strongly support the diagnosis of hypothyroidism.
   c. Additional diagnostic tests (i.e., endogenous TSH, thyroglobulin or thyroid hormone autoantibody) are indicated if serum T_4 concentration is normal but the initial evaluation of the dog strongly supports the diagnosis of hypothyroidism-or-the veterinarian is uncertain if hypothyroidism exists after evaluation of history, physical examination, routine bloodwork, and serum T_4 or free T_4 concentration.
3. Commonly used screening protocols utilizing two diagnostic tests include baseline serum T_4 or baseline serum free T_4 measured by MED and serum TSH concentration.
   a. Treatment is indicated if the serum T_4 or free T_4 concentration is low and the initial evaluation of the dog strongly supports the diagnosis of hypothyroidism, regardless of the serum TSH test result.
   b. Treatment is not indicated if all of these tests are normal and the initial evaluation of the dog does not strongly support the diagnosis of hypothyroidism.
   c. Treatment is not indicated and the tests should be repeated in 8 to 12 weeks if the serum free T_4 concentration is normal and the serum TSH concentration is increased.
   d. Evaluation of serum thyroglobulin or T_4 autoantibody test is indicated if serum T_4 concentration is normal, serum TSH concentration is increased, and the initial evaluation of the dog strongly supports the diagnosis of hypothyroidism.
4. Common components of a thyroid panel include serum T_4 concentration, serum T_4 concentration measured by MED, serum TSH concentration, and an antibody test for lymphocytic thyroiditis.
   a. Treatment is indicated if all of the tests for thyroid gland function are abnormal and the initial evaluation of the dog strongly supports the diagnosis of hypothyroidism, regardless of the thyroid hormone antibody test results.
   b. Treatment is not indicated if all of the tests for thyroid gland function are normal and the initial evaluation of the dog does not strongly support the diagnosis of hypothyroidism, regardless of the thyroid hormone antibody test results. Positive thyroid hormone antibody test results support the presence of lymphocytic thyroiditis and the need to monitor tests of thyroid gland function every 3 to 6 months.
   c. When discordant thyroid gland function test results are obtained, the decision to treat should be based on the initial evaluation of the dog, the clinician's index of suspicion for hypothyroidism, and a critical evaluation of each thyroid gland function test result. Serum free T_4 concentration by MED is the most accurate test of thyroid gland function.

The reference range for serum T_4 concentration may also vary between breeds. The reference range is usually established based on the mean plus and minus two standard deviations calculated from results of serum T_4 measured in a large population of dogs without regard for breed. The reference range for serum T_4 and free T_4 measured by modified equilibrium dialysis (see page 116) is now recognized to be lower in sight hounds, most notably Greyhounds, than in non-Greyhound pet dogs (Gaughan and Bruyette, 2001). These findings suggest that breed-specific reference range values for thyroid hormone tests may need to be established and used when evaluating thyroid gland function in the respective breed. Until such information is established for the breed, interpretation of thyroid hormone test results will have to follow the principles discussed below and on page 134.

We do not recommend use of an arbitrary serum T_4 value to separate euthyroidism from hypothyroidism. Rather, we recommend evaluating the serum T_4 result in the context of the history, physical examination findings, and other clinicopathologic data. All of this information yields an index of suspicion for euthyroidism or hypothyroidism. For the clinician, it is difficult to judge the effect extraneous factors, especially concurrent illness, have on the serum T_4 concentration. Because these variables can suppress a baseline serum T_4 concentration to less than 0.5 µg/dl in a euthyroid dog and because hypothyroid dogs rarely have serum T_4 concentrations greater than 1.5 µg/dl, we use the baseline serum T_4 concentration as a measure of

euthyroidism. The higher the T_4 concentration, the more likely the dog is euthyroid (Table 3-13). The one exception is the hypothyroid dog with circulating antithyroid hormone antibodies (see page 125). Conversely, the lower the T_4 value, the more likely the dog has hypothyroidism, assuming the history, physical examination findings, and clinicopathologic data are also consistent with the disease and severe systemic illness is not present. If the clinician's index of suspicion is not high for hypothyroidism but the serum T_4 concentration is low, then other factors such as the euthyroid sick syndrome must also be considered (see page 126).

INTERPRETATION: CONCURRENT THYROID HORMONE SUPPLEMENTATION. Occasionally, a clinician wants to determine whether a dog receiving thyroid supplementation is, in fact, hypothyroid. The exogenous administration of thyroid hormone, either T_4 or T_3, will suppress pituitary TSH secretion and cause pituitary thyrotroph atrophy, and subsequently thyroid gland atrophy in a healthy euthyroid dog (Panciera et al, 1990). Serum T_4, fT_4, and TSH concentrations are decreased or undetectable; the severity of the decrease is dependent on the severity of thyroid gland atrophy induced by the thyroid hormone supplement. Serum T_4 and fT_4 results are often suggestive of hypothyroidism, even in a previously euthyroid dog, if the testing is performed within a month of discontinuing treatment (Panciera et al, 1989). Thyroid hormone supplementation must be discontinued and the pituitary-thyroid axis allowed to regain function

TABLE 3–13 INTERPRETATION OF BASELINE SERUM THYROXINE (T₄) AND FREE THYROXINE (fT₄) CONCENTRATION IN DOGS WITH SUSPECTED HYPOTHYROIDISM

Serum T_4 Concentration (μg/dl)	Serum fT_4 Concentration (ng/dl)	Probability of Hypothyroidism
> 2.0 μg/dl	> 2.0 ng/dl	Very unlikely
1.5 to 2.0 μg/dl	1.5 to 2.0 ng/dl	Unlikely
1.0 to 1.5 μg/dl	0.8 to 1.5 ng/dl	Unknown
0.5 to 1.0 μg/dl	0.5 to 0.8 ng/dl	Possible
< 0.5 μg/dl	< 0.5 ng/dl	Very likely*

*Assuming that a severe systemic illness is not present.

before meaningful results of baseline serum T_4, fT_4, and TSH concentrations can be obtained. The time interval between the discontinuation of thyroid hormone supplementation and the acquisition of meaningful results regarding thyroid gland function depends on the duration of treatment, the dosage and frequency of administration of the thyroid hormone supplement, and individual variability. As a general rule, thyroid hormone supplements should be discontinued a minimum of 4 weeks and preferably 6 to 8 weeks before critically assessing thyroid gland function.

Baseline Serum Total Triiodothyronine Concentration

ASSAY TECHNIQUE. Baseline serum total T_3 concentrations are the sum of the protein-bound and free levels circulating in the blood. Almost all commercial laboratories currently use RIA techniques for measuring T_3 concentrations in the blood. Most human RIAs for T_3 are suitable for use in the dog because blood concentrations are similar for both species. Using the RIA technique, an approximate normal range for blood T_3 concentrations is 0.8 to 1.5 ng/ml, although the exact range varies from laboratory to laboratory because of differences in RIAs used, laboratory technique, and expertise.

STABILITY AND FACTORS INTERFERING WITH MEASUREMENT. Stability of serum T_3 and factors interfering with its measurement are as described for serum T_4. The incidence of anti-T_3 antibodies is greater than that of anti-T_4 antibodies in dogs with lymphocytic thyroiditis.

INTERPRETATION OF RESULTS. Measurement of baseline serum T_3 concentration is of minimal value in differentiating euthyroidism from hypothyroidism in the dog (Fig. 3-15). Essentially no difference exists in the mean or range of serum T_3 concentration between groups of healthy dogs, dogs with hypothyroidism, and euthyroid dogs with concurrent illness (Nelson et al, 1991; Miller et al, 1992). Serum T_3 concentration is a poor indicator of thyroid gland function, because the majority of circulating T_3 is produced from deiodination of T_4 at extrathyroidal sites; minimal amounts of T_3 are secreted by the thyroid gland in comparison with T_4. In addition, thyroidal secretion of T_3 and peripheral

tissue 5'-deiodination of T_4 to T_3 may increase with mild thyroid gland dysfunction (Utiger, 1980; Lum et al, 1984). The latter can result in "normal" serum T_3 and low serum T_4 concentrations in some hypothyroid dogs. Peripheral tissues may also autoregulate 5'-deiodination in humans with hypothyroidism in order to preserve blood T_3 concentration as long as possible (Lum et al, 1984). Blood T_3 concentrations are also affected by many of the same factors that affect blood T_4 levels (see page 126). We no longer measure serum T_3 concentrations as part of our evaluation of thyroid gland function and basically ignore results when serum T_3 is included as part of a thyroid panel obtained from commercial laboratories.

Some clinicians argue that measurement of serum T_3 concentration is justified because serum T_3 is a better marker than serum T_4 for thyroid hormone autoantibodies and lymphocytic thyroiditis. The prevalence of T_3 autoantibodies in canine serum samples submitted for determination of thyroid hormone concentrations has been reported to vary between 0.3% and 4.5% (Young et al, 1985; Nachreiner et al, 1990). The thyroglobulin autoantibody test has a greater sensitivity for lymphocytic thyroiditis than the T_3 or T_4 autoantibody test and is preferred in dogs (see page 124).

Similarly, some clinicians will argue that measurement of the serum T_3 concentration is helpful for identifying dogs with suspected problems with con-

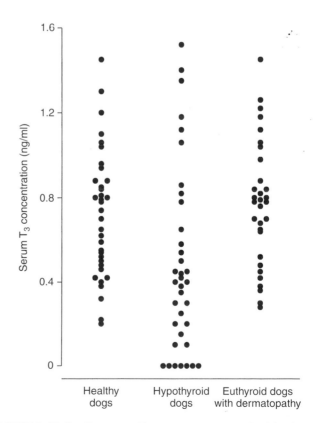

FIGURE 3–15. Baseline serum T_3 concentrations in 35 healthy dogs, 35 dogs with hypothyroidism, and 30 euthyroid dogs with concurrent dermatopathy. Note the overlap in serum T_3 results between the three groups of dogs.

version of T_4 to T_3, a syndrome which is suspected when the serum T_4 concentration is normal but the serum T_3 concentration is low or undetectable. Often labeled as "poor converters," these dogs have erroneously been deemed hypothyroid because of the low serum T_3 concentration. A selective absence of 5'-deiodinase activity, the enzyme responsible for conversion of T_4 to T_3, has not been documented as a cause of hypothyroidism in any species. The normal T_4 concentration is consistent with euthyroidism, whereas the low T_3 concentration is not an unexpected finding in dogs for reasons previously discussed. Undetectable serum T_3 concentrations may also be indicative of T_3 autoantibodies and lymphocytic thyroiditis (see page 125).

Baseline Serum Free Thyroxine Concentration

Serum fT_4 is currently measured by one of two methods: radioimmunoassay (RIA) using kits designed for use in human beings and a modified equilibrium dialysis (MED) technique that uses a short dialysis step to separate free from protein-bound T_4 followed by radioimmunossay for fT_4. The MED technique (Nichols Institute, San Juan Capistrano, CA) is the most accurate method for determining serum fT_4 concentrations and is the preferred fT_4 test for assessing thyroid gland function in dogs. Serum stored in plastic tubes can be shipped without cooling if assayed within 5 days (Behrend et al, 1998); however, we recommend freezing the serum sample and shipping it to the laboratory on ice packs. In one study, the sensitivity and specificity of the MED technique for fT_4 was 98% and 93%, respectively (Peterson et al, 1997). Accuracy of the MED assay has been greater than 90% in all studies in which it has

been critically evaluated, compared with an accuracy of 75% to 85% for serum T_4 (Nelson et al, 1991; Scott-Moncrieff et al, 1994; Peterson et al, 1997). In general, serum fT_4 values obtained by the MED technique that are greater than 1.5 ng/dl are consistent with euthyroidism and values less than 0.8 ng/dl (especially those less than 0.5 ng/dl) are suggestive of hypothyroidism, assuming the history, physical examination, and clinicopathologic abnormalities are also consistent with the disorder and severe systemic illness is not present (Table 3-13). Circulating antithyroid hormone antibodies do not affect the fT_4 results determined by the MED technique. Serum fT_4 is not affected by the suppressive effects of concurrent illness as much as serum T_4, although severe illness can cause fT_4 concentrations to decrease below 0.5 ng/dl (see Euthyroid Sick Syndrome, page 128). The reference range for serum fT_4 concentration measured by MED may vary between breeds, most notably sight hounds such as the Greyhound, which may also affect interpretation of results (see page 126) (Gaughan and Bruyette, 2001).

Results of serum fT_4 concentrations are often significantly less when determined by RIA, compared with results using equilibrium dialysis in the same blood samples (Fig. 3-16). Our studies have failed to identify any advantage to measuring serum fT_4 by RIA in lieu of serum T_4. The accuracy of RIAs for fT_4 measurement typically range from 65% to 85%, compared with an accuracy of 75% to 85% for serum T_4 and greater than 90% for fT_4 measured by MED (Nelson et al, 1991; Montgomery et al, 1991; Scott-Moncrieff et al, 1994; Peterson et al, 1997). Serum fT_4 measured by RIA and serum total T_4 concentrations also have similar sensitivities, specificities, and predictive values in assessing thyroid gland function (Nelson et al, 1991; Montgomery et al, 1991). Most of

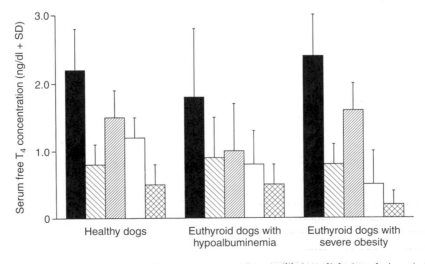

FIGURE 3–16. Results of serum free T_4 measurements using equilibrium dialysis technique (*solid bars*) and four commercially available radioimmunoassays for free T_4 in 54 healthy dogs, 12 euthyroid dogs with hypoalbuminemia (total albumin <2.0 g/dl), and 11 euthyroid dogs with severe obesity. Free T_4 by each method was determined from the same serum sample obtained from each dog. Note the discrepancy in results between equilibrium dialysis and the radioimmunoassays.

the weaknesses associated with the application of interpretation of serum total T_4 measurement are also found with serum fT_4 measured by RIA. A significant difference is found in mean serum fT_4 concentration in healthy dogs versus dogs with hypothyroidism; however, the range of fT_4 values overlaps between these two groups of dogs (Nelson et al, 1991). A single fT_4 concentration cannot be established to clearly separate euthyroid and hypothyroid dogs without altering the sensitivity or specificity of the test (Fig. 3-17). In addition, although significant differences in mean serum fT_4 concentration exist in groups of euthyroid dogs with specific concurrent illnesses (e.g., allergic inhalant dermatitis, flea-allergy dermatitis, idiopathic megaesophagus) compared with hypothyroid dogs, individual serum fT_4 values can fall within the hypothyroid range in euthyroid dogs, regardless of the type of concurrent illness (Fig. 3-17). The incidence of these false-positive results (i.e., hypothyroid values in euthyroid dogs) increases with the severity of the illness. The incidence of false-positive results is less and the sensitivity, specificity, and accuracy is higher when fT_4 is measured by MED, compared with RIA (Fig. 3-18). For these reasons, we always determine serum fT_4 concentrations using the MED technique.

Baseline Serum Free Triiodothyronine Concentration

Serum fT_3 is derived from intracellular 5'-deiodination of fT_4 in peripheral tissues and, to a lesser extent, in the thyroid gland. The theory behind measuring serum fT_3 is similar to that for fT_4. RIAs designed for measurement of serum fT_3 in humans have been used in the dog. Using an RIA technique, Nachreiner (1984) reported normal ranges for free T_3 (2.5 to 6.0 pg/ml) in the dog. A critical assessment of the sensitivity and specificity of these RIAs has not been reported in dogs, nor has the diagnostic usefulness of measuring serum fT_3 for evaluating thyroid gland function been reported. Presumably, many of the problems discussed for serum T_3 exist for serum fT_3. Currently, we do not measure serum fT_3 concentrations as part of our evaluation of thyroid gland function and basically ignore results when serum fT_3 is included as part of a thyroid panel obtained from commercial laboratories.

Baseline Serum Reverse Triiodothyronine Concentration

Reverse T_3 (rT_3) is a relatively inactive product of thyroxine 5'-deiodination. The vast majority of rT_3 is produced intracellularly from T_4; very little is secreted by the thyroid gland. Serum rT_3 concentration can be measured by specific RIAs that do not cross-react with T_4 or T_3. Normal baseline serum rT_3 concentrations are approximately one-fourth to one-half of the respective T_3 concentrations (i.e., 6 to 58 ng/dl) (Ferguson, 1984). The clinical benefit of measuring rT_3 has not yet been

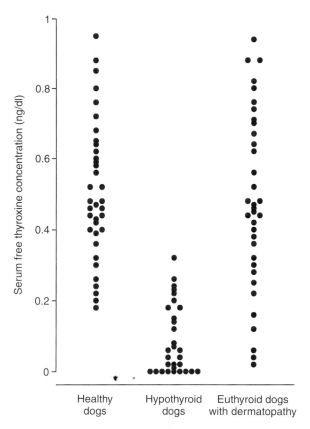

FIGURE 3–17. Baseline serum free T_4 concentrations measured by radioimmunoassay in 36 healthy dogs, 30 dogs with hypothyroidism, and 35 euthyroid dogs with concurrent dermatopathy. Note the overlap in serum free T_4 results between the three groups of dogs.

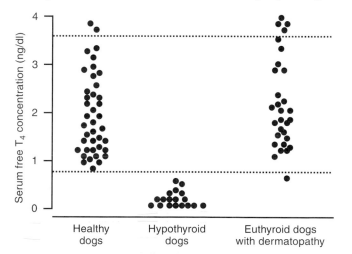

FIGURE 3–18. Baseline serum free T_4 concentrations measured by modified equilibrium dialysis in 40 healthy dogs, 18 dogs with hypothyroidism, and 30 euthyroid dogs with concurrent dermatopathy. Note the separation in serum free T_4 results between the euthyroid dogs and the hypothyroid dogs. *Dotted lines* represent upper and lower limits of the normal range.

demonstrated in dogs. In theory, dogs with hypothyroidism should have low basal total T_4, total T_3, and rT_3 concentrations, whereas euthyroid dogs with hormone alterations secondary to concurrent illness or drug therapy may have low basal T_4 and T_3 but normal or elevated rT$_3$ concentrations. Unfortunately, considerable overlap is seen in rT$_3$ values in euthyroid, hypothyroid, and euthyroid sick human patients (Kaplan et al, 1982). Measurement of serum rT$_3$ is not routine and is available through only a few laboratories.

Baseline Serum Thyrotropin (TSH) Concentration

An immunoradiometric assay (Coat-A-Count Canine TSH IRMA; Diagnostic Products Corp, Los Angeles, CA) was the first commercially available assay to be validated for measurement of canine TSH (Williams et al, 1996). Induction of hypothyroidism in six healthy Beagle dogs resulted in a 35-fold increase in the mean serum TSH concentration and treatment with sodium levothyroxine resulted in a return of the mean serum TSH concentration to baseline (Fig. 3-19). Administration of TRH resulted in a prompt and significant increase in TSH, with peak serum TSH concentrations occurring 10 to 30 minutes post-TRH administration (Fig. 3-20; Meij et al, 1996). These patterns of change supported the validity of this assay for measuring TSH concentrations in dogs. A chemiluminescent immunometric assay (Immulite Canine TSH; Diagnostic Products Corp, Los Angeles, CA) and an enzyme immunometric assay (Milenia Canine TSH; Diagnostic Products Corp, Los Angeles, CA) have since become available commercially. In a recent study evaluating the three analytical procedures, the highest precision for canine TSH analysis was obtained with the chemiluminescent assay (Marca et al, 2001). However, the correlation between the three assays in the analysis of canine serum TSH was satisfactory.

Clinical studies have shown that the serum TSH test has high specificity (90% or higher) when used for the diagnosis of hypothyroidism in dogs, so long as TSH concentration is interpreted in conjunction with baseline serum T$_4$ or fT$_4$ concentration (Dixon et al, 1996; Ramsey et al, 1997; Peterson et al, 1997; Scott-Moncrieff et al, 1998). Specificity is considerably lower when the TSH concentration is interpreted by itself, in part because of overlap in results between hypothyroid dogs and euthyroid dogs with concurrent illness (Fig. 3-21). In addition, depending on the study, approximately 20% to 40% of dogs with hypothyroidism have TSH concentrations within the reference range; therefore test sensitivity is only 63% to 82%. Possible reasons that hypothyroid dogs might have serum TSH concentrations within the reference range include random fluctuations in the serum TSH concentration (Fig. 3-22), secondary hypothyroidism, concurrent drug administration or disease suppressing pituitary TSH secretion, an inability of the current TSH assay to detect all isoforms of circulating TSH, and decreased pituitary TSH secretion with chronic hypothyroidism (Ramsey et al, 1997; Peterson et al, 1997; Bruner et al, 1998; Kooistra et al, 2000b). Prolonged periods with low thyroid hormone concentrations may result in disruption of the feedback pathway by down-regulation or exhaustion of TSH production by

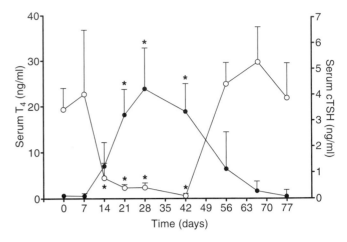

FIGURE 3–19. Mean serum thyroxine (T$_4$; o) and canine thyroid stimulating hormone (cTSH; ●) concentrations after experimental induction of hypothyroidism (Day 0) and treatment with levothyroxine (beginning on Day 42). Bars represent SD. *Significantly (P <0.05) different from day 0 values. (Williams DA, et al: JAVMA 209:1730, 1996).

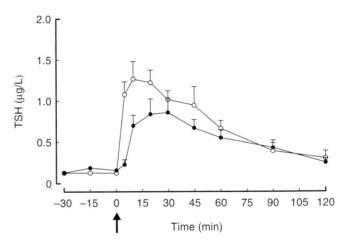

FIGURE 3–20. Plasma TSH response (mean ± SE) in eight healthy male Beagle dogs after the rapid (30-sec) intravenous injection *(arrow)* of a combination of four hypothalamic releasing hormones (●) compared with that after the injection of 10 µg of TRH/kg alone (o). In the combined test, the releasing hormones were injected in the following order and doses: 1 µg of CRH/kg, 1 µg of GHRH/kg, 10 µg of GnRH/kg, and 10 µg of TRH/kg. (From Meij BP, et al: Dom Anim Endocr 13:465, 1996.)

the pituitary thyrotrophs (Ramsey et al, 1997). In addition, comparing a single serum TSH measurement from an individual dog with the conventional population-based reference range may be too insensitive to detect small but important changes in the serum TSH concentration for that particular dog; that is, the serum TSH result may be abnormal for that dog despite falling within the reference range (Iversen et al, 1999). Fortunately, sample collection time does not appear to predictably influence serum TSH test results (Bruner et al, 1998).

Currently, a serum TSH concentration of 0.6 ng/ml is used by most clinical laboratories as the upper limit

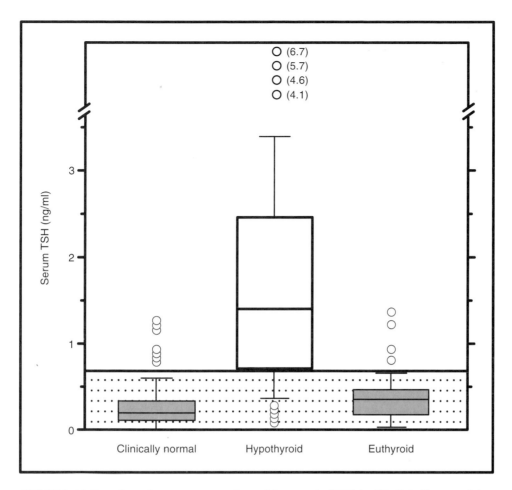

FIGURE 3–21. Box plots of serum concentrations of thyrotropin (TSH) in 150 clinically normal dogs, 54 hypothyroid dogs, and 54 euthyroid dogs with nonthyroidal disease. For each box plot, T-bars represent the main body of data, which in most instances is equal to the range. Each box represents the interquartile range (25th to 75th percentile or middle half of the data). The horizontal bar in each box is the median. Open circles represent outlying data points. Numbers in parentheses are exact values for outlying data points that are outside the range of the graph. The shaded area represents the reference range. (From Peterson ME, et al: JAVMA 211:1396, 1997.)

of the reference range. Although the sensitivity of the TSH assay is 0.1 ng/ml (Williams et al, 1996), the lower limit of the reference range is currently below the sensitivity of the assay. Current TSH assays cannot differentiate low from normal serum TSH concentrations, which impairs our ability to identify secondary hypothyrodism, suppression of pituitary TSH secretion by concurrent drugs and diseases, and excess administration of levothyroxine sodium during treatment of hypothyroidism (see page 139).

The serum TSH concentration should always be interpreted in conjunction with the serum T_4 or fT_4 concentration measured in the same blood sample and should never be used as the sole test for assessing thyroid gland function. A low serum T_4 or fT_4 concentration and a high TSH concentration in a blood sample obtained from a dog with appropriate history and physical examination findings supports the diagnosis of primary hypothyroidism, whereas a finding of normal serum T_4, fT_4, and TSH concentrations rules out hypothyroidism. Any other combination of

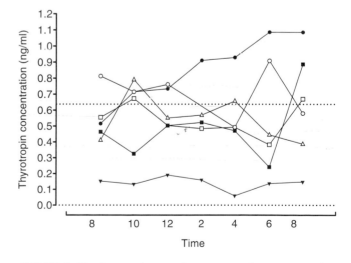

FIGURE 3–22. Serum thyrotropin concentrations measured at 2-hour intervals from 8 AM to 8 PM in 6 dogs with naturally developing hypothyroidism. Reference range is between the horizontal dotted lines. Each symbol represents values obtained for 1 hypothyroid dog. (From Bruner, et al: JAVMA 212:1572, 1998.)

serum T_4, fT_4, and TSH results is difficult to interpret. Based on the accuracy of the assays, reliance on fT_4 measured by MED technique is recommended. A normal serum T_4 or fT_4 concentration and an increased serum TSH concentration are found in the early stages of primary hypothyroidism in humans (Larsen et al, 1981). Although similar thyroid hormone and TSH results have been identified in dogs (see Table 3-2) it is not known what percentage of these dogs will progress to clinical hypothyroidism. Clinical signs of hypothyroidism are usually not evident in these dogs, in part because serum T_4 and fT_4 concentrations are in the normal range. Treatment with levothyroxine sodium is not indicated. Rather, assessment of thyroid gland function should be repeated in 3 to 6 months, especially if antibody tests for lymphocytic thyroiditis are positive. If progressive destruction of the thyroid gland is occurring, serum TSH will gradually increase, serum T_4 and fT_4 will gradually decrease, and clinical signs will eventually develop.

T_3 Resin Uptake Test (T_3 RU)

The T_3 RU test is an indirect method for estimating changes in thyroid hormone binding by plasma proteins. In humans, this test correlates well with the percentage of free T_4 in serum as determined by equilibrium dialysis (Belshaw, 1983; Ferguson, 1984). The product of serum T_4 and T_3 RU is called the *free thyroxine index* (FTI) and is used as a reliable substitute for the direct measurement of free T_4 concentration in humans. Because of the relative lack of high-affinity serum thyroid hormone–binding proteins (i.e., thyroid-binding globulin) in the dog, the T_3 RU test is an insensitive evaluator of thyroid function. Because the FTI depends on the T_3 RU test, it too is an insensitive indicator of free T_4 concentrations in the dog.

Thyrotropin (TSH) Stimulation Test

The TSH stimulation test evaluates the thyroid gland's responsiveness to exogenous TSH administration. The primary advantage of the TSH stimulation test is the differentiation of hypothyroidism from the euthyroid sick syndrome (see page 128) in a dog with low basal thyroid hormone concentrations. Unfortunately, TSH for injection has not been available at a reasonable cost for use in dogs and cats for several years, and there is no indication that it will become available in the foreseeable future. A brief synopsis of the TSH stimulation test is presented below. See the second edition of *Canine and Feline Endocrinology and Reproduction* for detailed information on this test.

Bovine or recombinant human TSH can be used for the TSH stimulation test. The canine thyroid gland can respond to bovine or recombinant human TSH because, unlike the immunologic activity of the TSH molecule, the biologic activity of the TSH molecule is not species-specific (Kaptein et al, 1982). Although a number of

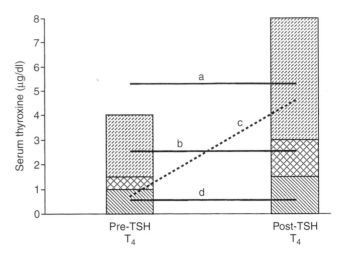

FIGURE 3–23. Interpretation of TSH stimulation test in the dog. Post-TSH T_4 values that fall into the normal range usually indicate normal thyroid gland function. Exceptions include high pre-TSH T_4 values with no increase in post-TSH T_4 *(line a)* and low pre-TSH T_4 values with normal response to TSH *(line c)*. Primary hypothyroidism with anti-T_4 antibodies *(lines a and b)* and secondary hypothyroidism or the suppressive effects of concurrent disease *(line c)* should be considered. Low pre-TSH and post-TSH T_4 values *(line d)* and post-TSH T_4 values in the nondiagnostic range may be indicative of hypothyroidism or the suppressive effects of concurrent disease. The more serious the disease, the more suppressive the effect on the post-TSH T_4 values. ▨, Normal; ▧, nondiagnostic range; ▨, hypothyroid range. (From Nelson RW, Couto GC: Essentials of Small Animal Internal Medicine. St. Louis, Mosby-Year Book, 1992, p 549, with permission.)

different protocols have been advocated in the literature, we prefer the following protocol when using bovine TSH: 0.1 IU of bovine TSH per kilogram of body weight (maximum, 5 IU TSH/dog) intravenously and blood for serum T_4 determination obtained before and 6 hours after TSH administration. Serum fT_4 concentrations increase in a manner similar to serum T_4, do not provide additional diagnostic information, and therefore are not routinely measured. The following protocol has been recommended when using recombinant human TSH (rhTSH) (Thyrogen; Genzyme Corporation, Cambridge, ME): 50 µg of rhTSH per dog intravenously and blood for serum T_4 determination obtained before and 6 hours after rhTSH administration (Sauvé and Paradis, 2000).

Interpretation of the TSH stimulation test should be based on a comparison of the pre- and post-TSH absolute T_4 results with the respective normal ranges for the laboratory being used. For our laboratory and using the bovine TSH protocol described above, euthyroid dogs have a post-TSH serum T_4 concentration greater than 3 µg/dl, whereas dogs with primary hypothyroidism have a post-TSH serum T_4 concentration below the normal baseline serum T_4 range (i.e., <1.5 µg/dl). Post-TSH serum T_4 concentrations between 1.5 and 3 µg/dl are nondiagnostic and may be found in the early stages of hypothyroidism or may represent suppression of thyroid gland function as a result of concurrent illness or drug therapy in an otherwise euthyroid dog (Fig. 3-23). Hypothyroidism is usually characterized by a gradual loss of thyroid function and a resultant gradual loss of thyroid responsiveness to TSH. Eventually a hypothyroid response (i.e., no response) is attained. Prior to that time, however, results of a TSH stimulation test may resemble findings in the euthyroid sick syndrome. Euthyroid dogs with decreased baseline thyroid hormone concentrations due to such factors as illness, drugs, and glucocorticoid administration (i.e., the euthyroid sick syndrome) usually respond to TSH, although the response is often suppressed (Fig. 3-24). Severe systemic illness, however, can result in post-TSH serum T_4 concentrations in the range considered diagnostic for primary hypothyroidism (i.e., <1.5 μg/dl; Fig. 3-25). Evaluation of rhTSH in a clinical setting has not been reported in dogs. However, results using rhTSH in healthy dogs were similar to those obtained in healthy dogs administered bovine TSH, suggesting that the interpretation of the TSH stimulation test should be similar for rhTSH and bovine TSH (Sauvé and Paradis, 2000).

Thyrotropin-Releasing Hormone (TRH) Stimulation Test

INDICATIONS. The TRH stimulation test evaluates the pituitary gland's responsiveness to TRH and the thyroid gland's responsiveness to TSH secreted in response to TRH administration. The TRH stimulation test is used to differentiate between hypothyroidism

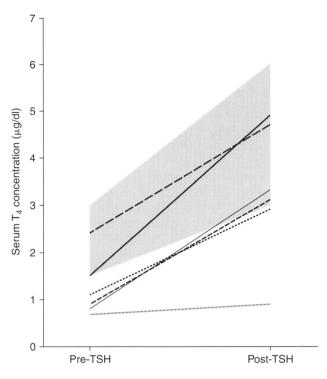

FIGURE 3–24. Mean serum T_4 concentration before and 6 hours after the intravenous administration of 0.1 IU of TSH/kg body weight in 34 dogs with hypothyroidism (⑊⑊⑊⑊⑊), 12 dogs with hyperadrenocorticism (..............), 10 euthyroid dogs with peripheral neuropathy (━ ━ ━), 10 euthyroid dogs with idiopathic megaesophagus (━━━), 8 euthyroid dogs with cardiomyopathy (━━━), and 5 euthyroid bitches with infertility (- - - -). Shaded area, normal range.

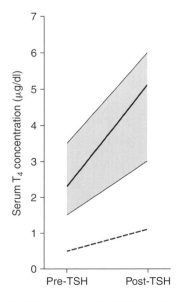
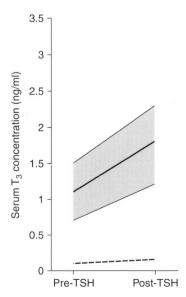

FIGURE 3–25. Mean results of a TSH stimulation test performed in five diabetic dogs at the time of initial presentation for severe diabetic ketoacidosis (━ ━ ━ ━) and 4 to 6 weeks after resolution of ketoacidosis and establishment of glycemic control with insulin therapy (━━━). Note the suppressive effects of concurrent illness (i.e., diabetic ketoacidosis) on thyroid function and the reversal of suppression following correction of the illness. Shaded area, normal range.

**TABLE 3–14   SOME OF THE PUBLISHED PROTOCOLS FOR PERFORMING
THE TRH STIMULATION TEST IN DOGS**

TRH Dose	Route of Administration	Blood Sampling Times (Hours)	Reference
0.2 mg/dog	IV	0, 4	Various authors
0.25 mg/dog	IV	0, 4	Kemppainen et al, 1983
0.05 mg/kg	IV	0, 6	Avgeris et al, 1990
0.1 mg/kg	IV	0, 6	Lothrop et al, 1984b
0.3 mg/kg	IV	0, 4	Kaufman et al, 1985
0.3–0.5 mg/kg	IV	0, 6–8	Li et al, 1986

and the euthyroid sick syndrome (see page 128) in a dog with low basal thyroid hormone concentrations and, in theory, to differentiate between primary and secondary hypothyroidism. Some investigators believe that the TRH stimulation test is a more sensitive thyroid function test than the TSH stimulation test (Lothrop et al, 1984b; Li et al, 1986). In our experience, the TRH stimulation test can be difficult to interpret because of the relatively minimal increase in serum T_4 concentration after TRH administration. Unfortunately, TRH for injection is becoming increasingly difficult to obtain and may soon become unavailable.

PROTOCOL. A number of different protocols have been recommended in the literature for the TRH stimulation test (Table 3-14). These protocols merely emphasize the importance of following the procedure recommended by the specific laboratory being used. Adverse effects observed at TRH dosages in excess of 0.1 mg/kg include increased salivation, urination, defecation, vomiting, miosis, tachycardia, and tachypnea (Lothrop et al, 1984a; Li et al, 1986). Lothrop et al have shown that increasing the dosage of TRH increases the duration, but not the magnitude, of T_4

stimulation. Therefore the protocol for the TRH stimulation test should use the lowest dose of TRH that maximally stimulates T_4 secretion without causing adverse reactions.

When performing the TRH stimulation test in our hospital, we administer 0.2 mg of TRH (Thypinone; Abbott Laboratories, Abbott Park, IL) intravenously; blood for serum total T_4 determination is obtained before and 4 hours after TRH administration (Evinger et al, 1985), and blood for serum TSH determination is obtained before and 30 minutes after TRH administration (Scott-Moncrieff and Nelson, 1998). Measurement of serum TSH concentration after TRH administration is used to assess pituitary responsiveness to TRH whereas measurement of serum T_4 concentration is used to assess the thyroid gland's responsiveness to the TRH-induced increase in pituitary TSH secretion. Serum fT_4 concentrations increase in a manner similar to serum T_4, do not provide additional diagnostic information, and therefore are not routinely measured.

INTERPRETATION. Interpretation of the TRH stimulation test is more subjective than that of the TSH

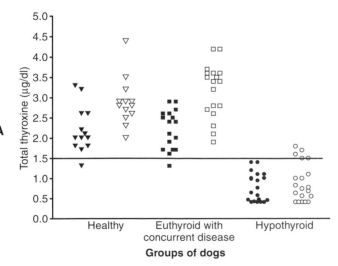
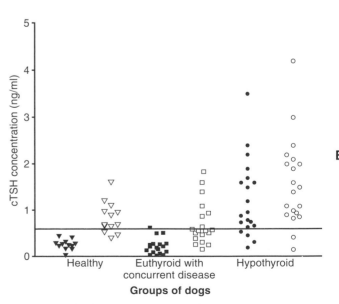

FIGURE 3–26. T_4 concentration *(A)* and TSH concentration *(B)* before *(solid symbol)* and 30 minutes (for TSH) and 4 hours (for T_4) after *(open symbols)* administration of TRH to healthy dogs, hypothyroid dogs, and euthyroid dogs with concurrent diseases. The horizontal line represents the upper limit of the reference range for T_4 *(A)* and TSH *(B)*. (From Scott-Moncrieff JCR, Nelson RW: JAVMA 213:1435, 1998.)

stimulation test, in part because the increase in serum total T_4 concentration is considerably less dramatic with TRH than with TSH (Frank, 1996). For our laboratory and when using the TRH protocol described above, euthyroid dogs should have a post-TRH serum T_4 concentration greater than 2 µg/dl. Alternatively, post-TRH serum T_4 should increase at least 0.5 µg/dl above baseline serum T_4 concentration in a euthyroid dog. In contrast, dogs with primary hypothyroidism should have a post-TRH serum T_4 concentration below the normal baseline serum T_4 range (i.e., <0.5 µg/dl) and less than 0.5 µg/dl increase in serum T_4 after TRH administration (Fig. 3-26). Post-TRH serum T_4 concentrations between 1.5 and 2.0 µg/dl are nondiagnostic and may be found in the early stages of hypothyroidism or may represent suppression of thyroid gland function as a result of concurrent illness or drug therapy in an otherwise euthyroid dog. Factors that affect the TSH stimulation test are believed to affect the TRH stimulation test in a similar manner.

In theory, differences in serum TSH response to exogenous TRH should be useful for diagnosing primary and secondary hypothyroidism and differentiating between hypothyroidism and the euthyroid sick syndrome. In healthy dogs, there is a significant increase in serum TSH concentration between 10 and 30 minutes after TRH administration (see Fig. 3-20; Meij et al, 1996). In one study evaluating the usefulness of the TSH response to TRH administration, mean baseline serum T_4 concentration was significantly less and mean baseline serum TSH concentration was significantly higher in dogs with hypothyroidism than concentrations in healthy dogs and in euthyroid dogs with concurrent illness, and TRH-stimulated mean serum TSH concentration was higher in hypothyroid dogs than the TRH-stimulated concentrations in healthy dogs and in euthyroid dogs with concurrent illness (Fig. 2-26; Scott-Moncrieff and Nelson, 1998). However, percentage of change in TSH concentration in response to TRH administration for hypothyroid dogs was significantly less than the percentage of change for healthy dogs and for euthyroid dogs with concurrent illness (Fig. 3-27). Using a greater than 100% increase in TSH concentration after TRH administration as a cutoff for diagnosis of euthyroidism, sensitivity was 85%, specificity was 94%, and overall accuracy was 90%, values that are similar to sensitivity, specificity, and accuracy of other tests of thyroid gland function. Thus measurement of change in TSH concentration in response to TRH administration does not offer any additional diagnostic advantage over measuring a combination of baseline serum T_4, fT_4, and TSH.

In humans with secondary hypothyroidism, TSH concentrations are low or low-normal and the TSH concentration fails to increase after TRH administration. Because the reference range for serum TSH concentration in dogs extends below the sensitivity of the assay, the current TSH assay does not distinguish between normal and low TSH concentrations. In addition, because most dogs with primary hypo-

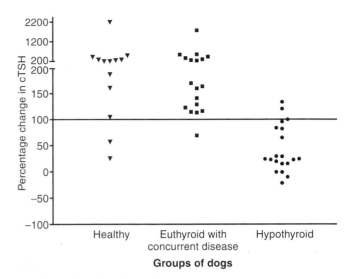

FIGURE 3–27. Percentage of change in TSH concentration after administration of TRH to healthy dogs, hypothyroid dogs, and euthyroid dogs with concurrent diseases. The horizontal line represents the assigned cutoff point for discrimination between euthyroid and hypothyroid dogs. (From Scott-Moncrieff JCR, Nelson RW: JAVMA 213:1435, 1998.)

thyroidism have decreased responses to TRH (see Fig. 3-27), it appears that measurement of percentage change in TSH concentration in response to TRH administration is not useful in distinguishing secondary from primary hypothyroidism in dogs (Scott-Moncrieff and Nelson, 1998).

The "K" Value

The K value is a number generated from a canonical discriminant analysis combining baseline serum T_4 concentration with response to TSH administration or baseline serum fT_4 with serum cholesterol concentration (Larsson, 1988). The intent was to improve the accuracy of assessing thyroid gland function by evaluating several diagnostic tests simultaneously. When using baseline serum fT_4 (as determined by Amerlex-M free T_4 RIA; Amersham Ltd, Amersham, Bucks, England) and cholesterol concentration, the K value is derived from the following formula (see Conversion Table for SI and Common Units on inside front cover of this textbook):

$$K = 0.7 \times fT_4 \ (pmol/L) - cholesterol \ (mmol/L)$$

If the K value is greater than 1, hypothyroidism is ruled out and if the K value is less than –4, hypothyroidism is likely. Values between –4 and 1 are nondiagnostic.

As with other tests of thyroid gland function, the K value is influenced by factors that affect baseline serum thyroid hormone concentrations (e.g., euthyroid sick syndrome). In addition, the K value is affected by diseases that alter serum cholesterol concentration and by the methodology used to assay serum cholesterol and especially fT_4. We prefer to interpret results of a thyroid panel (see page 134) in conjunction with history, physical findings, and clinical pathology when assessing thyroid gland function and do not recommend reliance on the K value.

TESTS FOR LYMPHOCYTIC THYROIDITIS

Circulating thyroglobulin (Tg) and thyroid hormone (T_3 and T_4) autoantibodies have been described in the dog (Haines et al, 1984; Young et al, 1985) and are believed to correlate with the presence of lymphocytic thyroiditis (Chastain et al, 1989; Beale and Torres, 1991; Gaschen et al, 1993). Thus tests for the presence of Tg, T_3, and T_4 autoantibodies in the serum of dogs can be used to identify lymphocytic thyroiditis in dogs, to explain unusual serum T_3 and T_4 test results, and possibly as a genetic screening test for hypothyroidism caused by lymphocytic thyroiditis in dogs. Autoantibodies predominately develop against Tg. T_3 and T_4 are haptens and not antigenic by themselves. Tg is the protein that provides the antigenic stimulus, and because T_3 and T_4 are attached to the Tg molecule, autoantibodies develop against them as well (Gaschen et al, 1993; Rajatanavin et al, 1989). Dogs with thyroid hormone autoantibodies typically have autoantibodies against Tg but the converse is not true (Kemppainen and Young, 1992). Thus the better screening test for lymphocytic thyroiditis is the Tg autoantibody test.

Serum Thyroglobulin Autoantibodies

Circulating Tg autoantibodies have been detected in 34% to 59% of hypothyroid dogs (Haines et al, 1984; Vollset and Larsen, 1987; Beale et al, 1990; Thacker et al, 1992) and, in one study using thyroid biopsy, six of seven dogs with lymphocytic thyroiditis and none of five dogs with thyroid atrophy (Beale and Torres, 1991). Tg autoantibodies frequently occur in conjunction with T_3 and T_4 autoantibodies (Thacker et al, 1992). Autoantibodies to Tg are also detected more frequently in samples with low serum concentrations of thyroid hormone (Beale et al, 1990; Thacker et al, 1992). These findings support a correlation between Tg autoantibodies, lymphocytic thyroiditis, and hypothyroidism in the dog.

Historically, a number of assays for Tg autoantibodies have been used, including passive hemagglutination, complement fixation, fluorescent antibody, enzyme-linked immunosorbent, and radioimmunoprecipitation assay (Nachreiner et al, 1998). Enzyme-linked immunosorbent assays (ELISAs) are currently the most commonly used technology. Studies performed in the 1980s identified an unacceptable prevalence of false-positive test results for the Tg autoantibody test, ranging from 14% to 47% of euthyroid dogs tested (Haines et al, 1980; Vollset and Larsen, 1987). Recent studies evaluating newer ELISAs for Tg autoantibodies have reported significant improvement in the prevalence of false-positive results (Iversen et al, 1998; Nachreiner et al, 1998). In one study evaluating an ELISA for Tg autoantibodies in dogs, sensitivity and specificity was 91% and 97%, respectively (Iversen et al, 1998). A commercially available ELISA (Oxford Biomedical Research Inc, Oxford, MI) for detection of Tg autoantibodies has been shown to be sensitive and specific for identification of Tg autoantibodies in dogs when positive results were defined as at least twice (200%) the optical density of the negative-control sample (Nachreiner et al, 1998). This ELISA is currently the most common Tg autoantibody assay used by commercial laboratories.

Results of the ELISA by Oxford Biomedical Research are reported as negative, positive, and inconclusive. Negative and positive controls are evaluated each day blood samples are analyzed for Tg autoantibodies. Positive, negative, and inconclusive test results are based on the results of the negative controls. A positive test result is defined as any value that is greater than two times the mean value of the negative controls; a negative test result is any value that is less than two standard deviations above the mean of the negative controls; and an inconclusive test result is any value that is greater than two standard deviations above, but less than twice the mean, of the negative controls.

Presence of serum Tg autoantibodies implies pathology in the thyroid gland but provides no information on the severity or progressive nature of the inflammatory response or the extent of thyroid gland involvement. Furthermore, this test is not an indicator of thyroid gland function. Tg autoantibodies should not be used as the sole criteria to establish the diagnosis of hypothyroidism. Dogs with confirmed hypothyroidism can be negative, and euthyroid dogs can be positive for Tg autoantibodies. Identification of Tg autoantibodies would support hypothyroidism caused by lymphocytic thyroiditis if the dog has clinical signs, physical findings, and thyroid hormone test results consistent with the disorder.

Tg autoantibodies may be used as a prebreeding screen for lymphocytic thyroiditis in valuable breeding dogs. Currently, a positive Tg autoantibody test is considered suggestive of lymphocytic thyroiditis and supports retesting in several months before breeding the dog. The value of serum Tg autoantibodies as a marker for eventual development of hypothyroidism remains to be clarified. A recent 1-year prospective study found that approximately 20% of 171 dogs with positive Tg autoantibody and normal serum fT_4 and TSH test results developed changes in fT_4 and/or TSH test results consistent with hypothyroidism, 15% reverted to a negative Tg autoantibody test with no change in fT_4 and TSH test results, and 65% remained Tg autoantibody–positive or had an inconclusive result with no change in fT_4 and TSH test results 1 year later (Graham et al, 2001b).

Serum Thyroid Hormone Autoantibodies

Thyroid hormone autoantibodies are also considered an indicator of lymphocytic thyroiditis and may also be an indicator of the potential for development of hypothyroidism in dogs. In a recent study, thyroid hormone autoantibodies were detected in 6.3% of 287,948 serum samples from dogs with clinical signs consistent with hypothyroidism (Nachreiner et al, 2002). T_3 autoantibodies alone were detected in 4.64%, T_4 autoantibodies alone were detected in 0.63%, and both T_3 and T_4 autoantibodies were detected in 1.03% of the serum samples. An inverse correlation existed between prevalence of thyroid hormone autoantibodies and age of the dogs, females had a significantly higher chance of being positive for thyroid hormone auto-antibodies than did males, and neutered males and females had a significantly higher prevalence of thyroid hormone autoantibodies than did sexually intact dogs. Breeds at increased risk for having thyroid hormone autoantibodies were also identified (see Table 3-3).

Measurement of serum T_4 and T_3 autoantibodies is offered by some commercial endocrine laboratories as part of an extensive thyroid panel. Testing for serum T_3 and T_4 autoantibodies is indicated in dogs with unexpected or unusual serum T_3 or T_4 test results. T_3 and T_4 autoantibodies may interfere with the RIAs used to measure serum T_3 or T_4 concentrations, causing unexpected and often confusing test results (Young et al, 1985; see Fig. 3-14). The type of interference depends on the separation system employed in the RIA. Falsely low results are obtained if non-specific separation methods are used (e.g., ammonium sulfate, activated charcoal); falsely increased values are obtained if single-step separation systems utilizing antibody-coated tubes are used. For most commercially available T_4 assays, T_4 autoantibodies will falsely increase the measured T_4 concentration. The false increase may be enough to raise a hypothyroid dog's result into the reference or hyperthyroid range. The same false increase occurs with nondialysis (direct) RIAs used for measuring serum fT_4 concentrations (Kemppainen et al, 1996). False elevations in serum fT_4 concentration do not occur if fT_4 is measured using a dialysis procedure (e.g., MED technique; see page 116), because autoantibodies cannot pass through the dialysis membrane and interfere with the assay. Thus evaluation of serum fT_4 concentration measured by MED should be done in lieu of serum T_4 in dogs suspected of having T_4 autoantibodies. Fortunately spurious T_4 values resulting from clinically relevant concentrations of T_4 autoantibody account for less than 1% of such results from commercial endocrine laboratories (Nachreiner et al, 2002).

Positive serum thyroid hormone autoantibody test results imply pathology in the thyroid gland but provide no information on the severity or progressive nature of the inflammatory response or the extent of thyroid gland involvement, nor are these tests an indicator of thyroid gland function. T_3 and T_4 auto-antibodies should not be used as the sole criteria for establishing the diagnosis of hypothyroidism. Dogs with confirmed hypothyroidism can be negative and euthyroid dogs can be positive for thyroid hormone autoantibodies (Rajatanavin et al, 1989). Identification of T_3 or T_4 autoantibodies supports hypothyroidism caused by lymphocytic thyroiditis if the dog has clinical signs, physical findings, and thyroid hormone test results consistent with the disorder.

FACTORS AFFECTING THYROID GLAND FUNCTION TESTS

Correct interpretation of tests of thyroid gland function is one of the primary diagnostic challenges in canine clinical endocrinology. There are many factors that affect baseline thyroid hormone and endogenous TSH concentrations (Table 3-15). Unfortunately, many of these factors decrease baseline thyroid hormone concentrations and may increase endogenous TSH in euthyroid dogs, potentially causing misdiagnosis of hypothyroidism if the clinician accepts the results out of context. In our experience the most common factors that result in lower baseline thyroid hormone concentrations in euthyroid dogs are concurrent illness (i.e., euthyroid sick syndrome), use of drugs (especially glucocorticoids), and random fluctuations in thyroid hormone concentrations. In any given dog, other factors may also influence baseline thyroid hormone concentrations. It is important to recognize the potential influence of these factors when interpreting thyroid hormone test results.

Age

Studies in groups of euthyroid dogs have identified age-related changes in the mean serum T_4 and T_3 concentrations. Mean serum T_4 concentration is increased in neonates less than 6 weeks of age compared with dogs between 6 weeks and 1 year of age (Fig. 3-28; Reimers et al, 1990; Ray and Howanitz, 1984; Weller et al, 1983). As dogs age, serum T_4 concentration decreases. In one study, mean serum T_4 concentration was 50% lower in dogs 6 to 11 years of age than in nursing puppies (Reimers et al, 1990). However, serum T_4 concentrations remained greater than 1.0 $\mu g/dl$ in most older dogs.

Similar trends with age do not seem to occur with serum T_3 concentration. In one study, mean serum T_3 concentrations were lowest in dogs less than 12 weeks old, increased in dogs between 3 and 12 months, and then decreased slightly in dogs greater than 1 year of age (Fig. 3-28; Reimers et al, 1990). However, differences in mean serum T_3 concentration were minimal in dogs between 3 months and 11 years of age and probably were not clinically significant.

The effect of age on serum fT_4 and TSH concentrations has not yet been reported in the dog.

TABLE 3-15 VARIABLES WHICH MAY AFFECT BASELINE SERUM THYROID HORMONE FUNCTION TEST RESULTS IN THE DOG

Age	Inversely proportional effect
neonate (< 3 mo)	increased T_4
aged (> 6 yr)	decreased T_4
Body size	Inversely proportional effect
small (< 10 kg)	increased T_4
large (> 30 kg)	decreased T_4
Breed	
Sight hounds (e.g. Greyhounds)	T_4 and free T_4 lower than normal range established for dogs; no difference for TSH
Gender	No effect
Time of day	No effect
Weight gain/obesity	Increased
Weight loss/fasting	Decreased T_4, no effect on free T_4
Strenuous exercise	Increased T_4, decreased TSH no effect on free T_4
Estrus (estrogen)	No effect on T_4
Pregnancy (progesterone)	Increased T_4
Surgery/anesthesia	Decreased T_4
Concurrent illness*	Decreased T_4 and free T_4; Depending on illness, TSH may increase, decrease or not change
Drugs	
Clomipramine	Decreased T_4, free T_4; No effect on TSH
Carprofen	Decreased T_4, free T_4 and TSH
Etodolac	No effect on T_4, free T_4 or TSH
Glucocorticoids	Decreased T_4 and free T_4; Decrease or no effect on TSH in majority of dogs
Furosemide	Decreased T_4
Methimazole	Decreased T_4 and free T_4; Increased TSH
Phenobarbital	Decreased T_4 and free T_4; Delayed increase in TSH
Phenylbutazone	Decreased T_4
Potassium bromide	No effect on T_4, free T_4, or TSH
Progestagens	Decreased T_4
Propylthiouracil	Decreased T_4, and free T_4; Increased TSH
Cephalexine	No effect on T_4, free T_4 or TSH
Sulfonamides	Decreased T_4 and free T_4; increased TSH
Ipodate	Increased T_4, decreased T_3
Dietary iodine intake	If excessive, decreased T_4 and free T_4; Increased TSH
Thyroid hormone autoantibodies	Increased or decreased T_4; no effect on free T_4 or TSH

*There is a direct correlation between severity and systemic nature of illness and suppression of serum T_4 and free T_4 concentration.

Breed/Body Size

Comparison of normal thyroid hormone values between groups of dogs based on body size has identified differences in mean serum T_4 and T_3 concentrations (Fig. 3-29; Reimers et al, 1990). Dogs were divided into three groups based on body size. Small dogs had a mean middle-aged body weight of 7.1 kg and included Poodles, Beagles, and Miniature Schnauzers; medium-sized dogs had a mean middle-aged body weight of 23.3 kg and included English Pointers, English Setters, and Siberian Huskies; large dogs had a mean middle-aged body weight of 30.6 kg and included Black and Tan Coonhounds, Labrador Retrievers, Doberman Pinschers, and German Shepherd dogs. Mean serum T_4 concentration was greater in small than in medium-sized and large dogs. However, mean serum T_3 concentration was greater in medium-sized than in small and large dogs. The effect of body size on serum fT_4 and TSH concentrations has yet not been reported in dogs.

The reference range for serum T_4 and fT_4 concentration may also vary between breeds. The reference range is usually established based on the mean plus and minus two standard deviations calculated from results of serum T_4 or fT_4 measured in a large population of dogs without regard for breed. The reference range for serum T_4 and free T_4 measured by MED is lower in sight hounds, most notably Greyhounds, than in non-Greyhound pet dogs (Gaughan and Bruyette, 2001; Hill et al, 2001). For example, in one study, mean ($\pm$ SD) baseline serum T_4 concentration was 13.9 $\pm$ 6.3 nmol/L in 61 healthy Greyhounds versus 25.7 $\pm$ 6.9 nmol/L in 19 healthy non-Greyhound pet dogs of assorted breeds (Gaughan and Bruyette, 2001; see Conversion Table for SI and Common Units on inside front cover). Serum TSH concentrations were similar between Greyhound and non-Greyhound pet dogs. These findings suggest that breed-specific reference ranges for thyroid hormone tests need to be established and used when evaluating thyroid gland function in the respective breed. Until breed-specific reference ranges are established, diagnosis of hypothyroidism should rely on results of multiple tests of thyroid gland function in addition to the history, physical examination findings, and results of the CBC and serum biochemistry panel (see page 134).

Gender and Reproductive Stage of the Female

When the specific stage of the female reproductive cycle is not considered and dogs are merely classified as male or female, gender has no apparent effect on serum thyroid hormone concentrations (Reimers et al, 1990). The mean ($\pm$ SE) serum T_4 and T_3 concentrations in approximately 550 female versus 515 male dogs were 2.11 $\pm$ 0.04 versus 2.08 $\pm$ 0.04 μg/dl and 0.94 $\pm$ 0.01 versus 0.92 $\pm$ 0.01 ng/ml, respectively.

Testosterone decreases thyroid-binding protein and can decrease serum T_4 while having little effect on serum fT_4 concentrations (Wenzel, 1981). The effect of testosterone on thyroid hormone test results in dogs is unclear. In one study, serum T_4 concentration increased significantly after male Greyhound dogs were castrated and when not in training (Hill et al, 2001). There was no effect of castration on serum fT_4 or TSH concentrations. However, in another study, serum T_4, fT_4, and

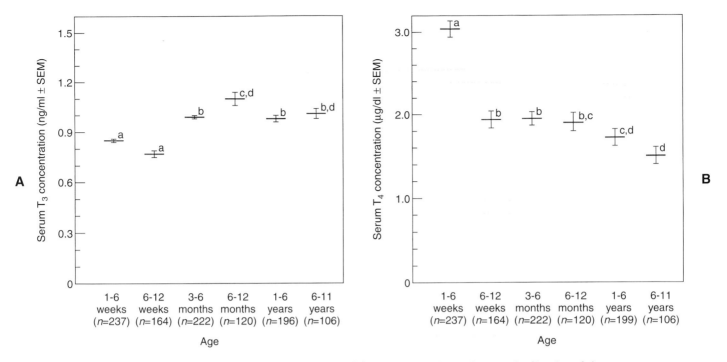

FIGURE 3–28. Mean (± SEM) serum T_3 *(A)* and T_4 *(B)* concentrations in nursing puppies (1 to 6 weeks), weanling puppies (6 to 12 weeks), juvenile dogs (3 to 6 months), young adults (6 to 12 months), middle-aged adults (1 to 6 years), and old dogs (6 to 11 years). Means having different superscripts are significantly (P <0.05) different. (Adapted from Reimers TJ, et al: Am J Vet Res 51:454, 1990.)

TSH concentrations were not different between testosterone-treated and untreated female Greyhound dogs, suggesting that exogenous testosterone administration may not affect thyroid hormone test results (Gaughan and Bruyette, 2001).

In the female dog, progesterone (but not estrogen) affects serum T_4 and T_3 concentrations. In one study, serum T_4 and T_3 concentrations were greater in serum from diestrus females than from anestrus, proestrus, and lactating females or male dogs (Reimers et al, 1984). In another study, dogs with hyperestrogenism did not reveal any alterations in baseline serum T_4 or T_3 concentrations, although the T_4 response to TSH administration was mildly depressed (Gosselin et al, 1980). It has been postulated that progesterone (elevated during diestrus with or without pregnancy) may enhance the binding affinity of plasma proteins for thyroid hormones, resulting in an increase in serum concentrations of total T_4 and T_3 (Wenzel, 1981).

Can hypothyroidism be masked in a diestrual female dog because of a progesterone-induced increase of serum T_4 into the normal range? Does a low-normal serum T_4 concentration in a diestrual female suggest hypothyroidism? Until the answers to these questions are known, the clinician must rely on other factors (e.g., history, physical findings, clinical pathology) in addition to evaluation of multiple tests of thyroid gland function when evaluating a diestrual female for hypothyroidism.

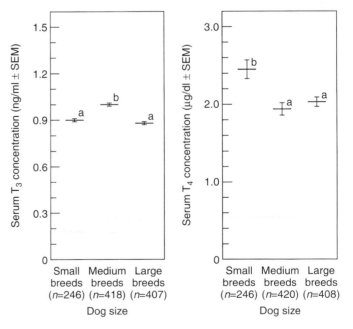

FIGURE 3–29. Mean (± SEM) serum T_3 and T_4 concentration in small breed dogs (mean body weight, 7.1 kg), medium breed dogs (mean body weight, 23.3 kg), and large breed dogs (mean body weight, 30.6 kg). Means having different superscripts are significantly (P <0.05) different. (Adapted from Reimers TJ, et al: Am J Vet Res 51:454, 1990.)

Diurnal Rhythm

Although a diurnal rhythm with a peak in serum thyroid hormone concentration at mid-day has been suggested in the dog, investigators have been unable to document its occurrence, at least during the sampling times of the studies (Kempainnen and Sartin, 1984; Miller et al, 1992). Similarly, a diurnal rhythm in TSH secretion has not been identified in the dog (Bruner et al, 1998). Sporadic and unpredictable fluctuations in blood thyroid hormone and TSH concentrations occur in the dog (see below). Presumably, the time of day when the blood is drawn should not influence the accuracy of assessing thyroid gland function.

Random Fluctuations

Random or pulsatile fluctuations in baseline serum T_4, T_3, and TSH occur in healthy dogs, euthyroid dogs with concurrent illness, and hypothyroid dogs (Fig. 3-22 and 3-30; Kemppainen and Sartin, 1984; Miller et al, 1992; Bruner et al, 1998; Kooistra et al, 2000b). Fluctuations in serum T_4 and TSH concentrations may be clinically significant because randomly obtained blood from a euthyroid dog could have serum T_4 and TSH results within the hypothyroid range (Miller et al, 1992; Brunner et al, 1998). Similarly, a random blood sample from a dog with hypothyroidism could have a serum TSH concentration within the normal range. Fluctuations of serum T_4 concentration, however, do not extend into the normal range (i.e., >1.5 μg/dl) in

dogs with hypothyroidism unless there is anti-T_4 antibody interference with the RIA used to measure T_4 (see page 125). Clinically misleading random fluctuations are more frequently found in euthyroid dogs with concurrent illness than in healthy dogs, a finding that probably relates, in part, to the mechanisms involved in the euthyroid sick syndrome (see below). The incidence of abnormal thyroid hormone values in euthyroid dogs or normal values in hypothyroid dogs also depends on the normal range set by the laboratory (see Interpretation of Serum T_4 Results, page 113). Random fluctuations in serum fT_4 measured by MED have not yet been reported in dogs.

Concurrent Illness (the Euthyroid Sick Syndrome)

OVERVIEW. The *euthyroid sick syndrome* refers to suppression of serum thyroid hormone concentrations in euthyroid dogs in response to concurrent illness. A decrease in serum thyroid hormone concentrations may result from a decline in TSH secretion secondary to suppression of the hypothalamus or pituitary gland, from decreased synthesis of T_4, from decreased concentration or binding affinity of circulating binding proteins (e.g., thyroid binding globulin), from inhibition of the deiodination of T_4 to T_3, or any combination of these factors (Wartofsky and Burman, 1982). The subsequent decrease in serum total T_4 and, in many cases, fT_4 concentrations is believed to represent a physiologic adaptation by the body, with the purpose to decrease cellular metabolism during periods of illness. It is not indicative of hypothyroidism, per se. Generally, the

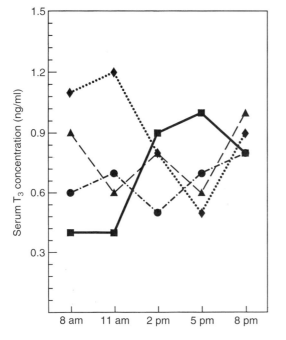
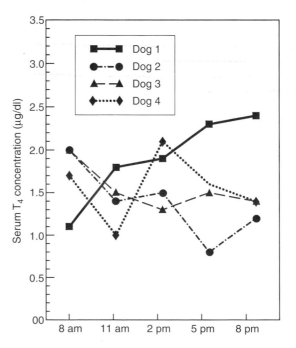

FIGURE 3–30. Sequential baseline serum T_3 and T_4 concentrations from blood samples obtained at 8 AM, 11 AM, 2 PM, 5 PM, and 8 PM in four healthy dogs. Note the random fluctuation in serum T_3 and T_4 concentrations throughout the day and the occasional low value, which could result in a misdiagnosis of hypothyroidism.

type and magnitude of most alterations in serum thyroid hormone concentrations are not unique to a specific disorder but reflect the severity of the illness or the catabolic state and appear to represent a continuum of changes (Kaptein, 1988; Kantrowitz et al, 2001). Systemic illness has more of an effect in lowering serum thyroid hormone concentrations than do, for example, dermatologic disorders (Nelson et al, 1991). In addition, the more severe the systemic illness, the more suppressive the effect on the serum thyroid hormone concentration (Fig. 3-31). With severe concurrent illness, results of TSH or TRH stimulation tests can also mimic hypothyroidism. Correction of the concurrent illness in these dogs results in normal TSH or TRH stimulation test results (see Fig. 3-25).

Unfortunately, euthyroid dogs with concurrent illness can have serum T_4 concentrations that often fall between 0.5 and 1.0 µg/dl and with severe illness (e.g., cardiomyopathy, severe anemia) can be less than 0.5 µg/dl. Alterations in serum concentrations of fT_4 and TSH are more variable and probably depend in part on the pathophysiologic mechanisms involved in the illness. In general, serum fT_4 concentrations tend to be decreased in dogs with concurrent illness but to a lesser extent than total T_4 concentrations (Peterson et al, 1997; Kantrowitz et al, 2001). However, fT_4 concentrations can be less than 0.5 ng/dl if severe illness is present. Serum TSH concentrations may be normal or increased, depending in part on the effect of the concurrent illness on fT_4 concentrations and on pituitary function. If pituitary function is suppressed, TSH concentrations will be in the normal range or undetectable. If pituitary response to changes in fT_4 concentration is not affected by the concurrent illness, TSH concentrations will increase in response to a decrease in fT_4. Serum TSH concentrations can easily exceed 1.0 ng/ml in dogs with the euthyroid sick syndrome. In general, serum TSH concentrations are more likely to stay within the reference range in euthyroid dogs with concurrent illness than T_4 or fT_4 concentrations (Fig. 3-31). In one study, approximately 8% of 223 dogs with nonthyroidal disease had high serum TSH concentrations suggestive of hypothyroidism, whereas 22% had low fT_4 and 31% had T_4 concentrations suggestive of hypothyroidism (Kantrowitz et al, 2001).

Studies performed in human hospitals suggest that the severity of suppression of serum thyroid hormone concentrations can be used as a prognostic indicator for humans with severe illness (Slag et al, 1981; Kaptein et al, 1982). The lower the serum thyroid hormone concentration, the greater the mortality rate. A similar correlation has been documented in euthyroid sick dogs and cats (Peterson and Gamble, 1990; Elliott DA et al, 1995).

Treatment of the euthyroid sick syndrome should be aimed at the concurrent illness. Serum thyroid hormone concentrations return to normal once the concurrent illness is corrected. Treatment of the euthyroid sick syndrome with levothyroxine sodium is controversial. Several studies in humans have shown no improvement when humans with systemic illness and the euthyroid sick syndrome are treated with either T_4 or T_3 (Becker et al, 1982; Brent and Hershman, 1986). Currently, no studies are available that document a clear benefit when euthyroid sick animals are treated with thyroid hormone. Because the euthyroid sick syndrome is believed to be a protective mechanism by the body, most investigators do not recommend treating affected humans with thyroid hormone. Although many dogs with euthyroid sick syndrome are inadvertently treated with levothyroxine sodium without obvious deleterious consequences, we do not routinely treat dogs suspecting of having the euthyroid sick syndrome, especially if the concurrent illness is severe and there is nothing in the history, physical examination, or blood work to support the existence of hypothyroidism.

DERMATOLOGIC DISORDERS. Hypothyroidism is frequently included in the differential diagnoses for many dermatologic disorders in the dog. Can skin disorders induce the euthyroid sick syndrome and falsely lower serum thyroid hormone concentrations into the hypothyroid range? If so, which dermatologic disorders are most likely to induce the euthyroid sick syndrome? Several studies suggest that common dermatologic disorders (e.g., pyoderma, flea hypersensitivity, allergic dermatitis) do not typically cause mean serum thyroid hormone concentrations to decrease into the hypothyroid range in euthyroid dogs (Slade et al, 1984; Nelson et al, 1991; Beale et al, 1992). Borderline serum T_4 and free T_4 concentrations occur in individual euthyroid dogs with skin disease. Depending on the lower limit of normal established by the laboratory (see Interpretation of Serum T_4 Results, page 113), it is also possible for an occasional serum T_4 or free T_4 concentration to fall into the hypothyroid range. It is not known whether this decrease is a result of the euthyroid sick syndrome, random fluctuation in serum thyroid hormone concentration, or some other factor.

SYSTEMIC DISORDERS. Systemic disorders can definitely induce the euthyroid sick syndrome in dogs and falsely lower serum T_4 and fT_4 and increase TSH concentrations into the hypothyroid range (Nelson et al, 1991; Peterson et al, 1997; Ramsey et al, 1997; Scott-Moncrieff et al, 1998; Kantrowitz et al, 2001). A direct correlation exists between the severity of illness and the magnitude of the decrease in serum thyroid hormone concentration. In our experience, disorders that are frequently associated with the euthyroid sick syndrome in the dog include renal and hepatic disease, cardiac failure, severe infections, immune-mediated disorders (e.g., hemolytic anemia), and diabetic ketoacidosis. It is difficult to be certain that the diagnosis of hypothyroidism is correct in dogs with these disorders, especially when relying on results of a single test of thyroid gland function. Normal test results are indicative of euthyroidism, but abnormal test results do not necessarily confirm the diagnosis of hypothyroidism. Abnormal thyroid hormone test results are common with systemic disorders; however, the simultaneous occurrence of low

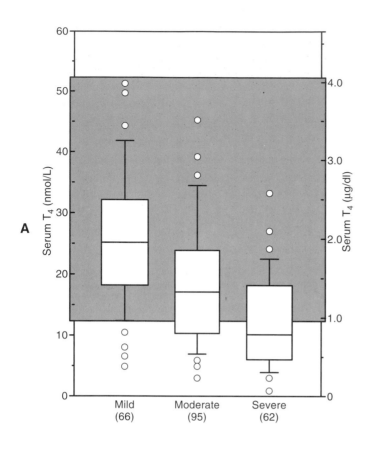

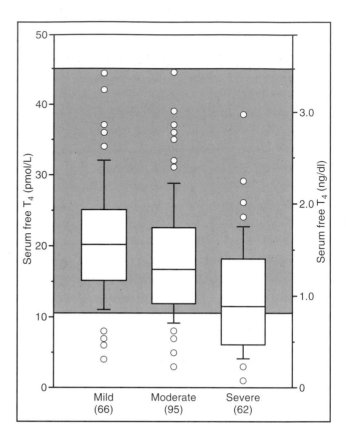

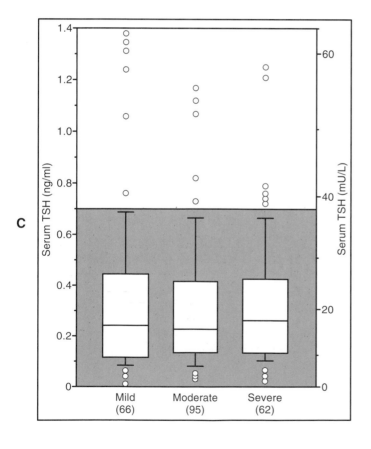

FIGURE 3–31. Box plots of serum concentrations of total T_4 (A), free T_4 (B), and thyrotropin (TSH) (C) in 223 dogs with nonthyroidal disease stratified according to severity of disease. For each box plot, T-bars represent the main body of data, which in most instances is equal to the range. Each box represents interquartile range (25th to 75th percentile). The horizontal bar in each box is the median. Open circles represent outlying data points. Numbers in parentheses indicate the numbers of dogs in each group. Reference range is indicated by the shaded area. (From Kantrowitz LB, et al: JAVMA 219:765, 2001.)

T_4, fT_4, and high TSH concentration is uncommon, occurring in only 1.8% of 223 dogs with nonthyroidal illness (Kantrowitz et al, 2001). Tests of thyroid gland function are most useful when they are interpreted in combination, which is especially important when systemic illness is present (see Establishing the Diagnosis, page 134).

DIABETES MELLITUS. An association between hypothyroidism and insulin-dependent diabetes mellitus (IDDM) has been identified in colony-raised Beagles, and a higher incidence of circulating thyroglobulin autoantibodies has been reported in dogs with IDDM versus healthy dogs (Haines et al, 1984). Concurrent hypothyroidism can also cause insulin resistance in diabetic dogs (Ford et al, 1993). Recognition of hypothyroidism may be difficult in dogs with poorly controlled diabetes mellitus. Many clinical signs (e.g., lethargy, weakness, endocrine alopecia) and abnormalities in clinical pathologic values (e.g., lipemia, hypercholesterolemia) associated with hypothyroidism can also be found in euthyroid dogs with poorly controlled diabetes. Reliance on baseline serum thyroid hormone concentrations can be misleading because of the euthyroid sick syndrome. Suppression of serum thyroid hormone concentration has been documented in euthyroid human beings with IDDM (Gilani et al, 1984), and in our experience, in euthyroid dogs with IDDM as well. Evaluation of baseline thyroid hormone and TSH concentrations in the diabetic dog should not be undertaken until after treatment for the diabetes has been initiated. Interpretation of test results should take into consideration the degree of success achieved in controlling hyperglycemia and the impact poorly controlled diabetes mellitus may have on serum T_4, fT_4, and TSH concentrations.

HYPERADRENOCORTICISM. Endogenously produced and exogenously administered glucocorticoids frequently lower baseline serum T_4, T_3, and free T_4 concentrations in the dog (Peterson et al, 1984; Nelson et al, 1991; Ferguson and Peterson, 1992). There are several proposed mechanisms for the alterations in serum thyroid hormone concentrations in dogs with hyperadrenocorticism (Table 3-16), including inhibition of TSH secretion, reduced serum protein binding of T_4, reduced T_3 production and degradation, and possibly inhibition of peripheral 5'-deiodination of T_4 (Kemppainen et al, 1983; Ferguson and Peterson,

1992). In essence, dogs with naturally acquired hyperadrenocorticism have the potential to develop acquired secondary hypothyroidism with baseline serum thyroid hormone concentrations in the hypothyroid range. In our experience, approximately 60% of our dogs with naturally acquired hyperadrenocorticism in which thyroid gland function is assessed have serum T_4 and fT_4 concentrations in the range consistent with hypothyroidism. Serum TSH concentration is variable in these dogs. Approximately 75% of dogs with naturally acquired hyperadrenocorticism and low thyroid hormone concentrations have undetectable serum TSH concentrations or values that are within the normal range, whereas 25% have serum TSH concentrations greater than 0.6 ng/ml. To date, all affected dogs have been negative for Tg autoantibodies. Treating the hyperadrenocorticism should resolve the secondary hypothyroidism, and serum thyroid hormone concentrations should return to normal. Treatment with levothyroxine sodium is not indicated unless the clinician is unable to control the hyperadrenocorticism and the dog is symptomatic for hypothyroidism or concurrent primary hypothyroidism is suspected.

A diagnostic dilemma exists in trying to differentiate hyperadrenocorticism from hypothyroidism in a dog with endocrine alopecia. Usually, the clinician is able to differentiate tentatively between these two disorders based on the history (e.g., polydipsia, polyuria, polyphagia in hyperadrenocorticism but not hypothyroidism), the presence of additional physical abnormalities, and the presence of abnormalities on a CBC, urinalysis, and serum biochemical panel (e.g., increased alkaline phosphatase activity). The value of obtaining and reviewing a thorough history and physical examination cannot be overemphasized when reviewing these two disorders. In most situations, hyperadrenocorticism and hypothyroidism can be differentiated in the examination room before obtaining any laboratory tests. Occasionally, however, the history, physical examination, and results of routine blood and urine tests do not help. In this situation, a screening test for hyperadrenocorticism (e.g., urine cortisol/creatinine ratio, ACTH stimulation test) should be considered in addition to tests of thyroid gland function to avoid a misdiagnosis of hypothyroidism in a cushingoid dog. If a cushingoid dog is inadvertently treated with levothyroxine sodium, a poor response to treatment or development of additional clinical manifestations (e.g., polyuria and polydipsia) will eventually lead the clinician back towards the diagnosis of hyperadrenocorticism.

TABLE 3–16 PROPOSED ALTERATIONS IN THYROID HORMONE PHYSIOLOGY CAUSED BY GLUCOCORTICOIDS

Decreased 5'-monodeiodination enzyme activity*
Decreased binding affinity of plasma proteins for T_4,T_3
Decreased cellular binding of T_4, T_3
Increased metabolic clearance rate of T_4
Decreased metabolic clearance rate of T_3, rT_3
Inhibition of TSH secretion (secondary hypothyroidism)†
Inhibition of TRH secretion

*Primary alteration in humans
†Primary alteration in dogs

Environmental and Body Temperature

Seasonal influence on thyroid hormone concentrations was evaluated in healthy outdoor dogs in Hokkaido, Japan (Oohashi et al, 2001). Serum T_4 concentration decreased in January and increased in August and September, fT_4 concentration increased in January and November, and there was no significant seasonal variation in serum TSH concentration. It is not known whether a similar seasonal variation occurs in dogs housed indoors or whether temperature variation, photoperiod, or region of the world may impact the results. Acute cold exposure may increase serum concentrations of TSH and thyroid hormones in the rat and possibly in humans, and acute exposure to heat may decrease serum TSH, T_4, and T_3 and increase serum rT_3 concentrations (Wartofsky and Burman, 1982). Hypothermia and hyperpyrexia may also alter serum T_4, T_3, rT_3, and TSH. It is not known, however, whether these alterations are a result of temperature fluctuations or other factors associated with the euthyroid sick syndrome.

Obesity

An increase in serum T_3 and T_4 concentrations has been reported in obese euthyroid dogs (Gosselin et al, 1980). Increased serum thyroid hormone levels are believed to correlate with increased caloric intake rather than obesity per se. Currently, obesity is not believed to have any specific effect on thyroid function (Wartofsky and Burman, 1982). In our experience, obese hypothyroid dogs have low serum T_4 and fT_4 concentrations and high TSH concentrations, suggesting that obesity does not mask the ability to identify hypothyroidism in dogs.

Fasting and Cachexia

In humans, fasting causes a significant, rapid decrease in serum concentrations of T_3 and an increase in serum rT_3 without affecting serum T_4 or TSH concentrations (Wartofsky and Burman, 1982). Refeeding with either a mixed-nutrient or carbohydrate-rich diet causes the fasting-induced changes to reverse quickly. Impaired conversion of T_4 to T_3 from inhibition of peripheral 5'-deiodinase has been proposed to account for these abnormalities (Borst et al, 1983), although studies in rats have also shown decreased thyroidal secretion of T_4. Fasting up to 36 hours did not affect baseline serum T_4 or T_3 concentrations in euthyroid Beagles (Reimers et al, 1986). However, fasting in excess of 48 hours did decrease T_3 concentrations in dogs (de Bruijne et al, 1981). Serum T_4 and T_3 but not fT_4 concentrations were significantly lower in dogs with chronic weight loss causing cachexia, compared with dogs that had not undergone weight loss (Vail et al, 1994). The decrease in serum T_4 and T_3 concentration was proportional to the degree of weight loss associated with their disease. The decline in serum T_4 and T_3 was believed to be related to the severity of the illness or an abnormal nutritional state.

Exercise

The effect of aerobic and anaerobic exercise on thyroid hormone concentrations is minimal in dogs. In one study, serum T_4 concentration increased in Greyhounds when measured 5 minutes after a short sprint race but fT_4 and TSH concentrations remained unchanged (Hill et al, 2001). In sled dogs that underwent severe endurance exercise during the Iiterod race, there was no change in T_4, T_3, or fT_4 concentrations before or after the race (Case et al, 1993). Resting T_4 concentrations were slightly (13%) lower in Beagles undergoing long-distance aerobic exercise on a treadmill, compared with sedentary dogs, but there was no change in fT_4 or T_3 concentrations (Arokoski et al, 1993).

Drugs

Our knowledge of the effect, if any, of various drugs and hormones on serum thyroid hormone and TSH concentrations in dogs is gradually expanding as investigators continue to examine the interplay between medications and thyroid hormone test results (Table 3-14). Undoubtedly, many more as yet unrecognized drugs also affect serum thyroid hormone and TSH concentrations. Until proved otherwise, any drug should be suspected of affecting thyroid hormone test results, especially if the drug has been shown to alter serum thyroid hormone concentrations in humans (Table 3-17) and the history, clinical signs, and clinicopathologic abnormalities do not support a diagnosis of hypothyroidism in the dog.

GLUCOCORTICOIDS. Glucocorticoids are the most commonly used drugs that affect serum thyroid hor-

TABLE 3–17 SOME DRUGS AND DIAGNOSTIC AGENTS THAT CAN ALTER BASAL SERUM THYROID HORMONE CONCENTRATIONS IN HUMANS AND POSSIBLY DOGS

Decrease T_4 and/or T_3	Increase T_4 and/or T_3
Amiodarone (T_3)	Amiodarone (T_4)
Androgens	Estrogens
Cholecystographic agents	5-Fluorouracil
Diazepam	Halothane
Dopamine	Insulin
Flunixin	Narcotic analgesics
Furosemide	Radiopaque dyes (e.g., ipodate) (T_4)
Glucocorticoids	Thiazides
Heparin	
Imidazole	
Iodide	
Methimazole	
Mitotane	
Nitroprusside	
Penicillin	
Phenobarbital	
Phenothiazines	
Phenylbutazone	
Phenytoin	
Primidone	
Propranolol	
Propylthiouracil	
Radiopaque dyes (ipodate) (T_3)	
Salicylates	
Sulfonamides (sulfamethoxazole)	
Sulfonylureas	

mone concentrations. The effect of exogenously administered glucocorticoids on serum thyroid hormone concentrations is similar to that seen with naturally occurring hyperadrenocorticism (see Chapter 6 and page 131). Serum T_4, fT_4, and T_3 concentrations are decreased, often into the hypothyroid range. Proposed mechanisms for this decrease include inhibition of colloid resorption in thyroid follicular cells, increased binding of T_4 to carrier proteins, decreased conversion of T_4 to T_3 at peripheral sites, and suppressed pituitary TSH secretion when exposure to glucocorticoids has been chronic (Woltz et al, 1984; Kaptein et al, 1992; Moore et al, 1993). Serum TSH concentrations typically remain in the reference range, in part, because the reference range for serum TSH extends below the sensitivity of the current TSH assay (i.e., extends to 0 ng/ml; see page 118). Thus identification of serum TSH concentrations below the reference range is not possible. The magnitude and duration of suppression of serum thyroid hormone concentrations depend on the type of glucocorticoid, dosage, route of administration, and duration of glucocorticoid administration. The higher the dosage, the longer the administration; and the more potent the glucocorticoid administered, the more severe the suppression of serum thyroid hormone concentrations.

Because of the common use of glucocorticoid therapy in the management of various internal medical and dermatologic disorders, a thorough history regarding prior glucocorticoid therapy is extremely important before evaluating thyroid gland function. Failure to identify prior glucocorticoid administration can result in a misdiagnosis of hypothyroidism. If glucocorticoids have been administered in the recent past, assay of baseline serum thyroid hormone concentrations should be delayed or must be interpreted carefully. Normal serum T_4, fT_4, and TSH concentrations in these dogs confirm normal thyroid function; low serum T_4 and fT_4 concentrations and high TSH concentrations, suggest hypothyroidism if clinical signs and physical examination findings are consistent with the disease; and any other combination of test results are not easily interpretable. Ideally, glucocorticoids should be discontinued and serum thyroid hormone and TSH concentrations assessed 4 to 8 weeks later if initial test results are not interpretable.

Typically, the administration of exogenous glucocorticoids does not result in clinical signs of hypothyroidism. The exceptions are dogs receiving relatively high dosages of glucocorticoids for prolonged periods to treat chronic steroid-responsive disorders (e.g., immune-mediated diseases). In these dogs, glucocorticoid-induced secondary hypothyroidism may become clinical and require treatment with levothyroxine sodium.

ANTICONVULSANTS. In dogs, phenobarbital treatment at therapeutic dosages decreases serum T_4 and fT_4 concentrations into the range consistent with hypothyroidism (Gaskill et al, 1999; Kantrowitz et al, 1999; Gieger et al, 2000; Muller et al, 2000). Although the mechanism remains unproven in dogs, increased metabolism and excretion of T_4 secondary to hepatic microsomal enzyme induction is believed to be primarily responsible for the decrease in serum thyroid hormone concentrations. A delayed increase in the serum TSH concentration may occur secondary to loss of negative feedback as serum T_4 and fT_4 concentrations decline. Increased serum TSH concentrations quickly return to the reference range following discontinuation of phenobarbital treatment, whereas serum T_4 and fT_4 concentrations may take up to 4 weeks to return to pretreatment values (Gieger et al, 2000).

Bromide, a halide similar to iodide, could potentially affect the thyroid axis by interfering with iodine uptake or with organification by the thyroid gland. However, in vitro studies have suggested that bromide is unlikely to be incorporated into thyroglobulin and is unlikely to affect thyroid hormone synthesis (Taurog and Dorris, 1991). In a recent study, potassium bromide treatment did not have a significant effect on serum T_4, fT_4, T_3, and TSH concentrations in eight dogs with a seizure disorder (Kantrowitz et al, 1999).

SULFONAMIDE ANTIBIOTICS. Sulfonamides interfere with thyroid hormone synthesis by means of dosage- and duration-dependent inhibition of thyroid peroxidase activity (Doerge and Decker, 1994). Thyroid peroxidase is responsible for oxidation of iodide, iodination of tyrosine residues on thyroglobulin, and coupling of tyrosines prior to thyroid hormone secretion. Decreases in serum T_4, fT_4, and T_3 and an increase in TSH concentrations have been documented in dogs treated with sulfonamides (e.g., sulfamethoxazole, sulfadiazine; Hall et al, 1993; Torres et al, 1996; Gookin et al, 1999). Serum T_4 concentrations can decrease into the hypothyroid range within 1 to 2 weeks, and serum TSH concentrations can increase above the reference range within 2 to 3 weeks after initiating sulfonamide therapy (Hall et al, 1993; Cambell et al, 1995; Williamson et al, 2002). Clinical signs of hypothyroidism can develop with chronic sulfonamide administration. The increase in the serum TSH concentration occurs secondary to loss of negative feedback as serum T_4 and fT_4 concentrations decline. The increase in serum TSH can lead to thyroid hyperplasia and goiter (Torres et al, 1996). Alterations in results of thyroid gland function tests may resolve within 1 to 2 weeks or last as long as 8 to 12 weeks after cessation of the antibiotic (Hall et al, 1993; Williamson et al, 2002). Administration of sulfadiazine in combination with trimethoprim during the last 4 weeks of pregnancy in female dogs does not affect the thyroid gland in the neonates (Post et al, 1993).

NONSTEROIDAL ANTI-INFLAMMATORY DRUGS. Nonsteroidal anti-inflammatory drugs (NSAIDs) may decrease serum T_4, fT_4, T_3, and TSH concentrations in humans and other species (Bishnoi et al, 1994). Proposed mechanisms include impaired protein binding of thyroid hormones, impaired hepatic uptake of thyroid hormones, and decreased thyroid hormone deiodination (Topliss et al, 1989; Wang et al, 1999). The effect of NSAIDs on thyroid function tests varies depending on the drug. In dogs, administration of etodolac for 4 weeks did not affect serum thyroid hormone or TSH concentrations (Panciera and Johnston, 2002). In contrast, administration of carprofen for 5 weeks caused a mild but significant decrease in serum T_4 and TSH concentrations, compared with pretreatment values (Ferguson et al, 1999). Serum fT_4 concentration also decreased, but the change was not significant.

Thyroid Hormone Autoantibodies

The presence of thyroid hormone autoantibodies in serum can interfere with the RIAs used to measure serum T_3 or T_4 concentrations, causing unexpected and often confusing test results (Young et al, 1985; see Fig. 3-14). The type of interference depends on the separation system employed in the RIA (see page 125). For most commercially available T_4 assays, T_4 autoantibodies will falsely increase the measured T_4 concentration. The false increase may be enough to raise a hypothyroid dog's result into the reference or hyperthyroid range. The same false increase occurs with nondialysis (direct) RIAs used for measuring serum fT_4 concentrations (Kemppainen et al, 1996). False elevations in serum fT_4 concentration do not occur if fT_4 is measured using a dialysis procedure (e.g., MED technique; see page 116), because autoantibodies cannot pass through the dialysis membrane and interfere with the assay. Measurement of serum T_4 and T_3 autoantibodies is offered by some commercial endocrine laboratories as part of an extensive thyroid panel. Testing for serum T_3 and T_4 autoantibodies is indicated in dogs with unexpected or unusual serum T_3 or T_4 values. Alternatively, evaluation of serum fT_4 concentration measured by MED can be done in dogs with unexpected or confusing T_4 test results. Fortunately, spurious T_4 values resulting from clinically relevant concentrations of T_4 autoantibody account for less than 1% of such results from commercial endocrine laboratories (Nachreiner et al, 2002).

THYROID BIOPSY

Histologic evaluation of a thyroid biopsy specimen is definitive for identifying pathology of the thyroid gland. Lymphocytic thyroiditis and severe thyroid atrophy are readily identified histologically, and in the dog with appropriate clinical signs and diagnostic test results, these findings confirm the diagnosis of primary hypothyroidism. Unfortunately, histologic evaluation of a thyroid biopsy does not always clarify the status of thyroid gland function, especially when clinical signs or diagnostic test results are vague and thyroid pathology is not readily apparent in the biopsy. Variants of normal can be difficult to differentiate from secondary hypothyroidism, primary atrophy, and follicular cell hyperplasia, especially when the last two conditions are in the early stages of development. The influence of concurrent illness on thyroid gland morphology may also affect biopsy results.

Biopsies of the thyroid gland are obtained surgically because of the typical dorsolateral location of the thyroid gland in relation to the trachea, the unpredictable location of the thyroid gland in relation to the long axis of the trachea, and the small size of thyroid lobes affected by lymphocytic thyroiditis and thyroidal atrophy. In our experience, cytologic evaluation of fine-needle aspiration biopsy specimens of the thyroid gland obtained using ultrasound guidance has been disappointing, in part because of the difficulty in obtaining a representative sample and contamination of the sample with blood during the aspiration procedure. If a surgical biopsy is performed, the surgeon must consider potential complications caused by general anesthesia (e.g., hypotension, prolonged anesthetic recovery from slowed drug metabolism) and must maintain the vascular integrity of at least one parathyroid gland to prevent hypocalcemia. Removal of one thyroid lobe and its parathyroid glands without manipulating the opposite thyroid lobe ensures an adequate biopsy specimen, minimal intraoperative hemorrhage, and two functioning parathyroid glands. Biopsy specimens should initially be placed in Bouin's fixative for 4 to 6 hours to reduce shrinkage artifacts. This should be followed by fixation in 10% neutral buffered formalin (Belshaw, 1983).

The disadvantages of thyroid gland biopsy include the invasiveness of the procedure, cost to the client, time commitment of the veterinarian, and lack of guarantee that diagnostically useful information will be obtained. We believe that the disadvantages outweigh the benefits of thyroid gland biopsy and, in a clinical setting, do not recommend surgical biopsy of the thyroid gland to establish a diagnosis of hypothyroidism.

ESTABLISHING THE DIAGNOSIS

Recommendations regarding the approach to the diagnosis of hypothyroidism, reached at an international symposium on canine hypothyroidism held in 1996 (*Canine Practice*, Vol 77, 1997) are provided in Table 3-12. The presence of appropriate clinical signs is imperative, especially when relying on baseline thyroid hormone concentrations for a diagnosis. Identification of a mild nonregenerative anemia on the CBC and especially an increased serum cholesterol concentration on a serum biochemistry panel adds further evidence for hypothyroidism. Baseline serum T_4 concentration is often used as the initial screening test for thyroid gland function, in part because it is widely available at low cost and can be measured in-house. It is important to remember that serum T_4 concentrations can be suppressed by a variety of factors, most notably the euthyroid sick syndrome. Thus measurement of the serum T_4 concentration should be used to confirm a euthyroid state. A normal serum T_4 concentration establishes euthyroidism in the vast majority of dogs. The exceptions are a very small number of hypothyroid dogs with lymphocytic thyroiditis and serum T_4

autoantibodies that interfere with the RIA used to measure T_4 (see page 125). A low serum T_4 concentration (i.e., less than 0.5 µg/dl), in conjunction with hypercholesterolemia and clinical signs strongly suggestive of the disease, supports the diagnosis of hypothyroidism, especially if systemic illness is not present. The definitive diagnosis must then rely on response to trial therapy with levothyroxine sodium. Additional diagnostic tests (i.e., fT_4 and TSH) are warranted (1) if the serum T_4 concentration is less than 1.0 µg/dl but clinical signs and physical examination findings are not strongly supportive of the disease and hypercholesterolemia is not present, (2) if severe systemic illness is present and the potential for the euthyroid sick syndrome is high, or (3) if drugs known to decrease serum T_4 concentration are being administered.

Although measurement of serum T_4 concentration can be used as an initial screening test, measuring a combination of thyroid gland tests is preferred because this provides a more informative analysis of the pituitary-thyroid gland axis and thyroid gland function. Many diagnostic laboratories offer a variety of options in thyroid panels that incorporate two or more of the following: serum T_4, fT_4 by RIA or MED, T_3, fT_3, rT_3, TSH, and antibody tests for lymphocytic thyroiditis. The thyroid panel at our hospital includes serum T_4, fT_4 by MED, TSH, and the thyroglobulin autoantibody test. A normal serum T_4, fT_4, and TSH concentration rules out hypothyroidism. Low serum T_4 and fT_4 and increased serum TSH concentrations in a dog with appropriate clinical signs and clinicopathologic abnormalities strongly supports the diagnosis of hypothyroidism, especially if systemic illness or drugs known to affect thyroid test results are not present. Concurrent presence of Tg autoantibodies suggests lymphocytic thyroiditis as the underlying etiology.

Unfortunately, discordant test results are common when multiple tests are evaluated, creating confusion. When this occurs, reliance on appropriateness of clinical signs, clinicopathologic abnormalities, and clinician index of suspicion become the most important parameters in deciding whether to treat the dog with levothyroxine sodium. Serum fT_4 concentration measured by MED is the single most accurate test of thyroid gland function and carries the highest priority when assessing thyroid gland function, followed by serum T_4 concentration. Results of TSH concentration increases the likelihood of euthyroidism or hypothyroidism when results are consistent with results of serum fT_4, but TSH test results should not be used as the sole indicator of hypothyroidism. Low serum fT_4 and normal TSH test results occur in approximately 20% of dogs with hypothyroidism and high TSH test results occur in euthyroid dogs with the euthyroid sick syndrome (Scott-Moncrieff et al, 1998; Kantrowitz et al, 2001). Normal serum fT_4 and high TSH may suggest early compensated hypothyroidism, but why would clinical signs develop if serum fT_4 is normal? A positive Tg autoantibody test merely suggests the possibility of lymphocytic thyroiditis; Tg autoantibody is not a thyroid function test. Positive results increase the suspicion for hypothyroidism if serum T_4 or fT_4 concentrations are low but have no bearing on generation of clinical signs if serum T_4 and fT_4 concentrations are normal. Positive serum T_4 and T_3 autoantibody test results are interpreted in a similar manner. When faced with discordant test results, the clinician must decide whether to initiate trial therapy with levothyroxine sodium or to repeat the tests sometime in the future, a decision that must ultimately be made based on the appropriateness of clinical signs and results of the serum fT_4 concentration measured by MED.

Admittedly, interpretation of serum T_4, fT_4, and TSH concentrations is not always simple. Because of expense and the frustration of working with tests that are not always reliable, many veterinarians and some clients prefer trial therapy as a diagnostic test. Trial therapy should be done only when thyroid hormone supplementation does not pose a risk to the patient. Response to trial therapy with levothyroxine sodium is nonspecific. A dog that has a positive response to therapy either had hypothyroidism or had "thyroid-responsive disease." Because of its anabolic nature, thyroid hormone supplementation can create an effect in a dog without thyroid dysfunction. This is perhaps most notable in the quality of the hair coat. Thyroid hormone supplementation stimulates telogen hair follicles into the anagen stage and improves the hair coat, presumably even in euthyroid dogs (Gunaratnam, 1986; Credille et al, 2001). Therefore, if a positive response to trial therapy is observed, thyroid supplementation should be gradually discontinued once clinical signs have resolved. If clinical signs recur, hypothyroidism is confirmed and the supplement should be reinitiated. If clinical signs do not recur, a "thyroid-responsive disorder" or a beneficial response to concurrent therapy (e.g., antibiotics, flea control) should be suspected.

DIAGNOSIS IN A PREVIOUSLY TREATED DOG. Occasionally, a clinician wants to determine whether a dog receiving thyroid hormone supplementation is, in fact, hypothyroid. The exogenous administration of thyroid hormone, either T_4 or T_3, will suppress pituitary TSH secretion and cause pituitary thyrotroph atrophy, and subsequently thyroid gland atrophy, in a healthy euthyroid dog. Serum T_4, T_3, and TSH concentrations are decreased or undetectable; the severity of the decrease is dependent on the severity of thyroid gland atrophy induced by the thyroid supplement. Serum T_4 and fT_4 results are often suggestive of hypothyroidism, even in a previously euthyroid dog, if testing is performed within a month of discontinuing treatment. Thyroid hormone supplementation must be discontinued and the pituitary-thyroid axis allowed to regain function before meaningful baseline serum T_4 concentrations can be obtained. The time between the discontinuation of thyroid hormone supplementation and the acquisition of meaningful results regarding thyroid gland function depends on the duration of treatment, the dose and frequency of administration of the thyroid hormone supplement, and individual variability. As a general rule, thyroid hormone supplements should be discontinued for a minimum of 4 weeks, but preferably 6 to 8 weeks, before thyroid gland function is critically assessed.

DIAGNOSIS IN PUPPIES. An approach similar to the one described above is used to diagnose congenital hypothyroidism. However, serum TSH concentrations are dependent on the etiology. Serum TSH concentrations will be increased in dogs with primary dysfunction of the thyroid gland (e.g., iodine organification defect) and an intact hypothalamic-pituitary-thyroid gland axis. However, serum TSH concentrations will be within the normal range or undetectable in dogs with pituitary or hypothalamic dysfunction as the cause of the hypothyroidism. Results of a TRH stimulation test with measurement of TSH and serum thyroid hormone concentrations may help localize the site of the problem.

TREATMENT

Thyroid hormone supplementation is indicated for the treatment of confirmed hypothyroidism and to tentatively diagnose hypothyroidism through clinical response to trial therapy. The initial therapeutic approach is similar for both situations and involves the administration of a synthetic thyroxine preparation (Table 3-18). For dogs with secondary hypothyroidism, additional therapy may be necessary, depending on the etiology.

TABLE 3–18   SOME OF THE THYROID HORMONE REPLACEMENT PRODUCTS CURRENTLY AVAILABLE FOR USE IN HUMANS AND DOGS

Synthetic Products

Levothyroxine
  AmTech Levothyroxine Sodium Tablets (Phoenix Scientific)
  Canine Thyroid Chewable Thyroid Tablets (Pala-Tech)
  Heska Chewable Thyroid Tablets (Heska)
  Levotabs (Vetus)
  Levothyroid (Forest)
  Levoxyl (Jones Pharma)
  Nutrived T-4 Chewable Tablets (Vedco)
  Soloxine (Jones Pharma)
  Synthroid (Knoll)
  Thyro-Form (Vet-A-Mix)
  Thyro-L (Vet-A-Mix)
  Thyro-Tab (Vet-A-Mix)
  Thyrosyn (Vedco)
  Thyroxine-L (Butler)
  Thyrozine (Phoenix)
  Unithroid (Jerome Stevens Pharma)
Liothyronine
  Cytomel (Jones Pharma)
Levothyroxine + Liothyronine
  Thyrolar (Rhone-Poulenc Rorer)

Animal Products

Desiccated Thyroid
  Armour Thyroid (Forest)
  S-P-T (Fleming)
  Thyroid USP (Several companies)

Initial Therapy with Levothyroxine Sodium (Synthetic T₄)

Synthetic levothyroxine is the initial therapy of choice for treating hypothyroidism (Table 3-19). The oral administration of synthetic T_4 should result in normal serum concentrations of T_4, T_3, and TSH, attesting to the fact that these products can be converted to the more metabolically active T_3 by peripheral tissues. A name brand levothyroxine sodium product approved for use in animals is recommended initially. Because the hormonal content of some thyroxine preparations may be considerably less than the amount stated on the label (Fish et al, 1987), only products known to be effective in dogs should be used. Untested thyroxine products can be tried once a clinical response has been observed, although the reason to do this is not readily apparent.

The consensus recommendation reached at an international symposium on canine hypothyroidism held in August 1996 (Canine Practice, vol 77, 1997) was to administer levothyroxine sodium at an initial dosage of 0.02 mg/kg of body weight (0.1 mg/10 lb; maximum dose, 0.8 mg) every 12 hours. This dosage is similar to the average calculated oral replacement dosage (0.018 mg/kg) determined in a study evaluating replacement T_4 requirements in thyroidectomized dogs (Ferguson and Hoenig, 1997). The oral absorption of levothyroxine is low in dogs, compared with humans, which explains why the dosage of levothyroxine is considerably higher in dogs versus humans. Some investigators believe that the dose of levothyroxine may correlate with metabolic rate better than with body weight (Chastain, 1982). Metabolic rate, in turn, is more closely related to body surface

TABLE 3–19   RECOMMENDATIONS FOR THE INITIAL TREATMENT AND MONITORING OF HYPOTHYROIDISM IN DOGS

Initial Treatment

Use a name brand synthetic levothyroxine sodium product approved for animal use.
The initial dosage per administration should be 0.02 mg/kg of body weight (0.1 mg/10–15 pounds), with a maximum dose of 0.8 mg.
The initial frequency of administration is every 12 hours.

Initial Monitoring

Response to treatment should be critically evaluated 6 to 8 weeks after initiating treatment.
Serum T_4 or free T_4 (measured by equilibrium dialysis) and TSH concentration should be measured 4 to 6 hours after administration of thyroid hormone.
  Serum T_4 or free T_4 concentration should be in the normal range or increased.
  Serum TSH concentration should be in the normal range.
Measuring serum T_4 or free T_4 (measured by equilibrium dialysis) concentration immediately prior to thyroid hormone administration (i.e., trough level) is optional but is recommended if thyroid hormone is being given once a day.
  Serum T_4 or free T_4 concentration should be in the normal range.

Adapted from consensus recommendations reached at an international symposium on canine hypothyroidism held in August 1996 (Canine Practice, vol 77, 1997).
T_4, thyroxine; *TSH*, thyrotropin.

area than to body weight. A smaller dog has a proportionately greater body surface area and metabolic rate and thus a greater levothyroxine requirement than a larger dog. The recommended dosage of levothyroxine based on body surface area is $0.5 mg/m^2$. We prefer to dose levothyroxine based on body weight rather than body surface area.

The plasma half-life of levothyroxine is variable and depends, in part, on the dosage and frequency of administration, with higher dosages and more frequent administration associated with a shorter half-life of levothyroxine (Nachreiner et al, 1993). In one study, the mean (± SD) serum half-life of levothyroxine was $9.0 ± 5.9$ and $8.6 ± 3.1$ hours when levothyroxine was administered at 22 µg/kg once and twice a day, respectively (Nachreiner et al, 1993). At this dosage, mean time to peak serum T_4 concentration was $3.8 ± 2.0$ hours after levothyroxine administration. It is interesting to note that maximal and minimal serum T_4 concentrations were higher and lower, respectively, with single versus twice-daily levothyroxine administration. As a result, serum T_4 concentrations were above the physiologic range for a number of hours with single levothyroxine administration, whereas concentrations closer to physiologic ranges were achieved by use of divided doses. The consensus recommendation reached at an international symposium on canine hypothyroidism held in 1996 was to administer levothyroxine sodium every 12 hours initially. Because of variability in its absorption and metabolism, the dose and frequency may have to be adjusted before a satisfactory clinical response is observed; this variability is one reason for the monitoring of therapy in dogs.

Initial treatment with levothyroxine sodium twice a day is especially important when trial therapy is being used to establish the diagnosis of hypothyroidism. Some dogs require levothyroxine twice a day to alleviate clinical signs, whereas others require it only once a day (Ferguson and Hoenig, 1997). Initially administering the hormone twice daily should benefit both groups of dogs. Conversely, once-daily therapy benefits only the group of dogs with slower metabolism and longer duration of effect of the hormone supplement (i.e., dogs that require the hormone once a day). Physiologic adaptations typically prevent thyrotoxicosis from developing in dogs that only need once-daily treatment but are receiving levothyroxine twice a day or in dogs receiving dosages higher than necessary to control the disorder. These adaptations include less efficient absorption of levothyroxine from the gastrointestinal tract; saturation of binding proteins, which increases clearance of thyroid hormone; and a change in hormone metabolism so that degradation is more rapid as the dog's basal metabolic rate increases (Nachreiner and Refsal, 1992; Nachreiner et al, 1993).

The initial dosage of levothyroxine sodium may need to be modified in dogs with concurrent illness in which thyroid hormone–induced alterations in cellular metabolic functions may have a deleterious effect. A classic example is the dog with concurrent cardiomyopathy. Thyroid supplementation increases basal metabolism and oxygen consumption, increases heart rate, and may reduce ventricular filling time. A sudden increase in demand for oxygen delivery to peripheral tissues, plus the chronotropic effects of the medication, may place undue stress on a poorly functioning heart, causing decompensation and worsening signs of heart failure. Initially using a lower dosage of levothyroxine sodium (e.g., 25% of recommended dose once daily) in a dog with concurrent illness allows the dog to "adapt" to the hormone and helps minimize the potential deleterious effects of the supplement. The dosage of levothyroxine sodium may then be gradually increased over the ensuing 3 to 4 weeks.

The majority of intestinal absorption of orally administered levothyroxine occurs in the ileum and colon. Absorption is influenced by the form in which the hormone is administered (e.g., gelatin capsule versus albumin carrier) and by intraluminal contents, including plasma proteins, soluble dietary factors, and intestinal flora. All of these intraluminal contents can bind levothyroxine and impair absorption. In humans, between 40% and 80% of orally administered levothyroxine is absorbed into the circulation. Although similar studies have not been reported in the dog, the greater dosage of levothyroxine used in dogs versus humans suggests that intestinal absorption of levothyroxine is less in dogs. Variability in absorption of levothyroxine is one reason for therapeutic monitoring of treated dogs. Excessive binding of levothyroxine to intraluminal intestinal contents could result in a poor clinical response to treatment (Table 3-20).

Response to Levothyroxine Sodium Therapy

Thyroid hormone supplementation should be continued for a minimum of 6 to 8 weeks before critically evaluating the effectiveness of treatment. With appropriate therapy, all of the clinical signs and clinicopathologic abnormalities associated with hypothyroidism are reversible (Fig. 3-32). An increase in mental alertness and activity usually occurs initially and is seen within the first week of treatment (Table 3-21); this is an important early indicator that the diagnosis of hypothyroidism was correct. Although some hair regrowth usually occurs within the first month in dogs with

---

TABLE 3–20 POTENTIAL REASONS FOR POOR CLINICAL RESPONSE TO TREATMENT WITH LEVOTHYROXINE SODIUM (SYNTHETIC T_4)

Owner compliance problems
Use of inactivated or outdated product
Use of some generic levothyroxine sodium preparations
Inappropriate levothyroxine sodium dose
Inappropriate frequency of administration
Low tablet strength*
Poor bioavailability (e.g., poor gastrointestinal absorption)
Inadequate time for clinical response to occur
Incorrect diagnosis of hypothyroidism
Concurrent disease causing clinical signs (e.g., allergic dermatitis)

*Tablet strength refers to actual amount of active drug in tablet as opposed to the stated amount.

TABLE 3–21 ANTICIPATED TIME OF CLINICAL RESPONSE TO SODIUM LEVOTHYROXINE TREATMENT IN DOGS WITH HYPOTHYROIDISM

Area of Improvement	Time to Improvement
Mentation and activity	2 to 7 days
Lipemia and clinical pathology	2 to 4 weeks
Dermatologic abnormalities	2 to 4 months
Neurologic abnormalities	1 to 3 months
Cardiac abnormalities	1 to 2 months
Reproductive abnormalities	3 to 10 months

endocrine alopecia, it may take several months for complete regrowth and a marked reduction in hyper-pigmentation of the skin to occur. Initially, the hair coat may worsen as large amounts of hair in the telogen stage of the hair cycle are shed. If obesity is caused by hypothyroidism, it should also begin to improve within 2 months after initiating levothyroxine sodium therapy along with adjustments in diet and exercise (Fig. 3-33). Initial improvement in neurologic manifestations is usually evident within 1 to 2 weeks of initiating treatment; complete resolution of neurologic signs is unpredictable and may take 3 months of treatment or longer before occurring. Improvement in cardiac function is usually evident by 4 to 8 weeks.

Failure to Respond to Levothyroxine Sodium Therapy

Problems with levothyroxine therapy should be suspected if clinical improvement is not seen within 8 weeks of the initiation of therapy. There are several

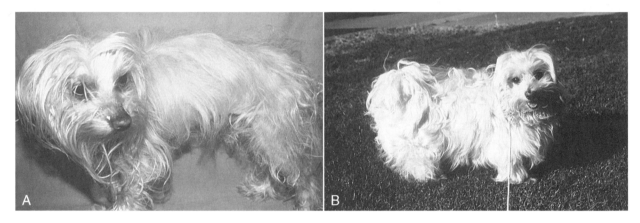

FIGURE 3–32. *A*, A 7-year-old male Maltese with hypothyroidism and diabetes mellitus. *B*, Same dog as in *A* after 3 months of levothyroxine sodium treatment. Note the marked improvement in appearance and hair coat.

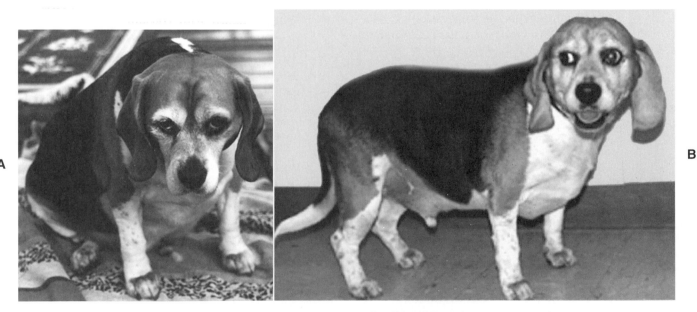

FIGURE 3–33. *A*, An 8-year-old male castrated Beagle with hypothyroidism. The primary owner complaints were obesity, lethargy, and weakness. The dog weighed 31 kg. *B*, Same dog as in *A* after 6 months of levothyroxine sodium treatment and adjustments in caloric intake and type of diet to promote weight loss. The owner reported marked improvement in the dog's alertness and activity, and its body weight had decreased to 19 kg.

possible reasons for a poor response to therapy (Table 3-19). An inappropriate diagnosis of hypothyroidism is the most obvious. Hyperadrenocorticism can be mistaken for hypothyroidism if other clinical signs (e.g., polyuria, polydipsia) commonly associated with hyperadrenocorticism are not present because of the suppressive effects of cortisol on serum thyroid hormone concentrations (see page 131). Failure to recognize the impact of concurrent illness on thyroid hormone test results is another common cause for misdiagnosing hypothyroidism. Concurrent disease (e.g., allergic skin disease, flea hypersensitivity) is also common in dogs with hypothyroidism and may affect the clinical impression of response to levothyroxine sodium therapy if the concurrent disease is not recognized. Whenever a dog shows a poor response to levothyroxine therapy, the history, physical examination findings, and diagnostic test results that prompted the initiation of levothyroxine therapy should be critically reevaluated and a thorough evaluation for concurrent disease that may be perpetuating clinical signs undertaken. In addition, problems with the treatment regimen should be investigated, including poor owner compliance in administering the hormone, the use of outdated preparations, an inappropriate dose or frequency of administration of levothyroxine sodium, the use of some generic levothyroxine products, or poor intestinal absorption of levothyroxine.

Therapeutic Monitoring

Therapeutic monitoring includes evaluation of the clinical response to thyroid hormone supplementation and measurement of serum T_4 and TSH concentrations before or after levothyroxine sodium administration, or both. Serum T_4 and TSH should be measured 4 to 8 weeks after initiating therapy, whenever signs of thyrotoxicosis develop, or when there has been minimal or no response to therapy. They should also be measured 2 to 4 weeks after an adjustment in levothyroxine therapy in dogs showing a poor clinical response to treatment.

Serum T_4 and TSH concentrations are typically evaluated 4 to 6 hours after the administration of levothyroxine in dogs receiving the medication twice daily and just before and 4 to 6 hours after administration in dogs receiving it once a day (Nachreiner and Refsal, 1992). This information allows the clinician to evaluate the dose, frequency of administration, and adequacy of intestinal absorption of levothyroxine sodium. Measurement of serum fT_4 by the MED technique can be done in lieu of T_4 but is more expensive and probably does not offer additional information except in dogs with serum T_4 autoantibodies (see page 125). If autoantibodies to T_4 are present in the serum of a dog receiving thyroid hormone supplementation, measurement of serum T_4 cannot be used to monitor therapy. Results of serum fT_4 measurements by assays that use a dialysis step (e.g., MED technique, see page 116) are not affected by thyroid hormone autoantibodies. The presence of thyroid hormone autoantibodies does not interfere with the physiologic actions of thyroid hormone supplements.

Postdosing serum T_4 and TSH results and recommendations for changes in therapy are given in Figure 3-34. If the dose of the thyroid hormone supplement and the dosing schedule are appropriate, the serum T_4 concentration should be in the upper half of or above the reference baseline range (i.e., 2.5 to 4.5 µg/dl) when measured 4 to 6 hours after thyroid hormone administration and the serum TSH concentration should be in the reference range (i.e., less than 0.6 ng/ml) in all blood samples evaluated. Postdosing serum T_4 concentrations measured at times other than 4 to 6 hours after levothyroxine sodium administration should be interpreted with the realization that serum T_4 may not be at peak concentrations. Conceptually, the serum T_4 concentration increases following levothyroxine administration, peaks approximately 4 to 6 hours after administration, and then declines until the next levothyroxine tablet is administered (Nachreiner et al, 1993). There is an inverse correlation between the time interval from actual blood sample collection to the 4- to 6-hour postdosing time and the postdosing serum T_4 concentration; that is, the greater the time interval, the lower the serum T_4 concentration, and vice versa. Ideally, all postpill serum T_4 concentrations should be greater than 1.5 µg/dl, regardless of the time interval between levothyroxine administration and postpill blood sampling. Postdosing serum T_4 concentration may also be affected by pharmaceutical preparation, concurrent drugs, and possibly diet. Preliminary studies suggest that peak serum T_4 concentrations are decreased with the administration of generic preparations and Heska Chewable Thyroid Supplement for Dogs (Heska Corp, Ft. Collins, CO), compared with Soloxine (King Pharmaceuticals Inc., Bristol, TN); decreased with concurrent glucocorticoid treatment; and decreased, albeit insignificantly, with consumption of high-fiber diets (Johnson et al, 1999; Graham, 2002).

Postdosing serum T_4 concentrations are frequently above the normal range. A retrospective evaluation of postpill serum T_4 and T_3 results from 100 hypothyroid dogs treated with levothyroxine sodium and randomly selected from our canine hypothyroid population revealed that the 6- ± 1-hour postpill T_4 concentration was within, above, and below the normal baseline range in 54%, 41%, and 5% of the dogs, respectively. All of the dogs had received levothyroxine sodium twice daily at a mean (± SD) dosage of 0.018 ± 0.007 mg/kg, and all dogs had responded to treatment. None of the dogs with abnormally increased postpill T_4 concentrations exhibited signs of thyrotoxicosis. The postpill T_3 concentration was within the normal baseline range in the dogs with increased postpill T_4 concentration, suggesting physiologic adaptations to prevent hyperthyroidism (Nachreiner and Refsal, 1992). The finding of an increased postdosing serum T_4 concentration is therefore not an absolute indication to reduce the dose of levothyroxine sodium, especially if there are no clinical signs of thyrotoxicosis. However, we recommend a reduction in the dose whenever serum T_4 concentrations exceed 6.0 µg/dl.

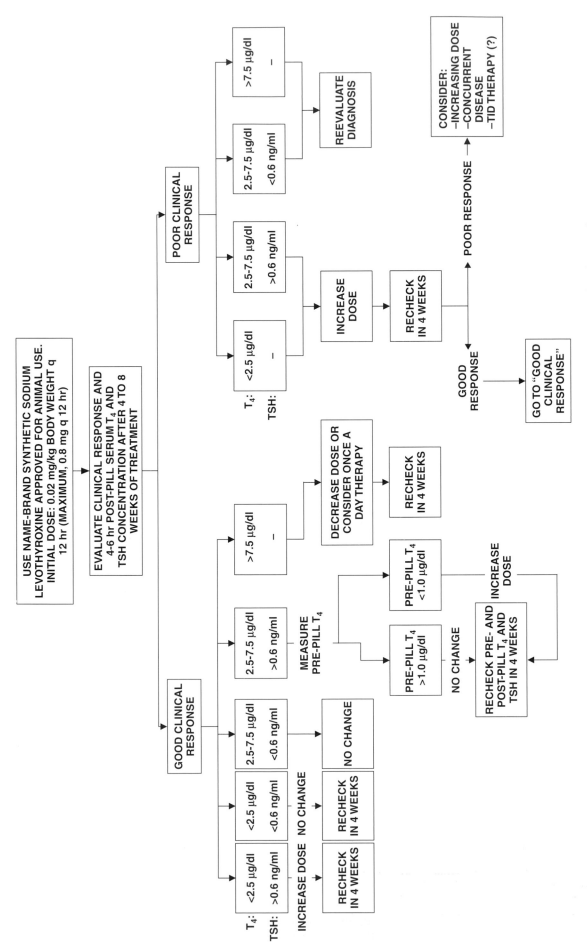

FIGURE 3–34. Initial therapeutic approach and monitoring recommendations for dogs with hypothyroidism. (From Nelson RW, Couto EC: Small Animal Internal Medicine, 3rd ed. St. Louis, Mosby-Year Book, 2003, p. 708.)

Perhaps the most problematic diagnostic dilemma occurs with the dog in which trial therapy is used to tentatively establish a diagnosis of hypothyroidism, the clinical response is poor to thyroid hormone supplementation, postdosing serum T_4 concentrations are within or above the reference range, and serum TSH concentrations are less than 0.6 ng/ml. A pretreatment serum T_4 concentration should be evaluated to determine the "trough" concentration. The poor response to therapy may be caused by inadequate thyroid hormone supplementation if the predosing serum T_4 concentration is less than 1.0 µg/dl, especially if the postdosing serum T_4 concentration is near the lower end of the reference range (e.g., less than 2.0 µg/dl). An increase in the dosage or frequency of administration of levothyroxine sodium should be considered, and the pre- and postdosing serum T_4 concentration and clinical response should be re-evaluated in 2 to 4 weeks. If the pre- and postdosing serum T_4 concentrations are greater than 1.5 µg/dl, euthyroidism has been obtained and another reason for the poor response should be sought. In our experience, the persistence of clinical signs in the majority of these dogs is caused by another disease that has not yet been diagnosed. Although trial therapy with liothyronine sodium may be attempted, it is usually ineffective in producing a beneficial response in a dog that has failed to respond to levothyroxine sodium and whose serum T_4 concentrations are in the normal range.

Thyrotoxicosis

It is unusual for thyrotoxicosis to develop as a result of the excessive administration of levothyroxine sodium in the dog, owing to physiologic adaptations that impair gastrointestinal tract absorption and enhance clearance of thyroid hormone by the liver and kidneys (Nachreiner and Refsal, 1992). Nevertheless, thyrotoxicosis may develop in dogs receiving excessive amounts of levothyroxine sodium; in dogs in which the plasma half-life for levothyroxine is inherently prolonged, especially in those receiving levothyroxine twice daily; and in dogs with impaired metabolism of levothyroxine (e.g., concurrent renal or hepatic insufficiency). Rarely, thyrotoxicosis develops in a dog given minute amounts of levothyroxine sodium. The reason for this marked sensitivity to the hormone is not known.

Clinical signs of thyrotoxicosis include panting, nervousness, aggressive behavior, polyuria, polydipsia, polyphagia, and weight loss. The documentation of increased serum thyroid hormone concentrations supports the diagnosis. However, these concentrations can occasionally be within the normal range in a dog with signs of thyrotoxicosis, and they are commonly increased in dogs with no signs of thyrotoxicosis. Adjustments in the dose or frequency of administration of thyroid hormone medication, or both measures, are indicated if appropriate clinical signs develop in a dog receiving thyroid hormone supplements. Supplementation may have to be discontinued

for a few days in such animals if the clinical signs are severe. Signs of thyrotoxicosis should resolve within 1 to 3 days if they are due to the thyroid medication and the adjustment in treatment has been appropriate. It is recommended that therapy be monitored 2 to 4 weeks after levothyroxine sodium treatment has been adjusted and the clinical signs have resolved.

Trial Therapy with Liothyronine Sodium (Synthetic T_3)

Liothyronine sodium (Cytomel; Jones Pharma, St. Louis, MO) is not the initial thyroid hormone supplement of choice for the treatment of hypothyroidism. Liothyronine sodium supplementation results in normal serum T_3 but low to nondetectable serum T_4 concentrations. The decrease in serum T_4 after initiation of liothyronine sodium therapy is often misinterpreted as support for the diagnosis of hypothyroidism. The decrease in serum T_4 is actually caused by decreased secretion of T_4 by the thyroid gland secondary to the inhibitory influence of liothyronine sodium on pituitary TSH secretion, in conjunction with an inability of liothyronine to be converted to T_4. A decrease in serum T_4 would occur in a normal dog treated with liothyronine sodium. In contrast, levothyroxine sodium therapy results in normal serum levels of both T_3 and T_4 because levothyroxine can be converted to T_3. Normalization of both serum T_4 and T_3 provides the most nearly normal intracellular concentrations of T_3 in all tissues, thus producing euthyroidism.

Liothyronine therapy is indicated when levothyroxine therapy has failed to achieve a response in a dog with confirmed hypothyroidism. The most plausible explanation for failure to respond to a T_4 supplement is impaired absorption of levothyroxine from the intestinal tract. Impaired absorption of levothyroxine sodium should be suspected when baseline serum T_4 concentrations are low, serum TSH is high, and no increase in serum T_4 concentration occurs following oral levothyroxine administration. Thyroid hormone autoantibodies that interfere with the RIA technique should also be considered. In contrast to T_4, T_3 is almost completely absorbed from the human intestine (95% versus 40% to 80%). This more complete absorption reflects less binding affinity of intestinal contents for T_3, especially plasma proteins secreted in the bowel lumen.

Historically, liothyronine sodium has been used in dogs with normal serum T_4 but low serum T_3 concentration. These dogs were often suspected of having a defect in the conversion of T_4 to T_3. It is now recognized that most of these dogs are either normal, have the euthyroid sick syndrome (see page 128), or have T_3 autoantibodies that cause a false lowering of the serum T_3 concentration (see page 125). Conversion abnormalities have not been documented in any species, including dogs. Conceptually, conversion defects are most likely to be congenital, and thus, affected puppies should have died shortly after birth or should have developed cretinism. If the decision is made to treat the dog with normal serum T_4 and low serum T_3 concentration, sodium levothyroxine should be used initially.

The initial dosage of liothyronine is 4 to 6 μg/kg body weight every 8 hours. As with levothyroxine sodium, the plasma half-life and time of peak plasma concentration after administration of liothyronine are variable among dogs. In most dogs, the plasma half-life of liothyronine is approximately 5 to 6 hours, with peak plasma concentrations occurring 2 to 5 hours after administration. Once clinical improvement is observed, the frequency of administration may be reduced to twice a day. If clinical signs recur, three daily doses should be reinstituted.

Blood for therapeutic monitoring should be obtained just before and 2 to 4 hours after administration of liothyronine sodium. Evaluation of serum T_3 is mandatory with this supplement. Serum T_4 concentrations are low to nondetectable with adequate T_3 supplements because of the negative feedback suppression on the remaining functional thyroid tissue and an inability of T_3 to be converted to T_4. Guidelines for adjustments in T_3 therapy are similar to those for T_4 supplements. Serum T_3 concentrations before and following T_3 administration should be within the normal range in a dog receiving an adequate dosage of a T_3 supplement.

Combination T_4/T_3 Products

Synthetic preparations are available that contain both levothyroxine and liothyronine (see Table 3-18). The T_4-to-T_3 ratio is generally 4 to 1, which is an attempt to mimic normal human thyroid secretion ratios (Rosychuk, 1982). We do not recommend combination T_4/T_3 products for the following reasons: (1) the rate of metabolism and thus the frequency of administration differ between levothyroxine and liothyronine; (2) levothyroxine therapy provides adequate serum concentrations of both T_4 and T_3; and (3) the use of synthetic combinations may result in serum concentrations of T_3 that could produce thyrotoxicosis. In addition, synthetic combination products tend to be more expensive than either synthetic levothyroxine or liothyronine alone.

Crude Animal-Origin Hormonal Preparations

Animal-origin preparations include desiccated thyroid and thyroglobulin. Desiccated thyroid is derived from cleaned, dried, and powdered thyroid glands of slaughterhouse origin (porcine and bovine), devoid of connective tissue and fat. Thyroglobulin is obtained from purified extracts of frozen hog thyroid.

The biologic activity of these preparations is variable and may result in a poor initial response to therapy or relapse of clinical signs despite owner compliance. There are several reasons for these problems. The United States Pharmacopeia states that the total iodine content of animal-origin products must be between 0.17% and 0.23% and that they may contain no other inorganic or otherwise extraneous iodine products. However, no requirement exists for bioassay or chemical analysis for T_4 or T_3 content (Rosychuk, 1982). Unfortunately, hormone potency and iodine content vary independently and are influenced by a number of factors, including species of origin, method of processing, and the impact of seasonal, geographic, and feeding characteristics on iodothyronine content of animal thyroid. Hog thyroid, for instance, contains greater quantities of T_3 than does that of beef or sheep origin. Increased quantities of hormonally inactive monoiodotyrosine and diiodotyrosine and iodinated casein in desiccated thyroid may also impair biologic activity. Finally, crude products that have been stored for long periods may become inert, suggesting a variable shelf life.

Crude animal-origin thyroid preparations are not recommended for the treatment of hypothyroidism in dogs. Nevertheless, these preparations have been used successfully. The recommended dosage is 15 to 20 mg of desiccated thyroid per kilogram of body weight once daily (Rosychuk, 1982). Ideally, the tablets should be crushed and administered with a small amount of food.

PROGNOSIS

The prognosis for dogs with hypothyroidism depends on the underlying cause. The life expectancy of an adult dog with primary hypothyroidism that is receiving appropriate therapy should be normal. Most, if not all, of the clinical manifestations will resolve in response to thyroid hormone supplementation. The prognosis for puppies with hypothyroidism (i.e., cretinism) is guarded and depends on the severity of skeletal and joint abnormalities at the time treatment is initiated. Although many of the clinical signs resolve with therapy, musculoskeletal problems, especially degenerative osteoarthritis, may develop as a result of abnormal bone and joint development (Saunders and Jezyk, 1991; Greco et al, 1991). Degenerative osteoarthritis is more prevalent in joints with adjacent epiphyseal dysgenesis (see page 108). Epiphyseal dysgenesis may result in increased susceptibility to trauma, articular cartilage damage, osteochondrosis-type lesions, and degenerative joint changes. Contributing to these changes are the biomechanical abnormalities caused by radial bowing with subsequent humeroradial joint widening and humeroulnar joint subluxation, which is seen in some dogs with congenital hypothyroidism.

The prognosis for dogs with secondary hypothyroidism caused by malformation or destruction of the pituitary gland is guarded to poor. The life expectancy is shortened in dogs with congenital malformation of the pituitary gland (i.e., pituitary dwarfism), primarily because of the multiple problems that develop in early life (see Chapter 2, page 48). Acquired secondary hypothyroidism is usually caused by destruction of the region by a space-occupying mass, which has the potential to expand into the brainstem.

FELINE HYPOTHYROIDISM

Naturally acquired primary hypothyroidism is a rare clinical entity in the cat, and secondary and tertiary forms of hypothyroidism have not been documented. Most clinical descriptions of feline hypothyroidism in the veterinary literature have been confined to anecdotal reports, with several early descriptions based on clinical impressions rather than measurement of blood thyroid hormone concentrations. To date, only a few case reports have adequately documented adult-onset (Rand et al, 1993) and congenital (Arnold et al, 1984; Sjollema et al, 1991; Jones et al, 1992) hypothyroidism in the cat. In contrast, iatrogenic hypothyroidism following any of the three common treatments for hyperthyroidism is well recognized.

Low serum T_4 concentrations are being recognized more and more frequently by veterinarians because of inclusion of serum T_4 concentration in the typical "feline blood panel" offered by many commercial laboratories. Unfortunately, the blood sample is usually submitted for evaluation of another problem (e.g., systemic illness) and the low T_4 concentration is an unexpected and sometimes confusing finding. For the vast majority of these cats, the low serum T_4 concentration is a result of the suppressive effects of nonthyroidal illness on serum T_4 concentration (i.e., euthyroid sick syndrome; see page 128) and not hypothyroidism.

ETIOLOGY

IATROGENIC HYPOTHYROIDISM. Iatrogenically induced hypothyroidism is usually a result of treating hyperthyroidism and is far more common than naturally acquired hypothyroidism in cats. Iatrogenically induced hypothyroidism can result from bilateral thyroidectomy, radioactive iodine treatment, or an overdose of antithyroid drugs. Depending on the treatment for hyperthyroidism, plasma thyroid hormone concentrations can decline to subnormal concentrations within hours (surgery), days (antithyroid drugs), or weeks to months (radioactive iodine). The only signs of hypothyroidism that develop in many of these cats are a decrease in activity (lethargy) and a tendency to gain weight. These changes often look good to the owner of a previously hyperthyroid cat. Thyroid hormone supplementation is usually not requested unless lethargy becomes severe, anorexia develops, or dermatologic signs occur.

ADULT-ONSET HYPOTHYROIDISM. Naturally acquired adult-onset primary hypothyroidism has not been well documented in the cat. One cat with lymphocytic thyroiditis and clinical hypothyroidism has been reported (Rand et al, 1993). Histopathologic studies of the feline thyroid gland have revealed several distinct alterations consistent with development of naturally acquired hypothyroidism, including atrophy, lymphocytic thyroiditis, amyloidosis, ultimobranchial cysts, cystic follicles, and goiter (see Feldman and Nelson, 1987, for further references); these findings suggest that hypothyroidism should be more commonly recognized clinically in the cat. Unfortunately, a correlation between histologic findings and clinical disease was not made in these pathologic studies.

CONGENITAL HYPOTHYROIDISM. Congenital primary hypothyroidism causing disproportionate dwarfism (see page 104) is recognized more frequently than adult-onset hypothyroidism in the cat. Reported causes of congenital hypothyroidism include a defect in thyroid hormone biosynthesis, most notably an iodine organification defect (Sjollema et al, 1991; Jones et al, 1992) and thyroid dysgenesis (Peterson, 1989). Goiter is common with defects in thyroid hormone biosynthesis. An inherited defect in iodine organification was documented in a family of Abyssinian cats with congenital hypothyroidism (Jones et al, 1992). Inbreeding of affected cats resulted in hypothyroidism in all offspring, whereas breeding affected cats to unrelated cats resulted in phenotypically normal kittens. These results suggest an autosomal recessive mode of inheritance for the disease in this family of cats. Although rare, iodine deficiency has been reported to cause hypothyroidism in kittens fed a strict all-meat diet.

CLINICAL SIGNS

ADULT-ONSET HYPOTHYROIDISM. The clinical signs that have been associated with feline hypothyroidism are listed in Table 3-22. Of these, the most commonly seen are lethargy, inappetance, and obesity. Lethargy and inappetance may become severe. Dermatologic signs are quite variable and often develop secondary to a decrease in grooming behavior by the cat. Affected cats often develop a dull, dry, unkempt hair coat with matting and seborrhea. Easily epilated and poor regrowth of hair may lead to alopecia affecting the pinnae, points of pressure, and the dorsal and lateral tail base region (Peterson, 1989; Rand et al, 1993; Scott et al, 2001). Asymmetric or bilaterally symmetric alopecia involving the lateral neck, thorax, and abdomen may also develop. Myxedema of the face, causing a "puffy" appearance, was also reported in one cat with naturally acquired adult-onset hypothyroidism (Rand et al, 1993). Bradycardia and mild hypothermia may be additional findings on physical examination.

CONGENITAL HYPOTHYROIDISM. The clinical signs of congenital hypothyroidism are similar to those in dogs (see page 104). Affected kittens typically appear normal at birth, but a decrease in growth rate usually

TABLE 3–22 CLINICAL MANIFESTATIONS OF FELINE HYPOTHYROIDISM

Adult-Onset Hypothyroidism	Congenital Hypothyroidism
Lethargy	Disproportionate dwarfism
Inappetence	Failure to grow
Obesity	Large head
Dermatologic	Short, broad neck
Seborrhea sicca	Short limbs
Dry, lusterless hair coat	Lethargy
Easily epilated hair	Mental dullness
Poor regrowth of hair	Constipation
Endocrine alopecia	Hypothermia
Alopecia of pinnae	Bradycardia
Thickened skin	Retention of kitten hair coat
Myxedema of the face	Retention of deciduous teeth
Reproduction	
Failure to cycle	
Dystocia	
Bradycardia	
Mild hypothermia	

becomes evident by 6 to 8 weeks of age. Disproportionate dwarfism develops over the ensuing months, with affected kittens developing large heads, short broad necks, and short limbs. Additional findings include lethargy, mental dullness, constipation, hypothermia, bradycardia, and prolonged retention of deciduous teeth (Arnold et al, 1984; Peterson, 1989; Sjollema et al, 1991; Jones et al, 1992). The hair coat may consist mainly of undercoat with primary guard hair scattered thinly throughout. Radiographic abnormalities are similar to those described for the dog (see page 108).

TESTS OF THYROID GLAND FUNCTION

Unlike the dog, the demand for accurate tests to assess thyroid gland function in the cat has been driven by the need to distinguish normal from hyperthyroid cats, not from those that might be hypothyroid. Measurement of baseline serum T_4 and fT_4 concentrations has been effective in diagnosing feline hyperthyroidism. Thus many of the tests used to assess thyroid gland function in the dog have not been critically evaluated or developed in the cat. In most situations, assessment of thyroid gland function relies on measurement of baseline serum T_4 and fT_4 concentrations.

BASELINE SERUM T_4 CONCENTRATION. Measurement of baseline serum T_4 concentration is perhaps the best screening test for hypothyroidism in a cat with appropriate clinical signs, especially if the cat has been previously treated for hyperthyroidism. The radioimmunoassays used to measure thyroxine in the dog are also useful in cats (see page 112; Reimers et al, 1981). An approximate normal range for the cat is 1 to 4 µg/dl, although this range varies among laboratories. Unlike puppies, kittens have adult cat values for serum T_4 concentration (Zerbe et al, 1998).

Cats with hypothyroidism should have baseline serum T_4 concentrations below the lower limit of normal for the laboratory used, ideally less than 0.5 µg/dl. Unfortunately, a low serum T_4 concentration does not, by itself, confirm hypothyroidism. Nonthyroidal factors, most notably concurrent illness and administration of drugs (e.g., glucocorticoids), can falsely lower serum T_4 concentration into the hypothyroid range (Fig. 3-35). Interpretation of baseline serum T_4 concentration is similar for the dog and cat (see page 113). The interpretation of the serum T_4 concentration must be done in conjunction with history and physical examination findings. All of this information gives the clinician an index of suspicion for euthyroidism or hypothyroidism. It is difficult for the clinician to judge what effect extraneous factors, especially concurrent illness, have on the serum T_4 concentration. Because these variables can suppress baseline serum T_4 concentration to less than 1 µg/dl and sometimes to less than 0.5 µg/dl in a euthyroid cat, we use baseline serum T_4 concentration as a measure of euthyroidism. If the T_4 concentration is within the reference range, it is likely that the cat is euthyroid. Conversely, the lower the T_4 value, the more likely it is that the cat has hypothyroidism, assuming that the history and physical findings are also consistent with the disease. If the clinician's index of suspicion is not high for hypothyroidism but the serum T_4 concentration is low, then other factors such as the euthyroid sick syndrome must also be considered.

BASELINE SERUM T_3 CONCENTRATION. Measurement of baseline serum T_3 concentration is not routinely done in the cat, in part because serum T_4 is effective in identifying hyperthyroidism in the cat and because serum T_3 is unreliable in identifying hypothyroidism in the dog (see page 115). Presumably, problems encountered with serum T_3 measurements in differentiating euthyroidism from hypothyroidism in the dog also exist in the cat. Nevertheless, serum T_3 concentration can be measured in the cat using the same radioimmunoassays used in the dog (see page 115; Reimers et al, 1981). An approximate normal range for the cat is 0.7 to 1.1 ng/ml, although this range varies among laboratories. Serum T_3 concentrations are lower in kittens than adult cats until 5 weeks of age (Zerbe et al, 1998).

Ideally, baseline serum T_3 concentration should be less than the lower limit of normal for the laboratory used in the cat with hypothyroidism. However, a normal serum T_3 concentration in a cat with appropriate history, physical examination findings, and low serum T_4 concentration does not rule out hypothyroidism. Similarly, a low serum T_3 concentration in a cat with normal serum T_4 concentration does not rule in hypothyroidism, especially if the remainder of the clinical picture does not support the diagnosis.

BASELINE SERUM FREE T_4 CONCENTRATION. Serum fT_4 concentrations have been reported in healthy cats using RIA (Sparkes et al, 1991), equilibrium dialysis (Mooney et al, 1996a), and MED (Peterson et al, 2001) techniques. Although a critical comparison between RIA and MED techniques for measurement of fT_4 has not been reported in cats, the MED technique (Nichols

Institute, San Juan Capistrano, CA) is currently the preferred fT_4 test for assessing thyroid gland function in dogs (see page 116) and presumably the same is true for cats. An approximate normal range for serum fT_4 concentration measured by MED in the cat is 1 to 4 ng/dl, although this range may vary among laboratories. Kittens have adult cat values for serum fT_4 concentration (Zerbe et al, 1998).

Cats with hypothyroidism should have baseline serum fT_4 concentrations below the lower limit of normal for the laboratory used, ideally less than 0.5 ng/dl. As with serum T_4, a low serum fT_4 concentration does not, by itself, confirm hypothyroidism. Nonthyroidal factors, most notably concurrent illness and administration of drugs (e.g., glucocorticoids), can falsely lower the serum fT_4 concentration into the hypothyroid range (Fig. 3-35). However, serum fT_4 is not as likely to be influenced by factors such as nonthyroidal illness and administration of drugs as serum T_4, and serum fT_4 concentrations may increase rather than decrease in some euthyroid cats with nonthyroidal illness (Mooney et al, 1996a; Peterson et al, 2001). Presumably, the sensitivity and specificity is better for serum fT_4 versus serum T_4 for assessing thyroid gland function in cats with suspected hypothyroidism, a finding that has been well documented in dogs.

BASELINE SERUM TSH CONCENTRATION. Currently, there is no feline-specific TSH assay. A few preliminary reports have evaluated the commercial canine TSH immunoradiometric assay (see page 118) for assessing thyroid gland function in the cat. In one preliminary study, a reference range of 0 to 0.32 ng/ml canine equivalent immunoreactivity was established in 50 healthy cats (Graham et al, 2000). Serum TSH concentration was decreased in 47 cats with hyperthyroidism and was undetectable in the majority of these cats (Graham et al, 2000; Otero et al, 2002). Serum TSH concentration was increased in hyperthyroid cats that had undergone thyroidectomy or been treated with radioactive iodine. There was an inverse correlation between serum T_4 concentration and prevalence of increased serum TSH concentration in hyperthyroid cats treated with methimazole. Although cats with naturally acquired hypothyroidism or euthyroid cats with nonthyroidal illness were not evaluated, the results of these preliminary studies suggest that the measurement of feline TSH using the commercial canine TSH immunoradiometric assay may be of value in assessing thyroid gland function in cats with suspected hypothyroidism.

TESTS FOR LYMPHOCYTIC THYROIDITIS. Tests for the presence of circulating thyroglobulin (Tg) and thyroid hormone (T_3 and T_4) autoantibodies (see page 124)

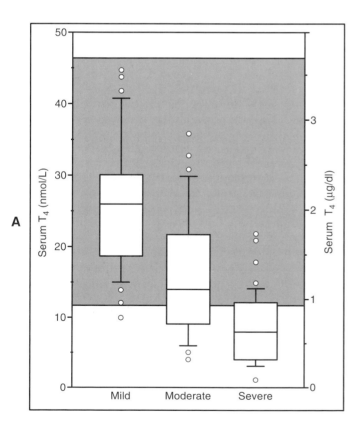
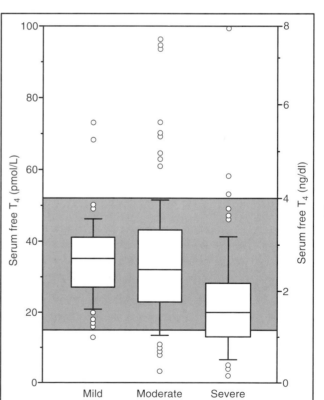

FIGURE 3–35. Box plots of serum total T_4 *(A)* and free T_4 *(B)* concentrations in 221 cats with nonthyroidal disease stratified according to severity of disease. Of the 221 cats, 65 had mild disease, 83 had moderate disease, and 73 had severe disease. For each box plot, T-bars represent the main body of data, which in most instances is equal to the range. Each box represents the interquartile range (25th to 75th percentile). The horizontal bar in each box is the median. Open circles represent outlying data points. The shaded area indicates the reference range. (From Peterson ME, et al: JAVMA 218:529, 2001.)

have not been reported, nor are they currently available in the cat.

FACTORS AFFECTING BASELINE THYROID HORMONE CONCENTRATIONS. Many of the nonthyroidal factors known to affect serum thyroid hormone concentrations in dogs have yet to be evaluated in cats (see page 126). The effects of age, gender, and breed on serum T_4 and T_3 concentrations in cats are controversial. In one study, serum T_4 and, to a lesser extent, serum T_3 concentrations in both genders tended to decrease until approximately 5 years of age and then increase again; females (intact and neutered) had significantly higher serum T_4 but not T_3 concentrations than males (intact or neutered); and serum T_3 but not T_4 concentration was significantly higher in pedigree cats than in Domestic Short- and Long-Haired cats (Thoday et al, 1984). Serum thyroid hormone concentrations remained within the normal range in these cats regardless of any influence of age, gender, or breed on blood thyroid hormone levels. In another study, Zerbe et al (1998) identified adult cat values for serum T_4 and fT_4 concentrations in kittens from birth to 12 weeks of age, whereas serum T_3 concentrations were low until kittens were 5 weeks of age. Still other investigators have not identified an effect of age, gender, and/or breed on serum thyroid hormone concentrations (see Feldman and Nelson, 1987 for references). A diurnal variation in blood thyroid hormone concentrations apparently does not occur in the cat (Hoenig and Ferguson, 1983), so the time of day that the blood is sampled should not affect the results.

The most worrisome nonthyroidal factors are those that have the potential to falsely lower serum T_4 concentration into the hypothyroid range, that is, the euthyroid sick syndrome and administration of drugs. The euthyroid sick syndrome refers to suppression of serum thyroid hormone concentrations in euthyroid animals in response to concurrent illness and is discussed on page 128. Nonthyroidal illness causing the euthyroid sick syndrome has been documented in the cat (Peterson and Gamble, 1990; Mooney et al, 1996a; Peterson et al, 2001). As with the dog, serum T_4 and T_3 concentrations are more likely to be decreased with nonthyroidal illness than serum fT_4 concentrations, and there is a direct correlation between the severity of illness and the magnitude of the decrease in serum thyroid hormone concentrations (Fig. 3-35). The more severe the nonthyroidal illness, the more likely serum thyroid hormone concentrations will decrease into the hypothyroid range. Serum T_4 values less than 0.5 µg/dl and fT_4 values less than 0.5 ng/dl may occur with severe systemic illness in a euthyroid cat. It is interesting to note that some euthyroid cats with nonthyroidal disease will have decreased serum T_4 concentrations but increased serum fT_4 concentrations when an equilibrium dialysis technique is used to measure fT_4. Increased serum fT_4 concentrations were found in 12% of 98 euthyroid cats with nonthyroidal illness in one study (Mooney et al, 1996a) and 6.3% of 221 euthyroid cats with nonthyroidal illness in another study (Peterson et al, 2001). Nonthyroidal illnesses in

these cats included diabetes mellitus, gastrointestinal tract disease, hepatic disease, renal insufficiency, and neoplasia. The reason for increased serum fT_4 concentrations in some cats with nonthyroidal illness is not known but may be related to decreased protein binding of circulating T_4 and/or impaired clearance of T_4 from the circulation.

The effects of drugs on serum thyroid hormone concentrations have not been extensively evaluated in the cat. Two classes of drugs that can decrease serum thyroid hormone concentrations into the hypothyroid range are glucocorticoids (see page 132) and antithyroid hormone drugs (i.e., methimazole, propylthiouracil; see page 195). Undoubtedly, many more as yet unrecognized drugs also affect serum thyroid hormone concentrations in cats. Until proven otherwise, any drug should be suspected of affecting thyroid hormone test results, especially if the drug has been shown to alter serum thyroid hormone concentrations in humans and dogs (see Table 3-17) and the history and clinical signs do not support a diagnosis of hypothyroidism in the cat.

TSH STIMULATION TEST. The indications, protocol, and interpretation of the TSH stimulation test are similar for the cat and dog and are discussed on page 120. Unfortunately, TSH for injection has not been available at a reasonable cost for use in dogs and cats for several years and there is no indication that it will become available in the forseeable future. A brief synopsis of the TSH stimulation test is presented below. See the second edition of *Canine and Feline Endocrinology and Reproduction* for detailed information on this test.

Several protocols have been recommended for performing the TSH stimulation test in the cat (Table 3-23). Our protocol is similar to that for the dog—that is, 0.1 IU of TSH/kg of body weight (typically 0.5 IU/cat) administered intravenously and blood sample for serum T_4 determination obtained before and 6 hours after TSH administration. Serum T_3 concentration is not routinely measured. In a euthyroid cat, the serum T_4 concentration should increase 2 to 3 µg/dl after TSH administration, and ideally, the post-TSH serum T_4 concentration should exceed 3 µg/dl. In contrast, there should be minimal increase (i.e., <1 µg/dl) in serum T_4 concentration after TSH administration in cats with hypothyroidism, and ideally, the post-TSH serum T_4 concentration should remain below the normal baseline serum T_4 range (i.e., <1 µg/dl). Post-TSH serum T_4 concentrations between 1 and 3 µg/dl are nondiagnostic and may be found in the early stages of hypothyroidism or may represent suppression of thyroid gland function as a result of concurrent illness or drug therapy in an otherwise euthyroid cat.

TRH STIMULATION TEST. The indications and interpretation of the TRH stimulation test are similar for the cat and dog and are discussed in detail on page 120. The TRH stimulation test can be used in place of the TSH stimulation test for evaluation of thyroid gland function. In our experience, adverse reactions following TRH administration are common in cats and the TRH stimulation test can be difficult to interpret

TABLE 3–23 SOME PUBLISHED RECOMMENDATIONS FOR PERFORMING THE TSH AND TRH STIMULATION TEST IN CATS

	Route of Administration	Blood Sampling Times (Hours)	Normal Results	Reference
TSH Dose				
5 IU/cat	IM, SC	Pre and 10-12 hr post	Doubling of T_4	Scott, 1980
1 IU/kg	IV	Pre and 6 hr post	Post T_4 > 4 µg/dl; post T_4 increase of 2.5 µg/dl over basal T_4	Hoenig and Ferguson, 1983
2.5 IU/cat	IM	Pre and 8-12 hr post	Doubling of T_4	Kemppainen et al, 1984
1 IU/cat	IV	Pre and 4 hr post	Doubling of T_4	Peterson et al, 1983
1 IU/cat	IV	Pre and 7 hr post	Doubling of T_4	Sparkes et al, 1991
5 IU/cat	IV	Pre and 4 hr post	Doubling of T_4	Di Bartola and Tarr, 1989
0.5 IU/kg	IV	Pre and 6 hr post	Doubling of T_4	Mooney et al, 1996b
TRH dose				
0.1 mg/cat	IV	0, 4	>40% increase in T_4	Sparkes et al, 1991
0.1 mg/kg	IV	0, 6	Doubling of T_4	Lothrop et al, 1984
0.1 mg/kg	IV	0, 4	>50% increase in T_4	Peterson et al, 1994

because of the relatively minimal increase in serum T_4 concentration after TRH administration and the potential suppressive effects of nonthyroidal illness on pituitary TSH response to TRH. In addition, TRH for injection is becoming increasingly difficult to obtain and may soon be unavailable.

The recommended protocol for the TRH stimulation test in the cat is 0.1 mg of TRH/kg of body weight intravenously and blood obtained before and 4 to 6 hours after TRH administration for evaluation of T_4 concentration (Table 3-23; Lothrop et al, 1984; Sparkes et al, 1991). Adverse effects may develop in cats given more than 0.1 mg TRH/kg body weight; these include panting, salivation, vomiting, defecation, urination, miosis, and tachycardia (Lothrop et al, 1984; Tomsa et al, 2001). In the cat with a functionally intact pituitary-thyroid axis, the serum T_4 concentration should increase 1 to 2 µg/dl or greater than 50% above baseline serum T_4 concentration after administration of TRH. Failure of serum T_4 concentration to increase after TRH administration suggests dysfunction of either the pituitary or the thyroid gland or suppression of the pituitary-thyroid axis by nonthyroidal factors (e.g., concurrent illness; Tomsa et al, 2001). If results of a previous TSH stimulation test were normal, an abnormal TRH stimulation test implies pituitary dysfunction.

ESTABLISHING THE DIAGNOSIS

The diagnosis of hypothyroidism in the cat should be based on a combination of history, clinical signs, physical examination findings, and baseline serum thyroid hormone concentrations. The incidence of hypercholesterolemia and normocytic, normochromic nonregenerative anemia is not known in adult cats with naturally acquired hypothyroidism, but it is occasionally identified in cats with iatrogenic hypothyroidism (i.e., postthyroidectomy, postradioactive iodine treatment) or cats with congenital hypo-

thyroidism. Therefore our initial screening blood tests for hypothyroidism in the cat are similar to those in the dog—CBC, serum cholesterol, and baseline serum T_4 concentration. A normal serum T_4 concentration supports euthyroidism. A low serum T_4 concentration in a cat that has undergone thyroidectomy or radioactive iodine treatment or a kitten with disproportionate dwarfism supports the diagnosis of hypothyroidism. The definitive diagnosis must then rely on response to trial therapy with levothyroxine sodium. For cats with iatrogenic hypothyroidism, treatment with levothyroxine sodium is indicated if appropriate clinical signs are also present. Asymptomatic cats with low serum T_4 concentration may not require therapy.

Because naturally acquired primary hypothyroidism is rare and, in our experience, a low serum T_4 concentration in an adult cat is almost always caused by the euthyroid sick syndrome (see page 128) or some other nonthyroidal factor, we are reluctant to diagnose hypothyroidism based solely on serum T_4 concentration in an adult cat that has not been previously treated for hyperthyroidism. A serum fT_4 concentration should be measured by equilibrium dialysis if the serum T_4 concentration is low. A serum fT_4 concentration that is less than 0.5 ng/dl in a cat with appropriate clinical signs and no concurrent severe nonthyroidal illness adds further support for the diagnosis of hypothyroidism. We also measure feline TSH using the commercial canine TSH immunoradiometric assay. Finding an increased serum TSH concentration in conjunction with a decreased serum T_4 and fT_4 concentration is further evidence for hypothyroidism. Although evaluation of a TSH or TRH stimulation test should be completed to prove the diagnosis, we prefer to evaluate response to trial therapy if all of the tests of thyroid gland function support hypothyroidism, especially if significant nonthyroidal disease is not present. It is important to remember that response to trial therapy with levothyroxine sodium is nonspecific and does not, by itself, prove the diagnosis. If a positive response is observed, thyroid supplementation should be gradually discontinued once clinical signs have resolved. Hypothyroidism is likely if clinical signs recur after thyroid hormone treatment is discontinued and resolve after treatment is reinitiated.

TREATMENT AND PROGNOSIS

Treatment of hypothyroidism is similar for the cat and dog and is described in detail on page 136. Levothyroxine sodium is the recommended thyroid hormone supplement. The initial dosage for cats is 0.05 or 0.1 mg once daily. A minimum of 4 to 6 weeks should elapse before critically assessing the cat's clinical response to treatment. Subsequent reevaluations should include history, physical examination, and measurement of serum thyroid hormone concentrations (see Therapeutic Monitoring, page 139). The goal of therapy is to resolve the clinical signs of hypothyroidism while avoiding signs of hyperthyroidism. This can usually be accomplished by maintaining serum T_4 concentration between 1.0 and 3.0 µg/dl. The dosage and frequency of levothyroxine sodium administration may need modification to achieve these goals. If serum thyroid hormone concentrations are normal after 4 to 6 weeks of treatment but there is no clinical response, the clinician should reassess the diagnosis.

The prognosis for feline hypothyroidism depends on the underlying cause and the age of the cat at the time clinical signs develop. With appropriate therapy, the life expectancy of an adult cat with primary hypothyroidism should be normal. Most, if not all, of the clinical manifestations resolve following thyroid hormone supplementation. The prognosis for kittens with congenital hypothyroidism is guarded and depends on the severity of skeletal changes at the time treatment is initiated. Although many of the clinical signs resolve with therapy, musculoskeletal problems may persist or develop as a result of abnormal bone and joint development.

REFERENCES

Canine Hypothyroidism

Allbritton AR: Autoimmune disease and vaccination? Vet Allergy Clin Immunol 4:16, 1996.

Arokoski J, et al: Effects of aerobic long distance running training (up to 40 km/day) of 1-year duration on blood and endocrine parameters of female Beagle dogs. Eur J Appl Physiol Occup Physiol 67:321, 1993.

Avgeris S, et al: Plasma von Willebrand factor concentration and thyroid function in dogs. JAVMA 196:921, 1990.

Barrie J, et al: Plasma cholesterol and lipoprotein concentrations in the dog: the effects of age, breed, gender and endocrine disease. J Small Anim Pract 34:507, 1993.

Beale KM, et al: Prevalence of antithyroglobulin antibodies detected by enzyme-linked immunosorbent assay of canine serum. JAVMA 196:745, 1990.

Beale K, et al: Serum thyroid hormone concentrations and thyrotropin responsiveness in dogs with generalized dermatologic disease. JAVMA 201:1715, 1992.

Beale K, et al: Correlation of racing and reproductive performance in Greyhounds with response to thyroid function testing. JAAHA 28:263, 1992.

Beale KM, Torres S: Thyroid pathology and serum antithyroglobulin antibodies in hypothyroid and healthy dogs. J Vet Intern Med 5:128, 1991.

Becker RA, et al: Hypermetabolic low triiodothyronine syndrome of burn injury. Crit Care Med 10:870, 1982.

Behrend EN, et al: Effect of storage conditions on cortisol, total thyroxine, and free thyroxine concentrations in serum and plasma of dogs. JAVMA 212:1564, 1998.

Belshaw BE: Thyroid diseases. In Ettinger SJ (ed): Textbook of Veterinary Internal Medicine, 2nd ed. Philadelphia, WB Saunders, 1983, p 1592.

Bichsel P, et al: Neurologic manifestations associated with hypothyroidism in four dogs. JAVMA 192:1745, 1988.

Bilezikian JP, Loeb JN: Increased myocardial beta-receptor and adrenergic responsiveness. Endocr Rev 4:3378, 1983.

Bishnoi A, et al: Effects of commonly prescribed nonsteroidal anti-inflammatory drugs on thyroid hormone measurements. Am J Med 96:235, 1994.

Borst GC, et al: Fasting decreases thyrotropin responsiveness to thyrotropin-releasing hormone: A potential cause of misinterpretation of thyroid function tests in the critically ill. J Clin Endocrinol Metab 57:380, 1983.

Bowen D, et al: Autoimmune polyglandular syndrome in a dog: A case report. JAAHA 22:649, 1986.

Branam JE, et al: Radioisotope imaging for the evaluation of thyroid neoplasia and hypothyroidism in a dog. JAVMA 180:1077, 1982.

Braund KG, et al: Hypothyroid myopathy in two dogs. Vet Pathol 18:589, 1981.

Brent GA, Hershman JM: Thyroxine therapy in patients with severe nonthyroidal illnesses and low serum thyroxine concentration. J Clin Endocrinol Metab 63:1, 1986.

Brömel C, et al: Ultrasonographic evaluation of the thyroid gland in Golden Retrievers (abstract). JVIM 15:297, 2001.

Brömel C, et al: Ultrasonographic evaluation of the thyroid gland in canine breeds predisposed for hypothyroidism (abstract). JVIM, 16:632, 2002.

Bruner JM, et al: Effect of time of sample collection on serum thyroid-stimulating hormone concentrations in euthyroid and hypothyroid dogs. JAVMA 212:1572, 1998.

Budsberg SC, et al: Thyroxine-responsive unilateral forelimb lameness and generalized neuromuscular disease in four hypothyroid dogs. JAVMA 202:1859, 1993.

Calvert CA, et al: Congestive cardiomyopathy in Doberman Pinscher dogs. JAVMA 181:598, 1982.

Calvert CA, et al: Thyroid-stimulating hormone stimulation tests in cardio-myopathic Doberman Pinschers: A retrospective study. JVIM 12:343, 1998.

Campbell KL, Davis CA: Effects of thyroid hormones on serum and cutaneous fatty acid concentrations in dogs. AJVR 51:752, 1990.

Campbell KL, et al: Effects of trimethoprim/sulfamethoxazole on thyroid physiology in dogs. Proceedings, 11th Annual AAVD/ACVD Meeting, 1995, p 55.

Case S, et al: Effects of the Iditarod Sled Dog Race on serum thyroid hormones and body composition. Arctic Med Res 52:113, 1993.

Castillo VA, et al: Changes in thyroid function in puppies fed a high iodine commercial diet. Vet Journal 161:80, 2001.

Chastain CB: Canine hypothyroidism. JAVMA 181:349, 1982.

Chastain CB, et al: Myxedema coma in two dogs. Canine Pract 9:20, 1982.

Chastain CB, et al: Congenital hypothyroidism in a dog due to an iodide organification defect. Am J Vet Res 44:1257, 1983.

Chastain CB, et al: Anti-triiodothyronine antibodies associated with hypothyroidism and lymphocytic thyroiditis in a dog. JAVMA 194:531, 1989.

Chastain CB, Schmidt B: Galactorrhea associated with hypothyroidism in intact bitches. JAAHA 16:851, 1980.

Chen Y: Effect of thyroxine on the immune response of mice in vivo and in vitro. Immunol Commun 9:260, 1980.

Conaway DH, et al: The familial occurrence of lymphocytic thyroiditis in Borzoi dogs. Am J Med Genet 22:409,1985a.

Conaway DH, et al: Clinical and histological features of primary progressive, familial thyroiditis in a colony of Borzoi dogs. Vet Pathol 22:439, 1985b.

Cortese L, et al: Hyperprolactinaemia and galactorrhoea associated with primary hypothyroidism in a bitch. J Small Anim Pract 38:572, 1997.

Credille KM, et al: The effects of thyroid hormones on the skin of Beagle dogs. JVIM 15:539, 2001.

Crocker AD, Cameron DL: Evidence for post-synaptic changes mediating increased behavioural sensitivity to dopamine receptor agonists in hypothyroid rats. Prog Neuro-Psychopharmacol Biol Psyciat 12:607, 1988.

Dalton RG, et al: Hypothyroidism as a cause of acquired von Willebrand's disease. Lancet 1:1007, 1987.

de Bruijne J, et al: Fat mobilization and plasma hormone levels in fasted dogs. Metabolism 30:190, 1981.

Delauche AJ, et al: Nemaline rods in canine myopathies: 4 case reports and literature review. JVIM 12:424, 1998.

Dewey CW, et al: Neuromuscular dysfunction in five dogs with acquired myasthenia gravis and presumptive hypothyroidism. Prog Vet Neurol 6:117, 1995.

Dixon RM, et al: Serum thyrotropin concentrations: A new diagnostic test for canine hypothyroidism. Vet Rec 138:594, 1996.

Dodds WJ: Estimating disease prevalence with health surveys and genetic screening. Adv Vet Sci Comp Med 39:29, 1995.

Dodman NH, et al: Animal behavior case of the month. JAVMA 207:1168, 1995.

Doerge DR, Decker CJ: Inhibition of peroxidase-catalyzed reactions by arylamines: Mechanism for the anti-thyroid action of sulfamethazine. Chem Res Toxicol 7:164, 1994.

Dowell RT, et al: Beta-adrenergic receptors, adenylate cyclase activation, and myofibril enzyme activity in hypothyroid rats. Am J Physiol 266:H2527, 1994.

Drvota V, et al: Downregulation of the thyroid hormone receptor subtype mRNA levels by amidarone during catecholamine stress in vitro. Biochem Biophys Res Commun 211:991, 1995.

Duclos DD, et al: Prognosis for treatment of adult onset demodicosis in dogs: 34 cases. JAVMA 204:616, 1994.

Eigenmann JE: Diagnosis and treatment of dwarfism in a German Shepherd dog. JAAHA 17:798, 1981.

Eisenbarth GS, Jackson RA: The immunoendocrinopathy syndromes. In Wilson JD, Foster DW (eds): Williams Textbook of Endocrinology, 10th ed. Philadelphia, WB Saunders, 1992, p 1555.

Elliott DA, et al: Thyroid hormone concentrations in critically ill canine intensive care patients. J Vet Emerg Crit Care 5:17, 1995.

Evinger JV, et al: Thyrotropin-releasing hormone stimulation testing in healthy dogs. Am J Vet Res 46:1323, 1985.

Extein IR, Gold MS: Thyroid hormone potentiation of tricyclics. Psychosomatics 29:166, 1988.

Ferguson DC: Thyroid function tests in the dog: Recent concepts. Vet Clin North Am 14:783, 1984.

Ferguson DC, Peterson ME: Serum free thyroxine concentrations in spontaneous canine hyperadrenocorticism. Fourth Annual Veterinary Medical Forum, Washington DC, 1986, p 14.

Ferguson DC, Peterson ME: Serum free and total iodothyroinine concentrations in dogs with hyperadrenocorticism. Am J Vet Res 53:1636, 1992.

Ferguson DC, Hoenig M: Re-examination of dosage regimens for L-thyroxine (T_4) in the dog: bioavailability and persistence of TSH suppression (abstract). JVIM 11:120, 1997.

Ferguson DC, et al: Carprofen lowers total T_4 and TSH, but not free T_4 concentrations in dogs (abstract). JVIM 13:243, 1999.

Fish LH, et al: Replacement dose, metabolism, and bioavailability of levothyroxine in the treatment of hypothyroidism. Role of triiodothyronine in pituitary feedback in humans. N Engl J Med 316:764, 1987.

Ford SL, et al: Insulin resistance in three dogs with hypothyroidism and diabetes mellitus. JAVMA 202:1478, 1993.

Frank LA: Comparison of thyrotropin-releasing hormone (TRH) to thyrotropin (TSH) stimulation for evaluating thyroid function in dogs. JAAHA 32:481, 1996.

Froelich PA, Meserve LA: Altered growth patterns and depressed pituitary growth hormone content in young rats: Effects of pre- and post-natal thiouracil administration. Growth 16:296, 1982.

Gaschen F, et al: Recognition of triiodothyronine-containing epitopes in canine thyroglobulin by circulating thyroglobulin autoantibodies. Am J Vet Res 54:244, 1993.

Gaskill CL, et al: Effects of phenobarbital treatment on serum thyroxine and thyroid-stimulating hormone concentrations in epileptic dogs. JAVMA 215:489, 1999.

Gaughan KR, Bruyette DS: Thyroid function testing in Greyhounds. AJVR 62:1130, 2001.

Gaynor AR, et al: Risk factors for acquired megaesophagus in dogs. JAVMA 211:1406, 1997.

Gerritsen RJ, et al: Relationship between atrial fibrillation and primary hypothyroidism in the dog. Vet Quart 18:49, 1996.

Gieger TL, et al: Thyroid function and serum hepatic enzyme activity in dogs after phenobarbital administration. JVIM 14:277, 2000.

Gilani B, et al: Thyroid hormone abnormalities at diagnosis of insulin-dependent diabetes mellitus in children. J Pediatr 105:218, 1984.

Gookin JL, et al: Clinical hypothyroidism associated with trimethoprim-sulfadiazine administration in a dog. JAVMA 214:1028, 1999.

Gosselin SJ, et al: Biochemical and immunological investigation on hypothyroidism in dogs. Can J Comp Med 44:158, 1980.

Gosselin SJ, et al: Lymphocytic thyroiditis in dogs: Induction with a local graft-versus-host reaction. Am J Vet Res 42:1856, 1981a.

Gosselin SJ, et al: Histopathologic and ultrastructural evaluation of thyroid lesions associated with hypothyroidism in dogs. Vet Pathol 18:299, 1981b.

Gosselin SJ, et al: Induced lymphocytic thyroiditis in dogs: Effect of intrathyroidal injection of thyroid autoantibodies. Am J Vet Res 42:1565, 1981c.

Graham PA: Thyroid replacement therapy: The numbers game. Proceedings, 20th ACVIM Forum, Dallas, TX, 2002, p 678.

Graham PA, et al: Lymphocytic thyroiditis. Vet Clin North Am 31:915, 2001a.

Graham PA, et al: A 12-month prospective study of 234 thyroglobulin antibody positive dogs which had no laboratory evidence of thyroid dysfunction (abstract). J Vet Intern Med 15:298, 2001b.

Greco DS: Polyendocrine gland failure in dogs. Vet Med 95:477, 2000.

Greco DS, et al: Juvenile-onset hypothyroidism in a dog. JAVMA 187:948, 1985.

Greco DS, et al: Congenital hypothyroid dwarfism in a family of Giant Schnauzers. J Vet Intern Med 5:57, 1991.

Greco DS, et al: The effect of levothyroxine treatment on resting energy expenditure of hypothyroid dogs. J Vet Intern Med 12:7, 1998.

Green ST, Ng J-P: Hypothyroidism and anaemia. Biomed Pharmacother 40:326, 1988.

Greenspan FS: The thyroid gland. In Greenspan FS and Gardner (eds): Basic and Clinical Endocrinology, 6th ed. New York, Lange Medical Books/ McGraw Hill, 2001, p 201.

Gross TL, Ihrke PJ, Walder EJ: Veterinary Dermatopathology. A Macroscopic and Microscopic Evaluation of Canine and Feline Skin Disease. St Louis, Mosby-Year Book, 1992.

Gunaratnam P: The effects of thyroxine on hair growth in the dog. J Small Anim Pract 27:17, 1986.

Haber RS, Loeb JN: Selective induction of high-oubain-affinity isoforms of Na^+–K^+–ATPase by thyroid hormone. Am J Physiol 255:E912, 1988.

Haines DM, et al: Survey of thyroglobulin autoantibodies in dogs. Am J Vet Res 45:1493, 1984.

Haines DM, Penhale WJ: Antibodies to pancreatic islet cells in canine diabetes mellitus. Vet Immunol Immunopathol 8:149, 1985.

Hall IA, et al: Effect of trimethoprim/sulfamethoxazole on thyroid function in dogs with pyoderma. JAVMA 202:1959, 1993.

Hamann F, et al: Pituitary function and morphology in two German Shepherd dogs with congenital dwarfism. Vet Rec 144:644, 1999.

Hargis AM, et al: Relationship of hypothyroidism to diabetes mellitus, renal amyloidosis, and thrombosis in pure-bred Beagles. Am J Vet Res 42:1077, 1981.

Hawthorn MH, et al: Effect of thyroid status on beta-adrenoreceptors and calcium channels in rat cardiac and vascular tissue. Naunyn Schmiedebergs Arch Pharmacol 337:539, 1988.

Hayashizaki Y, et al: Deoxyribonucleic acid analysis of five families with familial inherited thyroid stimulating hormone deficiency. Clin Endocrinol Metab 71: 792, 1990.

Henik RA, Dixon RM: Intravenous administration of levothyroxine for treatment of suspected myxedema coma complicated by severe hypothermia in a dog. JAVMA 216:713, 2000.

Henley WN, et al: Hypothyroidism increases serotonin turnover and sympathetic activity in the adult rat. Can J Physiol Pharmacol 69:205, 1991.

Hess RS, et al: Association between hypothyroidism, diabetes mellitus, and hyperadrenocorticism and development of atherosclerosis in dogs (abstract). JVIM 16:360, 2002.

Hill RC, et al: Effects of racing and training on serum thyroid hormone concentrations in racing Greyhounds. AJVR 62:1969, 2001.

Horney BS, et al: Evaluation of an automated, homogeneous enzyme immunoassay for serum thyroxine measurement in dog and cat serum. Vet Clin Path 28:20, 1999.

Hymes K, et al: Easy bruising, thrombocytopenia, and elevated platelet immunoglobulin G in Graves' disease and Hashimoto's thyroiditis. Ann Intern Med 94:27, 1981.

Indrieri RJ, et al: Neuromuscular abnormalities associated with hypothyroidism and lymphocytic thyroiditis in three dogs. JAVMA 190:544, 1987.

Iversen L, et al: Development and validation of an improved enzyme-linked immunosorbent assay for the detection of thyroglobulin autoantibodies in canine serum samples. Dom Anim Endocr 15:525, 1998.

Iversen L, et al: Biological variation of canine serum thyrotropin (TSH) concentration. Vet Clin Path 28:16, 1999.

Jaggy A, et al: Neurological manifestations of hypothyroidism: A retrospective study of 29 dogs. J Vet Intern Med 8:328, 1994.

Joffe RT: A perspective on the thyroid and depression. Can J Psychiatry 35:754, 1990.

Johnson C, et al: Effect of ^{131}I-induced hypothyroidism on indices of reproductive function in adult male dogs. JVIM 13:104, 1999.

Johnson RJ: A pharmacokinetic comparison of two commercially available L-thyroxine products (abstract). JVIM 13:245, 1999.

Johnstone JB, et al: Thyroid supplementation effect on plasma von Willebrand factor/factor VIII in Doberman Pinschers [abstract]. J Vet Intern Med 7:130, 1993.

Kantrowitz LB, et al: Serum total thyroxine, total triiodothyronine, free thyroxine, and thyrotropin concentrations in epileptic dogs treated with anticonvulsants. JAVMA 214:1804, 1999.

Kantrowitz LB, et al: Serum total thyroxine, total triiodothyronine, free thyroxine, and thyrotropin concentrations in dogs with nonthyroidal illness. JAVMA 219:765, 2001.

Kaplan MM, et al: Prevalence of abnormal thyroid function test results in patients with acute medical illnesses. Am J Med 72:9, 1982.

Kaptein EM: Thyroid hormone metabolism in nonthyroidal illness. Proceed ACVIM, Washington DC, 1988, p 643.

Kaptein EM, et al: Peripheral serum thyroxine, triiodothyronine, and reverse triiodothyronine kinetics in the low thyroxine state of acute nonthyroidal illness. J Clin Invest 69:526, 1982.

Kaptein EM, et al: Relationship of altered thyroid hormone indices to survival in nonthyroidal illnesses. Clin Endocrinol 16:565, 1982.

Kaptein EM, et al: Effects of prednisone on thyroxine and 3,5,3'-triiodothyronine metabolism in normal dogs. Endocrinology 130:1669, 1992.

Kelly MJ, Hill JR: Canine myxedema stupor and coma. Comp Cont Ed Pract Vet 6:1049, 1984.

Kemppainen RJ, et al: Effects of prednisone on thyroid and gonadal endocrine function in dogs. J Endocrinol 96:293, 1983.

Kemppainen RJ, Sartin JL: Evidence for episodic but not circadian activity in plasma concentrations of adrenocorticotrophin, cortisol, and thyroxine in dogs. J Endocrinol 103:219, 1984.

Kemppainen RJ, Young DW: Canine triiodothyronine autoantibodies. *In* Kirk RW, Bonagura JD (eds): Current Veterinary Therapy XI. Philadelphia, WB Saunders, 1992, p 327.

Kemppainen RJ, et al: Autoantibodies to triiodothyronine and thyroxine in a Golden Retriever. JAAHA 32:195, 1996.

Kern TJ, et al: Horner's syndrome in dogs and cats: 100 cases (1975–1985). JAVMA 195:369, 1989.

Kern TJ, Riis RC: Ocular manifestations of secondary hyperlipidemia associated with hypothyroidism and uveitis in a dog. JAAHA 16:907, 1980.

Kintzer PP, Peterson ME: Thyroid scintigraphy in small animals. Semin Vet Med Surg Small Anim 6:131, 1991.

Klein I: Thyroid hormone and the cardiovascular system. Am J Med 88:631, 1990.

Kooistra HS, et al: Polyglandular deficiency syndrome in a Boxer dog: Thyroid hormone and glucocorticoid deficiency. Vet Quart 17:59, 1995.

Kooistra HS, et al: Combined pituitary hormone deficiency in German Shepherd dogs with dwarfism. Domest Anim Endocrinol 19:177, 2000a.

Kooistra HS, et al: Secretion pattern of thyroid-stimulating hormone in dogs during euthyroidism and hypothyroidism. Dom Anim Endocr 18:19, 2000b.

Lantz GC, et al: Transsphenoidal hypophysectomy in the clinically normal dog. Am J Vet Res 49:1134, 1988.

Larsen PR, et al: Relationships between circulating and intracellular thyroid hormones: Physiological and clinical implications. Endocrinol Rev 2:87, 1981.

Larsen PR, et al: The thyroid gland. *In* Wilson JD, Foster DW, Kronenberg HM, Larsen PR (eds): Williams Textbook of Endocrinology, 9th ed. Philadelphia, WB Saunders, 1998, p 389.

Larsson MG: Determination of free thyroxine and cholesterol as a new screening test for canine hypothyroidism. JAAHA 24:209, 1988.

Lee DE, et al: Effects of hyperlipemia on radioimmunoassays for progesterone, testosterone, thyroxine, and cortisol in serum and plasma samples from dogs. Am J Vet Res 52:1489, 1991.

Li WI, et al: Effects of thyrotropin-releasing hormone on serum concentrations of thyroxine and triiodothyronine in healthy, thyroidectomized, thyroxine-treated, and propylthiouracil-treated dogs. Am J Vet Res 47:163, 1986.

Liu S, et al: Clinical and pathologic findings in dogs with atherosclerosis: 21 cases (1970–1983). JAVMA 189:227, 1986.

Lothrop CD, et al: Canine and feline thyroid function assessment with the thyrotropin-releasing hormone response test. Am J Vet Res 45:2310, 1984a.

Lothrop CD, et al: Diagnosis of canine pituitary-thyroid dysfunction with the thyrotropin releasing hormone (TRH) stimulation test. Proceedings of the 12th Annual Scientific Program, American College of Veterinary Internal Medicine, Washington DC, 1984b, p 32.

Lum SMC, et al: Peripheral tissue mechanism for maintenance of serum triiodothyronine values in a thyroxine-deficient state in man. J Clin Invest 73:570, 1984.

Lumsden JH, et al: Prevalence of hypothyroidism and von Willebrand's disease in Doberman Pinschers and the observed relationship between thyroid, von Willebrand, and cardiac status. JVIM 7:115, 1993 (abstract).

Lurye JC, et al: Evaluation of an in-house enzyme-lined immunosorbent assay for quantitative measurement of serum total thyroxine concentration in dogs and cats. JAVMA 221:243, 2002.

Marca MC, et al: Evaluation of canine serum thyrotropin (TSH) concentration: Comparison of three analytical procedures. J Vet Diag Invest 13:106, 2001.

Maruo T, et al: The role of maternal thyroid hormones in maintaining early pregnancy in threatened abortion. Acta Endocrinol 127:118, 1992.

Meij BP, et al: Thyroid-stimulating hormone responses after single administration of thyrotropin-releasing hormone and combined administration of four hypothalamic releasing hormones in Beagle dogs. Dom Anim Endocr 13:465, 1996.

Meij BP, et al: Results of transsphenoidal hypophysectomy in 52 dogs with pituitary-dependent hyperadrenocorticism. Vet Surg 27:246, 1998.

Meric SM, et al: Serum thyroxine concentrations after radioactive iodine therapy in cats with hyperthyroidism. JAVMA 188:1038, 1986.

Miller AB, et al: Serial thyroid hormone concentrations in healthy euthyroid dogs, dogs with hypothyroidism, and euthyroid dogs with atopic dermatitis. Br Vet J 148:451, 1992.

Miller CW, et al: Echocardiographic assessment of cardiac function in Beagles with experimentally produced hypothyroidism. J Ultrasound Med (Suppl) 3:157, 1984.

Milne KL, Hayes HM: Epidemiologic features of canine hypothyroidism. Cornell Vet 71:3, 1981.

Montgomery T, et al: Comparison of five analog RIAs for free thyroxine in dogs (abstract). J Vet Intern Med 5:128, 1991.

Monzani et al: Subclinical hypothyroidism: Neurobehavioral features and beneficial effect of L-thyroxine treatment. Clin Invest 71:367, 1993.

Mooney CT, Anderson TJ: Congenital hypothyroidism in a Boxer dog. J Small Anim Pract 34:31, 1993.

Moore GE, et al: Effects of oral administration of anti-inflammatory doses of prednisone on thyroid hormone response to thyrotropin-releasing hormone and thyrotropin in clinically normal dogs. AJVR 54:130, 1993.

Morkin E, et al: Studies on the use of thyroid hormone and a thyroid hormone analogue in the treatment of congestive heart failure. Ann Thorac Surg 56:54, 1993.

Moruzzi P, et al: Medium-term effectiveness of L-thyroxine treatment in idiopathic dilated cardiomyopathy. Am J Med 101:461, 1996.

Muller GH, et al: Cutaneous endocrinology. *In* Muller GH, et al (eds): Small Animal Dermatology, 3rd ed. Philadelphia, WB Saunders, 1983, p 492.

Muller PB, et al: Effects of long-term phenobarbital treatment on the thyroid and adrenal axis and adrenal function tests in dogs. JVIM 14:157, 2000.

Nachreiner RF: New thyroid function tests. Vet Diagn News (Michigan State University) 1:3, 1984.

Nachreiner RF, et al: Incidence of T_3 and T_4 autoantibodies in dogs using a sensitive binding assay. J Vet Intern Med 4:114, 1990.

Nachreiner RF, et al: Pharmacokinetics of L-thyroxine after its oral administration in dogs. Am J Vet Res 54:2091, 1993.

Nachreiner RF, Refsal KR: Radioimmunoassay monitoring of thyroid hormone concentrations in dogs on thyroid replacement therapy: 2,674 cases (1985–1987). JAVMA 201:623, 1992.

Nachreiner RF, et al: Prevalence of autoantibodies to thyroglobulin in dogs with nonthyroidal illness. Am J Vet Res 59:951, 1998.

Nachreiner RF, et al: Prevalence of serum thyroid hormone autoantibodies in dogs with clinical signs of hypothyroidism. JAVMA 220: 466, 2002.

Nelson RW, et al: Serum free thyroxine concentration in healthy dogs, dogs with hypothyroidism, and euthyroid dogs with concurrent illness. JAVMA 198:1401, 1991.

Nesbitt GH, et al: Canine hypothyroidism: A retrospective study of 108 cases. JAVMA 177:1117, 1980.

Neufeld M, et al: Two types of autoimmune Addison's disease associated with different polyglandular autoimmune (PGA) syndromes. Medicine 60:355, 1981.

Oohashi E, et al: Seasonal changes in serum total thyroxine, free thyroxine, and canine thyroid-stimulating hormone in clinically healthy Beagles in Hokkaido. J Vet Med Sci 63:1241, 2001.

Panciera DL: An echocardiographic and electrocardiographic study of cardiovascular function in hypothyroid dogs. JAVMA 205:996, 1994.

Panciera DL: Conditions associated with canine hypothyroidism. Vet Clin North Am 31:935, 2001.

Panciera DL, et al: Thyroid function tests in euthyroid dogs treated with L-thyroxine. Am J Vet Res 51:22, 1989.

Panciera DL, et al: Quantitative morphologic study of the pituitary and thyroid glands of dogs administered L-thyroxine. Am J Vet Res 51:27, 1990.

Panciera DL, Johnson GS: Plasma von Willebrand factor antigen concentration in dogs with hypothyroidism. JAVMA 205:1550, 1994.

Panciera DL, Johnson GS: Plasma von Willebrand factor antigen concentration and buccal mucosal bleeding time in dogs with experimental hypothyroidism. JVIM 10:60, 1996.

Panciera DL, Johnston SA: Thyroid function tests and plasma proteins in dogs administered etodolac (abstract). JVIM 16:374, 2002.

Penhale WJ, Young PR: The influence of microbial environment on susceptibility to experimental autoimmune thyroiditis. Clin Exp Immunol 72:288, 1988.

Peruccio C: Incidence of hypothyroidism in dogs affected by keratoconjunctivitis sicca. Proceedings of the American Society of Veterinary Ophthalmology, Las Vegas, 1982, p 47.

Peterson ME, et al: Effects of spontaneous hyperadrenocorticism on serum thyroid hormone concentrations in the dog. Am J Vet Res 45:2034, 1984.

Peterson ME, Ferguson DC: Thyroid diseases. *In* Ettinger SJ (ed): Textbook of Veterinary Internal Medicine, 3rd ed. Philadelphia, WB Saunders, 1989, p 1632.

Peterson ME, Gamble DA: Effect of nonthyroidal illness on serum thyroxine concentrations in cats: 494 cases (1988). JAVMA 197:1203, 1990.

Peterson ME, et al: Pretreatment clinical and laboratory findings in dogs with hypoadrenocorticism: 225 cases (1979–1993). JAVMA 208:85, 1996.

Peterson ME, et al: Measurement of serum total thyroxine, triiodothyronine, free thyroxine, and thyrotropin concentrations for diagnosis of hypothyroidism in dogs. JAVMA 211:1396, 1997.

Peterson ME, et al: Total thyroxine testing: Comparison of an in-house test kit with radioimmuno- and chemiluminescent assays (abstr). J Vet Intern Med 17:396, 2003.

Pisarev MA, Gartner R: Autoregulatory actions of iodine. *In* Braverman LE, Utiger RD (eds): The Thyroid, 6th ed. Philadelphia, Lippincott, 2000, p 85.

Post K, et al: Lack of effect of trimethoprim and sulfadiazine in combination in mid- to late gestation on thyroid function in neonatal dogs. J Reprod Fertil Suppl 47:477, 1993.

Rajatanavin R, et al: Thyroid hormone antibodies and Hashimoto's thyroiditis in mongrel dogs. Endocrinology 124:2535, 1989.

Ramsey IK, et al: Thyroid-stimulating hormone and total thyroxine concentrations in euthyroid, sick euthyroid and hypothyroid dogs. J Small Anim Pract 38:540, 1997.

Ray RA, Howanitz P: RIA in thyroid function testing. Diagn Med 7:55, 1984.

Reimers TJ, et al: Effects of storage, hemolysis, and freezing and thawing on concentrations of thyroxine, cortisol, and insulin in blood samples. Proc Soc Exp Biol Med 170:509, 1982.

Reimers TJ, et al: Effects of reproductive state on concentrations of thyroxine, 3,5,3?-triiodothyronine, and cortisol in serum of dogs. Biol Reprod 31:148, 1984.

Reimers TJ, et al: Effect of fasting on thyroxine, 3,5,3?-triiodothyronine, and cortisol concentrations in serum of dogs. Am J Vet Res 47:2485, 1986.

Reimers TJ, et al: Effects of age, sex, and body size on serum concentrations of thyroid and adrenocortical hormones in dogs. Am J Vet Res 51:454, 1990.

Rogers JS, et al: Factor VIII activity and thyroid function. Ann Intern Med 97:713, 1982.

Rogers WA, et al: Lipids and lipoproteins in normal dogs and in dogs with secondary hyperlipoproteinemia. JAVMA 166:1092, 1975.

Rosychuk RA: Thyroid hormones and antithyroid drugs. Vet Clin North Am [Small Anim Pract] 12:111, 1982.

Rosychuk RA: Dermatologic manifestations of canine hypothyroidism. Hypothyroidism: Diagnosis and Clinical Manifestations. St Petersburg, Daniels Pharmaceuticals Inc, 1998, p 18.

Sainteny F, et al: Thyroid hormones induce hematopoietic pluri-potent stem cell differentiation toward erythropoiesis through the production of pluri-poietin-like factors. Exp Cell Res 187:174, 1990.

Saunders HM, Jezyk PK: The radiographic appearance of canine congenital hypothyroidism: Skeletal changes with delayed treatment. Vet Radiol 32:171, 1991.

Sauvé F, Paradis M: Use of recombinant human thyroid-stimulating hormone for thyrotropin stimulation test in euthyroid dogs. Can Vet J 41:215, 2000.

Scott DW, Miller WH, Griffin CE (eds): Muller & Kirk's Small Animal Dermatology, 6th ed. Philadelphia, WB Saunders Co, 2001, p 780.

Scott-Moncrieff C, et al: Measurement of serum free thyroxine by modified equilibrium dialysis in dogs (abstract). J Vet Intern Med 8:159, 1994.

Scott-Moncrieff JCR, Nelson RW: Change in serum thyroid-stimulating hormone concentration in response to administration of thyrotropin-releasing hormone to healthy dogs, hypothyroid dogs, and euthyroid dogs with concurrent disease. JAVMA 213:1435, 1998.

Scott-Moncrieff JCR, et al: Comparison of serum concentrations of thyroid-stimulating hormone in healthy dogs, hypothyroid dogs, and euthyroid dogs with concurrent disease. JAVMA 212:387, 1998.

Scott-Moncrieff JCR, et al: Evaluation of antithyroglobulin antibodies after routine vaccination in pet and research dogs. JAVMA 221:515, 2002.

Shahrara S, et al: Upregulation of thyroid hormone receptor β_1 and β_2 messenger RNA in the myocardium of dogs with dilated cardiomyopathy or chronic valvular disease. AJVR 60:848, 1999.

Slade E, et al: Serum thyroxine and triiodothyronine concentrations in canine pyoderma. JAVMA 185:216, 1984.

Slag MF, et al: Hypothyroxinemia in critically ill patients as a predictor of high mortality. JAMA 245:43, 1981.

Smith CA: Are we vaccinating too much? JAVMA 207:421, 1995.

Strakosch CR, et al: Immunology of autoimmune thyroid diseases. N Engl J Med 307:1499, 1982.

Sullivan P, et al: Altered platelet indices in dogs with hypothyroidism and cats with hyperthyroidism. Am J Vet Res 54:2004, 1993.

Sunthornthepvarakul T, et al: Brief report: Resistance to thyrotropin caused by mutations in the thyrotropin-receptor gene. N Engl J Med 332:155, 1994.

Swanson JW, et al: Neurologic aspects of thyroid dysfunction. Mayo Clin Proc 56:504, 1981.

Szabadi E: Thyroid dysfunction and affective illness. Br Med J 302:923, 1991.

Taurog A, Dorris ML: Peroxidase-catalyzed bromination of tyrosine, thyro-globulin, and bovine serum albumin: Comparison of thyroid peroxidase and lactoperoxidase. Arch Biochem Biophys 287:288, 1991.

Thacker EL, et al: Prevalence of autoantibodies to thyroglobulin, thyroxine, or triiodothyronine and relationship of autoantibodies and serum concentrations of iodothyronines in dogs. Am J Vet Res 53:449, 1992.

Tomer Y: Anti-thyroglobulin autoantibodies in autoimmune thyroid diseases: Cross-reactive or pathogenic? Clin Immunol Immunopathol 82:3, 1997.

Topliss DJ, et al: Uptake of 3,5,3'-triiodothyronine by cultured rat hepatoma cells is inhibitable by nonbile acid cholephils, diphenylhydantoin, and non-steroidal anti-inflammatory drugs. Endocrinology 124:980, 1989.

Torres SMF, et al: Hypothyroidism in a dog associated with trimethoprim-sulfadiazine therapy. Vet Derm 7:105, 1996.

Utiger RD: Decreased extrathyroidal triiodothyronine production in non-thyroidal illness: Benefit or harm? Am J Med 69:807, 1980.

Vail DM, et al: Thyroid hormone concentrations in dogs with chronic weight loss, with special reference to cancer cachexia. JVIM 8:122, 1994.

Vajner L: Lymphocytic thyroiditis in Beagle dogs in a breeding colony: Findings of serum autoantibodies. Vet Med Czech 11:333, 1997.

Valdermarsson S, et al: Relations between thyroid function, hepatic and lipoprotein lipase activities and plasma lipoprotein concentrations. Acta Endocrinologica 104:50, 1983.

Verge CF: Immunoendocrinopathy syndromes. In Wilson JD, Foster DW, Kronenberg HM, Larsen PR (eds): Williams Textbook of Endocrinology, 9th ed. Philadelphia, WB Saunders Co, 1998, p 1651.

Vollset I, Larsen HJ: Occurrence of autoantibodies against thyroglobulin in Norwegian dogs. Acta Vet Scand 28:65, 1987.

Wang R, et al: Salsalate and salicylate binding to and their displacement of thyroxine from thyroxine-binding globulin, transthyretin, and albumin. Thyroid 9:359, 1999.

Wartofsky L, Burman KD: Alterations in thyroid function in patients with systemic illness: The euthyroid sick syndrome. Endocrinol Rev 3:164, 1982.

Weller RE, Kinnas TC, Stevens D: Basal serum thyroxine concentration and its response to thyroid-stimulating hormone administration decreases with chronologic age in Beagle dogs. Scientific Proceedings, American College of Veterinary Internal Medicine, New York, 1983, p 38.

Wenzel KW: Pharmacological interference with in vitro tests of thyroid function. Metabolism 30:717, 1981.

Werner SC: Normal thyroid physiology. Proceedings of the American Association of Clinical Chemists, July, 1982, p 1.

Williams DA, et al: Validation of an immunoassay for canine thyroid-stimulating hormone and changes in serum concentration following induction of hypothyroidism in dogs. JAVMA 209:1730, 1996.

Williamson NL, et al: Effects of short-term trimethoprim-sulfamethoxazole administration on thyroid function in dogs. JAVMA 221:802, 2002.

Woltz HH, et al: Effect of prednisone on thyroid gland morphology and plasma thyroxine and triiodothyronine concentrations in the dog. AJVR 44:2000, 1984.

Young DW, et al: Abnormal canine triiodothyronine-binding factor characterized as a possible triiodothyronine autoantibody. Am J Vet Res 46:1346, 1985.

Feline Hypothyroidism

Arnold U, et al: Goitrous hypothyroidism and dwarfism in a kitten. JAAHA 20:753, 1984.

DiBartola SP, Tarr MJ: Corticotropin and thyrotropin response tests in Abyssinian cats with familial amyloidosis. JAAHA 25:217, 1989.

Feldman EC, Nelson RW: Canine and Feline Endocrinology and Reproduction. Philadelphia, WB Saunders, 1987.

Graham PA, et al: The measurement of feline thyrotropin (TSH) using a commercial canine immunoradiometric assay (abstract). JVIM 14:342, 2000.

Hoenig M, Ferguson DC: Assessment of thyroid functional reserve in the cat by the thyrotropin-stimulation test. Am J Vet Res 44:1229, 1983.

Jones BR, et al: Preliminary studies on congenital hypothyroidism in a family of Abyssinian cats. Vet Rec 131:145, 1992.

Kemppainen RJ, et al: Endocrine responses of normal cats to TSH and synthetic ACTH administration. JAAHA 20:737, 1984.

Lothrop CD, et al: Canine and feline thyroid function assessment with the thyrotropin-releasing hormone response test. Am J Vet Res 45:2310, 1984.

Mooney CT, et al: Effect of illness not associated with the thyroid gland on serum total and free thyroxine concentrations in cats. JAVMA 208:2004, 1996a.

Mooney CT, et al: Serum thyroxine and triiodothyronine responses of hyper-thyroid cats to thyrotropin. AJVR 57:987, 1996b.

Otero T, et al: Serum TSH in hyperthyroid cats pre- and post-therapy (abstract). Proceedings, 12th ECVIM-CA/ESVIM Congress, Munich, Germany, September, 2002, p 173.

Peterson ME: Feline hypothyroidism. In Kirk RW (ed): Current Veterinary Therapy X. Philadelphia, WB Saunders, 1989, p 1000.

Peterson ME, et al: Feline hyperthyroidism: Pretreatment, clinical, and laboratory evaluation of 131 cases. JAVMA 183:103, 1983.

Peterson ME, et al: Use of the thyrotropin releasing hormone stimulation test to diagnose mild hyperthyroidism in cats. J Vet Intern Med 8:279, 1994.

Peterson ME, Gamble DA: Effect of nonthyroidal illness on serum thyroxine concentrations in cats: 494 cases (1988). J Vet Intern Med 197:1203, 1990.

Peterson ME, et al: Measurement of serum concentrations of free thyroxine, total thyroxine, and total triodothyronine in cat with hyperthyroidism and cats with nonthyroidal illness. JAVMA 218:529, 2001.

Rand JS, et al: Spontaneous adult-onset hypothyroidism in a cat. J Vet Intern Med 7:272, 1993.

Reimers TJ, et al: Validation of radioimmunoassays for triiodothyronine, thyroxine and hydrocortisone (cortisol) in canine, feline, and equine sera. Am J Vet Res 42:2016, 1981.

Scott DW: Hormonal and metabolic disorders. JAAHA 16:390, 1980.

Scott DW, Miller WH, Griffin CE (eds): Muller & Kirk's Small Animal Dermatology, 6th ed. Philadelphia, WB Saunders Co, 2001, p 780.

Sjollema BE, et al: Congenital hypothyroidism in two cats due to defective organification: Data suggesting loosely anchored thyroperoxidase. Acta Endocrinol 125:435, 1991.

Sparkes AH, et al: Thyroid function in the cat: Assessment by the TRH response test and the thyrotrophin stimulation test. J Small Anim Pract 32:59, 1991.

Thoday KL, et al: Radioimmunoassay of serum total thyroxine and triiodothyronine in healthy cats: Assay methodology and effects of age, sex, breed, heredity and environment. J Small Anim Pract 25:457, 1984.

Tomsa K, et al: Thyrotropin-releasing hormone stimulation test to assess thyroid function in severely sick cats. JVIM 15:89, 2001.

Zerbe CA, et al: Thyroid profiles in healthy kittens from birth to 12 weeks of age. Proc Annu Meet American College of Veterinary Internal Medicine 16:702, 1998.

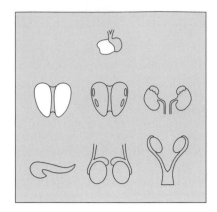

4

FELINE HYPERTHYROIDISM (THYROTOXICOSIS)

The thyroid gland was first described in detail by Vesalius in the sixteenth century. Thomas Wharton (1614-1673) named the gland from the Greek word *thyreos,* or shield, based on its physical appearance. One of the first described thyroid disorders was an association between iodine deficiency and enlargement of the thyroid (goiter), initially suspected in the 1500s to be a possible cause of cretinism. This description also represents the first mention of thyroid gland enlargement. Endemic cretinism in the region around Salzburg, Austria, was described by the Swiss-German physician Paracelsus (1493-1541).

Hyperthyroidism, caused by autonomous growth and function of the thyroid follicular cells, was initially described in humans by Henry Plummer in 1913. Clinical observations led him to characterize two types of hyperthyroidism: exophthalmic goiter (Graves' disease) and toxic adenomatous goiter. In Graves' disease, the hyperthyroidism appeared to be associated with diffuse hyperplasia of the thyroid glands. Toxic adenomatous goiter was associated with either single or multiple nodules and variable histologic patterns. The latter disease involved the slow growth of autonomous functioning follicles. Interestingly, toxic nodule syndrome (toxic adenomatous goiter) is believed to be most similar (homologous) to the disorder seen in most hyperthyroid cats, initially described as a clinical entity in 1979 by Peterson and in 1980 by Holzworth and colleagues.

DEFINITION

Naturally occurring hyperthyroidism (thyrotoxicosis) is a clinical condition that results from excessive production and secretion (and, subsequently, circulating concentrations) of thyroxine (T_4) and triiodothyronine (T_3) by the thyroid gland. Hyperthyroidism in cats is almost always the result of a primary autonomous condition (i.e., it arises independent of a hypothalamic or pituitary abnormality). Rarely, hyperthyroidism in people may be caused by a hypothalamic or pituitary disorder (Brucker-Davis, 1999). Theoretically, hyperthyroidism may also result from acute destruction of thyroid tissue, causing excessive release of thyroid hormone. Syndromes involving the hypothalamus, the pituitary, or thyroid destruction have not been described in cats. Hyperthyroidism in cats, therefore, is most often due to an intrinsic disease within one or both thyroid lobes.

HISTORY OF HYPERTHYROIDISM

The recognition of thyroid disease in cats by veterinary pathologists and clinicians has dramatically escalated in the past 20 years. In 1914 Carlson suggested that cats were less susceptible to thyrid hyperplasia than dogs. In a review of 3000 feline necropsies in 1927, Huquenin described three thyroid adenomas. In 1955, a report authored by Schlumberger from the Armed Forces Institute of Pathology included one thyroid adenocarcinoma in a cat. In a report published by Clark and meier in 1958, a review of the thyroids from 54 cats revealed five adenomas and two carcinomas. Clark and meier, however, suggested that these abnormal-appearing thyroid glands were functioning normally.

Necropsies from 75 geriatric cats, including a thorough evaluation of the thyroids, were reported by Lucke in 1964. The cats were from veterinary practices in one area of England, and in no cat was thyroid disease suspected clinically. However, 27 (36%) had obvious thyroid pathology, including thyroid adenomas (23 cats), nodular (adenomatous) goiter (3 cats), and thyroid carcinoma (1 cat). Two of three cats with nodular goiter had signs that would now be associated with hyperthyroidism. From a pathologic viewpoint, thyroid abnormalities in geriatric cats were potentially becoming more common by the mid-1960s.

In 1976 Leav and colleagues reviewed the clinical and pathology files on canine and feline thyroid tumors from the veterinary school in the Netherlands. This review included cats that had been necropsied between 1949 and 1973. Fifty-two tumors of the feline thyroid were studied (47 adenomas and 5 carcinomas). Most of these tumors were not believed to have caused clinical signs. However, benign tumors in five cats were thought to have been large enough to have been clinically detected, and in two cats, carcinomas had metastasized to regional lymph nodes and caused clinical signs prior to the animals' death. Leav and colleagues also noted, in retrospect, that some of the cats with thyroid neoplasia had signs that may have reflected an altered hormonal status. It was suggested that benign tumors of the feline thyroid were common, carcinomas rare, and that both occurred almost exclusively in old cats.

Veterinary clinicians were not aware of feline hyperthyroidism until two clinical reports were published (Peterson et al, 1979; Holzworth et al, 1980). With this information, practitioners began to recognize cats with signs suggestive of hyperthyroidism (thyrotoxicosis). Cats with clinical hyperthyroidism were not recognized at the University of California prior to 1980. Within a 5-year period after the studies published in 1979 and 1980 (1980 through 1985), 125 hyperthyroid cats with clinical disease were identified at our hospital. During a similar period, cats with the disease were being recognized at a rate of three per month at the Animal Medical Center in New York City (Peterson et al, 1983). In a 1993 survey conducted at the Animal Medical Center, approximately 22 cats with hyperthyroidism were recognized each month (Broussard et al, 1995; Peterson, 1995a and 2000). It is not clear whether the incidence of the condition continues to escalate, but there is no doubt that feline hyperthyroidism is now commonly recognized in Great Britain, Europe, and Japan, as well as throughout the United States.

PATHOLOGY

Background

A thorough review of feline thyroid pathology has not been published in the 20 to 25 years since the incidence of hyperthyroidism, as a clinical condition frequently diagnosed by veterinary practitioners, became common. However, previous publications do give some insight into the current situation. Also, review of surgically removed tissue and necropsy specimens provide additional information. As in the dog, microscopic evaluation of most feline thyroid tumors reveals a follicular, compact, or mixed cellular pattern. Benign tumors appear to be much more common than malignant tumors.

Benign Thyroid Tumors

MULTINODULAR ADENOMATOUS GOITER. In the 1976 review by Leav and colleagues, multinodular adenomatous tumors were not often associated with enlargement of the thyroid, but experience since then demonstrates that most hyperthyroid cats have a palpably enlarged gland. Multinodular adenomatous goiter is the most common histologically described thyroid lesion in thyrotoxic cats (Carpenter et al, 1987). Similarly affected cats have had thyroid tissue classified as *adenomatous hyperplasia*, and still others have been described as having *adenomas*. It will be interesting to learn whether all three conditions are the same and simply identified by a different set of "terms," or whether the three conditions (multinodular adenomatous tumors, adenomatous hyperplasia, and adenoma) are somehow distinct. It would appear that most cats (approximately 70% to 75%) have this "benign" adenomatous condition involving both thyroid lobes.

In affected thyroids, multifocal nodules are dispersed throughout the gland. The foci of hyperplastic tissue form nodules that range from less than 1 mm to greater than 3 cm in diameter (Peterson, 2000). The thyroid may have the appearance of a compressed cluster of grapes (Fig. 4-1). Most are solid, but a small percentage may be cystic or "cavitary" and filled with fluid (see Fig. 4-1). The lesions are histologically similar to nodular hyperplasia or multiple adenomatous goiter of humans. The foci are composed of irregularly arranged, colloid-filled follicles that are quite different from normal tissue. Occasionally the surrounding parenchyma is compressed, and in a few cases microfollicular or compact cellular patterns may be observed. Colloid-filled cysts are frequently found adjacent to nodules. The follicular cells are uniform and cuboidal in shape.

ADENOMA. Less common than multinodular adenomatous hyperplasia are glands that some pathologists describe as composed of a "thyroid adenoma," which cause the affected lobe to be enlarged and distorted. Adenomas are usually solitary and large, involving much of the lobe. Distinct capsules are rarely present. Microscopically, adenomas are usually composed of irregularly arranged follicles containing varying amounts of colloid. In some, papillary infolding of follicular epithelium is seen, and in others compact cellular foci are dispersed throughout the affected lobe. In some cases the tumor has a lobular appearance, but this feature is less distinct or absent in other cases.

ATYPICAL ADENOMA. This small group of tumors has a few histologic characteristics often associated with malignancy, but these adenomas lack the critical features of capsular and vascular invasion. The affected lobe usually is enlarged and distorted, but externally it has a smooth capsular surface rather than the lobulated pattern of adenomas or adenomatous hyperplasia. Microscopically, these atypical adenomas are characterized by foci of closely packed follicles that have merged with cells arranged in a compact cellular pattern. The follicles are usually devoid of colloid, and the cells of these masses are larger than those of typical adenomas.

Malignant Thyroid Tumors

INTRODUCTION. Thyroid carcinoma, the primary cause of hyperthyroidism in dogs, is recognized to cause hyperthyroidism in only 1% to 3% of hyperthyroid cats. These tumors may appear to be well encapsulated, solitary, and to involve one thyroid lobe. Carcinomas may involve both lobes and appear to be simple bilateral disease. However, there may be numerous masses throughout the cervical region. They may be locally invasive and there may be distant metastases. In other words, there is a variety of clinical presentations.

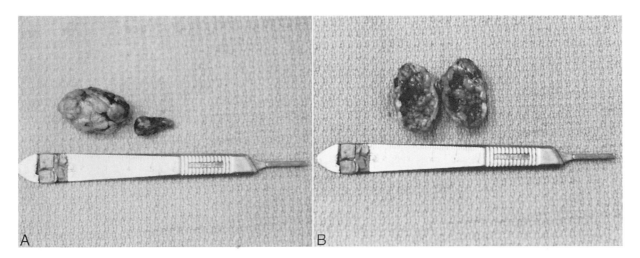

FIGURE 4–1. *A,* Multinodular adenomatous goiter, which has the gross appearance of a compressed cluster of grapes. This is an example of bilaterally asymmetric thyroid enlargement. *B,* After the larger mass is cut in half, the cavitary nature of the goiter is obvious.

FOLLICULAR CARCINOMA. These tumors cause enlargement and distortion of affected lobes. They are relatively uncommon and are usually nonfunctioning (i.e., they do not often cause hyperthyroidism). All of these tumors have a compact pattern in distinct follicles that contain little colloid. Some may be less differentiated, with small, dense follicles merging with cells in compact cellular foci. Capsular and vascular invasions are typical.

PAPILLARY CARCINOMA. This histologic pattern is detected less frequently than follicular carcinomas. The tumor does not cause gross alteration of the affected lobe and is usually detected only microscopically. It is characterized by papillary fronds of fibrovascular connective tissue lined by large, cuboidal neoplastic cells that invade the capsule.

ETIOLOGY

Historical Background

INCIDENCE. There is little doubt that the incidence of hyperthyroidism in cats steadily increased from the time the first reports describing this condition in 1979 and 1980 were published until the early to mid-1990s. Whether the incidence continues to expand is not yet known. Regardless, it is fair to question whether the current "common" status of this condition is due to increased awareness of owners, the diagnostic acuity of veterinarians, the longer life span and increased popularity of cats as pets, or a true increasing incidence of the disease. It is likely that all these explanations have merit, because it is now estimated that the disorder affects as many as 1 in 300 cats (Gerber et al, 1994).

PLAUSIBLE EXPLANATIONS. Although much has been learned about feline hyperthyroidism, its primary cause has not yet been elucidated. Because in approximately 70% to 75% of cats both thyroid lobes are involved and because there is no physical connection between the two lobes, it has been postulated that some circulating internal or external factor may influence development of thyrotoxicosis in a species that may be predisposed to this condition. Further, it is fascinating to realize that commercial cat foods were first test-marketed in East Coast and California cities in the mid-1960s. This means that the first generation of cats raised and maintained almost entirely on commercial foods was reaching middle and old age in the late 1970s and early 1980s, which coincides with the recognition of feline hyperthyroidism in Boston, New York, Philadelphia, Los Angeles and San Francisco. The question arises: Is there a correlation between a diet of commercial foods and the development of hyperthyroidism?

Possible Nutritional and Environmental Causes

GOITROGENS. Although most commercial cat foods contain relatively large amounts of iodine, studies have failed to demonstrate a correlation between dietary iodine and feline hyperthyroidism. Commercial cat foods and the environment contain a variety of other *goitrogens* (ingredients that might cause thyroid enlargement or hyperthyroidism, or both), including phthalates, resorcinol, polyphenols, and polychlorinated biphenyls. Most of these hydrocarbons are metabolized via glucuronidation, a process that is unusually slow in cats (Court and Greenblatt, 2000).

SOYBEANS. Inadvertent inclusion of goitrogenic compounds in diets is plausible. Soybean is a potential dietary goitrogen that is used as a source of high-quality vegetable protein in commercial cat food. Soy isoflavones genistein and daidzein have been implicated due to their inhibitory effect on thyroid peroxidase, an enzyme essential to thyroid hormone synthesis (Divi et al, 1997). Glucuronidation appears to be an important pathway for eliminating soy isoflavones via the liver, a process that is deficient in feline liver. These compounds, therefore, could play an etiologic role in feline thyrotoxicosis. Genistein and daidzein are common constituents of commercial cat foods, and soy isoflavones have been detected in amounts predicted to have a biologic effect (Court and Freeman, 2002). Further research on this subject is anticipated.

EPIDEMIOLOGY. An early epidemiologic study suggested that feeding of canned cat foods, living strictly indoors, being a non-Siamese breed, and having reported exposure to flea sprays, fertilizers, insecticides, and herbicides increased the risk of developing hyperthyroidism (Scarlett et al, 1988). In another study, two genetically related cat breeds (Siamese and Himalayan) were found to have a diminished risk of developing hyperthyroidism. In addition, there was a twofold to threefold increase in risk of developing hyperthyroidism among cats fed mostly canned cat food. There was also a threefold increase in risk among cats using cat litter (Kass et al, 1999). In a more recent study, there was no breed association with risk for developing hyperthyroidism. Exposure to fertilizers, herbicides, plant pesticides, or flea control products or the presence of a smoker in the home were not significantly associated with an increased risk for developing hyperthyroidism. Cats that preferred fish-flavored or liver and giblets–flavored canned cat food had an increased risk of hyperthyroidism (Martin et al, 2000).

SELENIUM. The thyroid gland contains more selenium per gram of weight than any other tissue, which suggests an important role for this trace element in homeostasis. Selenium exerts its biologic activity through the expression of selenoproteins, including glutathione peroxidases and thioredoxin reductase, which protect thyrocytes from oxidative damage. Because selenium is also a growth factor, this dietary element may play a role in development of toxic nodular goiter in cats. Cats were studied from two geographic areas with an allegedly high incidence of hyperthyroidism and two regions with a lower incidence. It was found that cats have higher concentrations of selenium in the plasma than do other species but that this does not appear to affect the incidence of hyperthyroidism. However, the authors concluded that high selenium concentrations may affect feline health if they are influenced by the amount included in diets (Foster et al, 2001).

Possible Autocrine or Paracrine Growth Factors

GENERAL. Growth factors, or peptides that stimulate cell proliferation, may have a role in normal growth and in carcinogenesis. *Autocrine* activity defines a cell reacting to a growth factor that it produces itself. *Paracrine* activity defines a cell reacting to growth factors produced by neighboring cells. Cells generally require multiple growth factors for optimal response. Several growth factors have been identified in thyroid cells, including platelet-derived factors, epidermal growth factors, and the insulin-like growth factors. It remains to be determined whether any of these families of growth factors contribute to the development of feline hyperthyroidism (Brown et al, 1992).

G PROTEINS. The synthesis and secretion of thyroid hormone are regulated by thyroid-stimulating hormone (TSH). TSH binds to a receptor (TSH-R) on the surface of thyroid cells. The receptors are bound to specific proteins that are members of a "superfamily" known as G proteins. Binding of TSH to the TSH-R stimulates growth and differentiation of thyroid cells via a G protein–mediated cyclic adenosine monophosphate (cAMP)-dependent signal transduction pathway. Alterations in the expression of G proteins could be involved in the pathogenesis of feline hyperthyroidism. In an in vitro study of thyroid adenomas obtained from hyperthyroid cats, a decreased amount of one G protein was identified (Hammer et al, 2000). When present, this G protein may inhibit growth and differentiation of thyroid cells. Decreased expression of this G protein from adenomatous thyroid glands, therefore, may reduce the inhibitory effect on the cAMP cascade in thyroid cells, leading to autonomous growth and hypersecretion of thyroxine. An understanding of the molecular mechanisms of hyperthyroidism in cats may lead to better treatment or ultimately to prevention of the disease (Hammer et al, 2000).

Circulating Thyroid Stimulators or Genetic Mutations

Although as yet not demonstrated, it is possible that hyperthyroidism in cats is caused by circulating factors similar to the immunoglobulins that bind to TSH receptors and stimulate thyroid hormone secretion, resulting in Graves' disease in people (Peterson et al, 1987b). Studies directed at finding mutations in the TSH receptor gene have failed to identify such abnormalities (Pearce et al, 1997). The structure of the feline TSH receptor is similar to that of the human TSH

receptor. Serum from humans with Graves' hyperthyroidism, but not serum from cats with hyperthyroidism, activates feline TSH receptors (Nguyen et al, 2002). However, future studies may yet elucidate "gain in function" mutations or circulating immunoglobulins that play a role in the development of this disease.

CLINICAL FEATURES

Signalment

Hyperthyroidism is probably the most common endocrinopathy affecting cats older than 8 years of age. The reported age range is 4 to 22 years, with a mean just under 13 years. A small number of cats younger than 4 years have been diagnosed with hyperthyroidism, although the disorder remains quite uncommon in this age group (Gordon et al, 2003). Fewer than 5% of cats diagnosed with hyperthyroidism are younger than 8 years of age (Fig. 4-2). There has been no breed or gender predilection, although the Siamese and Himalayan, as previously noted, may have a decreased risk of developing hyperthyroidism (Thoday and Mooney, 1992a; Broussard et al, 1995; Peterson, 1995a).

Signs and Their Physiopathology

HUMANS. Interestingly, the most common clinical signs diagnosed in elderly people (>70 years of age) with hyperthyroidism are quite similar to those observed in hyperthyroid cats: weight loss, thinness, atrial fibrillation, agitation, anxiousness, and muscle weakness and tremor. Less frequent findings (fewer

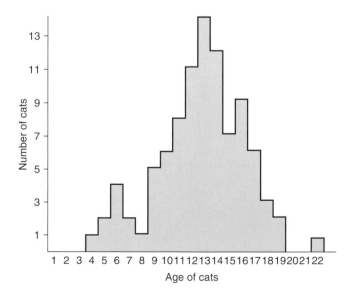

FIGURE 4-2. The ages of the initial 94 hyperthyroid cats at the University of California, Davis, at the time of diagnosis. The average was 12.9 years.

than 50% of humans) have included heat intolerance, confusion, apathy, and diarrhea (Martin et al, 1996). However, another report suggests that the diagnosis of hyperthyroidism in elderly people is a greater challenge than in younger people because the clinical manifestations may be more subtle and often suggest a single-organ condition (Maugeri et al, 1996). Subclinical hyperthyroidism is well documented in humans; it may be defined as abnormal test results in a person without clinical signs or as a condition of subtle clinical signs but normal serum T_3 and T_4 concentrations (Toft, 2001). Subclinical hyperthyroidism may be diagnosed in about 1% of people over the age of 60. It is not clear whether a comparable condition exists in cats. Most hyperthyroid cats have a variety of clinical signs that reflect multiple organ dysfunction, although some have one clinical sign that predominates (Mooney, 1998a and 1998b).

General overview: factors affecting clinical signs

DELAYED OWNER CONCERN. Signs of hyperthyroidism are insidiously progressive, which often delays owner recognition of a problem and therefore may allow the disease to progress before veterinary attention is considered. More than half of our hyperthyroid cats had clinical signs for longer than 6 months to 1 year before the owners sought veterinary assistance. The primary reason for this delay in owner action is the sequence of the development of clinical signs. Hyperthyroid cats initially maintain good (sometimes ravenous) appetites and are active (if not overactive) pets. These changes are usually interpreted as evidence of health, not disease. More worrisome signs also begin slowly, are seen infrequently, or remain subtle for prolonged periods (Table 4-1). The owner, therefore, typically observes a pet that "appears healthy" during the initial phases of hyperthyroidism. It is not until weight loss is severe or some of the other,

TABLE 4–1 OWNER OBSERVATIONS (HISTORICAL SIGNS) OF CATS WITH HYPERTHYROIDISM

Sign	Percent of Cats
Weight loss	92
Polyphagia	61
Polydipsia/polyuria	47
Increased activity/restless	40
Gastrointestinal (diarrhea, increased frequency, increased volume, steatorrhea)	39
Vomiting	38
Skin changes (patchy alopecia, matting, dry coat, greasy seborrhea, thin skin)	36
Respiratory signs (dyspnea, panting, coughing, sneezing)	23
Decreased appetite/anorexia	14
Decreased activity/lethargy	11
Weakness	10
Tremor/seizures	7
Seeks cool areas/heat intolerance	5
Hematuria	2
Ventroflexion of neck	<1

more worrisome clinical signs become frequent or more obvious that an owner realizes his or her cat may be ill. One common owner misconception, once the signs are appreciated, is that the cat is simply "aging" and these changes are to be expected. Sometimes it is only when the signs become intolerable that professional advice is sought. The most common reasons for owners to seek veterinary help are cats with obvious weight loss, polyphagia, polydipsia/polyuria, vomiting, and/or diarrhea.

CONCURRENT DISEASE. The clinical manifestations of hyperthyroidism in cats can be mild to severe. Clinical signs are affected by the duration of the hyperthyroid state and the presence or absence of nonthyroidal illness. Thyroid hormone affects virtually every organ system. In hyperthyroidism, this process is reflected in the variety of clinical signs exhibited. Some cats have signs suggesting dysfunction of several organ systems, whereas others have signs localized to one. Concurrent illness complicates the clinical picture and potentiates the chance for signs from one organ system to dominate. Because the signs are so variable, the presence or absence of any one clinical sign cannot be used to diagnose or exclude hyperthyroidism.

INCREASED VETERINARIAN AWARENESS. In the early 1980s, hyperthyroidism in cats was just beginning to be recognized as a clinical entity. As expected with any newly described syndrome, the incidence of the disease was uncommon, and cats diagnosed with hyperthyroidism usually had obvious if not classic clinical signs. Over the ensuing years, hyperthyroidism in cats became well described and practitioners became more familiar with the variable "presentations" associated with excesses in thyroid hormone, and the disease now is appreciated to be common. The index of suspicion among most veterinary practitioners is quite high.

Assays of the serum thyroxine concentration are now a routine component of feline serum biochemistry profiles, which helps clinicians recognize hyperthyroidism before signs become severe. As a result, cats with hyperthyroidism are being diagnosed earlier in the course of the disease, and therefore the clinical signs observed by owners and veterinarians may not be as obvious, severe, or frequent as those described in the 1980s (Broussard et al, 1995; Kintzer, 1995; Mooney, 1998a; Bucknell, 2000) (see Table 4-1). These factors do not diminish the importance of a thorough history and physical examination. On the contrary, these parameters gain value as the clinician attempts to diagnose a condition before serious complications develop.

Weight loss and polyphagia

SIGN. Weight loss and polyphagia are extremely common signs in cats with hyperthyroidism. Approximately 90% of hyperthyroid cats have some weight loss, according to their owners. The weight loss described by owners may be mild to severe, and a small percentage of hyperthyroid cats are severely cachectic (Fig. 4-3). The weight loss typically occurs

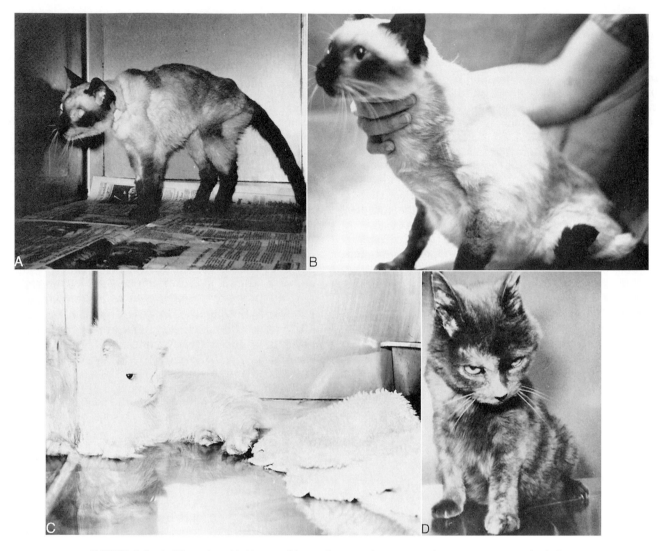

FIGURE 4–3. *A,* Hyperthyroid 13-year-old cat showing the emaciated appearance typical of the disease. *B,* Same cat as in *A* 2 months after return to a euthyroid condition. *C,* Hyperthyroid cat choosing the cool cage floor rather than a warm fleece pad. *D,* Hyperthyroid cat with marked ventroflexion of the head, a finding suggestive of concomitant thiamine or potassium deficency. (*D* Courtesy Dr. Jane Turrel, Pacifica, CA.)

gradually over a period of months. Owners may comment that the weight loss was not recognized until someone who had not seen the cat for several months noticed the change. It has been suggested that weight loss is usually evident if greater than 10% of body weight has been lost and is often described as emaciation if greater than 20% has been lost (Mooney, 1998b).

An increase in appetite may occur with a variety of disorders. This is an extremely important historical finding, because the combination of polyphagia and weight loss has fewer differential diagnoses than anorexia and weight loss (Mooney, 1998b; Table 4-2). Cats previously thought to be finicky eaters may develop excellent appetites, a change that may not be perceived as a problem by the owner. Other cats are described as "always hungry." They eat rapidly and then proceed to eat food put out for other household pets. One of our owners resorted to feeding her German Shepherd dog and hyperthyroid cat in separate rooms to avoid having the cat attack the dog for its food. Owners have described previously lazy or docile cats that had to be locked outdoors while the owners ate to avoid having the animal leap on the table and attempt to steal food.

TABLE 4–2 THE DIFFERENTIAL DIAGNOSIS FOR CATS WITH POLYPHAGIA AND WEIGHT LOSS

Hyperthyroidism
Diabetes mellitus
Poor quality or insufficient diet
Gastrointestinal disease
   Malabsorption
   Maldigestion
Hyperadrenocorticism [diabetes mellitus]

EXPLANATION. A major consequence of hyperthyroidism is increased energy expenditure. Physiologic functions and mechanical work are accomplished with reduced efficiency. To counterbalance these changes, increased food intake, utilization of stored energy, and increased oxygen consumption occur. Despite this increased food intake, however, the state of chronic caloric and nutritional inadequacy persists. In humans, both the synthesis and degradation of proteins are increased, the latter to a relatively greater extent than the former, with the result that there is net degradation of tissue protein. The negative nitrogen balance is evidenced by loss of weight, muscle wasting, weakness, and mild hypoalbuminemia. The exact mechanism for the increase in appetite is not known. Approximately 6% of hyperthyroid cats exhibit periods of decreased appetite (see Decreased Appetite [Apathetic Hyperthyroidism], page 160).

Polydipsia and/or polyuria (PD/PU)

SIGN. As with any sign associated with feline hyperthyroidism, remarkable variation in severity is common. Alterations in the amount of water consumed or urine excreted are highly variable. Although greater than 50% of owners did not notice changes in water intake or urine output (a smaller percentage than in the 1980s), others still report dramatic increases (Broussard et al, 1995). When present, these abnormalities can be quite striking and are an important diagnostic clue for the veterinary clinician. There are myriad causes of weight loss, but only a short list of diseases that result in significant polydipsia and polyuria.

EXPLANATION. Renal blood flow, the glomerular filtration rate (GFR), and renal tubular resorptive and/or secretory capacities are increased in hyperthyroidism (Peterson and Randolph, 1989; Mackovic-Basic and Kleeman, 1991). No specific renal pathology is attributed to hyperthyroidism, although azotemia is common among these cats. Renal failure represents one cause of PD/PU. However, increases in renal blood flow secondary to hyperthyroidism may delay the clinical and biochemical consequences of renal failure in cats with both thyroid and renal disease (see In-Hospital Diagnostic Evaluation, BUN, and Creatinine, page 166) (Peterson, 1995a). After resolution of hyperthyroidism, regardless of the treatment method, renal perfusion may acutely decrease in some cats, "unmasking" their existing renal failure.

Many hyperthyroid cats have signs of PD/PU without evidence of renal disease. Failure to concentrate urine in these cats is probably due to an increased renal medullary blood flow and resultant decline in the medullary solute concentration gradient (Spaulding and Utiger, 1981). Studies of water balance in thyrotoxic humans usually revealed impaired concentrating ability after water had been restricted to the point of clinical dehydration. Some people have decreases in serum osmolality, indicating a possible primary thirst disorder. Given these individuals' sensitivity to heat, plus the physical and personality lability seen in hyperthyroidism, primary (psychogenic) polydipsia is possible.

Nervousness, hyperactivity, aggressive behavior, and tremor

SIGNS. Increased circulating concentrations of thyroid hormone may cause hyperkinetic behavior and agitation, presumably by a direct effect on the nervous system. This is true in people as well as cats. In a recent study on hyperthyroid people, 76% had tremor and 38% had generalized hyperreflexia (Duyff et al, 2000). The "nervousness" of the thyrotoxic cat is characterized by restlessness, irritability, and/or aggressive behavior (see Table 4-1). Many hyperthyroid cats appear to have an intense desire to move about constantly. A smaller percentage have been observed on occasion to "shiver" or have "tremors." Surprisingly, this behavior is not apparent to many owners, even with careful questioning. Owners may note that their cats wander, pace, sleep for only brief periods, and waken easily. Although rare, focal or generalized seizures have also been described (Joseph and Peterson, 1993). To experienced veterinarians, many hyperthyroid cats appear "anxious." They often cannot be held for the short time required to complete a physical examination. Some become aggressive if an attempt is made to further restrain them (Joseph and Peterson, 1993).

EXPLANATION. Emotional lability is a prominent symptom of the thyrotoxic human. These people lose their tempers easily, and hyperkinesia is common. Such patients cannot sit still; they drum their fingers on the table, tap their feet, or shift position frequently. Movements are quick, jerky, exaggerated, and often purposeless (Utiger, 1987). Signs referable to the nervous system may reflect increased adrenergic activity, because some improvement occurs during treatment with adrenergic antagonists. Although the cerebral blood flow of thyrotoxic patients is increased, arteriovenous oxygen difference is diminished and oxygen extraction is unchanged. This correlates well with failure of thyroxine to increase oxygen consumption by brain tissue.

Diarrhea, vomiting, and bulky stool

SIGN. The most common signs referable to the gastrointestinal tract are polyphagia and weight loss. Stools may be soft and bulky (increased volume) and may be foul smelling. The frequency of defecation may be increased. Vomiting is relatively common, occurring in about 40% of hyperthyroid cats. Anorexia and watery diarrhea are less common but when present are usually seen in cats with severe hyperthyroidism or in those with coexistent primary intestinal problems. Abdominal pain has been noted in some thyrotoxic humans but has not been appreciated in cats. As with many of the signs attributed to hyperthyroidism, those associated with the gastrointestinal tract are noted less frequently than in the 1980s (Broussard et al, 1995). Their significance, however, is just as important.

EXPLANATION. Vomiting may result from direct action of thyroid hormone on the chemoreceptor trigger zone. Hyperthyroid cats that rapidly eat or overeat, or both, may vomit as a result of acute gastric distention. Vomiting is more common in hyperthyroid cats from multicat households, an environment that may contribute to rapid eating. One of the major gastrointestinal abnormalities is hypermotility with rapid gastric emptying and shortened small and large bowel transit times (Papasouliotis et al, 1993; Schlesinger et al, 1993). These disturbances contribute to both the increased frequency of defecation and the diarrhea.

Malabsorption with increased fecal fat excretion develops in approximately 25% of thyrotoxic humans but is less common in hyperthyroid cats. It is also likely that excessive fat intake resulting from polyphagia contributes to the increased fat excretion in some of these cats. Reversible abnormalities in pancreatic exocrine function may occur, although the exact mechanism for steatorrhea in hyperthyroidism is not always an enzyme deficiency. Pancreatic trypsin secretion has been reported to be reduced by as much as 50% in thyrotoxicosis. The catecholamine-like properties of thyroid hormone may account for depressed pancreatic enzyme secretion.

Hair loss/unkempt coat

SIGNS. Although an infrequent owner concern, hair coat changes (patchy alopecia, matted hair, lack of grooming behavior that may lead to matting or a seborrheic appearance, excessive grooming behavior with resulting alopecia) are found in a significant number of hyperthyroid cats. Problems of this nature have been identified in almost 40% of hyperthyroid cats (see Table 4-1). Like many signs associated with this disease, these problems are identified less frequently than a few years ago, with some investigators noting a dramatic decrease in incidence (from 50% in 1983 down to 9% in 1993) (Peterson, 1995a; Broussard et al, 1995). Typical bilaterally symmetric, nonpruritic "endocrine" alopecia is not often seen. Many cats have an unkempt, ungroomed hair coat. Some owners have reported seeing their cats pulling out hair in clumps, an unusual sign. Pulling out of hair may be a result of the heat intolerance seen in some cats. Heat intolerance is a classic sign of thyrotoxicosis in humans.

EXPLANATION. In humans with thyrotoxicosis, skin changes are caused by increased protein synthesis, vasodilation, and increased generation of heat. The heat causes a warm, moist feel to the skin, which results from the vasodilation occurring secondary to the hyperdynamic circulatory state. Thin, fine hair, sometimes with areas of alopecia, are typical of thyrotoxicosis in humans. Warm skin, which is typical of thyrotoxicosis, may be appreciated in the alopecic areas of cats (see Heat and Stress Intolerance, page 161).

Panting and respiratory distress

SIGN. Open-mouth breathing (panting) is rare in cats and is often associated with significant hyperthermia, congestive heart failure, respiratory disease, pleural effusion, pulmonary edema, or hyperthyroidism. Slightly more than 10% of hyperthyroid cats exhibit panting, dyspnea, or hyperventilation periodically at rest. Respiratory signs are more common (>20% of cats; see Table 4-1) with the stress of traveling, restraint, playing briefly with another cat or, potentially, heart failure.

EXPLANATION. Abnormalities in respiratory function described in humans with hyperthyroidism include decreased vital capacity, decreased pulmonary compliance, and increased minute ventilation (Ingbar, 1991). These changes are due to a combination of respiratory muscle weakness and increased carbon dioxide (CO_2) production. The alveolar and arterial partial pressures of oxygen (PO_2) and of carbon dioxide (PCO_2) are usually normal. Ventilatory responses to hypoxemia or hypercapnia are increased. Respiratory muscle weakness has been described in a hyperthyroid cat with hypokalemia, which again supports the recommendation that serum potassium concentrations be monitored in ill hyperthyroid cats (Nemzek et al, 1994).

Decreased appetite (apathetic hyperthyroidism)

SIGN. Although contradictory to the previously mentioned polyphagia, some hyperthyroid cats (about 14%) have been brought to veterinarians because of a diminished appetite (see Table 4-1). Some cats are polyphagic for months before progressing to inappetence or complete anorexia. This deterioration may correspond with the development of severe weight loss, muscle wasting, and weakness. The diminished appetite, therefore, is simply one component of progressive deterioration. Some cats have periods of polyphagia that alternate with periods of inappetence.

EXPLANATION. Humans with thyrotoxicosis uncommonly develop poor appetites or anorexia. There is a clinical form of human thyrotoxicosis called *apathetic hyperthyroidism* in which the typical hyperthyroid symptoms are replaced by apathy or extreme depression (Peake, 1986). These people are usually extremely ill, and their weight loss is associated with anorexia. Their condition is due in part to psychological disturbances associated with thyrotoxicosis. Severe cardiovascular disease may also be a common component of this syndrome. Thyrotoxic-induced thiamine deficiency may contribute to depression and anorexia (see Physical Examination, page 161).

Cats with a decreased appetite and profound weakness may have cardiac abnormalities that include arrhythmias or congestive heart failure. However, some other concurrent, severe, nonthyroidal illness may also be a complicating factor. It has been suggested that almost all cats with apathetic hyperthyroidism suffer from renal failure, cardiac disease, or neoplasia (Peterson, 2000). As discussed previously, a small number of these cats have pronounced ventroflexion of the head and neck, a condition that may result from thiamine deficiency, hypokalemia, or simply severe muscle weakness (Fig. 4-3, *D*) (Mooney, 1998a).

Weakness and lethargy

SIGN. Decreased activity, weakness, fatigability, and lethargy are variable findings in hyperthyroid cats, occurring in fewer than 15% of cats (see Table 4-1). Some cats are overactive and restless for 6 to 18 months before progressing to listlessness and weakness. With a few hyperthyroid cats, the first problem the owner notices is apparent weakness. Some chronically hyperthyroid cats have episodes of ataxia, whereas others can no longer jump as well or as high. A few cats develop severe cachexia and obvious weakness, requiring hand feeding and, in rare cases, tube feeding.

Weakness and fatigability are frequent complaints in humans with thyrotoxicosis. In a recent study, 67% of hyperthyroid people had complaints of muscle weakness, mainly in the proximal muscles of the legs, and 19% had symmetric distal sensory abnormalities and depressed distal tendon reflexes (Duyff et al, 2000). These patients often want to be active but are hampered by fatigue. They are often tired from "the neck down, rather than from the top of the head down." In most instances this weakness is not accompanied by objective evidence of local disease in the muscles, save for the generalized wasting seen with weight loss. In the extreme, these individuals may be unable to rise from a sitting or lying position and may be unable to walk.

EXPLANATION. The biochemical basis of the muscular weakness is uncertain, but the condition may simply be caused by weight loss and the catabolic state. Some hyperthyroid cats may be weak secondary to hypokalemia. Monitoring of serum potassium concentrations in weak hyperthyroid cats is strongly encouraged so that appropriate treatment can be instituted (Nemzek et al, 1994). Muscle weakness may also be related to the impaired ability of muscles in hyperthyroid individuals to phosphorylate creatine. On muscle biopsy, little if any inflammatory change is evident, but atrophy and infiltration by fat cells and lymphocytes have been reported. Electromyography reveals a decreased duration of mean action potentials and an increased percentage of polyphasic potentials. Thiamine deficiency may also explain the muscle weakness seen in some hyperthyroid cats.

Heat and stress intolerance

SIGN. Heat intolerance is a mild sign but one that may be obvious to some cat owners. The normal cat seems to seek a sunny spot on the floor to sleep, sleeps nestled against a heating register, curls itself within feet of a roaring fire, or lies on the hood of a car that is still warm from use. Cats that reverse heat-seeking behavior and are found sleeping in the bath tub or on cool tile floors are quickly noticed (Fig. 4-3, *C*). Although such behavior is observed in only 5% of hyperthyroid cats (see Table 4-1), some owners have claimed that their cats had always sought out cool areas.

In addition to heat intolerance, some hyperthyroid cats have an obvious impaired tolerance for stress. Brief car rides, bathing, and visits to boarding kennels or veterinary hospitals, for example, may cause some hyperthyroid cats to become severely weakened. Hyperthyroid cats can be extremely fragile, to the point that being held for a physical examination results in marked deterioration, respiratory distress, weakness, or even cardiac arrest. The clinician should always take into consideration this inability to cope with stress when diagnostic or therapeutic procedures are considered.

EXPLANATION. Heat intolerance and an inability to cope with stress are classic abnormalities in human thyrotoxicosis. The excess heat production can be manifested by a slightly elevated body temperature, a feature in some hyperthyroid cats. Many of the effects induced by increases in thyroid hormone are reminiscent of those induced by epinephrine, including calorigenesis, glycogenolysis, lipolysis, and tachycardia. Moreover, some of the clinical manifestations of thyrotoxicosis, among them heat intolerance, excessive sweating (in humans), tremor, and tachycardia, are at least partly alleviated by adrenergic antagonists that either deplete tissue stores or block the action of catecholamines. These observations may indicate that a state of increased adrenergic activity exists in thyrotoxicosis. However, no increase in catecholamine production occurs. The total serum catecholamine and dopamine β-hydroxylase concentrations are reduced in thyrotoxicosis. Catecholamine excretion and serum epinephrine concentrations are normal. In some tissues, however, thyroid hormone increases the number of adrenergic receptors, which could result in increased catecholamine sensitivity.

Ventroflexion of the head

Ventroflexion of the head is discussed under Decreased Appetite (Apathetic Hyperthyroidism), above, and in the following section, Physical Examination.

PHYSICAL EXAMINATION

General

Many of the signs described by an owner are also obvious to the veterinarian. Some changes may be more obvious or worrisome to the owner than to the veterinarian (e.g., weight loss, patchy alopecia/ unkempt hair coat; see Table 4-1), and others may be more obvious to the veterinarian (e.g., hyperactivity). Additional abnormalities may also be detected during a thorough physical examination. Some of these changes become obvious with experience, whereas others remain subtle (Table 4-3).

TABLE 4–3 PHYSICAL EXAMINATION FINDINGS ASSOCIATED WITH HYPERTHYROIDISM IN CATS

Finding	Percent of Cats
Palpable thyroid	91
Thin	71
Tachycardia (>240 beats/min)	48
Hyperactive/difficult to examine	48
Heart murmur	41
Skin changes (patchy alopecia, matting, dry coat, greasy seborrhea, thin skin)	36
Small kidneys	26
Increased rectal temperature	14
Gallop cardiac rhythm	12
Easily stressed	12
Dehydrated/cachectic appearance	11
Aggressive behavior	8
Premature cardiac beats	8
Increase nail growth	2
Depressed/weak	2
Ventroflexion of the neck	<1

Palpable Cervical Mass (Goiter)

NORMAL VERSUS HYPERTHYROID CATS. In healthy cats, the thyroid lobes are positioned just below the cricoid cartilage and extend ventrally over the first few tracheal rings; they lie dorsolateral to and on either side of the trachea. The thyroid lobes are not palpable in normal cats. Hyperthyroidism is invariably associated with enlargement of one or both thyroid lobes (goiter), an enlargement that is palpable in about 90% of hyperthyroid cats. Palpation of a cervical mass is not pathognomonic for hyperthyroidism, however, because some cats with palpable thyroids are *clinically* normal and because some cervical masses are not the thyroids. Nonetheless, because many clinically normal cats with thyroid gland enlargement eventually develop clinical hyperthyroidism, frequent monitoring of these cats is warranted (Graves and Peterson, 1990; 1992).

Because the thyroid lobes are only loosely attached to the trachea, the increased weight associated with the adenomatous hyperplasia or thyroid tumor causes migration of the lobes ventrally in the neck. In fact, the abnormal lobe (or lobes) may descend through the thoracic inlet and into the anterior mediastinum. This situation should be suspected in any hyperthyroid cat without a palpable goiter, although a small, non-palpable goiter is also possible. Careful palpation is required to locate a goiter, which can be difficult in a restless or agitated cat.

PALPATION TECHNIQUE. Palpation of the thyroid glands in the cat is analogous to assessing the size and shape of the popliteal lymph nodes (using thumb and index finger with gentle manipulation over the site). Evaluation of the thyroid area should be part of the physical examination of every cat seen by a veterinarian. This allows the clinician to develop expertise and confidence when palpating a cat suspected of having hyperthyroidism, and it occasionally allows identification of a mass that would otherwise go undetected.

For the evaluation, the cat's head should be gently extended. The thumb and index finger of one hand are gently placed on either side of the trachea in the jugular furrows at the thoracic inlet. The area is gently compressed, and the fingers are smoothly slid up to the larynx and back down again to the thoracic inlet. The fingertips should remain within the jugular furrows. Thyroid enlargement is usually felt as a somewhat movable, subcutaneous nodule approximately one half the size of the popliteal lymph node. Thyroid size in most hyperthyroid cats varies from the size of a lentil to the size of a lima bean. Occasionally, extremely large masses may be detected, such as one reported to be $4 \times 7 \times 10$ cm), but masses this large are rare (Hofmeister et al, 2001). Thyroid tissue, if present and enlarged, "slips" under the fingertips.

In many instances we have been able to have owners visualize a goiter by having them watch the neck of their cat after we have moistened the area with alcohol, as our fingers slide toward the thoracic inlet, causing the enlarged thyroid to "pop up." Success in this maneuver depends on not squeezing too hard; the pressure exerted must be gentle enough to allow the abnormal nodule to slide under the fingertips but firm enough to detect the mass. Also, for demonstration purposes, the ventrocervical area can be clipped free of hair and moistened. Occasionally this process allows easy visualization of a cervical mass (Fig. 4-4). Palpation of the neck is performed with greater confidence once a goiter can be seen.

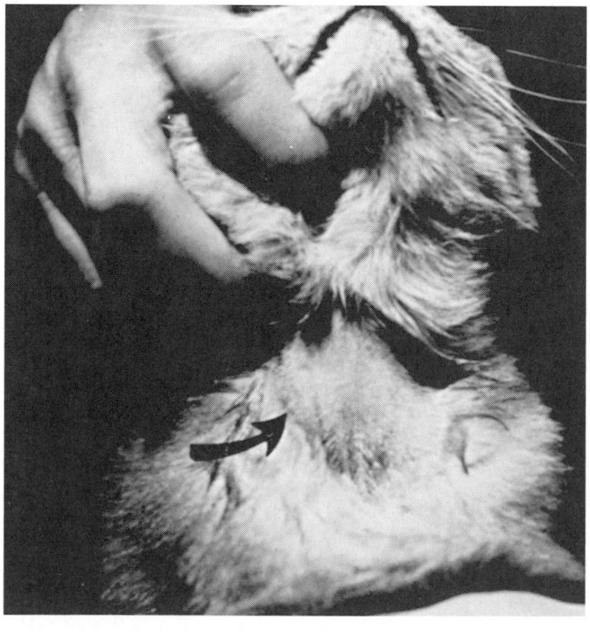

FIGURE 4–4. The clipped ventrocervical area of a cat with a large, obvious goiter *(arrow)*. Even when apparently obvious, a goiter can be missed on a physical examination.

Cardiac Disturbances

TACHYCARDIA, MURMURS, PREMATURE BEATS, AND GALLOP RHYTHM. Many hyperthyroid cats have clinical evidence of heart disease. In addition, the various findings ascribed to cardiac disease make identification of these abnormalities relatively common. The common cardiovascular abnormalities include systolic murmurs, tachycardia, and gallop rhythms. Less commonly, arrhythmias and signs of congestive heart failure may be detected. Signs of failure include dyspnea, muffled heart sounds, and ascites.

Because thin cats have relatively easily heard (loud) heart sounds, the clinician may develop a suspicion of heart disease. Furthermore, tachycardia in cats is a common finding, especially since veterinarians tend to compare the heart rates of cats with those of dogs. Heart rates greater than 240 beats per minute are typical of nervous cats, hyperthyroid cats, and some primary heart diseases. In addition, premature cardiac contractions associated with pulse deficits, gallop rhythms, murmurs, and pleural effusion (causing muffled heart sounds) are suggestive of primary heart disease, but these must also be considered consistent with thyrotoxicosis. Premature contractions are likely the result of myocardial irritation due to poor oxygenation, whereas murmurs may be exacerbated by either dilated or hypertrophic forms of cardiomyopathy associated with chronic thyrotoxicosis. Gallop rhythms may be associated with heart failure due to any cause. Many of the clinical findings suggestive of heart disease are also associated with hyperthyroidism (see Table 4-3). For these reasons, clinicians must maintain a high index of suspicion for hyperthyroidism in an aged cat with cardiac signs. Veterinarians must also be aware that these two diseases may occur concurrently.

Some hyperthyroid cats have predominating signs of cardiovascular or respiratory disease. Clinicians are challenged to remember a complete list of disorders that belong in the differential diagnosis (including hyperthyroidism). In addition to abnormalities directly associated with cardiac disease, other signs such as dyspnea, muffled heart sounds, and ascites may be detected and assumed to result from a primary cardiac disorder rather than from hyperthyroidism. Hyperthyroidism in cats can induce a variety of cardiac-related disturbances, most notably secondary cardiomyopathies. Hypertrophic cardiomyopathies are much more common in these cats than the dilated type. Either form of cardiomyopathy may result in heart failure, with severe failure more common among hyperthyroid cats with the dilated form of cardiomyopathy (Jacobs and Panciera, 1992).

As is true of the various signs and physical examination findings among hyperthyroid cats, cardiac-related abnormalities are less common now than in the 1980s. As the index of suspicion increases and as cats are diagnosed earlier in the course of the disease, many signs are less prominent and/or less severe than they were when affected cats were more severely debilitated because the disease was not as well recognized.

EXPLANATION. Hyperthyroidism can result in a high-output cardiac state in which vascular resistance is low and cardiac output high. This condition is due to the direct effects of thyroid hormone on cardiac muscle plus interactions between thyroid hormone and the sympathetic nervous system. The high-output state is also enhanced by increased metabolic rates and oxygen requirements in various tissues. Volume overload is created by low peripheral vascular resistance coupled with renal mechanisms to conserve fluid (sodium retention, which leads to water retention and then increases in blood volume). The principal cardiac compensatory mechanisms in high-output conditions are chamber dilation, in response to the increasing volumes of blood, and hypertrophy, in response to the increased work demand on the myocardium.

In humans with hyperthyroidism, heart rate, stroke volume, and cardiac output often increase but peripheral resistance decreases. These changes are due to the positive inotropic and chronotropic effects of thyroid hormone and to the increased peripheral oxygen requirements resulting from the thyrotoxicosis-induced increased basal metabolic rate. Peripheral arteriovenous oxygen differences may be normal or decreased (Spaulding and Utiger, 1981). Although cardiac output is increased, regional blood flow is not uniformly increased; skin (in an effort to dissipate the excess heat produced), muscle, cerebral, and coronary blood flows are increased, whereas hepatic blood flow is not. Other adaptive mechanisms that augment peripheral oxygen delivery include increases in red blood cell mass and in red blood cell 2,3-diphosphoglyceric acid concentrations.

Thyroid hormone was thought to exert inotropic and chronotropic effects largely through the adrenergic nervous system by sensitizing a catecholamine-responsive adenylate cyclase–cAMP system in the myocardium. However, inotropic and chronotropic effects appear to be directly mediated by activation of a thyroid hormone–specific adenylate cyclase–cAMP system. Nevertheless, catecholamine-dependent mechanisms may influence the development of many cardiac disturbances associated with hyperthyroidism, including sinus tachycardia and atrial arrhythmias. Some amelioration of the hemodynamic manifestations of thyrotoxicosis accompanies treatment with adrenergic antagonists that do not alter thyroid hormone concentrations. Excessive concentrations of circulating thyroid hormone may alter effective sympathetic drive, either by directly increasing the activity of the sympathetic nervous system or by increasing cardiovascular response to normal sympathetic stimulation. Catecholamine concentrations in the plasma and urine of thyrotoxic humans are normal, and an increased responsiveness to normal sympathetic stimulation is likely. Excess thyroid hormone increases cardiac responsiveness to circulating catecholamines by increasing the number or affinity of cardiac β-adrenergic receptors (Tse et al, 1980).

Excess thyroid hormone causes a switch in cardiac myosin isoenzyme distribution from a predominance of low adenosine triphosphatase (ATPase) activity to appreciably higher activity (Chizzonite et al, 1982; Litten et al, 1982). Because myosin ATPase activity is closely linked to the intrinsic contractile state of the heart, this may partly explain the increase in cardiac performance observed in hyperthyroidism.

Hyperactivity/"Easily Stressed"

Only about 40% of owners believe their hyperthyroid cats are hyperactive (see Table 4-1), whereas to veterinarians a larger percentage of these cats seem hyperactive (see Table 4-3). The objective opinion of an examining veterinarian is perhaps more valid. The owner observes the cat on a daily basis and is less likely to be aware of changes that take place gradually. An active cat is not usually considered abnormal; this sign is less likely to arouse an owner's concern than is severe weight loss, vomiting, or diarrhea. Some hyperactive cats are in fact quite fragile, and the use of restraint for examination, obtaining blood samples, or taking radiographs can cause collapse. This fragile condition must be respected.

Dehydration/Cachexia/Weakness

SIGN. Perhaps the most obvious sign of hyperthyroidism is weight loss. It is not surprising that weight loss continues to be observed in more than 90% of hyperthyroid cats. This sign is classic for the syndrome, easily detected, and considered worrisome by most owners. Over the past 10 to 15 years, however, the number of hyperthyroid cats considered *cachectic* (severely emaciated) and/or "dehydrated" has plummeted from greater than 60% in 1986 to approximately 10% over the past few years (see Table 4-3). This decrease in incidence most likely reflects the fact that hyperthyroidism now is diagnosed earlier in the course of the illness, with fewer cats allowed to become severely debilitated by the condition. Weakness is also associated with cachexia and is a sign of chronic hyperthyroidism or concurrent illness.

EXPLANATION. Weight loss is accompanied by progressive loss of skin elasticity and turgidity. Many severely hyperthyroid, cachectic cats appear moderately to markedly dehydrated based on lack of skin turgidity. Although the skin does not rapidly return to place in most of these cats, this is a reflection of severe weight loss, not dehydration. If fluid replacement therapy is deemed necessary, it should be accomplished slowly and with careful monitoring. Weakness may be due to chronic illness and muscle wasting, which are typical of hyperthyroidism. Weakness may also be due to cardiac dysfunction or may occur secondary to a variety of problems (e.g., renal or gastrointestinal disorders) commonly observed in this condition. Weakness may also be due to thiamine deficiency or significant hypokalemia.

Small Kidneys

SIGN. A decrease in kidney size on palpation is not suggestive of or consistent with feline hyperthyroidism. However, both thyrotoxicosis and chronic renal failure may be associated with polydipsia, polyuria, weight loss, vomiting, and anorexia. Thus an older cat with these signs and small kidneys on physical examination may be thought to have primary renal disease. Many older, hyperthyroid cats have concurrent impairment of renal function, which complicates the diagnostic picture. As with heart disease, older cats with signs and/or test results suggestive of renal failure should be checked for concurrent thyrotoxicosis.

IMPORTANCE. As described earlier in the section on polydipsia and polyuria, a dilemma arises regarding treatment of cats for hyperthyroidism when renal function test results are borderline or abnormal. It could be argued that reduction of serum thyroid hormone concentrations in older cats with mild hyperthyroidism and chronic renal disease should be avoided because treatment may reduce the GFR and allow the emergence of significant azotemia. However, if an increased GFR results in glomerular hyperfiltration in hyperthyroid cats, the endocrine disorder may contribute to progression of renal disease. If so, hyperthyroidism may predispose cats to chronic renal disease, and early effective treatment of the thyroid disorder may slow pathologic changes in the kidneys that could lead to progressive failure. These concerns are addressed in the therapy section of this chapter, but conservative, reversible oral treatment and monitoring of renal function are recommended before a more permanent form of therapy is considered.

Ventroflexion of the Head (Thiamine or Potassium Deficiency)

SIGN. A small number of hyperthyroid cats have pronounced ventroflexion of the head (see Fig. 4-3, *D*). This abnormality, although rare, is striking when present. The head of an affected cat can be lifted without difficulty, but the cat immediately resumes the abnormal posture when released. Signs usually seen in association with the ventroflexion are anorexia, mild ataxia, and mydriasis, which are signs consistent with thiamine or potassium deficiency. Ventroflexion has also been noted in hypertensive cats, but it is not known whether there is a cause-and-effect relationship between these two problems. If so, it is assumed that hypertension could cause a cerebrovascular accident with secondary ventroflexion (Maggio et al, 2000) (see Blood Pressure and Hypertension, page 169).

EXPLANATION. Hyperthyroidism may cause vitamin deficiencies secondary to polyuria, malabsorption, diarrhea, vomiting, and anorexia. Thiamine deficiency results in striking features seen on the physical examination, including ventroflexion of the head. Thiamine deficiency causes lesions in the periventricular gray matter of the brain stem, archicerebellum, and cerebral cortex. Treatment for thiamine deficiency should be instituted in any cat with appropriate clinical signs. Therapy with 1 to 2 mg of thiamine hydrochloride, given intramuscularly daily, usually results in clinical improvement. Parenteral thiamine therapy is warranted until the clinical signs resolve and the cat is eating normally. Oral vitamin supplementation with a multiple vitamin B complex preparation should be continued until the hyperthyroid state has been corrected.

Before thiamine therapy is begun, the serum potassium concentration should be assessed in weak cats with or without ventroflexion of the head. Potassium depletion can occur secondary to vomiting, diarrhea, anorexia, or excess urine loss and can result in the same clinical signs as thiamine deficiency. Hypokalemia can be quickly demonstrated with serum evaluations. Treatment is straightforward, using potassium-supplemented parenteral fluid therapy (Lievesly and Gruffydd-Jones, 1989; Willard, 1989; Nemzek et al, 1994).

Ocular Lesions

See also Blood Pressure and Hypertension, page 169.

BACKGROUND. Hyperthyroidism is one of the more common causes of systemic hypertension in cats. Retinopathy is indicative of substantial hypertension that warrants investigation into possible causes and specific treatment. In a study by Maggio and colleagues (2000) of 69 cats with hypertensive retinopathy, a clearly identifiable cause for hypertension was not detected in 38 cats; 26 of these 38 had mild azotemia, and 12 had normal renal function. Chronic renal failure was diagnosed in 22 cats and hyperthyroidism in five cats. For this reason, although not as common as "primary" hypertension or that occurring secondary to chronic renal failure, hyperthyroidism must be considered a differential diagnosis in cats brought to the veterinarian for treatment of acute blindness or retinal edema, hemorrhage, or detachment (see Blood Pressure and Hypertension, page 169).

PREVALENCE. Ophthalmic examinations, including slitlamp biomicroscopy and indirect ophthalmoscopy, was performed by a veterinary ophthalmologist in 100 hyperthyroid cats and 30 controls. There were no ophthalmologic abnormalities more common in hyperthyroid cats than in euthyroid cats. Two hyperthyroid cats had retinal changes consistent with hypertensive retinopathy, including retinal hemorrhage and focal retinal detachment with subretinal effusion. The authors concluded that ocular abnormalities are uncommon in hyperthyroid cats (Van der Woerdt and Peterson, 2000).

IN-HOSPITAL DIAGNOSTIC EVALUATION

Background

Cats with hyperthyroidism may have abnormalities involving several organ systems, and these abnormalities, on an individual basis, may or may not arise

TABLE 4–4 LABORATORY ABNORMALITIES ON ROUTINE TESTING OF HYPERTHYROID CATS

Test	Percent of Cats
Complete Blood Counts (CBC)	
Erythrocytosis	39
Increase in MCV	27
Leukocytosis	19
Lymphopenia	22
Eosinopenia	13
Serum Chemistry Profile	
Increased ALT	85
Increased SAP	62
Azotemia (Increased BUN)	26
Increased creatinine	23
Hyperphosphatemia	18
Electrolyte abnormalities	11
Hyperbilirubinemia	3
Hyperglycemia	5
Urinalysis	
Specific gravity >1.035	63
Specific gravity <1.015	4
Glucosuria	4
Inflammation/infection	2

secondary to thyrotoxicosis (Table 4-4). The veterinarian must be aware of concurrent disorders because some require immediate attention. Cats should be evaluated with screening tests to help identify concurrent disorders, in addition to ultimately determining a diagnosis of hyperthyroidism. Minimum testing should include a complete blood count (CBC), serum biochemistry profile, urinalysis, and serum T_4 concentration. Thoracic radiography, electrocardiography, blood pressure, and other studies are usually warranted. Despite the trend toward diagnosing hyperthyroidism earlier in the course of the disease, before owners have identified many serious problems, the relative frequency of laboratory abnormalities has not changed much over the past 5 to 10 years. Routine laboratory evaluation provides valuable indicators of thyrotoxicosis and helps detect concurrent problems. The specific hormone tests for thyroid status are reliable and relatively inexpensive.

Complete Blood Count (CBC)

RED BLOOD CELLS. The red blood cell count, hematocrit, and red blood cell indices are usually normal in hyperthyroid cats (see Table 4-4). Approximately 40% to 50% of hyperthyroid cats have a mild elevation in the packed cell volume (PCV) (Broussard et al, 1995). The increase in the red blood cell count may be directly related to thyrotoxicosis, because this has been seen in humans and in clinically normal dogs given large doses of thyroid hormone. The erythrocytosis of hyperthyroidism may result from a direct effect of thyroid hormone on bone marrow erythroid precursors, an effect mediated by a β-adrenergic receptor. Thyroid hormones may also stimulate the production of erythropoietin (Mooney, 1998a). By increasing the rate of red blood cell differentiation and decreasing total red blood cell maturation time, an excess of erythropoietin would cause release of macrocytic erythrocytes into the circulation (Peschle, 1980).

Approximately 20% of hyperthyroid cats have macrocytosis (Broussard et al, 1995). This helps explain why some cats have an elevated PCV but a normal red blood cell count and hemoglobin concentration. The red blood cell mass may increase in response to an increase in oxygen requirements or in the basal metabolic rate. Increased oxygen demand would be mediated by an increase in erythropoietin secretion. In addition, oxygen release from hemoglobin is increased in thyrotoxicosis due to an increase in the red blood cell content of 2,3-diphosphoglyceric acid. This substance enhances the dissociation of oxygen from hemoglobin by virtue of its ability to bind hemoglobin and stabilize its reduced form.

Anemia is a rare complication of hyperthyroidism that, in humans, can be related to bone marrow exhaustion, a deficiency in iron, or deficiencies in other micronutrients (Mooney, 1998a). Heinz body formation may be a complicating factor in cats (Christopher, 1989). If anemia is documented, a cause should be sought prior to treatment of the cat for hyperthyroidism, because anemia is an uncommon component of the syndrome.

WHITE BLOOD CELLS. Hyperthyroid cats tend to demonstrate a typical stress response with leukocytosis, neutrophilia, and an associated shift toward immaturity of the neutrophils, lymphopenia, and eosinopenia. In our hyperthyroid cats, a neutrophilic leukocytosis was not frequently seen, and when observed, it was not usually associated with an active bacterial infection.

PLATELETS AND CLOTTING. In humans with thyrotoxicosis, platelet counts and the intrinsic clotting mechanisms are normal. However, the concentration of Factor VIII is often increased, perhaps as a result of increased adrenergic activity. This may predispose a cat to intravascular thrombosis. Problems with hemorrhage, clotting, or thrombosis are not features of hyperthyroidism in cats. Hyperthyroid cats have been demonstrated to have larger platelets than normal controls, but differences were not observed in platelet counts or hematocrits (Sullivan et al, 1993).

Urinalysis

RESULTS. Urinalysis evaluation is an integral component of the attempt to determine why an animal is ill. Because approximately 33% of hyperthyroid cats have increases in the blood urea nitrogen (BUN) or serum creatinine concentration and because it is common for these cats to be described as polydipsic and polyuric and/or to appear dehydrated (see Tables 4-1, 4-3, and 4-4), renal problems are often suspected. These evaluations gain value as long as no result is taken out of context; that is, many abnormalities are explained

when hyperthyroidism is confirmed. The urine specific gravity has ranged from 1.006 to greater than 1.060 among hyperthyroid cats.

IMPORTANCE. Measurement of the specific gravity is useful for differentiating prerenal uremia from primary renal disease and for recognizing such disorders as diabetes mellitus and urinary tract infections. A significant number of hyperthyroid cats have some degree of renal insufficiency, and a smaller number have evidence of infection or diabetes mellitus on urinalysis. As discussed in the sections on polydipsia/polyuria and kidney size, determining which hyperthyroid cats have renal function abnormalities that are likely to improve with resolution of the hyperthyroid condition and which cats have renal abnormalities that will become worse remains a dilemma. Careful management and monitoring of these cats are warranted and recommended.

Serum Chemistry Profile

Liver enzyme activities

RESULTS. Abnormal liver enzymes are among the most frequently observed screening test alterations seen in hyperthyroid cats (see Table 4-4). More than 75% of hyperthyroid cats exhibit abnormalities in serum alanine aminotransferase (ALT) or serum alkaline phosphatase (SAP) activities, and more than 90% show increases of at least one of these enzymes. Most of these abnormalities are considered mild to moderate (normal values <100 IU/L; hyperthyroid cats, usually 100 to 400 IU/L). Hyperthyroid cats with liver enzyme activities greater than 500 IU/L should be considered likely candidates for serious concurrent disease. In these cats, abdominal (liver) ultrasonography should be recommended and liver biopsy strongly considered. A number of our cats with marked increases in liver enzyme activities were found on liver biopsy to have significant concurrent disease, such as cholangiohepatitis or lymphosarcoma. However, increases in SAP activities are as likely to occur secondary to changes in bone metabolism as they are to be due to hepatic abnormalities.

ALTERED BONE METABOLISM (BONE ISOENZYMES). People with hyperthyroidism, regardless of its etiology, have some degree of bone loss, as demonstrated via assessment of bone mineral density (Jodar et al, 1997). They commonly have increases in serum bone isoenzymes of alkaline phosphatase, osteocalcin, calcium, and phosphorus (Duda et al, 1988). These changes in the bone isoenzyme have been associated with increased bone metabolism attributed to the direct effects of thyroid hormones on bone cells.

In hyperthyroid cats, increases in serum alkaline phosphatase activities have been associated with increases in both bone and liver isoenzymes (Horney et al, 1994). In a study on 36 cats with naturally occurring hyperthyroidism, all had marked increases in the bone isoenzyme of their serum alkaline phosphatase activity. Osteocalcin was increased in 44% of the cats.

There were no correlations in magnitude of serum alkaline phosphatase bone isoenzyme, osteocalcin, and serum thyroxine concentrations. Increases in serum phosphorus was found in 35% of the cats. Total calcium concentrations were consistently within reference limits, but 50% of the cats had decreases in the serum ionized calcium concentration (Archer and Taylor, 1996). It was concluded, in this and subsequent studies, that hyperthyroid cats have altered bone metabolism and that hepatic abnormalities represent only one of two common sources of this enzyme (Foster and Thoday, 2000). However, no clinical signs attributed to altered bone metabolism have been reported in hyperthyroid cats.

LIVER DYSFUNCTION. Minor abnormalities in hepatic function test results are present in 33% to 60% of people with hyperthyroidism (Gurlek et al, 1997; Biscoveanu and Hasinski, 2000). Hepatic enzyme activity abnormalities may be due in part to malnutrition, congestive heart failure, infection, and direct toxic effects of thyroid hormones on the liver. Hepatic hypoxia is thought to be the major cause of abnormalities in liver enzyme values. Splanchnic bed oxygen consumption is increased, although its blood flow is essentially unchanged in thyrotoxicosis. As a result, the arteriovenous oxygen difference across the splanchnic bed is greater. This oxygen deficit, together with the increased metabolic rate and a relative state of caloric deprivation, may also account for depletion of hepatic glycogen stores.

Another explanation for abnormal hepatic test results is congestion that occurs secondary to cardiac dysfunction. In humans, because these abnormalities do not predict the occurrence of hepatotoxicity in patients treated with antithyroid drugs, it is recommended that no further action be taken regarding the finding of abnormal test results until the hyperthyroidism has been treated (Utiger, 2002a). In the absence of severe thyrotoxicosis or congestive heart failure, the liver is usually histologically unremarkable.

In the hyperthyroid cats we have studied, liver biopsies have revealed increased pigment within hepatocytes, aggregates of mixed inflammatory cells in the portal regions, and focal areas of fatty degeneration. Some have mild hepatic necrosis. In severe cases of thyrotoxicosis, centrilobular fatty infiltration may occur, together with patchy portal fibrosis, lymphocytic infiltration, and proliferation of bile ducts. The fatty infiltrate may indicate that some cats, especially those that are anorexic, may be developing hepatic lipidosis. Serum ALT activity is specific for hepatic necrosis in humans and in cats. Liver enzyme activities, regardless of their origin, usually return to normal with successful management of the hyperthyroidism (Mooney et al, 1992a).

Blood glucose

RESULTS. Cats have a remarkable ability to increase their blood glucose concentrations in response to acute stress. Acutely stressed cats can have blood glucose concentrations as high as 400 to 500 mg/dl. This hyperglycemia is believed to result from an acute release of epinephrine. Although hyperthyroid cats are definitely "stressed," their stress is chronic and persistent, perhaps accounting for a majority having normal blood glucose concentrations on random sampling (see Table 4-4). Those uncommon cats with blood glucose concentrations persistently greater than 200 mg/dl (5% of hyperthyroid cats) were found to have both diabetes mellitus and hyperthyroidism.

EXPLANATION. In humans, the increased energy expenditure of thyrotoxicosis is compounded by the inefficient maintenance of basic physiologic functions. To counterbalance these processes, increases in food consumption, utilization of stored energy, and enhanced oxygen expenditure alter the metabolism of carbohydrate, lipid, and protein. Intestinal absorption of glucose and the rate of glucose production from glycogen, lactate, glycerol, and amino acids are increased. Hepatic glycogen stores are decreased, owing to increased glucose utilization by muscle and adipose tissue. Plasma glucose and insulin responses to an oral glucose load are usually normal. However, hyperthyroid cats, like thyrotoxic humans, have some degree of glucose intolerance, possibly due to peripheral insulin resistance (Hoenig and Ferguson, 1989). Hyperthyroidism, like diestrus and hyperadrenocorticism, may exaggerate insulin secretory deficiencies. In cats with preexisting diabetes mellitus, accelerated insulin catabolism increases requirements for exogenous insulin (see Serum Fructosamine, page 169).

BUN and creatinine

RESULTS. Renal blood flow, the GFR, and renal tubular resorptive and secretory capacities may be increased or decreased in cats with hyperthyroidism. Which cats have increased blood flow to the kidneys and which have decreased flow is not easily determined prior to therapy. The only clinical sign usually referable to the urinary system is polyuria. Signs of polydipsia, weight loss, and apparent dehydration in an elderly cat are consistent with hyperthyroidism, diabetes mellitus, renal failure, and other disorders. Cats with increases in BUN and creatinine are a diagnostic challenge. More than 25% of hyperthyroid cats are mildly to severely azotemic (see Table 4-4). Management of the hyperthyroid cat that has abnormal or borderline renal function test results is both challenging and controversial. The reader is referred to the treatment section of this chapter for a complete discussion of this topic (see page 192).

EXPLANATION. A recognized single mechanism for the development of azotemia in hyperthyroid cats has not been appreciated. Thyroid hormones have a diuretic action, and the condition may impair urine concentrating ability by increasing total renal blood flow and decreasing renal medullary solute concentration. However, increased protein catabolism and prerenal uremia from reduced renal perfusion due to hyperthyroid-induced decreased cardiac output may also play a role. Some cats have primary renal disease concurrent with hyperthyroidism, and the renal problems may be masked by the thyroid problem. Others suffer complications of reduced cardiac output due to primary heart disease. The clinician must manage azotemic hyperthyroid cats as individuals rather than follow a "cookbook" protocol. Treatment using oral methimazole, which is reversible, is recommended because many cats have a reduced GFR and worsening renal function after successful treatment of hyperthyroidism (Graves et al, 1994; DiBartola et al, 1996). If renal parameters improve with resolution of the hyperthyroidism, more permanent treatment measures (surgery or radioactive iodine) can be considered. If renal parameters worsen, it is wise to tailor treatment to the needs of each cat and owner to minimize signs related to hyperthyroidism without worsening the azotemia.

Calcium, phosphorus, and parathyroid hormone (PTH)

RESULTS. In a study by Barber and Elliott (1996), 30 cats with untreated hyperthyroidism were documented to have blood ionized calcium and plasma creatinine concentrations below reference limits. Most hyperthyroid cats have a normal serum total calcium concentration, but these cats had significantly higher plasma phosphate and PTH concentrations (see Table 4-4). Hyperparathyroidism occurred in 77% of the cats, with PTH concentrations reaching up to 19 times the upper limit of the reference range. As previously discussed, osteocalcin and 1,25–vitamin D concentrations tend to be increased in hyperthyroid cats (Archer and Taylor, 1996). As cats with hyperthyroidism have come to be diagnosed earlier in the course of the disease, the percentage of cats with hyperphosphatemia has declined over the past 5 to 10 years from as many as 50% to current levels of 10% to 20%. As a group their serum phosphate concentrations remain significantly increased.

The finding of azotemia or hyperphosphatemia in an older cat with polydipsia, polyuria, and weight loss is consistent with chronic renal failure. However, these alterations also can occur secondary to hyperthyroidism. Azotemia was identified more frequently in hyperthyroid cats than were alterations in the serum calcium or phosphorus concentration. Not all cats with renal insufficiency had hyperphosphatemia.

EXPLANATION

Humans. The relationship between the thyroid gland, bone, and mineral metabolism is complex. Changes in the structure of bone and in the metabolism of calcium and phosphorus have been ascribed to direct effects of thyroid hormone. Thyrotoxic bone disease is explained in part by increases in osteoclastic activity and calcium release documented in bone culture systems. Histomorphometry of tetracycline-labeled bone biopsies from people with hyperthyroidism show increases in the number of active bone remodeling units, causing negative bone balance (Eriksen et al, 1985). The net bone loss leads to calcium

release, negative feedback to the parathyroid glands, and hypoparathyroidism (Fraser et al, 1991). The augmented skeletal calcium resorption may also induce a compensatory decrease in serum 1,25–vitamin D concentrations (Spaulding and Utiger, 1981). Decreases in parathyroid function would result in decreased gastrointestinal calcium absorption, increased excretion of calcium in the urine and stool, and increased renal tubular resorption of phosphate. The biochemical result is increased serum phosphate and normal to decreased serum calcium concentrations. Calcitonin, which is secreted by the thyroid gland and has effects generally antagonistic to those of parathyroid hormone, may also play a role.

Cats. In the study by Barber and Elliott (1996) on 30 cats with untreated hyperthyroidism, the syndrome appeared to be quite different from that in humans. It has been demonstrated that hyperparathyroidism is common in hyperthyroid cats. The condition appears to arise secondary to the hyperphosphatemia and decreases in serum ionized calcium. With hyperparathyroidism occurring in 77% of the hyperthyroid cats, the combined resorptive effects of excess PTH and thyroid hormones may have significant consequences for skeletal integrity. High phosphate concentrations may predispose cats to soft tissue calcification, which may in turn adversely affect renal function. However, bone problems and soft tissue calcification are not commonly reported in hyperthyroid cats, nor have such problems been recognized in our series of hyperthyroid cats. Therefore the significance of hyperparathyroidism in cats with hyperthyroidism remains to be established.

Cholesterol

Serum cholesterol concentrations are usually normal in hyperthyroid cats. The synthesis and especially clearance of cholesterol and triglycerides are increased in hyperthyroidism, resulting in modest reductions in both the serum cholesterol and triglyceride concentrations. Lipolysis is also accelerated, resulting in increased plasma free fatty acid concentrations.

Total protein and albumin

The concentrations of serum proteins are usually normal in hyperthyroid cats. Although not of particular value in arriving at a diagnosis, these findings are helpful in dismissing dehydration as a diagnosis in some thin and cachectic cats.

Sodium and potassium

Serum sodium and potassium concentrations have been normal in almost all our hyperthyroid cats. Abnormalities, when present, were usually mild, although hypokalemia, when severe, can cause significant muscle weakness, including ventroflexion of the head. For weak cats with hyperthyroidism, the serum electrolyte concentrations should be monitored and treatment should be directed at correcting detected abnormalities. Total body water and potassium are usually decreased, possibly because of a decrease in lean body mass, but sodium tends to be increased.

Fecal Fat (Steatorrhea)

Malabsorption with steatorrhea is recognized in many hyperthyroid cats that have diarrhea. Malabsorption with steatorrhea in thyrotoxic humans is thought to be related to a relative deficiency of pancreatic trypsin. Decreased pancreatic enzyme secretion is believed to result from the catecholamine-like properties of thyroid hormone. Fecal fat excretion also varies with dietary fat intake. Those cats that ingested the greatest amount of fat had the most marked steatorrhea (Peterson et al, 1983). The daily fecal fat excretion in these cats was two to 15 times higher than the upper limit of normal. The percentage of fat absorbed from the intestine remained constant regardless of the dietary intake. The mean percentage of fat digestibility, calculated as the difference between the amount of fat ingested and the amount excreted divided by the amount ingested, was significantly reduced in thyrotoxic cats (Peterson et al, 1983). Therefore the polyphagia seen in thyrotoxicosis contributes to the steatorrhea.

Plasma Cortisol

Adrenocortical hyperplasia, an uncommon finding in cats, was found in one third of hyperthyroid cats in one study (Liu et al, 1984). In thyrotoxic humans, the metabolic clearance rates of cortisol and aldosterone are increased, leading to increased rates of secretion. Therefore adrenocortical hyperplasia in thyrotoxicosis appears to represent a compensatory response. Studies on plasma cortisol concentrations in hyperthyroid cats have not been reported, although the combination of hyperthyroidism and hyperadrenocorticism is rare.

Serum Fructosamine

Fructosamine is produced by an irreversible reaction between glucose and plasma proteins. Serum fructosamine concentrations in cats are thought to reflect the mean blood glucose concentration during the preceding 1 to 2 weeks. However, fructosamine concentrations are also affected by the concentration and metabolism of serum proteins. Because hyperthyroidism can have a profound effect on protein metabolism, fructosamine concentrations may also be affected. This concept was evaluated and serum fructosamine concentrations were documented to be significantly lower in hyperthyroid cats versus healthy controls (Reusch and Tomsa, 1999). Fifty percent of hyperthyroid cats had serum fructosamine concentrations less than the reference range. Serum fructosamine concentrations in hyperthyroid, normo-

proteinemic cats did not differ from values in hypoproteinemic cats. During treatment for hyperthyroidism, an increase in serum fructosamine concentration was detected. It was concluded that the concentration of serum fructosamine in hyperthyroid cats may be low because of accelerated protein turnover, independent of blood glucose concentration. For these reasons, the serum fructosamine concentration should not be considered a reliable monitoring tool in hyperthyroid cats with concurrent diabetes mellitus. Additionally, serum fructosamine concentrations should not be considered reliable for differentiating between diabetes mellitus and transitory stress-related hyperglycemia in hyperthyroid cats (Reusch and Tomsa, 1999).

Blood Pressure and Hypertension

Hypertension (persistent systolic blood pressure readings of 160 to 170 mmHg or higher) is a recognized problem in older cats (Henik, 1997). It is not yet known how common hypertension may be in cats, especially considering the potential rise in blood pressure associated just with being brought to a veterinary hospital (the "white coat effect") (Belew et al, 1999). Regardless, hypertension has been well documented in cats with chronic renal failure, cardiac disease, or without an obvious underlying etiology (primary hypertension) and less commonly in cats with hyperthyroidism (Kobayashi et al, 1990; Littman, 1994; Bodey and Samson, 1998). Hypertension may be suspected clinically in cats with hyperemia of the ear pinnae and mucous membranes. More seriously, hypertensive cats are at risk for developing retinal hemorrhage, edema, partial or complete detachment, or degeneration (Stiles et al, 1994; Maggio et al, 2000; Elliott et al, 2001). Cerebrovascular thrombosis ("accidents") are possible and may explain the disorientation, vestibular signs, ataxia, seizures, stupor, tremors, paraparesis, and ventroflexion diagnosed in some hypertensive cats.

It has been recommended that blood pressure monitoring and funduscopic evaluations be performed routinely in cats "at risk" for hypertension. At-risk cats include those with hyperthyroidism with or without concurrent azotemia. It was suggested that hyperthyroidism can cause hypertension by means of increased β-adrenergic activity that induces tachycardia, increased myocardial contractility, systemic vasodilation, and activation of the renin-angiotensin-aldosterone system. Although mild to moderate increases in systemic blood pressure have been documented in as many as 87% of hyperthyroid cats (Kobayashi et al, 1990), studies on feline hypertension have identified a relatively small prevalence of hyperthyroidism. Additionally, in a large population of hyperthyroid cats, obvious ocular signs, such as blindness, were not reported (Peterson et al, 1983). The latter study, however, was conducted well before blood pressures were being assessed in those cats. More recently, ophthalmic examinations, including slitlamp biomicroscopy and indirect ophthalmoscopy, were

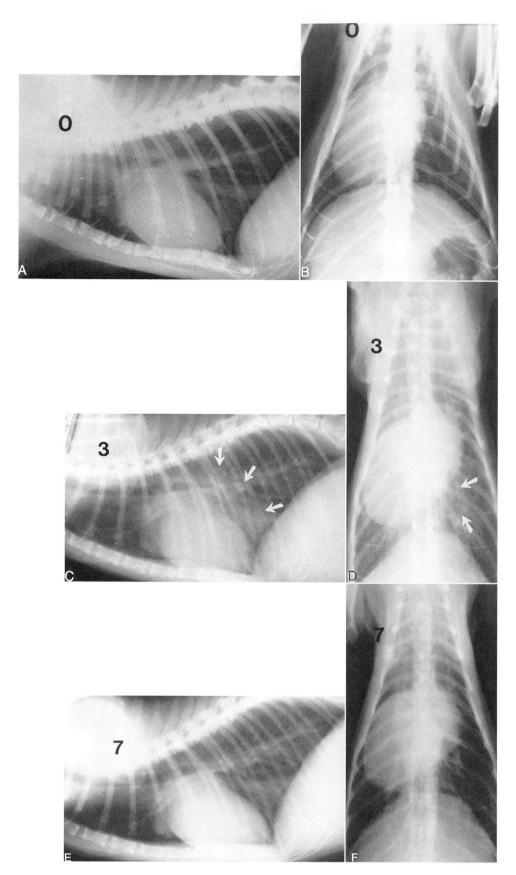

FIGURE 4–5. These radiographs illustrate that (1) thyrotoxic cats can deteriorate quickly, especially if stressed, and (2) the appearance of hyperthyroidism and heart failure can result in a confusing syndrome that is a challenge to diagnose and successfully treat. *A* and *B,* Lateral and dorsoventral radiographs of the thorax of a hyperthyroid cat. Mild cardiomegaly is present. *C* and *D,* Three days later, respiratory distress in the same cat prompted recheck radiographs. They reveal hilar density consistent with cardiogenic pulmonary edema *(arrows). E* and *F,* Seven days after the first radiographs had been obtained and 4 days after furosemide and propranolol therapy.

performed by a veterinary ophthalmologist in 100 hyperthyroid cats and 30 controls cats (Van der Woerdt and Peterson, 2000). No ophthalmologic abnormalities were more common in hyperthyroid cats than in euthyroid cats. Two hyperthyroid cats had retinal changes consistent with hypertensive retinopathy, including retinal hemorrhage and focal retinal detachment with subretinal effusion. The authors concluded that ocular abnormalities are uncommon in hyperthyroid cats.

Hypertension should remain a concern in any hyperthyroid cat, and blood pressure should be assessed whenever possible. If hypertension is demonstrated, it would be prudent to monitor the eyes and blood pressure during treatment directed at resolving the hyperthyroidism. In addition, oral amlodipine besylate has been reported to be an effective antihypertensive agent (0.625 to 1.25 mg q12-24h) (Henik et al, 1997; Maggio et al, 2000; Elliott et al, 2001). Other antihypertensive agents have been used and are currently under investigation.

Radiography

Signs associated with feline thyrotoxicosis may incriminate several organs, including the cardiovascular, pulmonary, hepatic and renal systems. Thoracic and abdominal radiographs may be used as screening tests to assess these structures. Thoracic radiographs are especially helpful because of the close relationship between hyperthyroidism and cardiovascular abnormalities. Thoracic radiographs should be obtained in cats with (1) obvious respiratory distress, (2) tachypnea or panting, (3) muffled heart sounds, (4) tachycardia, (5) arrhythmias, or (6) murmurs.

Overlapping signs associated with cardiomyopathy and hyperthyroidism can be both striking and confusing. Thoracic radiographs, although extremely valuable, do not differentiate between these two disorders. Cats with cardiomyopathy may have normal or abnormal thoracic films, and the same can be said of cats with thyrotoxicosis. As many as 50% of hyperthyroid cats have mild to severe cardiomegaly. A smaller percentage of these cats (<5%) have evidence of congestive heart failure with pulmonary edema and/or pleural effusion (Fig. 4-5) (Jacobs et al, 1986). Although thoracic radiographs may not be diagnostically specific, they are beneficial when attempting to understand the clinical signs in an individual cat and in formulating a therapeutic plan. Cats with pleural effusion, pericardial effusion, or pulmonary edema are in need of therapy regardless of the presence of primary or secondary cardiomyopathy. Administration of diuretics or direct drainage of the pleural space can be lifesaving (see Fig. 4-5).

Echocardiographic evaluation appears to be the most reliable diagnostic tool for identifying the type of cardiomyopathy present in individual cats (Bond, 1986; Jacobs et al, 1986; Jacobs and Panciera, 1992). Cats with hypertrophic cardiomyopathy usually benefit from diuretics and β-adrenergic blocking agents (e.g., propranolol). Those with dilated cardiomyopathy and congestive heart failure typically require diuretics and drug therapy to increase the strength of contraction (inotropic support; digoxin). Because many practices do not have the equipment for echocardiography, it would be wise for those practitioners to use radiography and then to treat cats that have pleural effusion with drainage and those that have pulmonary edema with diuretics. This approach benefits most afflicted cats. Referral of such cats to colleagues who are competent echocardiographers is indicated (see Echocardiography, below).

Electrocardiography (ECG)

FINDINGS. The cat with hyperthyroidism may have various problems that suggest primary heart disease, such as lethargy, panting, tachycardia, premature beats with pulse deficits, gallop rhythms, murmurs, cardiomegaly, and/or overt congestive heart failure. Any of these problems can be assessed in part by ECG. ECG is an important diagnostic tool, whether hyperthyroidism is confirmed, under consideration, or not yet in the differential diagnosis. Some alterations on the ECG may point to the diagnosis of thyrotoxicosis, whereas others may indicate a need for immediate treatment, regardless of any underlying disease.

The ECG changes seen in cats with thyrotoxicosis are listed in Table 4-5 and are illustrated in Figs. 4-6, 4-7, and 4-8. Tachycardia (heart rate above 240/min) and an increased R-wave amplitude in lead II (greater than 1.0 mV) are the abnormalities most frequently seen, although each is now detected less frequently than in the 1980s (Broussard et al, 1995). The arrhythmias identified included atrial premature contractions, atrial fibrillation, and ventricular premature contractions. In an earlier study, ventricular tachycardia, bigeminy, ventricular preexcitation, and atrial tachycardia were also identified (Peterson et al, 1982). More than 50% of hyperthyroid cats had at least one ECG abnormality, and more than 33% had two or more. A close correlation is found between rapid heart rate, increased

TABLE 4–5 PRETREATMENT ELECTROCARDIOGRAM FINDINGS IN CATS WITH HYPERTHYROIDSM

Finding	Percent of Cats
Sinus tachycardia	42
Increased R-wave amplitude (lead II)	22
Right axis deviation (right bundle branch block)	7
Atrial premature contractions	5
Left axis deviation (left anterior fascicular block)	4
Widened QRS complexes	4
Atrial tachycardia or atrial fibrillation	2
Ventricular preature contractions	1

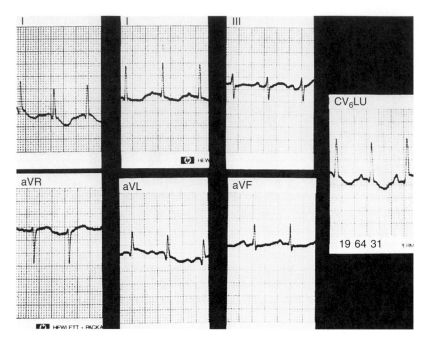

FIGURE 4–6. Electrocardiogram from a thyrotoxic cat showing R waves of increased amplitude in lead II (actually all leads) and deviation of the mean electrical axis to 30 degrees, suggestive of left heart enlargement.

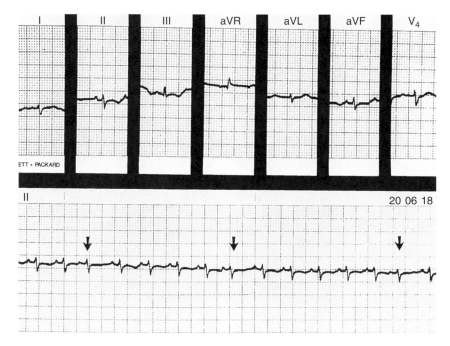

FIGURE 4–7. Electrocardiogram from a thyrotoxic cat showing normal P-QRS-T complex amplitudes. However, three atrial premature contractions can be seen in the rhythm strip *(arrows)*, and an abnormal heart rate of 300 beats per minute is present.

R-wave amplitudes, and the initial serum T_4 concentration. Most ECG abnormalities resolve with successful management of the thyrotoxicosis. However, a small percentage of cats continue to have cardiac problems and are subsequently shown to have either the hypertrophic or congestive (dilative) form of cardiomyopathy. Concurrent myocardial

disease and thyrotoxicosis is extremely challenging to manage.

Because cardiovascular signs may dominate the clinical picture of some hyperthyroid cats, the ECG becomes an important diagnostic tool. The results do not reliably distinguish primary from secondary cardiac disease but can be used to better understand

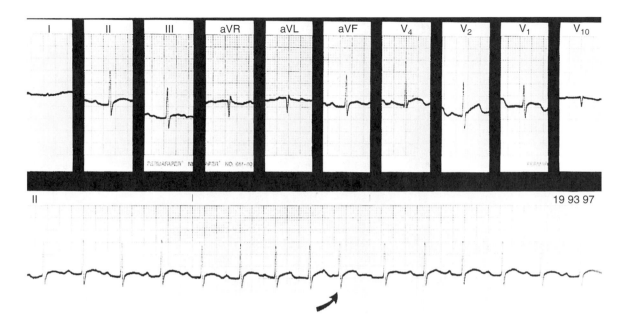

FIGURE 4–8. Electrocardiogram from a thyrotoxic cat showing both increased amplitude in the R waves and an atrial premature contraction *(arrow)*.

cardiovascular problems, especially arrhythmias. Older cats with myocardial disease should be evaluated for thyroid disease and vice versa. Certainly, if a middle-aged or older cat has clinical, ECG, and radiographic signs compatible with a diagnosis of hypertrophic cardiomyopathy, the serum T_4 concentration should be measured, especially if other signs of hyperthyroidism are present, such as weight loss, polyphagia, hyper-excitability, or diarrhea (see Tables 4-1 and 4-3).

EXPLANATION. Sinus tachycardia is the most common ECG alteration in thyrotoxic humans, as well as in cats (Williams and Braunwald, 1980). Factors that influence cardiac function in hyperthyroidism and thus alter the ECG include direct action of thyroid hormone on the heart, interactions with the sympathetic nervous system, and cardiac changes that compensate for changes in tissue metabolism. Catecholamine-dependent mechanisms may influence the development of many of these ECG disturbances. The ability of β-adrenergic blocking drugs to partly correct tachyarrhythmias without affecting abnormal thyroid hormone concentrations provides indirect evidence for the role of catecholamines in these ECG disturbances (Bond, 1986; Jacobs and Panciera, 1992). The thyrotoxic myocardium in humans and rats frequently contains foci of necrosis, round cell infiltration, and replacement fibrosis. Similar abnormalities, if present in cats, would account for the conduction disturbances occasionally identified on ECGs.

Echocardiography

Echocardiography has led to tremendous advances in the noninvasive diagnostic evaluation and treatment of cardiovascular problems in dogs and cats. Hyperthyroid cats can often be placed in one of four categories, depending on the presence of cardiac pathology, the type of heart disease, and/or the chamber/wall abnormalities recognized: (1) hyperdynamic function of the myocardium, (2) hypertrophic cardiomyopathy, (3) congestive cardiomyopathy, and (4) no abnormality (Bond et al, 1988; Jacobs and Panciera, 1992). Echocardiography allows visualization of myocardial wall thickness, the ventricular septum, the shape and function of the valves, the capacity of the ventricles and atria, and the velocity and force of contractions.

Echocardiographic abnormalities frequently identified in hyperthyroid cats include left ventricular hypertrophy, thickening of the interventricular septum, and left atrial and ventricular dilation. Myocardial hypercontractility is manifested by increased shortening fractions and increased velocity of circumferential fiber shortening (Fig. 4-9) (Bond et al, 1988). Less commonly, the dilated form of cardiomyopathy is observed. Evidence for this abnormality includes subnormal myocardial contractility and marked ventricular dilation. These cats often have radiographic evidence of congestive heart failure (Jacobs et al, 1986; Bond et al, 1988).

The finding of a "hyperdynamic myocardium" on echocardiography is consistent with hyperthyroidism. Echocardiography, when used in conjunction with thoracic radiography and ECG, improves the competence level in formulating a therapeutic plan. In one report using an objective evaluation system, including measurement of the ventricular dimensions, wall thickness, atrial dimensions, and velocity of contractions, 29 of 30 hyperthyroid cats had echocardiographic abnormalities (Bond et al, 1983). Long-term adminis-

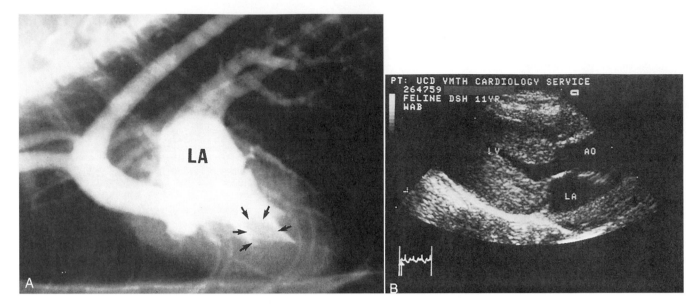

FIGURE 4–9. *A,* Nonselective angiogram of a cat with hypertrophic cardiomyopathy typical of hyperthyroidism. The left atrium (LA) is dilated, the left ventricular chamber is small, and the papillary muscles *(arrows)* and walls of the left ventricle are thick. *B,* Right parasternal long axis echocardiogram of a cat with hypertrophic cardiomyopathy demonstrating mild left atrial dilation (LA) and marked thickening of the septum and left ventricular wall. *LV,* Left ventricle; *AO,* aorta. (*A,* Fox PR: *In* Ettinger SJ [ed]: Textbook of Veterinary Internal Medicine, 3rd ed. Philadelphia, WB Saunders, 1989, p 1113; *B,* Sisson DD, Thomas WP: *In* Ettinger SJ, Feldman EC [eds]: Textbook of Veterinary Internal Medicine, 4th ed. Philadelphia, WB Saunders, 1995, p 1019.)

tration of high T_4 doses to normal cats caused massive biventricular hypertrophy, with right and left ventricular weights increasing 60% and 86%, respectively.

DIFFERENTIAL DIAGNOSIS

Hyperthyroid cats can be a diagnostic challenge to the veterinarian. A wide variety of signs may occur that are not specific for thyrotoxicosis. In addition, the physical examination often reveals abnormalities consistent with disorders of other organ systems that may represent primary or secondary problems. The results of blood tests, radiography, ECG, and echocardiography are usually not specific for hyperthyroidism. The clinician, therefore, must maintain a high index of suspicion for this common endocrinopathy, especially in cats older than 8 years of age. As seen in Table 4-6, the differential diagnosis list can be extensive.

SERUM THYROID HORMONE CONCENTRATIONS (CONFIRMING THE DIAGNOSIS)

Basal Total Serum Thyroxine (T_4) Concentration

VALUE OF THE TEST. Measurement of the serum total T_4 and T_3 concentrations is commonly used to assess thyroid gland function in veterinary medicine. Although the serum total T_4 and T_3 values can be altered in the absence of thyroid disease (Utiger, 1980; Larsen et al, 1981), measurement of random basal serum T_4 concentrations has been extremely reliable in identifying cats with hyperthyroidism. In our series, as well as in studies by others, random measurement of the basal serum T_4 concentration was more reliable than measurement of the basal serum T_3 level (Fig. 4-10) (Broussard et al, 1995; Peterson, 1995a). Commercial veterinary laboratories now include serum total T_4 concentrations as a component of feline chemistry profiles. This has been a valuable aid to practitioners.

As more experience has been gained in "screening" cats for hyperthyroidism, general agreement has evolved that hyperthyroidism can be diagnosed in most cats based on: (1) clinical signs consistent with the condition, (2) a palpable thyroid nodule, and (3) an abnormally increased serum total T_4 concentration. Thus the initial screening test of choice is assay of the serum total T_4. There is also general agreement that T_3 assay results do not have the sensitivity necessary for reliable screening tests. In a recent study, serum total T_4 concentrations were above the reference range in 91% of hyperthyroid cats and within the reference range in the remaining 9% (Peterson et al, 2001). In the same study, the serum T_3 concentration was above the reference range in 67% of hyperthyroid cats and within the reference range in the remaining 33%. As will be discussed, if a cat suspected of having hyperthyroidism has a serum total T_4 concentration within the reference range, the current recommendations are first, to repeat the test, and second, to assay the serum for the "free" T_4 concentration (Fig. 4-11).

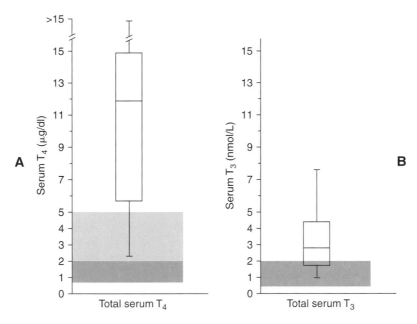

FIGURE 4–10. Mean and range of random total serum T_4 (A) and total serum T_3 (B) concentrations in hyperthyroid cats. Seventy-five percent of hyperthyroid cats have results within the box, and the balance are within the limitation bars above and below the box. Note that virtually all hyperthyroid cats have an abnormal or "borderline" serum T_4 concentration, whereas the results of the serum T_3 concentrations are less sensitive. Cross-hatching represents normal reference range, and the dot pattern the "borderline" or "nondiagnostic" range.

TABLE 4–6   DIFFERENTIAL DIAGNOSIS FOR HYPERTHYROIDISM IN CATS

Differential Diagnosis	Major Clinical Areas of Overlap with Hyperthyroidism*
Nonthyroid endocrine disease	
Diabetes mellitus	PD, PU, polyphagia, weight loss
Hyperadrenocorticism (rare)	PD, PU, polyphagia, weight loss
Diabetes insipidus (rare)	PD, PU, mild weight loss
Acromegaly (rare)	PD, PU, polyphagia
Renal disease	PD, PU, anorexia, weight loss, elevated BUN
Heart disease and failure	
Hypertrophic cardiomyopathy	Respiratory distress, weight loss, tachycardia, murmur, arrhythmia: radiography, ECG,
Congestive cardiomyopathy	echocardiogram abnormalities are not specific for hyperthyroidism
Idiopathic arrhythmia	
GI disease	
Pancreatic exocrine insufficiency	Bulky, foul-smelling stool, weight loss, polyphagia
Diffuse GI disorders	
Inflammatory	Diarrhea, vomiting, anorexia, chronic weight loss
Cancer (including lymphosarcoma)	
Hepatopathy	Elevated liver enzymes
Inflammatory	
Cancer	
Pulmonary disease	Respiratory distress, panting

*PD, Polydipsia; PU, polyuria; GI, gastrointestinal; BUN, blood urea nitrogen; ECG, electrocardiogram.

ASSAYS. Assays for serum T_4 concentrations are widely available. Although sophisticated laboratory procedures have been described for specific assays, most commercial veterinary laboratories use human T_4 radioimmunoassay (RIA) kits, and many of these kits have been validated for use in the cat. Nonisotopic and automated techniques are becoming increasingly popular and could prove valuable. Veterinarians are urged to establish reference feline values for their laboratory rather than rely on the results in the literature. Each laboratory and individual assay should be evaluated independently.

Semiquantitative assays for total thyroxine that are suitable for in-hospital testing also appear to be useful in the diagnosis of overt hyperthyroidism (Mooney, 1998a). However, substantial discrepancies between enzyme-linked immunosorbent assay (ELISA) and RIA results for T_4 concentrations were demonstrated

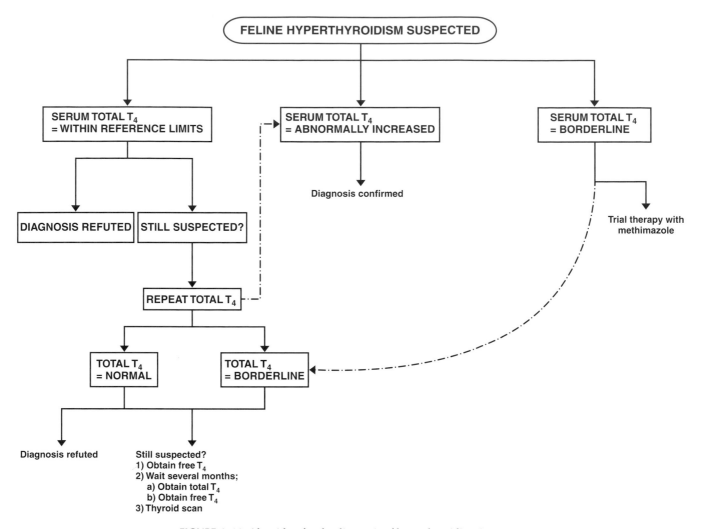

FIGURE 4–11. Algorithm for the diagnosis of hyperthyroidism in cats.

in one study (Lurye et al, 2002). These authors concluded that the in-house ELISA kit that they evaluated was not accurate for determining serum total T_4 concentrations in cats.

FLUCTUATING SERUM T_4 CONCENTRATIONS. Assessment of a single random serum T_4 concentration has been reliable in correctly confirming the diagnosis of hyperthyroidism in more than 90% of afflicted cats. An abnormally increased serum T_4 concentration strongly supports the diagnosis of hyperthyroidism, especially when appropriate clinical signs are present. Although thyroid hormone concentrations fluctuate considerably among hyperthyroid cats, those fluctuations tend to be persistently abnormal (Peterson et al, 1987a). In other words, in cats with fluctuating levels, the lowest detected serum T_4 concentration is well above the reference range (Fig. 4-12). Thus fluctuation of serum T_4 concentrations is not usually of diagnostic significance. An exception is the cat with mild hyperthyroidism (i.e., minimal clinical signs and serum T_4 values just above the reference range), in which the serum T_4 concentration may fluctuate both within and

above the reference range. The diagnosis of hyperthyroidism should not be excluded on the basis of one "normal" test result, especially with a cat that has appropriate clinical signs and a palpable mass in the neck. Rather, measurement of the serum total and "free" T_4 concentrations should be repeated once or twice before the diagnosis is excluded or other tests (e.g., T_3 suppression test) are considered.

Cats with Suspected Hyperthyroidism that Have a "Normal" T_4 Level

WHAT IS NORMAL? In recent surveys, approximately 2% to 10% of cats confirmed to have hyperthyroidism had a "normal" serum T_4 concentration on initial testing (McLoughlin et al, 1993; Broussard et al, 1995; Peterson et al, 2001). Failure to understand how "reference" or "normal" ranges are established for many laboratories can contribute to the confusion. For example, the feline T_4 reference range for our laboratory is 0.8 to 2.0 µg/dl. A small percentage of

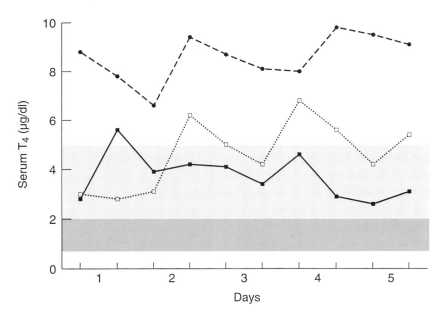

FIGURE 4–12. Serum T_4 concentrations fluctuate in normal and hyperthyroid cats. This figure demonstrates the amount of fluctuation typical of cats with hyperthyroidism. Cats with significantly increased serum T_4 concentrations usually have persistently abnormal results *(dashed line),* whereas cats with "borderline" values have serum T_4 concentrations that can be "nondiagnostic" and occasionally abnormally increased *(dotted line)* or *(solid line).* Dark gray area is the normal range, and the light gray area is the "nondiagnostic" range.

normal cats have serum T_4 concentrations greater than 2.0 but less than 5.0 µg/dl. Values strongly consistent with the diagnosis of hyperthyroidism exceed 5.0 µg/dl. Hyperthyroid cats, however, may have serum T_4 concentrations of 2.0 to 5.0 µg/dl. For this reason, values between 2.0 and 5.0 should be considered "nondiagnostic" or "borderline," because normal cats, hyperthyroid cats, and hyperthyroid cats with significant nonthyroidal disease may all have test results in this range. When the serum total T_4 values are in this nondiagnostic range, the decision to pursue the diagnosis of hyperthyroidism must depend on a review of the history, the physical examination findings, and the clinician's index of suspicion for the disease.

HOW CAN A HYPERTHYROID CAT HAVE A "NORMAL" TEST RESULT? Many cats with normal or "borderline" serum T_4 concentrations (1.5 to 4.0 or 5.0 µg/dl) that are subsequently diagnosed with hyperthyroidism have relatively early or mild features of the disease. It is presumed that allowing the disease to continue unabated would result in progressive increases in the serum T_4 concentration. Eventually these cats would have persistently increased and, therefore, "diagnostic" test results (Graves and Peterson, 1992; Peterson, 1995a).

It should be emphasized that no test result is as reliable and consistent as the results of the history and the physical examination. If, after reviewing the history and physical examination findings, a veterinarian is convinced that a particular cat is hyperthyroid, one nondiagnostic serum total T_4 value should not rule out the diagnosis, and a second serum T_4 concentration should be determined. Conversely, if

a cat demonstrates no evidence of hyperthyroidism on review of the history and physical examination findings, a positive test result should be viewed with skepticism.

Two concepts have been proposed to explain the contradictory concept of clinical hyperthyroidism in a cat with "normal" serum T_4 concentrations: (1) fluctuation of serum hormone concentrations and (2) suppression of increased hormone concentrations as a result of a serious concurrent nonthyroid disorder (Peterson, 1995a). The concept of fluctuating concentrations has been reviewed in a previous section. Concurrent hyperthyroidism should always be suspected in severely ill cats with middle to high reference range total serum T_4 concentrations (Mooney, 1998) (see next section).

EFFECT OF NONTHYROIDAL ILLNESS ON SERUM TOTAL T_4 CONCENTRATIONS. In a recent study that included 98 euthyroid ill cats, one cat had an abnormally increased serum total T_4 concentration (in the "borderline" range), 21 cats had values below the reference range, and 76 cats had values within the reference range (Mooney et al, 1996a). In another study that included 221 euthyroid ill cats, none had an abnormally increased serum total T_4 concentration, and 38% of those cats had a low concentration (Fig. 4-13) (Peterson et al, 2001). These studies demonstrate that illness can lower serum T_4 concentrations. However, the question arises whether concurrent illness decreases these hormone values in cats with hyperthyroidism, as has been suggested (Peterson and Gamble, 1990). In one study, 110 cats were diagnosed as having hyperthyroidism; 14 had serum T_4 concentrations of 2.5 to

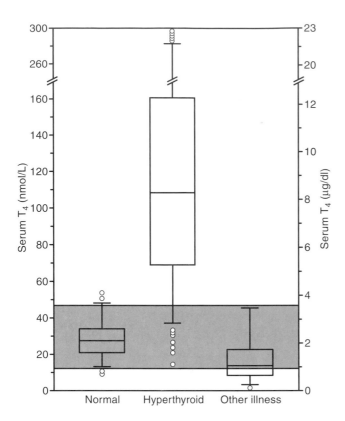

FIGURE 4–13. Box plots of serum total thyroxine (T₄) concentrations in 172 clinically normal cats, 917 cats with untreated hyperthyroidism, and 221 cats with nonthyroidal disease (other illness). The box represents the interquartile range (i.e., 25th to 75th percentile range, or the middle half of the data). The horizontal bar in the box represents the median value. For each box plot, the T bars represent the main body of data, which in most instances is equal to the range. Outlying data points are represented by open circles. The shaded area indicates the reference range for the serum T₄ concentration. (Peterson ME, et al: J Am Vet Med Assoc 218:529, 2001).

4.0 μg/dl, and 10 of those 14 had nonthyroid illnesses (McLoughlin et al, 1993). Successful management of the concurrent illness results in an increase of the serum total T₄ concentration into the diagnostic range for hyperthyroidism.

SUMMARY (SEE FIG. 4-11). If mild hyperthyroidism is suspected in a cat with a nondiagnostic serum T₄ concentration, the recommendation is to repeat the test and also to rule out nonthyroidal illness. Because thyroid hormone concentrations vary more over a period of days than over a period of several hours, repeat measurement of the serum T₄ concentration should be performed days to weeks after the initial result was obtained (Peterson et al, 1987a). If the serum T₄ concentration remains nondiagnostic and hyperthyroidism is still suspected, the most appropriate course of action in some cases may be to reassess thyroid function after resolution of any nonthyroidal illness, to assay the serum free T₄ concentration, to obtain a thyroid scan, to perform a T₃ suppression test, or to perform a thyrotropin-releasing hormone (TRH) stimulation test.

Basal Total Serum Triiodothyronine (T₃) Concentrations

Triiodothyronine (T₃) is the biologically "active" thyroid hormone. However, the primary hormone secreted from the canine and feline thyroid gland is thyroxine (T₄), which is metabolized to T₃ at the cellular level. Thyroxine, therefore, can be considered a "prohormone" or a reservoir for T₃ (see Chapter 3). Assessment of thyroid gland function in cats suspected of having hyperthyroidism has been most reliable with measurement of randomly obtained serum T₄ concentrations (Peterson et al, 1988; McLoughlin et al, 1993). As many as 25% to 33% of cats with confirmed hyperthyroidism have serum T₃ concentrations within the reference range (see Fig. 4-10) (Broussard et al, 1995; Peterson, 1995a; Peterson et al, 2001). Simultaneous measurement of the T₃ and T₄ concentrations offers no advantage; assessment of serum T₄ is recommended.

Basal Free Thyroid Hormone Determination

BACKGROUND. Most commercial laboratories performing thyroid hormone evaluations in dogs and cats assay and report the *total* serum thyroxine (T₄) concentrations. The *total* value includes both the protein-bound fraction (more than 99% of the total) and the free, unbound fraction of thyroid hormone (<1% of the total). Only the free fraction of thyroid hormone is available for entry into cells and, in that regard, represents the "active" hormone (or active "prohormone" for T₃). Measured serum thyroid hormone concentrations can be altered by many illnesses that do not directly affect the thyroid gland (nonthyroidal illness). Total T₄ concentrations can be affected by alterations in metabolism, hormone binding to plasma carrier proteins, transport into cells, and intracellular binding. It has been suggested that measurement of serum *free* thyroid hormone concentrations (fT₄) may circumvent the effects of nonthyroidal illness and provide a more consistent assessment of thyroid gland function than measurement of the total thyroid hormone concentration.

ASSAYS. It has been suggested that fT₄ concentrations be assayed by a method called *equilibrium dialysis.* Controversy surrounds alternative methods of assaying fT₄ concentrations, particularly systems involving analogs. Some authors have suggested that methods other than equilibrium dialysis be considered "estimates" (Paradis and Page, 1996; Mooney, 1998a). As the reliability of non-equilibrium dialysis assays improves, their expense will decline and their likely use will expand.

RESULTS: SPECIFICITY VERSUS SENSITIVITY. In one early study, all the hyperthyroid cats evaluated had abnormal total serum T₄ concentrations, but the results of fT₄ concentrations were not as consistent (Ferguson et al, 1989). In a subsequent report, however, serum fT₄ concentrations (reference range, 15 to 48 pmol/L; assay by equilibrium dialysis) proved to be a useful tool in the diagnosis of hyperthyroidism in cats with high-normal or borderline total T_4 results (Peterson et al, 1995). Sixty percent of 26 hyperthyroid cats had diagnostic (abnormal) total serum T_4 concentrations, and 96% had diagnostic (abnormal) fT_4 results (values, 41 to 144 pmol/L). In this same study, 5% of cats with normal thyroid function but serious disease had abnormally increased fT_4 results.

Two additional publications provide further insight into the value of assaying serum fT_4 concentrations in cats. Combining results from these two studies, 319 euthyroid ill cats were evaluated. The cats did not have hyperthyroidism, and only one had a total T_4 concentration that was incorrect (abnormal, or above the reference range) and that result was considered borderline (Mooney et al, 1996a; Peterson et al, 2001). Of the 319 cats, 25 (8%) had abnormally increased serum fT_4 concentrations (i.e., these 25 cats had test results that were incorrect). It must also be remembered that in one of the two studies, 91% of cats with confirmed hyperthyroidism had an abnormally increased serum total T_4 concentration (91% correct results, 9% incorrect results). However, 98.5% of those same cats had abnormally increased serum fT_4 concentrations (98.5% correct results, 1.5% incorrect results) (Peterson et al, 2001). The advantage of assaying the serum fT_4 concentration is that it is more *sensitive* than the serum total T_4 concentration in hyperthyroid cats; that is, cats with the disease are more likely to have an abnormal result. The disadvantage is that the serum fT_4 concentration is less *specific*, meaning that cats without the disease may also have an abnormal test result (Fig. 4-14).

SUMMARY. The fT_4 assay by equilibrium dialysis appears to be a useful tool for evaluating a select group of cats suspected of having hyperthyroidism; specifically, this assay should be used for cats strongly suspected of being hyperthyroid that repeatedly have serum *total* T_4 concentrations within the reference range (see Fig. 4-11). These cats, in general, have "mild" disease (Fig. 4-15) (Peterson et al, 2001). In this setting, the fT_4 result should identify hyperthyroidism. It should be kept in mind that this approach uses a test that is less specific. The abnormal result may be obtained from a cat with nonthyroidal disease. Regardless, this approach is widely and successfully used by practitioners (Peterson et al, 1995 and 2001.).

Thyroid Hormone (T_3) Suppression Test

HISTORY. Traditionally, humans suspected of having hormonal deficiencies are tested with provocative (stimulation) tests, and those suspected of having hormonal excesses are tested with suppression tests (Utiger, 1986). Inhibition of pituitary TSH via administration of thyroid hormone is characteristic of the normal inhibitory feedback from the thyroid to the pituitary. In other words, administration of thyroid hormone to an individual with a normal pituitary-thyroid axis should suppress pituitary TSH secretion and in turn suppress endogenous thyroid hormone secretion. Administration of T_3 to normal cats should suppress pituitary TSH secretion, causing a subsequent decrease in the serum T_4 concentration. Measurement of serum T_4 is a valid marker of thyroid gland function, because exogenous T_3 cannot be converted to T_4.

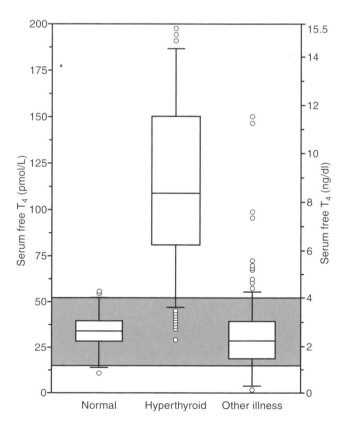

FIGURE 4–14. Box plots of serum free T_4 concentrations in 172 clinically normal cats, 917 cats with untreated hyperthyroidism, and 221 cats with nonthyroidal disease (see Fig. 4-13 for key). (Peterson ME, et al: J Am Vet Med Assoc 218:529, 2001.)

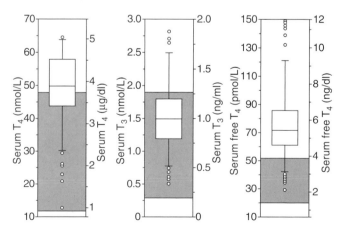

FIGURE 4–15. Box plots of serum total T_4, T_3, and free T_4 concentrations in 205 cats with mild hyperthyroidism (defined as total T_4 concentration <66 nmol/L). (see Fig. 4-13 for key). (Peterson ME, et al: J Am Vet Med Assoc 218:529, 2001.)

TABLE 4–7 COMMONLY USED PROTOCOLS FOR DYNAMIC THYROID FUNCTION TESTS IN CATS.*[†]

	T_3 Suppression	TSH Stimulation	TRH Stimulation
Drug	Cytobin	Bovine or human TSH	TRH
Dose	25 mg Q8hr × 7 doses	0.5 IU/kg (bovine)	0.1 mg/kg
		0.025 to 0.2 mg (human)	
Route	Oral	IV	IV
Sampling times	Before and 2–4hr after last dose	0 & 6 hours	0 & 4 hours
Assays	Total T_3 & T_4	Total T_4	Total T_4
Interpretation:			
a) Euthyroid	<20 nmol/L with >50% suppression	>100%	>60%
b) Hyperthyroid	>20 nmol/L ± <50% suppression	Minimal or no	<50%
		increase from baseline	
Reference	Peterson et al, 1990	Mooney et al, 1996	Peterson et al, 1994

*Values quoted are guidelines only. Each laboratory should furnish its own reference ranges.
[†]T_3, Triiodothyronine; T_4, thyroxine; *TSH*, thyroid stimulating hormone; *TRH*, thyrotropin-releasing hormone.

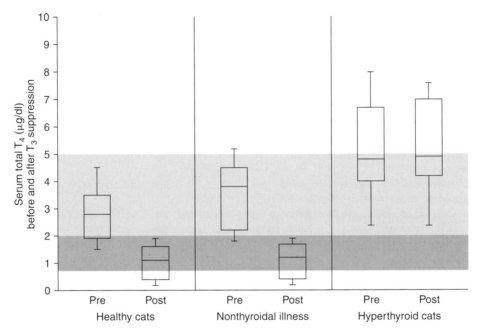

FIGURE 4–16. Serum total T_4 concentrations before and at completion of the T_3 suppression test. Note that normal and nonhyperthyroid ill cats suppress significantly. Hyperthyroid cats, however, do not suppress. Seventy-five percent of results are within the "boxes"; the bars represent the complete range of test results.

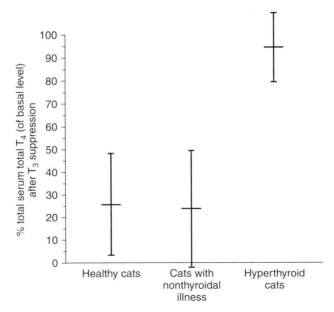

FIGURE 4–17. Percentage decrease in total serum T_4 concentrations after administration of seven doses of T_3 over 2.5 days. Note the significant decrease (>50%) in healthy cats and cats with nonthyroidal illness versus little to no change in hyperthyroid cats.

Cats with hyperthyroidism have *autonomous* secretion of thyroid hormone (i.e., hormone secretion is independent of pituitary control). Thus administration of T_3 to hyperthyroid cats should have little or no effect on the serum T_4 concentration because pituitary TSH secretion has already been chronically suppressed and T_3 administration has no further suppressive effect. The T_3 suppression test should allow discrimination between cats with a normal pituitary-thyroid axis from those with autonomous thyroid secretion and probable hyperthyroidism. A practical protocol has been developed for T_3 suppression testing in cats, using serum T_4 assessments and taking advantage of the relatively short (6 to 8 hours) serum half-life of T_3 in the feline (Broome et al, 1987; Hays et al, 1988; Peterson et al, 1990).

PROTOCOL. Initially, serum is obtained for determination of both serum T_3 and T_4 concentrations. Owners are then instructed to administer T_3 (liothyronine [Cytomel]; Jones Medical Industries, St. Louis, Mo.) beginning the next morning at a dosage of 25 µg given orally three times daily for two days. On the morning of day 3, a seventh 25 µg dose should be administered and the cat returned to the hospital so that a second blood sample can be obtained. This blood sample, to be assayed for both serum T_3 and T_4 concentrations, should be obtained 2 to 4 hours after administration of the seventh dose of liothyronine (Peterson et al, 1990). The pretreatment and posttreatment serum samples should be submitted to the laboratory together to eliminate any concern about a possible effect of interassay variation on the results (Table 4-7).

INTERPRETATION

Change in Serum T_4. Normal cats demonstrate a marked reduction in the serum T_4 concentration after seven doses of synthetic T_3. Cats with hyperthyroidism, however, demonstrate minimal or no decrease in serum T_4 concentrations. This is true even for cats with mild hyperthyroidism and high-normal or marginally increased resting T_4 concentrations (Figs. 4-16 and 4-17). Normal cats consistently have post-pill serum T_4 concentrations of less than 1.5 µg/dl. Hyperthyroid cats have post-pill T_4 concentrations greater than 2.0 µg/dl. Values between 1.5 and 2.0 µg/dl should be considered nondiagnostic. The percentage of decrease in the serum T_4 concentration is not as reliable a criterion as the absolute value, although suppression of greater than 50% below the baseline value was observed only in nonhyperthyroid cats (Peterson et al, 1990; Refsal et al, 1991). The use of complex formulas to determine whether a result is normal or abnormal (value = post-liothyronine T_4 – [0.5 × basal T_4]), as suggested by one group (Refsal et al, 1991), is not recommended because these formulas do not improve the reliability, sensitivity, or specificity of a diagnosis (Fig. 4-18). As for any endocrine test, it is important for each laboratory to establish reference ranges rather than to use values extracted from the literature.

Change in Serum T_3. Assay results for the serum T_3 concentration are not used to evaluate the status of the pituitary-thyroid axis. Rather, serum T_3 results are used to determine whether the owner successfully administered the T_3. The serum T_3 concentration should increase in all cats properly medicated, regardless of the status of thyroid gland function (Fig. 4-19). If the serum T_4 concentration fails to decline in a cat that does not demonstrate an increase in the serum T_3 concentration, problems with owner compliance could explain these results and the test results should not be trusted (Peterson, 1995a).

SUMMARY. The T_3 suppression test is particularly useful in distinguishing euthyroid from mildly hyperthyroid cats with vague or borderline resting serum T_4 concentrations. The disadvantages of the test are the 3 days required to complete the regimen and the need to rely on owners to administer the drug seven times (Peterson et al, 1990; Refsal et al, 1991). Although the test is reasonably reliable and potentially useful for veterinarians in practice, it is not often used. The explanation is "practicality"; in addition to the limitations just mentioned for the T_3 method, repeat measurement of the serum total T_4 concentration has been demonstrated to be reliable and, when repeated testing fails, assays of serum fT_4 concentration should be informative.

Thyroid-Stimulating Hormone (TSH) Response Test

PROTOCOL. The TSH response test is commonly recommended as a diagnostic aid in evaluating thyroid gland function in dogs. Similar tests have been recommended for studying thyroid function in cats (see Table 4-7). The test involves obtaining serum for determination of the T_4 level before and after TSH administration. Several protocols have been recommended. The most recent protocol uses recombinant human thyroid-stimulating hormone (rh TSH) by IV administration of 0.025 to 0.2 mg, measuring serum to total T_4 concentrations at the time of injection and 6 to 8 hours later (Stegeman et al, 2003).

INTERPRETATION. A TSH response test is not indicated when the basal serum total T_4 concentration is clearly increased and abnormal. It has been suggested that normal cats have greater responsiveness to TSH than hyperthyroid cats (Peterson, 1984). Therefore the cat with suspected hyperthyroidism that does not have a clearly abnormal T_4 concentration may have little or no response to exogenous TSH if hyperthyroidism is present. Further studies have demonstrated an overlap in test results comparing cats without thyroid disease to hyperthyroid cats when using absolute serum T_4 concentrations or "percent rise" in serum T_4 values after stimulation with TSH.

NOT RECOMMENDED. Several reports have demonstrated that many mildly hyperthyroid cats with normal resting serum T_4 concentrations respond to TSH in a manner indistinguishable from normal cats (Mooney et al, 1992b; Peterson, 1995a; Mooney et al, 1996b; Mooney, 1998a). The TSH response test may

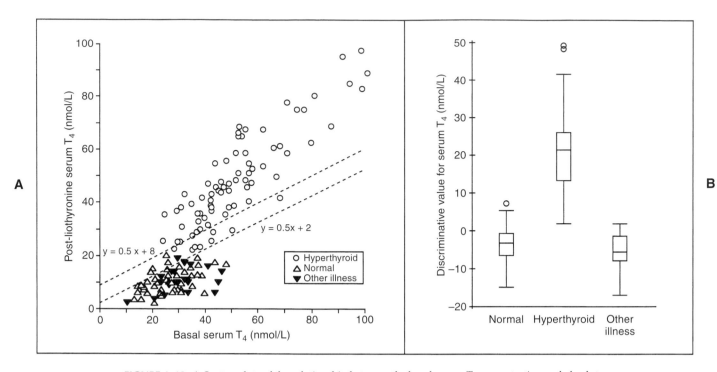

FIGURE 4–18. *A*, Scatter plots of the relationship between the basal serum T_4 concentration and absolute change in T_4 concentration after administration of T_3 (liothyronine) to 44 clinically normal cats, 77 cats with hyperthyroidism, and 22 cats with nonthyroidal illness. The dashed lines indicate canonical discriminant functions to distinguish hyperthyroid cats from normal cats and cats with nonthyroidal disease. *B*, Scores (D values) calculated by canonical discriminant analysis of the basal T_4 concentrations and response to liothyronine suppression in the three groups of cats. Formula used to calculate scores: D value = Post-liothyronine T_4 (nmol/L) - (0.5) Basal T_4 (nmol/L). "Boxes" represent the interquartile range from the 25th to the 75th percentile, the middle half of the data; the horizontal bar through the box is the median; the "whiskers" represent the main body of data, which in most cases is equal to the range; outlying data points are represented by open circles. To convert serum T_4 concentrations from nmol/L to μg/dl, divide the given values by 12.87.) (Peterson ME: *In* Ettinger SJ, Feldman EC [eds]: Textbook of Veterinary Internal Medicine, 4th ed. Philadelphia, WB Saunders, 1995, p 1974.)

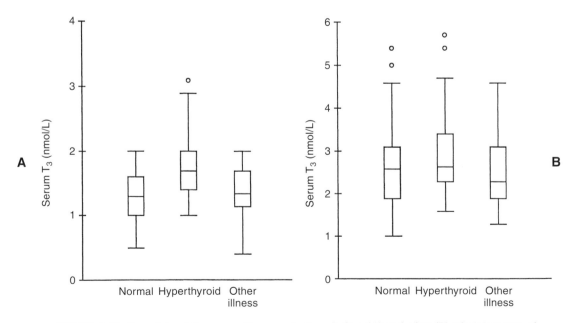

FIGURE 4–19. Box plots of the serum T_3 concentrations before *(A)* and after *(B)* administration of liothyronine to 44 clinically normal cats, 77 cats with hyperthyroidism, and 22 cats with nonthyroidal disease. Data plotted as described in Fig. 4-13. (Peterson ME, et al: J Vet Intern Med 4:233, 1990.)

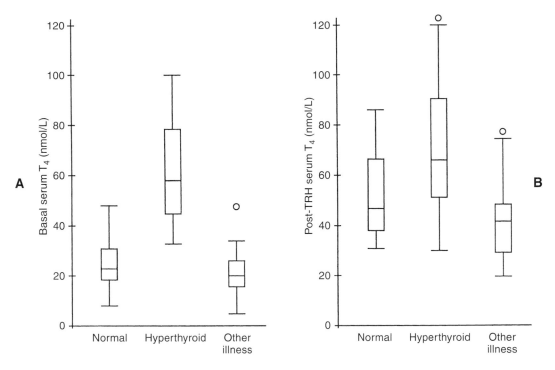

FIGURE 4–20. Box plots of the serum T_4 concentrations before *(A)* and after *(B)* TRH stimulation in 31 clinically normal cats, 35 cats with hyperthyroidism, and 15 cats with nonthyroidal illness. Data plotted as described in Fig. 4-13.(Peterson ME, et al: J Vet Intern Med 8:279, 1994.)

have value for evaluating dogs and cats suspected of having hypothyroidism, but it cannot be recommended for diagnosing hyperthyroidism.

Thyrotropin-Releasing Hormone (TRH) Stimulation Test

BACKGROUND. In humans the T_3 suppression test, considered by some to be cumbersome and time-consuming, has been replaced by the TRH stimulation test. This test can be completed in 1 day, and normal humans consistently demonstrate an increase in the serum TSH concentration. Hyperthyroid people have a blunted or absent response, presumably because endogenous TSH secretion has been chronically suppressed (Utiger, 1986).

PROTOCOL. Although a reliable TSH assay is being validated for cats, the TRH stimulation test (see Table 4-7) can be performed by evaluating changes in the serum T_4 concentration rather than evaluating the serum TSH concentration, as is done in people (Peterson, 1991; Peterson et al, 1994). Blood is collected for serum T_4 determination before and 4 hours after intravenous administration of TRH* at a dosage of 0.1 mg/kg body weight. Adverse reactions are common with intra-

venous administration of TRH, including salivation, vomiting, tachypnea, and defecation. Side effects usually begin immediately after TRH administration and may continue as long as 4 hours. Side effects are reported to be the result of activating central cholinergic and catecholaminergic mechanisms and direct neurotransmitter effects of TRH on specific binding sites (Holtman et al, 1986; Beleslin et al, 1987a and 1987b).

INTERPRETATION. Healthy cats and those with nonthyroidal disease usually have a twofold increase in the serum T_4 concentration 4 hours after intravenous administration of TRH. Cats with mild hyperthyroidism have little or no increase in the serum T_4 concentration (Figs. 4-20 and 4-21). Serum T_3 assessments have been less consistent and are not recommended. A percent increase in the post-TRH serum T_4 concentration of less than 50% above basal values was also consistent with the diagnosis of hyperthyroidism. Post-TRH T_4 values greater than 60% above basal concentrations were observed only in normal cats and in those with nonthyroidal illness. Increases of 50% to 60% should be considered nondiagnostic (Peterson et al, 1994; Tomsa et al, 2001).

In addition to evaluation of the percent change in the serum T_4 concentration, a discriminative function score (D value), in nanomoles per liter, can be calculated ([2.2 × basal T_4] – [TRH-stimulated T_4]). A "D" value less than 20 is considered normal, and one greater than 30 is consistent with the diagnosis of hyperthyroidism. Values between 20 and 30 should be considered nondiagnostic (Peterson et al, 1994; Peterson, 1995a).

---

*Relefact TRH (0.5 mg vials, injectable), Hoechst-Roussel Pharmaceuticals, Somerville, NJ 08876; Thypinone (0.5 mg vials, injectable), Abbott Diagnostics, Abbott Park, Ill. 60064; Thytropar, Armour Pharmaceutical, Tarrytown, NY 10591.

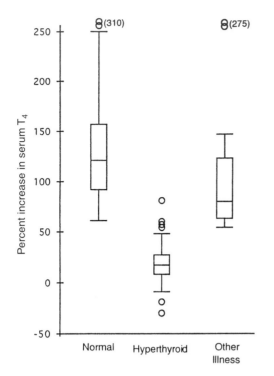

FIGURE 4–21. Box plots of the relative change in serum T_4 concentrations after TRH administration (percent increase) in 31 clinically normal cats, 35 cats with hyperthyroidism, and 15 cats with nonthyroidal disease. Data plotted as described in Fig. 4-13. (Peterson ME, et al: J Vet Intern Med 8:279, 1994.)

SUMMARY. The TRH stimulation test has been judged to be as reliable as the T_3 suppression test, with the TRH test having the advantages of being less time-consuming and not depending on someone administering pills to a cat (Sparkes et al, 1991; Peterson, 1995a). However, the combination of simply repeating the total serum T_4 concentration and, if necessary, assaying the serum fT_4 by equilibrium dialysis is easier, less expensive, has no side effects, and is superior to the TRH stimulation test. Although the TRH stimulation test can be used, we prefer using the previously mentioned total and free T_4 assays.

Confirming the Diagnosis of Hyperthyroidism

The clinician should gain a suspicion of hyperthyroidism based on careful review of the history and physical examination findings. Careful palpation of the cat's neck, especially in the area of the thoracic inlet, is quite important. Gradual pressure applied just below the thoracic inlet may move a thyroid mass located just inside the thoracic inlet back into the neck, where it can be palpated. Most cats with hyperthyroidism have a palpable thyroid mass. If a thyroid mass is not palpable, the clinician should consider that the abnormal thyroid tissue might be in the mediastinum, but other possible causes of the clinical signs observed by the owners should be considered (see Table 4-6).

The diagnosis of hyperthyroidism can usually be confirmed by evaluating a single, random, serum total T_4 concentration. If a cat that appears to be hyperthyroid does not have a diagnostic baseline serum total T_4 concentration, the test can be repeated days to weeks later, along with a serum free T_4 concentration. Other tests of the pituitary-thyroid axis can also be considered (e.g., T_3 suppression test). Waiting as long as 2 to 8 weeks before repeating the serum T_4 concentration measurement, although rarely necessary, should allow hyperthyroidism to progress and the serum T_4 concentrations (total or free, or both) to increase. Failure to observe an abnormally increased serum T_4 concentration, however, does not rule out the diagnosis of hyperthyroidism if the clinical signs and physical examination findings are consistent with the disease. The cat's clinical condition may progressively worsen, but this, too, is usually a gradual process. Waiting a short time should be reasonable.

If the serum T_4 concentrations (total and free) fail to confirm hyperthyroidism, the T_3 suppression test, TRH stimulation test, or a radionuclide thyroid scan should be considered. Finally, a positive response to methimazole therapy (see page 195) would also support the diagnosis. However, trial therapy should be considered a last resort and attempted only after all other possible causes of the clinical signs have been ruled out. Surgical exploration of the neck to identify a thyroid mass in an unconfirmed case is not recommended. As previously discussed, these are often aged, debilitated cats that are a definite surgical risk.

RADIONUCLIDE IMAGING: THYROID SCAN

Theory

Thyroid scans can provide helpful information for understanding the pathophysiology of hyperthyroidism, as well as contributing to the formulation of a therapeutic plan. Several radionuclides can be used for scanning (imaging) thyroid lobes. Like stable iodine, radioactive iodine (iodine-131 [^{131}I] and iodine-123 [^{123}I]) is trapped and concentrated within thyroid follicular cells. Any of these iodines are eventually incorporated into the tyrosine groups of thyroglobulin and then into T_3 and T_4.

Radioactive technetium-99m (pertechnetate; [99m]TcO$_4$) is also trapped and concentrated within thyroid follicular cells. The configuration of the pertechnetate ion mimics that of iodide to such a degree that it is trapped by the thyroidal iodide-concentrating mechanism but is not incorporated into the organic thyroid hormone and therefore is not retained in the thyroid gland. Thus [99m]TcO$_4$ uptake reflects the trapping mechanism but not function of the gland. Some other epithelial structures (salivary glands, gastric mucosa) can also concentrate pertechnetate without organic binding or storage within the tissue (Nap et al, 1994). Pertechnetate is excreted by the kidneys.

TABLE 4–8   RADIONUCLIDES USED IN THYROID IMAGING STUDIES

Isotope	Expense/Availability	Principal Gamma Energy (keV)	Time from Injection to Scanning Procedure	Physical Half-Life	Risk to Technicians
Iodine-131	Inexpensive/available	364	24 hours	8.1 days	Yes
Iodine-123	Expensive/less available	159	4 hours	13.3 hours	Little
$^{99m}TcO_4$ (pertechnetate)	Inexpensive/available	140	20 minutes	6.0 hours	Safe

Physiology of Scanning

CHOICE OF RADIONUCLIDE. All three radionuclides (^{131}I, ^{123}I, and pertechnetate) provide excellent thyroid images, but pertechnetate, for several reasons, is the material most commonly used (Table 4-8). Iodine-131 is inexpensive and readily available. However, because it has a long physical half-life (8.1 days), a wait of 24 hours is required after administration before the imaging procedure can be performed. In addition, ^{131}I emits a high-energy γ-photon (364 keV) that is inefficiently collimated by the camera. [131]I also emits β-particles that are not detected by the camera but that increase total body and thyroid radiation exposure. The increased risk to technicians administering ^{131}I makes this material less suitable for routine use (Beck et al, 1985).

In contrast to ^{131}I, iodine-123 has a short physical half-life (13.3 hours), emits low-energy γ-rays (159 keV) that are well suited for scanning, and has no β-emission. The imaging procedure can begin 4 hours after administration. For these reasons, ^{123}I is a good agent for thyroid scanning. In addition, it may be superior to ^{131}I in detecting thyroid carcinoma in people (Mandel et al, 2001). However, the high cost of ^{123}I limits its use (Beck et al, 1985).

Pertechnetate, a widely available and relatively inexpensive radionuclide, is considered by most investigators to be the best choice for routine imaging of thyroid glands in humans and cats (Beck et al, 1985). Pertechnetate has a short physical half-life (6 hours), and imaging procedures can begin 20 minutes after administration because of its rapid uptake by the thyroid. Pertechnetate emits low-energy γ-particles (140 keV), has no β-emission, and gives the lowest radiation dose to the thyroid of all available scanning agents.

The quality of thyroid scans done with ^{123}I, ^{131}I, or pertechnetate is excellent. However, when oral antithyroid drugs are used to treat hyperthyroidism, radioactive iodine may fail to image the thyroid gland well because these drugs inhibit both organification of iodide and coupling of iodotyrosyl groups. Because the antithyroid drugs do not affect the trapping mechanism of the thyroid pump, pertechnetate still concentrates in the thyroid gland to produce an image, even after complete blockade of thyroid hormone synthesis by antithyroid drugs. In a noteworthy result from a study on healthy cats, recent withdrawal of methimazole treatment actually enhanced uptake of radioiodine and pertechnetate, changes that could alter interpretation of scans (Nieckarz and Daniel, 2001).

PROTOCOL. Thyroid scanning is accomplished after intravenous administration of radiolabeled pertechnetate (5 to 35 MBq [0.1 to 1 mCi]). A specific amount of time is allowed to elapse so that thyroid (and other) tissue can concentrate the radionuclide, and the scan is then completed. The elapsed period can be as brief as 15 to 20 minutes to as long as 4 to 6 hours. It has been suggested that a 60-minute delay between injection and scanning is ideal (Nap et al, 1994). At the time of scanning, the cat is placed under (or on) a scintillation camera, which detects radioactivity and records it on film. The cat is usually held during scanning for about 30 seconds per view. The film is then developed, revealing the major locations of radioactivity in the body (Fig. 4-22).

Tissue Identified

Scanning of the thyroid provides a picture of all functioning thyroid tissue. It permits delineation and

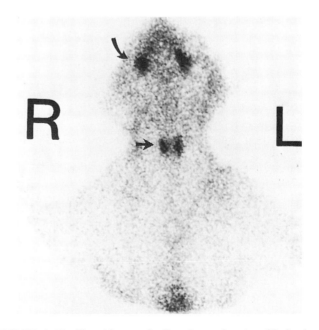

FIGURE 4–22. Thyroid scan (radioactive technetium-99m) of a normal cat. Note the similar size and density of the thyroids (*straight arrow*) and the salivary glands (*curved arrow*).

localization of functioning versus nonfunctioning areas of the thyroid. Pertechnetate concentrates primarily in three tissues, the thyroid lobes, salivary glands, and gastric mucosa. The similarity between the size and shape of the thyroids and those of the salivary glands in a normal cat is illustrated in Fig. 4-22. This 1:1 ratio of salivary glands to thyroid lobes is the standard for a normal study. Studies of most hyperthyroid cats are dramatically abnormal and usually easy to interpret (Peterson and Yoshioka, 1983; Beck et al, 1985; Kintzer and Peterson, 1991; Mooney et al, 1992c). In one study, in addition to concentrating in the tissues previously described, the imaging radionuclides accumulated in bronchogenic carcinomas in two cats (Cook et al, 1993).

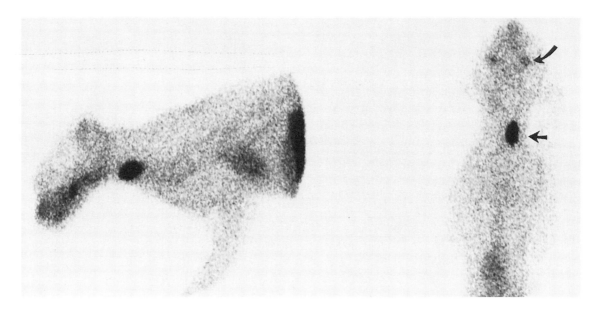

FIGURE 4–23. Thyroid ^{99m}Tc scan from a thyrotoxic cat with a unilateral thyroid tumor. Note the density of the thyroid *(straight arrow)* compared with that of the salivary glands *(curved arrow).*

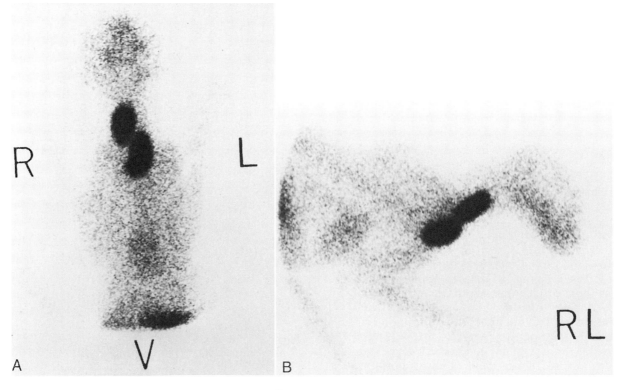

FIGURE 4–24. *A* and *B,*Thyroid ^{99m}Tc scan from a thyrotoxic cat with bilaterally symmetric adenomatous hyperfunctional thyroids.

Clinical Usefulness

UNILATERAL DISEASE. The clinical usefulness of thyroid scans is directly related to the treatment modalities available to the veterinarian (treatment methods are described in detail beginning on page 192). Approximately 15% to 20% of hyperthyroid cats have unilateral hyperthyroidism, in which one thyroid lobe is active and enlarged and causing the clinical signs. The lobe causing the disease usually contains a solitary adenoma, whereas the nondiseased lobe is nonfunctioning, atrophied, and not visualized (Fig. 4-23). Some cats with unilateral disease have adenomatous hyperplasia, but this is not usually a unilateral condition. Atrophy of the contralateral lobe is due to the suppressive effects of the hyperactive thyroid tissue on TSH secretion. It is recommended that cats with unilateral cervical hyperthyroidism be treated with surgical removal of the hyperactive thyroid lobe after an appropriate period of oral therapy.

BILATERAL DISEASE. More than 70% of hyperthyroid cats have both thyroid lobes involved. Only 10% to 15% of cats with both lobes involved have bilateral *symmetric* hyperthyroidism (Fig. 4-24). The veterinarian cannot always appreciate two distinct masses on palpation, but thyroid scans readily demonstrate this disorder. A large majority of hyperthyroid cats have bilateral *asymmetric* hyperthyroidism (Figs. 4-25 and 4-26). In more than 10% of hyperthyroid cats, one hyperactive gland is quite large and the other is extremely small but visible on a scan. On gross visual inspection of the thyroids, it may be difficult to distinguish cats with unilateral disease from those with bilateral asymmetric hyperthyroidism.

In some cats the smaller of two hypersecreting lobes may still be large, but in other cats the smaller lobe may contain slight amounts of adenomatous (hyperplastic) tissue and may be indistinguishable from an atrophied gland (Fig. 4-27). The thyroid scan, therefore, provides information that may prevent confusion at surgery. If a cat has one large, hyperfunctioning thyroid lobe on a scan, any additional thyroid tissue visualized on the contralateral side (above, parallel to, or below the larger gland) should also be assumed to be abnormal and probably adenomatous. Negative feedback to the pituitary from a unilateral adenoma should result in complete atrophy of the contralateral gland. Therefore any scintigraphic thyroid activity in a hyperthyroid cat, regardless of the number or size of the sites, should be interpreted as active adenomatous or cancerous tissue.

If surgery is performed after review of a radionuclide scan, the surgeon would know whether a cat requires unilateral or bilateral thyroidectomy, as well as the location of the tissue to be excised. Thus the surgeon would not need to rely on less accurate visual assessment. Oral antithyroid drugs or radioactive iodine therapy may be used instead of surgery for cats with bilateral hyperthyroidism. The ideal therapy for cats with bilateral hyperthyroidism is radioactive iodine.

MEDIASTINAL THYROID TISSUE. Approximately 3% of hyperthyroid cats have abnormal thyroid tissue in the anterior mediastinum and no palpable mass in the neck. Here again, thyroid scans have been an excellent diagnostic tool in locating the abnormal tissue (Fig. 4-28). Whether this tissue represents ectopic thyroid tissue or thyroids that migrated ventrally as they increased in weight and simply became "trapped" within the thorax is debated. Regardless, these cats should be treated with oral antithyroid drugs or radioactive iodine. Surgical exploration of the anterior mediastinum may be difficult and is not routinely recommended.

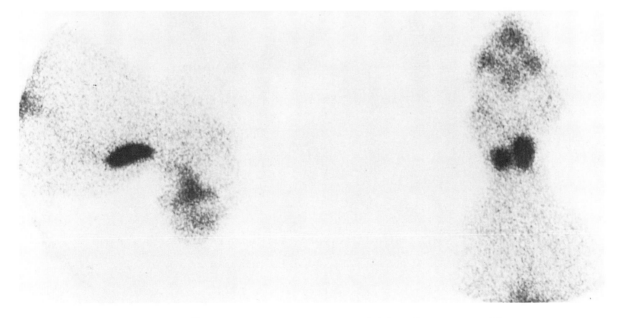

FIGURE 4–25. Thyroid ^{99m}Tc scan from a thyrotoxic cat with bilaterally asymmetric adenomatous hyperfunctional thyroids.

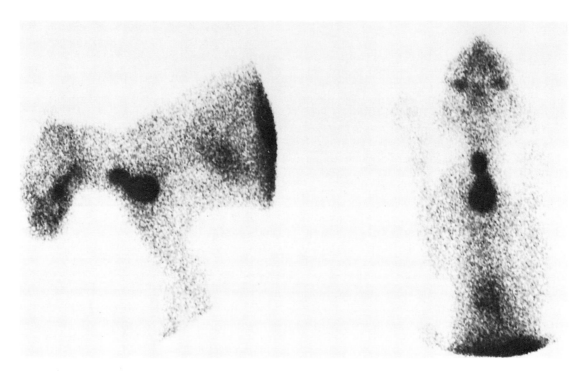

FIGURE 4–26. Thyroid ^{99m}Tc scan from a thyrotoxic cat with bilaterally asymmetric adenomatous hyperfunctional thyroids. Note that this scan shows the larger thyroid below the smaller rather than the side-by-side location seen in Fig. 4-25.

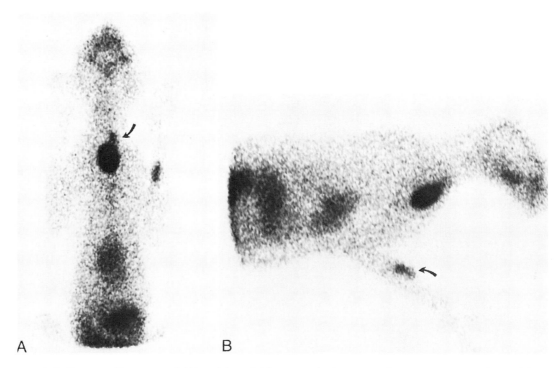

A   B

FIGURE 4–27. Dorsoventral *(A)* and lateral *(B)* views of a large intrathoracic anterior mediastinal thyroid mass with a small active gland just cranial to it *(arrow in A)*. This thyroid ^{99m}Tc scan is from a hyperthyroid cat that would be best treated with radioactive iodine. Also note that a small amount of pertechnetate leaked into the subcutaneous space during administration *(arrow in B)*.

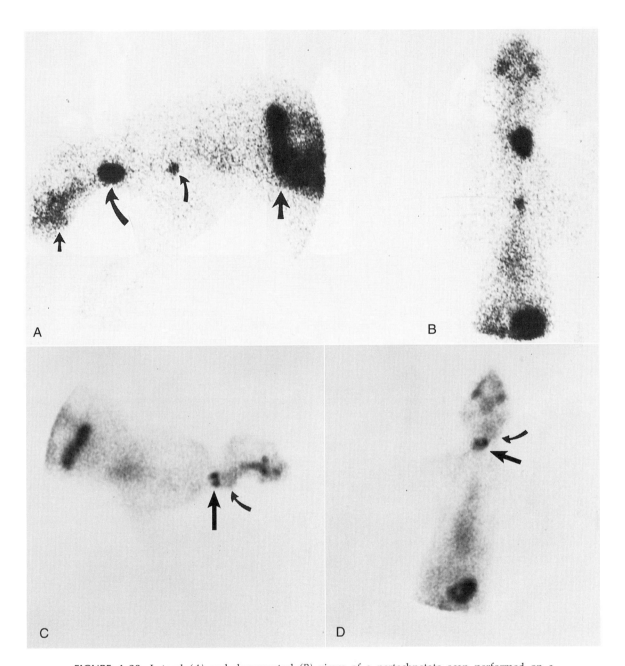

FIGURE 4–28. Lateral *(A)* and dorsoventral *(B)* views of a pertechnetate scan performed on a hyperthyroid cat. Note the large thyroid in the neck *(large curved arrow on lateral view)*; the small, adenomatous thyroid tissue in the anterior mediastinum *(small curved arrow)*; the salivary glands and the saliva, which concentrates pertechnetate *(small straight arrow)*; and the gastric mucosa, which concentrates pertechnetate *(large straight arrow)*. In the lateral *(C)* and dorsoventral *(D)* views of the pertechnetate scans from another cat, note the large intracervical mass *(curved arrows)* displacing the normal thyroid glands *(straight arrows)*. This mass was a salivary carcinoma, demonstrating that not all cervical masses are thyroid.

FUNCTIONING THYROID MALIGNANCY. When a cat has more than two thyroid masses, each of which exceeds the 1:1 ratio with the salivary glands, they are most likely to be functioning thyroid carcinomas (Fig. 4-29). The incidence of thyroid malignancy is approximately 3% of hyperthyroid cats. Some of these cats initially have only one or two thyroid masses, which emphasizes the importance of always obtaining histologic evaluation of surgically removed tissue. Malignancies

visualized on the scan are functioning and are sometimes called "hot." The incidence of nonfunctioning thyroid malignancies is not known; that is, they are hormonally inactive, do not trap pertechnetate, are seen on scans as areas within the thyroid devoid of radioactivity, and therefore are called "cold." These cells may be widely scattered or may have metastasized. However, as previously mentioned, two cats with bronchogenic carcinoma have been reported as

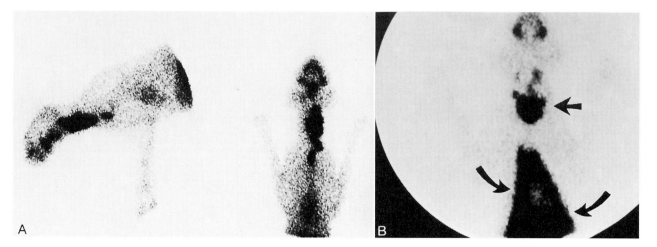

FIGURE 4–29. *A,* Thyroid ^{99m}Tc scan from a thyrotoxic cat with multiple functioning hyperactive thyroid masses. This may be representative of a cat with a functioning thyroid carcinoma that has undergone massive local invasion throughout the neck and anterior mediastinum. This also could represent multiple adenomatous tissue, some of which is ectopic. Radioactive iodine would be the most efficient therapy for this type of thyroid neoplasia. *B,* Thyroid ^{99m}Tc scan from a thyrotoxic cat with multiple functioning thyroid masses. This cat had a thyroid carcinoma with massive local invasion throughout the neck *(straight arrow)* and diffuse functioning carcinoma throughout the pulmonary parenchyma *(curved arrows).*

having pulmonary masses that concentrated radionuclide (Cook et al, 1993). Masses that concentrate pertechnetate, therefore, may not always be thyroid in origin.

Pertechnetate scans of the thyroid are the best tool available in veterinary medicine for recognizing metastasis of functioning thyroid malignancies. Treatment with the intent of "curing" a cat with metastatic thyroid carcinoma is difficult. Oral antithyroid drugs are not cytotoxic, which makes this therapeutic approach less than ideal. Surgery is not recommended as the sole therapy in these cats because it is not usually possible to remove all abnormal tissue. Radioactive iodine offers the best chance for successful management of the condition, because it concentrates in all hyperactive thyroid cells, regardless of location, and kills those cells. However, this tissue concentrates and retains iodine less efficiently than normal or adenomatous cells, requiring larger doses of radioactive iodine. The combination of surgical debulking followed by administration of high-dose radioactive iodine was successful in a small group of cats with functioning thyroid malignancies (Guptill et al, 1995).

THYROID TISSUE IN THE NECK AND MEDIASTINUM. Among the most confusing and frustrating of hyperthyroid cats, from a surgeon's point of view, are those with hyperthyroidism in which one large, hyperactive, palpable thyroid is located in the neck and another functioning mass is located within the anterior mediastinum (see Fig. 4-28). If treated without benefit of a scan, the palpable thyroid would be excised, no remaining thyroid tissue would be visible to the surgeon, and the hyperthyroidism would only partly resolve, fail to resolve, or recur.

SCANS AS A DIAGNOSTIC AID OR AN AID IN THERAPY. The thyroid scan may be used as a diagnostic test for cats with appropriate signs of hyperthyroidism but normal or borderline, nondiagnostic serum total and free T$_4$ concentrations. The thyroid gland to salivary gland ratio should normally be 1:1 (see Fig. 4-22), but in hyperthyroid cats the ratio is higher (Beck et al, 1985). In this setting the thyroid scan has the potential for diagnosing hyperthyroidism and locating the abnormal tissue. Investigators have also used scintigraphy to estimate thyroid mass volume and then have extended this information to help determine the dose of radioactive iodine to be administered for treatment (Forrest et al, 1996). Although estimation of thyroid volume can be accomplished with scintigraphy, it is not usually considered worthwhile.

CERVICAL (THYROID) ULTRASONOGRAPHY

Background

Ultrasonography is well established in small animal veterinary medicine as an excellent, noninvasive, highly informative diagnostic tool. Initial use of this tool focused on the evaluation of abdominal structures and the myocardium. Subsequently, ultrasonography of cervical structures became more commonly used (see Chapter 16, Hypercalcemia) (Wisner et al, 1991 and 1994). Cervical ultrasonography usually requires no anesthesia or sedation and is best performed with a 10 MHz transducer. As with any ultrasound evaluation, the value of cervical studies depends more on the skill of the operator than almost any other veterinary diagnostic tool.

Results

In a study on six healthy cats and 14 with confirmed hyperthyroidism, a significant difference was seen in the mean estimated thyroid volume of healthy cats compared with hyperthyroid cats. As experience in our clinic has increased, radiologists have become consistently able to locate both normal and abnormal thyroid lobes. Furthermore, correlation between thyroid scintigraphy and ultrasound has been excellent. We can consistently identify the single lobe causing hyperthyroidism in cats with "unilateral" disease and both lobes in cats with "bilateral" disease. Ultrasound cannot replace scintigraphy for locating distant ectopic or metastatic tissue, but it is considerably more available and less expensive.

Normal thyroid lobes are thin, fusiform-shaped structures that are moderately and uniformly echogenic (Fig. 4-30). Each lobe is located adjacent and medial to the common carotid arteries. The lobes are surrounded by a thin, hyperechoic fascia that can provide additional demarcation. The cranial and caudal ends of each lobe usually taper within this sheath, which sometimes makes the exact margins difficult to discern. Linear measurements of each lobe are easiest to make in the long axis plane. Normal lobes are usually 15 to 25 mm long, with calculated volumes of 40 to 140 mm^3 (Table 4-9) (Wisner et al, 1994).

Thyroid lobes from hyperthyroid cats are usually uniformly enlarged and have a tubular or sausage shape. Some lobes have mildly or moderately lobulated outer margins and/or poor delineation from surrounding tissue. Thyroid lobe parenchyma ranges from low to moderate echogenicity compared with surrounding tissue. In general, abnormal thyroids are also less echogenic than normal thyroid lobes. Although most abnormal glands are uniformly echogenic, a mottled echogenicity occasionally is seen. Although we are not certain of the incidence, we estimate that approximately 10% of hyperthyroid cats have large lobes containing cysts. Such cysts are easily visualized, anechoic structures on ultrasound examination. Cysts vary in shape and structure, some being unicameral and others containing one or several internal septae. It is not

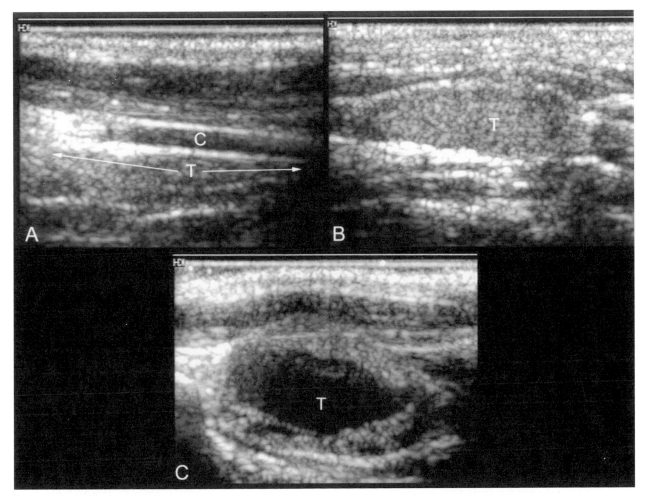

FIGURE 4–30. Cervical ultrasound of normal feline thyroid (*T*, thyroid; *C*, carotid artery) *(A)*; abnormal enlarged thyroid in a cat with hyperthyroidism *(B)*; and abnormal enlarged cystic thyroid in a cat with hyperthyroidism *(C)*.

TABLE 4–9 LINEAR MEASUREMENTS (mm) AND VOLUMETRIC ESTIMATIONS (mm³) FOR LEFT AND RIGHT THYROID LOBES OF CONTROL AND HYPERTHYROID CATS

	LEFT LOBE MEAN ± S.D.				RIGHT LOBE MEAN ± S.D.			
	Length	Height	Width	Volume*	Length	Height	Width	Volume*
Control (n = 6)	20.5 ± 1.6	3.3 ± 0.8	2.5†	89 ± 23	20.3 ± 1.6	3.0 ± 0.6	2.5†	80 ± 19
Hyperthyroid (n = 14)	20.2 ± 3.6	5.5 ± 2.4	5.7 ± 2.1	382 ± 312	21.9 ± 4.4	8.1 ± 3.0	7.7 ± 2.4	782 ± 449

*Volume estimation calculated using the formula for a prolate ellipsoid, $\pi/6$ (length * height * width).
†Width measurements for normal thyroid lobes defaulted to 2.5 mm because they could not be seen ultrasonographically.

unusual for abnormal thyroid lobes to be "normal" in length but obviously rounder and thicker; this accounts for the abnormal volume, which usually ranges from 140 to 1000 mm³ despite a length similar to that of the thyroid lobes of a healthy cat (see Fig. 4-30 and Table 4-9) (Wisner et al, 1994; Goldstein et al, 2001; Wells et al, 2001).

Uses for Thyroid Ultrasonography

Ultrasound was used initially as an adjunctive tool in locating cervical thyroid tissue, as a crude diagnostic aid for hyperthyroidism in some cats, and, more recently as a direct tool in novel therapies. We do not recommend that ultrasound be used in the diagnosis of hyperthyroidism; the history, physical examination findings, "database" laboratory testing, and total and free thyroxine measurements are excellent parameters for diagnosis. Ultrasound, by comparison, is not as reliable. However, for locating thyroid lobes and for injection procedures (see Novel "Ultrasound-Guided" Treatment Strategies, page 211), ultrasound has

provided an excellent, exciting approach to new management strategies.

GENERAL CONCEPTS IN TREATMENT

Background

The treatment of hyperthyroidism is directed at controlling or inhibiting excessive secretion of thyroid hormones. Three well-accepted methods of managing cats with this condition have emerged (Fig. 4-31). Each treatment modality has advantages, and each has some drawbacks (Table 4-10). Thyroid hormone synthesis can be inhibited medically, and this type of treatment can be tailored to the needs of each cat. However, medical therapy is not a permanent form of treatment. Medical therapy has the disadvantage of requiring continuing drug administration one to three times daily. Nonetheless, the transient nature of medical therapy can also be viewed as an advantage, because this form of treatment permits trial resolution

TABLE 4–10 ADVANTAGES AND DISADVANTAGES OF THE THREE MAJOR FORMS OF THERAPY FOR FELINE HYPERTHYROIDISM

Therapy	Advantages	Disadvantages
Surgery	1. Usually corrects the thyrotoxicosis 2. Thyroids easily accessible 3. Relatively inexpensive 4 Sophisticated equipment not required 5. Permanent "cure"	1. Risk of anesthesia in elderly and fragile cats 2. Anesthesia may decompensate other abnormal organ systems 3. Iatrogenic hypoparathyroidism 4. Iatrogenic hypothyroidism 5. Owner may refuse this form of treatment 6. Induction of thyrotoxicosis 7. Recurrent laryngeal nerve damage 8. Failure to remove all abnormal thyroid tissue 9. Permanent "cure"

Oral antithyroid drugs	1. Usually corrects the thyrotoxicosis
	2. Inexpensive
	3. Small tablet size
	4. No anesthesia or surgery
	5. No expensive facilities
	6. No hospitalization required
	7. Reversible
		1. Side effects of the medication:
		   a. Anorexia
		   b. Vomiting
		   c. Depression/lethargy
		   d. Thrombocytopenia
		   e. Granulocytopenia
		2. Daily medication required
		3. Iatrogenic hypothyroidism
		4. Not permanent

Radioactive iodine	1. Usually corrects the thyrotoxicosis 2. Only one treatment for most cats: no pills 3. No anesthesia or surgery 4. Rapid reduction in thyroid hormone concentrations 5. Permanent "cure"	1. Need for sophisticated facilities 2. Medication is dangerous to humans and not always available 3. Prolonged hospitalization before excretion of radioactivity is complete 4. Iatrogenic hypothyroidism 5. Re-treatment may be necessary in 2-5% 6. Permanent "cure"

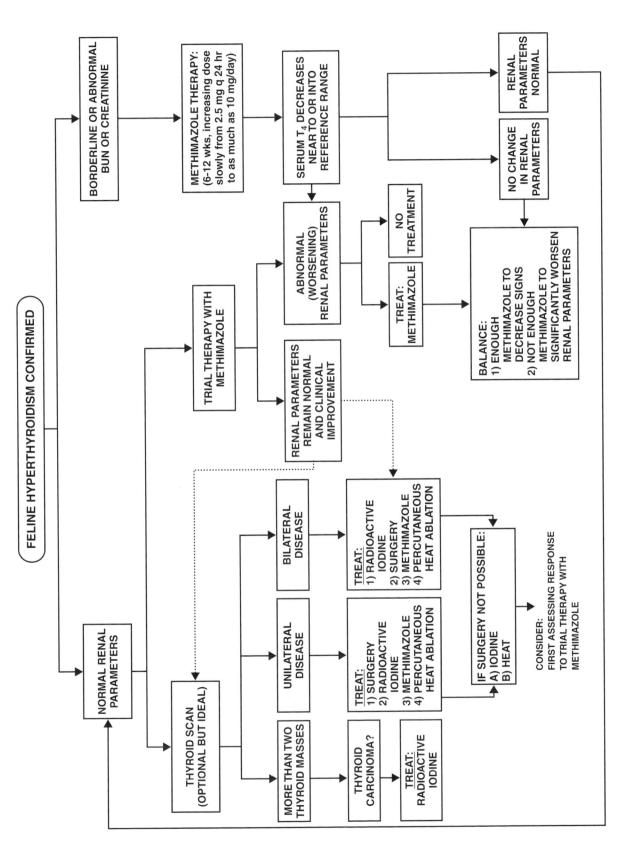

FIGURE 4–31. Algorithm for the treatment of cats with hyperthyroidism, emphasizing the potential negative effects of therapy on renal function.

of hyperthyroidism to be certain that a cat will not be harmed when euthyroid. The permanent forms of therapy include surgery and administration of radio-active iodine.

The treatment chosen for an individual cat depends on various factors, including the age of the cat and whether cardiovascular, renal, or other disorders are present. Other factors include the availability of a skilled surgeon or a facility with nuclear medicine capability for administering radioactive iodine. An owner may or may not choose to follow the advice of the veterinarian. In many cases, trial transient therapy with methimazole or carbimazole (oral or topical) should be evaluated prior to use of a permanent treatment method.

Hyperthyroidism versus Renal Function

BACKGROUND. Clinical evaluation and management of geriatric cats with concurrent hyperthyroidism and chronic renal failure (CRF) are challenging issues. The effect of nonthyroidal illnesses such as CRF in lowering serum thyroxine concentrations may mask hyperthyroidism. On the other hand, hyperthyroidism can increase the GFR and thereby decrease the serum creatinine and BUN concentrations, masking underlying renal disease. The progressive weight loss and reduction in muscle mass associated with hyperthyroidism may contribute to the reduction of serum creatinine concentrations, further "masking" any underlying renal disease. To make matters slightly more confounding, treatment of hyperthyroidism may not just "reveal" CRF, it may worsen that condition, making it a much greater risk to life than the hyperthyroidism.

PATHOPHYSIOLOGY. Hyperthyroidism increases cardiac output and decreases peripheral vascular resistance, leading to increased renal plasma flow (RPF) and an increase in the GFR. Both RPF and the GFR were increased in normal cats rendered hyperthyroid by administration of thyroxine for 30 days (Adams et al, 1997a). An increased GFR reduces serum creatinine, whereas an increased protein turnover associated with hyperthyroidism may increase BUN. Although emphasis has been placed on the adverse effects of treating a hyperthyroid cat that has CRF, it is also possible that hyperthyroidism contributes to the development of CRF in some older cats. In clinically normal cats, nearly 60% of renal perfusion pressure is transmitted to the glomerular capillary bed (DiBartola and Brown, 2000). Systemic hypertension frequently accompanies hyperthyroidism. If failure of auto-regulation occurs, a substantial portion of systemic hypertension may be transmitted to glomeruli, resulting in intraglomerular hypertension and hyperfiltration, factors that are recognized as contributing to glomerular sclerosis and progression of renal disease in cats.

These pathophysiologic relationships between hyperthyroidism and CRF raise important questions about the treatment of hyperthyroidism. It could be argued that reducing the serum thyroid hormone concentrations in older cats with mild hyperthyroidism and CRF should be avoided because such treatment may reduce the GFR and allow emergence of azotemia and uremia. Conversely, if an increased GFR results in glomerular hyperfiltration in hyperthyroid cats, it may contribute to progression of renal disease. If so, hyperthyroidism may predispose older cats to CRF, and early treatment may be important to prevent changes in the kidneys that could lead to progressive failure.

WORSENING RENAL FUNCTION AFTER RESOLUTION OF HYPERTHYROIDISM. It has been demonstrated that treatment of some cats for hyperthyroidism may have a profoundly negative effect on renal function (Graves et al, 1994). Treatment of hyperthyroidism by bilateral thyroidectomy in cats resulted in a decrease in the GFR from a mean of 2.5 ml/min/kg to 1.5 ml/min/kg, 30 days after surgery. In this same study, the mean serum creatinine and BUN concentrations increased from 1.3 to 2.0 mg/dl and from 27 to 35 mg/dl, respectively. In another study, the mean serum creatinine and BUN concentrations increased significantly, from 1.6 to 2.2 and then to 2.4 mg/dl and from 30 to 36 and then 37 mg/dl, respectively, 30 and 90 days after surgery or treatment with radioiodine or methimazole (DiBartola et al, 1996).

Changes in renal function were also studied in 22 cats with naturally occurring hyperthyroidism that were treated with radioactive iodine (Adams et al, 1997b). In this group, nine cats were classified as being in renal failure prior to treatment and 13 were so classified after treatment. In this study, renal failure was defined as a BUN greater than 30 mg/dl and/or a serum creatinine greater than 1.8 mg/dl with a concurrent urine specific gravity less than 1.035. It was determined that seven of the 22 cats that did not develop renal failure all had GFR measurements greater than 2.25 ml/min/kg prior to treatment. In contrast, 15 cats had GFR measurements less than 2.25 ml/min/kg. Two of these 15 did not respond to treatment and did not develop renal failure; however, the 13 cats that did respond to treatment all developed renal failure. Therefore not only was an association made between treatment for hyperthyroidism and worsening renal function test results, but it was suggested that pretreatment measurement of the GFR would be valuable in detecting subclinical renal disease and in predicting which cats may have clinically important decreases in renal function with treatment.

PREDICTING "MASKED" RENAL FAILURE BY DETERMINING THE GFR. BUN and serum creatinine concentrations vary inversely with the GFR and are used as indirect measures of the glomerular filtration rate. However, these two commonly used parameters are relatively insensitive indicators of renal disease, because at least 75% of functional renal mass needs to be lost before changes are noted. Significant renal disease, therefore, can be present in the absence of serum biochemical abnormalities. In addition, BUN and serum creatinine are affected by factors other than functional renal mass and blood flow. Estimation of the GFR, therefore, is more sensitive than routine serum biochemical analyses in assessing renal function. Furthermore, hyperthyroidism increases the GFR, and its treatment decreases the GFR. A study by Adams and colleagues (1997b) provided some parameters in the GFR that might help predict which cats will have worrisome increases in BUN and serum creatinine after treatment for hyperthyroidism.

The use of inulin or exogenous creatinine clearance to assess the GFR in cats is technically difficult, time-consuming, cumbersome, and requires anesthesia for urinary catheterization. Use of plasma clearance of radiolabeled diethylenetriamine penta-acetic acid (DTPA) requires approved nuclear medicine facilities. However, the use of plasma clearance of iohexol to estimate the GFR is reliable, simple, and requires no special equipment or facilities. Iohexol is an iodinated radiographic contrast agent, and the test has been validated for cats. An intravenous catheter must be placed for administration of the iohexol (2 ml/kg body weight, at a concentration of 300 mg iodine/ml) (Becker et al, 2000). Blood samples are taken 150, 195, and 240 minutes after iohexol administration; the serum iodine concentrations are assayed from each sample, and the GFR is calculated (Kruger et al, 1998; Braselton et al, 1997).

Using this protocol, the GFR was calculated before and after hyperthyroid cats were treated with methimazole (Adams et al, 1997b). The authors of this study demonstrated that 10 of 12 cats had a mean reduction in the GFR of about 50% after euthyroidism was established with treatment. Two of the 12 cats had increases in serum creatinine after treatment, and both had posttreatment reductions in the GFR to values less than 1 ml/min/kg. Arbitrarily, a pretreatment GFR less than 2.25 ml/min/kg was suggested to be worrisome (Adams et al, 1997b). However, use of this standard did not seem completely reliable in the iohexol study. Three of 12 cats had GFR values less than 2.25 ml/min/kg, and all three had BUN values above 30 with euthyroidism. However, five of the nine cats with values greater than 2.25 ml/min/kg also had BUN concentrations greater than 30 mg/dl with euthyroidism. The greatest BUN increase was noted in the cat with the second-highest GFR prior to treatment (Becker et al, 2000).

SUMMARY. Based on the studies completed to date, knowing the pretreatment GFR may be valuable. However, such studies do not consistently predict the development of renal failure after treatment re-establishes a euthyroid condition. Therefore a trial course of methimazole with follow-up serum bio-chemical and urine analyses may yet be the prudent initial steps in the treatment of hyperthyroid cats suspected of having renal dysfunction prior to electing "permanent therapy" (Becker et al, 2000). Unlike other modes of therapy, the methimazole effect seems to be completely reversible. For cats that develop overt renal failure, the hyperthyroidism should be left untreated or the dose of methimazole should be tailored to balance the two disorders. We recommend the methimazole treatment protocol discussed in the next section.

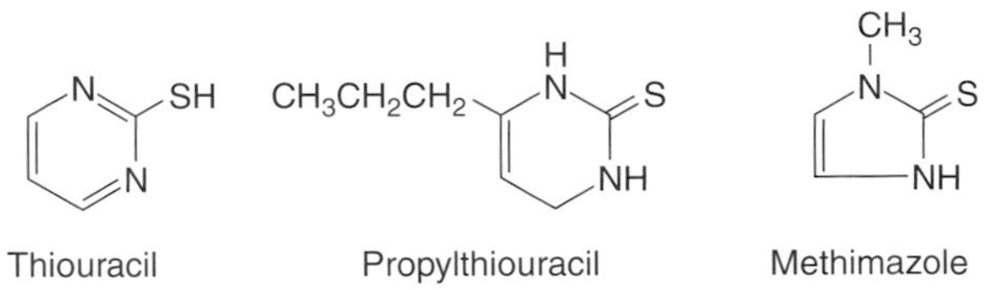

FIGURE 4–32. Chemical structures of the antithyroid drugs (thiocarbamides), which inhibit thyroidal iodide organification.

TREATMENT WITH ANTITHYROID DRUGS (THIOURYLENES)

Mode of Action

The structures of thiouracil, propylthiouracil (PTU), and methimazole (three commonly used thiourylenes) are shown in Fig. 4-32. These drugs are not cytotoxic and cannot permanently resolve hyperthyroidism. PTU and methimazole block the synthesis of thyroid hormones by inhibiting the organification of iodide and the coupling of iodothyronines to form T_4 and T_3 (Franklyn, 1994). There is some debate whether this is achieved by inhibition of the enzyme *thyroid peroxidase*. Antithyroid drugs also may attach to thyroglobulin and inhibit thyronine formation. PTU, in addition to its other effects, is known to impair peripheral deiodination of T_4 to T_3, an effect not attributed to methimazole. Neither of these drugs affects the iodide pump, which concentrates iodide in the thyroid cells, or the secretion of thyroid hormone formed prior to treatment (Peterson, 1995a). Carbimazole is metabolized to methimazole and therefore acts in a manner identical to methimazole.

When administered orally, antithyroid drugs are rapidly absorbed and have a volume of distribution close to that of total body water. PTU has a plasma half-life of 1 to 2 hours in humans, with 80% of the drug excreted into the urine within 24 hours (McDougall, 1981). Little of the drug is lost from the body except through the kidneys. Methimazole has a plasma half-life of 4 to 14 hours in humans, with two thirds of the medication recovered from the urine over 48 hours. The actions of PTU and methimazole appear to correlate with the dose administered and the *intrathyroidal* concentrations of the drugs, not with their plasma half-lives. Both drugs, therefore, have biologic effects that exceed their plasma half-lives. Also, both are selectively concentrated in the thyroid gland and are not recommended for administration more often than every 8 hours.

Propylthiouracil (PTU): No Longer Recommended

The use of PTU has been well reported in the veterinary literature. The drug is extremely effective in blocking the synthesis of thyroid hormones in cats and, therefore, in controlling hyperthyroidism

(Bradley and Feldman, 1982). However, PTU causes an unacceptable number of mild to severe adverse effects. These include anorexia, vomiting, lethargy, immune-mediated hemolytic anemia, and thrombocytopenia (Peterson et al, 1984; Aucoin et al, 1985 and 1988). Because of these side effects, and because methimazole is effective with fewer problems, PTU is not recommended for use in cats.

Methimazole (Tapazole)

INDICATIONS. Methimazole has three indications in the treatment of hyperthyroidism. *First,* it can be used to normalize serum T_4 concentrations, allowing assessment of the effect of resolution of hyperthyroidism on renal function ("test treatment"; see Fig. 4-31). After determining the effect of test therapy and being assured that renal function improved or remained static, the clinician could choose a more permanent means of treatment (surgery or radioactive iodine). *Second,* it can be used to prepare a cat for surgery or for

the prolonged hospitalization required for radioactive iodine treatment by allowing weight gain and improvement or resolution of any medical problem associated with hyperthyroidism. *Third,* it can be used as the only planned, short- and long-term treatment for hyperthyroidism (see Fig. 4-31 and Fig. 4-33).

ADVANTAGES. The advantages of oral methimazole therapy are numerous and are specifically compared with the advantages and disadvantages of surgery or radioactive iodine (see Table 4-10). Methimazole is quite popular because it is relatively inexpensive and readily available (usually through any veterinary distributor), and it does not require sophisticated training, facilities, or prolonged hospitalization. The medication is administered by owners, is relatively safe, and can be given to the oldest of hyperthyroid cats. Furthermore, with new compounding methodology, the drug not only can be given by the usual oral route, it can be administered topically as well (Trepanier et al, 2003b).

Methimazole carries no risks of permanent hypothyroidism or postsurgical hypoparathyroidism. Most

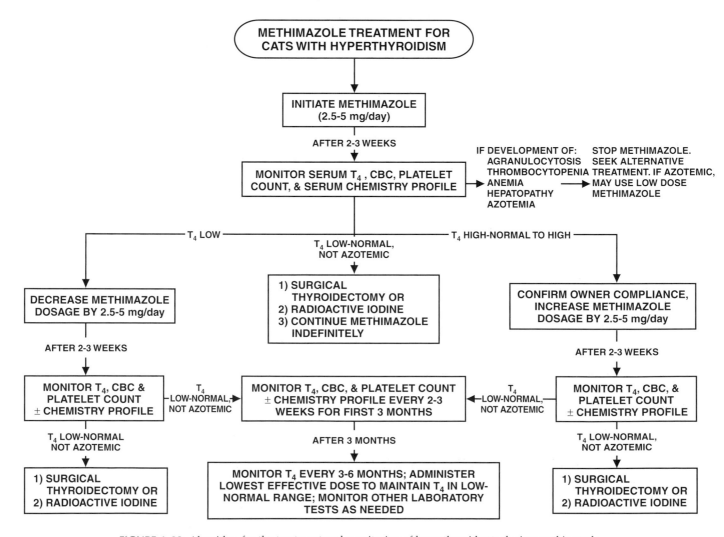

FIGURE 4–33. Algorithm for the treatment and monitoring of hyperthyroid cats during methimazole therapy.

importantly, the effects of the drug (positive or negative) are virtually always reversible upon its discontinuation. Methimazole is better tolerated and safer than PTU in cats and can be considered the antithyroid drug of choice for test therapy, preoperative control, and/or long-term management of feline hyperthyroidism. Carbimazole is equal to methimazole in efficacy and may be better tolerated by cats. Because methimazole is licensed for use in the United States and readily available, its use is emphasized here. In countries where carbimazole is available, its use is advisable.

ORAL DOSAGE PROTOCOL. The dosage protocol recommended here is a conservative variation of that suggested by others (Trepanier et al, 1991a and 1991b; Thoday and Mooney, 1992b; Peterson and Aucoin, 1993; Peterson, 1995a and 2000). The protocol is designed to gradually control the hyperthyroid syndrome while minimizing the incidence of side effects. Feline hyperthyroidism is a chronic and progressive disease syndrome. Acute resolution of the disease is almost never necessary. Furthermore, although the side effects associated with methimazole occur less commonly and are generally less severe than those due to PTU, minimization of any negative reaction is considered beneficial. Side effects are less frequently encountered and less severe at relatively low methimazole doses than with initial dosages of 10 to 15 mg/day.

Our recommended initial dose of methimazole is 2.5 mg (one half of a tablet) twice a day for 2 weeks. We have started numerous cats on 2.5 mg once daily (or 1.25 mg twice daily) when specific concerns about side effects warranted an even more conservative approach. We never recommend beginning with a dose greater than 5 mg/day. If an owner observes no untoward side effects, the dose should be increased to 2.5 mg three times a day (or 5.0 mg in the morning and 2.5 mg in the evening, or vice versa) for an additional 2 weeks.

After completion of these 4 weeks of "trial therapy," the cat should be assessed by the veterinarian. A history and physical examination should be completed, and blood should be obtained for a CBC, platelet count, serum biochemistry profile, and serum T_4 concentration measurement. Blood samples should be taken 4 to 6 hours after the most recent dose of methimazole. If the serum T_4 concentration is within or near the normal reference range, the dose may be maintained for an additional 2 to 6 weeks to allow determination of the need for any further dosage adjustments. If the serum T_4 concentration is below the reference range, the dose should be reduced. If the hyperthyroidism is not controlled, the dosage should continue to be increased every 2 weeks in increments of 2.5 mg a day. Once the hyperthyroidism is controlled, long-term dosing protocols can be initiated. If any adverse effect is likely from review of these assessments, methimazole should be discontinued, at least temporarily. Assuming that any adverse effect does resolve, a decision can then be made about choosing an alternative therapy or simply using lower doses of methimazole.

Most cats require 5 or 7.5 mg/day of methimazole to control hyperthyroidism. The drug is most effective given BID or TID (Trepanier et al, 2003a). Occasionally cats require 10 mg/day. It is unusual for cats to require more than 10 mg/day using this protocol. Rarely, cats are encountered that seem particularly resistant, requiring as much as 20 mg/day. In our experience, doses in excess of 12.5 to 15 mg/day are required by an extremely small percentage of hyperthyroid cats. The most common cause of *apparent* resistance to methimazole is owner inability to administer the drug to their cat. If doses of 10 mg/day or more do not reduce the serum T_4 concentrations, the veterinarian must assess owner compliance by watching the owner "pill" their cat.

TOPICAL METHIMAZOLE. With the new compounding laws for pharmacies, drugs such as methimazole can be placed in creams for topical administration. Creams can be made with methimazole at any concentration, although 20 mg/ml seems common and effective. The compounded drug is often available in 1 cc syringes, which allows the owner to place the appropriate dose on a fingertip. With this method, the owner wears a glove, removes the desired dose of methimazole from the syringe, and rubs the cream into the pinna of the ear. Anecdotal information has suggested that such topical formulations have been more effective, less effective, or equally effective compared with oral administration. In one study on healthy cats, a single lecithin/pluronic gel transdermal dose of methimazole resulted in generally low to undetectable bio-availabilities. However, one cat of five did achieve nearly 100% transdermal bioavailability relative to the oral route (Hoffman et al, 2002).

Overall, transdermal methimazole takes a little longer to become effective and doesn't work in as many cats as the oral form. The difference in efficacy is not significant by 4 weeks. There is no difference in liver, hematologic, or pruritus side effects, but fewer GI side effects occur with the transdermal form of methimazole. Some cats have mild crusting and erythema of the pinnae where the drug is applied. It is not common for the superficial irritation to prevent continuing use. Owners should be instructed to alternate ears, and to wipe away any residual drug/vehicle after each administration (Trepanier et al, 2003b). Until specific studies are conducted, we recommend that owners attempt to rub the gel in well and then remove any excess material 30 to 120 minutes later. We recommend a starting dose of 1 mg applied topically once daily for 2 weeks and then twice daily for an additional 2 weeks. The protocol followed is then the same as that recommended for oral administration. There is one warning, however. There is virtually no regulation of compounding pharmacies, therefore the cream used, the methimazole used, and the final product created vary. It is critical for veterinarians to understand these concerns. Although it has the potential to be extremely beneficial for owners of cats that are difficult to "pill," this form of therapy should be considered a trial until consistency in products can be assured.

HYPERTHYROID CATS WITH ABNORMAL RENAL PARAMETERS. Some hyperthyroid cats have abnormal BUN and creatinine concentrations. It does not appear possible to predict, even with assessment of the GFR, which cats will show improvement and which will demonstrate worsening renal parameters after therapy for hyperthyroidism. This dilemma has resulted in a modification of the treatment protocol for cats with hyperthyroidism and possible renal insufficiency; that is, before consideration is given to potentially permanent treatments (surgery or radioactive iodine), cats should be test treated with oral methimazole (see Figs. 4-31 and 4-33).

The recommended methimazole treatment protocol for hyperthyroid cats with concurrent renal insufficiency is 2.5 mg given once daily for 2 weeks (or 1.25 mg given twice daily for 2 weeks) and then 2.5 mg given twice daily for 2 weeks. The 4-week evaluation is completed as described above, but special attention is paid to the results of the serum T_4, BUN, creatinine, and phosphate determinations. If the serum T_4 concentration can be decreased to or toward normal levels and the renal parameters improve, continued oral antithyroid medications, surgery, or radioactive iodine treatments can be considered. However, if the renal parameters worsen with improved serum thyroid hormone concentrations, treating the hyperthyroidism may not be in the best interest of the cat. In this latter situation, oral therapy (which is completely reversible) should be discontinued, renal parameters monitored, and the entire syndrome explained to the owners. Some cats are undoubtedly healthier with hyperthyroidism than without (see Figs. 4-31 and 4-33). However, this is rarely the scenario at our hospital. The usual approach to worsening renal parameters after improvement or normalization of the serum T_4 concentration is to balance methimazole doses with knowledge of renal parameters. The goal is to minimize the clinical signs of hyperthyroidism as much as possible without causing escalation in renal failure. Continuing methimazole at doses below those needed for euthyroidism has proved extremely positive for both the cats and their owners.

MONITORING OF CATS DURING THE FIRST 1 TO 3 MONTHS OF THERAPY. Methimazole-treated cats may develop worrisome side effects (Table 4-11). These adverse reactions have become less and less common as we continue to use the conservative dose regimens outlined in the previous sections. However, because problems still occasionally occur, early detection may prevent catastrophic sequelae. It is recommended that baseline laboratory measurements (CBC, serum chemistry profile, and urinalysis) be done prior to initiation of treatment. Because side effects, if they occur, almost always develop in the first 4 to 8 weeks of treatment, repetition of these laboratory evaluations through the initial 8 to 12 weeks is recommended. It has been recommended that these parameters be rechecked after the initial 2 weeks of treatment; however, when methimazole is started at 2.5 or 5.0 mg/cat/day, no adverse reactions have been seen. We therefore phone owners after the first 2 weeks of treatment and recommend in-hospital rechecks after a total of 4 weeks on antithyroid medication. The serum T_4 concentration should also be monitored at each recheck. As mentioned in the discussion of the disadvantages of methimazole, careful review of liver enzyme activities, renal function parameters, red blood cell counts, white blood cell counts, and platelet counts is critical. Obvious changes consistent with methimazole toxicity in any of these parameters should be managed by discontinuation of treatment until normal results are again documented.

TABLE 4–11   ADVERSE REACTIONS ASSOCIATED WITH DRUGS USED THERAPEUTICALLY IN FELINE HYPERTHYROIDISM

Drug	Reaction	Approximate Percentage of Cats Affected	Time at Occurrence	Treatment Required
Methimazole	Vomiting, anorexia, depression	15	<4 wk	Usually transient
	Eosinophilia, leukopenia, lymphocytosis	15	<8 wk	Usually transient
	Self-induced excoriations	2	<4 wk	Withdrawal and glucocorticoid therapy
	Agranulocytosis, thrombocytopenia	<5	<3 mo	Withdrawal and symptomatic therapy
	Hepatopathy (anorexia, ↑ alanine aminotransferase, alkaline phosphatase)	<2	<2 mo	Withdrawal and symptomatic therapy
	Positive ANA	>50	>6 mo	Decrease daily dosage
	Acquired myasthenia gravis	Rare	<16 wk	Withdrawal or concomitant glucocorticoid therapy
Carbimazole	Vomiting, anorexia, depression	10	<3 wk	Usually transient
	Eosinophilia, leukopenia, lymphocytosis	5	<2 wk	Usually transient
	Self-induced excoriations	Rare	<4 wk	Withdrawal and glucocorticoid therapy
Stable iodine	Salivation and anorexia	Occasional	Immediate	Change formulation

After the first 3 months of therapy, cats treated with methimazole should be monitored every 3 to 6 months. Adverse side effects, although uncommon after 3 months of treatment, may occur. It is also possible for dosage requirements to vary with time. Monitoring of the serum T_4 concentration, therefore, is helpful. At any recheck the veterinarian should take advantage of the opportunity to check the body weight and to assess a complete history and physical examination. From this information decisions can be made regarding any additional tests that might be indicated.

TIME REQUIRED TO OBSERVE A RESPONSE. Serum T_4 concentrations respond to methimazole administration within a week. Rechecks 2 weeks after the start of therapy or after a change in dosage should reflect this response (e.g., no further response usually takes place with more time). If a dosage of methimazole is given that results in a euthyroid state, the serum T_4 concentrations will decline into the reference range within 1 to 2 weeks, or sooner. As suggested in the dosage protocol section, the effective dose requirement varies from cat to cat, with some needing only 2.0 to 2.5 mg/day and others requiring 10 to 12.5 mg/day. The drug is most efficacious if administered BID (Trepanier et al, 2003a). The protocol outlined above provides an excellent opportunity for treatment to be tailored to the needs of each cat, with only the necessary amount of medication given. Response to therapy is defined as improvement in or resolution of abnormal serum T_4 concentrations.

Although the effect on serum T_4 concentrations can be documented within days to weeks of initiation of methimazole therapy, *clinical* response is almost never observed this quickly (Fig. 4-34). Clinical improvement is usually noted by owners 2 to 6 weeks *after* good control of serum thyroid hormone concentrations has been achieved. Owners should be so informed in order to reduce their level of anticipation or frustration, especially when the conservative dosage protocol outlined above is used. With this low-dose regimen, clinical improvement may be delayed by weeks. Although we believe the benefits of this protocol outweigh the risks associated with more aggressive treatment regimens, good communication with owners is extremely important so that they understand what to expect.

LONG-TERM DOSING PROTOCOLS. Once control of hyperthyroidism has been achieved, usually by means of two or three doses per day, owners who plan to treat their cats long term usually prefer to administer pills once or twice daily. In this situation, the *total* daily dose required to reduce the serum T_4 concentrations into or below reference ranges should be maintained while the frequency of administration is cut back. For example, a regimen of 2.5 mg given three times daily often can be reduced to 5 mg given in the morning and 2.5 mg in the evening, or 7.5 mg given once daily. Owners often can provide insight into the success of a protocol after their cat has been maintained on a new schedule for 4 to 8 weeks. The response to therapy can be misjudged if enough time is not allowed.

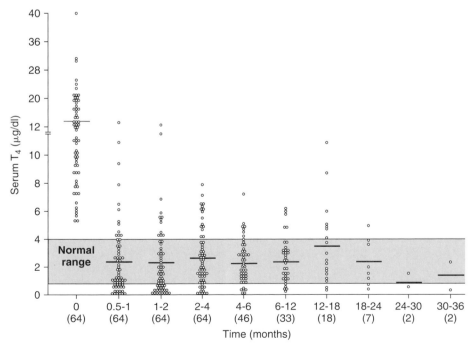

FIGURE 4–34. Serum T_4 concentrations in 64 cats with hyperthyroidism before and during long-term treatment with methimazole. The horizontal lines indicate mean values. The numbers in parentheses indicate the number of cats treated during each time period. (Peterson ME, et al: J Vet Intern Med 2:150, 1988.)

Owners should be warned to observe their cats for a gradual return of clinical signs that might result from administration of methimazole too infrequently. Good control usually can be maintained with twice-daily dosing. Once-daily administration is not as effective (Trepanier et al, 2003a). The serum half-life of methimazole is only 4 to 6 hours (Trepanier et al, 1991a and 1991b). However, studies in humans have demonstrated that methimazole is typically retained within thyroid tissue for as long as 20 hours (Cooper, 1984). Because antithyroid drugs act to inhibit hormone synthesis only after being concentrated in the thyroid, the serum half-life is not as valuable in determining dosing schedules as is the duration of effect.

Anytime an owner believes that the cat is deteriorating on a particular treatment regimen, a veterinary evaluation is warranted, and the owner should be questioned about his or her ability to administer the drug. If questions about owner compliance persist, a veterinarian or technician should evaluate the owner by watching the person administer a pill to their cat. If dose frequency is thought to be the problem, the best time for reevaluating the serum T_4 concentration is when the cat is due for its next dose. Such testing helps determine whether the duration of effect is sufficient to maintain the euthyroid state achieved with more frequent dosing. Appropriate adjustments in dose or frequency are relatively straightforward. If an owner cannot consistently administer methimazole orally, topical creams should be considered.

DISADVANTAGES

Daily Medication. The use of oral antithyroid drugs has several disadvantages, some of which include life-threatening problems. However, one of the most common complaints we receive from owners is the need for one, two, or three treatments per day. Owners simply become frustrated by the need to continually medicate their pets. This problem may worsen as the treatment period progresses. Ravenously hungry hyperthyroid cats, for example, may be easily treated by placing pills in quickly devoured food. However, as the hyperthyroidism resolves, these cats become less ravenous and do not readily consume pills; they usually just eat around the pill. The owner must then hold the cat and force it to accept the pills. "Pilling" cats is not easy and may cause a pet to begin hiding from its owner or hissing, biting, or scratching. When this occurs, the owner may return to the veterinarian for alternatives to daily oral medication, one of which is the use of compounded methimazole so that the drug can be given topically (see previous section).

Hypothyroidism. Subnormal serum T_4 concentrations commonly develop during short- and long-term methimazole treatment. However, most of those cats maintain serum T_3 concentrations within the reference range (Peterson et al, 1988). Clinical signs of hypothyroidism often are not recognized or do not concern the owners of these cats. Without worrisome signs, the dosage can be maintained. Unlike PTU, methimazole does not appear to inhibit the $5'$-deiodination of T_4 to T_3 (Utiger, 1987). Because T_3 is the biologically active hormone, normal circulating T_3 concentrations may explain the absence of clinical signs associated with subnormal serum T_4 concentrations. If signs of hypothyroidism are recognized, the methimazole doses may simply be reduced by 25% to 50% and the cat rechecked 4 to 8 weeks later.

Drug-Induced Clinical Side Effects. Relatively mild clinical side effects from methimazole therapy are common, occurring in approximately 10% to 15% of cats (Peterson, 1995a and 2000). Most side effects are observed during the first 4 to 6 weeks of treatment, and it is less common for a cat to develop methimazole-induced side effects after 2 to 3 months of treatment. Common side effects include anorexia, vomiting, and lethargy (Graves, 1995). These adverse reactions tend to be transient and may resolve with continued administration of the drug.

The conservative treatment protocol outlined in the previous sections dramatically reduces the incidence of side effects. Using small initial doses and slowly increasing the dosage as needed has rarely resulted in adverse reactions (<3% of treated cats). In most instances, gastrointestinal signs are managed by discontinuing the drug until all signs of toxicity have resolved for at least a week and then restarting the medication at a lower dose. It appears worthwhile to avoid these side effects from the outset by administering low initial doses.

Self-induced excoriation of the face and neck are unusual but alarming reactions to methimazole. Like most of the drug's adverse effects, this problem usually occurs within the first 4 to 8 weeks of therapy. Although these cutaneous lesions may be partly responsive to glucocorticoid treatment, methimazole should be discontinued until the signs resolve completely. Alternative treatment (surgery or radioactive iodine) should be considered for these cats.

Biochemical/Hematologic Side Effects. Because a variety of side effects have been recognized in cats treated with oral antithyroid drugs, monitoring of cats after the fourth week (every 2 weeks during the initial 8 to 12 weeks) is suggested, as outlined above. If adverse reactions to methimazole are identified, similar problems are likely to result with the use of other oral antithyroid drugs (PTU or carbimazole). Although antithyroid drugs are not thought to cause renal problems, renal problems may be exacerbated with control of the hyperthyroidism (see previous sections).

Apparent hepatic toxicity or injury occurs in a small number of cats treated with methimazole. This hepatopathy is characterized by clinical signs (anorexia, vomiting, lethargy), icterus, and abnormalities (sometimes marked) in serum ALT and SAP activities. Days to weeks may be required for all clinical and biochemical problems to resolve after the drug has been discontinued. Alternative therapies for hyperthyroidism should be considered for cats that develop these adverse reactions. If methimazole is the only acceptable treatment option, extremely low doses with conservative incremental increases should be used.

Mild hematologic changes caused by methimazole include eosinophilia, lymphocytosis, and transient leukopenia, each of which may be isolated abnormalities or may be related to the gastrointestinal signs that some of these cats develop (especially the eosinophilia). More worrisome alterations include severe thrombocytopenia (platelet counts <75,000 cells/mm^3), which can be associated with epistaxis, oral bleeding, or both. Agranulocytosis (total white blood cell counts <2000 cells/mm^3) is another serious complication that may be associated with fever, anorexia, lethargy, and localized or systemic infections (Peterson et al, 1988; Sheng et al, 1999). Fewer than 0.1% of cats treated with methimazole develop immune-mediated hemolytic anemia (Peterson, 1995a). As many as half the cats treated for longer than 6 months with antithyroid drugs have positive antinuclear antibody test results, but the importance of this finding is not known (Graves, 1995). Coagulopathy associated with methimazole administration to cats occurs rarely, if at all. If coagulopathy is suspected, protein induced by vitamin K absence or antagonism (PIVKA) testing may be more sensitive than the standard prothrombin time (PT) and activated partial thromboplastin time (APTT) in identifying these abnormalities. However, some hyperthyroid cats have abnormal coagulation profiles prior to treatment (Randolph et al, 2000).

If any of these serious complications is recognized, methimazole administration should be discontinued and supportive care given. The support required may include intravenous fluids, blood transfusions, and/or antibiotics. The adverse reactions typically resolve quickly (within 7 days) after discontinuation of the drug (Peterson et al, 1988). Because of the life-threatening nature of these side effects, surgery or radioactive iodine therapy should be considered rather than again exposing the cat to these medications.

Carbimazole

BACKGROUND. Methimazole is not available in Western Europe or the United Kingdom. The alternative to PTU is the carbethoxy derivative of methimazole, carbimazole (Neo-Mercazole, England), which is not available in the United States. Carbimazole is another thiourylene antithyroid drug that has been used successfully in humans for many years. This drug is converted to methimazole in vivo. A 5 mg dose of carbimazole is approximately equal to 3 mg of methimazole, which explains, in part, the differences in recommended dose and the frequency of side effects noted when comparing these two drugs (Mooney et al, 1992a; Peterson and Aucoin, 1993).

DOSE. A dosage of 5 mg given orally three times a day is recommended for carbimazole. Biochemical euthyroidism occurs within 1 to 2 weeks in most cats, and clinical improvement is usually noticed within 2 to 3 weeks (Mooney et al, 1992a). In contrast to methimazole, a once- or twice-daily treatment schedule appears to be less effective than a three times

a day regimen during the initial weeks of administration. However, long-term, twice-daily schedules are effective. Despite these recommendations, we recommend giving 2.5 mg twice a day for 7 days and then 5 mg twice a day for 3 weeks. At that time the serum T_4 concentrations should be assessed, along with other necessary parameters. Dose adjustments should then be made accordingly, but a regimen of 5 mg given twice a day has been recommended for the long-term management of hyperthyroid cats (Mooney, 1998a). Until conservative dosing schedules are demonstrated to be ineffective, we suspect that such a protocol will reduce the incidence and severity of side effects without adversely affecting efficacy.

ADVERSE SIDE EFFECTS. Most adverse reactions occur within the first 3 months of the start of carbimazole administration. In humans, carbimazole is described as tasteless, whereas methimazole is said to have a bitter taste; this difference may account for the lower incidence of anorexia and vomiting reported in cats treated with carbimazole. However, mild side effects of vomiting, with or without anorexia and depression, still are reported in approximately 10% of carbimazole-treated cats within the first 3 weeks of therapy at 5 mg three times a day. The percentage of cats exhibiting these side effects could be reduced with more conservative dosing schedules. Early in the course of therapy, mild and transient lymphocytosis, eosinophilia, or leukopenia occur in 5% of treated cats. Self-induced excoriation of the head and neck have been rarely described and usually occur during the first 6 weeks of treatment; this typically requires permanent withdrawal of the drug (Mooney, 1998a; Bucknell, 2000).

More serious adverse reactions have not yet been described with carbimazole (Mooney, 1998a). Agranulocytosis or thrombocytopenia (or both) remains a possibility, and monitoring of the CBC and platelet counts are recommended. It has been suggested that as an alternative to obtaining blood every 2 weeks, the cat could simply be observed for clinical signs and tested only if indicated. The hepatopathies and serum antinuclear antibodies without systemic signs of a lupuslike syndrome that have been described in cats treated with methimazole have not been observed with carbimazole. Cats treated with carbimazole have been described as frequently having serum T_4 concentrations below the reference range without associated clinical signs of hypothyroidism. It is assumed that clinical signs are not observed because corresponding serum T_3 concentrations tend to remain within the reference range due to extrathyroidal conversion from T_4 or because of preferential thyroidal production of T_3 (Mooney, 1998a).

TREATMENT WITH SURGERY

Presurgical Management

METHIMAZOLE. In an attempt to minimize perisurgical and postsurgical complications, hyperthyroid cats must be thoroughly evaluated for coexisting illness prior to surgery. Problems such as congestive heart failure, cardiac arrhythmias, renal failure (see previous section), and simple weight loss/cachexia should be identified and treated. In addition, the clinician can usually reduce surgical and anesthetic complications by controlling thyrotoxicosis prior to surgery.

Methimazole should be administered orally or topically for 6 to 12 weeks, until the cat is medically and clinically euthyroid. The conservative dose schedule outlined in previous sections is recommended. The stepwise increase in the methimazole dose delays obvious improvement in some cats but minimizes adverse side effects in most. Drug effectiveness should be demonstrated with a serum T_4 concentration within the reference range and by noting obvious clinical improvement. Clinical improvement, which is usually a subjective change, should be observed by the owner as well as the veterinarian. Successfully treated cats invariably gain weight. In severe hyperthyroidism, short-term oral antithyroid medication is safer than surgery. The 6- to 12-week treatment period is a guideline that has proved sufficient for most cats and that allows the veterinarian an opportunity to identify cats that have reduced renal function with resolution of the thyrotoxicosis (see Figs. 4-31 and 4-33).

ORAL POTASSIUM IODIDE, IODATE, AND PROPRANOLOL COMBINATIONS. In the 8 to 10 days preceding surgery, some cats benefit from 1 drop of saturated solution of potassium iodide (SSKI), which can be administered orally every day. This solution blocks the secretion of thyroid hormones and may reduce the vascularity of the thyroid, making surgical dissection easier (McDougall, 1981; Franklyn, 1994). Cats may salivate excessively after tasting this liquid. To avoid this problem, the drop of SSKI can be placed in a small gelatin capsule and immediately administered (Peterson, 1995a). We have no experience with this mode of therapy.

Combinations of propranolol and potassium iodate have been used to control hyperthyroidism and cardiac abnormalities prior to surgery (Foster and Thoday, 1999). However, a number of complications and side effects discourage the routine use of this combination of therapeutic agents. We recommend conservative methimazole or carbimazole treatment for presurgical management of hyperthyroid cats.

PROPANOLOL AND OTHER β-ANTAGONIST DRUGS. Propranolol is recommended for cats with severe tachycardia or supraventricular tachyarrhythmias. Propranolol should slow the heart rate, improve cardiac stroke volume, and increase cardiac output. In humans with hyperthyroidism, these drugs (including metoprolol, atenolol, and nadolol) ameliorate some of the symptoms and signs (e.g., tremor, anxiety, and palpitations) more rapidly than antithyroid drug therapy (Franklyn, 1994).

GENERAL GUIDELINES. On the day before surgery, the ventrocervical area should be clipped to minimize anesthesia time. Intravenous fluid should be administered immediately prior to and during surgery at or below maintenance rates to avoid fluid overload and decompensation of any cardiovascular compromise.

The goal of the above plan (including prior treatment with methimazole and propranolol) is to send to surgery as healthy and stable a cat as is medically possible. By attaining this goal, many of the complications associated with surgery are avoided. Surgery must be approached as an elective procedure, not one that must be performed hastily.

Anesthesia

GENERAL CONCERNS. Once hyperthyroidism has been controlled with oral agents, common anesthesia protocols are usually used. The rapid metabolic rate associated with hyperthyroidism increases the absorption, distribution, tissue uptake, and inactivation of anesthetic agents. In addition, some hyperthyroid cats are thin, even after 6 to 12 weeks of oral antithyroid therapy. These factors increase the importance of a careful check of body weight before any medication is administered.

PREMEDICATION AND ANESTHESIA INDUCTION. Drugs that stimulate or potentiate adrenergic activity capable of inducing tachycardia and arrhythmias should be avoided, whereas drugs that minimize these problems are preferred. The anesthetic procedure we have adopted is straightforward. Premedication with acepromazine (0.1 mg/kg IM) reduces the autonomic manifestations of hyperthyroidism. Anticholinergic agents such as atropine are avoided because they cause sinus tachycardia and are known to enhance anesthetic-induced cardiac arrhythmias. Some use glycopyrrolate instead of atropine.

Xylazine and ketamine are avoided, and some prefer isoflurane over halothane. We usually place the premedicated cat in an anesthesia induction chamber (box), and anesthesia is accomplished with halothane, nitrous oxide, and oxygen. Isoflurane has also provided excellent results as an inhalant anesthetic. It produces rapid induction of and recovery from anesthesia, which greatly shortens the anesthetic time. The major disadvantage of isoflurane is cost. Thiamylal sodium can also be used to induce anesthesia and allow intubation of these cats. Once anesthetized, the cat can be intubated and inhalation anesthesia continued. Minimizing anesthesia time is always advisable, and continuous monitoring is essential. For simple sedation, meperidine ([Demerol] 2 to 4 mg/kg IM) can be used. Demerol is useful for completing simple procedures in some fractious, hyperactive, or fragile hyperthyroid cats.

MONITORING. Careful monitoring of these cats is a must. Use of an esophageal stethoscope or continuous electrocardiography and repeated blood pressure measurements can prevent or aid in the recognition of catastrophe. Arrhythmias and subsequent cardiac arrest are the most common causes of mortality during surgery. It is imperative that injectable propranolol and lidocaine be available for emergencies. Propranolol can be diluted in sterile water (1 mg diluted in 10 ml of water) and 0.25 to 1.0 mg intravenous boluses administered to control tach-yarrhythmias (Mooney, 1998a). Usually one dose is beneficial and lasts for 10 to 30 minutes. If an arrhythmia recurs, the dose of propranolol can be repeated. Lidocaine is used only as a last resort, because it can cause methemoglobinemia in cats. The initial dose is 0.5 to 2.0 mg/kg given intravenously. If successful, lidocaine needs to be repeated every 10 to 30 minutes. It is also helpful to have someone other than the surgeon monitor the cat during anesthesia. Close observation should continue until the cat has completely recovered from anesthesia.

Surgical Techniques

GENERAL GUIDELINES. Surgical removal of abnormally active thyroid tissue is perhaps the most frequently used treatment for hyperthyroidism in veterinary practice. Exploratory surgery of the ventrocervical region is relatively simple, not time-consuming, and therefore not expensive. Normal thyroid lobes are pale tan, whereas thyroid adenomas or adenomatous hyperplasia is typically brown to reddish brown. The area from above the normal location of the thyroids (hyoid region) down to the thoracic inlet should be examined, with strict attention paid to hemostasis (Holzworth et al, 1980). After exposure and inspection of all visible thyroid tissue, the external parathyroid gland or glands should be identified and preserved (see section on parathyroid preservation, page 204) (Fig. 4-35). These external parathyroid glands are usually located in the loose fascia at the cranial pole of each lobe, although they may be located at the middle or distal part of the adjacent thyroid. The internal

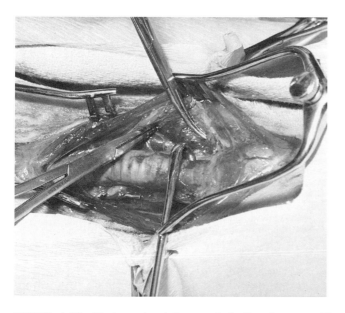

FIGURE 4–35. Photograph of the surgical site of a cat with hyperthyroidism undergoing thyroidectomy. Note the parathyroid gland located at the tip of the Alice tissue forceps.

parathyroids are usually embedded in the thyroid lobe parenchyma, and their location varies. The external parathyroids are much smaller than the thyroid lobes and can be distinguished from thyroid tissue by their lighter color and spherical shape. The thyroid lobes and their adjacent parathyroid glands lie within the cervical "gutters." In addition, each gutter contains the carotid artery, jugular vein, and recurrent laryngeal nerve (Birchard, 1998).

UNILATERAL VERSUS BILATERAL INVOLVEMENT. Bilateral lobe involvement occurs in more than 70% of hyperthyroid cats, therefore most hyperthyroid cats require bilateral thyroidectomy. However, in many cats, lobe enlargement is not symmetric and the smaller lobe may not be clearly palpable. For this reason, the decision regarding unilateral or bilateral thyroidectomy is usually made during surgery. In unilateral cases there is atrophy of the contralateral lobe, but the distinction between normal and atrophied may not always be obvious.

We have a tremendous advantage in our practice of virtually always having a presurgical thyroid scan. With the results of a scan available, the surgeon has the benefit of knowing exactly which tissue should be identified and extracted. Without a thyroid scan, we recommend removing only the enlarged gland whenever the surgeon is uncertain of the activity of a smaller, contralateral gland (see Figs. 4-23 to 4-29). If only one gland is visualized (Fig. 4-36), the decision is easy. If both glands are obviously enlarged, both should be excised. The suggestion has been made that 1.5 glands be removed in cats with bilateral thyrotoxicosis in an attempt to avoid hypoparathyroidism. However, the strong likelihood that hyperthyroidism will persist or recur detracts strongly from this recommendation.

INTRA(SUB)CAPSULAR VERSUS EXTRACAPSULAR THYROIDECTOMY. Two surgical techniques have been described and both have been successfully modified to enhance success rates for resolving hyperthyroidism and to preserve parathyroid tissue. The original intracapsular technique involved incision through the thyroid capsule and blunt dissection to separate and remove the thyroid lobe, leaving the capsule in situ. This technique did help preserve parathyroid tissue but was associated with recurrence due to regrowth of tissue adherent to the capsule (Swalec and Birchard, 1990; Mooney, 1998a). The original extracapsular technique involved removal of the intact thyroid lobe with its capsule after ligation of the cranial thyroid artery while attempting to preserve blood supply to the adjacent parathyroid gland. This technique reduced the recurrence rate but increased the risk of postsurgical hypoparathyroidism. Both these techniques have been modified (Fig. 4-37). The intracapsular modification involves removing most of the capsule after the thyroid tissue has been excised. If the extracapsular technique is chosen, use of bipolar "pinpoint" electrocautery rather than ligatures minimizes blunt dissection around the parathyroid glands (Welches et al, 1989). The modified extracapsular

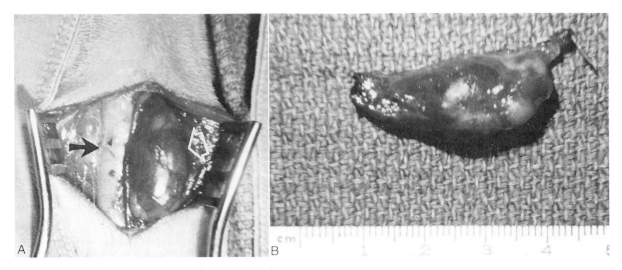

FIGURE 4-36. *A,* Photograph of the thyroid *(open arrow)* at surgery in a cat with unilateral hyperthyroidism. Note the trachea *(closed arrow). B,* The solitary adenoma after complete excision.

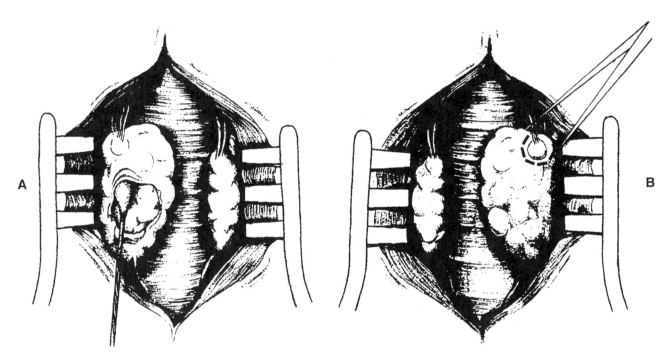

FIGURE 4-37. *A,* Intracapsular thyroidectomy. The thyroid capsule is incised and the thyroid lobe removed (the modified technique involves excision of the capsule). *B,* Extracapsular thyroidectomy. The thyroid lobe and capsule are removed, and the vascular supply to the external parathyroid glands is preserved (the modified technique involves bipolar cautery rather than ligatures). (Mooney CT: *In* Torrance AG, Mooney CT [eds]: Manual of Small Animal Endocrinology, 2nd ed. British Small Animal Veterinary Association, 1998a, p 115.)

technique is usually preferred because it is quicker and is associated with less hemorrhage that could obscure the surgical field (Mooney, 1998a).

POSTSURGICAL RECURRENCE OF HYPERTHYROIDISM. The disadvantage of any surgery, but more likely with the subcapsular method of thyroidectomy, is failure to remove all abnormal, adenomatous thyroid cells. With the modifications described, recurrence of hyperthyroidism due to less than complete removal of all

abnormal tissue is considered quite uncommon (Swalec and Birchard, 1990).

PARATHYROID AUTOTRANSPLANTATION TO PREVENT IATROGENIC HYPOPARATHYROIDISM (HYPOCALCEMIA)

Background. One of the most serious complications associated with bilateral thyroidectomy is postsurgical hypocalcemia. Hypocalcemia has been reported in 6% to 82% of cats, depending on the surgical method (Birchard et al, 1984; Flanders et al, 1987; Welches et al,

1989). In most cats that retain parathyroid gland activity, hypocalcemia is mild, transient, and usually attributed to the fact that thyrotoxicosis chronically depletes bone calcium. With successful surgery (even after unilateral tumor removal), the serum calcium concentration may decline below the normal or reference limits for several days as skeletal reserves are restored (McDougall, 1981). This mild hypocalcemia (serum calcium concentration of 7.0 to 9.0 mg/dl) must be differentiated from severe, acute hypocalcemia or the progressively worsening hypocalcemia associated with iatrogenic hypoparathyroidism, both of which require therapy. In these circumstances, the hypocalcemia is likely due to transient or permanent damage (or loss) of the parathyroid glands.

Parathyroid Autotransplantation. Autotransplantation involves transferring tissue from one site to another within an individual. In this case, an external parathyroid gland is placed in a site distant from its normal location. This procedure is well described and used in humans (Shaha et al, 1991). It involves carefully dissecting an external parathyroid gland free from surrounding tissues. It is critical to avoid transplanting thyroid adenoma cells. The parathyroid gland should then be sectioned so that no piece is greater than 3 mm in diameter. It is recommended that this sectioned tissue be placed in one sternohyoideus muscle bed, although tissue can be placed elsewhere. The muscle belly can be closed with a silk suture to mark the site. This procedure may not prevent severe hypocalcemia from occurring in the first week after surgery, but the transplant will likely begin functioning within 7 to 14 days of surgery (Padgett et al, 1998). We would recommend that this procedure be performed in any cat treated with bilateral thyroidectomy, but perhaps it should be considered for cats undergoing unilateral thyroidectomy as well.

Disadvantages of Surgery

Surgical treatment of hyperthyroidism has several drawbacks (see Table 4-10). First, thyrotoxic cats tend to be elderly, cachectic, fragile animals. Second, problems in other organ systems, particularly the cardiovascular and renal systems, tend to make these cats poor anesthetic risks. Third, some owners refuse surgery because of its expense or because they fear having their cat anesthetized. Fourth, the potential for a number of complications must be considered, including damage to the recurrent laryngeal nerve during surgery, causing laryngeal paralysis (with voice change); Horner's syndrome; postsurgical hypoparathyroidism, causing life-threatening hypocalcemia; and permanent hypothyroidism. Finally, lack of improvement or relapse of hyperthyroidism is a frustrating complication in cats that have undergone subtotal thyroidectomy (Flanders et al, 1987; Welches et al, 1989; Swalec and Birchard, 1990; Birchard, 1991). In humans, surgery without preoperative medical antithyroid therapy may result in a thyrotoxic crisis, a complication that has not been reported in cats.

The incidence of complications depends in large measure on the expertise of the surgeon, the thoroughness of preanesthetic evaluation, and presurgical management of the cat. Complications can be minimized if potential problems are identified and corrected; if the parathyroid glands are protected or salvaged and transplanted; and if the time under anesthesia is kept to a minimum. Some owners, however, simply refuse to allow their cats to undergo a surgical procedure. Therefore other modes of therapy may be necessary and should always be discussed with the owner.

Postsurgical Management

SHORT-TERM OBSERVATIONS. Postsurgically, fluid administration and urine output should be closely monitored. Fluid therapy should be discontinued as soon as possible. The cardiovascular system should be periodically evaluated by means of auscultation to detect pulmonary edema and, if possible, with electrocardiography and blood pressure measurements to detect arrhythmias and hypertensive or hypotensive disorders.

SERUM CALCIUM MONITORING/MANAGING TETANY
Background. The serum calcium concentration should be assessed at least once daily for 4 to 7 days if a bilateral thyroidectomy was performed. As discussed above, it is common for mild and transient hypocalcemia to follow surgery. Iatrogenic (postsurgical) hypoparathyroidism usually results in serum calcium concentrations less than 7.0 mg/dl. Careful observation for the onset of clinical signs consistent with hypocalcemic tetany is imperative for 4 to 7 days after bilateral thyroidectomy (Table 4-12). Ideally, hypocalcemia should be documented by measurement of the serum calcium concentration before therapy is begun. If an acute crisis with clinical signs of tetany develops, a blood sample should be obtained for later evaluation and immediate treatment with calcium should be instituted (Peterson, 1992). Severely hypocalcemic cats (serum calcium concentration <6.5 mg/dl), with or without clinical signs, should be treated with both oral vitamin D and calcium supplementation (a complete discussion of the diagnosis and management of hypocalcemia can be found in Chapter 17).

TABLE 4–12   SIGNS ASSOCIATED WITH HYPOCALCEMIA IN CATS

Restlessness
"Irritability"
Abnormal behavior
Muscle cramping or muscle pain
Muscle tremors, especially of face and ears
Tetany
Convulsions

Vitamin D₂. We have had experience with several different vitamin D products. Ergocalciferol (vitamin D_2 [Drisdol]; Winthrop-Breon Laboratories, New York, NY) is inexpensive and available in a liquid solution suitable for administration to cats. Usually 10,000 IU given orally once daily increases serum calcium concentrations, but it usually takes 5 to 21 days before an effect is seen. Because this vitamin preparation is fat soluble, tissue accumulation and subsequent hypercalcemia can occur. The ultimate dosage interval may decline to as little as once every 7 to 14 days. We do not recommend use of these drugs for cats with postsurgical hypocalcemia.

Dihydrotachysterol. Dihydrotachysterol (Roxane Laboratories, Columbus, Ohio; Hytakerol oral solution, Winthrop-Breon Laboratories, New York, NY) is more expensive than vitamin D_2, but the biologic action (increasing the serum calcium concentration) occurs more rapidly (1 to 7 days). Dihydrotachysterol also has a shorter duration of activity, which reduces the risk of tissue accumulation and prolonged iatrogenic hypercalcemia. A dose of 0.03 mg/kg given orally once daily for 3 days usually increases the serum calcium concentration. The dose should then be decreased to 0.02 mg/kg/day for the next 4 days, after which it should be tapered again. Successful treatment has been more consistent and has taken less time with the liquid solution than with the tablet formulations.

Vitamin D₃. The use of vitamin D_3 (calcitriol [Rocaltrol]; Roche, Nutley, NJ) has several advantages over the less expensive products. These advantages include quick onset of action, quick dissipation from the body if overdose occurs, and consistent effect. The recommended dose in cats is 2.5 to 10 ng/kg/day. The drug is supplied as 0.25 and 0.5 µg capsules, and authors have used one 0.25 µg capsule every 48 hours (Graves, 1995). Calcitriol is also available in an injectable form (see Chapter 17).

Calcium Supplementation. Calcium supplementation can be accomplished with several available calcium lactate or carbonate preparations. The dose is 0.5 to 3 g of calcium per day. One half or one tablet given two or three times a day is sufficient. If the cat is extremely tetanic and oral medication is not feasible, intravenous calcium gluconate may be administered slowly to effect, using ECG monitoring for bradycardia or arrhythmias. Calcium *gluconate* mixed in an equal volume of saline can then be given subcutaneously two to four times a day at a dose equal to that initially given intravenously to control tetany (usually 1 to 5 ml). Calcium chloride should never be given subcutaneously because it causes tissue irritation.

Transient Hypoparathyroidism. The persistence of apparent hypoparathyroidism is variable. Some cats may need medication for only a few days, whereas others require therapy for the rest of their lives. The transient nature of postsurgical hypoparathyroidism is difficult to predict. Recovery of parathyroid function may occur after days, weeks, or months of vitamin D and calcium supplementation. Whenever resolution of hypoparathyroidism is observed, it is assumed that reversible parathyroid damage occurred or that accessory parathyroid tissue may begin to compensate for glands damaged or removed at surgery. It is possible that accommodation of calcium-regulating mechanisms may occur despite absence of parathyroid hormone (Flanders et al, 1991).

Replacement vitamin D therapy can suppress recovery of endogenous parathyroid hormone secretion and can even cause hypercalcemia. Because it is difficult to predict the long-term need for vitamin D therapy in any cat, an attempt should be made to monitor the serum calcium concentration and to gradually wean all treated cats off medication. The tapering process can begin days to weeks after the start of vitamin D therapy and should continue over a period of at least 8 to 16 weeks. The goal is to maintain the serum calcium concentration within the low-normal range (8.5 to 9.5 mg/dl), concentrations adequate to prevent tetany but low enough to stimulate growth and function of any atrophied parathyroid tissue. If accessory parathyroid tissue is present and functional, the medications may be completely discontinued within weeks to months of surgery. If hypocalcemia recurs, therapy with vitamin D and calcium must be reinstituted.

HYPOTHYROIDISM

Subtotal Thyroidectomy. Cats that have undergone subtotal thyroidectomy may transiently develop low serum T_4 values. Thyroid hormone supplementation is not indicated in these cats. The remaining atrophied thyroid regains normal function within 1 to 3 months. Replacement thyroid medication only delays the growth and functional return of atrophied thyroid tissue.

Total Thyroidectomy. Plasma thyroid hormone concentrations decline, often to subnormal levels, within 24 to 72 hours of total thyroidectomy. However, this is not an absolute indication to initiate thyroid hormone supplementation. The common signs that develop are lethargy and obesity (see Chapter 3), signs that are often acceptable to the owner of a previously hyperthyroid cat. Dermatologic manifestations develop infrequently, and thyroid supplementation is rarely requested. This may be due in part to growth of accessory thyroid tissue in the neck or anterior mediastinum and subsequent secretion of thyroid hormone.

If thyroid replacement therapy is deemed necessary, synthetic thyroid replacement medication (Soloxine; Jones Medical Industries, St. Louis, Mo.) has proved satisfactory. The typical dosage for most cats is 0.05 to 0.2 mg/day. It should be remembered, however, that thyroid replacement therapy, like vitamin D and calcium therapy, may not be needed long term because cats may recover some endogenous thyroid function. Whether this represents the recovery of cellular function of cells left in situ or developing function in accessory tissue is not clear. Regardless, thyroid replacement therapy can suppress endogenous secretion of thyroid hormone; replacement therapy, therefore, should be tapered slowly and then discontinued after 1 to 3 months to determine the need for treatment.

RECURRENCE OF HYPERTHYROIDISM. Because of the potential for recurrence of hyperthyroidism, all cats treated surgically should have their serum thyroid hormone status monitored once or twice yearly (Welches et al, 1989; Swalec and Birchard, 1990). In cats with recurrence, treatment with oral antithyroid medication or with radioactive iodine is recommended. The incidence of surgical complications is considerably higher among cats undergoing a second surgery than among those undergoing their first surgery (Welches et al, 1989; Peterson, 1995a). A thyroid scan could be obtained to demonstrate the location of functioning thyroid tissue, information that would make a decision about surgery much easier.

PERSISTENCE OF HYPERTHYROIDISM. Rarely, clinical signs persist despite unilateral or bilateral thyroidectomy. This implies that abnormal (hyperplastic/neoplastic) thyroid tissue remains active. Such tissue would most likely be in the mediastinum, cranial to the heart. Radionuclide scans performed preoperatively identify this tissue and force the clinician to consider alternative treatments. Thyroid scans can be completed after surgery to confirm and locate abnormal thyroid tissue. We do not recommend surgical exploration of the thorax; rather, we prefer to localize the mass before attempting surgery. Administration of radioactive iodine is the ideal mode of therapy for such conditions. This possible complication reinforces the need for a thorough evaluation of the ventral neck during surgery, including the area of the thoracic inlet.

Results of Surgery

In most veterinary hospitals the results of surgery are excellent. Most treated cats respond well, with resolution of the hyperthyroidism. The exceptions to this trend are cats with concurrent disease (e.g., renal failure), cats with unrecognized mediastinal tissue secreting thyroid hormone, cats that undergo subtotal thyroidectomy but that have abnormal tissue in the contralateral gland, and cats with long-term recurrence. Problems with anesthesia, surgical complications, and the like have been limited by acquired experience and presurgical management protocols. The major advantages of surgery are that the procedure can be performed by most practitioners; it is relatively inexpensive; it can result in a permanent cure; and morbidity and mortality can be minimized by appropriate presurgical and postsurgical management protocols.

TREATMENT WITH RADIOACTIVE IODINE

Theory

Thyroid cells do not differentiate radioactive from stable (natural) iodine. In most thyrotoxic humans, the thyroid extracts more than 50% of a radioactive iodine dose from the circulation. That iodine is concentrated within the gland, and its emitted radiation destroys surrounding functioning thyroid cells. Radiation damage does not affect contiguous structures because the radiation travels an extremely limited distance. Also important, only functioning cells are killed. Atrophied thyroid cells receive a relatively small dose of radiation and for this reason are spared the radioiodines' killing effect. Thus, as these cells return to function, long-term hypothyroidism is avoided in most cats.

In January 1941, the first hyperthyroid human patient was treated with radioactive iodine, and about 40 years later, the first hyperthyroid cat was so treated. Radioactive iodine therapy is an excellent first-choice therapeutic modality for managing feline hyperthyroidism. Although its availability was limited during the first 10 to 15 years of its use in cats, it is now available in numerous locations throughout the United States and in various other countries. This form of treatment remains a valuable option in cats that would not be helped by surgery (i.e., cats with intrathoracic thyroid tumors or metastatic carcinomas, or those whose owners refuse surgery).

Choice of Radionuclide

Iodine-131 (half-life, 8.1 days) is the therapeutic radionuclide of choice. It emits both β-particles and γ-rays. The β-particles cause most of the radiation damage. These particles usually do not travel beyond 2 mm in tissue, their average path length being approximately 400 μm. β-Particles are locally destructive, causing pyknosis and necrosis of the follicular cells and, later, vascular and stromal fibrosis with disappearance of colloid. Cells that are not destroyed may develop abnormalities, leading to a shorter survival time and impaired replication. Thyroid damage, therefore, is both immediate and prolonged. The particles do not damage the parathyroid glands.

Goal of Therapy

The goal of ^{131}I therapy is to obtain a cure as quickly as possible with one dose. In humans, 60% to 70% of patients become euthyroid after the first dose, and approximately two out of three resistant patients respond satisfactorily to each subsequent dose. With conventional doses in cats, hormonal improvement occurs over a period of days to a few weeks (Figs. 4-38 to 4-40) (Meric et al, 1986; Peterson and Becker, 1995). The success rate in cats appears to be better than that in humans.

Dose Determination

CATS RECEIVING ANTITHYROID DRUGS PRIOR TO USE OF RADIOACTIVE IODINE. There has been discussion regarding the effect of oral antithyroid drugs given prior to

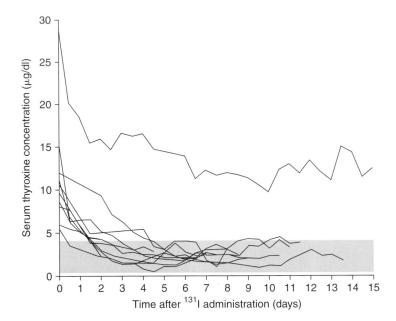

FIGURE 4–38. Serum T$_4$ concentrations in 10 hyperthyroid cats sampled every 12 hours following ^{131}I therapy. Note how quickly the T$_4$ concentrations decline. Shaded region represents the normal reference range. (Meric S, et al: J Am Vet Med Assoc 188:1038, 1986.)

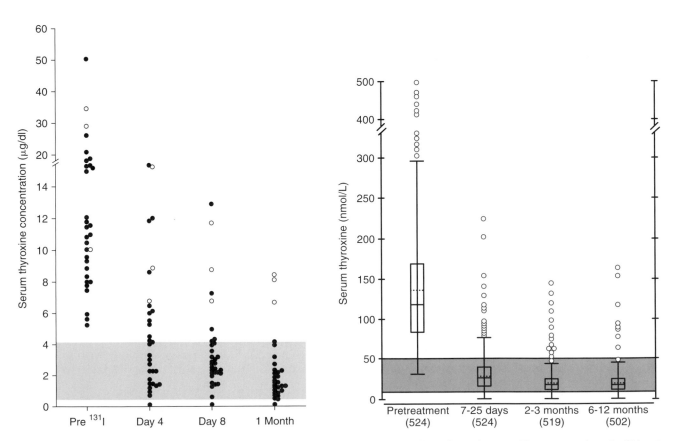

FIGURE 4–39. Serum T$_4$ concentrations in 31 hyperthyroid cats treated with ^{131}I. These cats were studied before therapy, 4 and 8 days after therapy, at the time of hospital discharge (variable), and 1 month after treatment. Note how quickly the T$_4$ concentrations decline. Open circles represent the three cats that remained hyperthyroid 1 month after treatment. Shaded area represents the normal reference range. (Meric S, et al: J Am Vet Med Assoc 188:1038, 1986.)

FIGURE 4–40. Box plots of serum T$_4$ concentrations in 524 cats before and at various times after administration of radioiodine for treatment of hyperthyroidism. (For key, please see Fig. 4-13.) (Peterson ME: *In* Ettinger SJ, Feldman EC [eds]: Textbook of Veterinary Internal Medicine, 5th ed. Philadelphia, WB Saunders, 2000, p 1400.)

administration of radioactive iodine. The concern has been that oral agents may interfere with an abnormal thyroid lobe's ability to "trap" iodine. Most radiation oncologists and endocrinologists believe that oral therapy does not interfere with the efficacy of radioactive iodine therapy. It has been stated that people with hyperthyroidism for whom treatment with ^{131}I is planned should not be pretreated with an antithyroid drug. For one thing, the time-line for onset of action with the two types of treatment does not differ significantly. For another, physicians question exposing patients to the potential side effects of an antithyroid drug if prolonged treatment to allow remission is not intended (Utiger, 2002b). However, based on the results of prospective and retrospective studies on hyperthyroid people, pretreatment with methimazole for weeks or months does not reduce the efficacy of ^{131}I therapy (Marcocci et al, 1990; Imesis et al, 1998; Andrade et al, 2001). It is assumed that methimazole therapy would not interfere with radioactive iodine therapy for cats (Smith et al, 1994 and 1995). In contrast, pretreatment with propylthiouracil does reduce the efficacy of ^{131}I therapy in people (Hancock et al, 1997; Imesis et al, 1998).

[131]I DOSE DETERMINED BY TRACER STUDIES. Prior to administration of iodine, uptake and excretion studies can be performed using a tracer dose of [131]I. The radiation dose delivered depends on the thyroid uptake of the tracer, the estimated size of the gland, and the effective half-life of the radionuclide. The goal in the treatment of cats is to deliver 150 Gy to the thyroid gland. A formula has been used to determine the correct dosage:

Dose of [131]I (μCi) =

$$\frac{20,000 \text{ rad/g} \times \text{Thyroid weight (g)} \times T_{1/2}{}^{131}I}{(160 \text{ rad}/\mu Ci) (\% \text{ Peak RAIU}) (100 \times T_{eff})}$$

where $T_{1/2}{}^{131}I$ is the half-life of iodine-131; *RAIU* is the radioactive iodine uptake by the thyroid; T_{eff} is the effective half-life of the iodine in the cat; and *160 rad/μCi* of iodine is the radiation level of [131]I. Despite this sophisticated approach to determining the appropriate dose, the ultimate dose received by the thyroid was remarkably erratic, varying between 7100 and 64,900 rad in one study (Turrel et al, 1984). It appears that the higher the pretreatment serum T_4 concentration, the lower the success rate of one dose of radioactive iodine. Using these calculations, the dose of ^{131}I may vary from as little as 1 mCi to as much as 10 mCi (37 to 370 mBq). This iodine may be administered orally, subcutaneously, or intravenously. With this protocol, approximately 80% of cats become euthyroid within 3 months, most within 1 week (see Figs. 4-38 and 4-39) (Turrel et al, 1984; Meric et al, 1986; Broome et al, 1988). Cats remaining hyperthyroid require a second ^{131}I dose or alternative therapy.

The disadvantages of evaluating thyroid gland kinetics are the various ancillary expenses needed for the extra procedure, which may require anesthesia or sedation and certainly adds several days to the hospitalization. Most of the cats we have treated require no sedation or anesthesia for tracer or treatment. In addition, as is suggested by the wide range of doses delivered, this protocol may provide results that are no more successful or not as successful as would be achieved using one standard dose. In humans, evidence indicates that giving a calculated dose of radioiodine has no advantage over a fixed dose of 5 or 10 mCi (Franklyn, 1994). For these reasons, fixed-dose radiation is also recommended for people with hyperthyroidism (Jarlov et al, 1995).

[131]I DOSE DETERMINED BY SERUM T_4 CONCENTRATION AND SEVERITY OF DISEASE. This method of ^{131}I dose determination omits evaluation of thyroid gland kinetics. The amount of ^{131}I administered to individual cats, orally, subcutaneously, or intravenously, is 2 to 6 mCi (74 to 222 mBq; 1 Ci = 3.7×10^{10} Bq) (Peterson and Becker, 1995). The dose of ^{131}I is determined by the severity of clinical signs, the subjective size of the abnormal thyroid(s), and the serum T_4 concentration. Based on these criteria, a low (2.5 to 3.5 mCi), moderate (3.5 to 4.5 mCi), or high (4.5 to 6.5 mCi) dose of ^{131}I was administered to hyperthyroid cats (Jones et al, 1991; Meric and Rubin, 1990; Peterson, 1995a and 1995b; Peterson and Becker, 1995; Peterson, 2000). Fewer than 2% of more than 500 cats remained hyperthyroid at 6 months and required a second dose of iodine (see Fig. 4-40). Only 2% developed signs and laboratory data consistent with a diagnosis of hypothyroidism. A similar number of cats (2%) had a relapse of hyperthyroidism within 1 to 6 years of treatment. This method of dose determination, therefore, can be quite efficacious and is more expedient than that required of the kinetic studies, because the kinetic study is eliminated. The need for extra sedation or anesthesia is also eliminated.

During the past 10 years, we have used a similar method of dose determination. Based on similar criteria (serum T_4 concentration at time of diagnosis, size of the thyroid lobe or lobes, and severity of clinical signs), we arbitrarily administer 3 to 8 mCi subcutaneously (Theon, 2002). Based on these criteria, a low (3 to 4 mCi), moderate (4 to 6 mCi), or high (6 to 8 mCi) dose of ^{131}I was administered to hyperthyroid cats. Most cats receive 4 to 5 mCi. The success rate in treating hyperthyroid cats with this slightly more aggressive regimen has been excellent. The incidence of failure to resolve hyperthyroidism or of recurrence is lower than with the less aggressive approach. Interestingly, the incidence of hypothyroidism also appears to be lower.

ROUTINE LARGE-DOSE ADMINISTRATION. Routine administration of an extremely large dose (10 to 30 mCi) of ^{131}I almost always results in destruction of all adenomatous and normal thyroid tissue. Such doses not only resolve hyperthyroidism, they also greatly increase the risk of hypothyroidism. Longer hospitalization usually is required because of the extra time needed for excretion of radioactive iodine. Such doses are typically reserved for cats with histologically confirmed functioning thyroid carcinoma because they offer the best chance of destroying all malignant tissue (Turrel et al, 1988; Theon, 2002).

HISTOLOGICALLY CONFIRMED THYROID CARCINOMA. Fewer than 2% to 3% of hyperthyroid cats have a thyroid carcinoma. Some of these cats, on thyroid scan, appear to have "typical" adenomatous hyperplasia or an adenoma, because a solitary mass or bilateral masses are detected. Many cats with carcinoma, however, have large, irregular masses, more than two masses, or obvious distant metastases. If carcinoma is confirmed, radioactive iodine is the preferred mode of therapy because it has the potential to be concentrated within and therefore to kill all carcinomatous tissue regardless of location. However, thyroid carcinomas concentrate and retain iodine less efficiently than adenomas or adenomatous hyperplasia. Most radiation oncologists use extremely large doses of radioactive iodine (10 to 30 mCi) (Guptill et al, 1995; Theon, 2002).

The combination of surgical debulking followed by administration of a high dose of radioactive iodine has also been reported to be a successful strategy for managing cats with thyroid carcinoma (Peterson and Becker, 1995; Guptill et al, 1995). Longer hospitalization can be anticipated if cats receive high doses of radioactive material due to the additional time required for excretion. However, because malignant cells are less efficient in "trapping" iodine, it may be quickly excreted, and cats may be returned to their owners after a relatively brief hospitalization. However, the prognosis correlates best with duration of hospitalization (i.e., the longer the required hospitalization, the better the prognosis).

Route of ^{131}I Administration

The intravenous versus the subcutaneous route of administering ^{131}I has been critically evaluated. Results from two groups of more than 80 cats demonstrated that the two routes were equally effective. It was further demonstrated that the subcutaneous route was safer for personnel and, subjectively, less stressful to the cats. Approximately 85% of the cats from each group were euthyroid 4 years after receiving the iodine. Approximately 6% became clinically hypothyroid afterward (Theon et al, 1994). Although commonly used in humans, oral ^{131}I is not often recommended because of the obvious increased risk of exposure to this radiation by the personnel dosing the cats. However, some treatment centers successfully employ use of oral ^{131}I placed in gelatin capsules (Weichselbaum et al, 2003).

Radiation Safety

IN-HOSPITAL. Radioactive iodine is hazardous material. As such, ^{131}I-treated cats are a potential source of hazardous radiation to humans and to other animals. Anyone using this material must adhere to national and state regulations (all regulations cannot be presented here). An attempt must be made to limit close contact of treated cats with humans for 1 to 3 weeks. Initially, each treated cat is hospitalized in a ward reserved solely for animals undergoing treatment with radioactive material. Each animal is kept in an individual metabolic cage. All urine and feces are disposed of as radioactive waste until the cat has a surface radioactivity level below 45 mR/hr. Personnel are restricted in the ward housing the cats; they are instructed to wear proper protective clothing; and they are required to carry closely monitored dosimeters. Disposable gloves are always used. Hospitalization for these cats averages 7 to 10 days from the first day of radioactive iodine therapy. When the cats are returned to their owners, the urine and stool are considered safe. It is difficult to estimate the duration of isolation needed from commonly used pretreatment parameters (Weichselbaum et al, 2003).

AFTER RELEASE FROM THE HOSPITAL. Owners should be given instructions on the proper care of their pet for the first few weeks after therapy. Each cat should wear a collar explaining that it has recently been treated with a radioactive substance and that it should not be handled. For the initial 2 to 3 weeks after release from the hospital, persons over 45 years of age are told to stay 3 feet or farther away from the cat except for brief periods needed for necessary care. Persons *under* 45 years of age should stay 6 feet or farther away from the cat, and children under 18 and pregnant women should have NO contact with these cats. The cat must be strictly confined to the home or kept on a leash. To further reduce any chance of unwanted exposure, it is recommended that owners line the litter pan with plastic. The used litter should be disposed of carefully, because radioactivity is excreted via urine. The hands should be washed thoroughly after handling of the cat, its food dishes, or the litter pan. The 2- to 3-week period of restricted owner contact should serve as a buffer for the hospitalization period, to avoid unnecessary human exposure to radioactive iodine.

LONG-TERM CARE, MONITORING, AND PROGNOSIS

Rechecks and Hypothyroidism. Initially, treated cats should be rechecked every 2 to 3 months after radioactive iodine administration. These visits should be used to obtain a complete history, perform a physical examination, and measure the serum T_4 concentrations. Overdose of radioactive iodine may result in hypothyroidism, which can be treated with 0.05 to 0.1 mg of L-thyroxine given orally once or twice daily. Cats that fail to improve clinically and continue to have abnormally increased serum T_4 concentrations 3 to 6 months after radioiodine therapy should be considered candidates for a second dose. The need for a third dose would be rare.

Prognosis for Resolution of Hyperthyroidism. The average number of radioiodine treatments required to control thyrotoxicosis in humans ranges from 1.4 to 2 doses (Holm et al, 1981). It would appear that ^{131}I therapy is more efficacious in cats, because 95% of cats were euthyroid 3 months after receiving one treatment. Only 5% of cats fail to respond completely and remain hyperthyroid. Most cats with persistent hyperthyroidism have large tumors, severe clinical signs, and extremely increased serum T_4 concentrations (Peterson and Becker, 1995). No adverse side effects to organs other than the thyroid lobes have been observed after ^{131}I therapy.

Predictors of Survival. One study evaluated long-term health and predictors of survival for hyperthyroid cats treated with radioactive iodine (Slater et al, 2001). More than 200 cats were followed, and most were relatively healthy at the time of treatment. Male cats were found to have a shorter life expectancy than females. Age at the time of treatment was also a prognostic factor, because older cats did not survive as long as younger cats. For example, 28% of 10-year-old male cats were alive 5 years after therapy and 4% of 16-year-old male cats were alive 5 years after treatment, whereas 42% of 10-year-old female cats were alive 5 years after treatment. The mean age of death was 15 years of age, with a range of 10 to 21 years. Clinical abnormalities documented just before death were renal disorders in 41% of cats, cancer in 16% of cats, minor problems only in 14% of cats, and then a variety of other concerns.

Advantages of Radioactive Iodine Therapy (See Table 4-10)

[131]I administration is not stressful for elderly cats, usually requiring no anesthesia, sedation, oral medication, or surgery (Peterson, 1995b; Peterson, 2000). With appropriate precautions, especially with subcutaneous administration of the radioactive iodine (Theon et al, 1994), human radiation exposure is avoided. This therapy has been successful in large numbers of cats, and the only recognized deleterious side effect has been hypothyroidism, which occurs in an extremely small number of cats and almost never requires therapy (Theon et al, 1994; Peterson and Becker, 1995). The response to therapy is rapid (Meric et al, 1986). In treating these cats, the precise dosage chosen does not need to be determined by means of computer technology. The effects of radioactive iodine therapy do not appear to be affected by previous and current oral antithyroid drugs.

Disadvantages of Radioactive Iodine Therapy (See Table 4-10)

As with the other major forms of therapy, there are disadvantages to the use of [131]I. This medication is not uniformly available and requires complete knowledge of radiation safety and the use of expensive and sophisticated equipment. The average cat requires 7 to 10 days of hospitalization after therapy, which may be an emotional problem for some owners, as well as expensive. A few cats require retreatment before thyrotoxicosis resolves.

Need for Retreatment

Approximately 2% to 5% of ^{131}I-treated hyperthyroid cats require a second treatment (Peterson, 1995a; 1995b; Peterson and Becker, 1995). As with any therapy, ^{131}I treatment is not perfect. Several factors may be involved in an incomplete response to an initial therapeutic dose of ^{131}I, such as errors in dosage, individual variation in disease status, gland size, gland activity, gland pathology (adenoma, adenomatous hyperplasia, or carcinoma), and excretion rates. A second dose is usually effective in treating these resistant cats.

NOVEL "ULTRASOUND-GUIDED" TREATMENT STRATEGIES

Percutaneous Ethanol Injection for Unilateral Hyperthyroidism

INTRODUCTION. Treatment with ultrasound-guided percutaneous ethanol injection (PEI) has been successfully used in recent years in humans with primary hyperparathyroidism or hyperthyroidism (Livraghi et al, 1990; Lippi et al, 1996; Monzani et al, 1997; Bennedbaek et al, 1997). Injected ethanol causes coagulation necrosis and vascular thrombosis within the parenchyma of exposed tissue. PEI has been used with excellent results in dogs with primary hyperparathyroidism (see Chapter 16). Based on the success in resolving hypercalcemia in those dogs, the brief anesthesia required (less than 30 minutes), and the decreased expense of treating dogs with primary hyperparathyroidism, it was decided to evaluate the efficacy of this treatment modality in hyperthyroid cats. Eight cats with "unilateral" hyperthyroidism were treated.

RESULTS. Each cat had a thyroid scan and cervical ultrasound that were consistent. The cats were placed under anesthesia, the cervical area was surgically prepared, the thyroid lobe was identified, and a needle was guided into the mass. The volume of the affected thyroid nodule had been estimated, and one half that volume of 100% ethanol was placed in a syringe, which was attached to the needle. More important, the dose injected was arbitrary and determined almost entirely by the lobe being completely infiltrated with ethanol, as determined by the radiologist viewing the injection with ultrasound. The needle was then removed and the cat allowed to awaken. Two of the eight cats had cystic thyroid nodules. In those two cats, the cystic fluid was aspirated prior to ethanol injection. The volume of ethanol injected ranged from 50% to 100% of the estimated thyroid volume.

Each of the 8 cats (four reported) had serum total T_4 concentrations decrease into the reference range within 48 hours of the procedure. Each cat was under anesthesia for less than 30 minutes, and no local or systemic adverse effects were noted in the 5 days after injection. However, two of the eight cats were noted to

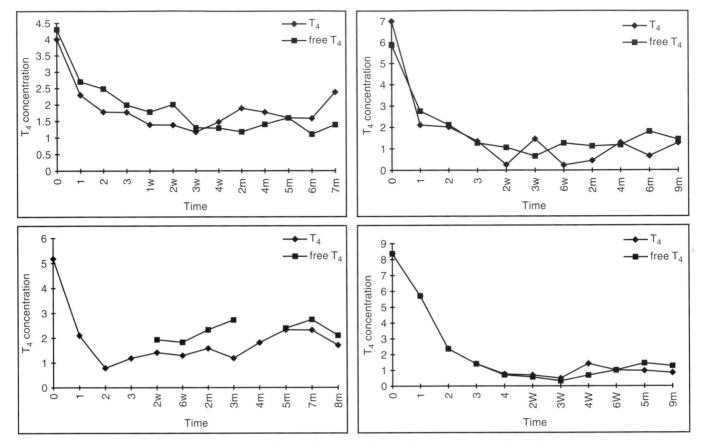

FIGURE 4–41. Serum thyroxine (T_4) (μg/dl) and free T_4 (ng/dl) concentrations before and over time (days 1, 2, and 3; weeks 2, 3, and 6; and months 2, 4, 6, and 9) after percutaneous ethanol injection (PEI). Each graph represents data from one cat. (Goldstein RE, et al: J Am Vet Med Assoc 218:1298, 2001.)

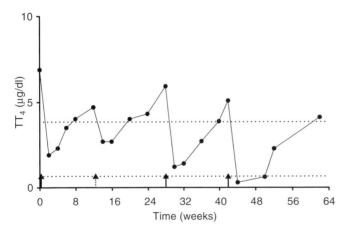

FIGURE 4–42. Serum total T_4 concentrations in one cat with hyperthyroidism over a 64-week period from the time of initial treatment with ethanol injection. Notice the transient response in total T_4 concentration after each injection. The solid arrows represent ethanol injection into the left thyroid lobe; the dashed arrow represents ethanol injection into the right thyroid lobe; and the horizontal dotted lines represent the reference range of 1.1 to 3.9 μg/dl. (Wells AL, et al: J Am Vet Med Assoc 218:1293, 2001.)

have a change in voice by their owners; the condition resolved in one cat after 6 weeks but persisted in the other. Each cat remained euthyroid for at least 18 months (Fig. 4-41). This treatment was considered efficacious (Goldstein et al, 2001).

Percutaneous Ethanol Injection for Bilateral Hyperthyroidism

After success in the treatment of cats with unilateral disease had been demonstrated, treatment of cats with bilateral disease was elected. The entire process was identical to that described for the cats with unilateral disease. Twelve hours after the first cat received ethanol injections into both thyroid lobes, the cat died. Retrospectively, after publication of the report of a cat suffering laryngeal paralysis after a similar method of treatment, it was realized that the ethanol had most likely caused bilateral laryngeal paralysis (Walker and Schaer, 1998). The next seven cats were treated in a staged manner, with the larger of the two thyroid lobes treated. Several cats did have transient unilateral laryngeal paralysis. Each cat responded to the ethanol injection, but euthyroidism lasted no longer than about 6 months in any cat (Fig. 4-42). PEI therefore was not considered efficacious because of failure to achieve long-term results and the occurrence of serious life-threatening side effects (Wells et al, 2001).

Percutaneous Radiofrequency Heat Ablation

INTRODUCTION. As a follow-up to our ultrasound-guided ethanol injection procedures, we elected to use radiofrequency heat ablation as an alternative. A similar use of this treatment modality had been evaluated for small hepatic, breast, and prostatic masses in people (Livraghi et al, 1999; Jiao et al, 1999; Djavan et al, 1999; Jeffrey et al, 1999). Radiofrequency heat destroys tissue by causing thermal necrosis at the needle tip; this offers several advantages compared with ethanol injection. The radiofrequency damages a discrete amount of tissue surrounding the noninsulated portion of the needle and does not damage regional vasculature. The operator, therefore, has much greater control over the tissue exposed, and there is no chance of "leakage." With experience, this modality has become our treatment of choice for dogs with primary hyper-parathyroidism (Pollard et al, 2001) (see Chapter 16).

A pilot study to assess the efficacy of unipolar heat ablation was conducted on nine hyperthyroid cats, four with unilateral and five with bilateral disease. The cats were evaluated with ultrasound as described for the ethanol procedure. The anesthesia, positioning, and preparation were the same. With ultrasound guidance, an insulated needle (over-the-needle catheter) was directed into the abnormal thyroid lobe in cats with unilateral disease or into the larger of two masses in cats with bilateral disease. Once location within thyroid tissue was assured, and radiofrequency pulses were applied, beginning with 10 watts of energy and progressing as needed to 30 watts. The goal of therapy was observed dramatic hyperechogenicity of tissue (Fig. 4-43). With appropriate levels of energy (enough to cause necrosis), the tissue turns white on the ultrasound screen and "bubbles." On the ultrasound video screen, the process is quite similar to watching corn pop.

RESULTS. Heat ablation was performed once on each of the thyroid nodules in the four cats with unilateral disease. Three of the four cats became euthyroid after the procedure for 4, 7, and 19 months, respectively. One of these three cats was treated a second time after recurrence and became euthyroid for an additional 9 months. One of the four cats had a reduction in total T_4 concentration but did not become euthyroid. After treatment of the larger of two thyroid masses in cats with bilateral disease, two cats became euthyroid for 7 and 9 months, respectively. Two of the five cats with bilateral disease did not become euthyroid after the initial treatment but did become euthyroid for 2 and 9 months, respectively, after a second procedure. Heat ablation was used three times in the fifth cat with bilateral disease, with dramatic improvement in the total T_4 concentration after the first treatment and euthyroidism for 5 months after each of the next two procedures. Horner's syndrome developed in two of the nine cats and resolved in both cats within 2 months. It appears that unipolar heat ablation is an effective short-term treatment for feline hyperthyroidism (Mallery et al, 2002). We are currently studying the use of "bipolar" heat ablation, and initial results appear superior to "unipolar" ablation.

MISCELLANEOUS THERAPIES

Propranolol

THEORY. Propranolol is a β-receptor blocking agent. In humans it is the β-adrenergic drug with the most beneficial effects in hyperthyroid individuals. Propranolol does not have any direct effects on the thyroid gland, therefore euthyroidism does not result from administration of this drug. A thyroid crisis has been described in people taking propranolol. Propranolol may inhibit the conversion of T_4 to T_3. In

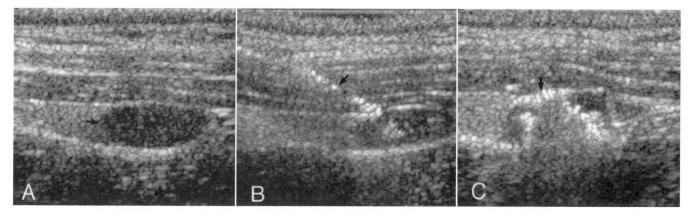

FIGURE 4–43. Ultrasound photograph demonstrating the hyperechogenicity associated with radiofrequency heat ablation tissue. *A,* The thyroid mass to be ablated. *B,* Needle placement into the thyroid. *C,* Increased echogenicity of the thyroid mass associated with heat application.

thyrotoxic humans, clinical improvement with propranolol results from control of the tachycardia, myocardial contractility problems, tremor, restlessness, anxiety, sweating, heat intolerance, myopathy, and weight loss associated with this disorder (McDougall, 1981).

Cats with thyrotoxicosis frequently are observed on echocardiography to have "hyperdynamic action" of the myocardium without significant chamber or myocardial enlargement. Many hyperthyroid cats with hyperdynamic hearts have cardiac problems that are due to tachycardia. Some cats (12%) have echocardiographic evidence of hypertrophic cardiomyopathy, and only a small number (3%) have evidence of congestive cardiomyopathy. Cats with hyperdynamic heart syndrome, hypertrophic cardiomyopathy, tachycardia, or supraventricular tachyarrhythmias may benefit from oral propranolol, which slows the heart rate, lowers the end-diastolic pressure of the left ventricle, prolongs the ventricular filling time, decreases the oxygen demand of the myocardium, acts as an antiarrhythmic agent, and reduces outflow pressure gradients.

The excessive concentration of thyroid hormones in hyperthyroid patients may increase the number of β-receptors in the heart, which probably accounts for the positive chronotropic and inotropic features of the disease. However, propranolol is useful in controlling the tachycardia, polypnea, hypertension, and hyperexcitability associated with hyperthyroidism. Propranolol may reduce the myocardial abnormalities in most hyperthyroid cats, but those with congestive cardiomyopathy would be best managed with digitalis rather than propranolol.

DOSE. The dosage of oral propranolol used in cats has ranged from 2.5 mg given twice daily to 5 mg given three times a day. Propranolol is rapidly absorbed from the gastrointestinal tract, and the plasma half-life is approximately 3 to 6 hours. For each cat given propranolol, the dosage should be adjusted to achieve specific goals. The dosage may need to be progressively increased to control tachycardia or arrhythmias associated with thyrotoxicosis (see Presurgical Management, page 201). Adjustments in the dosage should be based on the clinical response and periodic ECG monitoring. The ECG should reveal a decrease in the heart rate or a reduction in the frequency of atrial (supraventricular) premature contractions, or both. Propranolol is a potent myocardial depressant and should be used with extreme caution if heart failure is present. Congestive heart failure should be treated with furosemide in conjunction with other appropriate drugs.

In a study of induced hyperthyroidism, the half-life of propranolol was not affected by hyperthyroidism (Jacobs et al, 1997). After oral administration, total body clearance was lower and the peak plasma propranolol concentration, fractional absorption, and area under the curve were higher in hyperthyroid cats compared with euthyroid cats. This indicated increased bioavailability in thyrotoxicosis, which was calculated to exceed 100% and suggested enterohepatic recycling of the drug. The findings of this study indicate that commonly prescribed doses may need to be reduced in some hyperthyroid cats.

Atenolol

Atenolol offers some potential advantages over propranolol, including more selective β_1-adrenoreceptor blocking action, longer duration of activity, and availability in oral syrup form. Atenolol is used at a dosage of 6.25 to 12.5 mg/cat/day. The starting dose should be low and gradually increased to effect. This drug should not be started immediately prior to administration of anesthesia without a suitable period for dose titration (Mooney and Thoday, 2000).

Stable Iodine

Although the thyroid gland requires small amounts of iodide for hormone synthesis, large amounts given over a brief period (1 to 2 weeks) may result in transient hypothyroidism in normal individuals. Iodide can be rapidly effective in ameliorating increased serum thyroid hormone concentrations associated with hyperthyroidism. Beneficial effects are seen in 7 to 14 days and include improvement in signs, as well as reduction in the size and vascularity of the thyroid gland.

Unfortunately, it is rarely possible to achieve complete remission of hyperthyroidism or to maintain any degree of control for more than a few weeks with iodide. Iodide functions by inhibiting organification of thyroid hormone. It results in reduced secretion of formed hormone. Iodide administration may also inhibit other aspects of thyroid function, including the binding of iodine necessary for the formation of the thyroid hormones. Iodide has a small but definite role in the treatment of hyperthyroidism; 500 mg of iodide given orally is an important part of the treatment of thyroid crisis (storm) in humans. We have not used iodide to treat a cat in acute thyrotoxic crisis. SSKI has been used (see page 202), in addition to oral antithyroid drugs, to control the disease preoperatively. One or two drops are administered daily beginning 10 days prior to surgery. The SSKI is placed in a small gelatin capsule to avoid the aftertaste that bothers cats (Peterson and Turrel, 1986.

Iodinated Radiographic Contrast Agents

Oral cholecystographic agents (e.g., calcium ipodate) acutely inhibit peripheral conversion of T_4 to T_3 and may decrease T_4 synthesis and directly inhibit the effects of TSH. Blocking of the conversion of circulating thyroid hormone has been demonstrated in iatrogenic feline hyperthyroidism, and the drug appears to be well tolerated with few adverse side effects. In 12 cats with naturally occurring hyperthyroidism treated with calcium ipodate, eight exhibited a good response. The serum total T_3 concentrations decreased into the reference range within 2 weeks of the start of treatment and remained at those levels for a 14-week study period. In addition, improvement in clinical signs, body weight, heart rate, and blood pressure were documented. Four of the eight responders continued to do well for as long as 6 months, but two had relapses of hyperthyroidism by week 14. The serum total T_4 concentrations were not affected by treatment, and cats with severe disease were less likely to respond, even after the dose was doubled (Murray and Peterson, 1997). Calcium ipodate is an alternative to stable iodine for short-term preparation of hyperthyroid cats for surgery (Mooney and Thoday, 2000).

Glucocorticoids

One effect of excess glucocorticoids is inhibition of TSH secretion, which may result from direct effects at both the hypothalamic and the pituitary levels. Glucocorticoids may also promote the peripheral conversion of T_4 to reverse T_3 (rT_3) rather than to T_3. A direct inhibitory effect on the thyroid gland may also occur, particularly in hyperthyroidism. In hyperthyroid humans, the serum T_4, T_3, and thyroglobulin concentrations decrease after administration of glucocorticoids. This drug has not been evaluated for the therapy of feline hyperthyroidism.

Thiamine

Cats that have signs consistent with thiamine deficiency can improve dramatically with proper therapy. The syndrome and its treatment are discussed in an earlier section, Ventroflexion of the Head (Thiamine or Potassium Deficiency), page 164.

HYPERTHYROIDISM AND SIMULTANEOUS NONTHYROIDAL DISEASE

Perhaps one of the most challenging diagnostic problems in veterinary medicine is the cat with both thyrotoxicosis and another serious illness. Other diseases, such as primary heart disease, renal failure, intestinal neoplasia (especially lymphosarcoma), diabetes mellitus, and hyperadrenocorticism, can occur in association with hyperthyroidism in aged cats (see Table 4-5). More important, the signs of these disorders can mimic or accentuate some of the common clinical signs of hyperthyroidism. It is important, therefore, to maintain an index of suspicion for other diseases in an older cat even when a thyroid mass is palpable and hyperthyroidism has been confirmed. A thorough physical examination and diagnostic screening tests to evaluate other body systems should be performed in any ill, aged cat.

Abnormal increases in basal serum T_3 and T_4 concentrations confirm the diagnosis of hyperthyroidism. Appropriate therapy (methimazole, surgery, or radioiodine) should control the disease. If clinical signs persist after therapy, despite the finding of normal or low thyroid hormone concentrations, another disease mimicking thyrotoxicosis must be considered. Failure to correctly identify all diseases responsible for the clinical signs may result in incorrect diagnosis, frustration, and inappropriate therapy.

PROGNOSIS

The prognosis for a hyperthyroid cat depends on its physical condition at the time of diagnosis, as well as its age and gender, and whether simultaneous disease is present in another major organ system. Because all three major treatment modalities have been reasonably successful, we strongly encourage owners to treat their hyperthyroid cats. Life expectancy studies with each therapy suggest that these cats live approximately 2 years on average. There is, of course, tremendous individual variation, and survival studies are somewhat skewed because hyperthyroidism is a geriatric feline disease (Peterson, 1995a; Peterson and Becker, 1995; Slater et al, 2001).

Important prognostic factors are the histology and functional nature of the tumor. In contrast to thyroid tumors in dogs, which do not typically cause hyperthyroidism, thyroid tumors in cats usually secrete excessive amounts of thyroid hormone, causing clinical signs. The prognosis is obviously better in cats with adenomatous hyperplasia than in those with invasive or malignant carcinomas or both.

The therapeutic modalities available to the clinician may also determine the long-term prognosis. An older, cachectic cat with bilateral thyroid involvement is best treated with radioactive iodine. If this treatment is unavailable, the prognosis may worsen. The cat's tolerance of oral antithyroid drugs as the primary mode of therapy or as a presurgical agent also affects the ultimate prognosis. The skill of the surgeon, anesthetic complications, and myriad additional factors alter the success of treatment. Again, treatment is always recommended in an effort to effect the best prognosis.

REFERENCES

Adams WH, et al: Investigation of the effects of hyperthyroidism on renal function in the cat. Can J Vet Res 61:53, 1997a.
Adams WH, et al: Changes in renal function in cats following treatment of hyperthyroidism using [131]I. Vet Radiol Ultrasound 38:231, 1997b.
Andrade VA, et al: Methimazole pretreatment does not reduce the efficacy of radioiodine in patients with hyperthyroidism caused by Graves' disease. J Clin Endocrinol Metab 86:3488, 2001.
Archer FJ, Taylor SM: Alkaline phosphatase bone isoenzyme and osteocalcin in the serum of hyperthyroid cats. Can Vet J 37:735, 1996.
Aucoin DP, et al: Propylthiouracil-induced immune-mediated disease in cats. J Pharmacol Exp Ther 234:13, 1985.
Aucoin DP, et al: Dose dependent induction of anti-native DNA antibodies by propylthiouracil in cats. J Arthr Rheum 31:688, 1988.
Barber PJ, Elliott J: Study of calcium hemostasis in feline hyperthyroidism. J Small Anim Pract 37:575, 1996.

Beck KA, et al: The normal feline thyroid: Technetium pertechnetate imaging and determination of thyroid to salivary gland radioactivity ratios in 10 normal cats. Vet Radiol 26:35, 1985.

Becker TJ, et al: Effects of methimazole on renal function in cats with hyperthyroidism. J Am Anim Hosp Assoc 36:215, 2000.

Beleslin DB, et al: Nature of salivation produced by thyrotropin-releasing hormone (TRH). Brain Res Bull 18:463, 1987a.

Beleslin DB, et al: Studies of thyrotropin-releasing hormone (TRH)–induced defecation in cats. Pharmacol Biochem Behav 26:639, 1987b.

Belew AM, et al: Evaluation of the white-coat effect in cats. J Vet Intern Med 13:134, 1999.

Bennedbaek FN, et al: Percutaneous ethanol injection therapy in the treatment of thyroid and parathyroid diseases. Eur J Endocrinol 136:240, 1997.

Birchard SJ: Thyroidectomy and parathyroidectomy in the dog and cat. Probl Vet Med 3:277, 1991.

Birchard SJ: Thyroidectomy in the cat. In Peterson ME (ed): Hyperthyroidism. Daniels Pharmaceuticals Monograph, 1998, p 15.

Birchard SJ, et al: Surgical treatment of feline hyperthyroidism: Results of 85 cases. J Am Anim Hosp Assoc 20:705, 1984.

Biscoveanu M, Hasinski S: Abnormal results of liver function tests in patients with Graves' disease. Endocr Pract 6:367, 2000.

Bodey AR, Samson J: Epidemiological study of blood pressure in domestic cats. J Small Anim Pract 39:567, 1998.

Bond BR: Hyperthyroid heart disease in cats. In Kirk RW (ed): Current Veterinary Therapy IX. Philadelphia, WB Saunders, 1986, p 399.

Bond BR, et al: Echocardiographic evaluation of 30 cats with hyperthyroidism (abstract). American College of Veterinary Internal Medicine Science Proceedings, New York, 1983.

Bond BR, et al: Echocardiographic findings in 103 cats with hyperthyroidism. J Am Vet Med Assoc 192:1546, 1988.

Bradley RA, Feldman EC: Propylthiouracil treatment of feline hyperthyroidism (abstract). American College of Veterinary Internal Medicine Science Proceedings, 1982.

Braselton WE, et al: Measurement of serum iohexol by determination of iodine with inductively coupled plasma atomic emission spectroscopy. Clin Chem 43:1429, 1997.

Broome MR, et al: Peripheral metabolism of thyroid hormones and iodide in healthy and hyperthyroid cats. Am J Vet Res 48:1286, 1987.

Broome MR, et al: Predictive value of tracer studies for ^{131}I treatment in hyperthyroid cats. Am J Vet Res 49:193, 1988.

Broussard JD, et al: Changes in clinical and laboratory findings in cats with hyperthyroidism from 1983 to 1993. J Am Vet Med Assoc 206:302, 1995.

Brown RS, et al: Thyroid growth immunoglobulins in feline hyperthyroidism. Thyroid 2:125, 1992.

Brucker-Davis F, et al: Diagnosis and treatment outcome of patients with thyrotropin-secreting pituitary tumors. 84:476, 1999.

Bucknell DG: Feline hyperthyroidism: Spectrum of clinical presentations and response to carbimazole therapy. Aust Vet J 78:462, 2000.

Carpenter JL, et al: Tumors and tumorlike lesions. In Holzworth J (ed): Diseases of the Cat: Medicine and Surgery. Philadelphia, WB Saunders, 1987, p 406.

Chizzonite RA, et al: Isolation and characterization of two molecular variants of myosin heavy chain from rabbit ventricle: Change in their content during normal growth and after treatment with thyroid hormone. J Biol Chem 257:2056, 1982.

Christopher MM: Relation of endogenous Heinz bodies to disease and anemia in cats: 120 cases (1978-1987). J Am Vet Med Assoc 194:1089, 1989.

Cook SM, et al: Radiographic and scintigraphic evidence of focal pulmonary neoplasia in three cats with hyperthyroidism: Diagnostic and therapeutic considerations. J Vet Intern Med 7:303, 1993.

Cooper DS: Antithyroid drugs. N Engl J Med 311:1353, 1984.

Court MH, Freeman LM: Identification and concentration of soy isoflavones in commercial cat foods. Am J Vet Res 63:181, 2002.

Court MH, Greenblatt DJ: Molecular genetic basis for deficient acetaminophen glucuronidation by cats: UGT1A6 is a pseudo-gene, and evidence for reduced diversity of expressed hepatic UGT1A isoforms. Pharmacogenetics 10:355, 2000.

DiBartola SP, Brown SA: The kidney and hyperthyroidism. In Bonagura JD (ed): Kirk's Current Veterinary Therapy XIII. Philadelphia, WB Saunders, 2000, p 337.

DiBartola SP, et al: Effects of treatment of hyperthyroidism on renal function in cats. J Am Vet Med Assoc 208:875, 1996.

Divi RL, et al: Antithyroid isoflavones from soybean: isolation, characterization, and mechanisms of action. Biochem Pharmacol 54:1087, 1997.

Djavan B, et al: Outcome analysis of minimally invasive treatments for benign prostatic hypertrophy. Tech Urol 5:12, 1999.

Duda RJ, et al: Concurrent assays of circulating bone GLA-protein and bone alkaline phosphatase: Effects of age, sex, and metabolic bone disease. J Clin Endocrinol Metab 66:951, 1988.

Duyff RF, et al: Neuromuscular findings in thyroid dysfunction: A prospective clinical and electrodiagnostic study. J Neurol Neurosurg Psychiatry 68:750, 2000.

Elliott J, et al: Feline hypertension: clinical findings and response to antihypertensive treatment in 30 cases. J Small Anim Pract 42:122, 2001.

Eriksen EF, et al: Trabecular bone remodeling and bone balance in hyperthyroidism. Bone 6:421, 1985.

Ferguson DC, et al: Serum free and total iodothyronine concentrations in normal cats and cats with hyperthyroidism. J Vet Intern Med 3:121, 1989.

Flanders JA, et al: Feline thyroidectomy: A comparison of postoperative hypocalcemia associated with three different surgical techniques. Vet Surg 16:362, 1987.

Flanders JA, et al: Functional analysis of ectopic parathyroid activity in cats. Am J Vet Res 52:1336, 1991.

Forrest LJ, et al: Feline hyperthyroidism: Efficacy of treatment using volumetric analysis for radioiodine dose calculation. Vet Radiol Ultrasound 37:141, 1996.

Foster DJ, Thoday KL: Use of propranolol and potassium iodate in the presurgical management of hyperthyroid cats. J Small Anim Pract 40:307, 1999.

Foster DJ, Thoday KL: Tissue sources of serum alkaline phosphatase in 34 hyperthyroid cats: A qualitative and quantitative study. Res Vet Sci 68:89, 2000.

Foster DJ, et al: Selenium status of cats in four regions of the world and comparison with reported incidence of hyperthyroidism in cats in those regions. Am J Vet Res 62:934, 2001.

Franklyn JA: The management of hyperthyroidism. N Engl J Med 330:1731, 1994.

Fraser WD, et al: Intact parathyroid hormone concentration and cyclic AMP metabolism in thyroid disease. Acta Endocrinol 124:652, 1991.

Gerber H, et al: Etiopathology of feline toxic nodular goiter. Vet Clin North Am (Small Anim Pract) 24:541, 1994.

Goldstein RE, et al: Percutaneous ethanol injection for treatment of unilateral hyperplastic thyroid nodules in cats. J Am Vet Med Assoc 218:1298, 2001.

Gordon JM, et al: Juvenile hyperthyroidism in a cat. J Am Anim Hosp Assoc 39:67, 2003.

Graves TK: Complications of treatment and concurrent illness associated with hyperthyroidism in cats. In Bonagura JD (ed): Kirk's Current Veterinary Therapy XII. Philadelphia, WB Saunders, 1995, p 369.

Graves TK, Peterson ME: Diagnosis of occult hyperthyroidism in cats. Probl Vet Med 2:683, 1990.

Graves TK, Peterson ME: Occult hyperthyroidism in cats. In Kirk RW, Bonagura JD (eds): Current Veterinary Therapy XI. Philadelphia, WB Saunders, 1992, p 334.

Graves TK, et al: Changes in renal function associated with treatment of hyperthyroidism in cats. Am J Vet Res 55:1745, 1994.

Guptill L, et al: Response to high-dose radioactive iodine administration in cats with thyroid carcinoma that had previously undergone surgery. J Am Vet Med Assoc 207:1055, 1995.

Gurlek A, et al: Liver test abnormalities in hyperthyroidism before and during PTU therapy. J Clin Gastroenterol 24:180, 1997.

Hammer KB, et al: Altered expression of G proteins in thyroid gland adenomas obtained from hyperthyroid cats. Am J Vet Res 61:874, 2000.

Hancock LD, et al: The effect of propylthiouracil on subsequent radioactive iodine therapy in Graves' disease. Clin Endocrinol 47:425, 1997.

Hays MT, et al: A multicompartmental model for iodide, thyroxine, and triiodothyronine metabolism in normal and spontaneously hyperthyroid cats. Endocrinology 122:2444, 1988.

Henik RA, et al: Treatment of systemic hypertension in cats with amlodipine besylate. J Am Anim Hosp Assoc 33:226, 1997.

Hoenig M, Ferguson DC: Impairment of glucose tolerance in hyperthyroid cats. J Endocrinol 121:249, 1989.

Hoffman SB, et al: Bioavailability of transdermal methimazole in a pluronic lecithin organogel (PLO) in healthy cats. J Vet Pharmacol Therap p. 189, 2002.

Hofmeister E, et al: Functional cystic thyroid adenoma in a cat. J Am Vet Med Assoc 219:190, 2001.

Holm LE, et al: Cure rate after ^{131}I therapy for hyperthyroidism. Acta Radiol 20:161, 1981.

Holtman JR, et al: Central respiratory stimulation produced by thyrotropin-releasing hormone in the cat. Peptides 7:207, 1986.

Holzworth J, et al: Hyperthyroidism in the cat: Ten cases. J Am Vet Med Assoc 46:345, 1980.

Horney BS, et al: Agarose gel electrophoresis of alkaline phosphatase isoenzymes in the serum of hyperthyroid cats. Vet Clin Pathol 23:98, 1994.

Imesis RE, et al: Pretreatment with propylthiouracil but not methimazole reduces the therapeutic efficacy of iodine-131 in hyperthyroidism. J Clin Endocrinol Metab 83:685, 1998.

Ingbar DH: The respiratory system in thyrotoxicosis. In Braverman LE, Utiger RD (eds): The Thyroid: A Fundamental and Clinical Text, 6th ed. Philadelphia, JB Lippincott, 1991, p 744.

Jacobs G, Panciera D: Cardiovascular complications of feline hyperthyroidism. In Kirk RW, Bonagura JD (eds): Current Veterinary Therapy XI. Philadelphia, WB Saunders, 1992, p 756.

Jacobs G, et al: Congestive heart failure associated with hyperthyroidism in cats. J Am Vet Med Assoc 188:52, 1986.

Jacobs G, et al: Pharmacokinetics of propranolol in healthy cats during euthyroid and hyperthyroid states. Am J Vet Res 58:398, 1997.

Jarlov AE, et al: Calculated versus fixed dose of RAI for the treatment of hyperthyroidism. Clin Endocrinol 43:325, 1995.

Jeffrey SS, et al: Radiofrequency ablation of breast cancer: first report of an emerging technology. Arch Surg 134:1064, 1999.

Jiao LR, et al: Clinical short-term results of radiofrequency ablation in primary and secondary liver tumors. Am J Surg 177:303, 1999.

Jodar E, et al: Hyperthyroidism-induced bone loss. Clin Endocrinol 47:279, 1997.

Jones BR, et al: Radioiodine treatment of hyperthyroidism in cats. N Z Vet J 39:71, 1991.

Joseph RJ, Peterson ME: Review and comparison of neuromuscular and central nervous system manifestations of hyperthyroidism in cats and humans. Prog Vet Neurol 3:114, 1993.

Kass PH, et al: Evaluation of environmental, nutritional, and host factors in cats with hyperthyroidism. J Vet Intern Med 13:323, 1999.

Kintzer PP: Diagnosis of feline hyperthyroidism. Vet Previews 2:7, 1995.

Kintzer PP, Peterson ME: Thyroid scintigraphy in small animals. Semin Vet Med Surg (Small Anim) 6:131, 1991.

Kobayashi DL, et al: Hypertension in cats with chronic renal failure and hyperthyroidism. J Vet Intern Med 4:58, 1990.

Kruger JM, et al: Putting GFR into practice: Clinical applications of iohexol clearance. Proceedings of the 15th Annual Veterinary Medical Forum. American College of Veterinary Internal Medicine, 1998.

Larsen PR, et al: Relationships between circulating and intracellular thyroid hormones: Physical and clinical implications. Endocr Rev 2:87, 1981.

Lievesly P, Gruffydd-Jones TJ: Episodic collapse and weakness in cats. Vet Ann 29:261, 1989.

Lippi F, et al: Treatment of solitary autonomous thyroid nodules by percutaneous ethanol injection: Results of an Italian multicenter study. J Clin Endocrinol Metab 81:3261, 1996.

Litten RZ, et al: Altered myosin isozyme patterns from pressure overloaded and thyrotoxic rabbit hearts. Circ Res 50:856, 1982.

Littman MP: Spontaneous systemic hypertension in 24 cats. J Vet Intern Med 8:79, 1994.

Liu S, et al: Hypertrophic cardiomyopathy and hyperthyroidism in the cat. J Am Vet Med Assoc 185:52, 1984.

Livraghi T, et al: Treatment of autonomous thyroid nodules with percutaneous ethanol injection: preliminary results. Radiology 175:827, 1990.

Livraghi T, et al: Small hepatocellular carcinoma: Treatment with radiofrequency ablation versus ethanol ablation. Radiology 210:655, 1999.

Lurye JC, et al: Evaluation of an in-house enzyme-linked immunosorbent assay for quantitative measurement of serum total thyroxine concentration in dogs and cats. J Am Vet Med Assoc 221:243, 2002.

Mackovic-Basic M, Kleeman CR: The kidneys and electrolyte metabolism in thyrotoxicosis. In Braverman LE, Utiger RD (eds): The Thyroid: A Fundamental and Clinical Text, 6th ed. Philadelphia, JB Lippincott, 1991, p 771.

Maggio F, et al: Ocular lesions associated with systemic hypertension in cats: 69 cases (1985-1998). J Am Vet Med Assoc 217:695, 2000.

Mallery K, et al: Percutaneous ultrasonographically guided radiofrequency heat ablation for treatment of hyperthyroidism in cats. J Vet Intern Med 16:360, 2002 (abstract).

Mandel SJ, et al: Superiority of iodine-123 compared with iodine-131 scanning for thyroid remnants in patients with differentiated thyroid carcinoma. Clin Nucl Med 26:6, 2001.

Marcocci C, et al: A reappraisal of the role of methimazole and other factors on the efficacy and outcome of radioiodine therapy of Graves' hyperthyroidism. J Endocrinol Invest 13:513, 1990.

Martin FIR, et al: Hyperthyroidism in elderly hospitalized patients. Med J Australia 164:200, 1996.

Martin KM, et al: Evaluation of dietary and environmental risk factors for hyperthyroidism in cats. J Am Vet Med Assoc 217:853, 2000.

Maugeri D, et al: Elevated thyroid hormone levels and hyperthyroidism in the elderly. Arch Geront Geriat 22:145, 1996.

McDougall IR: Treatment of hyper- and hypothyroidism. J Clin Pharmacol 21:365, 1981.

McLoughlin MA, et al: Influence of systemic nonthyroidal illness on serum concentrations of thyroxine in hyperthyroid cats. J Am Anim Hosp Assoc 29:227, 1993.

Meric SM, Rubin SI: Serum thyroxine concentrations following fixed-dose radioactive iodine treatment in hyperthyroid cats: 62 cases (1986-1989). J Am Vet Med Assoc 197:621, 1990.

Meric SM, et al: Serum thyroxine concentrations after radioactive iodine therapy in cats with hyperthyroidism. J Am Vet Med Assoc 188:1038, 1986.

Monzani F, et al: Five-year follow up of percutaneous ethanol injection for the treatment of hyperfunctioning thyroid nodules: a study of 117 patients. Clin Endocrinol 46:9, 1997.

Mooney CT: Feline hyperthyroidism. In Torrance AG, Mooney CT (eds): Manual of Small Animal Endocrinology, 2nd ed. British Small Animal Veterinary Association, 1998a, p 115.

Mooney CT: The elderly cat with weight loss. In Torrance AG, Mooney CT (eds): Manual of Small Animal Endocrinology, 2nd ed. British Small Animal Veterinary Association, 1998b, p 31.

Mooney CT, Thoday KL: CVT Update: Medical treatment of hyperthyroidism in cats. In Bonagura JD (ed): Kirk's Current Veterinary Therapy XIII. Philadelphia, WB Saunders, 2000, p 333.

Mooney CT, et al: Carbimazole therapy of feline hyperthyroidism. J Small Anim Pract 33:228, 1992a.

Mooney CT, et al: The value of thyrotropin (TSH) stimulation in the diagnosis of feline hyperthyroidism. Proceedings of the British Small Animal Veterinary Association, 1992b.

Mooney CT, et al: Qualitative and quantitative thyroid imaging in feline hyperthyroidism using technetium-99m as pertechnetate. Vet Radiol 33:313, 1992c.

Mooney CT, et al: Effect of illness not associated with the thyroid gland on serum total and free thyroxine concentrations in cats. J Am Vet Med Assoc 208:2004, 1996a.

Mooney CT, et al: Serum thyroxine and triiodothyronine responses of hyperthyroid cats to thyrotropin. Am J Vet Res 57:987, 1996b.

Murray LAS, Peterson ME: Ipodate treatment of hyperthyroidism in cats. J Am Vet Med Assoc 211:63, 1997.

Nap AMP, et al: Quantitative aspects of thyroid scintigraphy with pertechnetate (^{99m}TcO$_4$) in cats. J Vet Intern Med 8:302, 1994.

Nemzek JA, et al: Acute onset of hypokalemia and muscular weakness in four hyperthyroid cats. J Am Vet Med Assoc 205:65, 1994.

Nguyen LQ, et al: Serum from cats with hyperthyroidism does not activate feline thyrotropin receptors. Endocrinology 143:395, 2002.

Nieckarz JA, Daniel GB: The effect of methimazole on thyroid uptake of pertechnetate and radioiodine in normal cats. Vet Radiol Ultrasound 42:448, 2001.

Padgett SL, et al: Efficacy of parathyroid gland autotransplantation in maintaining serum calcium concentrations after bilateral thyroparathyroidectomy in cats. J Am Anim Hosp Assoc 34:219, 1998.

Papasouliotis K, et al: Decreased orocaecal transit time, as measured by the exhalation of hydrogen in hyperthyroid cats. Res Vet Sci 55:115, 1993.

Paradis M, Page CT: Serum free thyroxine concentrations measured by chemiluminescence in hyperthyroid and euthyroid cats. J Am Anim Hosp Assoc 32:489, 1996.

Peake RL: Recurrent apathetic hyperthyroidism. Arch Intern Med 141:258, 1986.

Pearce SH, et al: Mutational analysis of the thyrotropin receptor gene in sporadic and familial feline thyrotoxicosis. Thyroid 7:923, 1997.

Peschle C: Erythropoiesis. Annu Rev Med 31:303, 1980.

Peterson ME: Feline hyperthyroidism. Vet Clin North Am (Small Anim Pract) 14:809, 1984.

Peterson ME: Use of a thyrotropin-releasing hormone (TRH) stimulation test as an aid in the diagnosis of mild hyperthyroidism in cats. J Vet Intern Med 5:129, 1991.

Peterson ME: Hypoparathyroidism and other causes of hypocalcemia in cats. In Kirk RW, Bonagura JD (eds): Current Veterinary Therapy XI. Philadelphia, WB Saunders, 1992, p 376.

Peterson ME: Hyperthyroidism. In Ettinger SJ, Feldman EC (eds): Textbook of Veterinary Internal Medicine. Philadelphia, WB Saunders, 1995a, p 1466.

Peterson ME: Radioactive iodine (Radioiodine) treatment for hyperthyroidism in cats. In Bonagura JD (ed): Kirk's Current Veterinary Therapy XII. Philadelphia, WB Saunders, 1995b, p 372.

Peterson ME: Hyperthyroidism. In Ettinger SJ, Feldman EC (eds): Textbook of Veterinary Internal Medicine, 5th ed. Philadelphia, WB Saunders, 2000, p 1400.

Peterson ME, Aucoin DP: Comparison of the disposition of carbimazole and methimazole in clinically normal cats. Res Vet Sci 54:351, 1993.

Peterson ME, Becker DV: Radioiodine treatment of 524 cats with hyperthyroidism. J Am Vet Med Assoc 207:1422, 1995.

Peterson ME, Gamble DA: Effect of nonthyroidal disease on serum thyroxine concentrations in cats: 494 cases (1988). J Am Vet Med Assoc 197:1203, 1990.

Peterson ME, Randolph JF: Endocrine diseases. In Sherding RG (ed): The Cat: Diagnosis and Clinical Management. New York, Churchill Livingstone, 1989, p 1095.

Peterson ME, Turrel JM: Feline hyperthyroidism. In Kirk RW (ed): Current Veterinary Therapy IX. Philadelphia, WB Saunders, 1986, p 1026.

Peterson SL, Yoshioka MM: The use of technetium-99m pertechnetate for thyroid imaging in a case of feline hyperthyroidism. J Am Anim Hosp Assoc 19:1015, 1983.

Peterson ME, et al: Spontaneous hyperthyroidism in the cat abstract. Am Coll Vet Intern Med 1979, p 108 (abstract).

Peterson ME, et al: Electrocardiographic findings in 45 cats with hyperthyroidism. J Am Vet Med Assoc 180:934, 1982.

Peterson ME, et al: Feline hyperthyroidism: Pretreatment clinical and laboratory evaluation of 131 cases. J Am Vet Med Assoc 103:103, 1983.

Peterson ME, et al: Propylthiouracil-associated hemolytic anemia, thrombocytopenia, and antinuclear antibodies in cats with hyperthyroidism. J Am Vet Med Assoc 184:806, 1984.

Peterson ME, et al: Serum thyroid hormone concentrations fluctuate in cats with hyperthyroidism. J Vet Intern Med 1:142, 1987a.

Peterson ME, et al: Lack of circulating thyroid stimulating immunoglobulins in cats with hyperthyroidism. Vet Immunol Immunopathol 16:277, 1987b.

Peterson ME, et al: Methimazole treatment of 262 cats with hyperthyroidism. J Vet Intern Med 2:150, 1988.

Peterson ME, et al: Triiodothyronine (T$_3$) suppression test: An aid in the diagnosis of mild hyperthyroidism in cats. J Vet Intern Med 4:233, 1990.

Peterson ME, et al: Use of the thyrotropin-releasing hormone (TRH) stimulation test to diagnose mild hyperthyroidism in cats. J Vet Intern Med 8:279, 1994.

Peterson ME, et al: Determination of free T$_4$ by dialysis as an aid in diagnosis of mild hyperthyroidism in cats. J Vet Intern Med 9:183, 1995 (abstract).

Peterson ME, et al: Measurement of serum concentrations of free thyroxine, total thyroxine, and total triiodothyronine in cats with hyperthyroidism and cats with nonthyroidal disease. J Am Vet Med Assoc 218:529, 2001.

Pollard RE, et al: Percutaneous ultrasonographically guided radiofrequency heat ablation for treatment of primary hyperparathyroidism in dogs. J Am Vet Med Assoc 218:1106, 2001.

Randolph JF, et al: Prothrombin, activated partial thromboplastin, and proteins induced by vitamin K absence or antagonists: Clotting times in 20 hyperthyroid cats before and after methimazole treatment. J Vet Intern Med 14:56, 2000.

Refsal KR, et al: Use of the triiodothyronine suppression test for diagnosis of hyperthyroidism in ill cats that have a serum concentration of iodothyronines within normal range. J Am Vet Med Assoc 199:1594, 1991.

Reusch CE, Tomsa K: Serum fructosamine concentrations in cats with overt hyperthyroidism. J Am Vet Med Assoc 215:1297, 1999.

Scarlett JM, et al: Feline hyperthyroidism: A descriptive and case-control study. Prev Vet Med 6:295, 1988.

Schlesinger DP, et al: Use of breath hydrogen measurement to evaluate orocecal transit time in cats before and after treatment for hyperthyroidism. Can Vet J 57:89, 1993.

Shaha AR, et al: Parathyroid autotransplantation during thyroid surgery. J Surg Oncol 46:21, 1991.

Sheng WH, et al: Antithyroid drug–induced agranulocytosis and infectious complications. Q J Med 92:455, 1999.

Slater MR, et al: Long-term health and predictors of survival for hyperthyroid cats treated with iodine-131. J Vet Intern Med 15:47, 2001.

Smith TA, et al: Pretreatment thyroxine concentrations and pertechnetate scans as a predictor of radioiodine treatment success. J Vet Intern Med 8:159, 1994 (abstract).

Smith TA, et al: Radioiodine treatment outcome in hyperthyroid cats: Effects of prior methimazole treatment. J Vet Intern Med 9:183, 1995 (abstract).

Sparkes AK, et al: Thyroid function in the cat: Assessment by the TRH response test and the thyrotropin stimulation test. J Small Anim Pract 32:59, 1991.

Spaulding SW, Utiger RD: The thyroid: Physiology, hyperthyroidism, hypothyroidism, and the painful thyroid. In Felig P, et al (eds): Endocrinology and Metabolism. New York, McGraw-Hill, 1981, p 281.

Stegemen JR, et al: Use of recombinant human thyroid-stimulating hormone for thyrotropin-stimulation testing of euthyroid cats. Am J Vet Res 64:149, 2003.

Stiles J, et al: The prevalence of retinopathy in cats with systemic hypertension and chronic renal failure or hyperthyroidism. J Am Anim Hosp Assoc 30:564, 1994.

Sullivan P, et al: Altered platelet indices in dogs with hypothyroidism and cats with hyperthyroidism. Am J Vet Res 54:2004, 1993.

Swalec KM, Birchard SJ: Recurrence of hyperthyroidism after thyroidectomy in cats. J Am Anim Hosp Assoc 26:433, 1990.

Theon AP: Personal communication, 2002.

Theon AP: A prospective randomized comparison of intravenous versus subcutaneous administration of radioiodine for treatment of feline hyperthyroidism: A study of 120 cats. Am J Vet Res 55:1734, 1994.

Thoday KL, Mooney CT: Historical, clinical and laboratory features of 126 hyperthyroid cats. Vet Rec 131:257, 1992a.

Thoday KL, Mooney CT: Medical management of feline hyperthyroidism. In Kirk RW, Bonagura JD (eds): Current Veterinary Therapy IX. Philadelphia, WB Saunders, 1992b, p 338.

Toft AD: Subclinical hyperthyroidism. N Engl J Med 345:512, 2001.

Tomsa K, et al: Thyrotropin-releasing hormone stimulation test to assess thyroid function in severely sick cats. J Vet Intern Med 15:89, 2001.

Trepanier LA, et al: Pharmacokinetics of intravenous and oral methimazole following single- and multiple-dose administration in normal cats. J Vet Pharmacol Ther 14:367, 1991a.

Trepanier LA, et al: Pharmacokinetics of methimazole in normal cats and cats with hyperthyroidism. Res Vet Sci 50:69, 1991b.

Trepanier LA, et al: Efficacy and safety of once versus twice daily administration of methimazole in cats with hyperthyroidism. J Am Vet Med Assoc 222:954, 2003.

Trepanier LA, et al: Efficacy and safety of transdermal versus oral methimazole. ACVIM Forum, 2003.

Tse J, et al: Thyroxine induced changes in characteristics in b-adrenergic receptors. Endocrinology 107:6, 1980.

Turrel JM, et al: Radioactive iodine therapy in cats with hyperthyroidism. J Am Vet Med Assoc 184:554, 1984.

Turrel JM, et al: Thyroid carcinoma causing hyperthyroidism in cats: 14 cases (1981-1986). J Am Vet Med Assoc 193:359, 1988.

Utiger RD: Decreased extrathyroidal triiodothyronine production in nonthyroidal illness: Benefit or harm? Am J Med 69:807, 1980.

Utiger RD: Tests of thyroregulatory mechanisms. In Ingbar SH, Braverman LE (eds): The Thyroid: A Fundamental and Clinical Text, 6th ed. Philadelphia, JB Lippincott, 1986, p 511.

Utiger RD: The thyroid: Physiology, hyperthyroidism, hypothyroidism, and the painful thyroid. In Felig P, et al (eds): Endocrinology and Metabolism, 2nd ed. New York, McGraw-Hill, 1987, p 389.

Utiger RD: Commentary on "Methimazole pretreatment does not reduce the efficacy of radioiodine in patients with hyperthyroidism caused by Graves' disease." Clinical Thyroidology 13:42, 2002a.

Utiger RD: Commentary on "Abnormal results of liver function tests in patients with Graves' disease." Clinical Thyroidology 13:42, 2002b.

Van der Woerdt A, Peterson ME: Prevalence of ocular abnormalities in cats with hyperthyroidism. J Vet Intern Med 14:202, 2000.

Walker MC, Schaer M: Percutaneous ethanol treatment of hyperthyroidism in a cat. Feline Pract 26:10, 1998.

Weichselbaum RC, et al: Evaluation of relationships between pretreatment patient variables and duration of isolation for radioiodine-treated hyperthyroid cats. Am J Vet Res 64:425, 2003.

Welches CD, et al: Occurrence of problems after three techniques of bilateral thyroidectomy in cats. Vet Surg 18:392, 1989.

Wells AL, et al: Use of percutaneous ethanol injection for treatment of bilateral hyperplastic thyroid nodules in cats. J Am Vet Med Assoc 218:1293, 2001.

Willard MD: Disorders of potassium homeostasis. Vet Clin North Am (Small Anim Pract) 19:241, 1989.

Williams GH, Braunwald E: Endocrine and nutrition disorders and heart disease. In Braunwald E (ed): Heart Disease: A Textbook of Cardiovascular Medicine. Philadelphia, WB Saunders, 1980, p 1835.

Wisner ER, et al: Normal ultrasonographic anatomy of the canine neck. Vet Radiol Ultrasound 32:185, 1991.

Wisner ER, et al: Ultrasonographic examination of the thyroid gland of hyperthyroid cats: comparison to 99mTc scintigraphy. Vet Radiol Ultrasound 35:53, 1994.

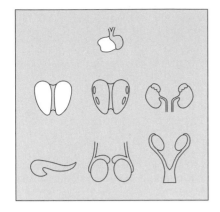

5

CANINE THYROID TUMORS AND HYPERTHYROIDISM

Thyroid nodules in humans are commonly encountered, being particularly frequent among women. The prevalence of people with thyroid nodules in the United States has been estimated to be about 4% of the adult population, with a female:male ratio of 4:1. In young children, the incidence is less than 1%; in persons ages 11 to 18 years, about 1.5%; and in persons over age 60, about 5%. In contrast to the common incidence of thyroid "nodules" in people, thyroid "cancer" is considered rare. According to the Third National Cancer Survey, the incidence of thyroid cancer affecting people within the United States is 0.004% of the populace per year. Thus most thyroid nodules are benign in people (Greenspan, 2001). In contrast to these statistics regarding humans, the statistics for dogs are quite different.

The thyroid gland, made up of two lobes, is not normally palpable in either dogs or cats. However, thyroid tumors are usually easy to feel in both species. Although benign thyroid masses are commonly detected in cats, especially those older than 8 years of age, thyroid masses are only occasionally encountered in dogs. Malignant tumors account for a large percentage of these thyroid nodules in dogs. It has been estimated that thyroid tumors account for approximately 1% to 4% of all canine neoplasms (Priester and McKay, 1980; Birchard and Roesel, 1981; Loar, 1986; Wheeler, 1989; Ogilvie, 1996; Waters and Scott-Moncrieff, 1998). Veterinarians have become well educated regarding thyroid disease in cats. Coincidental with the remarkable incidence of thyroid disease in cats and owner interest in their treatment, has been an increasing number of dog owners being interested in aggressive management of their pets with thyroid tumors. This combination of factors creates an interest for comparing the thyroid conditions affecting the two species. However, significant differences exist in their thyroid diseases (Table 5-1). A tremendous percentage of cats with thyroid disease have benign conditions and hyperthyroidism, whereas dogs with thyroid masses commonly have malignant disease and are usually euthyroid.

Virtually every "general pathology study" published on dogs includes a significant number of dogs with thyroid tumors. In contrast to the relatively recent identification of clinically significant thyroid disease in cats (since 1980), thyroid neoplasia has long been a recognized disorder in dogs. In general, the clinical syndrome caused by thyroid tumors is surprisingly different in these two species. Thyroid tumors in the cat tend to be functioning, noninvasive, relatively small adenomatous masses. In the dog, these tumors tend to be nonfunctioning, invasive, large, carcinomatous masses. In both species, therapeutic measures are warranted, but those that are effective in cats are not usually effective in dogs (see Table 5-1). More than 90% of the clinically detectable thyroid tumors in dogs are carcinomas. This remarkable prevalence concerning malignancy is related, in part, to the fact that most thyroid adenomas in dogs are nonfunctional, they cause no clinical signs, and they are too small to be palpable.

TABLE 5–1 COMPARISONS OF CANINE AND FELINE THYROID TUMORS

	Canine	Feline
Incidence	Not common	Quite common
% Malignant	80–90%	<5%
Local invasion	Common	Rare
Metastatic behavior	Common (more-so with large tumors)	Rare
% Hyperthyroid	<10%	>95%
Association with:		
Heart disease	Rare	Moderate
Kidney disease	Rare	Common
Therapeutic Modalities	Surgery	Surgery
	External beam radiation	Radioactive iodine
	Doxorubicin	Methimazole
	Cisplatin	Carbimazole

TUMOR CLASSIFICATION

Pathology (Necropsy) versus Clinical Experience

Benign thyroid tumors (adenomas) account for 30% to 50% of thyroid masses identified in studies published by veterinary pathologists (Brodey and Kelly, 1968; Leav et al, 1976). These benign tumors tend to be small, noninvasive, and clinically silent. Therefore, although it has been more than 25 years since these publications first appeared in the literature, it is generally assumed that their results remain valid. Benign tumors are usually described as being incidental findings on necropsy. Clinical studies, however, suggest that almost all thyroid tumors in dogs are malignant and that a significant percentage of those tumors are large, invasive, palpable, and the source of worrisome clinical signs (Mooney, 1998; Lurye and Behrend, 2001; Withrow and MacEwen, 2001). Benign tumors, like normal thyroid lobes, are described as not being palpable. They are mobile, ovoid, and typically involve only one lobe. In contrast, thyroid carcinomas are classically described as large and coarsely multinodular, not mobile, and easily palpable. About one-third of these carcinomas involve both thyroid lobes, and two-thirds are located in one lobe. They are poorly encapsulated and commonly extend into or around the trachea, esophagus, and muscles of the neck. They are highly vascular and may invade local blood vessels.

Physical Examination and Clinical Signs

It is assumed that most benign thyroid tumors (adenomas) are nonfunctional in dogs. Furthermore, since these tumors are small, mobile, noninvasive, and inactive, they are clinically silent. In other words, there is no reason for an owner or veterinarian to suspect that a dog has a benign thyroid tumor. Palpation of the cervical area is not a component of physical examinations performed on dogs by most veterinarians. If palpation of the cervical area is performed, it is typically cursory. Furthermore, benign thyroid tumors are described as being small enough to rarely be palpable, even if such a mass were suspected.

By comparison, most malignant thyroid tumors in dogs are large. Three of the more common reasons that dogs with malignant thyroid tumors are brought into a veterinary hospital are (1) the owner finds a large mass in the dog's neck; (2) the owner notices that the dog is having trouble swallowing; or (3) the owner notices respiratory signs—for example, the dog is breathing abnormally fast (even at times of rest), there is a change in the tone of the dog's bark, the dog exhibits surprisingly loud breathing or coughing, or the dog is in apparent respiratory distress (dyspnea), especially with excitement or exercise. Any of these owner observations should cause a veterinarian to carefully palpate the cervical area. Since thyroid masses in these situations are large, they are typically easy to palpate. Additional problems in dogs with thyroid carcinomas may be nonspecific (poor appetite, weight loss, vomiting, lethargy, etc.) and may or may not encourage a veterinarian to palpate the neck.

The Incidentally Discovered Thyroid Mass

The veterinary literature suggests that small benign or malignant thyroid masses in dogs are often clinically silent and usually go unnoticed on physical examination. However, the past few years have witnessed changes in the diagnostic approach to various clinical conditions in dogs, the result being the incidental discovery of a greater number of hither-to unsuspected and nondiagnosed thyroid masses. Specifically, the use of cervical ultrasonography will change the frequency of diagnosing thyroid masses in dogs.

In our hospital, cervical ultrasonography has become a routine component in the diagnostic evaluation of several conditions in dogs. This procedure is noninvasive, simple, readily available, and no more expensive than radiographs or "routine" blood and urine testing. Dogs with respiratory distress or tachypnea undergo cervical ultrasound, especially if the source of the problem is thought to be an upper respiratory condition. Dogs suspected of having laryngeal paralysis also undergo cervical ultrasonography. Certainly, dogs with hypercalcemia, especially those believed to have primary hyperparathyroidism, are evaluated with cervical ultrasonography. Furthermore, any dog with swallowing difficulties or evidence of regurgitation problems is evaluated with cervical ultrasonography. With these and a growing number of other indications for ultrasonography of the neck, we have identified a number of thyroid masses that were not anticipated.

Approximately 40% of the thyroid masses that were "incidentally discovered" with cervical ultrasonography have been benign adenomas. After such masses have been described by our radiologists, most clinicians remain unable to palpate them. Approximately 60% of the incidentally identified thyroid masses have been diagnosed with histologic evaluation as being thyroid carcinomas. The frequency of incidentally discovered thyroid masses diagnosed with cervical ultrasonography is expected to increase over the next 5 to 10 years. It is also anticipated that responses to surgery, radiation, and medical management of such tumors will improve, because they will be diagnosed earlier than ever before in the history of our profession. Keep these concepts in mind as you review this chapter. Veterinary medicine, like all such professions, is constantly evolving. The examples provided in the balance of this chapter may represent worst-case scenarios. Management practices and prognoses for thyroid tumors will improve if more of these tumors are diagnosed before they become large, easily palpable, and clinically catastrophic.

NONFUNCTIONING THYROID TUMORS (EUTHYROID OR HYPOTHYROID DOGS WITH NONTOXIC THYROID TUMORS)

Definition

The term *goiter* means enlargement of the thyroid gland, regardless of the cause. The two thyroid lobes are small and located dorsolateral to the trachea. They are not palpable in dogs under normal circumstances. Palpation of a thyroid lobe or any cervical mass implies the presence of a goiter or other worrisome problem and should raise immediate concern. If the palpated mass is thyroid tissue, there should be concern that neoplasia is the cause for the enlarged thyroid in any adult dog. The majority of goiters in dogs are unilateral, nonfunctioning carcinomas or "slightly functional" tumors that are not causing clinical signs of hyperthyroidism. Although extremely rare, goiter in neonates or juvenile dogs may be caused by iodine deficiency or be secondary to an inborn error in thyroid hormone synthesis and secretion. Immune-mediated thyroiditis rarely causes palpable goiter in dogs.

Pathogenesis

BACKGROUND. As with most neoplastic conditions, the exact cause of thyroid neoplasia is not known. Studies have suggested an association between thyroid neoplasia and (1) iodine deficiency or excess, (2) chronic excesses in thyroid-stimulating hormone (TSH) secretion, (3) ionizing radiation, and (4) gene abnormalities and oncogene expression. In addition to these potential pathogenic mechanisms, in some older humans, a long-standing, slowly growing papillary carcinoma may begin to grow rapidly and "convert" to an undifferentiated or anaplastic carcinoma. This condition is usually recognized, because small thyroid masses can be easily detected in people and any sudden change in size can be easily monitored. There may be some similarity between this well-defined process in people and the poorly defined process in dogs. Some

dogs will appear to have had a small thyroid mass that "suddenly" begins to expand, dramatically increasing in size. This "late anaplastic shift" is a potential cause of death from papillary carcinoma. Many of these papillary carcinomas secrete thyroglobulin, which can be used as a marker for recurrence or metastasis of the cancer (Greenspan, 2001).

IODINE DEFICIENCY OR EXCESS. Early epidemiologic data suggested that thyroid cancer in people was more frequent in iodine-deficient areas, but others have contested these findings (Konig et al, 1981). In areas where iodine excess prevails, such as Iceland and Hawaii, a high incidence of thyroid cancer, particularly of the papillary type, has been reported in humans (Verschueren and Goslings, 1992). Experimental data and clinical experience in dogs have neither confirmed nor denied these trends.

THYROTROPIN, THYROID-STIMULATING HORMONE (TSH), AND THYROID GROWTH FACTORS. The primary factor responsible for maintaining thyroid follicular cell function is TSH (Roger and Dumont, 1982). The role of TSH in thyroid growth is not as obvious, however. There are conflicting opinions regarding the importance of TSH in thyroid neoplasia in humans. In dogs, receptor affinity and concentration, as well as a functional response to TSH, are similar in both normal thyroids and thyroid carcinomas (Verschueren et al, 1992a). Thus some canine thyroid carcinomas appear to retain sensitivity to the growth-promoting effect of TSH, but poor correlation has been demonstrated between TSH binding and TSH dependence in humans (Darbre and King, 1987). Many tumors with TSH binding and adenylate cyclase response did not regress following suppression of serum TSH concentrations with L-thyroxine treatment (Saltiel et al, 1981).

IONIZING RADIATION. The relationship between ionizing radiation and thyroid cancer has been recognized in humans since the late 1940s and early 1950s. The causative effect of radioiodine on thyroid cancer development was further supported by its high incidence in areas of radioactive fallout, such as the Marshall Islands (Conard, 1984). The short-lived isotopes (^{132}I and ^{135}I) are of greater concern than the more commonly used isotope, ^{131}I (Verschueren, 1992a). Thyroid cancers resulting from radiation exposure are usually well-differentiated thyroid papillary or papillary-follicular carcinomas (Schneider, 1986). Irradiation has been demonstrated to be a cause of thyroid neoplasia in dogs (Verschueren, 1992a).

ONCOGENES. Extensive studies have been conducted on the expression of oncogenes in human thyroid cancers. This research has revealed evidence of gene mutations in both benign and malignant thyroid neoplasms (Fig. 5-1). Activating mutations in the *gsp* oncogene or TSH-R in the thyroid follicular cell have been associated with increased growth and function. Aberrant DNA methylation, activation of the *ras* oncogene, and mutation of the *MEN1* gene located at 11q13 are associated with benign follicular adenomas. Loss of the *3P* suppressor gene may then result in the development of follicular carcinoma, and further loss

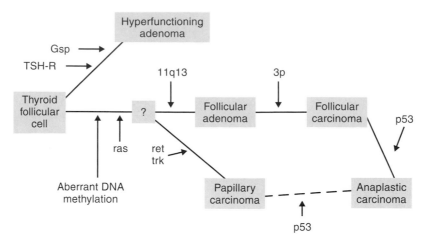

FIGURE 5–1. Molecular defects associated with development and progression of human thyroid neoplasms. The hypothetical role of specific mutational events in thyroid tumorigenesis is inferred from their prevalence in the various thyroid tumor phenotypes. (Reproduced with permission from Greenspan, 2001).

of suppressor gene *P53* may allow progression to an anaplastic carcinoma. Mutations in the *ret* and *trk* oncogenes are associated with the development of papillary carcinomas. Again, loss of the P53 suppressor gene may allow progression of this tumor to an anaplastic carcinoma. These hypotheses suggest progressions from benign to malignant tumors or from a "differentiated" carcinoma to an "undifferentiated" (and more lethal) carcinoma. Indeed, pathology specimens from older affected people that had long-standing goiters and recent rapid growth of the masses may demonstrate transition from papillary or follicular carcinoma to anaplastic carcinoma (Suarez et al, 1988; Bos, 1989; Lemoine et al, 1990; Wynford-Thomas, 1997; Komminoth, 1997; Schlumberger, 1998; Hanna et al, 1999; Greenspan, 2001). This phenomenon is referred to as "late anaplastic shift" and is mentioned in the introduction to this section. Similar studies have not yet been applied to canine thyroid neoplasia.

Pathology

PATHOLOGIC VERSUS CLINICAL SURVEYS. The percentages of malignant and benign canine thyroid tumors identified at *necropsy* are approximately equal. Malignant thyroid tumors occur with a greater frequency in the dog than in other species. Furthermore, the relatively frequent finding of benign tumors in the dog from *pathology* reports exceeds *clinical* experience. Benign thyroid tumors in the dog are usually unrecognized antemortem, because they are nonfunctional, quite small, and cause no clinical signs. In contrast, malignant thyroid tumors are relatively large, cause clinical signs that can be recognized by owners, and are easily palpated by veterinarians. As discussed earlier in this chapter, with the increased use of cervical ultrasonography as a diagnostic aid for dogs with a variety of conditions, it can be safely assumed

that the diagnosis of "incidentally discovered" thyroid tumors will escalate. Therefore clinical identification of benign thyroid tumors, as well as "small" malignant thyroid tumors, will increase.

RECOGNITION OF MALIGNANT VERSUS BENIGN THYROID TUMORS. As is typical of most endocrine tumors, pathologists sometimes have difficulty distinguishing benign from malignant thyroid tumors. Criteria such as cellular atypia and mitotic activity are not consistently reliable markers in discriminating between these two forms of neoplasia. Well-differentiated follicular carcinoma, in some cases, may be histologically distinguished from the benign condition only by demonstration of vascular or capsular invasion (Hedinger et al, 1988; Verschueren and Goslings, 1992). Owing to the recognized prevalence of malignant tumors seen by veterinary practitioners, most pathologists tend to identify thyroid masses that have been biopsied or surgically removed as "malignant until proven otherwise."

Benign Thyroid Tumors

PHYSICAL APPEARANCE AND CLINICAL FEATURES. The majority of benign canine thyroid tumors (adenomas) are small, solid, focal lesions that are not usually detected during life. The frequency with which these tumors are identified will be greatly enhanced by the increased use of cervical ultrasonography as a diagnostic tool. It is not understood why small, benign thyroid tumors in the cat tend to be functioning tumors that result in clinical hyperthyroidism whereas similar tumors in the dog are more commonly nonfunctioning or normally functioning. If a dog is diagnosed with a benign, nonpalpable thyroid tumor in our hospital, the most common reason is simple identification of an incidentally discovered mass with cervical ultrasonography. Much less commonly, a dog with a benign tumor may have the same clinical signs associated with any cervical mass: owner observation of the mass, respiratory signs, or difficulty swallowing (Loar, 1986; Lawrence et al, 1991).

Canine thyroid adenomas are often solitary, distinct, slightly soft masses. A well-delineated capsule is seldom noted. Solid adenomas are round or ovoid and measure a few millimeters to several centimeters in diameter. They are usually cream to reddish brown in color and may compress adjacent normal thyroid tissue. Large cystic adenomas can be turgid and filled with an amber or blood-tinged fluid (Belshaw, 1983; Capen, 1985). The central cavities of cystic adenomas have either a smooth or an irregular lining. The physical appearance of canine thyroid adenomas is distinct from the "adenomatous hyperplasia" typically identified in hyperthyroid cats. Although small focal masses similar to those seen in dogs are recognized in cats, the most frequently recognized feline hyperfunctioning thyroid resembles a compressed cluster of grapes involving the entire gland that may be cystic or cavitary upon cutting through the tissue.

HISTOLOGY. In dogs, most small solid thyroid adenomas are characterized as having follicles that are irregular and either small or large, microscopically. The cystic structures noted in some tumors are lined by dense fibrous tissues from which project fronds of uniform cells arranged in follicular and/or compact cellular patterns. Because cysts are seen in some small adenomas, it is likely that growth is inhibited occasionally by degenerative episodes and these patterns of development are responsible for the final gross and microscopic appearance of these tumors (Belshaw, 1983; Capen, 1985). Although canine thyroid adenomas are well recognized and thoroughly described in the literature, thyroid tumors observed by clinicians should be assumed to be malignant until proven otherwise. Some thyroid tumors may be benign, but the incidence of malignancy and the aggressive nature of these tumors dictate rapid action on the part of the veterinarian. This approach can assure the owners that their pet is being given the best chance for a cure.

Malignant Thyroid Tumors

INTRODUCTION. Carcinomas of the canine thyroid are usually large solid masses. Their malignant nature is often grossly evident at the time of surgery or necropsy as a result of invasion into adjacent structures. Extension of malignant thyroid tumors into or around the esophagus, trachea, cervical musculature, nerves, and thyroidal vessels is fairly common. However, invasion into the lumen of structures, such as the esophagus or trachea, is extremely unusual. Distant metastasis is quite common. It has been estimated that 40% to 60% of affected dogs have detectable distant metastases at time of clinical admission (Jeglum and Whereat, 1983; Harari et al, 1986; Withrow and MacEwen, 2001). Distant metastases are most likely

identified in the pulmonary parenchyma or in regional lymph nodes. By contrast, results of necropsy studies suggest that 60% to 80% of thyroid carcinomas had spread (Capen, 1985; Verschueren et al, 1992b). Of course, the typical necropsy takes place a significant amount of time after the average time of diagnosis. Thus the higher incidence of distant tumor spread is to be expected. In addition, metastases too small to be detected with radiographs, ultrasonography, or other diagnostic aids may be noted histologically.

DEMONSTRATION OF METASTASIS. Metastasis occurs most commonly to the lungs, retropharyngeal lymph nodes, and liver (Lurye and Behrend, 2001). Lymphatic drainage of the thyroid gland is primarily in the cranial direction, so lymph node enlargement is most likely to be detected cranial and medial to the primary tumor. Occasionally, both ipsilateral and contralateral cervical lymph nodes may be involved. Metastasis to other locations is also possible, including the adrenal gland, kidneys, liver, heart base, spleen, bone and bone marrow, prostate, brain, skeleton, and spinal cord (Harmelin et al, 1993; Verchueren et al, 1992b; Lurye and Behrend, 2001). The differentiation between benign and malignant thyroid neoplasia depends on the answers to two questions: (1) Is there evidence of similar tissue in regional lymph nodes, lungs, or other locations, as well as evidence of local invasion into surrounding structures? (2) What is the microscopic appearance of the tissue? Rarely, small malignant tumors may resemble adenomas. Histologic evaluation is imperative on any thyroid tumor removed by a veterinarian.

HISTOLOGY. Cellular pleomorphism may suggest malignant potential, but the diagnosis of carcinoma is dependent primarily on evidence of capsular and vascular invasion. These features may be subtle, and diagnosis of malignancy should not be assumed to be solely the job of the pathologist. Good communication between clinician (who can inform the pathologist regarding gross tissue invasion by the tumor, vascularity of the mass, and other pertinent clinical information) and pathologist can be quite helpful in gaining a full and complete understanding of the microscopic findings of submitted tissue.

Thyroid tumors of follicular cell origin are usually further subclassified as follicular, compact (solid), papillary, compact-follicular, or undifferentiated (anaplastic), depending on their pattern of growth (Table 5-2). In addition, veterinary oncologists use a clinical staging classification system initially developed by the World Health Organization (Table 5-3). The largest percentage of canine thyroid carcinomas contain both follicular and compact cellular patterns and are classified as "mixed-cellular," "compact-follicular," or "solid-follicular" carcinomas. Slightly less common are the pure follicular carcinomas. A smaller percentage of thyroid tumors are pure compact carcinomas. Undifferentiated (anaplastic) tumors are uncommon but recognized in about 10% of dogs with thyroid tumors. Papillary carcinomas are rare in the dog. Thyroid carcinomas may also arise

TABLE 5–2 HISTOLOGIC DIAGNOSIS OF THYROID TUMORS IN 237 DOGS RECOGNIZED AS HAVING A THYROID MASS ANTEMORTEM

Tumor Histology	Number	Percent
Compact follicular carcinomas	77	32
Follicular carcinomas	56	24
Compact (solid) carcinomas	41	17
Undifferentiated (anaplastic) carcinomas	28	12
Parafollicular (C-cell) carcinomas	20	9
Follicular adenoma	15	6
Obvious metastasis or local invasion	163	69

TABLE 5-3 CLINICAL STAGING OF CANINE THYROID TUMORS

T: Primary tumor
  T0 No evidence of tumor
  T1 Tumor <2 cm maximum diameter: T1a—not fixed, T1b—fixed
  T2 Tumor 2–5cm maximum diameter: T2a—not fixed, T2b—fixed
  T3 Tumor >5 cm maximum diameter: T3a—not fixed, T3b—fixed
N: Regional lymph nodes (RLN)*
  N0 No evidence of RLN involvement†
  N1 Ipsilateral RLN involved: N1a—not fixed, N1b—fixed
  N2 Bilateral RLN involved: N2a—not fixed, N2b—fixed
M: Distant metastasis
  M0 No evidence of distant metastasis
  M1 Distant metastasis detected

Stage Grouping	T	N	M
I	T1a, b	N0	M0
II	T0	N1	M0
	T1a, b	N1	
	T2a, b	N0 or N1a	
III	Any T3	Any N	M0
	Any T	Any Tb	
IV	Any T	Any N	M1

*The RLN are the mandibular and the superficial cervical lymph nodes.
†Involvement implies histologic evidence of tumor invasion.
Modified from Owen LN (ed): The TNM Classification of Tumours in Domestic Animals, Geneva, World Health Organization, 1980.

from parafollicular cells (C-cells, medullary carcinomas), but this cell type is uncommon in dogs. As discussed in the next section, medullary thyroid carcinoma has probably been underdiagnosed in the past, and the prevalence of this histologic type of tumor will increase with appropriate use of immunocytochemical stains. The least common thyroid tumors recognized by veterinary clinicians are benign tumors (adenoma). However, as previously discussed, it is anticipated that the prevalence of benign thyroid tumors will rise as cervical ultrasonography provides evidence of incidentally discovered cervical masses. Electron microscopy and immunohistochemistry may be helpful and/or necessary in defining the cell of origin.

IMMUNOHISTOCHEMISTRY. Immunochemical techniques have refined the pathologic diagnoses of virtually all neoplasms, including those of thyroid origin. Immunohistochemical analysis of thyroid neoplasms for thyroglobulin, calcitonin, calcitonin gene–related peptide (CGRP), and neuron-specific enolase has been studied in dogs and has been demonstrated to contribute to the diagnosis of medullary carcinoma (Moore et al, 1984; Holscher et al, 1986; Leblanc et al, 1991). Studies of these C-cell complexes have demonstrated four different cell types: those that stained for thyroglobulin, calcitonin and CGRP, somatostatin, or no marker. These data suggest the possibility of a common cell lineage for the follicular cell and the parafollicular cell. This finding concurs with the occurrence of mixed follicular and parafollicular tumors in humans, bulls, and horses, but not in dogs (Ljungberg et al, 1983; Ljungberg and Nilsson, 1985; Tateyama et al, 1988; Leblanc et al, 1990; 1991).

It has been accepted that medullary carcinoma may be difficult to distinguish from other thyroid tumors by light microscopy alone. This has probably resulted in a prevalence of underestimation regarding medullary carcinoma among dogs with thyroid malignancy. The incidence was thought to be <5% (Patnaik and Lieberman, 1991; Leblanc et al, 1991); however, when specific immunocytochemical stains were applied to thyroid tumors from dogs, the incidence of medullary thyroid carcinoma was 36%. This is obviously a much higher incidence than previously suggested (Carver et al, 1995). Furthermore, it was thought that histologic classification was not a useful prognostic factor (Brodey and Kelly, 1968; Mitchell et al, 1979; Harari et al, 1986; Klein et al, 1988; Ogilvie, 1996). The long-term prognosis may be better for dogs with medullary carcinoma of the thyroid compared with that in dogs with thyroid carcinomas of follicular origin. Medullary carcinomas have a lower rate of distant metastases, they are well encapsulated versus the incomplete encapsulation typical of follicular carcinomas, and they appear to be easier to surgically remove (83% successful removal of medullary carcinoma versus 52% successful removal of follicular carcinoma; Carver et al, 1995).

INCIDENCE. Several reports agree that thyroid tumors account for 1% to 4% of all tumors found in dogs. It is also understood that some thyroid tumors are not recognized by clinicians and are found only at necropsy, because they are too small to be palpated and do not cause clinical signs. Thyroid tumors may represent an isolated neoplastic "event," or they may occur in conjunction with the development of other tumors. The identification of more than one tumor in an individual dog is usually considered simply a coincidental finding.

MULTIPLE ENDOCRINE NEOPLASIA (MEN) SYNDROMES. Veterinary medicine has derived benefit, historically, from the experience of physicians in human medicine and from using human beings as our "animal model" of disease. Physicians often have the ability to track family histories relative to disease states and to determine the likelihood that an individual may or may not have certain problems based on "familial" tendencies. This is certainly true of thyroid disease and thyroid neoplasia. Therefore attempts to draw analogies from the human experience and to apply that information to veterinary patients may be helpful. About 80% of people with medullary carcinoma of the thyroid, for example, have "sporadic" disease. By contrast, 20% of those patients have a tumor that can be traced back as a "familial disorder," that is, one in which their genetic background predisposed them to this condition. Four familial patterns of disease occur with respect to medullary carcinoma of the thyroid. These familial conditions in people should be used to remind veterinary clinicians that a thorough evaluation of any dog is warranted, even after diagnosis of thyroid cancer. This is true because some dogs may have more than one problem. Before investing time, money, and emotion into treating one problem, we should attempt to ensure that a dog does not have other serious disease.

Of the four familial patterns associated with medullary carcinoma of the thyroid in humans, one or more may have analogous conditions in dogs. The four patterns recognized in people are (1) familial medullary thyroid carcinoma without associated endocrine disease (FMTC); (2) multiple endocrine neoplasia syndrome 2A (MEN 2A), consisting of medullary carcinoma, pheochromocytoma, and hyperparathyroidism; (3) multiple endocrine neoplasia syndrome 2B (MEN 2B), consisting of medullary carcinoma, pheochromocytoma, and multiple mucosal neuromas; and (4) MEN 2, consisting of MEN syndrome together with cutaneous lichen amyloidosis, a pruritic skin condition. The genes responsible for these familial syndromes have been mapped to the centromeric region of chromosome 10, which is the location of the *ret* proto-oncogene (a receptor-like tyrosine kinase gene), and mutations in exon 10, 11, or 16 of this location have been demonstrated in patients with these syndromes (Greenspan, 2001). If medullary carcinoma is diagnosed in a person, it is recommended that family members be screened for that tumor and that the patient and family members be screened for any of the other conditions found in MEN 2. In addition to tests designed to detect abnormalities suggestive of medullary carcinoma, gene mutations can be demonstrated in DNA from peripheral white blood cells by using polymerase chain reaction (PCR), restriction fragment-length polymorphism (RFLP), and family unit linkage analysis to identify gene carriers. In this manner, families can be screened for the carrier state, as well as for early diagnosis and treatment of serious disease states.

Dogs occasionally have tumors in several different endocrine organs (including the thyroid) simultaneously (Table 5-4). The answer as to whether these dogs have familial disorders analogous to the well-defined MEN syndromes in human beings awaits genetic study. It is suspected that many of these dogs simply have coincidental multiple problems. However, it is interesting to note that we have diagnosed seven dogs with concurrent medullary carcinoma of the thyroid, pheochromocytoma, and primary hyperparathyroidism due to a parathyroid adenoma. This does fit the criteria for MEN 2A. Also, a number of other dogs with thyroid tumors in our series have shown evidence of other glandular neoplasias (see Table 5-4).

TABLE 5–4 HISTOLOGIC EVIDENCE OF MULTIPLE ENDOCRINE NEOPLASIA (MEN) SYNDROME IN 63 DOGS WITH THYROID TUMORS

Tissue Description	Number of Dogs
Thyroid adenoma and chemodectoma	2
Thyroid follicular carcinoma and adrenocortical adenoma	4
Thyroid follicular carcinoma and adrenocortical carcinoma	4
Thyroid follicular carcinoma, pituitary adenoma, and adrenocortical hyperplasia	12
Thyroid follicular (3) or compact-follicular carcinoma (3) and parathyroid hyperplasia/adenoma	6
Thyroid compact-follicular carcinoma, pituitary adenoma, and adrenocortical hyperplasia	11
Thyroid follicular adenoma, pheochromocytoma, pituitary adenoma, and adrenocortical hyperplasia	3
Thyroid follicular adenoma and adrenocortical adenoma	4
Thyroid parafollicular (C-cell) carcinoma, pituitary tumor, and pheochromocytoma	4
Thyroid parafollicular (C-cell) carcinoma, pheochromocytoma, and parathyroid adenoma	7
Thyroid compact-follicular carcinoma and parathyroid adenoma	6

These 63 dogs include 27 different breeds. Multiple endocrine tumors do exist in dogs and cats, emphasizing the value of complete diagnostic evaluations even when a tumor, such as a thyroid mass, is palpable and recognized easily.

SIGNALMENT. Thyroid tumors in the dog typically develop in middle-aged and older animals. The average age for dogs with thyroid tumors, benign or malignant, is approximately 10 years. The age range is quite wide, but almost all dogs with thyroid tumors are 5 years of age or older (Fig. 5-2). One study conducted within a small colony of Beagles demonstrated an age-specific incidence of thyroid tumors of 1.1% per year in dogs 8 to 12 years of age and 4.0% per year in dogs 12 to 15 years of age (Haley et al, 1989).

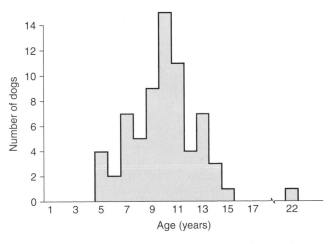

FIGURE 5–2. The ages of 69 dogs with thyroid neoplasia at the time of diagnosis. The average age is approximately 10 years.

There is no obvious gender predilection for thyroid neoplasia in the dog (Harari et al, 1986). By contrast, the incidence of human thyroid cancer is about four times greater in women than in men at most ages (Greenspan, 2001). The breeds thought to be at increased risk appear to include Boxers, Beagles, and Golden Retrievers (Harari et al, 1986; Verschueren, 1992), although our experience is slightly different, with mixed-breed dogs and Labrador Retrievers being most commonly afflicted. As seen in Table 5-5, Beagles, Boxers, and Golden Retrievers were among the 42 breeds represented in our series. Breed incidence in dogs with thyroid tumors, in our experience, tends to correlate with breed popularity.

CLINICAL SIGNS. Dogs with *nontoxic* (not *hyperthyroid*) thyroid tumors are usually brought to veterinarians because the owners have seen or felt a mass in the neck or because the mass is causing clinical signs. The signs reported by different authors vary slightly. Without doubt the most frequent owner concern is feeling or sometimes seeing a midcervical or ventrocervical mass. Owners, while petting and scratching their

TABLE 5–5 BREED DISTRIBUTION OF 237 DOGS WITH THYROID TUMORS

Breed	Number	Percent
Mixed-Breed Dogs	32	13
Labrador Retriever	22	9
Golden Retriever	17	7
Boxer	15	6
Australian Shepherd	14	6
German Shepherd Dog	14	6
Poodle	14	6
Dachshund	12	5
Rottweiler	12	5
Beagle	12	5
Doberman Pinscher	10	4
32 other breeds (<10 cases each)	63	27

dogs, may simply note the presence of a "swelling" in the throat area (Fig. 5-3). The mass may be unilateral or bilateral in location. Most thyroid tumors are felt to be just below the area of the larynx, but larger tumors may extend (common) or descend (uncommon) closer to the thoracic inlet.

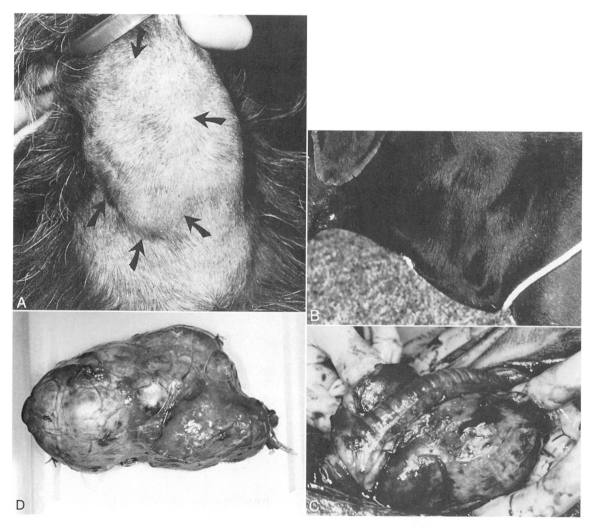

FIGURE 5–3. *A,* Photograph of the shaved ventral cervical area of a dog with a large, obvious goiter *(arrows).* (Photograph courtesy of Dr. Jane Turrel.) *B,* Lateral view of the dog with a large thyroid tumor. The mass is delineated ventrally by the leash. *C,* Large thyroid tumor, at surgery, displacing the trachea. *D,* The thyroid tumor following excision.

TABLE 5–6 OWNER-OBSERVED SIGNS IN 237 DOGS WITH THYROID TUMORS

Sign	Percent of Dogs
Visible mass in neck	78
Coughing	34
Rapid breathing (even at rest)	32
Dyspnea (difficulty breathing-distress)	28
Trouble swallowing (dysphagia)	23
Change in bark (dysphonia)	14
Weight loss	14
Listlessness/Depression	13
No observed signs	12
Vomiting/Regurgitation	11
Anorexia/Decrease in appetite	11
Polydipsia/Polyuria	10
Hyperactivity	9
Diarrhea	9
Increased appetite	3
Facial edema	2
Apparent cervical discomfort	2

Because most affected dogs remain healthy for some time, the swelling in the neck caused by tumor growth is often noted to develop slowly. In more than 75% of our dogs that were diagnosed antemortem as having a thyroid tumor, either the swelling was the only reason for seeking veterinary care or the swelling was pointed out by a veterinarian during an examination for some other problem (Table 5-6). Other clinical signs include coughing, rapid breathing (especially at times of rest), respiratory distress, difficulty in swallowing (dysphagia), alteration in the sound of a normal bark (dysphonia), weight loss, listlessness/depression, vomiting, regurgitation, anorexia or an obvious decrease in appetite, polydipsia, polyuria, hyperactivity, diarrhea, increased appetite, facial edema, and apparent pain or discomfort (see Table 5-6). Not surprisingly, the length of time between owner observation of the mass or clinical sign(s) and presentation of the dog for veterinary care is highly variable. In our series, some dogs were seen as quickly as the same day a mass was discovered, whereas others were not seen until as long as 36 months later. The average length of time was within 2 to 6 weeks.

A surprising percentage of owners fail to notice any clinical signs in their dogs with thyroid tumors. As stated previously, there has been a dramatic increase in the use of cervical ultrasonography as a diagnostic aid. For the most part, we had been using this tool for dogs suspected to have laryngeal paralysis and those suspected as having primary hyperparathyroidism. As we began to bring "healthy" middle-aged and older dogs (>5 years of age) to our hospital for cervical ultrasonography to serve as controls, a number of "incidentally discovered" thyroid masses were identified. Added to this group of "healthy dogs" were the dogs with primary hyperparathyroidism that had hypercalcemia identified as a serendipitous finding on routine screening blood work. These dogs had blood taken as part of a geriatric assessment and, like our apparently healthy controls, had no clinical signs and were thought to be well. These healthy control dogs and the dogs with primary hyperparathyroidism account for almost all the dogs in our series with thyroid tumors but no clinical signs.

PHYSICAL EXAMINATION. Most dogs with thyroid tumors have nontoxic thyroid malignancies. *Nontoxic*, in this context, means that the tumor is not functional and that the dog is not hyperthyroid. Physical examination reveals few abnormalities other than those problems noted by the owner. Many dogs are remarkably healthy, especially when compared with hyperthyroid cats. Two important aspects of a physical examination are emphasized: (1) The veterinarian should be certain that a complete physical examination is performed before making any recommendations to an owner regarding diagnosis, treatment, and prognosis. (2) The veterinarian must attempt to appreciate the size and invasive nature of the thyroid mass. If possible, the veterinarian should answer this question: Is this cervical mass (presumably thyroid until proven otherwise) freely movable?

Most thyroid masses are firm, asymmetrical, irregular in shape, and nonpainful. If both thyroid lobes are affected, the masses tend to be irregular and asymmetrical. Most thyroid tumors are located close to the typical normal thyroid region (at and ventral to the laryngeal area) in the neck and are not as ventral in location or as freely movable in the subcutaneous space as those in cats (see Fig. 5-3). Usually, the thyroid mass is nonmovable and obviously well embedded into surrounding tissue. It is usually not possible to palpate the interior or medial surface of the mass because of local invasion. An irregular shape is not always diagnostic of carcinoma, but an immovable mass usually implies local invasion and should raise a strong suspicion for malignancy at the time of examination.

Inspiratory and expiratory dyspnea has been identified in several dogs. Only a few dogs have been obviously cachectic (Fig. 5-4), depressed, or dehydrated. The noncachectic dogs are usually alert and active and have good mucous membrane color, normal capillary refill time, and no fever. A dry, lusterless hair coat is common, but alopecia is rare. Heart sounds are normal, and examination of the mouth, eyes, ears, and abdomen is unremarkable. Submandibular lymph nodes may be enlarged as a result of tumor spread or lymphatic obstruction.

IN-HOSPITAL EVALUATION. *Hemogram (CBC), Serum Chemistry Profile, and Urinalysis.* These preliminary "database" studies are rarely helpful or consistent in diagnosis or management of dogs with thyroid tumors. Less than 10% of dogs with thyroid tumors are anemic, and when identified, these anemias are typically mild, normocytic, normochromic, and nonregenerative. Leukocytosis was present in only a few dogs. Serum chemistry profiles have revealed a mild increase in blood urea nitrogen (BUN) and an increase in liver enzyme activity in 14% and 24% of the dogs we have evaluated, respectively. One report identified increased liver enzymes in 7 of 21 dogs, and this finding was not associated with a thyrotoxic state (Harari et al, 1986). Abnormal liver enzyme activities do not indicate hepatic metastasis. Hypercalcemia was identified in three dogs with thyroid carcinoma and believed to be a paraneoplastic condition. Urinalysis was usually unremarkable and not contributory to the final diagnosis.

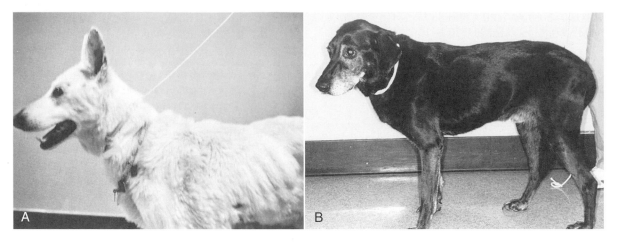

FIGURE 5–4. *A,* A cachectic 9-year-old German Shepherd dog with hyperthyroidism caused by a functioning thyroid carcinoma. *B,* A thin 12-year-old Labrador-mix with mild hyperthyroidism secondary to a functioning thyroid carcinoma.

Although a preliminary database was not beneficial in establishing a diagnosis of thyroid tumor, in differentiating benign from malignant tumors, or in tumor staging, these studies still have significant value. Dogs with thyroid tumors (known, suspected, or identified at a later date) are usually 8 years of age or older, with potential problems in more than one organ system. Concurrent disease and the potential for multiple primary tumors cannot be underestimated. Normal test results imply that a dog is a relatively safe anesthetic risk. Furthermore, when more than one abnormality is recognized, problems can be prioritized relative to the importance of resecting or debulking a thyroid mass. Consideration can be given to simultaneous therapy for each problem identified.

RADIOGRAPHY. Radiographs of the thorax should always be evaluated in a dog with a suspected thyroid mass. Thoracic radiographs successfully identified four of four dogs with pulmonary metastasis found at necropsy in one study (Birchard and Roesel, 1981). Thoracic radiographs were positive for metastasis in 38% of dogs with thyroid carcinoma in another report (Harari et al, 1986). Using radiography, we have recognized 11 dogs with metastasis to the region of the base of the heart, as well as 40 of 73 dogs with metastasis to the lungs. In our series, approximately 50% of dogs with pulmonary metastasis were identified by thoracic radiography. Many of the dogs with positive radiographs and some with unremarkable thoracic studies will have positive radioactive sodium pertechnetate scan results diagnostic for distant metastases. Radiography and careful lymph node palpation/biopsy have helped owners decide how aggressive to be regarding therapy. In part, it helps veterinarians "stage" thyroid tumors and provide advice to these owners.

Radiography of the cervical area may identify a small mass that was suspected but not definitively identified on physical examination, it may illustrate the severity of displacement of adjacent structures, and it may identify local invasion of the mass into the larynx and trachea. In our dogs, cervical or abdominal radiographs have not been routinely obtained, because we prefer ultrasonography. However, a few dogs with irregular hepatic silhouettes were shown to have hepatic metastasis, suggesting that abdominal radiography or ultrasonography be included in the routine database of any dog suspected of having thyroid neoplasia.

ELECTROCARDIOGRAM (ECG) AND/OR ECHOCARDIOGRAM. Evaluation of an ECG is imperative if cardiac arrhythmias are detected. Thoracic radiographs, echocardiography, and/or electrocardiography are indicated if murmurs are detected or if the dog is thought to be in heart failure. Dogs with nontoxic thyroid tumors usually have no cardiac disorders and have normal cardiac function. The exception are those dogs with heart disease unrelated to the thyroid tumor.

ULTRASONOGRAPHY. *Equipment and Positioning.* Examination of the thyroid lobes requires an ultrasound unit with a high-frequency, 7.5- to 10.0-MHz transducer. As transducer frequency increases, spatial resolution improves. Smaller structures and finer anatomic details can be appreciated. Even in the largest dog, thyroid depth rarely exceeds 4 cm, the depth to which a 10-MHz frequency transducer is limited. Our radiologists use a blended 5- to 10-MHz linear array transducer with a 38-mm scanning width for initial examination of the cervical area. More detailed examination is then completed with a 26-mm width transducer. Blended probes provide an advantage over standard single-frequency transducers, because they allow more superficial structures to be imaged at a higher frequency for improved spatial resolution. Deeper structures can then be imaged at the lower end of the frequency range to improve image quality in the far field (Wisner et al, 1991; Wisner and Nyland, 1998).

The ventral cervical area should be carefully clipped. Stubble and unclipped hair can reduce image quality. Dogs are positioned as straight as possible on a padded v-top table in dorsal recumbency. There should be little lateral or ventral flexion of the neck. Dogs almost never require sedation, and minimal restraint is usually all that is needed for study completion. However, dogs that have cervical masses large enough to produce upper airway obstruction, such as those with large thyroid masses, are at risk for developing severe dyspnea after being placed in dorsal recumbency and then having their cervical area compressed with a transducer. Therefore care is warranted in these dogs; it may be safer to examine some of them under anesthesia with an endotracheal tube in place (Wisner and Nyland, 1998).

Normal Anatomy, Imaging Planes, and Indications. The thyroid lobes are normally located just caudal to the arch of the cricoid cartilage. Healthy medium-sized dogs have flattened lobes measuring approximately $5.0 \times 1.5 \times 0.5$ cm (Fig. 5-5). The common carotid arteries lie lateral and slightly superficial to the thyroid lobes, serving as an important internal landmark. Two standard imaging planes are used in evaluating the thyroid lobes. If a particularly large cervical mass is present, additional imaging planes may be necessary (Wisner et al, 1991). The obvious indications for thyroid or cervical ultrasonography are to evaluate the origin, location, and margination of clinically undifferentiated cervical masses. Ultrasonography also may be useful in determining whether a mass is unilateral or bilateral, that is, whether it involves one or both lobes. Since many such masses are thyroid and, in dogs, thyroid carcinomas, ultrasound findings are an important component in the decision-making process regarding therapeutic alternatives for the owner (Wisner et al, 1994).

Differential Diagnosis of Neck Masses. Ultrasonography often allows thyroid tumors to be distinguished from other space-occupying masses. Common differential diagnoses for ventral cervical masses include thyroid adenoma or carcinoma; submandibular, medial retropharyngeal, or cervical lymphadenopathy; cellulitis; abscess or granuloma; salivary gland tumor or inflammation; and other neoplastic masses such as rhabdomyosarcomas, leiomyosarcomas, and carotid body tumors (Wisner et al, 1994). When evaluating a dog with a neck mass of unknown etiology, the veterinarian should begin the ultrasound examination by attempting to identify both thyroid lobes. This often allows quick identification of thyroid masses. Large cervical masses, however, can distort anatomy and make origin identification more difficult. On the other hand, lymph nodes and salivary masses are usually not difficult to distinguish from thyroid lobes based on location (usually cranial and lateral to the thyroid lobes) and echogenicity. Salivary glands, for example, are typically uniformly hypoechoic with characteristic internal linear arborization that likely represents the salivary duct system (Wisner and Nyland, 1998).

Ultrasound Appearance of a Thyroid Carcinoma. Because thyroid carcinomas are usually nonfunctional, they are typically quite large at the time of diagnosis. They vary from being well marginated with a definitive capsule to being poorly marginated (Fig. 5-6). Thyroid parenchyma is hypoechoic compared with normal thyroid tissue, and the character of this parenchyma may not be homogeneous. The parenchyma may be complex, sometimes containing multiple cysts, or may have foci of mineralization. Thyroid carcinomas are highly vascular, and a large arterial vascular plexus is often distributed in and around these masses. The vascular plexus can be verified by pulsed or color-flow Doppler ultrasonographic evaluation. Some dogs naturally develop arteriovenous malformations as a component of the carcinoma, or such abnormalities can develop after surgery (Wisner et al, 1994; Wisner and Nyland, 1998).

Thyroid carcinomas may be bilateral, may involve surrounding fascial sheaths, and may encroach on and invade the cervical vasculature. Careful examination of thyroid carcinoma margins is useful in determining whether surgical intervention is a plausible treatment option. Uncommonly, carcinomas do invade the esophageal wall, causing dysphagia. Esophageal involvement may be best demonstrated with a barium study. Although a diagnosis of thyroid carcinoma can be made with confidence in most dogs based on localization to one or both thyroid lobes and on qualitative ultrasonographic characteristics, such an impression can be confirmed by fine needle or tissue core biopsy. Because of the vascularity of these lesions, aspiration should be performed with ultrasound guidance to aid in avoiding larger blood vessels.

The Incidentally Discovered Thyroid Mass. As has been discussed earlier in this chapter, ultrasonography is being used as a diagnostic tool for a wide variety of concerns. Thus dogs with no palpable cervical mass are undergoing cervical ultrasonography. With the aid of ultrasound, unsuspected thyroid masses are being identified. Approximately 40% to 50% of these incidentally discovered masses have been adenomas and 50% to 60% have been thyroid carcinomas. Thorough evaluation of these masses is encouraged.

RADIOACTIVE PERTECHNETATE SCANS. *Protocol.* Thyroid gland scintigraphy in dogs can be completed following IV administration of 2 to 4 mCi of ^{99m}Tc-pertechnetate. Gamma camera imaging of the cervical region and thorax should be obtained within 1 hour of pertechnetate administration. The radiolabeled pertechnetate is trapped by any cells that concentrate iodine, as is typical of the thyroid. Usually, 1-minute static left lateral, right lateral, ventral, and dorsal images are recommended (Marks et al, 1994).

Interpretation. Pertechnetate is concentrated by thyroid tissue, salivary glands, and gastric mucosa (Fig. 5-7). Those tissues considered likely to contain thyroid cells (primary or metastatic sites) can be evaluated for size and for extent of invasion or metastasis. It has been suggested that pertechnetate scans do not provide information regarding thyroid function (euthyroid, hypothyroid, or hyperthyroid). In other words, thyroid scans should not be used as a thyroid function test but rather to locate thyroid tissue, both

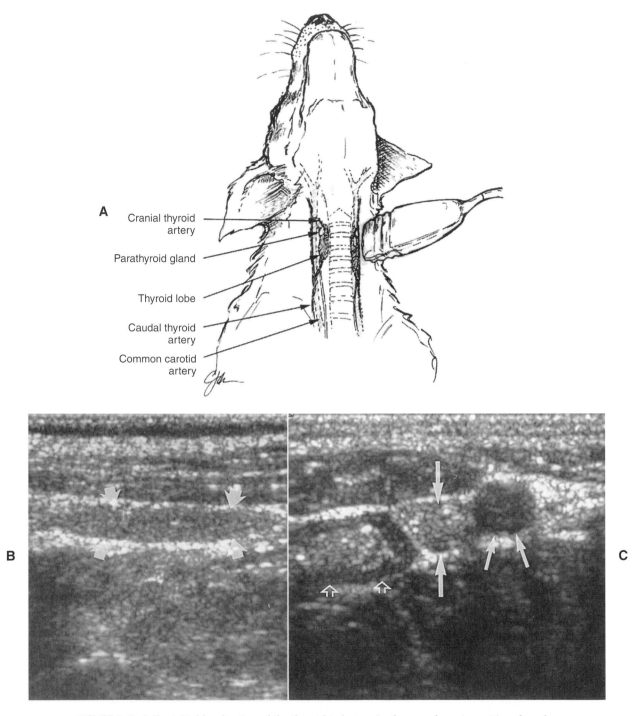

Cranial thyroid artery

Parathyroid gland

Thyroid lobe

Caudal thyroid artery

Common carotid artery

A

B

C

FIGURE 5–5. *A,* For initial localization of the thyroid in long axis, the transducer is positioned on the jugular groove with the imaging plane directed midway between the frontal and parasagittal planes. The ipsilateral common carotid artery serves as an anatomic landmark. *B,* the normal canine thyroid lobe appears as a uniformly moderately echoic ellipsoid structure *(arrows).* A thin hyperechoic fascial sheath surrounds and defines the thyroid lobe. *C,* In the short-axis view, the thyroid lobe *(large solid arrows)* appears as a roughly triangular structure adjacent and medial to the common carotid artery *(small solid arrows).* The esophagus can be seen when imaging the left thyroid lobe and appears as an irregularly shaped structure medial and dorsal to the thyroid lobe *(open arrows).* (From Wisner ER, Nyland TG: Ultrasonography of the thyroid and parathyroid glands. Vet Clin N Amer: Sm Anim Pract 28:973, 1998. Used with permission).

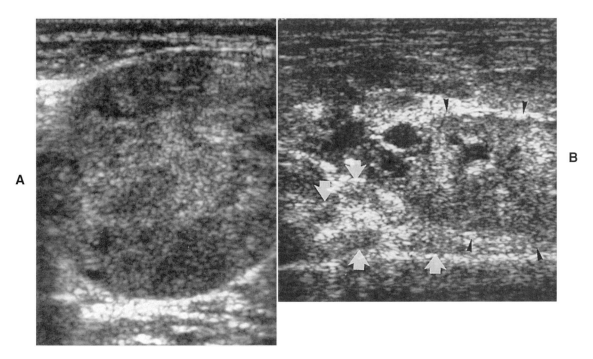

FIGURE 5–6. *A*, Encapsulated thyroid carcinoma in a dog. The thyroid is grossly enlarged, and thyroid parenchyma is heterogeneous, but the lesion appears to be well marginated. *B*, Poorly marginated thyroid carcinoma in a dog. The thyroid is enlarged, and thyroid parenchyma is heterogeneous *(arrowheads)*. In addition, lesion margins are poorly defined and appear to extend into surrounding tissues *(arrows)*. (From Wisner ER, Nyland TG: Ultrasonography of the thyroid and parathyroid glands. Vet Clin N Amer: Sm Anim Pract 28:973, 1998. Used with permission).

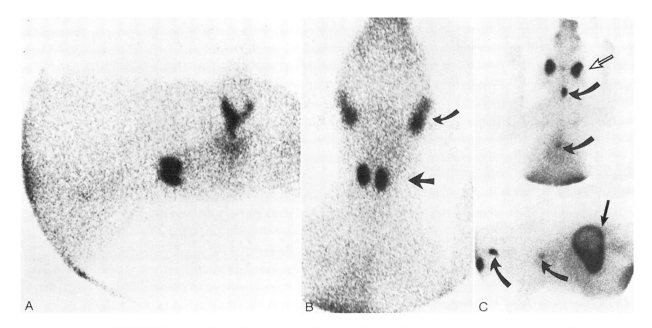

FIGURE 5–7. Lateral *(A)* and dorsoventral *(B)* views of a pertechnetate thyroid scan from a normal dog. The thyroids of a normal dog *(straight arrow)* are approximately the size of normal salivary glands (curved arrow). *C*, One normal cervical thyroid and one ectopic anterior mediastinal thyroid *(curved arrows)* in a dog that had one thyroid lobe surgically removed. Salivary glands *(open arrow)* and stomach *(straight arrow)* are also visualized because these tissues concentrate pertechnetate.

normal and abnormal and to help determine extent of local invasion or metastasis (Turrel et al, 1987; Rijnberk, 1996). However, recent studies and our experience suggest that thyroid scans do provide some information regarding thyroid function (Balogh et al, 1998).

Uptake is considered normal if radioactivity in the thyroid area is similar in size and density to that seen in the parotid salivary glands on the ventral image (see Fig. 5-7). Identification of two symmetrical, normal-sized masses in the neck with normal radioactive uptake implies that it is normal thyroid tissue. Two patterns of pertechnetate uptake were identified in dogs with thyroid tumors in one of our studies. Pattern I was characterized as a well-circumscribed, homogeneous area of uptake (Fig. 5-8). Pattern II was characterized as a poorly circumscribed, heterogeneous area of uptake (Fig. 5-9). Focal areas of uptake within the thorax or distributed in unusual areas of the neck should be interpreted as highly suspicious of metastases (Marks et al, 1994).

Results in Dogs with Thyroid Tumors. In our study, all 29 dogs with thyroid neoplasia had abnormal pertechnetate scans. Pattern I uptake was found in 11 dogs, whereas 18 dogs had a pattern II uptake. Of the 29 dogs, 24 had thyroid adenocarcinoma; 9 of those 24 dogs had pattern I uptake and 15 had pattern II uptake. Three dogs had undifferentiated thyroid carcinoma; one pattern I and two pattern II. One dog had a thyroid adenoma with pattern I uptake, and one dog had a C-cell carcinoma with pattern II uptake. The most common scintigraphic appearance (13 of 29 dogs) was a unilateral thyroid mass with increased radio-iodine uptake (Marks et al, 1994). Radionuclide uptake in one thyroid lobe was found in 21 of the 29 dogs; 5 dogs had uptake in both thyroid lobes, and 3 dogs had uptake in areas distant from the location of the normal thyroid gland (Fig. 5-10). Exploratory surgery in 24 of 29 dogs demonstrated thyroid neoplasia in sites that correlated with the areas demonstrated by scintigraphy.

If cells within metastasic sites retain the ability to trap iodine, those sites should be visualized on radioactive thyroid scintigraphy. Also, ectopic sites of thyroid function (neoplastic or normal) may be seen. Of 29 dogs, two had *radiographic* evidence of pulmonary metastasis, but only one of the two had evidence of pulmonary metastasis on pertechnetate scans (Fig. 5-11; Marks et al, 1994). Thus scintigraphy has demonstrated that the iodine trapping capability of thyroid neoplasia is variable. If a malignancy, especially a distant site of metastasis, does not trap iodine effectively, the scintigraphic study will fail to identify that site. For this reason, thyroid scintigraphy is considered a relatively *specific* tool for identification of metastasis, but it is not considered *sensitive*. Failure to identify distant metastatic sites with scintigraphy does not mean that distant metastasis does not exist.

Scintigraphic Results versus Histologic Results ("Hot" versus "Cold" Nodules). Follicular carcinomas are characterized by the maintenance of small follicles with minimal colloid formation. Follicular carcinoma may be indistinguishable from follicular adenoma except that carcinomas demonstrate capsular or vascular invasion. Follicular carcinomas are specifically mentioned, because in humans, and probably in dogs, these tumors often retain the ability to concentrate iodine and, less commonly, to synthesize T_3 and T_4. Thus "functioning thyroid cancer" is almost always follicular carcinoma in humans (Greenspan, 2001). These tumors, and possibly their metastases, are more likely to concentrate sodium pertechnetate and to be visualized on a scan.

In contrast to results in humans, pertechnetate scans in dogs with thyroid neoplasia, regardless of the histologic classification, are almost always abnormal. Tumors that concentrate pertechnetate and are visualized on a scan are often referred to as "hot" tumors. It has been proposed that these tumors (see Figs. 5-8 to 5-10) might be more responsive to radioactive iodine therapy than are "cold" thyroid tumors, that is, tumors that do not concentrate pertechnetate (see Fig. 5-11). Hot tumors are more likely to be functional, whereas cold tumors are usually not functional. Nonfunctional tumors are least likely to concentrate pertechnetate and least likely to concentrate iodine (see Fig. 5-11). In theory, cold tumors should be less responsive to radioactive iodine therapy. The correlation between hot and cold thyroid tumor and responsiveness to radioactive iodine therapy has not yet been thoroughly studied in dogs. In our experience, the ability of a thyroid tumor to concentrate pertechnetate (i.e., appear "hot") and its sensitivity to radioactive iodine may correlate. Use of radioactive iodine can be considered in the treatment plan of dogs with tumors that concentrate radioactive pertechnetate. In our experience, however, it is rare for a malignant canine thyroid tumor to be successfully ablated with radioactive iodine.

Most of the thyroid tumors we have diagnosed in dogs invade, destroy, or displace normal thyroid tissue. These canine thyroid tumors usually have been non-functioning (i.e., they do not secrete thyroid hormone), despite retaining the ability to concentrate pertechnetate. Thyroid adenomas are clinically rare and their appearance on a pertechnetate scan is not uniquely different from carcinoma or normal thyroid lobes. Adenomas concentrate pertechnetate in a manner similar to that of carcinomas, with a type I pattern (Fig. 5-12). However, as has been discussed in several sections within this chapter, the increased use of cervical ultrasonography and early diagnosis of thyroid neoplasia is dramatically increasing the antemortem diagnosis of benign thyroid neoplasia. Response of these tumors to radioactive iodine may be superior to that demonstrated by malignant thyroid tumors.

Of the 29 dogs with thyroid tumors we reported, 20 had radionuclide uptake that was interpreted as greater than that seen in the salivary glands. In eight dogs the radionuclide uptake of thyroid tissue was less than that of the salivary glands. In one dog with a thyroid tumor the uptake of salivary glands and thyroid tissue was considered comparable. It is interest-

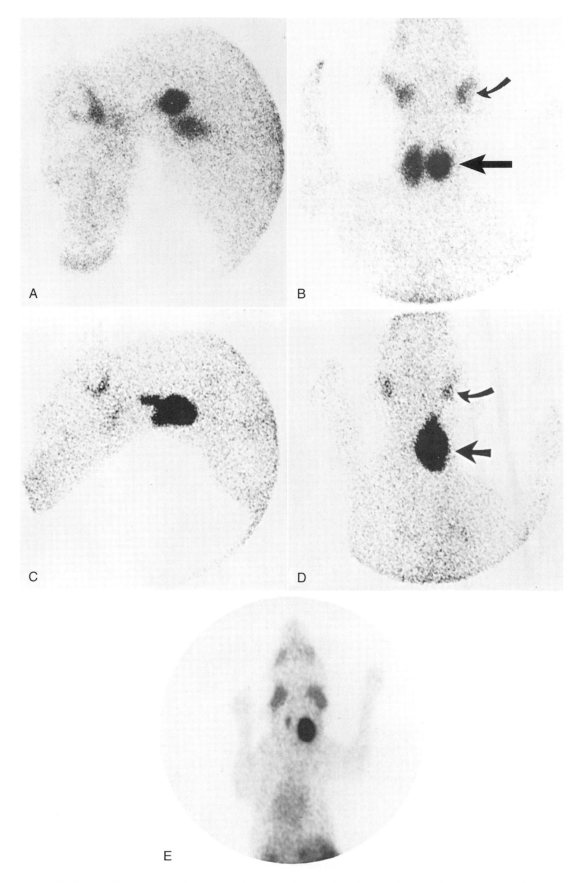

FIGURE 5–8. Pertechnetate thyroid scans from three dogs, each with thyroid tumors demonstrating well-circumscribed, homogeneous (pattern I) uptake. In the first two dogs *(B and D)* the thyroid tissue *(straight arrow)* and salivary tissue *(curved arrow)* are defined by uptake of the radioactive contrast. The first dog has bilateral thyroid follicular carcinomas, which were large (lateral *A* and dorsoventral *B* view) with partial ability to concentrate the radioactive material. The dog was euthyroid. Lateral *(C)* and dorsoventral *(D)* views of a pertechnetate thyroid scan from a dog with one large functioning thyroid follicular carcinoma *(straight arrow)*, which concentrated the pertechnetate to a much greater degree than the salivary glands *(curved arrow)*. This dog was hyperthyroid. *E,* Scan from a hypothyroid dog with a thyroid carcinoma.

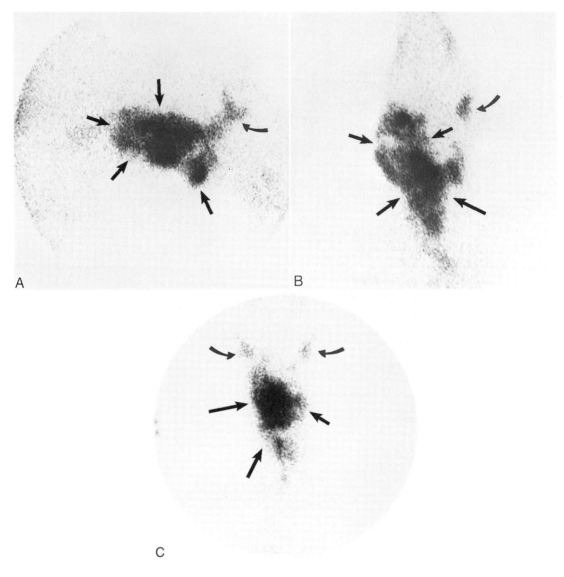

FIGURE 5–9. Pertechnetate thyroid scans from two dogs, each with thyroid carcinomas demonstrating poorly circumscribed, heterogeneous (pattern II) uptake in the cervical area. (thyroid—*straight arrows;* salivary tissue—*curved arrows*). Lateral *(A)* and dorsoventral *(B)* views of a pertechnetate thyroid scan from a dog with typical local invasion of neoplastic cells throughout the cervical area. The dog was euthyroid despite the appearance of the thyroid on the scan. *C,* Ventral scintiscan from a dog with a thyroid tumor causing hyperthyroidism.

ing to note that all six dogs that were hyperthyroid had increased radionuclide uptake. Additionally, 10 of 16 euthyroid dogs had increased uptake by the thyroid tumor, and 2 of 3 hypothyroid dogs had increased uptake (see Figs. 5-8 to 5-10; Marks et al, 1994). Therefore the amount of radionuclide uptake by a canine thyroid tumor is not a reliable indicator of its functional status, nor of benign versus malignant nature. As mentioned, ability to concentrate pertechnetate has not always translated to positive results with radioactive iodine treatment.

THYROID FUNCTION TESTS AND THEIR INFLUENCE ON THERAPY. *Basal Serum Thyroxine (T$_4$) and Triiodothyronine (T$_3$) Concentrations.* Results of serum thyroid function test results and radionuclide thyroid scans have provided inconsistent information in dogs afflicted with thyroid tumors. Although serum T$_3$ and T$_4$ concentrations are easily obtained, widely available through commercial laboratories, relatively inexpensive, and usually reliable, they are not a major component in the evaluation of human beings with thyroid malignancy. Similarly, though they are accurate for assessing canine thyroid function for veterinarians, they do not tend to be of much value for managing dogs with thyroid tumors, except in determining current status regarding euthyroidism, hypothyroidism, or hyperthyroidism. This information, although interesting, does not seem critical for developing a treatment strategy in humans (Greenspan, 2001); it does, however, influence our treatment recommendations.

Many thyroid tumors are only mildly destructive to nonneoplastic tissue, leaving enough normal thyroid

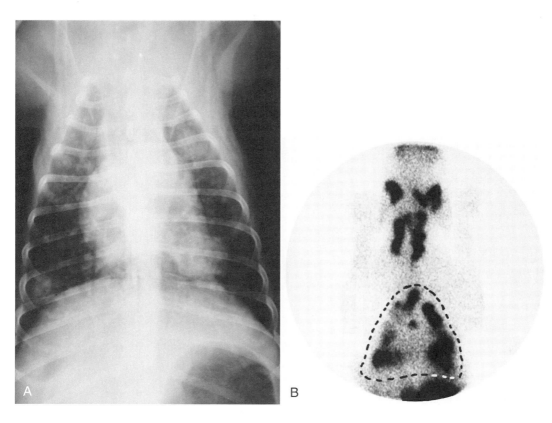

FIGURE 5–10. Radiographic *(A)* and scintigraphic *(B)* views of a dog with thyroid adenocarcinoma and pulmonary metastases. The location of the thorax is shown by *dotted lines* on the scintigraphic image.

tissue to maintain a euthyroid or mildly hypothyroid state. From our series of cases and from the literature, dogs with thyroid tumors usually have normal serum thyroid hormone concentrations (i.e., they are "euthyroid"). Approximately 55% to 60% of dogs with thyroid tumors are euthyroid, and 30% to 35% are hypothyroid secondary to destruction of normal glandular tissue by an expanding nonfunctioning tumor (Fig. 5-13). It has been suggested that hypothyroidism is rare in dogs with thyroid malignancy and that hypothyroidism, when diagnosed, may have been a preexisting condition (Mooney, 1998).

Our experience is that hypothyroidism is common and that it is a result of the thyroid malignancy destroying normal thyroid tissue, but that its significance is questionable. In addition to destruction of normal thyroid tissue by tumor invasion, hypothyroidism can occur with large thyroid tumors that produce significant amounts of inactive thyroid hormone. Although these iodoproteins are not biologically active, they may suppress TSH secretion, causing secondary atrophy of normal thyroid tissues (Loar, 1986). Although some investigators have described hyperthyroidism in as many as 20% of their cases, we have had only a 10% rate of hyperthyroidism (see Fig. 5-13).

Application of Serum Thyroid Hormone Concentrations. Basal serum T_3 and T_4 concentrations should be obtained from any dog suspected or known to have a thyroid tumor. The general care for these dogs or explanations for their clinical signs may be influenced by these serum thyroid hormone concentrations (i.e., lethargy and inappetence may be understood and easily treated if solely a result of hypothyroidism; weight loss, cardiac disorders, gastrointestinal signs, and the like might be explained by hyperthyroidism). The specific management of a cervical mass in a hyperthyroid dog may be altered from that for dogs with mildly functioning or nonfunctioning thyroid tumors. A TSH response test offers little additional information and is rarely indicated.

THYROID BIOPSY. Although most thyroid tumors detected in veterinary practice are readily palpable, they are not simple to biopsy. Thyroid tumors are highly vascular and hemorrhage associated with any biopsy procedure (fine-needle biopsy, as well as large-bore core biopsy) is common. It may be reasonable to suggest that the more hemorrhage associated with a biopsy attempt, the more likely that a neck mass is thyroid in origin (Thompson et al, 1980). The hemorrhagic potential of these masses precludes routine large-bore needle biopsy procedures. Rather, we recommend fine-needle aspiration, using a 21- to 23-gauge needle and performed only with ultrasound guidance. This technique is usually adequate for differentiating thyroid tumors from abscesses, cysts, salivary mucoceles, or lymph nodes.

The number of neoplastic cells obtained by needle aspiration is variable, and the sample is almost always contaminated with blood. Because neoplastic follicular cells are fragile, many isolated nuclei may be seen, but intact cells found in clusters resemble glandular

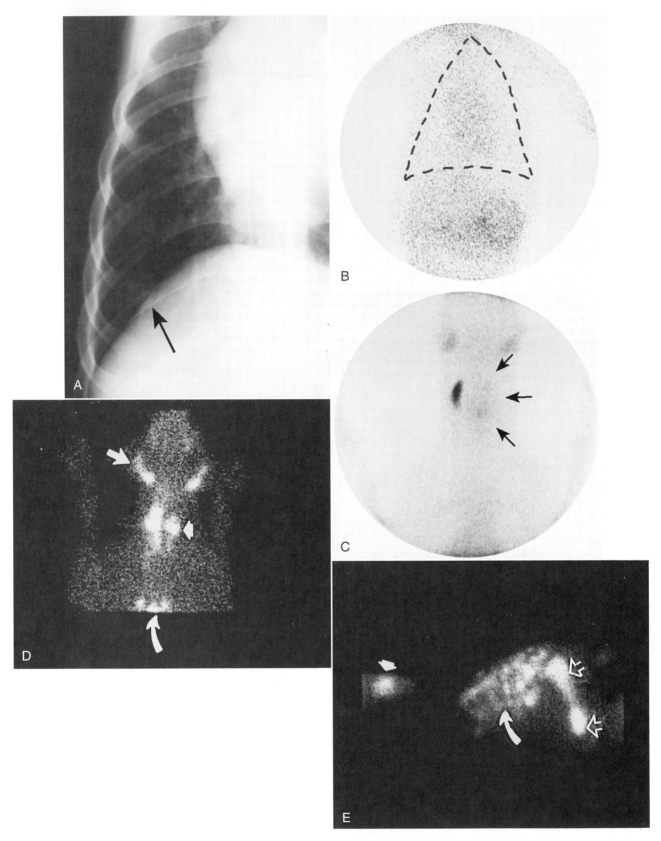

FIGURE 5–11. Radiographic *(A)* view of the thorax and scintiscan images of the thorax *(B)* and cervical region *(C)* in a dog with an undifferentiated thyroid carcinoma and pulmonary metastases. A metastatic nodule can be seen on the radiograph (arrow) but not on the thoracic scintiscan. The location of the thorax is shown by dotted lines on the scintigraphic image. The primary tumor had minimal pertechnetate uptake *(arrows)*. The dorsoventral area *(D)*, cervical area, and lateral thoracic area *(E)* on scintiscan of a hyperthyroid dog with a thyroid carcinoma and pulmonary metastases that concentrate pertechnetate. In this scan *(D and E)* radioactive uptake is white. The salivary tissue *(straight arrow)*, stomach *(open arrowheads)*, cervical thyroid *(closed arrowheads)* and pulmonary metastases *(curved arrows)* can be visualized.

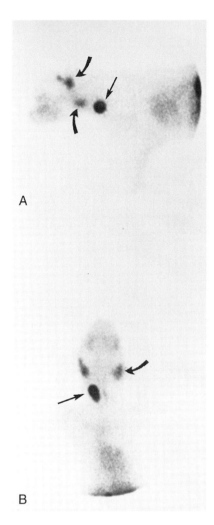

FIGURE 5–12. Lateral *(A)* and dorsoventral *(B)* scintiscans from a dog with hyperthyroidism secondary to a solitary functioning thyroid follicular adenoma. Note the parotid salivary glands *(curved arrows)* and the thyroid adenoma *(straight arrows)*. Surgical excision resulted in complete resolution of all clinical signs. Five-year follow-up was unremarkable.

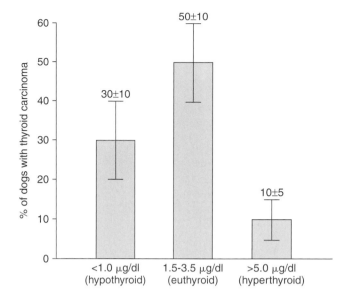

FIGURE 5–13. Percentage of dogs with thyroid tumors detected clinically that were hypothyroid, euthyroid, or hyperthyroid as determined from clinical signs and serum T_4 concentrations.

structures. Definitive recognition of malignancy is not often possible, but the tissue can usually be recognized as thyroid. If a diagnosis of thyroid neoplasia is made based on the cytologic study of an aspirate, therapeutic options can then be considered. If a diagnosis is not possible on an aspirate, the clinician may consider large-bore needle biopsy. However, our experience suggests not only that cervical ultrasonography is a safe, simple and non-invasive procedure, but also that this procedure often allows a strong tentative diagnosis in favor of or against the diagnosis of thyroid being the source of a mass. Thyroid scan can help confirm a diagnosis, but as previously discussed, this test is not always definitive.

Differential Diagnosis

Common differential diagnoses for ventral cervical masses in dogs include thyroid adenoma or carcinoma; submandibular, medial retropharyngeal, or cervical lymphadenopathy that may result from tonsillar squamous cell carcinoma or spread from tumors arising from other oral or cervical cancers; cellulitis; abscess or granuloma (such as that occurring secondary to a foreign body); salivary gland tumor or inflammation; and other neoplastic masses that would include rhabdomyosarcomas, leiomyosarcomas, and carotid body tumors (Wisner et al, 1994). Soft tissue masses in the pericardium or heart base include infectious and granulomatous diseases, neoplasms of the chemoreceptor and baroreceptor organs, hemangiosarcoma, mesothelioma, lymphosarcoma, and tumors of aberrant thyroid tissue (Loar, 1986).

Treatment: Large Invasive (Fixed) Tumor Without Visible Metastasis in Dogs That Are Euthyroid or Hypothyroid (Fig. 5-14)

BACKGROUND. In humans, external-beam irradiation is used for extensive (i.e., extraglandular) or invasive tumors, for gross postoperative residual cancer, and for unresectable tumors (Parsons et al, 1994). Treatment options for large and invasive thyroid carcinomas in dogs are limited. Complete surgical resection of such thyroid tumors is not possible without removing vital structures, such as the larynx, trachea, esophagus, recurrent laryngeal nerve, and the carotid sheath (Flanders, 1994). Treatment with radioactive iodine is not effective for control of large tumors, even when the tumor is hyperfunctional and appears to concentrate the radionuclide. Treatment of advanced functional thyroid carcinomas with large doses of radioiodine ($>2.22 \times 109$ Bq) is palliative, at best. In one study, *progression-free survival time* (PFST) in four dogs that were treated one to two times with radioiodine (^{131}I)

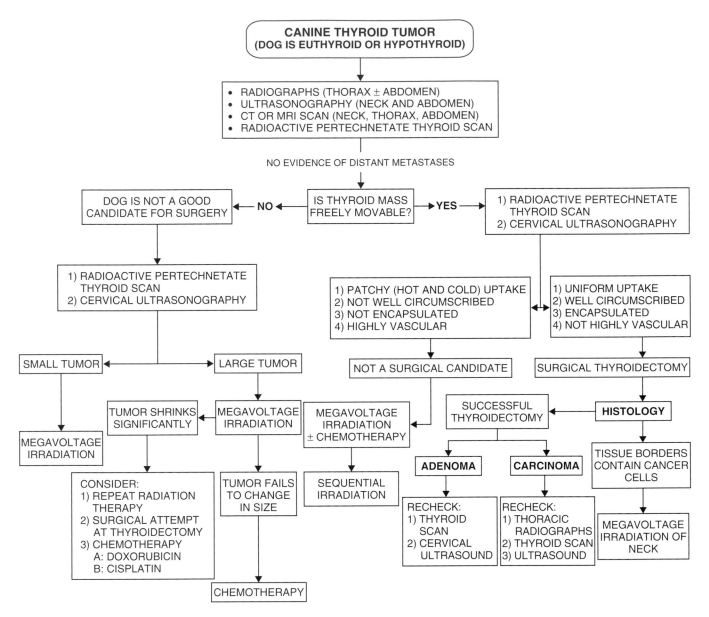

FIGURE 5–14. Algorithm demonstrating the various treatment options for managing euthyroid or hypothyroid dogs with thyroid tumors and no evidence of metastasis.

ranged from 3 to 29 months with a median PFS of 8 months (Adams et al, 1995). In another study, PFS time was 17 months in one dog treated three times with [131]I (Peterson et al, 1989). The use of various chemotherapeutic agents has also failed to result in cures or in long-term positive responses. The slow regression rate of thyroid carcinomas after irradiation, as well as the high metastatic risk for this type of tumor, has led to the misconception that external beam irradiation does not have a curative or palliative role in the management of such tumors.

Regardless of this apparent lack of efficacious treatment options, an attempt at therapy is recommended, because many treated dogs appear to be more comfortable and have the potential for increased longevity after treatment. Because the majority of clinically detected thyroid tumors are malignant, a decision regarding treatment should be made as quickly as possible. Staging of thyroid tumors usually places them among T1b, T2b, T3b categories (see Table 5-3). Surgery, chemotherapy, radioactive iodine, and cobalt therapy can be considered. The functional status of the thyroid tumor should not dramatically alter the treatment approach (see Fig. 5-14).

MEGAVOLTAGE IRRADIATION. ***Dogs Studied and Treatment Used.*** Our opinions regarding this form of treatment for dogs with invasive thyroid carcinoma are based on studies that we have completed (Theon et al, 2000). These results are complemented by other studies. In 13 dogs treated with external beam irradiation, the mean survival time was 96 weeks (range: 6 to 247 weeks; Brearley et al, 1999). Another retrospective study of eight dogs with thyroid carcinoma treated with external beam megavoltage irradiation resulted in a median survival time >2 years (Pack et al, 2001). These optimistic results can be coupled with our experience, in which we evaluated 25 dogs with histologically confirmed differentiated thyroid carcinoma that were treated with megavoltage irradiation. The radiation was administered with curative intent. In this study, dogs with histologic, cytologic, or radiographic evidence of regional or distant metastases, or in which the tumor had recurred, were not evaluated. Tumors were categorized as compact-cellular (nine dogs), follicular (eight dogs), and follicular-compact-cellular (eight dogs) adeno-carcinomas. The dogs were 3 to 18 years of age (median, 10 years), and various breeds were represented. All had been referred for irradiation because their tumors were unresectable on the basis of clinical findings such as palpation, ultrasonography, and radiography (11 dogs), or after unsuccessful attempts at resection (14 dogs). Bilateral enlargement of the thyroid lobes was present in 16 dogs, whereas 9 had unilateral enlargement. Of the 25 dogs, 6 had been diagnosed as hypothyroid; the other 19 were euthyroid (Theon et al, 2000).

Imaging studies with sodium pertechnetate Tc ^{99}m (^{99m}TcO$_4$) were performed in 20 of the 25 dogs. Five dogs were not studied with ^{99m}TcO$_4$ because of previous attempts at resection. The ^{99m}TcO$_4$ studies that were completed demonstrated that seven dogs had unilateral lobe involvement, eight had bilateral lobe involvement, and five had ventral midline masses with invasion of the laryngeal cartilages. A well-circumscribed area of homogeneous uptake was observed in seven dogs. Poorly circumscribed areas of uptake were demonstrated in 13 dogs; 9 of these dogs had diffuse uptake throughout their masses, and four of them had mixed areas of no uptake together with some areas of uptake. Each dog was treated using a telecobalt unit to deliver a radiation dose of 48 Gy administered in 12 fractions on a 3-day-per-week schedule. The treatment plan for each dog was based on a computerized protocol that used a variety of factors (neck contour, radiographs, CT scan or MRI image results, and ultrasonography).

Results. Mean PFST in these 25 dogs was 45 months. Age, sex, tumor histologic type, tumor stage, gland involvement (right versus left), and pattern of ^{99m}TcO$_4$ uptake did not affect response to therapy. Time to maximum tumor size reduction ranged from 8 to 22 months. Patterns of failure were identified in 14 of the 25 dogs (11 did not have evidence of failure despite being followed for more than 4 years). In three dogs, local tumor progression was the first cause of failure. In four dogs with no clinical evidence of tumor progression, metastasis was the first cause of failure. Pulmonary metastases were detected in five dogs, one of which also had bone metastasis. In two dogs, metastases were found in abdominal viscera. Dogs with bilateral tumors had 16 times the risk for metastasis. Previous attempts at resection did not affect risk of metastasis (Theon et al, 2000).

Long-Term Survival. Megavoltage irradiation was established to be an effective treatment for dogs with locally advanced thyroid carcinoma. Irradiation is not presented here as a cure for dogs with invasive thyroid carcinomas, but this form of treatment does enhance survival time by providing long-term control for a large percentage of the dogs. Progression-free survival rate of greater than 150 weeks after irradiation was 72%. In dogs with comparable disease, survival without treatment ranged from 2 to 38 weeks after diagnosis (Verschueren et al, 1992b). Dogs with thyroid carcinoma treated with cisplatin chemo-therapy had a mean survival time of 28 weeks and a median survival time of 14 weeks (Fineman et al, 1998). Only 3 of 13 dogs with thyroid carcinoma treated with doxorubicin had a 50% volume reduction in tumor size (Ogilvie et al, 1989). Mitoxantrone only provided short-term palliation (Ogilvie et al, 1991).

Veterinarians and owners are reminded that when megavoltage irradiation treatment was successful, there was little change in tumor size for months after treatment. Tumor disappearance or maximum tumor shrinkage was not observed for 8 to 22 months. These results emphasize the need for thorough client education prior to beginning irradiation, patience on the part of both veterinarian and client, and long periods between evaluations following treatment to determine therapeutic benefit. Slow tumor shrinkage may lead to the misconception that thyroid carcinomas are radio-resistant. Finally, human beings with papillary thyroid carcinomas have a better prognosis following mega-voltage irradiation than do people with follicular carcinomas. In contrast, tumor histologic type does not seem to have prognostic value in dogs.

Metastasis Following Irradiation. The treatment plan in this section has been formulated for dogs that do not have visible metastasis at the time of diagnosis. Following megavoltage irradiation, the proportion of dogs in our study with local failure (redevelopment of thyroid carcinoma in the irradiated cervical area) and distant metastasis was higher than the proportion of dogs with local control and no distant metastasis. In other words, local control appears to be of primary importance. In addition, effective local treatment with irradiation was found to affect late (>12 months), but not early (<6 months), development of metastasis. Early metastasis, which was observed in dogs with local tumor control, had most likely developed before diagnosis of thyroid carcinoma and was not affected by local irradiation. Alternatively, late development of metastases in dogs with tumor progression was assumed to reflect the development of distant meta-stasis from the persistent or recurring primary tumors.

Side Effects Caused by Irradiation. Irradiation did create some side effects. Acute reactions included esophageal, tracheal, or laryngeal mucositis that caused mild hoarseness and cough in 12 dogs and dysphagia in 8. These reactions tended to be well tolerated and self-limiting. Chronic radiation reactions included skin fibrosis and permanent alopecia in six dogs and chronic tracheitis causing a dry cough in four dogs. Of the 19 euthyroid dogs, 2 became hypo-thyroid 13 and 29 months after radiation, respectively, and 1 of these 2 dogs also became hypoparathyroid. This latent period for induction of hypothyroidism was longer than that previously reported for one dog that was treated with both radiation and surgery (Kramer et al, 1994). Case numbers are so small that meaningful conclusions will likely be misleading, but perhaps the combination therapy hastened or enhanced development of hypothyroidism. In humans, hypothyroidism is a common complication following irradiation of the head and neck regions when the thyroid gland is in the radiation field. Subclinical hypothyroidism is the most common complication (Nishiyama et al, 1996). Irradiation did not result in any life-threatening complications. This is in contrast to surgical tumor resection, which is associated with greater risk for complication. In a study of 20 dogs with large mobile thyroid carcinomas, 5 dogs (25%) died as a result of surgery-related complications (Klein et al, 1995).

USE OF RADIOACTIVE IODINE. Radioiodine treatment of unresectable or inoperative primary thyroid tumors in dogs does not appear to result in appreciable tumor regression. Furthermore, use of this treatment modality does not appear to prolong survival time unless treatments are repeated (Peterson et al, 1989; Adams et al, 1995). Our experience is similar to that of others: most dogs with differentiated thyroid tumors are euthyroid or hypothyroid and are poor candidates for radioiodine therapy. Candidates for radioiodine treatment must have a functional thyroid tumor defined as a tumor having prolonged iodine-trapping capacity, as assessed by a ^{131}I tracer study. In other words, the tumor must be able to trap and retain iodine for a sufficient length of time to allow the radioactivity to kill tumor cells. In our experience, most thyroid carcinomas in dogs do not adequately concentrate iodine, and therefore those dogs are not candidates for this form of therapy.

USE OF CHEMOTHERAPEUTIC AGENTS. *Background.* Dogs with thyroid carcinomas have been treated with various chemotherapeutic agents. Of those dogs treated with either doxorubicin or cisplatin, 30% to 50% may demonstrate a partial response, defined as a >50% reduction in tumor volume (Jeglum and Wherat, 1983; Post and Maudlin, 1992; Fineman et al, 1998). Survival times for a majority of these dogs have not been demonstrated to have been increased. Such response rates of thyroid carcinoma to chemotherapy suggest a secondary role for chemotherapy in the management of these masses, whereas megavoltage irradiation and surgery currently have more important roles (see Fig. 5-14). These latter forms of treatment have been more effective and offer the best chance for cure or long-term response. However, removal or destruction of all neoplastic tissue is not common. Therefore chemotherapy becomes an important and practical mode of adjunctive therapy for dogs with thyroid tumors. Chemotherapy is indicated when total surgical removal or destruction with external beam radiation is not successful, when distant metastatic lesions have been identified, or when the size of the primary tumor is such that local invasion or metastasis is likely even though it cannot be identified with diagnostic tests. When the thyroid mass exceeds approximately 4 cm in diameter, the probability of

metastasis becomes extremely high, (Verschueren et al, 1992b).

Doxorubicin and "Combination" Therapies. Doxorubicin (Adriamycin; Adria Laboratories, Inc, Dublin, OH 43017) has been the most effective chemotherapeutic drug for thyroid cancer in humans, either as a single agent or in combination with cisplatin (Shimaoka et al, 1985; Ahuja and Ernst, 1987). Tumor control has also been achieved in locally advanced thyroid cancer by combining low-dose doxorubicin chemotherapy with radiation therapy (Kim and Leeper, 1987). A combination of doxorubicin therapy and external beam irradiation in eight dogs resulted in a mean survival time of 11 months (Post and Mauldin, 1992). However, our results have been much better. This difference is likely a reflection of the selection criteria employed for the dogs treated. Inconsistent results were achieved with drugs such as cisplatin and mitoxantrone (Ogilvie GK, et al, 1991; Fineman et al, 1998) Alternative agents, such as bleomycin, vincristine, etoposide, and methotrexate, have not been reported to have promising results (Poster et al, 1981; Spanos et al, 1982; Hoskin and Harmer, 1987; Tallroth et al, 1987).

The response of canine thyroid tumors to chemotherapy is variable. For most dogs, doxorubicin delays further growth of the tumor and may result in a slight reduction in tumor size, but this is only rarely associated with total tumor remission. In one study, the median survival time for 10 dogs with thyroid tumors treated with doxorubicin alone was 37 weeks (Jeglum and Whereat, 1983). The dose of doxorubicin in dogs has been reported at 30 mg/m^2 body surface area IV every 3 to 6 weeks (Ogilvie et al, 1989). Treatment should be continued until total remission of the tumor is obtained or adverse reactions associated with chronic therapy develop. In these studies, approximately 25% of treated dogs had total remission or objective reduction in tumor size. Some dogs were treated with combinations of doxorubicin with cyclophosphamide (Cytoxan; Bristol-Myers Oncology Division, Syracuse, NY 13226) and/or vincristine (Oncovin; Eli Lilly and Company, Indianapolis, IN 46285). Combination chemotherapy using cyclophosphamide and vincristine in conjunction with doxorubicin may be tried when doxorubicin alone is ineffective.

Toxicity. One of the important forms of toxicity attributed to doxorubicin is that noted when the drug is given concurrently with megavoltage irradiation. Doxorubicin administration enhances radiation toxicity; this combination should be avoided. Cardiac toxicity is another well recognized side effect of doxorubicin. Additional acute adverse reactions to therapy with this drug include anaphylaxis, gastrointestinal dysfunction, hypotension, and cardiac arrhythmias (Susaneck, 1983a,b). Diphenhydramine hydrochloride (Benadryl; Parke-Davis, Morris Plains, NJ 07950) should be given if these acute reactions, especially anaphylaxis, occur. Chronic adverse reactions to doxorubicin include weight loss, anorexia, bone marrow hypoplasia, alopecia, testicular atrophy, and cardiomyopathy.

SUMMARY: TREATING FIXED THYROID TUMORS. No established guidelines exist for any specific treatment directed at canine thyroid tumors. There have been too few studies and too few dogs reported with any one type of thyroid neoplasia or therapy to achieve solid recommendations. In humans, external megavoltage irradiation is indicated for extensive inoperable disease and for gross residual disease in the operative field; it is also indicated if connective tissue is invaded or if there is extensive infiltration of the cervical lymph nodes (Grigsby and Luk, 1998). Our results suggest that megavoltage irradiation can play an important role in the management of dogs with differentiated inoperable thyroid tumors and dogs with no evidence of systemic metastases (see Fig. 5-14). These results are similar to those in humans with inoperable disease approached with curative intent. Postoperative irradiation for humans with differentiated thyroid carcinoma after incomplete resection resulted in a 5-year survival rate of 78% in one study (Tubiana et al, 1985). Thus, drawing from the human experience and the results of our experience, there is rationale for postoperative surgical-field-irradiation of incompletely resected differentiated thyroid tumors in dogs. In dogs that cannot have surgery because of the advanced nature of their tumor, external-beam irradiation should also be considered as a cytoreductive treatment, with reassessment of the tumor for resectability at a later time (see Fig 5-14).

Treatment: Small Invasive (Fixed) Tumor Without Visible Metastasis in Dogs That Are Euthyroid or Hypothyroid (Fig. 5-14)

There is strong temptation to attempt surgical extirpation of small thyroid tumors, even when they are fixed, that is, not movable, within the cervical area. These masses, however, are extremely difficult to remove completely. Most oncologists and surgeons actually agree that surgery is not ideal for any dog with a fixed thyroid tumor, regardless of size. Therefore the previous discussion regarding use of external beam megavoltage irradiation applies to dogs with small fixed thyroid tumors. However, if the tumor shrinks considerably after radiation and there continues to be no evidence of distant metastasis, an attempt at surgery can be considered. In contrast, if distant metastasis is identified, the veterinarian and owner can consider chemotherapy as a palliative approach to prolong survival as long as possible. Surgery in this setting should be considered only if there are signs of local distress from the mass (dysphagia or dyspnea). Here, surgery would be palliative, at best.

Treatment: Non-Invasive (Mobile) Tumor Without Visible Metastasis in Dogs That Are Euthyroid or Hypothyroid (Fig. 5-14)

Successful management of thyroid carcinomas in dogs requires controlling the primary tumor. For most dogs, as can be appreciated from previous discussions, surgical excision alone will not be sufficient to control the primary tumor because of local invasion into adjacent structures. However, in dogs with freely moveable tumors, surgical excision alone may be appropriate. Mobility is best determined when the dog is anesthetized, since attachment to deep structures is often overestimated when the dog is awake (Withrow and MacEwen, 2001). In a study of dogs with operable tumors and no evidence of metastasis, tumor resection resulted in long-term local control and decreased incidence of metastasis (Klein et al, 1995). In that study, the low incidence of metastasis after surgery (2 of 20 dogs) provides evidence that local tumor control had an impact on subsequent development of metastasis. Our findings also support this assumption. Therefore, if surgery is warranted based on careful use of specific criteria, as outlined in the next section, long-term survival is a reasonable and achievable goal.

CASE SELECTION. Initially, a dog with a thyroid tumor should be assessed with physical examination. A freely moveable mass, on careful palpation, is defined as not being attached to contiguous structures, as determined when the dog is awake and again when evaluated under anesthesia. Further assessment is best accomplished with both cervical ultrasonography and use of a radioactive pertechnetate thyroid scan. Ultrasonography is an excellent tool for determining how "deep" a tumor extends and whether such a mass is really "free" of invasion into nearby cervical structures. Furthermore, ultrasonography is an excellent tool for determining "vascularity" of a tumor. Assuming that ultrasonography indicates that a tumor does appear to be "mobile," encapsulated, and not highly vascular, the dog should then undergo the thyroid scan. If the mass demonstrates uniform uptake of pertechnetate, is well circumscribed, and seems to be well encapsulated, surgical thyroidectomy should be considered. However, surgery is not recommended for the dog with a highly vascular tumor that is not encapsulated or well circumscribed and that demonstrates patchy uptake of pertechnetate. These dogs should be managed as is recommended for dogs with fixed tumors.

SURGERY. Encapsulated, mobile (movable) thyroid tumors may be relatively easy to remove, and surgery alone may result in long-term survival. Mobility of the mass and absence of identifiable metastatic disease are important criteria for deciding in favor or against surgery. Age and breed are not important criteria, nor does specific tumor type seem to be critical, because survival time was not found to be significantly associated with histologic classification (Klein et al, 1995). Large tumors often require an incision directly over the mass to facilitate removal (see Fig. 5-3), and ligation of the cranial thyroid artery at the level of the carotid artery is imperative. Inferior thyroid artery and vein ligation is also recommended.

Growth into adjacent structures by highly malignant tumors usually prevents complete excision. This is true even of many thyroid tumors that appear to be well encapsulated and freely movable. Invasion of the vasculature usually results in difficulty with hemostasis and also prevents total mass removal. Regional coagulation abnormalities may become systemic coagulopathies following surgical manipulation. These complications should serve to emphasize the importance of client communication regarding prognosis before (and even during) surgery. Nevertheless, debulking of tumor mass has been beneficial in making some dogs more comfortable. It is possible to sacrifice the jugular vein, carotid artery, and vagosympathetic trunk unilaterally with acceptable morbidity (unilateral Horner's syndrome). Bilateral resection may result in laryngeal paralysis and/or megaesophagus.

Extensive tumor invasion and aggressive attempts at surgical removal, especially with bilateral tumors, threaten the recurrent laryngeal nerves, parathyroid glands, and normal thyroid tissue. It may be difficult to recognize and save these structures if they have been anatomically displaced. Debulking is helpful, but heroic attempts to remove all malignant tissue are not usually feasible and may be harmful. Even after stringent case selection criteria, authors of one study reported that several dogs required tracheostomies as attempts were being made to excise a freely movable thyroid tumor, indicating that some of the tumors must have invaded, or at least been closely adjacent to, the trachea or both recurrent laryngeal nerves. Case selection criteria are extremely important (see Fig. 5-14).

POSTSURGICAL MONITORING. **Calcium and Thyroid Hormones.** Monitoring serum calcium concentrations before and after surgery may be critically important if there is any chance of the parathyroid glands being excised or damaged. Hypoparathyroidism is uncommon following thyroid surgery (incidence <10%), but is always possible. With extensive bilateral surgery, the serum calcium concentration must be monitored at least once daily for 5 to 7 days. Vitamin D and calcium therapy should be instituted if any evidence of hypoparathyroidism (hypocalcemia) is present (see Chapter 17). We have rarely identified dogs with thyroid tumors that naturally resolved their calcium deficiencies via return of parathyroid function after presumed surgical damage. The aggressive surgeon must weigh benefit versus risk when attempting to excise a large invasive thyroid tumor. The serum T_4 concentration should initially be assessed 1 to 3 weeks after surgery and, depending on clinical signs, replacement therapy implemented accordingly.

Histology. Evaluation of tissue by a pathologist, after it has been surgically removed, is critically important in choosing a subsequent treatment plan (see Fig. 5-14). If the pathologist is convinced that the tumor is a benign adenoma and that it has been completely removed, there is an excellent chance that the dog has been cured. An aggressive approach after establishment of this diagnosis would be to recheck a thyroid scan and cervical ultrasound examination 6 and 12 months later. If the pathologist reports that the mass removed was a malignant thyroid tumor and that all borders are free of any such cells, one should strongly consider periodic (2 to 4 times yearly) physical examination, thoracic radiographs, cervical

and abdominal ultrasonography, and thyroid scans. If the pathologist diagnoses thyroid malignancy and "dirty borders" of the tissue removed (i.e., the surgery was incomplete and tumor cells are definitely remaining in the edges of the surgical field), a more aggressive approach is warranted. In this situation we recommend megavoltage irradiation of the entire tumor bed. This should be followed by chemotherapy, as well as periodic rechecks, including physical examinations, thoracic radiographs, cervical and abdominal ultrasonography, and thyroid scans.

Treatment: Thyroid Malignancy in Euthyroid or Hypothyroid Dogs with Metastases Identified (Fig. 5-15)

Metastasis is often present at the time of diagnosis and is considered the principal cause of death in affected dogs. In the literature, the number of dogs diagnosed as having distant metastasis at the time the thyroid tumor is diagnosed is quite variable (Harari et al, 1986; Miles et al, 1990). After metastases are diagnosed, we still encourage some owners to consider palliative therapy of their pet. It is important for owners to understand the meaning of palliative therapy. The goal of this form of therapy is to afford relief from pain or discomfort. Virtually no chance of cure is expected.

With understanding that metastases are present, the veterinarian must review the reasons that the dog has been brought to the hospital. If the dog is exhibiting signs associated with the mass itself (trouble breathing [dyspnea], trouble swallowing [dysphagia], cough, etc.), the management approach is directed at reducing the bulk of the mass. This can be accomplished, potentially, by any of three treatment strategies: (1) partial thyroidectomy, (2) external beam megavoltage irradiation, or (3) chemotherapy. It is possible for these therapies to be combined. Regardless, chances of a cure are remote at best. Again, the purpose of any one of these treatments or a combination of these treatments is to make the dog more comfortable. If the dog has no evidence of "distress," the most common mode of treatment is chemotherapy. Usually doxorubicin is used, although cisplatin and other chemotherapeutics can also be considered.

Prognosis in Euthyroid or Hypothyroid Dogs with Thyroid Neoplasia

HISTOMORPHOLOGIC GRADE. In dogs with thyroid cancer, it has been estimated that 30% to >60% have distant metastases at the time of diagnosis (Jeglum and Whereat, 1983; Harari et al, 1986). In dogs managed surgically, the histomorphologic malignancy grade for a tumor (including the presence of capsular and vascular invasion, degree of cellular and nuclear polymorphism, and frequency of mitoses) was found to be the only significant prognostic factors (Verschueren et al, 1992b). Histologic tumor classification, breed,

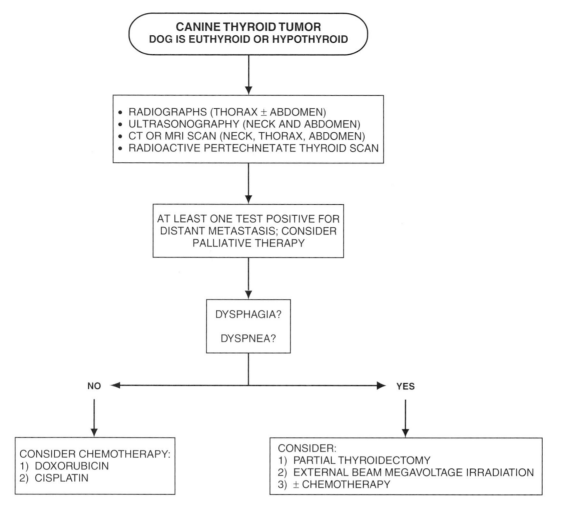

FIGURE 5–15. Algorithm demonstrating the various treatment options for managing euthyroid or hypothyroid dogs with thyroid tumors and evidence of metastasis.

gender, age, serum thyroid hormone concentrations, and serum thyroglobulin concentrations were not significant factors in determining prognosis (Klein et al, 1988; Verschueren et al, 1992b). The clinical staging of canine thyroid tumors has received some attention (see Table 5-3), although specific staging (other than recognition of distant metastases) is not often used by veterinary clinicians.

THYROID TUMOR SIZE. In one study, Leav et al (1976) demonstrated that when the tumor volume was less than 23 cm^3, the percentage of animals with metastasis at necropsy was only 14%. In dogs with carcinomas between 23 and 100 cm^3, 74% had metastasis; with tumor volumes greater than 100 cm^3, 100% had metastasis. Thus, smaller tumors carry a better prognosis, and an aggressive therapeutic approach is warranted with small to moderate-sized masses. In our series, however, "large" tumors were extremely common at the time that thyroid neoplasia was diagnosed. Surgical estimates of tumor size in 47 dogs has averaged more than 80 cm^3. It appears that clinical recognition of small thyroid carcinomas is not common. However, as has been discussed earlier in

this chapter, the increased use of cervical ultrasonography as a diagnostic aid will likely result in earlier diagnosis and, therefore, diagnosis when tumors are much smaller than they have been during the past few decades. A long-term prospective clinical study should answer many of the remaining questions concerning the prognosis for dogs with thyroid cancer treated with a variety of different modalities.

BENIGN VERSUS MALIGNANT. Surgical excision of thyroid *adenomas* is likely to be curative. Unfortunately, these tumors are rare in clinical practice, and recognition of a small, benign, nonfunctioning thyroid tumor has not been common (Lawrence et al, 1991). Most dogs with thyroid tumors have a large, nonfunctioning, invasive malignancy. Again, earlier diagnosis with cervical ultrasonography should result in more dogs being diagnosed prior to tremendous growth or spread. In general, the prognosis for dogs with nonfunctioning thyroid tumors is guarded to poor. The nonfavorable prognosis is related to the following factors: the invasive nature of these tumors; their frequent metastasis; age at the time of diagnosis; expense of surgery, chemotherapy, and radiation therapy; side effects of these modes of treatment; and the lack of statistics indicating any true cures. No distinction has been made regarding tumor type and prognosis. One study, on a small number of dogs, failed to demonstrate an obvious difference in life expectancy for dogs with compact tumors compared with those that had mixed tumors (Harari et al, 1986).

Recurrence of malignancy after attempts at surgical excision in dogs with thyroid neoplasia is frequently documented. Regrowth has been recognized 1 to 54 months following the first surgery. Regrowth may occur on the same side as the original mass or on the opposite side. Regrowth has been documented 6 to 24 months after a second surgery in a few dogs. Although recurrence, in itself, is discouraging, the length of time between these observations indicates that many dogs live well beyond 2 years from the time of initial diagnosis.

FUNCTIONING THYROID TUMORS (THYROTOXICOSIS, HYPERTHYROIDISM)

Background

Most dogs with thyroid tumors are euthyroid or hypothyroid, and only about 10% of dogs with thyroid tumors are hyperthyroid (see Fig. 5-13; Rijnberk, 1996; Verschueren, 1992). In dogs, hyperthyroidism is almost always associated with thyroid malignancy. Although functioning thyroid adenomas have been described, the incidence of benign tumors causing hyperthyroidism in dogs is low (Lawrence et al, 1991; Marks et al, 1994). A thyroid tumor causing hyperthyroidism should be presumed to be a carcinoma until proven otherwise. In contrast, malignant thyroid tumors account for less than 5% of hyperthyroidism in cats. The only naturally occurring cause of hyperthyroidism in the dog is an autonomous hypersecreting thyroid tumor. A disease entity similar to the immune-mediated thyroiditis and hyperthyroidism in humans, called *Graves' disease*, has not been recognized in dogs. In Graves' disease, anti-TSH antibodies bind to TSH receptors on the thyroid follicular cell and stimulate secretion of thyroid hormone. Diffuse hyperplasia and goiter of both thyroid lobes result.

Diffuse hyperplasia is not a histologic component in dogs with hyperthyroidism. Rather, neoplastic tissue can be identified and the nonneoplastic thyroid tissue appears atrophied. If hyperthyroidism is secondary to excess TSH secretion or secondary to excess stimulation of TSH receptors by antibodies, diffuse hyperplasia of the thyroids would be expected. In addition, nonneoplastic thyroid tissue does not concentrate iodine and hence is not visualized on radionuclide scans. However, injections of TSH for several days stimulate atrophied noncancerous thyroid cells to become active, thereby allowing visualization of normal tissue on a subsequent radionuclide scan. Logically, a dog must progress from normal thyroid function to a stage in which functioning normal and neoplastic cells secrete thyroid hormone (compensated toxic thyroid tumor) and then to a stage in which hormone secretion is by cancerous cells only, as TSH secretion is inhibited by negative feedback (decompensated toxic thyroid tumor).

Clinical Signs

The clinical signs of canine and feline hyperthyroidism are similar. These signs include weight loss, polydipsia, polyuria, polyphagia, vomiting, voluminous soft stools, increased activity or nervousness, weakness, poor hair coat, heat intolerance, panting, and shivering. One major clinical difference between feline and canine hyperthyroidism is the size of the thyroid gland causing these signs. It is extremely rare for owners of hyperthyroid cats to notice a goiter (enlarged thyroid), whereas owners of hyperthyroid dogs often report noticing a "swelling" in the neck. For a few hyperthyroid dogs, the cervical mass is the first abnormality noticed and the reason for seeking veterinary advice. Signs caused by the size of the mass may also result in a dog's owner seeking veterinary care. These include respiratory signs (coughing, rapid breathing, respiratory distress) or signs related to swallowing difficulties. Signs may be seen for days to months (in some cases, years), underlining the insidious nature of the disease in some dogs. (See Chapter 4 for a thorough clinical review and physiopathology of each abnormality.)

Physical Examination

Physical examination findings are similar for hyperthyroid dogs and cats. Hyperthyroid dogs are thin and may be cachectic (see Fig. 5-4). Muscle wasting is usually obvious and dehydration may be suspected, although lack of skin turgidity is most likely a reflection of severe weight loss and reduction in dermal fat. Tachycardia, with or without premature contractions, is typical. Affected dogs may pant without obvious reason, and examination may be difficult because of their restlessness. Panting, respiratory distress, and swallowing difficulties may result from the tumor mass compressing the trachea and/or esophagus. These signs may also be the result of thyrotoxicosis. Weakness may also be identified.

Careful palpation of the neck usually reveals the thyroid tumor. A normal thyroid gland is not palpable. Functioning thyroid tumors are reported to be smaller and less obvious to the owner and veterinarian than nonfunctioning thyroid tumors. Functioning thyroid tumors are usually 2 to 5 cm in diameter and movable in the neck on careful palpation (Verschueren, 1992). In our experience, it has not been possible to distinguish functioning thyroid tumors from nonfunctioning tumors based on palpable features of the mass. Rather, the appearance of the dog coupled with an owner's observations has often suggested the hyperthyroid state, later substantiated by serum thyroid hormone evaluations.

In-Hospital Evaluation

A complete in-hospital evaluation is recommended for dogs with a palpable cervical mass, especially if additional signs (e.g., weight loss, vomiting) are noted by the owner. Alterations in test results documented in hyperthyroid dogs are similar to those seen in cats. Abnormal increases in the serum T_4 concentration confirm the diagnosis of hyperthyroidism and presence of a functioning thyroid carcinoma should be presumed to be the cause. Final confirmation should be made via needle aspiration and cytology of the cervical mass or with histologic evaluation of tissue removed under ultrasound guidance or at surgery. Dogs with thyroid masses should be evaluated with radiographs of the thorax, with or without radiographs of the abdomen.

Ultrasonography of the neck is imperative, and if available, abdominal ultrasonography is also recommended. These studies are recommended to determine whether there is any evidence of tumor metastasis and to evaluate the mass itself. Size of the thyroid mass correlates with malignant potential. Masses 23 to 100 cm³ in volume have a 74% incidence of malignancy and 100% of those >100 cm³ have been malignant. Furthermore, ultrasonography is an excellent aid for determining whether a tumor is invasive and whether a tumor is highly vascular. In either of these situations, malignancy is more probable, and surgery becomes less likely to be curative.

Treatment Strategies (Fig. 5-16)

INITIAL DECISION PROCESS. Once a dog has been diagnosed as having a thyroid tumor and as being hyperthyroid, a variety of tests should be considered.

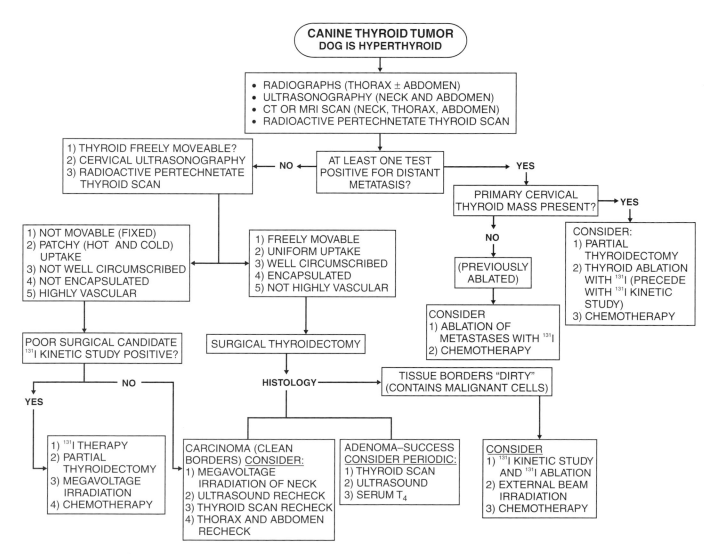

FIGURE 5–16. Algorithm demonstrating the various treatment options for managing hyperthyroid dogs with thyroid tumors.

The dog should be assessed for malignancy before any specific therapy is considered. The most common sites of metastasis are to the lungs and local lymph nodes, although spread to abdominal viscera and to the skeleton have also been reported (Bentley et al, 1990). Ideally, this assessment consists of thoracic radiographs coupled with cervical ultrasonography and then ultrasonography of the abdomen. In this situation, abdominal ultrasonography is superior to radiography in the diagnosis of metastasis. As has been discussed, tumor size, invasive nature, and vascularity can be assessed with ultrasonography. Although we do not often use CT or MRI scans in these dogs, we do utilize radioactive pertechnetate thyroid scans. In this regard, the assessment is directed at determining whether the thyroid mass has uniform or patchy uptake of radioactivity; whether the mass is well-circumscribed; whether the mass appears to be encapsulated; and whether there is any evidence of distant metastasis.

No Evidence of Metastasis—Mass Is Freely Movable. *Mass Has Uniform Uptake and Is Well Circumscribed and Encapsulated.* As would be anticipated, the title of this section creates the best scenario possible. The dog with a freely movable mass with uniform uptake of pertechnetate is an ideal surgical candidate. Surgery is the first choice for managing these dogs because any tumor could be malignant, and freely moveable tumors might be completely removable. Thyroid adenoma is possible, and the mass could also cause hyperthyroidism, but this is not common (Lawrence et al, 1991). Therefore, surgical mass removal is recommended. Following thyroidectomy, tissue evaluation by a pathologist becomes critically important. If the mass appears to have been removed totally and it appears to be an adenoma, the chances of a cure are excellent. In this situation, the owner and veterinarian can consider periodic (every 6 months?) evaluations. Each recheck should include a thorough history, physical examination, serum T_4 concentration, cervical ultrasound, and if possible, a thyroid scan. With each negative assessment, the duration between rechecks can be increased.

Oral antithyroid drugs are not recommended as the primary mode of therapy, because they are not cytotoxic. However, we have used antithyroid drugs as palliative therapy to control clinical signs of hyperthyroidism in untreated dogs or those that had recurrence of hyperthyroidism after surgery or treatment with ^{131}I or doxorubicin. Our therapeutic approach is similar to that used in hyperthyroid cats, that is, 2.5 mg of methimazole twice daily, with subsequent increases in the dosage as needed to control clinical signs and maintain serum T_4 concentrations between 1.0 and 2.0 g/dl.

Another possible scenario following surgery is that the pathologist finds "clean" borders around the tissue submitted; that is, there is no evidence of cancer at the edges of the tissue removed. However, the mass is diagnosed as a carcinoma. Again, the options regarding future management of such a dog are not always obvious. We would assume that metastases may yet be diagnosed. Therefore, at a minimum, we would conduct rechecks consisting of the same procedures recommended for a functioning adenoma. However, in this case, we would add thoracic radiographs and abdominal ultrasonography to diagnose metastasis as soon as possible. Some would recommend external beam megavoltage irradiation of the surgical bed, as well. The irradiation would commence as soon as the surgical site appeared to have healed.

The other likely scenario following surgery is that the pathologist diagnoses carcinoma and "dirty" borders of the tissue submitted; that is, the tissue removed indicates that cancer cells definitely remain within the surgical bed. Remember, this is not a reflection of inadequate performance by the surgeon. Rather, these tumors can be highly invasive with a myriad of invasive cancer "fingers" that cannot be distinguished, regardless of the surgeons' previous experience. In this situation there are several alternatives regarding the next steps in patient management. The veterinarian could consider completing a radioactive iodine (^{131}I) tracer study and, if positive, attempting to ablate all remaining tissue with radioactive iodine. Alternatives to iodine include external beam megavoltage irradiation and chemotherapy.

No Evidence of Metastasis—Mass Is "Fixed" in the Neck. *Mass Has Patchy Uptake and Is Poorly Circumscribed and Not Obviously Encapsulated.* Obviously, the title of this section indicates a scenario that is not ideal for the dog being evaluated. The fixed, nonmovable mass with patchy uptake of pertechnetate is a poor candidate for surgery, because these thyroid tumors tend to be highly invasive and almost impossible to surgically extirpate. Therefore surgery is not an ideal choice for a dog with a thyroid mass such as this. The recommended approach, since the dog is hyperthyroid, is to complete a kinetic study to determine whether the tumor can trap and retain radioactive iodine (^{131}I). If the ^{131}I kinetic study proves positive, radioactive iodine therapy should be recommended. Other options include partial surgical thyroidectomy (not ideal or recommended), use of external beam megavoltage irradiation of the cervical area, or chemotherapy. Assuming that radioactive iodine is used, rechecks should consist of a history, physical examination, serum T_4 concentration, and periodic radioactive pertechnetate thyroid scans. These studies are directed at answering two questions: Has the hyperthyroidism been resolved, and has the malignancy been controlled?

Radioactive iodine (^{131}I) irradiation of thyroid tumors in human beings and dogs is based on the assumption that the tumor cells trap, concentrate, and retain circulating radioactive iodine. This radioactive material, in turn, kills the neoplastic cells. Although cancerous cells are less effective than normal cells in iodine uptake (trapping, concentrating, and retaining), the former are more sensitive to the destructive effects of radiation. Iodine-131 therapy in human beings is used most effectively after subtotal to total thyroidectomy, reducing the number of tumor cells that need to be killed by the radioactive iodine.

Several treatment modalities using ^{131}I have been recommended, including frequent administration of low doses and higher doses administered less frequently (Beierwaltes et al, 1982; Gershengorn and Robbins, 1987). Radioactive iodine therapy seems to have the greatest efficacy in dogs with functioning thyroid tumors. As discussed in the radionuclide scan section, follicular carcinomas often retain the ability to concentrate iodine, even though they do not always cause a hyperthyroid (thyrotoxic) state. Thorough evaluation of this form of therapy is not currently available in the veterinary literature. However, the increased use of radionuclide scans will presumably be associated with increasing use of radioactive iodine therapy for tumors that concentrate pertechnetate and iodine (Peterson et al, 1989; Verschueren, 1992). It is strongly suggested that kinetic studies using ^{131}I be conducted before treatment, because most canine thyroid tumors do not adequately trap, concentrate, or retain the iodine. These factors limit the use of this mode of therapy in dogs.

If assessment with radioactive iodine kinetic studies indicate that this form of therapy would likely fail, veterinarians are encouraged to recommend palliative therapy. As mentioned in previous discussions, these dogs can be managed with cervical external beam megavoltage irradiation or chemotherapy. Use of both these forms of therapy can also be considered. However, remember that doxorubicin therapy enhances radiation toxicity. Therefore use of chemotherapy should be reserved for the period after the radiation sequence has been completed. Surgery remains a poor treatment alternative except when attempting to relieve discomfort due to the compressive effects of the mass itself (including respiratory or swallowing difficulties). These dogs have a poor prognosis; owners must be made aware that their opinion regarding their pet's quality of life determines how aggressive a veterinarian should be and whether (and when) euthanasia should be considered.

EVIDENCE OF METASTASIS (FIG. 5-15). As would be anticipated, evidence of metastasis creates an extremely poor prognosis. Surgery is not an option for a dog with a thyroid mass that has metastasized, except in attempting to relieve discomfort due to the compressive effects of the mass itself (e.g., respiratory or swallowing difficulties). The ideal approach to this dog is to conduct a kinetic study to determine whether the tumor (both the primary and the metastases) can trap and retain radioactive iodine (^{131}I). If the ^{131}I kinetic study proves positive, radioactive iodine therapy can be attempted. Chemotherapy can also be considered, although the chances for long-term survival with medical therapy are not as promising as they would be with ^{131}I treatment, assuming that both the primary tumor and the metastases trap iodine.

Prognosis

The prognosis for dogs with thyroid tumors causing hyperthyroidism is no better or worse than for euthyroid or hypothyroid dogs with thyroid tumors. Because the disorder is almost always due to a malignant tumor, the prognosis must be considered poor to grave. However, with more veterinarians aggressively managing these dogs with combination therapies, the prognosis for these dogs may be better than for dogs with nonfunctioning tumors. This optimism is based on the possibility that functioning tumors may trap and concentrate iodine, making these tumors more likely to respond to radioactive iodine treatment. Furthermore, as has been stressed throughout this chapter, increased use of cervical ultrasonography as a diagnostic aid for dogs with cervical masses, respiratory signs, swallowing difficulties, hypercalcemia, etc., will allow earlier diagnosis of thyroid masses and of clinical or subclinical hyperthyroidism. It is assumed that some of these incidentally discovered cervical (thyroid) masses will be adenomas. Thus the prognosis for dogs with thyroid tumors, regardless of whether or not the dogs are hyperthyroid, is expected to improve.

MEDULLARY CARCINOMA OF THE THYROID (C-CELL TUMORS, PARAFOLLICULAR CARCINOMAS, PRIMARY HYPERCALCITONINEMIA)

Medullary carcinomas are derived from the parafollicular or C-cells of the thyroid. Neoplasia involving this tissue comprises 4% to 12% of thyroid carcinomas in human beings. They are encapsulated and composed of solid masses of round, polyhedral, or elongated cells growing in a hyaline stroma containing amyloid (Gershengorn and Robbins, 1987). The incidence of C-cell tumors of the thyroid in dogs is uncertain. In one report, 7 of 200 thyroid gland tumors in dogs were derived from C-cells, and in another, 2 of 141 were C-cell derived, although another recent study provides evidence that this condition has probably been underdiagnosed for years (Carver et al, 1995). In our series, 12 of 75 thyroid tumors were parafollicular cell carcinomas or adenomas (see Table 5-2). It is now better understood that medullary carcinomas may be difficult to distinguish from other thyroid carcinomas by light microscopy alone. When specific immunocytochemical stains are used, the incidence of medullary carcinoma is much higher. These tumors may have a more favorable prognosis, because their distant metastatic spread is less common. They also appear to be well encapsulated and easier to remove during surgery (Carver et al, 1995).

Clinical syndromes associated with abnormalities in calcitonin secretion have been recognized rarely in veterinary medicine. Medullary carcinoma of the thyroid is the only known cause of persistent hypersecretion of calcitonin. Calcitonin was discovered in 1961 by Copp, who inferred its existence from studies he performed on dogs. However, medullary carcinoma of the human thyroid was first recognized as distinct from other primary thyroid tumors in 1951. The establishment of its histologic features occurred in 1959; since then, hundreds of cases have been reported in humans.

This tumor, in people, causes at least five recognized syndromes: (1) a sporadic nonfamilial type, (2) a familial type, (3) a familial type with associated pheochromocytoma, (4) a familial type with both pheochromocytoma and hyperparathyroidism (MEN types IIA and IIB), and (5) a neuroma phenotype (Gershengorn and Robbins, 1987).

The principal effect of prolonged excess secretion of calcitonin is on skeletal remodeling, with reduction in the rate of bone resorption and formation. With chronic excess secretion, the latter effect predominates, and bone formation and skeletal remodeling decline. Calcitonin is thought to decrease serum calcium concentrations acutely, but in humans and dogs with medullary carcinoma, the serum calcium concentration is normal or only slightly decreased. Thus mineral homeostasis can be maintained under conditions in which skeletal remodeling is slow. Of the few dogs described with medullary carcinoma of the thyroid, only one had significant hypocalcemia.

Diarrhea has been described as the most striking clinical feature of canine medullary carcinoma of the thyroid (Rijnberk, 1996). Diarrhea is believed to result from secretion of serotonin and/or prostaglandins by the neoplasm. Hypocalcemic tetany has also been reported as a primary reason for owners seeking veterinary care for their pets. In one dog, an owner simply noted a "swelling in the neck" (Patnaik et al, 1978). Perhaps the most important ideas to be gained from this section are that (1) careful cervical palpation should be a part of every physical examination and (2) medullary carcinoma is a rare cause of hypocalcemia in the dog. Treatment for medullary carcinoma is as described for other thyroid tumors in the dog.

ECTOPIC THYROID TUMORS

Thyroid tissue has been recognized in normal dogs outside the area of the normal thyroid lobes. Ectopic thyroid tissue may be present as far anterior as the base of the tongue and as far posterior as the base of the heart. Not surprisingly, thyroid neoplasia has been identified in these unusual areas, including such anatomic regions as within the pericardial sac or just anterior to the heart. We have observed a dog with a thyroid carcinoma (nonfunctioning) at the base of the tongue, unassociated with neoplasm of the cervical thyroid lobes. The oral tumor caused obvious clinical signs, including difficulty in eating and drinking. Thyroid tumors at the base of the heart cause respiratory symptoms if they compress the trachea or if they bleed into the pleural or pericardial space.

REFERENCES

Adams WH, et al: Treatment of differentiated thyroid carcinoma in seven dogs utilizing [131]I. Vet Radiol 36:417, 1995.

Ahuja S, Ernst H: Chemotherapy of thyroid cancer. J Endocrinol Invest 10:303, 1987.

Balogh L, et al: Thyroid volumetric measurement and quantitative thyroid scintigraphy in dogs. Acta Veterinaria Hungarica 46:145, 1998.

Beierwaltes WH, et al: Survival time and "cure" in papillary and follicular thyroid carcinoma with distant metastases: Statistics following University of Michigan therapy. J Nucl Med 23:561, 1982.

Belshaw BE: Thyroid diseases. In Ettinger SJ (ed): Textbook of Veterinary Internal Medicine, 2nd ed. Philadelphia, WB Saunders Co, 1983, p 1592.

Bentley JF, et al: Metastatic thyroid solid-follicular carcinoma in the cervical portion of the spine of a dog. JAVMA 197:1498, 1990.

Birchard SJ, Roesel OF: Neoplasia of the thyroid gland in the dog: A retrospective study of 16 cases. JAAHA 17:369, 1981.

Bos J: Ras-oncogenes in human neoplasms. Cancer Res 49:4682, 1989.

Brearley MJ, Hayes AM: Hypofractionated radiation therapy for invasive thyroid carcinoma in dogs: A retrospective analysis of survival. J Sm Anim Pract 40:206, 1999.

Brodey RS, Kelly DF: Thyroid neoplasms in the dog. A clinicopathologic study of 57 cases. Cancer 22:406, 1968.

Capen CC: The endocrine glands. In Jubb KVF, et al (eds): Pathology of Domestic Animals, 3rd ed. Orlando, FL, Academic Press, vol 3, p 237, 1985.

Carver JR, et al: A comparison of medullary thyroid carcinoma and thyroid adenocarcinoma in dogs: A retrospective study of 38 cases. Vet Surg 24:315, 1995.

Conard RA: Late effects in Marshall Islanders exposed to fallout 28 years ago. In Boice JD, Fraumeni JE (eds): Radiation Carcinogenesis: Epidemiology and Biological Significance. New York, Raven Press, 1984, p 54.

Darbre PD, King RJB: Progression to steroid insensitivity can occur irrespective of the presence of functional steroid receptors. Cell 51:521, 1987.

Fineman LS, et al: Cisplatin chemotherapy for treatment of thyroid carcinoma in dogs: 13 cases. J Am Vet Med Assoc 34:109, 1998.

Flanders JA. Surgical therapy of the thyroid. Vet Clin North Am: Sm Anim Pract 24:607, 1994.

Gershengorn MC, Robbins J: Thyroid neoplasia. In Green WL (ed): The Thyroid. New York, Elsevier, 1987, p 293.

Greenspan FS: The thyroid gland. In Greenspan FS, Gardner DG (eds): Basic and Clinical Endocrinology. 6th ed. San Francisco, Lange Medical Books/McGraw-Hill, 2001, p 201.

Grigsby PW, Luk KH: Thyroid. In Perez CA, Brady LW, (eds): Principles and practice of radiation oncology. 3rd ed. Philadelphia: Lippincott-Raven, 1998, p 1157.

Haley PJ, et al: Thyroid neoplasms in a colony of Beagle Dogs. Vet Pathol 26:438, 1989.

Hanna NN, et al: Advances in the pathogenesis and treatment of thyroid cancer. Curr Opin Oncol 11:42, 1999.

Harari J, et al: Clinical and pathologic features of thyroid tumors in 26 dogs. JAVMA 188:1160, 1986.

Harmelin A, et al: Canine medullary thyroid carcinoma with unusual distant metastases. J Vet Diagn Invest 5:284, 1993.

Hedinger C, et al: Histological typing of thyroid tumors. WHO International Histologic Classification of Tumours, 2nd ed. Berlin, Springer-Verlag, 1988.

Holscher MA, et al: Ectopic thyroid tumour in a dog: Thyroglobulin, calcitonin, and neuron-specific enolase immunocytochemical studies. Vet Pathol 23:778, 1986.

Hoskin PJ, Harmer C: Chemotherapy for thyroid cancer. Radiother Oncol 10:187, 1987.

Jeglum KA, Whereat A: Chemotherapy of canine thyroid carcinoma. Compend Contin Educ Pract Vet 5:96, 1983.

Kim JH, Leeper RD: Treatment of locally advanced thyroid carcinoma with combination doxorubicin and radiation therapy. Cancer 60:2372, 1987.

Klein MK, et al: Canine thyroid carcinomas: A retrospective review of 64 cases. Vet Cancer Soc Newsletter 12:7, 1988.

Klein MK, et al: Treatment of thyroid carcinoma in dogs by surgical resection alone: 20 cases (1981–1989). JAVMA 206:1007, 1995.

Komminoth P: The RET proto-oncogene in medullary and papillary thyroid carcinoma, molecular features, pathophysiology and clinical implications. Virchows Arch 431:1, 1997.

Konig MP, et al: Thyroid cancer in regions of endemic goitre. In Andreoli M, et al (eds): Advances in Thyroid Neoplasia. Rome, Field Education Italia, 1981, p 177.

Kramer RW, et al: Hypothyroidism in a dog after surgery and radiation therapy for a functional thyroid adenocarcinoma. Vet Radiol Ultrasound 35:132, 1994.

Lawrence D, et al: Hyperthyroidism associated with a thyroid adenoma in a dog. JAVMA 199:81, 1991.

Leav I, et al: Adenomas and carcinomas of the canine and feline thyroid. Am J Pathol 83:61, 1976.

Leblanc B, et al: Immunocytochemistry of thyroid C-cell complexes in dogs. Vet Pathol 27:445, 1990.

Leblanc B, et al: Immunocytochemistry of canine thyroid tumours. Vet Pathol 28:370, 1991.

Lemoine NR, et al: Partial transformation of human thyroid epithelial cells by mutant Ha-ras oncogene. Oncogene 5:1833, 1990.

Ljungberg O, et al: A compound follicular-parafollicular cell carcinoma of the thyroid: A new tumour entity? Cancer 52:1053, 1983.

Ljungberg O, Nilsson PO: Hyperplastic and neoplastic changes in ultimobranchial remnants and in parafollicular (C) cells in bulls: A histologic and immunohistochemical study. Vet Pathol 22:95, 1985.

Loar AS: Canine thyroid tumors. In Kirk RW (ed): Current Veterinary Therapy IX. Philadelphia, WB Saunders Co, 1986, p 1033.

Lurye JC, Behrend E: Endocrine tumors. Vet Clin N Amer: Sm Anim Pract 31:1095, 2001.

Marks SL, et al: ^{99}mTc-pertechnetate imaging of thyroid tumors in dogs: 29 cases (1980–1992). JAVMA 204:756, 1994.

Miles KG, et al: A retrospective evaluation of the radiographic evidence of pulmonary metastatic disease on initial presentation in the dog. Vet Radiol 31: 79, 1990.

Mitchell M, et al: Canine thyroid carcinomas: clinical occurrence, staging by means of scintiscans, and therapy of 15 cases. Vet Surg 8:112, 1979.

Mooney CT: Canine thyroid tumours and hyperthyroidism. In Torrence AG, Mooney CT (eds): BSAVA Manual of Small Animal Endocrinology, 2nd ed. United Kingdom, British Small Animal Veterinary Association, 1998.

Moore FM, et al: Thyroglobulin and calcitonin immunoreactivity in canine thyroid carcinomas. Vet Pathol 21:168, 1984.

Nishiyama K, et al: A prospective analysis of subacute thyroid dysfunction after neck irradiation. Int J Radiat Oncol Biol Phys 34:439, 1996.

Ogilvie GK, et al: Phase II evaluation of doxorubicin for treatment of various canine neoplasms. JAVMA 195:1580, 1989.

Ogilvie GK, et al: Toxicoses associated with administration of mitoxantrone to dogs with malignant tumors. JAVMA 198:1613, 1991.

Ogilvie GK: Tumors of the endocrine system. In Withrow SJ, MacEwen E (eds): Small Animal Clinical Oncology, 2nd ed. Philadelphia, WB Saunders Co, 1996, pp 316.

Owen LN: Clinical stages (TNM) of canine tumours of the thyroid gland. In Owen LN (ed): TNM Classification of Tumours in Domestic Animals. Geneva, World Health Organization, 1980.

Pack LA, et al: Definitive radiation therapy for infiltrative thyroid carcinoma in dogs. Vet Radiol Ultrasound 42:471, 2001.

Parsons JT, et al: Carcinoma of the thyroid. In Million RR (ed): Management of head and neck cancer: A multidisciplinary approach. 2nd edition. Philadelphia, JB Lippincott Co, 1994, pp 785.

Patnaik AK, et al: Canine medullary carcinoma of the thyroid. Vet Pathol 15:590, 1978.

Patnaik AK, Lieberman PH: Gross, histologic, cytochemical, and immunocytochemical study of medullary thyroid carcinoma in sixteen dogs. Vet Pathol 28:223, 1991.

Peterson ME, et al: Radioactive iodine treatment of a functional thyroid carcinoma producing hyperthyroidism in a dog. J Vet Intern Med 3:20, 1989.

Post GS, Mauldin GN: Radiation and adjuvant chemotherapy for the treatment of thyroid adenocarcinoma in dogs. In Proceedings of the 12th Annual Veterinary Cancer Society Conference, Asilomar, CA, 1992.

Poster DS, et al: Current status of chemotherapy in the treatment of advanced carcinoma of the thyroid gland. Cancer Clin Trials 4:301, 1981.

Priester WA, McKay FW: The occurrence of tumours in domestic animals. National Cancer Institute Monograph 54, NIH Publication No. 80-2046. Bethesda, National Institute of Health, 1980.

Rijnberk A: Thyroids. In Rijnberk A (ed): Clinical Endocrinology of Dogs and Cats. Dordrecht, The Netherlands, Kluwer Academic, 1996, pp 35.

Roger PP, Dumont JE: Epidermal growth factor controls the proliferation and differentiation of canine thyroid cells in primary culture. FEBS Let 144:209, 1982.

Saltiel AR, et al: Thyrotropin receptor–adenylate cyclase function in human thyroid neoplasms. Cancer Res 41:2360, 1981.

Schlumberger M: Papillary and follicular thyroid carcinoma. N Engl J Med 338:297, 1998.

Schneider AB: Radiation-related thyroid cancer. In Ingbar SH, Braverman LE (eds): Werner's The Thyroid. A Fundamental and Clinical Text, 5th ed. Philadelphia, JB Lippincott, 1986, p 801.

Shimaoka K, et al: A randomized trial of doxorubicin versus doxorubicin plus cisplantinum in patients with advanced thyroid carcinoma. Cancer 56:2155, 1985.

Spanos GA, et al: Pre-operative chemotherapy for giant cell carcinoma of the thyroid. Cancer 50:2252, 1982.

Suarez HG, et al: Detection of activated ras oncogenes in human thyroid carcinomas. Oncogene 2:403, 1988.

Susaneck SJ: Thyroid tumors in the dog. Comp Cont Educ Vet Pract 5:35, 1983a.

Susaneck SJ: Doxorubicin therapy in the dog. JAVMA 182:70, 1983b.

Tallroth E, et al: Multimodality treatment in anaplastic giant cell thyroid carcinoma. Cancer 60:1428, 1987.

Tateyama S, et al: The ultimobranchial and its hyperplasia or adenoma in equine thyroid gland. Jpn J Vet Sci 50:714, 1988.

Theon AP, et al: Prognostic factors and patterns of treatment failure in dogs with unresectable differentiated thyroid carcinomas treated with megavoltage irradiation. JAVMA 216:1775, 2000.

Thompson EJ, et al: Fine-needle aspiration cytology in the diagnosis of canine thyroid carcinoma. Can Vet J 21:186, 1980.

Tubiana M, et al: External radiotherapy in thyroid cancers. Cancer 55:2062, 1985.

Turrel JM, et al: Canine thyroid tumors. In Morgan R (ed): Handbook of Veterinary Medicine. New York, Churchill Livingstone, 1987.

Verschueren CP: Clinico-pathological and endocrine aspects of canine thyroid cancer. Ph.D. Thesis, Utrecht, The Netherlands, 1992.

Verschueren CP, Goslings BM: Comparative aspects of thyroid cancer. Ph.D. Thesis, Utrecht, The Netherlands, 1992, p 95.

Verschueren CP, et al: Thyrotropin receptors in normal and neoplastic (primary and metastatic) canine thyroid tissue. J Endocrinol 132:461, 1992a.

Verschueren CP, et al: Evaluation of some prognostic factors in surgically treated canine thyroid carcinomas. Ph.D. Thesis, Utrecht, The Netherlands, 1992b, p 11.

Waters CB, Scott-Moncrieff JC: Cancer of endocrine origin. In Morrison WB (ed): Cancer in Dogs and Cats: Medical and Surgical Management, 1st ed. Baltimore, Williams & Wilkins, 1998, pp 599.

Wheeler SL: Endocrine tumors. In Withrow SJ, MacEwen EG (eds): Clinical Veterinary Oncology. Philadelphia, JB Lippincott, 1989, p 253.

Wisner ER, et al: Ultrasonographic evaluation of cervical masses in the dog and cat. Vet Radiol Ultrasound 35:310, 1994.

Wisner ER, et al: Normal ultrasonographic anatomy of the canine neck. Vet Radiol 32:185, 1991.

Wisner ER, Nyland TG: Ultrasonography of the thyroid and parathyroid glands. Vet Clin N Amer: Sm Anim Pract 28:973, 1998.

Withrow SJ, MacEwen EG: Tumors of the endocrine system. In Withrow and MacEwen: Small Animal Clinical Oncology, 3rd ed. Philadelphia, WB Saunders Co, 2001, p 423.

Wynford-Thomas D: Origin and progression of thyroid epithelial tumors: Cellular and molecular mechanisms. Horm Res 47:145, 1997.

THE ADRENAL GLAND

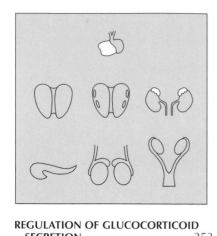

6

CANINE HYPERADRENOCORTICISM (CUSHING'S SYNDROME)

In 1932 Dr. Harvey Cushing described eight humans with a disorder that he suggested was "the result of pituitary-basophilism." Six of those eight patients had small, basophilic pituitary adenomas and clinical features of excess adrenocortical cortisol secretion. Careful study of these and other individuals diagnosed years ago suggests numerous primary causes for what was then considered a single condition. Chronic excesses in the serum cortisol concentration, however, represent the final common denominator of their illnesses. The eponym *Cushing's syndrome* is an "umbrella term" referring to the constellation of clinical and chemical abnormalities that result from chronic exposure to excessive concentrations of glucocorticoids. The eponym *Cushing's disease* is applied to cases of Cushing's syndrome in which hypercortisolism occurs secondary to inappropriate excessive secretion of adrenocorticotropic hormone (corticotropin, ACTH) by the pituitary; that is, pituitary-dependent hyperadrenocorticism (PDH). Canine hyperadrenocorticism (canine Cushing's syndrome [CCS]) also has various pathophysiologic origins, but all have that common denominator: chronic excesses in systemic cortisol.

A pathophysiologic classification CCS causes would include (1) pituitary tumors that synthesize and secrete excess ACTH, with secondary adrenocortical hyperplasia (common); (2) pituitary hyperplasia caused by excesses in corticotropin-releasing hormone secretion due to a hypothalamic disorder and, secondarily, adrenocortical hyperplasia (extremely rare in people and never reported in dogs or cats); (3) primary excesses in adrenal cortisol autonomously secreted by an adrenocortical carcinoma or adenoma (relatively common); and (4) iatrogenic causes resulting from excessive ACTH administration (extremely rare) or excessive glucocorticoid medication (quite common). Various tumors outside the hypothalamus or pituitary that produce excessive amounts of ACTH have been described in humans but not in dogs or cats.

REGULATION OF GLUCOCORTICOID SECRETION

Corticotropin-Releasing Hormone (CRH)

With an understanding of the portal circulation, which "connects" the hypothalamus and the pituitary, came an appreciation that the hypothalamus exerts control over secretion of ACTH by the anterior pituitary. ACTH, in turn, exerts control over adrenocortical secretion of cortisol. Cortisol, in part, then completes the circle by inhibiting secretion of hypothalamic and pituitary hormones (Fig. 6-1). The factor released by the hypothalamus is CRH, a polypeptide containing 41 amino acid residues. The CRH-secreting neurons are located in the anterior portion of the paraventricular nuclei in the hypothalamus. CRH has a long plasma half-life (approximately 60 minutes). Both arginine vasopressin and angiotensin II potentiate CRH secretion and, in turn, ACTH in humans. In contrast, oxytocin inhibits CRH-mediated ACTH secretion in humans. Regulatory roles in the physiology of ACTH secretion for arginine vasopressin, oxytocin, and angiotensin II have not been consistently demonstrated in dogs, but the importance of CRH in controlling normal ACTH release has been supported (Kemppainen and Sartin, 1987; Kemppainen et al, 1992).

Adrenocorticotropic Hormone (ACTH)

ACTH is a 39-amino acid peptide hormone (MW 4500) processed from a large precursor molecule, proopiomelanocortin (POMC) (MW 28,500). In the pituitary cells responsible for the synthesis of ACTH (corticotrophs), messenger ribonucleic acid (mRNA) directs the synthesis of POMC and its processing into smaller, biologically active fragments (Fig. 6-2). The function and importance of these peptide fragments— β-lipotropin (β-LPH), α–melanocyte-stimulating hormone (α-MSH), β-MSH, β-endorphin, and N-terminal

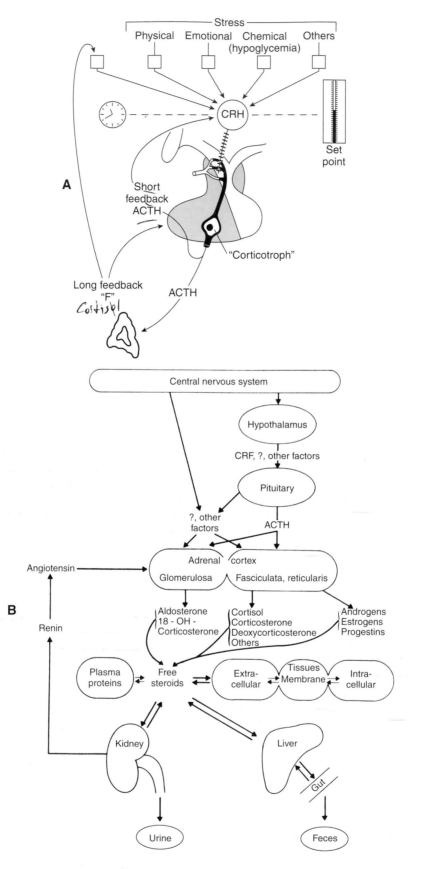

FIGURE 6–1. *A,* The hypothalamic-pituitary-adrenal axis, illustrating the various stimuli that enhance corticotropin-releasing hormone (CRH) secretion as well as negative feedback by cortisol ("F") at the hypothalamic and pituitary levels. A short negative feedback loop of ACTH on the secretion of CRH is also illustrated. *B,* Interrelationships between the various tissues and body compartments in the synthesis of adrenal steroids and their regulation, the peripheral uptake of the steroids, and their metabolism and excretion. (From Baxter JD, Tyrrell JB: *In* Felig P, et al [eds]: Endocrinology and Metabolism. New York, McGraw-Hill, 1981, p 396.)

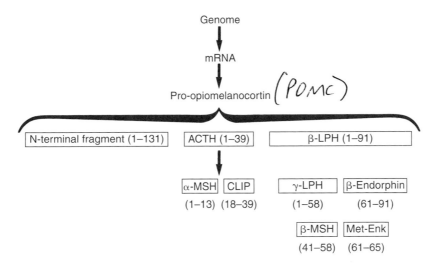

FIGURE 6–2. The processing of pro-opiomelanocortin (MW 28,500) into its biologically active peptide hormones. Abbreviations are expanded in the text.

fragment—constitute an evolving area of endocrine study. Most of these peptides are glycosylated to some extent, resulting in their various reported molecular weights. The basophilic staining characteristics of corticotrophs can be explained by the carbohydrate nature of these moieties (Aron et al, 2001a).

Two of the fragments depicted in Fig. 6-2 are contained within the structure of ACTH and therefore are byproducts of ACTH metabolism: α-MSH is identical to $ACTH_{1-13}$, and corticotropin-like intermediate-lobe peptide (CLIP) is identical to $ACTH_{18-39}$. Neither of these peptides is secreted as a separate hormone in humans. β-Endorphin may act as an "endogenous opiate," which suggests a role in pain sensation. It may also affect endocrine regulation of other pituitary hormones and may have a role in neural control of breathing (Aron et al, 2001a). Plasma concentrations of the N-terminal fragment have been demonstrated to increase in response to hypoglycemic stress; this fragment may also be an adrenal growth factor and/or may potentiate ACTH action on steroidogenesis. The physiologic function of β-LPH is not well understood. However, it is known that both β-LPH and β-endorphin have the same secretory dynamics as ACTH; that is, they increase in response to stress or hypoglycemia and are suppressed by glucocorticoids. These hormones also parallel ACTH in disease states. For example, concentrations increase in Addison's disease, pituitary Cushing's disease, and "Nelson's syndrome" (growing pituitary tumor after removal of the adrenals) (Peterson et al, 1986). Concentrations of β-LPH and β-endorphin decrease in dogs with autonomously secreting adrenocortical tumors.

Both CRH and ACTH are secreted in a pulsatile manner, with a diurnal rhythm in humans that results in a peak before awakening followed by a progressive decline in concentrations throughout the day. Diurnal rhythms have not been established in dogs (Kemppainen and Sartin, 1984 and 1987; Murase et al,

1988). ACTH secretion also increases in response to feeding in both humans and animals (Aron et al, 2001a). The primary function of ACTH is to stimulate the secretion of glucocorticoids from the adrenal cortex. The stimulatory properties of ACTH on adrenocortical mineralocorticoid secretion and on androgenic steroids are less important. The amino terminal end of the ACTH molecule (amino acids 1 to 18) is responsible for its biologic activity.

Many types of stress stimulate secretion of ACTH, often superseding normal daily fluctuations. Physical, emotional, and chemical stressors such as pain, trauma, hypoxia, acute hypoglycemia, cold exposure, surgery, and pyrogens have been demonstrated to stimulate ACTH and cortisol secretion (Aron et al, 2001a). The increase in ACTH concentrations during stress is mediated by vasopressin and CRH. Although physiologic cortisol levels do not blunt the ACTH response to stress, high doses of exogenous corticosteroids do suppress ACTH.

Negative feedback by cortisol and synthetic glucocorticoids on ACTH secretion occurs at both the hypothalamic and pituitary levels and appears to act by two mechanisms: "Fast feedback" is sensitive to the rate of change in the cortisol concentration, whereas "slow feedback" is sensitive to the absolute cortisol concentration. The first mechanism is probably nonnuclear; that is, this phenomenon occurs too rapidly to be explained by the influence of corticosteroids on nuclear transcription of specific mRNA responsible for ACTH. Slow feedback, which occurs later, may be explained by a nuclear-mediated mechanism and a subsequent decrease in the synthesis of ACTH. This latter form of negative feedback is the type probed by the dexamethasone suppression test. In addition to the negative feedback by adrenal steroid secretion, ACTH also exerts a negative feedback effect on (i.e., inhibits) its own secretion (short loop feedback), as depicted in Fig. 6-1 (Aron et al, 2001a).

TABLE 6–1   NOMENCLATURE OF STEROIDOGENIC ENZYMES

Enzyme	Gene Symbol	Trivial Name	Past Name
P450scc	CYP11A1	Cholesterol side chain cleavage enzyme	P450scc
3β-Hydroxysteroid dehydrogenase	HSD3B1 HSD3B2	3β-Hydroxysteroid dehydrogenase	3β-HSD
P450c17	CYP17	17α-Hydroxylase; 17,20-lyase	P450c17
P450c21	CYP21A2	21β-Hydroxylase	P450c21
P450c11b	CYP11B1	11β-Hydroxylase	P450c11
P450c11AS	CYP11B2	P450aldo; aldosterone synthase; corticosterone methyloxidase	P450c11AS

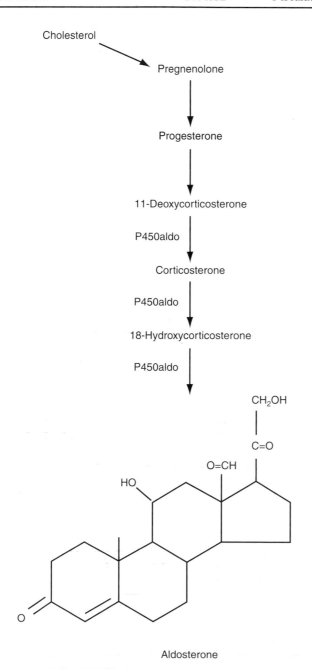

FIGURE 6–3. Steroid biosynthesis in the zona glomerulosa. The steps from cholesterol to 11-deoxycorticosterone are the same as in the zona fasciculata and zona reticularis. However, the zona glomerulosa lacks 17α-hydroxylase activity and thus cannot produce cortisol. Only the zona glomerulosa can convert corticosterone to 18-hydroxy-corticosterone and aldosterone. The single enzyme P450aldo catalyzes the conversion of 11-deoxycorticosterone to corticosterone and then to 18-hydroxycorticosterone and then aldosterone.

Steroids

ZONES OF THE ADRENAL CORTEX AND THEIR PRODUCTS. The major hormones secreted by the adrenal cortex are cortisol and aldosterone. Histologically, the adrenal cortex is composed of three zones. The scheme of adrenal steroidogenic synthesis has been clarified by analysis of the enzymes involved in the synthesis of these hormones. Most of the enzymes belong to the family of cytochrome P450 oxygenases (Table 6-1). Because of the enzymatic differences between the zona glomerulosa and the inner two zones, the adrenal cortex functions as two separate units, with differing regulation and secretory products.

The outer zona glomerulosa produces aldosterone and is deficient in 17α-hydroxylase activity (new enzyme name, CYP17), which renders this zone incapable of synthesizing cortisol or androgens. In contrast, only cells in the zona glomerulosa contain the enzymes necessary for dehydrogenation of 18-hydroxycorticosterone to synthesize aldosterone. Aldosterone synthesis is regulated primarily by the renin-angiotensin system and by serum potassium concentrations (see Fig. 6-1, B and Fig. 6-3). The middle zona fasciculata, the thickest of the three adrenocortical layers, functions as a unit with the narrow, inner zona reticularis; these are the two zones from which cortisol and androgens are produced. Only cells in these two layers of the adrenal cortex have 17α-hydroxylase (CYP17) activity and can synthesize 17α-hydroxypregnenolone and 17α-hydroxyprogesterone, precursors of cortisol and adrenal androgens (Fig. 6-4). These zones are regulated primarily by ACTH. The conversion of cholesterol to pregnenolone is the rate-limiting step in adrenal steroidogenesis and the major site of ACTH action, via activation of adenylate cyclase, which increases cyclic adenosine monophosphatase (AMP) and then activation of intracellular phosphoprotein kinases (Fig. 6-5) (Aron et al, 2001b).

STEROIDOGENESIS. Cortisol, aldosterone, androgens, and estrogens are "steroids." Synthesis of these steroids begins from enzymatic action on cholesterol (see Figs. 6-3 and 6-4). Plasma lipoproteins are the major source of adrenal cholesterol, though synthesis in the gland from acetate also occurs. Low-density lipoprotein (LDL) accounts for about 80% of cholesterol delivered to the adrenals, and a small pool of free cholesterol is available in the adrenals for rapid response to stimulation. When stimulation occurs,

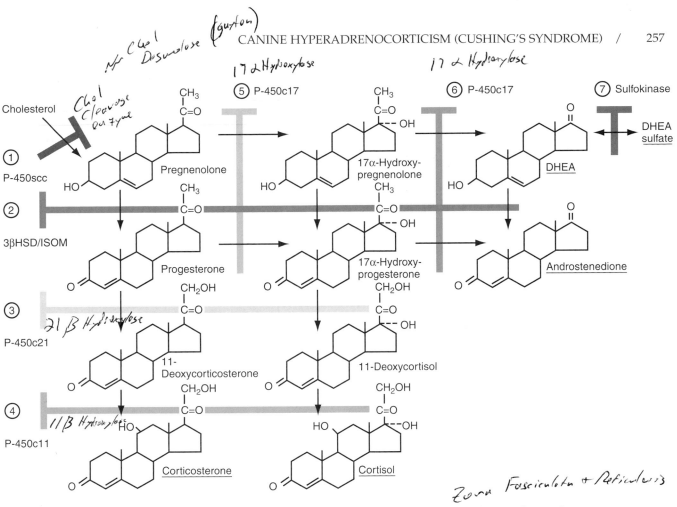

FIGURE 6–4. Steroid biosynthetic pathway in the adrenal cortex. The branching pathways for glucocorticoids, mineralocorticoids, and adrenal androgens and the structures of these steroids and their biosynthetic precursors are shown. The names of the biosynthetic enzymes are shown in the boxes. See Table 6-1 for the nomenclature of steroidogenic enzymes.

there is also increased hydrolysis of stored cholesteryl esters to free cholesterol, increased uptake from plasma lipoproteins, and increased cholesterol synthesis in the adrenals. The acute response to a steroidogenic stimulus is mediated by the steroidogenic acute regulatory (StAR) protein. This mitochondrial phosphoprotein enhances cholesterol transport from the outer to the inner mitochondrial membrane (Aron et al, 2001b).

The conversion of cholesterol to pregnenolone is the rate-limiting step in adrenal steroidogenesis and the major site of ACTH action on the adrenal. Conversion to pregnenolone occurs in the mitochondria and involves two hydroxylations, followed by the side-chain cleavage of cholesterol (see Fig. 6-5). A single enzyme, CYP11A1, mediates this process; each step requires molecular oxygen and a pair of electrons. After synthesis, pregnenolone is transported out of the mitochondria. Cortisol is the focus of this chapter, and its synthesis proceeds via 17α-hydroxylation in smooth endoplasmic reticulum (Aron et al, 2001b). By means of the steps outlined in Fig. 6-4, cortisol is continuously synthesized, and under basal conditions in the dog, this typically results in serum concentrations that range from 1 to 5 µg/dl.

REGULATION OF SECRETION. ACTH is the trophic hormone of the zonae fasciculata and reticularis. Delivery of ACTH to the adrenal cortex leads to rapid

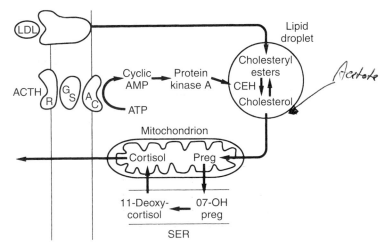

FIGURE 6–5. Mechanism of action of ACTH on cortisol-secreting cells in the inner two zones of the adrenal cortex. When ACTH binds to its receptor (R), adenylate cyclase (AC) is activated via Golgi structures (GS). The resulting increase in cyclic AMP activates protein kinase A, and the kinase phosphorylates cholesterol ester hydrolase (CEH), increasing its activity. Consequently, more free cholesterol is formed and converted to pregnenolone in the mitochondria. Note that in the subsequent steps in steroid biosynthesis, products are shuttled between the mitochondria and the smooth endoplasmic reticulum (SER). LDL, low-density lipoprotein.

synthesis and secretion of cortisol and androgens. Secretion of ACTH, in turn, is regulated by the hypothalamus and central nervous system via neurotransmitters, CRH, and arginine vasopressin. The plasma concentration of cortisol increases within minutes of ACTH administration. ACTH increases RNA, deoxyribonucleic (DNA), and protein synthesis. Chronic stimulation leads to adrenocortical hyperplasia and hypertrophy; conversely, ACTH deficiency results in decreased steroidogenesis and is accompanied by adrenocortical atrophy, decreased weight of the gland, and decreased protein and nucleic acid content (Aron et al, 2001b).

PATHOPHYSIOLOGY

Pituitary-Dependent Hyperadrenocorticism

PATHOLOGY IN HUMANS. "ACTH-secreting pituitary tumors exist in virtually all patients with (pituitary) Cushing's disease" (Aron et al, 2001a and 2001b). These tumors are usually benign adenomas less than 10 mm in diameter. About 50% of these tumors are 5 mm or smaller in diameter, and microadenomas as small as 1 mm have been described. The tumors identified in people with Cushing's disease are either basophilic or chromophobe adenomas and may be found anywhere in the anterior pituitary. About 15% to 25% of ACTH-secreting tumors are large and have invasive tendencies. Malignant tumors have been reported. Diffuse hyperplasia of anterior pituitary corticotrophs, or *adenomatous hyperplasia*, which is presumed to result from excess CRH, is poorly defined and occurs rarely. The adrenal glands in people with Cushing's disease are thickened due to hyperplasia of both the zona fasciculata and the zona reticularis; the zona glomerulosa is normal. In some cases, ACTH-secreting pituitary adenomas cause bilateral nodular hyperplasia. These adrenals are diffusely hyperplastic and have one or more nodules that vary in size from microscopic to several centimeters in diameter, although the most common presentation is multiple small nodules (Aron et al, 2001b).

PITUITARY CONTROL AND FEEDBACK. In normal individuals (humans and animals), ACTH secretion appears to be both random and episodic. This appearance is misleading, because although ACTH is secreted episodically, it functions exquisitely well in maintaining plasma cortisol concentrations at the levels required for homeostasis. Secretion, therefore, is not "random." The most common abnormality in pituitary-dependent hyperadrenocorticism (PDH) is the fact that both the frequency and amplitude of ACTH secretory "bursts" are chronically excessive. Chronic excesses in ACTH secretion result in excess cortisol secretion and, eventually, adrenocortical hyperplasia. Feedback inhibition of ACTH secreted from a pituitary adenoma by physiologic or excess levels of glucocorticoids is *relatively* ineffective (Fig. 6-6). If glucocorticoids were "normally" effective in negative feedback inhibition of ACTH secretion, PDH would not evolve. In dogs with naturally occurring Cushing's disease, episodic secretion of ACTH and, in turn, cortisol results in fluctuating plasma concentrations of both hormones that are often within the normal or reference ranges for most laboratories (Fig. 6-7).

"NORMAL" CORTISOL CONCENTRATIONS IN HYPERADRENOCORTICISM. Studies of cortisol production in dogs or people with hyperadrenocorticism, such as urine cortisol excretion over 24 hours, easily illustrate the existence of excessive cortisol secretion. The combination of excessive secretion and absence of diurnal variation (if it exists in dogs) in glucocorticoid secretion causes the clinical manifestations of Cushing's syndrome. The excessive secretion of cortisol is *not* readily appreciated by randomly assaying basal cortisol concentrations. As shown in Fig. 6-7, most dogs with hyperadrenocorticism usually have plasma cortisol concentrations within the reference or "normal" range at any given moment. The excess cortisol becomes readily apparent when one evaluates the "area under a plasma cortisol curve" over time for dogs with Cushing's syndrome, especially when those findings are compared with data from healthy dogs. The dog or cat with hyperadrenocorticism is exposed to more cortisol, on a daily

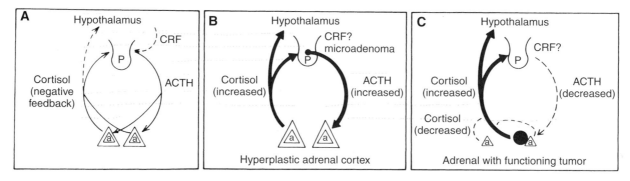

FIGURE 6–6. The pituitary-adrenal axis in normal dogs *(A)*, dogs with pituitary-dependent hyperadrenocorticism *(B)*, and dogs with a functioning adrenocortical tumor *(C)*. a, Adrenal; P, pituitary; CRF, corticotropin-releasing factor. (From Feldman EC: *In* Ettinger SJ [ed]: Textbook of Veterinary Internal Medicine, 2nd ed. Philadelphia, WB Saunders,1983, p 1673.)

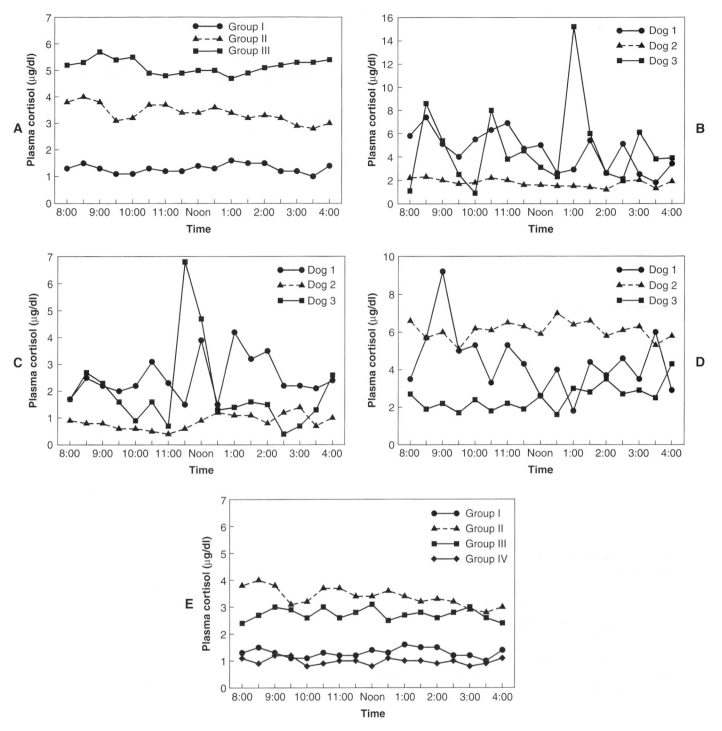

FIGURE 6–7. *A,* Mean plasma cortisol concentrations taken every 30 minutes for 8 hours from 15 normal dogs (Group I), 30 dogs with pituitary-dependent Cushing's syndrome (Group II), and 18 dogs with Cushing's syndrome secondary to an adrenocortical tumor (Group III). Note that the plasma cortisol concentrations in the dogs with Cushing's syndrome are much greater than in the normals, but all mean values are within normal limits. Demonstrating significant individual variation in plasma cortisol concentrations with time are values from three healthy dogs *(B),* three dogs with pituitary-dependent Cushing's syndrome *(C),* and three dogs with adrenocortical tumors *(D). E,* Mean plasma cortisol concentrations over time from 15 normal dogs (Group I); 30 untreated dogs with pituitary-dependent Cushing's syndrome (pituitary-dependent hyperadrenocorticism [PDH]) (Group II); 15 o,p'-DDD–treated but not controlled PDH dogs (Group III); and 25 o,p'-DDD–treated and well-controlled PDH dogs (Group IV).

basis, than is a normal animal. This chronic and persistent abnormality results in the clinical syndrome associated with cortisol excess.

LOSS OF HYPOTHALAMIC CONTROL.   One reflection of excessive ACTH secretion is the absence of stress responsiveness. Stimuli such as hypoglycemia or surgery fail to further stimulate ACTH and cortisol secretion. Chronic hyperadrenocorticism suppresses hypothalamic function and CRH secretion. Hypothalamic control of ACTH secretion is lost (Aron et al, 2001a), probably owing to suppression of hypothalamic function and CRH secretion as a result of chronic hypercortisolism. Thus chronic hypercortisolism causes a loss of hypothalamic control of ACTH secretion (Aron et al, 2001b; van Wijk et al, 1992).

INCIDENCE OF PITUITARY TUMORS.   Eighty percent to 85% of dogs with naturally occurring Cushing's syndrome have PDH; that is, excessive secretion of ACTH by the pituitary, causing bilateral adrenal hyperplasia and excessive secretion of glucocorticoids (Feldman, 1983a-c,). The reported incidence of recognized pituitary tumors in dogs with PDH varies tremendously but likely depends on the competence and persistence of the pathologist, as well as the microdissection capabilities and staining capacities of the laboratory performing the histologic examination. It has been reported that more than 90% of dogs with PDH have a pituitary tumor (Zerbe, 1992). Our experience is similar; virtually 100% of dogs with naturally occurring pituitary-dependent Cushing's syndrome have a pituitary tumor.

PARS DISTALIS VERSUS PARS INTERMEDIA.   In humans and dogs, the pituitary gland is distinctly divided into an anterior section (pars distalis) and a posterior section (pars nervosa). However, dogs, unlike humans, also have a distinct area that separates the anterior and posterior lobes of the pituitary, the pars intermedia (Peterson et al, 1982a). Furthermore, the pars intermedia has been shown to have two distinct cell types (Halmi et al, 1981; Jackson et al, 1981). The predominant cells (A cells) immunostain intensely for α-MSH but only weakly for ACTH. The second population of pars intermedia cells (B cells) stain strongly for ACTH and only weakly for α-MSH. The intense ACTH staining of pars intermedia B cells is similar to the staining characteristics of ACTH-producing pars distalis cells (Peterson et al, 1986).

Pars distalis POMC (the ACTH prohormone molecule; see Fig. 6-2) and, therefore, ACTH secretion are regulated primarily by the interaction of the stimulatory hypothalamic peptide (CRH) and, the inhibitory adrenocortical glucocorticoids. The pars intermedia, however, is under negative regulation by dopamine secreted from the arcuate nucleus, as well as by serotonin and CRH. Thus the pars distalis is devoid of a nerve supply and is controlled by hypothalamic CRH that reaches it through the hypophyseal portal vessels, whereas the relatively avascular pars intermedia is innervated and controlled by dopaminergic and serotoninergic fibers from the brain (Peterson et al, 1982a; Peterson, 1984).

Almost all dogs with PDH have a pituitary adenoma, most derived from the pars distalis. However,

some dogs with hyperadrenocorticism have been diagnosed with "A cell" pars intermedia adenomas and others with "B cell" pars intermedia adenomas. With extreme rarity, hyperadrenocorticism has been claimed to be caused by pituitary hyperplasia. Even more confusing are individual dogs with (1) two pituitary adenomas, each tumor apparently arising from a different pituitary lobe, or (2) both a tumor and hyperplasia of the pituitary. A small number of dogs have been described as having a functioning pituitary carcinoma. As is quickly appreciated, pituitary "hyperadrenocorticism" is a syndrome with the potential for multiple causes (Peterson et al, 1986; Peterson, 1987). The final common pathway for these disorders remains similar, however. Chronic systemic cortisol excess due to adrenocortical hyperplasia results from chronic and excessive secretion of pituitary ACTH. Clinically, the syndrome of cortisol excess is similar regardless of the underlying pathogenesis or the source of the cortisol.

Investigators have attempted to distinguish dogs with pars distalis tumors from those with pars intermedia A-cell or B-cell tumors. It has been suggested that dogs with pars distalis tumors and those with B-cell pars intermedia tumors have excess endogenous ACTH and that their plasma cortisol concentrations are suppressible with large doses of glucocorticoids. The A-cell pars intermedia tumors may not be suppressible (Peterson et al, 1986; Peterson, 1987). Our experience has been different; we have not found it possible to easily distinguish the cause based on antemortem testing (Fig. 6-8) (Leroy and Feldman, 1989). Furthermore, such antemortem testing is likely affected by numerous other factors (e.g., age, breed, duration of illness, tumor size, and benign or malignant nature of the tumor). These discussions currently are of academic interest and have not yet been demonstrated to have clinical significance.

ETIOLOGY OF PDH. Both a primary pituitary abnormality (ACTH-secreting adenoma) (Aron et al, 2001b) and a central nervous system (CNS) derangement with excessive stimulation of pituitary corticotrophs by CRH or other hypothalamic factors (Krieger, 1983) have been proposed in the past. It was suggested that chronic stimulation of pituitary corticotrophs by hypothalamic CRH could lead to excessive secretion of ACTH, pituitary "hyperplasia," and eventually neoplastic transformation of some corticotrophs, resulting in a "polyclonal" tumor. However, CRH concentrations in the cerebrospinal fluid of dogs with PDH have been demonstrated to be decreased, whereas ACTH concentrations were normal, despite the syndrome of excess cortisol secretion (van Wijk et al, 1992). Adenomas of the pars distalis are the most common histologic finding in canine PDH, and they represent the best evidence that pituitary tumors are a primary and autonomous cause of the disorder.

We also believe that humans with Cushing's syndrome represent an excellent and accurate model of the condition in dogs. Virtually all peer-reviewed evidence indicates that humans with pituitary-dependent Cushing's syndrome have a primary pituitary disorder and that hypothalamic abnormalities

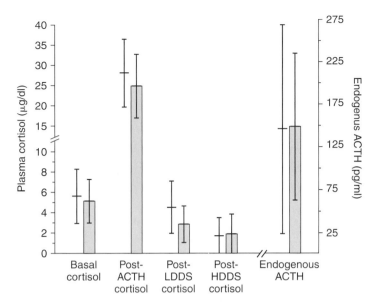

FIGURE 6–8. Mean (± SD) plasma cortisol and ACTH concentrations from 12 dogs with pituitary pars distalis tumors causing pituitary-dependent hyperadrenocorticism (PDH) (no shading) and another 12 dogs with pituitary pars intermedia tumors causing PDH (shaded values). No significant difference exists in the parameters from these two groups of dogs. Thus dogs cannot be classified regarding tumor location based on results of basal, post-ACTH, post low-dose dexamethasone (Post-LDDS) or post–high-dose dexamethasone (Post-HDDS) plasma cortisol concentrations. Plasma endogenous ACTH concentrations are also not significantly different between these two groups of dogs with pituitary-dependent Cushing's syndrome.

(when present) arise secondary to cortisol excess. The endocrine abnormalities in human pituitary-dependent Cushing's syndrome are (1) excess secretion of ACTH, with bilateral adrenocortical hyperplasia and hypercortisolemia; (2) absent circadian periodicity of ACTH and cortisol secretion; (3) absent responsiveness of ACTH and cortisol to stress (e.g., hypoglycemia or surgery); (4) abnormal negative feedback of ACTH secretion by glucocorticoids; and (5) subnormal responsiveness of growth hormone (GH), thyroid-stimulating hormone (TSH), and gonadotrophs to stimulation (Aron et al, 2001a).

Further evidence that pituitary Cushing's syndrome is a primary pituitary disorder is based on the high frequency of pituitary adenomas, the response to their removal (in people and dogs), and the interpretation of hypothalamic abnormalities as occurring secondary to hypercortisolemia. People and dogs in which pituitary tumors have been removed, with resolution of their condition, virtually never have a recurrence. Recurrences should be common if the underlying problem were hypothalamic, because regrowth of the tumors should occur. In addition, molecular studies have found that nearly all corticotroph adenomas are monoclonal (Gicquel et al, 1992; Biller, 1994; Faglia, 1994; Orth, 1995). These findings suggest that ACTH hypersecretion arises from a naturally developing pituitary adenoma and that the resulting hypercortisolism suppresses the normal hypothalamic-pituitary axis and CRH release, thereby abolishing hypothalamic regulation of ACTH and cortisol (Aron et al, 2001a).

The small number of dogs that have been claimed to have pituitary hyperplasia (which suggests a hypo-thalamic disorder that causes excessive stimulation of pituitary corticotrophs) remains rare or nonexistent. If pituitary hyperplasia exists, it has not been well documented in the literature. It is conceivable but unlikely that adenomas arise secondary to prolonged CNS stimulation of corticotrophs. It would be difficult for one hypothalamic disorder to account for tumors arising in either the pars distalis or the pars intermedia because regulation of the two lobes is so different.

Other support for the theory that pituitary Cushing's syndrome is a primary disorder in dogs can be traced to the results of various therapeutic trials that used agents directed at a hypothalamic disorder. In dogs, cyproheptadine, an antiserotonin agent, was therapeutically effective in only three of 24 dogs with PDH, and only one of the three was considered a complete treatment success (Drucker and Peterson, 1980; Stolp et al, 1984). Bromocriptine, a dopamine agonist, was successful in only one of seven dogs with PDH (Peterson, 1987). The dopamine agonists L-deprenyl and pergolide have failed to demonstrate efficacy in the treatment of dogs with pituitary Cushing's syndrome (Reusch et al, 1999; Tobin et al, 1998). Therefore the concept that such medications are safe and potentially effective, as has been suggested (Bruyette et al, 1997; Peterson, 1999), must be seriously questioned. It is safe to propose that PDH may result from several different physiopathogenic mechanisms but that a hypothalamic cause has not yet received strong scientific support.

EFFECT OF GLUCOCORTICOID EXCESS ON PITUITARY FUNCTION. In addition to its systemic effects, an excess of glucocorticoids also inhibits normal pituitary and hypothalamic function, including the release of TSH, GH, and gonadotropin (luteinizing hormone [LH] and follicle-stimulating hormone [FSH]). Inhibition of secretion of these trophic hormones results in reversible secondary hypothyroidism (TSH), failure to cycle in females or testicular atrophy in males (FSH and LH), and failure to grow in puppies (GH), as well as short stature in children.

Adrenal Tumor Hyperadrenocorticism (ATH)

Primary adrenocortical tumors, both adenomas and carcinomas, apparently develop autonomously. Functioning adrenocortical tumors secrete excessive amounts of cortisol independent of pituitary control. Thus the steroid products of these tumors suppress hypothalamic CRH and circulating plasma ACTH concentrations. Remaining POMC peptides (except α-MSH) are also suppressed by the negative feedback effects of the autonomously secreted glucocorticoids (Peterson et al, 1986). The result of this chronic negative feedback is cortical atrophy of the uninvolved adrenal and atrophy of all normal cells in the involved adrenal (see Fig. 6-6).

Little is known about the events leading to formation of adrenocortical tumors. Molecular defects, including activating mutations of receptors for corticotrophic factors, have been suspected as contributing to this process. Structural mutations of the corticotropin-receptor gene have not been detected in adrenocortical tumors (Reicke et al, 1997). However, some of these tumors have had gastric inhibitory polypeptide receptors, vasopressin receptors, receptors for β-adrenergic response and, more recently, receptors for immune cells and their cytokine products (Lacroix et al, 1997; Willenberg et al, 1998). For example, high local concentrations of interleukin-1 combined with aberrant expression of type I interleukin-1 receptors by a particular population of adrenocortical cells could have been followed by clonal expansion of those cells, thus providing a basis for tumor formation.

Cortisol secretion by adrenocortical tumors is episodic and random (see Fig. 6-7). However, most if not all of these tumors appear to retain ACTH receptors, because they respond to exogenous administration of ACTH by synthesizing and secreting cortisol. These adrenocortical tumors are typically unresponsive to manipulation of the hypothalamic-pituitary axis with pharmacologic agents such as dexamethasone. There have been no consistent clinical or biochemical features that aid in distinguishing dogs or cats with functioning adrenal adenomas from those with adrenal carcinomas. The only characteristic considered somewhat consistent is that adrenocortical carcinomas tend to be larger than adenomas (Reusch and Feldman, 1991).

Ectopic ACTH Syndrome

Ectopic ACTH syndrome has not yet been diagnosed in the dog. In humans it comprises a varying group of tumors that are capable of synthesizing and secreting ACTH, which in turn ultimately causes adrenocortical hyperplasia and hypercortisolism. Tumors with the potential for causing ectopic ACTH syndrome in humans include oat cell (small cell) carcinoma of the lung, thymoma, pancreatic islet cell tumors, carcinoid tumors (lung, gut, pancreas, and ovary), medullary carcinoma of the thyroid, pheochromocytoma, and pulmonary tumorlets (Arioglu et al, 1998; Aron et al, 2001b). When such tumors synthesize and secrete excessive amounts of biologically active ACTH, related β-LPH and β-endorphin peptides are also synthesized and secreted in excess, as are inactive ACTH fragments. CRH-like activity has also been demonstrated in ectopic tumors that secrete ACTH; however, secretion of CRH into plasma has not been demonstrated, and the role of tumor-derived CRH is unclear (Tyrrell et al, 1991; Bertagna, 1994; Becker and Aron, 1994).

Adrenocortical Nodular Hyperplasia

Macronodular hyperplasia of the adrenals occurs in about 20% of people with adrenocortical hyperplasia. Virtually all of these people are thought to have pituitary-dependent Cushing's disease. One or both adrenals are usually grossly enlarged and have multiple nodules of varying size in the cortex (Bertagna, 1992). Dogs and cats with bilateral adrenocortical nodular hyperplasia are also well recognized, accounting for 5% to 10% of hyperadrenocorticism cases. The exact pathogenesis of this syndrome is unclear, although, as in humans, virtually all these dogs and cats are presumed to represent an anatomic variant of PDH.

Rarely, humans have ACTH-*independent* bilateral nodular adrenocortical hyperplasia (Malchoff et al, 1989; Samuels and Loriaux, 1994). It is conceivable that some non-ACTH factor stimulates abnormal adrenocortical cells. On investigation, several humans with one subset of this syndrome had clinical features of hyperadrenocorticism, adrenocortical nodular hyperplasia, subnormal morning plasma cortisol concentrations, and suppressed responsiveness to exogenous ACTH (Lacroix et al, 1992; Reznik et al, 1992). Food intake stimulated cortisol secretion in these people (Hamet et al, 1987). Each showed inappropriate adrenocortical sensitivity to normal postprandial increases in the secretion of gastric inhibitory polypeptide (GIP). In view of the poor homology between GIP and ACTH, it was unlikely that the adrenocortical ACTH receptors were modified to bind GIP (Bertagna, 1992).

Unilateral versus Bilateral Adrenal Tumors

BILATERAL ADRENOCORTICAL TUMORS. Hyperadrenocorticism caused by bilateral adrenocortical neoplasia is rare in dogs. In four such dogs, three had bilateral adrenocortical adenomas and one had bilateral carcinomas. In a study of 15 dogs with Cushing's syndrome caused by functioning adrenocortical tumors, three (20%) had bilateral tumors (Hoerauf and Reusch, 1999). However, we believe that the incidence of bilateral adrenocortical tumors is far lower than is implied in the latter study. In such cases, the history, physical examination findings, clinicopathologic abnormalities, and results of ACTH stimulation and low-dose dexamethasone suppression tests should be compatible with a diagnosis of hyperadrenocorticism. Adrenocortical neoplasia can usually be differentiated from PDH by finding lack of plasma cortisol suppression after administration of a high dose of dexamethasone, undetectable endogenous ACTH concentrations, and identification of the adrenal masses on abdominal ultrasonography (Ford et al, 1993; Hoerauf and Reusch, 1999). A review of this condition is presented in the ultrasonography section of this chapter.

ADRENOCORTICAL TUMOR AND PHEOCHROMOCYTOMA. We have diagnosed several dogs with a pheochromocytoma (adrenal medullary tumor) in one adrenal and an *adrenocortical* tumor in the contralateral gland. This can be confusing, because ultrasonography may reveal bilateral adrenomegaly, and endocrine testing suggests an adrenocortical tumor (Von Dehn et al, 1995). This is a relatively uncommon, but not rare, condition. As adrenal ultrasonography continues to expand its role as a frequent and valuable diagnostic aid, these diagnoses likely will become more frequent. A review of this condition is presented in the ultrasonography section of this chapter.

Simultaneous Pituitary Tumor and Adrenal Cushing's Syndrome

Several dogs with both a functioning adrenocortical tumor and a pituitary microadenoma or macroadenoma (and bilateral adrenocortical hyperplasia) have been reported (Greco et al, 1999). Endocrine evaluation of such dogs has been diagnostic for hyperadrenocorticism. However, tests to distinguish between pituitary-dependent and adrenocortical tumor hyperadrenocorticism provide confusing or contradictory results. This must be considered an extremely rare condition. A review of this syndrome and its diagnosis and management is presented in the diagnosis section of this chapter.

PATHOLOGY

Pituitary

MICROADENOMAS. Eighty percent to 85% of dogs with naturally developing hyperadrenocorticism have pituitary-dependent disease. The reported incidence of histologically recognized pituitary tumors varies between 20% and 100% (Meijer, 1980; McNicol, 1987). Pituitary tumors in dogs, like those in humans, can be smaller than 1 mm in diameter. At the time of diagnosis, it is well documented that approximately 50% of dogs with pituitary Cushing's disease have tumors less than 3 mm in diameter. The remainder of evaluated dogs with PDH, specifically those without CNS signs, had tumors 3 to 12 mm in diameter (Bertoy et al, 1995). Recognition of some pituitary tumors requires careful microdissection, experience, special stains, and a great deal of patience. Because these criteria are not always met, the reported incidence of recognized pituitary tumors in dogs with PDH is underrepresented. Tumors larger than 3 mm in diameter should be grossly visible, easier to recognize, and more likely to be identified than the smaller masses.

Most ACTH-secreting pituitary tumors are defined as microadenomas because they are less than 1 cm in diameter (Aron et al, 2001a). They are not usually encapsulated but may be surrounded by a rim of compressed normal pituitary cells. With routine histologic stains, these tumors are typically composed of compact sheets of well-granulated basophilic cells in a sinusoidal arrangement. ACTH-secreting adenomas show Crooke's changes (a zone of perinuclear hyalinization that results from chronic exposure of corticotrope cells to hypercortisolism). Electron microscopy demonstrates secretory granules that vary in size from 200 to 700 nm. The number of granules varies in individual cells.

MACROADENOMAS. A significant percentage of dogs with PDH (at least 10% and more likely more than 20%) have large pituitary tumors (Duesberg et al, 1995). A macroadenoma is defined as a tumor visible on gross examination of the pituitary, or greater than 1 cm in diameter. These tumors have the potential to compress or invade adjacent structures as they expand dorsally beyond the confines of the sella turcica. The masses usually extend dorsally into the hypothalamus, often causing signs (see page 296). Because the canine sella turcica is shaped like a saucer rather than a cup (as in humans), bony destruction of the sella walls has not been observed in dogs with expanding tumors. Large, expanding masses need not contact bone to expand into the overlying structures of the brain. Such tumors may appear chromophobic on routine histologic study, but they typically contain ACTH and its related peptides. Malignant pituitary tumors occur but are uncommon.

PITUITARY HYPERPLASIA. Diffuse hyperplasia of corticotrope cells may occur. If so, it is extremely rare. Although such cases may result from excessive stimulation of the anterior pituitary by CRH, it is also possible that these histologic diagnoses are incorrect. Most dogs claimed to have pituitary hyperplasia also have pituitary tumors. The experience in humans is no different. With surgical removal of the tumor in afflicted humans, signs of hyperadrenocorticism typically resolve, negating the significance of histologically observed hyperplasia (Aron et al, 2001a). The presence of hyperplasia is important because the presence of hyperplasia secondary to a hypothalamic etiology of Cushing's syndrome is a controversial issue with significant financial implications regarding some medical therapies directed at correcting the hypothalamic disorder. If no hypothalamic disorder exists or if such disorders exist but are rare, use of these therapies should be discouraged. Such "controversial" drugs are not only expensive, they carry "expectations" that are unlikely to be fulfilled and could lead to owner frustration and euthanasia of pets that otherwise would be managed successfully (Braddock, 2002).

Adrenocortical Hyperplasia

TYPICAL BILATERAL HYPERPLASIA. This histologic diagnosis is made secondary to chronic ACTH hypersecretion associated with PDH. The combined adrenal weight is usually modestly increased. Histologically, there is equal hyperplasia of the compact cells of the zona reticularis and the clear cells of the zona fasciculata; consequently, the width of the cortex is increased. As previously discussed, the zona glomerulosa typically is normal in appearance. Electron microscopy reveals normal ultrastructural features (Aron et al, 2001b).

NODULAR HYPERPLASIA OF THE ADRENALS. As discussed in the section on physiopathology (see page 262), this is a poorly understood and uncommon finding in dogs or cats afflicted with hyperadrenocorticism. In humans with this disorder, the adrenals are enlarged, sometimes markedly. Grossly, multiple nodules are seen in the adrenal cortices, with widening of the intervening cortex. The nodules are typically yellow, and on histologic examination they resemble the clear cells of the normal zona fasciculata. The remainder of the adrenal cortices show the histologic features of simple adrenocortical hyperplasia. Long-standing ACTH hypersecretion, almost always associated with PDH, may cause this nodular, rather than the more common "diffuse," adrenocortical enlargement. In humans, dogs, and cats, these focal nodules may be visualized on ultrasound scans, computed tomography (CT) scans, or magnetic resonance imaging (MRI) scans. Once identified, they may be mistaken for adrenal neoplasms, an error that has led to unnecessary and unsuccessful unilateral adrenal surgery. In humans, removal of the ACTH-secreting pituitary tumor results in regression of the nodules and resolution of the hypercortisolism in almost all patients (Aron et al, 2001b). This syndrome probably accounts for at least a significant percentage of dogs and cats described as having both pituitary-dependent hyperadrenocorticism and an adrenocortical tumor.

Adrenal Tumors

PROBLEMS IN CLASSIFICATION. Histologic classification of endocrine tissue is known to be a challenge. It is not unusual for pathologists to have difficulty distinguishing between normal and hyperplastic tissue. It may also be difficult to distinguish diffuse hyperplasia from adenomatous hyperplasia (adenoma). Furthermore, it can be difficult to distinguish some adenomas from some carcinomas. It can also be challenging to distinguish an *adrenocortical* tumor from an adrenal *medullary* tumor (pheochromocytoma). Several dogs have been described as having an adrenocortical tumor

in one adrenal and a pheochromocytoma in the opposite adrenal, making both the clinical and pathologic diagnoses quite difficult (Von Dehn et al, 1995). For these reasons, excellent communication between clinician and pathologist, plus inclusion of laboratory and clinical impressions, may help the pathologist provide useful and correct information. New capabilities, including staining for specific hormones and cell types, have improved the diagnostic acumen of pathologists.

ADENOMAS. Adrenal adenomas are usually encapsulated, grossly visible, and range in size from 1 to 6 cm. They usually are equal to or less than 75% of the size of that dog's normal kidney. Microscopically, cells of the zona fasciculata predominate, although cells typical of the zona reticularis may also be seen. Approximately 50% of adrenocortical adenomas are partly calcified (Reusch and Feldman, 1991). Three dogs have been described with bilateral adrenocortical adenomas (Ford et al, 1993).

CARCINOMAS. Adrenal carcinomas can become quite large. They tend to be greater than 50% of the size of a normal kidney and are often equal in size to or larger than a normal kidney. Grossly, they may not be encapsulated, but they are highly vascular; necrosis, hemorrhage, and cystic degeneration are common. Partial calcification has been identified in approximately 50% of these masses (Reusch and Feldman, 1991). The histologic appearance of adrenocortical carcinomas varies considerably; they may appear to be benign, or they may exhibit considerable pleomorphism. Vascular or capsular invasion is predictive of malignant behavior, as is local extension. Adrenocortical carcinomas may invade local structures (kidney and/or its blood vessels, liver, vena cava, aorta, and retroperitoneum), or they may metastasize hematogenously to the liver and lungs. One dog has been described with bilateral adrenocortical carcinomas (Ford et al, 1993).

UNINVOLVED ADRENOCORTICAL TISSUE. The cortical tissue contiguous with a functioning adrenocortical adenoma or carcinoma and that of the contralateral gland are atrophic. Although the cortex of the opposite adrenal may be markedly thinned and the capsule thickened, the gland may yet be visualized with ultrasonography. This visualization can be explained in part by the remaining normal adrenal medullary and glomerulosa tissue, together with the ever-improving results of ultrasonography. Histologically, the zona reticularis is virtually absent, and the remaining cortex is composed of clear zona fasciculata cells. The architecture of the zona glomerulosa is usually normal.

SIGNALMENT

Age

Hyperadrenocorticism is a disease of middle-age and older dogs. It is generally agreed that almost all dogs with pituitary-dependent Cushing's syndrome (PDH) and those with functioning adrenocortical tumors are older than 6 years of age. More than 75% of dogs with

PDH are older than 9 years of age, and their median age is 11.4 years (Reusch and Feldman, 1991). The diagnosis of hyperadrenocorticism in any dog younger than 6 years of age must be viewed with skepticism, not because the diagnosis is incorrect, but because the condition is unusual in young dogs. Veterinarians, therefore, must be confident that their diagnosis is well documented before embarking on therapeutics. The differential diagnosis for hyperadrenocorticism should include disorders that have similar clinical or biochemical features (e.g., diabetes mellitus) and those that may cause cortisol excess (e.g., portosystemic shunts or iatrogenic Cushing's syndrome) (Sterczer et al, 1998). We have seen only five dogs with Cushing's syndrome younger than 2 years of age at the time of diagnosis (Figs. 6-9 and 6-10).

Dogs with hyperadrenocorticism caused by functioning adrenocortical tumors tend to be older than those with pituitary-dependent disease. Most of these dogs are 6 to 16 years of age at the time of diagnosis (Reusch and Feldman, 1991). The median age in dogs with adrenocortical tumors is 11.6 years, and more than 90% of dogs with this disease are older than 9 years of age.

Gender

Fifty-five percent to 60% of dogs with PDH are female, as are 60% to 65% of dogs with functioning adrenocortical tumors (Reusch and Feldman, 1991).

Breed/Body Weight

PITUITARY-DEPENDENT HYPERADRENOCORTICISM. Poodles (various Poodle breeds), Dachshunds, various Terrier breeds, Beagles, and German Shepherd dogs have been commonly represented among the breeds of dogs afflicted with PDH. The Boston Terrier

TABLE 6–2 DOG BREEDS MOST COMMONLY AFFLICTED WITH PITUITARY-DEPENDENT HYPERADRENOCORTICISM (TOTAL: 750 DOGS)

Percentage	Number	Breed
16%	119	Poodles (various breeds)
11%	84	Dachshunds
10%	76	Terriers (various breeds)
7%	54	Beagles
6%	48	German Shepherd dogs
5%	38	Labrador Retrievers
5%	36	Australian Shepherd
4%	30	Maltese
4%	28	Spaniel (various breeds)
3%	22	Schnauzer
3%	22	Lhasa Apso
2%	19	Chihuahua
2%	18	Boston Terrier
2%	15	Golden Retrievers
2%	14	Shih Tzu
2%	12	Boxer
16%	115	Other breeds (38 breeds)

and Boxer have been mentioned to be at increased risk. PDH has been diagnosed in virtually every breed (Table 6-2). Approximately 75% of dogs with PDH weigh less than 20 kg (Reusch and Feldman, 1991). This emphasizes the concept that PDH tends to occur more frequently in smaller dogs. In contrast, almost 50% of dogs with adrenocortical tumors weigh more than 20 kg.

ADRENAL-DEPENDENT HYPERADRENOCORTICISM. In our series of dogs with naturally occurring hyperadrenocorticism due to a functioning adrenocortical tumor, Toy Poodles (and other Poodle breeds), German Shepherd dogs, Dachshunds, Labrador Retrievers, and various Terrier breeds were most commonly represented (Table 6-3). Approximately 45% to 50% of dogs with functioning adrenocortical tumors weigh more than 20 kg. These body weight percentages are similar for both dogs with adrenocortical adenomas and those with carcinomas (Reusch and Feldman, 1991).

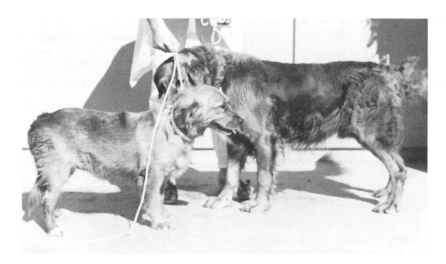

FIGURE 6–9. A 1-year-old dog with pituitary-dependent hyperadrenocorticism (left) and a normal adult. Note the short stature and immature hair coat in the young dog. (From Feldman EC: In Ettinger SJ [ed]: Textbook of Veterinary Internal Medicine, 2nd ed. Philadelphia, WB Saunders, 1983, p 1675.)

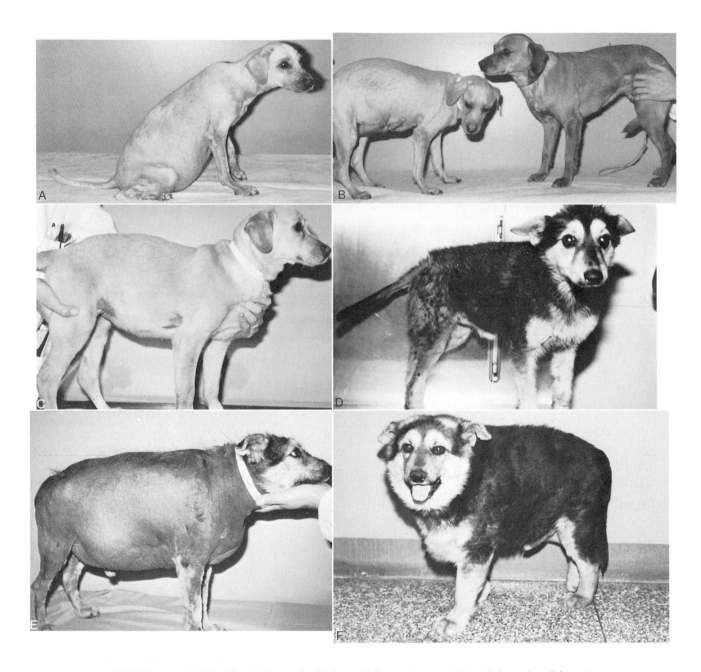

FIGURE 6–10. *A*, Mixed-breed 18-month-old dog with hyperadrenocorticism. *B*, Same dog *(left)* and a normal littermate. *C*, Same dog as in *A* 5 months after initiation of o,p'-DDD therapy. *D*, A 6-month-old German Shepherd dog with hyperadrenocorticism. *E*, Same dog as in *D* after 4 years without therapy. *F*, Same dog as in *D* and *E* 4 months after initiation of therapy with o,p'-DDD.

HISTORY

Items of Importance NOT in the History

Before embarking on a discussion of all the problems noted in dogs with hyperadrenocorticism, it may be valuable to review the problems these dogs do *not* have. Dogs with this syndrome are rarely believed to be critically or even seriously ill. Owners of these dogs almost never observe poor appetite, vomiting, diarrhea, coughing, sneezing, pain, seizures, or bleeding. The more than 2000 dogs in our series have almost never had pancreatitis, and the incidence of

renal failure is almost as unusual (Table 6-4). Most dogs with Cushing's syndrome have signs that progress slowly. Usually these are not problems of an acute nature or problems that frighten the owner.

General Review

ADULT-ONSET HYPERADRENOCORTICISM. Chronic exposure to excess cortisol often results in the development of a classic combination of clinical signs and lesions that can be subtle or dramatic. Many of the abnormalities we associate with excesses in plasma

TABLE 6–3 DOG BREEDS MOST COMMONLY AFFLICTED WITH FUNCTIONING ADRENOCORTICAL ADENOMA OR CARCINOMA CAUSING HYPERADRENOCORTICISM (TOTAL: 102 DOGS)

Percentage	Breed
15%	Poodles (various breeds)
12%	German Shepherd dogs
11%	Dachshunds
10%	Labrador Retrievers
8%	Terriers (various breeds)
5%	Cocker Spaniels
4%	Alaskan Malamute
4%	Boston Terrier
4%	Shih Tzu
3%	Boxer
3%	Shetland Sheepdog
3%	English Springer Spaniel
3%	Australian Shepherd
15%	Other breeds (12 breeds)

TABLE 6–4 PROBLEMS THAT DOGS WITH HYPERADRENOCORTICISM DO *NOT* HAVE

Poor appetite/anorexia
Vomiting
Diarrhea
Sneezing
Coughing
Icterus
Pruritus
Pain
Lameness due to inflammation
Seizures
Bleeding
Renal failure
Pancreatitis
Liver failure
Immune mediated diseases

TABLE 6–5 INITIAL HISTORY FOR DOGS WITH HYPERADRENOCORTICISM

Polydipsia/polyuria
Polyphagia
Abdominal enlargement
Decreased exercise tolerance (muscle weakness)
Increased respiratory rate or panting
Lethargy
Obesity
Alopecia (sparing head and distal extremities)
Calcinosis cutis
Anestrus
Testicular atrophy
Heat intolerance
Acne (skin infection, comedones)
Cutaneous hyperpigmentation
Exophthalmos

cortisol do create "dramatic" clinical signs. Among the common signs associated with cortisol excess (naturally occurring or iatrogenic) are polydipsia, polyuria, polyphagia, abdominal enlargement, alopecia, pyoderma, panting, muscle weakness, and lethargy. It must be remembered, however, that not all dogs with hyperadrenocorticism develop the same signs.

A small percentage of dogs with "Cushing's" have almost all described clinical signs. Most dogs, however, exhibit only one or several signs (Table 6-5). Hyperadrenocorticism is a *clinical* disorder, and animals with this disease have *some* associated clinical signs. The reason we emphasize this concept is that some veterinarians recommend treating dogs for Cushing's syndrome *before* clinical signs develop. Until this rationale is supported by peer-reviewed research, however, we believe such recommendations are inappropriate and dangerous. The primary reason for treating a dog for Cushing's syndrome is to resolve clinical signs. If a dog has no clinical signs, regardless of biochemical test results, Cushing's syndrome does not exist.

Signs result from the combined gluconeogenic, lipolytic, protein catabolic, antiinflammatory, and immunosuppressive effects of glucocorticoid hormones on various organ systems. The course of the disease is insidious and slowly progressive. Owners usually report observing some alterations typical of hyperadrenocorticism in their pet for 6 months to 6 years before the diagnosis is made. This amount of time elapses before owners seek veterinary attention for their pet because the abnormalities are usually quite gradual in onset and because most of the signs are believed to be simple "aging." Professional opinions are sought only when the signs become intolerable to the client or alterations are specifically pointed out by people who see the pet infrequently (and therefore objectively note obvious changes that have developed so slowly that the owners do not observe them). The most common reasons that owners give for finally seeking veterinary help for their dogs are usually polydipsia/polyuria, polyphagia, lethargy/panting, and/or hair coat changes. Uncommonly, clinical signs have been claimed to be intermittent, with periods of remission and relapse (Peterson et al, 1982b). This is a clinical phenomenon that we have not observed.

Occasionally, dogs with rapidly growing adrenocortical tumors and some with PDH may be reported by their owners to have rapid onset and progression of clinical signs. This situation is more likely the result of an owner not noticing changes for a period of time. Pets may compensate for some signs until this can no longer be accomplished or owners become aware and then realize that a problem is dramatic. The best example of this situation is a polyuric dog in which the problem goes unnoticed until the animal is no longer housebroken. Once the dog begins urinating in the home, it seems obvious, dramatic, and acute in onset to an owner. The polyuria is not truly acute in onset (in contrast to the polyuria in a diabetic). The duration of clinical signs and the type of signs noticed have not been reliable aids in distinguishing pituitary-dependent from adrenal-dependent hyperadrenocorticism.

HYPERADRENOCORTICISM IN YOUNG DOGS. This disease is most commonly diagnosed in dogs that are 6 to 8 years of age or older, with the mean age at the time of diagnosis being over 11 years. We have diagnosed only five dogs as having hyperadrenocorticism during the first 6 to 18 months of life (see Fig. 6-10). Young dogs have had growth retardation and abdominal enlargement in addition to the more typical signs (e.g., polyuria/polydipsia, alopecia). Children and adolescents, by comparison, also usually exhibit weight gain and growth retardation (Leinung and Zimmerman, 1994; Magiakou et al, 1994).

Polyuria and Polydipsia

Polyuria and polydipsia are extremely common signs associated with hyperadrenocorticism, and they are the most frequently cited reasons for an owner to bring a pet to the veterinarian. Actually, owners are not as concerned with polydipsia as they are with polyuria. As mentioned above, many previously housebroken animals are no longer able to go through the night without urinating. The pet pesters the owner to be let outside or urinates indoors, and the situation can quickly become intolerable for an owner. Polydipsia and polyuria have been documented in approximately 80% to 85% of dogs with CCS. Although there are many striking similarities between human and canine hyperadrenocorticism, polydipsia and polyuria are not typical clinical signs in people with cortisol excess.

Normal water intake for the average dog is less than 40 to 60 ml/kg of body weight per day. Owners usually report the water intake in their polydipsic, hyperadrenal pets to be two to 10 times normal. The cause of the polyuria remains obscure. Some investigators believe that it is the result of interference by cortisol with the action of antidiuretic hormone at the level of the renal collecting tubules (a form of nephrogenic diabetes insipidus). It has also been proposed that cortisol may increase the glomerular filtration rate, thus initiating a diuresis. It has been shown by one group of researchers that atrial natriuretic peptide is not a cause of the polyuria (Vollmar et al, 1991), although others have found that this peptide is increased in the serum of humans with Cushing's syndrome (Yamaji et al, 1988).

Our experience suggests that most (not all) dogs with polyuria and hyperadrenocorticism have a form of *central* diabetes insipidus (deficiency in antidiuretic hormone). These dogs often exhibit a positive response to administration of natural or, more recently, synthetic antidiuretic hormone, with a dramatic reduction in urine output and water intake. Therefore cortisol interference with release of antidiuretic hormone is the most plausible explanation for polyuria and polydipsia (Raff, 1987; Hughes, 1992). Direct compression of the posterior pituitary gland by an anterior pituitary tumor or compression of the hypothalamus or hypothalamic stalk is rarely the cause for diabetes insipidus, even in dogs with large pituitary tumors.

Polyphagia

Increased appetite is usually viewed by owners as a sign of health. However, polyphagia may be troublesome, because the dog with Cushing's syndrome may resort to stealing food, eating garbage, begging continuously, and occasionally aggressively attacking or protecting food. In most instances, however, the dog's continued excellent appetite, despite other abnormalities, convinces an owner that the pet is healthy and does not require veterinary attention. Increased appetite is assumed to be a direct effect of glucocorticoids, a unique effect in the dog. Polyphagia does not occur with cortisol excess in humans or cats. Polyphagia is present in more than 90% of dogs with Cushing's syndrome. The most common reason for a dog with Cushing's syndrome to have a poor appetite or anorexia would be a large pituitary tumor that compresses adjacent structures.

It is possible, but not common, for the glucocorticoid-induced antiinsulin effect to produce subclinical (sometimes overtly clinical) diabetes mellitus. This could result in an increased appetite as the dog attempts to compensate for "starvation." Our impression is that only about 5% of dogs with Cushing's syndrome have overt diabetes mellitus.

Abdominal Enlargement

The "potbellied" or pendulous abdominal profile in hyperadrenocorticism is a classic symptom in humans and is present in >80% of affected dogs. This sign is believed to be the cumulative result of increased weight of abdominal contents and decreased strength of the abdominal muscles due to the catabolic effects of cortisol. Part of the increased weight of the abdominal contents can be attributed to redistribution of fat from various storage areas to the omentum; part is due to hepatomegaly; and part is due to the sometimes overdistended urinary bladder.

The mechanism responsible for the redistribution of fat is not understood, but the result is a significant amount of abdominal fat deposition. When the weight of abdominal fat is added to the increased size and weight of the liver (secondary to cortisol's effect), the chronically full and large urinary bladder, and the muscle wasting that is a direct result of excess cortisol, a pendulous abdomen results. Urine accumulation is partly due to the increased volume produced (polyuria) and partly to a reduced ability to completely void a bladder weakened by cortisol's catabolic effect combined with the trained nature of most dogs not to urinate in the home. Protein catabolism accounts for muscle wasting and therefore muscle weakness. The abdominal muscles, weakened by glucocorticoid effects, simply cannot prevent bulging of the belly, as shown in Figs. 6-11 and 6-12.

Muscle Weakness, Lethargy, and Lameness

COMMON SIGNS. Muscle weakness, lethargy, and lameness are rarely major concerns to the owner. Hyperadrenal dogs are usually quite capable of rising from a prone position and of going for short walks.

Muscle weakness in small dogs is usually demonstrated by an inability to climb stairs, to jump onto furniture, or to jump into a car. Most dogs with these signs can descend stairs without hesitation and jump down from furniture or from a car. Many owners fail to even notice this phenomenon, perhaps thinking that their pet is spoiled, or they associate the problem with aging. Exercise tolerance is often reduced. Although dogs with hyperadrenocorticism can walk without problem, running may cause undue fatigue. Long walks are difficult for these dogs to complete. As with abdominal distention, muscle weakness is at least partly the result of muscle wasting caused by protein catabolism and has been noted in 75% to 85% of dogs with Cushing's syndrome. Lethargy is probably an expression of muscle weakness and muscle wasting. Hyperadrenal dogs are usually alert, but they are often not active. As mentioned before, this vague sign is certainly one that most owners attribute to simple aging.

MORE PROFOUND BUT LESS COMMON SIGNS. Infrequently, muscle weakness is so profound that dogs may not be capable of rising, may have difficulty standing for any length of time, and may develop decubital ulcers because they spend so much time down. Decubital ulcers are more common in large dogs with Cushing's syndrome, owing to their predisposition to remain recumbent in addition to the effect of their weight. Chronic hypercortisolism can result in an exaggeration of common problems such as anterior cruciate ligament rupture and patellar luxation lameness. One of our young dogs with Cushing's syndrome suffered a stress fracture across a tibial crest epiphysis, which had failed to close at a normal age (Fig. 6-13). Another dog suffered atraumatic rupture of both gastrocnemius muscles (Fig. 6-14), a problem that has also been seen with iatrogenic Cushing's disease (Rewerts et al, 1997).

LAMENESS DURING AND AFTER TREATMENT. Many older dogs suffer from chronic degenerative joint disease and arthritis. Hyperadrenocorticism may mask the signs related to these problems by inhibiting this inflammation. Successful management of Cushing's

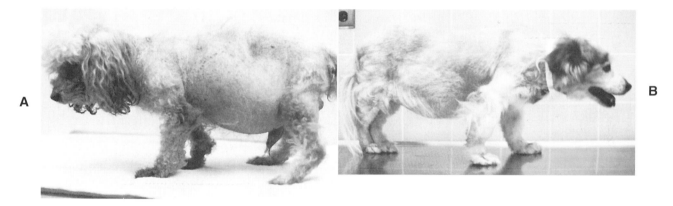

FIGURE 6–11. *A,* Poodle with pituitary-dependent hyperadrenocorticism, illustrating the potbellied appearance and diffuse alopecia sparing the head and distal extremities. *B,* This dog with pituitary-dependent hyperadrenocorticism illustrates the potbellied appearance seen in canine Cushing's syndrome (CCS). The dog's hair was clipped by the owner 1 year previously; note the lack of regrowth. (From Feldman EC: *In* Ettinger SJ [ed]: Textbook of Veterinary Internal Medicine, 2nd ed. Philadelphia, WB Saunders, 1983, p 1677.)

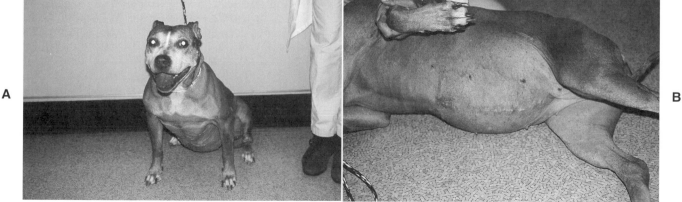

FIGURE 6–12. *A,* Dog with hyperadrenocorticism. *B,* Same dog as in *A* on its side, demonstrating potbelly typical of hyperadrenocorticism.

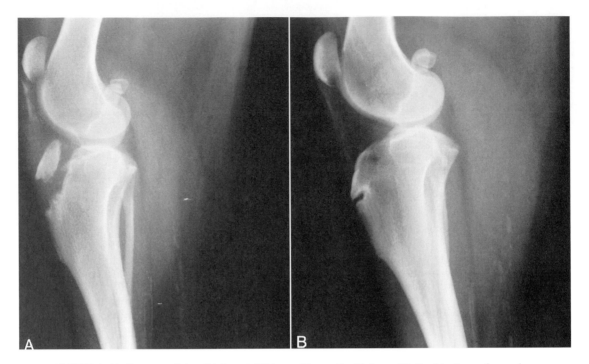

FIGURE 6–13. Fracture of the tibial crest *(A)* in an 18-month-old dog with Cushing's syndrome (see Fig. 6-10) with partially closed epiphyses. Hyperadrenocorticism delays epiphyseal closure in young dogs; note the normal stifle *(B)*.

syndrome has the potential for "unmasking" some of these occult, age-related joint diseases, and owners should be so warned prior to initiation of treatment.

Cutaneous Markers of Hyperadrenocorticism

ALOPECIA AND PRURITUS. The reported incidence of alopecia and other skin abnormalities in dogs with hyperadrenocorticism is affected by the interests of authors who publish on this subject. One group of

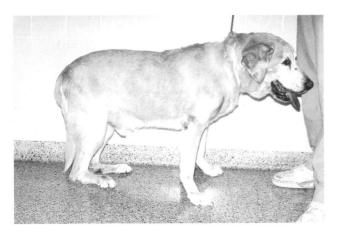

FIGURE 6–14. Dog with ruptured gastrocnemius muscles, a condition that may have occurred secondary to concurrent hyperadrenocorticism.

dermatologists described dermatologic signs in 100% of 60 dogs with hyperadrenocorticism, with 80% of the dogs having some form of alopecia and 25% described as pruritic owing to seborrhea, calcinosis cutis, demodicosis, or pyoderma (White et al, 1989). Internists note that some hyperadrenal dogs have no apparent dermatologic signs (Peterson, 1984; Reusch and Feldman, 1991). In any case, cutaneous signs are common and are usually *not* associated with pruritus.

The hair loss associated with Cushing's syndrome is a common owner concern. This is a slow and progressive problem that may begin with hair loss at points of wear (e.g., bony prominences) and eventually may involve the flanks, perineum, and abdomen. The result (Fig. 6-15) is severe alopecia, with only the head and distal extremities retaining a coat. The pinnae and the base of the ears may be alopecic, especially in the Dachshund. Atrophy of hair follicles and the pilosebaceous apparatus, with keratin accumulation in the atrophic hair follicle, is common.

"Endocrine alopecia" may be associated with thyroid, ovarian, testicular, and growth hormone disturbances, as well as with hypercortisolism (see Chapter 2). Each of these disorders, especially hyperadrenocorticism, has the potential to cause a bilaterally symmetric alopecia, which may be severe (see Fig. 6-15) or mild (Fig. 6-16) or may involve a poor and abnormal hair coat (Figs. 6-17 and 6-18). Bilaterally symmetric alopecia has also been noted in cats with Cushing's syndrome (Fig. 6-19), although this dermatologic abnormality is less common than in dogs. The alopecia

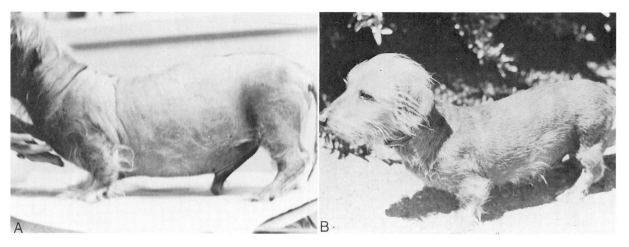

FIGURE 6–15. *A,* Dachshund with pituitary-dependent hyperadrenocorticism (PDH) showing severe, bilaterally symmetric alopecia. *B,* Same dog as in *A* 2 months after therapy with o,p'-DDD. (From Feldman EC: *In* Ettinger SJ [ed]: Textbook of Veterinary Internal Medicine, 2nd ed. Philadelphia, WB Saunders, 1983, p 1677.)

is not always bilaterally symmetric and may not involve the trunk.

FAILURE TO REGROW SHAVED HAIR. Atrophy of the hair follicles disrupts the attachment of the hair shaft to the follicle, causing hair loss and lack of hair regrowth. If the hair is shaved, regrowth is poor or nonexistent (see Figs. 6-11, *B,* and 6-18), and any new hair is brittle, sparse, and fine.

THIN SKIN, PYODERMA, SEBORRHEA, AND DEMODICOSIS. Thin skin, poor healing (Fig. 6-20), and susceptibility to infection are typical of hypercortisolism in dogs and cats. The skin of these animals is thin and easily wrinkled. Sometimes the subcutaneous blood vessels can be easily visualized. In addition, keratin-plugged follicles (comedones) are often found around the nipples and along the dorsal midline, although they may be present anywhere on the trunk. Pyoderma has been observed in as many as 55% of hyperadrenal dogs. Skin infection is especially common along the dorsal midline. At times it may be severe and may be worse in areas of hyperpigmentation. The suppressed immune system associated with hyperadrenocorticism exaggerates the problem.

Adult-onset demodicosis has been associated with coexistent iatrogenic and naturally occurring hypercortisolism. This condition is not common in adult

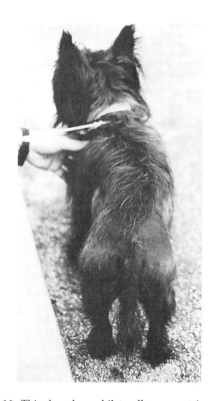

FIGURE 6–16. This dog shows bilaterally symmetric alopecia and hyperpigmentation of the flanks and thighs. (From Feldman EC: *In* Ettinger SJ [ed]: Textbook of Veterinary Internal Medicine, 2nd ed. Philadelphia, WB Saunders, 1983, p 1677.)

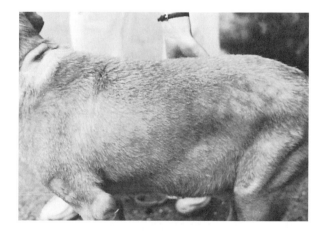

FIGURE 6–17. Labrador Retriever, which had hyperadrenocorticism caused by a functioning adrenal tumor, showing alopecia and a poor hair coat secondary to hyperadrenocorticism. Note the potbelly as well. (From Feldman EC: *In* Ettinger SJ [ed]: Textbook of Veterinary Internal Medicine, 2nd ed. Philadelphia, WB Saunders, 1983, p 1678.)

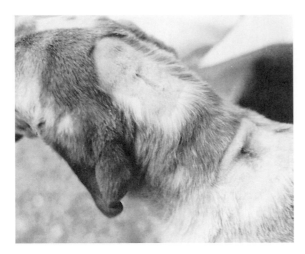

FIGURE 6–18. Close-up of the dog in Fig. 6-17. The area shown had been shaved 8 months earlier by the referring veterinarian prior to removal of a small skin tumor. Note the failure of the hair to grow back, as well as the obvious scars from the surgeries. These scars are the result of poor wound healing, with resultant "striae" formation. (From Feldman EC: *In* Ettinger SJ [ed]: Textbook of Veterinary Internal Medicine, 2nd ed. Philadelphia, WB Saunders, 1983, p 1679.)

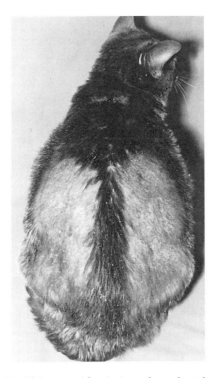

FIGURE 6–19. This cat with pituitary-dependent hyperadrenocorticism shows an unusual pattern (in cats) of bilaterally symmetric alopecia.

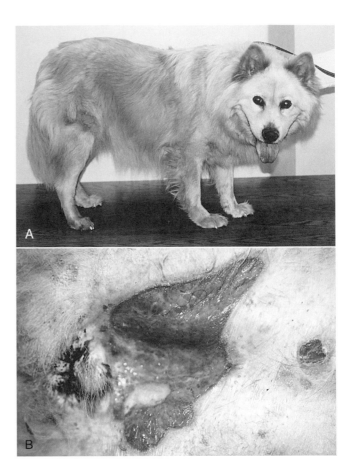

FIGURE 6–20. *A,* An 8-year-old mixed-breed dog that had been chronically treated with glucocorticoids. *B,* Open, nonhealing wounds on the ventral abdomen. The nonhealing nature of these wounds was likely secondary to the effects of chronic glucocorticoid therapy.

dogs and is uncommon to rare in dogs with Cushing's syndrome. However, one of the causes of this condition is immunosuppression, such as would occur with certain anticancer treatments and with cortisol excess. Therefore if an adult dog is diagnosed with *Demodex* infestation, it would be prudent to determine if any signs of Cushing's syndrome are present (Hillier and Deusch, 2002).

In one report, thin skin was observed in 13% of hyperadrenal dogs. More than 33% of dogs had a form of seborrhea, and comedones were observed in 5% (White et al, 1989). As previously discussed, many of the larger breed dogs with muscle weakness spend much of their time lying down, and these dogs tend to develop decubital ulcers, which are often infected and usually heal quite slowly if at all. Management of these lesions requires treatment of the Cushing's syndrome and diligent cleaning, as well as the use of soft bedding to minimize further trauma.

BRUISING, REDUCED SUBCUTANEOUS FAT, AND STRIAE. The fragility observed with thin skin is also present in the blood vessels. Excessive bruising can follow venipuncture (Fig. 6-21) or other minor trauma. We have had a number of dogs that underwent ovariohysterectomy years before developing Cushing's syndrome, only to have the metal sutures in the ventral midline begin to cause bruising after the dogs developed hyperadrenocorticism (Fig. 6-22, *A* and *B*). These abnormalities are worsened by the decrease in subcutaneous tissue that occurs secondary to Cushing's syndrome. Wounds that heal do so tenuously, with fragile, thin scar tissue equivalent to the striae seen in

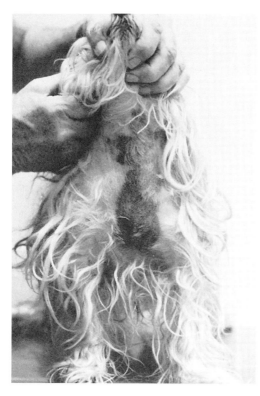

FIGURE 6–21. This dog with hyperadrenocorticism had two blood samples obtained from the jugular vein. The bruising was obvious 2 hours later. (From Feldman EC: *In* Ettinger SJ [ed]: Textbook of Veterinary Internal Medicine, 2nd ed. Philadelphia, WB Saunders, 1983, p 1679.)

humans (Fig. 6-22, *C*). Healing skin lesions often are subject to dehiscence because of the limited amount of fibrous tissue present.

CALCINOSIS CUTIS AND CUTANEOUS METAPLASTIC OSSIFICATION. Calcium deposition in the dermis and subcutis is an uncommon but well-described sign associated with canine Cushing's syndrome. On examination these areas may feel like firm, irregular plaques in or under the skin, almost as if bone were replacing normal skin or subcutaneous tissue. The common locations for this calcium deposition (called *calcinosis cutis*) are the temporal area of the head and the dorsal midline, neck, ventral abdominal, and inguinal areas (Fig. 6-23). Calcinosis cutis is characterized by dystrophic calcium deposition. The mechanisms of this process are not completely understood, but they involve phase transformation of calcium and phosphate ions from solution into crystalline aggregate with deposition in matrices of dermal collagen and elastin. A similar dermatologic condition in humans, known as metaplastic ossification, is characterized by metaplastic osteoid formation in the dermis.

Two dogs with cutaneous metaplastic ossification secondary to iatrogenic Cushing's syndrome have been described. Osseous metaplasia may represent a distinct syndrome or a variant of calcinosis cutis. One of the two dogs had areas of collagen mineralization (calcinosis cutis) that were superficial and separate

from deeper areas of osseous metaplasia. Both dogs had skin biopsies and later necropsies, which revealed multifocal spicules of osteoid or mineralized lamellar bone lined by osteoblasts and occasional osteoclasts. Some of these dermal osseous foci contained centrally located bone marrow elements or haversian canals containing blood vessels (Frazier et al, 1998).

Obesity

Owners of hyperadrenal dogs usually comment on their pet's apparent "weight gain." In fact, dogs with hyperadrenocorticism do not usually gain a large amount of weight. Rather, most have fat redistribution, as mentioned previously, and a potbellied appearance, which exaggerates the appearance of weight gain. Truncal obesity is a classic symptom of Cushing's syndrome (see Figs. 6-11, 6-12, and 6-15). In dogs and humans, this truncal obesity appears to occur at the expense of muscle and fat wasting from the extremities and subcutaneous stores; true obesity is present in less than half the dogs.

Respiratory Signs

PANTING
Differential Diagnosis. Dogs with hyperadrenocorticism are often noted to be short of breath or to have a rapid respiratory rate at rest (tachypnea). There are several explanations for these signs. One of the simple and logical propositions is based on the concept that dogs with Cushing's syndrome have increased fat deposition over the thorax, muscle wasting, and weakness of the muscles involved in respiration. Any or all these factors could contribute to tachypnea. The increased pressure placed on the diaphragm with fat accumulation in the abdomen, plus hepatomegaly, further accentuates disturbances in ventilatory mechanics. Coughing, however, is not a common owner complaint. Other causes include pulmonary interstitial mineralization, interstitial lung disease, and thromboembolism.

Signs of mild respiratory distress are believed to be exaggerated by a marked reduction in expiratory reserve volume and decreased chest wall compliance, which increase the work of breathing. If such a dog also has a collapsing trachea (a common problem in the smaller breeds), the combination of expiratory distress associated with the tracheal problem and the increased weight of abdominal contents pressing on the diaphragm can cause marked respiratory signs. Similar problems can easily be appreciated if the "potbellied" dog also has chronic mitral and/or tricuspid valvular disease. Signs are further exaggerated by the stress of excitement or exercise. The veterinary literature has alluded to a syndrome of marked obesity, alveolar hypoventilation, cyanosis, secondary polycythemia, and heart failure. In humans, this condition is called pickwickian syndrome, and changes

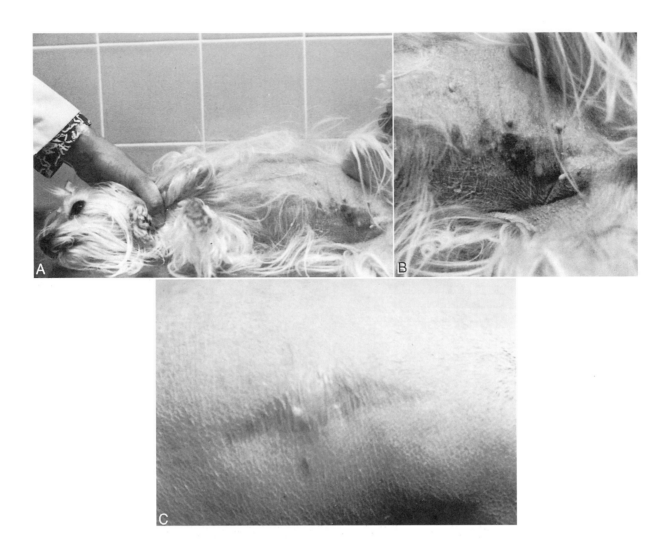

FIGURE 6–22. *A,* Bruising in the area of an ovariohysterectomy incision. This dog had had surgery 9 years earlier, but the bruising began 8.5 years later. *B,* Close-up of the bruising shown in A caused by metal sutures and a decrease in subcutaneous fat that normally "pads" the sutures. *C,* Thin, fragile, healed incision, typical of the poor healing process in a dog with hyperadrenocorticism. This fragile tissue is similar to striae in humans.

consistent with this syndrome are common in dogs with Cushing's syndrome.

Pulmonary Scintigraphy. Pulmonary interstitial mineralization can be detected microscopically in more than 90% of dogs with naturally occurring Cushing's syndrome. Four dogs with Cushing's syndrome had pulmonary mineralization based on thoracic radiographic changes or delayed bone phase scintigraphy on perfusion scans (Berry et al, 1994). Changes in the pulmonary interstitial connective tissue induced by persistent excesses in plasma cortisol were postulated to result in dystrophic mineralization, causing a diffusion impairment to blood oxygenation.

In a subsequent study, 21 dogs with PDH were evaluated with radiographs, blood gas analysis, and two different types of pulmonary scintigraphy scans (Berry et al 2000). Seven of the 21 dogs were documented to be hypoxemic. Fifteen of the 21 dogs had radiographic evidence of bronchial mineralization, and moderate to severe generalized interstitial lung

patterns were detected in six of the 21 dogs. Two of the six dogs were among the hypoxemic group and had severe interstitial pulmonary opacities consistent with pulmonary mineralization. Mineralization, therefore, may contribute to hypoxemia in some dogs with PDH.

THROMBOEMBOLISM. Thromboembolism is a recognized problem in humans and dogs with Cushing's syndrome (Burns et al, 1981; Small et al, 1983; Dennis, 1993). Dogs with pulmonary thromboembolism may have chronic signs or may develop acute, severe respiratory distress. The pathogenesis and treatment are described on page 293.

Testicular Atrophy in Males and Failure to Cycle in Females

Male dogs with Cushing's syndrome usually have bilaterally small, soft, spongy testicles. The female dog with Cushing's syndrome commonly ceases estrous

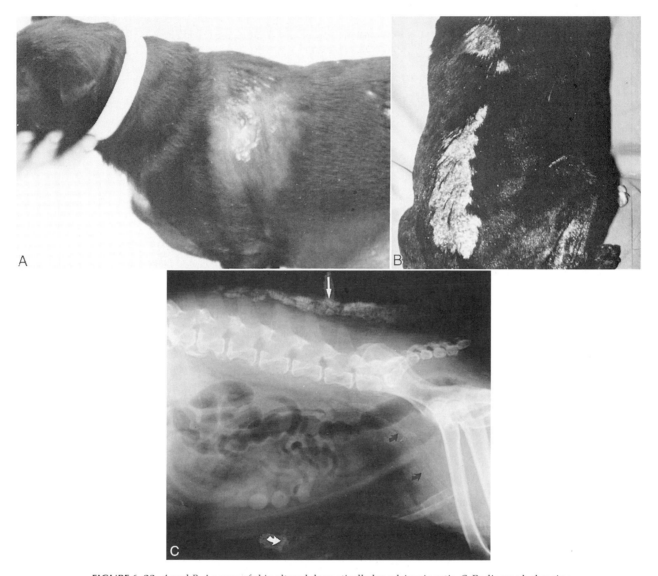

FIGURE 6–23. *A* and *B,* An area of skin altered dramatically by calcinosis cutis. *C,* Radiograph showing dorsal midline (*straight arrow*) and preputial (*curved white arrow*) calcinosis cutis, as well as calcified femoral arteries (*curved black arrows*).

cycle activity. Often the length of anestrus reflects the duration of hypercortisolism. Owner concerns related to the reproductive tract are extremely unusual, because so many pets are old, neutered, or both. If the pet is "intact," the owner is either unaware of the problem or associates the mentioned changes with age. Reproductive problems are discussed in greater detail in the physical examination section (page 277).

Myotonia (Pseudomyotonia)

Rarely, dogs with hyperadrenocorticism develop a distinct myopathy characterized by persistent, active muscle contraction after cessation of voluntary effort (this has been noted in eight of the more than 2000 dogs we have seen with Cushing's syndrome). Historically, these dogs have had a stiff gait (especially in the pelvic limbs), which coincides with develop-

ment of the other signs of Cushing's syndrome. One of our dogs could not ambulate at all with its rear legs (Fig. 6-24). Pelvic limb muscle stiffness is obvious on physical examination. Myotonic, bizarre, high-frequency discharges are noted on electromyography. Histologic, electron microscopic, and histochemical findings in the musculature of several dogs with "Cushing's myotonia" were characteristic of non-inflammatory degenerative myopathy. Clinical response to resolution of Cushing's syndrome is not predictable. The cause for this unusual phenomenon in hyperadrenocorticism is not known.

Facial Paralysis

Relatively infrequently, dogs with Cushing's syndrome have unilateral or bilateral facial nerve paralysis. This problem is not understood. The remaining

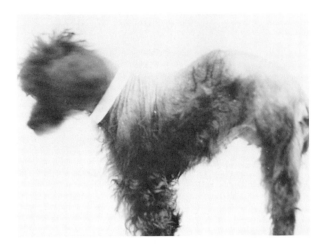

FIGURE 6–24. This 11-year-old dog had hyperadrenocorticism and pseudomyotonia, resulting in extreme rigidity of the pelvic limbs and inability to walk.

neurologic problems are reviewed in the section on central nervous system signs (page 296).

PHYSICAL EXAMINATION

General Review

The physical examination for a typical "Cushing's dog" reveals an animal that is stable and hydrated, has good mucous membrane color, and is not in distress. Veterinarians typically observe many of the signs seen by owners on physical examination of dogs with hyperadrenocorticism. Among these abnormalities are abdominal enlargement, panting, truncal obesity, bilaterally symmetric alopecia, skin infections, and comedones (hair follicles filled with keratin and debris, usually black in color and easily expressed). Changes noted specifically on examination that an owner would not usually mention might include hyperpigmentation, testicular atrophy, and hepatomegaly. Ectopic calcification, clitoral hypertrophy, and easy bruisability are much less common (Table 6-6). Remarkable variation exists in the number and severity of these signs. These dogs may have a single dominant sign or 10 signs.

Hyperpigmentation

Hyperpigmentation may be diffuse or focal (see Figs. 6-10, *E*, and 6-15, *A*). Histologically, increased numbers of melanocytes are found in the stratum corneum, basal epidermis, and dermal tissues. Because hyperpigmentation has been observed in dogs with either pituitary or adrenal causes of Cushing's syndrome, the likelihood that excess secretion of α-MSH as a byproduct of ACTH production (see Fig. 6-2) is the sole cause of hyperpigmentation would not be strongly supported (Aron et al, 2001a).

TABLE 6–6 PHYSICAL EXAMINATION FINDINGS IN DOGS WITH HYPERADRENOCORTICISM

Thin skin
Bilaterally symmetrical alopecia
Acne (skin infection, comedones)
Cutaneous hyperpigmentation
Calcinosis cutis
Abdominal enlargement
Muscle wasting of extremities
Hepatomegaly
Panting
Bruising
Exophthalmos
Testicular atrophy
Clitoral hypertrophy

Hepatomegaly

An enlarged liver, a classic sign with canine hyperadrenocorticism, contributes to any abdominal enlargement. The liver is typically swollen, large, pale, and friable. Hepatomegaly is easily palpated because of the weak abdominal muscles. The liver may be so large in some dogs that veterinarians may suspect an abdominal mass. In addition to detection of liver enlargement on the physical examination, hepatomegaly is typically documented radiographically or with abdominal ultrasonography. If a dog thought to have Cushing's syndrome does not have hepatomegaly or if the liver is small, another condition or a serious concurrent disease (e.g., a portovascular anomaly) should be suspected (Sterczer et al, 1998).

The histologic alterations seen on liver biopsy from dogs with naturally occurring or iatrogenic excesses in glucocorticoids are quite consistent. When this group of histologic alterations is present, few differential diagnoses other than steroid excess are likely. These changes include centrilobular hepatocytic vacuolation with a few, often single, large vacuoles that displace the nucleus of cells to the periphery. Hepatocellular glycogen accumulation is concentrated in periportal hepatocytes. Lipid deposits are not demonstrable with Sudan III stains. Hepatocellular necrosis, although present, is not a significant feature (Badylak and Van Vleet, 1981). Hepatic ultrastructural studies from dogs with "steroid hepatopathy" demonstrate progressive alterations to plasma membranes and other subcellular organelles, abundant glycogen accumulation, and few mitochondria in hepatocytes (Rutgers et al, 1955; Badylak and Van Vleet, 1982). Hepatic vacuolization alone can be caused by a variety of problems. "Steroid hepatopathy" does imply chronic elevation in circulating glucocorticoids. Not all dogs with Cushing's syndrome have steroid hepatopathy.

Testicular Atrophy, Anestrus, and Clitoral Hypertrophy

BACKGROUND. The direct biologic activity of the adrenal androgens (androstenedione, dehydroepiandrosterone [DHEA], and DHEA-sulfate) is usually minimal. These androgens function primarily as precursors for peripheral conversion to the active androgenic hormones testosterone and dihydrotestosterone. DHEA-sulfate secreted by the adrenal gland undergoes limited conversion to DHEA. Peripherally converted DHEA, plus that secreted by the adrenal cortex, can be further converted in peripheral tissues to androstenedione, which is the immediate precursor of active androgens (Aron et al, 2001b).

MALES. The negative feedback effects of hypercortisolism result in decreased secretion of pituitary gonadotropin (FSH and LH) (Meij et al, 1997a and 1997c). This explains the testicular atrophy, decreased libido, and depressed plasma testosterone concentrations typically seen in male dogs. Testicular androgen secretion is reduced, whereas adrenal androgen secretion is increased. However, conversion of adrenal androstenedione to testosterone accounts for less than 5% of the production rate of testosterone. Thus the physiologic effect of *adrenal* androgens is negligible in males, whereas the reduction in *testicular* androgen is significant. The final result is "feminization" of affected males. In one study, the plasma testosterone concentration averaged 4.7 ng/ml in normal males, compared with the significantly lower 1.2 ng/ml in male dogs with Cushing's syndrome (Feldman and Tyrrell, 1982).

FEMALES. In females, negative feedback effects of hypercortisolism decrease pituitary secretion of the same gonadotropins as in males. This causes suppression of normal ovarian function and prolonged anestrus. Dogs with PDH also have hyperprolactinemia (Meij et al, 1997a and 1997c). Excess prolactinemia was demonstrated to occur independent of excesses in plasma cortisol and probably contributes to the suppressed ovarian function in females. Ovarian androgen production is normal, but the adrenal gland substantially contributes to total androgen production in females. Abnormal adrenal function in Cushing's syndrome results in excessive secretion of adrenal androgens, and peripheral conversion of these androgens results in clinical androgen excess (virilization) in females. A small number of these dogs have clitoral hypertrophy, and one was described as having perianal adenomas and hypertestosteronemia secondary to hyperadrenocorticism (Dow et al, 1988). The average plasma testosterone concentration in normal female dogs was 20 pg/ml, whereas in females with CCS it was 30 pg/ml, a significant increase (Feldman and Tyrrell, 1982).

Ectopic Calcification

In addition to hyperadrenocorticism causing calcinosis cutis (see page 273), ectopic calcification may also involve the tracheal rings and bronchial walls (see Respiratory Signs, page 273), the kidneys and, rarely, the major arteries and veins of the body (Fig. 6-23, C). Ectopic calcification may be noted only histologically in some dogs but occasionally is visible radiographically or by ultrasonography. Calcific band keratopathy, a syndrome characterized by a grey-white superficial corneal opacity horizontally oriented in the interpalpebral opening, was reported in two dogs with hyperadrenocorticism (Ward et al, 1989).

Bruisability

Easy bruisability is one of the "classic" problems in people with Cushing's syndrome. It is not frequently observed in dogs, but it may be noted after venipuncture or any trauma (see Figs. 6-21 and 6-22). This problem reflects the poor wound healing associated with suppressed tissue granulation secondary to glucocorticoid excess (see Fig. 6-20 and Cutaneous Markers of Hyperadrenocorticism, page 270).

Sudden Acquired Retinal Degeneration Syndrome (SARDS)

SARDS is a retinal disorder of unknown cause that produces sudden and permanent blindness in adult dogs. The syndrome is characterized by noninflammatory degeneration and loss of retinal photoreceptors. An association has been suggested between SARDS and hyperadrenocorticism (Mattson et al, 1992). A series of 44 dogs with SARDS diagnosed during a 9-year period (1990 through 1998) were evaluated at our hospital. Sixteen of the dogs had at least one abnormality on the history, physical examination, or serum biochemistry profile consistent with Cushing's syndrome. Of those 16 dogs, eight (18% of the 44 total) had at least one endocrine screening test result consistent with Cushing's syndrome (Holt et al, 1999). It is possible that acute blindness causes some dogs to drink or eat excessively and that no link exists between these two conditions. Regardless, our results suggest that owners of dogs with SARDS be carefully questioned about signs of Cushing's syndrome and that a urinalysis and serum biochemical profile be performed on these dogs.

Acute Weakness Due to Nontraumatic Rupture of an Adrenal Mass

Nontraumatic rupture of an adrenal tumor is rare. In four dogs in which this occurred, each had acute development of severe lethargy, weakness, and pale mucous membranes. Signs of abdominal pain were detected during the physical examination. Two of the four dogs had adrenocortical carcinomas, and one of the two had a vague history consistent with hyperadrenocorticism prior to developing acute signs. Each dog had acute intraabdominal or retroperitoneal hemorrhage, required immediate supportive therapy, and then had emergency exploratory abdominal surgery (Whittemore et al, 2001). Although this scenario is rare, it is one of the few situations (along with pulmonary thromboembolism) in which a dog with Cushing's syndrome may develop an acute, life-threatening illness.

"ROUTINE" BLOOD AND URINE EVALUATIONS

General Approach

Any dog suspected of having hyperadrenocorticism (CCS) should be thoroughly evaluated before specific endocrine procedures are undertaken. Suspicion of CCS should always be based on the history and physical examination. Once a suspicion exists, each dog should undergo tests that should include clinicopathologic studies (complete blood count [CBC], urinalysis with culture, and a serum chemistry profile that includes liver enzymes, renal function tests, calcium, phosphorus, sodium, potassium, cholesterol, blood glucose, total plasma protein, plasma albumin, and total bilirubin). In addition to blood and urine testing, abdominal ultrasonography (preferred over radiography) should be performed.

If a large percentage of abnormalities consistent with Cushing's syndrome are seen in the initial screening test results, the veterinarian can make a presumptive diagnosis (Table 6-7). The more expensive and sophisticated studies needed to confirm a diagnosis and localize the cause of the syndrome can then be recommended to the client. The initial results not only ensure that the veterinarian is pursuing the correct diagnosis, they also might alert the clinician to any concomitant medical problems. These problems may be common for hyperadrenocorticism (urinary tract infection) or unexpected (congestive heart failure) but in any case should not be ignored.

Complete Blood Count (CBC)

Excessive production of cortisol results in neutrophilia and monocytosis due to steroid-enhanced capillary demargination of these cells and to the subsequent prevention of normal egress of cells from the circulation. Lymphopenia is most likely the result of steroid lympholysis, and eosinopenia results from bone marrow sequestration of eosinophils. These changes in the white blood cell differential are called a *stress response*. Approximately 80% of hyperadrenal dogs have reduced lymphocyte and eosinophil counts, and 20% to 25% have mild increases in total white blood cell numbers. The red blood cell count is usually normal, although mild polycythemia may occasionally be noted, owing to the previously described ventilatory problems or, in females, to androgenic stimulation of the bone marrow. Many dogs with CCS have increased platelet counts on CBC, some in

TABLE 6–7 HEMATOLOGIC, SERUM BIOCHEMICAL, URINE, AND RADIOGRAPHIC ABNORMALITIES TYPICAL OF HYPERADRENOCORTICISM*

Test	Abnormality
Complete blood count	Mature leukocytosis
	Neutrophilia
	Lymphopenia
	Eosinopenia
	Erythrocytosis; mild (females)
Serum chemistries	Increased alkaline phosphatase (sometimes extremely elevated)
	Increased ALT (SGPT)
	Increased cholesterol
	Increased fasting blood glucose
	Increased or normal insulin
	Abnormal bile acids
	Decreased BUN
	Lipemia
Urinalysis	Urine specific gravity <1.015, often <1.008
	Urinary tract infection
	Glycosuria (<10% of cases)
Radiography/ultrasonography	Hepatomegaly
	Excellent abdominal contrast
	Potbelly
	Distended bladder
	Osteoporosis
	Calcinosis cutis/dystrophic calcification
	Adrenal calcification (usually adrenal tumor)
	Congestive heart failure (rare)
	Pulmonary thromboembolism (rare)
	Calcified trachea and main stem bronchi
	Pulmonary metastasis of adrenal carcinoma
Miscellaneous	Low T_4/T_3 concentrations
	Response to TSH that parallels normal but both "pre" and "post" values may be decreased
	Hypertension

*It would be unusual for an individual animal to have all these abnormalities.

excess of 500,000 × $10^3/\mu l$. The significance of this thrombocytosis is unknown.

Blood Glucose and Serum Insulin

Glucocorticoids increase hepatic gluconeogenesis, increase blood glucose concentrations, and decrease peripheral utilization of glucose by antagonizing the effects of insulin. Dogs with hyperadrenocorticism, therefore, typically have mild increases in fasting plasma glucose concentrations that are not clinically worrisome. Modest antagonism of insulin with mild hyperglycemia is easily demonstrated physiologically by assessment of glycosylated hemoglobin concentrations. The amount of hemoglobin that becomes glycosylated correlates with mean blood glucose concentrations over time, and these values have been shown to be increased in dogs with naturally developing Cushing's syndrome that do not have overt diabetes mellitus (Elliott et al, 1997).

A small percentage of dogs with Cushing's syndrome have overt diabetes mellitus. Glycosuria occurs if the renal threshold for resorption of glucose (180 to 220 mg/dl) is exceeded. Comparisons have been made between fasted normal dogs and nondiabetic dogs with Cushing's syndrome (those without glucose in their urine). The mean morning serum insulin concentration in normal dogs was 12 μU/ml, whereas it was 38 μU/ml in the dogs with naturally developing hyperadrenocorticism. Plasma glucose concentrations averaged 85 mg/dl in the normal dogs and 111 mg/dl in the hyperadrenal dogs (Feldman and Tyrrell, 1982).

A subsequent study supported these findings with plasma C-peptide concentrations evaluated in dogs with Cushing's syndrome. C-peptide is the "connecting" peptide that joins insulin's two chains of amino acids during synthesis. Because C-peptide is part of the prohormone of insulin, it is synthesized and released simultaneously with insulin in equimolar amounts by pancreatic β-cells. In eight dogs with Cushing's syndrome, intravenous glucagon administration caused abnormal increases in blood glucose, plasma C-peptide, and serum insulin concentrations (Montgomery et al, 1996). These findings underscore the concept that the chronic excesses in circulating cortisol that cause CCS create a "prediabetic state" in dogs. In most dogs with Cushing's syndrome, the increased secretion of insulin partly controls carbohydrate intolerance but may not be adequate to completely normalize blood glucose parameters. These abnormalities usually resolve with successful therapy.

Despite these recognized tendencies, measurement of serum insulin concentrations in a fasted dog to help diagnose questionable cases of hyperadrenocorticism has no value. Fewer than half of dogs with hyperadrenocorticism have abnormal increases in the serum insulin concentration (Feldman and Tyrrell, 1982; Montgomery et al, 1996). Furthermore, any increase in serum insulin would have to be viewed as a nonspecific finding with a multitude of potential causes.

Blood Urea Nitrogen (BUN)

The diuresis stimulated by glucocorticoids causes a continual urinary loss of blood urea nitrogen. Polyuria is common and probably due to a reversible form of central diabetes insipidus in most dogs. One differential diagnosis for polydipsia, polyuria, and a urine specific gravity of 1.008 to 1.020 in any older dog would be renal insufficiency. Because a large percentage of dogs with Cushing's syndrome have a normal to *decreased* BUN concentration (similar results are seen in the creatinine concentration), the concern about renal function should be quickly dismissed after evaluation of a serum chemistry profile.

Rarely, a dog is diagnosed with renal failure and concurrent hyperadrenocorticism. If the Cushing's syndrome diagnosis is certain, there remain major concerns regarding treatment. The renal function of such a dog may be helped by having Cushing's syndrome. In other words, Cushing's syndrome may be the sole reason that the dog is eating and maintaining body weight and hydration. Treatment of these dogs may do more harm than good by removing their desire to eat, by reducing renal blood flow, and/or by simply removing their vague sense of "well-being." We do not treat dogs for Cushing's syndrome if they also have renal failure unless there is some critical reason to alter this philosophy.

Alanine Aminotransferase (ALT)

ALT activity is commonly increased in CCS. This is usually a mild increase (<400 IU/L), which is believed to occur secondary to damage caused by swollen hepatocytes, glycogen accumulation, or interference with hepatic blood flow. Hepatocellular necrosis, a minor but significant feature of "steroid hepatopathy," is also seen with enough frequency to account for mild increases in the serum ALT (Badylak and Van Vleet, 1981).

Serum Alkaline Phosphatase (SAP)

SOURCES. Serum alkaline phosphatases (SAPs) are a group of enzymes that catalyze the hydrolysis of phosphate esters. The main source of SAP is the liver, with bone alkaline phosphatase contributing smaller amounts to the circulation. SAPs from the liver and bone have serum half-lives of approximately 3 days. Intestinal, placental, and renal alkaline phosphatases are not detectable in serum because their half-lives are usually measured in minutes (Hoffmann et al, 1988).

As a result of hepatic glycogen deposition and vacuolization impinging on the biliary tract in dogs with hyperadrenocorticism, the rate of SAP production increases (Solter et al, 1994a). Although SAP increases in dogs under the influence of excess circulating cortisol, hepatic bile acid concentrations do not increase and therefore are not likely to be responsible for induction and release of SAP into the serum (Solter et al, 1994b). Other causes for increased concentrations of this enzyme in the serum include bone growth in young dogs, primary hepatopathies that cause cholestasis (inflammation, cirrhosis, lipidosis), pancreatitis, diabetes mellitus, abnormal bone osteolytic activity (hyperparathyroidism, neoplasia in bone: sarcomas, carcinomas), and isoenzymes induced by anticonvulsants and steroids.

CORTICOSTEROID-INDUCED ALKALINE PHOSPHATASE. The major contributor to the increase in SAP with canine hyperadrenocorticism is induction of a specific hepatic isoenzyme by either endogenous or exogenous glucocorticoids. In prednisone-treated dogs, synthesis of alkaline phosphatase is also increased in the kidneys and intestinal mucosa (Wiedmeyer et al, 2002). In dogs with hyperadrenocorticism, 70% to 100% of the SAP is specifically the steroid-induced hepatic fraction. The subcellular source of this isoenzyme was found to be on the bile canalicular membrane of hepatocytes. This corticosteroid-induced isoenzyme of SAP is unique to the dog (Teske et al, 1989). SAP is one of the most common biochemical measurements used to screen for the presence of liver disease, and the ability to discriminate between steroid-induced and liver isoenzymes of SAP may be important. Heat inactivation is a reliable method for distinguishing between these two isoenzymes of SAP (Teske et al, 1986). If a steroid-induced increase in SAP is established, further laboratory investigation to characterize a liver problem could be omitted.

An increase in SAP activity is the most common routine laboratory abnormality in CCS (Teske et al, 1989). SAP is increased in 90% to 95% of dogs with hyperadrenocorticism (see Table 6-7). Approximately 85% of hyperadrenal dogs have SAP activities that exceed 150 IU/L, values in excess of 1000 IU/L are common, and the mean concentration in our series of dogs is about 1100 IU/L. No correlation has been found between the SAP concentration and the severity of Cushing's syndrome, the response to therapy, or the prognosis. In addition, the SAP concentration is normal in some dogs with hyperadrenocorticism. The reason for the differences in SAP concentrations among dogs with Cushing's syndrome is unknown.

Several groups have evaluated the clinical application of assaying for steroid-induced alkaline phosphatase (SIAP). These studies have demonstrated rather uniform agreement. The greater the increase in SAP, the more reliable the results of SIAP. SIAP is present in increased concentrations in most dogs with Cushing's syndrome. As such, the test is considered quite *sensitive*. However, the finding of increases in SIAP is *nonspecific* (Fig. 6-25). SIAP is abnormal in dogs with primary hepatopathies and other endocrine problems (diabetes mellitus), as well as in those treated with anticonvulsants such as phenobarbital, phenytoin, and primidone (Muller et al, 2000a and 2000b). A major concern with an abnormal SIAP, however, is the inability to distinguish three disorders commonly confused with naturally developing hyperadrenocorticism: iatrogenic Cushing's syndrome, diabetes mellitus, and hypothyroidism (Fig. 6-25). The conclusion reached by most groups has been that finding no SIAP in the serum may have diagnostic value

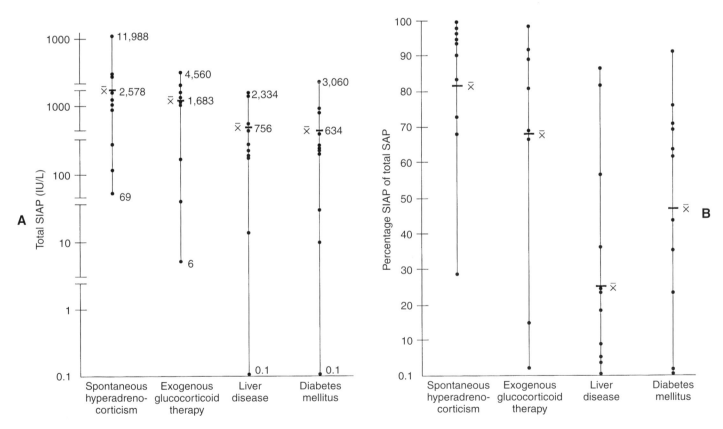

FIGURE 6–25. *A*, Mean and range of serum steroid-induced alkaline phosphatase (SIAP) activity in dogs with naturally occurring hyperadrenocorticism, dogs chronically treated with glucocorticoids, dogs with liver disease, and dogs with diabetes mellitus. *B*, The percentage of total serum alkaline phosphatase (SAP) concentrations, which is made up of the steroid-induced fraction in the same four groups described in *A*. These graphs show that SIAP is a sensitive indicator of Cushing's syndrome (dogs with the disease have an abnormal test result), but it is not a specific test (dogs with other conditions also can have an abnormal test result).

in ruling out hyperadrenocorticism, but an increase in SIAP can be caused by a variety of disorders and must be considered a nonspecific finding (Oluju et al, 1984; Teske et al, 1989; Jensen and Poulsen, 1992; Wilson and Feldman, 1992; Solter et al, 1994a and 1994b).

Cholesterol, Triglycerides, and Lipemia

Glucocorticoid stimulation of lipolysis causes an increase in blood lipid and cholesterol concentrations. Ninety percent of dogs with Cushing's syndrome have an increased plasma cholesterol concentration. Approximately 10% of dogs with Cushing's syndrome have serum cholesterol concentrations less than 250 mg/dl; 15% have concentrations of 250 to 300 mg/dl; and 75% have concentrations greater than 300 mg/dl (Fig. 6-26) (Ortega et al, 1995a). Lipemia (i.e., hypertriglyceridemia) is noted at least as frequently as the increases in serum cholesterol (Fig. 6-26) and may interfere with the accurate assessment of several serum tests (depending on the assays used). Parameters that can be altered by lipemia include red blood cell counts, hemoglobin, red cell indices, total plasma proteins, albumin, total bilirubin, alkaline phosphatase, calcium, phosphorus, amylase, lipase, sodium, and sulfobromophthalein (BSP) retention studies.

Serum Phosphate

Hypophosphatemia has been reported to occur in approximately one third of dogs with hyperadrenocorticism (Peterson, 1984). This may result from a glucocorticoid-induced increase in urinary excretion of phosphate. Our impression, however, is that the lower end of the reference range for serum phosphate varies remarkably among laboratories. Perhaps this is the explanation for serum phosphate concentrations being within reference limits among almost all the dogs with naturally developing Cushing's syndrome in our series. Of greater concern would be dogs thought to have Cushing's syndrome and an increase in the serum phosphate concentration. The most common explanation for increases in serum phosphate concentration is renal failure, an extremely uncommon feature in dogs with Cushing's. Management of the dog diagnosed with both renal failure and Cushing's syndrome is briefly discussed under Blood Urea Nitrogen (BUN), above.

Bile Acids

Bile acid measurements are considered to be equivalent to ammonia tolerance test results in many hepatic disorders. The bile acid test results may be mildly increased in as many as 30% of dogs with CCS (Reusch, 2005). Liver pathology, if present in dogs with Cushing's syndrome, is usually mild and of little clinical relevance and is reversible with successful treatment. Furthermore, liver function test results do not help differentiate dogs with primary liver disorders from dogs with hyperadrenocorticism.

Serum Electrolytes

Although of little diagnostic or clinical significance, mild abnormalities in the serum sodium concentration (increased) and the serum potassium concentration (decreased) are seen in a small percentage of dogs with

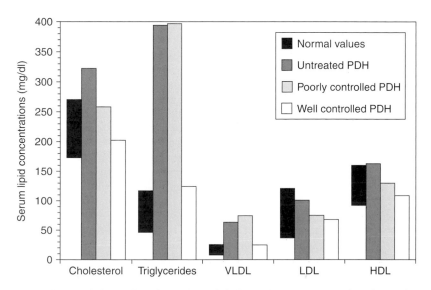

FIGURE 6–26. Serum cholesterol, triglyceride, and cholesterol content in very-low density lipoprotein (VLDL), low-density lipoprotein (LDL), and high-density lipoprotein (HDL) concentrations in normal dogs, dogs with untreated Cushing's syndrome, and poorly controlled and well-controlled treated dogs with naturally occurring Cushing's syndrome.

Cushing's syndrome. Assessment of serum electrolyte concentrations becomes extremely important if a dog with hyperadrenocorticism undergoing treatment develops anorexia, vomiting, or diarrhea, because changes in serum electrolyte concentrations typical of adrenal failure (Addison's disease) may become life-threatening.

Amylase and Lipase

Pancreatitis is extremely uncommon in dogs with Cushing's syndrome. If signs of pancreatitis occur, the gastrointestinal signs are more likely secondary to "garbage can gastritis," because these dogs are polyphagic and may eat anything. Inflammatory disease (pancreatitis) and antiinflammatory hormone excess (cortisol) creates an unlikely combination. Inflammatory diseases of any kind are uncommon in dogs with Cushing's syndrome, and their diagnosis should be viewed with skepticism or the Cushing's diagnosis may be incorrect. Serum lipase and amylase concentrations are not routinely measured.

Urinalysis

CONCENTRATION. Urinalysis is one of the most important initial studies in the evaluation of a dog with polyuria or polydipsia (PU/PD). It is strongly recommended that owners of any dog suspected of having PU/PD obtain a urine sample by clean-catch prior to bringing their pet to the hospital or that a urine sample be collected at the time of initial examination. The most frequent abnormality is dilute urine (specific gravity <1.020), which occurs in 85% of our cases. A large percentage of these dogs have randomly obtained urine with specific gravities less than 1.015.

Other investigators have found dilute urine less frequently, perhaps because samples were obtained after the dogs had been hospitalized for hours or even days. Dogs with Cushing's syndrome may *not* consume large amounts of water in a frightening environment (veterinary hospital), with the specific gravity reflecting this reduction in intake. It is usually not reliable to measure water intake in the hospital, and this practice is not encouraged. Most water-deprived dogs with Cushing's syndrome can concentrate the urine to an osmolality well above plasma osmolality (1.025 to 1.035), although the concentrating ability remains below normal. Having the owner bring a urine sample from the pet is a simple aid to documenting specific gravity; it also confirms the client's belief that the pet is PU/PD, makes the diagnosis of diabetes mellitus one that requires less than 30 seconds with a dipstick, and adds evidence to support the suspicion of Cushing's syndrome. This urine can also be used for determination of the urine cortisol:creatinine ratio, without the concern that a visit to the veterinary hospital altered test results.

GLUCOSE. In addition to determining the specific gravity, the veterinarian can assess the urine sample for glycosuria. This finding, which has been noted in about 5% of dogs with Cushing's syndrome, indicates that overt diabetes mellitus is present. Diabetes mellitus requires therapy regardless of whether the dog has hyperadrenocorticism.

PROTEINURIA/HYPERTENSION/GLOMERULOPATHY. Dogs with Cushing's syndrome frequently have proteinuria. One study involved 67 dogs with Cushing's syndrome that did not have pyuria or urinary tract infection (Hurley and Vaden, 1998). Among the dogs with untreated Cushing's syndrome, the mean urine protein to creatinine (UP:C) ratio was higher than in dogs with well-controlled pituitary-dependent Cushing's syndrome (PDH). The UP:C ratio was abnormally increased (>1) in 46% of dogs with untreated PDH, 31% of dogs with poorly controlled PDH, and 63% of dogs with untreated Cushing's syndrome secondary to an adrenocortical tumor. In untreated dogs with Cushing's syndrome, the mean UP:C ratio was 2.3. By comparison, the UP:C ratio was abnormal in only 21% of dogs with well-controlled PDH and 33% of dogs in which Cushing's syndrome resolved after surgical removal of an adrenal tumor. Only five dogs had a UP:C ratio that was "moderately" increased (5 to 13), and none had a ratio greater than 13. Thus the finding of proteinuria is common among dogs with Cushing's syndrome. Another group (Ortega et al, 1996) assessed a smaller group of 16 dogs and identified a similar percentage of dogs with proteinuria but found the severity of UP:C abnormalities to be less worrisome (mean UP:C of 1.2). Regardless, evidence of proteinuria should prompt the clinician to evaluate the dog's blood pressure and to submit urine for culture, because these problems could be associated with a urinary tract infection.

The incidence of protein-losing glomerulopathies in dogs with Cushing's syndrome is now documented to be common. The proteinuria is rarely severe (if it is, another cause should be considered) and almost never causes severe hypoalbuminemia or hypoproteinemia; it therefore has not been related to the development of edema, ascites, or pleural effusion. It remains to be seen whether protein losses relate to other documented problems in Cushing's syndrome (e.g., pyelonephritis [sepsis], thromboembolism). However, in one study (Ortega et al, 1996), blood pressure and UP:C ratio significantly declined in the group of dogs with well-controlled Cushing's syndrome but not in those with inadequately controlled disease. Kidney tissue was evaluated histologically in seven dogs from this study; five were identified to have diffuse glomerulosclerosis. The post–ACTH-stimulation plasma cortisol concentration significantly correlated with both blood pressure and the UP:C ratio; that is, the lower the stimulated plasma cortisol concentration, the lower the blood pressure and UP:C. Hypertension and proteinuria, therefore, are common in dogs with Cushing's syndrome, and they may represent a "cause-and-effect" relationship. These parameters should be evaluated in affected dogs, and successful resolution of the Cushing's syndrome should reduce their severity. However, some dogs remain hypertensive and proteinuric despite resolution of Cushing's syndrome.

INFECTION (UTI). Owner-collected *(outpatient)* urinalysis should be used to assess specific gravity and the presence of glucose, protein, and other urine contents. Because urinary tract infection (UTI) is a common sequela to Cushing's syndrome, urine for culture should be obtained by *cystocentesis*. Approximately 40% to 50% of dogs with Cushing's syndrome have a UTI at the time of initial examination (Forrester et al, 1999). One striking feature of Cushing's syndrome is that the excess concentration of circulating cortisol suppresses inflammation. For this reason, dogs with Cushing's syndrome that have a UTI often do not have stranguria, pollakiuria, discolored urine, or white blood cells in their urine. Most but not all have microscopic evidence of bacteria. The absence of these features should not reduce concern for infection or its consequences; rather, it simply indicates that urine culture in CCS should be a routine component of a "database" evaluation. The bacteria isolated are common, and the sensitivities are typical of any UTI (Forrester et al, 1999).

There are several potential explanations for this worrisome incidence of infection. First, glucocorticoid excess results in immunosuppression, with an increased risk for infection. Second, polyuria in many of these dogs causes remarkable volumes of urine, but the dogs attempt to remain housebroken. This combination of factors, added to the muscle weakness typical of Cushing's syndrome, creates a potential for chronic bladder overdistention, ultimately resulting in urine retention despite urination. Finally, it has been demonstrated that dilute urine increases susceptibility to lower urinary tract infection (Lulich and Osborne, 1994). In many dogs with Cushing's syndrome, the bladder may chronically contain dilute urine, which acts as a ready substrate for infection in an immunosuppressed dog. Control of UTI is important, although in some dogs the infection is difficult to resolve. Difficulty resolving an infection may be the consequence of choosing an antibiotic to which the bacteria are not sensitive; it may be the result of inadequate control of the Cushing's syndrome; or the dog may have underlying pyelonephritis.

Thyroid Function Tests

Abnormalities in thyroid function that suggest hypothyroidism are important in CCS because of the overlap in some clinical signs (i.e., listlessness; bilateral symmetric, nonpruritic alopecia; apparent weight gain; hypercholesterolemia). The overlap in signs can be a source of confusion to the veterinarian, especially if polyuria and polydipsia are not apparent. Treating a dog with Cushing's syndrome with thyroid replacement medication does not usually have a deleterious effect; in fact, many dogs become slightly more active. Because the primary disease is not treated, however, signs continue to develop (e.g., polyphagia, polyuria, polydipsia, panting), which should alert the veterinarian that hypothyroidism is not the complete explanation for the dog's problems.

Chronic hypercortisolism (iatrogenic or naturally occurring) suppresses pituitary secretion of TSH and causes secondary hypothyroidism (Torres et al, 1991; Meij et al, 1997c). Hypercortisolism may also alter thyroid hormone binding to plasma proteins, may enhance the metabolism of thyroid hormone, and may decrease peripheral deiodination of thyroxine (T_4) to triiodothyronine (T_3) (see Chapter 3). Approximately 70% of dogs with naturally occurring hyperadrenocorticism have decreases in the basal serum T_4 and/or T_3 concentrations. Administration of TSH increases the serum T_4 concentration in a manner parallel to normal but usually not to normal concentrations (Fig. 6-27) (Ferguson, 1984; Peterson et al, 1984) (see Chapter 3). Serum free T_4 concentrations have also been evaluated in dogs with Cushing's syndrome. Most of these dogs have reduced total T_4 and free T_4 concentrations, which suggests that reduced secretion and enhanced metabolism of thyroid hormones are likely mechanisms for the low serum thyroid hormone concentrations (Ferguson and Peterson, 1986).

RADIOGRAPHY

General Approach

Radiographs of the abdomen (if abdominal ultrasonography is not available; see page 286), and of the thorax should be evaluated in dogs with suspected or proven hyperadrenocorticism. In addition to looking for changes consistent with the diagnosis of Cushing's syndrome, the veterinarian should remember that these dogs are usually older and may have serious concurrent (perhaps subclinical) diseases that may be detected radiographically.

The Abdomen

HEPATOMEGALY AND CONTRAST. Approximately 80% to 90% of dogs afflicted with Cushing's syndrome have radiographically obvious hepatomegaly, with a relatively equal number of dogs having mild, moderate, or severe enlargement. There is no obvious association between the duration of illness and the degree of hepatomegaly (Huntley et al, 1982; Penninck et al, 1988). Good contrast, due to abdominal (primarily omental) fat deposition, is usually observed in dogs and cats with Cushing's syndrome. The potbellied appearance (60% of dogs with Cushing's syndrome) may be obvious.

URINARY BLADDER. Distention of the urinary bladder may be seen radiographically. As previously

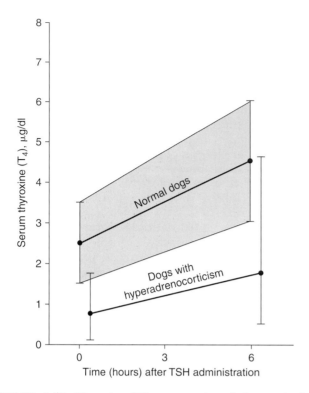

FIGURE 6–27. Thyroxine (T$_4$) concentrations before and after thyroid-stimulating hormone (TSH) administration in normal dogs and those with hyperadrenocorticism. The dogs with Cushing's syndrome may have normal or below (but parallel to normal) increases in serum T$_4$ concentrations.

discussed, some dogs with CCS have an atonic bladder and may not be capable of voiding completely. Many of these dogs, allowed to urinate "completely" before abdominal radiographs are obtained, still have a large and partly filled bladder (Fig. 6-28).

ADRENALS. Perhaps the most important but least common finding on abdominal radiography is visualization of an adrenal mass. Positive identification of such a mass occurs infrequently, because only 10% to 20% of dogs with naturally occurring hyperadrenocorticism have an adrenocortical tumor, and only about one half of these tumors are calcified, allowing them to be visualized radiographically. Approximately 50% of both adenomas and carcinomas are calcified.

In a review of 23 dogs with Cushing's syndrome caused by an adrenal tumor, 14 had adrenal masses that were visualized on radiography of the abdomen (Penninck et al, 1988). Thirteen of the 14 visualized masses were mineralized. Seven of the 13 calcified tumors were adrenal adenomas, and six were carcinomas (see Fig. 6-28 and Fig. 6-29). Another review of radiographic results included 35 dogs with adrenocortical tumors; 12 of 22 carcinomas were mineralized and visualized; one noncalcified carcinoma was visualized as a soft tissue mass; and seven of 13 dogs with adrenocortical adenomas had a mass identified, each of which was calcified. Sixteen dogs had noncalcified adrenal masses, and only one was visualized (Reusch and Feldman, 1991). One study demonstrated that tumors smaller than 2 cm were not likely to be visualized but that noncalcified tumors

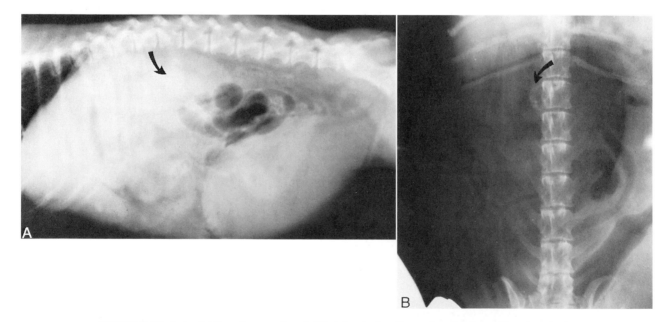

FIGURE 6–28. Lateral (A) and ventrodorsal (B) abdominal radiographs of a dog with a functioning adrenal tumor causing hyperadrenocorticism. Note the calcified adrenal tumor (arrows), hepatomegaly, distended (atonic) bladder, and excellent contrast due to fat mobilization. (From Feldman EC: In Ettinger SJ [ed]: Textbook of Veterinary Internal Medicine, 2nd ed. Philadelphia, WB Saunders, 1983, p 1683.)

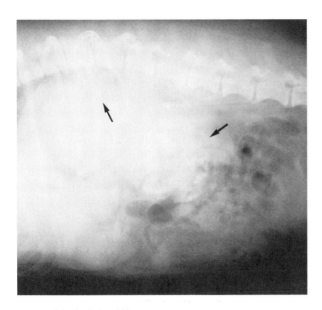

FIGURE 6–29. Lateral abdominal radiograph from a dog with a large, calcified, functioning adrenocortical carcinoma *(arrows).*

larger than 2 cm in diameter could be large enough to be identified (Voorhout et al, 1990a).

The Thorax

MINERALIZATION AND THE INTERSTITIUM. The most common thoracic radiographic abnormalities in dogs with Cushing's syndrome are bronchial mineralization, tracheal ring mineralization, and generalized interstitial lung patterns. These abnormalities are identified more commonly in dogs with tachypnea than in dogs without respiratory signs. In one study, almost 75% of dogs with Cushing's syndrome had bronchial mineralization, and about one quarter of the dogs had severe generalized interstitial lung patterns (Berry et al, 2000). A significant correlation was established between increases in interstitial lung opacities and the presence of hypoxemia. Another common finding on thoracic radiography is calcification of tracheal rings.

METASTASES AND THROMBOEMBOLISM. Radiographs must be evaluated for evidence of pulmonary metastases of an adrenocortical carcinoma, which can occur in a small percentage of these dogs. If an adrenocortical carcinoma is believed to have spread to the lungs, removal of the primary adrenal tumor would be expensive, life-threatening, and pointless. Metastases from unrelated cancers may be identified, and such problems must be recognized, understood, and explained to the owners before expensive, time-consuming diagnostics and therapeutics for CCS are undertaken. In such situations, the Cushing's syndrome may be far less important to the long-term health and well-being of a dog than the cause of pulmonary masses.

Another rare but major concern is pulmonary thromboembolism (see discussion of thromboembolism, page 293). Most dogs with pulmonary thromboembolism have abnormal thoracic radiographs. Two distinct pulmonary radiographic patterns have been described in these dogs: hypovascular lung regions and alveolar pulmonary infiltrates. Hypovascular lung fields appear as areas of increased radiolucency and represent regions of reduced vascular filling distal to sites of thrombosis. Alveolar infiltrates can be solitary or multiple. They correspond to areas of intrapulmonary atelectasis, hemorrhage, or infarction. Enlargement of the main pulmonary artery segment, right-sided cardiomegaly, and pleural effusion have been reported in dogs with pulmonary thromboembolism (Fluckiger and Gomez, 1984; Bunch et al, 1989; Klein et al, 1989; LaRue and Murtaugh, 1990).

The Skeleton

OSTEOPENIA. Osteopenia occurs with hyperadrenocorticism from hypercalciuria, suppressed intestinal absorption of calcium, and direct effects of cortisol on bone. The degree of osteopenia is usually mild and of no clinical importance in dogs. Radiographs are an insensitive tool for evaluating bone density. These concepts are discussed here because routine radiography of bone is an extremely crude means of determining the presence of osteopenia, yet this is frequently pursued. More than a third of bone density must be depleted before osteopenia is evident on routine radiography. It has been demonstrated that obesity, which is common among dogs with Cushing's syndrome, may give a false impression of osteopenia (Schwartz et al, 2000). Lameness due to bone pain or pathologic fractures virtually do not occur, with the exception of Cushing's syndrome in prepubertal animals. Failure of epiphyseal closure and epiphyseal fractures may occur in these rarely encountered dogs (see Fig. 6-13).

SKULL. Radiographs of the skull are not recommended. The studies are usually normal and require anesthesia. Bone destruction seen in the sella turcica of some humans with expanding pituitary tumors is not seen in dogs, in which the sella turcica is anatomically more shallow and open.

Dystrophic (Ectopic) Calcification

Calcinosis cutis and subcutaneous calcification may be visualized radiographically (see section on history, page 270; also see Fig. 6-23). Fewer than 5% of dogs with CCS have radiographic signs of calcinosis cutis. A smaller number have radiographic dystrophic calcification involving the renal pelvis, the liver, the gastric mucosa, or the branches of the abdominal aorta. Ectopic calcification is frequently seen involving the tracheal rings and mainstem bronchi. Calcification of these structures, however, can be seen in normally aging dogs and is not usually considered significant (Widmer and Guptill, 1995).

ABDOMINAL ULTRASONOGRAPHY

Visualization of the Adrenal Glands as a Test of Competency

Abdominal ultrasonography is used routinely to image the adrenal glands in humans, with as many as 85% of normal glands being visualized almost 20 years ago (Hamper et al, 1987). The percentage is much higher now (Aron et al, 2001b). The ability to visualize normal adrenal glands in dogs and cats has progressively improved over the past 10 years with the experience gained by radiologists and with improvements in equipment (Voorhout, 1990b; Nyland, 1995). Both adrenals now are routinely visualized in healthy dogs and cats, assuming that the pets' behavior allows thorough evaluation of the abdomen (Grooters et al, 1995). Perhaps more than with any other tool, the value of ultrasonography directly correlates with the skill of the operator (Widmer and Guptill, 1995; Grooters et al, 1996). With this in mind, practitioners can evaluate their colleagues or themselves on the basis of their ability to visualize adrenal glands, confidently, in healthy dogs.

Normal Dogs

A number of studies have been published regarding use of ultrasound to evaluate the adrenal glands in normal dogs. Transverse, longitudinal, and oblique scanning from the ventral abdomen must be performed to thoroughly evaluate each gland (Kantrowitz et al, 1986). Overlying bowel, especially when the pylorus or intestines contain gas, can compromise a study, as can the deep-chested body conformation typical of some breeds. The left adrenal, because it is located caudal to the right adrenal gland, is easier to visualize (Grooters et al, 1995). In general, ultrasonographers with expertise note that there is acceptable correlation between ultrasonographic and gross adrenal gland measurements, specifically regarding the thickness of both the left and right glands. In most cases, differentiation of the cortex from the medulla is possible. There does not appear to be any correlation between adrenal measurement and gender. Attempts have been made to correlate adrenal gland measurements with body weight and body surface area (Douglass et al, 1997); whether these correlations are helpful from a clinical perspective is not clear.

Dogs with Cushing's Syndrome and Those with an Incidentally Discovered Adrenal Mass

BACKGROUND. In our clinic, the "routine" evaluation of dogs with hyperadrenocorticism includes abdominal ultrasonography. Ultrasound evaluation of the abdomen has completely replaced radiography. There are several reasons for this evolution in using abdominal ultrasound scans rather than radiographic studies.

Ultrasound is far superior to radiographs in the amount of information gained. Our radiologists have a tremendous amount of experience due to case load, and they have developed remarkable expertise. The ultrasound equipment available to our radiologists is another factor to appreciate. The equipment they have used over the years has consistently been the most up-to-date in the industry. Another somewhat unique factor in our hospital is that ultrasound is readily available, with the cost to our clients being the same as that for abdominal radiographs. This situation is recognized to be in contrast to that in many private practices, in which the cost may be greater or a client and pet may need to be referred elsewhere for such studies.

LIMITATIONS, USE, AND MISUSE OF ULTRASONOGRAPHY. Numerous reports confirm the value of abdominal ultrasonography in the evaluation of Cushing's syndrome in dogs and cats (Poffenbarger et al, 1988; Voorhout, 1990b; Voorhout et al, 1990b; Reusch and Feldman, 1991; Barthez et al, 1995). In our opinion, it is extremely important for veterinarians to appreciate how much this field has changed over the past 5 to 10 years. Findings from 5 to 10 years ago may no longer reflect the state of the art. It seems that the expertise of radiologists and general practitioners using this tool continues to improve dramatically. When ultrasound was first used, recognition of the adrenal glands sonographically was an accomplishment; now it is routine. In the past, recognition of one or both adrenal glands meant that the gland or glands were abnormally enlarged and such dogs likely had Cushing's syndrome. This is no longer the case.

We believe that the adrenal appearance on ultrasound should be used as a test to help differentiate pituitary-dependent from adrenal tumor–dependent hyperadrenocorticism. Until proven otherwise, we strongly believe that abdominal ultrasound should *not* be used as a screening test for the diagnosis of Cushing's syndrome. The sensitivity and, more important, specificity of ultrasonography fail to meet the necessary standards for such use. Therefore, making a diagnosis of Cushing's syndrome from an ultrasound examination is improper, incorrect, and unfair to the pet and its owner. With this in mind, the confidence expressed in ultrasound findings will continue to improve. We consider abdominal ultrasonography to be an extremely valuable component of our *routine* database.

PRIMARY FUNCTIONS OF ABDOMINAL ULTRASONOGRAPHY. Abdominal ultrasonography serves two major functions:

1. It is part of the "routine database" used to evaluate the abdomen for expected abnormalities (hepatomegaly) and unexpected abnormalities (e.g., urinary calculi, masses within any organ, cysts) in a dog suspected of having Cushing's syndrome.
2. It is used to evaluate the size and shape of the adrenal glands. A finding of bilaterally normal sized or large adrenal glands that maintain, in

general, normal shape *in a dog otherwise diagnosed as having Cushing's syndrome* is considered strong evidence in favor of adrenal hyperplasia secondary to pituitary-dependent disease. A finding of a solitary and abnormally shaped adrenal mass that may be compressing or invading adjacent structures (e.g., vena cava, liver, or kidney) coupled with an opposite adrenal that is small, "thin," or not visualized is suggestive of a functioning adrenocortical tumor *in a dog otherwise diagnosed as having Cushing's syndrome.* If an adrenal tumor is suspected, ultrasonography is an excellent screening test for hepatic or other organ metastasis, tumor invasion of the vena cava or other structures, or compression of adjacent tissues.

PITUITARY VERSUS ADRENAL TUMOR CUSHING'S SYNDROME

Pituitary-Dependent Cushing's Syndrome (PDH).
Both adrenals are routinely visualized in dogs and cats with PDH. The adrenals are usually described as "relatively" equal in size, with normal or enlarged dimensions (Table 6-8). Adrenal size is best determined using the width of the left adrenal, with 7.5 mm representing the upper limit of normal. In one study, this parameter had a sensitivity of 81% and a specificity of 100% in detecting adrenal enlargement in dogs with hyperadrenocorticism (Barthez et al, 1995). However, as facilities and experience change and improve, these guidelines may not remain static.

Adrenal gland thickness in dogs with PDH is significantly greater than in healthy dogs. This thickening gives the hyperplastic gland a plump appearance. The normal peanut shape of the left adrenal gland and oval shape of the right adrenal gland is typically preserved in dogs with PDH (Grooters et al, 1996). In addition, the adrenal glands of dogs with PDH are homogeneous and hypoechoic compared with adjacent renal cortices (Gould et al, 2001). Sometimes the adrenal glands of dogs with PDH have a heterogenous parenchyma and focal areas of increased echogenicity. Such an appearance may indicate the presence of nodular hyperplasia, which must be distinguished from a tumor (Grooters et al, 1996). This discrimination may be better accomplished with endocrine testing, rather than by relying solely on ultrasound.

Visualization of a normal or slightly enlarged left adrenal and failure to visualize the right adrenal is not strongly specific for discriminating pituitary- from adrenal-dependent hyperadrenocorticism, because the left gland is easier to locate. Visualization of only the right adrenal is considered more suspicious for the presence of an adrenal mass, because the right adrenal is usually the more difficult to visualize.

Cushing's Syndrome Caused by an Adrenal Tumor.
If either adrenal is remarkably enlarged or irregular or is invading or compressing adjacent structures and the opposite adrenal cannot be visualized, suspicion of an adrenal tumor should be quite high (Fig. 6-30). In general, adrenal tumors tend to appear abnormally enlarged, rounded, or "irregularly rounded" on abdominal ultrasonography (Gould et al, 2001). As expertise and equipment have improved, ultrasonographers have been able to visualize the atrophied adrenal gland. Typically, when the contralateral adrenal is visualized (something we are noting more commonly), it tends to appear thin or narrow, although not significantly reduced in length. The medulla of this thin, contralateral gland may appear to be somewhat normal, but the cortex appears abnormally narrow. Location of adrenal tumors can involve either gland.

Determining the malignant potential of an adrenal mass is speculative. The results of a study by Besso and colleagues (1997) showed that adrenal masses with a thickness of more than 2 cm tended to be malignant, and all masses greater than 4 cm in thickness were malignant. Also, the shape of adrenal masses tended not to be helpful in distinguishing adrenocortical lesions from other histologic types. Nodular lesions were more common with adenomas, hyperplasia, and metastases. Echogenicity was not specific for the type of lesion. Mineralization and bilateral involvement occurred with both benign and malignant lesions. Vascular invasion occurred more often but was not restricted to malignant lesions.

In a study of 15 dogs with adrenal-dependent Cushing's syndrome, both adrenal glands were visualized in all cases (three of the 15 dogs had tumors involving both glands) (Hoerauf and Reusch, 1999). In the 12 dogs with unilateral adrenal tumors, the length and thickness of the contralateral adrenal was not significantly different from measurements in normal dogs. In this same study, unilateral adrenal tumors were identified more frequently in the right adrenal. These findings may reflect the small number of cases in the study, but they also reflect the fact that the knowledge base continues to expand, and new findings must be constantly evaluated. In a review of this report, concern was raised about the researchers' consistent finding of normal-size contralateral adrenal glands. The reviewer suggested that measurable adrenocortical atrophy would be expected in the contralateral adrenal before clinical signs of hyperadrenocorticism are evident. The reviewer also indicated that not only should the zona fasciculata and zona reticularis of the cortex atrophy secondary to chronic suppression of endogenous ACTH secretion, but also that cortical cortisol may have a trophic effect on its medulla by inducing the phenylethanomamine-N-methyl-transferase required for methylation of norepinephrine to epinephrine. It therefore seemed to the reviewer that both the cortex and the medulla in a nonneoplastic, contralateral adrenal should atrophy. Future reports likely will clarify this debate.

INCIDENTALLY DISCOVERED ADRENAL ENLARGEMENT OR A SOLITARY MASS.
With the increased use of sophisticated aids for evaluating the abdomen, unsuspected abnormalities are identified more and more frequently. It was estimated that in as many as 2% of humans evaluated with ultrasonography, CT scans, or MRI scans, an unsuspected adrenal mass was identified

TABLE 6–8   A. COMPARISON OF SIGNALMENT AND ADRENAL GLAND SIZE, DETERMINED BY MEANS OF ABDOMINAL ULTRASONOGRAPHY, IN 20 HEALTHY DOGS, 20 DOGS WITH NONENDOCRINE DISEASE, AND 22 DOGS WITH PITUITARY-DEPENDENT HYPERADRENOCORTICISM (PDH)

Variable	HEALTHY DOGS			DOGS WITH NONENDOCRINE DISEASE			DOGS WITH PDH	
	Mean	Range	SD	Mean	Range	SD	Mean	Range
Age (y)	5.2	0.6 to 13.2	4.1	11.7	7.6 to 15.4		10.2	7 to 13.3
Weight (kg)	19.6	4.4 to 38.8	9	18	2.4 to 40		17.3	3.8 to 43
Aortic diameter (mm)	9.3	6.1 to 12.4	1.8	9	4.9 to 12.4		8.9	5.2 to 13
Kidney length (mm)	58.5	36.8 to 80.5	12	57.7	26.8 to 76.7		58.1	37.5 to 82.7
Left adrenal gland								
Length (mm)	24.9	14.5 to 33.4	6	23	15.6 to 30.5		27.1	13.4 to 40.3
Maximum diameter (mm)	6.2	5.1 to 7.4	0.8	6.9	3.8 to 10.6		9.2	4.9 to 13.2
Minimum diameter (mm)	5.2	3 to 6.5	0.9	5.5	3.7 to 9		8	4.8 to 12.6
Right adrenal gland								
Length (mm)	22.4	14 to 31.1	5.2	22	12.2 to 28.1	4.3	26	2.8 to 34.6
Maximum diameter (mm)	5.7	3.6 to 8.1	1.2	6.5	3.8 to 11	1.9	8.6	3.9 to 13.9
Minimum diameter (mm)	4.1	1.8 to 6.7	1.2	5.2	3.4 to 9	1.4	6.8	3.4 to 12.1

B. SENSITIVITY AND SPECIFICITY OF USING ULTRASONOGRAPHIC MEASUREMENT OF ADRENAL GLAND SIZE AS A DIAGNOSTIC TEST FOR PDH, USING VALUES OBTAINED FOR 22 DOGS WITH PDH AND 20 DOGS WITH NONENDOCRINE DISEASES. FOR EACH DIMENSION (ADRENAL GLAND LENGTH, MAXIMUM DIAMETER, AND MINIMUM DIAMETER), THE CUTOFF VALUE BETWEEN A POSITIVE AND NEGATIVE RESULT WAS THE LARGEST VALUE OBTAINED FOR 20 HEALTHY DOGS

Dimension	Sensitivity (%)	Specificity (%)
Left Adrenal Gland		
Length	18	100
Maximum diameter	77	80
Minimum diameter	73	85
Right Adrenal Gland		
Length	24	100
Maximum diameter	68	80
Minimum diameter	55	90

(Aron and Ross, 1992). In humans, the optimal evaluation and treatment of patients with such lesions are being continuously assessed, because most of these people do not have a tumor that is secreting hormones nor do they have malignancies that require therapy (Ross and Aron, 1990; Bencsik et al, 1995).

If a dog or cat with enlarged adrenal glands or an adrenal mass has no historical, physical examination, or routine clinicopathologic findings suggestive of Cushing's syndrome, endocrine evaluation is not recommended. When Cushing's syndrome is not suspected, decisions must be made regarding an identified tumor and whether it should be monitored or removed. Some "adrenal masses" are normal tissue. Other differential diagnoses include adrenal cyst, myelolipoma, hemorrhage, nonfunctioning (non–hormone producing) primary tumor, pheochromocytoma, metastatic tumor, and granuloma. Our approach to the asymptomatic dog with an adrenal mass seen to be invading a vital structure (e.g., the vena cava) is to consider surgical removal.

If an asymptomatic dog has an adrenal mass without evidence of invasion, we usually recommend repeating an ultrasound study in 4 to 6 weeks. If the mass has changed little in appearance at that time, we recommend rechecking the dog 3 months later and then monitoring the animal every 6 to 12 months. We are currently following more than 30 such dogs. Those that have died and undergone necropsy have been documented to have nonfunctioning and clinically unimportant tumors or granulomas (40%); to have had no abnormalities (30%); or to have had a pheochromocytoma (30%). Whether pheochromocytoma in these dogs is clinically relevant (causing problems of any kind) is not known.

MEDICAL COMPLICATIONS ASSOCIATED WITH HYPERADRENOCORTICISM

Most dogs with hyperadrenocorticism are stable and not severely ill when initially examined. However,

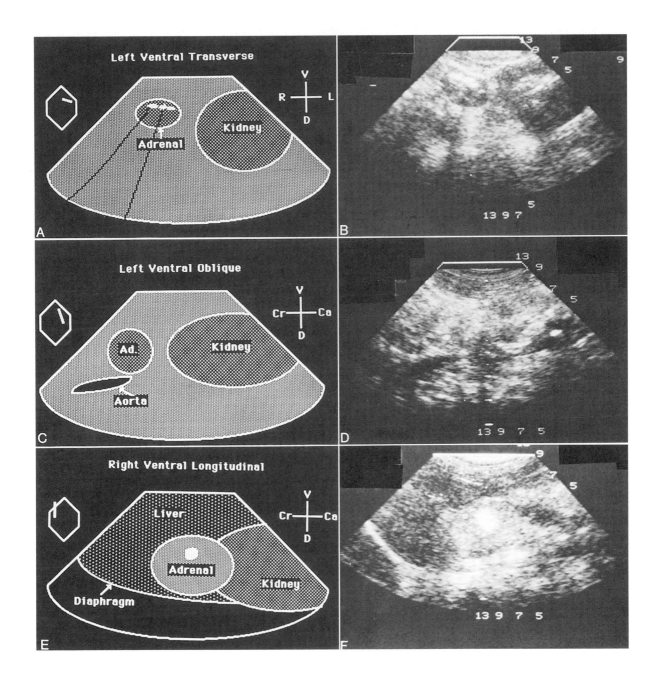

FIGURE 6–30. *A,* Diagrammatic illustration of the ultrasound image in *B,* showing the appearance of a calcified adrenal carcinoma in a dog with hyperadrenocorticism. *C,* Diagrammatic illustration of the ultrasound image in *D,* showing a hyperplastic adrenal gland in a dog with pituitary-dependent hyperadrenocorticism (PDH). *E,* Diagrammatic illustration of the ultrasound image in *F,* showing the opposite hyperplastic adrenal in the same dog with bilateral adrenal hyperplasia. *Continued*

various problems may arise secondary to prolonged steroid excess. In a few circumstances, such problems can be catastrophic.

Hypertension

HUMANS WITH CUSHING'S SYNDROME. Moderate, sustained hypertension has been documented in more than 90% of human beings with naturally occurring hyperadrenocorticism. Multiple factors have been implicated in the development of hypertension, including excessive secretion of renin (the circulating protein that acts to release angiotensin I), activation of the renin-angiotensin system via alternative stimulators, enhanced vascular sensitivity to pressors (such as catecholamines and adrenergic agonists), reduction of vasodilator prostaglandins, and increased secretion of non–zona glomerulosa mineralocorticoids (Melby, 1989). Plasma levels of deoxycorticosterone are

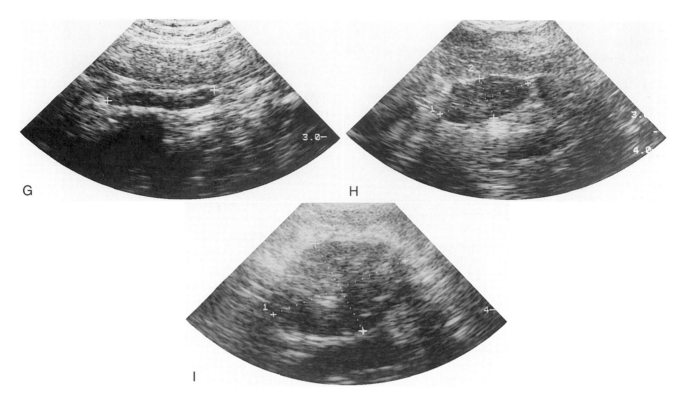

FIGURE 6–30.—cont'd *G*, Sagittal view of the left adrenal in a normal dog (2.40 cm long). *H*, Sagittal view of the right adrenal in a dog with PDH (1 = 2.41 cm long; 2 = 1.15 cm wide). *I*, Left adrenal tumor in a dog with Cushing's syndrome (1 = 4.48 cm long; 2 = 3.26 cm wide). *V*, Ventral; *D*, dorsal; *R*, right; *L*, left; *Cr*, cranial; *Ca*, caudal; the symbol in the upper left corner of *A*, *C*, and *E* is the location and orientation of the transducer in the ventral abdomen. (*A*, *C*, and *E* Courtesy Dr. Brett Kantrowitz, Davis, CA; *B*, *D*, and *F* from Kantrowitz BM, et al: Vet Radiol 27:15, 1986; *G*, *H*, and *I* courtesy Dr. Paul Barthez and Dr. Tom Nyland, Davis, CA.)

increased in humans with Cushing's syndrome (Yamaji et al, 1988).

ASSESSING BLOOD PRESSURE IN DOGS. Numerous studies have been performed to evaluate techniques for measuring blood pressure in dogs, including comparison of direct and indirect methods in awake, sedated, and anesthetized animals. Studies vary in animal positioning and type of indirect instrumentation used (Stepien and Rapoport, 1999). In a clinical setting, accurate, inexpensive, easy, practical, and rapid assessment of blood pressure is necessary. Use of anesthesia or sedation alters blood pressure readings and would make this tool of little clinical usefulness.

Recent studies have demonstrated that the mean values of systolic, diastolic, and mean arterial blood pressure measured in nonsedated, client-owned dogs using invasive and noninvasive methods in a clinical setting are comparable to those determined in dogs that have been acclimatized, trained, or sedated. However, results with noninvasive methods may not accurately reflect direct values (Stepien and Rapoport, 1999). Furthermore, although heart rates are more rapid in the hospital setting compared with the home setting, blood pressure readings were not significantly different in those two environments in one study (Remillard et al, 1991). It is also valuable to realize that research has demonstrated remarkable variation in

blood pressure readings due to age, breed, gender, temperament, disease state, exercise regimen and, to a minor extent, diet. Variation among different breeds was so dramatic that one group of authors suggested that normal ranges for dogs can be defined but that definition of hypertension demands attention to specific reference ranges established for a particular breed (Bodey and Michell, 1996).

DOGS WITH CUSHING'S SYNDROME. More than 50% of dogs with Cushing's syndrome are hypertensive on random testing (Nichols, 1992). Normal dogs in one study were defined to have average systolic, diastolic, and mean arterial blood pressures of approximately 150, 90, and 105 mmHg, respectively. Dogs with Cushing's syndrome had systolic, diastolic, and mean arterial blood pressures of 162 to 180, 116 to 120, and 135 to 145 mmHg, respectively (Kallet and Cowgill, 1982; Ortega et al, 1996).

In a study by Ortega and colleagues (1996), indirect measurements of systolic, diastolic, and mean systemic arterial blood pressures were evaluated in 77 dogs with Cushing's syndrome. The mean and diastolic blood pressures were highest in dogs with untreated or poorly controlled pituitary-dependent Cushing's syndrome, and all blood pressure measurements were higher in dogs with untreated adrenal tumor hyperadrenocorticism than were measurements in the same dogs after successful adrenalectomy. In this study, hypertension was arbitrarily defined as a systolic blood pressure greater than 160 mmHg, a diastolic pressure greater than 100 mmHg, and a mean systemic arterial pressure of greater than 120 mmHg. Using these standards, 86% of dogs with untreated Cushing's syndrome and 81% of inadequately treated dogs were hypertensive. Among these dogs, 12% were arbitrarily described as having "severe hypertension" (a systolic pressure >190 mmHg and a diastolic pressure >130 mmHg). These results were compared to the 40% of dogs with well-controlled pituitary-dependent Cushing's syndrome that had been hypertensive. Furthermore, no dog was hypertensive after surgical removal of the adrenocortical tumor.

Another finding of the study was a correlation between blood pressure and the urine protein: creatinine ratio; specifically, the higher the blood pressure, the greater the amount of protein lost in the urine and the more likely it was that the dog had glomerular damage. Hypertension resolved following successful management of the hyperadrenocorticism in some, but not all dogs (Ortega et al, 1996). It is assumed that some dogs do not have resolution of hypertension because it is caused by another disorder. Plasma aldosterone concentrations (before and after administration of exogenous ACTH) were highest in untreated dogs with pituitary-dependent Cushing's syndrome, near normal in dogs with well-controlled Cushing's syndrome, and intermediate to these values in dogs with poorly controlled Cushing's syndrome (Ortega et al, 1995b). These results imply an association between Cushing's syndrome, hyperaldosteronism, and systemic hypertension.

MANAGEMENT CONCERNS AND RECOMMENDATIONS. Hypertension causes concern because specific problems are related to this disorder. For example, hypertension-induced blindness may be due to intra-ocular hemorrhage or retinal detachment, or both (Littman et al, 1988). Hypertension may also exacerbate left ventricular hypertrophy and congestive heart failure. Hypertension may cause glomerulopathies, which in turn may lead to protein loss through the kidneys. Seventy-five percent of dogs with Cushing's syndrome have urine protein:creatinine ratios greater than 1.0, with a mean of 2.3 (normal, <1.0) (Ortega et al, 1996). Specifically, proteins important in coagulation (e.g., antithrombin III) may be lost, which could predispose a dog with CCS to thromboembolism. Although direct arterial blood pressure measurements are the most reliable and are relatively easy to obtain, the equipment for indirect monitoring is becoming more reliable and more widely used.

Assessment of blood pressure in dogs diagnosed as having Cushing's syndrome is warranted. Several groups agree that the hypertension in some of these dogs is severe enough to pose the risk of consequences such as retinal or renal vascular damage (Bodey and Michell, 1996; Ortega et al, 1996). On the other hand, vision loss is extremely rare in dogs with untreated hyperadrenocorticism. Although urine protein loss is common in these dogs (urine protein:creatinine ratios are often greater than 1.0), decreases in the serum total protein or serum albumin concentrations are extremely rare. With these factors in mind, our current recommendation is to monitor blood pressure in dogs with hyperadrenocorticism. We do not recommend therapy for hypertension until the hyperadrenocorticism has been controlled. In many treated dogs, hypertension resolves as the Cushing's syndrome resolves. In dogs with persistent hypertension despite resolution of the Cushing's syndrome, management of the hypertension depends on the severity and presence of worrisome abnormalities that could be attributed to this problem.

Pyelonephritis

Urinary tract infections are common in dogs with Cushing's syndrome, and such infections can ascend to the kidneys. Lowered resistance to infection may result from glucocorticoid-induced inhibition of neutrophil and macrophage migration into areas of infection. Dilute urine increases susceptibility to lower urinary tract infection but decreases susceptibility to pyelonephritis (Lulich and Osborne, 1994). Regardless of the urine specific gravity, severe chronic infections enhance the potential for pyelonephritis and renal failure in dogs with Cushing's syndrome. Clinical signs of pyelonephritis include pollakiuria, dysuria, and hematuria. However, it must be remembered that the antiinflammatory effects of glucocorticoids not only predispose dogs to pyelonephritis, but also mask many clinical signs. Suspicion of pyelonephritis should be raised if a urinary tract infection cannot be cleared. This is especially true if proper anti-biotic medication has been given to a dog in which CCS had resolved with therapy. Failure to resolve the Cushing's syndrome would predispose a dog to repeated urinary tract infections and may not indicate that an "upper" urinary tract problem exists. Anti-biotic selection should be based on the results of culture and sensitivity from a urine sample obtained by cystocentesis.

Urinary Calculi

In humans, hyperadrenocorticism may increase urinary calcium excretion, which in turn may increase the risk of development of calcium-containing uroliths. Furthermore, the increased incidence of urinary tract infection also contributes to a risk of calculi developing. Dysuria, a major sign resulting from urolithiasis and its associated inflammation, may not be obvious (i.e., may be masked) because the glucocorticoid excess may interfere with the inflammatory response. An extremely small percentage of dogs with Cushing's syndrome have calcium phosphate or calcium oxalate urinary calculi. In our series of cases, the percentage of dogs with cystic calculi is less than 2%. This is rather solid information, realizing that virtually all dogs with

Cushing's syndrome examined in our hospital undergo abdominal ultrasonography, an excellent tool for diagnosing calculi in the urinary tract.

In a study by Hess and colleagues (1998), of 20 dogs with both Cushing's syndrome and urolithiasis, 16 had calcium-containing uroliths (13 with calcium oxalate, one with calcium apatite, one with mixed carbonate-apatite struvite, and one with calcium hydrogen phosphate dihydrate), and four had struvite calculi. Statistically, dogs with Cushing's syndrome had a tenfold higher risk of developing calcium-containing uroliths than dogs without Cushing's syndrome. It was concluded that prompt diagnosis and treatment of Cushing's syndrome may reduce the prevalence of these uroliths. However, considering that the incidence of calculi is so small, this seems to be an unsound reason for treating any dog for Cushing's syndrome.

Congestive Heart Failure

One sequela of glucocorticoid excess is hypertension secondary to hypervolemia, which may increase the workload of the myocardium and result in myocardial hypertrophy. Congestive heart failure may occur as hypertension and fluid retention become severe. In addition, Cushing's syndrome frequently affects middle-age and older dogs of breeds commonly known to have acquired chronic mitral and tricuspid valvular disease. Theoretically, the combined effect of valvular insufficiency, hypertension, and hyper-cortisolism should result in myocardial overload. Despite this predisposition, congestive heart failure is rare in dogs with Cushing's syndrome. Radiographs of the thorax often reveal cardiomegaly associated with a prominent left ventricle. On the electrocardiogram, left ventricular hypertrophy, characterized by increased R wave amplitude and prolongation of the QRS complex, is a frequent finding. Pulmonary edema is rarely encountered.

Dogs that have both Cushing's syndrome and congestive heart failure respond poorly to therapy. Because many of these dogs are polydipsic and polyuric, diuretic therapy should be used with caution. Diuretics can predispose a dog with CCS to hypokalemia or alkalosis or both. Treatment of congestive heart failure and hypertension is best accomplished by initially focusing on the underlying cause of these disorders: the hyperadrenocorticism. With appropriate control of Cushing's syndrome, affected dogs may be rendered normotensive, leading to control of the cardiovascular complications without the need for specific heart failure therapy. For dogs that require cardiac therapy, improved response is observed with control of the Cushing's syndrome.

Pancreatitis

Dogs with hyperadrenocorticism have been described as being "predisposed" to the development of pancreatitis. Although various facets of Cushing's syndrome fit this impression (e.g., hyperlipidemia, hypercholesterolemia, and infection), it is our experience that pancreatitis is rare in dogs with Cushing's syndrome. Pancreatitis has uncommonly been observed after difficult adrenalectomy procedures. Given that dogs with hyperadrenocorticism have voracious appetites and histories of eating garbage and just about anything else they can swallow, it is surprising that more of them do not suffer from "garbage can gastritis." Although gastritis is not unheard of in these dogs, the incidence is not nearly as great as one would expect.

Diabetes Mellitus

Diabetes mellitus is a straightforward disease to diagnose in dogs. Hyperadrenocorticism is not as easily diagnosed, but the clinical picture of Cushing's syndrome is striking, which makes the diagnosis of Cushing's syndrome in most dogs with concurrent diabetes mellitus relatively uncomplicated. It is easy to recognize when a dog with established and well-controlled Cushing's syndrome develops diabetes mellitus, because there is a sudden increase in thirst, urine output, and glucose in the urine. However, a major dilemma arises in attempting to determine whether a dog with established diabetes mellitus has CCS.

For practitioners, the major clue is the presence of "insulin resistance." "Resistance," however, is a subjective phenomenon that has numerous differential diagnoses, most of which are more common than Cushing's syndrome (see Chapter 11). The clinician would be best served by relying on the dog's clinical presentation. Does it have an appearance consistent with the diagnosis of Cushing's syndrome? This question deserves careful consideration, because the clinical signs (polydipsia/polyuria, polyphagia, hepatomegaly), CBC (increase in the white blood cell count and "stress" leukogram), serum chemistry profile (increases in cholesterol, alkaline phosphatase, and alanine aminotransferase), radiographs (hepatomegaly), and ultrasound results of the two diseases are similar. The urine of the diabetic animal is usually more concentrated than that of the dog with both conditions, and both are prone to infection. These factors are emphasized here because we believe that more dogs with diabetes mellitus are diagnosed and treated for Cushing's syndrome than actually have CCS.

The ACTH stimulation test and low-dose dexamethasone test are relatively specific for hyperadrenocorticism and should help differentiate a dog with diabetes mellitus from one with diabetes mellitus and Cushing's syndrome. However, the urine cortisol: creatinine ratio is rather nonspecific, and the results of this test are neither reliable nor recommended. Appropriate use of screening tests enhances their reliability. Therefore the diagnosis of hyperadrenocorticism in a diabetic dog is more likely if the pet has clinical signs of the condition (bilaterally symmetric hair loss, calcinosis cutis, abdominal distention, low BUN and creatinine with a urine specific gravity of less than 1.020, adrenomegaly on abdominal ultrasonography, and unexpectedly high exogenous insulin requirements). It has been our belief that the most sensitive and specific test for the correct diagnosis of Cushing's syndrome in dogs is the history and physical examination. The insulin requirement, alone, is not sufficient reason to suspect that a diabetic dog has Cushing's syndrome.

Pulmonary Thromboembolism (PTE)

ETIOLOGY. Pulmonary thromboembolism (PTE) is a complication of hypercoagulability, stasis of blood flow, and damage to the endothelial lining of blood vessels (LaRue and Murtaugh, 1990). PTE and deep vein thrombosis should be considered part of the same pathologic process. Pulmonary embolism ranges in importance from incidental, clinically unimportant thromboembolism to massive embolism with sudden death. Hypercoagulability leads to the formation of thrombi in the leg, pelvis, and arm veins of people, with proximal extension as clots propagate. As thrombi form in these deep veins, they may dislodge and embolize to the pulmonary arteries. Pulmonary arterial obstruction and platelet release of vasoactive agents, such as serotonin, worsen pulmonary resistance. The resulting increase in alveolar dead space and redistribution of blood flow creates areas of decreased ventilation to perfusion, impairs gas exchange, and stimulates alveolar hyperventilation due to the release of irritant receptors. Reflex bronchoconstriction augments airway resistance. Lung edema (if present) decreases pulmonary compliance. As right ventricular afterload increases, tension rises in the right ventricular wall and may lead to dilation, dysfunction, and ischemia of the right ventricle (Goldhaber, 1998).

Pulmonary thromboembolism is a potential complication of hyperadrenocorticism and also several other disorders (e.g., various neoplasias, protein-losing nephropathies, renal failure, pancreatitis, sepsis, diabetes mellitus, immune-mediated hemolytic anemia, cardiac disease, heartworm disease, trauma, major surgery, and others) (Table 6-9). In both dogs and people with Cushing's syndrome, thromboembolism is at least partly related to the "hypercoagulable state" typical of this condition. People with Cushing's syndrome are four times more likely to suffer complications of thromboembolism than the general population (Small et al, 1983; Meaney et al, 1997). The incidence of deep vein thrombosis in nonhospitalized individuals is less than 1%; in nonhospitalized people with Cushing's syndrome, it is 7% to 25% (McLeod, 1991). Patients who undergo surgery for Cushing's disease are specifically predisposed to thrombosis (Reitmeyer et al, 2002). Predisposing factors in dogs with Cushing's syndrome are obesity, hypertension, increased hematocrit (resulting in vascular stasis), sepsis, and prolonged periods of recumbency.

TABLE 6–9 PRIMARY CLINICAL DISORDERS IN 29 DOGS WITH PULMONARY THROMBOEMBOLISM*

Immune mediated hemolytic anemia
Neoplasia
Systemic bacterial disease
   Sepsis
   Pneumonia
   Pyothorax
   Endocarditis
Hyperadrenocorticism
Amyloidosis (protein losing nephropathy)
Cardiomyopathy
Megaesophagus

*Modified from Johnson et al, 1999.

In a study of 56 dogs with naturally occurring Cushing's syndrome, levels of procoagulation factors II, V, VII, IX, X, XII, and fibrinogen were significantly increased (Jacoby et al, 2001). Natural antithrombotic antithrombin was significantly decreased, and the marker of subclinical thrombosis, thrombin-antithrombin complexes (TAT), was significantly increased (Fig. 6-31). These results are similar to those from a previous but less complete study (Feldman BF et al, 1982 and 1986), and they correlate with the results of studies completed in humans (Patrassi et al, 1985). TAT complexes are created rapidly after the production of thrombin and are used as a subclinical marker of thrombin formation. Several authors have recommended that this factor be used as a surrogate marker for clinical thromboembolism. Because previous studies have demonstrated inhibition of fibrinolytic activity in people with Cushing's syndrome, the lack of similar results in the dogs studied may suggest that this problem is not typical of the hypercoagulable state (Jacoby et al, 2001).

SIGNALMENT, HISTORY, AND PHYSICAL EXAMINATION. PTE can occur in dogs of any age, gender, or breed. The condition may be associated with various presenting clinical signs or physical examination abnormalities for two reasons: because it is almost exclusively a secondary disease (see Table 6-9) and because clinical signs may result from emboli formed concurrently in tissues other than the lung. Almost all the dogs with Cushing's syndrome in our series that developed PTE had an adrenocortical tumor surgically removed when the embolic episode began. A much smaller number of dogs in our series of those with PTE had recently undergone medical treatment with o,p'-DDD. In this setting, however, PTE is rare. Dogs with PTE would be expected to have acute respiratory distress, orthopnea and, less commonly, a jugular pulse. Panting may occur secondary to hypoxia and/or pleuritic pain (Burns et al, 1981; King et al, 1985). However, neurologic signs were among the most common clinical signs in dogs with PTE secondary to other causes. Only five of 29 were brought to veterinarians specifically for difficulty breathing, but 17 of the 29 had some relevant respiratory signs (Johnson et al, 1999).

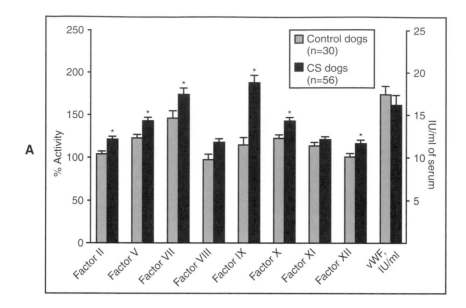

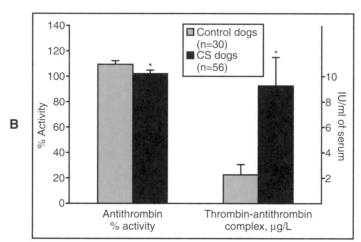

FIGURE 6-31. Coagulation assay results indicating that dogs with hyperadrenocorticism are predisposed to thromboemboli. *A,* Serum procoagulant factors as assayed from 30 healthy control dogs and 56 dogs with hyperadrenocorticism (CS). *B,* Antithrombin and thrombin-antithrombin complex results from 30 healthy control dogs and 56 dogs with hyperadrenocorticism. The asterisks (*) denote significance, and the bars indicate standard error.

LABORATORY RESULTS, THORACIC RADIOLOGY, AND ECHOCARDIOGRAPHY. A recent study found no laboratory test result pathognomonic for PTE. A number of laboratory abnormalities were noted, but these results either were caused by each dog's primary disease or were nonspecific. Some of the abnormalities included anemia and increases in white cell counts, alkaline phosphatase, alanine amino transferase, BUN, and creatinine. Decreases in sodium, potassium, and albumin were also noted (Johnson et al, 1999). Radiography of the thorax is an important component of the evaluation of any dyspneic animal. However, in this disease, results are not consistent. Radiography may reveal pleural effusion, loss of the pulmonary artery, alveolar infiltrates, cardiomegaly, hyperlucent lung fields, enlargement of the main pulmonary artery, or no abnormalities (Fluckiger and Gomez, 1984; Johnson et al, 1999). Alternatively, there may be an increased diameter and blunting of the pulmonary arteries, lack of perfusion of the obstructed pulmonary vasculature, and overperfusion of the unobstructed pulmonary vasculature (Fig. 6-32) (see discussion under Radiology, page 283). Normal thoracic radiographs in a dyspneic patient that lacks large airway obstruction may be consistent with pulmonary thromboembolism.

In humans with PTE, echocardiography with Doppler assessment provides relatively sensitive and specific information. Abnormal examinations were noted in 94% of cases with angiography-confirmed pulmonary embolism, whereas abnormal examinations were found in only 13% of people with similar

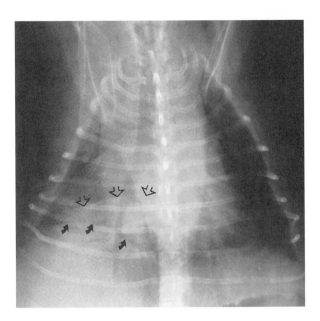

FIGURE 6–32. Dorsoventral thoracic radiograph of a dog with pulmonary thromboembolism that resulted in a focal area of density, which is outlined by the arrows.

clinical signs who did not have PTE. Right ventricular dilation (right ventricle/left ventricle diameter >0.6), high-velocity tricuspid regurgitation (>2.5 m/second), and paradoxic septal motion were found significantly more often in humans with proven embolization (Nazeyrollas et al, 1995). In dogs with PTE, echocardiography examination results have been normal, have demonstrated evidence of right ventricular pressure overload, or have given the impression of pulmonary hypertension based on a high-velocity tricuspid regurgitant jet. Detection of characteristic echocardiographic findings or right atrial thrombosis in dogs suspected of having PTE may provide a noninvasive means of supporting the diagnosis of PTE in veterinary medicine (Johnson et al, 1999).

BLOOD GAS ANALYSIS. PTE results in hypoxemia primarily from ventilation-perfusion mismatch, although physiologic shunting and increased dead space also contribute to reduced arterial oxygen content (West, 1992). Approximately 75% of affected humans show hypoxemia, and 95% have an increased alveolar-arterial oxygen gradient (Stein et al, 1991). Calculation of the alveolar-arterial gradient corrects for the contribution of alveolar hypoventilation to arterial hypoxemia but does not differentiate V-Q mismatch from other causes of hypoxemia. Dogs with PTE usually have hypoxemia and increased alveolar-arterial oxygen gradients while breathing room air. However, these findings are nonspecific indicators of inefficient gas exchange and cannot be the sole indicator of PTE. Dogs with PTE are also frequently hypocapnic.

Administration of oxygen corrects hypoxemia caused by V-Q mismatch, diffusion impairment, or alveolar hypoventilation; with PTE, the degree of improvement in the partial pressure of arterial oxygen

(PaO_2) depends on the percentage of the vascular bed obstructed, the concentration of inspired O_2 administered, and the distribution of ventilation-perfusion mismatching across the lung. This "oxygen responsiveness" has also demonstrated variable results in both people and dogs with PTE, presumably because as the degree of vascular obstruction exceeds 50% of the circulatory bed surface area, intrapulmonary shunting occurs, leading to venous admixture of blood and decreased oxygen responsiveness (Johnson et al, 1999).

DIAGNOSIS. A diagnosis of pulmonary thromboembolic disease can be supported by clinical signs and physical examination findings, hematologic and biochemical parameters, thoracic radiographs, echocardiographic results, blood pressure measurements, and arterial blood gas analysis. The results of these tests are not specific for PTE and may be normal. The value of these tests (except blood gas analysis) may be to exclude other disease processes that must be distinguished from thromboembolism. In people, the initial diagnostic study performed when PTE is suspected is ventilation-perfusion scanning. However, only 27% of patients had imaging results that permitted a definitive diagnosis. In most patients with indeterminate findings on ventilation-perfusion scans, pulmonary angiography is needed to confirm or rule out PTE. This approach, however, is invasive and expensive, even for people. More recently, magnetic resonance angiography has been demonstrated to be an excellent diagnostic aid, one that avoids the use of ionizing radiation or iodinated contrast material (Meaney et al, 1997).

Although they are not completely sensitive or specific, angiography of the lungs and radionuclear lung scans have been used to confirm thrombosis in dogs (Fig. 6-33). The absence of perfusion defects practically excludes the diagnosis of pulmonary thromboembolism. The greater the size and number of ventilated lung regions that demonstrate decreased perfusion on scintigraphy, the greater the probability of pulmonary thromboembolism. The presence of segmental or larger perfusion defects in lung regions with normal ventilation and no radiographic evidence of pulmonary disease is most diagnostic for pulmonary thromboembolism (Dennis, 1993).

THERAPY. The history of naturally acquired pulmonary thromboembolism in dogs is not well described. In experimental conditions, pulmonary thromboemboli begin to dissolve without treatment within hours of formation, and complete resolution has been documented within days (Dennis, 1993). In naturally occurring disease, a persistent prothrombotic tendency may exist. Consequently, the fibrinolytic mechanisms in these dogs may be hindered. The goals of therapy are to reverse the prothrombotic state and to alleviate the hemodynamic and pulmonary sequelae responsible for morbidity and mortality (Dennis, 1993).

In humans, aspirin therapy is begun before surgery to minimize the incidence of thrombosis (Reitmeyer, 2002). Therapy consists of general support and admin-

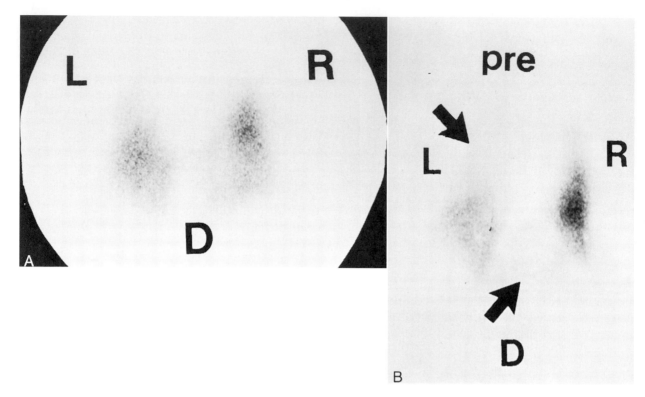

FIGURE 6–33. Lung scans from a normal dog (A) and from one with hyperadrenocorticism and pulmonary thromboembolism (B). Arrows point out areas with diminished uptake of radioactivity.

istration of oxygen and anticoagulants. The anticoagulant regimen is as follows: heparin (100 to 200 IU/kg IV, followed by the same dose SC q6h, adjusted to prolong the activated partial thromboplastin time by 1.5 to 2 times normal) and/or coumarin (warfarin, 0.2 mg/kg PO, followed by 0.05 to 0.1 mg/kg PO daily to achieve a prothrombin time of 1.5 to 2 times normal; this takes 2 to 7 days to become effective) (Rush, 1990; Dennis, 1993). Warfarin is potentially thrombogenic during the first few days, and this tendency can be counteracted by the anticoagulant effect of heparin. Antagonizing the coagulation system ideally prevents the growth of existing thrombi and the formation of new thrombi that may further compromise cardiovascular and respiratory function. Heparin and coumarin do not directly dissolve existing thrombi. Streptokinase and recombinant tissue plasminogen activator rapidly dissolve experimental pulmonary thromboemboli in dogs (Shiffman et al, 1988). The use of fibrinolytic agents to treat naturally acquired canine PTE was evaluated in four dogs and found to be effective and associated with few side effects (Ramsey et al, 1996), although the use of streptokinase in the treatment of large obstructing pulmonary emboli has not been established in veterinary studies (Johnson et al, 1999). As with anticoagulant therapy, the primary complication of fibrinolytic therapy is life-threatening hemorrhage (Dennis, 1993).

PROGNOSIS. The prognosis for PTE is guarded to grave. Recovery, if it occurs, usually requires at least

7 to 10 days before the dog can be safely removed from oxygen support. Thus treatment can be expensive, and the outcome is usually not promising.

Pituitary "Macrotumors" and Central Nervous System Signs

PATHOPHYSIOLOGY. Occasionally PDH results from a functioning large pituitary tumor (>1 cm in diameter), or small tumors can increase in size from the time of diagnosis and during therapy. Such masses, with dorsal expansion, may compress or invade the hypothalamus and other "suprasellar" structures; may invaginate the "pituitary stalk" that connects the hypothalamus with the pituitary; or may dilate the infundibular recess and third ventricle. Clinical signs exhibited by dogs with "macrotumors" often reflect both endocrine and space-occupying effects. The endocrine manifestations are those typical of Cushing's syndrome. Cortisone excess suppresses synthesis and/or secretion of the remaining pituitary hormones, making the diagnosis of hypopituitarism due to tumor destruction almost impossible to confirm.

Predicting which pituitary tumor will cause clinical signs because of its mass is difficult. We have evaluated more than 100 dogs with untreated, recently diagnosed PDH that had no clinical signs suggestive of a large intracranial mass. Each dog had a brain MRI or CT scan. Approximately 40% of these dogs had no visible pituitary mass, and 60% had pituitary tumors ranging in size from 4 to 13 mm at greatest vertical height. Most pituitary masses are easily visualized. Statistical studies completed by one group of researchers indicate that the size of the pituitary tumor correlates with endocrine test results (Kooistra et al, 1997). Although this is likely to be statistically correct, no clinical or endocrine tests *consistently* distinguish dogs with large tumors from those with tumors smaller than 4 mm (Fig. 6-34) (Kipperman et al, 1992; Bertoy et al, 1995). Therefore neither MRI nor CT scans should be obtained or recommended simply because of the results of endocrine testing. Rather, we recommend imaging studies for untreated and recently diagnosed dogs with PDH that have no clinical signs of a large pituitary tumor when (1) the facilities are available, (2) pituitary Cushing's syndrome is confirmed, and (3) the owner can afford testing. The treatment and long-term management of dogs with pituitary Cushing's syndrome can then be tailored to the individual dog (see Treatment sections beginning on page 325).

We have participated in several additional studies on dogs with PDH that have clinical signs caused by an enlarging pituitary tumor. Each dog with signs caused by an enlarging brain tumor had a mass 1 cm or greater in height, although signs have been noted in dogs with masses that were 8 to 9 mm in greatest diameter (Deusch, 2005). However, dogs with similar tumor masses were identified that had no clinical signs suggestive of an enlarging intracranial tumor. Again, no routine clinical pathology or endocrine test result consistently distinguished dogs with small pituitary tumors from those with large pituitary tumors, or dogs with clinical signs of an intracranial tumor from those without such signs (Fig. 6-35) (Kipperman et al, 1992; Duesberg et al, 1995).

CLINICAL SIGNS. When neurologic signs first begin to be recognized, they are almost always subtle, progressively more obvious to an owner but not usually obvious to a veterinarian. Therefore, knowing the owner and his or her observation skills is quite important. Common initial signs include a pet that seems to be "dull," listless, and inappetent. These signs may progress to anorexia, restlessness, loss of interest in normal household activities, delayed response to stimuli, and brief (or prolonged) episodes of disorientation. The differential diagnosis for these signs includes, among many others, o,p'-DDD overdose. More definitive signs exhibited by dogs with macrotumors include altered mentation (obtundation, stupor), ataxia, tetraparesis, and aimless pacing (Fig. 6-36 and Table 6-10). It is important to point out that a significant but small percentage of dogs with hyperadrenocorticism have facial paralysis. This abnormality is related to cortisol excess but not to a pituitary mass, even when the mass is quite large.

Less frequently observed problems include nystagmus, circling, head pressing, behavior changes, blindness, seizures, and coma. Anisocoria and strabismus are rare and may result from damage to cranial nerves. Some of these dogs may be misdiagnosed as blind because mental dullness results in inappropriate responses to visual stimuli (absent menace). With severe compression of the hypothalamus,

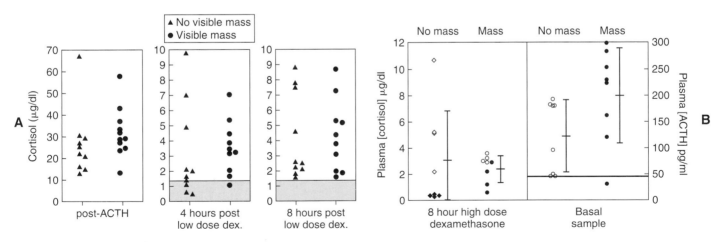

FIGURE 6–34. *A,* Plasma cortisol concentrations 1 hour after intramuscular administration of 0.25 mg of synthetic ACTH and 4 and 8 hours after intravenous administration of 0.01 mg/kg of dexamethasone in dogs with pituitary-dependent hyperadrenocorticism (PDH). (Triangles denote dogs without a visible pituitary mass on magnetic resonance imaging [MRI] scan; circles denote dogs with a visible pituitary mass on MRI scan. Shaded areas indicate reference ranges.) *B,* Plasma cortisol concentrations 8 hours after intravenous administration of 0.1 mg/kg of dexamethasone *(left),* and basal plasma endogenous ACTH concentrations *(right).* Diamonds on left denote dogs without a visible pituitary mass on MRI scan. Black diamonds and black circles denote dogs with values less than 50% of baseline cortisol concentrations after dexamethasone administration; open diamonds and open circles denote dogs with values greater than 50% of baseline cortisol concentrations after dexamethasone administration. The information on these graphs shows that endocrine test results are not reliable indicators of pituitary tumor size in dogs with PDH. (From Bertoy EH, et al: J Am Vet Med Assoc 206:651, 1995.)

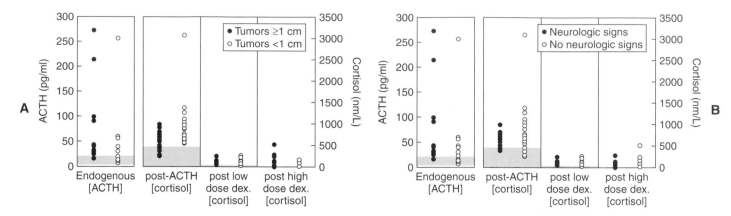

FIGURE 6–35. Basal plasma endogenous ACTH concentrations and plasma cortisol concentrations after administration of ACTH, after a low dose of dexamethasone, and after a high dose of dexamethasone in dogs with pituitary-dependent hyperadrenocorticism (PDH) attributed to pituitary tumors of 1 cm or more and less than 1 cm in diameter (*A*) and the same parameters from dogs with or without neurologic signs attributed to a growing pituitary tumor (*B*). These results show that endocrine test results are of no value in predicting pituitary tumor size in dogs with PDH.

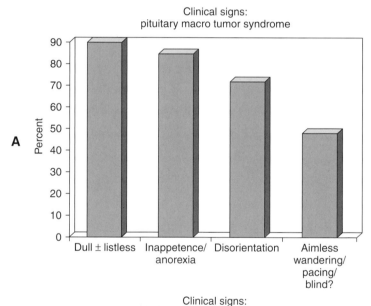

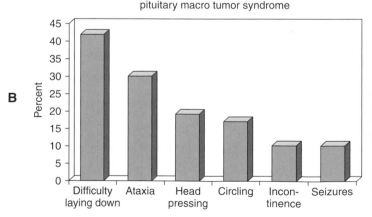

FIGURE 6–36. Bar graphs (*A* and *B*) illustrating the most common clinical signs owners and veterinarians observe in dogs with large pituitary tumors that cause central nervous system signs (note the difference in the vertical scale of the two graphs).

abnormalities related to dysfunction of the autonomic nervous system develop, but these are rare. They include adipsia, loss of temperature regulation, erratic heart rate, and inability to be roused from a "sleeplike" state. These are considered terminal signs.

DIAGNOSIS. Macrotumor syndrome may be present before Cushing's syndrome is diagnosed (<20% of dogs with macrotumors) or within 30 to 60 days of the start of treatment for Cushing's syndrome (20% to 30% of dogs with macrotumors), or it may be diagnosed 6 months or more after Cushing's syndrome has been treated (40% to 60% of cases) (Fig. 6-37). The diagnosis of macrotumor depends on elimination of the possibility of concurrent illnesses or overdose of o,p'-DDD, which might explain the clinical signs. No endocrine test result reliably correlates with the size of a pituitary tumor (see Figs. 6-34 and 6-35) (Kipperman et al, 1992; Bertoy et al, 1995; Duesberg et al, 1995). The diagnosis can be confirmed only with advanced imaging technology (CT or MRI). The results of these procedures

TABLE 6–10 CLINICAL SIGNS CAUSED BY AN ENLARGING PITUITARY TUMOR IN DOGS WITH HYPERADRENOCORTICISM*

Dullness, listlessness	Ataxia
Inappetence (poor appetite)/anorexia (no appetite)	Tetraparesis
	Nystagmus
Restlessness	Circling
Loss of interest in normal activities	Head pressing
	Behavior changes
Delayed response to various stimuli	Blindness
Disorientation/aimless pacing	Seizures
Altered mentation	Coma
Obtundation	Adipsia
Stupor	Loss of temperature regulation
	Erratic heart rate

*Listed in decreasing order of frequency.

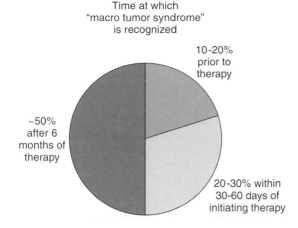

Time at which
"macro tumor syndrome"
is recognized

10-20%
prior to
therapy

~50%
after 6
months of
therapy

20-30% within
30-60 days of
initiating therapy

FIGURE 6–37. Pie chart showing when neurologic signs are detected in dogs with PDH due to a growing pituitary tumor, relative to the timing of PDH diagnosis and initiation of medical therapy for the disease.

and treatment with cobalt irradiation are discussed on pages 320 and 349, respectively.

DIFFERENTIAL DIAGNOSIS

General

The combination of clinical signs noted on the history and the results of the physical examination, in most dogs with hyperadrenocorticism, should be strongly consistent with the final diagnosis. As seen in Table 6-11, however, several diseases have some clinical signs and/or laboratory data that may overlap with those of CCS. The more obvious differential diagnoses are diabetes mellitus, acromegaly, diabetes insipidus, renal insufficiency, liver insufficiency, pyelonephritis, hypothyroidism, hyperthyroidism, Sertoli cell tumor, and hypercalcemia. The endocrine alopecia and hyperpigmentation found in dogs with "adult- onset growth hormone deficiency" may mimic the dermatologic signs of hyperadrenocorticism (see Chapter 2, page 270).

Congenital Portosystemic Shunts

Some dogs with portosystemic shunts have polyuria and polydipsia secondary to cortisol excess. In a study of 22 dogs with proven congenital portosystemic shunts, the urine cortisol:creatinine ratio prior to shunt closure was 13.4×10^{-6}; after surgical correction of the shunt, this ratio was 3.9×10^{-6} (Sterczer et al, 1998). The urine specific gravity increased after surgery, and the characteristics of cortisol binding by cortisol-binding globulin increased after surgical correction of the shunt. Thus congenital portosystemic shunt is not a differential diagnosis for hyperadrenocorticism as much as it is a cause for excesses in circulating cortisol.

TABLE 6–11 DIFFERENTIAL DIAGNOSES FOR CANINE CUSHING'S SYNDROME AND MAJOR AREAS OF OVERLAP

Differential Diagnosis	Overlap with Canine Cushing's Syndrome
Diabetes mellitus	PD/PU/polyphagia ↑ SAP, ↑ ALT, ↑ FBG, ↑ cholesterol Hepatomegaly Urinary tract infection
Renal disease	PD/PU
Liver disease	Hepatomegaly ↑ SAP, ↑ ALP, ↑ liver function test results
Hypothyroidism	Bilaterally symmetrical alopecia Apparent weight gain ↑ Cholesterol
Sertoli cell tumor	Bilaterally symmetrical alopecia
Pyelonephritis	Chronic recurring urinary tract infection PD/PU
Hypercalcemia	PD/PU
Diabetes insipidus	
Nephrogenic	PD/PU
Central	PD/PU
Primary (psychogenic) polydipsia	PD/PU
Acromegaly	PD/PU/polyphagia Poor hair coat ↑ SAP, enlarged abdomen Muscle weakness, inspiratory stridor ↑ Blood glucose, hepatomegaly
Ascites	Enlarged abdomen (may be difficult to palpate)
Anticonvulsant therapy	PD/PU; lethargy; polyphagia ↑ SAP; ↑ ALT; abnormal plasma cortisol concentrations

PD, polydipsia; *PU,* polyuria; *SAP,* serum alkaline phosphatase; *ALT,* alanine aminoransferase; *FBG,* fasting blood glucose.

Phenobarbital Administration

Dogs receiving phenobarbital may have side effects that result in clinical signs quite similar to those associated with the signs of naturally occurring hyperadrenocorticism. These signs include polydipsia, polyuria, and polyphagia. To make matters more confusing, phenobarbital administration can cause increases in serum alkaline phosphatase activity (Foster et al, 2000b; Muller et al, 2000b). Although it has been our impression that phenobarbital may interfere with serum cortisol concentrations, and therefore test results related to hyperadrenocorticism, these observations have been difficult to demonstrate in clinical studies (Dyer et al, 1994; Chauvet et al, 1995; Foster et al, 2000a; Muller et al, 2000a). It has also been our impression that chronic phenobarbital administration interferes with the effectiveness of o,p'-DDD treatment. It remains our recommendation that for any dog suspected of having naturally developing Cushing's syndrome that is receiving phenobarbital, the drug should be discontinued (with or without potassium bromide therapy as replacement) before diagnostic testing or therapy commences. On occasion, discontinuation of phenobarbital results in resolution of all clinical signs and laboratory abnormalities.

SPECIFIC EVALUATION OF THE PITUITARY-ADRENOCORTICAL AXIS

General Approach

DATABASE. After a presumptive diagnosis of canine or feline hyperadrenocorticism has been established from review of the owner's observations, the physical examination findings, the laboratory database (CBC, urinalysis, and serum biochemistry profile), radiographs, and/or ultrasonography, the clinician usually proceeds to attempt confirmation of the diagnosis. When necessary and if possible, an attempt can also be made to determine the source of the disorder (pituitary versus adrenal). As previously discussed, in dogs concurrently receiving phenobarbital, the drug should be discontinued (with or without potassium bromide replacement) prior to testing or treatment.

ENDOCRINE ASSAYS. The mainstay of diagnostic procedures is the measurement of plasma, serum, or urine cortisol concentrations. Assays for cortisol include fluorometric, radioimmunoassay (RIA), enzyme-linked immunosorbent assay (ELISA), chemiluminescent, and high-performance liquid chromatography assays. Commercially available RIAs are reliable, inexpensive, easily performed, and commonly used. Urine cortisol assays are similar to those used for plasma. Commercially available plasma ACTH assays are also being used more frequently, although ACTH is more fragile and the assays more expensive. Assays for aldosterone are also available commercially.

CORTISOL COLLECTION METHOD. Blood collected for cortisol determination should be placed in a tube containing heparin as the anticoagulant, although assays performed on serum are equally reliable. Heparinized blood should be centrifuged soon after the sample is obtained, with the separated plasma placed in a clean vial and frozen. Cortisol concentrations in *plasma* are stable, and cooling of the sample is not necessary; *serum,* however, should be shipped cold (Behrend et al, 1998). Because cortisol concentrations in frozen plasma are stable for long periods (months and perhaps years), it is recommended that all samples for cortisol be cold or frozen when sent to a laboratory. Cortisol is quite stable in plasma, and hemolysis or storage of samples at warm temperatures for short periods has little effect on assay results (Reimers et al, 1991). Hemolysis, lipemia, or hyperbilirubinemia do not significantly interfere with ELISA determinations of cortisol concentration (Lucena et al, 1998). A minimum of 1 ml of plasma should be sent to the laboratory from each blood sample, an amount that provides more than an adequate volume if

duplicate assays are to be performed. However, the individual laboratory recommendations should always be followed.

PLASMA ALDOSTERONE ASSAYS. Several commercially available RIA assay kits for aldosterone are valid for dogs and cats. Few situations, however, require this information for diagnosis of hyperadrenocorticism. Many dogs with hyperadrenocorticism demonstrate exaggerated plasma aldosterone responses to ACTH, paralleling the plasma cortisol response (Golden and Lothrop, 1988; Ortega et al, 1995b). When specific aldosterone-related disorders are suspected (see page 351), it is reasonable to assess plasma aldosterone concentrations. The diagnosis of primary hyperaldosteronism is rare in dogs.

Endocrine Testing

Generally, the evaluation of an animal suspected of having hyperadrenocorticism proceeds through two basic steps (Fig. 6-38). The first step is to confirm or rule out the existence of hyperadrenocorticism (Cushing's syndrome). This step is important and must be completed. The second step begins only after the diagnosis of hyperadrenocorticism has been confirmed. This latter step consists of differentiating PDH from adrenal tumor–dependent hyperadrenocorticism (ATH).

SCREENING TESTS: CONFIRMING A DIAGNOSIS OF HYPERADRENOCORTICISM

Background

"Screening" tests for hyperadrenocorticism or naturally occurring CCS are tests that aid in distinguishing dogs with CCS from dogs that do not have CCS. The choice of a screening test for hyperadrenocorticism is important because that test may determine whether a dog is treated. Routinely used screening tests include ACTH stimulation, low-dose dexamethasone, and the urine cortisol:creatinine ratio. However, it should be emphasized that our experience indicates that the most sensitive and specific screening tests for CCS are the history and physical examination. Treatment recommendations, therefore, should be based on the history, the physical examination findings, and the results of the initial database (i.e., CBC, serum chemistry profile, and urinalysis), as well as the results of an endocrine "screening" test. The decision to treat a dog for Cushing's syndrome should never be based solely on laboratory information. Cushing's syndrome is a *clinical* disorder with clinical signs. If a dog has no clinical signs, we do not recommend treatment.

Sensitivity and Specificity

The *sensitivity* of a test refers to the number of patients with a problem that have test results diagnostic of that

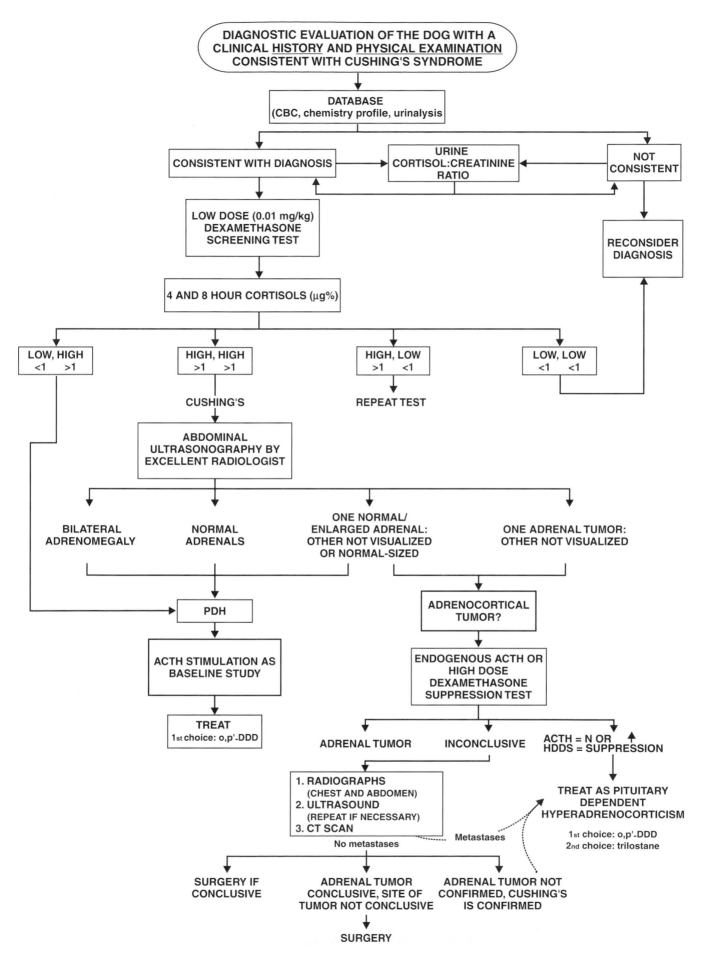

FIGURE 6–38. Flow chart for the diagnostic evaluation of a dog or cat with suspected hyperadrenocorticism.

TABLE 6–12 SENSITIVITY, SPECIFICITY AND DIAGNOSTIC ACCURACY OF ENDOCRINE SCREENING TESTS IN DOGS FOR THE DIAGNOSIS OF HYPERADRENOCORTICISM*

Test	Parameter (%)	STUDY				
		1	2	3	4	5
LDDS	Sensitivity	100	100	96	85	–
	Specificity	73	44	70	73	–
	Diagnostic accuracy	92	58	89	83	–
ACTH stimulation	Sensitivity	89	80	95	–	–
	Specificity	82	86	91	–	–
	Diagnostic accuracy	87	84	93	–	–
UCCR	Sensitivity	50	75	–	99	100
	Specificity	100	24	–	77	22
	Diagnostic accuracy	59	37	–	91	76

*ACTH, corticotrophin; LDDS, low-dose dexamethasone suppression; UCCR, urine cortisol:creatinine ratio; –, parameter not investigated.
Study 1: Zerbe et al 1987
2: Kaplan et al 1995
3: van Liew et al 1997
4: Rijnberk et al 1988
5: Feldman, Mack 1992

problem. The *specificity* of a test refers to the number of patients that do not have a problem but have test results diagnostic of that condition. This concept gains importance when it is understood that no screening test is correct all of the time; that is, sensitivity and specificity are never 100% for any test (Table 6-12). As has been reported, "dogs with nonadrenal disease may have false-positive test results for hyperadrenocorticism if tested with the commonly employed pituitary-adrenal function tests. Because false-positive test results were observed for all of the commonly used screening tests (ACTH stimulation test, low-dose dexamethasone test, urine cortisol: creatinine ratio), the definitive diagnosis of hyperadrenocorticism should never be based solely on the results of one or more of these screening tests, especially in dogs without classic clinical signs of the disease or in those with known nonadrenal disease (Kaplan et al, 1995).

Resting (Basal) Plasma Cortisol Concentrations

The basal (morning) plasma cortisol determination, by itself, is of virtually no diagnostic value in the attempt to confirm a diagnosis of hyperadrenocorticism in a dog. This is obvious when evaluating basal plasma cortisol concentrations in dogs that were ill or undergoing anesthesia (Church et al, 1994). The mean resting plasma cortisol concentration in dogs with naturally occurring Cushing's syndrome is significantly above the mean of normal dogs, but the results are usually still within reference ranges (see Fig. 6-7). This apparent discrepancy is explained by the fact that both ACTH and cortisol are secreted episodically. Bursts of secretion occur throughout the day, creating a myriad of peaks and valleys in the plasma cortisol concentration (see Fig. 6-7). These fluctuations account for the wide reference range for plasma cortisol concentration in dogs (usually 0.5 to 6.0 μg/dl).

Dogs with hyperadrenocorticism have a greater frequency of cortisol bursts, as well as increased amplitudes in these secretory patterns. For the most part, these bursts result in plasma cortisol concentrations that overlap with normal. During any 24-hour period, however, the hormonal secretory pattern in dogs with hyperadrenocorticism creates an excess in the amount of cortisol secreted. In other words, if one creates a mental picture of the area under the curve for cortisol concentrations in dogs with Cushing's syndrome, as seen in Fig. 6-7, there is a tremendous difference when comparing dogs that do not have Cushing's syndrome with those that do. Over a period of months or years, the clinical syndrome of hyperadrenocorticism results from this chronic and unrelenting pattern of cortisol excess.

Urinary Cortisol and Urine Cortisol:Creatinine Ratio (UC:CR)

24-HOUR COLLECTION AND ASSAY. Traditionally, the cortisol concentration is measured in an aliquot of urine from the volume collected over a 24-hour period. The result is then typically multiplied by the total volume collected in 24 hours to provide an integrated assessment of the amount of hormone produced over time. This has been the "gold standard" used in the diagnosis of hyperadrenocorticism in humans for decades, and it continues to be the most reliable means of confirming a diagnosis (Orth, 1995). This test was introduced after the first cortisol assays of any type were developed in the late 1940s. These first assays were for urine cortisol metabolites, and this test was a logical step once the syndrome carrying Dr. Cushing's name was understood to be one caused by cortisol excess.

It also should be remembered that the typical person with hyperadrenocorticism does not have the polyuria typically seen in CCS dogs. Thus human patients are not collecting enormous volumes of urine. Problems related to episodic release of cortisol, a factor with plasma assays, can be avoided. Assay of urine free cortisol is recommended because it is rapid and suitable for clinical use, and it has advantages over measurement of urine cortisol metabolites. The 24-hour urine specimen is collected in a suitable preservative and is stable when refrigerated (Baxter and Tyrrell, 1981). Despite the advantages of this diagnostic tool, it is rarely used in dogs and cats because of the cumbersome process of collecting urine. When used, however, the test results are quite reliable.

URINE CORTISOL:CREATININE RATIO

Background. Assay of the urine cortisol concentration in a sample collected over a 2-hour period may accurately assess the function of the pituitary-adrenal axis in humans (Allin et al, 1984). Further studies demonstrated that the ratio of the cortisol concentration to the creatinine concentration (UC:CR), from a single, randomly obtained, voided urine sample provided information that helped identify humans with hyperadrenocorticism (Atkinson et al, 1985; Contreras et al, 1986). Similar studies in dogs revealed that the measurement of UC:CR had potential as a screening test for canine hyperadrenocorticism (Stolp et al, 1983; Rijnberk et al, 1988a).

Sensitivity and Specificity. Several groups have evaluated the urine cortisol:creatinine ratio, arriving at different conclusions regarding its usefulness (see Table 6-12). There is general agreement that the UC:CR readily distinguishes between apparently healthy dogs and those with hyperadrenocorticism (i.e., it is a "sensitive" test) (Jones et al, 1990). One group recommends the UC:CR as the only necessary screening test for the diagnosis of Cushing's syndrome, based in part on a veterinarian's ability to rule out other diseases on review of the history, physical examination, and database testing and considering test sensitivity (Rijnberk et al, 1988a).

Other groups have demonstrated that the test is sensitive (although not perfect) (Kaplan et al, 1995) but lacks specificity. It has been demonstrated that 79% and 76% of dogs with moderate to severe *nonadrenal* disease had a UC:CR consistent with Cushing's syndrome (Smiley and Peterson, 1993; Kaplan et al, 1995, respectively). In our studies, the UC:CR was again demonstrated to be sensitive but nonspecific; that is, it was abnormal in dogs with Cushing's syndrome but was also abnormal in most dogs with diabetes mellitus, diabetes insipidus, pyometra, hypercalcemia, and liver failure, (Fig. 6-39) (Feldman and Mack, 1992).

Subsequent studies have evaluated the UC:CR using different cortisol assays, such as fluorescence polarization immunoassay (FPIA) (Kolevska and Svoboda, 2000) and ELISA methods (Jensen et al, 1997). In each case the UC:CR was determined to be highly sensitive for supporting the diagnosis of CCS. In one of these studies, specificity was 85%, but the reference range was much greater than in previous studies (Jensen et al, 1997). Differences in methodology have a significant effect on the measurement of urine cortisol concentrations, and they also affect the calculated reference range validated for each assay. Therefore each laboratory should always determine a reference range for the test offered. Regardless of the group evaluating the UC:CR, there has consistently been overlap between dogs with naturally developing hyperadrenocorticism and those with nonadrenal conditions; this overlap has prompted authors to recommend the ACTH stimulation or low-dose dexamethasone test for final confirmation of a diagnosis (Jensen et al, 1997; Kolevska and Svoboda, 2000).

Because of the high sensitivity reported in some studies, it has been recommended that this test be used for its negative predictive value. That is, if UC:CR results are within the reference range, CCS is unlikely. Thus it could be argued that the UC:CR is a reasonable test to screen for CCS in dogs in which the suspicion is low or in those that cannot be hospitalized for testing.

However, no test is perfect, and both false-positive and false-negative results are seen (Zerbe, 2000a).

Home versus Hospital Urine Collection. In one study, visitation to a veterinary hospital, in-hospital orthopedic examination, and hospitalization for several days was demonstrated to increase UC:CR results (Van Vonderen et al, 1998). The conclusion reached was that urine submitted for UC:CR must be collected by owners at home prior to arrival at the veterinary hospital, thereby avoiding a UC:CR consistent with hyperadrenocorticism when the dog is only stressed by transport to the hospital or by procedures done in the hospital prior to urine collection. However, it would appear that these authors forced their results to match their initial hypothesis. The results were published without placement of reference ranges on the graphed data, and placing a reference range on the graphs causes one to question the need for owner collection of urine (i.e., it completely reverses the conclusion) (Fig. 6-40).

Regardless, it is recommended that any owner of a dog that is exhibiting polyuria, frequency of urination, or inappropriate urination be encouraged to collect a urine sample from their pet prior to arrival at a veterinary hospital. Among the advantages of such a policy is that it allows rapid diagnosis of diabetes mellitus, polyuria, or urinary tract disorders. Furthermore, the UC:CR is not recommended as the sole confirmatory test for hyperadrenocorticism. The current recommendation is that the history, the physical examination findings, the clinicopathologic "database," and the ACTH stimulation or low-dose dexamethasone test be used as screening tests for Cushing's syndrome in dogs.

ACTH Stimulation Test

HISTORY. The ACTH stimulation test has been the most commonly used "screening" test to aid in confirming a diagnosis of hyperadrenocorticism in dogs. ACTH stimulation testing is safe, simple, relatively inexpensive, and not time-consuming (lasting 1 or 2 hours). However, it is interesting to point out that in humans suspected of having a hormone deficiency, *stimulation* testing is common. In contrast, people with hormone excess conditions undergo *suppression* testing. It is curious, therefore, that veterinary medicine elected to use a test for diagnosing Cushing's syndrome that is not used in people. During the past few years, the results of ACTH stimulation testing have undergone critical studies, which have revealed its weaknesses and strengths.

THEORY. Dogs with pituitary-dependent Cushing's syndrome (PDH) have adrenocortical hyperplasia secondary to chronic excessive stimulation by ACTH. These hyperplastic adrenals have the capacity to synthesize and secrete excessive (abnormal) amounts of cortisol. Dogs with functioning adrenocortical tumors (adenomas and carcinomas; ATH) have a similar abnormal capacity to synthesize and secrete excess cortisol. Therefore dogs with PDH or ATH have

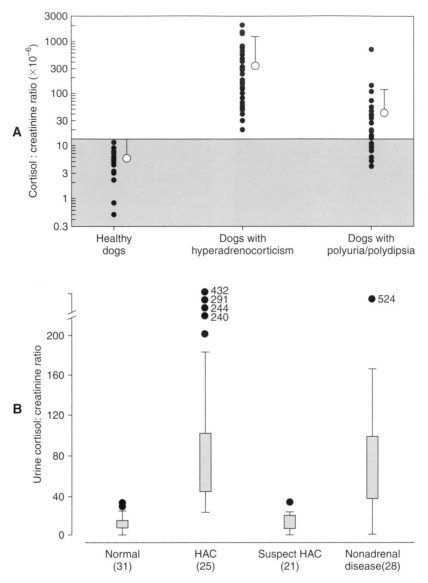

FIGURE 6–39. *A,* Urine cortisol:creatinine ratios (UC:CRs) from healthy dogs, dogs with naturally occurring hyperadrenocorticism, and dogs with polyuria/polydipsia due to disorders other than hyperadrenocorticism. These values show that the UC:CR is a sensitive test for Cushing's syndrome but is not specific and should not be used as the sole test in confirming a diagnosis. *B,* Box plots of the UC:CRs found in normal dogs; dogs with hyperadrenocorticism (HAC); dogs in which hyperadrenocorticism was initially suspected but that did not have the disease (suspect HAC); and dogs with a variety of severe, nonadrenal diseases. The number of dogs in each group is shown in parentheses. The "box" represents the interquartile range from the 25th to 75th percentiles (the middle half of the data). The horizontal bar through the box is the median. The "whiskers" represent the main body of data, which in most cases is equal to the range. Outlying data points are represented by the circles (exact value is given for these cases). These data show that the UC:CR is sensitive for the diagnosis of Cushing's syndrome but is not specific. (*A* from Mack RE, Feldman EC: J Am Vet Med Assoc 197:1603, 1990; *B* from Smiley LE, Peterson ME: J Vet Intern Med 7:163, 1993.)

the potential for an exaggerated response to ACTH stimulation. If this is true, and if the adrenals in both disorders maintain ACTH responsiveness, dogs with Cushing's syndrome can be distinguished from those that do not have the disorder based on the results of ACTH stimulation testing.

PROTOCOL. Numerous protocols for the ACTH stimulation test have been published (Table 6-13). The test can begin at any time of day and without patient preparation. Reliable results are obtained with ACTH

gel administered in doses of 1.0 or 2.2 IU/kg body weight given intramuscularly (Watson et al, 1998). Plasma samples (i.e., heparinized blood) for cortisol should be obtained prior to and 2 hours after injection of ACTH gel. Alternatively, synthetic ACTH (tetracosactrin, cosyntropin, Cortrosyn) can be used. Synthetic ACTH, however, is becoming quite expensive. We recommend administering this drug in a dose of 0.25 mg/dog (1 vial) given intramuscularly, regardless of body weight, and samples should be

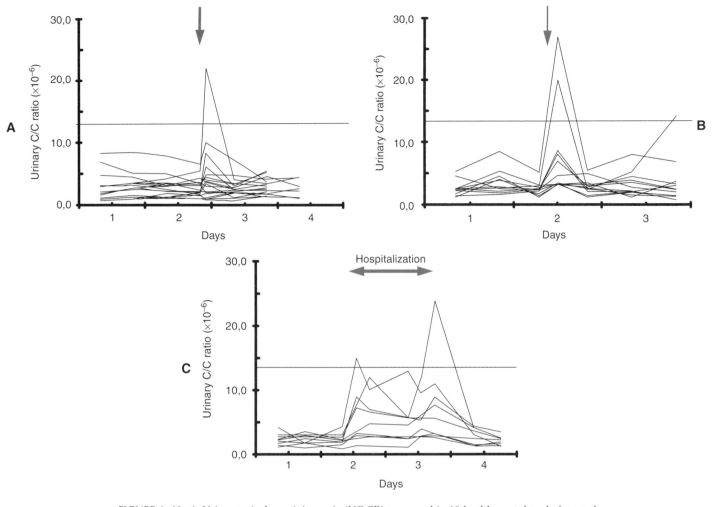

FIGURE 6–40. *A,* Urine cortisol:creatinine ratio (UC:CR) measured in 19 healthy pet dogs before and after a visit to a veterinary practice for yearly vaccination. The arrow indicates the time of the visit to the veterinary practice. The line indicates the upper reference limit of the assay. B, UC:CR measured in 12 pet dogs before and after a visit to a referral clinic for orthopedic examination. The arrow indicates the time of the visit to the referral clinic. The increase in the UC:CR on day 3 in one dog was most probably caused by an additional visit to a veterinary hospital. The line indicates the upper reference limit of the assay. C, UC:CR measured in nine healthy pet dogs before, during, and after a 1.5-day hospitalization at a referral clinic. The line indicates the upper reference limit of the assay.

TABLE 6–13 SOME ACTH (CORTICOTROPIN) STIMULATION TEST PROTOCOLS FOR ASSESSING ADRENOCORTICAL GLUROCORTICOID RESERVE

ACTH Preparation	Dose	Route of Administration	Timing of Post-Injection Cortisol	Reference
ACTH gel	1.0 IU/kg	IM	2 hours	Watson et al 1998
ACTH gel	2.2 IU/kg	IM	2 hours	Watson et al 1998
Synthetic ACTH	0.25 mg/dog	IM	1 hour	Feldman et al 1982
Synthetic ACTH	0.25 mg/dog	IV	1 hour	Hansen et al 1994
Synthetic ACTH	5 mg/kg	IV	1 hour	Greco et al 1998
				Frank et al 2000
Synthetic ACTH	5 or 10 mg/kg	IV	1 hour	Kerl et al 1999
				Frank & Oliver 1998

ACTH gel sources: HP ACTHar gel, 80 IU/ml, Rhone-Poulenc Rorer Pharm. Inc., Collegeville, PA; ACTH gel, Butler Co., Dublin, OH; Synthetic ACTH, Amphastar Pharm, Rancho Cucamonga, CA 91730.

obtained for cortisol before and 1 hour after administration. The drug can also be given intravenously (Hansen et al, 1994).

For cosyntropin, as an alternative to the standard 0.25 mg/dog dose, one can reliably use 1, 5, or

10 µg/kg given intravenously (Kerl et al, 1999; Frank et al, 2000). If one of these lower doses is used, partial vial use may result. Cosyntropin can be reconstituted and stored frozen at –20° C in plastic syringes for at least 6 months without adverse effects on the bio-

activity of the polypeptide (Frank and Oliver, 1998). However, because cosyntropin is provided in a single-use vial, it does not contain a preservative to inhibit bacterial growth. The risk of bacterial contamination must be weighed against the savings in using portions of a cosyntropin vial that have been stored frozen.

Both the ACTH gel and synthetic ACTH result in maximal stimulation of adrenocortical reserve. These two products and their respective protocols can be interchanged without altering test results or reducing one's confidence in the diagnosis (Feldman et al, 1982; Watson et al, 1998). Maximal adrenocortical stimulation is an important criterion that must be met by any stimulation test method. The exogenous ACTH must be more potent than the effects of traveling, hospital environment, handling, and venipuncture. With maximal exogenous stimulation, these important variables are eliminated. The advantage of using ACTH gel is its cost (it is less expensive), whereas a shorter stimulation period is used with synthetic ACTH (Greco et al, 1998). It appears that gel forms of ACTH are not consistently available nor have they been consistent in bioactivity. Synthetic ACTH has been more available (although it, too, can be back-ordered) and does provide consistent bioactivity.

RESULTS

Normal Dogs. Normal values must be established by each laboratory. Most laboratories, however, have reasonably similar results for plasma cortisol concentrations because most laboratories use similar assays and testing protocols. The normal or "reference range" for baseline cortisol concentrations is 0.5 to 6.0 µg/dl, and the normal poststimulation cortisol concentration is typically 6 to 17 µg/dl (Fig. 6-41). Poststimulation values between 17 and 22 µg/dl are considered

borderline, and values of 22 µg/dl or higher are consistent with a diagnosis of hyperadrenocorticism. However, as discussed previously in this section, the ACTH response test is not totally specific. Therefore it cannot replace a thorough history and physical examination for reliability in establishing a diagnosis.

Value of Basal Samples and Ratios. It is important to emphasize that ratios or percentage change, comparing the basal with the poststimulation cortisol concentration, is not informative. Only the post-ACTH plasma cortisol result should be evaluated. In fact, there is no reason to obtain a basal, or "pre," sample prior to starting this test. The only reason to obtain a basal sample for plasma cortisol is habit, and we are not convinced that it is a good habit. A normal dog can have a prestimulation cortisol concentration of 1.5 µg/dl and a poststimulation cortisol concentration of 14.0 µg/dl (greater than a ninefold increase), or it could have a prestimulation cortisol concentration of 6.5 µg/dl and a poststimulation concentration of 8.5 µg/dl (a 0.3-fold increase). In the same sense, a dog with Cushing's syndrome could have a prestimulation cortisol concentration of 3 µg/dl and a poststimulation level of 27 µg/dl (a ninefold increase) or prestimulation and poststimulation concentrations of 17.0 and 22.1 µg/dl, respectively (a 0.3-fold increase). A dog with hypoadrenocorticism could have a prestimulation cortisol value of 0.1 µg/dl and a post-ACTH cortisol value of 0.9 µg/dl (a ninefold increase). Ratios are always interesting, but their use with respect to interpreting ACTH stimulation studies is not recommended.

Pituitary-Dependent Hyperadrenocorticism (PDH). Of dogs with PDH, ACTH stimulation test results are greater than 22 µg/dl, and thus clearly abnormal, in approximately 30%; in the borderline range of 17 to 22 µg/dl in another 30%; and within the reference range in approximately 40%. Therefore the ACTH stimulation test is not, in our experience, highly sensitive for the diagnosis of dogs with naturally occurring PDH. Interestingly, these percentages are similar to results documented in people with PDH, and it is because of this poor sensitivity that the ACTH stimulation test is not used as a diagnostic aid in humans. Other studies have shown that the ACTH stimulation test has a greater sensitivity than is indicated here (Kaplan et al, 1995; Van Liew et al, 1997).

ACTH stimulation test results from dogs with PDH are not distinguishable from those from dogs ultimately shown to have functioning adrenocortical tumors. Thus the ACTH response test is a *screening* test in the diagnostic evaluation for Cushing's syndrome (Fig. 6-42). In addition to requiring little time, ACTH stimulation is the only test that can be used to identify dogs with iatrogenic Cushing's syndrome (they have low to low-normal plasma cortisol concentrations with little or no response to exogenous ACTH; see Fig. 6-41), and it remains the only test in veterinary medicine for monitoring response to treatment.

The ACTH stimulation test can be used as a screening test for CCS. If results are obviously abnormal, the veterinarian can pursue tests to differentiate pituitary-dependent from adrenocortical tumor–dependent

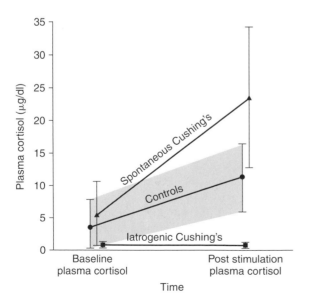

FIGURE 6–41. Mean radioimmunoassay (RIA) plasma cortisol concentrations (± 2 SD) determined before and 1 hour after administration of synthetic ACTH in control dogs, dogs with spontaneous hyperadrenocorticism, and those with iatrogenic hyperadrenocorticism.

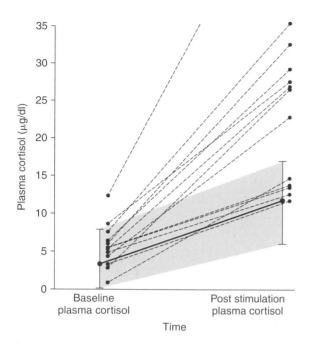

FIGURE 6–42. Plasma cortisol concentrations determined before and 1 hour after administration of synthetic ACTH in dogs with functioning adrenocortical tumors. These data show the variability in test results seen with functioning adrenal tumors. The shaded area represents results from control dogs.

disease. If the result is within reference limits or "borderline," the low-dose dexamethasone test is recommended. If the low-dose dexamethasone test is used initially to confirm a diagnosis of CCS, we commonly perform an ACTH stimulation test prior to initiating therapy to establish a "baseline" from which to monitor the patient.

Adrenocortical Tumors. Both production and secretion of endogenous ACTH are suppressed by the excessive secretion of cortisol from autonomously functioning adrenal tumors; low to undetectable concentrations of plasma ACTH are expected in dogs with hyperadrenocorticism caused by adrenal tumors (see Fig. 6-6). Suppression of endogenous ACTH results in atrophy of normal (nonneoplastic) adrenocortical tissue. However, despite their autonomous function, adrenocortical neoplastic cells retain surface ACTH receptors and the intracellular pathways integral to an ACTH response. Approximately 60% of dogs with hyperadrenocorticism caused by functioning adrenocortical tumors have exaggerated ("borderline" or obviously abnormal) ACTH stimulation test results. A significant percentage (about 40%) have results within reference limits (see Fig. 6-42). It is uncommon but possible for a small percentage of dogs with an adrenal tumor to demonstrate no response to exogenous ACTH. Dogs that demonstrate little or no response to ACTH may be dogs with tumors that synthesize non–cortisol steroids. For this reason, assay of 17α-OH-progesterone may be warranted (see section on this assay, page 311). It is recommended, however, that a low-dose dexamethasone test be completed first.

Basal and/or post-ACTH cortisol concentrations may vary if ACTH stimulation tests are repeated in individual dogs. Some dogs with an adrenocortical tumor had normal ACTH response test results on one trial but abnormal and totally different test results on another trial (Feldman, 1981; Peterson et al, 1982b). In one study, 44% of dogs with an adrenal adenoma had exaggerated (abnormal) responses to ACTH stimulation, whereas 69% of dogs with adrenal carcinoma had a hyperresponsive test result. Furthermore, the mean response of the dogs with carcinoma was approximately four times greater than that of the dogs with adenoma. The highest post-ACTH cortisol concentrations were from dogs with adrenal carcinoma (Peterson et al, 1982b). In another study, however, no consistent difference was noted in comparisons between ACTH responsiveness in dogs with adrenal adenoma and dogs with carcinoma (Feldman, 1983b).

The ACTH response test remains a good screening test. Dogs with adrenal tumors can be diagnosed as having Cushing's syndrome with this test. However, as in PDH, the test results may be normal. Test results do not distinguish between PDH and ATH.

IATROGENIC CUSHING'S SYNDROME. One advantage of obtaining an ACTH stimulation test as a screening test for dogs suspected of having Cushing's syndrome is the test's ability to readily identify animals with iatrogenic disease. Dogs chronically receiving glucocorticoid therapy can develop all the clinical features of naturally occurring hyperadrenocorticism; this has been seen with injectable, oral, topical, and even ophthalmic glucocorticoid preparations.* This remains a critically important aspect of testing, because not all owners understand, report, or realize the importance of their pet's medications.

A dog with clinical signs and routine laboratory test results suggestive of Cushing's syndrome, which also has a low-normal baseline cortisol concentration and little or no response to exogenous ACTH, is quite likely to have iatrogenic Cushing's syndrome (see Fig. 6-41). No other screening test differentiates naturally developing CCS from iatrogenic disease. It should be pointed out that pituitary-adrenal function in patients treated with glucocorticoids cannot be reliably estimated from the dose or duration of therapy nor from assaying basal plasma cortisol concentrations (Schlaghecke et al, 1992).

O,P'-DDD THERAPY. o,p'-DDD (mitotane, Lysodren) and Nizoral (ketoconazole) are commonly used in the treatment of dogs with hyperadrenocorticism, the former much more than the latter. In either case, the ACTH stimulation test is the only means of satisfactorily monitoring therapy. This is *the only* test that can assess adrenocortical reserve and provide reliable information regarding adequacy of therapy. The role of ACTH stimulation test results during medical treatment of Cushing's syndrome is discussed on page 343.

---

*Roberts et al, 1984; Zenoble and Kemppainen, 1987; Eichenbaum et al, 1988; Glaze et al, 1988; Murphy et al, 1990; Romantowski, 1990; Moore and Hoenig, 1992.

SUMMARY: GENERAL USE. The ACTH stimulation test aids in the identification of CCS in more than half of dogs with adrenocortical tumors (ATH) and in approximately 60% of dogs with PDH. Significant numbers of dogs with either PDH or ATH have normal test results. If hyperadrenocorticism is suspected clinically, the diagnosis should not be excluded because of normal or "borderline" ACTH stimulation test results (Feldman, 1983b). Furthermore, ACTH stimulation test results do not distinguish between PDH and ATH, nor do they reliably distinguish dogs with adrenal adenoma from those with adrenal carcinoma. The test is a relatively reliable, simple, and safe screening test in the diagnostic evaluation of dogs suspected of having hyperadrenocorticism and, if obtained prior to initiation of treatment, it readily provides information for posttreatment comparison. ACTH stimulation is the only test that readily identifies iatrogenic Cushing's syndrome (see Fig. 6-41).

DIABETES MELLITUS. Confusion about whether individual dogs with diabetes mellitus also have Cushing's syndrome is common. Well-regulated diabetics have normal endocrine test results (Zerbe et al, 1988). It has been proposed, however, that chronic illnesses (such as diabetes mellitus) may alter adrenocortical test results. Although that is possible, it has not been commonly demonstrated, as only 14% of dogs with nonadrenal illness had abnormal ACTH stimulation test results in one study (Kaplan et al, 1995), and only one abnormal and two borderline test results were documented in 42 stimulation tests obtained from dogs with lymphosarcoma (Gieger et al, 2002). Therefore, although the poorly regulated non–Cushing's syndrome diabetic can occasionally have misleading test results, screening test results are usually reliable. However, the diagnosis of hyperadrenocorticism in this situation should be supported by (1) abnormal results from two or more different screening tests *and* (2) clinical signs of Cushing's syndrome. "Insulin resistance" is nonspecific, and this condition alone should not provide sufficient impetus to treat an animal for Cushing's syndrome.

CHRONIC (NONENDOCRINE) DISEASE. As previously described, not all dogs with hyperadrenocorticism have abnormal or "diagnostic" ACTH stimulation test results (i.e., the test is "diagnostic" of hyperadrenocorticism in less than 35% of dogs and "borderline" in a similar percentage). However, not all "diagnostic" test results are found solely in dogs with hyperadrenocorticism. Nine of 59 dogs (15%) with nonadrenal disease had ACTH stimulation test results consistent with a diagnosis of Cushing's syndrome (Kaplan et al, 1995), and one of 42 stimulation test results was abnormal in dogs with chronic disease (lymphosarcoma) (Gieger et al, 2002). A single test result could always be spurious.

ANTICONVULSANT MEDICATION. See discussion in the Differential Diagnosis section of this chapter.

INCORRECT RESULTS. It is possible for an individual test result to be incorrect because of human error in handling or administering the ACTH, in processing the plasma, or in performing the cortisol assay. Dogs with clinical evidence of CCS that is supported by abnormalities in the routine in-hospital evaluation are likely to have that condition. If test results seem incorrect, the stimulation test can be repeated, or another screening test (low-dose dexamethasone test) can be performed.

Dexamethasone Screening Test (Low-Dose Dexamethasone Test)

THEORY

Normal Dogs. Pituitary ACTH, under hypothalamic control, stimulates adrenocortical synthesis and secretion of glucocorticoids, increasing the plasma glucocorticoid concentration, and these steroids, via negative feedback, suppress continued secretion of ACTH (see Fig. 6-6). Communication between the pituitary and the adrenal cortex is a continuous system of positive and negative stimulation. The result is maintenance of plasma cortisol concentrations in the physiologic range necessary for normal metabolic homeostasis.

Administration of relatively small doses of dexamethasone (identical to administration of any glucocorticoid) given intravenously (0.01 or 0.015 mg/kg body weight) inhibits pituitary secretion of ACTH and, in turn, decreases endogenous cortisol secretion for as long as 24 to 48 hours (Toutain et al, 1983). In normal dogs, plasma cortisol concentrations decrease within 2 to 3 hours of dexamethasone administration to values less than 1 to 1.4 µg/dl (depending on the laboratory used). Although these are the published upper limit of the reference range, almost all dogs that are not stressed or ill (remember, dogs with CCS are not "ill") and that do not have CCS suppress plasma cortisol concentrations to less than 0.7 µg/dl. Dexamethasone, a synthetic glucocorticoid, is used because it is not only potent, it also does not cross-react with cortisol assays, allowing documentation of its in vivo effect. Function of the normal pituitary-adrenal axis, therefore, can be demonstrated by administering dexamethasone and noting, within 2 to 3 hours, a reduction in the plasma cortisol concentration to values well below 1.4 µg/dl, which persists longer than 8 hours (Fig. 6-43, *A*). It is this 8-hour result, either less than 1.0 or less than 1.4 µg/dl, that is considered the reference value for most laboratories. A result greater than 1.4 µg/dl is considered consistent with a diagnosis of CCS.

Pituitary-Dependent Hyperadrenocorticism (PDH). ACTH secretion from functioning pituitary tumors causes adrenocortical hyperplasia through chronic and excessive stimulation of the adrenal cortex. Pituitary tumors in dogs with PDH, logically, must be somewhat resistant to the negative feedback action of cortisol. If this were not true, excess plasma cortisol concentrations would suppress ACTH secretion and PDH would not develop. Administration of a *small* dose of dexamethasone to an animal with PDH should not result in normal suppression of pituitary ACTH and therefore should not suppress plasma cortisol concentrations.

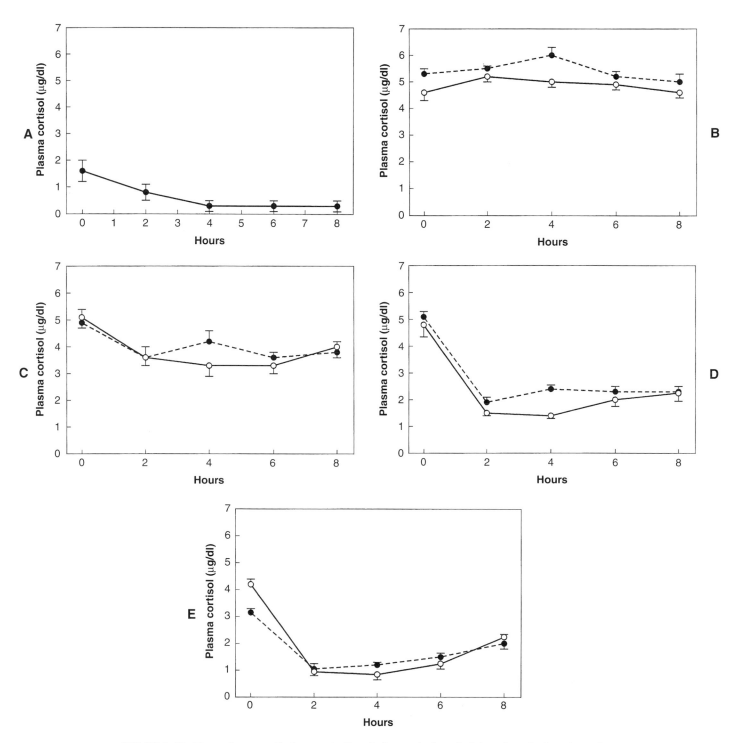

FIGURE 6–43. Mean plasma cortisol concentrations before and after administration of a low dose of dexamethasone in *(A)* 27 normal dogs; *(B)* 48 dogs with adrenocortical tumors; *(C)* 130 dogs with pituitary-dependent hyperadrenocorticism (PDH); *(D)* dogs from the 178 with Cushing's syndrome that had at least one plasma cortisol concentration less than 1.4 μg/dl after dexamethasone administration (total 54, each had PDH); and *(E)* dogs from the 178 with Cushing's syndrome that had at least one plasma cortisol concentration less than 50% of the baseline concentration after dexamethasone administration (total 95, each had PDH). Note that there are two curves for graphs *B, C, D,* and *E.* These represent the use of dexamethasone sodium phosphate *(dashed line)* or dexamethasone in polyethylene glycol *(solid line).* No significant difference in results is seen with these dexamethasone products.

Adrenocortical Tumor Hyperadrenocorticism (ATH). Functioning adrenocortical tumors secrete cortisol autonomously. Because this cortisol is typically synthesized and secreted in excess, it causes clinical signs of Cushing's syndrome and suppresses endogenous ACTH secretion. Cortisol secretion from these tumors occurs independent of ACTH control. Dexamethasone suppresses the plasma cortisol concentration by inhibiting pituitary ACTH secretion. ACTH synthesis and secretion are already inhibited by an autonomously secreting adrenocortical tumor. Thus dexamethasone administration to a dog with an adrenocortical tumor should not decrease plasma cortisol concentrations (Fig. 6-43, *B*).

RAPID DEXAMETHASONE CLEARANCE. In addition to "dexamethasone resistance," another explanation for the failure of plasma cortisol concentrations to decrease normally in dogs with Cushing's syndrome, specifically those dogs with PDH, is the clearance rate of dexamethasone. Rather than the normal 24- to 48-hour clearance rate, approximately 75% of dogs with Cushing's syndrome clear dexamethasone from plasma in less than 8 hours (usually in 3 to 6 hours). Thus dexamethasone clearance rates are more rapid in CCS. This allows plasma cortisol concentrations to transiently decrease (at 4 hours postadministration) but to escape the effects of dexamethasone (be abnormal) on samples obtained 8 hours postadministration (Lothrop and Oliver, 1984; Kemppainen and Peterson, 1993).

PROTOCOL. A morning baseline plasma or serum sample (whichever the laboratory requests) is obtained for cortisol determination, and dexamethasone (0.01 mg/kg body weight) then is administered intravenously. If a 0.015 mg/kg dose is used, the test results are virtually identical (Mack and Feldman, 1990). Dexamethasone sodium phosphate or dexamethasone in polyethylene glycol (Azium, Schering-Plough, Union, NJ) may be used interchangeably (Mack and Feldman, 1990). Samples should be taken 8 hours later for cortisol determination (Feldman, 1983a). Sampling between the basal sample and 8 hours is not necessary in the *screening* test; however, a 4-hour sample is recommended (see discrimination tests, page 314). Plasma or serum should be kept cold or frozen until sent to the laboratory for analysis.

TEST RESULTS

Nonstressed, Non–Cushing's Syndrome Dogs. Healthy dogs have plasma cortisol concentrations less than 1.0 µg/dl (usually <0.7 µg/dl) 8 hours after dexamethasone administration. As seen in Fig. 6-43, *A*, dexamethasone administration consistently suppresses plasma cortisol concentration in normal dogs, from 3 through 8 hours. Some studies of specificity have evaluated dogs that are ill from other conditions. Because we would not recommend performing this test on *any* ill dog, regardless of any suspicion of CCS, it is not clear why this test would be evaluated on ill dogs that do not have the condition. In our experience of evaluating test results from stable, nonstressed, and non–Cushing's syndrome dogs that have polyuria and polydipsia or that have alopecia, the test results are quite specific. This is a test that is both sensitive and specific.

Pituitary-Dependent Hyperadrenocorticism. Dogs with PDH consistently have plasma cortisol concentrations greater than 1.0 to 1.4 µg/dl 8 hours after dexamethasone administration. Cortisol concentrations between 1.0 and 1.4 µg/dl may be considered nondiagnostic, and the clinician should rely on other information to determine if hyperadrenocorticism is the correct diagnosis. However, such test results are certainly not "normal." The (low-dose) dexamethasone screening test has been extremely reliable in differentiating non–Cushing's syndrome dogs from those with hyperadrenocorticism. The results of this screening test are consistent with Cushing's syndrome in more than 99% of dogs with PDH (Feldman et al, 1996). Two distinct responses to a low dose of dexamethasone are commonly observed in dogs with PDH.

One result is that predicted through an understanding of the physiologic basis of the test; that is, the low dose of dexamethasone fails to suppress ACTH secretion from the autonomously functioning pituitary tumor, therefore plasma cortisol concentrations 4 and 8 hours after administration are relatively unchanged. The definition of "unchanged" is that plasma cortisol concentrations 4 and 8 hours after dexamethasone administration are greater than the basal plasma cortisol concentration, the same as the basal plasma cortisol concentration, or suppressed but still greater than 50% of the basal level. For example, a basal plasma cortisol concentration of 4 µg/dl and a 4- or 8-hour value of 2.5 µg/dl would indicate "lack of suppression." The interpretation would be the same whether the values at 4 and 8 hours were both 2.5 µg/dl, both 4.0 µg/dl, or both 5.5 µg/dl. These patterns in the plasma cortisol concentration are common and are noted in approximately 35% of dogs with PDH; that is, the 4-hour value did not decrease below 1.4 µg/dl (an absolute value) nor did it decrease to less than 50% of the basal cortisol concentration at either 4 or 8 hours. These results are consistent with the diagnosis of hyperadrenocorticism but do not help to distinguish PDH from ATH.

The second common response after administration of a low dose of dexamethasone in dogs with PDH is a "decrease" in the plasma cortisol concentration, as defined by any one of three criteria: (1) a plasma cortisol concentration less than 1.4 µg/dl at 4 hours; (2) a plasma cortisol concentration less than 50% of the basal concentration at the 4-hour sample period; or (3) a plasma cortisol concentration that is less than 50% of the basal cortisol concentration at the 8-hour sample period. These results are seen in approximately 65% of dogs with PDH; virtually 100% of the 8-hour results are greater than 1.4 µg/dl. Thus the results are "consistent" with the diagnosis of hyperadrenocorticism in almost all PDH dogs as defined by the 8-hour result (the test is highly sensitive). In this setting, dexamethasone suppresses pituitary ACTH synthesis and secretion but does so for only 3 to 6 hours. This duration of effect is far shorter than normal but typical of the increased rate of dexamethasone metabolism in dogs with Cushing's syndrome (Fig. 6-43, *C* to *E*) (Mack and Feldman, 1990; Feldman et al, 1996).

Adrenocortical Tumor Hyperadrenocorticism. Interpretation of the 8-hour postdexamethasone cortisol concentration is the same for ATH as for PDH; that is, plasma cortisol concentrations should be greater than or equal to 1.4 μg/dl. In contrast to most dogs with PDH, plasma cortisol concentrations do not suppress at any time after dexamethasone administration in dogs with ATH (Fig. 6-43, *B*). The only exception to this rule is "apparent suppression" due to an extremely unusual amount of fluctuation in plasma cortisol concentrations in which a transient nadir coincides with the timing of obtaining a blood sample (Feldman et al, 1996). Circulating cortisol concentrations do fluctuate, both in dogs with a normal pituitary-adrenal axis and in those with an abnormal axis. A recent report of eight dogs with adrenocortical tumors that did suppress after administration of dexamethasone is extremely atypical (Norman et al, 1999). It is our suspicion that none of these dogs had autonomously functioning cortisol-secreting tumors. This opinion is based on results from more than 300 dogs with naturally developing CCS secondary to confirmed adrenocortical adenoma or carcinoma. None of these dogs exhibited suppression on low-dose dexamethasone testing. It is not physiologically possible for dexamethasone to cause suppression if a dog has an autonomously secreting adrenocortical tumor causing CCS. Therefore, if test results do not match a veterinarian's expected results, either those expectations were incorrect or some mistake was made in the test.

DIABETES MELLITUS. As previously discussed, dogs that do not have Cushing's syndrome and that have well-controlled diabetes mellitus usually have normal adrenocortical endocrine test results. Poorly controlled diabetics also usually have test results within laboratory reference limits, but a small percentage may have abnormal results. We have evaluated several poorly controlled diabetic dogs with abnormal low-dose dexamethasone test results that had no clinical signs of Cushing's syndrome. These dogs never developed any clinical signs of Cushing's syndrome and at necropsy had no evidence of hyperadrenocorticism. This minority of diabetic dogs illustrates an important principle: the diagnosis of Cushing's syndrome should never be based solely on endocrine test results.

SENSITIVITY, SPECIFICITY, AND MISLEADING RESULTS. It is important to remember that no test is perfect, and low-dose dexamethasone screening tests are no exception. When dogs are chosen for this test that have history, physical examination, and "database" results consistent with Cushing's syndrome (CCS), the test has a sensitivity approaching 99%, (i.e., 99% of dogs with CCS have abnormal results). Unpublished data that we have accumulated indicates that the test is also sensitive. Fewer than 5% of "healthy" dogs with polyuria/polydipsia conditions (diabetes mellitus, diabetes insipidus, hypercalcemia, and chronic renal failure) had abnormal results. Thus, in combining sensitivity and specificity, it is our contention that the low-dose dexamethasone test is superior to ACTH stimulation or the UC:CR. It is also our recommendation that these three screening tests are "complimentary."

As with ACTH stimulation test results, dexamethasone screening test results can be misleading. Of 59 dogs with nonadrenal illness, 22 (37%) and 33 (56%) failed to demonstrate normal cortisol suppression at 4 and 8 hours, respectively (Kaplan et al, 1994). However, in our opinion, this study used an unfortunate study group. We do not recommend evaluating a clinically ill dog highly suspected of having CCS with endocrine tests. Our recommendation would be to postpone any endocrine testing in ill dogs until they are stable, partly because the test results would be more reliable then, and partly because ill dogs should not be treated for CCS.

Anticonvulsant medications can cause dogs to have unusual plasma cortisol concentrations, which may fail to be suppressed normally (Chauvet et al, 1995). The stress of bathing, hospitalization, illness, and numerous other factors may interfere with the suppressive effects of dexamethasone, although this is not common. Iatrogenic steroids may remain in the blood for long periods, causing an apparent failure to respond to dexamethasone because cortisol assays measure endogenous and iatrogenic glucocorticoids (not dexamethasone). Whenever iatrogenic disease is suspected, the ACTH stimulation test should be performed (see Fig. 6-41). The low-dose dexamethasone screening test is affected by more variables than the ACTH stimulation test. In the interpretation of either test, it is important to remember that neither is foolproof. The ACTH stimulation and low-dose dexamethasone screening tests are used to confirm a clinical suspicion; the most important initial screening tests are the history and physical examination.

Plasma 17-Hydroxyprogesterone Concentrations

BACKGROUND. Naturally occurring hyperadrenocorticism in dogs is considered a disease in which excess cortisol is produced secondary to one of two processes: either a pituitary tumor produces excess ACTH, stimulating secretion of abnormal amounts of adrenocortical cortisol and eventually causing hyperplasia of the adrenal cortices (PDH), or an adrenocortical adenoma or carcinoma functions autonomously, secreting cortisol in excess and causing abnormal increases in plasma cortisol concentrations (ATH). However, it is possible in either condition for steroid hormones other than cortisol to be synthesized and secreted. Through this mechanism, abnormal adrenal cortices may secrete 11-deoxycortisol, deoxycorticosterone, aldosterone, progesterone, 17α-OH-progesterone, estrogens, or androgens in excess. In almost every case, however, cortisol excess exists, and the increase in various cortisol precursors is an incidental occurrence. Perhaps this variation in physiologic processes explains why some dogs with CCS have hypertension and others do not, or why some have polyuria and polydipsia and others do not; or it may help explain the other "variations on the theme" of what we call canine Cushing's syndrome.

Dogs or cats with atypical Cushing's syndrome, therefore, could have one or several derangements in the steroid production pathway. These abnormalities could involve relative deficiencies in some enzymes that are integral to the synthesis of cortisol. If this occurs, there would develop a "blockade" in the steroid synthesis pathway that would result in abnormal increases in plasma concentrations of specific cortisol precursors, whereas cortisol responses to ACTH or dexamethasone administration may remain within the reference range. This has been proposed as an explanation for the occasional dog suspected of having CCS from the history and physical examination findings but in which the diagnosis cannot be confirmed on "routine" screening endocrine tests.

ADRENOCORTICAL TUMORS. An adrenocortical tumor, by definition, represents the development of a neoplasm from a single cell line. That cell line may be capable of synthesizing one steroid or several different steroid structures. Depending on the capabilities of the cell line, excesses in one or several steroid (hormonal) structures ensue. This theory is supported by the knowledge that although most adrenocortical tumors synthesize cortisol, some tumors do not synthesize cortisol but do synthesize aldosterone. There are also reports of adrenocortical tumors in humans secreting steroid structures (hormones) other than cortisol or aldosterone. For example, there are several reports of people who did not have clinical evidence of Cushing's syndrome but who had an incidentally discovered adrenal tumor and an exaggerated plasma 17-hydroxyprogesterone concentration after exogenous ACTH administration (Turton et al, 1992; Bondanella et al, 1997).

Progesterones are synthesized in the adrenal cortex from cholesterol via the intermediaries pregnenolone and 17-hydroxypregnenolone (see Figs. 6-3 and 6-4). Although only limited amounts of these progesterones normally reach circulation, some people have adrenocortical tumors with aberrant biosynthetic pathways that have been well characterized (Orth et al, 1998). Adrenal neoplasms may be deficient in enzymes involved in normal steroidogenic pathways. Such enzyme deficiencies result in an accumulation of precursor steroids proximal to the blockade (i.e., proximal to the enzyme deficit). In this manner, precursors may reach the circulation and cause clinical signs, or they may be shunted into alternative metabolic pathways and cause excesses in other steroid structures. Enzyme deficiencies of the nature described are most often thought to be a unique component of that particular tumor, with hormone synthesis in these individuals normal prior to their developing the tumor (Toth et al, 2000). However, in a few instances it is believed that an inherited partial enzyme deficiency present since birth remains clinically silent until tumor development.

Although some people with sex hormone–secreting adrenal tumors have no clinical signs, others have had clinical abnormalities that resolved after adrenalectomy (Bondanella et al, 1997). Some of these people have been reported to have normal responses to a low dose of dexamethasone (Orth et al, 1998). One dog that demonstrated suppression after dexamethasone administration was reported to have had a sex hormone–secreting adrenocortical tumor (Syme et al, 2001). Some progestins have considerable intrinsic glucocorticoid activity. Alternatively, increased progestin concentrations may result in clinical signs by displacing cortisol from cortisol-binding protein (Juchem et al, 1990; Selman et al, 1997). Displacement of cortisol results in excess concentrations of "free" cortisol, even though the total serum cortisol concentration may be normal or decreased. Free cortisol is metabolically active and could result in clinical signs that reflect these increases.

PITUITARY-DEPENDENT HYPERADRENOCORTICISM. Intuitively, synthesis and secretion of atypical steroid hormones seems less likely in dogs with PDH, simply because ACTH stimulates cortisol synthesis and secretion. Why would an adult animal have an inability to synthesize a vital hormone such as cortisol without developing signs of hypocortisolism early in life? It is also interesting to point out that chronic excesses in the plasma progesterone concentration are not a unique condition. All healthy bitches that progress through normal estrus and diestrus have tremendous increases in the plasma progesterone concentration for 60 to more than 90 days. These increases often approach or exceed 50 to 100 times anestrus concentrations. Furthermore, this physiologic condition normally persists for months. Dogs in diestrus do not typically have polydipsia, polyuria, polyphagia, muscle weakness, panting, hair loss, potbelly, and so on. However, others have claimed that such a pathogenesis exists for some dogs with PDH (Ristic et al, 2002). Thus 17-hydroxyprogesterone may have physiologic effects far different from progesterone.

VETERINARY REPORTS. One dog was described as having an adrenocortical tumor that secreted deoxycorticosterone (Reine et al, 1999). Two additional reports each described two dogs with adrenocortical tumors that had exaggerated concentrations of plasma 17-hydroxyprogesterone after stimulation with ACTH (Norman et al, 1999; Syme et al, 2001). These last four dogs each had clinical signs consistent with CCS; however, their cortisol concentrations were below reference limits after ACTH administration. The primary differential diagnosis for these clinical signs in dogs with test results of this nature would be iatrogenic cortisol excess, although it is theoretically possible for an adrenocortical tumor to lack ACTH receptors. Iatrogenic disease, however, would not explain the presence of an adrenal mass. Dogs with adrenocortical tumors that were unresponsive to ACTH administration had been previously reported (Reusch and Feldman, 1991).

Subsequent to reports on adrenocortical tumors causing excesses in circulating sex hormones came reports of plasma 17-hydroxyprogesterone concentrations being used as aids in the diagnosis of PDH. Five dogs with PDH were reported after diagnosis was based almost entirely on an exaggerated 17-hydroxyprogesterone response to exogenous ACTH (Frank et al, 2001).

Another report included several distinct groups of dogs (Ristic et al, 2002). One group comprised dogs with plasma cortisol concentrations that were abnormal on ACTH stimulation test results, another group had abnormal low-dose dexamethasone test results, a third group had equivocal screening test results, and a fourth group had all routine test results within reference limits. In this report, all dogs from all the groups had abnormal post-ACTH stimulation plasma 17-hydroxyprogesterone concentrations. Some of these dogs with CCS were considered "atypical" because their ACTH stimulation test results were within reference limits. However, because 40% of typical dogs with CCS have ACTH stimulation test results within reference ranges, this test does not possess the sensitivity necessary to claim that a result within reference limits would classify such dogs as "atypical." ACTH stimulation test results within reference limits are considered a common finding in humans, dogs, and cats with Cushing's syndrome, which is why ACTH stimulation is not used as a diagnostic aid in people suspected of having Cushing's syndrome. Seven dogs were considered atypical because they had borderline or "normal" stimulation and suppression test results. Four of these seven had adrenocortical tumors, again a situation we consider logical (they did not suppress after dexamethasone administration; rather, their cortisol concentrations were low throughout the study). However, three dogs were diagnosed as having PDH despite both ACTH stimulation and low-dose dexamethasone test results within reference limits. In these dogs, the diagnosis was supported by post-ACTH plasma 17-hydroxyprogesterone concentrations. Dogs with this condition require further scrutiny. Regardless, the addition of 17-hydroxyprogesterone concentrations as a screening test for CCS would appear to have potential for helping to diagnose some dogs, but it also has the potential to cause some dogs that do not have CCS to be treated incorrectly.

PROTOCOL AND REFERENCE VALUES. The protocol for using 17-hydroxyprogesterone as a diagnostic aid is straightforward. A routine ACTH stimulation test is performed as described earlier in this section. In addition to requesting serum or plasma cortisol measurements on the pre-ACTH and post-ACTH samples, the veterinarian should request that 17-hydroxyprogesterone be assessed as well. In one report, heparinized plasma was submitted, and the assay used was a solid-phase RIA (Coat-A-Count 17α-OH Progesterone, Diagnostic Products Corp.). The lower limit of sensitivity for this assay was 0.33 ng/ml. The reference range for the pre-ACTH sample was less than 0.33 to 0.63 ng/ml. The post-ACTH sample reference range was 0.33 to 1.82 ng/ml, and results greater than 1.32 ng/ml were considered a positive test result (Ristic et al, 2002). In another report, the reference ranges were slightly different, with a pre-ACTH range of 0 to 0.4 ng/ml and a post-ACTH range of 0.4 to 1.5 ng/ml (Frank et al, 2001). Dogs with CCS had post-ACTH values of 1.5 to 12.5 ng/ml, with a median well below 4 ng/ml, in one report (Ristic et al, 2002) and median pre-ACTH and post-ACTH values

TABLE 6–14 SERUM 17α-OH PROGESTERONE CONCENTRATIONS POST-ACTH IN HEALTHY DOGS AND DOGS WITH NATURALLY OCCURRING HYPERADRENOCORTICISM

	Male Dogs	Female Dogs
Normal range	($n = 21$) <3.58	($n = 20$) <7.98
Borderline range	3.58 to 4.40	7.98 to 10.48
Abnormal	>4.40	>10.48
PDH	($n = 12$)	($n = 13$)
Number normal	4	8
Number borderline	3	3
Number abnormal	5	2
ATH	($n = 10$)	($n = 7$)
Number normal	5	5
Number borderline	3	1
Number abnormal	2	1

of 1.3 and 4.2 ng/ml, respectively, in another report (Frank et al, 2001).

We have established reference ranges for post-ACTH serum 17α-OH progesterone concentrations for male and female dogs (Table 6-14). The ranges are based on the mean ±2 standard deviations (SD) from 21 healthy male dogs and 20 healthy female dogs. In 22 male dogs with naturally occurring CCS, 9 had results within the reference range, 6 were "borderline," and 7 were abnormal. In 20 female dogs with naturally occurring CCS, 13 had results within the reference range, 4 were "borderline," and 3 were abnormal. Therefore, 10 of 42 dogs (24%) had abnormal results (see Table 6-14). Further studies defining the value of this assay are anticipated.

Miscellaneous Screening Tests

ALKALINE PHOSPHATASE ISOENZYME. See Serum Alkaline Phosphatase (SAP), page 279, for a discussion on the use of isoenzymes as screening tests.

HIGH-PERFORMANCE LIQUID CHROMATOGRAPHY AND FREE CORTISOL CONCENTRATIONS IN PLASMA. These assays are not widely available, are expensive, are difficult to perform compared with commercially available RIA kits, and do not offer significant advantages over the more traditionally available tests.

COMBINED DEXAMETHASONE SUPPRESSION/ACTH STIMULATION. It was hoped that this test would provide information about pituitary gland and adrenal gland activity in a single, brief, relatively inexpensive trial (Zerbe, 2000a). However, we never recommend the combined test, nor do many laboratories. It is recognized to have combined two imperfect tests, with the result being a test less reliable than either of its components (Feldman, 1985 and 1986). If a clinician chooses to combine low-dose dexamethasone testing with ACTH stimulation testing (again, something we never recommend), a routine low-dose dexamethasone test is completed, and immediately after the 8-hour sample has been obtained, ACTH is administered. Others recommend a protocol that begins with a high-dose dexamethasone test and finishes the second arm of the test with an ACTH stimulation test (Zerbe, 2000a).

LIVER BIOPSY. Abnormal serum liver enzyme activities and abnormal liver function tests are common in CCS. For this reason, dogs with vague clinical features of CCS may be tentatively diagnosed as having a primary hepatopathy. With the increasing use of percutaneous liver biopsies, liver tissue from dogs with CCS might be submitted to pathologists with increasing frequency. Dogs with naturally occurring CCS or those given exogenous glucocorticoids usually have histologic evidence of "glucocorticoid-induced" or "steroid" hepatopathy. This hepatopathy is histologically characterized by centrilobular vacuolization, perivacuolar glycogen accumulation within hepatocytes, and focal centrilobular necrosis. It has been suggested that any dog with these histologic features on liver biopsy be evaluated for Cushing's syndrome. We would also recommend evaluation, but only if a dog has clinical signs of CCS. "Steroid hepatopathy" is unique to the dog; it has not been observed in any other species (Rutgers et al, 1995).

Vacuolar hepatopathies are associated with a variety of disorders (e.g., toxin exposure, bile stasis). "Steroid-induced hepatopathy," however, is rather specific for chronic exposure to glucocorticoids. Liver biopsy, therefore, could be used as a screening test to identify dogs with Cushing's syndrome. "Steroid hepatopathy," however, does not distinguish between naturally occurring and iatrogenic steroid excess. Other disadvantages to the routine use of liver biopsy as a screening test include potential complications of infection or inadequate healing after the procedure because of the systemic effects of CCS. The one obvious advantage is that the hepatomegaly typical of CCS makes for a straightforward percutaneous biopsy procedure.

DISCRIMINATION TESTS: DIFFERENTIATING PITUITARY-DEPENDENT FROM ADRENOCORTICAL TUMOR HYPERADRENOCORTICISM

Low-Dose Dexamethasone Suppression (LDDS) Test

BACKGROUND. Measurement of the plasma cortisol concentration 8 hours after administration of a low dose of dexamethasone is now recognized as a reliable, sensitive, and specific screening test for CCS. Most laboratories have reference values of less than 1.0 or less than 1.4 µg/dl for the 8-hour postdexamethasone cortisol concentration. Values equal to or greater than these reference ranges should be considered "consistent" with a diagnosis of CCS. Based on studies evaluating the low-dose dexamethasone test, a 4-hour sample is also recommended, not as a component of the screening test but as an aid in distinguishing pituitary-dependent CCS (PDH) from adrenal-dependent CCS (ATH) (Mack and Feldman, 1990; Feldman et al, 1996). Dexamethasone transiently suppresses pituitary secretion of ACTH in 60% to 65% of dogs with PDH. However, the duration of dexamethasone activity in dogs with PDH is only 3 to 6 hours, compared with the 24 to 48 hours noted in healthy dogs. Dexamethasone does not suppress ACTH secretion in dogs with ATH. Therefore demonstrated transient plasma cortisol suppression during the low-dose dexamethasone test is consistent with PDH and reliably rules out ATH.

PROTOCOL AND DEFINITIONS. As previously described, a basal plasma or serum sample for cortisol determination should be obtained, and then 0.01 mg/kg of dexamethasone is administered intravenously. Postadministration samples are obtained at 4 and 8 hours. Studies indicate that the 4-hour sample result should be used as a "discrimination" test, and the 8-hour sample result can be used for both "screening" and "discrimination" purposes. Use of the results of the LDDS test to distinguish PDH (suppression) from ATH requires that one or more of the following three criteria be met: (1) a 4-hour plasma cortisol concentration less than 1.4 µg/dl; (2) a 4-hour plasma cortisol concentration less than 50% of the basal level; or (3) an 8-hour plasma cortisol concentration less than 50% of the basal concentration (Fig. 6-44). Any dog with Cushing's syndrome with plasma cortisol concentrations that meet one or more of the criteria is extremely likely to have PDH (Feldman et al, 1996).

RESULTS. Approximately 25% of dogs with PDH have a 4-hour plasma cortisol concentration of less than 1.4 µg/dl and an 8-hour value greater than or equal to 1.4 µg/dl (i.e., consistent with the diagnosis of CCS) (Feldman et al, 1996). Approximately 50% of dogs with PDH have a 4-hour plasma cortisol concentration that is less than 50% of the baseline value, and approximately 25% have an 8-hour value that is less than 50% of baseline. Approximately 99% of dogs with CCS have an 8-hour plasma cortisol concentration that is consistent with the diagnosis (>1.4 µg/dl). Approximately 60% to 65% of dogs with PDH demonstrate suppression on the LDDS test as defined by meeting at least one of these three criteria (Fig. 6-45) (Feldman et al, 1996). In one study, two of 35 dogs with ATH demonstrated "suppression" as defined by these three criteria (Feldman et al, 1996). However, close analysis of these data suggest that the two dogs actually had borderline results that could easily be explained by fluctuating plasma cortisol concentrations.

Approximately 35% to 40% of dogs with PDH do not demonstrate suppression as defined by the three criteria established in the previous paragraph. The LDDS test results in these dogs are similar to those expected for adrenocortical tumor Cushing's syndrome. Lack of suppression, therefore, is considered a nonspecific result, consistent with the diagnosis of CCS but not informative with respect to pituitary versus adrenal origin. Dogs with a history, physical examination findings, and initial database consistent with CCS and an 8-hour LDDS test result equal to or greater than 1.4 µg/dl have CCS. Furthermore, those that demonstrate "suppression" on the LDDS test, by meeting at least one of the three criteria shown in Fig. 6-44, have PDH. This diagnosis can be further supported with other discrimination tests, but they are not likely to be needed. Dogs that meet all the above criteria for

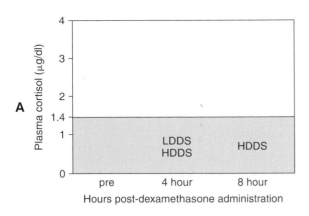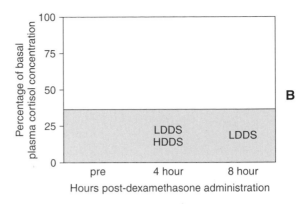

FIGURE 6–44. Definitions of "suppression" relative to distinguishing between pituitary-dependent and adrenal tumor–dependent hyperadrenocorticism in dogs after dexamethasone administration. *A,* Suppression is defined as a plasma cortisol concentration less than 1.4 µg/dl 4 hours after low-dose dexamethasone (LDDS) administration or less than 1.4 µg/dl at 4 or 8 hours after high-dose dexamethasone (HDDS) administration. *B,* Suppression can also be defined as a plasma cortisol concentration less than 50% of the basal level 4 or 8 hours after LDDS (0.01 mg/kg IV) or HDDS (0.1 mg/kg IV).

establishing the diagnosis of CCS but that fail to demonstrate "suppression" of plasma cortisol concentrations on the LDDS test must be considered candidates for either PDH or ATH.

Endogenous ACTH Concentrations

THEORY. In reviewing the underlying causes that lead to the development of naturally occurring or iatrogenic hyperadrenocorticism (see Fig. 6-6), the value of knowing the plasma endogenous ACTH concentration becomes obvious. Adrenocortical tumors

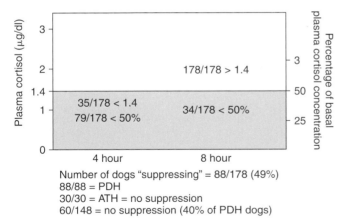

FIGURE 6–45. The shaded area of this graph represents results that indicate "suppression" on the low-dose dexamethasone (LDDS) test (<1.4 µg/dl at 4 hours or <50% of the basal level at 4 or at 8 hours), consistent with the diagnosis of PDH as opposed to one of adrenal tumor hyperadrenocorticism, in 178 dogs with naturally occurring disease. As can be seen, 88 of the 178 dogs "suppressed," as determined by at least one of the three criteria, and all 88 had PDH. Sixty percent of dogs with PDH demonstrated suppression, whereas none of the dogs with adrenal tumors had results suggestive of suppression. All 178 dogs had an 8-hour value greater than 1.4 µg/dl, a result consistent with the diagnosis of hyperadrenocorticism.

and iatrogenic Cushing's syndrome should suppress ACTH secretion, and pituitary-dependent Cushing's syndrome is the result of excessive ACTH secretion. In humans and dogs, assays for ACTH concentration are not used to diagnose hyperadrenocorticism, because a large number of test results are within reference ranges. However, plasma endogenous ACTH concentrations are valuable aids in distinguishing Cushing's syndrome patients with adrenocortical tumors (ATH) from those with pituitary-dependent disease (PDH) once the Cushing's syndrome diagnosis has been confirmed.

PROTOCOL. Pituitary secretion of ACTH occurs episodically (i.e., it is released in bursts). Plasma concentrations, therefore, fluctuate moment to moment. Overlying these fluctuations, in human beings, are diurnal variations, which cause more frequent bursts of a higher frequency in the early morning hours compared with the decreased frequency and amplitude in secretion seen at night (Van Cauter and Refetoff, 1985). The protocol for obtaining blood for endogenous ACTH determination is borrowed from the literature on humans, and in order to diminish the variables of stress and time of day, blood samples should be obtained between 8 and 9 AM, after the dog has been hospitalized for a night. If an ACTH stimulation test is performed and then an endogenous ACTH measurement is desired, it is recommended to wait 24 hours before collecting blood for the endogenous ACTH test.

Blood obtained for ACTH measurement must be handled quickly, because ACTH rapidly disappears from fresh whole blood. To prevent erroneous values, blood specimens should not be allowed to stand at room temperature for even short periods. Contact with glass (unless the interior of an ethylenediamine tetra-acetic acid [EDTA] tube is silicone coated) must be avoided during collection, separation, and storage, because plasma ACTH adheres to glass. We collect blood in chilled, silicone-coated EDTA tubes, centrifuge the tubes immediately, transfer the plasma to plastic tubes, and then freeze the samples until they are assayed. Other researchers have stated that aprotinin can be added to EDTA tubes as an effective preservative for ACTH and that glass contact or temperature is not critical (Kemppainen et al, 1994a and 1994b). Plasma ACTH levels can be effectively preserved by processing blood samples in plastic containers and storing them at –20° C for no longer than 1 month (Hegstad et al, 1990).

ASSAY METHODS AND REFERENCE RANGES. As endogenous ACTH assays have gained acceptance, their use in humans has increased dramatically. A number of RIA kits for human ACTH are currently marketed. Fortunately, several kits for human ACTH have excellent cross-reactivity in dogs and cats (Nelson et al, 1985; Hegstad et al, 1990). ACTH assays can be moderately expensive. Any assay used by veterinarians must be validated for the species being studied, and test results obtained from control animals must be made available. Basal plasma ACTH concentrations in healthy dogs average 25 to 35 pg/ml, and the reference range is 10 to 70 pg/ml (Fig. 6-46).

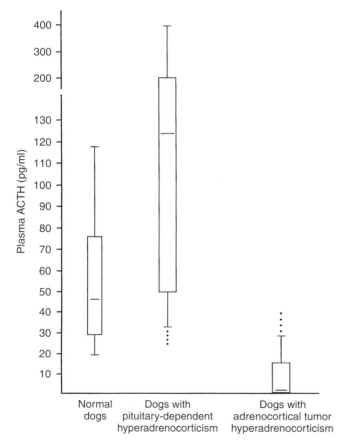

FIGURE 6–46. Endogenous plasma ACTH concentrations from clinically normal dogs, dogs with functioning adrenocortical carcinomas or adenomas, and dogs with pituitary-dependent hyperadrenocorticism (PDH). Each "box" represents the inter-quartile range from the 25th to 75th percentiles (the middle half of the data). The horizontal bar through the box is the median. The "whiskers" represent the main body of data, which in most cases is equal to the range. Outlying data points are represented by the circles.

RESULTS

Adrenocortical Tumor Hyperadrenocorticism (ATH). Endogenous ACTH concentrations less than 10 pg/ml (or that are undetectable) in dogs with naturally developing hyperadrenocorticism are strongly consistent with the presence of a functioning adrenocortical tumor (see Fig. 6-46). The plasma endogenous ACTH concentration would also be less than 10 pg/ml in a dog with iatrogenic hyper-adrenocorticism, but the ACTH stimulation test should reveal the underlying disorder (see Fig. 6-41). In one study, 62 endogenous ACTH concentrations were evaluated from 41 dogs with adrenocortical tumors causing Cushing's syndrome. In 36 (58%), the ACTH concentration was undetectable. The remaining 26 samples had values of 10 to 44 pg/ml. Twenty-nine of the 41 dogs (70%) had at least one sample in which the plasma ACTH concentration was undetectable. Twenty-two of 39 ACTH concentrations (56%) were undetectable in dogs with adrenocortical carcinomas. Fourteen of 23 ACTH concentrations (61%) were undetectable in dogs with adrenocortical adenomas (Reusch and Feldman, 1991). In the decade since publication of these data, plasma ACTH concentrations from dogs with ATH have usually been undetectable or in the low-normal range. Other studies have confirmed these findings (Gould et al, 2001).

Pituitary-Dependent Hyperadrenocorticism (PDH). ACTH concentrations of 45 pg/ml or greater are consistent with a diagnosis of PDH. Suspicion of the diagnosis should be based on the history and physical examination findings, and then appropriate screening tests must be used to confirm the diagnosis of CCS. The endogenous ACTH concentration is greater than 45 pg/ml in 85% to 90% of dogs with PDH (see Fig. 6-46). Approximately 35% to 45% of dogs with PDH have endogenous ACTH concentrations greater than the reference limits for assays commonly used in veteri-nary medicine. Approximately 55% of PDH dogs have an endogenous ACTH concentration of 45 to 70 pg/ml. As many as 15% of the dogs with PDH that we have evaluated have had endogenous ACTH con-centrations of 10 to 45 pg/ml, values that are con-sidered nondiagnostic. Dogs with PDH rarely, if ever, have endogenous ACTH concentrations less than 10 pg/ml.

NONDIAGNOSTIC RESULTS. Dogs with CCS that have endogenous ACTH concentrations greater than 10 pg/ml but less than 45 pg/ml have nondiagnostic results (see Fig. 6-46). If an animal has an endogenous ACTH concentration in that range, either the ACTH concentration should be rechecked or PDH should be distinguished from ATH using other tests described in this section. Dogs with values less than 10 pg/ml on recheck should be considered in the ATH group. Dogs with concentrations of 45 pg/ml or higher on recheck should be regarded as having PDH. Dogs with ACTH concentrations of 10 to 45 pg/ml on recheck cannot be given a firm diagnosis. In that group, the final therapeutic plan is determined by the results of abdominal ultrasonography, radiography, the three criteria that can be applied to results of the LDDS that allow its use as a discrimination test, or the post high-dose dexamethasone plasma cortisol level, or on the results of more sophisticated imaging studies (nuclear scan, MRI, CT).

High-Dose Dexamethasone Suppression Test (HDDS)

THEORY. The pituitary-adrenal axis in dogs with CCS is abnormally resistant to suppression by glucocorticoids and/or glucocorticoids are cleared from the circulation at an accelerated rate. Adrenocortical tumors function autonomously and therefore independent of pituitary control, as illustrated by their ability to completely suppress ACTH secretion yet continue to synthesize and secrete excessive quantities of cortisol. Regardless of the dose, dexamethasone theoretically would never suppress adrenocortical cortisol secretion when the source of that cortisol is an autonomously functioning adrenocortical tumor. PDH, in contrast, results from chronic excess secretion of ACTH. The source of that ACTH is a pituitary tumor. Glucocorticoid-induced suppressibility of ACTH secretion by a pituitary tumor is variable and may be dose dependent. Most but not all humans with PDH have pituitary tumors that are suppressible if the patient receives enough dexamethasone (a high dose). Administration of larger and larger doses of dexamethasone eventually should suppress pituitary ACTH secretion in most dogs with PDH.

PROTOCOL. The high-dose dexamethasone suppression (HDDS) protocol recommended involves the collection of plasma or serum samples before and 4 or 8 hours after intravenous administration of dexamethasone (0.1 mg/kg body weight) (Feldman, 1983b and 1985; Feldman et al, 1996). Either dexamethasone sodium phosphate or dexamethasone in polyethylene glycol is suitable. Suppression (Fig. 6-47) is defined by any of four criteria: a plasma cortisol concentration less than 50% of the baseline concentration 4 or 8 hours after dexamethasone administration or less than 1.4 µg/dl at 4 or 8 hours (Feldman et al, 1996).

RESULTS

Adrenocortical Tumors (ATH). Administration of a high dose of dexamethasone does not cause cortisol suppression in dogs with ATH (see Fig. 6-47) (Feldman, 1983b and 1985; Feldman et al, 1996). However, plasma cortisol concentrations fluctuate, and occasionally a "suppressed" plasma cortisol concentration could be seen as a result of a simple fluctuation in plasma cortisol concentrations. However, such test results are extremely unusual in a dog with ATH.

Pituitary-Dependent Hyperadrenocorticism (PDH). The HDDS test should suppress ACTH secretion from the pituitary, regardless of whether the source of the ACTH is a functioning neoplasm (adenoma or carcinoma) or hyperplastic pituitary cells. Approximately 60% of dogs with PDH have plasma cortisol

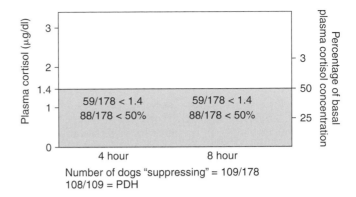

FIGURE 6–47. Results of the high-dose dexamethasone suppression (HDDS) test (0.1 mg/kg IV with samples obtained 4 and 8 hours later) in 178 dogs with naturally occurring hyperadrenocorticism. The shaded area defines "suppression" (a plasma cortisol concentration <1.4 µg/dl at 4 or 8 hours or a plasma cortisol concentration <50% of the basal value at 4 or 8 hours). Note that 109 of the 178 dogs demonstrated suppression and that 108 of the 109 dogs had PDH and one had an adrenal tumor. The HDDS test is reliable, but not perfect, for differentiating PDH from adrenal tumor dogs. Forty of 148 dogs with PDH and 29 of 30 dogs with adrenal tumors did not suppress.

concentrations less than 50% of the baseline concentration at 4 and/or 8 hours after administration of the high dose of dexamethasone (see Fig. 6-47). The percentage is not much different in dogs tested with the 1.0 mg/kg dose of dexamethasone. Approximately 40% of dogs with PDH have plasma cortisol concentrations less than 1.4 µg/dl 4 and 8 hours after the HDDS test (see Fig. 6-47). Approximately 75% of dogs with PDH meet at least one of the four criteria for "suppression" (less than 50% of basal values at 4 or 8 hours; less than 1.4 µg/dl at 4 or 8 hours) on the HDDS test, as shown in Fig. 6-44, *B* (Feldman et al, 1996). Dogs with naturally occurring Cushing's syndrome that "suppress" on the 0.1 mg/kg dose of dexamethasone, based on any one of these four criteria, are quite likely to have PDH. Among dogs with CCS that fail to demonstrate suppression are approximately 25% of dogs with PDH and virtually 100% of dogs with adrenocortical tumors (Feldman, 1985; Feldman et al, 1996).

It is not known why some dogs with PDH are resistant to dexamethasone suppression, whereas others suppress completely after administration of a high dose of dexamethasone. Pituitary tumors in some of these dogs arise from pars intermedia tissue, and this may account for a lesser degree of dexamethasone suppressibility because this area of the pituitary gland is under neural rather than hormonal control (Peterson, 1987). Additionally, several groups have reported that the larger the pituitary tumor, the less likely the dog is to suppress after receiving any dose of dexamethasone (Kemppainen and Zenoble, 1985; Safarty et al, 1988; Dow et al, 1990; Galac et al, 1997). We have seen partial but not total correlation between the size of a pituitary tumor and plasma cortisol response to dexamethasone (Nelson et al, 1989; Kipperman et al, 1992; Bertoy et al,

1995; Duesberg et al, 1995). Dogs with microsized pituitary tumors have been identified that "fail to suppress," and dogs with large macrotumors have been identified that "suppress," and vice versa. None of these results is definitive, and overlap in results regarding tumor size definitely exists (see Figs. 6-34 and 6-35).

MULTIPLE SAMPLES. Until recently, the literature neither supported nor rejected the need for samples to be obtained at 2, 3, 4, and 6 hours or at other times after administration of a high dexamethasone dose. Agreement is uniform that the 8-hour sample is important. In a study on 148 dogs with PDH, 108 demonstrated "suppression" on the HDDS test, as defined in Fig. 6-44, B. Ninety of those 108 dogs had suppressed plasma cortisol concentrations at both 4 and 8 hours after HDDS. Nine suppressed only at 8 hours, and nine suppressed only at the 4-hour sampling. Of the nine that suppressed only at 4 hours, six had previously "suppressed" on the 4-hour component of the LDDS. Thus the 4-hour HDDS sampling was informative in only three of 148 dogs with PDH (2%) that had been tested with both LDDS and HDDS and in only three of 178 total dogs with Cushing's syndrome studied (1.7%) (Fig. 6-48) (Feldman et al, 1996). Our experience strongly suggests that pretest and 8-hour samples should be obtained; others are not usually necessary.

SUMMARY. The low- and high-dose dexamethasone tests are usually performed in tandem; that is, on consecutive days. In a study on 178 dogs with naturally occurring Cushing's syndrome, 148 had PDH. Of the 148 dogs with PDH, 109 suppressed on HDDS testing. Of the 109 dogs that suppressed on HDDS testing, 86

(79%) had suppressed on LDDS tests using one of the three criteria in Fig. 6-44, A (Fig. 6-49) (Feldman et al, 1996). No dog with an adrenocortical tumor suppressed on LDDS testing. Therefore the recommendation is to perform the LDDS test. If the dog has Cushing's syndrome (8-hour cortisol level >1.4 µg/dl) and meets one of the three criteria for suppression in Fig. 6-44, A, a diagnosis of PDH is established, and the HDDS test is not necessary. If no suppression is noted on LDDS testing, a "discrimination test" can be done.

Dexamethasone suppression tests (low dose and high dose) are readily available to veterinarians. Any dog with Cushing's syndrome that demonstrates cortisol suppression on an HDDS test can be assumed to have PDH. Failure of dexamethasone to suppress plasma cortisol concentrations, using any of the seven criteria in Fig. 6-44, A and B, must be viewed as an inconclusive test result. Failure of suppression is typical of dogs with adrenocortical tumors and some dogs with pituitary-dependent Cushing's syndrome.

Urine Cortisol:Creatinine Ratio (UC:CR) in Distinguishing PDH from ATH

It is accepted that the UC:CR can be abnormally increased for reasons other than hyperadrenocorticism; that is, the results of this test are not highly specific. However, the test results are sensitive, and a protocol has been developed for using this test as a discrimination test in addition to using it for "screening" purposes.

In a study of 160 dogs with CCS (Galac et al, 1997), urine was collected by owners on two consecutive

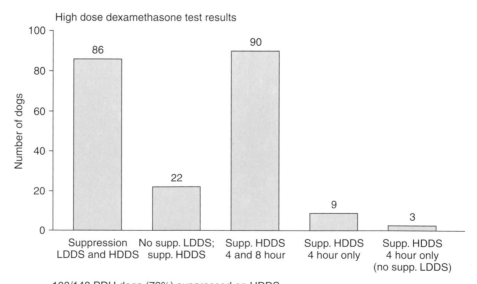

FIGURE 6–48. Of 148 dogs with PDH, 108 suppressed on the HDDS test. This graph shows that of those 108 dogs, 86 had demonstrated suppression on the LDDS test, making the HDDS test unnecessary in that group. Of the 22 dogs suppressing on HDDS but not LDDS testing, only three dogs suppressed at the 4-hour mark and no other, and 19 suppressed at 8 hours. Thus the HDDS test has limited but important value if the LDDS test is performed first, and only the 8-hour sample is needed during the HDDS test.

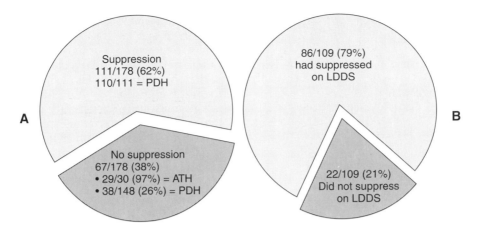

FIGURE 6–49. *A*, Of 178 dogs with naturally occurring hyperadrenocorticism that were tested with both LDDS and HDDS, 111 dogs suppressed using at least one of the seven criteria defined in Fig. 6-44. Of the 111 dogs, 110 had pituitary-dependent hyperadrenocorticism (PDH). Twenty-nine of 30 dogs (97%) with adrenal tumors (adrenal tumor hyperadrenocorticism [ATH]) did not suppress plasma cortisol concentrations using any of the seven criteria, and 38 of the 148 dogs with PDH (26%) did not suppress. *B*, Of the 109 dogs suppressing on the HDDS test, 86 (79%) had suppressed on the LDDS test. This shows that if the LDDS test is performed on dogs suspected of having hyperadrenocorticism, the HDDS test is not necessary in approximately 60% of dogs with PDH.

days for a "basal" UC:CR. After the second urine collection, 0.1 mg/kg of dexamethasone was given orally three times at 8-hour intervals. A third urine sample was collected 8 hours after administration of the third dexamethasone dose. (Typically, the first urine samples are collected on consecutive mornings, and immediately after collection of the second urine sample, the first dexamethasone dose is administered. The second and third doses are administered in the afternoon and evening of the same day, respectively, and the third urine sample is collected the next morning. Thus urine is collected on three consecutive mornings.) If the UC:CR in the third sample was suppressed by more than 50% of the mean value of the first two ratios (basal ratios), PDH was diagnosed. If suppression was less than 50%, no discrimination was possible (as is the case with any suppression test). Eighty of 111 dogs (72%) with PDH exhibited suppression. This percentage of dogs with PDH that "suppressed" with dexamethasone is similar to the results obtained with the previously described low-dose and high-dose dexamethasone tests. However, the UC:CR protocol depends on owner compliance regarding administration of the drug. All dogs with ATH, as well as 27% of those with PDH, failed to exhibit suppression (Galac et al, 1997).

It is important to remember that the basal UC:CR is quite sensitive in CCS but its specificity is poor, therefore a diagnosis of CCS should be supported by typical clinical signs and serum biochemistry, CBC, and urinalysis abnormalities, as well as by ACTH stimulation or low-dose dexamethasone test results. After the diagnosis of CCS has been confirmed, a reduction in the UC:CR to values less than 50% of basal values with the dexamethasone protocol described would be consistent with PDH. Failure to suppress must be considered nondiagnostic.

Corticotropin-Releasing Hormone (CRH) and Vasopressin (ADH) Response Testing

Dogs with PDH have an ACTH-secreting pituitary tumors. These ACTH-secreting cells typically retain some responsiveness to CRH and ADH, in contrast to nonresponsive adrenocortical tumors. Plasma ACTH and cortisol responses to CRH and ADH were assessed in 16 healthy dogs, 16 dogs with PDH, and five dogs with ATH (van Wijk et al, 1994). In this study, it was concluded that dogs with PDH had a greater response to ADH than to CRH and that these responses may be used to discriminate these dogs from those with ATH. However, the expense, the lack of availability of CRH and ADH, and the difficulties encountered with ACTH assays limit the use of these protocols.

Metyrapone Testing

Metyrapone is an enzyme blocker that inhibits the action of 11-β-hydroxylase in steroid synthesis. Thus, in normal dogs, plasma cortisol concentrations decline, whereas 11-desoxycortisol accumulates as ACTH stimulation continues. The suggested dose of metyrapone is 25 mg/kg given orally every 6 hours for four treatments, with plasma collected prior to the test and 6 hours after the final dose. Samples are assayed for both cortisol and 11-desoxycortisol. If metyrapone causes a decrease in the plasma cortisol concentration and a concomitant increase in the plasma 11-desoxycortisol level, a diagnosis of PDH can be made. If the plasma cortisol and 11-desoxycortisol concentrations both decline after the four metyrapone doses, an adrenal tumor is the likely cause of the hyperadrenocorticism (Zerbe et al, 1986 and 2000b).

Radiology

See page 283.

Abdominal Ultrasonography

See page 286.

Computed Tomography (CT) or Magnetic Resonance Imaging (MRI) Scans

DOGS WITH PDH THAT HAVE CLINICAL SIGNS OF PITUITARY MACROTUMOR.   The use of CT and MRI scans is increasing in veterinary medicine. The following sections focus on the use of these sophisticated diagnostic aids. The study recommended (CT or MRI) should simply be whichever is least expensive or most readily available. Although there are advantages to MRI scans in detecting subtle abnormalities, the purpose of either study in a dog with PDH and clinical signs of a large pituitary tumor is to detect an obvious abnormality (i.e., a pituitary tumor greater than 8 to 10 mm in greatest diameter; see page 296). At the time of writing, we have obtained either CT or MRI scans of the pituitary region from more than 200 dogs with PDH. As with any group of veterinarians, as our experience expands, our understanding of this disease and of CT or MRI pituitary scans continues to improve.

DOGS WITH RECENTLY DIAGNOSED PDH AND NO SIGNS OF MACROTUMOR.   The second group of dogs for which we recommend a pituitary imaging study comprises those with recently diagnosed, usually untreated PDH and no clinical signs suggestive of a pituitary macrotumor. Imaging is recommended from our experience of appreciating those dogs at greatest risk of developing a life-threatening pituitary macrotumor. In other words, CT or MRI scans can be used as part of the "database" in dogs with PDH. The limiting factors for this use are simple: expense, availability, and anesthetic risk. If these studies were free, readily available, and did not require anesthesia, we would recommend CT or MRI scanning for every dog diagnosed as having PDH. The thought process is simply based on the concept of a pituitary tumor having the potential to increase in size anywhere from 0 to 4 times in the 12 to 36 months following the diagnosis of PDH.

If a dog with PDH has no visible mass (i.e., the mass is less than 3 to 4 mm in greatest diameter), the chance of such a tumor causing clinical problems due to growth is remote. Even if the mass doubled or tripled in size, it would likely be less than 8 to 10 mm in greatest diameter, would cause no clinical signs, and would have little chance of expanding into critical structures. A repeat scan is not recommended for such dogs, and the owners are informed that the chance of their pet developing a large pituitary mass is remote.

If a dog with PDH has a visible mass 3 to 7 mm in greatest diameter, we recommend routine therapy for PDH with o,p'-DDD and a repeat scan 12 to 24 months after the first scan. If these tumors increase 2 to 4 times in size, they would be a significant hazard to the pet, and radiation therapy can be recommended at that time.

If a dog with PDH has a pituitary mass that is equal to or greater than 8 mm in greatest diameter, we recommend pituitary irradiation prior to medical therapy for PDH. Expansion of these tumors by 50% to 100% would likely result in serious to life-threatening problems. For masses that are not causing clinical signs and that are less than 12 mm in greatest diameter, irradiation offers the best chance of significant shrinkage (Goossens et al, 1998; Theon and Feldman, 1998). Although we have had excellent results in reducing pituitary tumor size in this latter group of dogs, irradiation has not consistently negated the need for medical therapy for the hyperadrenocorticism.

CT scans

AVAILABILITY.   The use of CT scans has been part of a minor revolution in the high technology of modern human and veterinary medicine (Bailey, 1986; Turrel et al, 1986). This sophisticated diagnostic aid was initially available primarily at veterinary schools and through a small number of veterinarians working in concert with local human hospitals. The availability of CT for veterinary patients continues to expand in accord with public demand. Although there is little question about the value of CT scan results in diagnosing pituitary tumor size, there are several drawbacks. In addition to the expense associated with the use of such equipment, CT scans require veterinarians or physician-radiologists with expertise to interpret results and manage the facilities. Traditional CT scans usually require 30 minutes to 2 hours of anesthesia. Use of newer helical CT units, however, reduces the time required for completing these studies, thus reducing anesthesia time as well.

HUMAN PITUITARY.   The normal appearance of the human pituitary gland in CT images was determined several decades ago, and these studies serve as the foundation for identification of pituitary abnormalities. The advent of high-resolution and rapid image acquisition CT equipment has resulted in the ability to identify pituitary microtumors in people. Changes associated with these masses include identification of a well-circumscribed region of hypoattenuation compared with the contrast-enhanced region of the gland; convexity of the upper margin of the gland; deviation of the infundibular stalk; displacement of the pituitary capillary bed (the "tuft sign"); and bony erosion to the floor of the sella turcica (Bonneville et al, 1983).

HEALTHY DOG PITUITARY.   CT scans are typically obtained on dogs under anesthesia before and after administration of a contrast agent, such as water-soluble iodinated agents. The use of CT scans by veterinarians preceded studies that defined normal or reference limits from healthy dogs and cats. Studies on healthy dogs, therefore, began to appear in the literature years after this tool was used by clinicians. In one study, peak pituitary enhancement was seen within 10 to 30 seconds of contrast injection (Love et al, 2000). Pituitary glands have variable appearances during the course of scanning. During the first 30 to 50 seconds, contrast enhancement was intense and the pituitary gland was described as having an inverted triangular appearance with an irregular dorsal margin. As imaging progressed, a peripheral rim of enhancement was seen surrounding a more hypoattenuated central region of the gland.

Dynamic CT of the pituitary was performed in 55 dogs with PDH in a recently reported study. The protocol revealed a distinct contrast enhancement of the neurohypophysis ("pituitary flush") in 36 dogs. In 24 dogs the flush was displaced, indicating the presence of an adenoma. This suspicion was confirmed surgically and histologically in 18 of the 24 dogs. In 19 dogs there was a diffusely abnormal contrast enhancement pattern. Results of surgery agreed with the results of CT in 13 of these 19 dogs and histology agreed with CT results in all 19 dogs. It was concluded that a "dynamic series of scans" should be included in CT scan protocols of the pituitary in dogs with PDH because it allows identification of either an adenoma or a diffusely abnormal pituitary (van der Vlugt-Meijer et al, in press).

ADRENALS. The CT scan is a noninvasive method of visualizing the anatomy of almost any area of the body; in Cushing's syndrome, it has been successful in distinguishing dogs and cats with normal adrenals from those with one large adrenal (Fig. 6-50) and those with two large adrenals (Fig. 6-51) (Emms et al, 1986; Widmer and Guptill, 1995). Abdominal radiography is not as sensitive as CT scanning in detecting adrenocortical tumors in dogs (Voorhout et al, 1990a). Abdominal ultrasonography has the same ability as nephrotomography to detect and localize most adrenocortical tumors (Voorhout, 1990b; Voorhout et al, 1990a).

CT OF THE PITUITARY IN PDH. Approximately 40% to 50% of dogs with PDH do not have visible abnormalities in the pituitary region because they have *microadenomas*. Interestingly, CT scanning has a diagnostic accuracy of about 40% for detecting tumors in people with PDH, a percentage similar to that for dogs (Klibanski and Zervas, 1991). Most dogs with PDH considered candidates for pituitary CT scanning have clinical signs suggestive of a large intracranial mass (see page 296). In this population of dogs (and cats), the CT scan results have been quite satisfactory, because the goal is to determine whether a large tumor is the cause of clinical signs. If such a dog has a small tumor that CT failed to detect, the diagnosis of large tumor is still adequately rejected as the cause for the clinical signs. CT is extremely accurate for visualization of large pituitary tumors (Fig. 6-52) or of cerebral ventricular dilation secondary to a pituitary/hypothalamic mass (Fig. 6-53).

At our hospital, we are fortunate to have both CT and MRI scanning facilities. CT is the less expensive with respect to owner cost. Therefore, CT is the recommended study for dogs with PDH, because we are evaluating these dogs for obvious abnormalities. The advantage of MRI scans in identifying subtle abnormalities is negated in dogs with PDH.

MRI scans

BACKGROUND. MRI has become an essential tool in humans for attempting to diagnose CNS disorders and is used increasingly for the evaluation of a variety of diseases in other organ systems. MRI is frequently compared with and has several advantages over CT: superior tissue contrast, absence of artifacts caused by bone, vascular imaging capability, absence of ionizing radiation, and safer contrast media. Longer scanning time was once a disadvantage, but new facilities are providing equipment capable of faster imaging. Gadolinium-enhanced T1-weighted images are preferred for the diagnosis of intracranial tumors. MRI is superior to CT in the detection of associated tumor features: edema, cysts, vascularity, hemorrhage, and necrosis (Edelman and Warach, 1993). Several reports of MRI scans in dogs have been published that demonstrate that the test is both sensitive and accurate (Kraft et al, 1989; Kornegay, 1990).

In one recent study, a group of 96 healthy dogs (weighing 13 to 45 kg) were evaluated with MRI scans (Kippenes et al, 2001). At necropsy, the pituitary gland from each dog was grossly and histologically normal. The pituitary was measured from transverse MRI T1-weighted scans after contrast (gadolinium) administration. The mean (± SD) pituitary gland height was 5.1 mm (± 0.9 mm), and the mean width was 6.4 mm (± 1.1 mm). Correlation coefficients comparing pituitary versus brain measurements, between pituitary measurement versus body weight, and brain measurements versus body weight were established. A hyperintense region was present on T1-weighted images in the center of the pituitary gland in 64% of dogs.

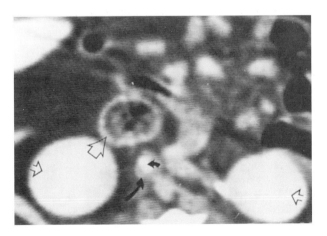

FIGURE 6-50. CT scan of the abdomen of a dog with a functioning adrenocortical tumor (*long black arrow*) with a calcified density (*short black arrow*). The kidneys, which are highlighted as a result of concentration of contrast material (*small open arrows*), and the colon (*large open arrow*) are easily identified.

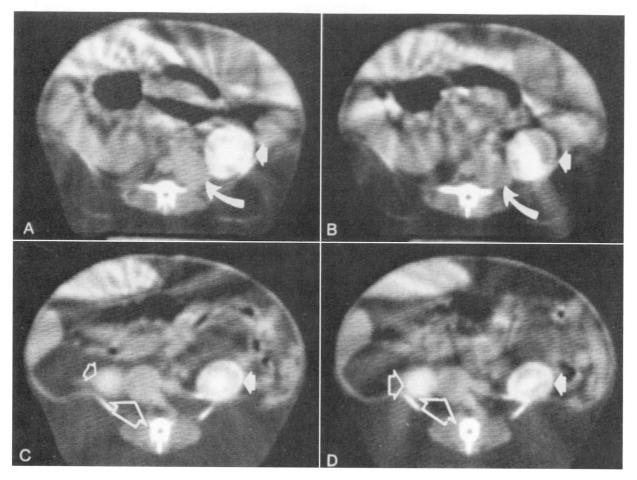

FIGURE 6–51. CT scan of the abdomen of a dog with bilateral adrenal hyperplasia. The sequential scans (*A* through *D*) are progressively moving from cranial to posterior, showing the right adrenal (*white curved arrow*) and right kidney (*small white arrow*) first; the left adrenal (*large open arrow*) and left kidney (*small open arrow*) are posterior to the right-sided structures.

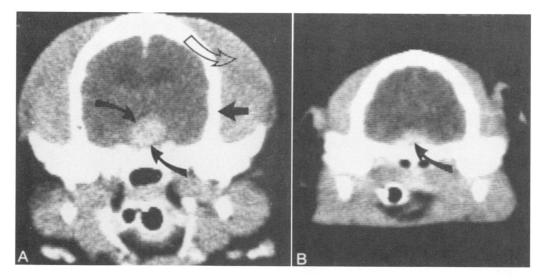

FIGURE 6–52. CT scan of the head, showing a large pituitary tumor (*curved black arrows*), in a dog (*A*) and a cat (*B*) with pituitary-dependent hyperadrenocorticism (PDH). The straight black arrow points to the cranium and the open curved arrow to the temporal muscles.

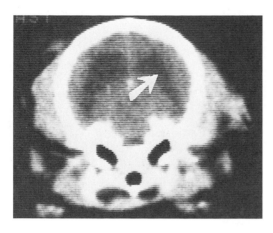

FIGURE 6–53. CT scan of the head showing dilated ventricles (*arrow*) in the brain of a hyperadrenal dog with obstruction of cerebrospinal fluid flow caused by a pituitary tumor.

PROTOCOL. The MRI scans that we have performed on dogs and cats were done at a local human hospital initially and then at our facility during the past 5 years. Most commonly, dogs were heavily sedated with an intravenous mixture of ketamine and diazepam. Each dog received small doses of the drug mixture every 10 to 15 minutes throughout the scanning period. The sedation allowed intubation, which reduced respiratory movement and improved scan quality. No acute or long-term problems have been associated with this mode of sedation, even in severely debilitated dogs with massive intracranial tumors. More recently, dogs undergoing MRI scan are placed under general anesthesia, again with virtually no morbidity.

DOGS WITH UNTREATED PDH AND NO CNS SIGNS. Approximately 40% to 50% of dogs with untreated PDH and no signs suggestive of an intracranial mass have normal MRI brain scans, and the remaining 50% to 60% have relatively small but easily visualized pituitary tumors on MRI. The visible masses measure 4 to 13 mm at greatest vertical height (Fig. 6-54). Most of the visible masses appear to extend beyond the dorsal confines of the sella turcica, and most are contrast enhancing. The lateral ventricles were enlarged in several dogs, but this finding was considered an age-related change rather than an indication of obstructive hydrocephalus (Bertoy et al, 1995 and 1996).

DOGS WITH UNTREATED PDH: ONE-YEAR FOLLOW-UP. In monitoring one group of 21 dogs with PDH that had had an MRI scan for the year after initial diagnosis, we had the opportunity to evaluate the effect of therapy and/or time on tumor growth. Eleven of the 21 dogs had a visible tumor at the time of diagnosis, and 20 of the 21 dogs were treated with o,p'-DDD (one dog that had a visible tumor was not treated). Three of the 11 dogs with a visible pituitary tumor died during the year after diagnosis; two of those three dogs had signs of an enlarging pituitary tumor, and both had tumors greater than 1 cm in diameter at the time that medical therapy was started.

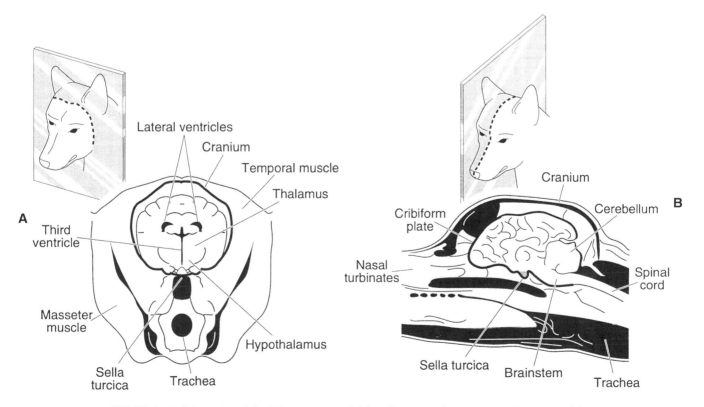

FIGURE 6–54. Orientation of the (*A*) transverse and (*B*) midline sagittal sections on MRI scans and the anatomic structures seen on each view.   *Continued*

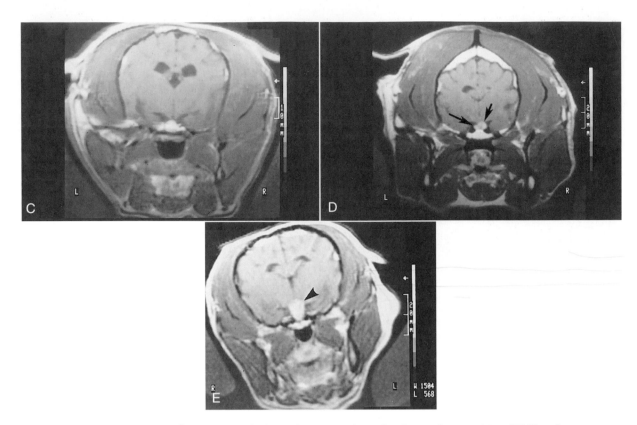

FIGURE 6–54.—cont'd *C*, MRI scan of a dog with pituitary-dependent hyperadrenocorticism (PDH) and a normal pituitary area. *D*, MRI scan of a dog with PDH and a relatively small (7 mm) pituitary mass *(arrows)*. *E*, MRI scan of a dog with PDH caused by an 11 mm mass *(arrow)*. (From Bertoy EH, et al: J Am Vet Med Assoc 206:651, 1995.)

Eight of the 11 dogs that had a visible pituitary tumor underwent a second MRI scan 1 year after the first scan. Four of the eight had no apparent change in tumor size (tumors ranged in size from 7 to 9 mm in greatest diameter before and after 1 year). Four of the eight dogs had pituitary tumor enlargement (5, 6, 8, and 11 mm at time of diagnosis; 10, 9, 11, and 14 mm 1 year later, respectively). The two dogs with the largest tumors (11 and 14 mm) developed clinical signs attributable to an enlarging pituitary tumor. The largest growth was in the dog that underwent no therapy (5 to 10 mm). Five of the 10 dogs that had no visible pituitary tumor at the time of diagnosis underwent a second scan, with two of those five dogs having a visible tumor 1 year later (6 and 7 mm, respectively).

Our conclusions from these studies were then and continue to be: (1) 15% to 25% of dogs with PDH are at risk of developing neurologic signs and life-threatening problems due to an enlarging tumor; (2) of the 15% to 25% at risk for developing a large and clinically worrisome tumor, most have problems within the first 6 to 18 months after PDH diagnosis due to continued tumor expansion; (3) o,p'-DDD treatment does not have a major effect on tumor growth rate; (4) neurologic signs are associated almost exclusively with tumors 10 mm or greater in diameter; (5) pituitary irradiation should be considered for any dog with PDH that has a pituitary tumor equal to or greater than 8 mm in greatest diameter; and (6) MRI or CT scans of the pituitary in dogs with PDH that have no clinical signs attributable to an enlarging pituitary mass are helpful in predicting dogs likely to develop problems due to an enlarging pituitary tumor (Bertoy et al, 1995 and 1996).

DOGS WITH PDH AND SIGNS OF AN INTRACRANIAL TUMOR. We have completed MRI scans in more than 100 dogs with PDH that had signs of an intracranial tumor (see page 296). These dogs had a mean age of 9.5 years (younger than the mean for all dogs with PDH) and a mean body weight of 24 kg (larger than the average dog with PDH). MRI scans were definitive in demonstrating the size and nature of the tumor in each dog. All masses were better visualized after administration of contrast (gadolinium DTPA). The masses measured 8 to 31 mm at greatest vertical height (Fig. 6-55). All tumors had expanded dorsally, well beyond the limits of the sella turcica. Some masses elevated the floor of the third ventricle, and some appeared to compress the hypothalamus. Obstructive hydrocephalus was suspected in a small minority of dogs. Tumor-associated necrosis or hemorrhage was not apparent on any scans (Duesberg et al, 1995).

EVALUATION OF THE PATIENT WITH AN INCIDENTALLY DISCOVERED ADRENAL MASS. See discussion in the ultrasonography section, page 286.

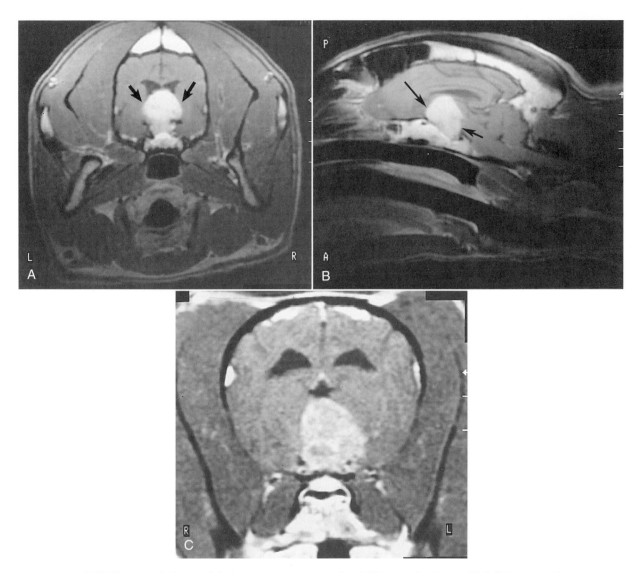

FIGURE 6–55. *A*, Post-gadolinium transverse view of an MRI scan of a 7-year-old Bull Terrier with pituitary-dependent hyperadrenocorticism (PDH) caused by a 2.4 cm mass *(arrows)*. The dog had developed signs of disorientation and ataxia. *B*, Midline sagittal view of the brain of the same dog (using MRI), showing the densely enhancing mass *(arrows)* arising from the pituitary fossa; the mass had caused compression of the floor of the overlying third ventricle. *C*, Post-gadolinium MRI scan of an 8-year-old Boston Terrier with PDH and signs of disorientation, ataxia, and circling.

Radioisotope Imaging of the Adrenals

γ-Camera imaging of the adrenal glands has been reported in normal dogs and in dogs with Cushing's syndrome. Dogs were given iodine-131-19-iodocholesterol intravenously. In normal dogs, both adrenal glands could be visualized separately. Distinguishing between the images of normal glands, hyperplastic glands, and functioning adrenal tumors presented no difficulty. In addition, γ-camera imaging allowed the correct surgical site to be selected for removal of adrenal tumors. The use of radioactive substances, the expense of γ-cameras, and the need for specialized facilities limit the use of this tool. The sensitivity and reliability of ultrasonography, CT, and MRI render this diagnostic test almost obsolete.

TREATMENT—GENERAL APPROACH

Background

Approximately 80% to 85% of dogs with naturally developing hyperadrenocorticism have PDH, and 15% to 20% have functioning adrenocortical tumors. Therapy may be selected on the basis of what has caused the Cushing's syndrome (pituitary or adrenocortical tumor), as well as the veterinarian's experience. Knowing whether a dog has PDH or an adrenocortical tumor, although ideal, is not always vital (see next section, Therapy without Defining the Underlying Cause). An attempt is made to determine this information, but it is recognized that a thorough diagnostic evaluation of every animal cannot always be completed. Several therapeutic options are available, including medical therapies and sophisticated surgeries.

Excellent rapport between veterinarian and owner is imperative during the long-term management of a dog or cat that has been diagnosed as having hyperadrenocorticism. The surgical and medical options should be discussed in detail, including what is expected of the owner. One hopes to return such dogs to a normal endocrine state, but this is not always possible, and all complications must be discussed. These dogs may have endocrine excesses or deficiencies after treatment, and the prepared owner can better accept these setbacks. Time spent explaining the pathophysiology in lay terms is well worth the effort to improve client understanding and to establish a good basis for communication.

Therapy without Defining the Underlying Cause

Naturally occurring hyperadrenocorticism is a common disorder. A veterinarian may suspect that a dog has CCS and complete an in-hospital evaluation, including database and screening tests, but may not proceed diagnostically to distinguish whether a dog has a pituitary or an adrenocortical tumor. This may occur because of unfamiliarity with tests that distinguish pituitary-dependent (PDH) from adrenocortical tumor (ATH) CCS, owner financial constraints, lack of facilities to perform some of the tests, or tests that are completed but inconclusive. How does the veterinarian proceed in these situations?

There are two major alternatives. One is to refer the dog to a colleague or institution that can proceed with more sophisticated testing. The second is to realize that most dogs with CCS have PDH with associated bilateral adrenocortical hyperplasia and are responsive to therapy with o,p'-DDD. Based on this diagnosis and treatment, the chance of achieving control is excellent. Furthermore, the veterinarian can make an educated guess about differentiation of PDH (easily controlled) from ATH (relative o,p'-DDD resistance) by monitoring the response to o,p'-DDD (see page 333).

TREATMENT—SURGERY

Adrenal Tumor Hyperadrenocorticism

PREOPERATIVE EVALUATION

Prognosis. Dogs diagnosed as having ATH have an excellent prognosis if the tumor can be surgically removed and if they survive the first 2 weeks after surgery. Obviously, those are rather large "ifs." Once the diagnosis of Cushing's syndrome and the presence of an adrenal tumor have been confirmed, an attempt should be made to localize the tumor and rule out metastasis. Abdominal radiography localizes approximately 50% of tumors via adrenal calcification or size (see Figs. 6-28 and 6-29), but abdominal ultrasonography

(see page 286) is the preferred tool for localizing tumors, identifying tissue or vascular invasion, and noting possible abdominal metastasis. In addition, ultrasonography is an excellent tool for identifying vessel or organ invasion or compression. Abdominal surgery should not be considered without prior ultrasound evaluation and should only be performed by a qualified and experienced surgeon.

Imaging and Metastases. Adrenal tumors that metastasize usually spread to the liver or lungs, or both. Radiographs of the thorax, therefore, are also mandatory (Fig. 6-56). Ultrasound evaluation of the liver has been quite valuable in predicting and detecting metastasis. If metastasis is suspected, an ultrasound-guided biopsy of the liver can be performed to confirm this suspicion. Approximately 10% of the dogs we have examined with Cushing's syndrome secondary to an adrenocortical tumor have had obvious metastases at the time of initial examination at our hospital.

Screening tests, such as radiographs, ultrasonography, and CT scans, may also provide valuable information about tumor size. Small tumors (Fig. 6-57; see also Fig. 6-28) are much more likely to be benign and easily removed than large tumors (Fig. 6-58; see also Fig. 6-29). In general, a "small" adrenocortical tumor is arbitrarily defined as being equal to or smaller than one half the size of a normal kidney. A "large" tumor can be arbitrarily defined as equal to or larger than a normal kidney in size. According to these arbitrary definitions, it is also possible to suggest that small tumors are usually adenomas, are well encapsulated, and are somewhat easier to remove surgically than large tumors, which are usually carcinomas, are not well encapsulated, and often are quite difficult to excise surgically. However, adrenocortical carcinomas may be "small." Histologic evaluation of any tumor is imperative.

CT scans are a noninvasive method of evaluating the size and shape of the adrenal glands and may also be used to identify metastatic disease (Voorhout et al, 1990a; Widmer and Guptill, 1995; Zerbe, 2000b; Hill and Scott-Moncrief, 2001). For accurate interpretation, experience in CT and a detailed knowledge of cross-sectional anatomy are essential. Anesthesia, expense, and availability of such facilities are the principal drawbacks to the routine use of this imaging modality. MRI scans may be more accurate than CT in the identification of adrenal masses and their metastasis or vascular invasion. As availability improves and costs decrease, this may become the imaging modality of choice.

Determining Reasonable Surgical Candidates. The initial preoperative evaluation should be directed at determining whether a particular dog is a reasonable surgical candidate. There is the obvious assessment based on the physical examination and the opinion of an experienced veterinarian. In addition, assessment should include an evaluation of systemic blood pressure, urine protein:creatinine ratio, and serum antithrombin III concentrations. If either of the first two parameters is significantly increased and/or

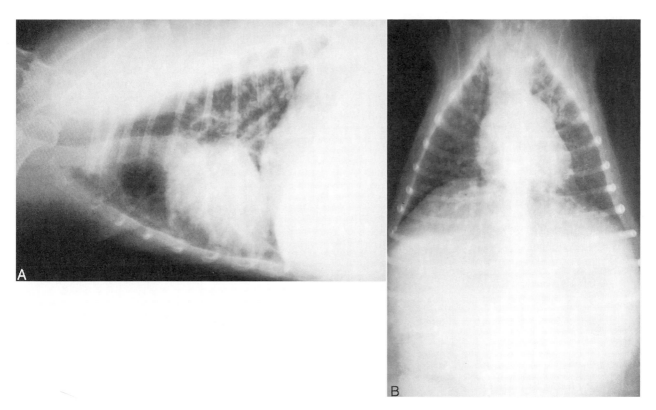

FIGURE 6–56. Lateral (*A*) and dorsoventral (*B*) thoracic radiographs from a dog with hyper-adrenocorticism caused by an adrenocortical tumor that has metastasized to the lungs.

if the antithrombin III concentration is significantly decreased, the dog may be at greater risk for thromboembolism than the typical dog with Cushing's syndrome (please see page 293) (Ortega et al, 1995; Jacoby et al, 2001). Without a doubt, the risk of thromboembolism in dogs with CCS is greatest when they are placed under anesthesia and undergo prolonged abdominal surgery. Treating the dog at increased risk for anesthetic, surgical, or postsurgical problems for 1 to

3 months before surgery with ketoconazole or o,p'-DDD could be beneficial in resolving many of the problems associated with Cushing's syndrome–related debilitation. This time can also be used to treat any other concurrent problems (infection). Although this approach is often mentioned, we rarely find dogs that need such therapy prior to surgery.

SURGICAL APPROACH. The recommended surgical approach is either paracostal (flank) or ventral midline laparotomy. A ventral midline celiotomy provides the best opportunity for exposure of both adrenal glands and complete evaluation of the abdominal contents, especially the liver, for metastasis or other problems (Scavelli et al, 1986; Emms et al, 1987; Anderson et al, 2001). Any abnormal tissue should be excised or biopsied. However, problems may be associated with wound healing in tissues that have been chronically exposed to excess concentrations of corticosteroids, and this would be exaggerated by a ventral weight-bearing incision. In addition, the large amount of abdominal fat found in dogs with Cushing's syndrome, coupled with the location of the adrenals dorsal and medial to the kidneys (Fig. 6-59), makes the ventral midline approach difficult. However, the ventral midline approach is routinely used in our practice. For dogs with large masses and for tumors that are difficult to visualize, are invading vascular structures (most commonly the vena cava or renal vein), or are invading or compressing the liver, our surgeons commonly improve exposure by adding a paracostal incision to the ventral midline approach.

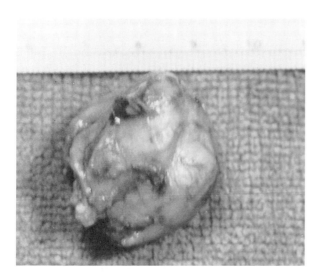

FIGURE 6–57. Photograph of a small, functioning adrenocortical adenoma.

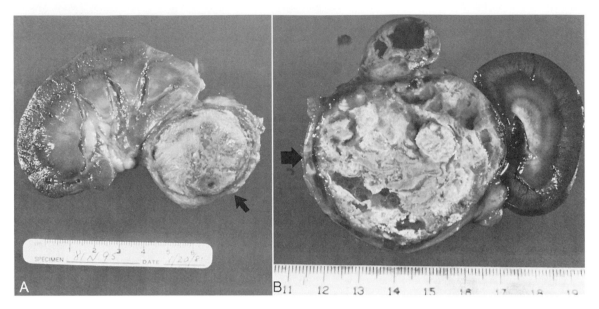

FIGURE 6–58. Photographs of moderate size *(A)* and large *(B)* adrenocortical carcinomas *(arrows)* closely adhered to the associated kidney.

The paracostal retroperitoneal approach to adrenalectomy provides adequate exposure of the adrenal gland on that side of the abdomen (Van Sluijs et al, 1995). This approach avoids the wound-healing problems with a weight-bearing ventral midline incision and the difficulties of traversing an abdomen filled with fat. Also, an adrenal located in the area of the vena cava and aorta may be more accessible via the paracostal approach (see Fig. 6-59). Marked disadvantages of the paracostal approach include (1) the area of only one adrenal can be explored (exploration of the opposite side requires closure of the first incision and a second surgical procedure) and (2) the liver and most of the abdomen cannot be evaluated for metastasis.

Both surgical approaches are well described in several veterinary surgery texts and are not reviewed here (Johnston, 1983). When an adrenal tumor is recognized, an attempt at total excision is usually made. However, the surgeon may encounter a large mass or one that has invaded surrounding tissues and cannot be excised. In this circumstance, as much tumor should be removed as possible, because the tissue provides histologic confirmation of the diagnosis, and debulking may improve the endocrine status of the dog or cat.

PATIENT MANAGEMENT DURING AND AFTER SURGERY (FIG. 6-60)

Glucocorticoid Therapy. The autonomous secretion of cortisol from an adrenocortical tumor causes suppression of pituitary ACTH via negative feedback, resulting in significant atrophy of normal cells within the zona reticularis and zona fasciculata (which synthesize cortisol) of the opposite adrenal and unaffected cells of the adrenal that contains the tumor. Suppression of endogenous ACTH by the tumor may also cause some atrophy of the zona glomerulosa,

which synthesizes aldosterone. Acute hypocortisolism is expected and should occur after surgery. At the time of anesthesia, intravenous fluids (saline or Ringer's solution) should be administered at a maintenance rate. When an adrenal tumor is recognized by the surgeon, dexamethasone should be placed in the IV infusion bottle at a dosage of 0.05 to 0.1 mg/kg body weight. This dose is given over a 6-hour period and then usually repeated two more times that day and then BID or TID, subcutaneously, until the dog can be safely given oral medication without danger of vomiting.

Alternatively, a continuous infusion of hydrocortisone hemisuccinate (625 µg/kg/hr) can be given during and after surgery by means of an infusion pump. In theory, the hydrocortisone provides both glucocorticoid and mineralocorticoid effects, although we have not been impressed with the mineralocorticoid effect of this drug. We do not recommend hydrocortisone; we do recommend dexamethasone. Although some investigators have recommended treating surgical patients with corticosteroids for 1 or 2 days *prior to* adrenalectomy, this protocol is unnecessary and actually potentially harmful. The iatrogenic steroids may predispose a dog to worsening hypertension and overhydration, as well as increasing the risk of thromboembolic problems.

After successful recovery from anesthesia, dogs should be continued on dexamethasone with or without mineralocorticoid medications using the treatment protocol described for hypoadrenocorticism (see Chapter 8). Dexamethasone can be administered at a tapering dose (0.01 to 0.1 mg/kg) in intravenous fluids or subcutaneously two to four times a day (we usually administer dexamethasone SQ twice after surgery and tid the day after surgery). Parenteral medication is usually not continued for more than 24 to 72 hours,

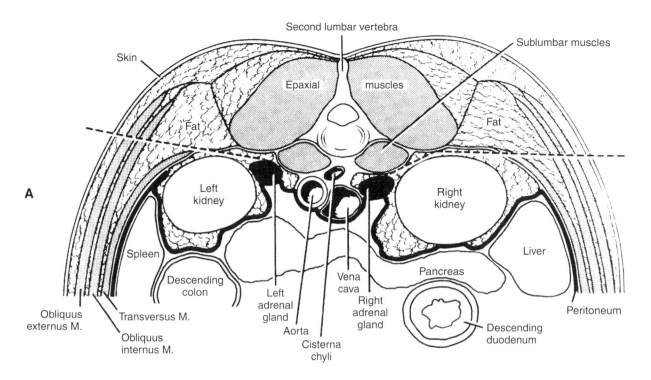

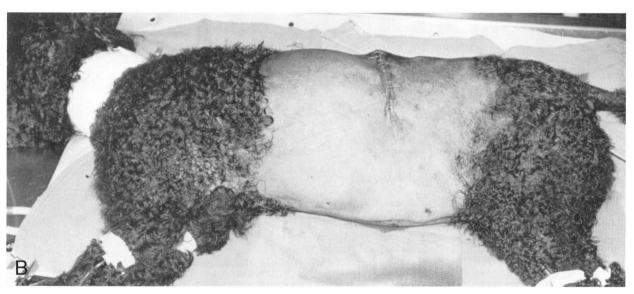

FIGURE 6–59. *A,* Anatomic diagram showing the location of the canine adrenals and the surgical approach *(dashed lines)* via paracostal incisions to each gland. *B,* Photograph of a dog with hyperadrenocorticism caused by an adrenal tumor that was removed via the paracostal approach. *(A* from Johnston D: J Am Vet Med Assoc 170:1093, 1977.)

because by that time most dogs are eating and drinking normally and are not receiving intravenous fluids. In that setting, oral medication can be initiated. Once the dog is eating and drinking on its own, it should receive approximately 0.25 to 1.0 mg/kg of prednisone orally twice daily for 2 days (the larger dose for small dogs and the smaller dose for large dogs). That dosage is then reduced as long as the dog maintains an appetite and has no problems with vomiting or diarrhea. For example, in small dogs, the

reduction regimen could be: 0.5 mg/kg twice daily for 2 days; then 0.25 mg/kg twice daily for 3 weeks; then 0.25 mg/kg once daily for 3 weeks, then 0.25 mg/kg every other day for 1 month, and finally 0.25 mg/kg every third day for 1 month. The glucocorticoid treatment period is usually tapered over a period of 3 to 6 months until the dose is extremely small. After every other day or every third day therapy has been achieved, a trial period with no medication can be undertaken.

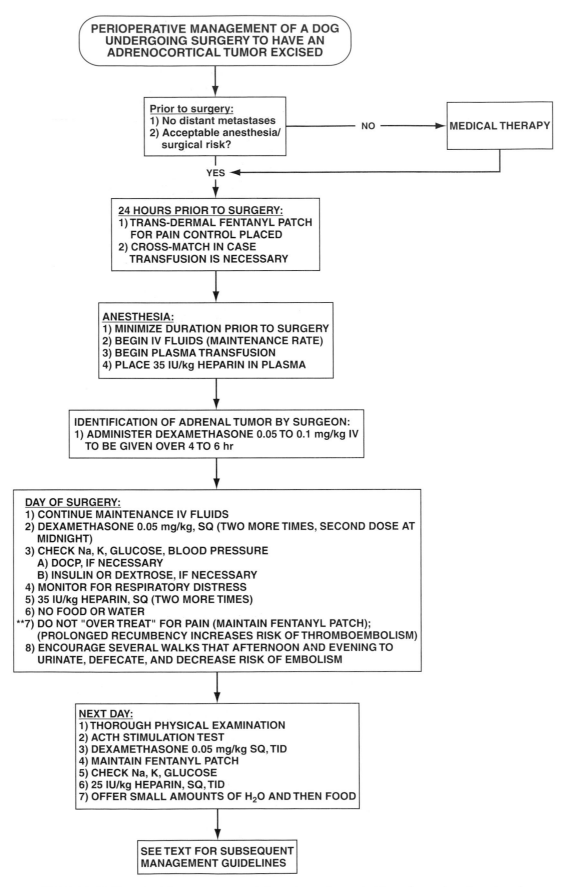

FIGURE 6–60. Flow chart for management of the perioperative period for a dog undergoing adrenal tumor resection.

Mineralocorticoid Therapy. Postoperatively, the blood pressure, BUN, serum electrolytes, and blood glucose concentrations should be closely monitored. Approximately 15% to 20% of our dogs have mild hypokalemia or hypernatremia, or both, after surgery. These abnormalities slowly resolve as exogenous steroid doses are reduced and the dog begins to eat. Serum sodium concentrations less than reference values and/or serum potassium concentrations greater than the reference range may indicate a need for mineralocorticoid therapy. Mild hyperkalemia and/or hyponatremia has been documented in 40% of our dogs in the 24- to 48-hour period after surgery. In almost all dogs, these abnormalities are transient and resolve within a day or two. Because mineralocorticoid therapy is rather benign and because it is not possible to determine which dogs will have transient problems and which will have serious mineralocorticoid deficits, treatment is recommended if these abnormalities become worrisome (serum sodium <135 mEq/L or serum potassium >6.5 mEq/L) or if they persist longer than 72 hours.

A small number of our dogs have been treated with oral fludrocortisone acetate (0.02 mg/kg; see maintenance therapy, Chapter 8). Oral mineralocorticoids can be given twice daily and the need for continuing treatment assessed prior to each administration. Oral mineralocorticoids can usually be discontinued after 2 to 7 days, to be given again only if hyperkalemia or hyponatremia recurs. The dose of fludrocortisone acetate usually can be slowly tapered, similar to the protocol suggested for prednisone. Although not common (~10%), the dogs thought to require mineralocorticoid therapy are given desoxycorticosterone pivalate (DOCP) as described in Chapter 8. It is extremely unusual for one of these dogs to need a second injection 25 days later. If needed, one half of the dose is administered at the next injection (day 25), and one fourth of the dose on day 50. With DOCP-treated dogs, the serum electrolyte concentrations should be checked every 7 to 10 days. It is rare for a dog to need more than two or three injections.

SUMMARY OF GLUCOCORTICOID AND MINERALOCORTICOID THERAPY. Glucocorticoid and mineralocorticoid medication must meet individual requirements; "cookbook" approaches must be avoided. It is recommended that an ACTH stimulation test be completed the morning after surgery, before that day's dose of dexamethasone is given. If the results are dramatically low (pre-ACTH and post-ACTH plasma cortisol concentrations <1 μg%), the surgery was likely a success, although nonfunctional metastases are always a possibility. If the results are no different than those prior to surgery, then surgery must be considered a failure and exogenous glucocorticoids are not necessary. Furthermore, if low cortisol concentrations are documented, these values provide proof of a need for glucocorticoid therapy and also a baseline for monitoring therapy. Glucocorticoid therapy should continue until ACTH stimulation test results are within a low-normal range (this may require 2 to 5 months).

Ideally, dogs should be on alternate-day glucocorticoid therapy within 4 to 8 weeks of surgery and off all medication within 3 to 6 months. This time period for tapering medication should be sufficient for return of normal pituitary-adrenal function. ACTH stimulation tests can be used as an adjunct to therapy in determining when to discontinue glucocorticoids. Anytime a dog becomes listless, anorectic, or ill during the tapering process, the glucocorticoid dose may need to be increased, or the results of serum electrolyte monitoring with or without an ACTH stimulation test can be assessed. If the dog has a normal ACTH stimulation test result, steroid medication should no longer be needed.

PROPHYLAXIS AGAINST PAIN. Twenty-four hours prior to surgery, every dog that is to undergo adrenal tumor excision should have a transdermal fentanyl patch placed. We have found this to be an excellent method of treating pain without causing depression. We strongly discourage any therapy that sedates a dog to the point that it remains recumbent for hours; such treatment tremendously increases the risk of thromboembolism.

PROPHYLAXIS AGAINST THROMBOEMBOLISM. Dogs with hyperadrenocorticism that undergo the prolonged anesthesia and recumbency associated with surgery are at increased risk of thromboembolism. We have evaluated four treatment strategies for these dogs. One group received only dexamethasone during and after surgery. The second group received a hydrocortisone infusion during surgery and during the 4- to 6-hour period after surgery, with dexamethasone given that evening and the next day. The third group was treated with dexamethasone and with plasma (a source of antithrombin III) and heparin during surgery (35 U/kg in the plasma infusion) and with 35 U/kg given twice subcutaneously after surgery. The subcutaneous heparin dose is then tapered over a period of 4 days. An infusion of hetastarch is administered intravenously on the fifth postsurgical day (10 to 20 ml/kg over a period of 6 hours). It is thought that the single infusion of hetastarch may reduce the potential for thromboembolism for a period of days (Smiley and Garvey, 1994). The fourth group was given a hydrocortisone infusion during surgery and after surgery in addition to the plasma, heparin, and hetastarch. The highest incidence of thromboembolism has been in the dogs receiving only the hydrocortisone infusion. The lowest incidence of thromboembolism was in the group receiving dexamethasone, plasma, heparin, and hetastarch. This latter regimen is our current recommendation.

RESULTS (PROGNOSIS). Of the 223 dogs that we have diagnosed with functioning adrenocortical tumors, 208 had a unilateral tumor, and 144 of those underwent surgery. Nine dogs were euthanized at surgery after an inoperable mass was identified. Twenty-nine dogs died during surgery or soon after as a result of direct complications from the surgery (hemorrhage) or of postoperative sepsis or thromboembolism. Of the 106 dogs that underwent successful surgery, 61 had carcinomas.

Dogs that undergo "successful" surgery have an excellent prognosis if metastasis has not occurred and if they survive the 1- to 4-week postsurgical period. Medical therapy was used in some of the dogs that had surgery (due to recurrence), as well as those not undergoing surgery. The average life expectancy of the dogs treated surgically is approximately 36 months. It must be remembered that the average age at the time of surgery was 11.1 years, therefore life expectancies much longer than this are not realistic. Most dogs that recover from surgery and survive the first 4 weeks after surgery die of problems unrelated to Cushing's syndrome and unrelated to having had an adrenocortical carcinoma. Dogs with adenomas have a better prognosis. Although dogs with adenoma do live longer as a group, the histology of some tumors has been misdiagnosed (adenomas ultimately diagnosed as carcinomas). As previously discussed, endocrine tumors are notorious for being difficult to correctly identify and classify. Because of this, rigid statements to owners about metastatic potential and life expectancy are unwise.

INOPERABLE MASS, POOR ANESTHETIC RISK, OR OBVIOUS METASTASIS. Surgery is not recommended for some dogs with Cushing's syndrome that have adrenocortical tumors. The reasons for avoiding surgery include finding a large, obviously inoperable mass on radiography, ultrasonography, or CT scan; finding metastatic lesions in the lungs, liver, or other tissue; a dog so debilitated that surgery would likely be terminal; and an owner who refuses surgery. In these dogs, medical therapy should be considered (see page 333).

INTRAPERITONEAL OR RETROPERITONEAL HEMORRHAGE. The causes of intraperitoneal or retroperitoneal hemorrhage are diverse but can be broadly classified into traumatic conditions and naturally occurring diseases. The most common causes of nontraumatic retroperitoneal hemorrhage are coagulopathies, rupture of vascular anomalies, migration of foreign bodies, or rupture of a renal neoplasia. We recently reported four dogs with intraabdominal or retroperitoneal hemorrhage secondary to nontraumatic rupture of an adrenal neoplasia. In an earlier report, one dog was examined after a 3-day history of trembling and a "hunched back," abdominal pain, and decreased mentation after hemorrhage of an adrenocortical tumor (Vandenbergh et al, 1992). Each of our four dogs had severe lethargy, weakness, pale mucous membranes, and abdominal pain. Each also had evidence of an abdominal mass or hemorrhage in the abdomen or retroperitoneal space on physical examination, radiographs, or ultrasonography (Whittemore et al, 2001). These five dogs represent abdominal emergencies that required surgery due to progressive deterioration in the clinical condition despite administration of intravenous fluids and additional supportive care.

Pituitary-Dependent Hyperadrenocorticism

HYPOPHYSECTOMY
Background. Ideally, the treatment of canine PDH should be directed at eliminating the cause for the condition (i.e., removal or destruction of the ACTH-secreting pituitary tumor). These tumors are primary in origin and not the result of a hypothalamic disorder (van Wijk et al, 1992). In humans, selective microsurgical removal via the transsphenoidal approach is considered the treatment of choice for pituitary tumors in the sella turcica causing Cushing's disease (Mampalam et al, 1988; Melby, 1988; Thorner et al, 1992). The pitfalls and complications of this procedure have been described in detail (Landolt, 1990).

Surgery to remove the pituitary gland, and thus the source of ACTH in PDH has been successfully performed in the dog (Lantz et al, 1988; Niebauer and Evans, 1988; Niebauer et al, 1990) and should be performed only by individuals with considerable experience. CT and MRI scans allow accurate preoperative localization and assessment of pituitary size. The surgical technique of transsphenoidal hypophysectomy in normal dogs has been refined with new developments in neurosurgical instrumentation (Meij et al, 1997b), and the complications have been described (Schwartz, 1996). In a prospective study, 52 dogs with PDH had this surgery, with the results (survival, disease-free interval, remission, and recurrence) and complications assessed. Also, the results in the first 26 dogs were compared to the results in the second group of 26 dogs (Meij et al, 1998).

Results (Meij et al, 1997a, 1997b, and 1998). Preoperative CT enabled assessment of pituitary size (24 nonenlarged and 28 enlarged) and localization relative to intraoperative anatomic landmarks. Preoperative pituitary localization with CT was considered essential, regardless of skull type. The surgical approach was hindered by the palatine bone but still possible in brachycephalic dogs with extreme rostral pituitary localization. Treatment failures included procedure-related mortalities (five dogs) and incomplete hypophysectomies (four dogs). The 1-year estimated survival rate was 84%, and the 2-year rate was 80%. In 43 of the 52 dogs, Cushing's syndrome went into remission. Recurrence was documented in five dogs.

The most serious complications of pituitary surgery were transient, mild postoperative hypernatremia (due to transient iatrogenic diabetes insipidus); transient reduction or cessation of tear production (25 eyes in 18 dogs); permanent (five dogs) or prolonged (nine dogs) diabetes insipidus; and secondary hypothyroidism. Normal tear production had resumed in all but one dog after a median period of 10 weeks. In the second series of dogs (numbers 27 through 52), the hospitalization period was shorter, the number of dry eyes fewer, the survival fraction greater, and the postoperative mortality lower than in the first 26 dogs. In comparing presurgical values with those 8 weeks after surgery, the basal plasma ACTH, cortisol, GH, LH, TSH, and prolactin concentrations had significantly decreased. However, return of normal function in the pituitary-adrenocortical axis was documented in this time period. Postoperative CT scan results did not correlate well with remission or subsequent recurrence of Cushing's syndrome.

The number of PDH dogs that have been treated surgically with hypophysectomy was increased to 84 dogs in a subsequent report. The overall response rate was 86%. These results not only compare favorably with medical treatment, but also include procedures performed before the surgeons had developed significant experience (Meij et al, 2002) where there was a greater incidence of mortality and incomplete resections (Meij et al, 2002).

Conclusions. Neurosurgeons who perform hypophysectomy must accept that a learning curve will be required to become confident and competent in this procedure. They must become familiar with the most frequent complications of the surgery and must be able to recognize them as early as possible so as to treat them immediately and effectively. Urine cortisol:creatinine ratios were sensitive for assessing remission and recurrence of Cushing's syndrome. Microsurgical transsphenoidal hypophysectomy for the treatment of dogs with PDH is an effective method of treatment. In our opinion, this procedure is the *treatment of choice* for dogs with PDH. The only explanation for not using this form of therapy as a "routine" procedure is the lack of experienced neurosurgeons willing to develop this expertise.

ADRENALECTOMY. PDH results in bilateral adrenocortical hyperplasia. Removal of both adrenals results in complete resolution of signs attributed to Cushing's syndrome. This surgery involves the risk of putting an ill animal, with a compromised immune system and poor wound healing, through a difficult surgical procedure. As with hypophysectomy, experience minimizes these risks. However, these dogs must be treated for hypoadrenocorticism (see Chapter 8) for the rest of their lives, and they always have the potential for developing a hypoadrenal crisis. Because "medical adrenalectomy" is relatively easy to accomplish in dogs using o,p'-DDD, the risk of surgery seems unwarranted.

TREATMENT—MEDICAL MANAGEMENT OF CUSHING'S SYNDROME USING o,p'-DDD

Pituitary-Dependent Hyperadrenocorticism

INITIAL CHEMOTHERAPY USING O,P'-DDD

Background. Since the treatment protocol first suggested by Schechter and colleagues in 1973, chemotherapy with o,p'-DDD has become the most common means of managing dogs with naturally occurring Cushing's syndrome. The systemic effects of o,p'-DDD (mitotane [Lysodren]), a chemical derived from the insecticide DDT, were first reported in 1949 by Nelson and Woodard. The agent was administered to dogs and found to be a potent adrenocorticolytic drug, causing severe progressive necrosis of the zona fasciculata and zona reticularis. A subsequent study by Kirk and Jensen in 1975 also demonstrated partial or complete necrosis of the zona glomerulosa. The only other pathologic processes included moderate to severe hepatic fatty degeneration, centrilobular atrophy,

and congestion. No other pathology in the liver or any other organ was considered significant.

It is interesting to note that normal dogs given o,p'-DDD appear relatively resistant to the adrenocorticolytic effects of the drug. In the 1940s study, four dogs received 50 mg/kg 5 days per week. Two of the four died after 20 and 21 *months* of therapy, respectively. The third dog was euthanized after 21 months of therapy, and the fourth dog was alive after 38 months of receiving the drug. In the 1975 study, 10 dogs were treated at a dosage of 50 mg/kg/day. One dog died after 124 consecutive days of treatment, and a second died after 147 days. The remaining eight dogs were clinically healthy at the time of euthanasia, after 36 to 150 consecutive days of drug therapy. These dogs, however, had biochemical evidence of decreased adrenocortical reserve and adrenocortical destruction after only 3 to 10 days of therapy despite appearing healthy clinically.

The implication from the research on o,p'-DDD is clear: the normal canine adrenal cortex is quickly damaged, but normal dogs survive long periods with minimal adrenocortical support. Dogs with adrenal hyperplasia appear to be more sensitive to the destructive effects of o,p'-DDD because they usually respond after 5 to 9 days of o,p'-DDD therapy and often become ill (hypoadrenal) if medication is not discontinued after the first hint of response. Any dog diagnosed as having PDH that requires more than 21 consecutive days of o,p'-DDD therapy must be carefully reevaluated. Possible explanations for "resistance" are (1) the dog is not receiving the drug; (2) the dog has an adrenocortical tumor; (3) the drug is not being absorbed from the intestinal tract; (4) the dog is receiving other medication that may interfere with the actions of o,p'-DDD (e.g., phenobarbital); (5) the diagnosis is incorrect; and, least likely, (6) the dog may have a resistant form of PDH (see Failure to Respond to o,p'-DDD, page 340).

Pretreatment Assessments: Appetite. There are several clinical signs that owners and veterinarians must appreciate and understand prior to initiation of o,p'-DDD therapy. These include the dog's attitude, activity, daily water intake, and appetite. Awareness of these factors aids in assessment of treatment success or failure and in recognition of adverse reactions or the development of new problems, such as those associated with a growing pituitary tumor. Veterinarians should remember that *NO dog with a poor appetite or with anorexia, vomiting, or diarrhea should EVER receive o,p'-DDD.*

Without doubt, the most important and reliable monitoring tool used in the initial (loading dose) phase of o,p'-DDD therapy is a dog's appetite. Dogs with PDH that are treated with o,p'-DDD, without exception, must be treated by owners at home. These dogs should *never* be treated in-hospital. Decreases in appetite will be noted by an owner prior to the occurrence of any other o,p'-DDD effect. Most important, dogs are more likely to eat normally in their home environment, owners know their pet best, and owners will detect changes in their pet sooner than a veterinary professional. As will be discussed, the most sensitive criterion for determining when to stop the "loading dose" phase of therapy is reduction in appetite. For approximately 80% to 85% of dogs with PDH, this "loading dose" phase lasts 5 to 9 days. A small percentage of dogs (~10%) respond to the drug in 3 to 5 days. Fewer than 10% of dogs with PDH require more than 9 consecutive days of o,p'-DDD therapy.

We instruct owners to feed their pet one third of its normal daily food intake twice daily (they should receive two thirds of their normal daily intake each day during this loading dose phase of therapy; Table 6-15). These dogs are usually ravenously hungry, and reducing their daily food allotment enhances appetite. The owner can then observe the dog for *any* reduction in appetite (usually just a pause when eating is reason to stop this induction phase). The goal of therapy is to discontinue o,p'-DDD administration long before the pet becomes anorectic. In addition to providing the most important monitoring tool, administration of o,p'-DDD to dogs twice daily, with or immediately after each meal, enhances drug absorption (Watson et al, 1987).

It would be *extremely unusual* (in our opinion, incorrect) to treat a dog with o,p'-DDD for Cushing's syndrome that did not have an excellent to ravenous appetite. Anorexia or poor appetite should cause the veterinarian to question the diagnosis. One must search for concurrent problems to explain any appetite described as less than "excellent." If the diagnosis of PDH is correct and no concurrent problem can be identified, the most common cause of poor appetite or anorexia would be a large pituitary tumor (macrotumor syndrome).

Water Intake. After in-hospital diagnostic studies have been completed, polydipsic dogs with hyperadrenocorticism can be returned to their owners for monitoring of water intake. If an owner has more than one pet, the water intake of the pets at home can be determined while the dog suspected of having Cushing's syndrome is being evaluated in the hospital. In this manner, the dog with Cushing's syndrome can be returned to its normal environment for water intake monitoring, and the owner will know the approximate amount of water to subtract from the total to determine the affected dog's water intake. Water intake is determined for several (two to four) 24-hour periods to eliminate errors in measurement and to achieve a reliable average figure from which therapy can begin.

Given proper instructions, owners usually provide reliable information. Any measuring device can be

TABLE 6–15   CLIENT INFORMATION

o,p'-DDD Treatment of Pituitary Cushing's

Hyperadrenocorticism (Cushing's syndrome) refers to a clinical condition that results from having excess cortisone in the system. A minority of dogs with this disease have a tumor in one of the two glands that produce cortisone (the adrenal glands). Your dog, like more than 80% of dogs with the naturally acquired form of this disease, has a small tumor at the base of the brain in an area called the pituitary gland. The pituitary gland controls adrenal function. A tumor in the pituitary can cause excess cortisone throughout the body and results in symptoms recognized by owners ("pituitary-dependent" Cushing's). The most common symptoms of Cushing's syndrome in dogs include excess urination and water consumption, a voracious appetite, hair loss, muscle weakness, a "pot-bellied" appearance, panting, thin skin, and lethargy. Virtually all dogs with Cushing's syndrome have at least one or two of these signs, but it would be uncommon for a dog to have all these symptoms. By evaluating a variety of test results, your veterinarian has diagnosed your dog as having pituitary-dependent Cushing's. Now, treatment with o,p'-DDD has been recommended.

During World War II, scientists did research on the insecticide DDT in an attempt to create an extremely toxic agent. One of the forms of DDT created was o,p'-DDD (Lysodren; Mitotane), a chemical which can destroy the cortisone producing cells of adrenal glands in dogs. The drug has been used successfully in thousands of dogs with Cushing's, but you must remember that it is a "poison" and that it must be respected and used appropriately. The protocol we use in treating dogs with this drug is straight-forward. A day or 2 before starting treatment, begin feeding your dog 1/3 of its normal food allotment twice daily (each 24 hours it should receive a total that equals 2/3 of the normal amount). This should make your dog even more hungry, but this is just for a brief time (we do not recommend use of this drug in dogs with a poor appetite). After 1 or 2 days of reduced feeding, begin giving the o,p'-DDD at a dose of 25 mg/kg of body weight twice daily (a dog weighing 22 pounds would receive 1/2 tablet twice daily; the tablets contain 500 mg). The drug should be given immediately after the dog eats. So, feed your dog, note how long it takes to finish the meal, and then give the medication (the drug is absorbed best from a stomach containing food).

The key to treating these dogs is watching them eat and knowing when to stop giving the o,p'-DDD. As long as their appetite is ravenous, give the medication. As soon as you see any reduction in appetite, STOP giving the drug. Reduction in appetite may be noted as taking longer to finish the meal, the dog may eat 1/2 of the food and wander away for a drink and then finish, the dog may simply look up at you (the owner) once or twice before finishing. In other words, we do not want your dog to stop eating entirely, we wish to see a "reduction" in appetite as a signal to stop the medication. Other signals to stop giving the medication include reduced water intake, vomiting, diarrhea, and listlessness. But, appetite reduction usually precedes there more worrisome symptoms. Most dogs respond to this drug in 5 to 9 days, a few in as little as 1 to 3 days and some may take longer than 14 days.

No dog should receive more than 8 days of o,p'-DDD without being tested on the effect of the drug. The test is done by your veterinarian and will take 1 to 2 hours. We typically start the treatment on a Sunday, plan the recheck test 8 days later (Monday) and more than 85% of owners have stopped medication on the Thursday, Friday, Saturday or Sunday before the test is performed on Monday. Once the o,p'-DDD has been demonstrated to have had effect, your dog no longer will require food restriction. Your dog will continue to receive o,p'-DDD the rest of its life. The initial maintenance dose is usually approximately 50 mg/kg per week (a 22 pound dog would receive 1/4 tablet, 4 times each week). That dose will likely be increased or decreased based on testing performed 1 month after maintenance treatment has been started and on testing performed every 2 to 4 months, thereafter. The average dog (11.5 years old when the syndrome is diagnosed) treated in this manner lives about 30 months (some live a few weeks and some for 6-10 years). The dogs with the longest survival have owners who are committed to helping their pet, diligent veterinarians, and luck. Close observation and frequent veterinary rechecks can only help in the long-term management of these dogs.

used, but we recommend a cup measuring in ounces because this is a common kitchen tool that provides quantities of fluid easily handled (1 cup = 240 ml; 1 ounce = 30 ml; normal water intake = <30 ml/lb/day or <66 ml/kg/day). Although the literature suggests that normal daily water intake in dogs can be as high as 100 ml/kg, in our experience this number is excessive. Approximately 20% of dogs with PDH are not polydipsic. Like the polydipsic dogs, they can and should be treated by their owners at home. Absence of polydipsia simply eliminates one of the parameters that can be monitored during the initial phases of therapy, but observation of food intake can continue. Before beginning therapy, the clinician may wish to obtain blood for BUN, sodium, and potassium determinations. These parameters may be monitored during therapy.

INITIATING THERAPY WITH o,p'-DDD: THE LOADING DOSE PHASE (FIG. 6-61). Therapy is begun *at home* with the owner administering o,p'-DDD (Lysodren, Bristol-Myers Oncology Division, Syracuse, N.Y.) at a dosage of 50 mg/kg/day, *divided and given twice daily.* Glucocorticoids are not advised, but some veterinarians choose to have the owner supplied with prednisolone or prednisone tablets for an emergency (we do not supply our owners with glucocorticoid medication). The owner should receive thorough instructions on the actions of o,p'-DDD and should also have specific instructions on when the drug should be discontinued (see Table 6-14). Lysodren administration should be stopped when (1) the dog demonstrates *any* reduction in appetite; this might mean just pausing slightly during meal consumption, stopping to drink some water, or stopping in response to the owner's voice; (2) the polydipsic dog consumes less than 66 ml/kg/day of water; (3) the dog vomits; (4) the dog has diarrhea; or (5) the dog is unusually listless. The first two indications for stopping the medication are strongly emphasized because they are common and they almost always precede worrisome overdose. Observation of any of these signs strongly indicates that the endpoint in therapy has been achieved.

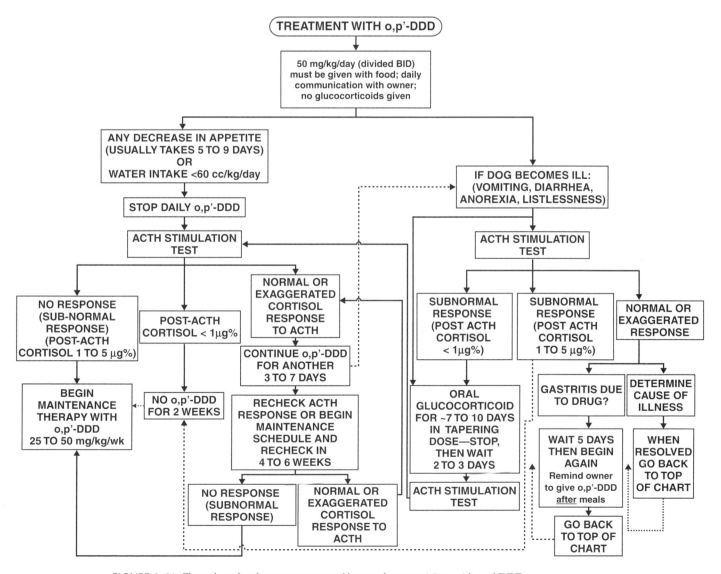

FIGURE 6–61. Flow chart for the management of hyperadrenocorticism with o,p'-DDD.

Because of the potency of o,p'-DDD, the veterinarian is encouraged *not* to rely on the instructions given to an owner. An owner should *never* be provided with more than 7 or 8 days of o,p'-DDD initially. This drug is highly successful in eliminating the signs of hyperadrenocorticism because of its potency coupled with *close communication between owner and veterinarian.* Either the veterinarian or a technician should contact the owner for a verbal report on the dog every day beginning with the second day of therapy. In this way, the owner is impressed with the veterinarian's concern and the need to observe the pet closely. It is wise for the owner to feed the dog two small meals each day, as previously described (each meal equal to one third of the dog's normal daily intake). The dog's appetite should be observed prior to giving each dose of Lysodren. If food is rapidly consumed (with or without polydipsia), medication is warranted. If food is consumed (1) slower than usual; (2) with an atypical pause; or (3) not at all, the medication should be discontinued until consultation with the veterinarian. Usually the initial loading dose phase is complete when a reduction in appetite is noted or after water intake approaches or falls below 66 ml/kg/day.

Water intake in polydipsic dogs may decrease to the normal range in as few as 2 days, or this may take as long as 30 to 45 days (average is 9 to 14 days). Owners must continue to monitor the water intake daily until it falls to or below 66 ml/kg/day. The water intake usually diminishes within a week or two of beginning o,p'-DDD treatment, but it does not usually become normal until *after* some reduction in appetite is observed. We place much greater reliance on owner observation of food intake and, in most cases, do not have owners measure the volume of water consumed.

Within 1 to 4 days of beginning treatment, a small percentage of dogs demonstrate mild gastric irritation or systemic signs of illness from the o,p'-DDD. These signs include anorexia, vomiting, diarrhea, weakness, and lethargy. If any of these signs are observed, the medication should be discontinued until the veterinarian can evaluate the dog. The most common explanations for these signs after only several days of treatment would be completed response to therapy or an owner who is giving o,p'-DDD to a dog with an empty stomach. Veterinarians should double-check when the medication is being given, and the owners should be reminded to administer the o,p'-DDD *after* the dog eats. Some owners withhold a small amount of food, wait until the meal is finished and, if the dog eats ravenously, place o,p'-DDD in the remaining food and give it to the dog. If signs of vomiting or inappetence are the result of drug sensitivity and not because the treatment is complete, dividing the dose further may be helpful; discontinuation of the medication for a few days may be necessary. It is recommended that o,p'-DDD treatment be initiated on a Sunday so that if illness develops after just a few days, the veterinarian would be available during the regular workweek.

VETERINARY MONITORING. In addition to making daily phone calls, the veterinarian should see the dog 8 to 9 days after the start of therapy, sooner if the dog shows a reduction in appetite before this length of time has passed. This recheck should include a thorough history and physical examination and an ACTH response test. Evaluation of the urine cortisol:creatinine ratio is not as reliable a monitoring tool (Reusch et al, 1995; Angles et al, 1997; Guptill et al, 1997; Randolph et al, 1998). Evaluation of the BUN, serum sodium, and serum potassium concentrations may also be warranted, although these test results are rarely abnormal, and we do not routinely request them. If the dog has responded clinically to the medication (or if the owner is not certain about response), therapy should be withheld until the ACTH response test results can be evaluated. If the dog has not responded clinically, an ACTH response test should be performed, but the dog can also remain on daily therapy (see Fig. 6-61).

GOAL OF THERAPY. The goal of therapy with o,p'-DDD is to have a dog become clinically normal. This goal can typically be achieved when the post-ACTH plasma cortisol concentration is less than the reference limit for the laboratory. In our laboratory, successful response to o,p'-DDD is indicated by a pre-ACTH plasma cortisol concentration less than 5 µg/dl and a post-ACTH plasma cortisol concentration equal to or greater than 1 µg/dl but less than 5 µg/dl (Fig. 6-62, *A* to *D*). Whenever the appetite declines or the water intake decreases to below 66 ml/kg/day, the ACTH response test results typically correspond and are dramatically decreased.

A dog that has a normal or exaggerated response to ACTH prior to therapy and a response to ACTH within reference limits (i.e., post-ACTH cortisol concentration of 6 to 15 µg/dl) (Fig. 6-62, *E* to *H*) after the initial phase of therapy is likely to demonstrate some clinical improvement but not become completely normal to an owner (i.e., it may continue to have some clinical evidence of Cushing's syndrome). This is due to the continuing presence of an abnormal pituitary-adrenal axis (see Fig. 6-7). Mitotane therapy has no effect on the ACTH-secreting pituitary tumor. Mild to severe excesses in ACTH secretion continue (Nelson et al, 1985), causing excess cortisol secretion for most of each 24-hour period. The goal of maintenance therapy in these dogs is to decrease and then maintain plasma cortisol concentrations (post–exogenous ACTH administration) at a level equal to or greater than 1 µg/dl and less than 5 µg/dl.

DETERMINING WHETHER TO CONTINUE O,P'-DDD AT THE "LOADING DOSE." If a dog with CCS has a normal or exaggerated response to ACTH after the initial 8 to 9 days of o,p'-DDD therapy, medication should be continued. Usually it is continued for 3 to 7 additional consecutive days, the shorter period being used for dogs that have shown significant (albeit inadequate) response. Repeat ACTH response tests are done every 7 to 10 days until an appropriate post-ACTH plasma cortisol response is achieved. Numerous repeat ACTH response tests are virtually never necessary, because most dogs (~95%) respond during the initial 5 to 9 days and almost all respond by day 14 of therapy.

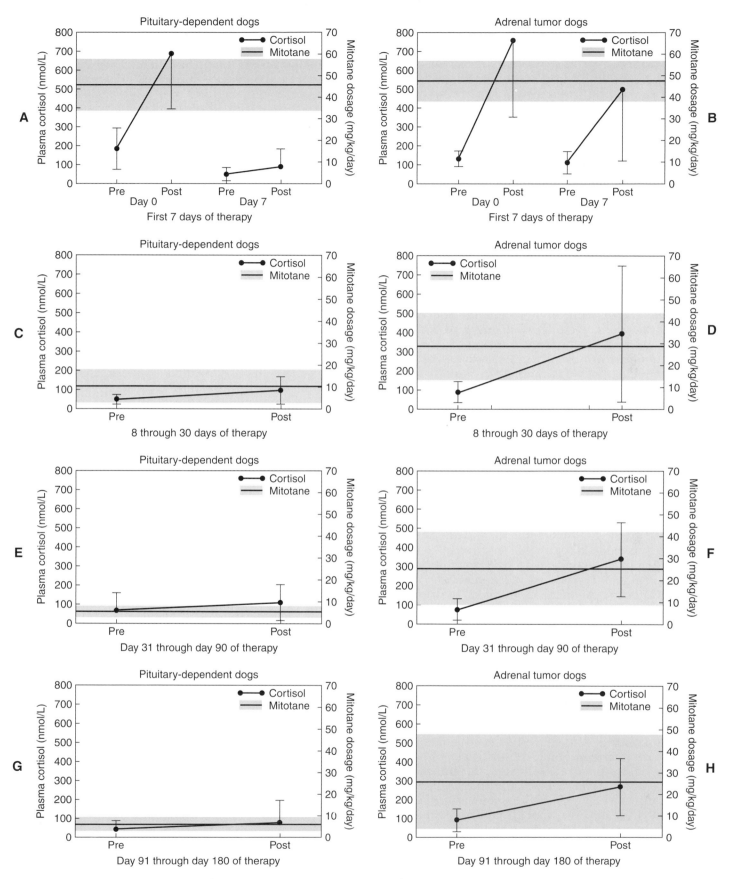

FIGURE 6–62. ACTH response test results and mean o,p'-DDD doses from a group of 12 dogs with pituitary-dependent hyperadrenocorticism *(A)* before and after 7 days of o,p'-DDD treatment and after *(B)* 30, *(C)* 90, and *(D)* 180 days of treatment. Compare with the results of the same tests from a group of 12 dogs with hyperadrenocorticism due to adrenocortical tumors that were matched for age, body weight, and dose *(E through H)*. The results show that dogs with PDH are more sensitive to o,p'-DDD than are dogs with adrenocortical tumors.

AVERAGE DURATION OF DAILY "LOADING DOSE" o,p'-DDD THERAPY. Most dogs with PDH respond to o,p'-DDD within 5 to 9 days. Less than 3% of dogs respond as quickly as 2 or 3 days, and less than 3% require more than 21 consecutive days of therapy. The average time for response is 6.4 days. More than 80% of our dogs respond within 5 to 9 days and more than 90% respond within 2 to 10 days. It is important to emphasize that each dog must be treated as an individual. There appears to be no reliable method of predicting the length of time a dog needs to respond or the amount of o,p'-DDD necessary to destroy enough of the adrenal cortices for response to be seen.

CONCOMITANT GLUCOCORTICOIDS DURING THE "LOADING DOSE" PHASE. The veterinary literature includes two distinct protocols for the induction or "loading dose" phase of o,p'-DDD therapy: no concurrent glucocorticoids versus concurrent administration of both glucocorticoids *and* o,p'-DDD. Both protocols have advantages and disadvantages.

No Administration of Glucocorticoids. We recommend against administration of glucocorticoids. Arguments for not giving these drugs include the following: (1) close communication between veterinarian and client, plus an understanding of when to discontinue medication, has been quite successful clinically; (2) if a dog receives glucocorticoids, it may not be possible for an owner or veterinarian to know if or when an adequate amount of, or too much, o,p'-DDD has been given; (3) because the endpoint of the induction phase cannot be seen clinically, the veterinarian must rely on the ACTH stimulation test—however, for the ACTH test, all glucocorticoid therapy must be withdrawn for 1 or 2 days to avoid having the cortisol assay detect the oral drug rather than the dog's endogenous glucocorticoid concentrations; (4) if glucocorticoids are needed because of o,p'-DDD overdose, a crisis may develop after their withdrawal; (5) simultaneous administration of glucocorticoids did not eliminate clinical signs of cortisol deficiency in many dogs treated with both drugs (Kintzer and Peterson, 1991); and (6) it is easier to determine a need for glucocorticoid therapy.

The incidence of o,p'-DDD overdose with clinical signs is actually less in dogs that do not receive simultaneous glucocorticoids than in dogs that do receive the drug. We believe this is true because the owners can appreciate mild clinical changes early in therapy and stop the medication before overdose occurs. Veterinarians must not underestimate the importance of home therapy by owners who know their pet well and who should have an appreciation for the potential toxicity of a drug derived from the insecticide DDT. Transient need for glucocorticoids has occurred in only about 7% of our dogs (versus 35% in glucocorticoid-treated dogs) (Kintzer and Peterson, 1991) and permanent Addison's disease has occurred in fewer than 2% of our dogs (versus 5.5% of glucocorticoid-treated dogs). If signs of cortisol deficiency develop, the veterinarian can be certain that the endpoint in therapy has been achieved. An ACTH response test may be performed immediately, and the dog then placed on glucocorticoids. However, response to glucocorticoid medication would also be diagnostic of surpassing the desired endpoint of therapy.

Administration of Glucocorticoids. The advantages of glucocorticoid use are (1) the use of both glucocorticoids (usually at a dosage of 0.5 mg/kg divided bid) and o,p'-DDD has been quite successful; (2) dogs may develop one or more adverse side effects to o,p'-DDD, and administration of glucocorticoids minimizes or eliminates these signs; (3) resolution of clinical signs has been obvious to owners despite glucocorticoid therapy; and (4) oral glucocorticoids do not interfere with assays if the medication is discontinued the day of testing (Kintzer and Peterson, 1991).

NEED FOR GLUCOCORTICOIDS. If signs of anorexia, vomiting, diarrhea, weakness, or listlessness develop, glucocorticoid therapy is warranted. If a dog has received no glucocorticoids during the initial phase of o,p'-DDD therapy, glucocorticoids should be started. If a dog has been treated with glucocorticoids, the dose may need to be increased, although a search for other causes of vomiting may be indicated. This is true during the maintenance phase of therapy or if a dog in which the disorder is well-controlled undergoes any major stress (e.g., illness, trauma, or elective surgery). Prednisone is administered at a dosage of 0.1 to 0.5 mg/kg twice daily for 2 days. If signs have developed as a result of o,p'-DDD overdose, the dog usually shows clinical improvement within hours of initiation of prednisone therapy. If oral therapy is not possible because of vomiting, parenteral fluids and glucocorticoids are warranted. After 2 days of glucocorticoid therapy at the recommended high dose, the dosage should be lowered by 50% for 2 days (still given bid), then to once daily for 3 days, every other day for 7 to 10 days, and then stopped. Recurrence of signs demands reinstitution of therapy or an increase in the dosage.

PLANNED INDUCTION OF PERMANENT HYPOADRENOCORTICISM: PLANNED MEDICAL ADRENALECTOMY. Favorable long-term results have sometimes been associated with accidental induction of permanent hypoadrenocorticism (assuming that the dog does not become extremely ill). Such a response prompted some veterinarians to suggest that all dogs with hyperadrenocorticism undergo treatment aimed at complete destruction of the adrenal cortices. Substitution therapy for the ensuing adrenocortical insufficiency would continue for the life of the dog. The treatment protocol involves 25 to 35 consecutive days of o,p'-DDD administration at a dosage of 50 to 75 mg/kg daily and as much as 100 mg/kg daily for toy breeds. The o,p'-DDD dosage is divided into three or four administrations per day, with food, to "minimize neurologic complications and ensure good intestinal absorption." Lifelong oral administration of cortisone (2 mg/kg bid), mineralocorticoid (fludrocortisone, 0.0125 mg/kg), and sodium chloride (0.1 g/kg) is begun on the third day of o,p'-DDD administration. The prednisone dosage should be tapered after the daily administration schedule has been completed (Rijnberk and Belshaw, 1988).

This protocol has several disadvantages (Den Hertog et al, 1999). First, adverse effects that resulted in temporary or permanent cessation of mitotane treatment or death occurred in 40% of dogs. Adverse effects in all dogs so treated in one report included anorexia (28%), vomiting (27%), weakness (19%), depression (11%), and diarrhea (4%). Fifteen of 129 dogs died during treatment (seven from hypoadrenocorticism). Approximately 40% of dogs so treated relapse with Cushing's syndrome within the first 12 to 18 months (Den Hertog et al, 1999), which suggests that periodic ACTH stimulation testing is still necessary, just as with the traditional modes of treatment. This treatment protocol is considerably more expensive than the conventional method of treatment because fludrocortisone and DOCP are costly. Finally, a dog with well-controlled Cushing's syndrome that receives o,p'-DDD several times a week or month is not in danger if the medication is not given; however, it is crucial to treat a dog with hypoadrenocorticism. We do not recommend use of this protocol.

NEED FOR BOTH GLUCOCORTICOIDS AND MINERALOCORTICOIDS. o,p'-DDD administration is reported to spare the zona glomerulosa, therefore mineralocorticoid secretion is maintained despite successful destruction of the zona fasciculata and zona reticularis. Dogs that develop signs of weakness, anorexia, and/or vomiting without electrolyte imbalances require immediate glucocorticoid therapy. Electrolyte disturbances suggestive of a deficiency in mineralocorticoids (increased serum potassium and/or decreased serum sodium concentrations) have resulted from o,p'-DDD administration; these dogs require both glucocorticoid and mineralocorticoid therapy (see Chapter 8). Severe, inadvertent overdose of this magnitude is rare (it is seen in fewer than 2% of our owner-monitored dogs). Glucocorticoid deficiency is usually transient in dogs treated with o,p'-DDD. Addison's disease (a deficiency of both glucocorticoids and mineralocorticoids) in dogs treated with o,p'-DDD is often permanent.

TIME SEQUENCE FOR IMPROVEMENT IN SIGNS AND BIOCHEMICAL ABNORMALITIES. Dogs with PDH that are treated with o,p'-DDD usually respond quickly. The first and most obvious response is reduction in appetite, usually noted within the first 5 to 9 days of therapy. Owners often comment that they see an increase in activity during the first or second week of treatment, and this is usually when reductions in water intake and urine output are observed. Other signs take longer to dissipate. Muscle strength improves within days to weeks, as does reduction in the potbellied appearance. Alopecia, thin skin, acne, calcinosis cutis, and panting often take weeks to months for significant improvement to be noted. Dogs with hair coat abnormalities may go through a phase of severe seborrhea associated with a terrible hair coat or worsening alopecia and pruritus, which may last 1 or 2 months, before a new, healthy hair coat replaces that lost. Some dogs go through a phase of

"puppy hair coat" before the normal adult coat returns (Fig. 6-63). A few dogs have dramatic changes in coat color after successful therapy (Fig. 6-64). Females may begin an estrous cycle within 1 or 2 months of successfully completing treatment, although virtually 100% of our female dogs were spayed long before they developed CCS.

The external appearance of a dog with Cushing's syndrome improves with therapy before internal changes are noted. Serum liver enzymes and cholesterol may take months to improve. Liver enzyme values may not appear to improve, however, because of the mild but continuing effects of o,p'-DDD on the liver. In humans, o,p'-DDD has been demonstrated to cause increases in the serum cholesterol concentration (Vassilopoulou-Sellin and Samaan, 1991; Maher et al, 1992; Gebhardt et al, 1993). For these reasons, serum liver enzyme activities should not be used as markers of response to therapy. Improvement in blood pressure can be detected within 3 to 6 months. Because hypertension may exist independent of the CCS, it does not dissipate in all treated dogs. Urinary tract infections may resolve quickly or may linger for prolonged periods as a result of pyelonephritis, bladder retention of urine, or calculi. Urine protein loss, as monitored by the urine protein:creatinine ratio, usually improves within 4 to 6 months of initiation of therapy (Ortega et al, 1996).

DEVELOPMENT OR REEMERGENCE OF CONCURRENT PROBLEMS DURING THERAPY. The antiinflammatory and immunosuppressive actions of cortisol often mask concurrent problems in dogs with CCS. Resolution of the CCS (due to o,p'-DDD or other therapy) may allow "masked" problems to recur or become clinically obvious. Perhaps the most common problems masked by hypercortisolism are degenerative arthritis and flea hypersensitivity. Some owners are extremely pleased to see that their pet is no longer polyuric and polydipsic, for example, but are also frustrated by the appearance of lameness, pruritus, or other allergies.

Problematic but uncommon disorders documented soon after correction of the hypercortisolemic state are acute autoimmune-mediated disorders in human beings (Colao et al, 2000) and similar conditions, such as hemolytic anemia and thrombocytopenia, in dogs. These immune-mediated disorders can seem to have been maintained in remission by the CCS, only to be "released" by the treatment. We have also had dogs that acutely developed lymphosarcoma or mast cell neoplasia after treatment for CCS. Recommended therapy for these dogs includes abandoning treatment of Cushing's syndrome and instituting appropriate therapeutic protocols for the new disease. Immune-mediated diseases should be treated with azathioprine, cyclophosphamide and, if needed, prednisone. There is no reason that a dog that had CCS could not be treated with glucocorticoids.

FAILURE TO RESPOND TO o,p'-DDD. It is rare for o,p'-DDD to fail to help resolve PDH. The drug is quite potent, and its ability to destroy the zona fasciculata and zona reticularis is consistent. There are several reasons for apparent treatment failures:

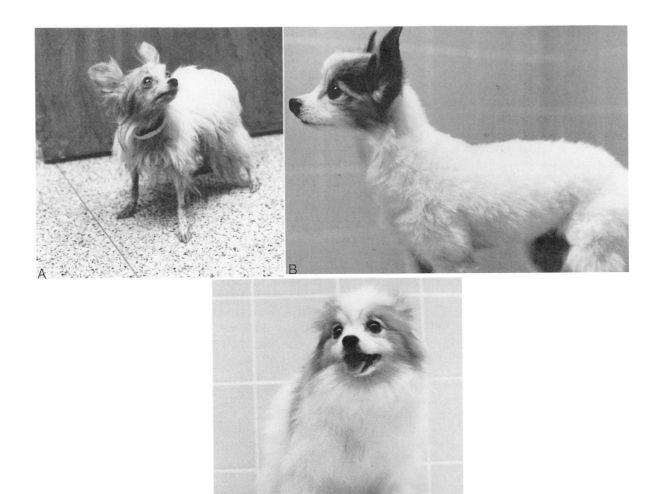

FIGURE 6–63. A Papillon with pituitary-dependent hyperadrenocorticism *(A)* before therapy; *(B)* 6 weeks after initiation of o,p'-DDD therapy, which resulted in the appearance of a new, puppylike hair coat; and *(C)* 10 weeks later, with a good, adult coat.

1. A dog thought to have PDH in fact may have an adrenocortical tumor (adenoma or carcinoma). Adrenocortical tumors are relatively resistant to the cytotoxic effects of o,p'-DDD (see Fig. 6-62).
2. The drug itself may not be potent, and replacing the owner's tablets with o,p'-DDD obtained from a new or different bottle may solve an apparent treatment failure.
3. If the drug is not given with food, absorption may be adversely affected (fatty meals improve absorption, but absorption is enhanced when the drug is given with any food). If the drug is being given with food and response is still lacking, we have owners crush the tablets, suspend the powder in lukewarm (not hot) corn oil, and then mix this suspension in the dogs'

food. Veterinarians are warned that a rapid response to o,p'-DDD may take place if this new protocol is followed.
4. Veterinarians often begin to worry about a treatment failure after 14 days without response, but an extremely small percentage of dogs require as long as 15 to 20 consecutive days of therapy, or they may require 100 to 150 mg/kg/day rather than the usual initial dosage of 50 mg/kg/day.
5. Dogs that are diagnosed incorrectly fail to respond; incorrect diagnoses may be reached in dogs with any illness that may mimic hyperadrenocorticism, including those being given anticonvulsant therapy (see Table 6-11).
6. The dog may have iatrogenic Cushing's syndrome.

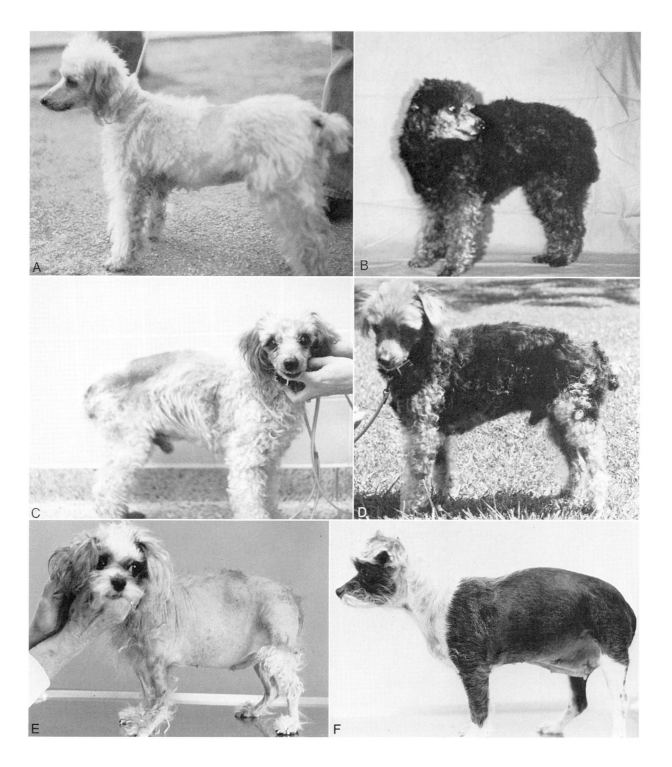

FIGURE 6–64. Photographs of a Poodle with pituitary-dependent hyperadrenocorticism *(A)* before therapy; *(B)* 2 months after completion of o,p'-DDD therapy, showing a dramatic change in the color of the hair coat; *(C)* after a relapse 4 years later; and *(D)* after reinstitution of o,p'-DDD therapy. *E,* A small, mixed-breed dog with PDH before o,p'-DDD therapy and *(F)* 2 months after completing therapy, showing a dramatic change in the hair coat color.

7. Any dog receiving phenobarbital may not respond to o,p'-DDD therapy. Typical response to o,p'-DDD, however, is noted if a dog is switched to an alternative anticonvulsant medication (e.g., potassium bromide).

The various causes of an apparent treatment failure must be considered before o,p'-DDD therapy is abandoned. It must be noted that we have virtually never needed to abandon use of o,p'-DDD. However, if treatment failure has occurred, trilostane or ketoconazole therapy may be tried, or bilateral adrenalectomy can be considered. Other medical therapies (described later in this chapter) can also be considered.

THERAPY OF CONCURRENT DIABETES MELLITUS AND PDH

Background. If a dog is diagnosed as having both diabetes mellitus and hyperadrenocorticism, both disorders must be treated. This combination of conditions is not common; only about 5% of dogs with CCS have concurrent diabetes mellitus. While completing the diagnostic evaluation for hyperadrenocorticism and awaiting test results, the clinician should initiate insulin therapy. Most diabetic dogs with Cushing's syndrome have insulin resistance due to the excesses in serum cortisol, and they therefore require relatively large doses of insulin. Dogs with CCS that require a conservative or low dose of insulin are occasionally seen, and dogs in this group have the best chance for being weaned from insulin after o,p'-DDD therapy. It is not recommended that a veterinarian attempt to achieve "excellent" control of diabetes mellitus in a dog that may have CCS. This suggestion is based on two concepts: (1) control of diabetes in a dog with known systemic insulin antagonism (cortisol) is extremely difficult to achieve and can become quite frustrating and (2) if excellent "glycemic control" were achieved, it should represent a worrisome overdose once the cortisol excess is resolved. For these reasons, a dose of insulin adequate to prevent ketoacidosis is advised (0.5 U/kg of NPH or lente insulin BID is a conservative initial dosage).

o,p'-DDD Dosage. Approximately 5% of dogs with Cushing's syndrome also have diabetes mellitus (i.e., persistent fasting hyperglycemia and glycosuria). We treat these dogs using the same protocol as that for nondiabetic dogs with CCS (administration of o,p'-DDD at 50 mg/kg/day, divided, and no glucocorticoids). However, it should be recognized that Cushing's syndrome results in insulin antagonism. Successful reduction of circulating cortisol concentrations should reduce insulin requirements by diminishing insulin resistance. Failure to plan for this enhanced insulin effectiveness could result in hypoglycemic reactions.

Treatment and Monitoring Protocol. Treatment of a dog with both diabetes mellitus and CCS requires more effort by both owner and veterinarian. These dogs often receive more than 2.0 U/kg/day of insulin. The complicated nature of the treatment of this combination of diseases should be carefully explained to the owner. Both owner and veterinarian must be aware that as a diabetic dog responds to o,p'-DDD and the CCS slowly resolves, insulin resistance should diminish. Both diseases must be monitored. Owners should be asked to obtain a urine sample from their pet at least two or three times daily during the "loading dose" phase of o,p'-DDD therapy. Each sample is checked for glucose. Anytime a urine sample tests negative for glucose, the subsequent insulin dose should be reduced by at least 10% to 20%. The hyperadrenocorticism in most of these dogs is controlled in the expected 5 to 9 days.

The ACTH stimulation test should be rechecked within 7 days of the start of o,p'-DDD therapy to determine if the endpoint has been achieved and to avoid overdose. The recheck protocol for these dogs should proceed as follows: (1) the owner feeds the dog at home; (2) the dog is brought to the veterinary hospital in the morning between 7 and 9 AM; (3) the blood glucose level is measured, and the owner then administers insulin while the veterinarian observes their technique; (4) the blood glucose level is monitored every 1 to 2 hours throughout the day; (5) 1 to 2 hours before the owner is due to pick up the pet in the late afternoon, an ACTH stimulation test is completed. This five-step protocol provides an opportunity to answer two critical questions: what effect has o,p'-DDD therapy had on glycemic control (blood glucose, insulin dosage), and what effect has o,p'-DDD therapy had on the hyperadrenocorticism?

One exception to this protocol deserves mention: if the first (morning) blood glucose concentration is less than 200 mg/dl, insulin should be withheld. Blood glucose concentrations can then be monitored over the course of the day, and a determination can made on whether insulin should be continued and, if so, at what dose. Most dogs with blood glucose concentrations less than 200 mg/dl either no longer require insulin or require a dramatic reduction in dose (we often reduce the dose by 50% from the last dose given).

Prognosis. Approximately 5% of dogs diagnosed with this combination of diseases require no insulin after successful o,p'-DDD therapy. An additional 80% require significantly less insulin, and their diabetes mellitus is easier to control. The insulin dose in the remaining dogs is minimally reduced by control of the PDH, but the insulin is more effective in lowering blood glucose concentrations. If none of these three results is observed, the original diagnosis of hyperadrenocorticism should be questioned.

Functioning Adrenocortical Tumors

BACKGROUND. Ideal treatment for dogs with functioning adrenocortical tumors causing hyperadrenocorticism (ATH) is surgical removal of that tumor. However, some of these dogs have inoperable tumors, some have metastases at the time of diagnosis, some are too debilitated for this type of major surgery, and some have owners who will not allow surgery for a variety of reasons. The adrenocorticolytic drug o,p'-DDD can be used (Rijnberk et al, 1993). We compared o,p'-DDD treatment of dogs with PDH with the same protocol used in dogs with adrenocortical tumors. Given similar doses of o,p'-DDD (50 mg/kg/day initially), dogs in the adrenal tumor group were significantly more resistant to the adrenocorticolytic effects of the drug (see Fig. 6-62) (Feldman et al, 1992). However, some dogs with adrenocortical tumors respond to traditional doses, and those that appear resistant often respond to higher dosages (Kintzer and Peterson, 1994).

PROTOCOL. We recommend the same o,p'-DDD treatment protocol for dogs with ATH tumors as that for dogs with PDH. The initial dose should be 50 mg/kg/day divided and given twice daily. If after the initial 7 to 10 days of treatment the ACTH response test result demonstrates improvement but post-ACTH cortisol concentrations are not in the ideal range (≥1 and <5 µg/dl), the original 50 mg/kg/day schedule should be continued for an additional several to 10 days. If the ACTH stimulation test result is similar to that obtained prior to therapy, an increase to 75 to 100 mg/kg/day of o,p'-DDD may be necessary. An ACTH stimulation test should again be assessed after this second 7 to 10 days. Lack of significant improvement in ACTH response testing after the second 7- to 10-day "loading dose" phase indicates a need to continue the o,p'-DDD at the same or twice the dosage for an additional 7 to 10 days. The duration of the "loading dose" phase and the dosage required are then determined on an individual basis.

RESULTS. With o,p'-DDD therapy, 43% of 32 dogs with adrenocortical tumors had exaggerated ACTH response test results after the first 10 to 14 days. Despite concurrent glucocorticoid therapy, 60% suffered adverse effects sometime during treatment as a result of direct drug toxicity associated with high-dose o,p'-DDD, low cortisol concentrations, or both. In one study, more than 60% of dogs with adrenocortical tumors that were treated with o,p'-DDD were considered to have a good to excellent response (Kintzer and Peterson, 1994). Sixty-three percent of the dogs suffered relapses, adverse effects were noted in 60% of the 32 dogs, and the mean survival period on therapy was only 16 months.

o,p'-DDD RESISTANCE AND HISTOLOGIC EVALUATION. Clinical response to therapy leaves little doubt that adrenocortical tumors are relatively resistant to the cytotoxic effects of o,p'-DDD compared with the response noted in dogs with adrenocortical hyperplasia due to PDH. This concept is supported by a review of histologic findings from these two groups of dogs. The adrenal cortices, specifically the zona fasciculata, of dogs with PDH evaluated soon after initiation of o,p'-DDD treatment typically exhibit acute collapse, necrosis, and hemorrhage. Fibrosis, atrophy, and degeneration of the adrenal cortices are seen in dogs given the drug chronically. In the latter group,

hyperplastic nodules occasionally are noted. In many, adrenocortical destruction is noted and hyperplasia is presumed to *have been* present.

In contrast, reports on dogs with adrenocortical tumors that were similarly treated with o,p'-DDD usually contain a clear description of tumor histology. The pathologist usually provides an impression with respect to the malignant potential of the tumor (adenoma or carcinoma) (Feldman et al, 1992; Kintzer and Peterson, 1994). Many of these evaluations contain no mention of destruction or necrosis. These observations lend support to the concept that adrenocortical tumors are more resistant to the cytotoxic effects of the drug.

Maintenance Therapy with o,p'-DDD

BACKGROUND. Once the initial daily "loading dose" phase of o,p'-DDD therapy has completed adequate destruction of the adrenal cortex, as determined by clinical signs (reduced appetite and water intake) and ACTH stimulation test results, maintenance therapy should begin. In dogs with PDH, o,p'-DDD does not affect the pituitary tumor, therefore excessive ACTH secretion continues or becomes exaggerated (Nelson et al, 1985). Failure to continue o,p'-DDD therapy usually results in regrowth of the adrenal cortices and return of clinical signs. This exacerbation of the disease may occur within weeks but typically takes place over a period of 2 to 24 months after cessation of therapy.

PROTOCOL

Routine Long-Term Care. Maintenance therapy involves choosing a regimen and altering that regimen as required by the patient. Dogs that respond to daily o,p'-DDD therapy and that have a post-ACTH plasma cortisol concentration less than 1 µg/dl should receive no medication for 2 weeks and should then be treated with the dose recommended for dogs with a post-ACTH plasma cortisol level greater than 1 µg/dl and less than 3 µg/dl. These dogs should begin a maintenance schedule of 25 mg/kg of o,p'-DDD per week. Those that have a post-ACTH plasma cortisol concentration greater than 3 µg/dl should be given 50 mg/kg of o,p'-DDD per week. In either situation, it is strongly advised that the weekly dose be divided into as many days of treatment each week as is logical and convenient. For example, if a dog is scheduled to receive one tablet weekly, we recommend giving the dog one-quarter tablet four days a week. With this approach, if the dog on a subsequent recheck appears to be slightly underdosed, we increase the dose to one-quarter tablet five days a week. If it appears to be overdosed, we reduce the dose from four to two or three doses weekly.

An ACTH response test should be completed 1 and 3 months after the start of maintenance therapy. If the plasma cortisol concentration after ACTH administration begins to rise to or above 5 µg/dl, the o,p'-DDD dosage can and should be increased, usually by about 25% weekly. Some dogs remain stable for months or years on conservative dosages, whereas others receive o,p'-DDD daily at rather large doses. It is important to tailor treatment to the needs of each dog. Return of clinical signs suggestive of hyperadrenocorticism should be managed by performing an ACTH stimulation test to confirm disease exacerbation and then increasing the dose of o,p'-DDD. Whenever an owner reports recurrence of polydipsia and/or polyuria, the dog should always be assessed for the development of diabetes mellitus, renal failure, or other such conditions (see Table 6-11). Obvious recurrence of CCS should be treated by increasing the maintenance dosage schedule or by using the "loading dose" regimen. We rarely find it necessary to repeat loading dose protocols.

Many dogs treated with o,p'-DDD remain quite stable on maintenance treatment. It is recommended that these dogs be rechecked with an examination and an ACTH response test every 3 or 4 months. Test results allow the veterinarian to adjust maintenance dosages if subclinical problems occur. Whenever the post-ACTH plasma cortisol concentration is less than 1 µg/dl, the dose of o,p'-DDD should be reduced, and whenever it exceeds 5 µg/dl, the dose should be increased. Whenever listlessness and anorexia are associated with low plasma cortisol results, even if the post-ACTH plasma cortisol concentration exceeds 1 µg/dl, o,p'-DDD should be transiently discontinued and the dose then reduced.

Stress. If a dog that is receiving o,p'-DDD undergoes any type of stress (e.g., illness, trauma, elective surgery), o,p'-DDD should be discontinued and the dog should be treated with glucocorticoids (usually at a dosage of 0.2 mg/kg, adjusted or tapered as needed). An adequately treated dog with PDH has sufficient adrenal reserve for day-to-day living but may not have enough to handle major stress. **No dog that requires glucocorticoid therapy should ever be given o,p'-DDD.**

O,P'-DDD OVERDOSE. Overdose with o,p'-DDD is common. Most overdosed dogs (20% to 50% of treated dogs in the literature) have mild and transient signs that resolve a few days after medication is withheld or within hours of glucocorticoid treatment. A minority of dogs (<2%) develop "permanent" Addison's disease. Permanent disease is associated not only with low plasma cortisol concentrations before and after ACTH administration, but also with hyperkalemia and hyponatremia. These dogs may require both mineralocorticoid and glucocorticoid treatment for life.

In the more typical and mild forms of o,p'-DDD overdose, the dog becomes weak or anorectic, lethargic or ataxic, or develops vomiting and/or diarrhea. The serum chemistry profiles, CBC results, and urinalysis findings are often unremarkable, but these assessments are warranted. The easiest method of confirming the diagnosis is to treat these dogs with about 0.2 mg/kg of prednisone. Clinical improvement in 1 to 3 hours (sometimes 6 to 12 hours) confirms that an overdose of o,p'-DDD has likely occurred. Treatment with o,p'-DDD should be transiently discontinued. Prednisone is initially administered to effect (to eliminate all signs),

and the dose then is slowly tapered over 10 to 21 days. As long as the dog needs prednisone, o,p'-DDD is withheld. When the prednisone is discontinued and the dog has been stable on no treatment for an additional 2 weeks, o,p'-DDD should be given again, but at a lower dosage.

O,P'-DDD–INDUCED CNS SIGNS. Rarely, dogs treated with o,p'-DDD develops CNS signs *induced by the drug.* These signs are reported to include apparent blindness, ataxia, dull appearance, unawareness of surroundings, circling, aimless walking, and head pressing. However, we believe such drug-induced signs are either rare or simply do not occur. The most likely reason for a dog treated with o,p'-DDD to have signs such as mental dullness, aimlessness, and inappetence is a growing pituitary tumor (see page 296 and Table 6-10). The drug-induced syndrome as described in the literature is transient, lasting 12 to 48 hours after each administration. Drug-induced signs occur after 3 to 24 months of therapy and are treated by lowering the dosage or by giving the drug more frequently in smaller increments.

Prognosis in Dogs with PDH Undergoing o,p'-DDD Therapy

We have been able to monitor more than 1500 dogs with PDH that have been treated with o,p'-DDD. Of the dogs that have died, the life span after diagnosis and institution of o,p'-DDD therapy averaged 31.6 months. This average includes the small percentage of dogs that lived only a few days, as well as several that lived longer than 10 years. It is important to remember that the average dog with PDH is older than 11 years of age when treatment is started. Therefore it is unlikely that any treatment protocol will result in survival much longer than these figures, because the average dog dies when it is about 14 years of age. Although most owners love to see their pet survive longer than this "established average," we remind them that our goal in therapy is to return each dog to health and to resolve the CCS. Furthermore, the goal in treating a dog younger than 10 years of age would certainly be a life span in excess of 30 months, whereas that goal may be unrealistic in a dog that is older than 12 or 13 at the time of diagnosis. Good owner observation and compliance appear to improve the prognosis.

Relapses are common; more than 35% of our 1500 dogs have had at least one period in which mild to moderate signs of hyperadrenocorticism recurred, requiring an increase in the maintenance dosage. We almost never need to treat a dog with a second "loading" dose of o,p'-DDD. Of the dogs that died, 37% had a problem that could have been or was related to the hyperadrenocorticism (e.g., thromboembolism, congestive heart failure, infection, diabetic ketoacidosis). However, more than 20% (perhaps as many as 30%) have died as the result of a growing pituitary tumor. Episodes of o,p'-DDD overdose were also common. Five percent of the dogs were mildly overdosed during the induction phase of therapy. A total of 32% were overdosed at some time during therapy. Death from overdose has been seen in fewer than 1% of the dogs.

TREATMENT—MEDICAL MANAGEMENT WITH KETOCONAZOLE

Background

Ketoconazole (Nizoral; Janssen Pharmaceutica, Inc., Piscataway, NJ), an imidazole derivative, is an orally active, broad-spectrum antimycotic drug. At picomolar concentrations, it inhibits C14-methylation of lanosterol to ergosterol and thus disturbs fungal membrane growth (Vanden Bossche et al, 1990). The drug has demonstrated efficacy in the treatment of deep mycotic infections. At higher serum concentrations, the drug also affects steroid biosynthesis by interacting with the imidazole ring and the cytochrome P450 component of various mammalian steroidogenic enzyme systems. In vivo, administration of low doses of ketoconazole leads to a significant reduction in serum androgen concentrations, whereas at higher doses cortisol secretion is suppressed (Engelhardt et al, 1991). This inhibitory effect of ketoconazole on steroid biosynthesis has led to its therapeutic use in the treatment of advanced prostatic cancer, hirsutism, precocious puberty, and Cushing's syndrome (Sonino et al, 1985; Contreras et al, 1985; Loli et al, 1986; McCance et al, 1987).

Protocol in Canine Cushing's Syndrome

Ketoconazole is administered initially at a dosage of 5 mg/kg twice daily for 7 days. If no problems with appetite or icterus are noted, the dose is increased to 10 mg/kg twice daily. After an additional 14 days, an ACTH response test should be completed within several hours of the dog being given the drug, in addition to a history and physical examination. If CCS is not being satisfactorily controlled, the dosage can be increased to 15 mg/kg twice daily. We have rarely used doses of 20 mg/kg twice daily. Some dogs can be maintained indefinitely at the 10 mg/kg dosage and others at the 15 mg/kg dosage. The dosage requirement is determined from owner opinion, physical examination results, blood chemistries, and ACTH stimulation test monitoring. The goals in ACTH stimulation results are pre-ACTH and post-ACTH plasma cortisol concentrations less than 5 µg/kg. Most dogs do not achieve clinical remission at doses less than 30 mg/kg/day.

Results

We have evaluated the use of this drug in more than 60 dogs with naturally occurring hyperadrenocorticism, including dogs with PDH and dogs with ATH. All underwent treatment using the protocol described and reaching doses of 30 mg/kg divided into two daily doses. The drug lasts 8 to 16 hours in most dogs and is most effective when administered twice daily. Laboratory data demonstrate that approximately 75% to 80% of treated dogs have a rapid reduction in the serum cortisol concentration and in cortisol responsiveness to ACTH (Fig. 6-65). In dogs treated for more than 2 months, there has been significant improvement in the clinical condition, as evidenced by a reduction in water intake, urine production, appetite, panting, and weight. Regrowth of hair and return of muscle strength are also noted. Signs of toxicity have rarely developed. Signs of overdose are usually those of hypocortisolism (Feldman et al, 1990).

It appears that 20% to 25% of dogs fail to respond to the drug as a result of poor intestinal absorption. Although this is true for many dogs that do not improve, other explanations must also be entertained, because some dogs demonstrate an *increase* in pre-ACTH and post-ACTH plasma cortisol concentrations when receiving ketoconazole. Plasma cortisol concentrations return to pretreatment levels when the drug is discontinued. The major drawbacks (Table 6-16) to the use of this drug are its expense, the failure of some dogs to respond, and the necessity for twice daily administration indefinitely.

Indications (see Table 6-16)

With its low incidence of toxicity and negligible effects on mineralocorticoid production, ketoconazole may be an attractive (albeit expensive) alternative in the medical management of canine hyperadrenocorticism. The drug is readily available through human pharmacies. The effects on enzyme blockage are completely reversible. Ketoconazole may be used as an alternative to o,p'-DDD in the medical management of dogs with malignant, large, or invasive adrenal tumors if surgical intervention is not an option but palliative therapy is desired. We have used ketoconazole in the preoperative stabilization of surgical candidates

TABLE 6–16   KETOCONAZOLE

Indications for Use

1. Preparation of a dog for surgery
2. Alternative therapy for a dog that has an adrenocortical tumor with metastasis or for any other reason is not a surgical candidate
3. Alternative for dogs not tolerating o,p'-DDD
4. Diagnostic aid—improvement points toward Cushing's syndrome
5. Sole mode of therapy

Drawbacks to Its Use

1. Must be given twice daily indefinitely
2. Expensive
3. 20–25% of treated dogs fail to respond (fail to absorb the drug?)
4. Overdosage problems can occur

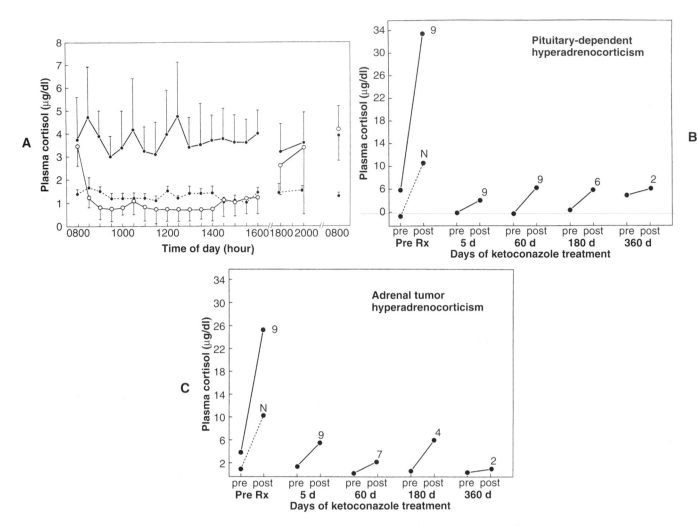

FIGURE 6–65. *A,* Mean plasma cortisol concentrations over a 24-hour period from 15 normal dogs *(dashed line);* from 18 dogs with untreated hyperadrenocorticism (nine with PDH and nine with adrenocortical tumors *[solid line with solid circles]);* and from the 18 dogs with hyperadrenocorticism after their first dose of ketoconazole *(solid line with open circles).* The results show the potent and rapid effect of ketoconazole in preventing cortisol synthesis. *B,* ACTH stimulation test results (mean plasma cortisol concentrations) from dogs with naturally occurring pituitary-dependent hyper-adrenocorticism before and 5, 60, 180, and 360 days after initiation of ketoconazole treatment. The numbers above each set of values indicate the number of dogs in each time period. The numbers decrease with time because of the expense associated with ketoconazole therapy, which prompted some owners to choose o,p'-DDD therapy instead. *C,* ACTH stimulation test results (mean plasma cortisol concentrations) from dogs with naturally occurring hyperadrenocorticism caused by functioning adrenocortical tumors before and 5, 60, 180, and 360 days after initiation of ketoconazole treatment. The numbers above each set of values indicate the number of dogs in each time period. The numbers decrease with time because of the expense associated with ketoconazole therapy, which prompted some owners to choose surgical therapy instead.

by providing a rapid decline in the hypercortisolemic state. Some dogs (extremely rare in our experience) do not tolerate o,p'-DDD at any dosage, and ketoconazole can be tried. Despite the number of screening tests for hyperadrenocorticism, response to therapy may be used as a diagnostic aid. In this situation, ketoconazole is an enzyme blocker with no long-term effects. Also, its effect can be assessed without causing tissue damage. All this being said, we have rarely used ketoconazole in the past several years, primarily because of the excellent and consistent results we achieve with o,p'-DDD therapy.

TREATMENT—MEDICAL MANAGEMENT WITH TRILOSTANE

Background: Humans

Trilostane is an orally administered, hormonally in-active steroid competitive inhibitor of 3β-hydroxysteroid dehydrogenase. This enzyme system mediates the conversion of pregnenolone to progesterone and of 17-hydroxypregnenolone to 17-hydroxyprogesterone in the adrenal cortices (see Fig. 6-4). Cortisol, aldosterone, and androstenedione are produced from progesterone and 17-hydroxypregnenolone via various biochemical pathways. Trilostane inhibits the production of progesterone and 17-hydroxyprogesterone, therefore the synthesis of various end products, including adrenal, gonadal, and placental steroids, is inhibited (Potts et al, 1978). Inhibition of adrenal steroidogenesis has been shown to occur at lower doses than those required to inhibit steroid synthesis in other organs. Trilostane is interconverted in vivo to the active metabolite 17-keto-trilostane, which has 1.7 times the biopotency of the parent compound (Robinson et al, 1984). Trilostane has proved effective in the treatment of people with some hormone-dependent neoplastic conditions and those with hyperaldosteronism (Griffing and Melby, 1989; Geldof et al, 1995; Ibrahim and Buzdar, 1995). The response noted in humans with hyperadrenocorticism, however, has been variable. Although some studies reported good efficacy with trilostane, others had inconsistent results. Currently, trilostane is not the drug of choice for the medical management of people with hyperadrenocorticism (Komanicky et al, 1978; Dewis et al, 1983).

Background: Dogs

The first report on the use of trilostane for treating naturally occurring hyperadrenocorticism in dogs was an abstract on four dogs with PDH and one with ATH. The dose used in these five dogs ranged from 2.6 to 4.8 mg/kg/day. All the dogs demonstrated a good clinical response, with resolution of clinical signs and no adverse effects noted during 3 to 7 months of therapy (Hurley et al, 1998). In a second report from the same group, six dogs with naturally occurring Cushing's syndrome received doses of 3 to 30 mg/kg/day given for as long as 7 months. Again, all dogs initially improved with therapy, but in this report three dogs suffered relapses despite continued administration (Ramsey and Hurley, 2000). In a third abstract, it was demonstrated that resting serum cortisol concentrations were decreased for as long as 13 hours and post-ACTH plasma cortisol concentrations were blunted for as long as 20 hours after trilostane administration to 10 dogs. There was some individual variation in response (Neiger and Hurley, 2001).

Several subsequent studies critically evaluated the use of trilostane therapy for dogs with PDH (Ruckstuhl, 2002; Neiger et al, 2002). In the study completed in Switzerland (Ruckstuhl et al, 2002), 11 dogs were treated. The initial dose was 30 mg/day for dogs that weighed less than 5 kg and 60 mg/day for dogs that weighed more. These doses calculated on a body weight basis were 3.9 to 9.2 mg/kg (median, 6.25 mg/kg). One objective of therapy was to achieve a post-ACTH serum cortisol concentration of 1.0 to 2.5 μg/dl. Trilostane dosages were adjusted as needed to meet this aim. In most dogs, dose adjustments were made in increments of 20 to 30 mg/dog and by the end of 6 months the doses ranged from about 4 to 16 mg/kg/day (median of about 6 mg/kg/day). All dogs responded well to treatment, with reductions in polyuria, polydipsia, and panting, and showed improvement in muscle strength. Polyphagia decreased in nine of 10 dogs, and nine of 11 showed improvement in coat quality. After 6 months of therapy, nine of the 11 were considered completely healthy, and two had improved. All dogs had an increase in adrenal gland size, as evaluated with abdominal ultrasonography. Seven dogs were treated for at least a year, three of the seven for at least 2 years. Adverse side effects were considered minor, with lethargy occurring in one dog and vomiting in another. These problems were managed by temporarily discontinuing treatment and providing prednisone. The conclusion reached in this study was that trilostane was an efficacious and safe medication for treatment of dogs with PDH.

In a study completed in Australia (Braddock, 2002), 31 dogs with PDH were treated with trilostane. The body weights of these dogs ranged from 4 to 42 kg. As in the Swiss study, these dogs responded quite well to trilostane therapy, and the average duration of treatment was about 1 year. This author also emphasized the concept that a wide range of doses (total or per kilogram of body weight) were required to induce and maintain adequate adrenocortical suppression. By the final test date, the dogs were receiving 1.4 to 8.7 times the initial "controlling" dose of trilostane. A frequent observation was that the dogs had an initial sensitivity to trilostane that was short-lived and that the dose then had to be increased until the appropriate "long-term dose" was achieved. The trend was for the dose to eventually plateau in each dog, not continually increase. It was pointed out that, as is true for any therapeutic protocol, veterinarian experience with the drug was important. In this case, it took an average of almost 90 days to achieve satisfactory control of PDH in the first 10 dogs treated, but it only took an average of 40 days to achieve a similar level of control in the last 10 dogs. The mean dose required to control PDH was 19.4 mg/kg given once daily, with a median of 16.7 mg/kg and a range of 5.3 to 50 mg/kg. It was suggested that veterinarians need to persist through the initial sensitive and insensitive periods before finding the appropriate long-term dose. The recommended starting dose was 10 mg/kg, with upward or downward adjustments (20 to 30 mg/dog) based on periodic ACTH stimulation test results performed 3 to 8 hours after trilostane administration. The doses most likely needed to control PDH are 16 to 19 mg/kg, with larger dogs requiring a lower dose per kilogram than smaller dogs. Clinical response, ACTH stimulation and urine cortisol:creatinine results can and should be used in monitoring therapy. One concern identified in this study was the cost of therapy, which was estimated to be two to four times the cost of o,p'-DDD therapy. It was also pointed out that trilostane may also be useful for dogs with an adrenocortical tumor causing hyperadrenocorticism.

In the United Kingdom, trilostane is officially registered for use in dogs under the trade name Vetoryl.

The product for use in humans is listed as Modrenal. The current recommendations from one group is to initially administer 30 mg/day to dogs weighing <5 kg; 60 mg/day to dogs weighing 5 to 20 kg; and 120 mg/day to dogs weighing >20 kg. Re-evaluations are suggested after 1, 3, 6, and 13 weeks, and then after 6 and 12 months. Each recheck should include a history, physical examination, and an ACTH stimulation test. The stimulation test should be completed 2 to 6 hours after administration of the trilostane. The target range for serum or plasma cortisol concentration should be 1 to 2 µg/dl. Since some dogs have been stable for prolonged periods with cortisol concentrations less than 1 µg/dl, it is assumed that such concentrations represent the daily nadir and that average daily concentrations are higher or that precursors accumulate in the serum and retain some biological activity, although these precursors are not assayed by the cortisol measurement (Reusch, in press).

TREATMENT—OTHER MEDICATIONS

Cyproheptadine

Increased CNS serotonin concentrations could theoretically be associated with excess pituitary secretion of ACTH and therefore increased adrenal secretory activity. Cyproheptadine (Periactin; Merck Sharp & Dohme, West Point, PA), a drug with antiserotonin, antihistamine, and anticholinergic effects, has been used with limited success in treating humans and dogs with PDH (Drucker and Peterson, 1980; Aron et al, 2001a). Although a few well-documented cases of clinical and biochemical remission of Cushing's disease have been reported with its use, cyproheptadine causes sedation, increased appetite, and weight gain and is usually ineffective in treating individuals with ACTH-secreting pituitary tumors. In one study (Peterson and Drucker, 1978), one of 10 dogs with PDH had a "complete remission," and in another study (Stolp et al, 1984), none of the nine dogs involved improved.

Bromocriptine

Bromocriptine (Parlodel; Sandoz, Inc., East Hanover, NJ), a dopamine agonist, lowers plasma ACTH concentrations and rarely produces remissions in people with pituitary-dependent Cushing's disease. In humans this drug is most commonly used in the treatment of hyperprolactinemia. Bromocriptine is not recommended for use in dogs or cats with Cushing's syndrome because of its relative ineffectiveness (Rijnberk et al, 1988b).

Metyrapone and Aminoglutethimide

Metyrapone, an 11β-hydroxylase inhibitor, and aminoglutethimide, which inhibits conversion of cholesterol to pregnenolone, have both been used to reduce cortisol hypersecretion. The drugs are expensive; their use is accompanied by increased ACTH concentrations that may overcome their enzyme inhibitory properties; and both cause gastrointestinal side effects in humans. More effective control of hypercortisolism with fewer side effects is obtained with combined use of the drugs. Several reports on the use of metyrapone as the sole therapy for people with Cushing's syndrome demonstrate effectiveness (Totani et al, 1990; Verhelst et al, 1991). No recommendations can be made regarding use of either or both drugs in dogs with Cushing's syndrome, but a report does describe aminoglutethimide as reducing circulating cortisol concentrations in normal dogs (Lacoste et al, 1989). The use of this drug in 12 dogs with PDH was reported to be beneficial (Castill et al, 1996). The use of metyrapone was reported in the management of two cats with hyperadrenocorticism (Daley et al, 1993; Moore et al, 2000). It should be pointed out that metyrapone has not been consistently available.

Etomidate

Etomidate is an imidazole derivative similar to ketoconazole. It is an ultra–short-acting anesthetic agent that is also a potent but transient inhibitor of adrenal cortisol synthesis in humans (Drake et al, 1998), dogs (Dodam et al, 1990), and cats (Moon, 1997). This drug is reported to be 10 times more potent than ketoconazole in blocking adrenocortical enzyme activity. Suppression is maintained for up to 6 hours after administration and can result in adrenal insufficiency (Absalom et al, 1999). Although this drug has been used for acute treatment of endocrine psychoses or severe hyperadrenal complications, its brief duration of action, potency, and need for parenteral administration limits its usefulness in dogs and cats.

L-Deprenyl

L-Deprenyl (selegiline, anipryl) is approved for use in humans with Parkinson's disease and is licensed for treatment of PDH in dogs. It acts as an irreversible inhibitor of the enzyme monoamine oxidase type B, thereby promoting normalization of dopamine in people with Parkinson's disease. ACTH secretion is controlled, in part, by hypothalamic CRH secretion via positive feedback and by dopamine via negative feedback. It is hypothesized that pituitary-dependent Cushing's syndrome may be caused by a lack of this negative suppression of ACTH, allowing its excess synthesis and secretion. By enhancing dopamine concentrations, L-deprenyl could "down-regulate" ACTH and control Cushing's syndrome. It is important to understand that L-deprenyl is degraded to amphetamine and methamphetamine. Thus the effects attributed to administration of this drug may be due to these metabolic byproducts and not to any effect on the pituitary-adrenocortical axis. It is interesting to note that the safety of L-deprenyl is also in question, because it ranked third in total human Possible Adverse Drug Experience reports filed with the U.S. Food and Drug Administration for 1998.

In a pilot study (Bruyette et al, 1993), seven dogs with PDH were treated with 2.0 mg/kg of L-deprenyl given orally once a day. Five of the seven demonstrated partial to complete resolution of the PDH within a 2-month period. This study was funded by the manufacturer and was not published in a peer-reviewed journal, therefore the results can and should be questioned. Several larger studies have been published that seriously question the efficacy of L-deprenyl in the treatment of dogs with PDH. In one independent, prospective evaluation (Reusch et al, 1999), treatment of 10 dogs with PDH with L-deprenyl was associated with some improvement in only two dogs, and even then the response was considered quite variable. The researchers' conclusion was that L-deprenyl could not be recommended for treatment of PDH in dogs (Reusch, in press). In an Australian prospective comparison study, an equal number of dogs were to have been treated with either trilostane or L-deprenyl. The choice of therapy that each dog received was random. However, after the first 13 dogs assigned to receive L-deprenyl failed to demonstrate any response to therapy, "this treatment was ceased for ethical reasons" (Braddock, 2002). Thirty-one dogs in this same study were treated with trilostane. L-Deprenyl should not be used in the treatment of dogs with PDH.

RU486

RU486 (mifepristone) is a 19-norsteroid that has antiprogesterone activity by virtue of its ability to inhibit progesterone binding competitively at the receptor level. This same mode of action explains its antiglucocorticoid effect; that is, the drug inhibits glucocorticoid binding at receptor levels. The result is blockage of the feedback effect of cortisol on ACTH secretion, as well as blockage of the systemic effects of cortisol. Thus, people treated with 4 to 6 mg/kg have *increases* in both plasma ACTH and cortisol concentrations, but they are prone to developing signs of cortisol deficiency (weakness, nausea, vomiting). Their serum cortisol concentrations are increased because the binding is inhibited, not hormonal synthesis or secretion. Treatment with mifepristone ameliorates the clinical manifestations of hypercortisolism in more than 50% of humans with Cushing's syndrome caused by adrenocortical tumor or in those in whom the source of ACTH is other than the pituitary ("ectopic"; not reported in dogs or cats). By contrast, humans with PDH do not respond with any consistency to mifepristone because their excesses in ACTH overwhelm the receptor

blockade (Laue et al, 1990; Silvestre et al, 1990; Spitz and Bardin, 1993).

TREATMENT—PITUITARY IRRADIATION

Dogs with PDH and Pituitary Masses that Do Not Cause Central Nervous System Signs

EXPERIENCE. Radiotherapy of pituitary tumors is reported to be an effective means of treatment in only 50% to 60% of people with PDH. Clinical signs resolve over a period of 2 to 5 years, and recurrence of the disease is rare (Halberg and Sheline, 1987; Littley et al, 1990; Tran et al, 1991; Murayama et al, 1992; Estrada et al, 1997). A group of six dogs with naturally developing PDH and a visible pituitary mass underwent pituitary irradiation as the primary mode of treatment for the condition (Goossens et al, 1998). No dog had any clinical signs suggestive of a large pituitary tumor, and the masses visualized with MRI scans were 3 to 14 mm (median, 6.5 mm) in greatest vertical height. Each dog received a radiation dose of 44 Gy divided into 11 equal fractions using a telecobalt 60 unit. No change in the clinical signs of hyperadrenocorticism were observed after radiation in one dog, and two dogs improved but did not "normalize." Three dogs normalized after the 4 weeks of radiation therapy, but recurrence of hyperadrenocorticism signs were noted 6, 9, and 12 months later, respectively. The results of ACTH stimulation testing and urine cortisol:creatinine ratios correlated with the clinical observations. In two dogs, the greatest vertical height of the pituitary tumors decreased from 8 mm prior to radiation to 6 mm 1 year after completion of the radiation. The other four dogs had tumors that ranged in size from 3 to 14 mm in greatest vertical height prior to radiation. No visible tumor was detectable with MRI scanning in these 4 dogs 1 year after completion of radiation (Goossens et al, 1998). Since completion of this study, 12 dogs with similar clinical features and pituitary masses equal to or greater than 8 mm in greatest vertical height have been treated with radiation. The results have been similar: a dramatic reduction in pituitary tumor size, but only transient resolution (none to as long as 2 years) of the hyperadrenocorticism.

RECOMMENDATIONS. Because the results from 18 dogs comprise a remarkably small number, conclusions must be made with care. At this time, we believe that pituitary CT or MRI scanning should be performed when PDH is diagnosed in a dog even if there is no clinical evidence of a large pituitary mass. We understand that CT or MRI scans are expensive, but for some clients this is feasible. The following suggestions are put forward: (1) if such a dog has no visible pituitary mass, o,p'-DDD or other suitable medical therapy should be initiated, and no further evaluation of the pituitary area is recommended; (2) if a mass is observed and measured to be 3 to 7 mm in greatest vertical height, o,p'-DDD or other suitable therapy should be initiated, and a repeat pituitary scan should be recommended 12 to 18 months later; and (3) if a pituitary mass is seen that is equal to or greater than 8 mm in greatest vertical height, pituitary irradiation is recommended, and medical therapy is used only if clinical hyperadrenocorticism fails to resolve within 3 to 6 months of completion of the radiation therapy or if the hyperadrenocorticism resolves but recurrence is noted.

The basis for these recommendations is hypothetical. One assumption is that the average dog treated medically for hyperadrenocorticism survives an average of 30 months. The second assumption is that the average pituitary tumor will double or triple in size during that time. If a dog has no visible pituitary mass (<3 mm in greatest vertical height) and that mass triples in size, the mass likely will never be large enough to be clinically significant, hence the recommendation for medical management of the Cushing's syndrome and no further follow-up for the pituitary. If a dog has a mass that is equal to or greater than 8 mm in greatest vertical height at the time of diagnosis, the mass would not even need to double in size before clinical signs occur. Thus the recommendation for irradiation as the primary mode of treatment. If a pituitary mass is 3 and 7 mm in greatest vertical height, doubling or tripling in size may or may not be problematic. Therefore the recommendation to treat the PDH medically but also to plan a recheck in 12 to 18 months. This waiting period is based on experience and should precede worrisome tumor growth in most dogs. The reader is reminded that this protocol is based on experience derived from a limited number of dogs. As experience in our hospital and that of others accumulates, these recommendations may change.

Dogs with PDH and Large Pituitary Tumors (Pituitary Macrotumor Syndrome)

BACKGROUND

Definitions. Approximately 50% of dogs with PDH and no CNS signs have visible pituitary tumors (masses usually >3 and <14 mm in greatest height) based on our experience with MRI (Bertoy et al, 1995) and CT scans. The term *macrotumor* in the context of PDH, however, should not imply *visible* tumor. Rather, this term suggests the presence of a tumor that causes CNS problems because of its size, location, and/or invasive properties. The clinical signs, endocrine testing, and diagnostic evaluation of dogs with *macrotumor syndrome* have been reviewed in the discussions under Pathology (page 263), Pituitary "Macrotumors" and Central Nervous System Signs (page 296), and Magnetic Resonance Imaging (MRI) Scans (page 320). Macrotumor syndrome is being recognized with increasing frequency as a result of an increasing index of suspicion and improved diagnostic capabilities (CT and MRI). Conservatively, 10% to 15% of dogs with PDH develop clinical problems due to their growing pituitary tumors; the more likely number is 20% to

30% of all dogs with PDH. The primary mode of treating these dogs is irradiation. Success, to date, has been variable. Most of the dogs undergoing radiation therapy have had significant clinical signs and extremely large intracranial masses. The response to treatment will improve as our ability to identify these dogs earlier in the course of their disease improves, so that the radiation is directed at smaller tumors in dogs less debilitated by the condition.

Diagnosis in Untreated and Newly Identified PDH. A dog with untreated PDH that is extremely "dull" or has a poor appetite but that also has other signs associated with Cushing's syndrome should be suspected of having a large intracranial tumor. A small number of our dogs (10% to 20%) with pituitary macrotumors have been diagnosed prior to therapy for PDH (see Figs. 6-37 and 6-55). Evaluations should confirm the diagnosis of PDH and attempt to identify any cause for the anorexia (e.g., renal failure, pancreatitis, severe hepatopathy). If the anorexia remains unexplained, evaluation of the pituitary with CT or MRI scanning is warranted.

Diagnosis in Dogs that Have Been Previously Identified and Treated for PDH. Signs of anorexia in a dog treated for PDH should always be assumed to be caused by hypocortisolism or a concurrent condition until proven otherwise. Medication (e.g., o,p'-DDD, ketoconazole, trilostane) should be discontinued, evaluation for unrelated systemic disease completed (e.g., renal failure, pancreatitis), an ACTH stimulation test performed, and prednisone therapy begun. If all the above information rules out concurrent conditions or drug overdose and if cortisone does not quickly resolve the signs, an intracranial mass should be considered. "Macrotumor syndrome" has been diagnosed within days of beginning therapy for PDH, as well as years into therapy (see Fig. 6-37).

EXPERIENCE. A significant correlation has been found between relative tumor size (i.e., the size of the tumor relative to the size of the calvarium) and the severity of neurologic signs. Significant inverse correlation was also noted between relative tumor size and remission of neurologic signs after irradiation (the larger the tumor, the less likely that resolution would be achieved). Although a significant correlation was also identified between relative tumor size and plasma endogenous ACTH concentrations, these statistically derived data certainly do not apply to every dog. The prognostic factor that independently affected overall survival time was severity of neurologic signs (i.e., the worse the neurologic signs, the poorer the prognosis). In our initial studies, dogs were treated with 44 to 48 Gy of radiation during 4 weeks of an alternate-day therapeutic schedule in which each dog received 4 Gy/fraction (Theon and Feldman, 1998). More recently, we have been treating dogs daily, Monday through Friday, for a total of 16 treatments while still delivering 48 Gy. This is a more aggressive mode of therapy that has the potential for improved rates of response but with the risk of causing greater damage to surrounding tissues.

Regardless of treatment protocol, it is safe to point out that veterinarians with an interest in hyperadrenocorticism should be well acquainted with the clinical signs of a growing pituitary tumor. The subtle nature of early signs must be appreciated. In other words, dogs with a completely unremarkable physical examination by the veterinarian but whose owners are concerned about unusual lethargy, inappetence, or a pet that sometimes appears "co nfused," "aimless," or "unaware of their surroundings" are dogs that have early signs of macrotumor and the best prognosis for response to pituitary irradiation.

CLINICAL IMPLICATIONS. Because radiation therapy was effective for treatment of relatively small tumors, early treatment of these masses improves prognosis. The suggestion that CT or MRI pituitary scans be done in as many dogs with PDH as possible, at the time of diagnosis, will improve longevity if dogs with pituitary masses equal to or greater than 8 mm at greatest vertical height undergo radiation as the primary mode of therapy. Until more of these dogs have been evaluated and followed long-term, this protocol remains arbitrary and unproven.

SUCCESS. Treatment success does not depend entirely on the source of photons (cobalt-60 versus linear accelerator), the dose per day, or the total dose of radiation delivered to the pituitary tumor. Although these factors are important, the most critical parameter is likely to be the time of diagnosis. A dog with severe clinical signs and a huge tumor (>2 cm in diameter) has a much poorer prognosis than a dog with subtle signs and a small tumor (1.2 to 1.5 cm in diameter). There is little doubt that brain CT or MRI scanning of all dogs with PDH, with subsequent radiation therapy for those with a visible pituitary tumor, has potential value. However, this is not currently feasible. We currently recommend radiation therapy for any tumor equal to or greater than 8 mm in diameter.

SPONTANEOUS REMISSION OF CUSHING'S SYNDROME

Spontaneous remission of Cushing's syndrome is a documented phenomenon in humans. It is possible for a dog with PDH to undergo spontaneous remission as well. We have had five dogs with histories, physical examination findings, and endocrine test results consistent with PDH. Treatment was withheld in each of these dogs because the owners believed their pets were already improving. Subsequent evaluations demonstrated resolution of all evidence supporting the diagnosis of PDH. It has been hypothesized that these dogs embolized their pituitary microadenomas, resulting in return of a normal endocrine state.

PRIMARY MINERALOCORTICOID EXCESS: PRIMARY HYPERALDOSTERONISM

Humans

ETIOLOGY. Primary hyperaldosteronism is usually caused by a solitary, unilateral adrenal adenoma or bilateral adrenal hyperplasia (Ganguly, 1998). Adrenal carcinoma is less common. The pathogenesis of zona glomerulosa hyperplasia is unknown. Humans with adrenal hyperplasia are typically classified as having idiopathic hyperaldosteronism (White, 1994). Primary hyperaldosteronism must be distinguished from the secondary type, which may be caused by cardiovascular failure, renal failure, or severe hepatocellular dysfunction.

PHYSIOPATHOLOGY. In humans, the increased production of aldosterone by abnormal zona glomerulosa tissue (adenoma, carcinoma, or hyperplasia) initiates a series of events that result in primary hyperaldosteronism. Aldosterone excess leads to increased sodium retention, expansion of the extracellular fluid volume, and increased total body sodium content. The expanded extracellular fluid and plasma volumes are registered by stretch receptors at the juxtaglomerular apparatus, and sodium retention is registered at the macula densa. With primary increases in aldosterone production, the renin system is suppressed. This is the hallmark of the disorder. Primary hyperaldosteronism is a disease of the zona glomerulosa. Cells of this zone do not have the capacity to make cortisol. There may or may not be abnormalities in cortisol production, the plasma cortisol concentration, or cortisol metabolism.

In addition to sodium retention (serum sodium concentrations are usually in the high-normal range), potassium depletion develops, decreasing the total body and plasma concentrations of potassium. The shift of potassium from the intracellular compartment to the extracellular fluid results in a reversed movement of hydrogen ions, increased renal excretion of hydrogen ions, and systemic alkalosis. Moderate potassium depletion reduces carbohydrate tolerance (shown by an abnormal glucose tolerance test), and resistance to antidiuretic hormone (vasopressin) occurs. Severe potassium depletion blunts baroreceptor function. Because aldosterone biosynthesis is intensified, the entire biosynthetic pathway becomes activated. Increased concentrations of precursor steroids such as desoxycorticosterone, corticosterone, and 18-hydroxycorticosterone can be present in the blood of humans with an aldosterone-producing adenoma.

CLINICAL SIGNS. The clinical features of primary hyperaldosteronism in people are not specific. The condition is more common in women than men, and it is rare in children. Some patients are completely asymptomatic. Others have symptoms related to hypertension (headache) or hypokalemia, (polyuria, nocturia, muscle cramps). Occasionally, serious muscle weakness, paresthesia, tetany, or paralysis resulting from profound hypokalemia can be prominent. Sometimes the medical history reveals no specific symptoms but often only nonspecific complaints of tiredness, loss of stamina, weakness, nocturia, and lassitude — all symptoms of potassium depletion. If potassium depletion is severe, alkalosis, thirst, and polyuria develop. Unsuspected hypertension may be diagnosed during the course of a physical examination. The blood pressure of patients with primary hyperaldosteronism can range from normal to severely increased (Ganguly, 1998).

DIAGNOSTIC TESTING. Assessment of the serum potassium concentration is an important initial screening procedure in humans with hypertension. Care must be taken to assess the state of sodium intake in the patient before serum electrolytes are obtained. The serum potassium concentration is determined to a great extent by the sodium chloride intake. A low-sodium diet, by sparing potassium loss, can correct serum potassium abnormalities and mask depletion of potassium. As the amount of sodium ion available for resorption is reduced, potassium secretion is retarded in the distal renal tubule. In the presence of normal renal function and aldosterone excess, salt loading reveals hypokalemia. Normokalemic hyperaldosteronism under these conditions has been reported but is considered rare. A normal (142 to 156 mEq/L) to increased serum sodium concentration in the presence of hypokalemia and a reduced hematocrit (due to increased extracellular fluid and plasma volume from sodium retention) are presumptive evidence of mineralocorticoid excess. Additional clues to the diagnosis of primary hyperaldosteronism, in addition to hypokalemia, are an inability to concentrate urine, an abnormal glucose tolerance test result, and alkalosis.

If hypokalemia is documented, the renin-angiotensin system must be evaluated. This is accomplished in humans by measuring random plasma renin activity. If plasma renin activity is normal or high in a patient who has been off diuretic therapy for 3 weeks, it is unlikely that primary aldosteronism is present. If the random plasma renin activity is suppressed, primary aldosteronism is a likely diagnosis.

Aldosterone production can best be assessed by measuring urinary aldosterone excretion over a 24-hour period under conditions of adequate sodium intake. Measurement of either the 18-glucuronide or the tetrahydroaldosterone metabolite is sufficient to assess the rate of total production. Plasma samples must be obtained under proper conditions to yield reliable diagnostic information. Although the value obtained for the *plasma* aldosterone concentration is the aldosterone level only at a given moment, in a properly prepared patient, it can provide an excellent assessment of mineralocorticoid production. Both plasma and urinary aldosterone measurements should be performed while the patient is eating a high-salt diet with sodium chloride supplementation. This is crucial, because with any diminution of salt intake, the plasma aldosterone concentration and aldosterone production normally increase. Although urinary measurements have been adequate for detecting abnormal production of aldosterone (and superior to plasma aldosterone concentration measurements), it has not been possible to use daily excretion of aldosterone to discriminate between adenoma and hyperplasia.

It is important to distinguish between adenoma and hyperplasia, because surgery is indicated for the former but not the latter. Plasma aldosterone concentrations in humans provide not only diagnostic information about the hyperaldosteronism but also differential diagnostic information about the pathologic process. After at least 4 days of sodium intake exceeding 120 mEq daily and after overnight (at least 6 hours) recumbency, the 8 AM plasma aldosterone concentration can be used to distinguish humans with an aldosterone-secreting adrenal adenoma from those with hyperplasia. A plasma aldosterone concentration greater than 20 ng/dl indicates adenoma, and a level less than 20 ng/dl usually indicates hyperplasia.

After 2 or 4 hours in the upright posture (which normally activates the renin system, with a rise in plasma aldosterone concentrations), the plasma aldosterone concentration either shows no significant change or decreases in 90% of humans with adenoma, but it almost always increases in humans with adrenocortical hyperplasia. This important differential maneuver is extremely accurate in identifying the specific disorder. The difference is due to the profound suppression of the renin system by excessive aldosterone production caused by an adrenal adenoma. In humans with adrenocortical hyperplasia, increased sensitivity of the hyperplastic gland to minute but measurable increases in renin that occur with assumption of the upright posture leads to an increased aldosterone level.

TREATMENT. Treatment depends for the most part on the precision of diagnosis. In humans with an aldosterone-producing adrenal adenoma and no contraindication to surgery, unilateral adrenalectomy is recommended. The reduction of blood pressure and correction of hypokalemia achieved with spironolactone provide a surprisingly close approximation to the actual response to surgery; in fact, greater reduction often occurs postoperatively, presumably because of a greater reduction of extracellular fluid. The surgical cure rate of hypertension associated with adenoma is excellent—over 50% in several series, with reduction of hypertension in the remainder.

In humans with aldosteronism of indeterminate type, spironolactone alone is usually effective in controlling both the hypertension and the potassium-depleted state. Because of the effectiveness of spironolactone in these patients, other antihypertensive medications can often be discontinued.

PATHOLOGY. Several pathologic abnormalities are associated with primary hyperaldosteronism. More than 50% of patients with the diagnosis who have undergone surgery have had unilateral adenoma. Bilateral tumors are rare. The characteristic adenoma is readily identified by its golden yellow color. In addition, small satellite adenomas are often found, and distinction from micronodular or macronodular hyperplasia is frequently difficult. In patients with adenoma, the contiguous adrenal gland can show hyperplasia throughout the gland. Hyperplasia is also present in the contralateral adrenal gland but is not associated with aldosterone abnormalities after removal of the primary adenoma (Biglieri and Kater, 1983).

Dogs

We have had experience with three dogs that have been diagnosed with primary hyperaldosteronism.

Each dog was 8 years of age or older at the time of diagnosis (8, 9, and 11 years of age, respectively). The breeds included a Beagle, a Miniature Poodle, and a Doberman Pinscher. The primary owner concern in each dog was episodic weakness, and each dog, on initial database blood evaluation, had a serum potassium concentration less than 3 mEq/L. Two of the three dogs have had extensive laboratory studies, including assessment of plasma aldosterone concentrations. These concentrations were consistently extremely increased (>3000 pmol/L) until surgical removal of the tumor, after which the hormone values decreased dramatically. Each dog had an adrenal tumor (one adenoma and two adenocarcinomas). One dog was euthanized before any attempt at treatment, and two became clinically and biochemically normal after surgery. One has been normal for more than 24 months (this dog had an adenoma), and one suffered a recurrence of severe hypokalemia and muscle weakness 24 months later, at which time widespread metastasis was recognized. Both of these dogs lived more than 4 years after surgery. We are aware of only two other dogs with primary hyperaldosteronism having been reported (Breitschwerdt et al, 1985; Rijnberk et al, in press).

REFERENCES

Absalom A, et al: Adrenocortical function in critically ill patients 24 hours after a single dose of etomidate. Anaesthesia 54:861, 1999.

Allin RE, et al: The elucidation of adrenal-cortical status by measuring 2-hour urinary free cortisol levels. Clin Chim Acta 143:17, 1984.

Anderson CR: Surgical treatment of adrenocortical tumors: 21 cases (1990-1996). J Am Anim Hosp Assoc 37:93, 2001.

Angles JM, et al: Use of urine corticoid:creatinine ratio versus adrenocorticotropic hormone stimulation for monitoring mitotane treatment of pituitary-dependent hyperadrenocorticism in dogs. J Am Vet Med Assoc 211:1002, 1997.

Arioglu E, et al: Cushing's syndrome caused by corticotropin secretion by pulmonary tumorlets. N Engl J Med 339:883, 1998.

Aron DC, Ross NS: Evaluation of patients with an incidentally discovered adrenal mass. Proceedings of the Tenth ACVIM Forum, San Diego, Calif, 1992, p 193.

Aron DC, et al: Anterior pituitary gland. In Greenspan FS, Gardner DG (eds): Basic and Clinical Endocrinology, 6th ed. New York, Lange Medical Books/McGraw-Hill, 2001a, p 100.

Aron DC, et al: Glucocorticoids and adrenal androgens. In Greenspan FS, Gardner DG (eds): Basic and Clinical Endocrinology, 6th ed. New York, Lange Medical Books/McGraw-Hill, 2001b, p 334.

Atkinson AB, et al: Cyclical Cushing's disease: Two distinct rhythms in a patient with a basophil adenoma. J Clin Endocrinol Metab 60:328, 1985.

Badylak SF, Van Vleet JF: Sequential morphologic and clinicopathologic alterations in dogs with experimentally induced glucocorticoid hepatopathy. Am J Vet Res 42:1310, 1981.

Badylak SF, Van Vleet JF: Tissue gamma-glutamyl transpeptidase activity and hepatic ultrastructural alterations in dogs with experimentally induced glucocorticoid hepatopathy. Am J Vet Res 42:649, 1982.

Bailey MQ: Use of x-ray–computed tomography as an aid in localization of adrenal masses in the dog. J Am Vet Med Assoc 188:1046, 1986.

Barthez P, et al: Ultrasonographic evaluation of the adrenal glands in normal dogs and in dogs with hyperadrenocorticism. J Am Vet Med Assoc 207:1180, 1995.

Baxter JD, Tyrrell JB: The adrenal cortex. In Felig P, et al (eds): Endocrinology and Metabolism. New York, McGraw-Hill, 1981, p 385.

Becker M, Aron DC: Ectopic ACTH syndrome and CRH-mediated Cushing's syndrome. Endocrinol Metab Clin North Am 23:585, 1994.

Behrend EN, et al: Effect of storage conditions on cortisol, total thyroxine, and free thyroxine concentrations in serum and plasma of dogs. J Am Vet Med Assoc 212:1564, 1998.

Bencsik ZS, et al: Incidentally detected adrenal tumours (incidentalomas): histological heterogeneity and differentiated therapeutic approach. J Intern Med 237:585, 1995.

Berry CR, et al: Pulmonary mineralization in four dogs with Cushing's syndrome. Vet Radiol Ultrasound 35:10, 1994.

Berry CR, et al: Frequency of pulmonary mineralization and hypoxemia in 21 dogs with pituitary dependent hyperadrenocorticism. J Vet Intern Med 14:151, 2000.

Bertagna X: New causes of Cushing's syndrome. N Engl J Med 327:1024, 1992.

Bertagna X: Pro-opiomelanocortin–derived peptides. Endocrinol Metab Clin North Am 23:467, 1994.

Bertoy EH, et al: Magnetic resonance imaging of the brain in dogs with recently diagnosed but untreated pituitary-dependent hyperadrenocorticism. J Am Vet Med Assoc 206:651, 1995.

Bertoy EH, et al: One-year follow-up evaluation of magnetic resonance imaging of the brain in dogs with pituitary-dependent hyperadrenocorticism. J Am Vet Med Assoc 208:1268, 1996.

Besso JG, et al: Retrospective ultrasonographic evaluation of adrenal lesions in 26 dogs. Vet Radiol Ultrasound 38:448, 1997.

Biglieri EG, Kater CE: Mineralocorticoids. In Greenspan FS, Forsham PH (eds): Basic and Clinical Endocrinology. Los Altos, Calif, Lange Medical Publications, 1983, p 295.

Biller BMK: Pathogenesis of pituitary Cushing's syndrome: Pituitary versus hypothalamic. Endocrinol Metab Clin North Am 23:547, 1994.

Bodey AR, Michell AR: Epidemiological study of blood pressure in domestic dogs. J Small Anim Pract 37:116, 1996.

Bondanella M, et al: Evaluation of hormonal function in a series on incidentally discovered adrenal masses. Metabolism 46:107, 1997.

Bonneville JF, et al: Dynamic computed tomography of the pituitary gland: the "tuft sign." Radiology 149:145, 1983.

Braddock JA: Investigation of some alternative therapies for management of pituitary-dependent hyperadrenocorticism in the dog. Master's Thesis, Sidney, Australia, 2002, University of Sydney.

Breitschwerdt EB, et al: Idiopathic hyperaldosteronism in a dog. J Am Vet Med Assoc 187:841, 1985.

Bruyette DS, et al: L-Deprenyl therapy of canine pituitary-dependent hyperadrenocorticism. J Vet Intern Med 7:114, 1993 (abstract).

Bruyette DS, et al: Management of canine pituitary-dependent hyperadrenocorticism with L deprenyl. Vet Clin North Am (Small Anim Pract) 27:273, 1997.

Bunch SE, et al: Idiopathic pleural effusion and pulmonary thromboembolism in a dog with autoimmune hemolytic anemia. J Am Vet Med Assoc 195:1748, 1989.

Burns MG, et al: Pulmonary artery thrombosis in three dogs with hyperadrenocorticism. J Am Vet Med Assoc 178:388, 1981.

Castill V, et al: Aminoglutethimide: Therapeutic alternative in canines with Cushing's disease (hypophysis dependent). [Spanish] Avan Cienc Vet 11:93, 1996.

Chauvet AE, et al: Effects of phenobarbital administration on results of serum biochemical analyses and adrenocortical function tests in epileptic dogs. J Am Vet Med Assoc 207:1305, 1995.

Church DB, et al: Effect of nonadrenal illness, anaesthesia and surgery on plasma cortisol concentrations in dogs. Res Vet Sci 56:129, 1994.

Colao A, et al: Successful treatment of Cushing's disease evokes thyroid autoimmunity. Clin Endocrinol 53:13, 2000.

Contreras LN, et al: Urinary cortisol in the assessment of pituitary-adrenal function: Utility of 24-hour and spot determinations. J Clin Endocrinol Metab 62:965, 1986.

Contreras P, et al: Adrenal rest tumor of the liver causing Cushing's syndrome: Treatment with ketoconazole preceding an apparent surgical cure. J Clin Endocrinol Metab 60:21, 1985.

Daley CA, et al: Use of metyrapone to treat pituitary-dependent hyperadrenocorticism in a cat with large cutaneous wounds. J Am Vet Med Assoc 202:956, 1993.

Den Hertog E, et al: Results of nonselective adrenocorticolysis by o,p'-DDD in 129 dogs with pituitary-dependent hyperadrenocorticism. Vet Rec 144:12, 1999.

Dennis JS: Clinical features of canine pulmonary thromboembolism. Compend Cont Ed Sm Anim Pract 15:1595, 1993.

Dewis P, et al: Experience with trilostane in the treatment of Cushing's syndrome. Clin Endocrinol 18:533, 1983.

Dodam JR, et al: Duration of etomidate-induced adrenocortical suppression during surgery in dogs. Am J Vet Res 51:786, 1990.

Douglass JP, et al: Ultrasonographic adrenal gland measurements in dogs without evidence of adrenal disease. Vet Radiol Ultrasound 38:124, 1997.

Dow SW, et al: Perianal adenomas and hypertestosteronemia in a spayed bitch with pituitary-dependent hyperadrenocorticism. J Am Med Assoc 192:1439, 1988.

Dow SW, et al: Response of dogs with functional pituitary macroadenomas and macrocarcinomas to radiation. J Small Anim Pract 31:287, 1990.

Drake WM, et al: Emergency and prolonged use of intravenous etomidate to control hypercortisolemia in a patient with Cushing's syndrome and peritonitis. J Clin Endocrinol Metab 83:3542, 1998.

Drucker WD, Peterson ME: Pharmacologic treatment of pituitary-dependent canine Cushing's disease. Program of the Sixty-Second Annual Meeting of the Endocrine Society, San Francisco, 1980, p 89 (abstract).

Duesberg CA, et al: Magnetic resonance imaging for diagnosis of pituitary macrotumors in dogs. J Am Vet Med Assoc 206:657, 1995.

Dyer KR, et al: Effects of short- and long-term administration of phenobarbital on endogenous ACTH concentration and results of ACTH stimulation tests in dogs. J Am Vet Med Assoc 205:315, 1994.

Edelman RR, Warach S: Magnetic resonance imaging. N Engl J Med 328:708, 1993.

Eichenbaum JD, et al: Effect in large dogs of ophthalmic prednisolone acetate on adrenal gland and hepatic function. J Am Anim Hosp Assoc 24:705, 1988.

Elliott DA, et al: Glycosylated hemoglobin concentrations in the blood of healthy dogs and dogs with naturally developing diabetes mellitus, pancreatic β-cell neoplasia, hyperadrenocorticism, and anemia. J Am Vet Med Assoc 211:723, 1997.

Emms SG, et al: Evaluation of canine hyperadrenocorticism using computed tomography. J Am Vet Med Assoc 189:432, 1986.

Engelhardt D, et al: The influence of ketoconazole on cortisol secretion in Cushing's syndrome. Acta Endocrinol (Suppl) (Copenh) 256:281, 1983 (abstract).

Estrada J, et al: The long-term outcome of pituitary irradiation after unsuccessful transsphenoidal surgery in Cushing's disease. N Engl J Med 336:172, 1997.

Faglia G: Epidemiology and pathogenesis of pituitary adenomas. Acta Endocrinol 129(suppl 1):1, 1994.

Feldman BF, et al: Thrombotic disease in canine Cushing's syndrome. American College of Veterinary Internal Medicine Scientific Proceedings, Salt Lake City, 1982, p 84 (abstract).

Feldman BF, et al: Hemostatic abnormalities in canine Cushing's syndrome. Res Vet Sci 41:228, 1986.

Feldman EC: The effect of functional adrenocortical tumors on plasma cortisol and corticotropin concentrations in dogs. J Am Vet Med Assoc 178:823, 1981.

Feldman EC: Comparison of ACTH response and dexamethasone suppression as screening tests in canine hyperadrenocorticism. J Am Vet Med Assoc 182:505, 1983a.

Feldman EC: Distinguishing dogs with functioning adrenocortical tumors from dogs with pituitary-dependent hyperadrenocorticism. J Am Vet Med Assoc 183:195, 1983b.

Feldman EC: The adrenal cortex. In Ettinger SJ (ed): Textbook of Veterinary Internal Medicine, 2nd ed. Philadelphia, WB Saunders, 1983c, p 1650.

Feldman EC: Evaluation of a combined dexamethasone suppression/ACTH stimulation test in dogs with hyperadrenocorticism. J Am Vet Med Assoc 187:49, 1985.

Feldman EC: Evaluation of a 6-hour combined dexamethasone suppression/ACTH stimulation test in dogs with hyperadrenocorticism. J Am Vet Med Assoc 189:1562, 1986.

Feldman EC, Mack RE: Urine cortisol:creatinine ratio as a screening test for hyperadrenocorticism in dogs. J Am Vet Med Assoc 200:1637, 1992.

Feldman EC, Tyrrell JB: Plasma testosterone, plasma glucose, and plasma insulin concentrations in spontaneous canine Cushing's syndrome. The Endocrine Society, Salt Lake City, 1982, p 343 (abstract).

Feldman EC, et al: Comparison of aqueous porcine ACTH with synthetic ACTH in adrenal stimulation tests of the female dog. Am J Vet Res 43:522, 1982.

Feldman EC, et al: Plasma cortisol response to ketoconazole administration in dogs with hyperadrenocorticism. J Am Vet Med Assoc 197:71, 1990.

Feldman EC, et al: Comparison of mitotane treatment for adrenal tumor versus pituitary-dependent hyperadrenocorticism in dogs. J Am Vet Med Assoc 200:1642, 1992.

Feldman EC, et al: Use of low- and high-dose dexamethasone tests for distinguishing pituitary dependent from adrenal tumor hyperadrenocorticism. J Am Vet Med Assoc 209:772, 1996.

Ferguson DC: Thyroid function tests in the dog: Recent concepts. Vet Clin North Am (Small Anim Pract) 14:783, 1984.

Ferguson DC, Peterson ME: Serum free thyroxine concentrations in spontaneous canine hyperadrenocorticism. American College of Veterinary Internal Medicine Scientific Proceedings, Washington, DC, 1986 (abstract).

Fluckiger MA, Gomez JA: Radiographic findings in dogs with spontaneous pulmonary thrombosis or embolism. Vet Radiol 25:124, 1984.

Ford SL, et al: Hyperadrenocorticism caused by bilateral adrenocortical neoplasia in dogs: Four cases (1983-1988). J Am Vet Med Assoc 202:789, 1993.

Forrester SD, et al: Retrospective evaluation of urinary tract infection in 42 dogs with hyperadrenocorticism or diabetes mellitus or both. J Vet Intern Med 13:557, 1999.

Foster SF, et al: Effect of phenobarbitone on the low-dose dexamethasone suppression test and the urinary corticoid:creatinine ratio in dogs. Aust Vet J 78:19, 2000a.

Foster SF, et al: Effects of phenobarbitone on serum biochemical tests in dogs. Aust Vet J 78:23, 2000b.

Frank LA, Oliver JW: Comparison of serum cortisol concentrations in clinically normal dogs after administration of freshly reconstituted versus reconstituted and stored frozen cosyntropin. J Am Vet Med Assoc 212:1569, 1998.

Frank LA, et al: Cortisol concentrations following stimulation of healthy and adrenopathic dogs with two doses of tetracosactrin. J Small Anim Pract 41:308, 2000.

Frank LA, et al: Steroidogenic response of adrenal tissues after administration of ACTH to dogs with hypercortisolemia. J Am Vet Med Assoc 218:214, 2001.

Frazier KS, et al: Multiple cutaneous metaplastic ossification associated with iatrogenic hyperglucocorticoidism. J Vet Diagn Invest 10:303, 1998.

Galac S, et al: Urinary corticoid:creatinine ratios in the differentiation between pituitary dependent hyperadrenocorticism and hyperadrenocorticism due to adrenocortical tumour in the dog. Vet Q 19:17, 1997.

Ganguly A: Primary hyperaldosteronism. N Engl J Med 339:1828, 1998.

Gebhardt DOE, et al: Mitotane (o,p'-DDD) administration raises the serum level of high-density lipoprotein (HDL) in normotriglyceridemia. Horm Metab Res 25:440, 1993.

Geldof AA, et al: Inhibition of 3b-hydroxysteroid-dehydrogenase: an approach for prostate cancer treatment? Anticancer Res 15:1349, 1995.

Gicquel C, et al: Monoclonality of corticotroph macroadenomas in Cushing's disease. J Clin Endocrinol Metab 75:472, 1992.

Gieger TL, et al: Lymphoma as a model for chronic illness: Effects on adrenocortical function tests. J Vet Intern Med 16:374, 2002 (abstract).

Glaze MB, et al: Ophthalmic corticosteroid therapy: Systemic effects in the dog. J Am Vet Med Assoc 192:73, 1988.

Golden DL, Lothrop CD: A retrospective study of aldosterone secretion in normal and adrenopathic dogs. J Vet Intern Med 2:121, 1988.

Goldhaber SZ: Pulmonary embolism. N Engl J Med 339:93, 1998.

Goossens MMC, et al: Efficacy of cobalt 60 radiotherapy in dogs with pituitary-dependent hyperadrenocorticism. J Am Vet Med Assoc 212:374, 1998.

Gould SM, et al: Use of endogenous ACTH concentration and adrenal ultrasonography to distinguish the cause of canine hyperadrenocorticism. J Small Anim Pract 42:113, 2001.

Greco DS, et al: Pharmacokinetics of exogenous corticotropin in normal dogs, hospitalized dogs with nonadrenal illness, and adrenopathic dogs. J Vet Pharmacol Therap 21:369, 1998.

Greco DS, et al: Concurrent pituitary and adrenal tumors in dogs with hyperadrenocorticism: 17 cases (1978-1995). J Am Vet Med Assoc 214:1349, 1999.

Griffing GT, Melby JC: Reversal of diuretic-induced secondary hyperaldosteronism and hypokalemia by trilostane, an inhibitor of adrenal steroidogenesis. Metabolism 38:353, 1989.

Grooters AM, et al: Ultrasonographic parameters of normal canine adrenal glands: Comparison to necropsy findings. Vet Radiol Ultrasound 36:126, 1995.

Grooters AM, et al: Ultrasonographic characteristics of the adrenal glands in dogs with pituitary dependent hyperadrenocorticism: Comparison with normal dogs. J Vet Intern Med 10:110, 1996.

Guptill L, et al: Use of the urine cortisol:creatinine ratio to monitor treatment response in dogs with pituitary-dependent hyperadrenocorticism. J Am Vet Med Assoc 210:1158, 1997.

Halberg FE, Sheline GE: Radiotherapy in the treatment of pituitary tumors. Endocrinol Metab Clin North Am 16:667, 1987.

Halmi NS, et al: Pituitary intermediate lobe in the dog: Two cell types and high bioactive adrenocorticotropin content. Science 211:72, 1981.

Hamet P, et al: Cushing's syndrome with food-dependent periodic hormonogenesis. Clin Invest Met 10:530, 1987.

Hamper UM, et al: Primary adrenocortical carcinoma: Sonographic evaluation with clinical and pathologic correlation in 26 patients. Am J Roentgenol 148:915, 1987.

Hansen BL, et al: Synthetic ACTH (cosyntropin) stimulation tests in normal dogs: comparison of intravenous and intramuscular administration. J Am Anim Hosp Assoc 30:38, 1994.

Hegstad RL, et al: Effect of sample handling on adrenocorticotropin concentration measured in canine plasma, using a commercially available radioimmunoassay kit. Am J Vet Res 51:1941, 1990.

Hess RS, et al: Association between hyperadrenocorticism and development of calcium containing uroliths in dogs with urolithiasis. J Am Vet Med Assoc 212:1889, 1998.

Hill K, Scott-Moncrieff JC: Tumors of the adrenal cortex causing hyperadrenocorticism. Vet Med pg 685, 2001.

Hillier A, Desch CE: Large-bodied Demodex mite infestation in 4 dogs, J Am Vet Med Assoc 220:623, 2002.

Hoerauf A, Reusch C: Ultrasonographic characteristics of both adrenal glands in 15 dogs with functional adrenocortical tumors. J Am Anim Hosp Assoc 35:193, 1999.

Hoffmann WE, et al: A technique for automated quantification of canine glucocorticoid-induced isoenzyme of alkaline phosphatase. Vet Clin Pathol 17:66, 1988.

Holt E, et al: The prevalence of hyperadrenocorticism in dogs with sudden acquired retinal degeneration (SARD). J Vet Intern Med 13:272, 1999 (abstract).

Hughes D: Polyuria and polydipsia. Compend Contin Educ 14:1161, 1992.

Huntley K, et al: The radiological features of canine Cushing's syndrome: A review of forty-eight cases. J Small Anim Pract 23:369, 1982.

Hurley KJ, Vaden SL: Evaluation of urine protein content in dogs with pituitary-dependent hyperadrenocorticism. J Am Vet Med Assoc 212:369, 1998.

Hurley KJ, et al: The use of trilostane for the treatment of hyperadrenocorticism in dogs. J Vet Intern Med 12:210, 1998 (abstract).

Ibrahim NK, Buzdar AU: Aromatase inhibitors: current status. Am J Clin Oncol 18:407, 1995.

Jackson S, et al: Nature and control of peptide release from the pars intermedia. *In* Evered (ed): Peptides of the Pars Intermedia. London, Pitman, 1981, p 141.

Jacoby RC, et al: Biochemical basis for the hypercoagulable state seen in Cushing's syndrome. Arch Surg 139:1003, 2001.

Jensen AL, Poulsen JSD: Preliminary experience with the diagnostic value of the canine corticosteroid-induced alkaline phosphatase isoenzyme in hypercorticism and diabetes mellitus. J Vet Med Series A 39:342, 1992.

Jensen AL, et al: Evaluation of the urinary cortisol:creatinine ratio in the diagnosis of hyperadrenocorticism in dogs. J Small Anim Pract 38:99, 1997.

Johnson LR, et al: Pulmonary thromboembolism in 29 dogs: 1985-1995. J Vet Intern Med 13:338, 1999.

Johnston DE: Adrenalectomy in the dog. *In* Bojrab MJ (ed): Current Techniques in Small Animal Surgery. Philadelphia, Lea & Febiger, 1983, p 386.

Jones CA, et al: Changes in adrenal cortisol secretion as reflected in the urinary cortisol/creatinine ratio in dogs. Dom Anim Endocr 7:559, 1990.

Juchem M, Pollow K: Binding of oral contraceptive progestogens to serum proteins and cytoplasmic receptor. Am J Obstet Gynecol 163:2171, 1990.

Kallet A, Cowgill LD: Hypertensive states in the dog. Proceedings of the American College of Veterinary Internal Medicine, Salt Lake City, 1982, p 79.

Kantrowitz BM, et al: Adrenal ultrasonography in the dog. Vet Radiol 27:15, 1986.

Kaplan AJ, et al: Effects of disease on the results of diagnostic tests for use in detecting hyperadrenocorticism in dogs. J Am Vet Med Assoc 207:445, 1995.

Kemppainen RJ, Peterson ME: Circulating concentration of dexamethasone in healthy dogs, dogs with hyperadrenocorticism, and dogs with nonadrenal illness during dexamethasone suppression testing. Am J Vet Res 54:1765, 1993.

Kemppainen RJ, Sartin JL: Evidence for episodic but not circadian activity in plasma concentrations of adrenocorticotropin, cortisol and thyroxine in dogs. J Endocrinol 103:219, 1984.

Kemppainen RJ, Sartin JL: Differential regulation of peptide release by the canine pars distalis and pars intermedia. Front Horm Res 17:18, 1987.

Kemppainen RJ, Zenoble RD: Non–dexamethasone-suppressible, pituitary-dependent hyperadrenocorticism in a dog. J Am Vet Med Assoc 187:276, 1985.

Kemppainen RJ, et al: Regulation of adrenocorticotropin secretion from cultured canine anterior pituitary cells. Am J Vet Res 53:2355, 1992.

Kemppainen RJ, et al: Aprotinin preserves immunoreactive adrenocorticotropin in canine plasma. J Vet Intern Med 8:163, 1994a (abstract).

Kemppainen RJ, et al: Preservative effect of aprotinin on canine plasma immunoreactive adrenocorticotropin concentrations. Dom Anim Endocr 11:355, 1994b.

Kerl ME, et al: Evaluation of a low-dose synthetic adrenocorticotropic hormone stimulation test in clinically normal dogs and dogs with naturally developing hyperadrenocorticism. J Am Vet Med Assoc 214:1497, 1999.

King RR, et al: Pulmonary function studies in a dog with pulmonary thromboembolism associated with Cushing's disease. J Am Anim Hosp Assoc 21:555, 1985.

Kintzer PP, Peterson ME: Mitotane (o,p'-DDD) treatment of 200 dogs with pituitary-dependent hyperadrenocorticism. J Vet Intern Med 5:182, 1991.

Kintzer PP, Peterson ME: Mitotane (o,p'DDD) treatment of dogs with cortisol-secreting adrenocortical neoplasia: 32 cases (1980-1992). J Am Vet Med Assoc 205:54, 1994.

Kippenes H, et al: Mensuration of the normal pituitary gland from magnetic resonance images in 96 dogs. Vet Radiol Ultrasound 42:130, 2001.

Kipperman BS, et al: Pituitary tumor size, neurologic signs, and relation to endocrine test results in dogs with pituitary-dependent hyperadrenocorticism: 43 cases (1980-1990). J Am Vet Med Assoc 201:762, 1992.

Kirk GR, Jensen HE: Toxic effects of o,p'-DDD in the normal dog. J Am Anim Hosp Assoc 11:765, 1975.

Klein MK, et al: Pulmonary thromboembolism associated with immune-mediated hemolytic anemia in dogs: Ten cases (1982-1987). J Am Vet Med Assoc 195:246, 1989.

Klibanski A, Zervas NT: Diagnosis and management of hormone-secreting pituitary adenomas. N Engl J Med 324:822, 1991.

Kolevska F, Svoboda M: Immunoreactive cortisol measurement in canine urine and its validity in hyperadrenocorticism diagnosis. Acta Vet Brno 69:217, 2000.

Komanicky P, et al: Treatment of Cushing's syndrome with trilostane (WIN 24,540), an inhibitor of adrenal steroid biosynthesis. J Clin Endocrinol Metab 47:1042, 1978.

Kooistra HS, et al: Correlation between impairment of glucocorticoid feedback and the size of the pituitary gland in dogs with pituitary-dependent hyperadrenocorticism. J Endocrinol 152:387, 1997.

Kornegay JN: Imaging brain neoplasms, computed tomography and magnetic resonance imaging. Vet Med Rep 2:372, 1990.

Kraft SL, et al: Canine brain anatomy on magnetic resonance images. Vet Radiol 30:147, 1989.

Krieger DT: Physiopathology of Cushing's disease. Endocr Rev 4:22, 1983.

Lacoste D, et al: Effect of 3-week treatment with [d-Trp, des-Gly-NH2] LHRH ethylamide, aminoglutethimide, ketoconazole, or flutamide alone or in combination on testicular, serum, adrenal and prostatic steroid levels in the dog. J Steroid Biochem 33:233, 1989.

Lacroix A, et al: Gastric inhibitory polypeptide-dependent cortisol hypersecretion: A new cause of Cushing's syndrome. N Engl J Med 327:974, 1992.

Lacroix A, et al: Propranolol therapy for ectopic b-adrenergic receptors in adrenal Cushing's syndrome. N Engl J Med 337:1429, 1997.

Landolt AM: Transsphenoidal surgery of pituitary tumors: Its pitfalls and complications. Prog Neurol Surg 13:1, 1990.

Lantz GC, et al: Transsphenoidal hypophysectomy in the clinically normal dog. Am J Vet Res 49:1134, 1988.

LaRue MJ, Murtaugh RJ: Pulmonary thromboembolism in dogs: 47 cases (1986-1987). J Am Vet Med Assoc 197:1368, 1990.

Laue L, et al: Effect of chronic treatment with the glucocorticoid antagonist RU 486 in man: Toxicity, immunological, and hormonal aspects. J Clin Endocrinol Metab 71:1474, 1990.

Leinung MC, Zimmerman D: Cushing's syndrome in children. Endocrinol Metab Clin North Am 23:629, 1994.

Leroy J, Feldman EC: Clinical comparison of dogs with pituitary-dependent hyperadrenocorticism of pars distalis versus pars intermedia origin. Proceedings of the Seventh ACVIM Forum, San Diego, Calif, 1989, p 1034 (abstract).

Littley MD, et al: Long-term follow-up of low-dose external pituitary irradiation for Cushing's disease. Clin Endocrinol (Oxf) 33:445, 1990.

Littman MP, et al: Spontaneous systemic hypertension in dogs: Five cases (1981-1983). J Am Vet Med Assoc 193:486, 1988.

Loli P, et al: Use of ketoconazole in the treatment of Cushing's syndrome. J Clin Endocrinol Metab 63:1365, 1986.

Lothrop CD, Oliver JW: Diagnosis of canine Cushing's syndrome based on multiple steroid analysis and dexamethasone turnover kinetics. Am J Vet Res 45:2304, 1984.

Love NE, et al: The computed tomographic enhancement pattern of the normal canine pituitary gland. Vet Radiol Ultrasound 41:507, 2000.

Lucena R, et al: Effects of haemolysis, lipaemia and bilirubinaemia on an enzyme-linked immunosorbent assay for cortisol and free thyroxine in serum samples from dogs. Vet J 156:127, 1998.

Lulich JP, Osborne CA: Bacterial infections of the urinary tract. *In* Ettinger SJ, Feldman EC (eds): Textbook of Veterinary Medicine. Philadelphia, WB Saunders, 1994, p 1775.

Mack RE, Feldman EC: Comparison of two low-dose dexamethasone suppression protocols as screening and discrimination tests in dogs with hyperadrenocorticism. J Am Vet Med Assoc 197:1603, 1990.

Magiakou MA, et al: Cushing's syndrome in children and adolescents. N Engl J Med 331:629, 1994.

Maher VMG, et al: Possible mechanism and treatment of o,p'-DDD–induced hypercholesterolemia. Q J Med 305:671, 1992.

Malchoff CD, et al: Adrenocorticotropin-independent bilateral macronodular adrenal hyperplasia: An unusual cause of Cushing's syndrome. J Clin Endocrinol Metab 68:855, 1989.

Mampalam TJ, et al: Transsphenoidal microsurgery for Cushing's disease: A report of 216 cases. Ann Intern Med 109:487, 1988.

Mattson A, et al: Clinical features suggesting hyperadrenocorticism associated with sudden acquired retinal degeneration syndrome in a dog. J Am Anim Hosp Assoc 28:199, 1992.

McCance DR, et al: Clinical experience with ketoconazole as a therapy for patients with Cushing's syndrome. Clin Endocrinol 27:593, 1987.

McLeod MK: Complications following adrenal surgery. J Natl Med Assoc 83:161, 1991.

McNicol AM: Pituitary morphology in canine pituitary-dependent hyperadrenocorticism. Front Horm Res 17:71, 1987.

Meaney JFM, et al: Diagnosis of pulmonary embolism with magnetic resonance angiography. N Engl J Med 336:1422, 1997.

Meij BP, et al: Residual pituitary function after transsphenoidal hypophysectomy in dogs with pituitary-dependent hyperadrenocorticism. J Endocrinol 155:531, 1997a.

Meij BP, et al: Transsphenoidal hypophysectomy in Beagle dogs: Evaluation of a microsurgical technique. Vet Surg 26:295, 1997b.

Meij BP, et al: Alterations in anterior pituitary function of dogs with pituitary-dependent hyperadrenocorticism. J Endocrinol 154:505, 1997c.

Meij BP, et al: Results of transsphenoidal hypophysectomy in 52 dogs with pituitary-dependent hyperadrenocorticism. Vet Surg 27:246, 1998.

Meij BP, et al: Progress in transsphenoidal hypophysectomy for treatment of pituitary-dependent hyperadrenocorticism in dogs and cats. Molec Cell Endocrinol 197:89, 2002.

Meijer JC: Canine hyperadrenocorticism. *In* Kirk RW (ed): Current Veterinary Therapy VII. Philadelphia, WB Saunders, 1980, p 975.

Melby JC: Therapy of Cushing's disease: A consensus for pituitary microsurgery. Ann Intern Med 109:445, 1988.

Melby JC: Clinical Review 1: Endocrine hypertension. J Clin Endocrinol Metab 69:697, 1989.

Montgomery TM, et al: Basal and glucagon-stimulated plasma C peptide concentrations in healthy dogs, dogs with diabetes mellitus, and dogs with hyperadrenocorticism. J Vet Intern Med 10:116, 1996.

Moon PF: Cortisol suppression in cats after induction of anesthesia with etomidate compared with ketamine-diazepam combination. Am J Vet Res 58:868, 1997.

Moore GE, Hoenig M: Duration of pituitary and adrenocortical suppression after long-term administration of antiinflammatory doses of prednisone in dogs. Am J Vet Res 53:716, 1992.

Moore LE, et al: Hyperadrenocorticism treated with metyrapone followed by bilateral adrenalectomy in a cat. J Am Vet Med Assoc 217:691, 2000.

Muller PB, et al: Effects of long-term phenobarbital treatment on the thyroid and adrenal axis and adrenal function tests in dogs. J Vet Intern Med 14:157, 2000a.

Muller PB, et al: Effects of long-term phenobarbital treatment on the liver in dogs. J Vet Intern Med 14:165, 2000b.

Murase T, et al: Measurement of serum glucocorticoids by high-performance liquid chromatography and circadian rhythm patterns of the cortisol value in normal dogs. Jpn J Vet Sci 50:1133, 1988.

Murayama M, et al: Long term follow-up of Cushing's disease treated with reserpine and pituitary irradiation. J Clin Endocrinol Metab 75:935, 1992.

Murphy CJ, et al: Iatrogenic Cushing's syndrome in a dog caused by topical ophthalmic medications. J Am Anim Hosp Assoc 26:640, 1990.

Nazeyrollas P, et al: Diagnostic accuracy of echocardiography-Doppler in acute pulmonary embolism. Int J Cardiol 47:273, 1995.

Neiger R, Hurley K: Twenty-four-hour cortisol values in dogs with hyperadrenocorticism on trilostane. J Small Anim Pract 42:376, 2001 (abstract).

Neiger R, et al: Trilostane treatment of 78 dogs with pituitary-dependent hyperadrenocorticism. Vet Rec 150:799, 2002.

Nelson AA, Woodard G: Severe adrenal cortical atrophy (cytotoxic) and hepatic damage produced in dogs by feeding 2,2-bis (parachlorophenyl)-1, 1-trichloroethane (DDD or TDE). Arch Pathol 48:387, 1949.

Nelson RW, et al: Effect of o,p'-DDD therapy on endogenous ACTH concentrations in dogs with hypophysis-dependent hyperadrenocorticism. Am J Vet Res 46:1534, 1985.

Nelson RW, et al: Pituitary macroadenomas and macroadenocarcinomas in dogs treated with mitotane for pituitary-dependent hyperadrenocorticism: 13 cases (1981-1986). J Am Vet Med Assoc 194:1612, 1989.

Nichols R: Concurrent illness and complications associated with canine hyperadrenocorticism. Proceedings of the Tenth ACVIM Forum, San Diego, Calif, 1992, p 357.

Niebauer GW, Evans SM: Transsphenoidal hypophysectomy in the dog: A new technique. Vet Surg 17:296, 1988.

Niebauer GW, et al: Study of long-term survival after transsphenoidal hypophysectomy in clinically normal dogs. Am J Vet Res 51:677, 1990.

Norman EJ, et al: Dynamic adrenal function testing in eight dogs with hyperadrenocorticism associated with adrenocortical neoplasia. Vet Rec 144:551, 1999.

Nyland T: Personal communication, May 2003.

Oluju MP, et al: Simple quantitative assay for canine steroid-induced alkaline phosphatase. Vet Rec 115:17, 1984.

Ortega T, et al: Evaluation of fasting serum lipid profiles in dogs with Cushing's syndrome. J Vet Intern Med 9:182, 1995a (abstract).

Ortega T, et al: Plasma aldosterone concentrations in dogs before and after o,p'-DDD therapy for pituitary-dependent hyperadrenocorticism. J Vet Intern Med 9:182, 1995b (abstract).

Ortega T, et al: Systemic arterial blood pressure and urine protein/creatinine ratio in dogs with hyperadrenocorticism. J Am Vet Med Assoc 209:1724, 1996.

Orth DN: Cushing's syndrome. N Engl J Med 332:791, 1995.

Orth DN, et al: The adrenal cortex. In Wilson JD, Forster DW (eds): Williams Textbook of Endocrinology. 9th ed. Philadelphia, WB Saunders, 1998, p 590.

Patrassi GM, et al: Further studies on the hypercoagulable state of patients with Cushing's syndrome. Thromb Haemost 54:518, 1985.

Penninck DG, et al: Radiologic features of canine hyperadrenocorticism caused by autonomously functioning adrenocortical tumors: 23 cases (1978-1986). J Am Vet Med Assoc 192:1604, 1988.

Peterson ME: Hyperadrenocorticism. Vet Clin North Am (Small Anim Pract) 14:731, 1984.

Peterson ME: Pathophysiology of canine pituitary-dependent hyperadreno-corticism. Front Horm Res 17:37, 1987.

Peterson ME: Medical treatment of pituitary-dependent hyperadreno-corticism in dogs: Should L deprenyl ever be used? J Vet Intern Med 13:289, 1999 (editorial).

Peterson ME, Drucker WD: Cyproheptadine treatment of spontaneous pituitary-ACTH dependent canine Cushing's disease. Clin Res 26:703A, 1978 (abstract).

Peterson ME, et al: Immunocytochemical study of the hypophysis in 25 dogs with pituitary-dependent hyperadrenocorticism. Acta Endocrinol 101:15, 1982a.

Peterson ME, et al: Plasma cortisol response to exogenous ACTH in 22 dogs with hyperadrenocorticism caused by an adrenocortical neoplasia. J Am Vet Med Assoc 180:542, 1982b.

Peterson ME, et al: Effects of spontaneous hyperadrenocorticism on serum thyroid hormone concentrations in the dog. Am J Vet Res 45:2034, 1984.

Peterson ME, et al: Plasma immunoreactive pro-opiomelanocortin peptides and cortisol in normal dogs and dogs with Addison's disease and Cushing's syndrome: Basal concentrations. Endocrinology 119:720, 1986.

Poffenbarger EM, et al: Gray-scale ultrasonography in the diagnosis of adrenal neoplasia in dogs: Six cases (1981-1986). J Am Vet Med Assoc 192:228, 1988.

Potts GO, et al: Trilostane, an orally active inhibitor of steroid biosynthesis. Steroids 32:257, 1978.

Raff H: Glucocorticoid inhibition of neurohypophyseal vasopressin secretion. Am J Physiol 252:R635, 1987.

Ramsey CC, et al: Use of streptokinase in four dogs with thrombosis. J Am Vet Med Assoc 209:780, 1996.

Randolph JF, et al: Use of the urinary corticoid:creatinine ratio for monitoring dogs with pituitary-dependent hyperadrenocorticism during induction treatment with mitotane (o,p'-DDD). Am J Vet Res 59:258, 1998.

Reicke M, et al: Deletion of the adrenocorticotropin receptor gene in human adrenocortical tumors: Implications for tumorigenesis. J Clin Endocrinol Metab 82:3054, 1997.

Reimers TJ, et al: Effects of hemolysis and storage on quantification of hormones in blood samples from dogs, cattle, and horses. Am J Vet Res 52:1075, 1991.

Reine NJ, et al: Deoxycortisone-secreting adrenocortical carcinoma in a dog. J Vet Intern Med 13:386, 1999.

Reitmeyer M, et al: The neurosurgical management of Cushing's disease. Molec Cell Endocrinol 197:73, 2002.

Remillard RL, et al: Variance of indirect blood pressure measurements and prevalence of hypertension in clinically normal dogs. Am J Vet Res 52:561, 1991.

Reusch CE: Hyperadrenocorticism. In Ettinger SE and Feldman EC (eds): Textbook of Veterinary Internal Medicine, 6th ed. Philadelphia, Saunders, 2005.

Reusch CE, Feldman EC: Canine hyperadrenocorticism due to adrenocortical neoplasia. J Vet Intern Med 5:3, 1991.

Reusch CE, et al: Monitoring of individual response to o,p'-DDD during initial therapy in dogs with pituitary dependent hyperadrenocorticism. J Vet Intern Med 9:186, 1995 (abstract).

Reusch CE, et al: The efficacy of L-deprenyl in dogs with pituitary-dependent hyperadrenocorticism. J Vet Intern Med 13:291, 1999.

Rewerts JM, et al: Atraumatic rupture of the gastrocnemius muscle after corticosteroid administration in a dog. J Am Vet Med Assoc 210:655, 1997.

Reznik Y, et al: Food-dependent Cushing's syndrome mediated by aberrant adrenal sensitivity to gastric inhibitory polypeptide. N Engl J Med 327:981, 1992.

Rijnberk A, Belshaw BE: An alternative protocol for the medical management of canine pituitary-dependent hyperadrenocorticism. Vet Rec 122:486, 1988.

Rijnberk A, et al: Assessment of two tests for the diagnosis of canine hyper-adrenocorticism. Vet Rec 122:178, 1988a.

Rijnberk A, et al: Effects of bromocriptine on corticotropin, melanotropin, and corticosteroid secretion in dogs with pituitary-dependent hyperadreno-corticism. J Endocrinol 118:271, 1988b.

Rijnberk A, et al: Corticoid production by four dogs with hyperfunctioning adrenocortical tumours during treatment with mitotane (o,p'-DDD). Vet Rec 131:484, 1993.

Rijnberk A, et al: Aldosteronoma in a dog with polyuria as the leading symptom. J Vet Intern Med (in press).

Ristic JME, et al: The use of 17-hydroxyprogesterone in the diagnosis of canine hyperadrenocorticism. J Vet Intern Med 16:433, 2002.

Roberts SM, et al: Effect of ophthalmic prednisolone acetate on the canine adrenal gland and hepatic function. Am J Vet Res 45:1711, 1984.

Robinson DT, et al: The bioavailability and metabolism of trilostane in normal subjects: A comparative study using high-pressure liquid chromatographic and quantitative cytochemical assays. J Steroid Biochem 21:601, 1984.

Romantowski J: Iatrogenic adrenocortical insufficiency in dogs. J Am Vet Med Assoc 196:1144, 1990.

Ross NS, Aron DC: Hormonal evaluation of the patient with an incidentally discovered adrenal mass. N Engl J Med 323:1401, 1990.

Ruckstuhl NS, et al: Results of clinical examinations, laboratory tests, and ultrasonography in dogs with pituitary-dependent hyperadrenocorticism treated with trilostane. Am J Vet Res 63:506, 2002.

Rush JE: Vascular disease. Proceedings of the Eighth ACVIM Forum, Washington, DC, 1990, p281.

Rutgers HC, et al: Subcellular pathologic features of glucocorticoid-induced hepatopathy in dogs. Am J Vet Res 56:898, 1995.

Safarty D, et al: Neurologic, endocrinologic, and pathologic findings associated with large pituitary tumors in dogs: Eight cases (1976-1984). J Am Vet Med Assoc 193:854, 1988.

Samuels MH, Loriaux DL: Cushing's syndrome and the nodular adrenal. Endocrinol Metab Clin North Am 23:555, 1994.

Scavelli TD, et al: Results of surgical treatment for hyperadrenocorticism caused by adrenocortical neoplasia in the dog: 25 cases (1980-1984). J Am Vet Med Assoc 189:1360, 1986.

Schechter RD, et al: Treatment of Cushing's syndrome in the dog with an adrenocorticolytic agent (o,p'-DDD). J Am Vet Med Assoc 162:629, 1973.

Schlaghecke R, et al: The effect of long-term glucocorticoid therapy on pituitary-adrenal responses to exogenous corticotropin-releasing hormone. N Engl J Med 326:226, 1992.

Schwartz A: Endocrine surgery. In Lipowitz AJ, et al (eds): Complications in Small Animal Surgery: Diagnosis, Management, Prevention. Baltimore, Williams & Wilkins, 1996, p 287.

Schwarz T, et al: Osteopenia and other radiographic signs in canine hyperadrenocorticism. J Small Anim Pract 41:491, 2000.

Selman PJ, et al: Effects of progestin administration on the hypothalamic-pituitary-adrenal axis and glucose homeostasis in dogs. J Reprod Fertil Suppl 51:345, 1997.

Shiffman F, et al: Treatment of canine embolic pulmonary hypertension with recombinant tissue plasminogen activator: Efficacy of dosing regimes. Circulation 19:214, 1988.

Silvestre L, et al: Voluntary interruption of pregnancy with mifepristone (RU486) and a prostaglandin analogue. N Engl J Med 322:645, 1990.

Small M, et al: Thromboembolic complications in Cushing's syndrome. Clin Endocrinol 19:503, 1983.

Smiley LE, Garvey MS: The use of hetastarch as adjunct therapy in 26 dogs with hypoalbuminemia: A phase two clinical trial. J Vet Intern Med 8:195, 1994.

Smiley LE, Peterson ME: Evaluation of a urine cortisol:creatinine ratio as a screening test for hyperadrenocorticism in dogs. J Vet Intern Med 7:163, 1993.

Solter PF, et al: Assessment of corticosteroid-induced alkaline phosphatase isoenzyme as a screening test for hyperadrenocorticism in dogs. J Am Vet Med Assoc 203:534, 1994a.

Solter PF, et al: Hepatic total 3-alpha-hydroxy bile acid concentration and enzyme activities in prednisone-treated dogs. Am J Vet Res 55:1086, 1994b.

Sonino N, et al: Prolonged treatment of Cushing's disease by ketoconazole. J Clin Endocrinol Metab 61:718, 1985.

Spitz IM, Bardin CW: Mifepristone (RU486): A modulator of progestin and glucocorticoid action. N Engl J Med 329:404, 1993.

Stein PD, et al: Clinical, laboratory, roentgenographic, and electrocardiographic findings in patients with acute pulmonary embolism and no preexisting cardiac or pulmonary disease. Chest 100:598, 1991.

Stepien RL, Rapoport GS: Clinical comparison of three methods to measure blood pressure in nonsedated dogs. J Am Vet Med Assoc 215:1623, 1999.

Sterczer A, et al: Fast resolution of hypercortisolism in dogs with portosystemic encephalopathy after surgical shunt closure. Res Vet Sci 66:63, 1998.

Stolp R, et al: Urinary corticoids in the diagnosis of canine hyperadrenocorticism. Res Vet Sci 34:141, 1983.

Stolp R, et al: Results of cyproheptadine treatment in dogs with pituitary-dependent hyperadrenocorticism. J Endocrinol 101:311, 1984.

Syme HM, et al: Hyperadrenocorticism associated with excessive sex hormone production by an adrenocortical tumor in two dogs. J Am Vet Med Assoc 219:1725, 2001.

Teske E, et al: Separation and heat stability of the corticosteroid-induced and hepatic alkaline phosphatase isoenzymes in canine plasma. J Chromatogr 369:349, 1986.

Teske E, et al: Corticosteroid-induced alkaline phosphatase isoenzyme in the diagnosis of canine hypercortism. Vet Rec 125:12, 1989.

Theon AP, Feldman EC: Megavoltage irradiation of pituitary macrotumors in dogs with neurologic signs. J Am Vet Med Assoc 213:225, 1998.

Thorner MO, et al: Approach to pituitary disease. In Wilson JD, Foster DW (eds): Williams Textbook of Endocrinology, 8th ed. Philadelphia, WB Saunders, 1992, p 246.

Tobin R, et al: Treatment of pituitary-dependent hyperadrenocorticism in dogs using pergolide mesylate. J Vet Intern Med 12:245, 1998 (abstract).

Torres SMF, et al: Effect of oral administration of prednisolone on thyroid function in dogs. Am J Vet Res 52:412, 1991.

Totani Y, et al: Effect of metyrapone pretreatment on adrenocorticotropin secretion induced by corticotropin-releasing hormone in normal subjects and patients with Cushing's disease. J Clin Endocrinol Metab 70:798, 1990.

Toth M, et al: Comparative analysis of plasma 17-hydroxyprogesterone and cortisol responses to ACTH in patients with various adrenal tumors before and after unilateral adrenalectomy. J Endocrinol Invest 23:287, 2000.

Toutain PL, et al: Pharmacokinetics of dexamethasone and its effect on adrenal gland function in the dog. Am J Vet Res 44:212, 1983.

Tran LM, et al: Radiation therapy of pituitary tumors: Results in 95 cases. Am J Clin Oncol 14:25, 1991.

Turrel JM, et al: Computed tomographic characteristics of primary brain tumors in 50 dogs. J Am Vet Med Assoc 188:851, 1986.

Turton DB, et al: Incidental adrenal nodules: Association with exaggerated 17 hydroxyprogesterone response to adrenocorticotropic hormone. J Endocrinol Invest 15:789, 1992.

Tyrrell JB, et al: Glucocorticoids and adrenal androgens. In Greenspan FS (ed): Basic and Clinical Endocrinology, 3rd ed. Los Altos, Calif, Lange Medical Publications, 1991, p 323.

Van Cauter E, Refetoff S: Evidence for two subtypes of Cushing's disease based on the analysis of episodic cortisol secretion. N Engl J Med 312:1343, 1985.

van der Vlugt-Meijer RH, et al: Dynamic computed tomography of the pituitary gland in dogs with pituitary-dependent hyperadrenocorticism (Cushing's disease). J Am Vet Med Assoc (in press).

Van Liew CH, et al: Comparison of results of adrenocorticotropic hormone stimulation and low dose dexamethasone suppression tests with necropsy finding in dogs: 81 cases (1985-1995). J Am Vet Med Assoc 211:322, 1997.

Van Sluijs FJ, et al: Results of adrenalectomy in 36 dogs with hyperadrenocorticism caused by adrenocortical tumour. Vet Q 17:113, 1995.

Van Vonderen IK, et al: Influence of veterinary care on the urinary corticoid:creatinine ratio in dogs. J Vet Intern Med 12:431, 1998.

van Wijk PA, et al: Corticotropin-releasing hormone and adrenocorticotropic hormone concentrations in cerebrospinal fluid of dogs with pituitary-dependent hyperadrenocorticism. Endocrinology 131:2659, 1992.

van Wijk PA, et al: Responsiveness to corticotropin-releasing hormone and vasopressin in canine Cushing's syndrome. Eur J Endocrinol 130:410, 1994.

Vanden Bossche H, et al: From 14a-demethylase inhibitors in fungal cells to androgen and estrogen biosynthesis inhibitors in mammalian cells. Biochem Soc Trans 18:10, 1990.

Vandenbergh GGD, et al: Haemorrhage from a canine adrenocortical tumour: A clinical emergency. Vet Rec 13:539, 1992.

Vassilopoulou-Sellin R, Samaan A: Mitotane administration: An unusual cause of hypercholesterolemia. Horm Metab 23:619, 1991.

Verhelst JA, et al: Short- and long-term responses to metyrapone in the medical management of 91 patients with Cushing's syndrome. Clin Endocrinol 35:169, 1991.

Vollmar AM, et al: Atrial natriuretic peptide concentration in dogs with congestive heart failure, chronic renal failure, and hyperadrenocorticism. Am J Vet Res 52:1831, 1991.

Von Dehn BJ, et al: Pheochromocytoma in 6 dogs with naturally acquired hyperadrenocorticism: 1982-1992. J Am Vet Med Assoc 207:322, 1995.

Voorhout G: Cisternography combined with linear tomography for visualization of the pituitary gland in healthy dogs. Vet Radiol 31:68, 1990a.

Voorhout G: X-ray-computed tomography, nephrotomography, and ultrasonography of the adrenal glands of healthy dogs. Am J Vet Res 51:625, 1990b.

Voorhout G, et al: Assessment of survey radiography and comparison with x-ray computed tomography for detection of hyperfunctioning adrenocortical tumors in dogs. J Am Vet Med Assoc 196:1799, 1990a.

Voorhout G, et al: Nephrotomography and ultrasonography for the localization of hyperfunctioning adrenocortical tumors in dogs. Am J Vet Res 51:1280, 1990b.

Ward DA, et al: Band keratopathy associated with hyperadrenocorticism in the dog. J Am Anim Hosp Assoc 25:583, 1989.

Watson ADJ, et al: Systemic availability of o,p'-DDD in normal dogs, fasted and fed, and in dogs with hyperadrenocorticism. Res Vet Sci 43:160, 1987.

Watson ADJ, et al: Plasma cortisol responses to three corticotrophic preparations in normal dogs. Aust Vet J 76:255, 1998.

West JB: Pulmonary Pathology: The Essentials, 4th ed. Baltimore, Williams & Wilkins, 1992, p51.

White PC: Disorders of aldosterone biosynthesis and action. N Engl J Med 331:250, 1994.

White SD, et al: Cutaneous markers of canine hyperadrenocorticism. Compend Contin Educ 11:446, 1989.

Whittemore JC, et al: Nontraumatic rupture of an adrenal gland tumor causing intraabdominal or retroperitoneal hemorrhage in four dogs. J Am Vet Med Assoc 219:329, 2001.

Widmer WR, Guptill L: Imaging techniques for facilitating diagnosis of hyperadrenocorticism in dogs and cats. J Am Vet Med Assoc 206:1857, 1995.

Wiedmeyer CE, et al: Alkaline phosphatase expression in tissues from glucocorticoid-treated dogs. Am J Vet Res 63:1083, 2002.

Willenberg HS, et al: Aberrant interleukin-1 receptors in a cortisol-secreting adrenal adenoma causing Cushing's syndrome. N Engl J Med 339:27, 1998.

Wilson SM, Feldman EC: Diagnostic value of the steroid-induced isoenzyme of alkaline phosphatase in the dog. J Am Anim Hosp Assoc 28:245, 1992.

Yamaji T, et al: Plasma levels of atrial natriuretic hormone in Cushing's syndrome. J Clin Endocrinol Metab 67:348, 1988.

Zenoble RD, Kemppainen RJ: Adrenocortical suppression by topically applied corticosteroids in healthy dogs. J Am Vet Med Assoc 191:685, 1987.

Zerbe CA: Etiology of pituitary dependent hyperadrenocorticism. Proceedings of the Tenth ACVIM Forum, San Diego, Calif, 1992, p 360.

Zerbe CA: Screening tests to diagnose hyperadrenocorticism in cats and dogs. Compend Contin Educ 22:17, 2000a.

Zerbe CA: Differentiating tests to evaluate hyperadrenocorticism in dogs and cats. Compend Contin Educ 22:149, 2000b.

Zerbe CA, et al: Use of metyrapone for differentiation of spontaneous hyperadrenocorticism in the dog. American College of Veterinary Internal Medicine Scientific Proceedings, Washington, DC, 1986 (abstract).

Zerbe CA, et al: Adrenal function in 15 dogs with insulin-dependent diabetes mellitus. J Am Vet Med Assoc 193:454, 1988.

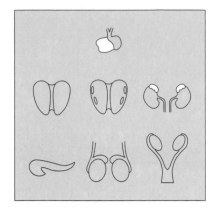

7

HYPERADRENOCORTICISM IN CATS (CUSHING'S SYNDROME)

In 1932, Dr. Harvey Cushing authored a report in which he described a group of people with a disorder that he suggested was "the result of pituitary basophilism." Subsequent study of the clinical, biochemical, and histologic features of these individuals indicate that each had been afflicted with a syndrome resulting from chronic exposure to excesses in circulating cortisol concentrations. The eponym *Cushing's syndrome* is an "umbrella" term referring to this condition (hyperadrenocorticism) in people and, more recently, in animals. Chronic cortisol excess may occur secondary to iatrogenic cortisol administration, or it may occur with naturally occurring disease. Thus a pathophysiologic classification of causes for Cushing's syndrome includes several different conditions. In addition to the iatrogenic condition, the naturally occurring disorder can be caused by a pituitary tumor secreting excess ACTH with subsequent adrenocortical hyperplasia and excess adrenocortical cortisol secretion. The other common naturally occurring condition in animals is that caused by an autonomously functioning, cortisol-secreting, adrenocortical tumor. As discussed later, adrenocortical tumors

possess the ability to synthesize steroid hormones other than cortisol. Such cortisol-secreting tumors have been documented in cats together with two additional syndromes (progesterone and aldosterone excess).

ACTH-secreting pituitary tumors have been demonstrated to be the result of an aberrant single cell line that autonomously secretes ACTH in excess, which in turn causes chronic cortisol excess and adrenocortical hyperplasia. This is a relatively uncommon but well-described disease in humans. Autonomous cortisol-secreting primary adrenocortical tumors are also well described in humans, cause cortisol excesses, and occur less frequently than the pituitary-dependent disease. Iatrogenic cortisol excess due to chronic administration of ACTH does not occur, but chronic administration of glucocorticoids is a common cause of Cushing's syndrome. Other forms of this syndrome have been described, but these are rare and of little importance in veterinary medicine.

Veterinary medicine, especially canine and feline veterinary medicine, has received support from studies describing conditions, diagnoses, and management of diseases acquired by human beings. Thus studies by physicians have been of great benefit to veterinarians. Human beings are the animal model most frequently studied by veterinarians. In many situations, what has been learned about people is then applied to dogs. Often, what has been learned and applied to dogs is then applied to cats. In some situations, illnesses in cats may be analogous to conditions in dogs, whereas other illnesses may be analogous to the conditions in people. Some feline diseases, of course, are unique. With respect to hyperadrenocorticism (Cushing's syndrome), there are more similarities when comparing cats with people than there are when comparing cats with dogs. One of the more obvious comparisons involves the incidence of hyperadrenocorticism. In dogs this endocrine disorder is surprisingly common, whereas in people and cats it is quite uncommon.

We assume that the underlying physiologic causes for hyperadrenocorticism are similar in people, dogs, and cats. Thus the reader interested in applied physiology and in mechanisms of disease is encouraged to review the appropriate sections in Chapter 6. The focus of this chapter is a review of the clinical condition of hyperadrenocorticism in cats. To aid in this discussion, information from the records of 46 cats diagnosed as having naturally occurring hyperadrenocorticism at our hospital were added to the information from an additional 24 cats described in the literature (Immink et al, 1992; Daley et al, 1993; Goossens et al, 1995; Watson and Herrtage, 1998; Moore et al, 2000a; Meij et al, 2001), for a total of 70 cats with hyperadrenocorticism. This literature includes only those reports published since 1992. We chose reports from this time period in order to be sure that valid and currently available assays were used in the assessment of each cat and that current concepts in diagnosis and treatment were used. Before 1990, only a few cats with this disease were mentioned in the literature (Meijer et al, 1978; Peterson and Steele, 1986; Zerbe et al, 1987; Nelson et al, 1998). Furthermore, in the reports we arbitrarily used, we set the following selection criteria: each cat must have had some clinical signs associated with Cushing's syndrome, each diagnosis must have been confirmed with appropriate screening test results, and each cat must have had advanced imaging (computed tomography [CT] or magnetic resonance imaging [MRI] scans) confirmation or histologic confirmation of the diagnosis. Reports that did not meet these inclusion criteria were not used.

ETIOLOGY

Iatrogenic Cushing's Syndrome

Among the major differences regarding Cushing's syndrome when comparing species is the relative frequency of iatrogenic disease. Iatrogenic Cushing's syndrome is extremely common among people and

dogs. By comparison, iatrogenic Cushing's syndrome in cats is rare. This can be explained, in part, by what appears to be a relative "insensitivity" to the negative or deleterious side effects of chronic glucocorticoid administration in cats. We are aware of only three cats described in recent literature within the past 10 years with iatrogenic Cushing's syndrome. By contrast, the number of people and dogs reported in the literature to have had iatrogenic Cushing's syndrome is considerable.

Several studies on laboratory cats experimentally treated with glucocorticoids have been published. Those treated for a 4-week period had few abnormalities on physical examination and no consistent hematologic or biochemical changes (Scott et al, 1979; Scott et al, 1982). When treated for 9 weeks or longer, some cats exhibited polydipsia, polyuria, polyphagia, abdominal enlargement, thin skin, and curling of their ear tips. Some of these cats also developed liver enlargement, muscle wasting, ecchymoses, and skin fragility (Scott et al, 1982). They also tended to develop mild hyperglycemia, mild hypercholesterolemia, glycogen accumulation in hepatocytes, and a vacuolar hepatopathy. Cataracts developed in some laboratory cats treated with topical glucocorticoids (Brightman, 1982; Zhan et al, 1992). The muscle weakness associated with glucocorticoid administration tends to be most pronounced in the muscles with fast twitch fibers (Robinson and Clamann, 1988).

Three privately owned cats have been described that had iatrogenic chronic glucocorticoid excesses. The cats had received steroids for stomatitis, feline infectious peritonitis (FIP), and pruritus (Greene et al, 1995; Schaer and Ginn, 1999; Ferasin, 2001). At the time of final presentation, one of the three cats was extremely ill as a result of FIP. Among the common features noted in these cats after chronic glucocorticoid exposure were abdominal enlargement, muscle wasting, poor hair coats, and skin fragility. The skin fragility included easy bruisability, skin tears, and thin skin. Two cats had increases in liver enzymes and hepatic vacuolar hepatopathy thought to be similar to those seen in dogs. The most important information derived from these three reports is the realization that iatrogenic Cushing's syndrome in cats is uncommon. In addition, some features seen in cats chronically treated with exogenous steroids are not seen in cats with naturally occurring Cushing's syndrome.

Naturally Occurring Feline Cushing's Syndrome (FCS)

The causes of naturally occurring feline Cushing's syndrome (FCS) are similar to those recognized in human beings and dogs. It has been suggested that resistance to glucocorticoid-induced side effects, likely to exist in cats, may help explain the relative low rate of naturally occurring disease diagnosis as compared with the incidence of the naturally occurring syndrome in dogs. In other words, if excess glucocorticoids cause few clinical signs in cats, how would the diagnosis ever be suspected in the first place? However, the incidence of the naturally occurring disease in cats (assessed nonscientifically) appears to be similar to the incidence of the syndrome in human beings; yet people are sensitive to the effects of glucocorticoids. Therefore it is our suspicion that naturally occurring FCS is simply less common among cats as compared with dogs.

Regardless, the majority of cats (~80%) with naturally occurring FCS have pituitary-dependent hyperadrenocorticism (PDH) and a minority (~20%) have adrenal tumor–dependent hyperadrenocorticism (ATH). Cats with PDH have autonomous secretion of ACTH synthesized by a pituitary adenoma, although several cats with a pituitary carcinoma have been diagnosed. About 50% of pituitary tumors are microscopic in size; the remaining tumors are large enough to be visualized with a CT scan or MRI scan, or they are grossly visible at necropsy or surgery (usually greater than 3 to 4 mm in greatest diameter). Approximately 50% of cats with an autonomously functioning adrenocortical tumor have had an adenoma, and 50% have had a carcinoma.

SIGNALMENT (AGE, SEX, BREED)

Hyperadrenocorticism is a disease of middle-aged and older cats. As can be seen in Table 7-1, the mean age of 39 cats diagnosed as having PDH was 10.7 years with a range of 5 to 16 years. The mean age among 12 cats with a functioning adrenocortical tumor was 12 years, with a range of 8 to 15 years. The mean age for all 51 cats was just under 11 years. Among these same 51 cats, there were 25 males and 26 females. Almost all cats that have been diagnosed as having naturally occurring FCS have been neutered. A variety of breeds are included among the cats diagnosed with hyperadrenocorticism. As seen in Table 7-2, the most commonly afflicted breed is the domestic short-haired cat (31 of 51 cats; 61%), and if domestic long-haired cats are added to that group, 38 of the 51 cats (75%) are represented. Cats representing various other breeds have been diagnosed with FCS.

DURATION OF CLINICAL SIGNS, CHIEF COMPLAINT, AND GENERAL HISTORY

Duration of Clinical Signs

In our review of records from cats diagnosed with FCS, the duration of clinical signs or the duration of specific owner concerns were available for 43 cats (Table 7-3). The range in duration of signs was from as little as 1 month to greater than 12 months. Forty-one of the 43 cats with either PDH or ATH had clinical signs for less than a year.

Owner Chief Complaints

It may be of interest to separate "owner chief complaints" from general "owner observations." The chief complaint is the primary reason that an owner seeks veterinary assistance. It should be obvious that an owners' primary concern does not always match the primary concern that a veterinarian may have after completion of an owner history. Certainly a veterinarian's major concern may be much different after completion of a thorough physical examination.

TABLE 7–1 AGE AT TIME OF HYPERADRENOCORTICISM DIAGNOSIS IN CATS (51 CATS)*

Age (Years)	Pituitary Dependent Number of Cats	Adrenocortical Tumor Number of Cats
5	1	–
6	5	–
7	2	–
8	3	1
9	3	2
10	4	–
11	4	1
12	5	3
13	3	1
14	4	2
15	2	2
16	3	–
Mean	10.7 years	12 years

*Mean age of all 51 cats was 10.9 years

TABLE 7–2 BREEDS OF CATS WITH NATURALLY OCCURRING CUSHING'S SYNDROME (TOTAL OF 51 CATS)

BREED	PITUITARY DEPENDENT		ADRENOCORTICAL TUMOR	
	Number	Percentage	Number	Percentage
Domestic Short Hair	23	59	8	67
Domestic Long Hair	6	15	1	8
Siamese	2	5	1	8
Persian	2	5	1	8
Abyssinian	2	5	–	–
European Short Hair	2	5	–	–
Devon Rex	1	3	–	–
Japanese Bobtail	–	–	1	8
Russian Blue	1	3	–	–
Total	39		12	

TABLE 7–3 DURATION OF CLINICAL SIGNS PRECEDING DIAGNOSIS OF HYPERADRENOCORTICISM IN CATS (43 CATS)

Duration (Months)	Number of Cats with Pituitary-Dependent Disease	Number of Cats with Adrenocortical Tumor
1	2	–
2	5	1
3	5	1
4	3	2
5	3	2
6	3	1
7	1	3
8	2	–
9	1	–
10	2	–
11	–	–
12	2	2
>12	2	–

The chief complaints noted in records from 48 cats with FCS included "difficult to regulate diabetes mellitus" in 26 cats (54%). Most commonly, diabetes mellitus was classified as difficult to regulate when owners felt that their pet had persistence of polyuria, polydipsia, and/or polyphagia despite administration of insulin (Table 7-4). Less frequently, owners believed their cats' diabetes mellitus was poorly controlled if their pet lost weight, failed to gain weight, remained lethargic, or had poor grooming habits. It was not always obvious from the records whether or not an owner believed that any of these problems was directly due to inadequate control of diabetes mellitus. Often, insulin dose and type had been altered numerous times by the primary care veterinarian in an effort to gain control of the diabetes mellitus prior to referral.

Of the 48 cats in this evaluation, 37 had diabetes mellitus. Eleven of the 37 diabetic cats were believed to be well controlled with insulin. Of the 11 nondiabetic

cats, 8 were believed to have polyuria and polydipsia (PU/PD); this problem was established as the owners' chief complaint. Other chief complaints varied and were relatively less common (see Table 7-4). Among the uncommon primary owner concerns were fragile (torn) skin in six cats (12%), lethargy in four cats, and alopecia or failure to regrow hair that had been previously shaved in four cats.

Owner Observations

SUMMARY OF OBSERVATIONS. Owner observations were available from 62 cats diagnosed as having FCS (Table 7-5). The most common concerns noted in the histories obtained from these owners was PU/PD in 51 cats (82%), polyphagia in 42 cats (68%), weight loss or failure to gain weight in 32 cats (52%), and lethargy or reports of "sleeps more" in 29 cats (47%). Concerns about skin problems were noted 61 times. These concerns ranged from the extremely worrisome fragile or torn skin noted in six cats, to a failure to grow hair after it had been shaved (usually for venipuncture or abdominal ultrasonography examination). There were also concerns over grooming excessively or not enough and concerns about a hair coat that had become unusually coarse. Multiple skin problems were noted in some cats, whereas others had none. The owners of 21 cats with PDH (from the total of 50, or 42%) and the owners of 3 cats with ATH (from the total of 12, or 25%) did not observe any problem relative to the skin or hair coat. Similar owner observations in cats with PDH as compared with those with ATH underscores the final common denominator of disease in these cats, that is, chronic exposure to excesses in circulating cortisol.

TABLE 7–4 CHIEF COMPLAINTS BY OWNERS OF CATS ULTIMATELY DIAGNOSED AS HAVING HYPERADRENOCORTICISM (48 CATS – TOTAL; 37 OF THESE 48 CATS HAD DIABETES MELLITUS AND 11 DID NOT HAVE DIABETES MELLITUS)

Complaint	Pituitary Dependent (36 Cats)	Adrenocortical Tumor (12 Cats)
Resistant diabetes mellitus (PD/PU/PP)*	22	4
Polyuria/polydipsia (of the 11 non-diabetic)	6	2
Fragile (torn) skin	3	3
Weight loss	2	–
Lethargy	2	2
Alopecia/failure to regrow hair	2	2
Diarrhea	2	–
Weakness	1	–
Vomiting	1	–
Abdominal enlargement	1	1
Not grooming	1	–

*PD, polydipsia; PU, polyuria; PP, polyphagia.

TABLE 7–5 OWNER OBSERVATIONS IN CATS WITH NATURALLY OCCURRING HYPERADRENOCORTICISM (TOTAL OF 62 CATS)

OBSERVATION	PITUITARY DEPENDENT (50 CATS)		ADRENOCORTICAL TUMOR (12 CATS)	
	Number	Percentage	Number	Percentage
Polyuria/polydipsia	40	80	11	92
Polyphagia	34	68	8	67
Weight loss	26	52	6	50
Lethargic/sleeps more	22	44	7	58
Weakness	18	36	3	25
Alopecia/failure to regrow hair	17	34	10	83
Stopped grooming	10	20	4	33
Coarse hair coat	9	18	2	17
Decreased appetite	4	8	2	17
Fragile (torn) skin	3	6	3	25
Weight gain/potbelly	3	6	2	17
Over grooming	2	4	–	–
Diarrhea	2	4	–	–
Not grooming	1	2	–	–
Vomiting	1	2	–	–

TABLE 7–6 PHYSICAL EXAMINATION ABNORMALITIES IN CATS WITH NATURALLY OCCURRING HYPERADRENOCORTICISM (TOTAL OF 62 CATS)

OBSERVATION	PITUITARY DEPENDENT (50 CATS)		ADRENOCORTICAL TUMOR (12 CATS)	
	Number	Percentage	Number	Percentage
Abdominal enlargement (potbelly)	32	64	9	75
Muscle atrophy	32	64	7	58
Thin skin	28	56	10	83
Unkempt hair coat	28	56	5	42
Hair loss	12	24	2	17
Hepatomegaly	9	18	3	25
Skin tears	7	14	1	8
Plantigrade stance	7	14	2	17
Bruising	6	12	3	25
Seborrhea	2	4	4	33
Palpable adrenal mass	–	–	2	17

It has been suggested that clinical signs of hyperadrenocorticism are not commonly detected by owners or veterinarians until cats with FCS develop diabetes mellitus. The results of this review suggest that this is true for a majority of afflicted cats. However, some of the signs in these cats did precede development of diabetes mellitus, and other cats never developed diabetes. Thus a suspicion of FCS may result from a history and physical examination in nondiabetic cats. Such abnormalities as thin skin, skin fragility, "potbelly" appearance, muscle atrophy, weakness, PU/PD, and various hair coat disorders might lead to the diagnosis of FCS in nondiabetic cats.

PHYSICAL EXAMINATION ABNORMALITIES

The physical examination abnormalities from 62 cats with naturally occurring hyperadrenocorticism are listed in Table 7-6. Observations from cats with

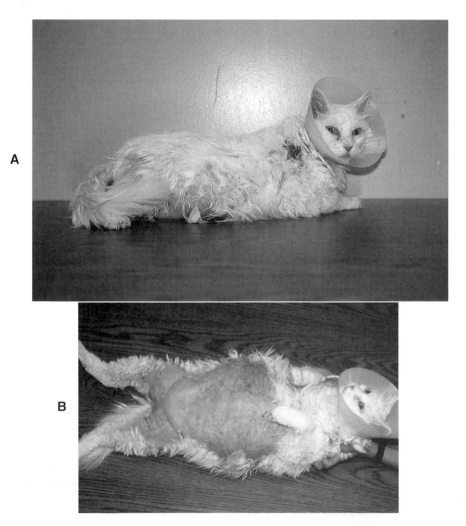

FIGURE 7-1. *A,* 12-year-old male cat with feline Cushing's syndrome (FCS). Note the "unkempt" appearance of the hair coat. *B,* Note the pot-bellied appearance and the thin skin. (The hair on the abdomen had been shaved for ultrasound evaluation.)

PDH are separated from cats with ATH. As can be appreciated, many of the previously described owner concerns were obvious to the veterinarian performing the physical examination. The most common abnormalities include obvious abdominal enlargement detected in 41 cats (66%; Fig. 7-1, A and B), muscle atrophy detected in 39 cats (63%), thin skin detected in 38 cats (61%), and an "unkempt" hair coat detected in 33 cats (53%). Less common abnormalities include hair loss, hepatomegaly, skin tears, plantigrade stance of the rear legs, bruising, and seborrhea. In one report, each of two cats with an adrenocortical tumor had palpable abdominal masses that were subsequently demonstrated to be neoplastic adrenal glands (Immink et al, 1992). The finding of a palpable adrenal tumor is considered quite unusual.

EXPLANATIONS FOR THE HISTORY AND PHYSICAL EXAMINATION ABNORMALITIES

Polyuria and Polydipsia

Polyuria and polydipsia (PU/PD), polyphagia, and weight loss are the cardinal signs of diabetes mellitus. Since a majority of cats with FCS also have diabetes mellitus (usually a result of excess cortisol causing insulin resistance), the explanation for signs such as PU/PD in diabetic cats is straightforward. However, some FCS cats with these clinical signs were not diabetic. Polyuria and polydipsia are extremely common clinical signs in dogs with excess circulating cortisol concentrations. Since it is not common for dogs with hyperadrenocorticism to have concomitant diabetes mellitus, it is thought that dogs have PU/PD secondary to central or nephrogenic diabetes insipidus caused by excess circulating cortisol. Despite being common in dogs (the single most common owner concern), PU/PD occurs uncommonly in human beings with naturally occurring or iatrogenic cortisol excess. This side effect is also not considered common in cats; however, the diabetes insipidus explanation remains a possibility in those cats that do not have glycosuria.

Eight of 11 nondiabetic cats were thought to have PU/PD by their owners. Confounding the issue is the realization that a huge majority of dogs with hyperadrenocorticism have randomly obtained urine samples with a specific gravity less than 1.024 and concomitant serum urea nitrogen or creatinine concentrations within or *below* the reference range. By contrast, only a small percentage of the urine samples obtained from 58 cats with FCS (50 with PDH and 8 with ATH) had a specific gravity less than 1.024 (5 cats, or 9%). Each of those five cats had an *increase* in their serum urea nitrogen, creatinine, or both. Thus the observation of PU/PD is noted almost exclusively in cats that had glycosuria or renal disease. It is also possible that some of these cats do have transient insulin resistance, glycosuria, and secondary PU/PD. This hyperglycemia and glycosuria may not be demonstrable at the time that in-hospital testing is carried out.

Polyphagia is common in nondiabetic dogs with hyperadrenocorticism. However, it is not a well-understood effect of excess circulating cortisol concentrations and is not a typical cortisol-induced problem in people or cats.

Weight Loss

In most cats with FCS, weight loss occurs secondary to diabetes mellitus. This is a classic clinical sign in individuals of any species after development of diabetes mellitus. The relative or absolute deficiency of insulin that occurs with diabetes mellitus causes an inability to utilize glucose and a physiologic condition analogous to starvation. The physiologic response to this problem is to synthesize glucose in the liver with products derived from the breakdown of muscle and fat. It is this breakdown of muscle and fat that causes weight loss. Since a majority of cats with FCS have diabetes mellitus and since a majority of these cats are poorly controlled, regardless of owner or veterinarian opinion, it is difficult for these cats to gain weight. Some remain thin (with a pot belly) and others continue to lose weight despite insulin therapy. Nearly every cat with FCS that has an owner concern of weight loss or remaining thin has concurrent diabetes mellitus. It is assumed that the non-diabetic cats have weight loss secondary to the protein catabolic effects of cortisol excess. Weight loss or remaining thin is an important feature of FCS because one differential diagnosis for insulin resistance in cats is acromegaly, a condition often associated with some weight gain.

Weakness, Lethargy, Pot Belly, and Bruising

Explanations for these clinical signs can be directly related to the physiologic effects of cortisol. Cortisol is protein-catabolic and therefore causes the breakdown of muscle. Muscle wasting results in weakness, which may be obvious to owners. Alternatively, weakness may appear to an owner to be lethargy or an increase in the amount of time spent sleeping. Furthermore, some cats with FCS have a plantigrade posture, which is often related to the neuropathy associated with diabetes mellitus in cats. Chronic cortisol excess is also well recognized to cause a redistribution of fat from areas throughout the body with specific increases in abdominal (mesenteric) fat deposition. This classic abnormality is common in human beings, dogs, and cats. The increase in abdominal fat content coupled with muscle wasting results in the pot belly appearance that is classic of Cushing's syndrome in all species. A pot belly is the clinical consequence of increased weight of abdominal content pressing down upon weakened abdominal musculature (see Fig. 7-1, A and B).

Cortisol also causes a relative decrease in the ability to heal because of blood vessel friability and a decrease in fibrous response to injury. Loss of subcutaneous fat (mobilized to the abdomen), friability of blood vessels that are more superficial because of loss of fat protection, and decreases in normal healing properties increase the predisposition to bruising in these cats. In many cats, bruising after venipuncture or clipping of hair can be dramatic.

Curled Ear Tips

As a component of the catabolic state that chronic cortisol excess creates, decreased strength of ligaments, tendons, and cartilaginous structures in general can be expected. Specifically, initial reports on iatrogenic Cushing's syndrome in cats included observations of "ear tip curling." However, not one comment regarding this clinical sign was retrieved from the records and reports of the 70 cats with FCS used in this review. Thus, although weakened cartilage was thought to be an explanation for this clinical observation, it must be quite uncommon or simply not considered significant by most veterinarians.

Dermatologic Abnormalities

Bilateral symmetric nonpruritic alopecia is a classic and common feature of Cushing's syndrome in dogs but not a typical abnormality in cats. The alopecia that most FCS cat owners observe is due to a failure to regrow hair that has been shaved by veterinarians or hair lost as a result of normal or excessive grooming (Fig. 7-2, A and B). It is difficult to know whether "excessive" grooming is truly an abnormality. Are these cats grooming normally but causing hair loss, thereby also causing owner concern? Or are they licking themselves more than normal? The failure to regrow lost hair is most likely secondary to atrophy of the hair follicles. This atrophy disrupts the hair shaft attachment to the follicle. Any new hair that does grow tends to be brittle, sparse, and fine.

Thin skin (Fig. 7-3, A and B), poor wound healing, and susceptibility to infection are typical sequelae to chronic excesses in circulating cortisol. Suppression of the immune system in individuals with Cushing's syndrome exaggerates these problems. Skin fragility is not typical of canine Cushing's syndrome but is well recognized in afflicted people and is well described but not common in cats (Fig. 7-4, A and B; see Tables 7-5 and 7-6). These dermatologic abnormalities are serious and can result in life-threatening overwhelming sepsis. Thin skin is an expression of the catabolic effects of cortisol.

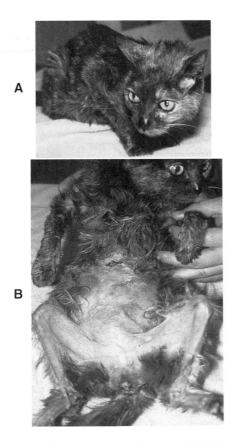

FIGURE 7-2. A, 10-year-old female cat with feline Cushing's syndrome (FCS). B, Note the hair loss sometimes associated with chronic exposure to excess cortisol.

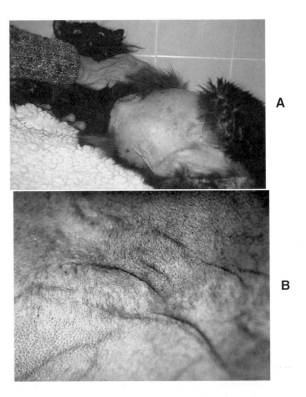

FIGURE 7-3. A, 11-year-old male cat with feline Cushing's syndrome (FCS). This cat had a progesterone-secreting tumor (see page 391). B, Note the thin skin sometimes associated with chronic exposure to excess cortisol.

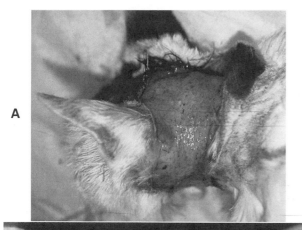

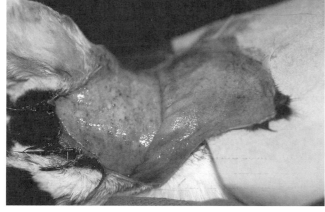

FIGURE 7-4. *A,* Skin tear in a 15-year-old male cat with feline Cushing's syndrome (FCS). *B,* Skin tear in a 10-year-old cat typical of the skin fragility sometimes associated with chronic exposure to excess cortisol.

ROUTINE CLINICAL PATHOLOGY (CBC, SERUM BIOCHEMISTRY, URINALYSIS)

Small animal (canine and feline) veterinarians are familiar with Cushing's syndrome. For the most part, this familiarity can be explained by the numerous indications for using corticosteroids in treating various canine conditions. Since glucocorticoids are commonly used, veterinarians are well aware of their attributes and side effects. These side effects also comprise the clinical signs and laboratory abnormalities that are associated with both iatrogenic and naturally occurring Cushing's syndrome in dogs. Therefore veterinary clinicians expect dogs with Cushing's syndrome to have PU/PD, isosthenuria/hyposthenuria, low-normal or low BUN, and low-normal serum creatinine concentrations. It is also assumed that affected dogs will have increases in serum alkaline phosphatase activities, serum cholesterol concentrations, and serum alanine aminotransferase activities. In fact, most veterinarians would be surprised if a steroid-treated dog or a dog with naturally occurring Cushing's syndrome failed to exhibit many, if not all, of these changes. Remember, the "final common denominator"

for naturally occurring Cushing's syndrome is the same as the iatrogenic syndrome, that is, chronic exposure to excesses in circulating glucocorticoids. With these changes in mind, we can state with confidence that, with regard to Cushing's syndrome, cats are not small dogs. The differences encountered when comparing the condition in these two species are at least equal to their similarities.

Complete Blood Count (CBC)

Complete blood count (CBC) results from 45 cats with naturally occurring hyperadrenocorticism can be found in Table 7-7. The most important feature of these results is the lack of consistent abnormalities. That is, none of the results seem "classic." A majority of afflicted cats had a "stress leukogram" (neutrophilia and reduction in lymphocyte and eosinophil percentages). Of the 45 cats, 24 (53%) had a neutrophil percentage of >86%, 25 (56%) had a lymphocyte percentage of <5%, and 26 (58%) had an eosinophil percentage of <2% of the total white cell count. As can be seen, therefore, stress leukograms were identified, but this was not a consistent feature of the CBC results. No cat was leukopenic, one was thrombocytopenic, and four were anemic. Of the four anemic cats, only one had a hematocrit below 24% (that result was 16%).

TABLE 7–7 COMPLETE BLOOD COUNT RESULTS FROM CATS WITH NATURALLY OCCURRING HYPERADRENOCORTICISM

	PITUITARY DEPENDENT (38 CATS)		ADRENOCORTICAL TUMOR (7 CATS)	
	Number	Percentage	Number	Percentage
White blood cell count				
<6000	–	–	–	–
6000 to 17,000	24	63	3	43
17,000 to 25,000	8	21	3	43
>25,000	6	16	1	14
% Neutrophils				
≤75	6	16	–	–
76 to 85	12	32	3	43
≥86	20	53	4	57
% Lymphocytes				
≤5	20	53	5	71
6 to 15	16	42	2	30
≥15	2	5	–	–
% Eosinophils				
≤2	22	58	4	57
3 to 6	10	26	3	43
≥7	6	16	–	–
Platelets				
<180,000	–	–	1	14
180,000 to 400,000	30	79	4	57
>400,000	8	21	2	30
Hematocrit				
≤27	2	5	2	30
28 to 35	22	58	2	30
36 to 46	14	37	3	43
≥47	–	–	–	–

Serum Biochemistry and Urinalysis

LIVER ENZYMES. The introduction to this section discusses the common routine biochemical test result abnormalities from *dogs* with naturally occurring or iatrogenic Cushing's syndrome. The results from cats with this endocrine disorder are strikingly different (Table 7-8). Although dramatic increases in serum alkaline phosphatase (SAP) activities (average >1,000 IU/L) are the most common biochemical abnormality in dogs, only 3 of 43 cats (7%) with naturally occurring Cushing's syndrome had an increase in serum alkaline phosphatase activity. Another common abnormality in dogs with Cushing's syndrome is mild to moderate increase in serum alanine aminotransferase (ALT) activity. This abnormality is identified in more than 50% of dogs, but occurred in only 12 of 43 cats (28%). Several of the cats with increases in ALT activity had significant hepatopathies that were not related to their Cushing's syndrome. Dogs with iatrogenic or naturally occurring excesses in serum cortisol concentration commonly develop "steroid hepatopathy," as well as significant circulating concentrations of the "steroid-induced" isoenzyme of SAP. Neither of these typical canine features of Cushing's syndrome is believed to occur in cats or human beings. However, "steroid hepatopathy" that included liver enlargement and a vacuolar appearance to hepatocytes has been occasionally described in cats with FCS.

SERUM CHOLESTEROL AND T_4. Increases in serum cholesterol concentration are identified in 60% to 70% of dogs with Cushing's syndrome. Fewer than 5% of those dogs have diabetes mellitus. In contrast, the serum cholesterol concentration was increased in only 13 of the 43 cats with FCS (30%), and all 13 had concurrent diabetes mellitus. Diabetes mellitus and hyperadrenocorticism are two of the classic causes for increases in serum cholesterol concentration. Excess serum cortisol concentrations also cause negative feedback to the pituitary, thereby decreasing TSH secretion and resulting in secondary hypothyroidism. Hypothyroidism is another classic cause of hypercholesterolemia. Hypothyroidism, together with the direct lipolytic actions of glucocorticoids exaggerated in Cushing's syndrome, are common explanations for the increases in serum cholesterol concentration typically identified in nondiabetic dogs with hyperadrenocorticism. However, serum T_4 concentrations were lower than the reference range in only 4 of the 43 cats (9%) with FCS, making this explanation for hypercholesterolemia unlikely. Cats with FCS were consistently euthyroid, and evidence of thyroid disease was identified in only three cats (all were hyperthyroid) at necropsy. Although thyroid disease

TABLE 7–8   SERUM BIOCHEMICAL AND URINALYSIS RESULTS FROM CATS WITH NATURALLY OCCURRING HYPERADRENOCORTICISM (43 CATS)

Test and Reference Range		PITUITARY DEPENDENT (32 CATS)			ADRENOCORTICAL TUMOR (11 CATS)		
		Number within Reference Range	Number Below	Number Above	Number within Reference Range	Number Below	Number Above
Serum							
Alkaline phosphatase	(14 to 71 IU/L)	31	–	1	9	–	2
ALT	(28 to 106 IU/L)	20	–	12	9	–	–
Albumin	(2.7 to 3.9 g/dl)	27	5	–	8	3	2
Globulin	(2.9 to 4.3 g/dl)	14	–	18	7	–	4
Total protein	(5.6 to 8.4 g/dl)	25	–	7	9	–	2
BUN	(18 to 33 mg/dl)	14	–	18	6	–	5
Creatinine	(0.9 to 1.8 mg/dl)	21	1	10	7	–	4
Cholesterol	(89 to 258 mg/dll)	20	–	12	10	–	1
Glucose	(73 to 134 mg/dl)	–	4	28	2	2	7
Calcium	(9.4 to 11.4 mg/dl)	28	4	–	8	3	–
PO_4	(3.2 to 6.3 mg/dl)	28	2	2	8	–	3
TCO_2	(15 to 25 mm/L)	25	4	3	11	–	–
K	(3.6 to 5.3 mm/L)	32	–	–	10	1	–
Na	(145 to 156 mm/L)	30	2	–	9	–	2
T_4	(1.0 to 2.5 µg/dl)	28	4	–	9	–	2
Urinalysis							
Specific gravity							
<1.010		–	–	–	1		
1.020 to 1.040		–	26	–	6		
>1.041		–	6	–	3		
Protein							
Negative		–	13	–	3		
Trace		–	11	–	2		
> Trace		–	8	–	5		
Bacteria							
Negative		–	31	–	9		
Positive		–	1	–	1		

remains possible in any cat, it would not be considered typical of cats with FCS.

BUN, SERUM CREATININE, URINE SPECIFIC GRAVITY. Perhaps one of the more consistent group of abnormalities seen in dogs that have Cushing's syndrome are those related to polyuria and polydipsia. A tremendous majority of these dogs have urine specific gravities <1.020 (especially on samples obtained by owners from dogs in their home environment), many are <1.014 and about 30% are <1.008. In other words, polyuria in this population of dogs is common and represents a frequent owner concern. Polyuria is one of the two most common reasons that owners seek veterinary care for their dog (the other is alopecia). If not resolved, polyuria is a frequent reason for owners to elect euthanasia. In addition to the PU/PD and the previously discussed isosthenuria/hyposthenuria in dogs with Cushing's syndrome are low-normal-to-*low* BUN and serum creatinine concentrations. These are classic features of canine Cushing's syndrome. Emphasizing this concept, increases in BUN or creatinine not only are rare in dogs with Cushing's syndrome but are a serious indication for avoiding treatment. Appetite in such dogs may be dependent on cortisol excess, and the concern in treating such dogs for Cushing's syndrome is unmasking both renal failure and its clinical signs (including poor appetite).

A review of the serum biochemical data presented in Table 7-8 from cats with naturally occurring FCS demonstrates remarkable differences in test results as compared with those from dogs that have Cushing's syndrome. None of the 43 cats had a BUN concentration below the reference range, and only 1 of the 43 had a serum creatinine concentration below the reference range. Only 1 of 43 cats had a randomly obtained urine specific gravity <1.020. That cat had both isosthenuria and renal failure. Furthermore, 23 of the 43 cats (53%) had abnormally *increased* BUN concentrations at the time of diagnosis, and 14 of those 23 cats (14 of the total 43 = 32%) also had abnormally increased serum creatinine concentrations. Thus it is likely that the polyuria and polydipsia recognized in most cats with FCS is either due to diabetes mellitus, chronic renal failure, or a combination of both conditions.

There have been descriptions of cats with FCS that have PU/PD but no clinical or laboratory evidence supporting concurrent renal failure or diabetes mellitus. The number of such cats is unknown, but the concept is that hypercortisolemia does occasionally cause PU/PD in some cats. On the one hand, it is possible that this does occur. On the other hand, we remain suspicious that some of these cats may have periodic hyperglycemia leading to episodic glycosuria and, thereby, episodic secondary polyuria. Stress-induced hyperglycemia is one explanation for hyperglycemia noted in some nondiabetic cats. This stress-induced condition interferes with our ability to distinguish those cats with persistent euglycemia except at times of stress from those with periodic physiologic hyperglycemia due to their hyper-

cortisolemia. Even use of glycosylated hemoglobin or fructosamine concentrations would not consistently identify cats with periodic hyperglycemia. There is no evidence, however, to suggest that any cat with FCS has a physiologic syndrome similar to the diabetes insipidus–like condition that occurs commonly in dogs with Cushing's syndrome, since such a situation would cause dilute urine. Cats with FCS rarely have dilute urine.

SERUM POTASSIUM AND SODIUM. Although cats with FCS are often described by their owners as being weak, the weakness is likely a direct result of glucocorticoid-induced catabolic effects on muscle. One suggested concern was that these cats may be predisposed to hypokalemia. However, only 1 of 43 cats had a serum potassium concentration lower than the reference range, and only 2 had serum sodium concentrations below the reference range.

PROTEINURIA, SERUM CALCIUM, ALBUMIN, GLOBULINS, AND TOTAL PROTEIN. Perhaps related to the frequent incidence of chronic renal failure in cats with hyperadrenocorticism, 7 of the 43 cats (16%) were mildly hypocalcemic (based on total serum calcium concentrations). However, each hypocalcemic cat also had mild decreases in serum albumin concentration. Proteinuria was common in this population of cats (26 of 43 cats, or 60%), and this is the most likely explanation for both their hypoalbuminemia and hypocalcemia. However, only 8 of 43 cats (17%) were hypoalbuminemic, and all 8 had serum albumin concentrations >2.2 g/dl. It is also of interest to point out that only 2 of 43 cats with FCS had serum albumin concentrations greater than their simultaneous serum globulin concentration. Furthermore, 22 of the 43 cats (52%) had serum globulin concentrations above the reference range. This hyperglobulinemia could be explained by a normal response to chronic antigen exposure, which occurs in any older individual. However, this degree of hyperglobulinemia was such that 9 of the 43 cats (22%) had hyperproteinemia.

URINARY TRACT INFECTION. Urinary tract infection was uncommon among the cats with FCS (2 of 43 cats, or 3%). Since many had been referred after being given antibiotics, perhaps the failure to identify infection was a result of this treatment. Once again, however, this is in contrast to our experience with dogs that have naturally occurring hyperadrenocorticism. In those dogs the incidence of infection is much greater, and most are also referred after being treated with antibiotics.

BLOOD GLUCOSE CONCENTRATIONS. Perhaps the most unpredictable routine biochemical test result, as compared with expectations, was the random blood glucose concentration. Since a majority of cats diagnosed with FCS have diabetes mellitus, increases in blood glucose concentration are expected. However, of the 43 cats with serum biochemical test results available at the approximate time of diagnosis, 10 cats were not diabetic. Of the 33 cats with diabetes mellitus whose serum chemistry results were available for inclusion in Table 7-8, 32 were being treated with exogenous insulin at the time of FCS diagnosis. It is not surprising, then, that six of the insulin-treated cats demonstrated hypoglycemia on random blood glucose testing. It is somewhat surprising, however, that only 2 of all 43 cats with FCS had blood glucose concentrations within reference limits. Furthermore, one of those two cats was diabetic and had received insulin prior to being tested that day. Ten of 11 FCS cats that had not been treated with insulin, therefore, demonstrated hyperglycemia when blood chemistry results were randomly obtained during the hospitalization in which the FCS was diagnosed. Therefore it does seem reasonable to suggest that finding a blood glucose concentration within reference limits is unusual in cats diagnosed with Cushing's syndrome.

HYPOGLYCEMIA VERSUS INSULIN DOSE.   Six of 43 FCS cats evaluated with a routine biochemical profile were hypoglycemic at the time that blood was obtained for the chemistry profile. All six hypoglycemic cats were diabetic and had received insulin prior to testing that day. Four of those six cats were described by their owners and referring veterinarians as "insulin-resistant." Insulin dose (per cat or per kilogram of body weight) varied tremendously. The occasional finding of hypoglycemia in any population of insulin-treated diabetic dogs or cats should never be viewed as unexpected. However, we believe that repeatedly increasing insulin dosage (as recommended by some veterinarians) in an attempt to "control" hyperglycemia in diabetic cats is dangerous. It is our experience that individual insulin doses in excess of 2.2 U/kg of body weight are unsafe. Although we do not doubt that some cats respond to extremely high insulin doses after appearing resistant to lower doses, "resistance" (if it exists in any particular cat) is not a continuum. In other words, insulin resistance seems to fluctuate, or "wax and wane." If this is true, the dose given when a cat appears resistant will be an overdose in that same cat at another time. We have had cats with FCS that had severe, life-threatening, hypoglycemic reactions to insulin. It is not recommended that any cat be given insulin doses in excess of 2.2 U/kg body weight.

HYPERGLYCEMIA.   Of the 43 cats with FCS whose laboratory data were included in Table 7-8, 35 were hyperglycemic at the time that blood was obtained for the chemistry profile. Twenty-six of the 35 hyperglycemic cats were diabetic, and 25 of the 26 were being treated with insulin and had received insulin that day. Since cats with FCS are commonly believed to be insulin-resistant, the finding of hyperglycemia would be expected in some of these cats. Resistance is not an acceptable explanation for all these hyperglycemic cats, however. An additional reason for the hyperglycemia could be inadequate control of the diabetes (with numerous causes ranging from owner error to FCS). Another possible explanation is that blood was obtained before or after the period of insulin effectiveness. Finally, any of these cats may have had stress-induced hyperglycemia in addition to their diabetes mellitus.

Nine of the 35 hyperglycemic cats were not diabetic. How many of the nine cats had simple stress-induced hyperglycemia at the time that blood was obtained? Of equal interest, how many of the nine hyperglycemic cats had some degree of glucose intolerance that had not been recognized as representing diabetes mellitus? The answers to these questions are unknown, but it is likely that at least some cats in this population fit into one of these two categories.

DIABETES MELLITUS.   Diabetes mellitus is among the more common conditions diagnosed in small animal practice, and it is, along with hyperthyroidism, one of the two most frequently diagnosed endocrine disorders in cats. In contrast, the diagnosis of feline hyperadrenocorticism, or FCS, is considered uncommon-to-rare. We cannot state that FCS is diagnosed only in diabetic cats with insulin resistance. To the contrary, FCS is diagnosed in nondiabetic as well as diabetic cats. It seems easier to suspect FCS in an insulin-resistant cat, however, than in a cat that is simply lethargic or pot-bellied. However, clinical signs of thin skin, skin fragility, alopecia, failure to regrow hair after it has been clipped, or PU/PD are also problems that could reasonably be explained should the cat be confirmed to have FCS.

One problem facing the veterinary practitioner is determining which *poorly controlled* diabetic cats are truly insulin-resistant and which of those truly insulin-resistant cats have FCS. Many of our diabetic cats have stress-induced hyperglycemia when examined at veterinary hospitals. Most of our poorly controlled diabetic cats have problems that can be traced to one or more of many potential owner errors. Although monitoring serum glycosylated hemoglobin or fructosamine concentrations may aid in identification of such cats, these tests are not perfect.

An additional group of poorly controlled diabetic cats are given insulin that has an extremely brief duration of action; these cats continue to exhibit clinical signs and have frequent hyperglycemia, since it is more likely to detect hyperglycemia than euglycemia at any given time of day in such cats. Another category of causes for poor control, or insulin resistance, in a diabetic cat includes many concurrent conditions that interfere with insulin action. These include pancreatitis, other nonseptic inflammatory conditions, infections, and other disorders (such as neoplasia and heart disease). Finally, problems such as acromegaly, anti-insulin antibodies, and hyperadrenocorticism are uncommon but popular conditions to diagnose.

We encourage veterinarians having difficulty controlling diabetes in any cat to prioritize the potential explanations for difficult control. The top of this priority list should be the fact that in-hospital testing may not reflect what is happening in the home environment. Owner history is the single most important monitoring tool in the long-term management of diabetes in cats, and if the owner is satisfied with the cat's response to therapy, in-hospital test results should not supersede this opinion unless hypoglycemia is documented. In-hospital stress-induced hyperglycemia is common, and this differential diagnosis should not be limited to "mean" (or obviously stressed) cats.

Next, veterinarians must consider all the potential owner errors that commonly take place. These errors include, but are not restricted to, using the incorrect insulin, mixing the insulin improperly, drawing insulin into the syringe incorrectly, using incorrect syringes, using out-dated insulin, and practicing improper administration techniques. Every time a diabetic cat is evaluated in the hospital, owners should be watched as they handle and administer *their* insulin. Once these potential problems have been dismissed, the veterinarian should consider the possibility that the insulin being used is either too weak (such as sometimes occurs with ultralente or PZI insulins) or too potent (which sometimes occurs with NPH or lente insulins) for the cat being evaluated. Additionally, one should consider the possibility that a concurrent disorder exists and may be interfering with insulin sensitivity. This could include any infection (urinary tract and skin infections are only two of the numerous potential infections that may or may not be obvious) or any source of inflammation (pancreatitis is just one of numerous potential inflammatory conditions that may or may not be obvious). Additional conditions that could cause insulin resistance include neoplasias, heart disease, and others. Last among the considerations of causes for insulin resistance should be anti-insulin antibodies, progesterone excess, acromegaly, and FCS.

HYPERTENSION. Blood pressure assessment is not commonly obtained from cats, and we have little data regarding the incidence of hypertension among cats with iatrogenic or naturally occurring hypercortisolism. However, hypertension is quite common among human beings with naturally occurring hyperadrenocorticism. Since there are more similarities between human beings and cats with this condition than between dogs and cats, we suspect that hypertension may be a common sequela to FCS. Long-term effects of hypertension in cats is also not well studied, but it is possible that chronic excesses in serum cortisol may have deleterious effects on the kidneys of cats.

ENDOCRINE SCREENING TESTS

Several endocrine tests are used for distinguishing cats that may have naturally occurring FCS from cats that do not have the disease. Those tests most commonly employed are the ACTH stimulation test, the low-dose dexamethasone screening test (LDDST), and the urine cortisol-to-creatinine ratio (UC:CR). Each of these tests has advantages and disadvantages. It is important to remember that no test is perfect. This concept gains significance when it is appreciated that cats with Cushing's syndrome do not have a good prognosis. Because of this poor prognosis, owners of cats diagnosed with FCS may elect to euthanize their pet rather than pursue therapy. Furthermore, the most effective treatment options appear to be pituitary surgery, adrenal surgery, or pituitary irradiation. Each of these therapeutic modalities is rather expensive, and special facilities and/or training are required, limiting availability. Neither surgery nor radiation therapy is a benign treatment. Thus it is recommended that the diagnosis of FCS be reserved for cats with clinical signs as well as endocrine test results consistent with the diagnosis.

Urine Cortisol-to-Creatinine Ratio (UC:CR)

BACKGROUND. The urine cortisol-to-creatinine ratio (UC:CR) has been recommended as a screening test to aid in separating patients *with* Cushing's syndrome from those *without* the condition. A thorough explanation of the test and the indications for its use are provided in Chapter 6. In summary, the "gold standard" screening test for Cushing's syndrome in human beings has been to assess total cortisol excreted in urine over a 24-hour period. Repeating this test several times further ensures validity of results. Cortisol excreted in urine reflects that secreted by the adrenal glands over time and negates concern of minute-to-minute pulsatile fluctuations in plasma concentrations. It is considered a reliable test for understanding whether the adrenal glands are producing normal or excessive quantities of cortisol.

The use of a randomly collected single urine sample, assessing it for cortisol concentration, and then creating a ratio of that cortisol to urine creatinine (UC:CR) is a short-cut to the more cumbersome 24-hour collection procedure. Although the UC:CR is much easier for patients and physicians, most physicians continue to use the 24-hour protocol. The UC:CR has been well studied in dogs. It is highly recommended by some veterinary endocrinologists but not by others because the test has both positive and negative traits. Those who recommend the UC:CR test usually point to several attributes: it is inexpensive, easy to perform and interpret, and sensitive (there is a high predictive value of a negative test result). Virtually all veterinarians who have critically evaluated the UC:CR in dogs with naturally occurring Cushing's syndrome agree that it is highly sensitive. In other words, a tremendous percentage (in the range of 97% to 99%) of dogs with the disease have an abnormal test result. Therefore if one is suspicious of Cushing's syndrome in a dog and the UC:CR test result is abnormal, there is a possibility that the dog has Cushing's syndrome.

However, the problem that others note with the UC:CR is that finding an abnormal result is not specific for dogs with Cushing's syndrome. For example, the UC:CR result is frequently abnormal in dogs with polyuria and polydipsia of any cause, such as those with diabetes mellitus, diabetes insipidus, renal failure, hypercalcemia, pyometra, and liver failure. Therefore, results of the UC:CR test may be consistent with a diagnosis of Cushing's syndrome in animals that do not have the disease.

PUBLISHED DATA. In the initial study evaluating the UC:CR in cats, it was suggested that there was a paradox in comparing reference ranges for dogs versus those for cats because of relative rates of urinary cortisol excretion when comparing the two species. The paradox is related to the relatively high reference UC:CR range in cats versus their low urinary excretion of administered radiolabeled cortisol. Healthy dogs excrete larger amounts of cortisol into urine than do healthy cats. It was suggested that the higher UC:CR in healthy cats, despite their lower overall excretion, may be explained by a higher glomerular filtration rate and/or a lower renal reabsorption of free cortisol. Thus the ratio between unaltered cortisol to conjugates and metabolites of cortisol in urine would be higher in cats than dogs (Goossens et al, 1995).

It is also wise to review the concerns that many veterinary clinical researchers have regarding specificity of UC:CR testing when it is used as the sole diagnostic aid for confirming Cushing's syndrome in cats. The results from one study indicate that health status of cats affects UC:CR (Henry et al, 1996). Test results in healthy cats were not affected by age, gender, or neuter status. Ill cats have higher UC:CR values than healthy cats, implying that specificity may be a problem (as in dogs). The UC:CR from 16 ill cats were evaluated. Three cats had test results consistent with hyperadrenocorticism ($\geq 3.6 \times 10^{-5}$), and another seven had results in the range we would consider "borderline" (i.e., between 1.0 and 3.6×10^{-5}. Thus 10 of 16 ill cats had UC:CR results that could be considered consistent with a diagnosis of hyperadrenocorticism. However, although the study demonstrated that sick cats had significantly higher UC:CR results than healthy cats, it did not include any results from cats with naturally occurring Cushing's syndrome, negating direct comparison of data from each of the three groups in question (healthy, ill, and FCS cats; Henry et al, 1996).

We are not aware of any additional studies evaluating specificity of the UC:CR in cats. Thus it is premature to suggest that the test should not be used. To the contrary, we do recommend use of the test, especially if owners can bring urine samples from home (perhaps using small quantities of litter or nonabsorbable litter to make urine easier to collect). Home-collected urine negates concern of spurious results due to the stress associated with in-hospital urine collection. Also, there is less concern about UC:CR results from ill cats than results from cats confirmed as not having hyperadrenocorticism but having some clinical signs suggestive of the disease. It is this group of cats that must be evaluated before concrete suggestions are made regarding use of the UC:CR.

TEST INTERPRETATION. Two studies have been published suggesting reference ranges for feline UC:CR. The reference range from the first report was $<3.6 \times 10^{-5}$ (Goossens et al, 1995), and from the second report it was $<2.8 \times 10^{-5}$ (Henry et al, 1996). If the initial reference range for cats ($<3.6 \times 10^{-5}$) is used, it should be remembered that this value is slightly higher than that for dogs (<1.0 or $<1.3 \times 10^{-5}$). It seems prudent to suggest, from the information published in these two reports coupled with our experience, that a UC:CR value $\geq 3.6 \times 10^{-5}$ in a cat with clinical signs consistent with hyperadrenocorticism (FCS) is consistent with that diagnosis. We also recommend that UC:CR values between 1.3 and 3.6×10^{-5} in cats with appropriate clinical signs be considered "borderline." It is possible for a cat with test results in this range to have naturally occurring hyperadrenocorticism.

RESULTS. As can be seen from the data presented in Tables 7-9 and 7-10, we were able to collate UC:CR data from a total of 37 cats that had confirmation of their naturally occurring hyperadrenocorticism. Twenty-four of the cats were from our series, and 13 were from cats from the literature with well-documented FCS (Goossens et al, 1995 [6 cats]; Meij et al, 2001 [7 cats]). Of these 37 cats, 29 had PDH and 8 had functioning adrenocortical tumor hyperadrenocorticism (ATH). Twenty-nine of the total of 37 cats

TABLE 7–9 ENDOCRINE SCREENING TEST RESULTS FROM CATS WITH NATURALLY OCCURRING PITUITARY-DEPENDENT CUSHING'S SYNDROME

	UC:CR*	PLASMA CORTISOL (µg%) LOW DOSE DEXAMETHASONE			PLASMA CORTISOL (µg%) ACTH STIMULATION		
		Pre	4 Hr	8 Hr	Pre	First Post	Second or Final Sample
Reference range	$<3.6 \times 10^{-5}$	0–5	<1.4	<1.4	0–5	5–15	5–15
"Borderline" range	$1.3–3.6 \times 10^{-5}$	–	0.9–1.3	0.9–1.3	–	15–19	15–19
Number of cats included	29	37	37	34	43	32	43
Number of results within reference range	1	–	2	0	17	21	27
Number of results in "borderline" range	4	–	0	0	–	3	3
Number of results consistent with Cushing's syndrome	24	–	35	34	–	8	13
Range of test results	$0.3–77 \times 10^{5}$	1.5–14.5	0.5–14.9	1.7–14.0	1.5–22.3	5.4–32.7	5–36
Mean ± S.D.	$11.5 \pm 14 \times 10^{-5}$	5.7 ± 2.8	4.9 ± 3.2	5.3 ± 3.0	6.6 ± 4	14.9 ± 6.7	16.5 ± 8.7
Median	8.0×10^{-5}	5.2	4.1	4.8	5.8	12.9	14.1

*UC:CR, Urine cortisol:creatinine ratio.

TABLE 7–10 ENDOCRINE SCREENING TEST RESULTS FROM CATS WITH HYPERADRENOCORTICISM CAUSED BY A FUNCTIONING ADRENOCORTICAL TUMOR

	UC:CR*	PLASMA CORTISOL (µg%) LOW DOSE DEXAMETHASONE TEST			PLASMA CORTISOL (µg%) ACTH STIMULATION TEST		
		Pre	4 Hr	8 Hr	Pre	First Post	Second or Final Sample
Reference range	$<3.6 \times 10^{-5}$	0.5	<1.4	<1.4	0–5	5–15	5–15
"Borderline" range	$1.3–3.6 \times 10^{-5}$	–	0.9–1.3	0.9–1.3	–	15–19	15–19
Number of cats included	8	8	6	8	8	6	8
Number of results within reference range	0	5	0	0	5	4	4
Number of results within "borderline" range	3	–	0	0	–	1	–
Number of results consistent with Cushing's syndrome	5	–	6	8	–	1	4
Range of test results	$1.1–16 \times 10^{-5}$	1.5–11.0	1.5–11.6	1.8–10.2	2.6–11.8	2.7–50.0	3.3–52.8
Mean ± S.D.	$6.4 \pm 5 \times 8$	4.9 ± 2.9	5.2 ± 3.5	4.9 ± 2.7	5.2 ± 3.4	17.3 ± 16.9	22.3 ± 18.2
Median	3.8	4.1	4.1	5.5	3.7	13.1	21.5

*UC:CR, Urine cortisol:creatinine ratio.

(78%; 24 from the PDH group and 5 from the ATH group) had results above the reference range of 3.6×10^{-5}. An additional 7 cats (19%) had results in the borderline range (4 from the PDH group and 3 from the ATH group). This now accounts for results from all 8 cats with ATH and for 28 of the 29 cats with PDH. Borderline values were defined as those above the approximate canine reference range ($<1.3 \times 10^{-5}$) but lower than the higher range established for cats in the previously mentioned study ($<3.6 \times 10^{-5}$). Only one cat had a UC:CR test result that was considered normal (that cat had PDH). Thus the UC:CR appears to be a sensitive test for confirming the diagnosis of Cushing's syndrome in cats, with a sensitivity approaching that demonstrated for dogs. We have not evaluated the specificity of the UC:CR but suspect that it may have similar problems to those noted in dogs.

CONCLUSIONS. The UC:CR is a sensitive diagnostic aid for helping to distinguish cats that have naturally occurring hyperadrenocorticism (FCS) from cats that do not have the disease. Since the specificity of the test has not been thoroughly evaluated, this may yet be a concern. Veterinarians are encouraged to place a great deal of importance on the history and physical examination and to use the evaluation of this information to decide whether to perform the UC:CR. Together, these could form the basis of diagnosing FCS. If there is doubt regarding the diagnosis, a low-dose dexamethasone test is recommended.

ACTH Stimulation Test

BACKGROUND. The ACTH stimulation test has been recommended as an aid in the diagnosis of Cushing's syndrome in dogs for more than 35 years. More recently, this test has been recommended as a diagnostic aid in the evaluation of cats suspected of having hyperadrenocorticism, presumably as an extension of its use in dogs. A complete discussion on the physiologic basis for this test and its usefulness is provided in Chapter 6. Briefly, it is important to point out that, in general, humans suspected of having endocrine deficiency syndromes (for example, hypoadrenocorticism [Addison's disease]), are typically evaluated with provocative or stimulation-type tests to help in confirming a diagnosis. Humans suspected of having endocrine excess syndromes (for example, hyperadrenocorticism [Cushing's syndrome]), are typically evaluated with suppression tests to help in confirming a diagnosis. These recommendations are based on the specificity and sensitivity of these testing protocols in confirmed cases.

Currently, the ACTH stimulation test is advocated for use in cats by some veterinary endocrinologists and not by others. Those who recommend using the test usually point out several attributes: the test requires little time (1 or 2 hours depending on the ACTH used) and only two venipunctures; results are easy to interpret; the test is relatively inexpensive; it is highly specific for hyperadrenocorticism when results are abnormal; it is the only test that can be used to distinguish iatrogenic from naturally occurring hyperadrenocorticism; and it is the only test used in the long-term monitoring of animals being medically treated for the disease. Detractors suggest that the test is neither as specific nor as sensitive as is required for its continued use.

Thus the ACTH stimulation test has both positive and negative traits that enhance or limit its usefulness. In our opinion, the primary negative trait of the ACTH stimulation test is exactly that problem which defines why it is not used in humans: it lacks sensitivity. That is, animals with naturally occurring hyperadrenocorticism often have test results within the reference range, and this can lead to the incorrect deletion of Cushing's syndrome from the list of differential diagnoses that might explain medical problems in a dog or cat.

PUBLISHED DATA. A number of studies have evaluated the ACTH stimulation test in either laboratory or privately owned cats. One of the earliest studies compared the use of two different doses of synthetic ACTH (cosyntropin) with the use of natural ACTH in stimulation tests conducted on privately owned healthy cats. The synthetic ACTH was administered at doses of 125 and 250 µg per cat, intramuscularly, with plasma samples obtained and then assayed for cortisol before administration and again at 15, 30, 60, 90, and 120 minutes after (Smith and Feldman, 1987). No significant difference was found between responses to the two doses of synthetic ACTH, although two cats vomited and remained depressed for several hours after receiving the higher dose. Since no difference in response to the two doses of exogenous ACTH was noted, the lower dose was recommended. Peaks in plasma cortisol concentration were most often documented 30 and 60 minutes after starting the test, and therefore both post-ACTH sampling times were recommended. Using the mean ±SD to establish the reference range for the post-ACTH plasma cortisols resulted in a plasma cortisol reference range of 6.2 µg% to 18.8 µg% at 30 or 60 minutes after the intramuscular injection.

Response to IV synthetic tetracosactrin (ACTH) was evaluated in laboratory cats by another group of researchers. In this study, 125 µg/cat was administered intravenously, and the conclusion was that cats demonstrated peak response 180 minutes after injection (Sparkes et al, 1990). The longer duration of action of IV versus IM administration was further supported in a subsequent study by yet another group. IM and IV routes were compared, again using 125 µg/cat. It was demonstrated that the intravenous route of ACTH administration induced significantly higher plasma cortisol concentrations and a more prolonged response than the intramuscular route. Peak cortisol response occurred between 60 and 90 minutes after starting the IV test (Peterson and Kemppainen, 1992a). No significant difference was noted in drug response after IV cosyntropin was compared with IV tetracosactrin in another study. Since several cats in this latter study demonstrated a later response to ACTH, it was recommended that blood for cortisol determinations be obtained 120 to 180 minutes after administration, as well as the previously recommended 60- and 90-minute samples (Peterson and Kemppainen, 1992b). These two studies were followed by another in which 1.25, 12.5, and 125 µg of cosyntropin were administered to cats. This study demonstrated comparable peak cortisol responses after each dose but more prolonged response with the highest dose (Peterson and Kemppainen, 1993).

A study specifically evaluating IV ACTH stimulation testing in overweight privately owned cats using 125 or 250 µg of tetracosactrin/cat was conducted. The authors had questioned whether previous work might be flawed since many studies had been completed on relatively young, relatively lean, laboratory cats, whereas cats with FCS tend to be older, obese, and privately owned. This study indicated, as had others, that a single blood sample collected at 60 minutes after ACTH administration would be appropriate. This study also suggested that higher doses of ACTH did not increase absolute cortisol concentrations but did prolong duration of effect. Most important, although the cats were overweight and privately owned, their peak cortisol concentrations after administration of ACTH were similar to those reported in the other studies (Schoeman et al, 2000). It has also been demonstrated that increases in hypothalamic-pituitary-adrenal activity occur as cats age (Goossens et al, 1995). ACTH stimulation test results do not appear to be significantly altered by this physiologic process.

Slight variations in post-ACTH cortisol concentration reference ranges may result from using cosyntropin versus tetracosactrin, from using small or larger doses, or from a protocol employing IV versus IM administration. The critical question, however, not addressed in any of these studies is simply whether or not the test should be employed at any time in cats suspected of having naturally occurring hyperadrenocorticism.

TEST INTERPRETATION. Based on the reports evaluating the ACTH stimulation tests cited previously, along with our own experiences, it seemed appropriate to arbitrarily assign "borderline" results in addition to statistically derived "normal reference" and "abnormal results" that would be consistent with a diagnosis of Cushing's syndrome for post-ACTH plasma cortisol concentrations. The "abnormal" cortisol value >19 µg% was derived from our initial study and from more than 100 privately owned cats assessed periodically over the years. Although some studies may utilize slightly lower or higher "abnormal" values, they are either not statistically derived or these ranges would not vary much from those we have employed. Further, lower reference ranges could be dangerous by losing specificity and causing more cats without the disease to be diagnosed as having FCS. As demonstrated in one study on privately owned cats that did not have FCS, baseline (pre-ACTH) plasma cortisol values ranged as high as 13 µg% and post-ACTH plasma cortisol values as high as 19.7 µg% (Schoeman et al, 2000). Just the basal values, therefore, might include some cats in the Cushing's syndrome group if lower plasma cortisol concentrations were considered diagnostic. The post-ACTH values in others would be best described as "borderline" since no cat in the Schoeman study was ever diagnosed as having FCS.

The "normal" post-ACTH reference range used in the evaluations included here was 5 µg% to 15 µg%, regardless of whether it was the first or second sample obtained. A "borderline" range was established as being 15 µg% to 19 µg% for either sample period. Results "consistent with Cushing's syndrome" were ≥19 µg%. Since 43 of the 51 cats included in this assessment were cats in our series, the ACTH used in each cat was cosyntropin (that form of synthetic ACTH most commonly employed in the United States) and post-ACTH samples were obtained at both 30 and 60 minutes from a large majority of tested cats.

RESULTS. ACTH stimulation test results were available from 51 cats with confirmed naturally occurring hyperadrenocorticism (FCS). The results were from cats in our series (43 cats), as well as from 8 cats reported in the literature (Immink et al, 1992 [1 cat]; Watson and Herrtage 1998 [5 cats]; Moore et al, 2000 [1 cat]). All 51 cats had confirmed FCS, and each of the 51 had at least one ACTH stimulation test result available for assessment. There were either two post-ACTH samples obtained (38 cats) or only one post-ACTH obtained (13 cats). If only a solitary post-ACTH test result was available, it was arbitrarily used for comparison with the second post-ACTH sample taken when two post-ACTH samples were obtained during testing (see Tables 7-9 and 7-10). Combining cats diagnosed as having PDH with those diagnosed as having ATH, 31 of 51 cats (61%) had post-ACTH plasma cortisol results within the reference range (61% of cats with FCS had normal ACTH stimulation test results). Three of the 51 cats (6%) had borderline results, and 17 (33%) had results that were ≥19 μg%. It should be pointed out that 5 of the 51 cats were from one study in which all 5 had strikingly abnormal results (Watson and Herrtage, 1998). In our experience, having five of five cats with FCS (100%) with strikingly abnormal ACTH stimulation test results is atypical. If the results from these five cats were not included in this evaluation, the ACTH stimulation test would be significantly less efficacious. The ACTH stimulation test was no more valuable in diagnosing PDH or ATH. Hence there seems to be little indication for using the ACTH stimulation test to evaluate cats for FCS.

In evaluations of the cats specifically diagnosed with PDH, 27 of 43 cats (63%) had results within the reference range, 3 (7%) had borderline test results, and 13 (30%) had clearly abnormal results. Combining the borderline and clearly abnormal results, 16 of 43 cats with PDH (37%) had abnormal results and 63% had results in the reference range. In evaluations of the cats specifically diagnosed with ATH, 4 of 8 cats (50%) had post-ACTH stimulation plasma cortisol concentration values within the established reference range and 4 cats had clearly abnormal results.

Thirty-eight cats with confirmed hyperadrenocorticism had two post-ACTH administration samples obtained during stimulation testing, allowing assessment of a "middle" result (see Tables 7-9 and 7-10). Of these 38 cats with either PDH or ATH, 25 cats (66%) had results within the reference range, 4 cats (10%) had borderline results and 9 cats (24%) had clearly abnormal results. Combining the clearly abnormal and borderline results, 13 of the 38 cats (34%) had results that were either borderline or clearly abnormal. Of the 32 cats that had PDH *and* an intermediate sample result, 21 of the 32 cats (66%) had results within the reference range and of the 6 cats with ATH, 4 (67%) had results within the reference range. Thus there was little diagnostic value associated with adding the intermediate sample during ACTH stimulation testing.

CONCLUSIONS. There are several attributes of ACTH stimulation testing. However, the concept that the test is brief, easy to complete, easy to interpret, and relatively inexpensive all lose value when two facts are considered. First, collated results indicate that the ACTH stimulation test lacks sensitivity and second, there are tests (UC:CR and LDDST) that are clearly superior. Thus the attributes associated with the ACTH stimulation test become trivial when it is realized that a majority of cats with FCS have normal results.

The ACTH stimulation test remains the only test that can confirm a diagnosis of iatrogenic Cushing's syndrome. However, although iatrogenic Cushing's syndrome is common in dogs, it is rare in cats. Its use in long-term monitoring of dogs treated medically is also negated since most cats are treated (or should be treated) with surgery or with radiation therapy. Finally, the concept that an abnormal test result is highly specific for confirming a diagnosis in dogs has never been fully evaluated in cats. The study on ACTH stimulation testing completed on 15 cats that did not have FCS at the time of evaluation or during the 12-month follow-up period is of interest (Schoeman et al, 2000). Using lower post-ACTH plasma cortisol concentrations as "diagnostic" would have resulted in several of those cats being misdiagnosed as having FCS. Thus the specificity of ACTH stimulation testing remains questionable. Our conclusion is simple: the ACTH stimulation test should not be used in the diagnostic evaluation of cats suspected as having hyperadrenocorticism.

Low-Dose Dexamethasone Testing

BACKGROUND. The low-dose dexamethasone screening test (LDDST) has been recommended as an aid in the diagnosis of Cushing's syndrome in dogs for more than 15 years. More recently, this test has been recommended as a diagnostic aid in the evaluation of cats suspected of having hyperadrenocorticism, presumably as an extension of its use in dogs. A complete discussion on the physiologic basis for this test and its usefulness is provided in Chapter 6. Typically, human beings suspected of having endocrine deficiency syndromes (for example, hypoadrenocorticism [Addison's disease]), are evaluated with provocative or stimulation-type tests to help in confirming a diagnosis. Human beings suspected of having endocrine excess syndromes (for example, hyperadrenocorticism [Cushing's syndrome]), are typically evaluated with suppression tests to help confirm a diagnosis. Therefore, use of the low-dose dexamethasone screening (suppression) test is well established in the evaluation of human beings suspected of having Cushing's syndrome, with a sensitivity and specificity approaching that of the 24-hour urine cortisol excretion test. In dogs the LDDST is also well accepted and is used commonly.

The physiology of low-dose dexamethasone testing is based on the effect of dexamethasone administration to healthy individuals (regardless of whether that individual is a human being, dog, or cat). Dexamethasone, following administration, circulates throughout the body. Included in the tissues encountered in this circulation pattern are the hypothalamus and pituitary gland. With receptor recognition and attachment by dexamethasone, suppression of hypothalamic synthesis, secretion of corticotropin, and in turn, suppression of synthesis and secretion of pituitary ACTH follows. Suppression of ACTH secretion thereby suppresses adrenocortical synthesis and secretion of cortisol. Suppression begins within 30 to 60 minutes and is dominant within 120 minutes. Suppression persists as long as the effects of dexamethasone persist. In the dog, dexamethasone suppresses the hypothalamic-pituitary-adrenal axis for an average of 30 hours. Therefore cortisol concentrations in the blood of a healthy dog will be quite low (suppressed) if assayed 4 and 8 hours after dexamethasone was administered. Dexamethasone has been the traditional glucocorticoid for suppression testing because early cortisol assays cross-reacted with prednisone or prednisolone but not with dexamethasone.

Consistent suppression of the hypothalamic-pituitary-adrenocortical axis, not only in healthy individuals but in any individual without disease involving these organs, is the single most important criterion of a reliable dexamethasone screening or suppression test. The reason for this requirement can be explained by the physiology of an individual that has PDH or ATH. The individual with an adreno-cortical tumor causing hyperadrenocorticism (ATH) has a neoplasm that autonomously secretes cortisol. That cortisol not only creates clinical signs but also chronically suppresses ACTH secretion from the normal hypothalamus and pituitary. Thus administration of dexamethasone to an individual with ATH cannot have any effect on cortisol secretion via dexamethasone-mediated suppression of pituitary ACTH, because that ACTH secretion was *already* suppressed by tumor secretion of cortisol. If an individual has pituitary-dependent hyperadreno-corticism (PDH), the individual has an autonomous functioning, ACTH-secreting tumor. Therefore the pituitary containing an ACTH-secreting tumor should be resistant to suppression by dexamethasone.

In summary, individuals with a healthy hypothalamic-pituitary-adrenal axis can be "suppressed" by low doses of dexamethasone, whereas those with naturally occurring Cushing's syndrome (ATH or PDH) are resistant to suppression. Furthermore, duration of dexamethasone activity is curtailed in individuals with hyperadrenocorticism. That is, dexamethasone has the previously mentioned 30-hour duration of activity in healthy dogs but that duration of activity is thought to be reduced to only 3 to 6 hours in dogs with hyperadrenocorticism. Thus, even if a pituitary tumor is sensitive to and therefore suppressed by dexa-methasone, it will be suppressed for only a brief time period. It is assumed that the effects of dexamethasone in cats are similar to those in dogs.

PROTOCOL AND PUBLISHED DATA. The low-dose or "screening" dexamethasone test that was initially recommended for cats used the protocol established in dogs. In this protocol, 0.01 mg/kg of dexamethasone was administered intravenously with plasma cortisol concentrations determined before and 4 and 8 hours after administration. However, because 15% to 20% of *healthy* cats failed to demonstrate suppression after being given this dose of dexamethasone, the dose was increased to 0.1 mg/kg (Smith and Feldman, 1987). As previously discussed, the primary criterion on which a low-dose dexamethasone suppression must be based is that it must consistently suppress the hypothalamic-pituitary-adrenocortical axis in virtually all normal individuals. The second critically important criterion that must be met is that the dose of dexamethasone must result in a test that demonstrates sufficient *sensitivity* for diagnosis of the disease in question. That is, the dose must not suppress plasma cortisol concentrations in individuals with naturally occurring Cushing's syndrome. Therefore, not only must cats with ATH be resistant to dexamethasone (logically, all must be resistant) but all or almost all cats with PDH must also be resistant. The resistance in cats with PDH may be due to true resistance, or it may be due to the brief duration of action of dexamethasone. Based on these criteria, the low dose of dexamethasone recommended for cats is 0.1 mg/kg, IV, with blood samples obtained before and 4 and 8 hours after administration.

TEST INTERPRETATION. As with evaluation of UC:CR and ACTH stimulation test results, reference ranges were established from more than 100 healthy cats. All healthy cats were privately owned and almost all were >5 years of age. Both genders were equally represented, and all cats were neutered. It was appropriate to arbitrarily assign "borderline" postdexamethasone plasma cortisol concentrations in addition to statis-tically derived "clearly abnormal results" that would be consistent with a diagnosis of Cushing's syndrome. The purpose of establishing borderline values was to improve both sensitivity and specificity. The potential cost of having borderline values is a loss of sensitivity in applying a clear diagnostic result, but the potential gain is an improvement in specificity. The statistically derived normal reference range for both 4 and 8 hour post–low-dose dexamethasone plasma cortisol con-centrations is ≤0.8 μg%, and the "clearly abnormal" value is ≥1.4 μg%. The borderline range we used in this analysis are post–low-dose dexamethasone plasma cortisol concentrations of 0.9 to 1.3 μg%.

Cats that satisfied our criteria for inclusion in this analysis had both clinical signs and histologic evidence of hyperadrenocorticism and had a low-dose dexamethasone suppression test completed using the 0.1 mg/kg dose protocol previously described. As previously discussed, we do not recommend using the 0.01 mg/kg low-dose dexamethasone protocol used in dogs.

RESULTS OF LDDST AS A "SCREENING" TEST. Forty-five cats met the criteria for inclusion for evaluating the low-dose dexamethasone test as a screening study for FCS. Thirty-seven of the 45 cats had confirmed

PDH, and 8 had confirmed ATH. Thirty-seven of the cats were from our series, and data from 8 cats were obtained from the literature (Immink et al, 1992 [2 cats]; Goossens et al, 1995 [3 cats]; Meij et al, 2001 [3 cats]). Two cats from our series (both with ATH) had basal and 8-hour samples but no 4-hour sample. Three cats from each of two reports (6 cats total) had data only from the basal and 4-hour samples (Goossens et al, 1995; Meij et al, 2001). Therefore 37 cats had basal, 4-hour, and 8-hour postdexamethasone plasma cortisol concentration results, 2 cats had basal and 8-hour postdexamethasone results, and 6 cats had basal and 4-hour test results (see Tables 7-9 and 7-10).

All 39 cats (100%) that had FCS and an 8-hour LDDS test result had clearly abnormal plasma cortisol concentrations (>1.4 µg%) after receiving 0.1 mg/kg of dexamethasone by IV. Forty-one of the 43 cats that had 4-hour postdexamethasone plasma cortisol concentrations assessed had values >1.4 µg%, and two cats had values <0.9 µg%. All cats with PDH and all cats with ATH had clearly abnormal 8-hour postdexamethasone test results, making this protocol not only "highly sensitive" but more sensitive than either the UC:CR or the ACTH stimulation test. All cats with ATH had clearly abnormal 4-hour postdexamethasone test results, and 35 of 37 cats with PDH had clearly abnormal test results on the 4-hour sampling. The 2 cats with 4-hour plasma cortisol concentrations <0.9 µg% both had PDH, results that are frequently obtained in dogs with PDH: that is, suppression at 4 hours and lack of suppression at 8 hours.

If an absolute plasma cortisol concentration at 4 hours of <0.9 µg% were used as a test to discriminate PDH (suppression) from ATH (lack of suppression), the conclusion would be that the low-dose dexamethasone failed in 35 of 37 cats with PDH (please see the following discussion on using percentage decrease rather than an absolute value). However, this would not be the recommended use of the test. When used as we recommend, that is, only as a screening test, the 0.1 mg/kg LDDS test has been superb. Although our results indicate 100% sensitivity, readers must understand that no test is perfect. Furthermore, although the test is obviously sensitive, this discussion does not address specificity.

RESULTS OF LDDS (0.1 MG/KG) AS A "DISCRIMINATION" TEST. Because the 0.1 mg/kg of dexamethasone test is the *discrimination* test for dogs (the test used as an aid in discriminating PDH from ATH), it seems fair to assess this test and dose as a discrimination test for cats with FCS. For a complete description, please see Chapter 6. To briefly review, the discrimination test is easiest to employ using >50% decrease in plasma cortisol concentration from baseline and at 4 or 8 hours postdexamethasone as criteria for suppression. Since adrenal tumors synthesize and secrete cortisol autonomously (independent of pituitary ACTH) and since dexamethasone functions by suppressing pituitary ACTH, cats with ATH should not exhibit decreases in plasma cortisol after they receive dexamethasone, regardless of the dose administered.

However, theoretically, some (not all) pituitary tumors may be suppressed by large doses of dexamethasone. Therefore, before using a discrimination test, it is assumed that a cat has been diagnosed as having Cushing's syndrome (FCS) based on clinical signs, routine laboratory results, and from results of appropriate screening test results. Then "suppression," as previously defined, would indicate that the cat has PDH. Failure to demonstrate suppression could further support the diagnosis of FCS but would not aid in discriminating PDH from ATH since not only will no cat with ATH demonstrate suppression but some cats with PDH will also fail to demonstrate suppression.

Based on evaluation of the 45 cats tested with the 0.1 mg/kg dose of dexamethasone, the test is an excellent "screening test" for FCS. However, of the 37 cats with PDH, only 8 (22%) demonstrated >50% suppression of plasma cortisol concentration at either the 4- or 8-hour postdexamethasone sampling. The 8 cats that did "suppress" all did so on the 4-hour plasma cortisol assay, and these included the 2 cats that also had plasma cortisol concentrations <0.9 µg%. Therefore 29 cats with PDH and all 8 cats with ATH failed to demonstrate suppression at either the 4- or 8-hour postdexamethasone sampling. Suppression, defined as >50% decrease from the baseline value, may well indicate PDH in a cat otherwise diagnosed as having FCS, but this test is not sensitive.

CONCLUSION. The 0.1 mg/kg dexamethasone test is an excellent screening test (100% sensitive) but was not remarkably effective as a discrimination test. Specificity of the LDDS test was not assessed. However, as a screening test, it outperformed both the UC:CR and the ACTH stimulation test. We strongly recommend this LDDS test as the test of choice in evaluating a cat for FCS. We also recommend the UC:CR (using urine obtained by owners from their cats in the home environment) as another excellent screening test either to confirm the diagnosis (not our choice) or to determine which cats are likely candidates for FCS and for LDDS screening (our choice).

TESTS TO "DISCRIMINATE" PITUITARY FROM ADRENAL TUMOR CUSHING'S SYNDROME

After the diagnosis of hyperadrenocorticism has been confirmed, several tests can be used to help discriminate those individuals that have pituitary-dependent hyperadrenocorticism (PDH) from those that have adrenocortical tumor hyperadrenocorticism (ATH). The primary reason for completing this exercise is based on the therapeutic options for the two conditions. Ideally, adrenocortical tumors should be surgically removed. Medical options for treating these individuals are limited. Ideally, pituitary tumors should also be surgically removed. Alternatively, pituitary tumors can be irradiated. Various medical therapies are available for managing cats with PDH, although in contrast to the experience in human beings and dogs, none has been consistently successful. In dogs, four discrimination tests can be used. These include the low-dose dexamethasone suppression (screening test; 0.01 mg/kg in dogs), the high-dose dexamethasone suppression test (0.1 mg/kg in dogs), plasma endogenous ACTH concentrations, and abdominal ultrasonography. Because of the expense and the need for specialized facilities and anesthesia requirements, CT and MRI scans, although potentially valuable, are not widely used as discrimination tests.

Each of the commonly used tests has both positive and negative traits when used in the evaluation of dogs. These traits may be different in cats. The effectiveness of the low-dose dexamethasone screening test (0.1 mg/kg in the cat) as a discrimination test for cats was reviewed in the previous section. It was not particularly effective, because only 8 of 37 cats with PDH that were reviewed would have been correctly identified. Results noted with the three remaining tests will be reviewed in this section. The cats included in this section represent those from our series as well as cats with confirmed hyperadrenocorticism, using similar protocols or assays from the literature.

High-Dose Dexamethasone Suppression Test

BACKGROUND. The high-dose dexamethasone suppression test (HDDST) is employed in human beings and in dogs with limited success. The physiologic basis for the test is that the administration of dexamethasone suppresses adrenocortical (endogenous) cortisol secretion by suppressing hypothalamic synthesis and secretion of corticotropin-releasing hormone (CRH), thereby decreasing pituitary ACTH synthesis and secretion. Dexamethasone also directly suppresses pituitary synthesis and secretion of ACTH. With decreases in ACTH, adrenocortical cells are not stimulated to synthesize or secrete cortisol. Plasma and urine cortisol concentrations decrease during the effective period of dexamethasone activity (30 hours in healthy dogs).

Adrenocortical tumors function autonomously and are therefore completely independent of pituitary control. In fact, pituitary ACTH-secreting cells atrophy in patients with functioning adrenocortical tumors. Therefore dexamethasone, regardless of dose administered, will not suppress cortisol secretion from an adrenocortical tumor in an individual with ATH. By contrast, although pituitary tumors in individuals with PDH function "somewhat" autonomously, secretion of ACTH by some (not all) pituitary tumors can be suppressed with large doses of dexamethasone. Thus individuals with confirmed Cushing's syndrome that demonstrate suppression of plasma or urine cortisol during an HDDST typically have PDH, whereas the group that fails to demonstrate suppression includes all those with ATH and a subpopulation of those with PDH. Any population of human beings or dogs with PDH will have 20% to 25% that cannot be suppressed by any dose of dexamethasone.

"IN-HOSPITAL" PROTOCOL. The protocol for the HDDST we employ is to administer 10 times the dose of dexamethasone used for the LDDST. In cats, the HDDST was performed using 1.0 mg/kg, IV, with blood samples obtained for plasma cortisol concentration before and 4 and 8 hours after dexamethasone administration. Remember, discrimination testing requires that the cat first have confirmed hyperadrenocorticism (FCS). Four criteria for suppression were applied to these test results: (1) >50% decrease in plasma cortisol concentration, from the basal value, at 4 hours; (2) a plasma cortisol concentration <1.4 µg% at 4 hours; (3) >50% decrease in plasma cortisol concentration, from the basal value, at 8 hours; and (4) a plasma cortisol concentration <1.4 µg% at 8 hours. If a cat met any one of these four criteria for suppression, the HDDST result was positive for PDH. Failure to meet any of these four criteria meant that the test result was inconclusive.

"AT-HOME" PROTOCOL. An alternative method of performing an HDDST employs the UC:CR (Goossens et al, 1995; Meij et al, 2001). Using this protocol, the entire test is carried out by the owner, without needing to bring the cat into the veterinary hospital. The owner is instructed to collect urine samples from the cat on two consecutive mornings. This can be easily accomplished by removing a majority of litter from the litter box or by replacing the cat's usual litter with nonabsorbable aquarium gravel when urine samples are needed. After the collection of the second urine sample, the owner should administer three doses of dexamethasone (0.1 mg/kg/dose) to the cat orally, at 8-hour intervals (i.e., at 8 AM, 4 PM, and midnight; Goossens et al, 1995) or two doses (at 4 PM and midnight; Meij et al, 2001). On the third morning, a final urine sample should be obtained by the owner and all three samples should then be delivered to the veterinarian. The interpretation of this HDDST initially requires assay of the first two morning samples for the UC:CR. These first two samples are the screening UC:CRs used in confirming a diagnosis of FCS. The mean of these two results are then used as the "basal value" for the HDDST. The cat is described as having responded to dexamethasone ("suppressed") if the third morning UC:CR result is <50% of the basal value. Cats meeting this criteria have results consistent with PDH, whereas those failing to demonstrate suppression could have either ATH or PDH.

RESULTS: IN-HOSPITAL HDDST. As can be reviewed in Table 7-11, HDDST results were available from 40 cats with confirmed FCS. All 40 cats included in this evaluation were from our series and all had the 1.0 mg/kg study performed at our hospital. Basal and 4-hour post-HDDST results were available from 24 cats with confirmed PDH and 4 cats with confirmed ATH. Eight-hour results were available from an additional 11 cats with PDH and an additional cat with ATH. These latter 12 cats did not have blood samples taken at 4 hours. The HDDST results were either classified as diagnostic for PDH based on suppression being documented or classified as nondiagnostic

TABLE 7–11   HIGH DOSE DEXAMETHASONE SUPPRESSION TEST AND PLASMA ENDOGENOUS ACTH RESULTS FROM CATS WITH NATURALLY OCCURRING HYPERADRENOCORTICISM

	PLASMA CORTISOL (µg%) HIGH DOSE DEXAMETHASONE TEST			ENDOGENOUS ACTH
	Pre	4 Hr	8 Hr	(pg/ml)
Pituitary Dependent Hyperadrenocorticism (PDH)				
Reference range	0–5	<1.4	<1.4	10–60
Borderline range for PDH	–	–	–	10–45
Results consistent with PDH (definition)	–	<1.4 or <50% baseline	–	>45
Number of cats	35	24	35	45
Number of results inconclusive (consistent with PDH or ATH)	–	11	20	3
Number of results consistent with PDH	–	13	15	42
Range of test results	2.4–39.0	0.2–15	0.1–25.8	38–3653
Mean (± S.D.)	8.8 ± 8.8	3.0 ± 3.6	4.9 ± 6.2	457 ± 619
Median	5.3	0.9	2.4	221
Adrenocortical Tumor Hyperadrenocorticism (ATH)				
Reference range	0–5	4.4	<1.4	10–60
Borderline range for ATH	–	–	–	10–45
Results consistent with ATH	–	> 1.4 *and* > 50% borderline	–	undetectable
Number of cats	5	4	5	6
Number of results inconclusive	–	0	0	0
Number of results consistent with ATH	–	4	5	6
Range of test results	3.0–7.1	3.7–6.1	4.4–6.1	all undetectable
Mean (± S.D.)	5.1 ± 1.6	5.0 ± 0.8	5.0 ± 0.7	–
Median	4.9	4.7	4.7	–

based on a lack of suppression, indicating that the cat could have either ATH or PDH.

Thirteen of 24 cats (54%) had 4-hour HDDST results that demonstrated suppression, results consistent with PDH. All 13 cats had PDH. Thus suppression on the 4-hour test result was specific for PDH. The 4 cats with ATH and a 4-hour HDDST result failed to demonstrate suppression, as was expected. Also as expected, some cats (11 of 24; 46%) with PDH failed to respond to the HDDST at 4 hours. Thus failure to suppress plasma cortisol concentration at 4 hours was a nonspecific finding that included cats with ATH and PDH.

Fifteen of 40 cats (38%) had 8-hour HDDST results that demonstrated suppression, results consistent with PDH. All 15 of those cats did have PDH, correctly identifying 15 of 35 cats (43%) with PDH. Thus suppression on the 8-hour test result was specific for PDH. The 5 cats with ATH and an 8-hour HDDST result failed to demonstrate suppression, as was expected. Also as expected, some cats (20 of 35; 57%) with PDH failed to respond to the HDDST at 8 hours. Failure to suppress plasma cortisol concentration at 8 hours was a nonspecific finding that included cats with ATH and PDH. It is also of interest to note that the 8-hour test was available from all 24 PDH cats tested at 4 hours plus an additional 11 cats with PDH. However, only 2 additional cats with PDH demonstrated suppression at 8 hours. All 13 cats that met at least one of the two criteria for suppression at 4 hours met at least one of the two criteria for suppression at 8 hours. Thus one consideration would be the necessity for obtaining blood at both 4 and 8 hours. As in the dog, it seems reasonable to suggest that only a 4-hour post-HDDST

blood sample be obtained, because the 8-hour sample does not offer significant chance of providing additional information.

RESULTS: AT-HOME URINE HDDST. As can be reviewed in Table 7-12, 13 cats were tested using the "at-home" protocol previously described in this section. All 13 cats had PDH and all 13 cats were from the literature (Goossens et al, 1995 [6 cats]; Meij et al, 2001 [7 cats]). Ten of the 13 cats (77%) did demonstrate suppression on the UC:CR from the sample obtained postdexamethasone, using the mean of two basal urine samples for the comparison. This result, as suggested by the authors of the first study, was significantly more reliable than results from the 0.1 mg/kg dexamethasone suppression test (Goossens et al, 1995). In addition, these results were an improvement over the results from the 1.0 mg/kg dexamethasone test we assessed in 35 cats with PDH. More important, the entire test could be carried out by an owner, decreasing cost and stress.

CONCLUSION. The in-hospital HDDST is relatively easy to perform, easy to interpret, not expensive, and not harmful. Suppression, when demonstrated, is consistent with PDH. It is recommended that the protocol consist of obtaining a basal blood sample for cortisol determination, administering 1.0 mg/kg of dexamethasone IV, and then obtaining a second blood sample 4 hours later. Since the 0.1 mg/kg dexamethasone dose resulted in suppression in only 8 of 37 PDH cats (22%), it is noted that the 1.0 mg/kg dexamethasone dose was more effective in identifying PDH at 4 hours (13 of 24 cats, 54%) and at 8 hours (15 of 35 cats, 43%). No cat with ATH demonstrated

TABLE 7–12 HIGH DOSE DEXAMETHASONE SUPPRESSION TEST RESULTS FROM 13 CATS UTILIZING THE "AT-HOME UC:CR" PROTOCOL. SUPPRESSION IS DEFINED AS A POST-DEXAMETHASONE UC:CR <50% OF THE MEAN OF 2 BASAL UC:CR. (ALL UC:CR RESULTS ARE × 10^{-5})*

Cat #	First Basal UC:CR	Second Basal UC:CR	Mean UC:CR	Post-Dexamethasone UC:CR	Positive for PDH
1	13.9	14.5	14.2	1.3	Yes
2	3.7	6.4	5.1	0.5	Yes
3	7.5	8.2	7.8	9.2	No
4	12.5	15.5	14.0	4.1	Yes
5	10.4	10.3	10.35	2.6	Yes
6	22.8	31.6	27.2	1.8	Yes
7	–	–	27.2	1.8	Yes
8	–	–	8.0	11.7	No
9	–	–	11.9	0.5	Yes
10	–	–	7.3	1.7	Yes
11	–	–	7.2	2.7	Yes
12	–	–	10.5	11.9	No
13	–	–	7.7	0.7	Yes

*All results compiled from Goossens et al, 1995, and Meij et al, 2001.
UC:CR, urine cortisol: creatinine ratio; *PDH*, pituitary dependent hyperadrenocorticism.

suppression at either 4 or 8 hours of the HDDST, but some cats with PDH also fail to suppress. Therefore, failure to demonstrate suppression should be considered an inconclusive result and is similar to results in human beings and dogs.

The at-home HDDST is easier to perform and interpret than the in-hospital protocol. In addition, results from 13 cats with PDH (77% suppressed) were better than those obtained from 24 cats with PDH tested at 4 hours (54% suppressed) or from 35 cats with PDH tested at 8 hours (43% suppressed) using the in-hospital protocol. Therefore, assuming that the owner can administer the dexamethasone, it seems reasonable to recommend the at-home protocol for both screening and discrimination testing since this protocol is generally easier to perform, less expensive, easier to interpret, safer (less bruising and no chance of skin trauma), and more reliable than the in-hospital protocols. Although the in-hospital LDDST results were slightly more reliable as a screening test than the protocol using urine collected at home for UC:CR, the at-home protocol has more advantages than the in-hospital protocols.

Plasma Endogenous ACTH Concentration Determination

BACKGROUND. Plasma endogenous ACTH concentrations have been used to help discriminate PDH from ATH in human beings that have Cushing's syndrome for more than 30 years. The first report using this hormonal assay as a discrimination test for dogs with Cushing's syndrome was published in 1981 (Feldman, 1981). Several reports on cats with FCS have included results of endogenous ACTH concentrations. The physiologic basis for use of this test is the underlying disease process in ATH versus that in PDH. Individuals with ATH have autonomously functioning adrenocortical tumors that suppress circulating plasma endogenous ACTH concentrations, whereas those with PDH should have excess concentrations that cause adrenocortical hyperplasia and excess

cortisol secretion. Among the positive traits of this test are that it requires only one blood sample, it is easy to interpret, and it has been relatively reliable. The negative traits of the test include the following: it is expensive, blood must be collected in plastic or silicone lined tubes with appropriate anticoagulant, the blood must be centrifuged immediately, the plasma must be transferred to tubes without touching glass, samples must be maintained frozen until assayed, and the hormone is labile, causing results from shipped samples to be less reliable. Furthermore, results of the test are not always definitive. Because of these drawbacks, in addition to the growing value of abdominal ultrasonography, the endogenous ACTH assessment has never gained wide usage.

INTERPRETATION OF TEST RESULTS. We have had experience in testing plasma endogenous ACTH concentrations in dogs. In our experience, results are often, but not always, definitive. The reference range in dogs is 10 to 80 pg/ml. Dogs with PDH have plasma endogenous ACTH concentrations of 45 to 450 pg/ml, and those with ATH have results that range from undetectable to 45 pg/ml. Therefore potential overlap exists in the range of 10 to 45 pg/ml that includes healthy, PDH, and ATH dogs. This is the most obvious reason that the test is considered a discrimination test and not a screening test. In addition, undetectable concentrations are obtained in dogs with iatrogenic Cushing's syndrome, as well as those with ATH.

The reference range for plasma endogenous ACTH concentrations was determined from our initial work (Smith and Feldman, 1987) and results from an additional 140 healthy cats that were >5 years of age and of either gender (all were neutered). That reference range for cats is 10 to 60 pg/ml. Undetectable plasma endogenous ACTH concentrations (<10 pg/ml) are considered consistent with ATH. Plasma endogenous ACTH concentrations >45 pg/ml are consistent with a diagnosis of PDH in dogs; arbitrarily, this definition was assigned to cats as well. Therefore plasma endogenous ACTH concentrations of 10 to 45 pg/ml in cats with FCS are considered nondiagnostic.

RESULTS. Plasma endogenous ACTH concentrations were available from 51 cats with FCS. Thirty-eight of these cats were from our series, and 13 were from the literature (Goossens et al, 1995 [6 cats]; Meij et al, 2001 [7cats]). All 13 cats from the literature had PDH, 32 cats from our series had PDH, and 6 cats from our series had ATH. As can be seen from Table 7-11, the results of endogenous ACTH testing were excellent. All 6 cats (100%) with ATH had undetectable concentrations of ACTH. Forty-two of 45 cats (93%) with PDH had concentrations consistent with that diagnosis (>45 pg/ml). The 3 PDH cats with non-diagnostic results had values of 38, 40, and 41 pg/ml, respectively. These values were distinct from the results obtained from cats with ATH. Considering that the range for nondiagnostic results was arbitrary and that all ATH cats had undetectable concentrations, it may be reasonable to change the range of results classified as consistent with PDH. In any case, the results were quite promising, with at least 48 of 51 cats with FCS (94%) having diagnostic and correct results.

Dogs with PDH usually have plasma endogenous ACTH concentrations that range from 45 to 450 pg/ml. Approximately 40% of PDH dogs have results within the reference range (45 to 80 pg/ml), and 40% have results between 80 and 450 pg/ml. About 20% of dogs with PDH have plasma endogenous ACTH concentrations that are not diagnostic (usually with results that range from 20 to 45 pg/ml). About 50% of dogs with ATH have undetectable (diagnostic) plasma endogenous ACTH concentrations, and 50% have non-diagnostic results. By comparison, dogs with naturally occurring hypoadrenocorticism (Addison's disease) have plasma endogenous ACTH concentrations of 500 to 5000 pg/ml. Dogs with PDH and those with Addison's disease have distinctly different endogenous ACTH concentrations (i.e., the results rarely overlap).

Twenty-five of the 45 cats with PDH had results typical of those noted in dogs (45 to 450 pg/ml). However, 17 of the 45 cats with PDH (38%) had plasma endogenous ACTH concentrations in excess of 450 pg/ml (range: 487 to 3850 pg/ml; mean: 1002 pg/ml ± a standard deviation of 731). Why so many cats with PDH had extremely increased plasma endogenous ACTH concentrations (>450 pg/ml) is not well understood. Is it that their pituitary tumors produce more ACTH, is the assay less reliable in cats, or is there some other explanation? The extremely high concentrations of ACTH, as noted in many cats from our series, was also noted by Meij and colleagues (2001). These authors pointed out that in one cat, the ACTH assay results as measured by an IRMA assay was only about 20% of the value obtained with an assay employing a polyclonal antibody. It is possible, therefore, that the polyclonal antibody assay recognized molecules as ACTH that were not ACTH. In other words, perhaps these pituitary tumors secreted precursor-molecule pro-opiomelanocortin (POMC) or POMC-derived peptides recognized as ACTH by the assay. This would be similar to what has been reported in the dog (Goossens et al, 1995).

In both dogs and cats, pituitary pars intermedia (PI) cells are immunocytochemically heterogenous. Some cells stain immunopositive for being capable of synthesizing ACTH similar to the corticotropic cells of the pars distalis (PD). In addition, there are PI cells that cleave ACTH to α-MSH and corticotropin-like intermediate lobe peptide. These melanotropic cells immunostain for α-MSH and not for ACTH (Halmi and Krieger, 1983); they are commonly found in PI of cats (Rijnberk, 1996). The authors then suggest that one would expect high plasma α-MSH concentrations in cats with PI adenomas (Meij et al, 2001). However, they note that the cats with the highest α-MSH concentrations were those with PD adenomas. For an explanation, they suggest that the gene encoding the enzyme responsible for the cleavage of ACTH (proconvertase 2) may have become "de-repressed" in the course of neoplastic transformation of PD corticotropes (Low et al, 1993). Alternatively, they suggest that some of the PD adenomas may have originated from a sparsely present melanocyte population of cells in the PD, as has been shown to occur in humans (Coates et al, 1986). In dogs, however, only occasional PD adenomas stain positively for α-MSH (Peterson et al, 1982). In contrast to what has been noted in dogs, origin of PI versus PD adenomas could not be traced by immunocytochemistry in cats, because their adenomas stained positively for both ACTH and α-MSH.

CONCLUSIONS. Correct diagnosis of ATH or PDH, based on plasma endogenous ACTH concentrations were assigned to 48 of 51 cats (94%) with FCS. All 6 cats with ATH had diagnostic plasma endogenous ACTH concentrations. Since the total number of ATH cats is so small, further studies will likely determine the sensitivity of this assay in providing correct information. Three of the 45 cats with PDH that were included in this evaluation had endogenous ACTH concentrations of 38 to 45 pg/ml (slightly less than the "diagnostic value"). However, 42 of 45 PDH cats had "correct" results; of the 51 cats in total, 48 had "correct" results; and no cat had "incorrect" results. These findings suggest that this test has value for discriminating cats with PDH from those with ATH.

Abdominal Radiography

Changes noted on radiography of cats with FCS are similar to those seen in dogs. These changes include excellent contrast as a result of fat deposition into the mesentery, hepatomegaly (which is usually secondary to diabetes mellitus in cats, as opposed to being more frequently secondary to steroid-induced hepatomegaly in dogs), and a pot-bellied appearance. Readers interested in radiography are encouraged to review the section on abdominal radiography in Chapter 6, which describes changes identified in dogs with Cushing's syndrome. The description here is brief because abdominal radiography has been replaced, for the most part, by abdominal ultrasonography as the

TABLE 7–13   LENGTHS AND WIDTHS OF ADRENAL GLANDS MEASURED ULTRASONOGRAPHICALLY IN 20 HEALTHY AWAKE CATS*

Number of Cats	Parameter	Length of R Adrenal	Width of R Adrenal	Length of L Adrenal	Width of L Adrenal
20	Range (cm)	0.7–1.4	0.3–0.45	0.45–1.3	0.3–0.5
	Median (cm)	1.0	0.4	0.9	0.4

*From Zimmer et al, 2000.
R, Right adrenal gland; L, left adrenal gland.

key abdominal study for evaluating cats known to have or suspected of having naturally occurring hyperadrenocorticism (feline Cushing's syndrome; FCS). The reason for this increased use of ultrasonography is simply that adrenal glands are not able to be visualized via radiography unless the gland(s) is calcified or extremely enlarged (both situations are rare). By contrast, canine and feline adrenal glands can be routinely visualized by experienced ultrasonographers. Understanding that the expense of ultrasound to the client need not be much greater than that of radiography, the tool that provides the greatest amount of information should be chosen.

Abdominal Ultrasonography

BACKGROUND.   Until recently, ultrasonographic examination of feline adrenal glands was rarely discussed or reported. In part, this is simply a reflection of adrenal disease being relatively uncommon in cats. In addition, ultrasound visualization of adrenal glands in general and feline adrenal glands specifically has had a reputation of being quite difficult. Regardless, abdominal ultrasonography has continued to gain importance over the past 10 to 15 years as a valuable diagnostic aid in small animal medicine. As practitioners have become more dependent on results of abdominal ultrasonography in the evaluation of numerous disorders in dogs and cats, experience and expertise has improved.

With respect to naturally occurring hyperadrenocorticism (Cushing's syndrome), visualization of adrenal glands has become an excellent tool for helping to discriminate PDH from ATH. Dogs with PDH tend to have adrenal glands that are relatively equal in size and that may or may not be enlarged. On the other hand, dogs with ATH tend to have one adrenal gland that has the obvious appearance of a "mass" with the opposite adrenal gland usually being undetectable or small. It is assumed that these same traits apply to the evaluation of adrenal glands in cats suspected or known to have FCS.

PUBLISHED INFORMATION.   Imaging of the adrenal glands in dogs has progressed with better knowledge of tissue orientation, improved operator experience, and use of better equipment (Barthez et al, 1995; Horauf and Reusch, 1995). One study on cats was completed on anesthetized healthy cats (Cartee and Finn-Bodner, 1993). Since anesthesia is virtually never used in general practice for ultrasound, a study on cats that had not been anesthetized was conducted on 20 healthy cats. The adrenal glands of all cats could be

imaged and measured reliably. Both glands were able to be visualized in all cats without the need for anesthesia or sedation. Further, both left and right adrenal glands were virtually identical in size and shape, with both being oblong and oval-to-bean–shaped (Table 7-13; Zimmer et al, 2000). In general, these authors found feline adrenal glands to be less echogenic than the surrounding tissues and the right adrenal to be technically more difficult to image. Two zones within the adrenal glands could be seen in 6 of the 20 cats, with the center of the glands being more echogenic than the periphery. These authors stated that the adrenal glands of healthy cats were easier to image than adrenal glands of healthy dogs.

RESULTS.   The results of abdominal ultrasonography and attempts at visualizing the adrenals in cats with FCS are summarized in Table 7-14. Forty-one cats were evaluated. They include 35 cats from our series and 6 cats with results taken from the literature (Daley et al, 1993 [1 cat]; Watson and Herrtage, 1998 [4 cats]; Moore et al, 2000 [1 cat]). In contrast to reviewing results of endocrine data, results of ultrasonographic studies must be assessed differently. Ultrasonography is the most "operator-dependent" diagnostic tool (other than history and physical examination) in small animal practice. In other words, these results are subjective and dependent on the skill and experience of the ultrasonographer, as well as on the equipment used.

With this limitation understood, the abdominal ultrasound examination results were good. It was assumed that cats with FCS and PDH should have equal-sized, normal-to-enlarged adrenal glands and that cats with

TABLE 7–14   ABDOMINAL ULTRASOUND INTERPRETATIONS FROM 41 CATS WITH NATURALLY OCCURRING HYPERADRENOCORTICISM

	Possible Finding	Number of Cats
Cats with ATH (9 cats)	R mass, L small	3
	L mass, R small	0
	R mass, L not seen	2
	L mass, R not seen	2
	Both adrenals enlarged	1
	No adrenals seen	1
Cats with PDH (32 cats)	Both adrenals normal	5
	Both adrenals enlarged	22
	L normal or enlarged, R not seen	2
	R normal or enlarged, L not seen	1
	No adrenals seen	2

ATH, Adrenal tumor hyperadrenocorticism; PDH, pituitary dependent hyperadrenocorticism; R, right adrenal gland; L, left adrenal gland.

ATH should have one adrenal mass, with the opposite gland being small or not visualized. Using these parameters, 34 of the 41 cats (83%) had correct abdominal ultrasound results (see Table 7-14). Three of the 41 cats (7%) had inconclusive studies because no adrenal tissue was identified (2 of these cats had PDH, and 1 had ATH). Four of the 41 cats (10%) had potentially misleading results. Three of the 32 cats (9%) with PDH had one normal to increased-sized adrenal gland, with the other gland not visible. These results would be consistent with ATH, but all 3 cats had PDH. One of the 9 cats with ATH had a report stating that both adrenal glands were enlarged, but at surgery the cat had one obvious adrenal mass (later it was histologically confirmed to be an adrenocortical carcinoma) and the opposite adrenal was abnormally small and atrophied.

Twenty-seven of the 32 cats (84%) with PDH had adrenal glands that were visualized and described as being relatively equal-sized. Thus ultrasound was a successful discrimination test in these 27 cats. A unilateral adrenal mass with the opposite gland being small or not visible was observed in 7 of 9 cats (78%) with ATH. Again, ultrasound was a successful discrimination test in these 7 cats. As stated previously, ultrasound correctly identified PDH or ATH in a total of 34 of 41 cats with FCS (83%). Realizing the subjective nature of ultrasonography, had all the studies been performed by one experienced radiologist, the results might have been much better. The same statement could be made had all the cats been examined with the newest equipment. Regardless, it seems reasonable to state that abdominal ultrasonography is an excellent discrimination test for separating ATH cats from those with PDH. It also seems reasonable to remind the reader that ultrasound examination results are subjective and success will vary. It would be quite unlikely that any large study would have uniformly correct results.

Ultrasound-Guided Biopsy

Several reports on cats with FCS mention successful percutaneous biopsy of suspected masses. However, each cat was already suspected as having FCS. Although percutaneous biopsy can be completed with ultrasound guidance, we question the value of such test results as weighed against risk of hemorrhage.

COMPUTED TOMOGRAPHY (CT) AND MAGNETIC RESONANCE IMAGING (MRI) SCANS

Background

In cats with diabetes mellitus, persistent hyperglycemia may result from the use of too low a dose of insulin, owner error in insulin handling or administration, rebound hyperglycemia secondary to insulin-induced hypoglycemia (Somogyi effect), rapid metabolism of insulin, or insulin resistance usually secondary to an underlying or concurrent illness. "Insulin resistance" (real or misdiagnosed) is one of the most common reasons that veterinarians develop a suspicion of Cushing's syndrome (FCS) in cats. As has been reviewed earlier in this chapter, there are other reasons to establish FCS as a potential differential diagnosis in cats (fragile skin, PU/PD, easy bruisability, etc). Insulin-resistant diabetes mellitus usually refers to a clinical syndrome in which a typically adequate dose of insulin fails to induce an acceptable decrease in blood glucose concentration. There is no absolute dose of insulin that clearly defines a resistant condition. However, cats with diabetes mellitus are generally considered to have resistance if serum glucose concentrations routinely fail to decrease below 300 mg/dl at any time after administering ≥ 2.2 U/kg/dose of insulin.

Two hormonal causes of insulin resistance in cats with diabetes mellitus are acromegaly and hyperadrenocorticism (FCS). The most common cause for either condition in cats is a functional pituitary tumor. The diagnostic approach to acromegaly is reviewed in Chapter 2, and that for FCS is reviewed in this chapter. We would recommend confirmation of either condition before pursuing sophisticated diagnostic imaging such as CT and MRI scanning. These techniques provide a noninvasive means of visualizing intracranial tumors; however, each technique requires specialized facilities, cats must be anesthetized, and such studies are expensive. We have little experience with abdominal CT or MRI scanning in cats with FCS. Therefore abdominal scans will not be discussed.

The magnetic resonance imaging (MRI) scan is the technique of choice for diagnostic imaging of the pituitary gland area in people (Chakere et al, 1989; Stein et al, 1989). Compared with computed tomography (CT) scans, MRI scans have superior anatomic resolution and soft tissue contrast. Also, MRI scans are less likely to create distracting artifacts when the middle and caudal fossae of the brain are imaged (Kaufman, 1984). MRI scanning also allows for acquisition of images oriented in any plane, an important feature when examining the pituitary fossa. However, the purpose of considering a sophisticated diagnostic aid such as CT or MRI in a cat suspected of having Cushing's syndrome (FCS) is to determine whether or not an obvious pituitary mass can be visualized. In our experience, both CT and MRI scans consistently allow visualization of pituitary masses >3 mm in greatest diameter. Therefore, if a veterinarian wants to perform such a study and only one of these two modalities is available, we would encourage using the tool available. Alternatively, if both imaging modalities are available, we encourage veterinarians to choose whichever tool is less expensive or whichever tool requires the shortest duration of anesthesia.

Healthy Cats

A recent study has been published in which the size range of the pituitary gland in healthy cats was reported. The pituitary gland was measured from transverse and sagittal MRI postgadolinium (postcontrast) studies in 17 cats. The cats were 1 to 15 years of age and weighed between 2.9 and 6.5 kg. Mean (± standard deviation [±SD]) pituitary length was 0.54 cm (±0.06 cm) and the mean width was 0.5 cm (±0.08 cm). Mean pituitary gland height measured on sagittal and transverse images was about 0.33 cm (±0.05). Mean pituitary volume was about 0.05 cm^3. There were no significant correlations between cat weight or age and pituitary volume. The pituitary gland appearance on the precontrast scan had a "mixed signal intensity," whereas on postcontrast scans the pituitary appeared to have uniform enhancement (Wallack et al, 2003).

Results

The results available from our series and from the literature were limited. Pituitary/brain scan results were available from 27 cats with FCS with confirmed PDH (Table 7-15). There were a total of 14 scan results from our series of cats with FCS with PDH and 13 scan results from a series of PDH cats in two reports from the veterinary school in Utrecht, The Netherlands (Goossens et al, 1995 [6 cats]; Meij et al, 2001 [7 cats]). A visible mass (5 to 11 mm in greatest diameter) was identified in 15 of the 27 PDH cats (56%; Fig. 7-5). This is quite similar to the percentage of dogs with PDH that have a visible pituitary tumor at the time of diagnosis. All 13 cats from Utrecht were evaluated with CT scans and visible masses were observed in 6 cats (46%). Fourteen PDH cats in our series were evaluated, and visible masses were observed in 9 (64%). Nine of our 14 cats were evaluated with a CT scan (mass noted in 6 cats), and 5 were evaluated with a MRI scan (mass noted in 3 cats). The cats with confirmed PDH and no obvious mass are assumed to have pituitary tumors that were simply too small for the detection limits of either CT or MRI scanning.

Conclusion

Pituitary imaging serves several potential roles. Either CT or MRI scans could be used to help confirm a diagnosis of FCS. This would be an expensive and

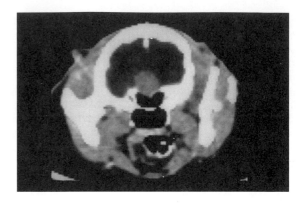

FIGURE 7-5. Computed tomography (CT) scan of the pituitary brain region from a cat with pituitary-dependent hyperadrenocorticism demonstrating a pituitary mass.

insensitive approach, considering that UC:CR or LDDS test results are much more sensitive, require no anesthesia, and are less expensive. Either CT or MRI scanning could be used as a discrimination test to help distinguish FCS cats with PDH from those with ATH. This, too, seems like an expensive and insensitive approach to the problem since cats with ATH would have normal scans and almost 50% of cats with confirmed PDH also have normal scans. Thus a normal scan would yield virtually no information other than suggesting that if a cat has PDH, the tumor is small.

Thus the recommendation is that CT or MRI scans be used as a presurgical screen for cats scheduled to undergo hypophysectomy or as a pretreatment screen for cats scheduled to undergo pituitary radiation. Either scan could be used to evaluate cats with FCS that also have central nervous system signs. However, central nervous system problems due to an enlarging pituitary tumor, as documented in human beings and dogs with PDH, have not yet been observed in a cat.

TREATMENT OF PITUITARY-DEPENDENT HYPERADRENOCORTICISM

The clinical signs and routine laboratory abnormalities identified in cats with hyperadrenocorticism (FCS) are becoming better appreciated. In addition, appropriate screening tests to confirm such a diagnosis, and discrimination tests to distinguish PDH from ATH are also being successfully employed. Thus veterinarians have a better opportunity to understand when FCS should be included in the differential diagnosis, and they have a better chance of correctly diagnosing this condition. The following discussion reviews several therapeutic strategies. These treatments include surgery of the pituitary or adrenals, radiation of the pituitary, and medical therapies. However, successful treatment protocols for FCS have not been established. None of these treatment modalities have been employed in a large enough group of cats to allow solid recommendations for or against any. Rather, this is an area of

TABLE 7–15 COMPUTED TOMOGRAPHY (CT) AND MAGNETIC RESONANCE IMAGING (MRI) SCAN RESULTS FROM 27 CATS* WITH FELINE CUSHINGS'S SYNDROME (FCS) AND CONFIRMED PITUITARY-DEPENDENT DISEASE (PDH)

Results	CT Scan	MRI Scan
Normal study (no mass seen)	10 cats	2 cats
Visible mass (5–11 mm in greatest diameter)	12 cats	3 cats
Total	22 cats	5 cats

* 14 cats from UC Davis series; 7 cats from Meij et al, 2001; 6 cats from Goossens et al, 1995.

veterinary practice that is in its infancy. We believe some of these treatments have great potential for becoming routinely successful (hypophysectomy), some have little chance of being routinely successful (mitotane [o,p'-DDD]), and the potential value of others is not yet known. Diagnosis of FCS by a veterinarian may be somewhat exciting, in part because the condition is so uncommon and in part because it is a disorder that has received some attention. However, for most cats FCS is a terrible disease and one that will more than likely be terminal, expensive to treat, or both.

Hypophysectomy

BACKGROUND. In humans, the treatment of choice for individuals with pituitary-dependent hyperadrenocorticism (PDH) is surgical removal of the pituitary tumor, thus eliminating the causative lesion, that is, the pituitary lesion causing the excess secretion of ACTH (Melby, 1988; Thorner et al, 1992). In human beings and dogs with PDH, there is increasing evidence that the pituitary tumors are primarily pituitary in origin and not the result of excessive hypothalamic stimulation (Scholten-Sloof et al, 1992; Van Wijk et al, 1992). If pituitary tumors are primary in origin, their removal should result in permanent resolution of the condition. If etiology of PDH were the result of a hypothalamic disorder, recurrence of the PDH would often follow successful pituitary surgery. Recurrence of PDH has not been the experience in people after successful surgical removal of a pituitary tumor. As in humans, the ideal treatment of dogs or cats with PDH would also be a similar surgical procedure. The procedure has been described, and the initial report of a microsurgical protocol used in 52 dogs with PDH illustrates great promise (Meij et al, 1997; Meij et al, 1998).

Hypophysectomy in cats has been used for both physiologic and pharmacologic research studies (Reaves et al, 1981; Sallanon et al, 1988). In addition, transsphenoidal selective anterior hypophysectomy in cats has been described in detail for advanced microsurgical training of physician neurosurgeons (Snyckers, 1975). With the recent progress made in microsurgical hypophysectomy for treatment of dogs with PDH by the researchers in The Netherlands, they have begun to evaluate use of this surgery in cats. Progress has been made for several reasons. First, credit must be given to the surgeon (Bjorn Meij) and to the institution (Utrecht University in The Netherlands) that have dedicated their combined research efforts to this treatment modality. They give credit for their progress, in part, to presurgical visualization of the pituitary gland using computed tomography (CT) scans. They also suggest that the surgical technique has been refined and improved as a result of new developments in neurosurgical instrumentation and to the recognition of complications that can result from this procedure (Meij et al, 1997).

TECHNIQUE. The group from Utrecht University has reported their initial results of transsphenoidal hypophysectomy in seven cats with naturally occurring PDH (Meij et al, 2001). It must be remembered that these results are not representative of those anticipated after more experience has been gained with a larger group of patients. On the one hand, seven cats with any disorder is a small number. On the other hand, feline PDH is quite uncommon and research inevitably begins with a small number of individuals (as did Dr. Cushing with his small number of patients). Thus we applaud this work as representing some of the first steps taken in employing a procedure with great potential.

These first seven cats were managed surgically between 1994 and 1998 (Meij et al, 2001). Six of the seven cats were male, and their body weights ranged from 2.6 to 6.5 kg. The diagnosis of hyperadrenocorticism and then PDH in each cat was made using previously discussed screening and discrimination tests. CT scans were obtained on each cat prior to surgery, with pituitary height and width measured on contrast-enhanced images. Pituitary length was estimated from the number of images that contained a section of the gland. For intraoperative localization of the pituitary, CT images were viewed sequentially, and the distance between the gland and surgical landmarks was determined (Meij et al, 1997). The imaging greatly facilitated the surgical procedure by indicating the exact location of the burr slot within the surgical field (Meij et al, 2001). Cats were placed in sternal recumbency, and after incision of soft palate and then mucoperiosteum, the sphenoid bone was exposed. Access to the pituitary fossa was completed using a burr and punches, the dura mater was incised, and the pituitary carefully extracted.

RESULTS. There was no intraoperative mortality. However, one cat did not recover from anesthesia, remained comatose, and died. After necropsy and histologic evaluation of tissues obtained, this cat was diagnosed as having had FCS, polycystic renal disease, and severe pancreatic fibrosis. A second cat was readmitted to the hospital 2 weeks after surgery for recurrence of chronic diarrhea. That cat developed neurologic abnormalities and died. After necropsy and histologic evaluation of tissues obtained, this cat was diagnosed as having had malignant lymphoma of the intestinal tract. Five cats had resolution of their clinical and chemical hyperadrenocorticism (FCS). One of these five cats had a recurrence of FCS 19 months after surgery, remained in good condition, but died unexpectedly 28 months after surgery. Another cat had a persistent oronasal fistula after surgery that was not treated, because it seemed to cause no problems to the cat. That cat became anemic and anorexic 6 months after surgery and was euthanized at the owner's request. Another cat also developed an oronasal fistula and then purulent rhinitis. Despite attempts to surgically correct this defect, recurrent infections of the nose and middle ear developed, and the cat was euthanized 8 months after hypophysectomy. Two cats were alive 15 and 46 months after surgery, respectively, at the time that the report was written and were in complete remission. Two of the 5 long-term survivors had resolution of diabetes mellitus after surgery (Meij et al, 2001).

CONCLUSION. The number of cats treated with hypophysectomy has been limited. However, as more experience is gained, there is no doubt that this will be the treatment of choice for cats with PDH, as it is for similarly afflicted human beings and dogs. There are, however, limiting factors. Those limiting factors include the necessary expertise to perform the surgery, the equipment needed for the surgery, and the facilities needed for postoperative medical care. As expertise improves, it is anticipated that specific removal of ACTH-secreting tumors will be accomplished while the healthy portion of the pituitary is preserved.

Pituitary Radiation

BACKGROUND. Radiation therapy refers to the use of ionizing radiation for local or regional treatment of patients with malignant and, occasionally, benign tumors. It is usually a consultative discipline in which a veterinary radiation oncologist evaluates an animal referred for therapy. The objective of radiation therapy is tumor eradication with preservation of normal tissue structure and function (Theon, 2000). Facilities typically needed are a cobalt-60 photon irradiation unit or a linear accelerator photon unit. Treatment usually involves delivery of a predetermined total dose of radiation given in fractions over a period of several weeks. Currently, we are evaluating delivery of 48 Gy, usually given in 3- to 4-Gy fractions, 5 days a week, with a total of 15 treatments. Since each treatment requires that the cat or dog be absolutely still, anesthesia is necessary.

The basic principle of clinical radiation therapy is that it should always have potential benefit for the pet, even though outcome may not be entirely predictable. The only contraindication, therefore, is inability of a dog or cat to tolerate the 15 anesthesia protocols in a 3-week time period. We have also learned the importance of rapid anesthesia recovery of cats and dogs, providing them with enough "conscious time" for them to eat prior to the obligatory cessation of food hours before the next scheduled anesthesia.

EXPERIENCE (DOGS). Our experience with irradiation of pituitary tumors in PDH dogs has been varied. Complete discussion of this topic is provided in Chapter 6. It is safe to state that PDH dogs without CNS signs that have tumors 4 to 12 mm in greatest diameter have an excellent prognosis for surviving therapy and for dramatic shrinkage of their pituitary mass. Resolution of hyperadrenocorticism, however, has not been a consistent response to radiation therapy in these dogs. Some have had complete but transient resolution of their Cushing's syndrome for as long as 6 to 12 months. However, our experience to date is that the clinical syndrome almost always recurs. In other dogs there has been clinical improvement but not complete resolution of their Cushing's, and in still others the radiation therapy, although dramatically

shrinking a tumor, does not alter the clinical Cushing's condition. Thus a large percentage of PDH dogs treated with pituitary radiation that shrinks the tumor must also be treated medically to manage the Cushing's syndrome. In dogs with CNS signs due to large pituitary tumors, tumor shrinkage is less predictable. Some dogs dramatically improve, and others do not. Some dogs with large pituitary masses have not survived the radiation treatment period.

EXPERIENCE (CATS). Our experience in treating PDH cats with pituitary radiation is extremely limited. Only four cats have been treated with sufficient follow-up to determine their response. Each of the four had obvious clinical signs, and two of the four had insulin-resistant diabetes mellitus. In addition to screening and discrimination testing to confirm the diagnosis of FCS and then PDH, each cat was evaluated either with a CT scan (three cats) or an MRI scan (one cat). Each of the four cats had a visible pituitary mass (5 to 11 mm in greatest diameter), and each was treated with 15 fractions of radiation divided over a period of 3 weeks. One cat demonstrated no response and was euthanized 7 months after radiation because of continuing signs of diabetes mellitus and fragile skin. The two nondiabetic cats appeared to improve by losing weight, becoming more active, and demonstrating healthier skin. However, one of these two cats died of unknown reasons 3 months after completion of treatment, and the other died 14 months after completing radiation as a result of renal failure. The fourth and youngest cat (8 years old at the time of diagnosis) responded quite well to pituitary radiation with improvement in various parameters plus complete resolution of its diabetes mellitus. This cat has been alive for more than 26 months. However, a population of four cats is far too few to draw any conclusions (two additional cats have been recently treated, but it is too soon to note a response). Pituitary radiation has potential to become a reasonable approach to management of PDH, but many more cats will need to be treated before opinions can be established.

Medical Therapy

MITOTANE. A number of different protocols using mitotane (Lysodren; o,p'-DDD) for the medical management of cats with PDH have been used with varying levels of short-term success. Long-term results have generally been discouraging (Peterson, 1998). It is interesting to point out that human beings with PDH, like their feline counterparts, are not nearly as sensitive nor as consistently responsive to o,p'-DDD as are dogs (see Chapter 6 for a complete discussion of o,p'-DDD). When o,p'-DDD was administered to clinically normal cats, only 50% demonstrated any adrenocortical suppression (Zerbe et al, 1987). Thus dogs are the unusual species by being so sensitive to a drug that does not induce a similar response in people or cats. Although concerns about feline sensitivity to chlorinated hydrocarbons are often mentioned, our experience is not that this drug makes cats ill; rather, the problem is that this drug does little. We have experience in treating only 4 cats with mitotane. Together with a small number of similarly treated cats that we are aware of from personal discussions, there are still only a limited number. Almost all have been treated orally with mitotane at a dose of 50 mg/kg, divided twice daily. This dose did not effectively suppress adrenocortical function, nor did it alleviate clinical signs of FCS (Peterson et al, 1994; Duesberg and Peterson, 1997). Doubling the dose did not improve efficacy. We do not recommend use of this drug for treatment of cats with FCS.

KETOCONAZOLE. Ketoconazole, an imidazole derivative, is an orally active broad-spectrum antimycotic drug that has been used successfully in treating fungal disease in humans beings and animals by inhibiting, at picomolar concentrations, C14-methylation of lanosterol to ergosterol. This disturbs fungal membrane growth. At higher serum concentrations, the drug also inhibits mammalian steroid biosynthesis (action of this drug is fully discussed in Chapter 6). Administration of this drug at doses typically recommended for mycotic infection can lead to significant reduction in serum androgen concentrations, and at higher doses, cortisol synthesis is suppressed (Engelhardt et al, 1991). Ketoconazole is the most efficacious oral medication for the treatment of human beings with PDH. Efficacy of ketoconazole, although "good," has not been as consistent nor as complete in dogs. It is believed that this reduced effectiveness is due, at least in part, to an inability of about 20% to 25% of dogs to absorb this drug from the GI tract.

Ketoconazole does not seem to consistently suppress adrenocortical function in either normal cats or cats with hyperadrenocorticism. A study on four healthy male cats given 30 mg/kg/day for 30 days failed to demonstrate significant changes in plasma testosterone or cortisol concentrations. Serum testosterone concentrations tended to decrease after the first 7 days of treatment, but in two of the four cats values returned to near-pretreatment concentrations by day 30 (Willard et al, 1986). This dose was the amount previously demonstrated to be effective in dogs. Our experience has been limited to using this drug in five cats with naturally occurring PDH. Three of the five cats responded moderately well but not completely. One cat demonstrated no response, and the fifth cat developed severe thrombocytopenia several weeks after treatment was initiated. Whether or not this thrombocytopenia was caused by the ketoconazole is not known. Regardless, use of ketoconazole for the treatment of cats with FCS is not highly recommended.

ETOMIDATE. Etomidate is a short-acting IV administered anesthetic agent used for induction of anesthesia in a variety of species. Because it has been shown to have minimal deleterious effect on the cardiovascular system, this drug is most often used to induce anesthesia in high-risk patients that are critically ill, hypovolemic, in shock, or have preexisting cardio-

vascular disease. It has been shown that administration of this drug, however, does suppress adrenocortical function in people, dogs, and cats. One study on cats demonstrated profound suppression of adrenocortical function during 2 hours of halothane anesthesia and 1 hour of recovery (Moon, 1997). Use of this drug for anesthesia induction could place critically ill cats at further risk. Use of a sustained-release form of this drug may become an effective mode of therapy for cats with hyperadrenocorticism.

METYRAPONE AND AMINOGLUTETHIMIDE. Metyrapone (Novartis; East Hanover, NJ) is an orally active drug that, when effective, inhibits the action of the enzyme 11-β-hydroxylase. This is the enzyme that converts 11-deoxycortisol to cortisol. Aminoglutethimide (Cytadren; CIBA Pharmaceutical Company, Summit, NJ) is another enzyme-blocking agent that prevents conversion of cholesterol to pregnenolone (we have used this drug on only one cat, although several veterinarians have used this drug under our direction). Since cortisol precursors have little or no biologic activity, inhibition of cortisol synthesis has the potential to resolve the excesses in circulating cortisol concentrations associated with naturally occurring Cushing's syndrome. In human beings with Cushing's syndrome, medical management (with drugs such as metyrapone) has been recommended to prepare patients for surgery, to resolve hypercortisolism while awaiting for radiation therapy to take effect, and to provide palliative treatment for metastatic disease (Verheist et al, 1991). Metyrapone has been documented to be effective in people with PDH and those with functioning adrenocortical tumors (ATH). Although adverse effects have been encountered rarely in humans chronically treated with this drug, one of the most common problems has been transient hypocortisolemia. The major problem with chronic use of metyrapone has been compensatory increases in endogenous ACTH concentrations resulting in an "override" of the adrenal blockade of cortisol synthesis (Orth, 1978).

We are not aware of reports describing use of metyrapone for treatment of dogs with naturally occurring Cushing's syndrome. Reports of several cats with FCS treated with metyrapone have been published, and we have had experience with only four additional cats. Clinical response without side effects (other than hypoglycemia) have been achieved in our cats and in two cats reported in the literature using 30 to 70 mg/kg orally, twice daily (Daley et al, 1993; Moore et al, 2000b). Whenever possible, we recommend starting at the lower end of the dose range for 2 to 4 weeks, rechecking the cat and possibly completing an ACTH stimulation test. Remember, the cat should remain on therapy if a stimulation test is obtained. As needed, the dose can be increased by small increments. We do not recommend doses greater than 70 mg/kg, twice daily. Higher doses have been mentioned, although these higher doses have been associated with a strong suspicion of drug-induced vomiting and inappetence that necessitated discontinuing therapy. We have not encountered these side effects using the doses mentioned here. (Aminoglutethimide dose and usage is described in this chapter section entitled Primary Progesterone-Secreting Adrenocortical Tumors in Cats).

Subjective clinical improvement was observed in at least three cats treated with metyrapone. One was lost to follow-up after 10 months of treatment (Nelson et al, 1988), and another cat in our series was treated for 6 months, but the owners would not allow further testing. This latter cat successfully underwent bilateral adrenalectomy at another hospital and survived without clinical signs of hyperadrenocorticism for several years. The third cat with FCS and diabetes mellitus was treated for only 21 days. Within that time period the owner had noticed a possible hypoglycemic reaction and had lowered the cat's insulin dose. This cat also had subjective improvement in hair coat, reduction in abdominal size, a smaller liver, and resolution of a facial abscess. Repeated ACTH stimulation testing did not demonstrate obvious change, but liver enzyme values had improved. This cat then underwent successful bilateral adrenalectomy (Moore et al, 2000a). One of two additional cats was treated and reported to have had slight improvement (Peterson, 1988). Another cat demonstrated transient reduction in baseline and ACTH-stimulated cortisol concentrations, had resolution of clinical signs, and underwent subsequent successful adrenalectomy (Daley et al, 1993).

If metyrapone is effective, there should be a reduction in baseline and ACTH-stimulated cortisol concentrations and an amelioration of clinical signs. Since virtually all treated cats were managed for short time periods, there has not been a well-documented case of rising endogenous ACTH concentrations and an override of adrenocortical blockade. Therefore, if a cat does improve clinically and can then be managed with surgery for a permanent resolution of the condition, treatment with metyrapone should be considered a success. Overall, the use of metyrapone in cats with FCS does continue to offer promise for short-term resolution of hypercortisolemia in preparation for surgery. Since long-term use has yet to be described, we await experience on this approach.

TRILOSTANE. See Chapter 6 for review of the actions of trilostane after administration to human beings and dogs with hyperadrenocorticism. Reports on its use in cats have not yet appeared.

Bilateral Adrenalectomy

BACKGROUND. In our experience, bilateral adrenalectomy has provided the best long-term response in managing FCS cats with PDH. This statement, it should be understood, is made with the understanding that we have not had the opportunity to experience either short- or long-term response after hypophysectomy, and experience with pituitary radiation is limited. As previously stated, hypophysectomy is the "treatment of choice" for patients with PDH, regardless of the species involved. Since hypophysectomy has not been an option for us, bilateral adrenalectomy remains the treatment that has provided the best chance for long-term response. This surgery is generally available in North America. The surgery protocol and medical management of cats during and after the procedure are similar to those used in dogs (please see Chapter 6) and are only briefly reviewed here.

PROTOCOL: PRE- AND POSTSURGICAL MANAGEMENT. Food is usually withheld for the 12-hour period preceding surgery. Conservative volumes of IV fluids (2.5% or 5% dextrose if the cat is diabetic) should be administered during the procedure and use of parenteral antibiotics seem to be inevitable, although specific antibiotics for specific infection represents a wiser approach. If the cat is an insulin-requiring diabetic, 50% of the usual morning dose should be given that morning. At the time that the surgeon begins the first adrenalectomy, it is recommended that dexamethasone be administered intravenously at a dose of 0.2 mg/kg. That dose should be repeated intramuscularly when surgery is complete, and 0.1 mg/kg should be given between 10 PM and midnight. The next day, 0.1 mg/kg should be given twice a day, SQ, until oral prednisone can be given. Oral medication should begin about 24 hours after the cat begins to eat without vomiting. Also when surgery is completed, desoxycorticosterone pivalate (DOCP; Novartis, East Hanover, NJ) should be administered (2.2 mg/kg, IM). That dose should be repeated 21 to 25 days later, SQ. Subsequent doses and timing should be individualized (see Chapter 8). Serum electrolyte concentrations should be assessed at the end of surgery, that evening, the next morning, and then daily until the cat is returned to the owner or until it is eating on its own without vomiting.

PROTOCOL: SURGERY. Adrenalectomy procedures are well described elsewhere. If discrimination test results are definitive for PDH, both adrenal glands must be removed during surgery. If discrimination tests are not performed or if they are inconclusive, the surgeon should be prepared to make decisions: if a cat has an obvious adrenal tumor, especially if the opposite adrenal gland appears atrophied, the surgeon should remove only the tumor; if both adrenal glands appear normal in size and shape, the surgeon must have an understanding regarding the confidence with which a diagnosis of PDH was made. In our opinion, no cat should undergo this surgery as "exploratory" to determine whether hyperadrenocorticism is the diagnosis. Rather, screening test results (especially the UC:CR and the LDDST) considered together with history and physical examination should be definitive for Cushing's. With this approach to diagnosis and decision making, the situation of "normal-appearing adrenal glands" should simply be supportive of PDH, and both glands should be extirpated.

PROTOCOL: POSTSURGERY. Postoperative complications are always a concern in a dog or cat with hyperadrenocorticism. Complications that can be terminal or that can lead a veterinarian to recommend euthanasia can be extremely disheartening to the owner, veterinarians, technicians, and nontechnical personnel. Therefore potential complications must be thoroughly explained to all involved, especially to the owner, who is invariably more emotionally and financially committed than all others. Some of the most serious potential complications include sepsis, pancreatitis, thromboembolic phenomena, wound dehiscence (surgical site or previous skin wounds due to fragility), and adrenocortical insufficiency (Duesberg et al, 1995). Sepsis continues to be a frequent occurrence because of the underlying disease (Cushing's syndrome predisposes patients to infection via immunosuppression), the animal's skin condition, and the abdominal surgery. Sepsis has been encountered in 40% of our cats despite extreme caution in tissue handling and in wound care before, during, and after surgery. Sepsis and skin fragility have been responsible for most of our problems leading to morbidity or mortality among these cats. Preoperative management of Cushing's with drugs such as metyrapone should be helpful in reducing complication rates.

EXPERIENCE. Experience with the surgical management of bilateral adrenocortical hyperplasia in FCS cats with PDH is limited and responses to surgery have varied tremendously. Almost all cats have survived surgery, and surgery has usually been successful. Postsurgical complications are common but they are not the cause of death in most of these cats. We have reviewed 21 cats that had PDH and bilateral adrenalectomy. These include 15 cats in our series and 6 cats from the literature (Watson and Herrtage, 1998 [4 cats]; Daley et al, 1993 [1 cat]; Moore et al, 2000a [1 cat]). Eight of the cats from our series have been reported in the literature (Duesberg et al, 1995).

Thirteen of 21 cats survived surgery, had complete resolution of the FCS, and lived for months or more than a year. Of these 13 long-term survivors, 9 seemed healthy when last examined, which was the final statement available. This includes four cats from our series that are currently alive and well and one cat from each of the three reports we consulted (Watson and Herrtage, 1998; Daley et al, 1993, and Moore et al, 2000). Three cats in our series and one from another (Watson and Herrtage, 1998) had complete resolution of their FCS, survived more than a year, and were thought to have died from unrelated conditions (renal failure in two, pancreatic carcinoma in one, and unknown in another).

Five cats did not survive an appreciable period of time after surgery. One cat was found dead in its cage within 24 hours of surgery, and another died 20 days after surgery from renal failure (Watson and Herrtage, 1998). Of three additional cats, two died of sepsis within a month of surgery. Both these cats had severe fragile skin disease that became overwhelmingly infected. Both were aggressively treated without success. The fifth cat died of confirmed pulmonary thromboembolism within 3 weeks of surgery. Three additional cats from our series survived the surgery and had complete resolution of their FCS but died

within months of surgery. One cat died 4 months following surgery after becoming extremely ill and being diagnosed as having a large abdominal mass; after euthanasia, this cat was documented to have had a pancreatic carcinoma. Two cats in our series each died from apparent hypoadrenal crisis, one 3 months and the other 6 months after surgery.

CONCLUSION. Total resolution of FCS by successfully completing a bilateral adrenalectomy is problematic. Certainly the risk of exposing one of these cats to celiotomy is significant. Risk can be reduced with a combination of patient selection, preoperative therapy, minimal time taken for anesthesia and surgery, and thorough care after surgery. However, these remain older cats that often have serious problems involving other organ systems. Perhaps this is the reason that a majority of the cats with FCS in our series were never treated. Regardless, bilateral adrenalectomy continues to represent the best long-term therapeutic strategy until hypophysectomy becomes more widely available or unless pituitary radiation proves efficacious. Alternatively, new medical therapies (trilostane?) may be used with improved success over those currently available.

TREATMENT OF ADRENAL TUMOR HYPERADRENOCORTICISM

Background

The ideal mode of therapy for human beings, dogs, or cats with Cushing's syndrome caused by an adrenocortical tumor is its surgical removal. Unfortunately, there are numerous reasons that this mode of therapy may not be available. Perhaps the most common reasons for an owner to decline this treatment option is cost coupled with prognosis. The surgery and perioperative treatment necessities can be quite expensive. When expenses are placed in the context of overall prognosis, many of our owners refuse surgery. In part, those of us who practice within "teaching hospitals" work with clients who are the most aggressive and who therefore choose treatments for their pets that others may not select as frequently. Thus the percentage of our cats that are treated is not a true reflection of what happens in the private practice situation. Patient selection is also critically important, and many cats with FCS simply are not reasonable candidates for this type of invasive procedure. Additional reasons for eliminating surgery as a treatment option would include presence of metastases or serious concurrent disease. Some adrenal masses may not be amenable to surgery because of size, tissue or vascular invasion or location. Therefore medical therapies may be the only option.

Surgery and Perioperative Management

Unilateral adrenalectomy in FCS cats with an adrenocortical tumor has provided the best long-term response. The entire perioperative protocol is the same as that used for bilateral adrenalectomy. Dexamethasone (0.2 mg/kg, IV) should be administered after the surgeon has isolated the adrenal mass and at the time that the mass is actually beginning to be removed. Glucocorticoids should not be administered earlier, since hypercortisolemia persists until mass removal is complete and the actions of dexamethasone begin immediately following administration. It is assumed, however, that all cats will be hypocortisolemic after adrenocortical tumor removal as a result of atrophy of glucocorticoid-secreting cells of the opposite (and remaining) adrenal gland. Once the cat is eating and drinking on its own without vomiting, parenteral dexamethasone should be replaced with oral prednisone. The initial prednisone dose should be approximately 1 to 2 mg/cat/day. The tapering process should begin within a week and be completed within 2 to 3 months.

In contrast to the routine need for glucocorticoids after removal of an adrenocortical tumor, since one adrenal gland is left *in situ*, it is not possible to predict need for mineralocorticoid replacement. Our experience in dogs, which far exceeds but is similar to our experience in cats, is that most do not require mineralocorticoid replacement. Therefore it is our recommendation that serum (or plasma) sodium and potassium concentrations be assessed when surgery has been completed and again between 10 PM and midnight that day. Assuming that the results are within reference limits for the laboratory, serum electrolytes should be rechecked once daily until the cat is eating and drinking on its own without vomiting. If decreases in serum sodium concentration or increases in serum potassium concentration (or both) are identified at any time, desoxycorticosterone pivalate (DOCP) should be administered at an initial dose of 2.2 mg/kg, IM. This dose should not need to be repeated for a minimum of 21 days and more commonly should not be needed for 25 days. Since these cats still have one normal (albeit atrophied) adrenal gland, permanent replacement should not be necessary. Therefore the second dose should be about 50% of the first dose, and a third dose should either not be necessary or should be tapered again by 50%.

In addition to managing the adrenal-dependent aspects of these cats, various other conditions should be addressed. This includes fluid therapy directed at maintaining hydration, being aggressive in the assumption that some of these cats will develop post-surgical pancreatitis, but not overloading a compromised cardiovascular system. We recognize that it is much easier to write generalizations than to actually treat one of these cats, but because specific statements will not apply to all cats, general vague guidelines suggesting individualization of therapy are the only reasonable recommendations that can be made. Management of the diabetes mellitus (if present) can be confusing. Reduction of insulin resistance should correlate with tapering glucocorticoid therapy, and the veterinarian must anticipate changes in insulin requirement to avoid potentially severe hypoglycemic reactions due to excessive insulin administration. Wound management and infection control is critically important. Tender loving care cannot be overemphasized, but these cats must be allowed to recover. Therefore the veterinarian must be certain that proper care is provided without preventing a cat from resting. We prophylactically attempt to prevent thromboembolism in these cats by using the protocol outlined in Chapter 6.

Experience

We have had the opportunity to surgically manage only eight cats that had adrenocortical tumors. Five of these cats were not treated medically before surgery to control their FCS. Two cats were treated with metyrapone, and one was given aminoglutethimide. All eight cats survived surgery; however, one died within a week from incision dehiscence and overwhelming wound infection, and another died within a week from pancreatitis. One cat died of renal failure 3 months after surgery, but this cat did have complete recovery from the procedure and appeared to have resolution of its hyperadrenocorticism. Two cats survived more than 6 but less than 12 months, both having completely recovered from surgery and both having complete resolution of the FCS. One of these cats died of heart failure, and the other was euthanized following severe illness secondary to development of a pancreatic carcinoma. Three of the eight cats lived well beyond a year. Each had complete resolution of FCS, although one did have a recurrence of clinical signs about 10 months after surgery, was diagnosed as having a second adrenocortical tumor, and underwent a second adrenalectomy. These cats, therefore, had a total of nine adrenocortical tumors: four adenomas and five carcinomas. In no cat was the histologic diagnosis made prior to surgery. None of these cats had or later developed local or distant metastasis.

Prognosis

Hyperadrenocorticism must be considered a serious disease in cats, one that carries a guarded to grave prognosis. The deleterious effects of chronic hypercortisolism on skin fragility, pancreatic endocrine function (diabetes mellitus), and the immune system are frequently responsible for morbidity and death of both treated as well as untreated cats. Treatment can be expensive, emotional (to the owner), and stressful (to the cat) without guarantee of success. Medical therapeutics have had limited or only short-term success. Abdominal surgery has not been routinely successful because it is difficult to perform in light of the previously described debilitated condition of most cats with FCS. Pituitary radiation is limited by facilities required, expense, and the multiple anesthetic procedures that are part of these protocols. Hypophysectomy is limited by the few veterinarians who have this expertise. Again, there are the problems of expense and patient debilitation. Experience with "successful" therapies (adrenalectomy [unilateral or bilateral], radiation, hypophysectomy) has resulted in less than 50% of cats surviving well beyond a year. Remember, most cats that have FCS are not treated. Most of the treated cats are those considered most stable. Therefore, 50% survival at a year (an optimistic number) does not include those cats never treated.

PRIMARY HYPERALDOSTERONISM IN CATS (ALDOSTERONE-SECRETING ADRENAL TUMOR)

Background

The primary function of aldosterone is the regulation of serum sodium and potassium homeostasis and maintenance of normal vascular fluid volume. Aldosterone is the principle mineralocorticoid synthesized and secreted by the zona glomerulosa of adrenal cortices and is mainly controlled by serum potassium concentrations and the renin-angiotensin system. An increase in serum potassium stimulates release of aldosterone. Decreases in blood pressure, primarily sensed by cells within the kidneys, stimulates synthesis and release of renin which, in turn, stimulates the angiotensins to secrete aldosterone. After synthesis and secretion, aldosterone promotes potassium excretion and stimulates conservation of sodium. In causing conservation of sodium, aldosterone indirectly causes conservation of water, which raises blood volume and increases blood pressure.

Excess production of aldosterone may be the result of primary or secondary causes. *Primary hyperaldosteronism* is defined as the "autonomous secretion of the hormone by abnormal cells within the adrenal cortex." In human beings, these abnormal cells are most commonly found within an adrenocortical adenoma, although carcinomas and autonomously secreting hyperplastic adrenals have been reported (White, 1994). Secondary hyperaldosteronism is the result of some disorder, such as kidney or heart disease, that stimulates normal adrenocortical cells to synthesize the hormone excessively. Therefore, in people, primary hyperaldosteronism is characterized by circulating excesses in aldosterone concentration, decreases in renin concentration, hypokalemia, potassium diuresis, and hypertension. Aldosterone excess leads to increased sodium retention, expansion of the extracellular fluid volume, and increased total body sodium content, although serum sodium concentrations may be within reference limits. The expanded extracellular fluid and plasma volumes are registered by stretch receptors at the juxtaglomerular apparatus, and sodium retention is registered at the macula densa. Therefore, with primary increases in aldosterone production, synthesis and secretion of renin is suppressed. This is the hallmark of the disorder.

Since primary hyperaldosteronism is a disease originating within the zona glomerulosa, it must be remembered that cells of this zone do not have the capacity to synthesize cortisol and, therefore, afflicted patients have no abnormalities in cortisol production, plasma cortisol concentrations, or in cortisol metabolism. However, as aldosterone synthesis progresses in excess, the entire biosynthetic pathway is enhanced. This causes increases in serum concentrations of precursor steroids, as well as in aldosterone concentrations. Thus human beings with aldosterone-secreting adrenal adenomas typically also have increased serum concentrations of desoxycorticosterone, corticosterone, and 18-hydroxycorticosterone.

In addition to serum sodium retention and potassium depletion, there are decreases in total body stores of potassium. There is a shift of potassium from its typical intracellular storage site to the extracellular fluid as the system attempts to maintain serum concentrations. The result is an intracellular movement and increased renal excretion of hydrogen ions with development of systemic alkalosis. It is also of interest to point out that moderate losses of potassium may decrease carbohydrate tolerance (as could be demonstrated with glucose tolerance testing) and could decrease sensitivity to antidiuretic hormone (vasopressin; ADH).

Clinical Experience in Cats

Human beings with primary hyperaldosteronism require medical attention usually because of symptoms that can be traced to hypokalemia. These signs include fatigue, loss of stamina, weakness, nocturia, and "lassitude." If hypokalemia is severe, afflicted individuals may have worsening thirst and signs of alkalosis. Hypertension, the other serious condition associated with primary hyperaldosteronism, is usually unsuspected and is diagnosed only serendipitously on physical examination. Blood pressure in these people can be normal to severely increased.

Five cats described in the literature and documented to have had primary hyperaldosteronism are used here to review their clinical signs (Eger et al, 1983; Flood et al, 1999; Moore et al, 2000b; Rijnberk et al, 2001). It is appreciated that the number of cats with this condition are limited; however, analogies to human beings exist. Although primary hyperaldosteronism is rare, veterinarians may encounter cats with this condition. More important, increased use of abdominal ultrasound as a routine screening test for geriatric healthy and ill cats results in the occasional observation of a possible adrenal mass. This endocrine disorder should be included among the differential diagnoses for cats with an undefined adrenal mass.

The five cats with primary hyperaldosteronism (Table 7-16) were 10, 12, 13, 17, and 20 years of age, respectively. Two were female, three were male, and all were neutered. The most common clinical signs noted by owners of these five cats included weakness

TABLE 7–16 SOME CLINICAL AND TESTING RESULTS FROM 5 CATS DIAGNOSED AS HAVING PRIMARY HYPERALDOSTERONISM (CAT #1: EGER ET AL, 1983; CATS #2 AND #3: FLOOD ET AL, 1999; CAT #4: MOORE ET AL, 2002; CAT #5: RIJNBERK ET AT, 2001)*

| Cat # | Age | Sex | CLINICAL SIGNS OR PHYSICAL EXAMINATION | | | | | SERUM | | | | Blood Pressure | Mass on U.S.? | Sx? | Histology |
			Weak	Ventroflexion	PU/PD	Blind	Mydriasis	K	Na	Aldosterone	Renin				
1	17	F/S	✓					↓	N	↑↑	N.D.	N.D.	N.D.	No	AC+M
2	20	F/S	✓			✓		↓	↑	↑↑	N	230	Yes	Yes	AC
3	10	M/N			✓	✓	✓	↓	N	↑↑	N	250	Yes	No	FNA: endo tumor
4	13	M/N	✓	✓	✓			↓	N	↑↑	↓	135	Yes	No	FNA: endo tumor
5	12	M/N	✓	✓			✓	↓	N	↑↑	N/↓	190	Yes	Yes	AC+M

*F/S, Female/spayed; M/N, male/neutered; ✓, cat had sign; ↓, below reference limit; ↑, above reference limit; N, normal; AC+M, adrenocortical carcinoma and metastases; FNA, fine needle aspirate; Na, serum sodium concentration; K, potassium concentration; U.S., ultrasound; Sx, surgery; PU/PD, polyuria/polydipsia; N.D., not done. Blood pressure was an indirect measurement in mmHg in each cat.

TABLE 7–17 SOME CLINICAL AND LABORATORY DATA FROM 3 CATS, EACH DIAGNOSED AS HAVING A PROGESTERONE-SECRETING ADRENOCORTICAL CARCINOMA (CAT #1 FROM BOORD AND GRIFFIN, 1999; CAT #2 FROM ROSSMEISL ET AL, 2000)*

| Cat # | Age (Years) | Sex | ACTH STIMULATION CORTISOL (µg%) | | | LDDST CORTISOL (µg %) | | | ACTH STIMULATION PROGESTERONE (ng/ml) | | [ACTH] | U.S. Identified Mass? | Sx? | AGT Rx? | Histology |
			Pre	30 Min	60 Min	Pre	4 Hr	6–8 Hr	Pre	Post					
1	7	M/N	2.2	–	4.4	1.7	1.3	1.1	3.6	27.6	–	Yes	Yes	No	A.C.
2	7	M/N	1.0	2.7	2.4	2.7	–	1.2	13.2	15.5	–	Yes	No	Yes	A.C.
3	9	M/N	2.8	2.7	3.3	1.5	1.5	1.8	4.7	N.A.	<1	Yes	Yes	Yes	A.C.

*M/N, Male/neutered; LDDST, low dose dexamethasone test; [ACTH], plasma endogenous ACTH; U.S., ultrasonography; Sx, surgery; AGT, aminoglutethimide; Histo, histology; A.C., adrenocortical carcinoma.

(four cats); cervical ventroflexion, polyuria and/or polydipsia, weight loss, decreased appetite (two cats each); ataxia, vision loss, nocturia, and abdominal enlargement (one cat each). Physical examination abnormalities included muscle atrophy, pendulous abdomen, cervical ventriflexion, detached retinas, mydriasis, and heart murmur (two cats each). All five cats were hypokalemic, three were hypertensive, two were alkalotic, two had concurrent diabetes mellitus, two had increases in BUN, and two of four cats had isosthenuria, as defined as a random urine specific gravity of 1.008 to 1.015 (1.009, 1.015, 1.022, and 1.031, respectively). All cats had remarkable increases in serum aldosterone concentration (Yu and Morris, 1998). Three of four cats had results within the reference range, and two had decreases in serum renin activity (one cat was evaluated twice). Abdominal ultrasound was performed in four cats, each had an adrenal mass identified, and three underwent ultrasound-guided fine-needle aspiration (FNA) of the adrenal mass. In all three cats, the FNA was consistent with endocrine tumor. Only two cats underwent surgery to remove the mass, and only one of those two cats had a successful surgery. The other cats were treated for varying time periods with potassium supplementation and for hypertension. At least two of the five cats had metastasis of their adrenal tumor.

Conclusion

Primary hyperaldosteronism is a rare disease that affects middle-aged to geriatric cats. The most common clinical sign is muscle weakness. The diagnosis should be suspected after repeated hypokalemia is documented in a cat with an adrenal mass visualized with abdominal ultrasonography. The prognosis must be considered guarded to grave because of the associated problems with hypertension and muscle weakness, the realization that the condition can be treated only with surgery, and the understanding that surgery is not only expensive but also may not be curative because of mass location, invasion of surrounding tissue, or the presence of metastasis.

PRIMARY PROGESTERONE-SECRETING ADRENAL TUMORS IN CATS

Background

As has been discussed in Chapter 6, it is known that adrenocortical tumors in human beings have the potential for secreting a variety of steroid substances in addition to cortisol and aldosterone. Therefore reports of people with endocrine problems caused by circulating excesses in "less-than-common" steroid products derived from such tumors are relatively rare but well documented. Progesterone-secreting adrenocortical tumors have been diagnosed in people and dogs (refer to the appropriate sections in Chapter 6 for review of these syndromes). Natural progesterone has a half-life in the blood of only a few minutes and serves as a precursor for androgens, estrogens, and cortisol in many mammals. Progesterone also binds to albumin, as well as cortisol-binding and sex-hormone-binding proteins. Chronic increases in progesterone concentrations may result in excess "free" cortisol by competitively binding to cortisol-binding proteins in the circulation, and in this manner, excess progesterone can simulate the actions of glucocorticoids. Whether or not this actually occurs in cats is not known, but it has been demonstrated to take place in human beings and dogs (Selman et al, 1996). In cats, progesterone appears to act as a glucocorticoid antagonist by suppressing the hypothalamic-pituitary-adrenocortical axis (Selman et al, 1994). However, progesterone-type drugs can simulate glucocorticoid activity. For example, progesterone is a potent insulin antagonist.

Clinical Experience in Cats

We are aware of three cats that have been diagnosed as having progesterone-secreting adrenocortical carcinomas. Two of the cats have been reported in the literature (Boord and Griffin, 1999; Rossmeisl et al, 2000), and one is from our series of cats with adrenocortical tumors. Some of the clinical information on these three cats is provided in Table 7-17. All three cats were male, neutered, and relatively young (7, 7, and 9 years of age, respectively). All three cats had similar skin problems consisting of nonpruritic, progressive, symmetric alopecia; thin fragile skin that easily bruised and, in one case, was torn after mild restraint was applied; and a hair coat in the nonalopecic areas that was considered greasy and unkempt in all three cats. One of the three cats had skin scrapings that were positive for Demodex cati. The chief owner complaint in one cat was the alopecia, whereas in the other two cats the primary owner concern was poorly controlled diabetes mellitus. The third cat did have periodic hyperglycemia and glycosuria. The combination of dermatologic signs and concurrent metabolic disease resulted in hyperadrenocorticism being included as a possible underlying disease process in the differential diagnosis of each cat.

None of the three cats had serious CBC or routine serum biochemistry abnormalities other than the two cats that had persistent hyperglycemia and glycosuria. One of the two cats had mild increases in BUN. Endocrine testing (see Table 7-17) was of interest since all three cats had ACTH stimulation test results that documented low-normal basal plasma cortisol concentrations and poststimulation plasma cortisol concentrations that were less than reference ranges. These results are not, in our experience, unusual in cats with adrenocortical tumors, and low or normal ACTH stimulation test results occur in more than 50% of cats with hyperadrenocorticism regardless of cause (see Tables 7-9 and 7-10). Note that the results in Table 7-10 from cats with functioning, cortisol-secreting, adreno-cortical tumors demonstrate that these eight cats include some with exaggerated test results and others with results that were less than the reference range. Thus we do not recommend use of ACTH stimulation testing for the diagnosis of hyperadrenocorticism in cats. Each of the three cats that had a progesterone-secreting tumor had abnormal basal progesterone concentrations, negating the need for stimulation. In one report, a healthy cat had a basal serum progesterone concentration of 0.06 ng/ml as compared with the value of 3.6 in the cat with an adrenal tumor (Boord and Griffin, 1999). In the other report, the reference range for basal progesterone concentration was listed as <0.03 to 0.35 ng/ml as compared with the cat with an adrenocortical tumor, which had a basal progesterone concentration of 13.2 ng/ml (Rossmeisl et al, 2000). The cat in our series had a basal plasma progesterone concentration of 4.7 as compared with the reference range we used, which was <0.3 ng/ml. Thus stimulation testing does not appear to be necessary.

Low-dose dexamethasone screening test (LDDST) results from these three cats were also interesting. Using the reference range that has been established in our laboratory of ≤0.8 g% at 4, 6, and 8 hours, all three cats had results that were consistent with hyperadrenocorticism. One cat, however, did have greater than 50% suppression in plasma cortisol concentration after dexamethasone administration, a result that would not be consistent with presence of a functioning adrenocortical tumor. Another cat did have an undetectable endogenous ACTH concentration. All three cats had an adrenal mass identified on abdominal ultrasonography. This information underscores the value of an abdominal ultrasound examination in any dog or cat suspected of having adrenal disease.

Two of the three cats were treated with amino-glutethimide (AGT; Cytadren; CIBA Pharmaceutical Company, Summit, NJ). Both were treated with about 6 mg/kg body weight, BID, orally. One was treated for approximately 2 months (Rossmeisl et al, 2000), and the cat from our series was treated for about 1 month, in preparation for abdominal surgery. AGT is an inhibitor of the cholesterol side-chain cleavage enzyme, desmolase (CYP11A1; see Chapter 6). This enzyme is responsible for conversion of cholesterol to pregnenolone during synthesis of adrenocortical steroids. Because AGT inhibits steroid synthesis at an early stage in the synthesis cascade, it should decrease synthesis of estrogens, androgens, glucocorticoids, and mineralocorticoids. The drug is used rarely in human beings for medical management of hyperadrenocorticism. Adverse effects in people are considered mild and may include anorexia, nausea, and rashes. In humans, long-term use of this drug is limited by increasing pituitary secretion of ACTH, which can override its enzyme blocking effects. Similarly, one cat did demonstrate response after 2 weeks of therapy. Response was not as significant at 6 weeks. The cat in our series was treated only for a total of about 6 weeks with a fascinating

response. First, the cat did clinically improve dramatically with resolution of thin fragile skin. This cat's diabetes mellitus resolved. What surprised us was that as this male cat improved, there was dramatic mammary gland enlargement. This effect, we assume, was due to the rapid decrease in plasma progesterone concentrations that stimulated, in turn, synthesis and secretion of prolactin. After AGT was discontinued, our surgeons were able to successfully remove the adrenal tumor. Successful surgery was also reported in one of the other cats (Boord and Griffin, 1999). Both cats lived well beyond a year after surgery without diabetes mellitus or other long-term problems.

Conclusion

Progesterone-secreting adrenocortical tumors are quite unusual in cats. Diagnosis can be suspected in any cat with clinical signs consistent with hyperadrenocorticism. If UC:CR or low-dose dexamethasone screening test results are close to or within reference ranges, having a progesterone assay run on a basal blood sample would be both reasonable and cost-effective. This would be emphasized as a logical step to take should the cat in question have an apparent adrenal mass on abdominal ultrasonography. Surgical removal of such a mass is the treatment of choice, and presurgical control of the condition, if needed, can be attempted with drugs such as aminoglutethimide.

REFERENCES

Barthez PY, et al: Ultrasonographic evaluation of the adrenal glands in dogs. J Am Vet Med Assoc 207:1180, 1995.

Boord M, Griffin C: Progesterone secreting adrenal mass in a cat with clinical signs of hyperadrenocorticism. J Am Vet Med Assoc 214:666, 1999.

Brightman AH: Ophthalmic use of glucocorticoids. Vet Clin North Am Small Anim Pract 12:33, 1982.

Cartee RE, Finn-Bodner ST: Ultrasound examination of the feline adrenal gland. J Med Sonography 9:327, 1993.

Chakere DW, et al: Magnetic resonance imaging of pituitary and parasellar abnormalities. Radio Clin North Am 27:265, 1989.

Coates PJ, et al: The distribution of immunoreactive-melanocyte-stimulating hormone cells in the adult human pituitary gland. J Endocrinol 111:335, 1986.

Daley CA et al: Use of metyrapone to treat pituitary-dependent hyperadrenocorticism in a cat with large cutaneous wounds. J Am Vet Med Assoc 202:956, 1993.

Duesberg CA et al: Adrenalectomy for treatment of hyperadrenocorticism in cats: 10 cases (1988-1992). J Am Vet Med Assoc 207: 1066, 1995.

Duesberg CA, Peterson ME: Adrenal disorders in cats. Vet Clin North Am Small Anim Prac 27:321, 1997.

Eger CE, et al: Primary aldosteronism (Conn's syndrome) in a cat: A case report and review of comparative aspects. J Small Anim Pract 24:293, 1983.

Engelhardt D, et al: The influence of ketoconazole on human adrenal steroidogenesis: Incubation studies with tissue slices. Clin Endocrinol 35:163, 1991.

Feldman EC: The effect of functional adrenocortical tumors on plasma cortisol and corticotropin concentrations in dogs. J Am Vet Med Assoc 178:823, 1981.

Ferasin L: Iatrogenic hyperadrenocorticism in a cat following a short therapeutic course of methylprednisolone acetate. J Feline Medicine and Surgery 3:87, 2001.

Flood SM, et al: Primary hyperaldosteronism in two cats. J Am Anim Hosp Assoc 35:411, 1999.

Goossens MMC, et al: Urinary excretion of glucocorticoids in the diagnosis of hyperadrenocorticism in cats. Domestic Anim Endocrinol 12:355, 1995.

Green CE, et al: Iatrogenic hyperadrenocorticism in a cat. Feline Pract 23:7, 1995.

Halmi NS, Krieger D: Immunocytochemistry of ACTH-related peptides in the hypophysis. *In* Bhatnagar AS (ed): The Anterior Pituitary Gland. New York, Raven Press, 1983, pp 1-15.

Henry CJ, et al: Urine cortisol:creatinine ratio in healthy and sick cats. J Vet Int Med 10:123, 1996.

Horauf A, Reusch C: Darstellung der nebennieren mittels ultraschall: Untersuchungen bei gesunden hunden, hunden mit nicht endokrinen Erkrankungen sowie mit Cushing-Syndrom. Kleintierpraxis 40: 337, 1995.

Immink WFGA, et al: Hyperadrenocorticism in four cats. Veterinary Quarterly 14:81, 1992.

Kaufman B. Magnetic resonance imaging of the pituitary gland. Radio Clin North Am 22:795, 1984.

Low MJ, et al: Post-translational processing of pro-opiomelanocortin (POMC) in mouse pituitary melanotroph tumors induced by a POMC-Simian virus 40 large T antigen transgene. J Biol Chem 268:24967, 1993.

Meij BP, et al: Transsphenoidal hypophysectomy in beagle dogs: Evaluation of a microsurgical technique. Vet Surg 26:295, 1997.

Meij BP, et al: Results of transsphenoidal hypophysectomy in 52 dogs with pituitary-dependent hyperadrenocorticism. Vet Surg 27:246, 1998.

Meij BP, et al: Transsphenoidal hypophysectomy for treatment of pituitary-dependent hyperadrenocorticism in 7 cats. Veterinary Surgery 30:72, 2001.

Meijer JC, et al: Cushing's syndrome due to adrenocortical adenoma in a cat. Tijdschr Diergeneesk 103:1048, 1978.

Melby JC: Therapy of Cushing's disease: A consensus for pituitary microsurgery. Ann Int Med 109:445, 1988.

Moon PF: Cortisol suppression in cats after induction of anesthesia with etomidate, compared with ketamine-diazepam combination. Am J Vet Res 58:868, 1997.

Moore LE, et al: Hyperadrenocorticism treated with metyrapone followed by bilateral adrenalectomy in a cat. J Am Vet Med Assoc 217:691, 2000a.

Moore LE, et al: Use of abdominal ultrasonography in the diagnosis of primary hyperaldosteronism in a cat. J Am Vet Med Assoc 217:213, 2000b.

Nelson RW et al: Hyperadrenocorticism in cats: Seven cases (1978-1987). J Am Vet Med Assoc 193:245, 1988.

Orth DN: Metyrapone is useful only as adjunctive therapy in Cushing's disease. Ann Intern Med 89:128, 1978.

Peterson ME: Endocrine disorders in cats: four emerging diseases. Compend Contin Educ Pract Vet 10:1353, 1988.

Peterson ME: Feline hyperadrenocorticism. *In* Manual of Small Animal Endocrinology, 2nd ed. Torrance AG, Mooney CT (eds). British Small Animal Veterinary Association, Cheltenham, 1998, pp 215.

Peterson ME, Kemppainen RJ: Comparison of intravenous and intramuscular routes for administering cosyntropin for corticotropin stimulation testing in cats. Am J Vet Res 53:1392, 1992a.

Peterson ME, Kemppainen RJ: Comparison of the immunoreactive plasma corticotropin and cortisol responses to two synthetic corticotropin preparations (tetracosactrin and cosyntropin) in healthy cats. Am J Vet Res 53:1752, 1992b.

Peterson ME, Kemppainen RJ: Dose response relation between plasma concentrations of corticotropin and cortisol after administration of incremental doses cosyntropin for corticotropin stimulation testing in cats. Am J Vet Res 54:300, 1993.

Peterson ME, Steele P: Pituitary-dependent hyperadrenocorticism in a cat. J Am Vet Med Assoc 189:680, 1986.

Peterson ME, et al: Immunocytochemical study of the hypophysis in 25 dogs with pituitary-dependent hyperadrenocorticism. Acta Endocrinol (Copenh) 101:15, 1982.

Peterson ME, et al: Endocrine diseases. *In* Sherding RG (ed): The Cat: Diagnosis and Clinical Management, 2nd ed. New York, Churchill Livingstone, pp 1404.

Reaves TA Jr, et al: Vasopressin release by nicotine in the cat. Peptides 2:13, 1981.

Rijnberk A: Pituitary-dependent hyperadrenocorticism. *In* Rijnberk A (ed): Clinical Endocrinology of Dogs and Cats. Dordrecht, The Netherlands, Kluwer Academic Publishers, 1996, pp 74-83.

Rijnberk A, et al: Hyperaldosteronism in a cat with metastasised adrenocortical tumour. Vet Quart 23:38, 2001.

Robinson AJ, Clamann HP: Effects of glucocorticoids on motor units in cat hindlimb muscles. Muscle and Nerve 11:703, 1988.

Rossmeisl JH, et al: Hyperadrenocorticism and hyperprogesteronemia in a cat with an adrenocortical adenocarcinoma. J Am Anim Hosp Assoc 36:512, 2000.

Sallanon M, et al: Hypophysectomy does not disturb the sleep-waking cycle in the cat. Neurosci Lett 88:173, 1988.

Schaer M, Ginn PE: Iatrogenic Cushing's syndrome and steroid hepatopathy in a cat. J Am Anim Hosp Assoc 35:48, 1999.

Schoeman JP, et al: Cortisol response to two different doses of intravenous synthetic ACTH (tetracosactrin) in overweight cats. J Small Anim Pract 41:552, 2000.

Scholten-Sloof BE, et al: Pituitary-dependent hyperadrenocorticism in a family of Dandie Dinmont terriers. J Endocrinol 135:535, 1992.

Scott DW, et al: Some effects of short-term methylprednisolone therapy in normal cats. Cornell Vet 69:104, 1979.

Scott DW, et al: Iatrogenic Cushing's syndrome in the cat. Fel Pract 12:30, 1982.

Scott DW, et al: Iatrogenic Cushing's syndrome in the cat. Feline Pract 12:30, 1982.

Selman PJ, et al: Progestin treatment in the dog, II. Effects on the hypothalamic-pituitary-adrenocortical axis. Eur J Endocrinol 131:422, 1994.

Selman PJ, et al: Binding specificity of medroxyprogesterone acetate and proligestone for the progesterone and glucocorticoid receptor in the dog. Steroids 61:133, 1996.

Smith MC, Feldman EC: Plasma endogenous ACTH concentrations and plasma cortisol responses to synthetic ACTH and dexamethasone sodium phosphate in healthy cats. Am J Vet Res 48:1719, 1987.

Snyckers FD: Transsphenoidal selective anterior hypophysectomy in cats for microsurgical training. Technical note. J Neurosurgery 43:774, 1975.

Stein AL, et al: Computed tomography versus magnetic resonance imaging for the evaluation of suspected pituitary adenomas. Obstet Gynecol 73:996, 1989.

Theon A: Practical Radiation Therapy. *In* Ettinger SJ, Feldman EC (eds): Textbook of Veterinary Internal Medicine, 5th ed. Philadelphia, WB Saunders Co, 2000, pp 489.

Thorner MO, et al: Approach to pituitary disease. *In* Wilson JD, Foster DW (eds): Williams Textbook of Endocrinology, 8th ed. Philadelphia, WB Saunders Co, 1992, pp 246.

Van Wijk PA, et al: Corticotropin-releasing hormone and adrenocorticotropic hormone concentrations in cerebrospinal fluid of dogs with pituitary-dependent hyperadrenocorticism. Endocrinology 131:2659, 1992.

Verheist JA, et al: Short and long-term responses to metyrapone in the medical management of 91 patients with Cushing's syndrome. Clin Endocrinol 35:169, 1991.

Wallach ST, et al: Mensuration of the pituitary gland from magnetic resonance images in 17 cats. Vet Radiol Ultrasound 44:278, 2003.

Watson PJ, Herrtage ME: Hyperadrenocorticism in six cats. J Small Anim Pract 39:175, 1998.

White PC: Disorders of aldosterone biosynthesis and action. N Engl J Med 331:250, 1994.

Willard MD et al: Effect of long-term administration of ketoconazole in cats. Am J Vet Res 47:2510, 1986.

Yu S, Morris JG: Plasma aldosterone concentration of cats. The Veterinary Journal 155:63, 1998.

Zerbe CA, et al: Hyperadrenocorticism in a cat. J Am Vet Med Assoc 190:559, 1987a.

Zerbe CA, et al: Effect of nonadrenal illness on adrenal function in the cat. Am J Vet Res 48:451, 1987b.

Zhan GL, et al: Steroid glaucoma: Corticosteroid-induced ocular hypertension in cats. Exp Eye Research 54:211, 1992.

Zimmer C, et al: Ultrasonographic examination of the adrenal gland and evaluation of the hypophyseal-adrenal axis in 20 cats. J Small Anim Pract 41:156, 2000.

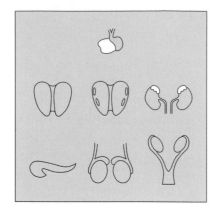

8

HYPOADRENOCORTICISM (ADDISON'S DISEASE)

BACKGROUND

The presence of the "suprarenal glands" was recognized by early anatomists, but their importance was not apparent until Thomas Addison described a clinical syndrome in humans that he associated with their dysfunction (Addison, 1855). Included in his description were "anemia, general languor, debility, remarkable feebleness of the heart's action, and irritability of the stomach." Autopsies usually revealed either tuberculous destruction or atrophy of the adrenal glands. At that time, no therapy was known, and patients who developed the disease died. About the same time that Thomas Addison described the clinical picture of adrenal insufficiency, Brown-Sequard (1856) demonstrated that adrenalectomy resulted in death in experimental animals, thus documenting the necessity of the adrenal glands for maintaining life.

In 1930, crude lipid extracts from the adrenal cortex were demonstrated to contain substances that maintained the lives of adrenalectomized cats. Similar extracts were then administered to humans to treat their adrenocortical insufficiency. Unfortunately, the extracts were of little help, because they were short-acting and contained little cortisol (although this was not known at the time). In 1933, sodium deficiency was demonstrated by Loeb to be a major component of Addison's disease, and the beneficial effects of oral or rectal saline solutions were demonstrated.

Synthetic desoxycorticosterone acetate (DOCA) was shown to be of benefit in the maintenance therapy of patients with adrenal insufficiency by Thorn and his co-workers in 1942. The beneficial effects of salt and desoxycorticosterone administration were related to correction of electrolyte disturbances and associated dehydration. Although these treatments were helpful for patients with partial adrenal insufficiency, they did not provide protection from severe stress (Nelson, 1980).

Furthering the understanding of adrenal insufficiency, cortisol and corticosterone were isolated from beef and porcine adrenal glands. The isolations, reported in 1937, were time-consuming and expensive, but they demonstrated the importance of these substances in carbohydrate metabolism and maintenance of life, which had not been demonstrated with desoxycorticosterone. Eventually, laboratory synthesis and the availability of cortisone and cortisol revolutionized the treatment of hypoadrenocorticism. These substances not only maintained the lives of individuals who had undergone adrenalectomy and those with naturally occurring adrenal insufficiency, in large enough doses, they also protected against stressful situations. By the mid-1950s, cortisol had been isolated from blood and demonstrated to be one of the major secretory products of the adrenal cortex in dogs and humans.

Knowledge of cortisol's structure quickly led to the development of methods to assay serum and urine concentrations. Understanding of adrenocortical function was further enhanced with the recognition of a salt-retaining hormone and, less important, androgenic

substances in the early 1950s. The three major types of hormones produced by the adrenal cortex were then classified: glucocorticoids (cortisol); mineralocorticoids (aldosterone); and the androgens.

Naturally occurring adrenocortical insufficiency in a dog was initially reported as a clinical entity in 1953. In the 1970s, brief accounts and then several series appeared in the veterinary literature. Since 1980, the veterinary literature has continued to expand this knowledge base with regard to the pathogenesis, diagnosis, and treatment of canine Addison's disease. The feline counterpart was described in the 1980s, and knowledge about the disease in this species is expanding.

ETIOLOGY

Hypoadrenocorticism is a syndrome that usually results from disease affecting both adrenal cortices (Fig. 8-1). Loss of more than 85% to 90% of adrenocortical cells appears to be required before clinical signs of deficient glucocorticoid and mineralocorticoid secretion (*primary* adrenocortical failure) become obvious. Less commonly, abnormalities in the hypothalamic-pituitary axis can result in reduced

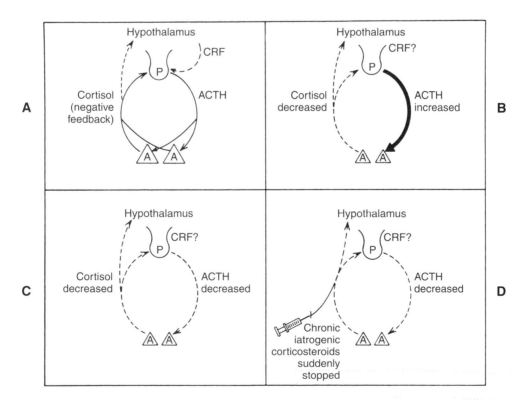

FIGURE 8-1. The pituitary-adrenal axis in normal dogs *(A)*; in dogs with loss of adrenocortical function and excess ACTH secretion due to a lack of negative feedback (the most common form of hypoadrenocorticism) *(B)*; in dogs with failure to secrete ACTH and secondary atrophy of the adrenal cortex, specifically the zona fasciculata and zona reticularis *(C)*; and in dogs that are chronically overtreated with exogenous glucocorticoids, causing insufficiency in pituitary ACTH secretion and secondary atrophy of the adrenal cortex *(D)*. *A*, Adrenal; *P*, pituitary; *CRF*, corticotropin-releasing factor (hormone). (From Feldman EC: *In* Ettinger SJ [ed]: Textbook of Veterinary Internal Medicine, 2nd ed. Philadelphia, WB Saunders, 1983, p 1667.)

secretion of the "trophic" hormone, adrenocorticotropic hormone (ACTH). Loss of ACTH has the potential to cause atrophy of the adrenal cortices (sparing the zona glomerulosa) and impaired secretion of glucocorticoids (*secondary* adrenocortical failure). Isolated hypo-aldosteronism is a recognized but rare syndrome in humans usually due to inadequate secretion by the kidneys. Reninemic hypoaldosteronism without gluco-corticoid deficiency has been described in a dog that also had a heart base chemodectoma (Lobetti, 1998).

Primary Adrenocortical Failure

IMMUNE-MEDIATED (AUTOIMMUNE) DISEASE. *Idiopathic* adrenal insufficiency is the most common diagnostic "label" for dogs with adrenocortical failure, because the cause of the disease is usually not obvious. However, the disease is most common in young to middle-age female dogs, and many of the features of the disease resemble those in humans. The most common cause of human hypoadrenocorticism is immune-mediated destruction of the adrenal cortices (Table 8-1), which affects four times as many women as men (Findling and Tyrell, 1991). In the active phase of the disease, histologic examination of the adrenals reveals wide-spread but variable infiltrates consisting of lympho-cytes, plasma cells, and macrophages. In advanced stages, the cortex is replaced by fibrous tissue (Findling et al, 1997).

It is likely that most dogs and cats with naturally occurring hypoadrenocorticism also have immune-mediated destruction of the adrenal cortices (Schaer et al, 1986; Reusch, 2000). Idiopathic atrophy of all the layers of the adrenal cortex continues to be the most frequently observed histologic lesion in dogs with hypoadrenocorticism. Necropsy of recently afflicted dogs is not common, which decreases the possibility of visualizing an active inflammatory process. Most dogs afflicted with hypoadrenocorticism either die without necropsy or are diagnosed and treated. Dogs and cats treated for any length of time have no immune-mediated infiltrates and are left with atrophied/fibrotic glands. The pituitary gland is normal in primary immune-mediated adrenocortical atrophy (Boujon et al, 1994).

Humans who would formerly have been considered to have idiopathic adrenal insufficiency can now be evaluated for the presence of antiadrenocortical anti-bodies. In this way, immune-mediated destruction of human adrenal cortices can be confirmed with readily available laboratory testing. Similar tests have not yet been applied and reported from a large series of dogs with the syndrome, although antiadrenal antibody testing is occasionally mentioned (Kooistra et al, 1995).

MULTIPLE IMMUNE-MEDIATED DISORDERS

Humans. Immune-mediated destruction of the adrenal glands in humans is commonly associated with other immune disorders. Two distinct immuno-endocrinopathic syndromes that involve the adrenal glands in humans, autoimmune polyglandular disease

TABLE 8-1 CAUSES OF PRIMARY AND SECONDARY ADRENAL INSUFFICIENCY IN HUMANS

Primary Adrenal Insufficiency	Secondary Adrenal Insufficiency
Slow Onset	
Autoimmune adrenalitis (alone or as a component of type I or II autoimmune polyglandular syndrome*)	Pituitary or metastatic tumor[†]
Tuberculosis	Craniopharyngioma[†]
Adrenomyeloneuropathy	Pituitary surgery or radiation
Systemic fungal infections (e.g., histoplasmosis, cryptococcosis, blastomycosis)	Lymphocytic hypophysitis[†]
	Sarcoidosis[†]
	Histiocytosis X[†]
	Empty-sella syndrome
	Hypothalamic tumors[†]
AIDS (opportunistic infections with cytomegalovirus, bacteria, or protozoa; Kaposi's sarcoma)	Long-term glucocorticoid therapy
Metastatic carcinoma (lung, breast, kidney), lymphoma	
Isolated glucocorticoid deficiency (often familial)	
Abrupt Onset	
Adrenal hemorrhage, necrosis, or thrombosis in meningococcal or other kinds of sepsis, in coagulation disorders or as a result of warfarin therapy, or in antiphospholipid syndrome	Postpartum pituitary necrosis (Sheeham's syndrome)
	Necrosis or bleeding into pituitary macroadenoma
	Head trauma, lesions of the pituitary stalk[†]
	Pituitary or adrenal surgery for Cushing's syndrome (transient)

From Oelkers (1996); used with permission.
*Type I autoimmune polyglandular syndrome consists mainly of adrenal insufficiency, hypoparathyroidism, and mucocutaneous candidiasis. Type II autoimmune polyglandular syndrome consists mainly of adrenal insufficiency, autoimmune thyroid disease, and insulin-dependent diabetes mellitus.
[†]Diabetes insipidus is often present.

type I and type II, have been described. Type I disease, typically an autosomal recessive disorder, usually begins during childhood; it involves adrenal insufficiency, hypoparathyroidism, and chronic mucocutaneous candidiasis. The more common type II disease, also called Schmidt's syndrome, involves adrenal insufficiency, thyroiditis, and insulin-dependent diabetes mellitus (see Chapter 3). Ovarian failure occurs in both syndromes. Alopecia, malabsorption syndromes, chronic hepatitis, vitiligo, and pernicious anemia are also associated with autoimmune hypo-adrenocorticism. One or more of these associated dis-orders are found in 40% to 53% of humans with Addison's disease (Baxter and Tyrrell, 1981; Oelkers, 1996).

The incidence of circulating antibodies to various endocrine organs and other tissues is greater than that of overt clinical disease (Table 8-2). Enzymes involved in steroidogenesis are target autoantigens in auto-immune Addison's disease. Of the three enzymes (17α-hydroxylase, 21α-hydroxylase, and the side-chain cleavage enzyme), 21α-hydroxylase appears to be the

TABLE 8-2 INCIDENCE OF CIRCULATING AUTOANTIBODIES IN HUMANS WITH AUTOIMMUNE ADRENOCORTICAL INSUFFICIENCY*

Cell Type	Percentage
Adrenal	64
Thyroid	
Cytoplasm	45
Thyroglobulin	22
Stomach	
Parietal cells	30
Intrinsic factor	9
Parathyroid	26
Gonad	17
Islet cell	8

*Adapted from Tyrrell JB, et al: Glucocorticoids and adrenal androgens. *In* Greenspan FS (ed): Basic and Clinical Endocrinology, 3rd ed. Philadelphia, WB Saunders Co, 1991, p 323.

most important autoantigen in isolated Addison's disease, as well as in the polyglandular syndromes (Chen et al, 1996; Soderbergh et al, 1996; Reusch, 2000). These findings suggest the potential for a genetic component in the pathogenesis of polyglandular failure. In our series of 187 dogs with primary adrenocortical insufficiency, 28 have had at least one other endocrinopathy. These problems included hypothyroidism in 16 dogs, diabetes mellitus in 14, hypoparathyroidism in three, and azoospermia in two (several dogs had more than one associated disorder). The incidence of hepatopathies has been much more significant in our hypoadrenal population (see page 415). Also of interest are dogs with naturally occurring hypoadrenocorticism and lymphocytic/plasmacytic (immune mediated? autoimmune?) gastrointestinal disorders and/or renal glomerular pathology (immune complex glomerulonephropathy).

Autoimmune polyglandular disease has been documented in a few veterinary cases (Bowen et al, 1986; Kooistra et al, 1995). Any endocrine deficiency syndrome may occur secondary to immune-mediated (autoimmune) destruction. It remains to be proved whether true immune-mediated disease accounts for a significant percentage of the dogs with hypoadrenocorticism, whether there is a familial association, and whether those dogs are predisposed to other immune-mediated disorders.

OTHER CAUSES OF PRIMARY HYPOADRENOCORTICISM. Uncommon (rare?) causes of canine adrenocortical insufficiency include destruction of the adrenal cortices by granulomatous diseases such as histoplasmosis and blastomycosis; hemorrhagic infarctions (secondary to trauma, warfarin-type toxicity, or other coagulopathies), metastases of cancer to the adrenal glands; amyloidosis of the adrenal cortices; trauma (accidents); and iatrogenic causes (surgical removal of the adrenals, rapid withdrawal of a dog from chronic glucocorticoid therapy, or overdose with the adrenocorticolytic drug o,p'-DDD, which is used in the treatment of hyperadrenocorticism). Interestingly, in humans with hypoadrenocorticism secondary to hemorrhage or metastases

to the glands, bilateral adrenal enlargement (sometimes massive enlargement) is often detected with ultrasonography or computed tomography (Tyrrell et al, 1991).

Secondary Adrenocortical Failure

NATURALLY OCCURRING DISEASE. In addition to disease processes specifically affecting the adrenal glands, reduced secretion of ACTH by the pituitary gland results in decreased synthesis and secretion of adrenocortical hormones, especially glucocorticoids (see Fig. 8-1). Reduced secretion of corticotropin-releasing hormone (CRH) by the hypothalamus may also result in secondary adrenocortical failure. Destructive lesions in the pituitary or hypothalamus that would result in ACTH or CRH insufficiency (or both) are usually caused by neoplasia; inflammation and trauma are less common causes (Velardo et al, 1992; Thodou et al, 1995) (see Table 8-1). Among humans with secondary disease, especially those with space-occupying lesions, few have only adrenal insufficiency. Other hormonal systems are usually involved, and neurologic or ophthalmologic symptoms may accompany, precede, or follow adrenal insufficiency (Vance, 1994).

IATROGENIC CAUSES

General. Adrenal insufficiency secondary to exogenous corticosteroid administration is seen commonly in small animal veterinary practice, although it only rarely results in clinical signs (see Fig. 8-1). Any pet chronically receiving amounts of corticosteroids sufficient to suppress the hypothalamic-pituitary axis is susceptible to secondary adrenal atrophy. Adrenal suppression can occur within a few days of administration of ACTH-inhibiting doses of corticosteroids, although suppression is markedly variable among individuals. This individual variation is reflected in the fact that some dogs quickly develop iatrogenic Cushing's syndrome from relatively low doses, whereas others show no effect from higher doses. If suppression is demonstrated, adrenal function usually recovers gradually (over a period of weeks) after hormone administration is stopped, perhaps taking more time if long-acting depot forms of glucocorticoids were used (see Table 8-2).

Glucocorticoids that Cause Suppression. A wide variety of glucocorticoids are used in veterinary practice. It must be remembered that any glucocorticoid can suppress pituitary secretion of ACTH, potentially leading to adrenocortical atrophy. Such effects usually follow chronic glucocorticoid administration, regardless of the specific drug or route. Pituitary suppression has been documented not only with injectable and oral glucocorticoids, but also with topical dermatologic, ophthalmic, and otic preparations (Roberts et al, 1984; Moriello et al, 1988; Murphy et al, 1990). Pituitary suppression caused by glucocorticoids can also occur in cats. Furthermore, cats also may suffer adrenocortical atrophy after receiving megestrol acetate (progestogens) (Chastain et al, 1982).

Although estimates of the relative biologic effectiveness of the clinical analogs vary, studies have shown prednisone/prednisolone to be five times more potent than cortisol in suppressing ACTH secretion, and dexamethasone to be 50 to 150 times more potent. Relatively small dosages of dexamethasone, therefore, may be sufficient to produce adrenal atrophy. The long-acting "depot" injectable corticosteroids (e.g., betamethasone), however, are the most potent drugs used in small animal practice for suppressing both the pituitary-adrenal axis and the immune system. One injection of such long-acting agents has been shown to suppress the pituitary-adrenocortical axis of dogs for as long as 5 weeks (Kemppainen et al, 1981 and 1982).

How Long to Wait before Testing the Pituitary-Adrenal Axis. Fortunately, most dogs receiving glucocorticoids for any length of time do not develop any problems after cessation of therapy. The results of an ACTH stimulation test can be used to demonstrate iatrogenic suppression of the pituitary-adrenal axis. To avoid confusion in test result interpretation or suppression of cortisol secretion associated with drug therapy, it is wise to wait at least 2 weeks but sometimes as long as 2 months after discontinuation of glucocorticoid medications before performing an ACTH stimulation test (Moore and Hoenig, 1992).

PATHOPHYSIOLOGY

Background

From a physiologic viewpoint, the adrenal cortices are composed of two important functional zones. The outer zone, the zona glomerulosa, synthesizes and secretes aldosterone and is under the primary control of angiotensin. The inner zone synthesizes and secretes glucocorticoids. This zone is actually composed of two histologically distinct areas, the zona fasciculata and the zona reticularis (Fig. 8-2) (Reusch, 2000).

Mineralocorticoids

PHYSIOLOGIC ACTIONS. Mineralocorticoids function to control sodium, potassium, and water homeostasis. They promote sodium, chloride, and water resorption, as well as potassium excretion in epithelial tissues, including the intestinal mucosa, salivary glands, sweat glands, and kidneys. The primary site of aldosterone effect is the renal tubule, where aldosterone promotes proximal convoluted renal tubular resorption of sodium and chloride and distal convoluted tubular resorption of sodium by exchange with potassium (Nelson, 1980).

RENIN-ANGIOTENSIN SYSTEM. Secretion of aldosterone is under primary control of the renin-angiotensin system. This system is closely associated with the renal juxtaglomerular apparatus, which consists of the juxtaglomerular cells surrounding the afferent arterioles of the renal cortical glomeruli and a group of special staining cells, the macula densa, situated in the distal convoluted tubule. The juxtaglomerular cells are specialized myoepithelial cells cuffing the afferent arterioles that act as miniature pressure transducers. They monitor renal perfusion by perceiving pressure changes as distortions of the existing stretch on the arteriolar walls. Volume depletion caused by events such as hemorrhage, diuretic administration, or salt restriction are perceived by the juxtaglomerular cells as decreased stretch. These cells respond to this stimulus by synthesizing and secreting renin.

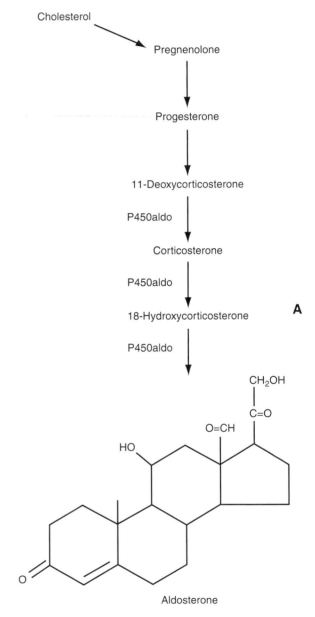

FIGURE 8-2. *A,* Steroid biosynthesis in the zona glomerulosa. The steps from cholesterol to 11-deoxycorticosterone are the same as in the zona fasciculata and zona reticularis. However, the zona glomerulosa lacks 17α-hydroxylase activity and thus cannot produce cortisol. Only the zona glomerulosa can convert corticosterone to 18-hydroxycorticosterone and aldosterone. The single enzyme P450aldo catalyzes the conversion of 11-deoxycorticosterone → corticosterone → 18-hydroxycorticosterone → aldosterone.

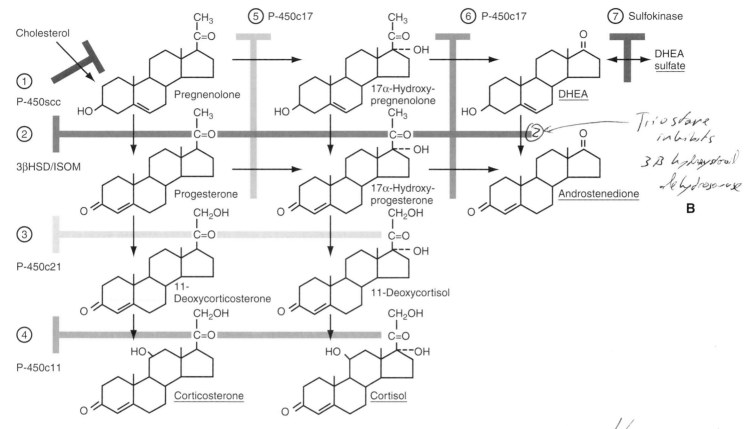

(handwritten annotations in right margin): Triostane inhibits 3β hydroxysterol dehydrogenase

B

(handwritten annotation lower right): Human auto immune targeted enzymes

FIGURE 8-2—cont'd *B*, Major biosynthetic pathways of adrenocortical steroid biosynthesis. The major secretory products are underlined. 1, Cholesterol desmolase (side-chain cleavage enzyme, P450scc); 2, 3β-hydroxysteroid dehydrogenase; 3, 21β-hydroxylase (P450c21); 4, 11β-hydroxylase (P450c11); 5, aldosterone synthetase; 6, 17α-hydroxylase (P450c17). The zona glomerulosa, which produces aldosterone, lacks 17α-hydroxylase and therefore cannot synthesize 17α-hydroxypregnenolone and 17α-hydroxyprogesterone, which are the precursors of cortisol and the adrenal androgens. The zona fasciculata and zona reticularis produce cortisol, androgens, and small amounts of estrogens. These zones do not contain the aldosterone synthetase and therefore cannot convert 11-deoxycorticosterone to aldosterone.

Renin, in turn, acts on a plasma α_2-globulin produced by the liver, releasing the decapeptide angiotensin I. Converting enzyme in the lung splits off two amino acids from angiotensin I, producing angiotensin II, which is a potent vasoconstrictor and a primary stimulant for aldosterone secretion. Increased plasma aldosterone concentrations enhance sodium retention, thereby expanding the extracellular fluid volume, increasing renal perfusion, and suppressing the initiating signal for release (Fig. 8-3) (Ganong, 1981; White, 1994).

NORMAL EFFECT OF PLASMA POTASSIUM CONCENTRATION. Aldosterone secretion can be regulated independent of the renin-angiotensin system as a function of the plasma potassium concentration. When a solution of potassium ions is injected into adrenal arteries, the adrenal venous aldosterone concentration immediately increases. Thus potassium appears to have a direct stimulatory effect on adrenocortical production of aldosterone, presumably through a transmembrane effect. This potassium-mediated aldosterone control system operates parallel to the renin-angiotensin system and is of comparable potency, although the

importance of this process in vivo is probably not as significant as that associated with renal perfusion.

NORMAL EFFECT OF ACTH. The release of aldosterone can be stimulated by ACTH, but ACTH is not the dominant force in stimulation of secretion of mineralocorticoids by the zona glomerulosa. Apparently, ACTH is not important in most physiologic conditions, but rather exerts a "permissive" influence over aldosterone secretion (Tyrrell et al, 1991).

PHYSIOPATHOLOGY OF MINERALOCORTICOID DEFICIENCY

Hyponatremia and Hypochloremia. With adrenocortical insufficiency, lack of aldosterone secretion results in impaired ability to conserve sodium and chloride and to excrete potassium, leading to hyponatremia, hypochloremia, and hyperkalemia. With an adequate sodium-chloride intake, mild aldosterone deficiencies may have few if any consequences. However, if sodium intake diminishes with the onset of anorexia or a change in diet or if sodium loss increases because of vomiting and/or diarrhea, the animal's health may quickly deteriorate. Continued loss of sodium and chloride through the gastrointestinal tract and kidneys may lead to severe depletion of total

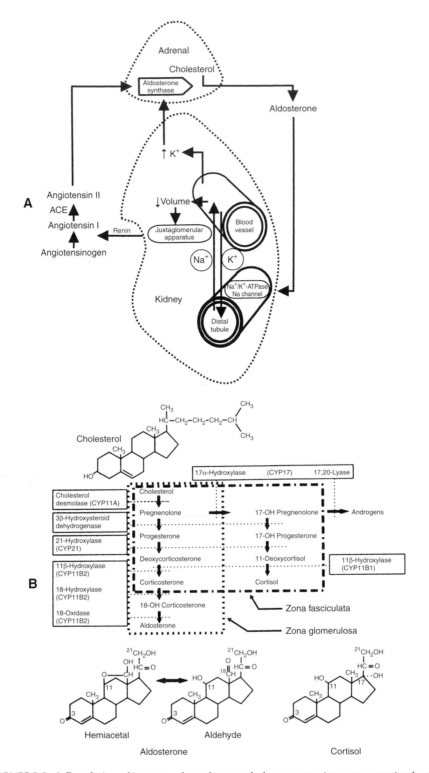

FIGURE 8-3. *A,* Regulation of intravascular volume and plasma potassium concentration by the renin-angiotensin-aldosterone system. A decrease in intravascular volume increases the secretion of renin by the juxtaglomerular apparatus, leading to increased conversion of angiotensinogen to angiotensin I and then to angiotensin II. Angiotensin II acts on the adrenal zona glomerulosa to increase the activity of aldosterone synthetase and therefore the secretion of aldosterone. Hyperkalemia also increases the activity of aldosterone synthase. Aldosterone acts on renal distal tubules to increase the resorption of sodium (Na excretion of potassium [K]). ACE denotes angiotensin-converting enzyme, and the arrows pointing up or down before a word or symbol indicate an increase or decrease, respectively. *B,* Pathways of adrenal steroid biosynthesis. The pathways of biosynthesis of aldosterone and cortisol from cholesterol are shown. The chemical structures of these substances appear at the bottom and top of the figure, respectively. Aldosterone exists in two conformations (18-aldehyde and hemiacetal) that are freely interconvertible; the hemiacetal predominates under physiologic conditions. The enzymes responsible for each biosynthetic step are shown at the left; the last three enzymatic conversions required for aldosterone biosynthesis are mediated by a single enzyme, aldosterone synthetase (CYP11B2). The conversions that take place in the zona glomerulosa and the zona fasciculata are indicated. (From White PC: N Engl J Med 331:250, 1994.)

body salt stores and, simultaneously, severe volume depletion.

Physiologically, sodium and chloride losses cannot take place without concurrent loss of water. Thus inability to retain sodium and chloride causes a reduced extracellular fluid volume that leads to progressive development of hypovolemia, hypotension, reduced cardiac output and, finally, decreased perfusion of the kidneys and other tissues. A decreased glomerular filtration rate (GFR) causes prerenal azotemia, increased renin production, and mild metabolic acidosis. Weight loss, weakness, microcardia, and depression are commonly associated with this syndrome.

Antidiuretic Hormone and Urine Concentration. The hypotension and dehydration that develop secondary to aldosterone deficiency stimulate secretion of pituitary vasopressin (AVP; antidiuretic hormone [ADH]) as the system attempts to compensate for fluid losses. Vasopressin causes water retention, potentially worsening the hyponatremia and hypochloremia by dilution. This physiologic process is not considered a major factor in hypoadrenocorticism, because these dogs tend to have relatively dilute urine (urine specific gravity of 1.010 to 1.025) despite dehydration and prerenal azotemia. Hyponatremia contributes to the development of dilute urine because sodium is an important component of the renal medullary concentration gradient. Furthermore, hyponatremia probably interferes with stimulation of ADH secretion by reducing serum osmolality. Thus decreases in sodium (and chloride) ions impair natural osmotic stimuli and promote dilute urine despite the dehydration (Tyler et al, 1987).

Hyperkalemia. Progressively worsening hyperkalemia develops as a result of diminished renal perfusion, which reduces glomerular filtration and depresses cation exchange by the distal convoluted renal tubules. Hyperkalemia can be exaggerated by metabolic acidosis, which promotes a shift of potassium ions from the intracellular to the extracellular space. The most prominent manifestation of hyperkalemia is the deleterious effect this anion has on cardiac function. Hyperkalemia causes decreased myocardial excitability, an increase in the myocardial refractory period, and slowed conduction. Hypoxia, which occurs secondary to hypovolemia and poor tissue perfusion, contributes to myocardial irritability. These abnormalities may be demonstrated on an electrocardiogram (see page 417). Ventricular fibrillation or cardiac standstill may eventually occur as the plasma potassium concentration exceeds 10 mEq/L.

Acidosis. Mild metabolic acidosis develops as a result of impaired ability to reabsorb bicarbonate and chloride ions in the renal tubules, as well as from failure of the poorly perfused kidneys to excrete metabolic waste products and hydrogen ions.

Glucocorticoids

BACKGROUND: PHYSIOLOGIC ACTIONS. Glucocorticoid secretion is controlled by the hypothalamic-pituitary axis via a simple negative feedback loop. CRH is synthesized and secreted by the hypothalamus, and it then stimulates the secretion of ACTH by the pituitary gland. ACTH stimulates the synthesis and secretion of adrenal glucocorticoids. As plasma concentrations of glucocorticoids increase, they exert negative feedback on the secretion of CRH and ACTH (see Fig. 8-1) (Ganong, 1981). A major physiologic factor that influences the secretion of ACTH is cortisol metabolism, which reduces negative feedback and releases CRH. A second major factor in ACTH release results from stress (Nelson, 1980). Diurnal fluctuation of ACTH secretion, considered a well-documented phenomenon in humans, is not well documented in dogs.

Glucocorticoids (cortisol) affect almost every tissue in the body. Cortisol has a vital supportive role in the maintenance of vascular tone, endothelial integrity, vascular permeability, and the distribution of total body water in the vascular compartment (Lamberts et al, 1997). Cortisol potentiates the vasoconstrictor actions of catecholamines and controls the secretion of corticotropin (ACTH), CRH, and vasopressin (ADH) by negative feedback inhibition. Cortisol is vital to the metabolism of carbohydrates and protein, at least in part by stimulating gluconeogenesis and glycogenesis by liver and muscle. It suppresses peripheral cellular uptake and utilization of plasma glucose. It has some control over the immune system by suppressing inflammatory responses and lymphoid tissue. Cortisol stimulates erythrocytosis, maintains normal blood pressure, and counteracts the effects of stress (Oelkers, 1996). Pain, fever, and hypovolemia all result in a sustained increase in the secretion of ACTH and cortisol. During surgical procedures, for example, serum ACTH and cortisol concentrations rise quickly, slowly returning to basal values within 24 to 48 hours. Patients receiving steroid treatment for chronic autoimmune or inflammatory disease need less additional corticosteroid during severe illness and perioperatively than those receiving replacement therapy for adrenal insufficiency (Lamberts et al, 1997).

PHYSIOPATHOLOGY OF SIGNS ATTRIBUTED TO INSUFFICIENT CORTISOL SECRETION

Cortisol Deficiency. Inadequate glucocorticoid secretion may result from destruction of the adrenal cortex or from dysfunction of the hypothalamus or pituitary gland, with insufficient secretion of CRH or ACTH, respectively. Regardless of the underlying cause, cortisol is necessary physiologically for a number of functions. Lack of cortisol secretion may result in any of a variety of gastrointestinal signs, including anorexia, vomiting, abdominal pain, and weight loss. Energy metabolism is diminished, owing to impaired gluconeogenesis, impaired fat metabolism, decreased fat utilization, and depletion of liver glycogen stores. As a result, fasting hypoglycemia may occur. Associated with these processes could be mental changes, such as diminished vigor and lethargy. Impaired ability to excrete water free of sodium may result in hyponatremia. With primary adrenal insufficiency, there is an unrestrained secretion of ACTH from the pituitary. One of the hallmark signs of hypocortisolism is impaired tolerance to stress, and clinical signs often become more pronounced when the animal is placed in stressful situations.

ACTH Deficiency. In adrenal insufficiency secondary to pituitary or hypothalamic disease, the renin-angiotensin-aldosterone system should be preserved, therefore plasma electrolyte homeostasis is maintained. The same is true in dogs chronically treated with corticosteroids if the medication is acutely discontinued. Exogenously administered corticosteroids inhibit ACTH secretion through negative feedback, resulting in secondary adrenocortical atrophy that spares the zona glomerulosa. Clinical signs, which result from cortisol deficiency, include some or all of the following: lethargy, inappetence, vomiting, diarrhea, weight loss, and weakness.

Iatrogenic Cortisol Deficiency Secondary to Administration of o,p'-DDD. Hypoadrenocorticism produced iatrogenically, such as with the adrenocorticolytic drug mitotane (o,p'-DDD) can produce physiologic changes identical to the natural disease in dogs. Normal dogs quickly become hypocortisolemic when treated with this drug, as demonstrated by ACTH stimulation test results. However, they may not exhibit typical clinical signs of hypoadrenocorticism as quickly as the test results would suggest. In contrast, dogs concurrently treated with the anticonvulsant drug phenobarbital appear to be relatively resistant to the effects of o,p'-DDD.

Dogs with pituitary-dependent hyperadrenocorticism (PDH) are relatively sensitive to o,p'-DDD. These dogs exhibit signs of cortisol deficiency quickly and consistently. Drug-induced complete destruction of the adrenal cortex can follow o,p'-DDD administration, but it is not common if accepted treatment protocols are followed (see Chapter 6). Ketoconazole, an enzyme blocker that interrupts the synthesis of cortisol, can cause severe but reversible cortisol deficiency at doses of approximately 30 mg/kg/day.

Sex Hormones

The zona reticularis of the adrenal cortex synthesizes and secretes androgens, estrogen-like compounds, and glucocorticoids. The physiologic importance of the androgens and/or estrogens secreted by the adrenals is not clear. Clinical manifestations as a result of impaired secretion of androgens and estrogens are not apparent in animals with primary adrenal insufficiency.

Severity of Adrenocortical Glandular Destruction

PATHOGENESIS. Development of the clinical syndrome associated with adrenocortical insufficiency is believed to require at least 90% destruction of adrenal cortices. Naturally occurring, immune-mediated destruction of the adrenal cortices is usually a gradual process, initially resulting in a "partial deficiency syndrome" characterized by inadequate adrenal reserve,

with symptoms manifest only during times of stress (see Table 8-1). Stress may be associated with surgery, trauma, infection, or even psychologic distress, such as when dogs are placed in boarding kennels. However, basal hormone secretion in the unstressed state may be adequate to maintain near-normal plasma electrolyte concentrations and minimal clinical signs. For these dogs, the diagnosis can be confirmed only with tests that assess adrenocortical reserve. As destruction of the adrenal cortices continues, hormone secretion becomes inadequate even under nonstressful conditions, and a true metabolic crisis without any obvious inciting event can result.

TIMING OF EFFECT ON ZONES OF THE ADRENAL CORTEX. In dogs with primary adrenal insufficiency, each of the three adrenocortical zones seems to become damaged at about the same rate. In other words, aldosterone deficiency (with its associated clinical signs and electrolyte abnormalities) and glucocorticoid deficiency (with its associated clinical signs) occur in tandem. Therefore the ACTH stimulation test (assaying plasma cortisol concentrations) is used to directly assess the capacity for cortisol synthesis and indirectly assess the capacity for aldosterone synthesis. It is extremely rare (but possible) for the zona glomerulosa (aldosterone secretion) to be significantly more or less damaged than the zona fasciculata and zona reticularis (cortisol secretion) (Lobetti, 1998). In contrast, insufficient cortisol response to exogenous ACTH administration in a dog with normal serum electrolyte concentrations could be explained by chronic glucocorticoid administration (common) or pituitary failure to secrete ACTH (rare).

SIGNALMENT

Incidence

The incidence of hypoadrenocorticism (Addison's disease) suggests the approximate rate at which new cases might be diagnosed. It has been estimated that the average veterinarian in private practice sees about 1400 to 1600 dogs per year and that Addison's disease occurs in about 0.5 dogs per 1000. Thus the average two-veterinarian practice should expect to diagnose at least one new case yearly (Kelch et al, 1998). The prognosis for treated dogs is excellent, and the average dog should have a normal life span, about 7 years from the average age of diagnosis. The average veterinary practice, therefore, is likely to have a number of addisonian dogs under treatment at any given time.

Dogs Used for Discussion

Hypoadrenocorticism is an uncommon endocrine disorder in dogs, and it is rare in cats. Data have been accumulated from our current series of 205 dogs with naturally occurring hypoadrenocorticism and arbitrarily from 76 and 225 dogs included in two reviews (Willard et al, 1982; Peterson et al, 1996). This collection of

506 dogs with hypoadrenocorticism likely represents a typical group for making generalizations concerning this condition.

Gender

Female dogs account for 349 cases (69%) of the 506 dogs with hypoadrenocorticism. Ninety-one dogs (18%) were castrated males. Predilection for the female is typical for immune-mediated disorders in the dog and may provide crude but further evidence of an immune-mediated pathogenesis for hypoadrenocorticism in most cases (Melian and Peterson, 1996). In a study critically evaluating these parameters, females were about twice as likely to develop Addison's disease as males. Neutered females and neutered males were each about three times more likely to develop the disease than their intact counterparts (Kelch et al, 1998).

Age

Although hypoadrenocorticism can be diagnosed in dogs of any age, it continues to be a disease mostly of young and middle-aged dogs. The age range for the 506 dogs reviewed was 4 weeks to 16 years. The average age at the time of diagnosis is about 4 to 5 years. Statistically, dogs up to 4 years of age are less likely and dogs 7 to 14 years of age are more likely to develop Addison's disease. However, a review of the information on the 506 dogs in the representative group showed that approximately 76% were younger than 7 years of age at diagnosis.

Breed

Significant breed predilections probably exist for this disease. However, virtually every report has documented that mixed-breed dogs are most prevalent and a wide variety of breeds are represented in the case reports and case series that have been published. In our representative dogs, 122 of 506 (24%) were mixed breed. Furthermore, many of the breeds represented reflect those that are simply popular (Table 8-3).

When appropriate statistical analysis is applied to the data, however, several breeds appear to be at increased risk for developing hypoadrenocorticism (see Table 8-3). This implication is based on breeds diagnosed as having Addison's disease compared with the prevalence of each breed in the overall population. When odds ratios are calculated, the Great Dane, Poodle (Toy, Miniature, and Standard), and West Highland White Terrier are among the breeds with a higher risk. Breeds at lower risk include Lhasa Apsos, Yorkshire Terriers, Boston Terriers, and those of mixed breeding. The Basset Hound, Saint Bernard, and Portuguese Water Dog may be at increased risk, but their lesser popularity, coupled with a small number of cases, precludes a high degree of certainty. Whether the Labrador Retriever is predisposed is not clear. Although reported

TABLE 8-3 BREED CHARACTERISTICS IN CANINE HYPOADRENOCORTICISM*

A. Breeds Most Commonly Diagnosed

Mixed breed	24%
Toy or miniature poodle	10%
Labrador Retriever	9%
Rottweilers	9%
Standard Poodle	8%
German Shepherd Dog	6%
Doberman Pinscher	4%
Golden Retriever	4%
West Highland White Terrier	4%
Great Dane	3%

B. Breeds at Increased Risk

Great Dane
West Highland White Terrier
Bearded Collie
Poodle (standard, mini, toy)
Basset hound

C. Breeds at Decreased Risk

Boston Terrier
Dalmatian
Pit Bull Terrier
Boxer
Pomeranian
Yorkshire Terrier
Shetland Sheepdog
Lhasa Apso

D. Breeds That May Have a Genetic Predisposition

Standard Poodle
Portuguese Water Dog
Bearded Collie
Labrador Retriever

*From Kelch, W.J. (1996); used with permission

to be at higher risk in one study, a more rigorous evaluation did not find the breed to be at higher or lower risk (Kelch et al, 1998).

Genetic predispositions for several breeds have been implicated. In one study, hypoadrenocorticism in the Bearded Collie was demonstrated to be highly heritable (Oberbauer et al, 2002). The other breeds that have been claimed to have a genetic predisposition include the Portuguese Water Dog, Standard Poodle, and Labrador Retriever (see Table 8-3). There have also been various reports of canine families afflicted with Addison's disease. Familial predisposition to hypoadrenocorticism has been suggested in Standard Poodles, Portuguese Water Dogs, Leonbergers, Labrador Retrievers, and other breeds (Auge, 1985; Shaker et al, 1988; Smallwood and Barsanti, 1995). In work underway, a genetic predisposition of Standard Poodles to hypoadrenocorticism, for example, seems to be likely.

HISTORY

Subjectivity of Owner Opinions

The ability to obtain from an owner all information pertinent to providing proper care for the pet is perhaps the most underrated but valuable diagnostic aid in medicine. The veterinarian must realize that some owners, even though quite observant, are not aware of what constitutes a "normal" pet. The best example would be the owners who brought in a severely ill, 2-year-old female Saint Bernard, claiming she had been sick for 2 days. They said that she had been perfectly healthy prior to the present illness. This dog was diagnosed and treated for hypoadrenocorticism. One week after discharge from the hospital, the owners described her as aggressive, playful, filled with energy, possessing an excellent appetite, and more active than she had ever been before. The owners then realized that the dog had been "ill" much of her life but had not demonstrated the type of signs necessary to warrant examination by a veterinarian. This example illustrates the importance to the veterinarian of developing an ability to ask questions and analyze answers without assuming that the owner will mention all relevant information.

Variability in Severity of Clinical Signs

The severity of any given sign can vary dramatically, and "worrisome" problems depend completely on subjective owner opinion. Owner concerns for dogs ultimately diagnosed as having hypoadrenocorticism commonly include poor appetite or anorexia, lethargy or depression, the dog being thin or losing weight, weakness, vomiting and/or regurgitation, diarrhea (sometimes with melena or obvious hematochezia), and/or collapse (Table 8-4). These signs are vague and often suggestive of more common small animal disorders, especially renal, gastrointestinal, and infectious diseases. There are no pathognomonic signs. As previously discussed, any and all signs vary in severity from dog to dog. The suspicion of hypoadrenocorticism is confirmed only when the clinician maintains a differential diagnosis that includes this illness. Correlating the signalment, history, and physical examination findings with a suspicion of adrenal insufficiency allows most practitioners the opportunity to diagnose and treat dogs for this disease.

TABLE 8-4   HISTORICAL OWNER CONCERNS FOR 506 DOGS WITH HYPOADRENOCORTICISM

Sign	Percentage
Poor appetite/anorexia	88
Lethargy/depression	85
Thin	82
Vomiting/regurgitation	68
Weakness	51
Weight loss	40
Diarrhea	35
Waxing-waning course of illness	25
Polyuria	17
Shaking/shivering	17
Collapse	10
Painful abdomen	8

Correlating Signs with Hormonal Deficiencies

Each clinical sign described in Table 8-4 can be directly related to a deficiency in glucocorticoid and/or mineralocorticoid secretion. Anorexia, vomiting, regurgitation, lethargy, weakness, loose stools, melena and/or hematochezia, and abdominal pain can be the result of glucocorticoid deficiency alone. These signs, however, are exaggerated if alterations in the plasma sodium and potassium concentrations also exist. Weight loss is a sequela of the problems described, and the "waxing-waning" course is a reflection of progressive but not necessarily absolute deficiency of adrenocortical hormones. Polyuria may be the result of excessive sodium loss into the urine, which causes "washout" of one solute component comprising the renal medullary concentration gradient. The shivering or shaking in dogs with hypoadrenocorticism is believed to be one expression of muscle weakness resulting from depletion of plasma sodium.

Classic Waxing-Waning Course of Illness

One clue in the history that a dog may have Addison's disease is the description of an illness that "waxes and wanes" or appears to affect the dog "episodically." However, this classic alteration has been observed in only about 25% of the dogs described with this disorder. A waxing-waning course of illness is simply not obvious to most owners of affected dogs. In some dogs with naturally occurring hypoadrenocorticism, the owners did observe episodic illness, weakness, and depression that lasted variable periods during the 2 to 52 weeks preceding a diagnosis. These dogs vacillated between appearing normal and quite ill, with illness developing either suddenly or gradually. The periods of apparent good health often followed nonspecific veterinary therapy, usually consisting of corticosteroid medication and/or parenteral fluid administration.

Dogs with adrenal insufficiency are usually brought to a veterinarian either in an acute "addisonian" crisis or for progressive, often intermittent, problems. Most dogs with hypoadrenocorticism, regardless of the duration of their illness, have chronic rather than acute disease. The period of time that owners observe signs, whether progressive or episodic, is often 2 weeks or longer. Most dogs that are initially brought to a veterinarian in an acute adrenal crisis have had progressive, untreated chronic adrenal or pituitary disease in which mild signs either were not observed or did not concern the owner. The history from owners whose dogs were brought to the hospital in acute crisis is similar to that provided when the dog is mildly ill. The only difference is the degree of depression, weakness, or other signs. Some dogs are so weak they have to be carried.

PHYSICAL EXAMINATION

Physical examinations completed on the hypoadrenal dogs in our series have not revealed consistent abnor-

TABLE 8-5 ABNORMALITIES NOTED ON PHYSICAL EXAMINATION OF 506 DOGS WITH HYPOADRENOCORTICISM

TABLE 8-5 ABNORMALITIES NOTED ON PHYSICAL EXAMINATION OF 506 DOGS WITH HYPOADRENOCORTICISM

Sign	Percentage
Depression/lethargy	87
Thinness	82
Weakness	66
Dehydration	41
Shock/collapse	24
Bradycardia	22
Weak femoral pulse	22
Melena/hematochezia	17
Hypothermia	15
Abdominal pain	7

malities, except that the dogs are usually "ill." Therefore, it should not be surprising that the vague signs of "depression," lethargy, and appearing thin and weak were the most common abnormalities described among 506 dogs with Addison's disease (Table 8-5). Dehydration, shock-or-collapse, hypothermia, bradycardia, and weak femoral pulses were detected in only a small number of dogs. Melena and/or hematochezia was occasionally observed after rectal temperature assessment or on rectal examination. Abdominal pain, hypothermia, and emaciation have been mentioned in the veterinary literature but have only rarely been seen by us or in the reports used in this series (Willard et al, 1982; Peterson et al, 1996).

A thorough physical examination is of paramount importance in evaluating any animal. In this disorder, as in others, the severity of an illness can be assessed on physical examination. The clinician may not understand the cause of a problem without additional information. Obtaining and evaluating a good medical history, as well as carefully choosing diagnostic tests, are imperative for a definitive diagnosis.

CLINICAL PATHOLOGY

Erythrocyte Parameters

In adrenal insufficiency, a normocytic normochromic anemia accompanied by little or no reticulocyte response secondary to bone marrow suppression from hypocortisolism is common. However, if an animal becomes hemoconcentrated secondary to dehydration, the underlying anemia may not be obvious on the initial complete blood count (CBC) (Table 8-6). Once rehydrated, these dogs usually exhibit the typical mild anemia of hypoadrenocorticism, with hematocrits of 20% to 35% being typical.

If the anemia at the time of initial physical examination is significant and the dog is in an "addisonian" crisis, rehydration may reduce the circulating red blood cell count to life-threatening levels. Severe anemia is usually associated with chronic bone marrow suppression and/or acute and significant gastrointestinal hemorrhage. Gastrointestinal hemorrhage can be specifically caused by glucocorticoid deficiency. Transfusion of red cells (fresh whole blood or packed cells) in these situations may be a critical component of patient management (Medinger et al, 1993).

Leukocyte Parameters

TOTAL WHITE BLOOD CELL (WBC) COUNTS. Total WBC counts in hypoadrenal dogs vary from low normal to mildly increased. Most of these dogs have normal total WBC counts. No consistent WBC differential count was obvious in our series of dogs. An increase in the WBC count may reflect a granulocytic response to concurrent bacterial infection (see Table 8-6).

EOSINOPHILS. The presence of an absolute eosinophilia in hypoadrenal dogs is not commonly reported in the veterinary literature. Some veterinarians have suggested that eosinophilia is common, but most have observed eosinophilia to be an inconsistent feature of the disease. Eosinophils were absent on CBCs obtained on admission in 14% of 506 dogs, whereas only 10% of these dogs had an absolute eosinophilia. The remaining dogs had eosinophil counts that were within the reference range, both on relative and absolute tabulations.

The presence of a normal absolute eosinophil count in an ill dog may be significant because a stress pattern with no or few eosinophils is expected in such dogs if they have normal adrenocortical function. The finding of a normal eosinophil count in a stressed or ill dog should be viewed with a suspicion for hypoadrenocorticism. It must be remembered that a relative or

TABLE 8-6 COMPLETE BLOOD COUNT VALUES IN DOGS WITH HYPOADRENOCORTICISM

Parameter	Normal Value	ADDISON'S DISEASE			
		Mean	Percent Decreased	Percent Increased	Range
Packed cell volume					
–at admission	37–55%	39%	34	10	15–57
–after 24 hrs	37–55%	28%	71	0	8–40
White blood cell count	6–17×10³	11	2	12	4–32
Neutrophils	60–77%	62%	4	13	45–84
Lymphocytes	12–30%	28%	7	13	8–44
Eosinophils	2–10%	8%	14	10	0–41%

TABLE 8-7 POTENTIAL CAUSES OF EOSINOPHILIA IN DOGS AND CATS

Parasitism
    Heartworm disease
    Gastrointestinal
    Dermatologic
    Other
Asthma
Nonparasitic dermatologic disease
Mast cell tumor
Hypoadrenocorticism (Addison's disease)
Uterine disease
Eosinophilic myositis
Eosinophilic pneumonitis/rhinitis/conjunctivitis
Eosinophilic enterocolitis (allergic colitis)
Eosinophilic leukemia
Eosinophilic granuloma complex
Eosinophilic vasculitis
Drug reaction

absolute eosinophilia may also occur with many other diseases and, when present, eosinophilia can be used in developing a differential diagnosis that may lead to an explanation or cause for the illness (Table 8-7) (Rothenberg, 1998). The presence or absence of eosinophils should be considered a nonspecific and insensitive means of deciding the likelihood that any animal may or may not have hypoadrenocorticism.

LYMPHOCYTES. Animals with normal adrenal function respond to stress in part by secreting cortisol. Glucocorticoids decrease lymphocyte numbers in the circulation. Therefore ill and untreated hypoadrenal dogs should have a relative or absolute lymphocytosis. However, as with eosinophils, lymphocyte numbers or percentages have not provided consistent, sensitive, or specific alterations that can be considered classic for hypoadrenocorticism (see Table 8-6). This parameter could be used as a "clue" to adrenocortical health. Hypoadrenocorticism should be suspected when normal or increased lymphocyte counts are present in an ill dog. Thirteen percent of our 506 hypoadrenal dogs had lymphocytosis, and 80% had normal absolute counts.

MODIFIED THORN TEST. Before assays were readily available to easily measure plasma cortisol concentrations, indirect tests of adrenocortical function were used. Included were tests that assessed changes in WBC numbers and/or percentages of certain WBCs present in the circulation after an injection of ACTH. A "modified Thorn test" (named after Dr. G. W. Thorn, who described such a protocol in 1948) has been reviewed. The recommendation for dogs was to obtain blood samples before and 4 hours after ACTH administration. Dogs with normal adrenocortical function demonstrate an increase in the neutrophil: lymphocyte ratio of at least 30%, and eosinophils decrease by at least 50% from pre-ACTH values (Chastain et al, 1989). This test was recommended as simple and readily available for determining the need for plasma cortisol measurements. We do not use this test.

Serum Electrolytes: "Classic" Hyponatremia and Hyperkalemia

PATHOPHYSIOLOGY OF SERUM ELECTROLYTE ALTERATIONS. The classic electrolyte alterations in Addison's disease are hyponatremia, hypochloremia, and hyperkalemia. These abnormalities are due primarily to aldosterone deficiency causing failure of the kidneys to conserve sodium or to excrete potassium. Hyponatremia is primarily caused by renal sodium wasting. Sodium lost via the kidneys is accompanied by water, resulting in both hyponatremia and dehydration should fluid intake not compensate for urinary losses. To some extent this dehydration may mask sodium depletion (mild or severe). Deficiency in adrenocortical hormones allows greater amounts of sodium to pass into the intracellular compartment as intracellular potassium concentrations decrease. Hyperkalemia results from both a shift of potassium from intracellular to extracellular compartments and from a decrease in renal excretion. The former condition results from a loss of cortisol effects on the sodium-potassium pump, which normally maintains a gradient across cellular membranes (Nelson, 1980).

Hypoaldosteronism and acidosis enhance the shift of potassium from intracellular to extracellular compartments. Decreased potassium exchange for sodium in the distal renal tubule leads to decreased urinary potassium excretion and increased sodium excretion. The shift in electrolytes between body compartments may be partly corrected by the administration of cortisol, but aldosterone or another mineralocorticoid is necessary to prevent renal loss of sodium and retention of potassium (Tyrrell et al, 1991).

SODIUM. Serum sodium concentrations have varied from normal to as low as 106 mEq/L at the time of diagnosis of Addison's disease in dogs (Table 8-8). Of 483 dogs with primary hypoadrenocorticism, 417 (86%) had serum sodium concentrations less than 142 mEq/L at the time of diagnosis. In addition, eight of the 23 dogs with apparent ACTH deficiency (secondary adrenocortical deficiency) were hyponatremic at the time of diagnosis. In 60 hypoadrenal dogs described in a separate study, the mean serum sodium concentration at the time of diagnosis was 128 mEq/L (Lynn et al, 1993), a value similar to the mean value for the 506 dogs.

POTASSIUM. Serum potassium concentrations in dogs at the time hypoadrenocorticism is diagnosed vary from normal to extremely increased levels that induce clinically obvious cardiac rhythm disturbances (see Table 8-8). Of the 483 hypoadrenal dogs in this review, 460 (95%) had serum potassium concentrations greater than 5.5 mEq/L at the time of diagnosis. In 60 of our more recently diagnosed hypoadrenal dogs, the mean serum potassium concentration was 7.2 mEq/L, and in the 506 dogs it was 7.0 mEq/L. None of the 23 dogs with apparent ACTH deficiency had hyperkalemia.

SODIUM:POTASSIUM RATIO: VALUE AND LIMITATIONS. The sodium to potassium ratio has frequently been used as a diagnostic tool to aid in gaining a suspicion

TABLE 8-8   SELECTED SERUM BIOCHEMISTRY VALUES FROM 506 DOGS WITH HYPOADRENOCORTICISM

| Parameter | Normal Value | ADDISON'S DISEASE | | | |
		Mean	Percent Decreased	Percent Increased	Range
Serum sodium (mEq/L)	142–155	128	84	0	106–150
Serum potassium (mEq/L)	4.1–5.5	7.0	0	92	4.7–10.8
Sodium potassium ratio	≥27	18	91	0	11.2–34.1
BUN (mg/dl)					
pretreatment	13–28	81	3	90	7–321
after 24 hr	13-28	26	4	24	8–194
Serum creatinine (mg/dl)	0.8–1.9	3.1	0	61	1.5–8.3
Serum glucose (mg/dl)	70–110	80	23	8	10–547
Venous total CO_2 (mEq/L)	18–24	16	46	3	9–21
Serum total protein (mg/dl)	5.4–7.8	6.4	14	10	4.3–8.2
Serum albumin (mg/dl)	2.8–3.9	2.9	14	4	1.6–4.4
Serum cholesterol (mg/dl)	140–240	166	11	11	31–788
Serum calcium (mg/dl)	9.6–11.7	11.1	12	29	6.6–15.9
Urine specific gravity	—	1.018	88% <1.030	0	1.005–1.044

or in specific identification of dogs with adrenal insufficiency. The normal ratio varies between 27:1 and 40:1. Values are often below 27:1 and may be below 20:1 in dogs with primary hypoadrenocorticism. Determination of serum electrolyte concentrations from dogs suspected of having adrenal insufficiency is of paramount importance. The finding of the classic electrolyte abnormalities, or of hyperkalemia without a decrease in the serum sodium concentration or vice versa (decreases in serum sodium without an increase in the serum potassium concentration) should prompt immediate therapy. The assumption that the clinician may be treating Addison's disease is warranted and may be lifesaving.

If the provisional diagnosis of hypoadrenocorticism made on the basis of serum electrolyte concentrations is incorrect, emergency therapy is rarely harmful. Aggressive management of hypoadrenocorticism is not significantly different from that for life-threatening renal or gastrointestinal diseases. However, the limitations of a diagnosis based solely on serum electrolyte determinations must be realized. Reliance on serum electrolyte concentrations as the sole criterion for diagnosing adrenal insufficiency can be misleading if three factors are not kept in mind (see next three sections): first and most important is the slow, progressive nature of the development of primary adrenal insufficiency in many dogs; second, dogs with pituitary failure continue to secrete aldosterone; and third, hyperkalemia and hyponatremia are not pathognomonic for adrenal insufficiency (Figs. 8-4 and 8-5).

SERUM ELECTROLYTE ASSESSMENT IS NOT ALWAYS DEFINITIVE

Insidious Illness. Adrenal insufficiency may be insidious in onset and gradually progressive, although an acute adrenal crisis seems more common clinically. Acute illness may be precipitated by any concurrent stress. The results of serum electrolyte assessments depend on the severity of clinical signs at the time such tests are evaluated. If a dog with Addison's disease is severely ill, typical serum electrolyte abnormalities usually exist. However, had that same dog been assessed immediately prior to development of obvious illness, it may have had normal serum electrolyte concentrations. Note that a small number of dogs with primary disease have normal serum electrolyte concentrations and that a small percentage of dogs with secondary disease have hyponatremia.

Only 17 of the 483 dogs (4%) with *primary* adrenocortical failure from our series and the two additional studies used had normal serum electrolyte concentrations at the time of diagnosis (see Table 8-8). Twelve of those 17 dogs developed typical electrolyte abnormalities weeks to months after glucocorticoid therapy (without mineralocorticoid support) was initiated. This uncommon finding of normal serum electrolyte concentrations has also been recognized by other investigators (Rogers et al, 1981; Bartges and Nielson, 1992; Schaer, 1994; Peterson et al, 1996). This does not include dogs with secondary adrenocortical atrophy due to pituitary ACTH deficiency. The diagnosis of Addison's disease in dogs with normal serum electrolyte parameters may be more obvious once the results of an ACTH stimulation test are available. The challenge rests in maintaining a clinical suspicion for hypoadrenocorticism and deciding to perform an ACTH stimulation test when the serum electrolyte concentrations are not suggestive of the diagnosis.

Pituitary ACTH Deficiency (Secondary Adrenocortical Failure). For the most part, electrolyte alterations are attributed to inadequate secretion of mineralocorticoids. Therefore an animal that has pituitary deficiency of ACTH may have a clinical syndrome that reflects only glucocorticoid deficiency. The gastrointestinal, mental, and metabolic changes typical of hypocortisolemia may become obvious to the owner and veterinarian, whereas those changes ascribed to hypoaldosteronism are absent.

Volume depletion, dehydration, and serum potassium abnormalities are usually absent because aldosterone is only minimally affected by ACTH. Hypotension is usually not present except in acute presentations. Hyponatremia was documented in 8 of 23 dogs in the

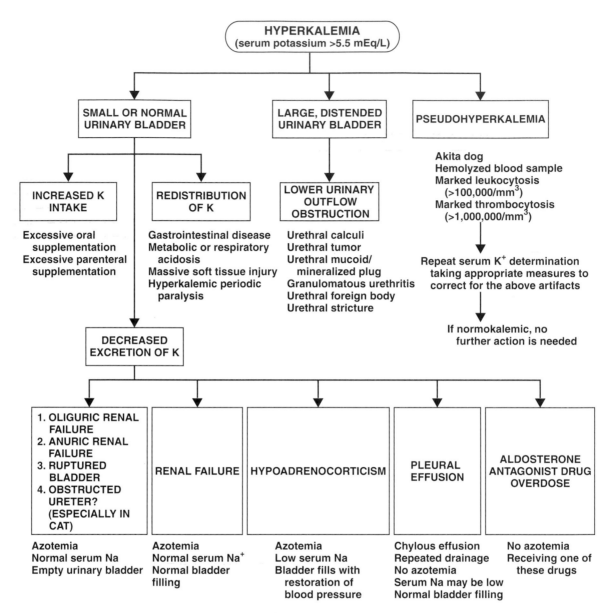

FIGURE 8-4. Algorithm for the differential diagnosis of hyperkalemia and for determining its cause.

series included here, and it may have been the result of water retention, anorexia, and vomiting and/or diarrhea. Inability to excrete a water load is not typically accompanied by hyperkalemia. Prominent clinical features are weakness, lethargy, anorexia, and occasionally vomiting. Joint, muscle, and/or abdominal pain may be apparent. Hypoglycemia is occasionally the presenting feature (Table 8-9). Acute decompensation and shock may occur.

ACTH deficiency may occur as a result of a primary pituitary problem (trauma, infection, cancer) or secondary to long-term corticosteroid medication that is acutely discontinued (see Fig. 8-1). Clinically, these dogs may be indistinguishable from dogs with primary adrenal insufficiency or those with renal or gastrointestinal problems. Only a thorough medical history can alert the veterinarian to the possibility of secondary adrenal insufficiency.

TABLE 8-9   SELECTED SERUM BIOCHEMISTRY VALUES IN 23 DOGS WITH NATURALLY OCCURRING SECONDARY HYPOADRENOCORTICISM

Parameter	Normal Value	Mean	Percent Decreased	Percent Increased	Range
Serum sodium (mEq/L)	142–155	135	34	0	122–150
Serum potassium (mEq/L)	4.1–5.5	5.1	0	4	4.9–5.7
Sodium:potassium ratio	≥27:1	26	43	0	24–28
BUN (mg/dl)	13–28	32	3	57	22–44
Glucose (mg/dl)	70–110	68	43	0	18–84

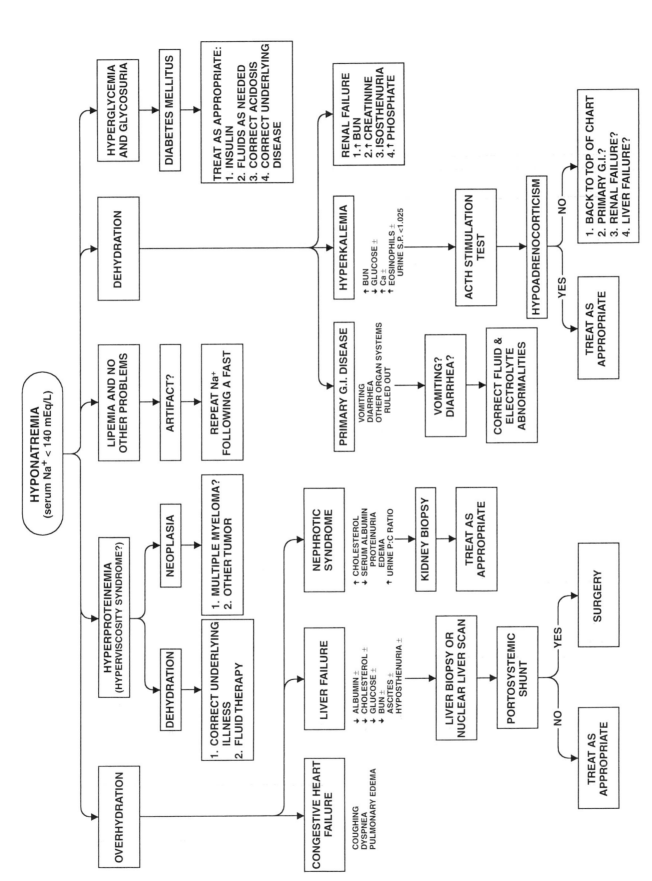

FIGURE 8-5. Algorithm for the differential diagnosis of hyponatremia and for determining its cause.

Hypocortisolism Secondary to Mitotane (o,p'-DDD) Therapy. Dogs with hyperadrenocorticism (Cushing's syndrome) that are overdosed with o,p'-DDD develop hypocortisolemia. This may be the most common cause of hypocortisolemia in veterinary practice and one with which most veterinarians are familiar. Clinical signs include depression, anorexia, vomiting, and diarrhea; serum electrolyte concentrations usually (but not always) remain within the normal range. The zones of the adrenal cortex (zonae fasciculata and reticularis), which produce cortisol, are more sensitive to the cytotoxic effects of o,p'-DDD than is the zona glomerulosa, which is responsible for producing aldosterone. Classic "Addison's disease" secondary to destruction of all three adrenocortical zones, with resultant hyponatremia and hyperkalemia, can result from o,p'-DDD overdose.

DIFFERENTIAL DIAGNOSIS FOR HYPERKALEMIA (SEE FIG. 8-4). Dogs and cats with nonadrenal causes of hyperkalemia must be distinguished from those with hypoadrenocorticism. Although the acute management of hyperkalemia is similar regardless of its cause (except that animals with urinary obstructions must have that specific problem relieved), the clinician must be certain of a diagnosis before pursuing lifelong therapy.

Urinary Tract Disorders. The most common nonadrenal causes of hyperkalemia are renal failure, urethral obstruction, and rupture of the bladder or ureter. These problems prevent excretion of potassium. Hyperkalemia is less common in chronic renal failure unless the dog or cat is terminally anuric or oliguric. Severe hyperkalemia can be associated with rupture of the urinary bladder and/or avulsion of a ureter. The resultant urine leakage into the peritoneal cavity prevents excretion of potassium and urea, two parameters that quickly become severely increased (Roth and Tyler, 1999).

Gastrointestinal Disease. Gastrointestinal disorders may also result in serum electrolyte abnormalities consistent with Addison's disease. These electrolyte disturbances were reported in dogs with intestinal parasitism (trichuriasis, ancylostomiasis), intestinal infection (salmonellosis), perforated duodenal ulcers, and gastric torsion (DiBartola, 1989; DiBartola et al, 1985; Roth and Tyler, 1999). Similar serum electrolyte abnormalities have been encountered in some of our puppies with parvovirus infection or canine distemper. Severe malabsorption syndromes occasionally cause hyperkalemia or hyponatremia or both. Dogs with trichuriasis, hyponatremia, and hyperkalemia do not have decreased serum concentrations of aldosterone (Graves et al, 1994).

Acidosis, Pancreatitis, and/or Trauma. Rapid cellular release of potassium and resultant hyperkalemia may occur as a result of severe acidosis or increased tissue destruction after surgery, crush injury, or extensive infection. Although not common, examples of disorders that can cause hyperkalemia are pancreatitis, diabetic ketoacidosis, aortic thrombosis in cats, and rhabdomyolysis secondary to heat stroke or prolonged exercise in dogs or cats. These conditions may also be associated with impaired renal excretion of potassium.

Pleural Effusions. Hyperkalemia and hyponatremia have been identified in some dogs with chylous pleural effusion after repeated pleural drainage procedures (Willard et al, 1991). Similar serum electrolyte abnormalities were identified in a dog with nonseptic, nonchylous effusion (Zenger, 1992). The incidence of these serum electrolyte abnormalities appears to be low, because only two of 17 dogs with experimentally induced chylothorax had hyperkalemia and hyponatremia (Fossum and Birchard, 1986; Willard et al, 1991). Hyperkalemia and hyponatremia may result from the failure of renal tubular sodium to enter cells in the distal nephron, thereby diminishing sodium resorption and subsequently decreasing potassium excretion into the renal tubule (Rose, 1984; Willard et al, 1991).

Miscellaneous Disorders. Low sodium:potassium ratios have been described in dogs with pyometra, perhaps as a result of acidosis, gastrointestinal signs, and severe dehydration. Hyperkalemia and hyponatremia have also been described in three near-term pregnant Greyhounds (Schaer et al, 2000), as well as in three dogs with disseminated neoplasia, two dogs with congestive heart failure, and one dog with mushroom toxicity (Roth and Tyler, 1999). Liver failure could cause similar electrolyte abnormalities, perhaps secondary to interference with the renin-angiotensin-aldosterone system, because angiotensin I is synthesized in the liver (Church, personal communication, 2002).

Iatrogenic and/or Drug Therapy. Excess potassium intake is an uncommon cause of hyperkalemia except in patients with renal insufficiency. Hyperkalemia can develop with overzealous potassium supplementation in intravenous fluids, using salt substitutes, or giving parenteral feeding solutions high in potassium. Potassium-sparing diuretics, angiotensin-converting enzyme inhibitors, and nonsteroidal antiinflammatory drugs also have the potential to cause mild hyperkalemia (Willard, 1989). Hypothyroidism in humans has been reported to cause decreased renal blood flow, reduced glomerular filtration rates, and hyponatremia (Baajafer et al, 1999).

Artifact. In vitro increases in the human serum potassium concentration may occur when a blood sample is hemolyzed or refrigerated or if separation of red blood cells from plasma is delayed. Another artifact is associated with severe hypernatremia, that may falsely increase potassium measurements performed with dry-reagent analysis (Ames, 1986). Hypertonicity has been suggested as a cause for hyperkalemia (Willard, 1989). Extreme leukocytosis ($>100,000$ mm^3) or thrombocytosis ($>1,000,000$ mm^3) may allow sufficient amounts of potassium to be released into the serum during clotting to falsely elevate the serum potassium value. In the latter situation, potassium increases in the serum as blood is clotting, an in vitro phenomenon.

Artifact: the Akita. The Akita breed appears to have unusually large concentrations of potassium in the red blood cells. In one study, six of eight Akitas had high erythrocyte potassium concentrations, and plasma from affected dogs displayed pseudohyperkalemia after

TABLE 8-10 ELECTROLYTE VALUES OF RED CELLS, PLASMA, AND STORED PLASMA*

Dog #	Breed	Age	Gender	RBC [K⁺] (mEq/L)	PLASMA (NA⁺/K⁺) Storage (0 Hr) (mEq/L)	Storage (24 Hr) (mEq/L)
1	Akita	2½ yr	M	69	161/3.9	148/16.4
2	Akita	4 yr	M	71	160/4.1	142/23.8
3	Akita	5 yr	F	65	159/4.5	145/17.2
4	Akita	2 yr	M	6.0	166/4.0	164/5.6
5	Akita	2 yr	F	4.0	158/3.9	159/4.9
6	Akita	5 yr	M	76	152/3.4	131/21.0
7	Akita	5 yr	M	68	154/4.4	147/14.2
8	Akita	6 yr	F/S	70	151/5.1	146/17.0
9	Japanese Tosa	2 yr	F	5.0	154/4.0	152/4.2
10	German Shepherd X	7 yr	M/C	3.5	156/4.6	152/5.2
11	Springer Spaniel	9 yr	FS	3.5	151/3.9	152/4.4
12	English Bulldog	9 yr	M	4.5	152/4.0	152/5.3
13	Labrador Retriever X	9 yr	F/S	5.0	152/4.7	149/5.5
14	Keeshound	3 mo	F	5.5	145/4.4	147/5.6

*Courtesy of Lisa Degen, DVM.
X, Mixed-breed dog; F/S, spayed female; M/C, castrated male; RBC[K⁺], red blood cell potassium concentration.

being refrigerated in contact with red cells for longer than 4 hours (Rich et al, 1986). The rise in the plasma potassium concentration (pseudohyperkalemia) was progressive with prolonged red cell contact and was accompanied by a fall in plasma sodium (Table 8-10).

DIFFERENTIAL DIAGNOSIS FOR HYPONATREMIA (TABLE 8-11 AND FIG. 8-5).

Naturally Occurring Diseases. In addition to hypoadrenocorticism, conditions associated with hyponatremia include renal tubular diseases, nephrotic syndrome, and postobstructive diuresis. Excessive urinary sodium losses can follow an osmotic diuresis such as occurs with diabetes mellitus. Hyperglycemia may also exacerbate hyponatremia as water shifts from the intracellular to the extracellular fluid compartment. Hyponatremia may develop from inadequate sodium intake, especially when coupled with excessive losses (Adrogue and Madias, 2000). Severe hyponatremia has been documented in dogs with severe gastrointestinal disease causing anorexia, vomiting, and/or diarrhea. These disorders include parasitism, ulcerative disease, viral disorders, and any condition that causes hemorrhagic gastroenteritis. All cause excessive loss of sodium.

Hyponatremia may also occur secondary to conditions that result in edema (in addition to nephrotic syndrome), such as congestive heart failure and myxedema in severe hypothyroidism. Hyponatremia can occur in association with any primary polydipsic disorder or with inappropriate secretion of ADH (see Chapter 1).

Iatrogenic Causes. Hyponatremia may be caused by delivery of excessive amounts of intravenous fluids containing inadequate amounts of sodium, by administration of drugs that cause an osmotic diuresis (e.g., glucose), or by frequent drainage of pleural effusion. Fourteen consecutive daily phlebotomies (approximately 15 ml/kg/day) and feeding a low-salt diet were also reported to cause severe hyponatremia (120 mEq/L) in a dog (Tyler et al, 1987).

Lipemia. Lipemia may cause a false decrease in the plasma sodium concentration by displacing a significant amount of the aqueous plasma phase in which sodium ions are found. When lipemic plasma is sampled, a less aqueous phase is obtained, resulting in an erroneous decrease in the plasma sodium concentration. If the sodium concentration is expressed as plasma water rather than as whole plasma, it is often normal. The problem is much less common in serum samples.

SUMMARY. Serum electrolyte profiles from dogs suspected of having hypoadrenocorticism are extremely valuable. They can be used to support a tentative diagnosis and are tremendously useful in modifying therapy. However, they do not provide a definitive diagnosis for hypoadrenocorticism (see Table 8-11). A definitive diagnosis can be obtained only by evaluating adrenocortical hormone concentrations and adrenocortical reserve. The differential diagnosis for hyperkalemia and hyponatremia is outlined in Table 8-11, and algorithms are provided in Figs. 8-4 and 8-5.

Blood Urea Nitrogen, Creatinine, and Urinalysis

BLOOD UREA NITROGEN (BUN). Reduced renal perfusion is a direct result of hypovolemia that, in turn, causes hypotension and diminished cardiac output. These problems develop secondary to chronic fluid losses through the kidneys via sodium diuresis, acute fluid losses due to vomiting, diarrhea, and inadequate fluid intake. Prerenal azotemia occurs in dogs with hypoadrenocorticism secondary to reduced renal perfusion and an associated decrease in the glomerular filtration rate. Increases in BUN are also attributed to gastrointestinal hemorrhage, which is common in Addison's disease. Gastrointestinal bleeding enhances ammonia production in the large bowel; the ammonia is absorbed into the portal system and converted to urea in the liver. The BUN in hypoadrenal dogs is highly variable, with values in excess of 200 mg/dl possible.

TABLE 8-11 DIFFERENTIAL DIAGNOSIS OF SIGNIFICANT HYPERKALEMIA AND/OR HYPONATREMIA IN DOGS AND CATS*

I. Hypoadrenocorticism
II. Renal and urinary tract disease
  A. Primary acute renal failure
  B. Chronic severe oliguric or anuric renal failure
  C. Urethral obstruction longer than 24 hours duration
  D. Osmotic or diuretic-induced diuresis
  E. Urine leakage into the peritoneal cavity
III. Severe liver failure
  A. Cirrhosis
  B. Neoplasia
IV Severe gastrointestinal disease, including
  A. Parasitic infestation
    1. Whipworms
    2. Ascarid overload
    3. Salmonellosis
  B. Viral enteritis (parvovirus)
  C. Gastric torsion
  D. Duodenal perforation
V. Severe metabolic or respiratory acidosis, including
  A. Diabetic ketoacidosis
  B. Pancreatitis
VI. Pleural effusion
  A. Specifically chylous effusion?
  B. Associated with repeated drainage?
VII. Congestive heart failure (hyponatremia)
  A. Advanced
  B. Acute
VIII. Massive tissue destruction
  A. Crush injury
  B. Extensive infection
  C. Hemolysis
IX. Primary polydipsia
X. Artifact
  A. Hyperkalemia
    1. Blood storage and hemolysis (especially from Akitas)
    2. Extreme leukocytosis or thrombocytosis
    3. Severe hypernatremia
  B. Hyponatremia
    1. Lipemia
    2. Low salt diet coupled with repeated phlebotomies

*Most of these diagnoses (other than hypoadrenocorticism) are not associated with electrolyte alterations, but such changes have been documented.

Of 483 dogs with primary hypoadrenocorticism, 435 (90%) were azotemic when first examined. Of the 23 dogs with secondary adrenocortical deficiency, 13 (57%) had an increase in BUN at the time of diagnosis (see Tables 8-8 and 8-9). With rehydration and the return of an adequate blood volume, the BUN should rapidly return to normal. Occasionally, however, rapid normalization may not occur, which suggests inadequate fluid therapy, primary renal dysfunction, or renal damage secondary to prolonged impaired renal perfusion and subsequent renal ischemia (see Table 8-8).

SERUM CREATININE. Relative to BUN concentrations, serum creatinine concentrations are less often abnormal and when abnormal are not increased to the same degree. One possible explanation for this disparity is hemorrhage into the gastrointestinal tract, which is commonly observed in Addison's disease. Gastrointestinal bleeding provides substrate for the production of ammonia, which is then absorbed into the portal circulation and converted to urea (BUN) by the liver. In such animals, BUN will be higher than predicted when evaluating the serum creatinine concentration. In the 506 dogs included in this evaluation, at the time of diagnosis, 90% were azotemic, whereas 61% had an increase in serum creatinine. In addition, the mean BUN of 81 mg/dl is approximately 300% of the reference range upper limit compared with a mean creatinine of 3.1 mg/dl, representing an increase of approximately 50% from its reference range upper limit. It is important to evaluate the BUN and the creatinine concentration in conjunction with the urinalysis.

URINALYSIS. The urine specific gravity in a dog with normal renal function and prerenal uremia secondary to dehydration and decreased cardiac output should be increased (>1.030). Urine specific gravity in a dog with primary renal failure is within or near the isosthenuric range (1.008 to 1.020). However, most dogs with hypoadrenocorticism have an impaired ability to concentrate urine because their chronic urinary sodium loss causes a reduction in the renal medullary sodium content, loss of the normal medullary concentration gradient, and impaired capacity for water resorption by the renal collecting tubules. As a result, some dogs with hypoadrenocorticism and prerenal azotemia have a urine specific gravity consistent with that expected in a dog with primary renal failure (1.008 to 1.020) (see Table 8-8). Of the 506 dogs used in this evaluation, 88% had a urine specific gravity less than 1.030 at the time of diagnosis, and 90% had concurrent azotemia. Therefore, the combination of an ill dog with an increase in BUN and isosthenuria presents a diagnostic dilemma. Ultimately, maintaining an index of suspicion regarding Addison's disease is important in order to remember that assessment of plasma cortisol concentrations is required to confirm or rule out the presence of adrenal disease, because there is similarity in "database" test results from dogs with renal versus adrenal failure.

RENAL PARAMETERS AND RESPONSE TO THERAPY. Increases in serum BUN and creatinine in a dog described by an owner as having clinical signs consistent with either hypoadrenocorticism or renal failure can be both misleading and challenging for a veterinary practitioner. Confusion may be exacerbated if the practitioner suspects hypoadrenocorticism but the BUN and creatinine fail to decline rapidly after institution of aggressive fluid therapy (within 12 to 24 hours), as has been reported to occur. There is no doubt that abnormalities in BUN tend to resolve quickly in most dogs with hypoadrenocorticism, but some dogs suffer intrinsic renal damage due to poor perfusion and hypoxia associated with the primary disease. This renal damage can be slow to resolve in some dogs. A small percentage of dogs have both hypoadrenocorticism and renal disease, which provides a second explanation for increases in the BUN and creatinine levels that fail to resolve despite aggressive fluid therapy.

Failure of a hypoadrenal dog to increase urine output after aggressive fluid therapy is rare and should be of concern. Most of these dogs are actually polyuric. Oliguria or anuria would most likely be secondary to severe dehydration, hypotension, and a critical reduction in renal perfusion. Restoration of extracellular fluid volume toward normal usually improves renal perfusion and urine output. However, in the unusual circumstance of oliguria or anuria, concomitant renal or cardiac disease may exist. In other dogs, however, diuresis may be delayed until normal blood pressure is attained and maintained with fluid therapy. The measurement of indirect venous blood pressure, direct arterial blood pressure, or central venous pressure may aid in understanding the cause for anuria or oliguria. Oliguria in conjunction with a low central venous pressure or hypotension suggests inadequate fluid therapy and continued poor renal perfusion. However, oliguria/anuria in conjunction with an increased central venous pressure or hypertension suggests overzealous fluid administration. In these animals, primary renal or cardiac dysfunction should be suspected.

Serum Glucose (Hypoglycemia)

PATHOPHYSIOLOGY. Glucocorticoids increase hepatic glycogen and glucose production (gluconeogenesis) while decreasing glucose uptake and utilization in peripheral tissues (Tyrrell et al, 1991). In glucocorticoid deficiency, glucose production by the liver is decreased and peripheral cell receptor sensitivity to insulin is increased. Together, these factors predispose the hypoadrenal animal to hypoglycemia. In human Addison's disease, hypoglycemia is more common in children than in adults and is more common in association with fasting, fever, infection, nausea, and/or vomiting (Tyrrell et al, 1991). A relative decrease in insulin secretion due to low blood sugar and resumption of eating helps to blunt hypoglycemia.

INCIDENCE. Of 483 dogs with primary hypoadrenocorticism, 106 (22%) were hypoglycemic at the time Addison's disease was diagnosed (blood glucose <70 mg/dl). Ten of 23 dogs (43%) with secondary disease were hypoglycemic (see Tables 8-8 and 8-9). Hypoglycemic convulsions were much less common; they were observed by owners or veterinarians in only 14 of 506 dogs. Sixteen dogs had other clinical signs (e.g., ataxia, disorientation) that may have been caused by hypoglycemia. Forty dogs had blood glucose levels in excess of 200 mg/dl at the time of diagnosis due to concurrent diabetes mellitus.

DIFFERENTIAL DIAGNOSIS. Hypoglycemia always represents a diagnostic challenge. When documented, the differential diagnosis for hypoglycemia is relatively short (Table 8-12; also see Chapter 14). In an adult dog, the disorders that can result in low blood glucose include sepsis, hepatopathy, insulin-secreting tumor, nonendocrine tumor (e.g., hepatic tumor, leiomyoma, leiomyosarcoma), hypoadrenocorticism, and insulin overdose.* The blood glucose concentration should always be measured in a dog known to have or suspected of having adrenal hypofunction. A 2.5% to 5% dextrose infusion, typically made by adding adequate amounts of 50% dextrose to Ringer's or normal

TABLE 8-12 CLASSIFICATION OF FASTING HYPOGLYCEMIA

I. Endocrine
  A. Excess insulin or insulin-like factors
    1. Insulin-producing islet cell tumors
    2. Extrapancreatic tumors producing and secreting insulin-like substances
    3. Iatrogenic-insulin overdose
  B. Growth hormone deficiency
    1. Hypopituitarism affecting several tropic hormones (e.g., ACTH, GH)
    2. Monotropic growth hormone deficiency
  C. Cortisol deficiency
    1. Hypoadrenocorticism
    2. Hypopituitarism
    3. Isolated ACTH deficiency
II. Hepatic
  A. Congenital
    1. Vascular shunts
    2. Glycogen storage diseases
  B. Acquired
    1. Vascular shunts
    2. Chronic fibrosis (cirrhosis)
    3. Hepatic necrosis: toxins, infectious agents
    4. Infiltrative diseases: neoplasia
III. Substrate
  A. Extrapancreatic tumors that use large quantities of glucose
  B. Puppy hypoglycemia
  C. Infection
    1. Significant sepsis
    2. Significant leukocytosis
  D. Uremia
  E. Gastrointestinal
    1. Starvation due to parasites, malabsorption, etc.
    2. Maldigestion
  F. Severe polycythemia
IV. Miscellaneous
  A. Artifact: sample held on erythrocytes
  B. Severe renal glycosuria
  C. Drugs: salicylates, ethanol, sulfonylurea

saline solution, should be administered as soon as hypoglycemia is documented. Hypoglycemia typically resolves within 24 to 48 hours of initiation of glucocorticoid treatment.

Serum Calcium (Hypercalcemia)

PATHOPHYSIOLOGY. A clear physiologic explanation for the hypercalcemia occasionally noted in dogs with Addison's disease is not available. There seems to be a strong but not complete correlation between hyperkalemia and hypercalcemia in dogs with naturally occurring disease, in those that have undergone adrenalectomy, and in those overdosed with o,p'-DDD. Thus there is a correlation between severity of disease, dehydration, hyperkalemia, and the presence of hypercalcemia. Possible mechanisms for hypercalcemia include hemoconcentration of calcium-binding proteins,

*Bennish et al, 1990; Walters and Drobatz, 1992; Levy, 1994; Beaudry et al, 1995; Thompson et al, 1995; Bagley et al, 1996.

increased avidity of binding proteins, diminished renal clearance, and increased mobilization of calcium through osteocyte activation (Montoll et al, 1992; Peterson et al, 1996).

Hypercalcemia decreases rapidly after administration of glucocorticoids, which suggests a possible relationship between hypercalcemia and glucocorticoid deficiency. Corticosteroids in large doses have been noted to decrease intestinal absorption of calcium by antagonizing the effects of vitamin D. Lack of cortisol, therefore, may cause increased intestinal absorption of calcium, resulting in hypercalcemia. However, studies of adrenalectomized dogs fed calcium-rich or calcium-free diets showed little difference in the degree of hypercalcemia (Feldman and Nelson, 1987).

Excess parathyroid gland activity is an unlikely etiology for hypercalcemia because parathyroidectomy does not prevent hypercalcemia in adrenalectomized dogs. Hyperproteinemia resulting from dehydration and hemoconcentration also appears to be an unlikely cause. Studies in animals have demonstrated an increase in both free ionic calcium and nonionic calcium bound to protein. In addition, there has been no correlation between the total serum calcium concentration and the total protein or albumin concentration in hypoadrenal dogs (Peterson and Feinman, 1982).

Diminished renal excretion of calcium may be the most likely contributor to the hypercalcemia of adrenal insufficiency. In adrenalectomized dogs, renal tubular resorption of calcium is excessive, as is shown by consistently depressed urinary excretion of calcium despite hypercalcemia. Humans with hypoadrenocorticism do not excrete normal amounts of calcium via the kidneys, and they have increased renal tubular resorption (Tyrrell et al, 1991). Finally, cortisone administration lowers the serum calcium concentration by increasing urinary calcium excretion.

DIFFERENTIAL DIAGNOSIS. It is important to recognize the relationship between hypercalcemia and adrenocortical insufficiency, because many clinical signs (vomiting, weight loss, anorexia, dehydration, polydipsia, and polyuria) are identical to those associated with other causes of hypercalcemia, including hypercalcemia of malignancy, primary hyperparathyroidism, and renal disease (Table 8-13). Adrenocortical failure should always be included in the differential diagnosis of hypercalcemia, especially if other electrolyte disturbances consistent with adrenocortical insufficiency are present.

INCIDENCE. Of 483 dogs with primary hypoadrenocorticism, 142 (29%) were hypercalcemic at the time of initial examination and diagnosis (see Table 8-8). Hypercalcemia develops most frequently in extremely ill hypoadrenal dogs, and the severity of hypercalcemia is usually but not always proportional to the severity of dehydration or serum electrolyte abnormalities. In a study of 40 dogs with hypercalcemia, Addison's disease was the second most common cause and accounted for 25% of the cases (Elliott et al, 1991; Herrtage, 1998). In our series of dogs with hypercalcemia, it occurs less commonly than in dogs with lymphosarcoma, chronic

TABLE 8-13 DIFFERENTIAL DIAGNOSIS OF HYPERCALCEMIA

Young growing animals
Primary renal failure
Lymphosarcoma
Apocrine gland (anal sac) tumors
Some malignancies that have metastasized to bone
  Mammary tumors
  Multiple myeloma
Primary hyperparathyroidism
  Adenoma
  Carcinoma
Variety of carcinomas (rare)
  Thyroid
  Vaginal
  Lung
  Liver
Hypoadrenocorticism
Hypervitaminosis D (iatrogenic)
Lipemia

renal failure, and primary hyperparathyroidism, but it remains common.

Acid-Base Status

PATHOPHYSIOLOGY. Hypoaldosteronism impairs renal tubular hydrogen ion secretion (Nelson, 1980). This impairment, in conjunction with hypotension and poor perfusion of tissues, most likely accounts for the mild acidosis documented in many dogs suffering from a hypoadrenal crisis. Evaluations of arterial blood gases and venous total carbon dioxide concentrations are adequate methods of determining acid-base status. The acidosis documented in hypoadrenocorticism rarely requires specific treatment. Adequate fluid and mineralocorticoid replacement therapy should restore renal perfusion, which in turn enhances urinary hydrogen ion excretion. Typically, this negates the need for parenteral administration of bicarbonate.

INCIDENCE. Mild to moderate metabolic acidosis is a frequent complication in ill hypoadrenal dogs. Slightly fewer than 50% of 506 hypoadrenal dogs had serum bicarbonate concentrations less than 17 mEq/L (see Table 8-8). Most dogs had relatively mild acidosis, with serum bicarbonate concentrations of 13 to 17 mEq/L. Fewer than 10% had severe metabolic acidosis (serum bicarbonate concentrations of 9 to 12 mEq/L), which required bicarbonate therapy.

TREATMENT. If the acid-base status cannot be assessed in a dog with adrenocortical insufficiency, bicarbonate therapy is not recommended. If the serum bicarbonate concentration is determined to be equal to or less than 12 mEq/L, one quarter of the calculated bicarbonate deficit should be added to the intravenous fluids and administered over a 6-hour period. The serum bicarbonate concentration should then be reevaluated; if it is still equal to or less than 12 mEq/L, the bicarbonate dose should be recalculated and, again, one quarter administered over a 6-hour period. This is the treatment protocol we use to manage diabetic ketoacidosis, and it has proved effective in the management of the acidosis of adrenocortical insufficiency as well. (Bicarbonate dosage formulas are provided in detail in Chapter 13).

Blood Pressure

Approximately 90% of humans with untreated hypoadrenocorticism are hypotensive. Hypotension may cause orthostatic symptoms or syncope or both. In severe chronic disease and in acute crisis, recumbent hypotension or shock is almost invariably present (Tyrrell et al, 1991). The veterinary profession is on the threshold of routinely measuring blood pressure in dogs and cats. The major limitation for decades has been the lack of inexpensive, reliable, easily applied equipment suitable for cats and dogs (especially considering their significant variation in size). There is little doubt that the ill hypoadrenal dog or cat is commonly hypotensive and that hypotension in a "crisis" can be life-threatening. We have documented hypotension in addisonian dogs that are severely ill when brought to our hospital, as well as in some dogs after maintenance treatment has been initiated. Hypotension is invariably associated with inadequate mineralocorticoid replacement and, occasionally, with inadequate glucocorticoid therapy.

Liver Function: Albumin, Cholesterol, BUN, and Glucose

GENERAL. Some dogs with severe kidney or gastrointestinal disease are recognized to have a history, physical examination findings, and/or clinical pathologic abnormalities similar to those of hypoadrenocorticism, and vice versa (Table 8-14). It is this potential confusion, together with the realization that kidney and gastrointestinal diseases are relatively common compared with hypoadrenocorticism, that makes confirmation of the latter diagnosis in a dog particularly exciting. Confusion may also arise in the case of dogs with hypoadrenocorticism that have abnormalities in clinical pathology or radiographic or ultrasonographic evaluations that are suggestive of a hepatopathy.

LIVER FUNCTION TEST RESULTS

Criteria. Not including serum liver enzyme activities, most veterinarians use five criteria to aid the identification of dogs that may be suffering from a significant hepatopathy. The five criteria are hypoalbuminemia (<2.8 g/dl), hypocholesterolemia (<140 mg/dl), hypoglycemia (<70 mg/dl), low BUN (<13 mg/dl), and microhepatia, as subjectively determined by abdominal radiography or ultrasonography.

Results. A review of the records of the 205 hypoadrenal dogs in our series showed that 44 (21%) were identified as having two or more of the previously described five abnormalities considered suggestive of a liver problem (see Table 8-14). Thirty-six dogs had hypoalbuminemia (mean, 2.1 mg/dl; range, 1.4 to 2.5 mg/dl); 35 had hypocholesterolemia (mean, 111 mg/dl; range, 72 to 125 mg/dl); nine had hypoglycemia (mean, 28 mg/dl; range, 11 to 44 mg/dl), seven had decreased BUN (mean, 10 mg/dl; range, 7 to 12 mg/dl), and 37 had microhepatia. Many of these dogs also had increased serum liver enzyme activities (alanine aminotransferase [ALT] or serum alkaline phosphatase [SAP] or both). Four dogs had abnormal preprandial and postprandial bile acid concentrations, and four dogs had abnormal ammonia tolerance test results. Nine dogs underwent liver biopsy, with nonspecific (lymphocytic/plasmacytic) hepatitis diagnosed in six and fibrosis in three. Similar problems (microhepatia and/or low serum albumin concentrations) have been alluded to by other authors (van den Broek, 1992; Levy, 1994; Hardy, 1995; Langlais-Burgess et al, 1995).

Interpretation. Hypoglycemia, as previously discussed, is considered a potential abnormality in any hypocortisolemic dog because lack of glucocorticoids decreases mobilization of glucose from the liver. Similarly, abnormal liver enzyme activities are considered potential sequela to any chronic hypovolemic or hypotensive condition that would cause tissue hypoxia. The other four abnormalities (albumin, cholesterol, BUN, and liver size) are not as easily explained in dogs with hypoadrenocorticism. The hypoalbuminemia could be caused by gastrointestinal blood loss, protein-losing enteropathy, malassimilation, or hepatopathy.

The combination of liver and adrenocortical problems may be explained by concurrent immune-mediated attack directed at both organs. Autoimmune Addison's disease in humans is frequently accompanied by other immune disorders (e.g., polyglandular autoimmune [PGA] syndrome, see page 396), including chronic hepatitis (Bethune, 1989). The nonspecific hepatitis identified in several of our dogs with hypoadrenocorticism may support this concept, and the fibrosis noted in three dogs could be the end result of chronic hepatitis. Alternatively, the liver may be

TABLE 8-14 OVERLAPPING CLINICAL AND IN-HOSPITAL INFORMATION: HYPOADRENOCORTICISM VERSUS OTHER DISEASES

I. Renal disease
  A. Weight loss, poor appetite, vomiting, diarrhea
  B. Increased BUN, creatinine, acidosis; low albumin
  C. Urine specific gravity 1.008–1.020, when ill
  D. Responsive to IV fluids
II. Gastrointestinal disease
  A. Weight loss, poor appetite, vomiting, diarrhea
  B. Decreased serum albumin
  C. Abnormal serum biochemistries correct with IV fluids
  D. Abnormal biopsies may be obtained
III. Hepatic disease
  A. Weight loss, poor appetite, vomiting, diarrhea
  B. Decreased albumin, cholesterol, glucose ± BUN
  C. Microhepatia: radiography or ultrasonography
  D. Abnormal liver enzyme activity ± liver function test results
  E. Ascites (seldom)
  F. Abnormal liver biopsy results

secondarily affected by chronic, subclinical adrenal insufficiency with its associated hypotension, impaired tissue perfusion, and/or glucocorticoid/mineralocorticoid insufficiency. In some dogs, liver insufficiency may be an independent problem. Regardless of the cause, it is important for clinicians to recognize the relationship between adrenal insufficiency and apparent hepatopathy in some dogs.

Of 36 dogs with glucocorticoid-deficient hypoadrenocorticism (18 of our 205 dogs plus 18 in a recent report), 24 had abnormally decreased serum cholesterol concentrations (Lifton et al, 1996). It was suggested that without glucocorticoid mediation, decreased fat absorption may contribute to this abnormality. Also, ACTH is known to increase free cholesterol by increasing cholesterol esterase activity while decreasing cholesteryl synthetase (Tyrrell et al, 1991). With low concentrations of ACTH typical of secondary hypoadrenocorticism, hypocholesterolemia may result. In these 36 dogs, 21 also had a decrease in serum albumin, 11 had hypoglycemia, and 15 had a decrease in serum total protein. Only five had a decrease in BUN.

Management. The dogs in our series with apparent hepatic abnormalities were treated only for hypoadrenocorticism. No specific treatment was directed at the hepatopathy. On reevaluation of each dog, all parameters related both to the Addison's disease and to the hepatopathy had improved. Because initial treatment invariably included glucocorticoid supplementation, it can only be presumed that this drug helped in the treatment of both conditions. The results of long-term follow-up assessment of the dogs with both conditions were no different from those observed in dogs that had no evidence of hepatic disease.

RADIOGRAPHY

Microcardia

Hypoadrenal dogs with severe hypovolemia often have microcardia, a flattened and decreased diameter of the descending aorta, and a narrow posterior vena cava, as seen in lateral radiographs of the thorax (Fig. 8-6). Similar radiographic appearances may be seen in some dogs with more insidious signs, such as depression, lethargy, and weakness. These findings support the tentative diagnosis of adrenal insufficiency and are observed in approximately 25% to 35% of afflicted dogs (Peterson et al, 1996). However, it should be remembered that microcardia is simply a general sign of hypovolemia or shock. Also, caution is needed in interpreting lateral thoracic radiographs of dogs with a deep thorax, such as the Irish Wolfhound or Borzoi. In these breeds, the heart is frequently not long enough to contact the sternum.

Megaesophagus

One study of 225 dogs with hypoadrenocorticism reported one dog with megaesophagus (Peterson et al, 1996), whereas seven of our 205 hypoadrenal dogs had radiographic and fluoroscopic evidence of aperistaltic esophageal dilation. Why some dogs with Addison's disease develop esophageal dilation is not clear. It has been proposed that the condition might be attributable to the effect of abnormal serum sodium and potassium concentrations on membrane potential and neuromuscular function (Burrows, 1987). In each of our dogs with hypoadrenocorticism, megaesophagus resolved with treatment for the hypoadrenocorticism. However, in 2 dogs with both hypoadrenocorticism and megaesophagus, abnormal serum electrolyte concentrations were never documented (Bartges and Nielson, 1992; Whitley, 1995). In a study of dogs with secondary hypoadrenocorticism, four of 11 that had thoracic radiographs taken were diagnosed with megaesophagus (Lifton et al, 1996), whereas none of our 18 dogs with secondary disease were so diagnosed. Cortisol deficiency and its associated muscle weakness was suggested as a cause of megaesophagus because the condition resolved with glucocorticoid therapy.

ELECTROCARDIOGRAPHY

Physiology of Hyperkalemia and the Heart

With modest hyperkalemia (potassium concentrations of 5.7 to 6.5 mEq/L), a transient and minor acceleration of cardiac conduction can be demonstrated. However, as the serum potassium (K^+) concentration rises above this level, depression of conduction occurs. Examination of the electrocardiogram (ECG) occasionally reveals "peaking" of T waves during modest elevations in the serum potassium concentration. Also, as the serum K^+ concentration rises (6.5 to 7.5 mEq/L), the P-R interval lengthens. The P wave ultimately disappears when the concentration exceeds 7.5 to 8.0 mEq/L. At these serum potassium concentrations, the QRS complex widens and R-R intervals become irregular. "Sinoventricular" conduction may be observed at this stage.

Sequential changes in myocardial electrical conduction with serum potassium concentrations above 7.5 to 8.0 mEq/L include atrioventricular junctional delay, followed by acceleration of junctional pacemakers, conduction delays in the His-Purkinje system, and delays in ventricular muscle contraction. As potassium concentrations continue to increase, asystole and cardiac arrest ensue. His bundle and bundle branch recordings indicate that asystole typically results from a block in the distal conducting system. The resultant peripheral ECG shows regular or irregular rhythm with widened QRS complexes. Although the morphology of the QRS complex may suggest that the arrhythmias are of ventricular origin, these rhythms have been shown to be junctional or sinus rhythms. Because hyperkalemia is seldom seen as an isolated finding, it must be remembered that other electrolyte disturbances, especially in sodium and calcium concentrations, modify pure potassium-mediated alterations.

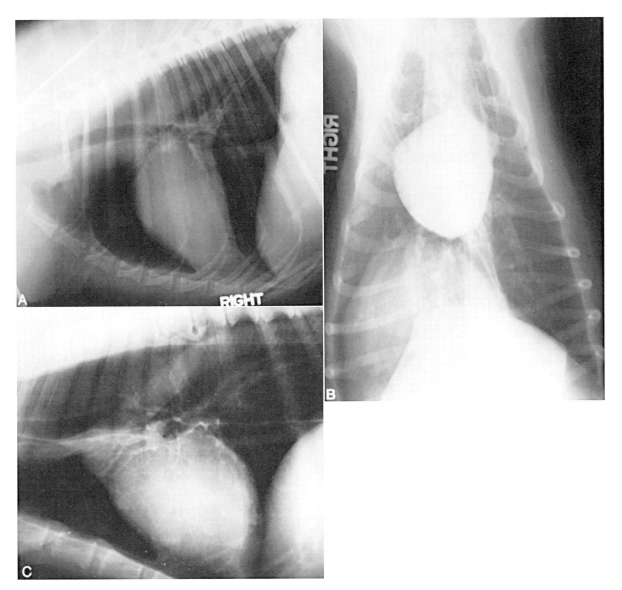

FIGURE 8-6. *A,* Radiographs of a 3-year-old Rhodesian Ridgeback that was brought to the hospital in a shocklike state secondary to hypoadrenocorticism. Note the small heart on both views and the poor pulmonary vascular pattern caused by poor cardiac output. This dog also has a somewhat flattened thoracic aorta, also caused by hypovolemia and poor cardiac output. *B,* Lateral thoracic view of a 5-year-old hypoadrenal dog with microcardia, a flattened caudal vena cava, and a dilated, air-filled esophagus. The esophageal dilation, seen occasionally in hypoadrenocorticism, may reflect the muscle weakness seen with severe hyperkalemia and is reversible with appropriate hormonal therapy for the primary disease.

Use of the Electrocardiogram

BACKGROUND. Hyperkalemia usually causes recognizable changes in an ECG (Fig. 8-7). The most prominent manifestations of hyperkalemia are seen on the ECG, which can be a vital aid for estimating the severity of hyperkalemia. However, veterinarians must always keep in mind that hypoadrenocorticism is only one of several potential causes of hyperkalemia. Once hyperkalemia has been diagnosed, however, potentially lifesaving measures can be initiated. No in-hospital screening test is as simple and rapid as an ECG, and none is as easily used for monitoring a patient during treatment.

Early diagnosis of hyperkalemia, accomplished in many cases with the ECG, allows rapid institution of therapy without waiting for the laboratory report on serum electrolyte concentrations. Regardless of its cause, marked hyperkalemia is an emergency situation that demands a quick therapeutic response. In addition to providing a tool for early recognition of hyperkalemia, the ECG also allows the clinician to easily, reliably, and inexpensively monitor therapy. As the hyperkalemia is treated, the various abnormalities present on an ECG resolve.

MILD HYPERKALEMIA (SERUM [K⁺]: 5.6 TO 6.5 MEQ/L). The earliest visible ECG alterations are slowing of the heart rate and peaking of the T wave, which occur

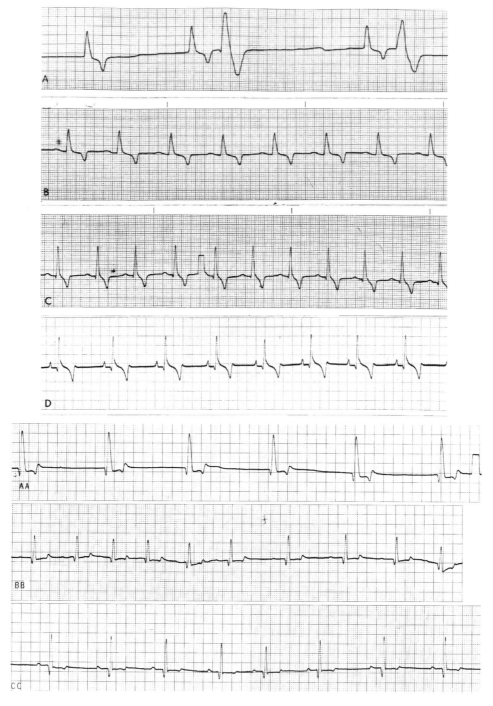

FIGURE 8-7. Serial ECG segments obtained from two dogs with hypoadrenocorticism and hyperkalemia. *A* and *AA* both illustrate the effect of severe hyperkalemia, with the former dog having a serum potassium concentration of 8.6 mEq/L and the latter a measurement of 9.4 mEq/L. Note the lack of visible P waves, the short and wide QRS complexes, and the T waves, which are not of excessive amplitude. The ECG in A also reveals a bizarre-looking QRS complex following a more normal-appearing QRS complex. This bizarre wave represents a ventricular escape beat that could be the result of hypoxia or hyperkalemia or both. *B* and *BB* are ECGs from the same dogs as in *A* and *AA*, respectively. They were each obtained approximately 1 hour after institution of intravenous normal saline administration as the only treatment. The serum potassium concentrations had decreased to 7.6 mEq/L and 7.9 mEq/L, respectively. Two important factors to note: (1) improvement is seen in each case, with the return of P waves, a more rapid heart rate, and disappearance of ventricular escape beats; and (2) abnormalities are still present, most obviously the prolonged P-R intervals (first-degree heart block), which alone suggest hyperkalemia, especially when associated with a widened QRS complex and a short Q-T interval. There are numerous other causes of P-R interval prolongation. In *C* and *CC*, the serum potassium concentrations are considerably lower, 6.2 mEq/L and 5.9 mEq/L, respectively. The P-R interval and P, QRS, and T waves are of shorter duration, and the R waves are taller. *D*, ECG from the dog in *A;* the serum potassium concentration is 5.6 mEq/L and a more spiked T wave is seen. (From Feldman EC: *In* Ettinger SJ [ed]: Textbook of Veterinary Internal Medicine, 2nd ed. Philadelphia, WB Saunders, 1983, p 1664.)

when the serum potassium concentration exceeds 5.5 mEq/L. These changes are not easily observed because of their subtle nature but when noted are frequently associated with shortening of the Q-T interval. The characteristic tall and narrow T waves occur before the ECG shows any measurable alteration of the QRS complex. Slowing of the heart rate and T-wave changes are *not* seen in all cases of mild hyperkalemia. The T-wave changes have been observed in 15% of our dogs with hyperkalemia, and bradycardia (heart rate <80 beats per minute) has been documented in 33% of our hyperkalemic dogs. As the serum potassium concentration rises above 7.0 mEq/L, the T wave may lose its classic "peaked" shape, if present, because abnormalities that take place secondary to intraventricular conduction disturbances obscure the primary T-wave changes. Bradycardia, if present, may resolve as the serum potassium concentration increases above 7.0 to 7.5 mEq/L because hypoxia may begin to increase the rate.

MODERATE HYPERKALEMIA (SERUM [K+]: 6.6 TO 7.5 MEQ/L). Slowed intraventricular impulse conduction is responsible for the QRS complex alterations that occur as the serum potassium concentration exceeds 6.5 mEq/L. At this juncture, T-wave abnormalities and the uniformly widened QRS complex could lead to a presumptive diagnosis of hyperkalemia. Widened QRS complexes and decreased R-wave amplitudes have been observed in 32% and 47% of our cases, respectively. With increasing serum potassium concentrations, the QRS duration increases progressively. Thus a rough correlation can be made between the duration of the QRS complex and the severity of the hyperkalemia.

MODERATE TO SEVERE HYPERKALEMIA (SERUM [K+]: 7.0 TO >8.5 MEQ/L). As the serum potassium concentration increases above 7.0 mEq/L, the P-wave amplitude decreases and its duration becomes prolonged secondary to slowed impulse conduction through the atria. The P-R interval also increases in duration as a result of slower atrioventricular transmission. When serum potassium concentrations exceed 8.5 mEq/L, the P wave frequently becomes invisible. This is the *classic* abnormality cited as easily recognized and presumptive for hyperkalemia. Prolongation of the P-R interval has been observed in 45% of our cases, and absent P waves have been observed in an additional 47% (total of 92%) of our dogs with hypoadrenocorticism. When P waves are absent, an erroneous diagnosis of atrial fibrillation may be made, particularly when the ventricular rate is irregular.

SEVERE HYPERKALEMIA (SERUM [K+]: >8.5 MEQ/L). Continued increases in the serum potassium concentration can be associated with deviation of the S-T segment from baseline. When potassium concentrations reach 11 to 14 mEq/L, the electrocardiographer may see ventricular asystole or ventricular fibrillation. These ECG alterations have only rarely been observed in our dogs with hypoadrenocorticism, perhaps because the highest serum potassium concentration in our series was 10.8 mEq/L (see Table 8-8).

HORMONE STUDIES: CONFIRMING THE DIAGNOSIS

Plasma Cortisol Concentrations

BASAL PLASMA CORTISOL CONCENTRATIONS. Cortisol concentrations in plasma and urine are generally decreased in hypoadrenocorticism. Because partial degrees of adrenal insufficiency occur and because most reference ranges for the basal cortisol concentration are as low as the detection limits of assays commonly used to measure cortisol, basal concentrations of plasma cortisol should not be used to diagnose this disease. Tests that measure adrenocortical reserve (plasma cortisol assayed from blood samples collected before *and after* ACTH administration; that is, ACTH stimulation tests) are necessary to establish the diagnosis.

URINARY STEROIDS. Determination of 24-hour urinary excretion of 17-hydroxycorticosteroids is an accurate means of confirming a diagnosis of hypoadrenocorticism, but obtaining the necessary 24-hour urine samples from housebroken pets in metabolism cages can be awkward, if not impossible, for veterinarians. In addition, these determinations do not assess adrenocortical reserve. The same problem is encountered with random urine cortisol:creatinine ratios; that is, the results may be low, but this is not a test of adrenocortical reserve. Random urine cortisol:creatinine ratios are not considered reliable for confirming a diagnosis of hypoadrenocorticism. The ACTH stimulation test is considered the only reliable method of confirming a diagnosis of hypoadrenocorticism (Addison's disease).

ACTH STIMULATION TESTING: THE "GOLD STANDARD"

Protocol. Measurement of the plasma cortisol concentration before and after stimulation of the adrenal cortices with exogenous ACTH has been used commonly, is reliable, and is considered the "gold standard" for the diagnosis of hypoadrenocorticism in humans, dogs, and cats suspected of having Addison's disease. The ACTH stimulation test is equally practical for out-patient and in-patient use because it requires little time (1 or 2 hours) and only two venipunctures.

The procedure for a stimulation study includes use of either synthetic ACTH (Cortrosyn; Amphastar Pharm., Rancho Cucamonga, CA) or natural ACTH (porcine extract: Cortigel 40; Savage Laboratories, Melville, NY). In dogs, blood should be obtained before and 1 hour after administration of synthetic ACTH (0.25 mg IM or IV, regardless of weight) or before and 2 hours after administration of ACTH gel (2.2 IU/kg IM). Various studies have demonstrated that the dose of 0.25 mg of synthetic ACTH is an excess; however, that dose represents one vial and, given intramuscularly, it remains our recommended dose. In cats, blood samples are collected before, 30, and 60 minutes after administration of synthetic ACTH (0.125 mg IM or IV, regardless of weight) or before, 60, and 120 minutes after administration of ACTH gel (2.2 IU/kg IM).

Test results using either source of ACTH (synthetic or natural) can be interpreted interchangeably (Table

TABLE 8-15 ACTH (CORTICOTROPIN) STIMULATION TEST PROTOCOLS FOR ASSESSING ADRENOCORTICAL GLUCOCORTICOID RESERVE*

ACTH Preparation	Dose	Route of Administration	Preinjection Cortisol	Timing of Postinjection Cortisol
Synthetic ACTH (Cortrosyn[†])	0.25 mg (dog)	IM	Yes	1 hr
Synthetic ACTH (Cortrosyn[†])	0.125 mg (cat)	IM or IV	Yes	30 + 60 min
Procine ACTH (Cortigel-40[‡])	2.2 IU/kg (1 IU/lb) (dog)	IM	Yes	2 hr
Procine ACTH (Cortigel-40[‡])	2.2 IU/kg (cat)	IM	Yes	1 and 2 hr

*Test should begin whenever a dog or cat is in "crisis," regardless of the time of day.
[†]Cortrosyn (cosyntropin), Organon Pharmaceuticals, West Orange, NJ 07052.
[‡]Cortigel-40 (repositol corticotropin injection, USP), Savage Laboratories, Melville, NY 11747.

8-15) (Feldman et al, 1982). Stimulation studies are reliable at any time of the day. The venous blood for cortisol determination should be placed in heparinized tubes and centrifuged, and the plasma should then be frozen until it is assayed. If a dog or cat is suspected to be in a hypoadrenal crisis, the test should be performed upon admission to the hospital, regardless of the time of day. Practitioners are urged to follow the instructions provided by their laboratory concerning the amount of serum or plasma needed and its handling. Cortisol degradation is minimal in serum or plasma stored at room temperature for up to 5 days; however, beyond this time, degradation may be significant (Olson et al, 1981). Cortisol concentrations in canine plasma can be determined with a variety of commercially available assays. Radioimmunoassays (RIAs) are the most commonly used assays in North America. Each laboratory should establish its own reference ranges. In-hospital enzyme-linked immunosorbent assay (ELISA) test systems are not yet recommended in the diagnosis of Addison's disease.

Results. One criterion is used in confirming the diagnosis of adrenocortical insufficiency: an abnormally decreased post-ACTH plasma cortisol concentration revealed by an appropriate, reliable stimulation protocol (see Table 8-15). A normal plasma cortisol concentration after ACTH administration is proof that adrenal insufficiency is not present. An abnormally inadequate response to this provocative test (post-ACTH plasma cortisol concentration <2.0 µg/dl) confirms the diagnosis (Table 8-16).

Between January 1988 and January 2002, we diagnosed naturally occurring hypoadrenocorticism in 205 dogs (18 of these 205 dogs had pituitary failure to secrete ACTH and secondary failure to secrete cortisol). The years beginning with 1988 are used because the plasma cortisol concentrations from these dogs were assayed using one RIA (normal pre-ACTH cortisol level, 0.5 to 5.5 µg/dl; normal post-ACTH cortisol level, 5.0 to 17.0 µg/dl).

If the 220 dogs with *primary* hypoadrenocorticism from the study by Peterson and colleagues (1996) are added to our 187 dogs with naturally occurring primary hypoadrenocorticism, every one of the 407 dogs had pre-ACTH and post-ACTH plasma cortisol concentrations equal to or less than 2.0 µg/dl. More than 75% of these dogs had post-ACTH plasma cortisol concentrations less than 1.0 µg/dl (see Table 8-16; also Fig. 8-8). Because the normal or reference value for the post-ACTH plasma cortisol concentration is approximately 5.0 to 17.0 µg/dl, it is obvious that none of the 407 dogs diagnosed as Addisonian had a value between 2.1 and 5.0 µg/dl. Test results in this range must be viewed as suspicious for *not* being diagnostic of hypoadrenocorticism. Furthermore, of the 407 dogs with primary adrenal insufficiency, approximately 75% had post-ACTH plasma cortisol concentrations that were equal to or less than the basal value. Those that did demonstrate a rise in the plasma cortisol concentration after ACTH administration had an extremely blunted response (see Table 8-16).

Of the five dogs with *secondary* adrenal insufficiency reported by Peterson and colleagues (1996) and the 18

TABLE 8-16 PLASMA CORTISOL CONCENTRATIONS BEFORE AND AFTER SYNTHETIC EXOGENOUS ACTH STIMULATION AND ENDOGENOUS PLASMA ACTH CONCENTRATIONS IN DOGS* WITH NATURALLY OCCURRING ADRENOCORTICAL INSUFFICIENCY

		PLASMA CORTISOL CONCENTRATIONS (µg/dl)		PLASMA ACTH CONCENTRATIONS (pg/ml)	
	Number of Dogs	Before Stimulation	After 60 Minutes	Before Treatment	After Treatment
Group I	407				
Mean values		0.9	1.0	1134	105
Ranges		0.1–2.0	0.1–2.0	≥1000 (52%)	<3–240
				253–3740	
Group II	23				
Mean values		0.9	1.1	12.7	
Ranges		0.1–2.0	0.1–3.1	<3–53	
Normal range		0.5–5.5	5.0–17.0	10–80	
Normal mean		2.2	9.6	38	

*Dogs include 205 from the continuing series at the University of California plus 220 from the report by Peterson et al (1996).
Group I, Dogs with primary adrenocortical disease; Group II, dogs with pituitary disease.

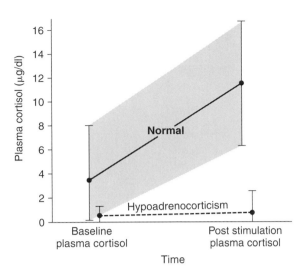

FIGURE 8-8. Radioimmunoassay plasma cortisol concentrations before and after exogenous ACTH stimulation from normal dogs and those with hypoadrenocorticism. The ranges are means ± 2 SD.

in our series, the basal plasma cortisol concentration in all 23 dogs was equal to or less than 2.0 µg/dl. The highest post-ACTH plasma cortisol concentration in these 23 dogs was only 3.1 µg/dl, slightly higher than the dogs with primary adrenocortical disease. However, 21 of the 23 dogs had post-ACTH plasma cortisol concentrations equal to or less than 2.0 µg/dl. Therefore, of 430 dogs with primary or secondary adrenocortical insufficiency, 428 had both pre-ACTH and post-ACTH plasma cortisol concentrations equal to or less than 2.0 µg/dl. Although individual data were not reported in a publication on 18 dogs with secondary disease, the mean post-ACTH plasma cortisol concentration was less than 2.0 µg/dl, and the highest value was 4.4 µg/dl (Lifton et al, 1996).

Limitations. The results of ACTH stimulation testing do not distinguish between dogs with naturally occurring *primary* adrenocortical disease and those with *secondary* insufficiency due to pituitary failure, secondary insufficiency due to chronic iatrogenic corticosteroid administration, or dogs with primary adrenocortical destruction caused by o,p'-DDD overdose (Fig. 8-9). Primary adrenocortical disease implies cellular destruction of the adrenal cortex leading to abnormal test results.

Secondary adrenal insufficiency severe enough to cause clinical signs is associated with significant atrophy of the adrenal cortex due to chronic ACTH deficiency caused by disease (e.g., autoimmune destruction, trauma, or tumor) in the pituitary or secondary to chronic glucocorticoid administration (see Fig. 8-9). Regardless of the cause, the atrophied cells do not have the capacity to respond to one injection of ACTH. However, these adrenocortical cells eventually should respond to repeated injections or to a chronic infusion of ACTH (Lamb et al, 1994). Chronic infusion of ACTH would not enhance cortisol secretion in dogs with primary causes of destruction of the adrenal cortices.

Serum or Plasma Aldosterone Concentrations

BACKGROUND. Measurement of the plasma cortisol concentration (before and after ACTH administration) as a diagnostic aid for confirming the diagnosis of hypoadrenocorticism has been used to indirectly assess function of the entire adrenal cortex. However, the plasma cortisol concentration may not always reflect the concentration of aldosterone in the circulation. Theoretically, direct measurement of aldosterone might provide information about primary disease (a reduction in both aldosterone and cortisol levels) versus secondary disease (a normal aldosterone level but a reduced cortisol level).

Measurement of blood aldosterone concentrations has not been used simply because cortisol assays have provided the information required for a diagnosis and because aldosterone assays have not been widely available until relatively recently. Cortisol assays have been commercially available for decades. It should also be pointed out that circulating aldosterone concentrations in people are affected by sodium intake and whether the patient is standing or recumbent. These are factors that veterinarians cannot easily control, which makes evaluation of aldosterone concentrations potentially less reliable.

TEST PROTOCOL, ASSAYS, AND RESULTS IN HUMANS. Several RIAs for the measurement of aldosterone are commercially available. We are currently using a solid-phase RIA designed for the quantitative measurement of aldosterone concentrations in unextracted serum (Coat-A-Count Aldosterone, Diagnostic Products Corp., Los Angeles, Calif.). The dog or cat need not be fasted, and no special preparations are necessary prior to performing the ACTH stimulation test. ACTH stimulates aldosterone secretion and is used to assess adrenocortical capacity for aldosterone synthesis and secretion. The protocol for ACTH stimulation assaying of aldosterone is the same as that previously described for cortisol, except that blood is collected into clot tubes. Serum should be separated from the cells. Serum and heparinized plasma yield comparable results, and blood can be obtained for both aldosterone and cortisol determination prior to and after ACTH administration.

Samples may be stored refrigerated at 2° to 8° C for 7 days, or they may be stored frozen at -20° C for up to 2 months. Results are not affected by severe icterus, hemolysis, lipemia, or the serum protein concentration. In humans, a high sodium intake tends to suppress serum aldosterone, whereas a low sodium intake may increase values. Reference baseline aldosterone concentrations in standing humans range from 40 to 310 pg/ml and in recumbent humans from 10 to 160 pg/ml. (Picograms per milliliter [pg/ml] can be converted to nanograms per milliliter [ng/dl] by dividing the result by 10. Picograms per milliliter [pg/ml] can be converted to picomoles per liter [pmol/L] by multiplying the result by 2.775; see the inside front cover).

RESULTS IN DOGS

Healthy Dogs. There are few reports of plasma aldosterone concentrations in dogs (Willard et al, 1987;

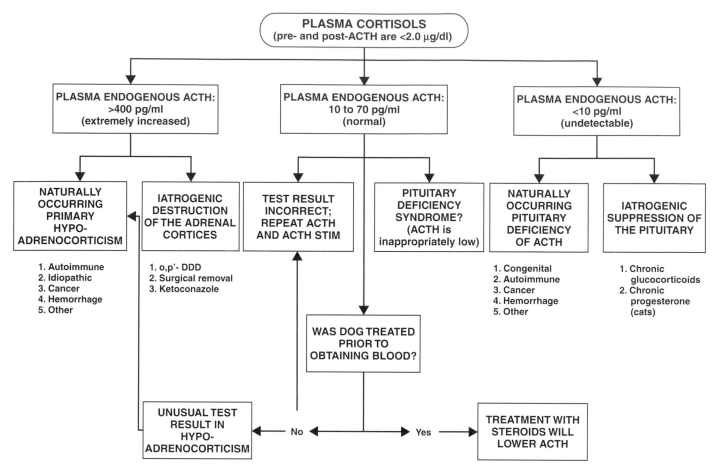

FIGURE 8-9. Algorithm for differentiating the various causes of abnormally decreased plasma cortisol concentrations on an ACTH stimulation test, using the endogenous plasma ACTH concentration.

Golden and Lothrop, 1988). In our laboratory, 32 healthy dogs were evaluated (Ortega et al, 1995). The mean basal serum aldosterone concentration was 49 pg/ml, with a range of 2 to 96 pg/ml. After ACTH administration, the mean concentration was 306 pg/ml, and the range was 146 to 519 pg/ml (Fig. 8-10).

Primary Hypoadrenocorticism. In 55 dogs with naturally occurring primary hypoadrenocorticism, hyponatremia, and hyperkalemia, the mean basal serum aldosterone concentration was 0.2 pg/ml, with a range of 0.1 to 1.0 pg/ml (42 of 55 results were 0.1 pg/ml, which is the detection limit for the assay). The mean post-ACTH serum aldosterone concentration for these dogs was 12 pg/ml, with a range of 0.1 to 91 pg/ml (36 of 55 results were 0.1 pg/ml, and 19 had results that ranged from 9 to 91 pg/ml; see Fig. 8-10).

Primary Hypoadrenocorticism, Normal Serum Electrolytes. We have had the opportunity to assay serum aldosterone concentrations from five dogs with primary hypoadrenocorticism that had normal serum electrolyte concentrations at the time of diagnosis (the time of the ACTH stimulation test). Within 1 month of the diagnosis in three dogs and within 3 months of the diagnosis in the other two dogs, the serum electrolyte concentrations demonstrated the expected abnormalities (hyponatremia and hyperkalemia). However, when the

electrolytes were normal, the serum aldosterone concentrations were similar to those in dogs with the classic serum electrolyte abnormalities. Basal serum aldosterone concentrations were 0.1 to 6.0 pg/ml, and post-ACTH serum aldosterone concentrations ranged from 0.1 to 87 pg/ml. These values were greater than the mean for the more typical addisonian dogs but were abnormally decreased (see Fig. 8-10). All five dogs eventually required mineralocorticoid treatment.

Secondary Hypoadrenocorticism. Fourteen of 18 dogs that had signs of hypoadrenocorticism, normal serum electrolyte concentrations, and low plasma cortisol concentrations before and after ACTH administration, but plasma endogenous ACTH concentrations that were extremely low, also underwent aldosterone evaluation. None of these dogs has required mineralocorticoid treatment. Interestingly, in 10 of these dogs, the serum aldosterone concentrations were abnormally low. The basal aldosterone concentrations were 0.1 to 11 pg/ml. The post-ACTH aldosterone concentrations were 1 to 94 pg/ml (see Fig. 8-10). The other four dogs had plasma aldosterone concentrations before and after stimulation within the reference range.

Summary. Serum or plasma aldosterone concentrations appear to be of academic interest in dogs suspected of having or known to have hypoadreno-

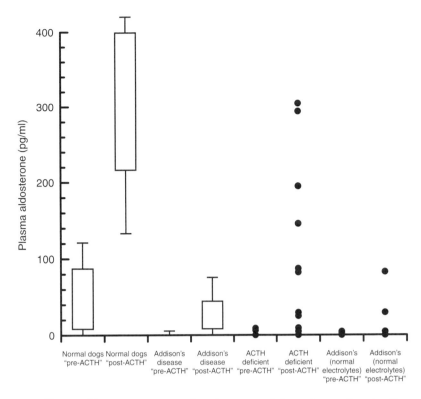

FIGURE 8-10. Plasma aldosterone concentrations from normal dogs, dogs with naturally occurring primary hypoadrenocorticism, dogs with apparent ACTH deficiency, and dogs with primary hypoadrenocorticism but normal serum electrolyte concentrations at the time of diagnosis.

corticism. Logic suggests that this assay would be of value in attempting to distinguish dogs with primary adrenal disease from those with secondary adrenal atrophy due to a pituitary or hypothalamic deficiency. Although we have evaluated only a few dogs, the aldosterone results from these different subgroups have not been of value. Further testing involving a larger number of dogs with classic Addison's disease, dogs with Addison's disease but without electrolyte abnormalities, and dogs with pituitary/hypothalamic dysfunction will be of interest.

Plasma Endogenous ACTH

BACKGROUND. Plasma endogenous ACTH concentrations can provide information about the location of failure in the pituitary-adrenocortical axis. For the most part, endogenous ACTH results are of academic rather than clinical value. As can be seen in Figs. 8-1 and 8-9, a dog with primary adrenocortical failure has little negative feedback to the pituitary, which results in markedly increased plasma ACTH concentrations. The same is true of dogs treated with the adrenocorticolytic drug o,p'-DDD. However, a dog with secondary adrenal insufficiency caused by pituitary disease should have insufficient ACTH secretion, reflected in low to low-normal plasma ACTH concentrations. Chronic ACTH deficiency (due to pituitary disease or chronic steroid treatment) also causes adrenocortical atrophy.

ASSAY AVAILABILITY AND SAMPLE HANDLING. The plasma ACTH concentration can now be routinely determined using commercially available RIAs (Nichols Institute, San Juan Capistrano, Calif.). The assay is one that we have used for more than a decade. An N-terminal antibody for ACTH is prepared in rabbits using corticotropin zinc as antigen. This antibody reacts strongly with the 19 to 24 amino acid sequence of ACTH. Blood collected for ACTH assays must be handled with urgency because the disappearance rate of ACTH from fresh whole blood is rapid, the biologic half-life being approximately 25 minutes. To avoid erroneously low values, blood specimens should not be allowed to stand at room temperature for even short periods. Contact with glass must be avoided during collection, separation, and storage, because the ACTH molecule adheres to glass and this may cause erroneously low results. Blood should be collected in *siliconized* tubes with EDTA as the anticoagulant (lavender-top Vacutainers). Siliconized tubes are recommended because use of nonsiliconized tubes generally gives lower ACTH values. Heparinized plasma samples are *not* used for the Nichols Institute assay. Plasma ACTH concentrations can be effectively preserved by processing blood samples in plastic containers and freezing them at extremely low temperatures. Each laboratory that performs endogenous ACTH assays is strongly encouraged to establish its own reference range.

RESULTS

***Normal Dogs and Dogs with Primary Hypoadreno-
corticism.*** The normal range for canine plasma
endogenous ACTH concentrations from our laboratory
is 10 to 80 pg/ml. The sensitivity of the assay is 3 pg/ml.
Of 180 dogs with naturally occurring primary hypoadrenocorticism diagnosed since 1988 in which plasma
ACTH was measured, 165 had plasma endogenous
ACTH concentrations that were extremely increased
(Fig. 8-11). These 165 dogs had endogenous ACTH
concentrations greater than 450 pg/ml, and 141 of
these 165 dogs had values greater than 1000 pg/ml.
The 450 pg/ml value is highlighted because dogs with
pituitary tumors that secrete ACTH, resulting in *hyperadrenocorticism,* typically have endogenous ACTH
concentrations of 45 to 450 pg/ml. Thus dogs with
normal pituitary glands but without negative feedback (primary hypoadrenocorticism) have much higher
endogenous ACTH concentrations than dogs with
ACTH-secreting pituitary tumors.

It is interesting to note that 15 of 180 dogs with
naturally occurring primary hypoadrenocorticism had
plasma endogenous ACTH concentrations between
100 and 450 pg/ml. Because ACTH is secreted episodically, these values may reflect that physiology. No
distinguishing features have been noted that would
separate dogs with relatively mild increases in plasma
ACTH from dogs with dramatic increases.

***Increased Endogenous ACTH and Normal Electro-
lytes.*** Eight dogs diagnosed as having primary
hypoadrenocorticism with increased plasma ACTH

concentrations had normal serum electrolyte concentrations at the time of diagnosis. Five dogs developed
typical electrolyte abnormalities (hyponatremia and
hyperkalemia) within 1 to 3 months of the initial
diagnosis and required mineralocorticoid replacement
therapy. However, three dogs received only glucocorticoid therapy and continue to maintain normal
serum electrolyte concentrations. Therefore, the finding
of abnormally decreased plasma cortisol concentrations before and after ACTH administration and an
increased plasma endogenous ACTH concentration
almost always indicates that a dog will require both
glucocorticoid and mineralocorticoid therapy because
it most likely has primary adrenal failure (Addison's
disease) (see Fig. 8-11). However, not 100% of those
dogs will require mineralocorticoid replacement.
Furthermore, all eight dogs described above had
abnormally decreased serum aldosterone concentrations, indicating that result of this assay does not
consistently prove a need for mineralocorticoid
replacement therapy.

Secondary Hypoadrenocorticism. We have defined
secondary hypoadrenocorticism as a condition of
adrenocortical insufficiency confirmed by abnormally
decreased plasma cortisol concentrations before and
after ACTH administration, a plasma endogenous
ACTH concentration that is low-normal or low, normal
serum electrolyte concentrations, and a demonstrated
need for chronic glucocorticoid but not mineralocorticoid therapy. To be certain of this unusual diagnosis, the dog must not have received *any* form of

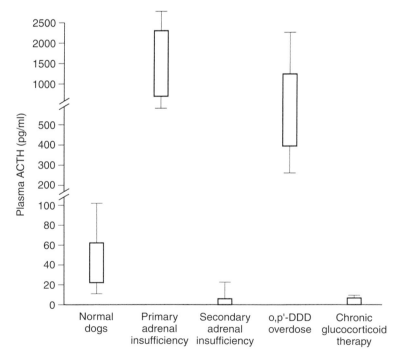

FIGURE 8-11. Plas-ma endogenous ACTH concentrations in normal dogs, dogs with primary
adrenocortical failure causing lack of negative feedback to the pituitary, dogs with pituitary failure to
secrete ACTH (secondary adrenal insufficiency) causing adrenocortical atrophy, dogs overdosed with
the adrenocorticolytic agent o,p'-DDD, and dogs chronically treated with glucocorticoids.

steroid treatment in the weeks preceding the diagnosis, because similar test results could be created by chronic administration of glucocorticoids (or other steroids) that are acutely discontinued.

Of 205 dogs in our series, 18 met all these criteria and were diagnosed as having secondary hypoadrenocorticism; 10 had undetectable plasma endogenous ACTH concentrations, and 8 had values of 7 to 35 pg/ml. All 18 dogs became stable after receiving glucocorticoid support. However, serum aldosterone concentrations were abnormally decreased in 10 of 14 dogs studied. This suggests that ACTH deficiency may have a significant effect on aldosterone secretion, that cortisol deficiency somehow results in aldosterone deficiency, or that these diagnoses are incorrect. As with any hypoadrenal animal, the key to long-term survival is a reliable owner who administers medication on time and who allows monitoring to ensure that the dog is stable.

EFFECT OF TREATMENT. Treatment for hypoadrenocorticism should lower the extremely elevated ACTH concentration in dogs with Addison's disease. Values checked in some dogs several months after treatment revealed that the endogenous ACTH concentration had decreased dramatically, presumably owing to negative feedback to the pituitary from the medication each dog had received (see Table 8-16).

SUMMARY. Knowing a hypoadrenal dog's plasma endogenous ACTH concentration is primarily of academic interest. However, if the dog with hypoadrenocorticism has normal serum electrolytes and an extremely increased plasma endogenous ACTH concentration, primary adrenocortical disease is present. Such a dog is likely to develop mineralocorticoid as well as glucocorticoid insufficiencies. If at the time of diagnosis the dog had normal plasma sodium and potassium concentrations, the practitioner could anticipate future development of electrolyte abnormalities. Monitoring of serum electrolytes is recommended once every 2 or 3 months, sooner if a dog exhibits worrisome clinical signs. Mineralocorticoid therapy could then be instituted when needed. By contrast, the dog with hypoadrenocorticism, normal serum electrolyte concentrations, and insufficient endogenous ACTH concentrations should maintain secretion of mineralocorticoids. These dogs should maintain normal serum electrolyte homeostasis and require only glucocorticoid therapy.

TREATMENT OF THE DOG IN "CRISIS"

Background

GENERAL. Rapid institution of therapy is vital for a dog or cat known to be or suspected of being in a hypoadrenal crisis. The term "crisis" is typically used for dogs or cats that are critically ill from severe hypotension, hyperkalemia, hyponatremia and dehydration. If the serum electrolyte concentrations, ECG, history, or physical examination findings are strongly

suggestive of Addison's disease, treatment should be directed toward this condition. Treatment in acute adrenal insufficiency is directed toward (1) correcting hypotension and hypovolemia, (2) improving vascular integrity and providing an immediate source of glucocorticoid, (3) correcting electrolyte imbalances, (4) correcting acidosis, (5) treating hypoglycemia, if present, and (6) providing confirmation of the diagnosis (Table 8-17).

IATROGENIC: O,P'-DDD–INDUCED HYPOADRENOCORTICISM. *Hyperadrenocorticism* is much more common in dogs than *hypoadrenocorticism,* and o,p'-DDD therapy is the preferred mode of treatment for the former condition. As with any drug, overdose can and does occur. Dogs receiving this drug may become ill during either the induction or the maintenance phases of treatment. Overdose can be confirmed by demonstrating plasma cortisol concentrations less than 1.0 to 1.5 µg/dl before and after ACTH administration.

If the dog has clinical signs of cortisol deficiency (i.e., anorexia, vomiting, diarrhea, and/or weakness) and normal serum sodium and potassium concentrations, it should respond to glucocorticoid treatment, which can then be tapered over a period of several

TABLE 8-17 TREATMENT OF ACUTE ADRENAL INSUFFICIENCY (HYPOADRENOCORTICISM)

Initial Therapy

1. Fluids: sodium chloride injection, USP (normal saline; use "shock" doses initially)
   a. 40 to 80 ml/kg/hr, first 1 to 2 hr
   b. 90 to 120 ml/kg/24 hr, next 1 to 2 days
2. Baseline cortisol and post-ACTH stimulation cortisol
3. Glucocorticoids (after completion of ACTH stimulation test)
   a. Prednisolone sodium succinate, 4 to 20 mg/kg IV
   b. Hydrocortisone sodium succinate, 0.5 to 0.625 mg/kg/hr IV infusion
   c. Dexamethasone, 0.05 to 0.1 mg/kg into infusion bottle
4. Mineralocorticoid: desoxycorticosterone pivalate (DOCP), 2.2 mg/kg IM
5. Consider IV glucose and insulin to rapidly lower serum potassium concentration (if serum K⁺ is above 8.5 mEq/L; rarely needed)
6. Acidosis: bicarbonate, 25% of calculated dose IV during first 6 hours of therapy if bicarbonate concentration of serum is <12 mEq/L (rarely needed)

Guidelines

1. Repeat serum electrolyte, glucose, and CO_2 concentrations at 6- to 8-hr intervals
2. Monitor urine production
3. Monitor ECG, if possible
4. Observe direct blood pressure or central venous pressure, if possible

Subsequent Therapy

1. Fluids: maintain until oral alimentation if possible
2. Glucocorticoids: injectable dexamethasone should be used until oral prednisone (usually low-dose) can be initiated
3. Mineralocorticoid: DOCP should be used once every 25 days, or oral fludrocortisone can be given
4. Bicarbonate: adjust dosage depending on subsequent blood CO_2 levels

weeks. If the same signs are observed in a dog receiving o,p'-DDD that has hyperkalemia and hyponatremia, mineralocorticoid as well as glucocorticoid therapy should be initiated. The treatment protocol for these dogs is no different from that recommended for naturally occurring hypoadrenocorticism. Although o,p'-DDD–induced mineralocorticoid deficiency may be reversible, most dogs require treatment for life (see Chapter 6).

Hypovolemia/Hypotension

PROTOCOL (FIG. 8-12). Because death from hypoadrenocorticism is often attributed to vascular collapse and shock (not hyperkalemia), rapid correction of hypovolemia is the first priority. An indwelling intravenous catheter should be placed in the jugular or cephalic vein. In order to both treat the patient and ultimately arrive at a diagnosis, a blood sample should

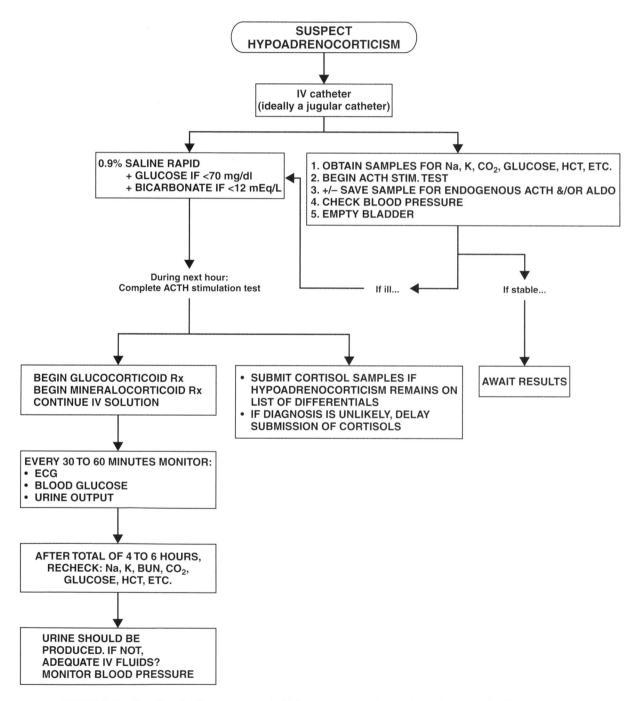

FIGURE 8-12. Algorithm for the emergency (crisis) management of a dog (or cat) suspected of having hypoadrenocorticism.

be obtained for serum electrolyte determinations, as well as for plasma cortisol measurement, before or immediately after the catheter is placed. ACTH for an ACTH stimulation test (0.25 mg Cortrosyn IM; see Table 8-15) should then be given intramuscularly, and 0.9% normal saline should be administered intravenously at an initial rate of 40 to 80 ml/kg/hr for the first 1 or 2 hours. After that, fluids should be administered at a rate of 90 to 120 ml/kg/24 hr (1.5 to 2 times the maintenance needs) for the next 36 to 48 hours (Reusch, 2000).

One dog has been reported to have had neurologic signs after intravenous saline administration for hypoadrenocorticism (Brady et al, 1999). However, the evidence that saline therapy caused these neurologic signs is weak. Furthermore, for unexplained reasons, that dog failed to receive mineralocorticoid therapy for at least 7 days and remained on saline persistently. Once serum sodium concentrations approach reference limits (often within 12 to 24 hours), the intravenous solution should be changed to Ringer's solution. We continue to recommend aggressive intravenous saline therapy as a lifesaving procedure in dogs suffering from an addisonian crisis.

VOLUME. The total volume of fluid delivered to an ill dog or cat should be determined and adjusted from an estimate of the degree of dehydration, urine output, insensible fluid losses, and other losses, such as those due to vomiting or diarrhea or both. Blood pressure measurement is a superb monitoring tool. Urine production should be closely monitored to ensure that anuric or oliguric renal failure is not present. This often requires placement of an indwelling urinary catheter to allow accurate determination of hourly urine production. Once the post-ACTH stimulation plasma cortisol sample has been obtained, additional hormone therapy (i.e., mineralocorticoids and glucocorticoids) can be administered (see Fig. 8-12).

FLUID OF CHOICE. Normal saline (0.9% sodium chloride) is the intravenous fluid of choice because it aids in the correction of hypovolemia, hyponatremia, and hypochloremia and increases intravascular volume, blood pressure, and tissue perfusion. Hyperkalemia is reduced by simple dilution (because saline contains no potassium) and by improved renal perfusion and glomerular filtration. Potassium-containing fluids are a relative contraindication but should be used in lieu of not giving intravenous fluids. Ringer's and lactated Ringer's solutions contain trivial amounts of potassium (4 mEq/L). Their use in hyperkalemic patients will decrease plasma potassium concentrations through dilutional effects and enhanced renal perfusion. If the dog is anuric, therapy with dopamine or other agents may be indicated. As previously discussed, once serum electrolyte concentrations approach or are within reference ranges, Ringer's solution is recommended.

If hypoglycemia is suspected or known to be present, 50% glucose should be added to the intravenous fluids to produce a 5% dextrose solution. The addition of dextrose to isotonic solutions produces a hypertonic solution, which ideally is administered through a jugular vein rather than the smaller cephalic vein. The ability to measure central venous pressure also makes the use of a jugular catheter preferable to a cephalic or saphenous catheter. It must be emphasized that normal saline alone, given intravenously, is the most important component of the entire therapeutic regimen (see Fig. 8-12).

Glucocorticoids

To provide glucocorticoids to dogs in an addisonian crisis, we prefer administration of dexamethasone solution or dexamethasone sodium phosphate, given intravenously, at a dosage of 0.5 to 2 mg/kg, repeated every 2 to 6 hours. Methylprednisolone sodium succinate can be administered intravenously (1 to 2 mg/kg) and then repeated every 2 to 6 hours. Alternatively, hydrocortisone hemisuccinate or hydrocortisone phosphate can be administered at dosages of 2 to 4 mg/kg given intravenously over 2 to 4 minutes and repeated every 8 hours. Hydrocortisone sodium succinate should be infused at a rate of 0.5 to 0.625 mg/kg/hr. Such an infusion will result in appropriate plasma cortisol concentrations. It is not certain whether this drug will provide adequate mineralocorticoid activity (Church et al, 1999). The ACTH stimulation test should be completed before administration of glucocorticoids (see Fig. 8-12).

Infusion of intravenous saline is sufficient therapy during the first hour (while ACTH response is completed). If initial glucocorticoid therapy included administration of a rapid-acting, water-soluble drug, we then subsequently recommend using dexamethasone. An initial dose of 0.5 to 1 mg/kg given intravenously should be adequate. Subsequent doses of 0.05 to 0.1 mg/kg given two to three times a day can be added to the intravenous solution. This should provide an adequate and continuous source of glucocorticoid for the dog until oral medication can be safely given (see Table 8-17).

Electrolyte Imbalance

RECOGNIZING THE PROBLEM. Direct assay of serum electrolyte concentrations is specific and sensitive for diagnosing hyperkalemia and hyponatremia. An alternate and rapid method of identifying severe hyperkalemia (the most worrisome electrolyte alteration) is with an ECG; (see page 417 and Fig. 8-7). If P waves are not seen and the heart rate is slow, severe hyperkalemia should be suspected. Invariably the serum potassium concentration with these ECG alterations is greater than 7.5 mEq/L. The major differential diagnosis is atrial fibrillation, which is usually associated with tachycardia and not vomiting or diarrhea. Adrenal insufficiency or atrial fibrillation can cause weakness, lethargy, anorexia, and weight loss.

SALINE TREATMENT. Therapy need not be overzealous when serum potassium concentrations are less than 6.5 mEq/L, whereas intensive therapy must be instituted in dogs and cats with serum potassium concentrations greater than 7.5 mEq/L. With marked hyperkalemia, rapid institution of treatment may be lifesaving. Intravenous 0.9% normal saline is a reliable treatment for attempting to lower the serum potassium concentration rapidly. Virtually every dog in hypoadrenocortical crisis that we have treated has received only rapid administration of 0.9% normal saline (with or without glucose) during the first hour of treatment. This approach *alone* has resulted in dramatic clinical, biochemical, and ECG improvement. Intravenous saline rapidly corrects the life-threatening complications of hypoadrenocorticism (e.g., hyponatremia, hypochloremia, hypovolemia, hypotension, hyperkalemia, and azotemia).

PRACTICAL THERAPY. Rapid intravenous infusion of saline (with or without glucose and/or bicarbonate) over the first hour of therapy has uniformly resulted in marked improvement of each dog's clinical status by increasing the blood volume, blood pressure, and serum sodium concentration while lowering the serum potassium concentration and moving ECG abnormalities toward normal. The serum potassium concentration decreases because of the dilutional effect provided by saline (which contains no potassium) and by improved renal perfusion. Increased renal blood flow allows further excretion of potassium into the urine. If sodium bicarbonate therapy is used, it will also increase the serum sodium concentration and shift potassium ions into the intracellular space. We have not needed to use insulin or calcium therapy for dogs or cats in hypoadrenal crisis.

MINERALOCORTICOID TREATMENT

General. In addition to intravenous fluids with or without bicarbonate and glucose, mineralocorticoids should be administered to maintain electrolyte balance. We administer mineralocorticoids immediately *after* completing the ACTH response test.

Desoxycorticosterone Pivalate (DOCP). This is the recommended drug for maintenance treatment of dogs and cats with hypoadrenocorticism. The dosage we use is 2.2 mg/kg of body weight, given either intramuscularly or subcutaneously every 25 days. In an emergency hypoadrenal crisis, we administer this same drug intramuscularly and have found it to be effective and reliable. Intravenous normal saline and DOCP given intramuscularly have corrected electrolyte abnormalities in virtually every hypoadrenal dog within 6 to 24 hours. We are not aware of harmful side effects if the drug is administered to a dog subsequently demonstrated to have normal adrenocortical function. Natural protection against overdose is the result of atrial natriuretic peptide secretion (Ramsay, 1991; Chow et al, 1993; Kaplan and Peterson, 1995). Therefore, for a severely ill dog suspected of having hypoadrenocorticism, short-term management with intravenous fluids and DOCP administered intramuscularly is warranted.

Hydrocortisone. In humans, injectable cortisol (hydrocortisone hemisuccinate or hydrocortisone phosphate) is a reliable drug in the management of a hypoadrenocortical crisis. Injectable cortisol is a glucocorticoid with sufficient sodium-retaining potency to also serve as a replacement for mineralocorticoid insufficiency (Tyrrell et al, 1991). We have used hydrocortisone hemisuccinate in several hypoadrenal dogs based on these observations in humans.

In dogs, the recommended dosage is 1.25 mg/kg given intravenously initially, followed by 0.5 to 1.0 mg/kg given intravenously every 6 hours. On the second day, the dosage is further tapered, ultimately reaching 0.1 to 0.25 mg/kg given four times a day, and then 0.1 to 0.25 mg/kg in two oral doses of hydrocortisone per day with mineralocorticoid as needed (see section on long-term treatment, page 431). We have *not* been convinced that the mineralocorticoid effect demonstrated in humans with hydrocortisone is consistently achieved in dogs. We have achieved more consistent mineralocorticoid activity using DOCP and glucocorticoid activity using dexamethasone.

Fludrocortisone Acetate (Florinef). This drug is commonly used for the long-term maintenance of dogs with hypoadrenocorticism. Although the absorption capacity for this drug in dogs is poorer than in humans (see page 434), it is a relatively effective mineralocorticoid. However, Florinef is rarely useful in a hypoadrenal crisis. The drug is available only in tablet form, and most of these dogs are much too ill (e.g., vomiting, obtundation) to receive oral therapy. In a crisis situation, injectable DOCP is the mineralocorticoid of choice.

GLUCOSE AND INSULIN TREATMENT. In the unusual circumstance that intravenous 0.9% normal saline is not successful in quickly lowering serum potassium concentrations and death from hyperkalemia is believed to be imminent, lowering of the serum potassium concentration can be further aided by intravenous infusion of a 10% glucose solution. In the first 30 to 60 minutes, 4 to 10 ml/kg of glucose solution should be given, usually added to the saline infusion. Glucose uptake by cells is accompanied by potassium uptake from the vascular compartment.

Subcutaneous or intravenous infusions of regular insulin (crystalline) at a dosage of 0.06 to 0.125 U/kg of body weight enhances the cellular uptake of glucose. For each unit of regular insulin, at least 20 ml of 10% glucose should be given to avoid precipitation of hypoglycemia. Although this therapy lowers serum potassium concentrations, intravenous saline alone has negated the need for this additional medication, in our experience. We have not used glucose or glucose and insulin in the management of hypoadrenal dogs or cats.

CALCIUM TREATMENT. An intravenous infusion of 10% calcium gluconate has been recommended in the management of acute hyperkalemia. A dose of 0.5 to 1.0 mg/kg given slowly over a period of 10 to 20 minutes appears to function by "protecting" the myocardium from the deleterious effects of hyperkalemia. This protection provides time for other modes of therapy to lower the serum potassium concentration. During a calcium infusion, the ECG must be monitored continuously and treatment must be stopped if any new arrhythmia is observed. Again, in our experience, intravenous saline alone has negated the need for this additional medication.

SODIUM BICARBONATE TREATMENT. Sodium bicarbonate, as discussed below, can be used to decrease serum potassium concentrations. The combination of 0.9% normal saline with adequate dextrose to make a 5% glucose solution and sodium bicarbonate are the immediate methods of treatment recommended for severe hyperkalemia in hypoadrenocorticism.

Acidosis

NEED FOR THERAPY. Dogs in an addisonian crisis usually have a mild metabolic acidosis that does not require bicarbonate therapy. Acidosis, when present and worrisome, can be corrected by adding sodium bicarbonate to the intravenous solutions. Fluid therapy alone corrects mild acidosis as hypovolemia, tissue perfusion, and renal GFR improve. Bicarbonate therapy is usually not used unless the serum bicarbonate concentration is less than 12 mEq/L. When arterial blood gas analysis is not available, total venous CO_2 concentrations can be used to estimate the base deficit by subtracting the patient's venous CO_2 concentration from the normal venous CO_2 concentration (approximately 22 mEq/L). In a severely ill dog or cat, a base deficit of 10 mEq/L can be assumed to be present while awaiting blood gas results. The number of milliequivalents of bicarbonate needed to correct the acidosis is then determined from the following equation:

$$\text{Deficit (mEq)} = (\text{Body weight [kg]}) (0.3) (\text{Base deficit})$$

Dogs and cats with Addison's disease seldom require the complete bicarbonate replacement dosage. Therefore it is recommended that 25% of the calculated dose be added to the intravenous fluids and administered during the initial 6 to 8 hours of therapy. At the end of this time, the dog's acid-base status should be reassessed. It would be rare for a dog to require additional parenteral sodium bicarbonate. We do not recommend indiscriminate use of sodium bicarbonate. If the total venous CO_2 or the serum bicarbonate concentration is greater than 12 mEq/L, sodium bicarbonate therapy is not necessary.

ADDITIONAL BENEFITS OF BICARBONATE ADMINISTRATION. Intravenous administration of sodium bicarbonate not only aids in correcting metabolic acidosis but also increases the serum sodium concentration while decreasing the serum potassium concentration. Sodium bicarbonate buffers hydrogen ions, decreases the *intracellular* hydrogen ion concentration, increases the intracellular potassium concentration, and thereby decreases the *(extracellular)* potassium concentration (Fig. 8-13).

Response to Therapy

FIRST FEW HOURS. Virtually every hypoadrenal dog treated initially with intravenous saline (first hour)

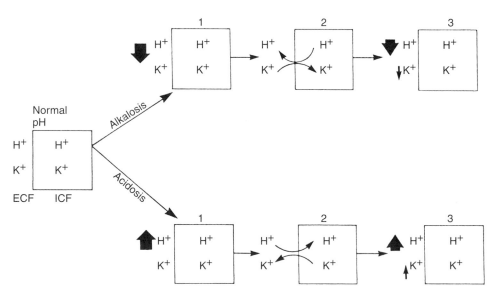

FIGURE 8-13. Redistribution of extracellular fluid (ECF) and intracellular fluid (ICF) potassium and hydrogen ions in response to changes in ECF pH. Alkalosis: *1*, The H^+ concentration decreases; *2*, H^+ moves out of cells and down its concentration gradient, and K^+ moves into cells to maintain electrical neutrality; *3*, this contributes to the hypokalemia associated with alkalosis. Acidosis: *1*, The H^+ concentration increases; *2*, H^+ moves into cells and down its concentration gradient, and K^+ moves out of cells to maintain electrical neutrality; *3*, the result of electrolyte shifts, that is, the hyperkalemia associated with acidosis. The size of the arrow represents the degree of change from normal. (From Gabow P: *In* Schrier RW [ed]: Renal and Electrolyte Disorders. Boston, Little, Brown & Co, 1976.)

and subsequently with glucocorticoids and mineralo-corticoids has shown rapid improvement. Within 1 to 2 hours of aggressive fluid therapy, these dogs are often able to stand and walk, even when they were initially extremely weak. They quickly regain an interest in their owners, food, water, and their environment. Typically, the ECG and the serum electrolyte and BUN concentrations correlate well with the clinical response by rapidly returning toward or to normal. The response to fluid therapy alone is highly suggestive of and consistent with adrenocortical insufficiency, because dogs with most other illnesses (severe renal, gastrointestinal, or hepatic diseases) do not usually have as dramatic a reversal of signs or laboratory abnormalities.

FIRST 24 TO 48 HOURS. If a dog is initially examined and thought to be in critical condition, with a tentative diagnosis of hypoadrenocorticism, intravenous fluids should be maintained for at least 48 hours. Access to food or water should be withheld for at least 24 hours, even if dramatic clinical improvement is observed. Assuming that the dog has significantly responded to therapy during the initial 24-hour treatment period, the rate of fluid administration can then be reduced by 50% while water is offered in small amounts every 1 to 2 hours.

FIRST 2 TO 7 DAYS

Fluids. Assuming that the dog is not vomiting after the first 24 hours of aggressive fluid and hormonal support, water (in small amounts every few hours) should be offered. If the water is consumed and vomiting is not seen for 12 additional hours, food may be offered in small amounts and the intravenous fluids decreased further. Typically, we offer a 50:50 or 25:75 mixture of low-fat cottage cheese and cooked white rice. If vomiting is not observed after 12 to 24 hours of consuming food, intravenous fluid administration may be discontinued.

If vomiting recurs, all oral intake should be stopped and intravenous fluid therapy reinstituted at or in excess of "maintenance" requirements. If there is no vomiting but the dog has no appetite and/or refuses to consume water, the clinician is encouraged to continue intravenous fluid therapy in volumes required to maintain hydration. The dog can then be offered food and/or water every 12 to 24 hours until the appetite returns. A search for problems slowing recovery may be rewarding. Most often, dogs that are slow to recover have lingering gastrointestinal problems (ulcerations, hemorrhage) or renal problems (azotemia) that resolve with time.

Glucocorticoids. Daily intravenous dexamethasone injections (in the IV solution or SQ) should be continued until the dog is eating and drinking normally and can be safely converted to oral prednisone therapy. The dexamethasone dosage we use is 0.01 to 0.05 mg/kg given twice daily. Prednisone is typically begun at a dosage of approximately 0.22 mg/kg given twice daily. This dosage can be slowly tapered to determine the required long-term needs of the individual. For maintenance, the typical 20 kg dog usually requires as little as 1.25 mg every other day to as much as 2.5 mg daily.

Mineralocorticoids. If the mineralocorticoid given was DOCP, serum electrolytes should be rechecked 12 and 25 days after administration and the next dose administered on that 25th day. Adjustments in dosage or frequency are based on the results of serum electrolyte determinations. If oral fludrocortisone acetate is used, it must be given daily. The initial dosage is approximately 0.02 mg/kg, divided and given twice daily (see section on long-term treatment, page 433, for information on both these drugs).

General. Each dog should remain hospitalized and under observation for at least 24 to 48 hours after discontinuation of intravenous therapy. After this time, if the dog continues to appear well on oral therapy, it can be returned to the owner. The dog should then be checked 7 and 14 days later. These evaluations should include a thorough history, complete physical examination, ECG, and blood tests, including BUN, sodium, potassium, and glucose concentrations. If the dog is well and the test results are normal, monthly rechecks can be scheduled for the next 6 months. Finally, rechecks every 3 to 6 months are strongly encouraged.

Concurrent Problems

GLUCOCORTICOID DEFICIENCY. The dog with hypoadrenocorticism that is treated only with the mineralocorticoid DOCP may encounter vague problems (inappetence, lethargy, depression). Such concerns may be subtle but are easily noted by owners. Common blood tests may not identify the cause of this incomplete response to treatment because serum electrolyte concentrations and renal parameters test normal, yet the dog does not appear to the owner to be in satisfactory condition. DOCP has no glucocorticoid activity, in contrast to Florinef. A trial period (2 to 4 weeks) of low-dose prednisone therapy (0.22 mg/kg bid), in addition to the mineralocorticoids, usually results in dramatic improvement.

If such vague problems do not respond to glucocorticoid treatment, numerous other conditions may be the cause. Lingering gastrointestinal or renal conditions may contribute. Significantly anemic dogs and cats may require several weeks to return to normal. This would also be true of dogs that had severe weight loss or muscle weakness. Therefore, if database evaluations are not worrisome, sometimes a bit of additional time may be necessary for complete response. However, the properly treated dog should become completely normal, and this should be the goal of therapy.

GASTROINTESTINAL HEMORRHAGE/ANEMIA. Dogs with hypoadrenocorticism usually have gastrointestinal signs, including anorexia, vomiting, and diarrhea. The vomitus and stools may contain significant amounts of blood, which may appear fresh or as melena. Ulceration in the gastrointestinal tract can be severe in dogs with Addison's disease, leading to prolongation of the recovery period or severe blood loss or both. Rarely, dogs require blood transfusions, which illustrates the potential severity of these problems. Furthermore, it has been recommended that ulcerogenic drugs be avoided in dogs with Addison's disease (Medinger et al, 1993). In some dogs, progression to disseminated intravascular coagulation (DIC; "Death Is Coming") can be documented, a fact that further supports the need for aggressive treatment of dogs suspected of having Addison's disease.

RENAL DISEASE. Abnormal renal parameters are classically associated with Addison's disease. These abnormalities are the result of hypovolemia, hypotension, and compromised renal perfusion. Abnormal renal test results usually quickly correct with therapy and are often normal within 24 to 48 hours. The severity and/or chronicity of Addison's disease may cause damage to the kidneys, which can be slow to resolve, but permanent renal failure is not a common sequela of Addison's disease. Furthermore, gastrointestinal bleeding results in a greater increase in BUN than in serum creatinine. Therefore evaluating both parameters allows the veterinarian to assess renal function and gastrointestinal bleeding. In the latter case, the BUN may be abnormal and the serum creatinine within the reference range or the BUN-to-creatinine ratio will exceed 20:1.

HEPATOPATHY. Dogs with Addison's disease and concurrent hepatopathy have been documented (see page 415). It is not known whether both problems are caused by concurrent autoimmune disease. The hepatopathies appear to resolve with treatment of the Addison's disease. Because this treatment involves glucocorticoids, it has not been possible to document any long-term liver disorder. To the contrary, most liver parameters are normal after 1 to 2 months of treatment for Addison's disease.

NEUROLOGIC DISEASE. Myelinolysis has been documented in two dogs that had severe hyponatremia due to whipworm infestations. It was suggested that the myelinolysis was due to overzealous treatment of the hyponatremia (O'Brien et al, 1994). This problem has not been documented in dogs with Addison's disease. However, the reported rate of correction of the hyponatremia did not appear overzealous; rather, it was slow relative to our recommendations.

LONG-TERM (MAINTENANCE) TREATMENT OF DOGS WITH PRIMARY HYPOADRENOCORTICISM

Initiation

Maintenance therapy can be initiated once a dog or cat is stable with parenteral medication. The dog should have a good appetite and no continuing evidence of vomiting, diarrhea, weakness, or depression. In addition, the serum electrolyte concentrations should be within the normal range. The veterinary practitioner and the owner have few alternatives in choosing long-

TABLE 8-18 LONG-TERM TREATMENT OF PRIMARY ADRENOCORTICAL INSUFFICIENCY

Mineralocorticoid	Desoxycorticosterone pivalate injectable, approximately 2 mg/kg IM or SC every month
Glucocorticoid	Prednisone as needed, 2.5–10 mg daily or every other day
OR	
Mineralocorticoid	Approximately 0.1 mg fludrocortisone/5 kg body weight (divided BID)
Glucocorticoid	Prednisone as needed, 2.5–10 mg daily, or every other day
OR	
Hydrocortisone	Approximately 0.125 mg/kg body weight daily, divided 3/4–2/3 AM: remainder PM
Fludrocortisone	As needed, approximately 0.05 mg/5 kg body weight (divided BID)
Divide oral mineralocorticoid replacement to protect dog against vomiting entire dose should an acute gastrointestinal problem arise.	
Clinical follow-up	Recheck every 3–6 months. Maintain normal weight and activity. Electrolytes and BUN should be normal.
Salt	No special addition if dog food diet
Times of stress	Increase glucocorticoid therapy
Owner education is imperative.	

term mineralocorticoid medications: injections every 25 days or daily oral therapy (Table 8-18).

Mineralocorticoids

INJECTIONS OF DESOXYCORTICOSTERONE (DOCP) EVERY 25 DAYS

Dosage. DOCP (Percorten-V; Novartis Animal Health, Greensboro, NC) is a long-acting trimethylacetate ester of desoxycorticosterone that is formulated in a microcrystalline suspension. When given intramuscularly (Fig. 8-14), DOCP provides mineralocorticoid activity for approximately 25 days. It was used for the treatment of people with Addison's disease beginning in the 1950s until the development of oral fludrocortisone. The initial recommended dosage is 2.2 mg/kg given intramuscularly or subcutaneously every 25 days (see Table 8-18 and Figs. 8-14 and 8-15) (Lynn and Feldman, 1991; Lynn et al, 1993; McCabe et al, 1995). Most owners have been taught to administer the drug to their pets, with emphasis placed on the importance of successful subcutaneous injection protocols. Most dogs receiving DOCP also require a low dose of glucocorticoids (prednisone, 0.22 mg/kg bid, initially).

Some authors have suggested a lower initial starting dose of DOCP (approximately 1.7 mg/kg every 25 days) rather than the manufacturer-recommended 2.2 mg/kg every 25 days (Kintzer and Peterson, 1997). The only reason for such an approach would be to reduce expense. Our experience, however, is that the manufacturer's recommendation results in consistent normalization of serum electrolytes. Although lower

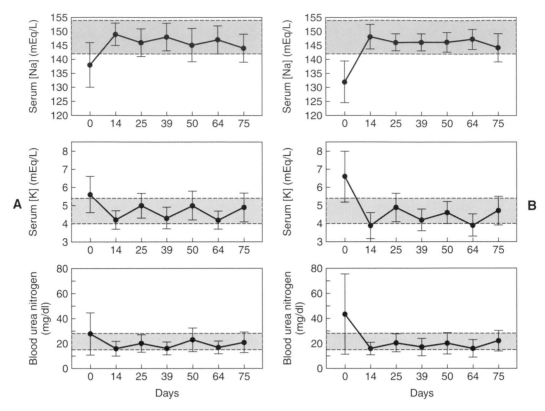

FIGURE 8-14. Serum biochemical values from 60 dogs given desoxycorticosterone pivalate (DOCP) intramuscularly for treatment of hypoadrenocorticism. *A, Top,* Serum sodium concentrations; *middle,* serum potassium concentrations; *bottom,* blood urea nitrogen concentrations. *B,* Serum biochemical values (top, middle, and bottom same as for *A*) for nine dogs given DOCP for treatment of recently diagnosed hypoadrenocorticism. *Shaded areas* indicate reference ranges for each value. Results are reported as mean ± SD. (From Lynn R, et al: J Am Vet Med Assoc 202:392, 1993.)

doses may be successful in some dogs, one episode of illness caused by underdosing would negate all the financial savings.

Monitoring. Every dog treated with DOCP should be monitored with a history, physical examination, and measurement of blood sodium, potassium, and BUN concentrations. Rechecks should be completed approximately 12 and 25 days after each of the first two or three DOCP injections. The goals of therapy are normal blood parameters and a completely healthy dog. The 12-day recheck, as well as the 40-day recheck, are viewed as "dose" assessments. If the serum electrolyte concentrations are not normal, an increase of 5% to 10% in the next dose should be considered. However, because this is so uncommon, the practitioner might also consider the possibility that the drug was not mixed appropriately or that an incorrect dose was drawn into the syringe.

The 25-day recheck, as well as the 50-day recheck, are "assessments" of dose frequency. In the unlikely situation of normal serum electrolyte concentrations at 12 days but abnormal levels at 25 days, the clinician must consider decreasing the interval between injections. However, if the serum electrolytes are within the reference range at 25 days, an attempt can be made to increase the interval between injections by 1 day each

cycle. Our experience with more than 175 treated dogs, however, is that fewer than 10% consistently do well receiving injections once monthly.

After the appropriate dose has been demonstrated, twice yearly rechecks are recommended. In this manner, the dog can be assessed and the owner can keep the veterinarian up-to-date on the dog's progress. Changes in body weight, for example, may require changes in DOCP dosage.

DOCP is a mineralocorticoid, and it contains virtually no glucocorticoid activity. Therefore it is recommended that all dogs and cats treated with DOCP also receive glucocorticoids as part of the maintenance regimen. It is strongly suggested that veterinarians remember that the dose of glucocorticoids needed for maintenance should be physiologic. In other words, the doses used for immunosuppression or to reduce inflammation are far in excess of the needs of an addisonian dog or cat.

Advantages. DOCP is an extremely effective mineralocorticoid. In virtually all treated dogs (we have treated more than 175 dogs and have participated in studies involving more than 100 additional dogs), the serum sodium and potassium concentrations returned to normal levels by the first "day 12" evaluation (see Fig. 8-14). Most dogs have been started on

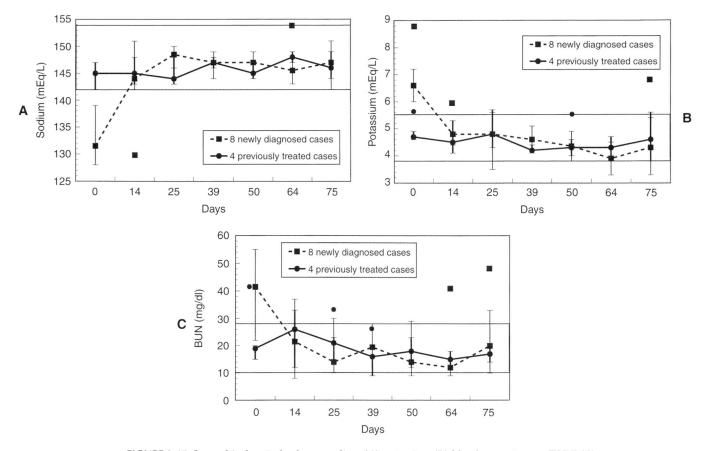

FIGURE 8-15. Serum biochemical values—sodium *(A)*, potassium *(B)*, blood urea nitrogen (BUN) *(C)*—from 12 dogs given DOCP subcutaneously for treatment of hypoadrenocorticism. Mean values (± range) from newly diagnosed dogs *(dashed line)* and previously treated dogs *(solid line)* are separated; normal values are indicated by the solid horizontal lines. Outliers are indicated by squares (newly diagnosed dogs) or dots (previously diagnosed dogs) above or below the range lines. On day 75, one dog was hyperkalemic and the same dog was azotemic on days 64 and 75. These abnormalities were resolved by administering the DOCP every 21 days rather than every 25 days.

the recommended dose, and that dose requirement has not changed over a period of years except for adjustments made to account for weight gain, which is common among treated addisonian dogs. Overdose has been weakly documented in one dog, in which polydipsia and polyuria resolved after the dose of DOCP had been reduced.

Owners have discovered that subcutaneous injections every 25 days are easy. The expense has been similar to or less than that of oral medication. Side effects, such as those associated with fludrocortisone, are not observed. If polydipsia, polyuria, and incontinence are noted, they are usually due to prednisone overdose and can be quickly resolved by reducing that dose.

Disadvantages. The dose of DOCP is variable, as is typical of most replacement hormone therapies. The DOCP dose must be titrated to the needs of each dog. In 58 of the first 60 dogs treated, the recommended dose was effective. However, in two dogs, the specified dosage was sufficient for only 22 or 23 days before signs of hypoadrenocorticism began to be observed. Decreasing the injection interval to 21 days was effective (Lynn et al, 1993).

The drug apparently failed in two of 175 dogs in our series. Those two dogs were subsequently controlled with oral fludrocortisone. "Failures" occur so infrequently that we suspect that this is a problem associated with mixing or injection technique, or both. Owners, therefore, must become competent at mixing the drug, drawing it into a syringe, and injecting it. Alternatively, the dog would need to be treated by a veterinarian when due for an injection, a distinct disadvantage compared with oral therapy.

DAILY ORAL THERAPY WITH FLUDROCORTISONE ACETATE

Dosage. Fludrocortisone acetate (Florinef; E.R. Squibb & Sons, Princeton, NJ) is the most commonly used treatment for humans with hypoadrenocorticism (Tyrrell et al, 1991), and it has been recommended for the treatment of canine hypoadrenocorticism for more than 20 years (Feldman and Nelson, 1987). Each tablet contains 0.1 mg of mineralocorticoid. The initial recommended dosage is 0.02 mg/kg, divided and given twice daily. The average 20 kg dog requires three to six tablets daily (see Table 8-18). Interestingly, the average dose in a human with Addison's disease is 0.05 to 0.1 mg (one half to one tablet) daily. Because humans require a dramatically lower dose than dogs, it is presumed that dogs fail to absorb the drug as effectively or that they metabolize the drug more rapidly than humans.

Monitoring. Initially, serum electrolyte concentrations should be monitored every 1 to 2 weeks until the dog or cat is stable. The goal in therapy is to have the serum electrolyte concentrations within the reference range. Rechecks consisting of a physical examination, progress report, and serum analysis of sodium, potassium, and BUN (the BUN is used as a crude evaluation of blood volume and tissue perfusion) are recommended two to three times per year. Monitoring of systemic blood pressure is also recommended, if available.

It has been our experience that the dosage of fludrocortisone acetate often needs to be moderately increased during the first 6 to 18 months of therapy. This adjustment may reflect continuing destruction of the adrenal cortex or changes in the absorption or metabolism (or both) of the drug. After the initial 6 to 18 months, the dosage usually remains relatively stable.

Advantages. The major advantage of tablet administration is the ease of diagnosing and adjusting an incorrect dosage (i.e., daily administration is easily altered). Tablet administration is easily accomplished by most owners. Daily therapy also serves as a constant reminder to the dog owner that the animal is afflicted with a serious, life-threatening disease and that it depends on the owner for survival. The drug is readily available at almost any human pharmacy.

Disadvantages. There are several major drawbacks to use of this oral therapy. Fludrocortisone has potent glucocorticoid activity as well as mineralocorticoid activity, which may complicate proper titration of the drug dose. The glucocorticoid effects may cause clinical signs of overdose, whereas the mineralocorticoid actions may be inadequate to normalize the serum electrolyte concentrations. Thus the development of clinical signs typical of iatrogenic Cushing's syndrome (i.e., polydipsia, polyuria, and incontinence) are noted in some dogs while either their serum sodium or potassium concentration is not within the reference range. In a random evaluation of serum electrolyte concentrations from 51 dogs we treated and considered well controlled with fludrocortisone, 84% had hyponatremia, hyperkalemia, and/or a subnormal sodium:potassium ratio. In addition, compared with humans, dogs require extremely high dosages of fludrocortisone, which makes this form of therapy expensive.

Abnormal serum electrolyte values may be attributed to inconsistent daily owner compliance; failure to administer adequate amounts of fludrocortisone because of expense, side effects, or infrequent monitoring; or simply subtle differences in physiologic effect. Complications may arise if normal serum electrolyte concentrations are used as the goal of treatment. In this situation, the fludrocortisone dose may be increased until the treated dog begins to manifest signs of glucocorticoid excess, with polydipsia, polyuria, and urinary incontinence being most common. Also, as the dose is increased, treatment of a dog can become quite expensive. These problems often can be resolved by using DOCP rather than fludrocortisone. When switching medications, we routinely taper the fludrocortisone over a period of 4 to 5 days beginning with the day that DOCP is given. DOCP has a rapid onset of action (hours), and we have not observed recurrence of clinical signs suggestive of hypoadrenocorticism during this transition period.

HYDROCORTISONE. We have not experienced success with hydrocortisone preparations in the chronic maintenance of dogs with hypoadrenocorticism (see Table 8-18).

Glucocorticoids

GENERAL THERAPEUTIC MEASURES. Virtually every dog and cat with Addison's disease that we treat with DOCP also is treated with low doses of prednisone. However, fewer than 50% of our dogs receiving fludrocortisone as a mineralocorticoid replacement require glucocorticoid medication. Some dogs receiving only mineralocorticoids may be reported not to be in perfect health yet may have normal serum electrolyte concentrations. In this situation, a minimal dose of prednisone or prednisolone (0.1 to 0.22 mg/kg bid, initially) often improves the dog's well-being. Owners quickly note improvement, the medication is inexpensive, and adverse reactions are minimal at these low dosages (see Table 8-18).

MANAGEMENT OF STRESS: WORKING DOGS; BREEDING. Some dogs with Addison's disease are "working" dogs" (e.g., hunters and field trial participants). In general, we encourage owners to allow their dogs to participate in activities to which they are accustomed. However, the owners must be made aware that addisonian dogs must be monitored more closely than the typical healthy pet and that activity should be discontinued if a dog appears to be unduly fatigued. On days of planned increased exercise or stress, it is convenient to recommend doubling any glucocorticoid dose being administered. Such dogs are likely predisposed, among other problems, to hypoglycemia. Chances for such complications would be reduced with additional glucocorticoid therapy (Syme and Scott-Moncrief, 1998). We do not strongly discourage use of addisonian dogs in breeding programs.

Salt Supplementation

Salt tablets or salting of food is only rarely needed to aid in controlling hyponatremia. Most dogs fed commercial diets receive adequate amounts of salt. The use of additional salt supplementation has been reported to be beneficial (Schaer, 1980). Salt supplementation may be useful in reducing unusually high doses of fludrocortisone. We do not routinely recommend use of salt.

LONG-TERM TREATMENT OF DOGS WITH SECONDARY HYPOADRENOCORTICISM

Naturally Occurring Disease

Dogs with secondary hypoadrenocorticism do not typically demonstrate mineralocorticoid deficiency, although measured aldosterone concentrations in several such dogs have been less than normal. Therefore daily doses of glucocorticoids, as described previously, are usually sufficient to control the signs associated with this disease. Veterinarians should periodically monitor serum electrolyte concentrations (i.e., three to four times yearly), because some animals that are believed to be pituitary deficient ultimately develop hyponatremia and hyperkalemia. These dogs have primary adrenal insufficiency (Rogers et al, 1981; Sadek and Schaer, 1996; Dunn and Herrtage, 1998).

Iatrogenic: o,p'-DDD Overdose

Dogs that develop signs of Addison's disease after o,p'-DDD therapy usually can be successfully treated with glucocorticoids, although this treatment is usually needed only transiently. The diagnosis can be supported with an ACTH stimulation test result. Management of these dogs has been reviewed in the section on treatment of the dog in crisis (page 425). Mineralocorticoid deficiency must be ruled out by measurement of serum electrolyte concentrations.

Iatrogenic: Withdrawal of Chronic Glucocorticoid Therapy

Iatrogenic hypocortisolism caused by chronic use of glucocorticoids that have been acutely discontinued is treated by placing the dog back on a glucocorticoid, such as prednisone, and then slowly tapering the dose over a period of 1 to 2 months. We usually decrease glucocorticoid therapy to a physiologic dose (approximately 0.25 mg/kg/day) as quickly as possible (within a week). If that dose is tolerated for a week without recurrence of clinical signs, the dosage is reduced by administering the drug every other day rather than daily. After 2 weeks at this dose, the frequency is again reduced by giving the drug every 3 days. After 2 to 3 weeks at this dose, the prednisone can be discontinued. If signs recur after any dose reduction, the previous amount is usually reinstituted. If clinical signs continue to recur, complete reevaluation of the dog is recommended.

PROGNOSIS

The prognosis in dogs with hypoadrenocorticism has been excellent, regardless of the mineralocorticoid supplement chosen, when diligent owners and veterinarians have teamed to manage these pets. Such dogs have led normal lives, with few if any restrictions. The most important factor in the long-term response to therapy is owner education. This disease must be carefully described, and owners must be warned of the consequences of apparently mild illnesses. All owners should have glucocorticoids available to administer to their dogs in times of stress. Some owners keep parenteral, rapid-acting glucocorticoids on hand should the need arise. Veterinarians should be aware of the increased glucocorticoid requirements of hypoadrenal dogs that undergo surgery, that experience other forms of stress, or that are ill with a non-adrenal-related disease.

HYPOADRENOCORTICISM IN CATS

Etiology

Primary hypoadrenocorticism is a rare disease in cats. Since the first report in 1983, fewer than 40 cases have been described in the veterinary literature (Johnessee et al, 1983; Freudiger, 1986; Peterson et al, 1989; Berger and Reed, 1993; Parnell et al, 1999). The University of Minnesota has reported seven cats with naturally occurring hypoadrenocorticism (Hardy, 1995), and our hospital has eight documented cases. The cause has been described as idiopathic adrenocortical atrophy in one cat with traumatically induced disease (Berger and Reed, 1993), and the condition occurred secondary to lymphoma of the adrenals in two cats (Parnell et al, 1999). Iatrogenic secondary hypoadrenocorticism may follow long-term use of either exogenous glucocorticoids or megestrol acetate, although these two causes are also considered rare.

Signalment and Clinical Signs

The age of cats with Addison's disease has varied from 1.5 to 14 years. All have been Domestic Long-Haired or Domestic Short-Haired cats. An equal number of males and females have been described, although all cats have been neutered.

The clinical signs and physical examination abnormalities are similar to those described for dogs (Table 8-19). The duration of signs noted by owners has been as short as a few days and as long as 3 to 4 months. The most common owner observations include lethargy, depression, anorexia, and weight loss. Less frequently noticed signs include vomiting, waxing-waning course of illness, polyuria, polydipsia, and previous response to nonspecific therapy, such as intravenous fluids or glucocorticoids. Diarrhea has not been reported (Peterson et al, 1989).

The most common physical examination abnormalities identified in these cats are depression, weakness, dehydration, hypothermia, slow capillary refill time, and weak femoral pulses. Less commonly observed examination findings included collapse, inability to rise, bradycardia, and painful abdomen (Peterson et al, 1989).

TABLE 8-19 CLINICAL FINDINGS IN 10 CATS WITH PRIMARY HYPOADRENOCORTICISM*

Clinical Findings	Number of Cats (%)
Historic Owner Complaints	
Lethargy/depression	10 (100)
Anorexia	10 (100)
Weight loss	9 (90)
Vomiting	4 (40)
Waxing-waning course of illness	4 (40)
Previous response to therapy	3 (30)
Polyuria/polydipsia	3 (30)
Physical Examination Findings	
Depression	10 (100)
Weakness	9 (90)
Dehydration	9 (90)
Hypothermia	8 (80)
Slow capillary refill time	5 (50)
Weak pulse	5 (50)
Collapse/unable to rise	3 (30)
Bradycardia	2 (20)
Painful abdomen	1 (10)

*From Peterson ME, et al: Primary hyperadrenocorticism in ten cats. J Vet Intern Med 3:55, 1989.

Laboratory, Radiographic, and ECG Abnormalities

Hematologic abnormalities were not common but included mild anemia. Rarely, lymphocytosis or eosinophilia has been noted. All the cats have been hyponatremic, and all but one were hyperkalemic (Table 8-20). Hypochloremia, azotemia, and hyperphosphatemia were identified in almost all cats. Each cat had an abnormal sodium:potassium ratio (<24:1). The hyperkalemia was not as severe as has been observed in dogs, with values of 5.4 to 7.6 mEq/L reported. Three of 10 cats were mildly acidotic, and one was hypercalcemic (serum calcium concentration of 14 mg/dl). Hypoglycemia has been observed in one cat seen in our series. The differential diagnosis for hypoglycemia in cats is similar to that noted in dogs (Thompson et al, 1995).

The urine specific gravity was less than 1.030 in seven of 10 cats with naturally occurring Addison's disease. All 10 cats were dehydrated and azotemic. The BUN concentration ranged from 31 to 80 mg/dl, with a mean of 55 mg/dl. Thus a tentative but incorrect diagnosis of renal failure in a cat with test results such as these would be well supported. As with dogs, similarities between the clinical descriptions, physical

TABLE 8-20 RESULTS OF LABORATORY TESTS IN 10 CATS WITH HYPOADRENOCORTICISM*

Test	Mean SD	Range	Normal Range
Packed cell volume (%)	29.5 ± 5.8	21.2–39.2	25–38
Erythrocyte count × 10⁶/mm³	6.4 ± 1.5	4.6–9.0	6–8.5
Hemoglobin (g/dl)	10.3 ± 1.7	7.3–12.6	8–15
Leukocytes/mm	11.656 ± 4335	7200–20,100	7000–15,000
Mature neutrophils	7586 ± 3514	4320–15,875	3500–11,250
Band neutrophils	144 ± 151	0–344	0–450
Lymphocytes	3348 ± 2233	1118–8410	1400–6000
Eosinophils	598 ± 935	145–3015	140–1400
Monocytes	178 ± 204	0–612	70–600
Serum glucose (mg/dl)	99.2 ± 24.9	71–139	70–150
Alanine aminotransferase (IU/L)	62.0 ± 21.0	43–100	10–80
Alkaline phosphatase (IU/L)	36.0 ± 29.7	10–108	10–80
Total bilirubin (mg/dl)	0.39 ± 0.23	0.1–0.8	0–0.5
Total protein (mg/dl)	6.5 ± 0.8	5.6–7.5	5.3–7.9
Albumin (mg/dl)	2.9 ± 0.5	2.3–3.5	2.3–3.8
Blood urea nitrogen (mg/dl)	55.6 ± 16.5	31–80	5–30
Creatinine (mg/dl)	3.2 ± 1.5	1.6–6.0	0.5–1.5
Total CO_2 (mEq/L)	18.6 ± 3.8	13–24	16–25
Inorganic phosphorus (mg/dl)	7.3 ± 0.94	6.1–9.1	3.0–6.0
Calcium (mg/dl)	10.7 ± 3.4	8.6–14.0	7.6–11.0
Sodium (mEq/L)	130.6 ± 8.1	111–138	140–155
Potassium (mEq/L)	6.2 ± 0.6	5.4–7.6	3.5–5.5
Chloride (mEq/L)	96.3 ± 9.7	74–108	100–120
Sodium:potassium ratio	21.0 ± 1.7	17.9–23.7	>26
Urine specific gravity	1.028 ± 0.014	1.008–1.045	1.001–1.080
Serum cortisol (µg/dl)			
Basal	0.26 ± 0.28	0.1–0.8	0.5–5.0[†]
1-hour post-ACTH	0.29 ± 0.37	0.1–1.1	4.5–13.0[†]
2-hour post-ACTH	0.39 ± 0.44	0.1–1.3	4.0–14.5[†]
Plasma ACTH (pg/ml)	3767 ± 2667	500–8000	10–125[‡]

*From Peterson ME, et al: Primary adrenocorticism in ten cats. J Vet Intern Med 3:55, 1989; used with permission.
[†]ACTH stimulation tests were performed in 33 clinically normal cats; mean ± SD: basal, 1-hour post-ACTH, and 2-hour post-ACTH cortisol concentrations were 2.1 ± 1.5 µg/dl, 7.9 ± 2.9 µg/dl, and 8.1 ± 2.7 µg/dl, respectively.
[‡]Immunoreactive plasma ACTH concentrations were determined in 50 clinically normal cats; the mean (± SD) value was 36.7 ± 36.0 pg/ml.
SD, Standard deviation; ACTH, adrenocorticotropic hormone.

findings, and test results for cats with renal disease (which is common) and those with hypoadreno-corticism (which is rare) make diagnosis of the latter condition difficult.

Microcardia was identified on thoracic radiographs of five cats. This nonspecific finding supports the observed dehydration, hypovolemia, and hypotension thought to be present in these cats. Other cardio-vascular abnormalities were not observed. Identified ECG abnormalities consisted of sinus bradycardia in two cats and atrial premature contractions in one cat. The characteristic changes in the T wave, P wave, P-R interval, and QRS complexes seen with hyperkalemia in dogs were not identified in these cats. The lack of these *classic* abnormalities on ECG are probably due to the relatively mild hyperkalemia documented in each of the cats.

Confirming the Diagnosis: Plasma Cortisol Concentrations

PROTOCOL. The ACTH stimulation test is the "gold standard" for diagnosis in cats, just as it is in humans and dogs. However, the protocol in cats is slightly different from that used in dogs. With syn-thetic ACTH (Cortrosyn), one-half vial (0.125 mg) should be administered intramuscularly, with blood samples obtained immediately before and 30 and 60 minutes after injection. If ACTH gel is used, 2.2 U/kg should be administered intramuscularly, with blood samples obtained before and 60 and 120 minutes after injection.

RESULTS. As is true in humans and in dogs, the diagnosis of hypoadrenocorticism in cats can be confirmed or refuted with the results of an ACTH stimulation test. The expected results in hypoadrenal cats are no different from those for hypoadrenal dogs: the pre-ACTH plasma cortisol concentration is usually undetectable or low-normal and the post-ACTH plasma cortisol concentration is similar to the pre-ACTH value. As in dogs, all plasma cortisol results (both pre-ACTH and post-ACTH) from addisonian cats were less than 2.0 µg/dl (see Table 8-20). The basal plasma cortisol con-centrations ranged from 0.1 to 0.8 µg/dl (normal is 0.5 to 5.0 µg/dl). The 1- and 2-hour results were 0.1 to 1.1 µg/dl and 0.1 to 1.3 µg/dl, respectively (normal is 4.5 to 13.0 µg/dl) (see Table 8-20) (Peterson et al, 1989).

DIFFERENTIAL DIAGNOSIS. The differential diagnosis for abnormal serum sodium and potassium concen-trations should include gastrointestinal disease, renal disease, and ascites (Bissett et al, 2001). The differential diagnosis for low plasma cortisol concentrations includes naturally occurring hypoadrenocorticism, chronic glucocorticoid administration, chronic megestrol acetate administration (Chastain et al, 1982), and failure to administer ACTH. The differential diagnosis of hypoadrenocorticism should include lymphoma, because this form of cancer is common and adrenal involvement has now been demonstrated to be possible (Parnell et al, 1999).

Plasma Endogenous ACTH

RESULTS. Plasma ACTH concentrations were measured in 7 of 10 cats with naturally occurring disease. Each cat had abnormally increased concentra-tions consistent with the diagnosis of primary adreno-cortical destruction and lack of negative feedback to the pituitary. The values ranged from 500 to 8000 pg/ml, with a mean of 3767 pg/ml (reference range for that assay is <10 to 125 pg/ml; see Table 8-20).

DIFFERENTIAL DIAGNOSIS. The differential diagnosis for cats with abnormally low plasma cortisol concen-trations and an abnormally increased endogenous ACTH concentration includes any disorder that causes destruction of the adrenal cortices (e.g., naturally occur-ring autoimmune destruction, trauma, and lymphoma). This pattern of endocrine test results is also obtained with inhibition or blockage of cortisol synthesis and/or secretion, which could be the result of treatment with drugs, such as ketoconazole, that block the synthesis of cortisol.

Cats treated chronically with glucocorticoids or progestogens (megestrol acetate) also have low to nondetectable levels of cortisol in the circulation (Middleton et al, 1987). These cats, however, have low plasma cortisol concentrations because the drugs block pituitary secretion of ACTH, resulting in adrenocortical atrophy. Thus they have low cortisol concentrations *and* low ACTH concentrations. They have *secondary* adrenocortical atrophy, and they usually have normal serum electrolyte concentrations because the renin-angiotensin-aldosterone system has not been inter-rupted; this system is minimally affected by ACTH. Any process that interferes with pituitary secretion of ACTH (e.g., pituitary trauma, tumor, inflammation) would result in similar endocrine test results.

Treatment

MANAGEMENT OF THE CAT IN HYPOADRENAL CRISIS. The principles of therapy for this condition in cats are no different from those in dogs. Initial therapy includes aggressive intravenous administration of 0.9% normal saline (40 ml/kg for 2 to 4 hours) to replace fluid deficits and restore blood pressure. After that has been accomplished, maintenance fluid (approximately 60 ml/kg/day) should be administered and slowly tapered until the cat is eating and drinking with no vomiting or diarrhea. Glucocorticoid deficits should be replaced with dexamethasone (0.1 to 2 mg/kg IV or IM q6-12h). Ideally, the ACTH stimulation test is completed prior to administration of glucocorticoids. Mineralocorticoids can be administered in the form of DOCP (2.2 mg/kg IM every 25 days).

One feature of hypoadrenocorticism that is some-what different in cats than in dogs is the slow response to therapy. Cats appear to remain weak, lethargic, and depressed for 3 to 5 days despite institution of appro-priate therapy. Three of 10 cats were euthanized after only 2 to 5 days of treatment because of poor response.

It is possible that they may have survived had they been treated for a longer period.

LONG-TERM (CHRONIC) THERAPY. As with acute management, chronic therapy is no different from that recommended for dogs. Chronic mineralocorticoid therapy involves oral fludrocortisone acetate (0.05 to 0.10 mg bid) or injectable DOCP. Glucocorticoid replacement, as needed, is usually accomplished with prednisone (0.5 to 2 mg/day, divided bid). Regular physical examinations, in addition to periodic monitoring of owner opinion regarding clinical response; serum electrolyte concentrations; and BUN levels are strongly recommended, as for dogs, to ensure that proper dosages are being given.

Prognosis

The long-term survival of cats with hypoadrenocorticism is excellent. As with dogs, owners who are aggressive and committed to helping their cats tend to have the best success. Frequent rechecks to ensure that drug dosing and frequency are optimal is valuable. Six of seven cats that survived the hypoadrenal crisis were alive for a mean of 34 months (Peterson et al, 1989).

REFERENCES

Addison T: On the constitutional and local effects of disease of the suprarenal capsules. London, Highley, 1855.

Adrogue HJ, Madias NE: Hyponatremia. N Engl J Med 342:1581, 2000.

Ames Technical Information on Seralyzer Reflectance Photometer: A quantitative strip test for potassium in serum or plasma. 1986.

Auge P: Addison's disease in littermates. Vet Med 80:43, 1985.

Baajafer FS, et al: Hyponatremia and hypercreatinemia in short-term uncomplicated hypothyroidism. J Endocrinol Invest 22:35, 1999.

Bagley RS, et al: Hypoglycemia associated with intraabdominal leimyoma and leimyosarcoma in six dogs. J Am Vet Med Assoc 208:69, 1996.

Bartges J, Nielson D: Reversible megaesophagus associated with atypical primary hypoadrenocorticism in a dog. J Am Vet Med Assoc 201:889, 1992.

Baxter JD, Tyrrell JB: The adrenal cortex. In Felig P, et al (eds): Endocrinology and Metabolism. New York, McGraw-Hill, 1981, p 385.

Beaudry D, et al: Hypoglycemia in four dogs with smooth muscle tumors. J Vet Intern Med 9:415, 1995.

Bennish ML, et al: Hypoglycemia during diarrhea in childhood. N Engl J Med 322:1357, 1990.

Berger SL, Reed J: Traumatically induced hypoadrenocorticism in a cat. J Am Anim Hosp Assoc 29:337, 1993.

Bethune JE: The diagnosis and treatment of adrenal insufficiency. In DeGroot LJ (ed): Endocrinology, 2nd ed. Philadelphia, WB Saunders, 1989, p 1647.

Bissett SA, et al: Hyponatremia and hyperkalemia associated with peritoneal effusion in four cats. J Am Vet Med Assoc 218:1590, 2001.

Boujon CE, et al: Pituitary gland changes in canine hypoadrenocorticism: A functional and immunocytochemical study. J Comp Pathol 111:287, 1994.

Bowen D, et al: Autoimmune polyglandular syndrome in a dog: A case report. J Am Anim Hosp Assoc 22:649, 1986.

Brady CA, et al: Severe neurologic sequelae in a dog after treatment of hypoadrenal crisis. J Am Vet Med Assoc 215:222, 1999.

Burrows C: Reversible megaesophagus in a dog with hypoadrenocorticism. J Small Anim Pract 28:1073, 1987.

Chastain CB, et al: Adrenocortical suppression in cats administered megestrol acetate. American College of Veterinary Internal Medicine Scientific Proceedings, Salt Lake City, 1982, p 54 (abstract).

Chastain CB, et al: A screening evaluation for endogenous glucocorticoid deficiency in dogs: A modified Thorn test. J Am Anim Hosp Assoc 25:18, 1989.

Chen S, et al: Autoantibodies to steroidogenic enzymes in autoimmune polyglandular syndrome, Addison's disease, and premature ovarian failure. J Clin Endocrinol Metab 81:1871, 1996.

Chow E, et al: Toxicity of desoxycorticosterone pivalate given at high dosages to clinically normal Beagles for six months. Am J Vet Res 54:1954, 1993.

Church DB: personal communication, 2002.

Church DB, et al: Plasma cortisol concentrations in normal dogs given hydrocortisone sodium succinate. Aust Vet J 77:316, 1999.

DiBartola SP: Hyponatremia. Vet Clin North Am (Small Anim Pract) 19:215, 1989.

DiBartola SP, et al: Clinicopathologic findings resembling hypoadrenocorticism in dogs with primary gastrointestinal disease. J Am Vet Med Assoc 187:60, 1985.

Dunn KJ, Herrtage ME: Hypoadrenocorticism in a Labrador retriever. J Small Anim Pract 39:90, 1998.

Elliott J, et al: Hypercalcemia in the dog: A study of 40 cases. J Small Anim Pract 32:564, 1991.

Feldman EC, Nelson RW: Canine and Feline Endocrinology and Reproduction. Philadelphia, WB Saunders, 1987.

Feldman EC, et al: Comparison of aqueous porcine ACTH with synthetic ACTH in adrenal stimulation tests of the female dog. Am J Vet Res 43:522, 1982.

Findling JW, Tyrrell JB: Anterior pituitary gland. In Greenspan FS (ed): Basic and Clinical Endocrinology, 3rd ed. San Mateo, Calif, Appleton & Lange, 1991, p 79.

Findling JW, et al: Glucocorticoids and adrenal androgens. In Greenspan FS, Strewler GJ (eds): Basic and Clinical Endocrinology, 5th ed. Stamford, Conn, Appleton & Lange, 1997, p 317.

Fossum TW, Birchard SJ: Lymphangiographic evaluation of experimentally induced chylothorax after ligation of the cranial vena cava in dogs. Am J Vet Res 47:976, 1986.

Freudiger U: Literaturubersicht uber Nebennierenrinden - Erkrankungen der Katze und Beschreibung eines Falles von primarer Nebennierenrinden - Insuffizienz. Schweiz Arch Tierheilk 128:221, 1986.

Ganong WF: Review of Medical Physiology, 10th ed. Los Altos, Calif, Lange Medical Publications, 1981.

Golden D, Lothrop CJ: A retrospective study of aldosterone secretion in normal and adrenopathic dogs. J Vet Intern Med 2:121, 1988.

Graves TK, et al: Basal and ACTH-stimulated plasma aldosterone concentrations are normal or increased in dogs with trichuriasis-pseudohypoadrenocorticism. J Vet Intern Med 8:287, 1994.

Hardy RM: Hypoadrenocorticism. In Ettinger SJ, Feldman EC (eds): Textbook of Veterinary Internal Medicine, 4th ed. Philadelphia, WB Saunders, 1995.

Herrtage ME: Hypoadrenocorticism. In Torrence AG, Mooney CT (eds): BSAVA Manual of Small Animal Endocrinology, 2nd ed. BSAVA, United Kingdom, 1998, pp 75-82.

Johnsessee JS, et al: Primary hypoadrenocorticism in a cat. J Am Vet Med Assoc 183:881, 1983.

Kaplan AJ, Peterson ME: Effects of desoxycorticosterone pivalate administration on blood pressure in dogs with primary hypoadrenocorticism. J Am Vet Med Assoc 206:327, 1995.

Kelch WJ, et al: Canine hypoadrenocorticism (Addison's disease). Comp Small Anim Pract 20:921, 1998.

Kemppainen RJ, et al: Adrenocortical suppression in the dog after a single dose of methylprednisolone acetate. Am J Vet Res 42:822, 1981.

Kemppainen RJ, et al: Adrenocortical suppression in the dog given a single intramuscular dose of prednisone or triamcinolone acetonide. Am J Vet Res 43:204, 1982.

Kintzer PP, Peterson ME: Treatment and long-term follow-up of 205 dogs with hypoadrenocorticism. J Vet Intern Med 11:43, 1997.

Kooistra HS, et al: Polyglandular deficiency syndrome in a Boxer dog: Thyroid hormone and glucocorticoid deficiency. Vet Q 17:59, 1995.

Lamb WA, et al: Effect of chronic hypocortisolemia on plasma cortisol concentrations during intravenous infusions of hydrocortisone sodium succinate in dogs. Res Vet Sci 57:349, 1994.

Lamberts SWJ, et al: Corticosteroid therapy in severe illness. N Engl J Med 337:1285, 1997.

Langlais-Burgess L, et al: Concurrent hypoadrenocorticism and hypoalbuminemia in dogs: A retrospective study. J Am Anim Hosp Assoc 31:307, 1995.

Levy JK: Hypoglycemic seizures attributable to hypoadrenocorticism in a dog. J Am Vet Med Assoc 204:526, 1994.

Lifton SJ, et al: Glucocorticoid-deficient hypoadrenocorticism in dogs: 18 cases (1986-1995). J Am Vet Med Assoc 209:2076, 1996.

Lobetti RG: Hyperreninaemic hypoaldosteronism in a dog. J S Afr Vet Assoc 69:33, 1998.

Lynn R, Feldman EC: Treatment of hypoadrenocorticism with microcrystalline desoxycorticosterone pivalate. Br Vet J 147:478, 1991.

Lynn R, et al: Efficacy of microcrystalline desoxycorticosterone pivalate for treatment of hypoadrenocorticism in dogs. J Am Vet Med Assoc 202:392, 1993.

McCabe M, et al: Subcutaneous administration of desoxycorticosterone pivalate for the treatment of canine hypoadrenocorticism. J Am Anim Hosp Assoc 31:151, 1995.

Medinger TL, et al: Severe gastrointestinal tract hemorrhage in three dogs with hypoadrenocorticism. J Am Vet Med Assoc 202:1869, 1993.

Melian C, Peterson ME: Diagnosis and treatment of naturally occurring hypoadrenocorticism in 42 dogs. J Am Anim Pract 37:268, 1996.

Middleton D, et al: Suppression of cortisol response to exogenous adrenocorticotropic hormone and the side effects of glucocorticoid excess in cats during therapy with megestrol acetate and prednisolone. Can J Vet Res 51:60, 1987.

Montoll A, et al: Hypercalcemia in Addison's disease: Calciotropic hormone profile and bone histology. J Intern Med 232:535, 1992.

Moore G, Hoenig M: Duration of pituitary and adrenocortical suppression after long-term administration of antiinflammatory doses of prednisone to dogs. Am J Vet Res 53:716, 1992.

Moriello K, et al: Adrenocortical suppression associated with topical administration of glucocorticoids in dogs. J Am Vet Med Assoc 193:329, 1988.

Murphy CJ, et al: Iatrogenic Cushing's syndrome in a dog caused by topical ophthalmic medications. J Am Anim Hosp Assoc 26:640, 1990.

Nelson DH: The Adrenal Cortex: Physiological Function and Disease. Philadelphia, WB Saunders, 1980, p 113.

Oberbauer AM, et al: Inheritance of hypoadrenocorticism in Bearded Collies. Am J Vet Res 63:643, 2002.

O'Brien DP, et al: Myelinolysis after correction of hyponatremia in two dogs. J Vet Intern Med 8:40, 1994.

Oelkers W: Adrenal insufficiency. N Engl J Med 335:1206, 1996.

Olson PN, et al: Effects of storage on concentration of hydrocortisone (cortisol) in canine serum and plasma. Am J Vet Res 42:1618, 1981.

Ortega TM, et al: Plasma aldosterone concentrations in dogs before and after o,p'-DDD therapy for pituitary-dependent hyperadrenocorticism. J Vet Intern Med 9:182, 1995 (abstract).

Parnell NK, et al: Hypoadrenocorticism as the primary manifestation of lymphoma in two cats. J Am Vet Med Assoc 214:1208, 1999.

Peterson ME, Feinman JM: Hypercalcemia associated with hypoadrenocorticism in 16 dogs. J Am Vet Med Assoc 181:802, 1982.

Peterson ME, et al: Primary hypoadrenocorticism in ten cats. J Vet Intern Med 3:55, 1989.

Peterson ME, et al: Pretreatment clinical and laboratory findings in dogs with hypoadrenocorticism: 225 cases (1979-1993). J Am Vet Med Assoc 208:85, 1996.

Ramsay DJ: Renal hormones and endocrine hypertension. In Greenspan FS (ed): Basic and Clinical Endocrinology, 3rd ed. San Mateo, Calif, Appleton & Lange, 1991, p 400.

Reusch CE: Hypoadrenocorticism. In Ettinger SJ, Feldman EC (eds): Textbook of Veterinary Internal Medicine, 5th ed. Philadelphia, WB Saunders, 2000, pp 1488-1499.

Rich LJ, et al: Elevated serum potassium associated with delayed separation of serum from clotted blood in dogs of the Akita breed. Vet Clin Pathol 15:12, 1986.

Roberts S, et al: Effect of ophthalmic prednisolone acetate on the canine adrenal gland and hepatic function. Am J Vet Res 45:1711, 1984.

Rogers W, et al: Atypical hypoadrenocorticism in three dogs. J Am Vet Med Assoc 179:155, 1981.

Rose BD: Clinical Physiology of Acid-Base Disorders, 2nd ed. New York, McGraw-Hill, 1984, p 567.

Roth L, Tyler RD: Evaluation of low sodium:potassium ratios in dogs. J Vet Diagn Invest 11:60, 1999.

Rothenberg ME: Eosinophilia. N Engl J Med 338:1592, 1998.

Sadek D, Schaer M: Atypical Addison's disease in the dog: A retrospective survey of 14 cases. J Am Anim Hosp Assoc 32:159, 1996.

Schaer M: Hypoadrenocorticism. In Kirk RW (ed): Current Veterinary Therapy VIII. Philadelphia, WB Saunders, 1980, p 983.

Schaer M: The atypical addisonian dog. Proceedings of the North American Veterinary Conference, Orlando, FL, 1994, p 219.

Schaer M, et al: Autoimmunity and Addison's disease in the dog. J Am Anim Hosp Assoc 22:789, 1986.

Schaer M, et al: Combined hyponatremia and hyperkalemia mimicking an addisonian crisis in three near-term pregnant Greyhounds. J Vet Intern Med 14:121, 2000.

Shaker E, et al: Hypoadrenocorticism in a family of Standard Poodles. J Am Vet Med Assoc 192:1091, 1988.

Smallwood LJ, Barsanti J: Hypoadrenocorticism in a family of Leonbergers. J Am Anim Hosp Assoc 31:301, 1995.

Soderbergh A, et al: Adrenal autoantibodies and organ-specific autoimmunity in patients with Addison's disease. Clin Endocrinol 45:453, 1996.

Syme HM, Scott-Moncrieff JC: Chronic hypoglycemia in a hunting dog due to secondary hypoadrenocorticism. J Small Anim Pract 39:348, 1998.

Thodou E, et al: Lymphocytic hypophysitis: Clinicopathological findings. J Clin Endocrinol Metab 80:2302, 1995.

Thompson JC, et al: Observations on hypoglycaemia associated with a hepatoma in a cat. N Z Vet J 43:186, 1995.

Tyler R, et al: Renal concentrating in dehydrated hyponatremic dogs. J Am Vet Med Assoc 191:1095, 1987.

Tyrrell JB, et al: Glucocorticoids and adrenal androgens. In Greenspan FS (ed): Basic and Clinical Endocrinology, 3rd ed. Philadelphia, WB Saunders, 1991, p 323.

van den Broek A: Serum protein values in canine diabetes mellitus, hypothyroidism and hypoadrenocorticism. Br Vet J 148:259, 1992.

Vance ML: Hypopituitarism. N Engl J Med 330:1651, 1994.

Velardo A, et al: Isolated adrenocorticotropic hormone deficiency secondary to hypothalamic deficit of corticotropin-releasing hormone. J Endocrinol Invest 15:53, 1992.

Walters PC, Drobatz KJ: Hypoglycemia. Comp Small Anim Pract 14:1149, 1992.

White PC: Disorders of aldosterone biosynthesis and action. N Engl J Med 331:250, 1994.

Whitley NT: Megaesophagus and glucocorticoid-deficient hypoadrenocorticism in a dog. J Am Anim Pract 36:132, 1995.

Willard MD: Disorders of potassium homeostasis. Vet Clin North Am (Small Anim Pract) 19:241, 1989.

Willard MD, et al: Canine hypoadrenocorticism: Report of 37 cases and review of 39 previously reported cases. J Am Vet Med Assoc 180:59, 1982.

Willard MD, et al: Evaluation of plasma aldosterone concentrations before and after ACTH administration in clinically normal dogs and dogs with various diseases. Am J Vet Res 48:713, 1987.

Willard MD, et al: Hyponatremia and hyperkalemia associated with idiopathic or experimentally induced chylothorax in four dogs. J Am Vet Med Assoc 199:353, 1991.

Zenger E: Persistent hyperkalemia associated with nonchylous pleural effusion in a dog. J Am Anim Hosp Assoc 28:411, 1992.

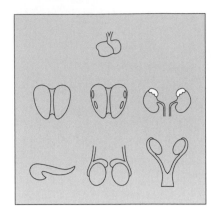

9

PHEOCHROMOCYTOMA AND MULTIPLE ENDOCRINE NEOPLASIA

PHEOCHROMOCYTOMA

Pheochromocytoma is a catecholamine-secreting tumor arising from the adrenal medulla. Historically, pheochromocytoma was most commonly identified as an incidental finding at necropsy; an antemortem diagnosis was uncommon in dogs and rare in cats (Schaer, 1980; Twedt and Wheeler, 1984; Bouayad et al, 1987; Henry et al, 1993; Gilson et al, 1994). This was due, in part, to a low index of suspicion for pheochromocytoma by veterinarians, the often vague and episodic nature of the clinical signs which were frequently attributed to other more common disorders, and the lack of a good diagnostic screening test for the disease. With the establishment of abdominal ultrasound as part of the routine diagnostic evaluation of the ill dog or cat, the identification of adrenal masses and consequently the consideration of pheochromocytoma has increased tremendously during the past decade. To illustrate this point, pheochromocytoma was suspected antemortem in only 11 confirmed cases seen at our hospital between 1984 and 1994 but was suspected antemortem in 33 confirmed cases between 1996 and 2002.

Etiology

The endocrine cells of the adrenal medulla are called chromaffin cells. They are derived from the neuroectoderm and are capable of synthesizing, storing, and secreting catecholamines (epinephrine and norepinephrine). Although most chromaffin cells are in the adrenal medulla, small numbers of extra-adrenal chromaffin cells also exist in and about sympathetic ganglia. The function of the extra-adrenal chromaffin cells is not known. Most regress early in postnatal development, although remnants may become the site of subsequent tumor formation (Young and Landsberg, 1998).

Pheochromocytoma is a catecholamine-producing tumor derived from the chromaffin cells. Pheochromocytoma arising from the chromaffin cells in the adrenal medulla is most common, may occur in one or both adrenal glands, and may be part of the multiple endocrine neoplasia syndrome (see page 459). Approximately 10% of catecholamine-secreting tumors in humans arise from extra-adrenal chromaffin cells and are called paragangliomas. Paragangliomas are located primarily within the abdomen but may also be found in the heart, the posterior mediastinum, along the aorta, in and around the kidney, and the urinary bladder wall (Goldfien, 2001; Young and Landsberg, 1998). Paragangliomas are rare in the dog and cat (Patnaik et al, 1990; Hines et al, 1993; Barthez et al, 1997; Buchanan et al, 1998).

Pheochromocytomas are usually solitary, slow-growing, vascular tumors ranging in size from nodules of less than 0.5 cm in diameter to masses greater than 10 cm in diameter. Pheochromocytomas affecting both adrenal glands and pheochromocytoma with an adrenocortical tumor in the contralateral adrenal gland have also been reported (Bouayad et al, 1987; Gilson et al, 1994; von Dehn et al, 1995; Bennett and Norman, 1998). Pheochromocytomas should be considered a malignant tumor in dogs (Bouayad et al, 1987). Approximately 40% of our dogs with pheochromocytoma had invasion or extension of the tumor into the lumen of the adjacent vena cava or phrenico-abdominal vein and/or entrapment and compression of the caudal vena cava. Mural invasion and/or luminal narrowing of the aorta, renal vessels, adrenal vessels, and hepatic veins may also occur (Bouayad et al, 1987). Approximately 30% of our dogs had metastasis of the tumor at the time of necropsy. Distant sites of metastasis include the liver, lung, regional lymph nodes, spleen, heart, kidney, bone, pancreas, CNS, and spinal canal (Gilson et al, 1994; Barthez et al, 1997).

Gross and histologic differentiation of pheochromocytoma from adrenocortical neoplasia can be difficult, especially with large tumors. Immuno-histochemical staining for chromogranin A and synaptophysin can be used to determine the site of origin (i.e., adrenal cortex vs medulla) of the tumor; techniques which are routinely performed on suspected adrenal medullary tumors in our hospital. Synaptophysin is a membrane component of synaptic vesicles in neurons and neuroendocrine cells. Chromogranin A is a protein present in the secretory granules of endocrine cells and functions in hormone packaging, secretory granule stabilization, and regulation of hormone secretion (Winkler and Fischer-Colbrie, 1992). Chromogranin A is a major constituent of secretory granules of the adrenal medulla, pituitary, parathyroid, thyroid C cells, pancreatic islets, endocrine cells of the gastrointestinal tract, and sympathetic nerves (Doss et al, 1998). Chromogranin A is not present in the cells of the adrenal cortex. In dogs, tumors with the strongest and most consistently positive chromogranin A staining are the pheochromocytoma and chemodectoma. Parathyroid, pituitary, and islet cell tumors yield inconsistent results. Endocrine tumors that produce chromogranin A may also co-secrete immunoreactive chromogranin A into the circulation, along with their characteristic hormone (Deftos et al, 1989). Documentation of increased concentrations of plasma chromogranin A has been proposed as a screening test to identify peptide-producing endocrine neoplasms in humans (O'Connor and Deftos, 1986; Hsiao et al, 1991), and changes in plasma chromogranin A concentrations have been used as a marker for treatment response (Moattari et al, 1989). Measurement of circulating chromogranin A concentration as a means to identify pheochromocytoma has not yet been reported in dogs or cats.

Pathophysiology

Pheochromocytoma is a tumor of the sympathetic nervous system. Preganglionic fibers of the sympathetic nervous system are cholinergic and liberate acetylcholine as their neurotransmitter. Postganglionic fibers are adrenergic and liberate norepinephrine and dopamine. The adrenal medulla can be viewed as sympathetic postganglionic neurons without axons. Normally, norepinephrine and epinephrine are both secreted by the adrenal medulla. However, the normal adrenal gland harbors high concentrations of the N-methylating enzyme, which converts norepinephrine to epinephrine, so that epinephrine is the predominant catecholamine produced by the adrenal medulla (Werbel and Ober, 1995). In cats, dogs, and humans,

60%, 70%, and 80% of catecholamine output from the adrenal medulla is epinephrine, respectively (Goldfien, 2001). Circulating norepinephrine is also derived from autonomic nerve endings. In contrast, most pheochromocytomas in humans contain predominantly norepinephrine or a mixture of norepinephrine, epinephrine, and dopamine (Prys-Roberts, 2000). Tumors rarely produce epinephrine exclusively (Young and Landsberg, 1998). Paragangliomas usually secrete norepinephrine. Evaluation of catecholamine secretory patterns for pheochromocytoma in the dog and cat have not been reported.

Although the biosynthesis and storage of catecholamines in pheochromocytomas may be different than in the normal adrenal medulla, chromaffin granules from pheochromocytomas are morphologically, physically, and functionally similar to chromaffin granules of the adrenal medulla (Johnson et al, 1982; Roizen et al, 1984). The increase in tissue turnover of catecholamines in vitro and in vivo in some tumors suggests an alteration in the regulation of catecholamine biosynthesis, possibly because of an impairment in feedback inhibition of tyrosine hydroxylase. The primary rate-limiting step in the synthesis of catecholamines is the hydroxylation of tyrosine by the enzyme tyrosine hydroxylase (Fig. 9-1). Cytoplasmic concentrations of norepinephrine normally act directly to inhibit the activity of tyrosine hydroxylase and thereby control catecholamine production (Young and Landsberg, 1998). With sympathetic nerve stimulation, the negative feedback inhibition of norepinephrine on tyrosine hydroxylase is removed, as newly formed and stored norepinephrine is released from the cell into the extracellular space. Increased enzyme activity

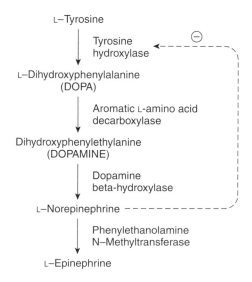

FIGURE 9–1. Biosynthetic pathway for the catecholamines. The formation of epinephrine takes place in the adrenal medulla, in neurons of the central nervous system, and in peripheral ganglia that use epinephrine as a neurotransmitter. Norepinephrine is the primary control of catecholamine synthesis via feedback inhibition of tyrosine hydroxylase. (From Twedt DC, Wheeler SL: Vet Clin North Am [Small Anim Pract] 1984; 14:767.)

then promotes further norepinephrine synthesis. In pheochromocytomas, ordinary intracellular concentrations of norepinephrine do not inhibit tyrosine hydroxylase. In addition, the turnover rate of catecholamines may be markedly increased, thereby preventing negative feedback inhibition of tyrosine hydroxylase.

The mechanisms of catecholamine release from pheochromocytoma are poorly understood. Unlike the normal adrenal gland, pheochromocytomas are not innervated and catecholamine release is not initiated by neural impulses. Stimulation of catecholamine secretion in response to physiologic stressors such as hypotension, low tissue perfusion, hypoxia, hypoglycemia, fear, and stress is variable and unpredictable. Direct pressure, manipulation of the tumor during surgery, and a variety of pharmacologic agents may initiate catecholamine release. Why some tumors release excessive hormone constantly and others do so paroxysmally is not understood.

The clinical manifestations of pheochromocytoma are predictable from the known physiologic and pharmacologic effects of catecholamines (Tables 9-1 and 9-2). The catecholamines epinephrine, norepinephrine, and dopamine exert their physiologic effects by interactions with appropriate receptors at the target tissue. Two classes of receptors (alpha [α] and beta [β]) exist which are capable of responding to epinephrine and norepinephrine. α-receptors are further subdivided into α1 and α2 receptors, and β-receptors into β1-, β2-, and β3-receptors. α1-receptors mediate a wide variety of effects, most prominently involving smooth muscle and including vasoconstriction, intestinal relaxation, uterine contraction, and pu pillary dilation (Young and Landsberg, 1998; Goldfien, 2001). α2-receptors are located on presynaptic sympathetic neurons, on cholinergic neurons within the gut, on CNS neurons involved in the regulation of cardiovascular function, on platelets, and on blood vessels. The α2-receptor mediates inhibition of norepinephrine release from adrenergic neurons, inhibition of acetylcholine release from cholinergic neurons, potentiation of the baroreceptor vasodepressor response mediated through central regulatory neurons, platelet aggregation, and vasoconstriction. β-receptors primarily mediate cardiac stimulation, bronchodilatation, and vasodilatation. The β1-receptor mediates cardiac stimulation and lipolysis; the β2-receptor mediates bronchodilatation, vasodilatation, and prejunctional stimulation of norepinephrine release from sympathetic neurons; and the β3-receptors primarily regulate energy expenditure and lipolysis.

TABLE 9-1 SELECTED PHARMACOLOGIC ACTIONS OF CATECHOLAMINES ON VARIOUS EFFECTOR ORGANS*

Effector Organ	Receptor Type	Response
Eye		
Radial muscle of iris	Alpha-1	Contraction (mydriasis)
Heart		
SA node	Beta-1	Increase heart rate
Atria	Beta-1	Increase contractility, conduction velocity
AV node and conduction system	Beta-1	Increase conduction velocity
Ventricles	Beta-1	Increase contractility, conduction velocity
Arterioles		
Coronary, skeletal muscle, renal, abdominal viscera	Alpha-1	Vasoconstriction
Skin and mucosa, cerebral, pulmonary, salivary glands	Beta-2	Vasodilatation
	Alpha-1	Vasoconstriction
Systemic veins	Alpha-1	Vasoconstriction
	Beta-2	Vasodilatation
Bronchial smooth muscle	Beta-2	Bronchodilation
Stomach		
Motility	Alpha, beta-2	Decreased motility
Sphincters	Alpha	Increased tone
Intestine		
Motility	Alpha, beta-2	Decreased motility
Sphincters	Alpha	Increased tone
Exocrine pancreas	Alpha	Inhibit secretion
Liver	Alpha-1, beta-2	Stimulate glycogenolysis and gluconeogenesis
Kidney	Alpha-1	Stimulate gluconeogenesis
	Alpha-2	Inhibit vasopressin response
	Beta	Stimulate renin secretion
Urinary bladder		
Detrusor muscle	Beta-2	Relaxation
Trigone and sphincter	Alpha	Contraction
Uterus	Alpha	Contraction
	Beta-2	Relaxation
Adipose tissue	Beta-2, beta-3	Stimulate lipolysis
	Alpha-2	Inhibit lipolysis
Muscle	Beta-2	Stimulate glycogenolysis

*Adapted from Goldfien A: Adrenal medulla. *In* Greenspan FS, Gardner DG (eds): Basic and Clinical Endocrinology, 6th ed. New York, Lange Medical Books/McGraw-Hill, 2001, p 407.

TABLE 9–2 MAJOR EFFECTS OF CATECHOLAMINES ON HORMONE SECRETION*

Endocrine Gland	Hormone	Catecholamine Receptor	Effect on Secretion
Pancreatic islets			
Alpha cell	Glucagon	Alpha	Increase
		Beta	Increase
Beta cell	Insulin	Alpha	Decrease
		Beta	Increase
Delta cell	Somatostatin	Alpha	Decrease
		Beta	Increase
PP cell	Pancreatic polypeptide	Alpha	Decrease
		Beta	Increase
Thyroid			
Follicles	T_4, T_3	Alpha	Decrease
		Beta	Increase
C cell	Calcitonin	Alpha	Decrease
		Beta	Increase
Parathyroid	Parathyroid hormone (PTH)	Alpha	Decrease
		Beta	Increase
Adrenal cortex			
Zona fasciculata	Cortisol	?	Increase
	Androstenedione	Beta	Increase
Zona glomerulosa	Aldosterone	Dopamine	Decrease
		Beta	Increase
Gastric antrum and duodenum	Gastrin	Beta	Increase
Kidney			
Juxtaglomerular apparatus	Renin	Beta	Increase
Peritubular cells (?)	Erythropoietin	Beta	Increase
Ovary and placenta	Progesterone	Beta	Increase
Granulosa cells or corpus luteum	Oxytocin	Beta	Increase
Theca cells	Androgens	Beta	Increase
Testis	Testosterone	Beta	Increase
Pineal gland	Melatonin	Beta	Increase
Heart, atrium	Atrial natriuretic factor	Alpha, beta	Increase

*Adapted from Young JB, Landsberg L: Catecholamines and the adrenal medulla. *In* Wilson JD, Foster DW, Kronenberg HM, Larsen PR (eds): Williams Textbook of Endocrinology, 9th ed. Philadelphia, WB Saunders Co, 1998, p. 695.

The mode of action of catecholamines is related to their potency at specific receptors. Epinephrine and norepinephrine are considered equipotent at sites with α1-, α2-, and β1-receptors, whereas β2-receptors are stimulated more by epinephrine than by norepinephrine and β3-receptors are stimulated more by norepinephrine than by epinephrine. Tissue response to catecholamines is dependent on the number and type of catecholamine receptors present on the cell membrane, and the proportion of α- and β-receptors and their respective thresholds for response in the particular tissue in question (Tables 9-1 and 9-2). For example, the smooth muscle surrounding blood vessels contains both α1- and β2-receptors. α1-receptors predominate when elevated plasma concentrations of catecholamines are present, resulting in vasoconstriction and the development of hypertension, a common problem associated with pheochromocytoma.

Catecholamine action is terminated by active reuptake of catecholamines by nerve endings or metabolic transformation of the hormone into inactive metabolites which are excreted by the kidney. Two hepatic enzyme systems, monoamine oxidase and catechol-O-methyl transferase metabolize norepinephrine and epinephrine into metanephrine, normetanephrine, and finally vanillylmandelic acid (Young and Landsberg, 1998). These urinary metabolites reflect the amount of catecholamines released by adrenergic and pheochromocytoma tissue.

Signalment

Pheochromocytoma has been identified most commonly in older dogs. The mean age of 98 dogs with pheochromocytoma seen at our hospital was 11 years, with a range of 1 to 18 years (Fig. 9-2). There is no apparent sex predisposition. Fifty-seven of our dogs were male or male castrate and 41 were female or

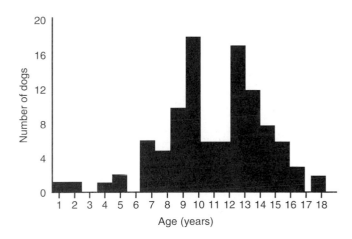

FIGURE 9–2. The age distribution of 98 dogs with pheochromocytoma. The mean and median age at the time of diagnosis was 11 years.

TABLE 9–3 BREED DISTRIBUTION AMONG 98 DOGS WITH PHEOCHROMOCYTOMA

Breed	Number of Dogs
Miniature Poodle	10
German Shepherd dog	10
Boxer	7
Golden Retriever	6
Labrador Retriever	5
Doberman Pinscher	5
Shetland Sheepdog	5
Mixed Breed	5
Miniature Schnauzer	4
Dachshund	3
Great Dane	3
Siberian Husky	2
Chow Chow	2
Dalmatian	2
Rottweiler	2
Springer Spaniel	2
Weimeraner	2
Other (1 each)	23

TABLE 9–4 FREQUENCY OF CLINICAL SIGNS IN 40 DOGS WITH PHEOCHROMOCYTOMA AND IDENTIFICATION OF NO OTHER CONCURRENT DISORDER

Clinical Sign	Number of Dogs	Percentage of Dogs
Collapsing episodes*	13	33%
Weakness*	12	30%
Panting/tachypnea*	12	30%
Polyuria/polydipsia	10	25%
Lethargy	10	25%
Vomiting	9	23%
Inappetence	8	20%
Anxiety/agitation/pacing*	6	15%
Diarrhea	4	10%
Abdominal distention	4	10%
Hemorrhage (nasal, ocular, gingival)	4	10%
Acute blindness	3	8%
Tremors*	3	8%
Weight loss	3	8%
Tachycardia/"pounding" heart*	2	5%
Rear limb edema	2	5%
Tender or painful abdomen	2	5%
Adipsia	1	3%
No clinical signs	4	10%

*Usually reported to be intermittent by the owner.

female spayed. There also does not appear to be a breed predisposition, although the Miniature Poodle, German Shepherd dog, Boxer, Golden Retriever, Labrador Retriever, Doberman Pinscher, and Sheltie were the most frequently affected breeds in our group of dogs (Table 9-3). However, the higher frequency in these breeds may merely represent their current popularity in our area of the country.

An adrenal pheochromocytoma has been reported in an 11-year-old female domestic shorthair cat (Henry et al, 1993) and was an incidental finding on abdominal ultrasound in a 15-year-old domestic shorthair cat with concurrent apocrine gland adenocarcinoma (Chun et al, 1997). An extra-adrenal pheochromocytoma (paraganglioma) has been reported in an 18-year-old spayed domestic shorthair cat (Patnaik et al, 1990). The paraganglioma was located close to but not involving the left adrenal gland, and was closely adhered to the renal capsule of the left kidney.

Clinical Manifestations

Clinical signs and physical examination findings develop as a result of the space-occupying nature of the tumor and its metastatic lesions or as a result of the excessive secretion of catecholamines (Table 9-4). The most common clinical signs are generalized weakness and episodic collapse. Additional signs that may be observed by the owner or be evident during the physical examination include intermittent agitation, pacing, excessive panting, tachypnea, a 'pounding' heart, polyuria, and polydipsia. Polyuria and polydipsia may be caused by excessive catecholamine secretion or develop secondary to renal failure caused by tumor thrombus-induced interference with renal blood flow. Excess catecholamine secretion may also cause severe systemic hypertension, which can result in sudden blindness due to retinal hemorrhage and

detachment, clinical signs resulting from spontaneous hemorrhage into the retroperitoneal space, abdominal cavity or an organ, most notably neurologic signs as a result of cerebrovascular hemorrhage, or bleeding from the nasal or oral cavity (Gilson et al, 1994; Williams et al, 2001; Whittemore et al, 2001).

Catecholamine secretion is sporadic and unpredictable. As such, clinical manifestations and systemic hypertension tend to be paroxysmal and are usually not evident at the time the dog is examined. Because clinical signs are often vague, nonspecific, and easily associated with other disorders, pheochromocytoma is often not considered a possible differential diagnosis until an adrenal mass is identified with abdominal ultrasound (see Incidental Adrenal Mass, page 458). Pheochromocytoma may also be an unexpected or incidental finding at necropsy, may result in acute collapse and death from a sudden, massive, and sustained release of catecholamines by the tumor, or may cause periodic clinical signs (e.g., collapsing episodes, tachypnea, pounding heart rate) which strongly suggest pheochromocytoma at the time of initial examination.

A retrospective evaluation of 98 dogs with pheochromocytoma seen at our hospital revealed that pheochromocytoma was an incidental finding at necropsy in 22% of the dogs, was an unexpected finding at necropsy in 33% of dogs that were euthanized because of concurrent disease, resulted in acute death in 14% of dogs, was an unexpected finding during abdominal ultrasound or anesthesia (i.e., sudden surge in blood pressure) in 5% of dogs, and was the primary differential diagnosis in 26% of the 98 dogs. These later dogs had clinical manifestations (e.g., intermittent collapsing episodes, agitation, pacing, severe tachycardia, tachypnea) that strongly suggested pheochromocytoma at the time of initial examination. The suspicion for pheochromocytoma was further enhanced by identifying an adrenal mass with abdominal ultrasound.

Unfortunately, many of the clinical signs caused by pheochromocytoma are vague and usually associated with other, more common disorders. In addition, pheochromocytoma typically occurs in conjunction with other, often serious disorders (Table 9-5). Clinicians tend to focus on the more recognizable disorders and often overlook the possibility of concurrent pheochromocytoma; an oversight which can have catastrophic consequences.

There may be a correlation between the size of a pheochromocytoma and the presence or severity of clinical signs (Bouayad et al, 1987). In our experience, small, well-demarcated pheochromocytomas, often causing minimal enlargement of the adrenal gland, are more commonly identified as incidental findings during an abdominal ultrasound or at necropsy. In contrast, dogs with clinical signs suggestive of pheochromocytoma typically have an easily identified adrenal mass, often with concurrent compression or invasion of surrounding blood vessels. Pheochromocytoma was an unexpected finding during abdominal ultrasound or at necropsy in 11 of our recently diagnosed 54 dogs. In 9 (82%) of these 11 dogs, the pheochromocytoma was either not identified during abdominal ultrasound or was a small (<1.5 cm diameter), well-demarcated mass. In contrast, only 8 (19%) of 43 dogs with clinical signs consistent with pheochromocytoma had a mass less than 2.0 cm in diameter on abdominal ultrasound.

Thirty-five of 43 dogs with clinical signs had an easily recognizable, large adrenal mass which was distorting the adrenal gland, often compressing or invading surrounding structures.

Physical Examination

Physical examination findings in dogs with pheochromocytoma are quite variable and dependent, in part, on the secretory activity of the tumor at the time of the examination, the size of the tumor, and the presence of concurrent problems. In our experience, the physical examination is often unremarkable and any abnormalities identified are more likely related to the older age of the dog (e.g., dental disease, lipomas, low-grade mitral murmurs) than to the presence of a pheochromocytoma. When identified, abnormalities are usually a result of excessive catecholamine secretion by the tumor and typically involve the respiratory (i.e., tachypnea, excessive panting), cardiovascular (i.e., tachycardia, cardiac arrhythmias, weak femoral pulses), and musculoskeletal systems (i.e., weakness, muscle wasting) (Table 9-6). Cardiac arrhythmias include premature ventricular contractions, third degree heart block, and atrial tachycardia.

An abdominal mass was palpable in only 5%, peripheral edema or ascites was present in 10%, and pain on palpation of the abdomen was identified in 10% of 40 dogs. None of the dogs with abdominal pain had a palpable abdominal mass. Fluid retention most likely results from local invasion and obstruction of the caudal vena cava by the tumor, a phenomenon that was documented at surgery or necropsy in 40% of our

TABLE 9–5 CONCURRENT DISORDERS IDENTIFIED IN 58 OF 98 DOGS WITH PHEOCHROMOCYTOMA

Generalized Disorders	Neoplasms
Diabetes mellitus	Adrenocortical adenoma*
Cushing's syndrome*	Astrocytoma
Megaesophagus	Biliary adenocarcinoma
Hepatic insufficiency	Fibrosarcoma
Pancreatitis	Hemangioma
Renal failure	Hepatocellular carcinoma
Pyelonephritis, cystitis	Histiocytoma
Congestive heart failure	Leiomyoma
Atherosclerosis	Lymphoma
Intervertebral disc disease	Mammary adenocarcinoma
Cervical spondylopathy	Mast cell tumor
Degenerative myelopathy	Melanoma
Otitis media	Nasal adenocarcinoma
Suppurative rhinitis	Osteosarcoma, chondrosarcoma
Pneumonia	Pancreatic adenocarcinoma*
Trauma-fractures	Pituitary macroadenoma*
Degenerative joint disease	Primary hyperparathyroidism*
	Rhabdomyosarcoma
	Seminoma
	Sertoli cell tumor
	Squamous cell carcinoma
	Thymoma
	Thyroid adenocarcinoma*

*Consistent with multiple endocrine neoplasia (MEN) seen in humans.

TABLE 9–6 FREQUENCY OF ABNORMAL FINDINGS ON PHYSICAL EXAMINATION OF 40 DOGS WITH PHEOCHROMOCYTOMA AND IDENTIFICATION OF NO OTHER CONCURRENT DISORDER*

Physical Finding	Number of Dogs	Percentage of Dogs
Panting, tachypnea	15	38%
Weakness	9	23%
Tachycardia	7	18%
Thin, muscle wasting	6	15%
Cardiac arrhythmias	6	15%
Hemorrhage (nasal, gingival, ocular)	6	15%
Weak pulses	4	10%
Pale mucous membranes	4	10%
Abdominal pain	4	10%
Ascites	4	10%
Lethargy	3	8%
Palpable abdominal mass	2	5%
Shocky	2	5%
Blindness, retinal detachment	2	5%
Rear limb edema	1	3%
Shaking, muscle tremors	1	3%
Lateral recumbency	1	3%
Anterior uveitis	1	3%
Unremarkable	15	38%

*Excluding common geriatric findings such as lipomas, dental disease, and incidental cardiac murmurs.

98 dogs and in each of the dogs with ascites or peripheral edema (Schoeman and Stidworthy, 2001). Obstruction of the posterior vena cava may also cause distention of the superficial veins of the ventral abdominal wall (Twedt and Wheeler, 1984).

Mydriasis, retinal hemorrhage, retinal detachment, and blindness may develop following sustained severe hypertension, although these were infrequent findings in our dogs. Interestingly, 2 dogs had persistent mild epistaxis, 2 dogs had persistent mild hemorrhage from sites of minor surgery performed within a week of being brought to our hospital, and 1 dog had persistent mild gingival bleeding; problems which were presumably a result of hypertension. Neurologic signs, including seizures, head tilt, nystagmus, and strabismus, have also been reported (Twedt and Wheeler, 1984; Gilson et al, 1994). Neurologic signs (spinal pain, rear limb ataxia and paresis) have also been described in 4 dogs with metastatic extra-adrenal paraganglioma (Hines et al, 1993) and 2 dogs with metastatic pheochromocytoma (Platt et al, 1998).

Clinical Pathology

There are no consistent abnormalities in the CBC, serum biochemical panel, or urinalysis which would raise suspicion of pheochromocytoma. There were no abnormalities identified on the CBC and serum biochemical panel in approximately 30% of our dogs with pheochromocytoma and no significant concurrent disease. Failure to identify abnormalities on routine bloodwork is helpful in differentiating a catecholamine-secreting from a cortisol- or aldosterone-secreting adrenal tumor (see page 458). Mild thrombocytopenia, typically ranging from 150,000 to 200,000/μL, was the most consistent abnormality on a CBC, identified in approximately 20% of our dogs. There was no correlation between identification of hemorrhage on the physical examination and thrombocytopenia on the CBC. A mild non-regenerative anemia (PCV, 25 to 35%), mild hemoconcentration (PCV, 45 to 55%), and neutrophilic leukocytosis were identified in less than 10% of our dogs. The cause and effect relationship between pheochromocytoma and these findings is not known. The non-regenerative anemia may be an anemia associated with chronic disease or be a result of other concurrent disease. The increase in the hematocrit most likely is a reflection of a decrease in plasma volume but could also result from either catecholamine-stimulated erythropoietin release from the kidney or an erythropoietin-like peptide produced and secreted by the pheochromocytoma (Young and Landsberg, 1998).

An increase in serum alkaline phosphatase and alanine aminotransferase activity, hypoalbuminemia, hypercholesterolemia, and azotemia are the most common abnormalities on the serum biochemical panel, being identified in approximately 80%, 60%, 45%, 25%, and 25% of 61 dogs in one retrospective study (Barthez et al, 1997). However, when results of the serum biochemistry panel are evaluated in dogs with pheochromocytoma and no significant concurrent disease, the prevalence of these abnormalities decreases to 40%, 10%, 5%, 15%, and 10%, respectively. Unfortunately, abnormalities identified on the serum biochemical panel are not helpful in establishing a diagnosis of pheochromocytoma. In our experience, there does not appear to be any correlation between changes in serum liver enzyme activities and metastatic disease within the liver. Elevations in liver enzymes were not present in most of our dogs with necropsy-confirmed hepatic metastasis of a pheochromocytoma.

The blood glucose concentration was between 120 mg/dl and 180 mg/dl and the urine was negative for the presence of glucose in approximately 20% of our dogs with pheochromocytoma, a finding reported to occur by others (Twedt and Wheeler, 1984; Barthez et al, 1997). Carbohydrate intolerance and elevated fasting blood glucose concentrations have been reported in humans with pheochromocytoma (Young and Landsberg, 1998). Epinephrine has both direct and indirect effects to stimulate hepatic glycogenolysis and hepatic and renal gluconeogenesis; provide muscle tissue with an alternative source of fuel by mobilizing muscle glycogen and stimulating lipolysis; mobilize gluconeogenic precursors (e.g., lactate, alanine, and glycerol); and inhibit glucose utilization by insulin-sensitive tissues like skeletal muscle (Fig. 9-3) (Cryer, 1993; Karam, 2001). The carbohydrate intolerance that develops in humans with pheochromocytoma is usually mild and does not require therapy. Interestingly, 3 of our 98 dogs with pheochromocytoma had concurrent insulin-dependent diabetes mellitus and 2 of these dogs developed severe diabetic ketoacidosis. In one dog, the diabetic state was well-controlled at the time pheochromocytoma was diagnosed. What role, if any, catecholamine-induced insulin antagonism may have played in the development of diabetes or ketoacidosis in these dogs is not known. It is possible that our dogs with carbohydrate intolerance and clinical diabetes were in a subclinical diabetic state (i.e., islet pathology and decreased beta cell numbers) at the time the pheochromocytoma developed. Catecholamine-induced insulin resistance increased the demand for insulin secretion; a demand which could not be adequately met in dogs with impaired insulin secretory capabilities. The severity of the ensuing hyperglycemia would be dependent on the severity of the islet pathology and the insulin resistance. We always include pheochromocytoma in the differential diagnoses for causes of poor glycemic control and ketoacidosis in diabetic dogs and cats.

The only consistent abnormality identified in the urinalysis was proteinuria, which was identified in approximately 15% of our dogs with pheochromocytoma and no significant concurrent disease. Mean urine specific gravity was 1.022, with a range of 1.004 to 1.041. Identification of hyposthenuria and isosthenuria in some dogs supports owner's observations of polydipsia and polyuria in their dogs (see Table 9-4).

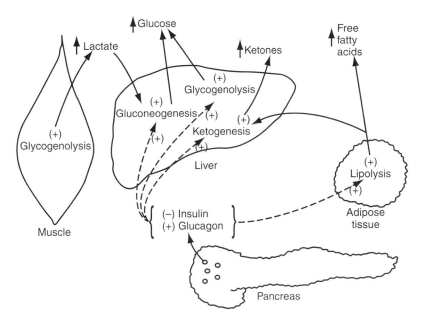

FIGURE 9–3. Schematic representation of catecholamine effects on fuel mobilization in liver, adipose tissue, and skeletal muscle. Direct effects are reinforced by (but do not require) catecholamine-mediated suppression of insulin and stimulation of glucagon. +, stimulation; –, inhibition. (From Landsberg L, Young JB: Catecholamines and the adrenal medulla. *In* Bondy PK, Rosenber LE (eds): Metabolic Control and Disease, 8th ed. Philadelphia, WB Saunders Co, 1980:1621-1693.)

Catecholamines, most notably norepinephrine, inhibit pituitary vasopressin secretion via a nonpressor interaction with arterial baroreceptors (Young and Landsberg, 1998). Hemodynamic factors and catecholamine-induced inhibition of vasopressin responses in the renal collecting tubules may also contribute to the development of polyuria and polydipsia (Krothapalli et al, 1983).

Diagnostic Imaging Techniques

ABDOMINAL ULTRASOUND. Abdominal ultrasound plays a critical role in the diagnosis of pheochromocytoma. Clinical signs of pheochromocytoma are episodic and often vague, findings on physical examination are usually non-contributory, and the clinician's index of suspicion for the disease is usually low. Pheochromocytoma is often considered only after an adrenal mass is identified on abdominal ultrasound performed as part of the routine diagnostic evaluation of any sick dog or cat. Ultrasound is an effective diagnostic tool for identifying an adrenal mass. Once identified, the clinician can then review the history, physical findings, and initial blood tests and perform the necessary diagnostic tests to determine the functional status of the mass and its most likely origin (i.e., cortex or medulla; see Incidental Adrenal Mass, page 458).

The most common ultrasound finding with pheochromocytoma is adrenomegaly (i.e., an adrenal mass) with a normal-sized contra lateral adrenal gland (Fig. 9-4). In contrast, dogs with adrenal-dependent hyperadrenocorticism should have unilateral adrenomegaly and a decreased size (i.e., atrophy) of the contralateral adrenal gland (Fig. 9-5) (see Chapter 6). An obvious adrenal mass was identified in approximately 85% of our dogs with pheochromocytoma, and the majority of the remaining dogs had asymmetry in adrenal gland size with a mass suspected in the larger adrenal gland. Pheochromocytoma may develop in both adrenal glands, resulting in bilateral adrenal masses (see Fig. 9-8) (Gilson et al, 1994; Barthez et al, 1997). Pheochromocytoma and an adrenocortical tumor can also occur simultaneously, which can pose a difficult diagnostic and therapeutic challenge (von Dehn et al, 1995; Bennett and Norman, 1998). Although finding normal-sized adrenal glands does not rule out pheochromocytoma, in our experience, there is a direct correlation between size of the tumor and severity of clinical signs and small pheochromocytomas (i.e., less than 1 cm in size) are usually incidental findings at necropsy.

Abdominal ultrasound can also provide useful information regarding metastasis or local invasion of the mass into surrounding structures, such as the caudal vena cava or kidney. Invasion of surrounding blood vessels, most notably the caudal vena cava and phrenicoabdominal vein, with subsequent development of a tumor thrombus is common with pheochromocytoma in dogs (Fig. 9-6) (Twedt and Wheeler, 1984; Bouyad et al, 1987; Kyles et al, 2003). In one study, the sensitivity and specificity of abdominal ultrasonography for detecting tumor thrombi in dogs with adrenal neoplasia was 82% and 86%, respectively (Kyles et al, 2003). Ascites may develop as a

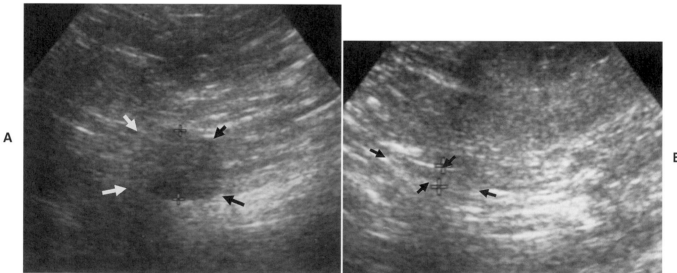

FIGURE 9–4. Ultrasound images of the adrenal glands in a 10-year-old female spayed Bichon Friese presenting for acute onset of vomiting. *A,* An unexpected mass involving the right adrenal gland was identified *(arrows),* measuring 1.4 cm in maximum diameter. *B,* The left adrenal gland was normal in size and shape *(arrows);* the maximum diameter was 0.6 cm. The normal-sized left adrenal gland suggests that the right adrenal mass is either a pheochromocytoma or is nonfunctional. Results of routine blood work and tests for hyperadrenocorticism were normal. Histologic examination of the right adrenal gland identified pheochromocytoma. (From Nelson RW: Disorders of the adrenal gland. *In* Nelson RW, Couto CG (eds): Small Animal Internal Medicine, 3rd ed. St Louis, Mosby Inc, 2003, p. 786.)

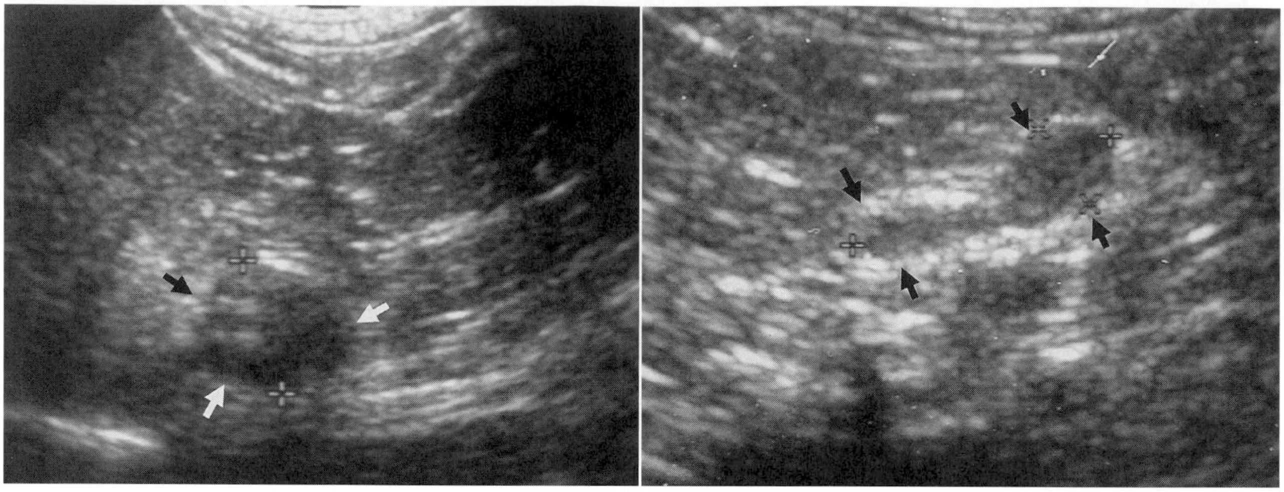

FIGURE 9–5. Ultrasound images of the adrenal glands in an 11-year-old male castrated Golden Retriever with adrenal-dependent hyperadrenocorticism. *A,* Cortisol-secreting tumor affecting the right adrenal gland *(arrows).* The maximum diameter of the adrenal mass was 1.6 cm. *B,* The left adrenal gland has undergone marked atrophy *(arrows* and *crosses)* has a result of suppression of pituitary ACTH secretion following negative feedback inhibition caused by the adrenocortical tumor. The maximum diameter of the left adrenal gland was less than 0.2 cm. (From Nelson RW: Disorders of the adrenal gland. *In* Nelson RW, Couto CG (eds): Small Animal Internal Medicine, 3rd ed. St Louis, Mosby Inc, 2003, p. 785.)

consequence of the tumor thrombus and be identified on abdominal ultrasound.

ABDOMINAL AND THORACIC RADIOGRAPHS. Abdominal radiographs are less effective than ultrasonography in identifying adrenomegaly. In 30 of our dogs with pheochromocytoma, abdominal radiographs revealed a cranial abdominal mass in the region of the adrenal gland in 11 (37%) dogs and calcification of the adrenal mass in 2 (7%) dogs. Additional findings on survey abdominal radiographs in these 30 dogs included hepatomegaly, renal displacement, abnormal renal contour, ascites, and enlargement of the caudal vena

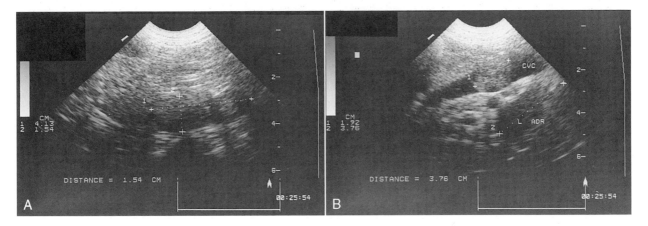

FIGURE 9–6. Abdominal ultrasound of a 14-year-old male standard Poodle. A nodular mass was identified in one pole of the left adrenal gland *(A)* with extension of the mass into the caudal vena cava *(B)*. Histologic evaluation of the mass confirmed pheochromocytoma. CVC, caudal vena cava; *ADR*, adrenal.

cava. Calcification of adrenal glands has been reported in 50% of dogs with adrenocortical tumors but is rarely observed in dogs with pheochromocytoma (Lamb et al, 1991). Abnormalities on thoracic radiographs included generalized cardiomegaly, right or left ventricular enlargement, pulmonary congestion, and pulmonary edema; abnormalities presumably resulting from systemic hypertension. Pulmonary nodules compatible with pulmonary metastasis is identified in approximately 10% of dogs (Gilson et al, 1994; Barthez et al, 1997).

COMPUTED TOMOGRAPHY AND MAGNETIC RESONANCE IMAGING. CT and MRI are noninvasive techniques for visualizing the adrenal glands and surrounding structures and assessing shape, architecture, size, and symmetry of the glands and to determine margination of a mass and invasion of adjacent structures (Rosenstein, 2000). Both imaging modalities can be used to identify the presence and location of an adrenal mass; to determine size, shape, architecture, and symmetry of the glands; to determine margination of the mass and invasion of the mass into surrounding blood vessels and organs (e.g., kidney); and to identify sites of metastasis (Fig. 9-7 and Fig. 9-8) (Rosenstein, 2000). In humans, MRI has been shown to be more sensitive for delineating the extent of venous thrombosis than CT imaging (Goldfarb et al, 1990). We consider performing a CT or MRI scan of the abdomen to confirm an adrenal mass in dogs where abdominal ultrasound has failed to establish the diagnosis and to identify tumor thrombus or tumor invasion of surrounding organs prior to adrenalectomy. The reader is referred to page 320 for more information on these sophisticated imaging techniques.

SPECIALIZED STUDIES. Historically, intravenous urography or arteriography has been used to identify an adrenal mass that has either invaded the cranial pole of the kidney or caused renal displacement. Venography has also been used to identify compression, deviation, or occlusion of the caudal vena cava (Twedt and Wheeler, 1984; Barthez et al, 1997). These techniques have been largely replaced by ultrasonography, computed tomography, and magnetic resonance imaging.

Metaiodobenzylguanidine (MIBG) is a structural analog of quanethidine derivative with a molecular structure similar to norepinephrine, is selectively taken up by adrenergic neurons and the adrenal medulla, concentrates in neurosecretory storage granules of chromaffin cells, shows little binding to postsynaptic receptors and causes little or no pharmacologic response (Sisson, 1986). Labeling MIBG with iodine-131 or iodine-123 allows the chromaffin tissue to be imaged, using a gamma camera (Sisson et al, 1981). Nuclear scintigraphy utilizing radiolabeled MIBG has been used to localize adrenal, ectopic, and disseminated pheochromocytomas in humans (Sisson et al, 1981; Fischer et al, 1984; Thompson et al, 1984; Hanson et al, 1991). Sensitivity and specificity of MIBG scans for identifying pheochromocytoma in humans have been reported to range from 77% to 88% and 88% to 100%, respectively (Shapiro et al, 1985; Werbel and Ober, 1995). False positive results are primarily a result of concentration of MIBG in normal adrenal glands (Gough et al, 1985). False negative results are attributed to either rapid uptake and secretion of the neurosecretory granules or lack of norepinephrine accumulation and decreased neurosecretory granule concentration within tumor cells (Tobes et al, 1985; Hanson et al, 1991). 123I-MIBG scintigraphy was effective in identifying a pheochromocytoma in the right adrenal gland in a Yorkshire terrier (Berry et al, 1993). p-[18F]Fluorobenzylguanidine ([18F]PFBG) is a norepinephrine analog that has been developed as a positron emission tomography (PET) imaging radiopharmaceutical for use in imaging tumors of neuroendocrine origin, including pheochromocytoma. [18F]PFBG was effective in identifying a pheochromocytoma in 2 dogs and was normal in a third dog suspected of having a pheochromocytoma who was subsequently shown to have normal adrenal glands at

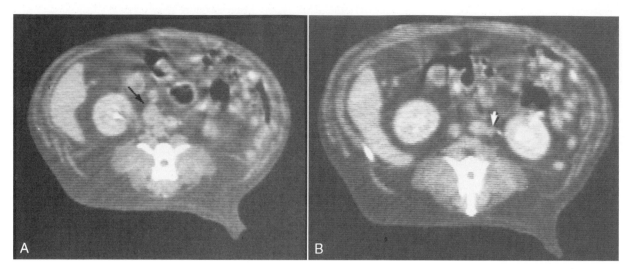

FIGURE 9–7. *A,* CT scan of the region of the left adrenal gland in a 10-year-old spayed female Rottweiler, illustrating an irregular soft tissue mass located medial to the left kidney *(arrow).* The mass was excised surgically, and histologic examination confirmed a pheochromocytoma. *B,* CT scan of the region of the right adrenal gland from the dog in *A,* illustrating the normal right adrenal gland *(arrow).*

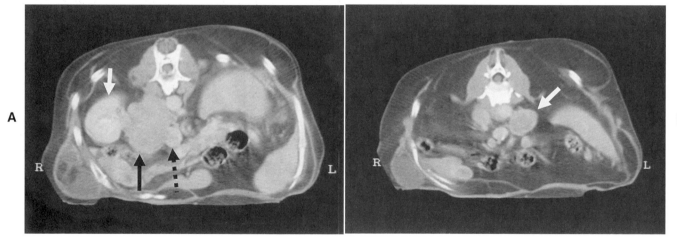

FIGURE 9–8. *A,* CT scan of the region of the right adrenal gland in a 10-year-old male castrate Afghan Hound with multiple endocrine neoplasia, illustrating a 6- by 7-cm irregular soft tissue mass *(solid black arrow)* medial to the right kidney *(solid white arrow)* and invading the caudal vena cava *(dashed black arrow)* and the kidney. *B,* CT scan of the region of the left adrenal gland from the dog in *A,* illustrating adrenomegaly. The left adrenal gland was oval with a smooth contour and measured 3 × 3 cm. Bilateral pheochromocytomas, adrenocortical adenoma of the left adrenal gland, thyroid carcinoma, and hyperplasia of the parathyroid gland were identified at necropsy.

surgery and on histologic examination of an adrenal gland biopsy (Berry et al, 2002).

Arterial Blood Pressure Measurements

Determination of systemic arterial blood pressure is indicated in any dog or cat with suspected pheochromocytoma. Several methods can be used to measure systemic arterial blood pressure, including direct measurement using a needle or fluid-filled catheter system connected to a pressure transducer and indirect noninvasive measurement using an inflatable cuff placed around a limb or the tail and either an oscillometric transducer (e.g., Dinamap Veterinary Blood Pressure Monitor, Critikon Inc, Tampa, FL) or Doppler ultrasound (e.g., Ultrasonic Doppler Flow Detector, Model 811, Parks Medical Electronics, Inc, Aloha, OR; Arteriosonde 1010, Hoffman-LaRoche, Nutley, NJ). Blood pressure results obtained by Doppler ultrasound and oscillometric methods correlate closely with direct blood pressure measurements. Multiple measurements (e.g., 5 to 10) should be taken and averaged to increase accuracy. Anxiety and stress related to the clinical setting may falsely increase blood pressure in some animals (i.e., "white-coat effect"). Using the least restraint possible in a quiet environment and before performing a physical examination or other diagnostic tests is recommended.

Defining normal arterial blood pressure is somewhat difficult in dogs, in part, because age, breed, gender, and other factors in healthy dogs, as well as concurrent disease, affects arterial blood pressure (Bodey and Mitchell, 1996). However, investigators agree that hypertension should be suspected with sustained systolic pressures >160 mm Hg and/or with sustained diastolic pressures >100 mm Hg. Documentation of hypertension in the non-azotemic dog with an adrenal mass and normal adrenocortical function would be consistent with various disorders, including the presence of a pheochromocytoma (Table 9-7). Unfortunately, catecholamine secretion by the tumor, and thus systemic hypertension, tends to be episodic. Failure to document systemic hypertension in a dog with appropriate clinical signs does not rule out pheochromocytoma. Blood pressure was increased in 11 (38%) of our 29 dogs with pheochromocytoma only, i.e. there was no concurrent disease which could affect arterial blood pressure results (e.g., hyperadrenocorticism, renal insufficiency, diabetes mellitus). In other studies, hypertension was documented in 43 to 50% of dogs in which blood pressure was measured (Twedt and Wheeler, 1984; Barthez et al, 1997). These findings correlate closely with human patients with pheochromocytoma, 25 to 40% of whom experience intermittent rather than sustained hypertension (Young and Landsberg, 1998). Ideally, blood pressure should be measured at the time owners believe clinical signs are present in their dog. Unfortunately, most dogs are asymptomatic at the time they are presented to the veterinary hospital. An alternative is to obtain serial blood pressure measurements either throughout the day or on sequential days in normotensive dogs with suspected pheochromocytoma in an effort to document hypertension.

In dogs with documented systemic hypertension, average systolic, diastolic, and mean arterial blood pressures were 193, 119, and 145 mm Hg, respectively, with corresponding ranges of 160 to 230, 102 to 145, and 133 to 166 mm Hg. Treatment in these dogs was aimed at the pheochromocytoma; none of these dogs were treated with antihypertensive drugs. In humans with pheochromocytoma, the response to conventional antihypertensive treatment is usually unsatisfactory. This refractoriness may be a clue to the diagnosis of pheochromocytoma. Humans with pheochromocytoma, however, respond to α-adrenergic blocking drugs, such as phenoxybenzamine, prazosin, and labetalol (Young and Landsberg, 1998).

Hormonal Testing

In humans, assessment of catecholamine production and excretion is important in the laboratory detection and diagnosis of pheochromocytoma. Biochemical evaluations typically include measurement of plasma or urinary catecholamine concentrations or their metabolites under basal conditions. Because pheochromocytomas are a heterogeneous group of hormone-secreting tumors, no single analyte achieves 100% sensitivity nor is there a universally agreed-on best test among pheochromocytoma experts. Many consider measurement of free catecholamines (i.e., epinephrine, norepinephrine, dopamine) in a 24 hour urine collection using high performance liquid chromatography with electrochemical detection the current best confirmatory test for pheochromocytoma in humans (Prys-Roberts, 2000). Others consider 24-hour urinary measurements of metanephrines and free catecholamines equivalent (Young and Landsberg, 1998). Unfortunately, the availability, technical difficulty, and expense involved with these tests have limited their use in veterinary medicine. As a result, the antemortem diagnosis of pheochromocytoma in a dog usually relies on surgical exploration and histopathologic examination of the adrenal mass. Nevertheless, these tests will be discussed briefly, as they are commonly performed in humans, have appeared in the veterinary literature, and may become more routinely performed in the future.

PLASMA CATECHOLAMINE CONCENTRATIONS. The value of basal plasma catecholamine determinations for establishing the diagnosis of pheochromocytoma is dependent, in part, on the persistence of hypertension and clinical signs. In humans with continuous hypertension or clinical signs, concentrations of plasma catecholamines and their metabolites are usually clearly increased. However, in humans having brief and infrequent paroxysms with symptom-free intervals, confirmation of the diagnosis may be more difficult. Although large amounts of catecholamines are produced during the brief episodes, abnormal plasma

TABLE 9–7 CAUSES OF PERSISTENT HYPERTENSION IN HUMANS, DOGS, AND CATS

Documented in Humans	Documented in Dogs and Cats
"Essential" or primary	"Essential" or primary
Renal parenchymal disease	Renal parenchymal disease
Renal vascular disease	Renal vascular disease
Hyperadrenocorticism	Hyperadrenocorticism
Primary hyperaldosteronism	Primary hyperaldosteronism
Hyperthyroidism	Hyperthyroidism
Hypothyroidism	Hypothyroidism
Pheochromocytoma	Pheochromocytoma
Diabetes mellitus	Diabetes mellitus
SIADH	SIADH
Liver disease	Liver disease
Obesity	Obesity
High salt intake	High salt intake
Hypercalcemia, hyperparathyroidism	Chronic anemia (cats)
Renin-secreting tumor	
Acromegaly	
CNS disease	
Hyperviscosity/polycythemia	
Coarctation of the aorta	
Hyperestrogenism	
Pregnancy	
Oral contraceptives	

SIADH, Syndrome of inappropriate antidiuretic hormone secretion.

TABLE 9–8   GUIDELINES USED IN THE INTERPRETATION OF BIOCHEMICAL TESTS FOR PHEOCHROMOCYTOMA IN HUMANS

Test	Normal Results	Diagnostic Levels	Sensitivity	Specificity
Plasma norepinephrine	<0.5 ng/ml	>2 ng/ml	58%–85%	88%–99%
Plasma epinephrine	<0.1 ng/ml	>0.4 ng/ml	33%–62%	79%–94%
24 hour excretion of:				
Norepinephrine	<75 ng/24 h	1.5- to 2-fold increase	70%–90%	54%–98%
Epinephrine	<25 ng/24 h	1.5- to 2-fold increase	50%–75%	84%–98%
Metanephrine	<0.4 mg/24 h	1.5- to 2-fold increase	58%–97%	96%–99%
Normetanephrine	<0.9 mg/24 h	1.5- to 2-fold increase	90%–97%	58%–98%
Metanephrine + normetanephrine	<1.3 mg/24 h	1.5- to 2-fold increase	97%–100%	84%–98%
Vanillylmandelic acid	<8.0 mg/24 h	1.5- to 2-fold increase	64%–90%	87%–98%

Adapted from Werbel SS, Ober KP: Pheochromocytoma. Update on diagnosis, localization, and management. Med Clin N Amer 79:131, 1995.

catecholamine concentrations may not be present at the time of evaluation (Duncan et al, 1988; Goldfien, 2001). Likewise, stress or excitement at the time of blood sampling and the existence of concurrent diseases may transiently increase plasma catecholamine concentrations into the range compatible with pheochromocytoma (Jones et al, 1980). In humans, basal plasma catecholamine determinations are occasionally indicated in the patient with borderline urinary assay results (see below). In normotensive humans, total plasma catecholamine concentrations are usually in the range of 0.1 to 0.5 ng/ml. Basal plasma catecholamine concentrations in excess of 2 ng/ml (12 nmol/L) support the diagnosis of pheochromocytoma, whereas values below 0.5 ng/ml (3 nmol/L) make the diagnosis unlikely (Table 9-8) (Werbel and Orber, 1995; Young and Landsberg, 1998). Similar determinations have not been reported in the dog or cat.

URINARY CATECHOLAMINES AND CATECHOLAMINE METABOLITES. Measurement of urinary catecholamines and their metabolites is the most commonly utilized diagnostic test for pheochromocytoma in humans. The diagnosis of pheochromocytoma is established by demonstrating increased urinary excretion of catecholamines or catecholamine metabolites. The metabolites of catecholamines that are measured in the urine include metanephrine, normetanephrine, and vanillylmandelic acid (VMA) (Fig. 9-9) (Werbel and Orber, 1995; Young and Landsberg, 1998). Urinary catecholamines and their metabolites are measured as total excretion/24 hours or on a random urine sample, expressing the values in µg/ml of creatinine. Because catecholamine secretion is usually episodic, determination of catecholamines and metabolites from a 24-hour urine collection is preferable to random urine sampling (Duncan et al, 1988). The ability to establish a diagnosis confidently is enhanced when 2 or more of these urinary compounds are determined at the same time (see Table 9-8). The amount of excreted free catecholamine and its metabolites varies, depending on the level of synthesizing and metabolizing enzymes within the tumor and the excretory function of the kidneys. These factors help account for reported false-positive and false-negative test results.

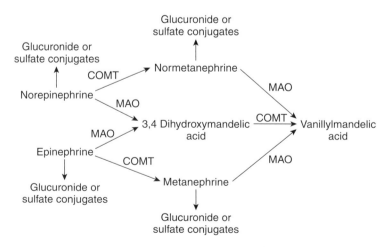

FIGURE 9–9. The primary metabolic breakdown pathways for norepinephrine and epinephrine. Conjugation of the catecholamines and their metabolites occurs in the liver and gastrointestinal tract. Catecholamines and their metabolites are primarily excreted in the urine, although the liver may also play a role. *COMT,* Catechol-*o*-methyl transferase; *MAO,* monoamine oxidase. (From Levine RJ, Landsberg L: *In* Bondy PK, Rosenberg LE: Duncan's Diseases of Metabolism, 7th ed. Philadelphia, W.B. Saunders Co, 1974, p 1196.)

In humans, certain precautions in patient preparation and collection techniques are followed to ensure accuracy and reliability when determining urinary catecholamines and their metabolites (Young and Landsberg, 1998). Ideally, urine should be collected with the patient at rest, on no medications, and without recent exposure to radiographic contrast agents. Most assays are reasonably specific, requiring minimal dietary restrictions. The VMA assay is the least specific, and a 10% to 15% false-positive test result has been reported in some laboratories when humans have been consuming food or beverages containing vanilla, such as bananas, nuts, and fruits. Finally, the urine must be acidified (pH below 3.0) and kept cold during and after collection. Urine is usually collected in 15 ml of 6 N hydrochloric acid, which can be obtained from any clinical laboratory performing these assays.

Total 24-hour urinary excretion of epinephrine, norepinephrine, and dopamine is usually below 0.02 mg/24h, 0.08 mg/24h, and 0.4 mg/24h, respectively, in normal humans (Goldfien, 2001). Most human patients with pheochromocytoma have values greater than two-fold above these normal values. Normal metanephrine, normetanephrine, and VMA excretion is usually less than 0.4 mg/24h, 0.9 mg/24h, and 8 mg/24h, respectively. Humans with pheochromocytoma typically excrete these metabolites in excess, often exceeding the normal range by three-fold. However, in some humans with brief and infrequent periods of hypertension and clinical signs and prolonged symptom-free intervals, confirmation of the diagnosis may be difficult because the total amount of catecholamines excreted during the 24-hr urine collection period may not be clearly abnormal, in contrast to humans whose tumors secrete continuously (Goldfien, 2001).

Evaluation of urinary catecholamines and their metabolites has been infrequently performed in veterinary medicine. In two reported dogs, the values were of questionable significance. The one dog in our series in which these parameters were measured had elevated urinary catecholamine concentrations that declined following surgical removal of the tumor. The accuracy of these urinary determinations in diagnosing pheochromocytoma in dogs or cats has not yet been critically examined.

SUPPRESSION AND PROVOCATIVE TESTING. Prior to the availability of accurate biochemical measurements of catecholamines and their metabolites, testing for pheochromocytoma in humans involved the administration of various agents designed to differentiate pheochromocytoma-related from stress-provoked increases in plasma catecholamines (e.g., clonidine suppression test) or provoke a striking increase in blood pressure by stimulating catecholamine secretion by the pheochromocytoma (e.g., histamine or glucagon administration) (Young and Landsberg, 1998). Most of these tests lack sensitivity and specificity, can cause serious adverse reactions and, as such, have been rendered obsolete by measurement of catechol-

amines and catecholamine metabolites in urine. The reader is referred to the second edition of *Canine and Feline Endocrinology and Reproduction* for more information on these tests.

Establishing the Diagnosis

A diagnosis of pheochromocytoma requires a high index of suspicion on the part of the clinician. No consistent abnormalities in the CBC, serum biochemical panel, or urinalysis findings are seen that would raise suspicion of pheochromocytoma. A history of acute or episodic collapse, generalized weakness, or excessive panting, tachypnea, or a 'pounding' heart rate (which are often episodic), identification of appropriate respiratory, cardiac, or ocular abnormalities (e.g., retinal hemorrhage from systemic hypertension) during the physical examination, the documentation of systemic hypertension (particularly if it is paroxysmal), and identification of an adrenal mass by abdominal ultrasonography are most helpful in establishing a tentative diagnosis of pheochromocytoma. Documentation of hypertension in the nonazotemic dog with an adrenal mass and normal adrenocortical function would be consistent with various disorders, including a pheochromocytoma. Unfortunately, catecholamine secretion by the tumor, and thus systemic hypertension, tends to be episodic. Failure to document systemic hypertension in a dog with appropriate clinical signs does not rule out a diagnosis of pheochromocytoma.

The ultrasound identification of adrenomegaly (i.e., adrenal mass) with a normal-sized contra lateral adrenal gland is further evidence of a pheochromocytoma. In dogs and cats with systemic hypertension, abdominal ultrasound assessment of adrenal size is perhaps the best screening test for pheochromocytoma, keeping in mind that a normal-sized adrenal gland does not rule out the diagnosis (von Dehn et al, 1995). Ultrasonography may also provide information regarding metastatic or local invasion of the mass into surrounding structures, such as the caudal vena cava. However, identification of local invasion of the mass or presence of a tumor thrombus is not, by itself, indicative of pheochromocytoma. In a recent retrospective study, 6 (56%) of 11 dogs with pheochromocytoma had tumor thrombi and 6 (21%) of 28 dogs with an adrenocortical tumor had tumor thrombi (Kyles et al, 2003). It is critically important to remember that abdominal ultrasonography, perhaps more than any other commonly used diagnostic aid in veterinary medicine, is extremely "operator dependent." A skilled radiologist or internist with experience in assessing adrenal glands should be consulted whenever an adrenal tumor is suspected.

Other possibilities must be considered if an adrenal mass is identified, most notably an adrenocortical tumor causing hyperadrenocorticism or a nonfunctional adrenal mass (see Table 9-10, page 459). Pheochromocytoma and an adrenocortical tumor can also occur simultaneously (von Dehn et al, 1995), which can pose a difficult diagnostic and therapeutic challenge. Many of the clinical signs (e.g., panting, weakness) and blood pressure alterations seen in dogs with hyperadrenocorticism (common) are similar to those seen in dogs with pheochromocytoma (uncommon). Therefore it is important to rule out hyperadrenocorticism through the performance of appropriate hormonal tests (see Chapter 6) before focusing on pheochromocytoma in a dog with an adrenal mass.

Measurement of urinary catecholamine concentrations or their metabolites can strengthen the tentative diagnosis of a pheochromocytoma. Unfortunately, these tests are not commonly performed in dogs and cats. As a result, the antemortem definitive diagnosis of a pheochromocytoma in a dog or cat ultimately relies on the findings yielded by histologic evaluation of the surgically excised adrenal mass.

Surgical Management

OVERVIEW. A period of medical therapy to reverse the effects of excessive adrenergic stimulation followed by surgical removal of the tumor is the treatment of choice for pheochromocytoma. Chemotherapy and radiation therapy have had limited success in humans with pheochromocytoma (Keiser et al, 1985; Averbuch et al, 1988) and results of the treatment of malignant pheochromocytoma with chemotherapy or radiation therapy has not been reported in dogs or cats. Mitotane (i.e., o,p'DDD) is ineffective for treating tumors arising from the adrenal medulla and is not recommended. Chronic medical therapy is primarily designed to control excessive catecholamine secretion rather than to lessen the risk of local invasion or metastasis of the tumor to other organs.

Criteria for selection of dogs to undergo surgical excision of a pheochromocytoma have not been established. Factors to consider include the age of the dog, size of the tumor, presence or absence of tumor invasion into surrounding structures (e.g., the vena cava) or metastatic disease, and the effect of concurrent disease on anesthetic risk. The chance of cure is enhanced if a dog does not have concurrent disease, metastasis of the tumor, or local tissue invasion. Twenty-three (33%) of 70 of our dogs with pheochromocytoma had histologically confirmed metastatic disease at the time of necropsy. Sites of metastasis included the caudal vena cava, liver, lung, regional lymph nodes, heart, spleen, kidney, bone, pancreas, and CNS (Barthez et al, 1997). As with many endocrine tumors, even if metastasis is identified during surgery, surgical debulking of the tumor may enhance the effectiveness of medical therapy, may improve the dog or cat's quality of life, and may prolong survival time. Similarly, identification of a tumor thrombus is not, by itself, an absolute contraindication for adrenalectomy and venotomy. In a recent study, 9 of 11 dogs with a pheochromocytoma that underwent adrenalectomy

survived the perioperative period, including 5 of 5 dogs without a tumor thrombus and 4 of 6 dogs with a tumor thrombus (Kyles et al, 2003).

PREOPERATIVE MANAGEMENT. Potentially life-threatening complications are common, especially during the induction of anesthesia and manipulation of the tumor during surgery (Fig. 9-10; von Dehn et al, 1995) The most worrisome complications include episodes of acute, severe hypertension (systolic arterial blood pressure of more than 300 mm Hg), episodes of severe tachycardia (heart rate of more than 250 beats/min) and arrhythmias, and hemorrhage. Preoperative α-adrenergic blockade is indicated to prevent severe clinical manifestations of hypertension in the preoperative period, to reverse the hypovolemia which is frequently present, and to promote a smooth anesthetic induction (Desmonts and Marty, 1984; Hull, 1986). In humans, perioperative mortality associated with the excision of pheochromocytoma was reduced from a range of 13% to 45% without preoperative medication to 0 to 6% when α-adrenergic blockade was introduced as preoperative therapy (Roizen et al, 1983; Lucon, 1997). This therapy was also demonstrated to be helpful when it was recognized that pheochromocytoma patients were often hypovolemic preoperatively (Roizen, 1981).

Phenoxybenzamine (Dibenzyline; SmithKline Beecham) is a non-selective, non-competitive α-adrenoreceptor antagonist that is widely used for α-adrenergic blockade. In humans, the initial dosage is 0.25 mg/kg PO bid and the dosage is gradually increased every few days as needed until control of blood pressure is achieved and clinical signs reduced. Our current protocol for the management of hypertension in dogs with pheochromocytoma includes preoperative phenoxybenzamine and intraoperative phentolamine. Our initial dosage of phenoxybenzamine is 0.25 mg/kg bid. Unfortunately, many of our dogs with pheochromocytoma have episodic clinical signs and hypertension making dosage adjustments based on improvement in clinical signs and blood pressure difficult. In addition, this dosage is often ineffective in preventing severe hypertension during surgery. As such, we gradually increase the phenoxybenzamine dosage every few days until clinical signs of hypotension (e.g., lethargy, weakness, syncope), adverse drug reactions (e.g., vomiting) or a maximum dosage of 2.5 mg/kg bid is attained. Surgery is recommended 1 to 2 weeks later. The drug should be continued until the time of surgery. Complications may still occur despite prior treatment with α-adrenergic blocking drugs; close monitoring of the dog during the perioperative period is critical for a successful outcome following adrenalectomy.

Doxazosin (Cardura, Pfizer Inc, New York, NY) is a competitive and selective α1-adrenoceptor agonist that has been successfully used for the preoperative treatment of humans with pheochromocytoma (Prys-Roberts, 2000). Doxazosin has a high bioavailability (>70%) and long duration of action that allows once-a-day dosing in humans. Because doxazosin selectively

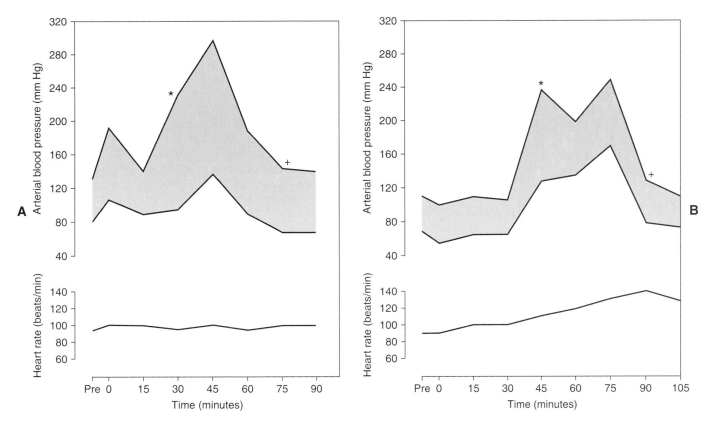

FIGURE 9–10. Direct arterial systolic and diastolic blood pressure measurements and heart rate prior to anesthesia (pre), during anesthetic induction (time 0), and during removal of a pheochromocytoma in a 16-year-old male castrate Border Collie *(A)* and a 12-year-old male West Highland White Terrier *(B)*. Note the sudden development of hypertension during anesthetic induction in the Border Collie and during manual manipulation of the pheochromocytoma in both dogs and the resolution of hypertension after the tumor is removed. *, Onset of tumor manipulation by surgeon; +, completion of tumor excision.

blocks α1-adrenoreceptors, adverse effects affiliated with blockade of α2-adrenoreceptors, such as loss of inhibition of norepinephrine release at cardiac sympathetic nerve endings, do not occur. In a recent study, pre-operative control of blood pressure was at least as good as that achieved with phenoxybenzamine in humans with pheochromocytoma and there were fewer undesirable side effects with doxazosin (Prys-Roberts and Farndon, 2002). We have not yet used doxazosin for the treatment of pheochromocytoma in dogs or cats.

If severe tachycardia is identified, β-adrenergic antagonist therapy (e.g., propranolol: 0.2 to 1 mg/kg, per os, TID; atenolol: 0.2 to 1 mg/kg, per os, SID to BID) should be utilized during the preoperative period. Propranolol should be given only after α-adrenergic blockade has been initiated because severe hypertension may develop following blockade of β-receptor-mediated vasodilation in skeletal muscle (Young and Landsberg, 1998).

ANESTHESIA AND INTRAOPERATIVE COMPLICATIONS. If a pheochromocytoma is suspected, it is imperative that the anesthetist be informed prior to induction of anesthesia. Potentially life-threatening complications are common, especially during induction of anesthesia

and manipulation of the tumor (von Dehn et al, 1995). The most worrisome complications include episodes of acute, severe hypertension (systolic arterial blood pressure > 300 mm Hg; see Fig. 9-10), episodic severe tachycardia (heart rate > 250 beats/min), cardiac arrhythmias, and hemorrhage. These complications may occur despite prior treatment with α-adrenergic blocking drugs. An electrocardiogram and arterial blood pressure should be monitored closely during the entire time the dog is anesthetized and for 24 to 48 hours post-operative. These parameters allow rapid recognition and initiation of appropriate therapy if cardiac arrhythmias, hypovolemia, and/or blood pressure problems develop.

Theoretically, drugs that release histamine, are vagolytic or sympathomimetic, sensitize the myocardium to catecholamines, or have been reported to cause pressor responses in humans with pheochromocytoma should be avoided (Table 9-9; Hull, 1986). Despite the potential problems with many preanesthetic and anesthetic drugs, virtually all anesthetic agents and techniques have been used successfully in humans with pheochromocytoma, and all have been associated with transient intraoperative dysrhythmias (Roizen et al, 1982). Choice of anesthetic

TABLE 9–9 PREANESTHETIC AND ANESTHETIC DRUGS CONSIDERED SAFE AND POTENTIALLY UNSAFE FOR USE IN HUMANS WITH PHEOCHROMOCYTOMA

Safe	Potentially Unsafe
Alfentanil	Atracurium
Benzodiazepines	Atropine
Enflurane	Chlorpromazine
Etomidate	Curare
Fentanyl	Droperidol
Isoflurane	Gallamine
Nitrous oxide	Halothane
Pentothal	Metocurine
Sufentanil	Morphine
Vecuronium	Pancuronium
	Succinylcholine
	Suxamethonium

technique is not the crucial factor determining patient outcome after resection of pheochromocytoma. Rather, optimal preoperative preparation, especially regarding α-adrenergic blockade; careful and gradual induction of anesthesia; appropriate patient monitoring, especially during induction of anesthesia and manipulation of the tumor; and good communication between surgeon and anesthesiologist are most important to the successful outcome of the operation.

Our current anesthetic protocol includes oxymorphone and atropine or glycopyrrolate for preanesthesia, fentanyl citrate and diazepam or midazolam for induction of anesthesia, and maintenance with a balanced anesthetic technique including isoflurane and fentanyl citrate. Using this anesthetic technique, complications were uncommon during induction of anesthesia in our dogs undergoing surgical excision of pheochromocytoma. However, intraoperative complications were common and included paroxysmal hypertension and hypotension, paroxysmal tachycardia, and cardiac arrhythmias. Our experiences emphasize the importance of appropriate patient monitoring, especially during manipulation of the tumor or occlusion of the caudal vena cava, and good communication between surgeon and anesthesiologist if a successful outcome is to be obtained.

Continuous monitoring of central venous pressure and direct arterial blood pressure will help identify hypertension and hypotension. Intraoperative hypotension is managed by decreasing the dose of or discontinuing phentolamine, decreasing the inhalant concentration and/or rapidly expanding the vascular volume by administration of crystalloid fluids, plasma volume expanders, or blood. Because hypotension generally responds better to volume replacement than to administration of vasoconstricting agents, pressor therapy such as the administration of the short-acting α1-adrenergic drug phenylephrine is generally withheld unless hypotension persists (Young and Landsberg, 1998).

Intraoperative hypertension is managed with the intravenous administration of phentolamine (Novartis, East Hanover, NJ), a short-acting, competitive α-adrenergic blocking drug. An initial loading dosage of 0.1 mg/kg IV is followed by a constant rate infusion of phentolamine at an initial dosage of 1-2 µg/kg/minute. Intraoperative hypotension is managed by decreasing the dose of or discontinuing phentolamine, administering the short-acting α1-adrenergic agonist phenylephrine, and/or expanding vascular volume by administering crystalloid fluids, plasma volume expanders, or blood.

If hypertension, tachycardia, or ventricular arrhythmias persists despite adequate α-adrenergic blockade, short-acting α1-adrenergic antagonist esmolol can be administered at an initial loading dosage of 0.1 mg/kg IV followed by a constant rate infusion at an initial dosage of 50 to 70 µg/kg/minute during surgery.

Unfortunately, dogs with pheochromocytoma often have concurrent disorders (see Table 9-5), some requiring anesthesia and surgery for treatment. For many of these dogs, pheochromocytoma is not suspected until life-threatening complications develop unexpectedly during maintenance of anesthesia. We have had several dogs with unsuspected pheochromocytoma acutely develop severe systemic hypertension, cardiac arrhythmias or both during induction of anesthesia for another problem (e.g., radiation therapy for neoplasia; lens extraction for cataracts). These experiences further emphasize the importance of appropriate patient monitoring whenever a dog is anesthetized.

SURGICAL CONSIDERATIONS, POSTOPERATIVE COMPLICATIONS, AND OUTCOME. The surgical approach and techniques for excision of an adrenal mass have been described in veterinary surgical textbooks and will not be discussed here. Surgery for pheochromocytoma can be technically demanding. The extent of surgical exploration depends on the results of pre-operative studies employed to localize the tumor and on intraoperative findings. Although most pheochromocytomas in dogs are associated with only one adrenal gland, complete exploration of both suprarenal areas and the sympathetic chain around the abdominal aorta is recommended. In addition, careful evaluation of the caudal vena cava, phrenicoabdominal vein, regional lymph nodes, and other abdominal organs, especially the liver, should be undertaken to identify sites of metastasis. The malignant potential of a pheochromocytoma can be difficult to predict based on histologic appearance. Therefore, an investigation for malignancy at the time of surgery should always be carried out. Fluctuations in arterial blood pressure and heart rate usually decrease and hypertension and tachycardia improve following removal of the tumor. Metastatic tissue should be suspected if the blood pressure fails to decline or erratic and severe spikes in blood pressure persist. If both adrenal glands are removed, the clinician must be prepared to initiate therapy for adrenal insufficiency (see Chapter 8).

Postoperative complications are common and include hypertension, cardiac arrhythmias, respiratory distress, and hemorrhage (Kyles et al, 2003). Eight of 17 dogs undergoing adrenalectomy for pheochromocytoma in our hospital died during or within 10 days of surgery (Barthez et al, 1997). During surgery, 2 dogs died of cardiovascular arrest, 2 dogs were euthanized because of widespread metastatic disease, and 1 dog was euthanized because the primary tumor could not be resected. Three dogs died from surgical complications (respiratory distress, sepsis) or were euthanized (poor postsurgical recovery) within 10 days of surgery. Two dogs were lost to follow-up after being discharged from the hospital, 1 dog died 6 months and 2 dogs died 3 years after surgery from unrelated causes, 1 dog died 3.25 years after surgery of metastatic pheochromocytoma, and 3 dogs were alive and free of disease 3 years after surgery.

Medical Management

CONTROL OF BLOOD PRESSURE AND ARRHYTHMIAS. Medical therapy before surgery should stabilize the metabolic status of the animal, minimize the development of cardiac arrhythmias and severe hypertension during surgery, and control signs attributable to excessive catecholamine secretion in the animal with metastatic or non-resectable neoplasia. The first 2 goals for medical therapy have been reviewed in the section on surgical management. Chronic medical management is primarily designed to control excessive catecholamine secretion rather than local invasion or metastasis of the tumor to other organs. The α-adrenergic blocking drug phenoxybenzamine is used to control the clinical signs caused by excessive catecholamine secretion (see page 454). The dosage needed to control clinical signs in dogs is variable and unpredictable. As such, we usually begin treatment at a dosage of 0.25 mg/kg bid and gradually increase the dose, as needed, until clinical signs are controlled or adverse reactions to phenoxybenzamine develop (see Preoperative Management, page 454). In some dogs, β-adrenergic antagonist therapy (e.g., propranolol, atenolol) is also required to control persistent tachycardia but these drugs should not be administered without prior β-adrenergic blockade. α-adrenergic antagonist therapy in the absence of an α-antagonist may cause severe hypertension.

Active suppression of catecholamine synthesis should theoretically be an effective way to control excess catecholamine secretion by the pheochromocytoma. α-methylmetatyrosine (Metyrosine; DemserR, Merck Sharp and Dohme, West Point, PA) inhibits tyrosine hydroxylase and blocks the rate-limiting conversion of tyrosine to dopa in the catecholamine synthetic pathway (see Fig. 9-1, page 441) (Fraser, 1979). α-methylmetatyrosine has been used to inhibit catecholamine biosynthesis by the pheochromocytoma. Using doses of 0.3 to 4 g/day, 40% to 80% inhibition of catecholamine biosynthesis has been produced in humans with pheochromocytoma (Fraser, 1979). However, renal and neurologic toxicity limits

the use of this drug in humans to those with metastatic pheochromocytoma who cannot be cured by surgery. Use of this drug for the treatment of pheochromocytoma in the dog has not been reported.

RADIATION AND CHEMOTHERAPY. Because approximately 90% of pheochromocytomas are benign in humans, adrenalectomy is the treatment of choice and is usually curative (Young and Landsberg, 1998). The treatment of malignant pheochromocytoma also revolves around surgical removal, if possible. Apart from surgical therapy, no other forms of therapy are curative for malignant pheochromocytoma. Radiation therapy may be of value for providing relief of pain and controlling symptomatic involvement of bone (Keiser et al, 1985). 131I-metaiodobenzylguanidine (MIBG) has been used for radioimmunotherapy in some humans with malignant pheochromocytoma. In one comprehensive review of 116 humans treated with multiple doses of 131I-MIBG, improvement in clinical signs was achieved in 76% of patients, a decrease or normalization of plasma and urinary catecholamines and metabolites was achieved in 45%, and a reduction in tumor size by 50% or more was achieved in 30% of patients (Loh et al, 1997). Although MIBG has been used to image pheochromocytoma in dogs (see page 449), use for MIBG for treatment of pheochromocytoma has not yet been reported in dogs or cats.

Limited success has been reported with combination chemotherapy using cyclical cyclophosphamide, vincristine, and dacarbazine in humans (Keiser et al, 1985; Averbuch et al, 1988). In one study, combination chemotherapy produced a partial to complete response rate of 57% (median duration, 21 months; range, 7 to greater than 34 months) in 14 humans with metastatic pheochromocytoma (Averbuch et al, 1988). Partial to complete biochemical responses were seen in 79% of these patients. Results of treatment of malignant pheochromocytoma with chemotherapy has not been reported in the dog or cat.

Prognosis

The prognosis is dependent, in part, on the size of the adrenal mass, presence of metastasis or local invasion of the tumor into adjacent blood vessels or organs (e.g., kidney), avoidance of perioperative complications if adrenalectomy is performed, and the presence and nature of concurrent disease. Surgically-excisable tumors carry a guarded to good prognosis. Survival time in our dogs that underwent adrenalectomy and survived the immediate post-operative period ranged from 2 months to greater than 3 years. If metastatic disease is not present, perioperative complications are avoided, and serious concurrent disease not present, the dog has the potential to live a significant length of time (i.e., >1 to 2 years). Pre-treatment with an α-adrenergic blocking drug prior to surgery and involvement of an experienced anesthesiologist and surgeon with expertise in adrenal surgery helps minimize potentially serious perioperative complications associated with anesthesia and digital manipulation of the tumor. Medically-treated dogs can live longer than a year from the time of diagnosis if the tumor is relatively small (less than 3 cm diameter), vascular invasion is not present, and treatment with an α-adrenergic blocking drug is effective in minimizing the deleterious effects of episodic excessive catecholamine secretion by the tumor. Most dogs die or are euthanized because of complications caused by excessive catecholamine secretion, complications caused by tumor-induced venous thrombosis, or complications caused by invasion of the tumor or its metastases into surrounding organs.

THE INCIDENTAL ADRENAL MASS

During the past decade, ultrasound has become a routine diagnostic tool for the evaluation of soft tissue structures in the abdominal cavity. One consequence of abdominal ultrasound is the unexpected finding of a seemingly incidental adrenal mass (Fig. 9-11). The clinical relevance of an incidentally discovered adrenal mass is related to its etiology and, if a tumor, its malignant potential and functional status. Most incidentally discovered adrenal masses in an otherwise healthy dog or cat are benign non-functional tumors or non-neoplastic lesions (e.g., granuloma). Most functional adrenal masses are either adrenocortical tumors secreting cortisol or adrenal medullary tumors secreting catecholamines. As a general rule of thumb, an adrenal mass should be considered neoplastic until proven otherwise. Adrenalectomy is the treatment of choice if the mass is functional or malignant but adrenalectomy may not be indicated if the mass is benign, small, and hormonally inactive.

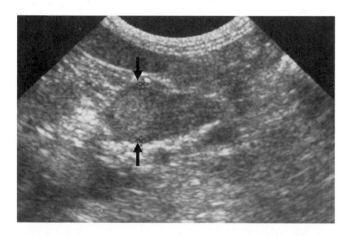

FIGURE 9–11. Abdominal ultrasound image of a 13-year-old female spayed Silky Terrier that presented to the veterinary hospital with a primary owner complaint of acute vomiting. A 1.2-cm diameter mass in one pole of the left adrenal gland *(arrows)* was unexpectedly found during the ultrasound examination. The right adrenal gland was normal in size. Results of routine blood work, tests for hyperadrenocorticism, and arterial blood pressure were normal. The etiology of the mass remains unknown.

Unfortunately, it is not easy to determine if an adrenal mass is malignant or benign prior to surgical removal and histopathologic evaluation. Guidelines to suggest malignancy include size of the mass, invasion of the mass into surrounding organs and blood vessels, and identification of additional mass lesions with abdominal ultrasound and thoracic radiographs. The bigger the mass the more likely it is malignant and the more likely metastasis has occurred, regardless of findings on abdominal ultrasound and thoracic radiographs. Cytologic or histologic evaluation of specimens obtained by ultrasound-guided fine needle aspiration or core biopsy of the adrenal mass, respectively, may provide guidance regarding malignancy and origin of the mass, i.e., adrenal cortex versus medulla (Chun et al, 1997; Rosenstein, 2000).

An adrenal tumor may be functional (i.e., producing and secreting a hormone) or nonfunctional. Excess secretion of cortisol, catecholamines, aldosterone, progesterone, and steroid hormone precursors have been documented in dogs and cats (Table 9-10). The most common functional adrenal tumors secrete cortisol (i.e., adrenal-dependent hyperadrenocorticism, see page 262) or catecholamines (i.e., pheochromocytoma, see page 440). Aldosterone-secreting adrenal tumors causing primary hyperaldosteronism (Conn's Syndrome) are rare in the dog and cat, and should be suspected in dogs and cats with lethargy, weakness, hypernatremia, severe hypokalemia (less than 3.0 mEq/L), and systemic hypertension (see page 351). Functional tumors arising from the zona reticularis of the adrenal cortex can secrete excessive amounts of estrogen, progesterone or testosterone but, to date, progesterone-secreting adrenocortical tumors have been most commonly identified (Boord and Griffin, 1999; Rossmeisl et al, 2000; Syme et al, 2001). Excessive progesterone secretion in affected cats caused diabetes mellitus and feline fragile skin syndrome, which was characterized by progressively worsening dermal and epidermal atrophy, patchy endocrine alopecia, and easily torn skin (see page 391). The clinical features mimicked feline hyperadrenocorticism, which is the primary differential diagnosis (see page 360). Results of tests of the pituitary-adrenocortical axis are normal to suppressed in cats with progesterone-secreting adrenal tumors and the contra lateral adrenal gland is normal in size and shape on abdominal ultrasound. Diagnosis requires documenting an increased plasma progesterone concentration.

Functional tumors producing excessive amounts of an intermediary in the biosynthetic pathway of adrenocortical steroids are rare in dogs and cats. A deoxycorticosterone-secreting adrenocortical carcinoma has been documented in a dog (Reine et al, 1999). Deoxycorticosterone is a precursor of aldosterone, has mineralocorticoid activity and acts on the same receptors as does aldosterone. The major clinical features were weakness, marked hypokalemia, and systemic hypertension. Increased plasma deoxycorticosterone and nondetectable plasma aldosterone concentrations were documented in the dog. Adrenal

TABLE 9–10   ADRENAL TUMORS REPORTED IN DOGS AND CATS

	Hormone Secreted	Species	Clinical Syndrome	Tests to Establish Diagnosis
Nonfunctional adrenal tumor	None	Dog*, Cat	- - -	Diagnosis by exclusion Histopathology
Functional adrenocortical tumor	Cortisol	Dog*, Cat	Hyperadrenocorticism Cushing's syndrome	ACTH stimulation test - measure cortisol. Low dose dexamethasone suppression test
	Aldosterone	Cat*, Dog	Hyperaldosteronism Conn's syndrome	Serum K/Na. ACTH stimulation - measure aldosterone
	Progesterone	Cat*, Dog	Mimics hyperadrenocorticism	Serum progesterone
	Steroid hormone precursors 17-OH-progesterone	Dog	Mimics hyperadrenocorticism	ACTH stimulation test - measure steroid hormone precursors
	Deoxycorticosterone	Dog	Mimics hyperaldosteronism	ACTH stimulation test - measure steroid hormone precursors
Functional adrenomedullary tumor	Epinephrine	Dog*, Cat	Pheochromocytoma	Diagnosis by exclusion Histopathology

*Species most commonly affected.
From Nelson RW, Couto CG: Small Animal Internal Medicine. St Louis, Mosby, 2003, p. 811.

tumors secreting 17-OH-progesterone and progesterone have also been documented in dogs (Ristic et al, 2002). 17-OH-progesterone is a precursor of cortisol. Affected dogs had clinical signs and physical examination findings suggestive of hyperadrenocorticism, results of tests to assess the pituitary-adrenocortical axis were normal or suppressed, and pre- and post-ACTH stimulation plasma 17-OH-progesterone concentrations were increased.

A thorough review of the clinical signs, physical examination findings, results of routine blood and urine tests and performance of appropriate hormonal tests should be done to determine the functional status of an incidental adrenal mass. Urine cortisol/creatinine ratio, ACTH stimulation test and low dose dexamethasone suppression test are used to rule out hyperadrenocorticism. If weakness and severe hypokalemia are present, plasma aldosterone concentrations can be measured in addition to plasma cortisol concentrations during the ACTH stimulation test. We do not routinely perform specific hormonal tests to identify pheochromocytoma. If hormonal tests for hyperadrenocorticism and serum electrolyte concentrations are normal and clinical signs suggestive of pheochromocytoma are present, we assume the adrenal mass is a pheochromocytoma and begin treatment with an α-adrenergic antagonist (see page 457).

If hormonal tests for hyperadrenocorticism and serum electrolyte concentrations are normal, clinical signs suggestive of pheochromocytoma are not present, and adrenalectomy is planned, we still assume the adrenal mass is a pheochromocytoma and begin phenoxybenzamine treatment prior to adrenalectomy.

Adrenalectomy may or may not be indicated if hormonal tests for hyperadrenocorticism and serum electrolyte concentrations are normal and clinical signs

and systemic hypertension suggestive of pheochromocytoma are not present. In theory, adrenalectomy offers the best chance for long-term survival of the dog or cat, assuming the mass is a malignant tumor. However, when considering adrenalectomy the clinician should also consider the age and health of the dog or cat, the size and invasive nature of the mass, and the probability for metastasis. Surgery is generally not indicated in old dogs and cats, especially if concurrent illness raises the anesthetic risk to an unacceptable level, when metastasis has been identified or if serious complications are likely because of the size or invasive nature of the mass. In addition, adrenalectomy may not be indicated when the mass is small (<3 cm diameter) and presumed to be nonfunctional, and the dog or cat is healthy. An alternative approach in these cases is to determine the rate of growth of the mass by repeating abdominal ultrasound initially at 1, 2, 4, and 6 months (Fig. 9-12). If the adrenal mass does not change in size, the time between ultrasound evaluations can be increased to every 4 to 6 months. However, if the adrenal mass is increasing in size, adrenalectomy should be considered.

MULTIPLE ENDOCRINE NEOPLASIA (MEN)

A group of heritable syndromes characterized by aberrant growth of benign or malignant tumors in a subset of endocrine tissues have been given the collective term multiple endocrine neoplasia (MEN) (Gardner, 2001). The tumors may be functional (i.e., capable of elaborating hormonal products that result in specific clinical findings characteristic of the hormone excess state) or nonfunctional. There are three major syndromes: MEN 1, MEN 2A, and MEN 2B (Table 9-11) (Gagel, 1998; Gardner, 2001). Mixed-type

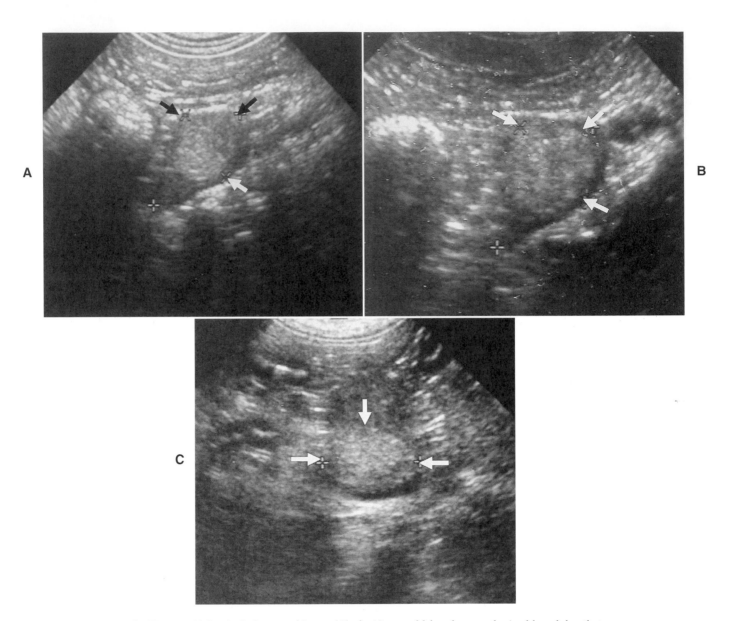

FIGURE 9–12. Abdominal ultrasound image *(A)* of a 10-year-old female spayed mixed-breed dog that presented to the veterinary hospital with a primary owner complaint of acute onset of lethargy, vomiting, and diarrhea. A 1.4-cm diameter mass in one pole of the left adrenal gland *(arrows)* was unexpectedly found during the ultrasound examination. The right adrenal gland was normal in size. Results of routine blood work, tests for hyperadrenocorticism, and arterial blood pressure were normal. Ultrasound evaluations of the adrenal mass were repeated various times during the next 2 years. At 1 year *(B)* and 2 years *(C)* later, the diameter of the adrenal mass measured 1.8 cm and 2.0 cm, respectively. During this time, the dog remained healthy and tests of adrenocortical function remained normal. The dog is alive and doing well 3 years after the initial discovery of the adrenal mass. The etiology of the mass remains unknown.

MEN syndromes with some of the features of MEN1, MEN 2A, and MEN 2B have also been reported in humans (Cance and Wells, 1985; Gagel, 1998).

MEN 1 and MEN 2 share certain characteristics in humans. First, the cell type involved in the neoplastic process is usually composed of one or more specific polypeptide- or biogenic-amine–producing cell types (i.e., amine precursor uptake and decarboxylation or APUD cells). The exceptions are lipomas associated with MEN 1 and mucosal neuromas and colonic polyps associated with MEN 2B. A second feature shared by these syndromes is the histological progression from hyperplasia to adenoma, and, in some cases, to carcinoma. Third, the development of hyperplasia is probably a multicentric process, with each focus of tumor derived from a single clone (Arnold et al, 1988). Last, each of these syndromes has an autosomal dominant pattern of inheritance. However, the MEN syndromes have different mechanisms of tumorigenesis. MEN 1 is caused by an

TABLE 9–11 COMPARISON OF THE CLINICAL FEATURES OF THE MAJOR SYNDROMES CHARACTERIZED BY MULTIPLE ENDOCRINE GLAND HYPERFUNCTION IN HUMANS

Endocrine Abnormality	MEN 1	MEN 2A	MEN 2B
Hyperparathyroidism	90%–95%	25%	Rare
Endocrine pancreatic tumors	30%–80%	——	——
Pituitary adenomas	20%–25%	——	——
Subcutaneous lipomas	30%	——	——
Thyroid adenoma	Rare	——	——
Adrenal adenomas	40%	——	——
Carcinoid tumor	20%	——	——
Medullary carcinoma of the thyroid gland	——	80%–100%	100%
Pheochromocytoma	——	40%	50%
Mucosal neuromas	——	——	100%
Intestinal ganglioneuromas	——	——	> 40%
Marfanoid habitus	——	——	75%
Inheritance	Autosomal dominant	Autosomal dominant	Autosomal dominant

inherited mutation of a tumor suppressor gene, menin, on the long arm of chromosome 11 (Gardner, 2001). Tumor suppressor genes control some important aspects of growth, differentiation, or cell death, and loss of both copies (alleles) results in unregulated growth. In contrast, MEN 2A and MEN 2B syndromes are caused by activation of the RET proto-oncogene located on chromosome 10 (Marsh et al, 1996; Pasini et al, 1996). The two most common RET mutations activate the tyrosine kinase receptor, thereby causing unregulated growth of the cells associated with MEN 2 (Gagel, 1998). Expression of a mutated RET gene in transgenic mice has been reported to precipitate C-cell hyperplasia and C-cell carcinomas morphologically similar to those seen in humans with MEN 2 syndromes (Michiels et al, 1997).

MEN TYPE 1. The familial association of parathyroid, pancreatic islet, and pituitary hyperplasia or neoplasia is called MEN 1 (see Table 9-11). Hyperparathyroidism causing hypercalcemia is the most common manifestation of MEN 1 (Gagel, 1998). Multiglandular parathyroid hyperplasia is the most common histological lesion, although in those humans where the disease is diagnosed late, adenomatous changes may also be present. Surgery is the treatment of choice for hyperparathyroidism associated with MEN 1. Recurrence of hypercalcemia is common, presumably because of the "hyperplastic" nature of the parathyroid disorder rather than solitary, functioning adenomas (Rizzoli et al, 1985).

Neoplasia of the pancreatic islet cells is the second most common manifestation of MEN 1. Although the pancreatic islet cell tumor is frequently identified by the clinical syndrome caused by a single hormone product (e.g., insulin), most of these tumors demonstrate hyperplasia of multiple cell types and produce several different peptides and biogenic amines (Pilato et al, 1988; Gardner, 2001). Gastrinoma causing the Zollinger-Ellison syndrome (i.e., gastric acid hypersecretion caused by excessive production of gastrin; see Chapter 15) is a major cause of morbidity and mortality in humans with MEN 1. Increased gastrin production has been demonstrated in approximately

50% to 60% of humans with functional pancreatic tumors associated with MEN 1 (Eberle and Grun, 1981). Insulinoma causing hypoglycemia is the second most common pancreatic islet cell tumor; accounting for about 20% of functional pancreatic neoplasms in MEN 1 (Gardner, 2001). Pancreatic tumors secreting excess glucagon (glucagonoma), vasoactive intestinal polypeptide (watery diarrhea syndrome), and pancreatic polypeptide (pancreatic polypeptide-oma) are uncommon components of MEN 1 (see Chapter 15).

Pituitary tumors occur in more than half of humans with MEN 1 (Eberle and Grun, 1981). The tumors are multicentric and include prolactinoma (most common), growth hormone-producing tumors, and adrenocorticotropin (ACTH)-producing tumors. Clinical manifestations include galactorrhea, acromegaly, and Cushing's syndrome, respectively.

MEN TYPE 2A. The clinical syndrome of MEN 2A is characterized by bilateral and multicentric medullary thyroid carcinoma, unilateral or bilateral pheochromocytoma, and, less commonly, parathyroid hyperplasia or adenomatosis (see Table 9-11; Gagel, 1998). Medullary thyroid carcinoma is a multicentric neoplasm of the parafollicular or C cell of the thyroid gland. The earliest demonstrable abnormality in the thyroid gland of humans with this syndrome is hyperplasia of C cells, followed by progression to nodular hyperplasia, microscopic medullary thyroid carcinoma, and finally frank medullary thyroid carcinoma (DeLellis et al, 1986). These changes are multicentric, with the frequent occurrence of more than one type of histological lesion in one or both lobes of the thyroid.

Adrenal chromaffin tissue in humans with MEN 2A undergoes the same type of histological progression as that observed for the C cell, including hyperplasia, diffuse expansion of the adrenal medulla, and pheochromocytoma (Gagel, 1998). The usual finding is single or multiple pheochromocytomas, with a background of hyperplastic chromaffin tissue. The pheochromocytomas may be unilateral or bilateral. Clinical signs are caused by excessive secretion of catecholamines (see page 444).

Hyperparathyroidism causing hypercalcemia occurs in 10 to 20% of humans with the mature form of MEN 2A (Cance and Wells, 1985). Histologic evaluation of parathyroid glands from affected humans usually reveals occasional adenomatous formation with a background of parathyroid hyperplasia (Carney et al, 1980), a finding that is analogous to that observed for C cell abnormalities.

MEN TYPE 2B. The association of medullary thyroid carcinoma and pheochromocytoma with multiple mucosal neuromas and intestinal ganglioneuromas is termed MEN 2B (see Table 9-11). The hallmark of this syndrome is the presence of characteristic mucosal neuromas on the distal portion of the tongue, on the lips and subconjunctival areas, and throughout the gastrointestinal tract (Gagel, 1998). The clinical course of humans with medullary thyroid carcinoma in this syndrome is more aggressive than that in MEN 2A; metastatic disease can occur in children younger than 1 year of age (Telander et al, 1986). Unilateral or bilateral pheochromocytoma occurs in approximately half of individuals with this disorder and is histologically similar to that in MEN 2A (Hubner and Holschneider, 1987).

MEN IN DOGS AND CATS. Syndromes resembling MEN in humans are uncommon to rare in dogs and cats, but have been described. Peterson et al (1982) described a 15 year old Wire-Haired Fox Terrier with medullary carcinoma of the thyroid gland, pheochromocytoma, and parathyroid hyperplasia. These findings would be consistent with MEN 2A of humans. Variants of MEN syndromes have also been described in the literature, including 4 dogs with thyroid neoplasia and adrenal adenoma (Hayes and Fraumeni, 1975), a 14 year old Yorkshire Terrier with pheochromocytoma and primary hyperparathyroidism (Wright et al, 1995), a 10 year old standard Schnauzer with a pituitary corticotrophic tumor, bilateral adrenocortical tumors, and pheochromocytoma (Thuróczy et al, 1998), and a 12 year old mixed-breed dog with pituitary-dependent hyperadrenocorticism and primary hyperparathyroidism (Walker et al, 2000). In our series of dogs with thyroid neoplasia, 63 dogs had tumors involving one or more endocrine glands in addition to the thyroid gland (see Table 5-4, page 225). Whether these dogs had familial disorders analogous to the MEN syndromes, had disorders similar to MEN of mixed type (i.e., overlap syndromes) or simply had multiple problems that were purely coincidental is not known. However, recognition that multiple endocrine tumors can occur in the same dog or cat, regardless of whether the finding is indicative of MEN or not, emphasizes the value of a complete diagnostic evaluation of animals with endocrine neoplasia.

In humans, each component of the various syndromes develop independently, and the clinical expression of the components within each form of MEN is variable, although hyperparathyroidism usually predominates in MEN 1, and medullary thyroid carcinoma predominates in MEN 2A and 2B (Leshin, 1985). A similar tendency has been observed in our dogs and cats diagnosed with MEN, i.e., each endocrine tumor expresses its own clinical signs and clinicopathologic abnormalities independent of concurrent endocrine tumors. Management of the various manifestations of MEN is, for the most part, similar to management of the identical manifestations when they occur in sporadic form.

REFERENCES

Arnold A, et al: Monoclonality and abnormal parathyroid hormone genes in parathyroid adenomas. N Engl J Med 318:658, 1988.

Averbuch SD, et al: Malignant pheochromocytoma: Effective treatment with a combination of cyclophosphamide, vincristine, and dacarbazine. Ann Intern Med 109:267, 1988.

Barthez PY, et al: Pheochromocytoma in dogs: 61 cases (1984-1995). J Vet Intern Med 11:272, 1997.

Bennett PF, Norman EJ: Mitotane (o,p'-DDD) resistance in a dog with pituitary-dependent hyperadrenocorticism and phaeochromocytoma. Aust Vet J 76:101, 1998.

Berry CR, et al: Use of ^{123}iodine metaiodobenzylguanidine scintigraphy for the diagnosis of a pheochromocytoma in a dog. Vet Rad Ultrasound 34:52, 1993.

Berry CR, et al: Imaging of pheochromocytoma in two dogs using p-[^{18}F]fluorobenzylguanidine. Vet Rad Ultrasound 43:183, 2002.

Bodey AR, Michell AR: Epidemiological study of blood pressure in domestic dogs. J Small Anim Pract 37:116, 1996.

Boord M, Griffin C: Progesterone secreting adrenal mass in a cat with clinical signs of hyperadrenocorticism. J Am Vet Med Assoc 214:666, 1999.

Bouayad H, et al: Pheochromocytoma in dogs: 13 cases (1980-1985). J Am Vet Med Assoc 191:1610, 1987.

Buchanan JW, et al: Left atrial paraganglioma in a dog: Echocardiography, surgery, and scintigraphy. J Vet Intern Med 12:109, 1998.

Cance WG, Wells SA, Jr. Multiple endocrine neoplasia type IIa. Curr Probl Surg 22:1, 1985.

Carney JA, et al: The parathyroid glands in multiple endocrine neoplasia type 2b. Am J Pathol 99:387, 1980.

Chun R, et al: Apocrine gland adenocarcinoma and pheochromocytoma in a cat. J Am Anim Hosp Assoc 33:33, 1997.

Cryer PE: Catecholamines, pheochromocytoma and diabetes. Diabetes Rev 1:309, 1993.

Deftos LJ, et al: Human pituitary tumors secrete chromogranin-A. J Clin Endocrinol Metab 68:869, 1989.

DeLellis RA, et al: Multiple endocrine neoplasia (MEN) syndromes: cellular origins and interrelationships. Int Rev Exp Pathol 28:163, 1986.

Desmonts JM, Marty J. Anaesthetic management of patients with phaeochromocytoma. J Anaesth 56:781, 1984.

Doss JC, et al: Immunohistochemical localization of chromogranin A in endocrine tissues and endocrine tumors in dogs. Vet Pathol 35:312, 1998.

Duncan MW, et al: Measurement of norepinephrine and 3,4-dihydroxyphenylglycol in urine and plasma for the diagnosis of pheochromocytoma. N Engl J Med 319:136, 1988.

Eberle F, Grun R. Multiple endocrine neoplasia, type I (MEN I). Ergeb Inn Med Kinderheilkd 46:76, 1981.

Fischer M, et al: Scintigraphic localization of phaeochromocytomas. Clin Endocrinol 20:1, 1984.

Fraser DG. Alpha-MPT and pheochromocytoma. Drug Intel Clin Pharm 13:597, 1979.

Gagel RF: Multiple endocrine neoplasia. In Wilson JD, Foster DW, Kronenberg HM, Larsen PR (eds): Williams Textbook of Endocrinology, 9th ed. Philadelphia, WB Saunders Co, 1998, p 1627.

Gardner DG: Multiple endocrine neoplasia. In Greenspan FS, Gardner DG (eds): Basic and Clinical Endocrinology, 6th ed. New York, Lange Medical Books/McGraw Hill, 2001, p 792.

Gilson SD, et al: Pheochromocytoma in 50 dogs. J Vet Int Med 8:228, 1994.

Goldfarb DA, et al: Magnetic resonance imaging for assessment of vena caval tumor thrombi: A comparative study with venacavography and computerized tomography scanning. J Urol 144:1100, 1990.

Goldfien A: Adrenal medulla. In Greenspan FS, Gardner DG (eds): Basic and Clinical Endocrinology, 6th ed. New York, Lange Medical Books/McGraw-Hill, 2001, p 399.

Gough IR, et al: Limitations of I-MIBG scintigraphy in locating pheochromocytomas. Surgery 98:115, 1985.

Hanson MW, et al: Iodine^{131}-labeled metaiodobenzylguanidine scintigraphy and biochemical analysis in suspected pheochromocytoma. Arch Intern Med 151:1397, 1991.

Hayes HM, Fraumeni JF: Canine thyroid neoplasms: Epidemiologic features. J Natl Cancer Inst 55:931, 1975.

Henry CJ, et al: Adrenal pheochromocytoma. J Vet Int Med 7:199, 1993.

Hines ME, et al: Metastasizing extra-adrenal paraganglioma with neurological signs in four dogs. J Comp Path 108:283, 1993.

Hsiao RJ, et al: Chromogranin A storage and secretion: Sensitivity and specificity for the diagnosis of pheochromocytoma. Medicine 70:33, 1991.

Hubner A, Holschneider AM. Multiple endocrine neoplasias in three generations. Langenbecks Arch Chir 372:747, 1987.

Hull CJ. Phaeochromocytoma. Diagnosis, preoperative preparation and anaesthetic management. Br J Anaesth 58:1453, 1986.

Johnson RG, et al: Catecholamine transport and energy-linked function of chromaffin granules isolated from a human pheochromocytoma. Biochem Biophys Acta 716:366, 1982.

Jones DH, et al: The biochemical diagnosis, localization and follow up of pheochromocytomas: The role of plasma and urinary catecholamine measurements. Q J Med 49:341, 1980.

Karam JH: Hypoglycemic disorders. In Greenspan FS, Gardner DG (eds): Basic and Clinical Endocrinology, 6th ed. New York, Lange Medical Books/McGraw-Hill, 2001, p 699.

Keiser HR, et al: Treatment of malignant pheochromocytoma with combination chemotherapy. Hypertension 7(suppl):118, 1985.

Krothapalli RK, et al: Modulation of the hydro-osmotic effect of vasopressin on the rabbit cortical collecting tubule by adrenergic agents. J Clin Invest 72:287, 1983.

Kyles AE, et al: Evaluation of the surgical management of adrenal tumor-associated tumor thrombi in dogs: 40 cases (1994-2001). J Am Vet Med Assoc 223:654, 2003.

Lamb CR, et al: Diagnosis of calcification on abdominal radiographs. Vet Radiol 32:211, 1991.

Leshin M: Multiple endocrine neoplasia. In Wilson JD, Foster DW (eds): Williams Textbook of Endocrinology, 7th ed. Philadelphia, WB Saunders Co, 1985, p. 1274.

Loh KC, et al: The treatment of malignant pheochromocytoma with iodine-131 metaiodobenzylguanidine (^{131}I-MIBG): A comprehensive review of 116 reported patients. J Endocrinol Invest 20:648, 1997.

Lucon AM, et al: Pheochromocytoma: Study of 50 cases. J Urol 157:1208, 1997.

Marsh DJ, et al: The identification of false positive responses to the pentagastrin stimulation test in RET mutation negative members of MEN 2A families. Clin Endocrinol 44: 213, 1996.

Michiels FM, et al: Development of medullary thyroid carcinoma in transgenic mice expressing the RET protooncogene altered by a multiple endocrine neoplasia type 2A mutation. Proc Natl Acad Sci USA 94:3330, 1997.

Moattari AR, et al: Effects of Sandostatin on plasma chromogranin-A levels in neuroendocrine tumors. J Clin Endocrinol Metab 69:902, 1989.

O'Connor DT, Deftos LJ. Secretion of chromogranin A by peptide-producing endocrine neoplasms. N Engl J Med 314:1145, 1986.

Pasini B, et al: RET mutations in human disease. Trends Genet 12: 138, 1996.

Patnaik AK, et al: Extra-adrenal pheochromocytoma (paraganglioma) in a cat. J Am Vet Med Assoc 197:104, 1990.

Peterson ME, et al: Multiple endocrine neoplasia in a dog. J Am Vet Med Assoc 180:1476, 1982.

Pilato FP, et al: Nonrandom expression of polypeptide hormones in pancreatic endocrine tumors. An immunohistochemical study in a case of multiple islet cell neoplasia. Cancer 61:1815, 1988.

Platt SR, et al: Pheochromocytoma in the vertebral canal of two dogs. J Am Anim Hosp Assoc 34:365, 1998.

Prys-Roberts C: Phaeochromocytoma-recent progress in its management. Br J Anaes 85:44, 2000.

Prys-Roberts C, Farndon JR: Efficacy and safety of doxazosin for perioperative management of patients with pheochromocytoma. World J Surg 19:26, 2002.

Reine NJ, et al: Deoxycorticosterone-secreting adrenocortical carcinoma in a dog. J Vet Intern Med 13:386, 1999.

Ristic JME, et al: The use of 17-hydroxyprogesterone in the diagnosis of canine hyperadrenocorticism. J Vet Intern Med 16:433, 2002.

Rizzoli R, et al: Primary hyperparathyroidism in familial multiple endocrine neoplasia type I. Long-term follow-up of serum calcium levels after parathyroidectomy. Am J Med 78:467, 1985.

Roizen MF: Preoperative evaluation of patients with diseases that require special preoperative evaluation and intraoperative management. In Miller RE (ed): Anesthesia (Vol 1). New York, Churchill Livingstone, 1981, p. 21.

Roizen MF, et al: A prospective randomized trial of four anesthetic techniques for resection of pheochromocytoma. Anesthesiology 57:A43, 1982 (abstract).

Roizen MF, et al: The effect of alpha-adrenergic blockade on cardiac performance and tissue oxygen delivery during excision of pheochromocytoma. Surgery 94:941, 1983.

Roizen MP, et al: Characterization of the monoamine uptake system in catecholamine storage vesicles isolated from a pheochromocytoma taken from a child. Biochem Pharmacol 33: 2245, 1984.

Rosenstein DS: Diagnostic imaging in canine pheochromocytoma. Vet Rad Ultrasound 41:499, 2000.

Rossmeisl JH, et al: Hyperadrenocorticism and hyperprogesteronemia in a cat with an adrenocortical adenocarcinoma. J Am Anim Hosp Assoc 36:512, 2000.

Schaer M. Pheochromocytoma in a dog: A case report. J Am Anim Hosp Assoc 16:583, 1980.

Schoeman JP, Stidworthy MF: Budd-Chiari-like syndrome associated with an adrenal phaeochromocytoma in a dog. J Small Anim Pract 42:191, 2001.

Shapiro B, et al: Iodine-131 metaiodobenzylguanidine for the locating of suspected pheochromocytoma: experience in 400 cases. J Nucl Med 26:576, 1985.

Sisson JC, Wieland DM: Radiolabeled meta-iodobenzylguanidine: pharmacology and clinical studies. Am J Physiol Imaging 1:96, 1986.

Sisson JC, et al: Scintigraphic localization of pheochromocytomas. N Engl J Med 305:12, 1981.

Syme HM, et al: Hyperadrenocorticism associated with excessive sex hormone production by an adrenocortical tumor in two dogs. J Am Vet Med Assoc 219:1725, 2001.

Telander RL, et al: Results of early thyroidectomy for medullary thyroid carcinoma in children with multiple endocrine neoplasia type 2. J Pediatr Surg 21:1190, 1986.

Thompson NW, et al: Extra-adrenal and metastatic pheochromocytomas, the role of ^{131}I-meta-iodobenzyl-guanidine in localization and management. World J Surg 8:605, 1984.

Thuróczy J, et al: Multiple endocrine neoplasias in a dog: Corticotrophic tumour, bilateral adrenocortical tumours, and pheochromocytoma. Vet Quart 20: 56, 1998.

Tobes MC et al: Comparison of the in vitro pharmacodynamics of meta-iodobenzylguanidine (MIBG) to the in vivo scintigraphy. Nucl Med Commun 6:585, 1985.

Twedt DC, Wheeler SL. Pheochromocytoma in the dog. Vet Clin North Am [Small Animal Pract] 14:767, 1984.

von Dehn BJ, et al: Pheochromocytoma and hyperadrenocorticism in dogs: Six cases (1982-1992). J Am Vet Med Assoc 207:322, 1995.

Walker MC, et al: Multiple endocrine neoplasia type 1 in a crossbred dog. J Small Anim Pract 41:67, 2000.

Werbel SS, Ober KP: Pheochromocytoma. Update on diagnosis, localization, and management. Med Clin N Amer 79:131, 1995.

Whittemore JC, et al: Nontraumatic rupture of an adrenal gland tumor causing intra-abdominal or retroperitoneal hemorrhage in four dogs. J Am Vet Med Assoc 219:329, 2001.

Williams JE, et al: Pheochromocytoma presenting as acute retroperitoneal hemorrhage in a dog. J Vet Emerg Critic Care 11:221, 2001.

Winkler H, Fischer-Colbrie R: Chromogranin A and B: The first 25 years and future perspectives. Neuroscience 49:497, 1992.

Wright KN, et al: Diagnostic and therapeutic considerations in a hypercalcemic dog with multiple endocrine neoplasia. J Am Anim Hosp Assoc 31: 156, 1995.

Young JB, Landsberg L: Catecholamines and the adrenal medulla. In Wilson JD, Foster DW, Kronenberg HM, Larsen PR (eds): Williams Textbook of Endocrinology, 9th ed. Philadelphia, WB Saunders Co, 1998, p. 665.

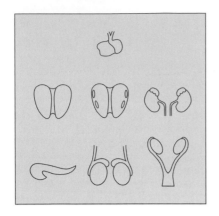

10

GLUCOCORTICOID THERAPY

The products secreted by the adrenal cortex, or outer portion of the adrenal gland, are hormones necessary for normal metabolic function. Although it is possible for life to continue for a transient period of time in the complete *absence* of adrenocortical function, serious metabolic derangements usually ensue, and the capacity of the individual to respond to physiologic or environmental stress is completely lost. Chances of survival are critically compromised in any animal with severe adrenocortical hormone deficiency. Life may also be sustained despite *excesses* in adrenocortical secretion. Again, severe metabolic derangements ensue that interfere with chances for normal survival. The vital role of the adrenal cortex is due to the production and regulated secretion of a group of hormones, all *steroid* in nature. Two major groups of hormones are synthesized and secreted by the adrenal cortex: mineralocorticoids and glucocorticoids. Glucocorticoids are perhaps the most widely used therapeutic agents in veterinary practice.

THE CHEMISTRY OF GLUCOCORTICOIDS

More than 50 natural steroids are synthesized and secreted by the adrenal cortex, but only a few have identified significant biologic actions. All adrenocortical hormones are derivatives of the cyclopentanoperhydrophenanthrene nucleus (Fig. 10-1).

These steroids include androgens, glucocorticoids, and mineralocorticoids. All of the adrenocortical steroids, except the androgens, contain 21 carbon atoms, an α,β-unsaturated ketone in ring A, and an α-ketol chain ($-COCH_2OH$) attached to ring D. They differ in the extent of oxygenation or hydroxylation at carbon 11, 17, or 19. Depending on whether the predominant biologic effect is related to electrolyte and water metabolism or to carbohydrate and protein metabolism, the adrenocortical steroids are classified as *mineralocorticoid* or *glucocorticoid,* respectively.

Clinical experience suggests that the antiinflammatory activity of adrenocortical steroids in humans correlates well with their glucocorticoid activity. The undesirable side effects (sodium retention, edema) are associated with mineralocorticoid activity. Synthetic steroids possessing higher glucocorticoid and lower mineralocorticoid activity than cortisol are commonly marketed. All adrenal corticoids require the 3-keto group and 4-5 unsaturation (see Fig. 10-1).

Additional unsaturation in ring A enhances antiinflammatory properties while reducing the sodium-retaining effect. Prednisolone, therefore, has four times the antiinflammatory activity of cortisol, yet only 0.8 the mineralocorticoid activity (Fig. 10-2). The presence of oxygen at position 11 is necessary for significant glucocorticoid activity but not for mineralocorticoid activity; the 11β-hydroxy group is more potent than the 11-keto group, which is converted into the active

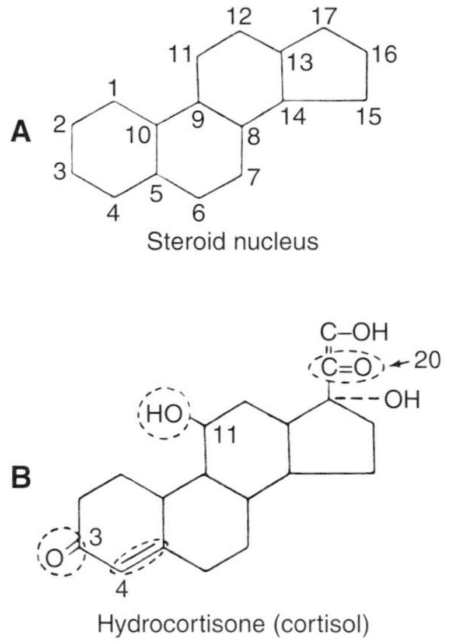

FIGURE 10–1. *A*, Steroid nucleus. *B*, Structure of cortisol. *Circled structures* are essential for glucocorticoid activity.

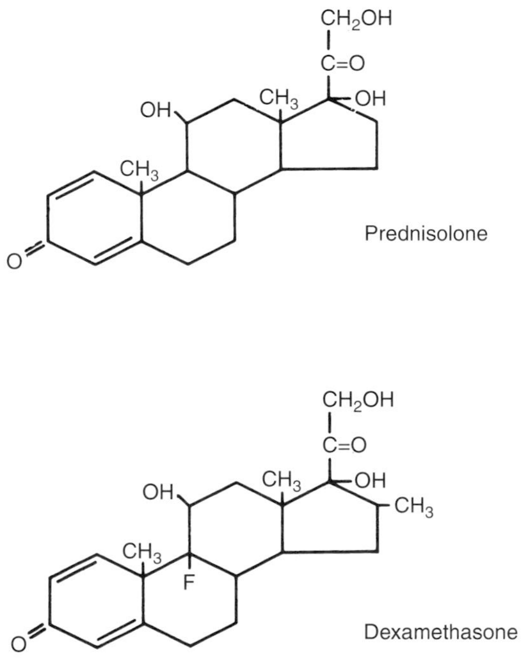

FIGURE 10–2. Synthetic corticosteroids. Structural differences between synthetic prednisolone and dexamethasone.

β-hydroxy group in the body. The 17α-hydroxy group is also important to glucocorticoid activity. The 21-hydroxy group is essential for mineralocorticoid activity; it favors but is not required for glucocorticoid activity. Introduction of either methyl or hydroxyl groups at position 16 markedly reduces mineralocorticoid activity but only slightly decreases glucocorticoid and antiinflammatory activity. Thus paramethasone (16α-methyl), betamethasone (16β-methyl), dexamethasone (16α-methyl), and triamcinolone (16α-hydroxy) have no significant mineralocorticoid

activity (see Fig. 10-2). 6α-Methylation has unpredictable effects. It enhances the mineralocorticoid activity of cortisol but virtually abolishes that of prednisolone. The 9α-fluoro group enhances both glucocorticoid and mineralocorticoid activity, but the effect of substitutions at the 6 and 16 positions overrides this effect (Osol, 1980).

BIOLOGIC EFFECTS

Molecular Mechanisms

Glucocorticoids were so-named because of their influence on glucose metabolism. They are currently recognized as *steroids* that exert their effect by binding to specific cytosolic receptors, which mediate their actions. Glucocorticoid receptors are present in virtually all tissues, and the glucocorticoid-receptor interaction is responsible for most of their known effects. Alterations in the structure of synthetic glucocorticoids have led to the development of compounds with greater glucocorticoid activity. The increased activity of these compounds is due to increased affinity for glucocorticoid receptors and delayed plasma clearance, which increases tissue exposure. Many of these synthetic glucocorticoids have negligible mineralocorticoid activity and thus do not cause sodium retention, hypertension, or hypokalemia.

Once a steroid hormone has permeated a cell membrane, it binds with a cytosolic glucocorticoid receptor protein (Fig. 10-3). These proteins probably originate in the nucleus but migrate into the cytosol in the presence of steroids. After binding, the steroid-protein complex enters the cell nucleus and interacts with nuclear chromatin acceptor sites. The 90 kDa heat shock protein hsp90 may be involved in hormone-induced glucocorticoid receptor activity. The DNA binding domain of the receptor is a cysteine-rich region that assumes a conformation known as a "zinc finger" after chelating zinc. The receptor-glucocorticoid complex binds to specific sites in nuclear DNA, the *glucocorticoid regulatory elements*. This results in the expression of specific genes and the transcription of specific messenger ribonucleic acids (mRNAs). The resulting proteins elicit the glucocorticoid response, which may be inhibitory or stimulatory depending on the specific gene and tissue affected.

Although glucocorticoid receptors are similar in many tissues, the proteins synthesized in response to glucocorticoids vary widely and are the result of specific gene expression. The mechanisms underlying this specific regulation are not known. Analyses of cloned complementary deoxyribonucleic acids (DNAs) for human glucocorticoid receptors have revealed marked structural and amino acid sequence homology between glucocorticoid receptors and receptors for other steroid hormones (e.g., mineralocorticoids, estrogen, progesterone), as well as for thyroid hormone and the oncogene v-*erb* A (Aron et al, 2001). Although the steroid-binding domain of the

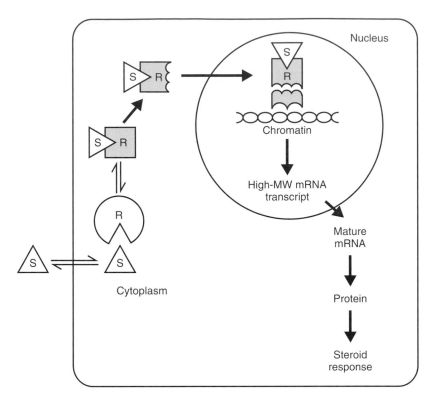

FIGURE 10–3. Steps in steroid hormone action. Activation of the intracellular receptors by steroid hormones is followed by nuclear binding of the complex and stimulation of mRNA synthesis. *R,* Receptor; *S,* steroid hormone. (From Aron DC, et al: *In* Greenspan FS, Gardner DG [eds]: Basic and Clinical Endocrinology, 6th ed. New York, Lange Medical Books/McGraw-Hill, 2001, p 334.)

glucocorticoid receptor confers specificity for glucocorticoid binding, glucocorticoids such as cortisol and corticosterone bind to the mineralocorticoid receptor with an affinity equal to that of aldosterone. Mineralocorticoid receptor specificity is maintained by the expression of 11β-hydroxysteroid dehydrogenase in classic mineralocorticoid-sensitive tissues. The expression of this glucocorticoid-inactivating enzyme in other tissues may serve to protect those tissues from excessive glucocorticoid action (Aron et al, 2001).

Mechanisms distinct from those described here are likely responsible for unique glucocorticoid actions. The most significant example is that of glucocorticoid-induced "fast feedback" inhibition of ACTH secretion. This effect occurs within minutes of glucocorticoid administration, which suggests that it is not due to the typical induction of RNA and protein synthesis. Rather, the feedback is probably related to changes in secretory function or cell membranes (Aron et al, 2001).

Intermediary Metabolism

Glucocorticoids, in general, inhibit DNA synthesis. In addition, in most tissues they inhibit RNA and protein synthesis and accelerate protein catabolism. These actions provide substrate for intermediary metabolism; however, accelerated catabolism also accounts for the deleterious effects of glucocorticoids on muscle, bone,

connective tissue, and lymphatic tissues. In contrast, RNA and protein synthesis in the liver are stimulated (Aron et al, 2001).

The effect of glucocorticoids on intermediary metabolism can be summarized as follows: (1) effects are minimal in the fed state; however, during fasting, glucocorticoids contribute to the maintenance of plasma glucose concentrations by increasing gluconeogenesis, glycogen deposition, and the peripheral release of substrate; (2) hepatic glucose production is enhanced, as is hepatic RNA and protein synthesis; (3) the effects on muscle are catabolic (i.e., decreased glucose uptake and metabolism, decreased protein synthesis, and increased release of amino acids); (4) in adipose tissue, lipolysis is stimulated; and (5) in glucocorticoid deficiency, hypoglycemia may result, whereas in states of glucocorticoid excess, there may be hyperglycemia, hyperinsulinemia, muscle wasting, and weight gain with abnormal fat distribution (Tyrrell et al, 1991).

Effects on Other Tissues

CONNECTIVE TISSUE. Glucocorticoids in excess inhibit fibroblasts, lead to loss of collagen and connective tissue, and thus result in thinning of the skin, easy bruising, and poor wound healing.

BONE. The physiologic role of glucocorticoids in bone metabolism and calcium homeostasis is not well understood. However, in excess, they directly inhibit bone formation by decreasing cell proliferation and the synthesis of RNA, protein, collagen, and hyaluronate. Glucocorticoids also directly stimulate bone-resorbing cells, leading to osteolysis and increased urinary hydroxyproline excretion. They also potentiate the actions of parathyroid hormone (PTH) and 1,25-dihydroxycholecalciferol (1,25[OH]$_2$D$_3$) on bone, and this may further contribute to net bone resorption.

CALCIUM METABOLISM. Glucocorticoids markedly reduce intestinal calcium absorption, which tends to lower the serum calcium concentration. This effect results in secondary increases in PTH secretion, in order to maintain the serum calcium concentration in the normal range by stimulating bone resorption. In addition, glucocorticoids may directly stimulate PTH release. The mechanism of decreased intestinal calcium absorption is unknown, although studies have demonstrated that it is not decreased synthesis or decreased serum concentrations of the active vitamin D metabolites; in fact, 1,25-vitamin D concentrations are normal or even increased in the presence of glucocorticoid excess. Increased 1,25-vitamin D synthesis may result from decreased serum phosphorus concentrations, increased serum PTH concentrations, and direct stimulation of renal 1α-hydroxylase. Glucocorticoids also increase urinary calcium excretion, and hypercalciuria is a consistent feature of cortisol excess in humans. Reduced tubular resorption of phosphate, leading to phosphaturia and decreased serum phosphorus concentrations, also occurs (Aron et al, 2001).

GROWTH AND DEVELOPMENT. Glucocorticoids accelerate the development of various systems and organs in fetal and differentiating tissues, although the mechanisms are unclear. As previously discussed, glucocorticoids are generally inhibitory, and stimulatory effects may be due to glucocorticoid interaction with other growth factors. Examples of development-promoting effects include increases in fetal lung surfactant production and accelerated development of hepatic and gastrointestinal enzyme systems.

Excess glucocorticoids inhibit growth in children, puppies, and kittens. This adverse effect could be a major complication of glucocorticoid therapy in immature individuals. Growth inhibition may be a direct effect of glucocorticoids on bone cells, although decreases in growth hormone (GH) secretion and somatomedin (insulin-like growth factor) generation also contribute.

CARDIOVASCULAR FUNCTION. Glucocorticoids may increase cardiac output and vascular tone by augmenting the effects of other vasoconstrictors, such as the catecholamines. Thus refractory shock may occur when a glucocorticoid-deficient individual is subjected to stress. Excess glucocorticoids may cause hypertension independent of their mineralocorticoid effects.

RENAL FUNCTION. Steroids affect water and electrolyte balance by actions mediated either by mineralocorticoid receptors (sodium and water retention, hypokalemia, and hypertension) or glucocorticoid receptors. The polydipsia and polyuria associated with glucocorticoid excess are rather unique to dogs and may be due to inhibition of vasopressin (ADH) secretion and/or interference with ADH action in renal tubular cells. Polyuria and polydipsia are not typical effects of glucocorticoid excess in cats or humans. Also of interest is the lack of renal concentrating ability associated with adrenocortical insufficiency in dogs.

CENTRAL NERVOUS SYSTEM (CNS). Glucocorticoids readily enter the brain, and although their physiologic role in CNS function is unknown, an excess or deficiency may profoundly alter behavior and cognitive function in humans (Tyrrell et al, 1991).

RED BLOOD CELLS. Glucocorticoids have little effect on erythropoiesis or hemoglobin concentration. Although mild polycythemia and anemia may be observed in dogs with Cushing's syndrome and Addison's disease, respectively, these alterations are more likely secondary to changes in androgen metabolism or secretion.

LEUKOCYTES. Glucocorticoids influence both white cell movement and function. Under the influence of glucocorticoids, white blood cell counts increase due to an increased rate of neutrophil (polymorphonuclear neutrophil [PMN]) release from the bone marrow, an increased circulating half-life of PMNs, and by inhibiting PMN movement out of the vascular space. Glucocorticoids reduce the numbers of circulating lymphocytes, monocytes, and eosinophils by increasing their movement out of the circulation. Glucocorticoids also reduce migration of inflammatory cells (PMNs, monocytes, and lymphocytes) to sites of injury. This is probably the primary mechanism of the anti-inflammatory action and increased susceptibility to infection associated with chronic steroid administration (Aron et al, 2001).

Effects on the Function of Endocrine Organs

IATROGENIC ADRENAL SUPPRESSION. The hypothalamic-pituitary-adrenal (HPA) axis of healthy dogs can be suppressed for an average of 32 hours after one intravenous injection of dexamethasone at a dosage of 0.1 mg/kg. Smaller doses result in a shorter mean duration of HPA suppression, which demonstrates that this suppressive effect is dose dependent (Kemppainen and Sartin, 1984). Cortisol typically suppresses the HPA axis for approximately 12 to 24 hours, whereas prednisolone is suppressive for 12 to 36 hours (Table 10-1). Adrenal suppression can follow treatment with almost any form of glucocorticoid. Ocular and topical skin formulations are examples of steroids that can be administered for several days or longer, can be absorbed systemically, and subsequently can suppress the HPA axis for weeks (Roberts et al 1984; Zenoble and Kemppainen, 1987).

Glucocorticoids given for days to weeks rarely have any prolonged significant clinical effects, but more chronic administration of any corticosteroid could cause

TABLE 10–1 DURATION OF ACTION OF NATURAL AND SYNTHETIC GLUCOCORTICOIDS FOLLOWING ORAL OR IV ADMINISTRATION

Drug	Duration of Action
Short-Acting	
Hydrocortisone	<12 hr
Cortisone	<12 hr
Intermediate-Acting	
Prednisone	12–36 hr
Prednisolone	12–36 hr
Methylprednisolone	12–36 hr
Triamcinolone	12–36 hr
Long-Acting	
Betamethasone	>48 hr
Dexamethasone	>48 hr
Flumethasone	>48 hr
Paramethasone	>48 hr

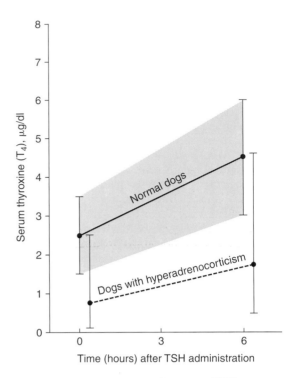

FIGURE 10–4. Thyroid-stimulating hormone (TSH) response test results in normal dogs and in dogs with spontaneous hyperadrenocorticism.

adrenocortical atrophy (iatrogenic hypoadrenocorticism). However, the degree of individual variation in response to glucocorticoid administration among dogs and cats is so pronounced that each dog and cat must be evaluated independently (Brockus et al, 1999).

Recovery of adrenocortical function occurs relatively quickly in dogs and cats after discontinuation of chronic steroid administration. Adrenocorticotropic hormone (ACTH) response test results usually return to normal within weeks. We almost never "taper" dogs or cats off steroids when administration of these drugs has been demonstrated to be unnecessary. Rather, the steroids are simply stopped. If there is concern about clinical signs caused by iatrogenic hypoadrenocorticism, steroids can be given at doses slowly tapered over a period of weeks, but this approach is almost never used. (Further discussion on suppression of the HPA axis is provided under Adverse Reactions, page 477.)

THYROID FUNCTION. Although basal thyroid-stimulating hormone (TSH) concentrations in humans are usually normal, TSH responsiveness to thyrotropin-releasing hormone (TRH) is frequently subnormal after chronic glucocorticoid therapy. Serum total thyroxine (T_4) concentrations are usually low-normal because of a decrease in thyroxine-binding globulin, but free T_4 concentrations are normal. Both the total and free T_3 concentrations may be low, because glucocorticoid excess decreases conversion of T_4 to T_3 and increases conversion to reverse T_3. Despite these alterations, manifestations of hypothyroidism are not apparent (Aron et al, 2001).

The serum total and free T_4 concentrations may be low normal or decreased both in dogs treated with glucocorticoids and in those with naturally occurring hyperadrenocorticism. Serum T_4 response to TSH may parallel but remain below normal reference limits (Fig. 10-4). The clinical and biochemical changes associated with chronic glucocorticoid excess in dogs are similar to those observed in hypothyroidism (lethargy, weakness, dermatologic alterations, hyper-

cholesterolemia). However, none of these require direct therapy, because correcting the cortisol excess resolves these problems (Woltz et al, 1983).

GONADAL FUNCTION. Glucocorticoids affect gonadotropin and gonadal function. In males, glucocorticoids inhibit gonadotropin secretion, as demonstrated by decreased circulating testosterone concentrations and testicular atrophy. In females, hypothalamic-pituitary suppression is also suggested by the interruption of estrus cycle activity.

Antiinflammatory Properties

OVERVIEW. The capacity of glucocorticoids to prevent or suppress inflammatory reactions not only is grossly visible by limiting heat, redness, swelling, and tenderness, but also can be documented microscopically. Glucocorticoids inhibit the early inflammatory phenomena of edema, fibrin deposition, capillary dilation, migration of leukocytes, and phagocytic activity. Glucocorticoids also limit later manifestations of inflammation such as capillary proliferation, fibroblast proliferation, deposition of collagen and, still later, cicatrization (Gilman et al, 1980; Aron et al, 2001).

Glucocorticoids inhibit inflammation whether the inciting agent is radiant, mechanical, chemical, infectious, or immune mediated. Such therapy is palliative in that the underlying cause of a disorder may remain, but its clinical manifestations are suppressed. This ability to suppress inflammation, regardless of its cause, has made glucocorticoids valuable therapeutic agents. However, these encompassing properties also make glucocorticoid therapy dangerous, because it can mask the clinical expression of a disease process. The inflammation that allows the clinician to recognize and monitor any nonsteroidal course of therapy can be completely suppressed, allowing a disease to continue or worsen while preventing this process from being identified. As with any therapy, the benefits of glucocorticoid medication must be weighed against the risks of their use.

Relative to dogs and cats, the rabbit, rat, mouse, and human being are relatively more sensitive to the antiinflammatory and/or immunosuppressive effects of glucocorticoids. Thus the results of research completed in the last four species, on in vitro models, and even in healthy animals may not apply to dogs and cats with naturally occurring diseases (Papich and Davis, 1989).

With these caveats established, several general effects of glucocorticoids have been documented. Polymorphonuclear neutrophils demonstrate decreased migration and egress into inflammatory tissue. The circulation of T-cell lymphocytes is decreased, and lymphocyte activation is suppressed. Glucocorticoids decrease vascular permeability and also the rate of synthesis of prostaglandins, prostacyclin, thromboxane, and leukotriene (Papich and Davis, 1989).

NEUTROPHILS

Membrane Effects. The classic antiinflammatory effect of glucocorticoids is decreased migration of PMNs into inflamed tissue. Soon after administration of a pharmacologic dose of glucocorticoids, neutrophilia occurs as a result of both increased release of cells from the maturation pool of the bone marrow and prolongation of PMN half-life (MacDonald, 2000). In addition, the egress of cells from blood vessels via diapedesis decreases. Because neutrophils mature within hours, inhibition of their egress results in a rapidly developing mature neutrophilia. The mechanism for decreased egress may be related to a cell surface configuration change that results in decreased vessel margination and adherence. Lysosomal membrane stabilization is probably a true antiinflammatory effect of glucocorticoids (Cupps and Fauci, 1982; Meuleman and Katz, 1985; Papich and Davis, 1989).

Phagocytosis. Glucocorticoids may impair the ability of neutrophils to phagocytize and destroy bacteria. Steroids may also hinder microbicidal activity by decreasing oxidative metabolism, by decreasing fusion of neutrophil granules to lysosomes, or by affecting the pH in the lysosomes of phagocytes. Regardless of the mechanism, corticosteroids increase susceptibility to infection because of an impaired ability to kill bacteria (Papich and Davis, 1989).

LYMPHOCYTES.

The lymphocyte population is composed of a circulating pool and a noncirculating pool. The circulating pool freely moves between the intravascular compartment and the extravascular compartment (lymph nodes, spleen, bone marrow, and thoracic duct). After glucocorticoid administration, lymphocytes of the circulating pool redistribute to the extravascular compartment. T-cell lymphocytes are affected more

than B cells (T cells constitute approximately 70% of the circulating pool). The discrepancy in the lymphocyte response is not easily explained, but the ability of B cells to metabolize glucocorticoids faster than T cells may be involved (Cupps and Fauci, 1982; Kehrl and Fauci, 1983; Papich and Davis, 1989). Furthermore, helper or inducer lymphocytes (CD4) are more sensitive than the cytotoxic suppressor cells (CD8). Steroids also inhibit the production of interleukin-2, resulting in inhibition of lymphocyte proliferation and cytotoxic function. Glucocorticoids also cause suppression of B-cell growth factors (BCGFs), affecting the proliferation of this cell type (MacDonald, 2000). Decreased numbers of circulating lymphocytes and decreased proliferative response of lymphocytes reduce these cells' ability to participate in immunologic and/or inflammatory reactions. Additional observations include a decreased response to mitogens, suppressed lymphokine synthesis, and decreased transformation and antigen recognition (Cupps and Fauci, 1982; Meuleman and Katz, 1985; Papich and Davis, 1989).

Glucocorticoids have few direct effects on B cells, but they indirectly alter B-cell function by modulating accessory cells. A complex series of interactions between T cells, macrophages, antigens, and cell mediators is required for full expression of lymphocyte function (Nossal, 1987). Commonly used doses of glucocorticoids do not prevent an animal from mounting a normal immunologic response to vaccinations or other antigens (Meuleman and Katz, 1985), but as doses of corticosteroids increase, concentrations of immunoglobulins IgG, IgA and, to a lesser extent, IgM are decreased. Synthesis of IgE is not affected. Studies in humans suggest that repeated daily doses of long-acting corticosteroids, such as dexamethasone, suppress antibody synthesis but that alternate-day administration of antiinflammatory doses of an intermediate-acting steroid, such as prednisolone, does not (Papich and Davis, 1989). Glucocorticoids induce eosinopenia, which is most likely a consequence of changes in distribution to various tissues. Evidence for a lytic or toxic effect on eosinophils has not yet been proven (MacDonald, 2000).

MACROPHAGES.

Mononuclear cells have several critical functions. They serve as antigen-presenting accessory cells during the induction of cell-mediated and humoral immune responses. They also function as "professional" phagocytes against bacteria, fungi, and viruses. In combination with antibodies, they may have tumor cell–killing capacity. They are also essential in clearing senescent cells, particularly erythrocytes, and in bone remodeling, wound healing, and lung surfactant turnover (MacDonald, 2000).

Monocytes and macrophages (lymphocyte accessory cells) appear to be more sensitive to the effects of glucocorticoids than neutrophils. Therapeutic corticosteroid doses decrease phagocytosis and bactericidal activity. Steroids also diminish macrophage and monocyte ability to process antigens for presentation to B cells. Synthesis of cell mediators, such as interleukin-1 (IL-1), also may be suppressed. Corticosteroids inhibit both lymphokine synthesis and the cellular response to lymphokines (Cupps and Fauci, 1982; Dinarello and Mier, 1987; Papich and Davis, 1989). Glucocorticoids also inhibit production of tumor necrosis factor (TNF), thereby affecting a wide variety of inflammatory processes. The major antiinflammatory effect of glucocorticoids is related also to decreased accumulation of mononuclear phagocytes at inflammatory foci. This may be a consequence of decreased chemotactic factors by other cells, including T lymphocytes outside the mononuclear cell population. Antienzymatic effects of steroids may also be a factor. Inhibition of cytokines such as IL-1, interferon-γ (IFN-γ), and TNF/cachectin also has been documented (Cohn, 1991; Scott et al, 1995).

BASOPHILS AND MAST CELLS.   Glucocorticoids reduce the number of circulating basophils, most likely through reduced production. Glucocorticoids reduce the number of mucosal mast cells, although the subtype of mast cell found in connective tissue is less sensitive. The reduction of mast cells most likely is a result of inhibition of IL-3 or mast cell growth factor. A direct effect may also occur. Migration of basophils is significantly reduced by steroids. Some suggest that steroids directly inhibit production and release of mast cell inflammatory mediators, or that this may be the simple result of a smaller number of mast cells causing degranulation. Topical glucocorticoids decreasing response to antigen may also involve decreased cell numbers or decreased access of antigen to tissue mast cells (Butterfield and Gleich, 1989; Munck and Guyre, 1989).

ARACHIDONIC ACID METABOLISM.   Injury to cell membranes stimulates the prostaglandin-leukotriene cascade, which in turn activates phospholipase A_2 in cell membranes to form arachidonic acid. The enzymes cyclooxygenase and lipooxygenase form prostacyclin, thromboxane, and leukotrienes from arachidonic acid. The antiinflammatory action of glucocorticoids is believed to be mediated by proteins synthesized in target tissues. Part of this action is related to reduced production of proinflammatory metabolites, especially those derived from arachidonic acid. Prostaglandins I_2 and E_2 plus leukotrienes B_4, C_4, D_4, and E_4 may be responsible for the end-inflammatory response modified by decreased metabolism of arachidonic acid.

In general, glucocorticoids induce an antiphospholipase effect by using second-messenger proteins called lipocortins. These proteins inhibit cellular phospholipase A, thus reducing the release of arachidonic acid and all subsequent proinflammatory mediators (prostaglandins, prostacyclines, thromboxanes, and leukotrienes). Lipocortins regulate cellular metabolism of phospholipases as well. Many cells release arachidonic acid when stimulated by neurotransmitters and certain drugs. Lipocortins are naturally digested by proteases. They promote the maturation of suppressor T cells and inhibit proliferation response to T cells by mitogens. β-Lipocortins

have a dose-dependent inhibitory effect on the acute phase of cytotoxic T cells. They also inhibit antibody-dependent cytotoxicity by natural killer cells and protect cells from complement-mediated lysis (Cupps, 1989; Flower, 1989; Hirata, 1989).

EFFECTS ON BLOOD VESSELS.   The beneficial effects of glucocorticoids when administered to animals in shock, to animals with CNS edema, and to those with various other inflammatory conditions are related to "stabilization of microvascular integrity." This phenomenon reduces edema formation and extravasation of cells from the vasculature to tissues. These effects may be attributed to suppressed neutrophil action and to reductions in prostaglandin synthesis. It has also been suggested that corticosteroids antagonize vasoactive substances such as histamine and kinins, thereby providing protection against the toxic effects of free oxygen radicals released during inflammation. Because it is known that macrophages release plasminogen activators as part of the cascade of reactions during inflammation, it is of interest that glucocorticoids likely inhibit this reaction. This is an important effect of glucocorticoids, because activated plasmin digests supporting tissue of vessels and enhances vascular permeability (Papich and Davis, 1989).

SUMMARY.   The immunosuppressive and antiinflammatory effects of glucocorticoids are attributed to their ability to interfere with complex interactions of cells and cell mediators. Most of the antiinflammatory activity of glucocorticoids is related to their effects on leukocytes. These same effects are immunosuppressive in nature, and as a result this class of drugs is excellent for the management of immune-mediated diseases. However, glucocorticoids enhance susceptibility to infection.

SOURCE

Although natural corticosteroids can be obtained from animal adrenals, they are usually synthesized from cholic acid (obtained from cattle) or steroid sapogenins, diosgenin in particular, found in plants of the Liliaceae and Dioscoreaceae families (Meyers et al, 1980). Further modifications of steroids at the carbon 1, 2, 6, 9, 16, and other positions (see Fig. 10-1) have led to the marketing of a large group of synthetic steroids with special characteristics that are pharmacologically and therapeutically important. The chemistry of each steroid synthesized is important in determining its biologic effects and duration of action (see Fig. 10-2). The route of administration and vehicle in which it is delivered are also critical to the final determination of the pharmacology of a drug.

DURATION OF ACTION

Duration of action is commonly assessed in terms of plasma half-life: the amount of time required for 50% of a drug's concentration to disappear from plasma.

This assumes that all individuals are similar in their ability to clear these drugs. It is suspected, however, that individual variation, especially among dogs and cats, can be considerable. Furthermore, in the case of glucocorticoids, a distinction must be made between plasma half-life and the more important "biologic half-life." The *biologic half-life* refers to the duration of effect. Because glucocorticoids usually act by induction of protein synthesis, their biologic effect correlates best with the half-life of the induced protein or proteins. It is the biologic half-life that must be considered when determining a dose regimen (see Table 10-1).

Cortisone and hydrocortisone are accepted as having biologic half-lives of less than 12 hours, whereas prednisone, methylprednisolone, and triamcinolone have half-lives of 12 to 36 hours. Paramethasone, flumethasone, betamethasone, and dexamethasone are all believed to have half-lives in excess of 48 hours. The route of administration, the preparation used, the patient's health, and various other factors influence the duration of action (Behrend and Kemppainen, 1997).

ABSORPTION

Modification Factors

The manner in which drugs are absorbed affects the duration and intensity of drug action. A change in these rates may dictate alteration of the dosage or the interval between doses to achieve the desired effects (Gilman et al, 1980). Variation in drug potency represents a difference in the properties of each compound in receptor binding and duration of activity on the receptor with respect to a specific tissue. Receptors do not respond differently to each glucocorticoid; rather, potency differences between prednisolone and dexamethasone, for example, are a reflection of the fact that less dexamethasone is required to attain an equipotent effect to that of prednisolone.

Variables that influence absorption of a drug include the drug's solubility, dissolution, concentration, circulation to the site of absorption, absorbing surface, and route of administration. Drugs administered in an aqueous solution are more rapidly absorbed than those given in oil, a suspension, or solid form. Drugs that are in high concentration are more rapidly absorbed than those that are diluted. Decreased blood flow, produced by vasoconstrictor agents, shock, or other disease factors, can slow absorption, especially from subcutaneous sites. Drugs are absorbed rapidly from large surface areas such as the pulmonary alveolar epithelium or intestinal mucosa, in contrast to agents injected into an intramuscular site (Gilman et al, 1980).

Route of Administration

Different routes of drug administration have individual advantages and disadvantages. Some characteristics of the major routes used to achieve systemic drug effects are compared in Table 10-2.

ORAL. Oral ingestion is the most common method of drug administration. It is also the safest, most convenient, and most economical. Disadvantages of the oral route include emesis as a result of irritation to the gastrointestinal mucosa, destruction of some drugs by low gastric pH, irregularities in absorption in the presence of food or other drugs, and the need for cooperation on the part of both the client and the pet. In addition, drugs in the gastrointestinal tract may be metabolized by the enzymes of the gastrointestinal mucosa, the intestinal bacterial flora, or the liver before they gain access to the general circulation.

INJECTABLE. Injection of drugs has certain distinct advantages over oral administration. In some instances, parenteral administration is essential for the drug to be absorbed in active form. Absorption is usually more rapid and predictable than when a drug is given by mouth, and the effective dose therefore can be more accurately selected. In emergency therapy, parenteral administration may be required. Injection also has its disadvantages. Asepsis must be maintained to avoid

TABLE 10–2 SOME CHARACTERISTICS OF COMMON ROUTES OF DRUG ADMINISTRATION

Route	Absorption Pattern	Special Utility	Limitations and Precautions
Intravenous	Absorption circumvented Potentially immediate effects	Valuable for emergency use Permits titration of dosage Suitable for large volumes and for irritating substances, when diluted	Increased risk of adverse effects Must inject solutions *slowly*, as a rule Not suitable for oily solutions or insoluble substances
Subcutaneous	Prompt, from aqueous solution Slow and sustained, from repository preparations	Suitable for some insoluble suspensions and for implantation of solid pellets	Not suitable for large volumes Possible pain or necrosis from irritating substances
Intramuscular	Prompt, from aqueous solution Slow and sustained, from repository preparations	Suitable for moderate volumes, oily vehicles, and some irritating substances	Precluded during anticoagulant medication May interfere with interpretation of certain diagnostic tests (e.g., creatine phosphokinase)
Oral ingestion	Variable, depends upon many factors (see text)	Most convenient and economical; usually safer than other routes	Requires patient cooperation Absorption potentially erratic and incomplete for drugs that are poorly soluble, slowly absorbed, or unstable

infection. Intravascular injection may occur when it is not intended, or pain may accompany administration. Cost is another consideration (Gilman et al, 1980).

TOPICAL. Topical glucocorticoids are used in dermatologic therapy in a variety of formulations and active steroid compounds. Topical therapy can provide high concentrations of a potent glucocorticoid at a specific site while minimizing systemic effects. It is important to remember that topically administered steroids are systemically absorbed and may create deleterious effects. Absorption from topical sites is increased by inflammation, use of occlusive wraps, and possibly clipping of affected skin. Other factors include the preparation vehicle, concentration of the glucocorticoid, anatomic site, frequency of administration, and size of the area treated (Behrend and Kemppainen, 1997).

Acetonide and valerate esters bind to affected tissue, enhancing the glucocorticoid effect. Because of their potency, fluorinated products (betamethasone, dexamethasone, triamcinolone, and fluocinolone) should be used only for short-term therapy. Short-acting medications should be used for chronic treatment. Topical steroids are available in creams, lotions, foams, gels, solutions, shampoos, rinses, and ointments. They are frequently incorporated into otic and ophthalmic antibacterial medications for their anti-inflammatory effect.

GLUCOCORTICOID PREPARATIONS

Structure versus Activity

The essential features of the structure for glucocorticoid activity are the C11 hydroxyl, a ketone at C3 and at C20, and a double bond between the fourth and fifth carbons (see Figs. 10-1 and 10-2). Addition of a double bond between the first and second carbons, methyl groups at C6 or C16, and florine to C9 are changes that can increase the biologic half-life of glucocorticoids, decrease their mineralocorticoid activity, and substantially increase their antiinflammatory potency.

Glucocorticoids are among the most commonly used (abused?) drugs in veterinary medicine. Much is known about the actions, indications, side effects, and toxicity of these compounds. However, there seems to be considerable confusion about the characteristics and pharmacokinetics of the various preparations available to veterinary practitioners. Corticosteroids are not active unless they possess the proper functional groups. For example, two commonly used compounds, cortisone and prednisone, have a ketone group at the 11 carbon position. The hydroxyl group at the 11 carbon position is essential for antiinflammatory activity. These compounds are reduced to the active hydroxyl forms (i.e., hydrocortisone and prednisolone) in the liver. Thus prednisolone is used in preference to prednisone in dogs with confirmed or suspected hepatopathy. Steroids that have the 11-hydroxyl group do not depend on metabolism for their activity; these

include dexamethasone (see Fig. 10-2). The conversion to active forms is rapid, and the 11-keto compounds are certainly effective when used systemically. Drugs that require hepatic alteration prior to their action cannot be used for topical or local application.

Oral Preparations

The oral route for glucocorticoid therapy is preferred in most systemic illnesses. Oral dose forms are usually tablets containing the free steroid alcohol. Oral absorption is usually quite rapid, and plasma half-lives are relatively brief. As previously discussed and unlike many other drugs, the duration of glucocorticoid biologic action (as measured by suppression of the hypothalamus or pituitary or both) does not directly parallel the plasma half-life, but rather persists for some time after plasma levels decline. Glucocorticoids act by enhancing transcription of both messenger RNA and ribosomal RNA in individual cells, thus creating a wide array of results, as well as different durations of action.

Comparison of glucocorticoid duration of action allows categorization of these compounds into short-, intermediate-, and long-acting agents (see Table 10-1). Duration of action is determined in part by the route of administration. Intravenous administration of drugs usually is associated with the quickest onset of action and the shortest half-life. Oral administration, by contrast, usually has a delayed onset of action and a much longer half-life. Duration of action is also affected by the absorption characteristics of any drug administered. For example, the duration of action of injectable suspensions is much longer owing to their delayed absorption.

Parenteral Preparations

Three parenteral glucocorticoid preparations are commonly used in veterinary medicine: aqueous solutions of soluble steroid esters; solutions of free steroid alcohols; and suspensions of insoluble steroid esters.

AQUEOUS SOLUTIONS OF SOLUBLE STEROID ESTERS. These solutions can be administered intravenously or intramuscularly. Absorption from intramuscular sites is quite rapid (Table 10-3). The sodium phosphate and sodium succinate esters are the commonly available forms (Fig. 10-5). These water-soluble, rapidly acting preparations are the preferred medications for treatment of acute conditions requiring large doses, such as endotoxic shock, cerebral edema, and CNS trauma. These glucocorticoids have a rapid onset of action (minutes) and last 12 to 72 hours. Two commonly used veterinary products are dexamethasone sodium phosphate (4 mg/ml sterile solution) and prednisolone sodium succinate (SoluDeltaCortef; The Upjohn Co., Kalamazoo, Mich.).

SOLUTIONS OF FREE STEROID ALCOHOLS. Solutions of free steroid alcohols are unique to veterinary medicine.

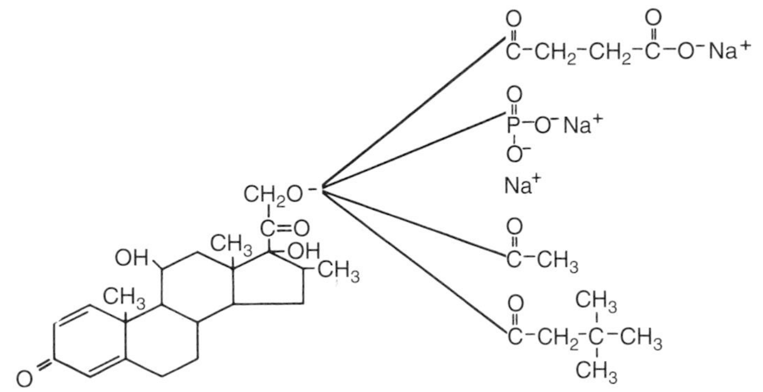

FIGURE 10–5. Esters of glucocorticoids. Glucocorticoid structure illustrating various esters that may bind to carbon 21.

TABLE 10–3   GENERAL DURATION OF ACTION OF VARIOUS STEROID ESTERS TYPICALLY ADMINISTERED IM

Steroid Ester	Absorption Period Following IM Dose	Duration of Action	Commonly Used Bases
Sodium succinate	Minutes to hours	Hours	Dexamethasone, betamethasone, hydrocortisone, methylprednisolone, prednisolone, prednisone
Sodium phosphate			
Acetate	Days to weeks	Days to weeks	Fluocinolone, isoflupredone, triamcinolone, methylprednisolone, betamethasone
Diacetate			
Acetonide	Weeks	Weeks	Desoxycorticosterone, triamcinolone
Privalate			

The relatively insoluble free steroid alcohols are prepared in sterile, dilute solution. Approximately 40% polyethylene glycol is used as a solubilizing vehicle. These preparations can be administered intramuscularly or intravenously. Intramuscular absorption is quite rapid (minutes) but may be slightly slower than with the soluble ester preparations, and the duration of effect is 12 to 72 hours. Although these preparations can be given intravenously, large doses may result in CNS side effects from the polyethylene glycol. Because of the potential for side effects, the aqueous solutions of soluble steroid esters are recommended for treating acute disorders requiring large doses. Two commonly used free steroid alcohol preparations are dexamethasone (Azium; Schering Corp., Kenilworth, NJ, and other preparations made by various pharmaceutical companies), at a formulation of 2 mg/ml, and flumethasone (Flucort Diamond Laboratories, Des Moines, Iowa), 0.5 mg/ml (Table 10-4).

SUSPENSIONS OF INSOLUBLE STEROID ESTERS. Suspensions are indicated primarily for intralesional and intraarticular administration, providing long-term therapy. Unfortunately, such long-acting, injectable glucocorticoids are frequently used for systemic effect and therefore represent some of the most abused and overused medications in veterinary medicine. Absorption of these insoluble esters is limited by the rate of their dissolution in tissue fluids at the injection site. With suspensions of insoluble steroid esters, the dissolution of the particles is the rate-limiting step, and absorption from these injection sites is quite slow. The glucocorticoids in these preparations have relatively short half-lives, but the slow absorption due to the vehicle used provides long-term, low-level therapy. These preparations are not to be used intravenously, and they do not provide adequate treatment of conditions in which quick effect and high plasma levels are needed (e.g., shock). The most common ester preparations are acetates, diacetates, acetonides, and pivalates.

The steroid ester suspensions should be handled and stored with care. Extremes of heat or cold may result in the development of large crystals at the expense of small ones, which decreases surface area and slows dissolution of suspended particles. Larger crystals also contribute to irritation when injected intraarticularly. Commonly used injectable steroid ester preparations include methylprednisolone acetate suspension (DepoMedrol; The Upjohn Co., Kalamazoo, MI), 20 mg/ml and 50 mg/ml; isoflupredone acetate (9-d-fluoroprednisolone acetate) suspension (Predef 2X; The Upjohn Co., Kalamazoo, MI), 2 mg/ml; triamcinolone acetonide suspension (Vetalog Parenteral; E.R. Squibb & Sons, Princeton, NJ), 6 mg/ml; and triamcinolone diacetate suspension (Aristocort Forte; Lederle Laboratories, Wayne, NJ), 40 mg/ml (see Table 10-4).

Other than for intralesional or intraarticular therapy, these ultra-long-acting glucocorticoid preparations are

TABLE 10–4   COMMONLY USED PRODUCTS CONTAINING GLUCOCORTICOIDS

Compound	Systemic Preparation	Topical Preparation
Betamethasone	Betasone*	Gentocin Durafilm, * Gentocin Topical,* or Gentocin Otic* Otomax* Topagen*
Dexamethasone	Azium* Voren†	Tresaderm‡
Flumethasone	Flucort§	Anaprime§
Fluocinolone		Synalar,§ Synalar Otic,§ Neo-Synalar§
Hydrocortisone	Cortef ‖ ‖ ‖ Hydrocortone‡ ‖ ‖ ‖	Cortisoothe¶ Cortispray** Forte-topical ‖ Epi-Otic HC¶ Neobacimyx-H* Neo-Predef ‖
Isoflupredone		
Methylprednisolone	Medrol, ‖ Solu-medrol, ‖ ‖ ‖ Depo-medrol ‖	
Prednisone/prednisolone	Deltasone ‖ ‖ ‖ Meticorten* Prelone‡ ‡ ‖ ‖ Solu-Delta-Cortef ‖	Chlorasone‡ ‡ Liquichlor with cerumene‡ ‡
Triamcinolone	Vetalog§ §	Panolog § § Vetalog § §

From Behrend EW and Kemppamen RJ, 1997 (used with permission).
*Schering.
†Bio-Ceutic.
‡Merck AgVet (veterinary product) or Merck (human product).
§Syntex.
‖ Upjohn.
¶Allerderm.
**DVM.
† †Muro.
‡ ‡EVSco.
§ §Solvay.
‖ ‖ Approved for human use only.

rarely indicated (see Table 10-3). There are few acceptable reasons for use of these agents for problems such as pruritus in dogs or cats. Exceptions include fractious cats and cats that live exclusively outdoors and may be seen by the owner only occasionally. The same antiinflammatory effects can be achieved with much shorter-acting oral agents. Use of short-acting products allows doses to be altered as needed, minimizes suppression of the normal pituitary-adrenal axis, allows a dose to be tapered prior to discontinuation, and avoids the trap of repeated injections, with their attendant deleterious side effects.

Combination Products

The controversy surrounding administration of a single, fixed-dose preparation containing one or more antimicrobial agents and a corticosteroid appears to be based on three issues: (1) dose discrepancy: administration based on the recommended dose of one constituent drug that may result in underdosing or overdosing of other drugs in the product; (2) variable durations of effectiveness and toxicity of constituent drugs; and (3) lack of data documenting clinical efficacy of fixed-dose preparations. Despite the controversy, fixed-dose combination products are used

extensively in small animal practice (Ford, 1984). Their use is not recommended.

Novel Steroids

The general suppression of the hypothalamic-pituitary axis and various other systemic side effects caused by administration of steroids have led to attempts to find "safer" formulations. Budesonide has been used for years as an inhaled drug for asthma in humans. It has been reformulated for use in dogs and cats. The supposed advantage of budesonide is that it is almost completely degraded first pass in the portal circulation through the liver. In humans it has been reported to have 10% of the systemic effects of equipotent doses of prednisolone.

Budesonide has been given to dogs and cats with inflammatory bowel disease with some success. Proper dosing, however, is not yet known. Furthermore, "steroid hepatopathy" still seems to occur in dogs, even with fewer systemic effects. It should be remembered that "steroid hepatopathy" is unique to dogs and does not occur in people or cats. Steroid hepatopathy does not result in liver failure or in any known clinical signs; it is simply an enlargement of the liver with typical histologic alterations.

An empirical oral dose of 3 mg of budesonide given twice daily in dogs and 1 mg given twice daily in cats has been recommended. Pharmacokinetic data are not available to support these recommendations. In Europe, an enteric-coated formulation has been developed for humans with inflammatory bowel disease (Crohn's disease). The enteric coating protects the budesonide until it is released in the distal small intestine. The value of this preparation for use in animals is unclear, because the intestinal inflammation in animals is more frequently diffuse compared with the condition in humans (Hall, 2002).

THERAPEUTIC INDICATIONS

Nonadrenal Disorders

Table 10-5 provides a partial list of disorders in which glucocorticoids have been found to be efficacious. This list is modified from a similar list in a text devoted to therapy of diseases in humans, but the use of glucocorticoids does apply to many species (Goldfein, 1994; Behrend and Kemppainen, 1997).

Goals in Glucocorticoid Therapy

The clinician should always attempt to bring a disease process under control using the lowest dose necessary of short-acting oral agents. Whenever possible, alternate-day therapy should be used (Spencer et al, 1980). There is no solid evidence that the time of day is critical for administration of medication (Kemppainen et al, 1981 and 1982). Whenever possible, specific treatment of an underlying disease (e.g., flea allergy) should be undertaken while the glucocorticoid is controlling the external signs.

Inflammation/Allergies

A variety of allergic or mild inflammatory diseases are encountered in veterinary practice. Although generalities can be made regarding treatment, information regarding specific conditions should be reviewed. In general, prednisone or prednisolone (0.55 mg/kg PO q12h) is commonly used in small animals for antiinflammatory effect (Ferguson and Hoenig, 1995). Cats may be more resistant to the effects of glucocorticoids, requiring twice the dosage that dogs need for the management of similar conditions. Dogs and cats usually respond quickly but may require 5 to 7 days of medication for full induction (Behrend and Kemppainen, 1997).

Immune-Mediated Disease

Frequently encountered immune-mediated (autoimmune?) conditions include joint disease, glomerulopathies, hemolytic anemia, thrombocytopenia, sys-

TABLE 10–5 PARTIAL LIST OF THERAPEUTIC INDICATIONS FOR GLUCOCORTICOID IN NONADRENAL DISORDERS

Allergic disease
Angioneurotic edema
Asthma
Contact or parasitic dermatitis
Drug reactions

Arthritis, bursitis, tenosynovitis

Collagen vascular disorders
  (musculoskeletal)
  Systemic lupus erythematosus
  Polymyositis
  Rheumatoid arthritis
  Idiopathic polyarthritis

Hematologic disorders/immune-
  mediated diseases
  Autoimmune hemolytic anemia
  Leukemia
  Idiopathic thrombocytopenia
  Multiple myeloma
  Glomerulonephritis

Eye diseases
  Acute uveitis
  Allergic conjunctivitis
  Choroiditis
  Optic neuritis

Gastrointestinal diseases
  Inflammatory bowel disease
  Regional enteritis
  Ulcerative colitis
  Chronic hepatitis
  Lymphangiectasia
  Feline gingivitis/stomatitis

Hypercalcemia
  Lymphosarcoma
  Multiple myeloma

Infection
  Gram-negative septicemia
  Excessive inflammation

Multisystemic
  Heat stroke
  Shock

Neoplasia
  CNS tumors
  Insulinoma
  Mast cell tumor
  Leukemia, lymphosarcoma,
    multiple myeloma

Neurologic disorders
  Acute trauma
  Cerebral edema
  Granulomatous
    meningoencephalitis
  Intervertebral disc disease
  Vestibular disorders

Pulmonary diseases
  Aspiration pneumonia
  Bronchial asthma
  Chronic/allergic bronchitis
  Heartworm sensitivity
  Eosinophilic granuloma
  Inhalation injury
  Pulmonary infiltrates with
    eosinophils

Renal disorders
  Certain nephritic syndromes
  Certain protein losing
    nephropathies

Skin disorders
  Atopic dermatitis
  Mycosis fungoides
  Pemphigus/other immune-
    mediated problems
  Seborrheic dermatitis
  Pyotraumatic skin disease
  Feline eosinophilic
    granuloma complex

temic lupus erythematosus, skin disease, and others. Recommended glucocorticoid doses for these conditions are usually prednisolone or prednisone, 2.2 to 6.6 mg/kg/day in divided doses, given orally twice to three times a day. Some have suggested superior results using dexamethasone at dosages of 0.6 to 2.2 mg/kg divided. The oral route is acceptable for most dogs and cats because gastrointestinal signs are minimal and treatment is easy to administer. The initial dose is continued until significant improvement is documented, which usually takes a few days. It has been suggested that 10 to 28 days may be required for induction of immunosuppression (Behrend and Kemppainen, 1997).

After the condition has resolved, the dose can be slowly tapered. There are as many protocols for diminishing a steroid dose as there are veterinarians who treat these conditions. One of our protocols typically involves a 50% reduction in the initial twice daily dose, while maintaining the twice daily frequency, for 2 weeks. Then, at 2-week intervals, the dose is reduced by 50% increments, then to once daily, 50% once daily, every other day, then every third day (see Glucocorticoid Preparations and Dose Schedules, page 481). Prior to each dose reduction, the dog or cat can be rechecked to ensure that the disease remains in remission. If relapse occurs, a higher dose or the original dose may be needed.

If glucocorticoid therapy does not result in significant improvement, additional therapy is often recommended. In this situation, more potent immunosuppressive therapy is added to glucocorticoid treatment protocols. The more common adjunctive therapies include cyclophosphamide, azathioprine and, more recently, cyclosporine (Cook et al, 1994).

Neoplasia, Hypercalcemia, and Chronic Palliation

Glucocorticoids are used as a form of "chemotherapy" for various tumors. These include lymphosarcoma, multiple myeloma, and mast cell tumors. Glucocorticoids may directly affect these tumor cell types. Although in dogs and cats glucocorticoids are probably not toxic to normal lymphocytes, they do cause lymphocytolysis in neoplastic cells (Papich and Davis, 1989). Two other nonendocrine indications for glucocorticoids, chronic palliation and hypercalcemia, may also be responsive to this mode of therapy. Glucocorticoids, used at antiinflammatory doses, can palliate the inflammation and/or pain associated with many cancers (Behrend and Kemppainen, 1997). It is extremely important to remember that initiation of glucocorticoid treatment should follow proof of neoplasia or cause of hypercalcemia. These drugs can alter the cytologic properties of cells such as lymphocytes, obscuring future chances of diagnosis. Dogs are also much more resistant than people to the deleterious effects of hypercalcemia (see Chapter 17), negating the need for "emergency" treatment in many cases.

Shock

GENERAL APPROACH. Shock is characterized by an acute condition that compromises blood pressure and subsequently tissue perfusion. The most important components of treatment for shock are (1) administration of intravenous fluids to restore blood volume, blood pressure, and tissue perfusion and (2) identification of the underlying cause so that steps can be taken to treat or correct the problem. Glucocorticoids are considered adjunctive and controversial in the management of hemorrhagic and septic shock.

HEMORRHAGIC SHOCK. Glucocorticoid therapy for this condition is considered beneficial because glucocorticoids may improve the vascular integrity of the microcirculation in major organs and stabilize the cell membranes against the toxic effects of oxygen radicals produced during any ischemic event (Papich and Davis, 1989). Typical treatments include intravenous prednisone or methylprednisolone (15 to 30 mg/kg) or intravenous dexamethasone (4 to 8 mg/kg). The beneficial actions of glucocorticoids are enhanced if the drugs are administered as soon after the onset of shock as possible.

SEPTIC SHOCK. If glucocorticoids are administered concomitantly with antibiotics to dogs or cats in septic shock, improvement in microvascular circulation may enhance delivery of antibiotics to those tissues. Furthermore, glucocorticoids may improve vascular integrity and decrease synthesis of arachidonic acid metabolites (Greisman, 1982; Hinshaw et al, 1982). The doses used by most practitioners are similar to those recommended for hemorrhagic shock, as is the critical nature of treating the animal as soon as the condition is recognized. Shock is an acute, life-threatening condition. Therefore realization that corticosteroids might enhance development of bacteremia or worsen sepsis in the long term is tempered by their potential lifesaving attributes in the short term.

Central Nervous System (CNS) Disorders

ACTIONS AND INDICATIONS. Glucocorticoids have been demonstrated to be beneficial in several CNS disorders. The benefits have been attributed to protection of cellular membranes from the toxic effects of oxygen-derived free radicals, improvement in microvascular integrity, stabilization of CNS intercellular tight junctions, decreased edema formation, and decreased intracranial pressure as a result of decreased cerebrospinal fluid formation (Papich and Davis, 1989). Corticosteroids interfere with norepinephrine-mediated ischemia and prevent oxygen free radical peroxidation in myelin, neuronal, glial, and vessel membranes. Owing to their various actions, glucocorticoids are used in a variety of brain and spinal cord problems.

Perhaps the most common use of corticosteroids in neurologic conditions is for "vasogenic edema" secondary to trauma. The most common traumatic injuries follow intervertebral disk protrusion or collapse. "Trauma" to the CNS may also be associated with accidents, neoplasia, hemorrhage, and abscesses. Corticosteroids have also been considered beneficial when given to dogs with aseptic meningitis, including granulomatous meningoencephalitis, steroid-responsive suppurative meningitis, and necrotizing vasculitis of the CNS (Meric et al, 1986; Meric, 1988). The cause of these three conditions has not yet been determined.

DOSE. Not surprisingly, neurologists do not agree on the most effective glucocorticoid preparation, consequently there are many recommended treatment protocols. Hydrocortisone (300 mg/kg); methylprednisolone, prednisone, or prednisolone (10 to 30 mg/kg); or dexamethasone (4.0 to 8.0 mg/kg) typically is given intravenously (Haskins, 1992). Dogs and cats may be treated two to six times daily, with remarkable variation in the total dose administered (Braughler and Hall, 1982; Hall and Braughler, 1982; Hankes et al, 1985; Hoerlein et al, 1985). Dogs with aseptic meningitis usually respond to tapering doses of prednisolone after an initial 2 to 4 mg/kg/day. Their response to treatment can be quite dramatic, with improvement sometimes observed within hours of the first dose (Meric, 1988).

ADVERSE REACTIONS

The benefits of glucocorticoid therapy must be weighed against their deleterious effects. Some of the major undesirable effects are not toxic; rather, they are exaggerations of expected actions and therefore result in a form of canine Cushing's syndrome. Other negative responses (e.g., sepsis, gastrointestinal mucosal damage, or abortion) can be attributed to known actions of corticosteroids that, again, would not be considered toxic but rather expected and physiologic.

Gastric and Intestinal Bleeding/Perforation

PATHOPHYSIOLOGY. Glucocorticoids may alter mucosal defense mechanisms and thereby place an animal at risk for gastric or intestinal ulceration and/or perforation. Corticosteroids are believed to predispose domestic animals to gastrointestinal tract ulcers by decreasing mucus production, altering the biochemical structure of gastric mucus, decreasing mucosal cell turnover, and increasing acid output (Toombs et al, 1980 and 1986; Piper et al, 1991; Rohrer et al, 1999a and 1999b). It is unlikely, however, that glucocorticoids act as the sole cause of these gastrointestinal problems. Experimental studies in dogs indicate that glucocorticoids lead to a breakdown of the mucus barrier (Sorjonen et al, 1983). Glucocorticoids may also stimulate gastrin secretion by the G cells in the stomach and impair blood flow to the mucosal region of the stomach. Hypergastrinemia, gastric hyperacidity, and gastric ischemia may in turn promote gastric erosion and ulcer formation. In dogs with prolonged intestinal transit (e.g., spinal cord disorders or primary intestinal pathologic conditions), fecal retention increases the physicochemical trauma to the intestinal mucosal cells. In addition, glucocorticoids decrease mucosal cell renewal. These factors plus glucocorticoid effects on connective tissue and on the inflammatory response result in an increased potential for catastrophic gastrointestinal erosion (Toombs et al, 1980).

CLINICAL FEATURES. Corticosteroid therapy in canine neurosurgical patients has been associated with gastrointestinal complications in 50 of 257 dogs from one study and in 20 of 72 dogs in another study (Moore and Withrow, 1982; Sorjonen et al, 1983). Recent studies concur (Rohrer et al, 1999a and 1999b). Such complications have included pancreatitis and gastrointestinal hemorrhage, ulceration, and perfo-

ration. Although infrequently seen, the most catastrophic of these complications is colonic perforation. Colonic perforation in 13 dogs treated with corticosteroids was uniformly fatal (Toombs et al, 1986). Ten of the 13 dogs were neurosurgical patients, and 12 of the 13 dogs had undergone recent major surgery.

Dexamethasone was the most frequently used corticosteroid, and 12 dogs received a mean cumulative dose of 6.4 mg/kg/day over a period of 5 days (Toombs et al, 1986). The most common clinical signs in dogs were depression, anorexia, and vomiting. Signs preceded death by about a day, and death occurred 4 to 8 weeks after surgery. Since publication of these experiences, subsequent problems have diminished as a result of concern that similar complications may occur secondary to corticosteroid treatment. Veterinarians are dosing their patients as conservatively as possible and monitoring for any signs of gastrointestinal complications. However, one study using methylprednisone sodium succinate again demonstrated gastric hemorrhage in all treated dogs (Behren and Kemppainen, 1997).

Dexamethasone and methylprednisone sodium succinate are potent antiinflammatory steroids that often cause gastrointestinal complications in any dog receiving more than 2 or 3 days of medication. Signs expected with a perforated viscus may be so modified by steroid effects that detection may be limited or not observed until late in the course of therapy (Leramo et al, 1982). Abscess formation is unusual in these patients, and generalized peritonitis, gram-negative septicemia, and endotoxic shock generally ensue. The use of nonsteroidal antiinflammatory drugs increases the likelihood of gastrointestinal hemorrhage and ulceration in steroid-treated dogs by impairing prostaglandin-mediated defense mechanisms of the bowel wall (Stewart et al, 1980). Use of the synthetic prostaglandin analog misoprostol did not prevent gastric hemorrhage in one study, nor was the H_2 blocker ranitidine an effective protectant (Daley, 1993; Rohrer et al, 1999a and 1999b).

Recommendations for avoiding gastrointestinal complications in high-risk patients (nonambulatory neurosurgical patients treated with dexamethasone or other steroids) include (1) using prednisolone or prednisone rather than dexamethasone; (2) limiting treatment with corticosteroids to as short a time as possible; (3) avoiding successive or concurrent use of multiple drugs with known ulcerogenic potential; (4) correcting fecal retention problems before surgery; (5) avoiding enemas during the first week after surgery; and (6) managing urine retention problems by continuous bladder decompression (closed urine drainage system) rather than by repeated manual expression of the bladder (Toombs et al, 1986).

Sepsis

PATHOPHYSIOLOGY. Corticosteroids block the acquisition and expression of cell-mediated immunity by reducing the numbers of circulating lymphocytes and monocytes. The total number of T lymphocytes is also selectively reduced. Steroids block antigen-induced sensitization of lymphocytes and decrease monocyte response to lymphocyte chemotactic substances. Glucocorticoid-induced suppression of phagocytosis could reduce the killing and removal of bacteria. Corticosteroids decrease interferon synthesis in some animals with naturally acquired viral infections. It should be obvious that host defense mechanisms can be severely impaired in the patient treated with steroids and that the outcome of these effects cannot be predicted (Calvert and Greene, 1986; Bone et al, 1987; Hinshaw et al, 1987).

INDICATIONS. Administration of corticosteroids to dogs or cats also receiving antimicrobial therapy may be justified in steroid-treated animals with acquired infection or in antimicrobial-treated dogs with a compromising inflammatory response to an infection. However, the prevalence of complicating infections in dogs and cats receiving long-term glucocorticoid therapy does not justify the routine use of anti-microbial therapy in *any* animal receiving corticosteroids. In the event that infection does occur in a steroid-treated animal, glucocorticoid therapy need not be discontinued. Because corticosteroids mask many of the clinical signs of an infection, these animals should be examined regularly.

The inflammatory component of the host defense mechanism, although important, can sometimes be harmful, such as in encephalitis, meningitis, myocarditis, pneumonitis, and myositis. Because corticosteroids can inhibit inflammation, their therapeutic role during the early stages of some infectious processes is supported. Guidelines regarding the use of these agents in animals with known or suspected infection are not well defined, and their use depends on the clinician's interpretation of the animal's status (Ford, 1984). The role of corticosteroid therapy in animals with infection centers on the need for intervention during acute, severe, and potentially life-threatening inflammation. To be most effective, treatment should be started during the early phases of inflammation and should be maintained for less than 7 days (Ford, 1984). Usually the corticosteroid used is a short- or intermediate-acting agent. One exception is the use of dexamethasone in animals with acute CNS inflammation.

LIMITATIONS. Simultaneous administration of an antimicrobial agent and a corticosteroid to a patient represents a pharmacologic dichotomy (Ford, 1984). Antimicrobial drugs are used to treat infection, whereas corticosteroids compromise normal host defense mechanisms. There are few clinical indications for the use of concurrent antimicrobial/corticosteroid therapy in small animal practice. Although concurrent therapy does have a place in clinical practice, it should be reserved for situations in which the infecting organism is known, specific antimicrobial therapy is available, and short-term (up to 7 days) corticosteroid therapy may attenuate or even prevent tissue injury associated with infection and inflammation. Indiscriminate use of corticosteroids in patients with known or suspected infections is clearly not indicated (Ford, 1984). Because natural indicators of and defenses against infection are attenuated by glucocorticoid therapy, careful and routine patient monitoring is required regardless of concomitant antibiotic administration. Infections of the genitourinary tract, skin, and lungs are particularly common in dogs receiving chronic glucocorticoid therapy.

Pancreatitis

A relationship between the use of glucocorticoids and the development of pancreatitis has been promoted. Much of the evidence regarding this association is related to an increase in the viscosity of pancreatic secretions in rabbits (Steinberg and Lewis, 1981). In dogs, however, increased viscosity of pancreatic secretions has been demonstrated only when pancreata were perfused with 400 mg of methylprednisolone; 200 mg of the same drug (a huge dose itself) did not alter the viscosity of secretions (Kimura et al, 1979). Reports in the literature have been sporadic and inconclusive (Behrend and Kemppainen, 1997). Furthermore, none of 24 experimental dogs treated with dexamethasone at various "clinically common" doses developed pancreatitis (Parent, 1982).

Anecdotally, the incidence of pancreatitis in dogs being treated with glucocorticoids by oncologists is rare. The incidence of pancreatitis in dogs with naturally occurring hyperadrenocorticism is rare. Because serum lipase concentrations may increase secondary to glucocorticoid administration in the absence of pancreatitis, measurement of this serum enzyme may be misleading. Finally, the combination of glucocorticoid treatment and neurologic disease may be a risk factor for pancreatitis, but no evidence exists that directly links this medication with pancreatitis (Behrend and Kemppainen, 1997).

Iatrogenic Cushing's Syndrome/Addison's Disease

CLINICAL SIGNS. Most dogs receiving glucocorticoid medication for 1 or 2 weeks (sometimes within hours of the first dose) develop polydipsia, polyuria, polyphagia, and panting. These are common steroid-induced side effects that dissipate as the dosage is tapered or discontinued. More chronic signs of glucocorticoid excess (alopecia, urinary tract infection, hepatomegaly, weakness, and poor wound healing, to name but a few) require longer drug exposure, usually weeks to months.

BIOCHEMICAL CHANGES. In addition to the development of obvious clinical signs, changes in complete blood counts, chemistry profiles, urinalyses, and radiographs also reflect the systemic effects of chronic glucocorticoid excess. The biochemical alterations consistent with iatrogenic Cushing's syndrome may begin within days of beginning corticosteroid therapy. Alternatively, some dogs receiving chronic pharmacologic doses of glucocorticoids have little or no clinical or laboratory evidence of these drugs. There is dramatic individual variation in response to these drugs.

STEROID PREPARATIONS COMMONLY AT FAULT. Iatrogenic Cushing's syndrome *most commonly* occurs after repeated injections of long-acting glucocorticoid preparations. This is an unfortunate problem because these parenteral sustained-release medications are not physiologic, and they are unnecessary, undesirable, and in most instances contraindicated in clinical medicine. These preparations are absolutely contraindicated in the long-term management of systemic disease. Iatrogenic Cushing's syndrome, however, may develop in dogs after therapy with almost any glucocorticoid preparation. This includes both the necessary and the overzealous use of short-acting oral and injectable forms of glucocorticoids, as well as topical and even ophthalmic preparations (Roberts et al, 1984).

CONFIRMING THE DIAGNOSIS. The presence of iatrogenic Cushing's syndrome can be confirmed with an ACTH stimulation test. Administration of glucocorticoids suppresses pituitary ACTH secretion and, with time, results in atrophy of the adrenal cortex. The ACTH response test in the patient with iatrogenic Cushing's syndrome, therefore, often reveals a suppressed or low-normal baseline plasma cortisol concentration with a subnormal response to ACTH (Fig. 10-6). The degree of adrenal unresponsiveness is a function of the dose, duration of therapy, and individual variation. If a dog or cat undergoing chronic steroid therapy has such a test result, it has iatrogenic Cushing's syndrome.

MANAGEMENT. If a dog's exogenous corticosteroid therapy is abruptly stopped or if it is receiving a conservative glucocorticoid dose and is acutely stressed, it may quickly develop signs of iatrogenic hypocortisolism. Iatrogenic Cushing's syndrome and iatrogenic hypocortisolism are, in this sense, different aspects of one condition: chronic glucocorticoid therapy. With rare exceptions, recovery eventually occurs in the dog with iatrogenic Cushing's syndrome when the drug is withdrawn. After prolonged suppression due to chronic glucocorticoid administration, full recovery may take as little as 1 month to as long as several months. These dogs should either have their medication acutely discontinued (if no clinical signs of hypocortisolism are observed) or be placed on progressively smaller (tapering) doses of glucocorticoids (if acute discontinuation of glucocorticoids resulted in anorexia, vomiting, or unusual listlessness). Ideally, if tapering is to be instituted, they should receive medication on an alternate-day schedule for 1 to 3 months and be given supplementary therapy at times of severe stress (e.g., illness, trauma, surgery, or boarding). If a tapering medication approach is undertaken, the dog should receive an amount of glucocorticoid that is slightly *less* than the physiologic replacement dose. Such a dose does not prevent the return of adrenocortical function but provides support in the interim.

CATS. Suppression of the feline HPA axis with exogenous glucocorticoids can and does occur (Scott, 1980 and 1982). Clinical development of iatrogenic Cushing's syndrome in cats is unusual, as are signs related to hypoadrenocorticism after glucocorticoids have been discontinued. Nevertheless, administration of supraphysiologic doses of methylprednisolone for as little as 7 days can suppress plasma cortisol concentrations (Crager et al, 1994). The use of progestagens (another *steroid*) also results in hypoadrenocorticism in cats (see Chapter 8).

Vaccinations

As previously discussed, glucocorticoid medication is a potent antiinflammatory agent. However, these preparations do not significantly interfere with antibody formation. Therefore dogs and cats receiving glucocorticoids and due for vaccinations should be vaccinated (Cohn, 1991).

Liver Parameters

The most common biochemical change in dogs treated with glucocorticoids is an increase in the serum alkaline phosphatase activity. There is no "upper limit" to the increase that results from naturally occurring or iatrogenic glucocorticoid therapy. Any glucocorticoid can acutely and dramatically cause an increase in this activity by means of induction of a unique hepatic isoenzyme (see Chapter 6). Although this change may

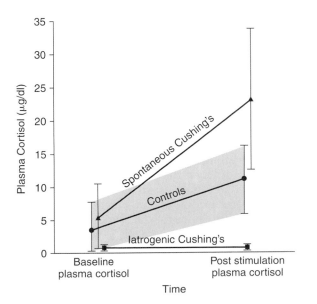

FIGURE 10-6. ACTH response test results in normal dogs, dogs with spontaneous hyperadrenocorticism, and dogs with iatrogenic Cushing's syndrome. Note that iatrogenic Cushing's syndrome is synonymous with iatrogenic hypoadrenocorticism.

be dose dependent, the tremendous amount of variation among dogs makes this concept difficult to predict. The same can be said of the duration of therapy or the route of administration. It is simply safe to state that glucocorticoids cause increases in alkaline phosphatase activity regardless of steroid type, dose, duration, or route of administration. In addition, steroid therapy typically, but not as dramatically, results in increases in serum alanine aminotransferase (ALT), γ-glutamyl transferase (GGT), and cholesterol concentrations. The blood urea nitrogen (BUN) typically decreases, partly because of the induced polyuria and polydipsia (with isosthenuria or hyposthenuria). Abnormalities in liver function test results (e.g., fasting and postprandial bile acid concentrations) may be abnormal. All these changes can begin within days of initiation of therapy, and all are reversible after discontinuation of glucocorticoids.

Interference with Therapy for Diabetes Mellitus

Glucocorticoids have potent antiinsulin actions (insulin antagonism) that are certain to interfere with the control of diabetes mellitus. In some cases, steroids have appeared to "induce" the diabetic state, although a "prediabetic state" probably existed (Jeffers et al, 1991). In addition, steroid-mediated breakdown of protein and the catabolic diversion of amino acids to glucose production increase the need for insulin. Interference with diabetic control may occur with topical glucocorticoid preparations (e.g., ophthalmic ointments and dermatologic creams), as well as with oral or parenterally administered preparations. Most dogs with naturally occurring Cushing's syndrome are glucose intolerant and insulin resistant (Feldman and Tyrrell, 1982). However, administration of glucocorticoids to normal dogs for 3 to 4 weeks did not produce hyperglycemia, glucose intolerance, or insulin resistance (Wolfsheimer et al, 1986). This is not surprising, because it is assumed that healthy dogs would likely require long-term glucocorticoid administration before these effects could be documented. It has been estimated that the average dog with naturally occurring Cushing's syndrome has had the condition for 12 months at the time of diagnosis.

Some diabetic pets develop disorders that require short-term or long-term glucocorticoid therapy. If glucocorticoid therapy is needed in a dog or cat with concomitant diabetes mellitus, steroids with a short duration of action are imperative. The dose given should always be the lowest needed to control a disorder. If short-term therapy is undertaken (1 or 2 weeks), good control of the diabetic state may be lost, but the owner should be made aware of the transient nature of this interference and of the obvious problems of induced polydipsia, polyuria, and polyphagia. These dogs and cats may develop insulin resistance, but ketoacidosis is rare unless infection or some other major problem develops. The insulin dose need not be altered; rather, it is recommended that the dose be maintained while patiently awaiting withdrawal of the interfering but necessary medication. If long-term glucocorticoid therapy is needed, an increase in the insulin dose is necessary to maintain control over the diabetic state. The amount of increase in daily insulin required is variable and should be based on parameters used to evaluate control of the diabetic patient, as described in Chapters 11 and 12.

Cats treated with glucocorticoids appear to develop glucose intolerance more readily than dogs. Most cats with naturally occurring Cushing's syndrome are also diabetic. Exogenous glucocorticoid therapy is associated with hyperglycemia even with administration of low doses of short-acting forms of these drugs (Middleton and Watson, 1985; Middleton et al, 1987).

Sodium Retention/Hypertension

Most glucocorticoids have so little mineralocorticoid effect that problems related to sodium retention are not worrisome. However, glucocorticoids may cause hypertension, which in turn could cause a variety of problems. Hypertension could have deleterious effects on glomeruli, leading to protein loss, or could cause problems such as hemorrhage, retinal detachment, or cardiac disorders.

Pregnancy and Fertility

Pregnant bitches that have progressed beyond 20 days of gestation are likely to suffer an abortion within 2 to 5 days of being given glucocorticoid medication. The entire litter or portions of a litter can be aborted. It is presumed that glucocorticoids exert strong negative feedback activity, thereby suppressing pituitary gonadotropin secretion, resulting in a loss of the ability to maintain pregnancy. The doses of glucocorticoids used in treating immune-mediated disorders, acute allergic problems, and other major diseases can be expected to terminate pregnancy. As with other corticosteroid-induced side effects, individual variation in response is extreme.

Dexamethasone has been advocated as a reliable agent for terminating pregnancy in dogs. Abortion was induced in 20 of 20 dogs estimated to be 28 to 51 days into gestation after they were given dexamethasone. The orally administered medication was tapered over 7.5 to 10 days, starting at 0.4 to 0.6 mg/kg (Zone et al, 1995).

The same inhibitory action on pituitary gonadotropin secretion may also interfere with fertility. Suppressed secretion of follicle-stimulating hormone and luteinizing hormone results in failure to cycle in the bitch and testicular atrophy and oligospermia in the male (see Biologic Effects, page 464). Fortunately, these effects are usually reversible after withdrawal of the glucocorticoid therapy.

Thyroid Function

See Biologic Effects, page 465.

Retardation of Growth

See Biologic Effects, page 465.

USE OF GLUCOCORTICOIDS IN DIAGNOSTIC TESTING

HYPERADRENOCORTICISM. Glucocorticoids, specifically dexamethasone, are used in screening and suppression tests in the diagnostic evaluation of dogs and cats suspected of having hyperadrenocorticism. The protocols for these tests are fully described in Chapters 6 and 7.

LYMPHOSARCOMA. Occasionally, dogs with non-specific illnesses or specific biochemical alterations (e.g., significant hypercalcemia) with no obvious cause are seen in veterinary practice. One potential cause for this dilemma is lymphosarcoma. A small percentage of these dogs and cats may not have any other screening test abnormalities. Although this situation is frustrating, occasionally the diagnosis cannot be made using radiographs, lymph node biopsies, bone marrow aspirates, liver biopsies, or splenic aspirates. A combination diagnostic and therapeutic trial of glucocorticoids in high doses can be attempted. If the dog or cat quickly improves or if the serum calcium concentration falls into the normal range, a diagnosis of lymphosarcoma, multiple myeloma, or some other steroid-responsive tumor is likely (see Chapter 17).

Use of corticosteroids in this manner, however, is strongly discouraged. This is *not* a recommended protocol. A specific diagnosis should be confirmed before corticosteroids are ever administered to a dog or cat (Rosenthal, 1982; Rosenthal and Wilke, 1983).

GLUCOCORTICOID PREPARATIONS AND DOSE SCHEDULES

As seen in Table 10-6, glucocorticoid preparations vary with respect to antiinflammatory potency and mineralocorticoid effect. These factors, plus the duration of action, cost, dosage forms available, and client compliance, must be considered when choosing a course of therapy. In determining a dosage protocol, the clinician considers the disorder being treated, past experience, and the individual animal (Coppoc, 1984). In many instances the amount of glucocorticoid required to maintain a therapeutic effect is less than that required to initiate a desired response. The lowest possible dose for the needed effect is usually determined by gradually lowering the dose until an exacerbation of disease occurs (McDonald and Langston, 1995).

Because numerous disorders are treated solely or in part with glucocorticoids, precise dosage recommendations cannot be made. The recommended duration of therapy may be only 5 to 14 days when treating such problems as asthma or acute allergic skin disorders, compared with 2 to 6 months of therapy initially undertaken when treating autoimmune hemolytic anemia, systemic lupus erythematosus, or other serious immune-mediated diseases.

In immune-mediated disease, we often begin *pharmacologic* therapy with prednisolone at a dosage of 2.2 to 6.6 mg/kg of body weight per day. The larger the animal, the lower the initial dose on a per weight basis. If dexamethasone is chosen, usually one fourth to one tenth of the prednisolone dose is used. Tapering then proceeds on a weekly or biweekly basis. For example, for a patient receiving 50 mg of prednisolone daily, the schedule would be:

Week 1: 50 mg/day (may be divided)
Week 2: 25 mg/day
Weeks 3 and 4: 50 mg every other day
Weeks 5 and 6: 25 mg every other day
Weeks 7 and 8: 12.5 mg every other day
Weeks 9 and 10: 7.5 mg every other day
Weeks 11 and 12: 2.5 mg every other day

Some dogs and cats require *physiologic* replacement glucocorticoid doses, such as the dog that has had a functioning adrenocortical tumor removed, leaving the pet with only nonfunctioning, atrophied adrenocortical cells. With dexamethasone, an approximate dose of 0.01 to 0.02 mg/kg given IM or SQ two to four times a day should be administered initially and then gradually tapered. Once the dog or cat is eating and drinking it should be switched to oral prednisone and tapered (see Chapter 6).

In virtually all internal medicine disorders, oral short-term medications are strongly advocated. The long-term injectables have little place in the therapy of seriously ill patients. We usually administer oral medications divided twice daily. Although other investigators have advocated morning therapy in dogs and evening therapy in cats, this advice seems academic.

TABLE 10–6 COMPARISON OF THE ACTION OF CORTICOSTEROID PREPARATIONS

| Preparation | RELATIVE POTENCIES | | | Equivalent Oral Dose (mg) | PREPARATIONS AVAILABLE | | |
	Glucocorticoid	Topical	Mineralo-corticoid		Oral	Injectable	Topical
Short-Acting							
Hydrocortisone	1	1	1	20	Syrup: 2 mg/ml Tablets: 5, 10, 20, 25 mg	25, 50, 125 mg/ml	Many forms
Cortisone	0.8	0	0.8	25	Tablets: 5, 10, 25 mg	25, 50 mg/ml	Ophthalmic ointment Ophthalmic drops
Intermediate-Acting							
Prednisone	4	0	0.3	5	Tablets: 1, 2.5, 5, 10, 20, 50 mg Capsules: 1.25 mg	—	—
Prednisolone	5	4	0.3	5	Tablets: 5 mg	20, 25, 40, 50, 100 mg/ml Powder: 50 mg/vial	Creams, ophthalmic ointment, and solutions; aerosols
Methylprednisolone	5	5	0	5	Tablets: 2, 4, 16 mg Medules: 2, 4 mg	20, 50, 62.5, 80 mg/ml Powder: 500, 1000 mg/vial	Creams and ointments
Triamcinolone	5	5–100	0	4	Tablets: 1, 2, 4, 8, 16 mg Syrup: 0.4, 0.8 mg/ml	5, 10, 20, 25, 40 mg/ml	Ointments, lotion, foam, spray, cream
Long-Acting							
Betamethasone	25–40	10	0	0.6	Tablets: 0.5, 0.6 mg Syrup; pellets	4, 6 mg/ml	Ointment, cream, gel, aerosol, lotin
Dexamethasone	30	10	0	0.75	Elixir: 0.05, 0.1 mg/ml Tablets: 0.25, 0.5, 0.75, 1.0, 1.5, 4 mg	1, 2, 4, 5, 8 mg/ml	Same as betamethasone
Paramethasone	10	—	0	2	Tablets: 1, 2, 6 mg	5, 20 mg/ml	—
Mineralocorticoids							
Fludrocortisone	10	10	250	2	Tablets: 0.1 mg	3 mg/ml	Otic suspension
Desoxycorticosterone	0	0	20	0	Linguets: 1, 5 mg	In oil: 5, 10, 50 mg/ml Pellets	Ointment

REFERENCES

Aron DC, et al: Glucocorticoids and adrenal androgens. *In* Greenspan FS, Gardner DG (eds): Basic and Clinical Endocrinology, 6th ed. New York, Lange Medical Books/McGraw-Hill, 2001, p 334.

Behrend EN, Kemppainen RJ: Glucocorticoid therapy. Vet Clin North Am 27:187, 1997.

Bone RC, et al: A controlled clinical trial of high-dose methylprednisolone in the treatment of severe sepsis and septic shock. N Engl J Med 317:653, 1987.

Braughler JM, Hall ED: Correlation of methylprednisolone levels in cat spinal cord with its effects on sodium potassium ATPase, lipid peroxidation, and alpha motor neuron function. J Neurosurg 56:838, 1982.

Brockus CW, et al: Effect of alternate-day prednisolone administration on hypophyseal-adrenocortical activity in dogs. Am J Vet Res 60:698, 1999.

Butterfield JH, Gleich GJ: Antiinflammatory effects of glucocorticoids on eosinophils and neutrophils. *In* Schleimer RP, Claman HN, Oronsky A (eds): Antiinflammatory Steroid Action: Basic and Clinical Aspects. New York, Academic Press, 1989, p 13.

Calvert CA, Greene CE: Bacteremia in dogs: Diagnosis, treatment, and prognosis. Compend Contin Educ 8:179, 1986.

Cohn LA: The influence of corticosteroids on host defense mechanisms. J Vet Intern Med 5:95, 1991.

Cook AK, et al: Effect of oral cyclosporine in dogs with refractory immune-mediated anemia or thrombocytopenia. J Vet Intern Med 8:170, 1994 (abstract).

Coppoc GL: Relationships of the dosage form of a corticosteroid to its therapeutic efficacy. J Am Vet Med Assoc 185:1098, 1984.

Crager CS, et al: Adrenocorticotropic hormone and cortisol concentrations after corticotropin-releasing hormone stimulation testing in cats administered methylprednisolone. Am J Vet Res 55:704, 1994.

Cupps TR: Effects of glucocorticoids on lymphocyte function. *In* Schleimer RP, Claman HN, Oronsky A (eds): Antiinflammatory Steroid Action: Basic and Clinical Aspects. New York, Academic Press, 1989, p 132.

Cupps TR, Fauci AS: Corticosteroid-mediated immunoregulation in man. Immunol Rev 65:133, 1982.

Daley CA: Effects of ranitidine on prednisone-induced hemorrhagic gastritis in dogs, master's thesis, Auburn, Ala, 1993, Auburn University.

Dinarello CA, Mier JW: Lymphokines. N Engl J Med 317:940, 1987.

Feldman EC, Tyrrell JB: Plasma testosterone, plasma glucose, and plasma insulin concentrations in spontaneous canine Cushing's syndrome. The Endocrine Society, Salt Lake City, 1982, p 343 (abstract).

Ferguson DC, Hoenig M: Glucocorticoids, mineralocorticoids, and steroid synthesis inhibitors. *In* Adams HR (ed): Veterinary Pharmacology and Therapeutics, 7th ed. Ames, Iowa, Iowa State University Press, 1995, p 622.

Flower RJ: Glucocorticoids and the inhibition of phospholipase A. *In* Schleimer RP, Claman HN, Oronsky A (eds): Antiinflammatory Steroid Action: Basic and Clinical Aspects. New York, Academic Press, 1989, p 409.

Ford RB: Concurrent use of corticosteroids and antimicrobial drugs in the treatment of infectious diseases in small animals. J Am Vet Med Assoc 185:1142, 1984.

Gilman AG, et al: The Pharmacologic Basis of Therapeutics, 6th ed. New York, Macmillan, 1980, p 1470.

Goldfein A: Adrenocorticosteroids and adrenocortical antagonists. *In* Katzung BG (ed): Basic and Clinical Pharmacology, 5th ed. Norwalk, Conn, Appleton & Lange, 1994, p 543.

Greisman SE: Experimental gram-negative bacterial sepsis: Optimal methylprednisolone requirements for prevention of mortality not preventable by antibiotics alone. Proc Soc Exp Biol Med 170:436, 1982.

Hall ED, Braughler JM: Effects of intravenous methylprednisolone on spinal cord peroxidation and sodium and potassium ATPase reactivity. J Neurosurg 57:247, 1982.

Hall EJ: Inflammatory bowel disease: Recent advances. Proceedings of the North America Veterinary Conference, Orlando, FL, 2002, pp 264-266.

Hankes GH, et al: Pharmacokinetics of prednisolone sodium succinate and its metabolites in normovolemic and hypovolemic dogs. Am J Vet Res 46:476, 1985.

Haskins SC: Management of septic shock. J Am Vet Med Assoc 200:1915, 1992.

Hinshaw LB, et al: Review update: Current management of the septic shock patient—experimental basis for treatment. Circ Shock 9:543, 1982.

Hinshaw LB, et al: Effect of high-dose glucocorticoid therapy on mortality in patients with clinical signs of systemic sepsis. N Engl J Med 317:659, 1987.

Hirata F: The role of lipocortins in cellular function as a second messenger of glucocorticoids. *In* Schleimer RP, Claman HN, Oronsky A (eds): Antiinflammatory Steroid Action: Basic and Clinical Aspects. New York, Academic Press, 1989, p 67.

Hoerlein BF, et al: Evaluation of naloxone, crocetin, thyrotropin-releasing hormone, methylprednisolone, partial myelotomy, and hemilaminectomy in the treatment of acute spinal cord trauma. J Am Anim Hosp Assoc 21:67, 1985.

Jeffers JG, et al: Diabetes mellitus induced in a dog after administration of corticosteroids and methylprednisolone pulse therapy. J Am Vet Med Assoc 199:77, 1991.

Kehrl JH, Fauci AS: The clinical use of glucocorticoids. Ann Allergy 50:2, 1983.

Kemppainen RJ, et al: Adrenocortical suppression in the dog after a single dose of methylprednisolone acetate. Am J Vet Res 42:822, 1981.

Kemppainen RJ, et al: Adrenocortical suppression in the dog given a single intramuscular dose of prednisone or triamcinolone acetonide. Am J Vet Res 42:204, 1982.

Kemppainen RJ, Sartin JL: Effects of single intravenous doses of dexamethasone on baseline cortisol concentration and responses to synthetic ACTH in healthy dogs. Am J Vet Res 45:742, 1984.

Kimura T, et al: Steroid administration with acute pancreatitis: Studies with an isolated, perfused canine pancreas. Surgery 85:520, 1979.

Leramo OB, et al: Massive gastroduodenal hemorrhage and perforation in acute spinal cord injury. Surg Neurol 17:186, 1982.

MacDonald JM: Glucocorticoid Therapy. *In* Ettinger SJ, Feldman EC (eds): Textbook of Veterinary Internal Medicine. Philadelphia, WB Saunders, 2000, p 307.

McDonald RK, Langston VC: Use of corticosteroids and nonsteroidal antiinflammatory agents. *In* Ettinger SJ, Feldman EC (eds): Textbook of Veterinary Internal Medicine. Philadelphia, WB Saunders, 1995.

Meric S: Canine meningitis: A changing emphasis. J Vet Intern Med 2:26, 1988.

Meric S, et al: Necrotizing vasculitis of the spinal pachyleptomeningeal arteries in three Bernese Mountain Dog littermates. J Am Anim Hosp Assoc 22:459, 1986.

Meuleman J, Katz P: The immunologic effects, kinetics, and use of glucocorticoids. Med Clin North Am 69:805, 1985.

Meyers FH, et al: Review of Medical Pharmacology, 7th ed. Los Altos, Calif, Lange Medical Publications, 1980, p 353.

Middleton DJ, Watson ADJ: Glucose intolerance in cats given short-term therapy of prednisolone and megestrol acetate. Am J Vet Res 46:2623, 1985.

Middleton DJ, et al: Suppression of cortisol responses to exogenous adrenocortical hormone, and the occurrence of side effects attributable to glucocorticoid excess, in cats during therapy with megestrol acetate and prednisolone. Can J Vet Res 51:60, 1987.

Moore RW, Withrow SJ: Gastrointestinal hemorrhage and pancreatitis associated with intervertebral disk disease in the dog. J Am Vet Assoc 180:1443, 1982.

Munck A, Guyre PM: Glucocorticoid actions on monocytes and macrophages. *In* Schleimer RP, Claman HN, Oronsky A (eds): Antiinflammatory Steroid Action: Basic and Clinical Aspects. New York, Academic Press, 1989, p 199.

Nossal GJV: The basic components of the immune system. N Engl J Med 316:1320, 1987.

Osol A: Remington's Pharmaceutical Sciences, 16th ed. Easton, Pa, Mack Publishing, 1980, p 898.

Papich MG, Davis LE: Glucocorticoid therapy. *In* Kirk RW (ed): Current Veterinary Therapy X. Philadelphia, WB Saunders, 1989, p 54.

Piper JM, et al: Corticosteroid use and peptic ulcer disease: role of nonsteroidal antiinflammatory drugs. Ann Intern Med 114:735, 1991.

Roberts SM, et al: Effect of ophthalmic prednisolone acetate on the canine adrenal gland and hepatic function. Am J Vet Res 45:1711, 1984.

Rohrer CR, et al: Gastric hemorrhage in dogs given high doses of methylprednisolone sodium succinate. Am J Vet Res 60:977, 1999a.

Rohrer CR, et al: Efficacy of misoprostol in prevention of gastric hemorrhage in dogs treated with high doses of methylprednisolone sodium succinate. Am J Vet Res 60:982, 1999b.

Rosenthal RC: Hormones in cancer therapy. Vet Clin North Am (Small Anim Pract) 12:67, 1982.

Rosenthal RC, Wilke JR: Glucocorticoid therapy. *In* Kirk RW (ed): Current Veterinary Therapy VIII. Philadelphia, WB Saunders, 1983, p 854.

Scott DW: Systemic glucocorticoid therapy. *In* Kirk RW (ed): Current Veterinary Therapy VII. Philadelphia, WB Saunders, 1980, p 988.

Scott DW: Iatrogenic Cushing's syndrome in the cat. Feline Pract 12:30, 1982.

Scott DW, et al: Dermatologic therapy: Hormonal agents. *In* Small Animal Dermatology. Philadelphia, WB Saunders, 1995, p 240.

Sorjonen DC, et al: Effects of dexamethasone and surgical hypotension on the stomach of dogs: Clinical, endoscopic, and pathologic evaluations. Am J Vet Res 44:1233, 1983.

Spencer KB, et al: Adrenal gland function in dogs given methylprednisolone. Am J Vet Res 41:1503, 1980.

Steinberg WM, Lewis JH: Steroid-induced pancreatitis: Does it really exist? Gastroenterology 81:799, 1981.

Stewart THM, et al: Ulcerative enterocolitis in dogs induced by drugs. J Pathol 131:363, 1980.

Toombs JP, et al: Colonic perforation following neurosurgical procedures and corticosteroid therapy in four dogs. J Am Vet Med Assoc 177:68, 1980.

Toombs JP, et al: Colonic perforation in corticosteroid-treated dogs. J Am Vet Med Assoc 188:145, 1986.

Tyrrell JB, et al: Glucocorticoids and adrenal androgens. *In* Greenspan FS (ed): Basic and Clinical Endocrinology, 3rd ed. San Mateo, Calif, Appleton & Lange, 1991, p 323.

Wolfsheimer KJ, et al: Effects of prednisolone on glucose tolerance and insulin secretion in the dog. Am J Vet Res 47:1011, 1986.

Woltz HH, et al: Effect of prednisone on thyroid gland morphology and plasma thyroxine and T$_3$ levels in dogs. Am J Vet Res 44:2000, 1983.

Zenoble RD, Kemppainen RJ: Adrenocortical suppression by topically applied corticosteroids in dogs. J Am Vet Med Assoc 191:685, 1987.

Zone M, et al: Termination of pregnancy in dogs by oral administration of dexamethasone. Theriogenology 43:487, 1995.

THE ENDOCRINE PANCREAS

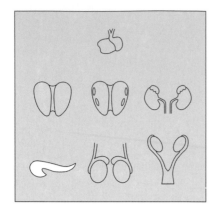

11

CANINE DIABETES MELLITUS

The endocrine pancreas is composed of the islets of Langerhans, which are dispersed as "small islands" in a "sea" of exocrine-secreting acinar cells. Four distinct cell types have been identified within these islets on the basis of staining properties and morphology—alpha cells, which secrete glucagon; beta cells, which secrete insulin; delta cells, which secrete somatostatin; and F cells, which secrete pancreatic polypeptide. Dysfunction involving any of these cell lines ultimately results in either an excess or a deficiency of the respective hormone in the circulation. In the dog and cat, the most common disorder of the endocrine pancreas is diabetes mellitus, which results from an absolute or relative insulin deficiency due to deficient insulin secretion by the beta cells. The incidence of diabetes mellitus is similar for the dog and cat, with a reported frequency varying from 1 in 100 to 1 in 500 (Panciera et al, 1990).

CLASSIFICATION AND ETIOLOGY

Diabetes mellitus is classified according to the disease in humans, that is, as type 1 and type 2 based on the pathophysiologic mechanisms and pathogenic alterations affecting the beta cells.

TYPE 1 DIABETES MELLITUS. Type 1 diabetes mellitus is characterized by a combination of genetic susceptibility and immunologic destruction of beta cells with progressive and eventually complete insulin insufficiency (Eisenbarth, 1986; Palmer and McCulloch, 1991). Autoantibodies are directed against several islet components, including insulin, beta cell, and glutamic acid decarboxylase (GAD) (Srikanta et al, 1985; Verge et al, 1996; Gorus et al, 1997). Serum anti-insulin, anti-beta cell, and/or anti-GAD autoantibodies are commonly identified at the time diabetes is diagnosed and are also detected early in the development of type 1 diabetes, prior to the onset of hyperglycemia or clinical signs (Verge et al, 1996; Gorus et al, 1997). Screening individuals for serum anti-insulin, anti-beta cell, and anti-GAD autoantibodies is used to identify individuals at risk for development of type 1 diabetes. Identification of anti-GAD autoantibodies or positive results for all three autoantibodies has the highest predictive value for development of type 1 diabetes (Tuomilehto et al, 1994; Schatz et al, 1994; Hagopian et al, 1995).

Immune-mediated destruction of the islets has been conceptually divided into six stages in humans, beginning with genetic susceptibility (Table 11-1) (Eisenbarth, 1986). Stage 2 involves a triggering event that leads

TABLE 11-1   STAGES IN THE DEVELOPMENT OF IMMUNE-MEDIATED INSULIN-DEPENDENT DIABETES MELLITUS IN HUMANS

Stage 1	Genetic susceptibility
Stage 2	Triggering event
Stage 3	Active autoimmunity and normal insulin secretion
Stage 4	Active autoimmunity and impaired insulin secretion
Stage 5	Overt diabetes with residual insulin secretion
Stage 6	Overt diabetes with complete beta-cell destruction

to beta-cell autoimmunity. Environmental factors that trigger the development of beta-cell immunity are poorly defined but probably include drugs and infectious agents. One interesting environmental factor that has been proposed in humans involves consumption of cow's milk during infancy. Some humans with newly diagnosed insulin-dependent diabetes mellitus (IDDM) have antibodies to bovine serum albumin and a 17-amino acid bovine serum albumin peptide. It has been hypothesized that the ingestion of cow's milk in early life can initiate beta-cell destruction through molecular mimicry between these proteins in cow's milk and a beta-cell protein (Karjalainen et al, 1992; Savilahti et al, 1993; Gerstein, 1994), although there is skepticism concerning an etiologic role of these antibodies (Atkinson et al, 1993). Stage 3 is the period of active autoimmunity,

but normal insulin secretion is maintained. During stage 4, immunologic abnormalities persist, but glucose-stimulated insulin secretion is progressively lost, despite maintenance of euglycemia. Overt (clinical) diabetes develops in stage 5, although some residual insulin secretion remains. Stage 6 is characterized by complete beta-cell destruction. As a result, individuals with type 1 diabetes are dependent on insulin to control glycemia, avoid ketoacidosis, and survive. Based on our current understanding of the disorder, it seems likely that the pathogenesis of diabetes mellitus in dogs progresses through similar stages. Unfortunately, we do not typically identify diabetes in dogs until stage 5 or 6, at which time insulin therapy is mandatory (Fig. 11-1).

TYPE 2 DIABETES MELLITUS.   Type 2 diabetes mellitus is characterized by insulin resistance and "dysfunctional" beta cells (Reaven, 1988; Leahy, 1990), defects that are believed to be genetic in origin, evident for a decade or longer before hyperglycemia and clinical signs of diabetes develop, and with deleterious effects that can be accentuated by environmental factors such as obesity (Warram et al, 1990; Martin et al, 1992). Debate still continues among human diabetologists about which defect—insulin resistance or impaired insulin secretion—initiates the cascade of events leading to overt diabetes mellitus. Hepatic resistance to insulin, potentially induced by increased free fatty

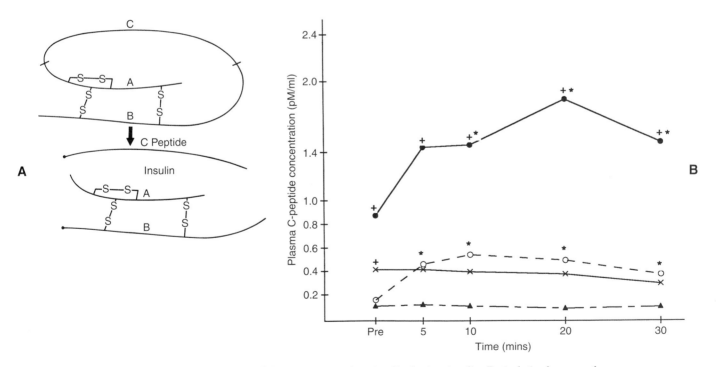

FIGURE 11-1. *A,* Schematic of the conversion of proinsulin *(top)* to insulin. Proteolytic cleavage of proinsulin forms equimolar concentrations of C peptide and insulin, which are stored in secretory granules of beta cells. *B,* Mean plasma C-peptide concentration before and after IV administration of 1 mg glucagon in 24 healthy dogs *(broken line-open circles),* 35 dogs with diabetes mellitus and low baseline C-peptide concentration *(broken line-triangles),* 7 dogs with diabetes mellitus and increased baseline C-peptide concentration *(solid line-Xs),* and 8 dogs with naturally acquired hyperadrenocorticism *(solid line-solid circles).* * = significantly (P<0.05) different from baseline value; + = significantly (P<0.05) different from corresponding time in healthy dogs. (*B* from Nelson RW: Diabetes mellitus. *In* Ettinger SJ, Feldman EC (eds): Textbook of Veterinary Internal Medicine, 4th ed. Philadelphia, WB Saunders Co, 1995, p 1511.)

acids in the portal circulation, results in excessive basal hepatic glucose production and fasting hyperglycemia (DeFronzo et al, 1989; Groop et al, 1989; Bergman and Mittleman, 1998; Massillon et al, 1997). Muscle insulin resistance impairs the ability of endogenously secreted insulin to augment muscle glucose uptake in response to a meal, resulting in an excessive postprandial increase in the blood glucose concentration (Mitrakou et al, 1990). Defects in insulin receptor function, insulin receptor–signal transduction pathway, glucose transport and phosphorylation, glycogen synthesis, and glucose oxidation contribute to muscle insulin resistance (DeFronzo, 1997). Impaired insulin secretion also plays a major role in the pathogenesis of glucose intolerance in humans with type 2 diabetes (Polonsky, 1995). Total amounts of insulin secreted during glucose tolerance testing may be increased, decreased, or normal compared with the *normal* fasting animal. However, relative to the severity of insulin resistance and prevailing hyperglycemia, even elevated serum insulin concentrations are deficient (Saad et al, 1989). As the fasting blood glucose concentration increases, insulin secretion decreases progressively, and by the time the fasting blood glucose concentration is greater than 180 to 200 mg/dl, the insulin response to glucose tolerance testing is deficient in absolute terms.

Humans with type 2 diabetes are typically not dependent on insulin to control the disease. Control of the diabetic state is usually possible through diet, exercise, and oral hypoglycemic drugs. However, insulin treatment may be necessary in some type 2 diabetics if insulin resistance and beta cell dysfunction are severe. As such, humans with type 2 diabetes can have IDDM or non–insulin-dependent diabetes mellitus (NIDDM). Insulin resistance and impaired insulin secretion have been identified in dogs and cats with obesity (Nelson et al, 1990; Appleton et al, 2001), and obesity is accepted as a contributing factor for the development of diabetes mellitus in dogs and cats (Panciera et al, 1990; Scarlett and Donoghue, 1998). Low insulin sensitivity has also been identified in a group of lean cats subsequently identified to be at greater risk for developing impaired glucose tolerance with obesity than lean cats with higher insulin sensitivity that subsequently developed obesity (Appleton et al, 2001). The authors speculated that these cats may be more at risk for progressing to overt diabetes mellitus. The role of genetics, if any, for variations in insulin sensitivity and risk for developing diabetes in cats remains to be determined.

INSULIN-DEPENDENT AND NON–INSULIN-DEPENDENT DIABETES MELLITUS. The classification of human diabetics as type 1 or type 2 is based on familial history, clinical presentation, and results of immunologic (e.g., identification of serum anti–beta cell and anti-insulin autoantibodies) and insulin secretagogue tests (Unger and Foster, 1998). In contrast, classifying diabetes as IDDM and NIDDM is based on the need for insulin therapy to control glycemia, avoid ketoacidosis, and survive. Individuals with IDDM must receive insulin to avoid ketoacidosis, whereas control of glycemia and

avoidance of ketoacidosis can be accomplished through diet, exercise, and oral hypoglycemic drugs in individuals with NIDDM. Approximately 10% of diabetic humans in the United States have type 1 diabetes, which is insulin-dependent. Approximately 90% of diabetic humans have type 2 diabetes, which may be insulin-dependent or non–insulin-dependent, depending on the severity of insulin resistance and beta cell dysfunction.

It is more clinically relevant and perhaps more accurate to classify diabetes in dogs and cats as IDDM or NIDDM rather than as type 1 or type 2. Familial history is rarely available in diabetic dogs and cats; the clinical presentation is usually not helpful in differentiating type 1 and type 2 diabetes, especially in cats (Nelson et al, 1993); insulin secretagogue tests are not routinely performed, and their results may be misleading (Kirk et al, 1993); and autoantibody tests for type 1 diabetes are not readily available. Therefore, as clinicians, we usually classify diabetic dogs and cats as either IDDM or NIDDM based on their need for insulin treatment. This can be confusing because some diabetics, especially cats, can initially appear to have NIDDM progressing to IDDM, or flip back and forth between IDDM and NIDDM as severity of insulin resistance and impairment of beta-cell function waxes and wanes. Apparent changes in the diabetic state (i.e., IDDM and NIDDM) are understandable when one realizes that islet pathology may be mild to severe and progressive or static; that the ability of the pancreas to secrete insulin depends on the severity of islet pathology and can decrease with time; that responsiveness of tissues to insulin varies, often in conjunction with the presence or absence of concurrent inflammatory, infectious, neoplastic, or hormonal disorders; and that all these variables affect the animal's need for insulin, insulin dosage, and ease of diabetic regulation. Use of serum insulin concentrations to differentiate between IDDM and NIDDM is discussed on page 495.

INSULIN-DEPENDENT DIABETES IN DOGS. In our experience, virtually all dogs have IDDM at the time diabetes mellitus is diagnosed. IDDM is characterized by hypoinsulinemia, essentially no increase in endogenous serum insulin concentration following administration of an insulin secretagogue (e.g., glucose or glucagon) at any time following diagnosis of the disease, failure to establish glycemic control with diet and/or oral hypoglycemic drugs, and an absolute necessity for exogenous insulin to maintain glycemic control. The cause of IDDM has been poorly characterized in dogs but is undoubtedly multifactorial (Table 11-2). Genetic predispositions have been suggested by familial associations in dogs and by pedigree analysis of Keeshonds (see Table 11-3) (Guptill et al, 1999; Hess et al, 2000a). The most common pathologic lesions in dogs with diabetes mellitus are a reduction in the number and size of pancreatic islets, a decrease in the number of beta cells within islets, and hydropic ballooning degeneration of beta cells (see Fig. 12-1, page 541). In some dogs, an extreme form of the disease may occur, represented by a congenital absolute deficiency of beta cells and pancreatic islet hypoplasia or aplasia (Alejandro et al, 1988; Atkins et al, 1988). Less severe changes of pancreatic islets and beta cells may predispose the adult dog to diabetes mellitus after it has been exposed to environmental factors, such as infectious agents, insulin-antagonistic diseases and drugs, obesity, and pancreatitis. Environmental factors may induce beta cell degeneration secondary to chronic insulin resistance or may cause release of beta cell proteins that induce immune-mediated destruction of the islets (Nerup, 1994). Studies evaluating for anti-beta cell autoantibodies in diabetic dogs have been conflicting, having been identified in newly diagnosed diabetic dogs with IDDM in one study (Hoenig and Dawe, 1992) but not in another (Haines, 1986). Immune-mediated insulitis has also been described in diabetic dogs (Alejandro et al, 1988). Seemingly, autoimmune mechanisms, in conjunction with environmental factors, may play a role in the initiation and progression of diabetes in dogs.

Clinically, pancreatitis is often seen in dogs with diabetes mellitus and has been suggested as a cause of diabetes after destruction of the islets. However, the incidence of histologically identifiable pancreatitis in diabetic dogs is only 30% to 40%. Although destruction of beta cells secondary to pancreatitis is an obvious explanation for the development of hypoinsulinemic diabetes mellitus, other perhaps more complex factors are involved in the development of diabetes mellitus in dogs without obvious exocrine pancreatic lesions.

NON–INSULIN-DEPENDENT DIABETES IN DOGS. Obesity-induced carbohydrate intolerance has been documented in dogs (Mattheeuws et al, 1984), and minute amounts of amyloid have been identified in the islets of some dogs with diabetes mellitus. Despite these findings, clinical recognition of NIDDM is very uncommon in the dog. A juvenile form of canine diabetes mellitus that closely resembles human maturity-onset diabetes of the young, a subclassification of NIDDM, has been described. Measurement of plasma C-peptide concentrations during insulin response testing also suggests the presence of some continuing beta-cell function in a small percentage of diabetic dogs (see Fig. 11-1). C-peptide is the connecting peptide found in the proinsulin molecule and is secreted into the circulation in equimolar concentrations as insulin. Increased plasma C-peptide concentrations in these latter dogs suggest either a severe form of type 2 diabetes mellitus or residual beta-cell function in dogs with type 1 diabetes mellitus. Unfortunately, clinical characteristics of juvenile canine NIDDM and the presence of some C-peptide secretory capabilities resemble IDDM, in that dogs with these conditions are treated with insulin to manage hyperglycemia.

TRANSIENT DIABETES IN DOGS. Transient or reversible diabetes is extremely uncommon in dogs and usually occurs in dogs with subclinical diabetes treated with insulin antagonistic drugs (e.g., glucocorticoids) or in the very early stages of an insulin-antagonistic disorder (e.g., diestrus in the bitch, hyperadrenocorticism). Such

TABLE 11-2 POTENTIAL FACTORS INVOLVED IN THE ETIOPATHOGENESIS OF DIABETES MELLITUS IN DOGS AND CATS

Dog	Cat
Genetics	Islet amyloidosis
Immune-mediated insulitis	Obesity
Pancreatitis	Pancreatitis
Obesity	Concurrent hormonal disease
Concurrent hormonal disease	Hyperadrenocorticism
Hyperadrenocorticism	Acromegaly
Diestrus-induced excess of growth hormone	Hyperthyroidism
	Drugs
Hypothyroidism	Megestrol acetate
Drugs	Glucocorticoids
Glucocorticoids	Infection
Infection	Concurrent illness
Concurrent illness	Renal insufficiency
Renal insufficiency	Cardiac disease
Cardiac disease	Hyperlipidemia (?)
Hyperlipidemia	Genetics (?)
Islet amyloidosis (?)	Immune-mediated insulitis (?)

TABLE 11-3 BREED RISKS FOR DEVELOPING DIABETES MELLITUS DERIVED FROM ANALYSIS OF THE VETERINARY MEDICAL DATABASE (VMDB) FROM 1970 TO 1993*[†]

Breed	Cases	Control	Odds Ratio
Australian Terrier	33	3	9.39
Standard Schnauzer	96	14	5.85
Miniature Schnauzer	526	88	5.10
Bichon Frise	39	11	3.03
Spitz	34	10	2.90
Fox Terrier	88	28	2.68
Miniature Poodle	712	244	2.49
Samoyed	159	56	2.42
Cairn Terrier	61	23	2.26
Keeshond	47	18	2.23
Maltese	42	20	1.79
Toy Poodle	186	90	1.76
Lhasa Apso	85	47	1.54
Yorkshire Terrier	96	57	1.44
Mixed Breed	1755	1498	1.00 (Reference group)
English Springer Spaniel	62	77	0.69
Irish Setter	66	84	0.67
Beagle	70	94	0.64
English Setter	29	41	0.60
Basset Hound	28	43	0.56
Rottweiler	37	62	0.51
Boston Terrier	27	45	0.56
Doberman Pinscher	103	180	0.49
Labrador Retriever	199	375	0.45
Australian Shepherd	32	62	0.44
Cocker Spaniel	77	186	0.35
Golden Retriever	91	274	0.28
Shetland Sheepdog	27	109	0.21
Collie	25	104	0.21
German Shepherd	68	317	0.18

*From Guptill L, et al: Is canine diabetes on the increase? In Recent Advances in Clinical Management of Diabetes Mellitus, Iams Company, Dayton, Ohio, 1999, p 24.
[†]The VMDB comprises medical records of 24 veterinary schools in the United States and Canada. VMDB case records analyzed included those from first hospital visits of 6078 dogs with a diagnosis of diabetes mellitus and 5922 randomly selected dogs with first hospital visits for any diagnosis other than diabetes mellitus seen at the same veterinary schools in the same year. Only breeds with more than 25 cases of diabetes mellitus are included.

dogs have a reduced but adequate mass of functional beta cells to maintain carbohydrate tolerance when insulin resistance is not present, but they are unable to secrete an adequate amount of insulin to maintain euglycemia in the presence of insulin antagonism. Early recognition and correction of the insulin antagonism may reestablish euglycemia without the long-term need for insulin therapy. Failure to quickly correct the insulin antagonism will result in progressive loss of beta cells, eventual development of IDDM, and the life-long requirement for insulin treatment to control the hyperglycemia. Additional causes of transient or reversible IDDM include NIDDM and the "honeymoon period" of IDDM. A transient increase in insulin secretion and reduced insulin dosage requirements may occur during the initial weeks to months after the diagnosis of IDDM in humans; this is called the honeymoon period (Rossetti et al, 1990). A syndrome similar to the honeymoon period occurs in some newly diagnosed diabetic dogs and is characterized by excellent

glycemic control using dosages of insulin considerably less than what would be expected (i.e., <0.2 U/kg per injection) (Fig. 11-2). Presumably, the existence of residual beta-cell function when diabetes is diagnosed (see Fig. 11-1) and correction of *glucose toxicity* (see page 544) after initiation of insulin therapy account for the initial ease of treating the diabetic state. Continuing progressive destruction of residual functioning beta cells results in worsening loss of endogenous insulin secretory capacity and a greater need for exogenous insulin to control the diabetes. As a result, glycemic control becomes more difficult to maintain, and insulin dosages increase to more commonly required amounts (0.5 to 1.0 U/kg per injection). This increase in insulin requirements usually occurs within the first 6 months of treatment.

SECONDARY DIABETES IN DOGS. Secondary diabetes mellitus is carbohydrate intolerance secondary to concurrent insulin antagonistic disease or medications. Examples include the bitch in diestrus and the cat

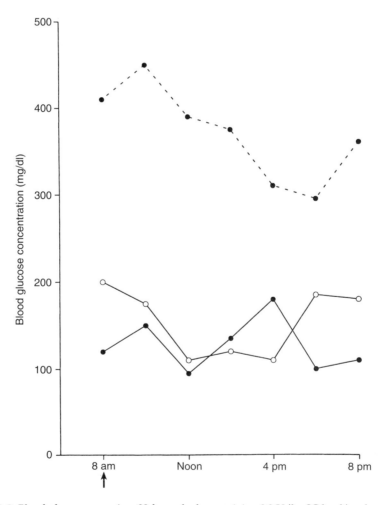

FIGURE 11-2. Blood glucose curve in a 32-kg male dog receiving 0.3 U/kg SC beef/pork source NPH insulin *(solid line-solid circles)*. The blood glucose curve was obtained shortly after initiating insulin therapy. Five months later, glycemic control deteriorated and clinical signs recurred despite increasing the insulin dosage to 0.6 U/kg *(broken line-solid circles)*. The dog was referred for possible insulin resistance. Insulin underdosage was pursued initially and glycemic control was reestablished at an insulin dosage of 1.0 U/kg *(solid line-open circles)*. ↑ = insulin injection and food.

treated with megestrol acetate (progesterone). Hyperinsulinemia may be initially present in these animals. However, with persistence of the insulin antagonistic disorder, beta-cell function becomes impaired, and permanent diabetes mellitus, typically IDDM, may develop. If the insulin antagonistic disorder resolves while some beta-cell function is still present, permanent overt diabetes mellitus may not develop. However, animals that become euglycemic after treatment of the insulin antagonistic disorder or discontinuation of the insulin antagonistic drug remain candidates to become "subclinical" diabetics, and an attempt should be made to avoid insulin antagonistic drugs and disorders to prevent overt diabetes mellitus from developing.

Older bitches occasionally develop diabetes during diestrus or pregnancy, presumably as a result of the insulin antagonistic actions of progesterone (see page 526). The diabetic state may resolve once the progesterone concentration declines to anestrual levels or may persist and require life-long insulin therapy. Development of diabetes during diestrus or pregnancy resembles gestational diabetes in humans. In humans, gestational diabetes is restricted to pregnant women in whom the onset or recognition of diabetes or impaired glucose tolerance occurs *during* pregnancy (Unger and Foster, 1998). After pregnancy termination, the woman may remain clinically diabetic, may revert to a subclinical diabetic state with impaired glucose tolerance, or may revert to a normal glucose-tolerant state. For the latter groups, the risk for developing overt diabetes later in life ranges from 10% to 40%, depending on severity of obesity. Bitches with transient diabetes caused by diestrus have a high likelihood of developing permanent IDDM during the next estrus. For this reason, all bitches with "gestational" diabetes should be spayed as soon as possible after diabetes is diagnosed.

Once the diagnosis of diabetes is established, dogs should be considered to have IDDM, and treatment with insulin should be initiated, even if secondary diabetes mellitus is suspected. Measurement of baseline serum insulin concentration or evaluation of serum insulin concentrations following administration of an insulin secretagogue (e.g., glucose, glucagon; see Table 12-1, page 547) are generally not recommended in newly diagnosed diabetic dogs because of the high prevalence of IDDM. The vast majority of newly diagnosed diabetic dogs will have either undetectable serum insulin concentrations or serum insulin concentrations in the lower half of the normal reference range (i.e., less than 12 µU/ml); findings consistent with IDDM and hypoinsulinemia. Measurement of serum insulin concentration may provide prognostic information in newly diagnosed diabetic dogs in which there is a strong suspicion of secondary diabetes mellitus (e.g., intact bitch in diestrus; severe acute pancreatitis). Serum insulin concentrations greater than one SD above the reference mean (>18 µU/ml in our laboratory) suggest the existence of functional beta cells and the possibility for secondary diabetes mellitus and the potential for reversion to a non-insulin-requiring state if the underlying cause of the insulin antagonism can be identified and corrected. Insulin treatment is still recommended in these situations to correct hyperglycemia and decrease the "stress" placed on the beta cells while waiting for the insulin antagonism to resolve. In theory, glucose toxicity may interfere with accurate assessment of serum insulin concentrations in diabetic dogs in a manner similar to that in diabetic cats (see page 544) (Nelson et al, 1998a). However, the syndrome of glucose toxicity has not yet been clearly established in diabetic dogs, in part because most dogs are truly hypoinsulinemic at the time diabetes mellitus is diagnosed.

PATHOPHYSIOLOGY

Diabetes mellitus results from a relative or absolute deficiency of insulin secretion by the beta cells. Insulin deficiency, in turn, causes decreased tissue utilization of glucose, amino acids, and fatty acids, accelerated hepatic glycogenolysis and gluconeogenesis, and accumulation of glucose in the circulation, causing hyperglycemia. Glucose obtained from the diet also accumulates in the circulation. As the blood glucose concentration increases, the ability of the renal tubular cells to resorb glucose from the glomerular ultrafiltrate is exceeded, resulting in glycosuria. In dogs, this typically occurs whenever the blood glucose concentration exceeds 180 to 220 mg/dl. The threshold for glucose resorption appears more variable in cats, ranging from 200 to 280 mg/dl. Glycosuria creates an osmotic diuresis, causing polyuria. Compensatory polydipsia prevents dehydration. The diminished peripheral tissue utilization of ingested glucose results in weight loss as the body attempts to compensate for perceived "starvation."

The interaction of the "satiety center" in the ventromedial region of the hypothalamus with the "feeding center" in the lateral region of the hypothalamus is responsible for controlling the amount of food ingested (Ganong, 1991). The feeding center, responsible for evoking eating behavior, is chronically functioning but can be transiently inhibited by the satiety center after food ingestion. The amount of glucose entering the cells in the satiety center directly affects the feeling of hunger; the more glucose that enters these cells, the less the feeling of hunger and vice versa (Ganong, 1991). The ability of glucose to enter the cells in the satiety center is mediated by insulin. In diabetics with a relative or absolute lack of insulin, glucose does not enter satiety center cells, resulting in failure to inhibit the feeding center. Thus these individuals become polyphagic despite hyperglycemia.

The four classic signs of diabetes mellitus are polyuria, polydipsia, polyphagia, and weight loss. The severity of these signs is directly related to the severity of hyperglycemia. As these signs become obvious to the owner, the pet is brought to the veterinarian for care. Unfortunately, some dogs and cats are not identified by their owners as having signs of disease, and these untreated animals may ultimately develop diabetic ketoacidosis (DKA). See Chapter 13 for a detailed discussion of the pathophysiology of DKA.

SIGNALMENT

Most dogs are 4 to 14 years old at the time diabetes mellitus is diagnosed, with a peak prevalence at 7 to 10 years of age. Juvenile-onset diabetes occurs in dogs less than 1 year of age and is uncommon. Female dogs are affected about twice as frequently as male dogs. Genetic predispositions for or against the development of diabetes have been suggested by familial associations in dogs and by pedigree analysis of Keeshonds (see Table 11-3; Guptill et al, 1999; Hess et al, 2000a). Breed popularity can also affect perceptions of predisposition. For example, epidemiologic studies suggest that the Labrador retriever is at decreased risk for development of diabetes mellitus; yet this is one of the most frequently affected breeds in our practice, presumably because of their popularity in our region.

ANAMNESIS

The history in virtually all diabetic dogs includes the classic signs of polydipsia, polyuria, polyphagia, and weight loss. Polyuria and polydipsia do not develop until hyperglycemia results in glycosuria. Occasionally an owner brings in a dog because of sudden blindness caused by cataract formation (Fig. 11-3). The classic signs of diabetes mellitus may have gone unnoticed or been considered irrelevant by the owner. If the clinical signs associated with uncomplicated diabetes are not observed by the owner and impaired vision caused by cataracts does not develop, a diabetic dog is at risk for the development of systemic signs of illness as progressive ketonemia and metabolic acidosis develop

(see page 584). The time sequence from the onset of initial clinical signs to the development of DKA is unpredictable, ranging from days to weeks.

A complete history is extremely important even in the "obvious" diabetic dog to explore for concurrent disorders, which are almost always present at the time diabetes mellitus is diagnosed. The clinician should always ask, "Why has the dog developed clinical signs of diabetes now?" In many dogs the insulin antagnism caused by concurrent disorders such as pancreatitis, bacterial infections, recent estrus, congestive heart failure, or hyperadrenocorticism is the final insult leading to overt diabetes. Identification and treatment of concurrent disorders plays an integral role in the successful management of the diabetic dog, and a thorough history is the first step toward identification of these disorders.

PHYSICAL EXAMINATION

Performance of a thorough physical examination is imperative in any dog suspected to have diabetes mellitus, in part because of the high prevalence of concurrent disorders that can affect response to treatment. The physical examination findings in a dog with newly diagnosed diabetes depend on whether DKA is present and its severity, on the duration of diabetes prior to its diagnosis, and on the nature of any other concurrent disorder. The nonketotic diabetic dog has no classic physical examination findings. Many diabetic dogs are obese but are otherwise in good physical condition. Dogs with prolonged untreated diabetes may have lost weight but are rarely emaciated unless concurrent disease (e.g., pancreatic exocrine insufficiency) is present. Lethargy may be evident; the haircoat may be sparse, with dry, brittle, and lusterless hair; and scales from hyperkeratosis may be present. Diabetes-induced

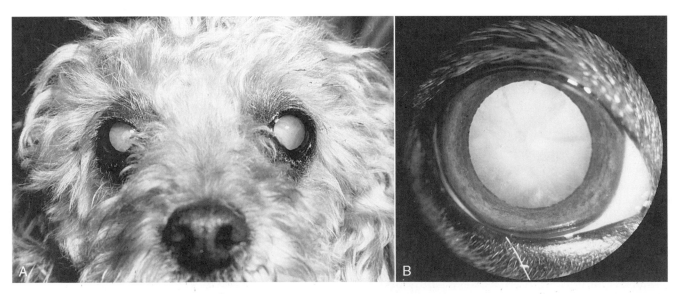

FIGURE 11-3. *A,* Bilateral cataracts causing blindness in a diabetic dog. *B,* Mature cataract with suture lines in a diabetic Collie.

hepatic lipidosis may cause hepatomegaly. Lenticular changes consistent with cataract formation are another common clinical finding in diabetic dogs. Additional abnormalities may be identified in the dog with diabetic ketoacidosis (see page 584).

ESTABLISHING THE DIAGNOSIS OF DIABETES MELLITUS

A diagnosis of diabetes mellitus requires the presence of appropriate clinical signs (i.e., polyuria, polydipsia, polyphagia, weight loss) and documentation of persistent fasting hyperglycemia and glycosuria. Measurement of the blood glucose concentration using a portable blood glucose monitoring device (see page 512) and testing for the presence of glycosuria using urine reagent test strips (e.g., KetoDiastix; Ames Division, Miles Laboratories Inc., Elkhart, Ind.) allows the rapid confirmation of diabetes mellitus. The concurrent documentation of ketonuria establishes a diagnosis of diabetic ketosis or ketoacidosis.

It is important to document both persistent hyperglycemia and glycosuria to establish a diagnosis of diabetes mellitus, because hyperglycemia differentiates diabetes mellitus from primary renal glycosuria, whereas glycosuria differentiates diabetes mellitus from other causes of hyperglycemia (Table 11-4). Stress-induced hyperglycemia is a common problem in cats and occasionally occurs in dogs, especially those that are very excited, hyperactive, or aggressive. Refer to page 567 for more information on stress-induced hyperglycemia.

Mild hyperglycemia (i.e., 130 to 180 mg/dl) is clinically silent and is usually an unexpected and unsuspected finding. If the dog with mild hyperglycemia is examined for polyuria and polydipsia, a disorder other than clinical diabetes mellitus should be sought, most notably hyperadrenocorticism. Mild

TABLE 11-4 CAUSES OF HYPERGLYCEMIA IN DOGS AND CATS

Diabetes mellitus*
"Stress" (cat)*
Postprandial (diets containing monosaccharides, disaccharides, and propylene glycol)
Hyperadrenocorticism*
Acromegaly (cat)
Diestrus (bitch)
Pheochromocytoma (dog)
Pancreatitis
Exocrine pancreatic neoplasia
Renal insufficiency
Drug therapy*
  Glucocorticoids
  Progestagens
  Megestrol acetate
  Thiazide diuretics
Dextrose-containing fluids*
Parenteral nutrition*
Head trauma

*Common cause

hyperglycemia can occur up to 2 hours postprandially in some dogs following consumption of soft moist foods (Holste et al, 1989), in "stressed" dogs, in early diabetes mellitus, and with disorders causing insulin resistance (see page 524). A diagnostic evaluation for disorders causing insulin resistance is indicated if mild hyperglycemia persists in the fasted, unstressed dog. Insulin therapy is not indicated in these animals, because clinical diabetes mellitus is not present.

CLINICAL PATHOLOGIC ABNORMALITIES

OVERVIEW OF PATIENT EVALUATION. A thorough evaluation of the dog's overall health is recommended once the diagnosis of diabetes mellitus has been established to identify any disease that may be causing or contributing to the carbohydrate intolerance (e.g., hyperadrenocorticism), that may result from the carbohydrate intolerance (e.g., bacterial cystitis), or that may mandate a modification of therapy (e.g., pancreatitis). The minimum laboratory evaluation in any "healthy" nonketotic diabetic dog should include a CBC, serum biochemical panel, and urinalysis with bacterial culture. Serum progesterone concentration should be determined if diabetes mellitus is diagnosed in an intact bitch, regardless of her cycling history. If available, abdominal ultrasound is indicated to assess for pancreatitis, adrenomegaly, pyometritis in an intact bitch, and abnormalities affecting the liver and urinary tract (e.g., changes consistent with pyelonephritis or cystitis). Because of the relatively high prevalence of pancreatitis in diabetic dogs, measurement of serum lipase or serum trypsin–like immunoreactivity (TLI) should be considered if abdominal ultrasound is not available. Measurement of the baseline serum insulin concentration or an insulin response test is not routinely done. Additional tests may be warranted after obtaining the history, performing the physical examination, or identifying ketoacidosis. The laboratory evaluation of dogs with glycosuria and ketonuria is discussed in detail in Chapter 13, page 586. Potential clinical pathologic abnormalities are listed in Table 11-5.

COMPLETE BLOOD COUNT. Results of a CBC are usually normal in the uncomplicated diabetic pet. A mild polycythemia may be present if the dog is dehydrated. An elevation of the white blood cell count may be caused by either an infectious process or severe inflammation, especially if an underlying pancreatitis is present. The presence of toxic or degenerative neutrophils or a significant shift toward immaturity of the cells supports the presence of an infectious process as the cause of the leukocytosis.

SERUM BIOCHEMICAL PANEL. The prevalence and severity of abnormalities identified in the serum biochemistry panel are dependent on the duration of untreated diabetes and the presence of concurrent disease, most notably pancreatitis. The serum biochemical panel is often unremarkable in "healthy" diabetic dogs without significant concurrent disease, aside from hyperglycemia and hypercholesterolemia.

TABLE 11-5 CLINICOPATHOLOGIC ABNORMALITIES COMMONLY FOUND IN DOGS AND CATS WITH UNCOMPLICATED DIABETES MELLITUS

Complete Blood Count

Typically normal
Neutrophilic leukocytosis, toxic neutrophils if pancreatitis or
 infection present

Biochemistry Panel

Hyperglycemia
Hypercholesterolemia
Hypertriglyceridemia (lipemia)
Increased alanine aminotransferase activity (typically <500 IU/L)
Increased alkaline phosphatase activity (typically <500 IU/L)

Urinalysis

Urine specific gravity typically >1.025
Glycosuria
Variable ketonuria
Proteinuria
Bacteriuria

Ancillary Tests

Hyperlipasemia if pancreatitis present
Hyperamylasemia if pancreatitis present
Serum trypsinlike immunoreactivity usually normal
  Low with pancreatic exocrine insufficiency
  High with acute pancreatitis
  Normal to high with chronic pancreatitis
Variable serum baseline insulin concentration
  IDDM: low, normal
  NIDDM: low, normal, increased
  Insulin resistance induced: low, normal, increased

IDDM, Insulin-dependent diabetes mellitus; *NIDDM*, non-insulin-dependent diabetes mellitus.

The most common abnormalities are an increase in serum alanine transaminase and alkaline phosphatase activities and hypercholesterolemia. The increase in liver enzyme activities is usually mild (less than 500 IU/L) and a result of hepatic lipidosis. Serum alkaline phosphatase activities in excess of 500 IU/L should raise suspicion for concurrent hyperadrenocorticism, especially if other abnormalities consistent with hyperadrenocorticism are identified in the laboratory data (see Chapter 6). Serum alanine transaminase activities in excess of 500 IU/L should raise suspicion for hepatopathy other than hepatic lipidosis, especially if additional abnormalities in endogenous liver function tests (e.g., low urea nitrogen, hypoalbuminemia, increased serum bile acids) are identified. An increase in the serum total bilirubin concentration should raise suspicion for extrahepatic biliary obstruction caused by concurrent pancreatitis. When appropriate, abdominal ultrasound and histologic evaluation of a liver biopsy specimen may be indicated to establish concurrent liver disease.

The BUN and serum creatinine concentrations are usually normal in the uncomplicated diabetic. An elevation in these parameters may be due to either primary renal failure or prerenal uremia secondary to dehydration. Primary renal failure as a result of

glomerulosclerosis, damage specifically related to hyperglycemia, is a well-recognized complication in humans but is uncommon in dogs (see Diabetic Nephropathy, page 532). Evaluation of urine specific gravity should help differentiate primary renal failure from prerenal uremia.

Alterations in serum electrolytes and acid-base parameters are common in pets with DKA and are discussed in the section dealing with therapy for the severe ketoacidotic diabetic (see page 596).

URINALYSIS. Abnormalities identified in the urinalysis that are consistent with diabetes mellitus include glycosuria, ketonuria, proteinuria, and bacteriuria with or without associated pyuria and hematuria. The dog with uncomplicated diabetes usually has glycosuria without ketonuria. However, a relatively healthy diabetic may also have trace to small amounts of ketones in the urine. If large amounts of ketones are present in the urine, especially in an animal with systemic signs of illness (e.g., lethargy, vomiting, diarrhea, or dehydration), a diagnosis of DKA should be made and the animal treated appropriately.

The presence and severity of glycosuria should be considered when interpreting the urine specific gravity. Despite polyuria and polydipsia, urine specific gravities typically range from 1.025 to 1.035 in untreated diabetic dogs, in part because of the large amount of glucose in the urine. As a general rule of thumb, 2% or 4+ glycosuria as measured on urine reagent test strips will increase the urine specific gravity 0.008 to 0.010 when urine specific gravity is measured by refractometry. As such, identification of a urine specific gravity less than 1.020 in combination with 2% glycosuria suggests a concurrent polyuric/polydipsic disorder, most notably hyperadrenocorticism or renal insufficiency.

Proteinuria may be the result of urinary tract infection or glomerular damage secondary to disruption of the basement membrane (Struble et al, 1998). Because of the high incidence of infection, the urine sediment should be carefully inspected for changes consistent with infection, including white blood cells, red blood cells, and bacteria. Failure to identify pyuria and hematuria does not rule out urinary tract infection (McGuire et al, 2002). Because of the relatively high prevalence of concurrent urinary tract infections in diabetic dogs, urine obtained by antepubic cystocentesis using aseptic technique should be submitted for bacterial culture and sensitivity testing in all dogs with newly diagnosed diabetes mellitus, regardless of the findings on urinalysis (Hess et al, 2000b).

SERUM CHOLESTEROL AND TRIGLYCERIDE CONCENTRATIONS. Hyperlipidemia and obvious lipemia are common in the untreated diabetic. Uncontrolled diabetes is accompanied by an increase in the blood concentration of triglycerides, cholesterol, lipoproteins, chylomicrons, and free fatty acids (DeBowes, 1987). Hypertriglyceridemia is responsible for the lipemia, which can be seen in a peripheral blood sample. Hypertriglyceridemia with increases in chylomicrons and very low density lipoprotein (VLDL) triglycerides results from insulin deficiency and the associated curtailment in lipoprotein lipase activity (Eckel, 1989). The enzyme lipoprotein lipase aids in the metabolism of the triglyceride-rich VLDLs and chylomicrons. Increased concentrations of VLDL triglyceride also result from excess hepatic production (induced by increased circulating free fatty acids), obesity, and a high caloric intake (Massillon et al, 1997; Unger and Foster, 1998).

Overall, blood cholesterol concentrations are increased in diabetics, but to a much lesser degree than is hypertriglyceridemia. In humans, several factors contribute to an increase in LDL cholesterol concentrations, including increased LDL synthesis from VLDLs; reduced activity of LDL receptors, impairing LDL clearance; and excess consumption of saturated fatty acids (Howard et al, 1987; Unger and Foster, 1998). In humans, high density lipoprotein (HDL) cholesterol levels are often low, presumably as a result of accelerated catabolism (Witzum et al, 1982). The combination of high LDL and low HDL cholesterol concentrations may play a role in the accelerated development of atherosclerotic vascular disease and coronary heart disease, which is the major long-term complication of diabetes in humans (Garg and Grundy, 1990). Similar vascular complications have been infrequently documented in diabetic dogs and cats (Hess et al, 2002). Fortunately, most lipid derangements can be improved with insulin and dietary therapy.

PANCREATIC ENZYMES. Blood tests to assess for the presence of pancreatitis should always be considered in the newly diagnosed diabetic dog, especially if abdominal ultrasound is not available. Measurement of serum lipase concentration and serum TLI are most commonly recommended. In theory, dogs with concomitant active pancreatitis should have an increase in serum lipase concentration and serum TLI. Unfortunately, serum lipase concentrations and serum TLI do not always correlate accurately with the presence or absence of pancreatitis (Hess et al, 1998). Pancreatic enzyme concentrations can be increased in dogs with a histologically confirmed normal pancreas and normal in dogs with histologically confirmed inflammation of the pancreas, especially when the inflammatory process is chronic and mild. For these reasons, interpretation of serum lipase and TLI results should always be done in context with the history, physical examination findings, and additional findings on the laboratory tests. In our experience, abdominal ultrasound is the single best diagnostic test for identifying pancreatitis in the dog and should be considered if pancreatitis is suspected after evaluation of the history, physical examination, and laboratory test results. The concomitant presence of pancreatitis may necessitate the instigation of intensive fluid therapy and a highly digestible, low-fat diet, which may otherwise not have been done. Identification of chronic pancreatitis also has important prognostic implications regarding success of establishing and maintaining control of glycemia and long-term survival (see page 528).

Measurement of serum TLI is also used to diagnose exocrine pancreatic insufficiency; an uncommon complication of diabetes mellitus that presumably develops as a sequela of chronic pancreatitis (Wiberg et al, 1999; Wiberg and Westermarck, 2002). Exocrine pancreatic insufficiency should be suspected in diabetic dogs that are difficult to regulate with insulin and are thin or emaciated despite polyphagia (see page 528).

SERUM THYROXINE CONCENTRATION. The veterinarian may periodically have to interpret a serum thyroxine (T_4) concentration in a diabetic dog, either because serum T_4 is a routine part of the serum biochemistry panel or because hypothyroidism is suspected after a review of the history, clinical signs, and physical examination findings. Interpretation of serum T_4 results must be done cautiously, especially in a dog with newly diagnosed diabetes mellitus and concurrent illness such as pancreatitis or infection. "Healthy" diabetic dogs without concurrent illness usually have normal serum T_4 concentrations. However, the more severe the diabetic state and the more severe the concurrent illness, the more likely serum T_4 concentrations will be decreased because of the euthyroid sick syndrome rather than because of hypothyroidism (see Fig. 3-25, page 121). As a general rule, in a newly diagnosed diabetic dog with a concurrent low serum T_4 concentration, we treat the diabetes and reevaluate the serum T_4 concentration once control of glycemia has been established. If hypothyroidism is strongly suspected at the time diabetes is diagnosed, we evaluate serum free T_4 and thyrotropin (TSH) concentrations before initiating sodium levothyroxine treatment. See Chapter 3 for a more detailed discussion of the effects of concurrent illness and drug therapy on serum thyroid hormone concentrations and the tests used to diagnose hypothyroidism in dogs.

SERUM INSULIN CONCENTRATION. Measurement of serum insulin concentration, either baseline or after the administration of an insulin secretagogue (see Table 12-1, page 547), is not a routine part of our diagnostic evaluation of the newly diagnosed diabetic dog. In theory, identifying increased endogenous serum insulin concentrations (i.e., >18 µU/ml) in a newly diagnosed diabetic dog would suggest the early stages of secondary diabetes, especially if an underlying insulin antagonistic disorder can be identified and treated (see page 490). Unfortunately, the suppressive effects of hyperglycemia on beta-cell function (i.e., glucose toxicity) may interfere with accurate interpretation of serum insulin results (Nelson et al, 1998a). Although increased serum insulin concentrations suggest the existence of functional beta cells, finding low serum insulin concentrations (i.e., <12 µU/ml) may not rule out the existence of functional beta cells, a problem commonly encountered in diabetic cats (see page 544). However, because the vast majority of dogs with newly diagnosed diabetes have IDDM and serum insulin concentration is typically in the lower half of normal or undetectable, routine measurement of serum insulin concentration is not a cost-effective diagnostic procedure. The exception are dogs suspected to be in the early stages of secondary diabetes, most notably intact bitches in diestrus.

TABLE 11-6 DIFFERENCES IN THE AMINO ACID SEQUENCE OF THE INSULIN MOLECULE IN THE DOG AND CAT VERSUS SOURCES OF COMMERCIAL INSULIN

| | COMPARISON WITH DOG | | | | | COMPARISON WITH CAT | | | |
| | AMINO ACID POSITION | | | | | AMINO ACID POSITION | | | |
	A8	A10	A18	B30		A8	A10	A18	B30
Dog	Thr	Ile	Asn	Ala	Cat	Ala	Val	His	Ala
Pig	Thr	Ile	Asn	Ala	Cow	Ala	Val	*Asn*	Ala
Human	Thr	Ile	Asn	*Thr*	Pig	*Thr*	*Ile*	*Asn*	Ala
Cow	*Ala*	*Val*	Asn	Ala	Human	*Thr*	*Ile*	*Asn*	*Thr*

Differences between the dog or cat and commercial insulins are italicized.

It is imperative that the radioimmunoassay (RIA) for insulin be validated for the species in which it is being used and that normal reference ranges for the species in question have been established. Commercial endocrine laboratories use RIAs designed for use in humans. Fortunately, the amino acid sequence of human and dog insulin are almost identical (Table 11-6), so RIAs designed for measurement of serum insulin concentrations in humans work well in dogs. The same is not true for cats.

TREATMENT OF NONKETOTIC DIABETES MELLITUS

GOALS OF THERAPY. The primary goal of therapy is elimination of the owner-observed signs occurring secondary to hyperglycemia and glycosuria. A persistence of clinical signs and the development of chronic complications (Table 11-7) are directly correlated with the severity and duration of hyperglycemia. Limiting blood glucose concentration fluctuations and maintaining near-normal glycemia will help minimize the severity of clinical signs and prevent the complications of poorly controlled diabetes. In the diabetic dog, this can be accomplished through proper insulin therapy, diet, exercise, and the prevention or control of concurrent inflammatory, infectious, neoplastic, and hormonal disorders.

Although it is worthwhile attempting to normalize the blood glucose concentration, the veterinarian must also guard against the development of hypoglycemia,

TABLE 11-7 COMPLICATIONS OF DIABETES MELLITUS IN DOGS AND CATS

Common	Uncommon
Iatrogenic hypoglycemia	Peripheral neuropathy (dog)
Persistent polyuria, polydipsia, weight loss	Glomerulonephropathy, glomerulosclerosis
Cataracts (dog)	Retinopathy
Bacterial infections, especially in the urinary tract	Exocrine pancreatic insufficiency
Pancreatitis	Gastric paresis
Ketoacidosis	Diabetic diarrhea
Hepatic lipidosis	Diabetic dermatopathy (dog)
Peripheral neuropathy (cat)	(i.e., superficial necrolytic dermatitis)

a serious and potentially fatal complication of therapy. Hypoglycemia is most apt to occur as the result of overzealous insulin therapy. The veterinarian must balance the benefits of tight glucose control obtainable with aggressive insulin therapy against the risk for hypoglycemia.

Insulin Therapy

OVERVIEW OF INSULIN TYPES. Commercial insulin is categorized by promptness, duration, and intensity of action after subcutaneous administration (Table 11-8). Commonly used insulins for the long-term management of diabetics include isophane (NPH), lente, ultralente, and protamine zinc (PZI) insulins. NPH and PZI insulin preparations contain the fish protein protamine and zinc to delay insulin absorption and prolong the duration of insulin effect (Davidson et al, 1991). The lente family of insulins rely on alterations in zinc content and the size of zinc-insulin crystals to alter the rate of absorption from the subcutaneous site of deposition. The larger the crystals, the slower the rate of absorption and the longer the duration of effect. The lente insulins contain no foreign protein (i.e., protamine). Ultralente is a microcrystalline, long-acting insulin preparation. Lente insulin is a mixture of three parts of short-acting, amorphous insulin and seven parts of long-acting, microcrystalline insulin. Lente insulin is considered an intermediate-acting insulin, although plasma insulin concentrations may remain increased for longer than 14 hours following subcutaneous administration in some dogs (Graham et al, 1997).

Insulin Mixtures. Mixtures of short- and long-acting insulin have been developed in an attempt to mimic the increase in portal insulin concentrations during and immediately following consumption of a meal, thereby minimizing postprandial hyperglycemia. NPH insulin can be mixed with regular crystalline insulin, and if injected immediately, the regular insulin remains rapid-acting. Stable premixed 70% NPH/30% regular and 50% NPH/50% regular preparations are available (e.g., Humulin 70/30, Eli Lilly and Co., Indianapolis, IN; Mixtard HM 70/30, Nordisk-USA, Princeton, NJ). In our experience, these premixed preparations are quite potent, causing a rapid decrease in blood glucose concentration within 60 to 90 minutes of subcutaneous administration (Fig. 11-4). In addition,

TABLE 11-8   PROPERTIES OF RECOMBINANT HUMAN INSULIN PREPARATIONS USED IN DIABETIC DOGS AND CATS* AND BEEF/PORK PZI INSULIN USED IN DIABETIC CATS

Type of Insulin	Route of Administration	Onset of Effect	TIME OF MAXIMUM EFFECT (HR)		DURATION OF EFFECT (HR)	
			Dog	Cat	Dog	Cat
Regular crystalline	IV	Immediate	½–2	½–2	1–4	1–4
	IM	10–30 min	1–4	1–4	3–8	3–8
	SC	10–30 min	1–5	1–5	4–10	4–10
NPH (isophane)[†]	SC	½–2 hr	2–10	2–8	6–18	4–12
Lente[†‡]	SC	½–2 hr	2–10	2–10	8–20	6–18
Ultralente	SC	½–8 hr	4–16	4–16	8–24	6–24
PZI[‡]	SC	½–4 hr	–	4–14	–	6–20

*Purified pork insulin has similar properties; beef/pork insulin mixtures are less potent and may have a longer duration of action than recombinant human insulins.
[†]Initial insulins of choice for the diabetic dog.
[‡]Initial insulins of choice for the diabetic cat.

the duration of effect has usually been short (<8 hours). We generally use these insulin mixtures only as a last resort when more conventional insulin preparations have been ineffective in establishing control of glycemia. Although regular insulin remains fast acting when added to NPH, when added to lente insulin, regular insulin binds to excess zinc in the lente, blunting regular insulin's quick effect (Galloway, 1988).

Insulin Analogs. Recently, recombinant DNA technology has been applied for the production of insulin analogs with faster and slower absorption characteristics than human insulin. Rapid-acting insulin analogs include insulin lispro (Humalog, Eli Lilly, Indianapolis, IN) and insulin aspart (Novolog, NovoNordisk, Princeton, NJ). The rate-limiting step in the absorption of human insulin is a hexamer formation of insulin molecules that occurs at high concentrations of insulin such as those obtained in the injectable fluid (Brange et al, 1988). The hexamers of insulin molecules slowly dissociate before absorption into the circulation occurs. By replacing certain amino acids in the insulin molecule, the tendency to self-associate can be reduced without affecting the insulin-receptor kinetics. Insulin lispro is produced by inverting the natural amino acid sequence of the B-chain at B28 (proline) and B29 (lysine), and insulin aspart is produced by substituting aspartic acid for proline in position B28 (Maarten et al, 1997; Lindholm et al, 2002). As a consequence of these alterations, insulin lispro and insulin aspart exhibit monomeric behavior in solution and display a rapid absorption, faster pharmacodynamic action, and shorter duration of effect than short-acting regular crystalline insulin (Howey et al, 1994; Home et al, 1997; Lindholm et al, 1999). Insulin lispro and insulin aspart are the current prandial insulins (i.e., insulin administered before each meal) of choice for control of postprandial blood glucose concentrations in human diabetics and are typically administered three times a day before each of the three main meals (breakfast, lunch, dinner). The role, if any, of these insulins for the treatment of diabetes in dogs or cats remains to be determined. Because of their extremely short duration of effect, insulin lispro and insulin aspart would have to be

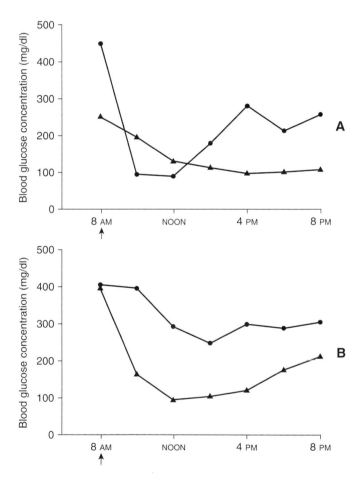

FIGURE 11-4. *A,* Blood glucose curve in a miniature poodle receiving recombinant human lente insulin, 6 U/kg body weight (▲) and recombinant human 70/30 NPH/regular insulin, 3 U/kg body weight (●) SC. *B,* Blood glucose curve in an 8-kg cat receiving 4 U recombinant human ultralente insulin (●) and 4 U of recombinant human 70/30 NPH/regular insulin (▲) SC. ↑ = insulin injection and food. (From Nelson RW: Diabetes mellitus. *In* Ettinger SJ, Feldman EC (eds): Textbook of Veterinary Internal Medicine, 4th ed. Philadelphia, WB Saunders Co, 1995, p 1528.)

used in conjunction with a longer-acting insulin preparation to maintain control of glycemia.

Insulin glargine (Lantus, Aventis Pharmaceuticals, Bridgewater, NJ) is a long-acting insulin analog that differs from human insulin by the replacement of asparagine with glycine at position A21 on the A-chain and the addition of two arginines to the C-terminus of the B-chain of the insulin molecule (Pieber et al, 2000). These modifications result in a shift of the isoelectric point from a pH of 5.4 toward a neutral pH, which makes insulin glargine more soluble at a slightly acidic pH and less soluble at a physiological pH than native human insulin. As a consequence, insulin glargine forms microprecipitates in the subcutaneous tissue at the site of injection from which small amounts of insulin glargine are slowly released. In humans, the slow sustained release of insulin glargine from these microprecipitates results in a relatively constant concentration/time profile over a 24-hour period with no pronounced peak in serum insulin. The glucose-lowering effect of insulin glargine is similar to that of human insulin, the onset of action following subcutaneous administration is slower than NPH insulin, and the duration of effect is prolonged, compared with NPH insulin (Owens et al, 2000). Insulin glargine is currently recommended as a basal insulin (i.e., sustained long-acting insulin used to inhibit hepatic glucose production) administered once a day at bedtime and used in conjunction with either rapid-acting insulin analogs or oral hypoglycemic drugs in human diabetics (Rosenstock et al, 2000; Rosenstock et al, 2001).

In a preliminary study evaluating the pharmacokinetics and pharmacodynamics of insulin glargine, PZI, and porcine lente insulin in nine healthy cats, most of the parameters evaluated (i.e., onset of action, glucose nadir, time for blood glucose concentration to return to baseline, mean daily blood glucose concentration, and area under the 24-hour blood glucose curve) were similar for insulin glargine and PZI (Marshall and Rand, 2002). Similar studies performed in diabetic cats have yet to be reported. In our experience, insulin glargine has a duration of effect ranging from 10 to 16 hours in most diabetic dogs and cats in which it was used. We have not yet encountered problems with inadequate absorption of insulin glargine, as described with ultralente insulin (see page 571), although it seems likely that this problem will be encountered as we gain more experience with insulin glargine. Currently, we consider using insulin glargine in diabetic dogs and cats with problems of short duration of effect of NPH, lente, and in cats, PZI insulin (see pages 520 and 570). Based on our current experiences, we do not consider insulin glargine a first choice insulin for the treatment of diabetes in dogs or cats.

SPECIES OF INSULIN. For each type of insulin (i.e., NPH, lente, ultralente), the clinician must also choose the species of insulin to be administered. Historically, insulin preparations were available as beef/pork combinations (e.g., Iletin I, Eli Lilly Co, Indianapolis,

IN), purified beef or pork (e.g., Iletin II, Eli Lilly and Co), and recombinant human insulin (e.g., Humulin, Eli Lilly and Co). Approximately 90% of beef/pork insulin preparation is beef insulin. Currently, more than 95% of human diabetics requiring insulin injections are treated with recombinant human insulin preparations and the majority of the rest are treated with purified pork insulin preparations. Commercial production of beef/pork and purified beef insulin for use by diabetic humans has been severely curtailed in the United States. Because the human market essentially dictates the insulin preparations available for use in diabetic dogs and cats, almost all diabetic dogs and most diabetic cats are treated with recombinant human insulin preparations. Fortunately, the development of anti-insulin antibodies following chronic administration of recombinant human or porcine insulin to diabetic dogs appears uncommon (see page 522) (Feldman et al, 1983; Harb-Hauser et al, 1998). In contrast, bovine insulin is antigenic in diabetic dogs and stimulates formation of anti-insulin antibodies in 40% to 65% of diabetic dogs in which it is used (Feldman et al, 1983; Haines, 1986; Harb-Hauser et al, 1998; Davison et al, 2003).

Presumably, the structure and amino acid sequence of the injected insulin relative to the native endogenous insulin influences the development of anti-insulin antibodies. Although differences exist in the amino acid sequence of human, bovine, and canine insulin (see Table 11-6) (Hallden et al, 1986; Ganong, 1991), studies suggest that conformational insulin epitopes are more important than linear subunits of the insulin molecule. Anti-insulin antibodies induced by exogenous insulin in humans cross-react with homologous insulin and require intact conformation of the insulin molecule for binding (Thomas et al, 1985; Thomas et al, 1988; Nell and Thomas, 1989). In a recent study evaluating anti-insulin antibody formation in diabetic dogs treated with bovine insulin, the greatest anti-insulin antibody reactivity was directed against the whole insulin protein rather than the A- or B-chain (Davison et al, 2003). Cross-reactivity with homologous insulin was also identified. Surprisingly, the insulin B-chain rather than the A-chain was the more reactive component of the insulin molecule. The reason for differences in A-chain versus B-chain antigenicity is not clear, especially considering that the amino acid sequence of the A-chain, not the B-chain, differs between the cow and dog.

Anti-insulin antibodies may affect the pharmacokinetics of the exogenously administered insulin by several mechanisms, which may either enhance or reduce the pharmacodynamic response. Antibodies may enhance and prolong the pharmacodynamic action by serving as a carrier, or they may reduce insulin action by neutralization (Bolli et al, 1984; Marshall et al, 1988; Lahtela et al, 1997). Antibodies may also have no apparent clinical effect on insulin dosage or status of glycemic control (Lindholm et al, 2002). In our experience, anti-insulin antibody production in diabetic dogs can alter the duration of insulin activity and prolong its duration of action or have a deleterious impact on insulin effectiveness, reduce the ability to maintain control of glycemia, and in extreme cases, cause severe insulin resistance (see page 522). Short duration of insulin effect is a more prevalent problem with recombinant human insulin than with beef-containing insulin preparations, presumably because of lack of anti-insulin antibody production. However, the deleterious impact of anti-insulin antibodies on control of glycemia associated with beef-containing insulin far outweighs any potential benefits related to duration of insulin effect.

Recently, beef/pork PZI insulin became commercially available for use in diabetic cats (see page 550). This insulin preparation is not routinely recommended for use in diabetic dogs because of concerns for anti-insulin antibody production directed at the beef insulin component of the insulin preparation, as discussed above. Purified porcine lente insulin (Caninsulin, Intervet, Ontario, Canada) is marketed for use in diabetic dogs in Canada and Europe but is not yet approved by the FDA for use in the United States. The amino acid sequences of canine and porcine insulin are identical (see Table 11-6) (Hallden et al, 1986; Ganong, 1991). The immunogenicity and duration of effect of porcine insulin preparations is similar to recombinant human insulin preparations (Feldman et al, 1983; Harb-Hauser et al, 1998). In theory, the effectiveness of purified porcine lente insulin and recombinant human lente insulin should be similar.

INITIAL INSULIN TREATMENT RECOMMENDATIONS. Intermediate-acting insulin (i.e., lente, NPH) is the initial insulin of choice for establishing control of glycemia in diabetic dogs (see Table 11-8). Recombinant human-source insulin should be used to avoid problems with insulin effectiveness presumably caused by circulating insulin antibodies (see page 522) Insulin therapy is begun with lente or NPH insulin of recombinant human origin at an approximate dosage of 0.25 U/kg twice a day. Dietary therapy is initiated concurrently (see below). Because greater than 90% of diabetic dogs require recombinant human lente or NPH insulin twice daily, we prefer to start with twice-a-day insulin therapy (Hess and Ward, 2000). Establishing control of glycemia is easier and problems with hypoglycemia and the Somogyi effect (see page 519) are less likely when twice daily insulin therapy is initiated while the insulin dose is low, that is, at the time insulin treatment is initiated. Glycemic regulation is more problematic and development of hypoglycemia and the Somogyi effect more likely when poorly controlled diabetic dogs receiving a high dose of insulin once daily are switched to insulin twice a day but the dose per injection is arbitrarily chosen.

Dietary Therapy

Dietary therapy plays an important role in the successful management of the diabetic dog. Adjustments in diet and feeding practices should be directed at correcting

TABLE 11-9 RECOMMENDATIONS FOR DIETARY TREATMENT OF DIABETES MELLITUS IN DOGS

I. Dietary composition
   Increased fiber content (see Table 11-10)
   Digestible carbohydrate content >45% of metabolizable energy
   Fat content <30% of metabolizable energy
   Protein content <30% of metabolizable energy
II. Feed canned and/or dry kibble foods; avoid diets containing monosaccharides, disaccharides, and propylene glycol
III. Caloric intake and obesity
   Average daily caloric intake in geriatric pet: 40-60 kcal/kg
   Adjust daily caloric intake on individual basis
   Eliminate obesity, if present, by:
     Increasing daily exercise
     Decreasing daily caloric intake
     Feeding low-calorie-dense, low-fat, high-fiber (preferred in diabetics) or low-calorie-dense, low-fat, low-fiber diet designed for weight loss
IV. Feeding schedule
   Maintain consistent caloric content of the meals
   Maintain consistent timing of feeding
   Feed within time frame of insulin action
   Feed one-half the total daily caloric intake at time of each insulin injection
   Let "nibbler" dogs continue to nibble throughout day and night

or preventing obesity, maintaining consistency in the timing and caloric content of the meals, and furnishing a diet that helps minimize the postprandial increase in blood glucose concentration (Table 11-9; Nelson and Lewis, 1990). Correction of obesity and increasing the fiber content of the diet are perhaps the two most beneficial steps that can be taken to improve control of glycemia.

DIETARY FIBER. Diets containing increased fiber content are beneficial for treating obesity and improving control of glycemia in diabetics (Nelson et al, 1991; Nelson et al, 1998b). Several mechanisms have been proposed to explain the fiber-induced slowing of intestinal glucose absorption and the corresponding improvement in glycemic control of the diabetic dog. These include a delay in the gastric emptying of nutrients; a delay in the intestinal absorption of nutrients, mostly likely resulting from an effect on the diffusion of glucose toward the brush border of the intestine; and a fiber-induced effect on the release of regulatory gastrointestinal tract hormones into the circulation (Meyer et al, 1988; Anderson et al, 1991; Nuttall, 1993). The ability of the food fiber to form a viscous gel and thus impair convective transfer of glucose and water to the absorptive surface of the intestine appears to be of greatest importance (Nuttall, 1993). The more viscous soluble fibers (e.g., gums, pectins) slow glucose diffusion to a greater degree than do the less viscous insoluble fibers (e.g., lignin, cellulose) and, as such, are believed to be of greater benefit in improving control of glycemia in diabetic human beings (Anderson and Akanji, 1991; Nuttall, 1993). Others have found both fiber types to be beneficial in diabetic human beings (Villaume et al, 1984; Vaaler, 1986). Studies in diabetic dogs have documented glycemic improvement in response to the consumption of diets containing increased amounts of soluble and insoluble fiber (Fig. 11-5) (Nelson et al, 1991; Graham et al, 1994; Nelson et al, 1998b). Most commercial high-fiber diets predominantly contain insoluble fiber, although diets containing mixtures of soluble and insoluble fiber are becoming available (Table 11-10). The amount of fiber varies considerably among products, ranging from 3% to 25% of dry matter (normal diets contain less than 2% fiber on a dry matter basis). In general, diets containing 12% or more insoluble fiber or 8% or more of a mixture of soluble and insoluble fiber are most likely to be effective in improving glycemic control in diabetic dogs.

The dog's susceptibility to the complications of high-fiber diets, its body weight and condition, and the presence of a concurrent disease (e.g., pancreatitis, renal failure) in which diet is an important aspect of therapy ultimately dictate which, if any, fiber diet is fed. Common clinical complications of high insoluble fiber diets include excessive frequency of defecation; constipation and obstipation; hypoglycemia 1 to 2 weeks after the increase in fiber content of the diet; and refusal to eat the diet (Table 11-11). Complications of soluble fiber-containing diets include soft to watery stools; excessive flatulence; hypoglycemia 1 to 2 weeks after the increase in fiber content of the diet; and refusal to eat the diet. If firm stools or constipation become a problem with high insoluble fiber diets, a mixture of insoluble and soluble fiber diets can be fed or soluble fiber (e.g., sugar-free Metamucil, canned pumpkin) can be added to the diet to soften the stool. Alternatively, if soft or watery diarrhea or flatulence become a problem with soluble fiber-containing diets, an insoluble fiber diet can be added and the quantity of the soluble fiber diet decreased.

Refusal to consume diets containing increased amounts of fiber may occur initially or develop after several months of eating the diet. If palatability is a problem initially, the dog can be gradually switched from its regular diet to a diet containing small amounts of fiber, followed by a gradual switch to diets containing more fiber. Refusal to consume high-fiber diets months after their initiation is usually a result of boredom with the food. Periodic changes in the types of high-fiber diets and mixtures of diets have been helpful in alleviating this problem. Diets containing an increased amount of fiber should always be considered in the list of differential diagnoses for inappetence in a diabetic dog.

Diets containing an increased amount of fiber should not be fed to thin or emaciated diabetic dogs, because high-fiber diets have a low caloric density, which can interfere with weight gain and may result in further weight loss. For thin diabetic dogs to gain weight, usually glycemic control must be reestablished through insulin therapy and the feeding of a higher-calorie–dense, lower-fiber diet designed for maintenance. Once a normal body weight has been attained, a diet containing more fiber can be gradually substituted for the previous diet.

DIETARY PROTEIN. The protein content of the diet remains controversial in humans with diabetes because of the potential for both restricted and liberal protein intakes to exert beneficial and adverse effects (Wylie-Rosett, 1988; Malik and Jaspan, 1989). Although protein is a much less potent insulin secretagogue than glucose,

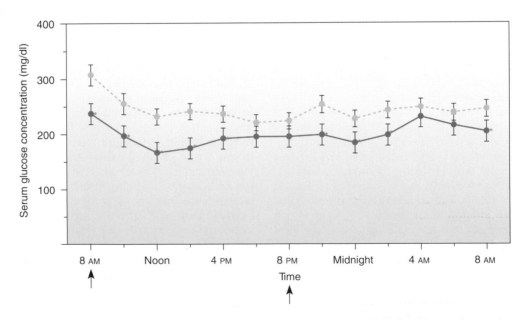

FIGURE 11-5. Mean (± standard error of the mean) serum concentrations of glucose in 11 dogs with naturally occurring diabetes mellitus fed high-insoluble fiber (i.e., cellulose; *solid line*) and low-fiber *(broken line)* diet. ↑ = Insulin administration and consumption of half of daily caloric intake; * = p<0.05, compared with low fiber diet. (From Nelson RW et al: Effect of dietary insoluble fiber on glycemic control in dogs with naturally occurring diabetes mellitus, JAVMA 212:280, 1998.)

TABLE 11-10 APPROXIMATE NUTRIENT CONTENT OF SOME COMMERCIALLY AVAILABLE HIGH-FIBER DOG FOODS

	Crude Fiber*	Carbohydrates†	Fat†	Protein†	Calories (Can/Cup)‡
Prescription Diet r/d					
Canned	26	45	22	33	249
Dry	24	49	21	30	205
Prescription Diet w/d					
Canned	14	54	29	16	390
Dry	17	62	19	19	226
Purina OM					
Canned	19	17	28	55	189
Dry	11	47	16	37	276
Science Diet Light					
Canned	10	58	24	18	364
Dry	14	62	18	20	295
Purina DCO					
Dry	8	45	32	24	320
Waltham Glucomodulation Control Diet					
Canned	10	55	11	34	339
Dry	5	62	10	28	316
Iams Eukanuba Optimum Weight Control					
Dry	3	53	21	26	253

*Expressed as a percent of the diet dry matter.
†Expressed as percent metabolizable energy derived from carbohydrate, fat, or protein.
‡Expressed as kilocalories of metabolizable energy per can (15 oz.) or for the dry diets per standard (8 oz. volume) measuring cup full.

TABLE 11-11 COMMON COMPLICATIONS ASSOCIATED WITH FEEDING DIETS CONTAINING INCREASED QUANTITIES OF FIBER

Inappetence caused by poor palatability or boredom with food
Increased frequency of defecation
Constipation and obstipation (insoluble fiber)
Soft stools and diarrhea (soluble fiber)
Increased flatulence (soluble fiber)
Weight loss
Hypoglycemia

variation in dietary protein may influence metabolic control of diabetes by altering gluconeogenic substrate availability and counterregulatory hormone secretion (Spillar et al, 1987; Krezowski et al, 1986; Henry, 1994). Prolonged consumption of excessive dietary protein, especially in conjunction with excessive phosphorus and sodium, may contribute to the progression of diabetic nephropathy in humans (Hostetter et al, 1982; Brenner et al, 1982), and consumption of low-protein diets may impede or delay the rate of development of diabetic renal disease (Friedman, 1982). The impact, if any, of liberal dietary protein consumption on renal function is controversial in dogs and cats, although dietary protein restriction is recommended once renal insufficiency is identified (Harte et al, 1994; Devaux et al, 1996). Because diabetes mellitus and renal insufficiency commonly occur together, it seems prudent to recommend a dietary protein intake that meets daily requirements but is not excessive (i.e., less than 30% protein on a metabolizable energy basis in dogs). Lower protein intake is indicated when evidence of renal insufficiency exists.

DIETARY FAT. Derangements in fat metabolism are common in diabetic dogs and include increased serum concentrations of cholesterol, triglycerides, lipoproteins, chylomicrons, and free fatty acids, hepatic lipidosis, atherosclerosis, and a predisposition for development of pancreatitis (DeBowes et al, 1987; Hess et al, 2002). Feeding high-fat diets may also cause insulin resistance, promote hepatic glucose production, and in healthy dogs, suppress β-cell function (Massillon et al, 1997; Kaiyala et al, 1999). These findings strongly support feeding diets that are relatively low in fat content, that is, less than 30% fat on a metabolizable energy basis. Feeding lower-fat diets will help minimize the risk for pancreatitis, control some aspects of hyperlipidemia, and reduce overall caloric intake to favor weight loss or maintenance (Remillard, 1999). A higher fat content may be needed for weight gain in thin or emaciated diabetic dogs.

CALORIC INTAKE AND OBESITY. Obesity can cause impaired glucose tolerance in dogs (Mattheeuws et al, 1984) and may be an important factor accounting for variations in response to insulin therapy in diabetic dogs. Weight reduction improves glucose tolerance in obese dogs, presumably via improvement in obesity-induced insulin resistance (Wolfsheimer et al, 1993). Successful weight reduction usually requires a combination of restriction of caloric intake, feeding low-calorie dense diets (i.e., high fiber content), and increasing caloric expenditure through exercise.

The dog's current body weight should be recorded, and the final ideal body weight of the dog should be calculated. The ideal body weight can be estimated either by reviewing the medical record for the body weight when the dog was in an ideal body condition, or by using breed-specific body weight charts. It is very important to set realistic and obtainable goals for weight loss in order to maintain client compliance. If the ideal body weight is below 15% of the current body weight, it is crucial to use a stepwise process to gradually achieve ideal body weight. The pet's initial goal should be set at 15% body weight loss. Once this goal has been achieved, a new target body weight can be selected until the dog has reached an ideal body weight. To achieve 15% body weight loss, dogs can be fed $55 \times$ [initial body weight (kg) $^{0.75}$] kcal per day (Elliott, 2003). When fed at this level, dogs will achieve 15% body weight loss in approximately 12 weeks. The calculated amount of calories to achieve 15% body weight loss should be compared with the current daily caloric intake obtained from the dietary history. Most pets will be consuming more calories than required for 15% body weight loss. However, if the number of calories to achieve weight loss is actually less than the current daily caloric intake, then the dietary history should be reevaluated to search for additional calories. If no additional daily calories are identified, then the daily caloric intake of the pet should be reduced by 15% to 20%. Although there are several diets specifically formulated for weight reduction in dogs, diets that utilize fiber are recommended in obese diabetic dogs for reasons previously discussed. The quantity of food to be fed is determined by dividing the daily caloric requirement by the number of calories per can or cupful of the diet. The amount fed per meal and the timing of the meals are dictated, in part by the pet's insulin treatment regimen and by the owner's schedule (see Feeding Schedule, right column). In addition to reducing the daily caloric intake, every effort should be made to increase the daily energy expenditure by encouraging exercise.

Dogs on weight reduction programs should be reevaluated every 2 weeks. Body weight should be recorded and the dietary history reviewed. Ideally, dogs should achieve 1% to 2% body weight loss per week. If the rate of weight loss exceeds 2% body weight loss per week, the number of calories fed to the pet should be increased by 10% to 15%. If there has not been any weight loss, the dietary history should be reevaluated for additional calories. If none are found, the daily caloric intake should be further reduced by 10% to 15%. Once the ideal body weight of the dog has been achieved, the daily caloric intake can be adjusted to maintain optimal body weight and a diet intended for maintenance of the diabetic dog initiated (e.g., Prescription Diet W/D, Hill's Pet Products, Topeka, KS;

Iams Eukanuba Optimum Weight Control, Iams Co., Dayton, Ohio).

FEEDING SCHEDULE. The feeding schedule should be designed to enhance the actions of insulin and minimize postprandial hyperglycemia. The development of postprandial hyperglycemia depends, in part, on the amount of food consumed per meal, the rate at which glucose and other nutrients are absorbed from the intestine, and the effectiveness of exogenous and endogenous insulin during this time. The daily caloric intake should be ingested when insulin is still present in the circulation and is capable of disposing of glucose absorbed from the meal. If the meals are consumed while exogenous insulin is still metabolically active, the postprandial increase in blood glucose concentration is minimal or absent. In contrast, feeding the diabetic dog after insulin action has waned results in increasing blood glucose concentration beginning 1 to 2 hours postprandially (Fig. 11-6). If this occurs, either the type of insulin, frequency of insulin administration, or timing of the meals in relationship to the insulin injection should be adjusted.

Typically, dogs receiving exogenous insulin twice a day are fed equal-sized meals at the time of each insulin injection. If the dog is receiving exogenous insulin once a day, one half of the daily caloric intake is fed at the time of the insulin injection and the remaining half approximately 8 to 10 hours later. Unfortunately, the eating behaviors of dogs vary considerably, from finicky eaters that nibble on food periodically throughout the day to gluttonous dogs that quickly consume everything placed in their food dish. Gluttonous dogs are fed as discussed above. Finicky dogs generally resist attempts by owners to convert them to a "gluttonous" type of eating behavior, which can be frustrating to the owner instructed to have their pet eat all of its food at the time of the insulin injection. However, if one adheres to the principle that feeding multiple small meals rather than one large meal within the time frame of insulin action helps minimize the hyperglycemic effect of each meal, then allowing a finicky eater to eat whenever it wants should help control fluctuations in blood glucose. For this reason, dogs that are finicky and nibble throughout the day should be allowed to continue their pattern of eating. For these dogs, the food should remain available beginning at the time of each insulin injection and the dog allowed to choose when and how much to eat. The process is repeated at the time of the next insulin injection.

MODIFICATIONS IN DIETARY THERAPY. Diabetes mellitus often occurs in conjunction with other diseases (e.g., renal failure, heart failure). Dietary therapy is used in the management of various diseases. Whenever possible, dietary therapy for all disorders should be "blended"; however, if this is not possible, dietary therapy for the most serious disorder should take priority. For example, dietary therapy for chronic renal failure, heart failure, or recurring pancreatitis is a higher priority than dietary therapy for diabetes mellitus. Dietary therapy for diabetes mellitus should

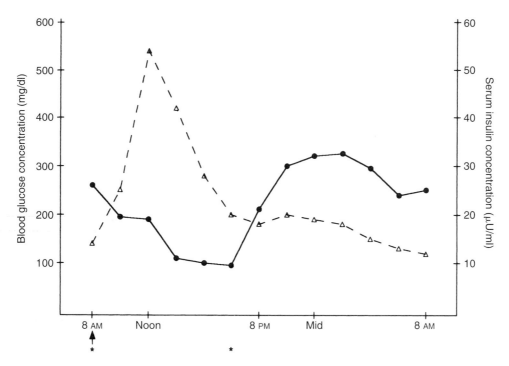

FIGURE 11-6. Mean blood glucose *(solid line)* and serum insulin *(broken line)* concentrations in eight dogs with diabetes mellitus treated with beef/pork source NPH insulin SC once daily. The duration of NPH effect is too short, resulting in prolonged periods of hyperglycemia beginning shortly after feeding the evening meal. ↑ = insulin injection; * = equal-sized meals consumed. (From Nelson RW: Diabetes mellitus. *In* Ettinger SJ, Feldman EC (eds): Textbook of Veterinary Internal Medicine, 4th ed. Philadelphia, WB Saunders Co, 1995, p 1525.)

be considered adjunctive; glycemic control can be maintained with insulin, regardless of the diet fed.

Acute and chronic pancreatitis and exocrine pancreatic insufficiency (EPI) are closely associated with diabetes mellitus in the dog. Fortunately, many of the dietary principles for diabetes, pancreatitis, and EPI are similar (Table 11-12). Many diabetic dogs with concurrent pancreatitis tolerate high-fiber diets once pancreatitis has subsided with the feeding of low-fat, highly digestible diets. Such diets are also recommended for dogs with EPI (Lewis et al, 1987). In vitro studies indicate that some fiber sources impair pancreatic enzyme activity, although cellulose, the fiber most commonly used in commercial high-fiber dog foods, did not affect pancreatic enzyme activity (Dutta and Hlasko, 1985). Clinical trials documenting deleterious effects of dietary fiber in vivo have not been reported in diabetic dogs or cats with EPI. The ability of oral pancreatic enzyme supplements to counter any such

effect is unknown. Although we have successfully fed diets containing increased amounts of fiber to several diabetic dogs and cats with EPI, studies are needed to critically assess the effects of dietary fiber on this combination of disorders.

Exercise

Exercise plays an important role in maintaining glycemic control in the diabetic dog by helping promote weight loss and by eliminating the insulin resistance induced by obesity. Exercise also has a glucose-lowering effect by increasing the mobilization of insulin from its injection site, presumably resulting from increased blood and lymph flow, by increasing blood flow (and therefore insulin delivery) to exercising muscles, by stimulating translocation (i.e., upregulation) of glucose transporters (primarily GLUT-4) in muscle

TABLE 11-12 COMPARISON OF GENERAL GUIDELINES FOR DIETARY TREATMENT OF DOGS AND CATS WITH DIABETES MELLITUS, PANCREATITIS, AND EXOCRINE PANCREATIC INSUFFICIENCY

Dietary Factor	Diabetes Mellitus	Pancreatitis	Exocrine Pancreatic Insufficiency
Digestibility	Normal	High	High
Fat content	Low	Low	Low
Carbohydrate content	High	Normal to low	Normal to low
Protein content	Normal to moderate restriction	Moderate restriction	Normal
Feeding schedule	Twice a day with insulin injection	Small meals often	Small meals often
Caloric intake	Correct and avoid obesity	Correct and avoid obesity	Correct and avoid weight loss

cells, and by increasing glucose effectiveness (i.e., ability of hyperglycemia to promote glucose disposal at basal insulin concentrations) (Fernqvist et al, 1986; Galante et al, 1995; Phillips et al, 1996; Nishida et al, 2001). The daily routine for diabetic dogs should include exercise, preferably at the same time each day. Strenuous and sporadic exercise can cause severe hypoglycemia and should be avoided. The insulin dose should be decreased in dogs subjected to sporadic strenuous exercise (e.g., hunting dogs during hunting season) on those days of anticipated increased exercise. The reduction in insulin dose required to prevent hypoglycemia is variable and determined by trial and error. We recommend reducing the insulin dose by 50% initially and making further adjustments based on the occurrence of symptomatic hypoglycemia and the severity of polyuria and polydipsia that develops during the ensuing 24 to 48 hours. In addition, owners must be aware of the signs of hypoglycemia and have a source of glucose (e.g., Karo syrup, candy, food) readily available to give their dog should any of these signs develop.

Oral Hypoglycemic Drugs

OVERVIEW. In the United States, five classes of oral hypoglycemic drugs are approved for the treatment of NIDDM in human beings: sulfonylureas, meglitinides, biguanides, thiazolidinediones, and α-glucosidase inhibitors. These drugs work by stimulating pancreatic insulin secretion, enhancing tissue sensitivity to insulin, or slowing postprandial intestinal glucose absorption (DeFronzo, 1999). In addition, chromium and vanadium are trace minerals that may also enhance tissue sensitivity to insulin. Oral hypoglycemic drugs are not routinely used to treat diabetes in dogs, in part because dogs develop IDDM and most dogs are hypoinsulinemic at the time diabetes is diagnosed. Drugs that stimulate pancreatic insulin secretion are ineffective because the beta cells have been destroyed. Insulin-sensitizing drugs require the presence of circulating insulin for efficacy and, as such, are ineffective as the primary mode of treatment in hypoinsulinemic diabetic dogs. Drugs that slow postprandial intestinal glucose absorption improve control of glycemia in diabetic dogs but are ineffective as the primary mode of treatment, are expensive, and adverse reactions are common (see Acarbose below). To date, only the α-glucosidase inhibitors and chromium have been critically evaluated in diabetic dogs. Refer to Chapter 12, page 555 for more information on oral hypoglycemic drugs.

ALPHA-GLUCOSIDASE INHIBITORS. Acarbose (Precose, Bayer, West Haven, CT) and miglitol (Glyset, Pharmacia & Upjohn Inc, Peapack, NJ) are complex oligosaccharides of microbial origin that competitively inhibit α-glucosidases (glucoamylase, sucrase, maltase, and isomaltase) in the brush border of the small intestinal mucosa (Lembcke et al, 1985; Balfour and McTavish, 1993). Inhibition of these enzymes delays digestion of complex carbohydrates and disaccharides to monosaccharides. This inhibition causes increased carbohydrate digestion within the ileum and, to a lesser extent, colon. Most important, it delays absorption of glucose from the intestinal tract and decreases postprandial blood glucose and insulin concentrations. Controlled clinical studies involving acarbose-treated human beings with NIDDM and IDDM have documented significant improvement in glycemic control (Rios, 1994; Coniff et al, 1995; Kelley et al, 1998). Improvements were characterized by significant reductions in postprandial blood glucose concentrations, blood glycated protein concentrations, and daily insulin requirements. Placebo-controlled clinical studies recently completed in healthy and diabetic dogs documented a decrease in postprandial total glucose absorption and total insulin secretion when healthy dogs were treated with acarbose, compared with placebo, and a decrease in daily insulin dose, mean blood glucose concentration during an 8-hour blood sampling period, and blood glycated protein concentrations in diabetic dogs treated with acarbose, compared with placebo (Fig. 11-7; Robertson et al, 1999; Nelson et al, 2000).

Results of these studies suggest that acarbose may be beneficial in improving control of glycemia in some dogs with IDDM. However, diarrhea and weight loss as a result of carbohydrate malassimilation were common adverse effects, occurring in approximately 35% of dogs (Robertson et al, 1999; Nelson et al, 2000). Diarrhea was more prevalent at higher doses of acarbose (i.e., 100 and 200 mg/dog) and typically resolved within 2 to 3 days of discontinuing the medication. Because of cost and prevalence of adverse effects, acarbose should probably be reserved for treating poorly controlled diabetic dogs in which the cause for poor control of glycemia cannot be identified and insulin treatment, by itself, is ineffective in preventing clinical signs of diabetes. The initial acarbose dosage is low (i.e., 12.5 to 25 mg at each meal) regardless of the body weight of the dog. The benefit of this drug is dependent on its interaction with the meal; it should only be given at the time of feeding. A stepwise increase to 50 mg/dog and, in large dogs (>25 kg) a further increase to 100 mg/dog, can be considered in dogs that fail to show improvement in control of glycemia after 2 weeks using the 12.5 to 25 mg/meal dosage regimen. However, adverse reactions (especially diarrhea) are more likely to occur at these higher doses.

CHROMIUM. Chromium is a ubiquitous trace element that exerts insulin-like effects in vitro. The exact mechanism of action is not known but the overall effect of chromium is to increase insulin sensitivity, presumably through a post-receptor mechanism of action (Anderson, 1992; Striffler et al, 1995). Chromium does not increase serum insulin concentrations. Chromium is an essential cofactor for insulin function and chromium deficiency results in insulin resistance. The effects of chromium treatment on glucose tolerance and control of glycemia in humans with diabetes is controversial. Some studies have identified improved control of glycemia when humans with NIDDM were

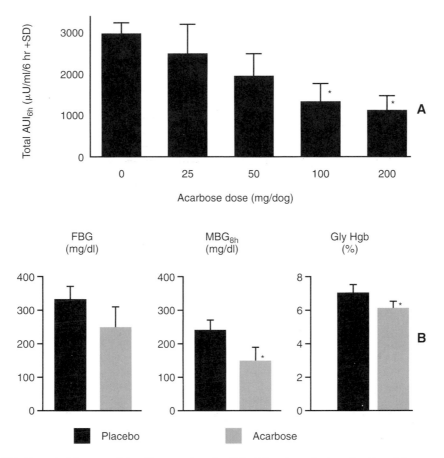

FIGURE 11-7. *A,* Mean total insulin secretion for 5 healthy dogs during the first 6 hours after consumption of a meal and a placebo or 25, 50, 100, or 200 mg of acarbose. Error bars represent standard error of the mean. * = p<0.05, compared with value obtained after treatment with the placebo. (From, Robertson J, et al: Effects of the α-glucosidase inhibitor acarbose on postprandial serum glucose and insulin concentrations in healthy dogs. Am J Vet Res 60:541, 1999.) *B,* Fasting blood glucose (FBG), mean blood glucose over an 8-hour time period (MGB$_{8h}$), and blood total glycosylated hemoglobin (Gly Hgb) in 5 dogs with insulin-dependent diabetes mellitus treated with insulin and placebo *(solid bars)* and insulin and acarbose *(hatched bars)* for 2 months each in a randomly assigned treatment sequence. Error bars represent standard deviation. *p = <0.05, compared with placebo value.

treated with chromium picolinate (Mossop, 1983; Evans, 1989; Anderson et al, 1997); other studies have failed to identify an effect in human diabetics (Rabinowitz et al, 1983; Abraham et al, 1992). In one study, dietary chromium picolinate supplementation improved results of an intravenous glucose tolerance test in healthy dogs, compared with healthy dogs not treated with chromium (Spears et al, 1998). Other studies failed to identify an effect of dietary chromium picolinate supplementation on glucose tolerance in obese dogs during weight reduction (Gross et al, 2000) or in obese and non-obese cats after 6 weeks of chromium picolinate supplementation (Cohn et al, 1999). The effect of oral chromium picolinate on control of glycemia in insulin-treated diabetic dogs was recently studied at our hospital (Schachter et al, 2001). Glycemic control was evaluated monthly for 6 months; chromium picolinate (200 to 400 µg per os twice daily) was administered during the last 3 months. Chromium picolinate did not affect the results of the complete blood count, serum biochemistry panel or urinalysis,

nor did it improve control of glycemia in the diabetic dogs (Fig. 11-8). Similar studies have not been reported in diabetic cats.

Chromium picolinate is considered a nutraceutical in the United States and can be purchased in health food and drug stores. It is inexpensive, and there are no known toxic effects associated with its ingestion. Although preliminary studies failed to identify an effect on control of glycemia, chromium picolinate treatment may be considered in poorly controlled diabetic dogs when the cause for poor control of glycemia cannot be identified and when insulin treatment, by itself, is ineffective in preventing clinical signs of diabetes. One commercial diet (Eukanuba Optimum Weight Control, Iams Co, Dayton, OH) currently marketed for the treatment of diabetes in dogs in the United States contains chromium picolinate.

HERBS, SUPPLEMENTS, AND VITAMINS. An increasing number of humans, primarily with type 2 diabetes, are trying alternative therapies that include herbs, supplements, and vitamins in conjunction with or in lieu of

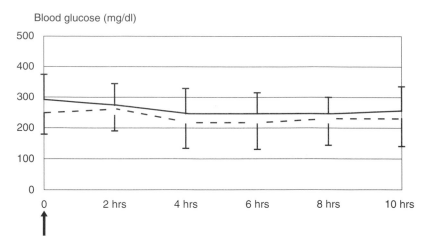

FIGURE 11-8. Mean (± standard deviation) blood glucose concentrations obtained from 13 dogs with insulin-dependent diabetes mellitus before insulin and feeding (Time 0) and for 10 hours after insulin administration only *(broken line)* or after insulin and chromium tripicolinate administration *(solid line)*. Dogs were treated for 3 months with insulin and then 3 months with insulin and chromium tripicolinate. Mean blood glucose concentrations are the mean of all corresponding blood glucose values obtained during the 10-hour blood sample collection period for each dog at 1, 2, and 3 months of each treatment period. *Arrow* indicates time of insulin or insulin and chromium picolinate. (From, Schachter S, et al: Oral chromium picolinate and control of glycemia in insulin-treated diabetic dogs. J Vet Intern Med 15:379, 2001.)

the more conventional treatment options for diabetes discussed above. The goals for using herbs, supplements, and vitamins are primarily centered around decreasing blood glucose, triglyceride, and cholesterol concentrations, delaying the onset of long-term complications of diabetes (e.g., coronary artery disease, retinopathy), and improving the overall well-being of the patient (Table 11-13; Roszler, 2001). Proposed beneficial effects vary with the herb, supplement, or vitamin used and include delaying nutrient absorption from the gastrointestinal tract, stimulating insulin secretion, improving insulin sensitivity, altering lipid metabolism, improving circulation, and benefits attributed to antioxidant properties. Some herbs, supplements, and vitamins, such as ginseng, chromium, fish oils, and psyllium, have been critically evaluated for efficacy whereas others are recommended based primarily on folk lore and testimonials (Pastors et al, 1991; Striffler et al, 1995; Vuksan et al, 2001). To date, chromium and vanadium are the only two supplements that have been critically evaluated in diabetic dogs and cats (see page 504). Critical studies assessing the effects of herbs, supplements, and vitamins on diabetic control and complications are needed before these alternative therapies can be recommended. Intuitively, it seems doubtful that the herbs, supplements, and vitamins listed in Table 11-13 could have much of an impact in diabetic dogs, in part because these therapies are primarily used for treating type 2 diabetes and delaying chronic diabetic complications, both of which are uncommon in dogs. Although type 2 diabetes and peripheral neuropathy do occur in cats, the chronic administration of herbs, supplements, and vitamins to a carnivore whose metabolism of the active ingredients in these supplements may differ tremendously from omnivores is worrisome without prior studies evaluating their efficacy and safety.

Identification and Control of Concurrent Problems

Concurrent disease and administration of insulin-antagonistic drugs are commonly identified in the dog with newly diagnosed diabetes mellitus (Hess et al, 2000b; Peikes et al, 2001). Concurrent disease and insulin-antagonistic drugs can interfere with tissue responsiveness to insulin. Tissue responsiveness to insulin may be impaired as a result of decreased number of insulin receptors at the surface of the cell membrane, alterations in insulin receptor binding affinity, or impairment in one of several postreceptor steps responsible for activation of glucose transport systems (Unger and Foster, 1998). Loss of tissue responsiveness results in insulin resistance and the severity of insulin resistance is dependent, in part, on the underlying etiology (see page 524). Insulin resistance may be mild and easily overcome by increasing the dosage of insulin or may be severe, causing sustained and marked hyperglycemia regardless of the type and dosage of insulin administered. Some causes of insulin resistance are readily apparent at the time diabetes is diagnosed, such as obesity and the administration of insulin-antagonistic drugs (e.g., glucocorticoids). Other causes of insulin resistance are not readily apparent and require an extensive diagnostic evaluation to be identified. In general, any concurrent inflammatory, infectious, hormonal, or neoplastic disorder can cause insulin resistance and interfere with the effectiveness of insulin therapy. Identification

TABLE 11-13 HERBS, SUPPLEMENTS, AND VITAMINS THAT HAVE BEEN USED TO TREAT DIABETES MELLITUS IN HUMANS. DOSAGES LISTED ARE RECOMMENDATIONS FOR HUMAN DIABETICS

Improve Hyperglycemia

Alpha-lipoic acid (100-600 mg daily)
Vitamin C (250-1000 mg daily)
Vitamin E (800 IU daily)
Chromium (400 µg daily)
Vanadium (5 to 25 mg daily)
Fenugreek seeds (5 to 30 g daily)
American and Asian ginseng (200 mg daily)
Gymnema sylvestre (200 mg twice daily)
Psyllium seeds
Cinnamon ($\frac{1}{4}$ to 1 tsp daily)

Prevent Coronary Artery Disease

Vitamin C
Vitamin E
Quercetin (100 mg three times daily)

Improve Circulation

Gingko biloba
Pycnogenol

Prevent/Control Pain from Neuropathy

Alpha-lipoic acid
Vitamin B$_6$ (<100 mg daily)
Capsaicin (cayenne pepper) (Topical ointment)
Evening primrose oil

Improve Hyperlipidemia

Vitamin E
Evening primrose oil (200 to 500 mg daily)
Fish oils (e.g., omega-3 fatty acids)
Selenium (400 µg daily)

Prevent Cataracts

Alpha-lipoic acid
Vitamin C

Prevent Retinopathy

Vitamin E
Pycnogenol (pine bark extract)

Antioxidant

Alpha-lipoic acid
Vitamin A (100 to 400 IU daily)
Vitamin C
Vitamin E
Pycnogenol
Quercetin
Selenium

From Roszler J: Herbs, supplements and vitamins: What to try, what to buy. Diabetes Interviews August, 2001, p. 45.

and treatment of concurrent disease plays an integral role in the successful management of the diabetic dog. A thorough history, physical examination, and complete diagnostic evaluation is imperative in the newly diagnosed diabetic dog (see Clinical Pathologic Abnormalities, page 493).

Initial Adjustments in Insulin Therapy

Diabetic dogs require several days to equilibrate to changes in insulin dosage or preparation. Therefore newly diagnosed diabetic dogs are typically hospitalized for no more than 24 to 48 hours to finish the diagnostic evaluation of the dog and to begin insulin therapy. During hospitalization, blood glucose concentrations are typically determined at the time insulin is administered and at 11 AM, 2 PM, and 5 PM. The intent is to identify hypoglycemia (blood glucose <80 mg/dl) in those dogs that are unusually sensitive to the actions of insulin. If hypoglycemia occurs, the insulin dosage is decreased before sending the dog home. The insulin dosage is not adjusted in those dogs that remain hyperglycemic during these first few days of insulin

therapy. The objective during this first visit is *not* to establish perfect glycemic control before sending the dog home. Rather, the objective is to begin to reverse the metabolic derangements induced by the disease, allow the dog to equilibrate to the insulin and change in diet, teach the owner how to administer insulin, and give the owner a few days to become accustomed to treating the diabetic dog at home. Adjustments in insulin therapy are made on subsequent evaluations, once the owner and pet have become accustomed to the treatment regimen.

Diabetic dogs are typically evaluated once weekly until an effective insulin treatment protocol is identified. We inform the owner at the time insulin therapy is initiated that it will take approximately one month to establish a satisfactory insulin treatment protocol, assuming unidentified insulin antagonistic disease is not present. The goals of therapy are also explained to the owner. During this month, changes in insulin dosage, type, and frequency of insulin administration are common and should be anticipated by the owner. At each evaluation, the owner's subjective opinion of water intake, urine output, and overall health of their pet is discussed; a complete physical examination is performed; change in body weight is noted; and serial blood glucose measurements between 7–9 AM and 4–6 PM are assessed. Adjustments in insulin therapy are based on this information, the pet is sent home, and an appointment is scheduled for the next week to reevaluate the response to any change in therapy. Glycemic control is attained when clinical signs of diabetes have resolved, the pet is healthy and interactive in the home, its body weight is stable, the owner is satisfied with the progress of therapy, and if possible, the blood glucose concentrations range between 100 and 250 mg/dl throughout the day.

Many factors affect the dog's glycemic control from day to day, including variations in insulin administration and absorption, dietary indiscretions and caloric intake, amount of exercise, and variables that affect insulin responsiveness (e.g., stress, concurrent inflammation, infection). As a consequence, the insulin dosage required to maintain glycemic control typically changes (increase or decrease) with time (Fig. 11-9). Nevertheless, a fixed dosage of insulin is administered at home during the first few months of therapy and changes in insulin dosage are made only after the owner consults with the veterinarian.

Adjustments in insulin dosage are common, and eventually a range of "safe" insulin dosages effective in maintaining glycemic control are established. Insulin dosages outside of the "safe" range usually cause signs of hypoglycemia or hyperglycemia. As the insulin dosage range becomes apparent and as confidence is gained in the owner's ability to recognize signs of hypoglycemia and hyperglycemia, the owner is eventually allowed to make *slight* adjustments in the insulin dosage at home based on clinical observations of their pet's well-being. However, the owner is instructed to stay within the agreed-upon insulin

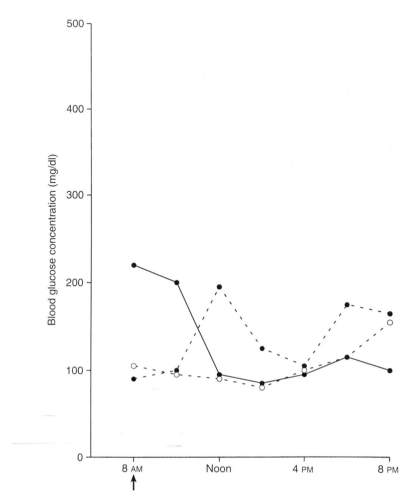

FIGURE 11-9. Blood glucose curves in a 7-kg spayed cat receiving 1.2 U/kg beef/pork source lente insulin *(solid line-solid circles)* 1 month after initiating insulin therapy, 0.6 U/kg beef/pork source lente insulin *(broken line-solid circles)* 4 months later, and 0.8 U/kg beef/pork source lente insulin *(broken line-open circles)* 10 months later. Note the fluctuation in insulin dosage required to maintain good glycemic control. ↑ = SC insulin injection and food.

dosage range. If the insulin dosage is at the upper or lower end of the established range and the pet is still symptomatic, the owner is instructed to call us before making further adjustments in the insulin dosage.

TECHNIQUES FOR MONITORING DIABETIC CONTROL

The basic objective of insulin therapy is to eliminate the clinical signs of diabetes mellitus while avoiding the common complications associated with the disease. Common complications in dogs include blindness caused by cataract formation, weight loss, hypoglycemia, recurring ketosis, and poor control of glycemia secondary to concurrent infection, inflammation, neoplasia, or hormonal disorders. The devastating chronic complications of human diabetes (e.g., nephropathy, vasculopathy, coronary artery disease) require several decades to develop and are uncommon in diabetic dogs. As such, the need to establish near

normal blood glucose concentrations is not necessary in diabetic dogs. Most owners are happy, and most dogs are healthy and relatively asymptomatic if most blood glucose concentrations are kept between 100 mg/dl and 250 mg/dl.

History and Physical Examination

The most important initial parameters to assess when evaluating control of glycemia are the owner's subjective opinion of severity of clinical signs and overall health of their pet, findings on physical examination, and stability of body weight (Briggs et al, 2000). If the owner is happy with results of treatment, the physical examination is supportive of good glycemic control, and the body weight is stable, the diabetic dog is usually adequately controlled. We prefer to talk to the owner and perform the physical examination of the dog at the beginning of the day (between 7:30 and 9:00 AM) prior to or within 1 hour of insulin administration, and we obtain blood for determination of glucose and serum fructosamine concentration (see below) at that time. In most well-regulated diabetic dogs, the blood glucose concentration measured between 7:30 and 9:00 AM and prior to or within 1 hour of insulin administration will be between 150 and 250 mg/dl. An early morning blood glucose concentration less than 150 mg/dl in a presumably well-controlled diabetic dog raises concern for development of hypoglycemia several hours after insulin administration, which either produces no symptoms or produces clinical signs that are not recognized by the owner. Measurement of serum fructosamine concentration is indicated in this situation; identification of a low serum fructosamine concentration (i.e., <350 μmol/L) suggests periods of hypoglycemia and a need to reduce the insulin dosage. Poor control of glycemia should be suspected, and additional diagnostics (i.e., serial blood glucose curve; serum fructosamine concentration; tests for concurrent disorders) or a change in insulin therapy considered if the owner reports clinical signs (i.e., polyuria, polydipsia, lethargy, signs of hypoglycemia), the physical examination identifies problems consistent with poor control of glycemia (e.g., thin or emaciated, poor hair coat), the dog is losing weight, or the blood glucose concentration measured in the early morning is greater than 300 mg/dl (Briggs et al, 2000).

Documenting an increased blood glucose concentration does not *by itself* confirm poor control of glycemia. Stress or excitement can cause marked hyperglycemia that does not reflect the patient's responsiveness to insulin and can lead to the erroneous belief that the diabetic dog is poorly controlled (see page 567). If a discrepancy exists between the history, physical examination findings, and blood glucose concentration or if the dog is fractious, aggressive, excited, or scared and the blood glucose concentration is known to be unreliable, measurement of serum fructosamine concentration should be done to further evaluate status of glycemic control.

Serum Fructosamine Concentration

Fructosamines are glycated proteins found in blood that are used to monitor control of glycemia in diabetic dogs and cats (Reusch et al, 1993; Crenshaw et al, 1996; Elliott et al, 1999). Fructosamines result from an irreversible, nonenzymatic, insulin-independent binding of glucose to serum proteins. All humans and animals have circulating fructosamines. Serum fructosamine concentrations are a marker of mean blood glucose concentration during the circulating lifespan of the protein, which varies from 1 to 3 weeks, depending on the protein (Kawamoto et al, 1991). The extent of glycosylation of serum proteins is directly related to the blood glucose concentration; the higher the average blood glucose concentration during the preceding 2 to 3 weeks, the higher the serum fructosamine concentration, and vice versa. Serum fructosamine concentration is not affected by acute increases in the blood

glucose concentration, as occurs with stress or excitement-induced hyperglycemia (Lutz et al, 1995; Crenshaw et al, 1996). Serum fructosamine concentrations can be measured during the routine evaluation of glycemic control performed every 3 to 6 months; to clarify the effect of stress or excitement on blood glucose concentrations; to clarify discrepancies between the history, physical examination findings, and serial blood glucose concentrations; and to assess the effectiveness of changes in insulin therapy (see page 567). Serum fructosamine concentrations increase when glycemic control of the diabetic dog or cat worsens and decrease when glycemic control improves (see Fig. 12-17, page 563).

Fructosamine is measured in serum, which should be frozen and shipped on cold packs overnight to the laboratory. Although freezing does not cause a significant change in results, storage of serum at room temperature overnight can decrease serum fructosamine results by 10%; storage of serum in the refrigerator can also decrease the serum fructosamine result (Jensen, 1992). An automated colorimetric assay using nitroblue tetrazolium chloride is used for measurement of fructosamine concentrations in serum (Baker et al, 1985). A linear relationship between serum total protein, albumin, and fructosamine concentration has been identified, and hypoproteinemia (total protein <5.5 g/dl) and hypoalbuminemia (albumin <2.5 g/dl) can decrease the serum fructosamine concentration below the reference range in healthy dogs and presumably diabetic dogs as well (Fluckiger et al, 1987; Loste and Marca, 1999; Reusch and Haberer, 2001). A similar decrease in serum fructosamine results has been identified with hyperlipidemia (cholesterol >380 mg/dl and triglycerides >150 mg/dl) and azotemia (blood urea nitrogen >28 mg/dl and serum creatinine >1.7 mg/dl) (Reusch and Haberer, 2001). A significant change in serum fructosamine results was not detected in healthy dogs with hyperproteinemia or hyperbilirubinemia.

In our laboratory, the normal reference range for serum fructosamine in dogs is 225 to 365 μmol/L, a range determined in healthy dogs with persistently normal blood glucose concentrations (Briggs et al, 2000). Serum fructosamine concentration in newly diagnosed diabetic dogs ranged from 320 to 850 μmol/L. The normal serum fructosamine concentration in a few diabetic dogs suggests that hyperglycemia severe enough to cause clinical signs had been present for only a short time before diagnosis.

Interpretation of serum fructosamine in a diabetic dog must take into consideration the fact that hyperglycemia is common, even in well-controlled diabetic dogs (Table 11-14). Most owners are happy with their pet's response to insulin treatment if serum fructosamine concentrations can be kept between 350 and 450 μmol/L. Values greater than 500 μmol/L suggest inadequate control of the diabetic state, and values greater than 600 μmol/L indicate serious lack of glycemic control. Serum fructosamine concentrations in the lower half of the normal reference range (i.e., <300 μmol/L) or below the normal reference range

TABLE 11-14 SAMPLE HANDLING, METHODOLOGY, AND NORMAL VALUES FOR SERUM FRUCTOSAMINE CONCENTRATIONS MEASURED IN OUR LABORATORY IN DOGS

	Fructosamine
Blood sample	1-2 ml serum
Sample handling	Freeze until assayed
Methodology	Automated colorimetric assay using nitroblue tetrazolium chloride
Factors affecting results	Hypoproteinemia and hypoalbuminemia (decreased), hyperlipidemia (decreased), azotemia (decreased), storage at room temperature (decreased)
Normal range	225 to 365 µmol/L
Interpretation in diabetic dogs:	
Excellent control	350-400 µmol/L
Good control	400-450 µmol/L
Fair control	450-500 µmol/L
Poor control	>500 µmol/L
Prolonged hypoglycemia	<300 µmol/L

should raise concern for significant periods of hypoglycemia in the diabetic dog. The Somogyi phenomenon (i.e., glucose counterregulation) should be suspected if clinical signs (i.e., polyuria, polydipsia, polyphagia, weight loss) are present in a diabetic dog with a serum fructosamine concentration less than 400 µmol/L, assuming hypoproteinemia or hypoalbuminemia is not present (see Table 11-14). Increased serum fructosamine concentrations (i.e., >500 µmol/L) suggest poor control of glycemia and a need for insulin adjustments; however, increased serum fructosamine concentrations do not identify the underlying problem (Fig. 11-10). Evaluation of serial measurements of blood glucose concentration is required to determine how to adjust insulin therapy (see Serial Blood Glucose Curve, page 511).

Blood Glycated Hemoglobin Concentration

Glycated hemoglobin (Gly Hb) is a glycated protein that results from an irreversible, nonenzymatic, insulin-independent binding of glucose to hemoglobin in red blood cells. Blood Gly Hb is a marker of mean blood glucose concentration during the circulating lifespan of the red blood cell, which is approximately 110 days in the dog (Jain, 1993). The extent of glycosylation of hemoglobin is directly related to the blood glucose concentration; the higher the average blood glucose concentration during the preceding 3 to 4 months, the higher the blood Gly Hb, and vice versa. Gly Hb rather than fructosamine is used to monitor long-term effectiveness of treatment in human diabetics, in part because diabetic humans self-monitor their blood glucose and adjust their insulin dose daily and Gly Hb assesses a longer treatment interval than fructosamine (i.e., 3 to 4 months versus 2 to 3 weeks, respectively). In contrast, measurement of serum fructosamine is used more commonly to assess control of glycemia in diabetic dogs and cats, in part because the assay is readily available commercially and is better for assessing the impact of changes in insulin therapy on control of glycemia in fractious dogs and cats because concentrations of fructosamine change more quickly than Gly Hb (i.e., 2 to 3 weeks versus 3 to 4 months, respectively).

In the dog and cat, there are three fractions of Gly Hb: one major fraction (Gly HbA$_{1c}$) that binds glucose and two minor fractions (Gly HbA$_{1a}$ and Gly HbA$_{1b}$) that do not (Hasegawa et al, 1991; 1992). Measurement of Gly HbA$_{1c}$ is typically used to evaluate status of

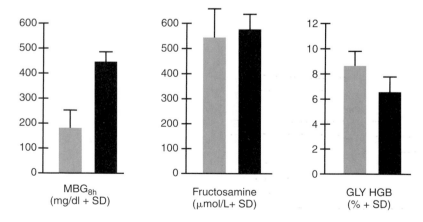

FIGURE 11-10. Mean blood glucose concentration determined over an 8-hour period (MBG$_{8h}$), serum fructosamine concentration, and blood total glycosylated hemoglobin (Gly Hgb) in 10 diabetic dogs with poor control of glycemia caused by the Somogyi phenomenon *(hatched bars)* and 12 diabetic dogs with poor control of glycemia caused by hyperadrenocorticism-induced insulin resistance *(solid bars).* Note the similar glycated protein results in both groups of dogs. Although the average blood glucose concentration is lower on the day hypoglycemia is identified in dogs with the Somogyi phenomenon, high blood glucose concentrations on subsequent days result in high glycated protein concentrations.

glycemic control in human diabetics, whereas studies in diabetic dogs have used assays that measure all three fractions, that is, total Gly Hg (Elliott et al, 1997) or Gly HbA$_{1c}$ (Marca et al, 2000; Marca and Loste, 2001). Most techniques that measure total Gly Hg have been shown to be clinically valid for assessing degree of diabetic control (Mahaffey and Cornelius, 1982; Elliott et al, 1997). Depending on the methodology, however, acute hyperglycemia may cause an increase in the concentration of total Gly Hb. Similar studies using Gly HbA$_{1c}$ to assess status of glycemic control have not yet been reported in diabetic dogs.

Gly Hb is measured in whole blood collected in EDTA. Blood samples can be refrigerated up to a week without significant change in the Gly Hb concentration. In dogs, blood Gly Hb has been measured by affinity chromatography (Wood and Smith, 1982; Elliott et al, 1997), colorimetric analysis (Mahaffey and Cornelius, 1981), ion-exchange high performance liquid chromatography (Hasegawa et al, 1991), and immunoturbidometric assay (Marca and Loste, 2001). We measure total Gly Hb using an affinity chromatography technique whose results are not affected by acute hyperglycemia (Elliott et al, 1997). Assays for measuring Gly Hb are designed for use in humans. As such, it is important that the Gly Hb assay be validated for use in the dog and that a normal reference range is established for the dog. In our experience, several Gly Hb assays, especially in-house automated analyzers for rapid measurement of Gly HbA$_{1c}$ in human diabetics, have not provided valid results in dogs or cats. Any condition that affects red cell life span may affect Gly Hb concentration. Anemia and polycythemia can falsely decrease and increase Gly Hb concentrations, respectively (Elliott et al, 1997). The hematocrit should be taken into consideration when interpreting Gly Hb concentrations.

In our laboratory, the normal reference range for total Gly Hb as measured by affinity chromatography in dogs is 1.7% to 4.9%; a range determined in healthy dogs with persistently normal blood glucose concentrations (Elliott et al, 1997). Blood total Gly Hb in newly diagnosed diabetic dogs ranged from 6.0% to 15.5%. Interpretation of blood Gly Hb in a diabetic dog must take into consideration the fact that hyperglycemia is common, even in well-controlled diabetic dogs (Table 11-15). Most owners are happy with their pet's response to insulin treatment if blood total Gly Hb can be kept between 4% and 6%. Values greater than 7% suggest inadequate control of the diabetic state and values greater than 8% indicate serious lack of glycemic control. Blood total Gly Hb less than 4% should raise concern for significant periods of hypoglycemia in the diabetic dog, assuming anemia is not present. Increased total Gly Hb (i.e., >7%) suggests poor control of glycemia and a need for insulin adjustments; however, increased total Gly Hb does not identify the underlying problem (see Fig. 11-10). Evaluation of serial measurements of blood glucose concentration is required to determine how to adjust insulin therapy (see Serial Blood Glucose Curve, right column).

TABLE 11-15 SAMPLE HANDLING, METHODOLOGY, AND NORMAL VALUES FOR BLOOD TOTAL GLYCOSYLATED HEMOGLOBIN CONCENTRATIONS MEASURED IN OUR LABORATORY IN DOGS

	Total Glycosylated Hemoglobin
Blood sample	1-2 ml whole blood in EDTA
Sample handling	Refrigerate until assayed
Methodology	Affinity chromatography and hemolysates derived from canine red blood cells
Factors affecting results	Storage at room temperature (decreased); storage at 4° C for longer than 7 days (decreased); anemia (Hct<35%) (decreased)
Normal range	1.7% to 4.9%
Interpretation in diabetic dogs:	
Excellent control	4% to 5%
Good control	5% to 6%
Fair control	6% to 7%
Poor control	>7%
Prolonged hypoglycemia	<4%

Urine Glucose Monitoring

Occasional monitoring of urine for glycosuria and ketonuria is helpful in those diabetic dogs that have problems with recurring ketosis or hypoglycemia to determine whether ketonuria or persistent negative glycosuria is present, respectively. We do not have the owner adjust daily insulin dosages based on morning urine glucose measurements in diabetic dogs, except to decrease the insulin dose in dogs with recurring hypoglycemia and persistent negative glycosuria. In our experience, the vast majority of diabetic dogs develop complications as a result of owners being misled by morning urine glucose concentrations. On occasion we recommend evaluation (e.g., on the weekends) of multiple urine samples obtained throughout the day and early evening. The well-controlled diabetic pet should have urine that is free of glucose for most of each 24-hour period. Persistent glycosuria throughout the day and night suggests inadequate control of the diabetic state and the need for a more complete evaluation of diabetic control using techniques discussed in this section.

Serial Blood Glucose Curve

If an adjustment in insulin therapy is deemed necessary after reviewing the history, physical examination, changes in body weight, and serum fructosamine concentration, then a serial blood glucose curve should be generated to provide guidance in making the adjustment unless blood glucose measurements are unreliable because of stress, aggression, or excitement (see page 567). The serial blood glucose curve provides guidelines for making rational adjustments in insulin therapy. Evaluation of a serial blood glucose curve is mandatory during the initial regulation of the diabetic dog, is periodically of value to assess glycemic control despite the fact that a dog may appear to be doing well in the home environment, and is necessary to reestablish glycemic control in the dog in which clinical manifestations of hyperglycemia or hypoglycemia have developed. Reliance on history, physical examination, body weight, and serum fructosamine concentration to determine when a serial blood glucose curve is needed help reduce the frequency of performing serial blood glucose curves, reduce the number of venipunctures, and shorten the time the dog spends in the hospital, thereby minimizing the dog's aversion (and stress) to these evaluations and improving the chances of obtaining meaningful blood glucose results when a serial blood glucose curve is needed.

PROTOCOL FOR GENERATING THE SERIAL BLOOD GLUCOSE CURVE IN THE HOSPITAL. When assessing glycemic control, the veterinarian or clinician should follow the insulin and feeding schedule used by the owner and blood should be obtained every 1 to 2 hours throughout the day for glucose determination. Owners of finicky diabetic dogs should feed their pets at their home, not at the hospital. Inappetence can profoundly alter the results of a serial blood glucose curve (Fig. 11-11). If insulin is usually given within 1 hour prior to the pet's presentation to the clinic, insulin is given by the owner (using their insulin and syringe) in the hospital *after* an initial blood glucose is obtained. The entire insulin administration procedure should be closely evaluated by a veterinary technician. If the owner usually administers insulin before 6 AM, we recommend that the owner give the insulin at 6 AM and bring the pet to the hospital at the first appointment of the day. It is more important to maintain the pet's daily routine than to risk inaccurate blood glucose results caused by inappetence in the hospital or insulin administration at an unusual time. The exception are those instances where the clinician wants to evaluate owner administration technique using insulin rather than physiologic saline.

Blood glucose concentrations are typically determined by either a point-of-care glucose analyzer or hand-held portable blood glucose monitoring device. Commercially available portable blood glucose monitoring devices provide blood glucose concentrations reasonably close to those obtained with reference methods (i.e., glucose oxidase and hexokinase methods), although results may consistently overestimate or underestimate actual glucose values (Fig. 11-12; Cohn et al, 2000; Wess and Reusch, 2000a). In our experience, blood glucose values determined by the majority of portable blood glucose monitoring devices are typically lower than actual glucose values determined by reference methods. This may result in an incorrect diagnosis of hypoglycemia or the misperception that glycemic control is better than it actually is. Failure to consider this "error" could result in insulin underdosage and the potential for persistence of clinical signs despite what appears to be "acceptable" blood glucose results.

By evaluating serial blood glucose measurements every 1 to 2 hours throughout the day, the clinician will be able to determine whether the insulin is effective and to identify the glucose nadir, time of peak insulin effect, duration of insulin effect, and severity of fluctuation in blood glucose concentrations in that particular diabetic dog. Obtaining only 1 or 2 blood glucose concentrations has not been reliable for evaluating the effect of a given insulin dose (Fig. 11-13). Persistent poor control of the diabetic state often stems from misinterpretation of the effects of insulin that is based on assessment of only 1 or 2 blood glucose concentrations.

The *ideal* goal of insulin therapy in diabetic dogs is to maintain the blood glucose concentration between 100 mg/dl and 250 mg/dl throughout the day and night. This goal can be very difficult, and in some diabetic dogs, impossible to attain. The ultimate decision on whether to adjust insulin therapy must always take into consideration the owner's perception of how the pet is doing at home, findings on physical examination, changes in body weight, serum fructosamine concentrations, as well as results of serial blood glucose measurements. Many diabetic dogs do well despite blood glucose concentrations consistently in the high 100s to low 300s.

PROTOCOL FOR GENERATING THE SERIAL BLOOD GLUCOSE CURVE AT HOME. Hyperglycemia induced by stress, aggression, or excitement is the single biggest problem affecting accuracy of the serial blood glucose curve, especially in cats. Stress can override the glucose-lowering effect of the insulin injection, causing high blood glucose concentrations despite the presence of adequate amounts of insulin in the circulation and leading to a spiraling path of insulin overdosage, hypoglycemia, Somogyi phenomenon, and poor control of glycemia. The biggest factors inducing stress hyperglycemia are hospitalization and multiple venipunctures. An alternative to hospital-generated blood glucose curves is to have the owner generate the blood glucose curve at home using the ear or lip prick technique and a portable home glucose monitoring device that allows the owner to touch the drop of blood on the ear or lip with the end of the glucose-test

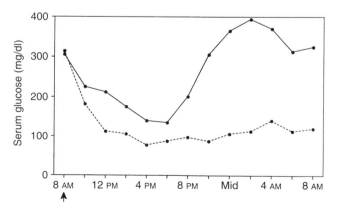

FIGURE 11-11. Mean blood glucose concentrations in 8 diabetic dogs following administration of NPH insulin (↑) and feeding equal-sized meals at 8 AM and 6 PM (*solid line*) or feeding nothing (*broken line*) during the 24 hours of blood sampling. (From Nelson RW, Couto CG: Essentials of Small Animal Internal Medicine. St Louis, Mosby-Year Book, 1992, p 572.)

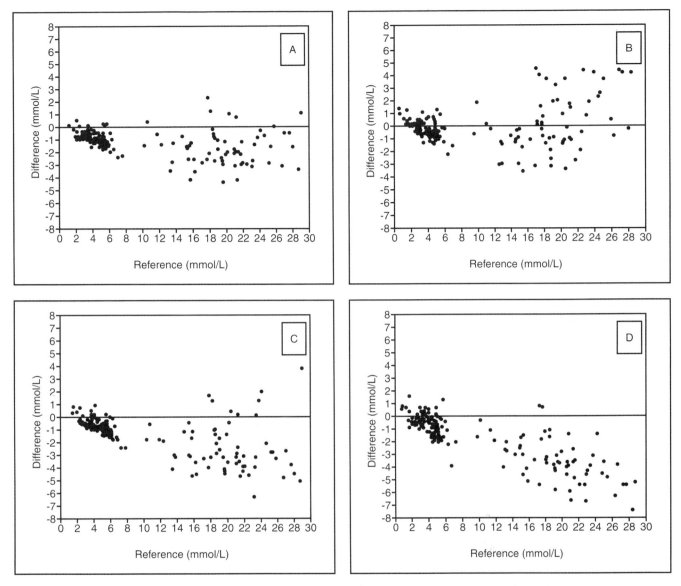

FIGURE 11-12. Scatterplots of the difference between blood glucose concentration obtained with four portable blood glucose meters and concentration obtained with a reference method versus concentration obtained with the reference method for blood samples from 170 dogs. (From Wess G, Reusch C: Evaluation of five portable blood glucose meters for use in dogs. JAVMA 216:203, 2000.).

strip (Wess and Reusch, 2000b). This technique is usually reserved for diabetic dogs in which the reliability of blood glucose results generated in the veterinary hospital is questionable. See page 565 for more information on monitoring blood glucose concentrations at home.

INTERPRETING THE SERIAL BLOOD GLUCOSE CURVE. Results of the blood glucose curve will allow the veterinarian to assess the effectiveness of the administered insulin to lower the blood glucose concentration and determine the glucose nadir and the duration of insulin effect (Fig. 11-14). Ideally, all blood glucose concentrations should range between 100 and 250 mg/dl during the time period between insulin injections. Typically, the highest blood glucose concentrations occur at the time of each insulin injection, but this does not always occur.

Insulin effectiveness, glucose nadir, and duration of insulin effect are the critical determinations from the serial blood glucose curve. The effectiveness of insulin is the first parameter to assess. Is the insulin effective in lowering the blood glucose concentration? The insulin dosage, the highest blood glucose concentration, and the difference between the highest and lowest blood glucose concentrations (i.e., blood glucose differential) must be considered simultaneously when assessing insulin effectiveness. For example, a blood glucose differential of 50 mg/dl is acceptable if the blood glucose ranges between 120 and 170 mg/dl but is unacceptable if the blood glucose ranges between 350 and 400 mg/dl. Similarly, a blood glucose differential of 100 mg/dl indicates insulin effectiveness if the patient receives 0.4 U of insulin per kilogram of body weight but suggests insulin

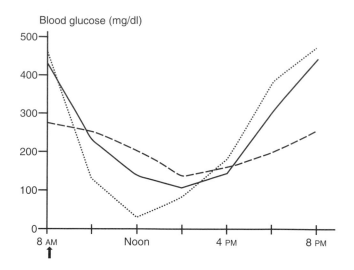

FIGURE 11-13. Blood glucose concentration curve in a Dachshund receiving 0.8 U of recombinant human lente insulin per kilogram body weight twice a day *(solid line)*, a Miniature Poodle receiving 0.6 U of recombinant human lente insulin per kilogram body weight twice a day *(broken line)*, and a Terrier-mix receiving 1.1 U of recombinant human lente insulin per kilogram body weight twice a day *(dotted line)*. Insulin and food was given at 8 AM for each dog. Interpretation of the blood glucose curves suggest short duration of insulin effect in the Dachshund, insulin underdosage in the Miniature Poodle, and the Somogyi effect in the Terrier-mix. Notice that the blood glucose concentrations were similar in all dogs at 2 PM and 4 PM and the glucose results at these times do not establish the diagnosis in any of the dogs. (From Nelson RW, Couto CG: Small Animal Internal Medicine, 3rd ed. St Louis, Mosby Inc, 2003, p 741.)

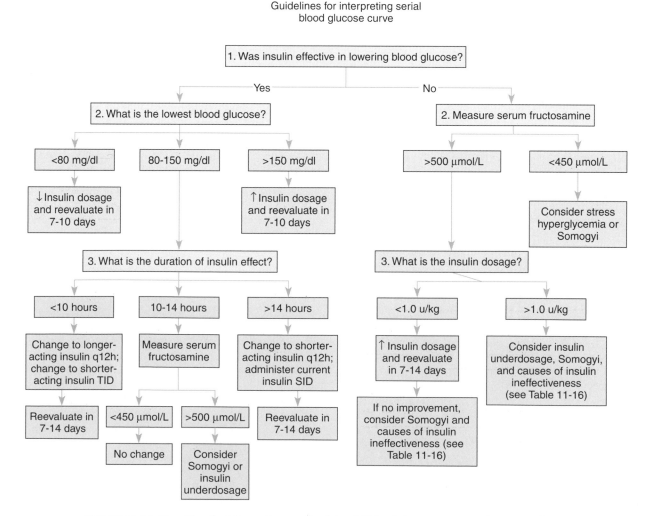

FIGURE 11-14. Algorithm for interpreting results of a serial blood glucose concentration curve. (From Nelson RW, Couto CG: Small Animal Internal Medicine, 3rd ed. St Louis, Mosby Inc, 2003, p 742.)

resistance if the patient receives 2.2 U of insulin per kilogram.

If the insulin is not effective in lowering the blood glucose concentration, the clinician should consider insulin underdosage and the differentials for insulin ineffectiveness and resistance (see Recurrence or Persistence of Clinical Signs, page 518). In general, insulin underdosage should be considered if the insulin dosage is less than 1.0 U/kg per injection in the diabetic dog and insulin ineffectiveness and resistance should be considered if the insulin dosage exceeds 1.0 to 1.5 U/kg per injection. The veterinarian should always be wary of the Somogyi phenomenon, especially in toy and miniature breeds, and the effect of stress on the blood glucose results.

If insulin is effective in lowering the blood glucose concentration, the next parameter to assess is the lowest blood glucose (i.e., glucose nadir). The glucose nadir should ideally fall between 100 and 125 mg/dl. If the glucose nadir is greater than 150 mg/dl, the insulin dosage may need to be increased, and if the nadir is less than 80 mg/dl, the insulin dosage should be decreased. For the latter, the insulin dosage is typically decreased approximately 10% to 25%. If the dog is receiving a large amount of insulin (e.g., >2.2 U/kg/injection), concurrent insulin resistance or the Somogyi phenomenon should be considered. A diagnostic evaluation for insulin resistance may be warranted (see page 524), and/or glycemic regulation started over again using the insulin dose recommended for the initial regulation of the diabetic dog (see page 496). Control of glycemia should be reevaluated 7 to 14 days after initiating the new dose of insulin and adjustments in the insulin dose made accordingly.

Duration of insulin effect can be assessed if the glucose nadir is greater than 80 mg/dl and there has not been a rapid decrease in the blood glucose concentration after insulin administration. Assessment of duration of insulin effect may not be valid when the blood glucose decreases to less than 80 mg/dl or decreases rapidly because of the potential induction of the Somogyi phenomenon, which can falsely shorten the apparent duration of insulin effect (see page 519). The duration of effect is roughly defined as the time from the insulin injection through the lowest glucose and until the blood glucose concentration exceeds 200 to 250 mg/dl (Fig. 11-15). Duration of effect of lente and NPH insulin is 10 to 14 hours in approximately 90% of diabetic dogs, necessitating twice daily insulin treatment. Dogs are usually symptomatic for diabetes if the duration of insulin effect is less than 10 hours (see page 520) and may develop hypoglycemia or the Somogyi phenomenon if the duration of insulin effect is greater than 14 hours and the insulin is being administered twice a day (Fig. 11-16).

Alterations in the dosage of insulin are often necessary at the same time as alterations in type of insulin. Adjustments in insulin dosage are usually dictated by the change in type of insulin and the glucose nadir. Longer-acting insulin (i.e., ultralente, PZI, glargine) is less potent than intermediate-acting

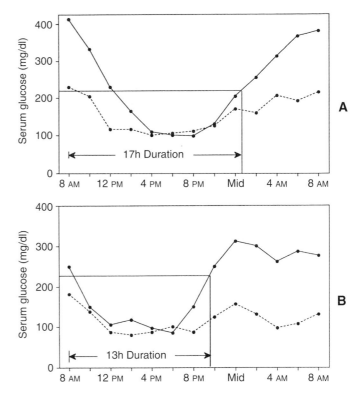

FIGURE 11-15. *A,* Blood glucose curve in a Poodle mix receiving beef/pork source NPH insulin, 1.1 U/kg body weight *(solid line).* Insulin is given at 8 AM, and the dog is fed at 8 AM and 6 PM. Hyperglycemia in excess of 225 mg/dl redevelops around midnight. The duration of insulin action is approximately 17 hours. Switching to beef/pork source ultralente insulin, 1.3 U/kg once daily, improved glycemic control *(broken line)* in this dog. *B,* Blood glucose curve in a Terrier mix receiving beef/pork source NPH insulin, 1 U/kg body weight *(solid line).* Insulin is given at 8 AM, and the dog is fed at 8 AM and 6 PM. Notice the postprandial hyperglycemia following the evening meal. Hyperglycemia in excess of 225 mg/dl redevelops around 9 PM. The duration of insulin action is approximately 13 hours. Switching to beef/pork source NPH insulin, 1 U/kg twice daily at 12-hour intervals and feeding at the time of the insulin injection improved glycemic control *(broken line)* in the dog. (From Nelson RW, Couto CG: Essentials of Small Animal Internal Medicine. St Louis, Mosby-Year Book, 1992, p 570.)

insulin (i.e., NPH, lente). It takes more of a less potent insulin to get a comparable decrease in the blood glucose concentration, compared with a more potent insulin (see Fig. 12-11, page 551). When switching from a more potent to a less potent insulin, the dose of insulin is usually not changed if the glucose nadir is between 80 and 120 mg/dl and is increased approximately 10% if the glucose nadir is greater than 120 mg/dl. When switching from a less potent to a more potent insulin, the dose of insulin is increased approximately 10% if the glucose nadir is greater than 150 mg/dl, is usually not changed if the glucose nadir is between 120 and 150 mg/dl, and is decreased approximately 10% if the glucose nadir is between 80 and 120 mg/dl. Control of glycemia should be reevaluated 7 to 14 days after initiating the new type of insulin and adjustments in the insulin dose made accordingly.

REPRODUCIBILITY OF THE SERIAL BLOOD GLUCOSE CURVE. The reproducibility of serial blood glucose

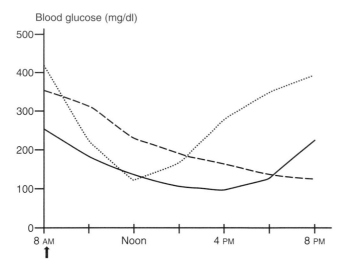

Blood glucose (mg/dl)

FIGURE 11-16. Blood glucose concentration curves obtained from 3 diabetic dogs treated with recombinant human lente insulin twice a day, illustrating a difference between dogs in the duration of insulin effect. The insulin is effective in lowering the blood glucose concentration in all dogs and the blood glucose nadir is between 100 and 175 mg/dl for the dogs. However, the duration of insulin effect is approximately 12 hours *(solid line)* in one dog with good control of glycemia (ideal duration of effect), approximately 8 hours *(dotted line)* in one dog with persistently poor control of glycemia (short duration of effect), and greater than 12 hours *(broken line)* in one dog with a history of good days and bad days of glycemic control (prolonged duration of effect); a history suggestive of the Somogyi phenomenon. (From Nelson RW, Couto CG: Small Animal Internal Medicine, 3rd ed. St Louis, Mosby Inc, 2003, p 743.)

curves varies from dog to dog. In some dogs, results of serial blood glucose curves may vary dramatically from day to day or month to month, depending, in part, on the actual amount of insulin administered and absorbed from the subcutaneous site of deposition, and the interaction between insulin, diet, exercise, stress, excitement, presence of concurrent disorders, and counterregulatory hormone secretion (i.e., secretion of glucagon, epinephrine, cortisol, growth hormone). In other dogs, serial blood glucose curves are reasonably consistent from day to day and month to month. Lack of consistency in results of serial blood glucose curves creates frustration for many veterinarians. However, it is important to remember that this lack of consistency is a direct reflection of all the variables that affect the blood glucose concentration in diabetics. Daily self-monitoring of blood glucose concentrations and daily adjustments in insulin dose are recommended in human diabetics to minimize the effect of these variables on control of glycemia. A similar approach for diabetic dogs and cats will undoubtedly become more common in the future, as home glucose monitoring techniques are refined. For now, initial assessment of control of glycemia is based on the owner's perception of their diabetic pet's health combined with periodic examinations by the veterinarian. Serial blood glucose measurements are indicated if poor control of glycemia is suspected. The purpose of serial blood glucose measurements is to obtain a glimpse at the actions of

insulin in that diabetic animal and ideally identify a reason (e.g., short duration of insulin effect) that could explain why the diabetic dog is poorly controlled.

We prefer to adjust insulin therapy based on interpretation of a single serial blood glucose curve and typically rely on owner perceptions of clinical response and change in serum fructosamine concentration to initially assess the impact of the adjustment on control of glycemia (see page 509). If problems persist, we consider repeating the serial blood glucose curve. We rarely perform serial blood glucose curves on multiple, consecutive days because it promotes stress-induced hyperglycemia. In addition, information gained from a prior serial blood glucose curve should never be assumed to be reproducible on subsequent curves, especially if several weeks to months have passed or the dog has developed recurrence of clinical signs. The protocol for the serial blood glucose curve should be followed each time a glucose curve is generated.

Role of Serum Fructosamine in Aggressive, Excitable, or Stressed Dogs

Serial blood glucose curves are unreliable in aggressive, excitable, or stressed dogs because of problems related to stress-induced hyperglycemia. In these dogs, the clinician must make an educated guess as to where the problem lies (e.g., wrong type of insulin, low dose), make an adjustment in therapy, and rely on changes in serum fructosamine to assess the benefit of the change in treatment. Refer to page 567 for more information on use of serum fructosamine in diabetic pets with stress-induced hyperglycemia.

INSULIN THERAPY DURING SURGERY

Generally, surgery should be delayed in diabetic dogs until the animal's clinical condition is stable and the diabetic state is controlled with insulin. The exception are those situations in which surgery is required to eliminate insulin resistance (e.g., ovariohysterectomy in a diestrus bitch) or to save the animal's life. The surgery itself does not pose a greater risk in a stable diabetic animal than in a nondiabetic animal. The concern is the interplay between insulin therapy and the lack of food intake during the perioperative period. The stress of anesthesia and surgery also causes the release of diabetogenic hormones, which in turn promotes ketogenesis (see Chapter 13, page 580). Insulin should be administered during the perioperative period to prevent severe hyperglycemia and minimize ketone formation. To compensate for the lack of food intake and prevent hypoglycemia, the amount of insulin administered during the perioperative period is decreased and IV dextrose is administered, when needed. To correct marked hyperglycemia (i.e., blood glucose concentration greater than 300 mg/dl), regular crystalline insulin is administered intramuscularly or by continuous IV infusion. Frequent blood glucose monitoring and appropriate adjustments in therapy are the key to avoiding hypoglycemia and severe hyperglycemia during the perioperative period.

We use the following protocol during the perioperative period in dogs and cats undergoing surgery. The day before surgery, the animal is given its normal dose of insulin and fed as usual. Food is withheld after 10 PM. On the morning of the procedure the blood glucose concentration is measured before the animal is given insulin. If the blood glucose concentration is less than 100 mg/dl, insulin is not given and an IV infusion of 2.5% to 5% dextrose is initiated. If the blood glucose concentration is between 100 and 200 mg/dl, one quarter of the animal's usual morning dose of insulin is given and an IV infusion of dextrose is initiated. If the blood glucose concentration is more than 200 mg/dl, one-half of the usual morning dose of insulin is given but the IV dextrose infusion is withheld until the blood glucose concentration is less than 150 mg/dl. In all three situations the blood glucose concentration is measured every 30 to 60 minutes during the surgical procedure. The goal is to maintain the blood glucose concentration between 150 and 250 mg/dl during the perioperative period. A 2.5% to 5% dextrose infusion is administered IV and regular crystalline insulin administered intermittently as needed to eliminate or prevent hypoglycemia and severe hyperglycemia, respectively. When the blood glucose concentration exceeds 300 mg/dl, the dextrose infusion should be discontinued and the blood glucose concentration evaluated 30 and 60 minutes later. If the blood glucose concentration remains greater than 300 mg/dl, regular crystalline insulin is administered intramuscularly at approximately 20% of the dosage of long-acting insulin being used at home. Subsequent doses of regular crystalline insulin should be given no more frequently than every 4 hours, and the dosage should be adjusted based on the effect of the first insulin injection on the blood glucose concentrations.

On the day after surgery the diabetic dog or cat can usually be returned to the routine schedule of insulin administration and feeding. An animal that is not eating can be maintained with IV dextrose infusions and regular crystalline insulin injections given subcutaneously every 6 to 8 hours. Once the animal is eating regularly, it can be returned to its normal insulin and feeding schedule.

COMPLICATIONS OF INSULIN THERAPY

Symptomatic and Asymptomatic Hypoglycemia

Hypoglycemia is a common complication of insulin therapy. Hypoglycemia may be symptomatic or asymptomatic. Asymptomatic hypoglycemia is more prevalent than symptomatic hypoglycemia in diabetic dogs and cats. Symptomatic hypoglycemia is most apt to occur following sudden large increases in the insulin dose, with excessive overlap of insulin action in dogs receiving insulin twice a day, during unusually strenuous exercise, and following prolonged inappetence. In these situations, severe hypoglycemia may occur before glucose counterregulation (i.e., secretion of glucagon, cortisol, epinephrine, and growth hormone) is able to compensate for and reverse the hypoglycemia. Signs of hypoglycemia include lethargy, weakness, head tilting, ataxia, seizures, and coma. The occurrence and severity of clinical signs is dependent on the rate of blood glucose decline and the severity of hypoglycemia. Symptomatic hypoglycemia is treated with glucose administered as food, sugar water, or dextrose IV (see Chapter 14, page 638). Whenever signs of hypoglycemia occur, the owner should be instructed to stop insulin therapy until hyperglycemia and glycosuria recur. Urine glucose testing by the owner with the dog in its home environment is useful for identifying when glycosuria recurs. The adjustment in the subsequent insulin dosage is somewhat arbitrary; as a general rule of thumb, the insulin dosage initially should be decreased 25% to 50% and subsequent adjustments in the dosage based on clinical response and results of blood glucose measurements. Failure of glycosuria to recur following a hypoglycemic episode suggests reversion to a non–insulin-dependent diabetic state or impaired glucose counterregulation (see below).

Asymptomatic hypoglycemia is typically identified during evaluation of a serial blood glucose curve. Serum fructosamine concentration less than 350 µmol/L (normal range, 225 to 365 µmol/L) is also suggestive of hypoglycemia. However, failure to identify hypoglycemia during a blood glucose concentration curve or low-normal serum fructosamine concentration does not rule out asymptomatic hypoglycemia, in part because of hypoglycemia-induced glucose counterregulation (Somogyi phenomenon) and transient insulin resistance (see page 519). Treatment of asymptomatic hypoglycemia involves decreasing the dose of insulin, typically 10% to 20%, and assessing the clinical response, change in serum fructosamine concentration, and in nonstressed dogs, blood glucose concentrations.

If hypoglycemia remains a reoccurring problem despite reductions in the insulin dose, excessive overlap in insulin action or reversion to a non–insulin-dependent diabetic state should be considered. Excessive overlap of insulin action results from twice-a-day administration of insulin with a duration of effect considerably longer than 12 hours in that diabetic animal (see page 521). Reversion from an insulin-dependent to a non–insulin-dependent diabetic state should be suspected if hypoglycemia remains a persistent problem despite administration of small doses of insulin once a day, blood glucose concentrations remain below 200 mg/dl prior to insulin administration, serum fructosamine concentrations are less than 350 µmol/L, or urine glucose test strips are consistently negative. These findings suggest the presence of endogenously derived circulating insulin, partial but not complete loss of pancreatic beta cells, and concurrent disease causing transient insulin resistance. Resolution of an apparent insulin-dependent diabetic state is uncommon in dogs and usually indicative of secondary diabetes (see page 490).

IMPAIRED GLUCOSE COUNTERREGULATION. Secretion of the diabetogenic hormones, most notably epinephrine and glucagon, stimulates hepatic glucose secretion and helps counter severe hypoglycemia. A deficient counterregulatory response to hypoglycemia has been identified as early as 1 year after diagnosis of IDDM in humans (White et al, 1983). As a consequence, when the blood glucose concentration approaches 60 mg/dl, there is no compensatory response by the body to increase the blood sugar, and prolonged hypoglycemia ensues. An impaired counterregulatory response to hypoglycemia has also been documented in dogs with IDDM (Duesberg et al, 1995). Dogs with impaired counterregulation had more problems with hypoglycemia than diabetic dogs without impaired counterregulation. Impaired counterregulation should be considered in a diabetic dog exquisitely sensitive to small doses of insulin or with problems of prolonged hypoglycemia after administration of an acceptable dose of insulin.

INAPPETENCE. A healthy, well-regulated diabetic dog or cat should maintain an excellent appetite. Occasional inappetence at mealtime is not, by itself, an indication to stop insulin therapy. Most diabetic dogs and cats eat within a couple of hours of the insulin injection, as the blood glucose begins to decline. If the inappetence persists or if other signs of gastrointestinal dysfunction develop (e.g., vomiting), insulin therapy should be modified or discontinued until the veterinarian has examined the dog or cat. Common causes of inappetence in diabetic dogs include pancreatitis, ketoacidosis, bacterial infection (especially involving the urinary system), neoplasia, finicky eaters, and boredom with high-fiber diets. Appropriate diagnostic and therapeutic steps should be initiated, depending on results of the physical examination.

Recurrence or Persistence of Clinical Signs

Recurrence or persistence of clinical signs (i.e., polyuria, polydipsia, polyphagia, weight loss) is perhaps the most common "complication" of insulin therapy in diabetic dogs. Recurrence or continuing clinical signs suggest insulin ineffectiveness or resistance. In diabetic dogs, insulin ineffectiveness is usually caused by problems with biologic activity of the insulin or with owner technique in administering insulin; problems with insulin therapy relating to the insulin type, dose, species, or frequency of administration; or problems with responsiveness to insulin caused by concurrent inflammatory, infectious, neoplastic, or hormonal disorders (i.e., insulin resistance). Discrepancies in the parameters used to assess glycemic control, resulting in an erroneous belief that the diabetic dog is poorly controlled, should also be considered. This is usually caused by erroneously high blood glucose concentrations that suggest insulin ineffectiveness; these high values may be stress-induced and may not reflect

the patient's responsiveness to insulin (see page 567). When a diabetic dog is evaluated for suspected insulin ineffectiveness, it is important that all parameters used to assess glycemic control be critically analyzed, most notably the owner's perceptions of how the pet is doing in the home environment, findings on physical examination, and changes in body weight (see Techniques for Monitoring Diabetic Control, page 508). If the history, physical examination, change in body weight, and serum fructosamine concentration suggest poor control of the diabetic state, a diagnostic evaluation to identify the cause is warranted, beginning with evaluation of the owner's insulin administration technique and the biologic activity of the insulin preparation.

PROBLEMS WITH OWNER ADMINISTRATION AND ACTIVITY OF THE INSULIN PREPARATION. Administration of biologically inactive insulin (e.g., outdated, overheated, mixed by shaking), use of inappropriate insulin syringes for the concentration of insulin (e.g., U-100 syringe with U-40 insulin), and problems with insulin administration technique (e.g., misunderstanding how to read the insulin syringe, inappropriate injection technique) will result in recurrence or persistence of clinical signs and an increase in serum fructosamine and blood glucose concentrations because of an inadequate dosage of insulin. Problems with owner administration and insulin action are identified by evaluating the owner's insulin administration technique and by administering new, undiluted insulin and measuring several blood glucose concentrations throughout the day. In addition, the skin and subcutaneous tissues should be assessed in the area where insulin injections are given. Some diabetic dogs develop low-grade inflammation, edema, and thickening of the dermis and subcutaneous tissues in areas of chronic insulin administration, and these changes can interfere with insulin absorption following subcutaneous administration (see Allergic Reactions to Insulin, page 524).

Freezing and heat inactivates insulin in the bottle. Although "room temperature" does not inactivate insulin, we instruct owners to store insulin in the door of the refrigerator to maintain a consistent environment for the insulin preparation. It is common practice for humans with diabetes to replace their insulin with a new bottle every month to avoid problems with loss of activity or sterility. Some veterinarians advocate similar recommendations for owners of diabetic dogs and cats. We have not appreciated a clinically significant loss of insulin action with time when insulin preparations are maintained in a constant environment (i.e., refrigerator) and handled appropriately. We do not routinely recommend purchasing a new bottle of insulin every month, especially if the diabetic dog or cat is doing well. However, we do evaluate the effectiveness of a new bottle of insulin if clinical signs recur in a diabetic dog or cat, especially if more than 75% of the owner's insulin preparation has been used.

Dilution of insulin is a common practice, especially in very small dogs and cats whose insulin requirements can be quite small. Although studies evaluating the shelf-life of diluted insulin have not been published, we recommend replacing diluted insulin preparations every 4 to 8 weeks. Even using these guidelines, insufficient amounts of insulin are administered when diluted insulin is used in some dogs, despite appropriate dilution and insulin administration techniques, inadequacies that are corrected when full-strength insulin is used. Small-volume insulin syringes (U-100, 0.3 ml) should be used with full strength U-100 insulin for dogs receiving small amounts of insulin.

PROBLEMS WITH THE INSULIN TREATMENT REGIMEN. The most common problems causing poor control of glycemia in this category include insulin underdosage, the Somogyi phenomenon, short duration of effect of lente and NPH insulin, and once-a-day insulin administration. The insulin treatment regimen should be critically evaluated for possible problems in these areas, and appropriate changes made to try to improve insulin effectiveness, especially if the history and physical examination do not suggest a concurrent disorder causing insulin resistance.

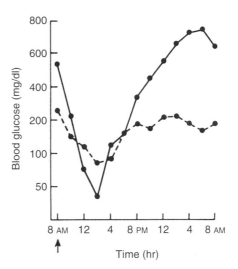

FIGURE 11-17. Blood glucose concentrations in a 6.1-kg Cairn terrier after receiving beef/pork source NPH insulin at 8 AM. The dog was fed at 8 AM and 6 PM. *Solid line* = 20 units; *broken line* = 4 units. ↑ = insulin injection. (From Feldman EC, Nelson RW: Insulin-induced hyperglycemia in diabetic dogs. JAVMA 180:1432, 1982.)

Insulin Underdosage

Control of glycemia can be established in most dogs using less than 1.0 U of insulin/kg of body weight administered twice each day. An inadequate dose of insulin in conjunction with once-a-day insulin therapy is a common cause for persistence of clinical signs. In general, insulin underdosage should be considered if the insulin dosage is <1.0 U/kg and the animal is receiving insulin twice a day. If insulin underdosage is suspected, the dose of insulin should be gradually increased by 1 to 5 units/injection (depending on the size of the dog) per week. The effectiveness of the change in therapy should be evaluated by client perception of clinical response and measurement of serum fructosamine or serial blood glucose concentrations. Other causes for insulin ineffectiveness and resistance should be considered once the insulin dosage exceeds 1.0 to 1.5 units/kg/injection, the insulin is being administered every 12 hours, and control of glycemia remains poor. Inducing hypoglycemia and the Somogyi phenomenon are the primary concerns when increasing the insulin dosage to rule out insulin underdosage as the cause of the poor control of glycemia, especially in toy and miniature breeds (see below). A gradual increase in the insulin dosage and close monitoring helps minimize the development of these problems.

Insulin Overdosing and Glucose Counterregulation (Somogyi Phenomenon)

A high dose of insulin may cause overt hypoglycemia or induce glucose counterregulation (Somogyi phenomenon) and transient insulin resistance. The Somogyi phenomenon results from a normal physiologic response to impending hypoglycemia induced by excessive insulin. When the blood glucose concentration declines to less than 65 mg/dl or when the blood glucose concentration decreases rapidly regardless of the glucose nadir, direct hypoglycemia-induced stimulation of hepatic glycogenolysis and secretion of diabetogenic hormones, most notably epinephrine and glucagon, increase the blood glucose concentration, minimize signs of hypoglycemia, and cause marked hyperglycemia within 12 hours of glucose counterregulation, in part because the diabetic dog cannot secrete sufficient endogenous insulin to dampen the continuing rise in the blood glucose concentration (Fig. 11-17; see Hypoglycemia and the Counterregulatory Response, page 617) (Cryer and Polonsky, 1998; Karam, 2001). By the next morning, the blood glucose concentration can be extremely elevated (400 to 800 mg/dl), and the morning urine glucose concentration is consistently 1 to 2 g/dl as measured with urine glucose test strips. If the owners of a diabetic dog are adjusting the daily insulin dose based on the morning urine glucose concentration, they interpret these readings as indicating the dog received insufficient amounts of insulin, especially if hypoglycemic signs (i.e., weakness, ataxia, bizarre behavior, or convulsions) are not observed. The owners invariably increase the insulin dose the following morning, and a continuous cycle of worsening insulin-induced hyperglycemia occurs. Unrecognized short duration of insulin effect combined with insulin dose adjustments based on morning urine glucose concentrations is historically the most common cause for the Somogyi phenomenon and a major reason why we do not recommend insulin dose adjustments based on morning urine glucose readings.

Clinical signs of hypoglycemia are typically mild or not recognized by the owner; clinical signs caused by hyperglycemia tend to dominate the clinical picture. The insulin dose that induces the Somogyi phenomenon is variable and unpredictable. The Somogyi phenomenon is often suspected in poorly controlled diabetic dogs whose insulin dosage is approaching 2.2 U/kg body weight/injection but can also occur at insulin dosages less than 0.5 U/kg/injection. Toy and miniature breeds of dogs are especially susceptible to development of the Somogyi phenomenon with lower-than-expected doses of insulin. The Somogyi phenomenon should always be suspected in any poorly controlled diabetic dog or cat, regardless of the amount of insulin being administered.

The diagnosis of the Somogyi phenomenon requires demonstration of hypoglycemia (<65 mg/dl) followed by hyperglycemia (>300 mg/dl) following insulin administration (Feldman and Nelson, 1982). The Somogyi phenomenon should also be suspected when the blood glucose concentration decreases rapidly regardless of the glucose nadir (e.g., a drop from 400 to 100 mg/dl in 2 to 3 hours). If the duration of insulin effect is greater than 12 hours, hypoglycemia often occurs at night following the evening dose of insulin and the serum glucose concentration is typically greater than 300 mg/dl the next morning (Fig. 11-18). Serum fructosamine concentrations are unpredictable in dogs with the Somogyi phenomenon, ranging from 300 to greater than 600 µmol/l (see Fig. 11-10). Values below 400 µmol/l in diabetic dogs with suspected poor control of glycemia suggest the Somogyi phenomenon. High serum fructosamine values identify poor control of glycemia but are not helpful in identifying the cause. The Somogyi phenomenon should be included in the list of causes for high serum fructosamine concentrations.

Unfortunately, the diagnosis of the Somogyi phenomenon can be elusive, in part because of the effects of the diabetogenic hormones on blood glucose concentrations following an episode of glucose counter-regulation. Secretion of diabetogenic hormones during the Somogyi phenomenon may induce insulin resistance, which can last 24 to 72 hours after the hypoglycemic episode. If a serial blood glucose curve is obtained on the day glucose counterregulation occurs, hypoglycemia will be identified and the diagnosis established. However, if the serial blood glucose curve is obtained on a day when insulin resistance predominates, hypoglycemia will not be identified and the insulin dose may be incorrectly increased in response to the high blood glucose values (see Fig. 12-21, page 570). Sometimes the diagnosis is established through response to treatment, that is, improvement in clinical signs when the insulin dose is decreased despite the high blood glucose values identified on the serial blood glucose curve. See page 617 for more information on insulin resistance induced by the Somogyi phenomenon.

Therapy involves reducing the insulin dose. The reduction in insulin dosage depends on the amount of insulin given at the time the Somogyi phenomenon is diagnosed. If the diabetic dog is receiving an "acceptable" dose of insulin (i.e., ≤1.0 U/kg/injection), the insulin dosage should be decreased 10% to 25%. If the insulin dose exceeds these amounts, glycemic regulation should be reinitiated using the insulin dosage recommended for the initial regulation of the diabetic dog (i.e., 0.25 U/kg given twice daily).

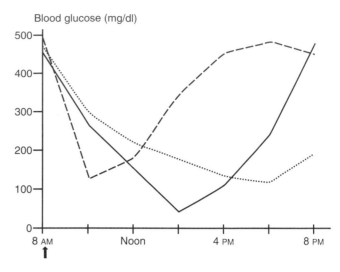

FIGURE 11-18. Blood glucose concentration curves obtained from 3 poorly controlled diabetic dogs treated with recombinant human lente insulin twice a day, illustrating the typical blood glucose curves suggestive of the Somogyi phenomenon. In one dog (*solid line*), the glucose nadir is less than 80 mg/dl and is followed by a rapid increase in the blood glucose concentration. In one dog (*dashed line*), a rapid decrease in the blood glucose concentration occurs within 2 hours of insulin administration and is followed by a rapid increase in the blood glucose concentration; the rapid decrease in blood glucose stimulates glucose counterregulation despite maintaining the blood glucose nadir above 80 mg/dl. In one dog (*dotted line*), the blood glucose curve is not suggestive of the Somogyi phenomenon, per se. However, the insulin injection causes the blood glucose to decrease by approximately 300 mg/dl during the day, and the blood glucose concentration at the time of the evening insulin injection is considerably lowering than the 8 AM blood glucose concentration. If a similar decrease in the blood glucose occurs with the evening insulin injection, hypoglycemia and the Somogyi phenomenon would occur at night and would explain the high blood glucose concentration in the morning and the poor control of the diabetic state. (From Nelson RW, Couto CG: Small Animal Internal Medicine, 3rd ed. St Louis, Mosby Inc, 2003, p 745.)

Evaluation of glycemic control (see page 508) should be done 1 to 2 weeks after initiating the new dose of insulin and further adjustments in the insulin dose made accordingly.

Short Duration of Insulin Effect

For most dogs, the duration of effect of recombinant human lente and NPH insulin is 10 to 14 hours and twice-a-day insulin administration is effective in controlling blood glucose concentrations (see Fig. 11-6). However, in some diabetic dogs, the duration of effect of lente and NPH insulin is less than 10 hours, a duration that is too short to prevent periods of hyperglycemia and persistence of clinical signs. Diabetic dogs with the problem of short duration of insulin effect have persistent morning glycosuria (>1 g/dl on urine glucose test strips). Owners of these pets usually mention continuing problems with evening polyuria and polydipsia or weight loss. If owners are adjusting the daily insulin dosage based on the morning urine glucose concentration, they usually induce the Somogyi phenomenon as the insulin dosage is gradually increased in response to persistent morning glycosuria. Serum fructosamine concentrations are variable but typically greater than 500 μmol/L. The diagnosis of short duration of insulin effect is made by demonstrating recurrence of hyperglycemia (>250 mg/dl) within 6 to 10 hours of the insulin injection, whereas the lowest blood glucose concentration is maintained above 80 mg/dl (see Fig. 11-16). The clinician must evaluate multiple blood glucose concentrations obtained throughout the day to establish the diagnosis (see page 511). One or two afternoon blood glucose determinations consistently fail to identify the problem. They may identify normal glucose concentrations or mild hyperglycemia, findings that are not consistent with the worries of the owner and do not identify the underlying problem. Alternatively, one or two afternoon blood glucose determinations may reveal severe hyperglycemia, findings that do not differentiate short duration of insulin effect from the Somogyi phenomenon or insulin resistance. Diabetic dogs that have a short duration of insulin effect can be diagnosed only by determining serial blood glucose concentrations. Treatment involves changing to a longer-acting insulin given twice daily (e.g., switching to ultralente or insulin glargine) (Fig. 11-19) or increasing the frequency of insulin administration (i.e., initiating TID therapy) if the duration of effect is less than 8 hours. PZI insulin of beef/pork source is not recommended in dogs because of potential problems with insulin antibodies (see below). Evaluation of glycemic control (see page 508) should be done 1 to 2 weeks after initiating the new dose of insulin and further adjustments in the insulin dose made accordingly. Refer to Interpretation of the Serial Blood Glucose Curve, page 514, for more information on the diagnosis and treatment of short duration of insulin effect.

Prolonged Duration of Insulin Effect

In some diabetic dogs, the duration of effect of lente and NPH insulin is greater than 12 hours, and twice-a-day insulin administration creates problems with hypoglycemia and the Somogyi phenomenon. In these dogs, the glucose nadir following the morning administration of insulin typically occurs near the time of the evening insulin administration, and the morning blood glucose concentration is usually greater than 300 mg/dl (see Fig. 11-16). Gradually decreasing blood glucose concentrations measured at the time of sequential insulin injections is another indication of prolonged duration of insulin effect. The effectiveness of insulin in lowering the blood glucose concentration is variable from day to day, presumably because of varying concentrations of diabetogenic hormones whose secretion was induced by prior hypoglycemia. Serum fructosamine concentrations are variable but typically greater than 500 μmol/L. An effective treatment depends, in part, on the duration of effect of the insulin. A 24-hour blood glucose curve should be generated following administration of insulin once in the morning and feeding the dog at the normal times of the day. This will allow the clinician to estimate the duration of effect of the insulin (see Interpreting the Serial Blood Glucose Curve, page 514). If the duration of effect is less than 16 hours, a shorter-acting insulin given twice a day or a lower dose of the same insulin given in the evening, compared with the morning insulin dose, can be tried (see Fig. 11-19). If the duration of effect is 16 hours or longer, switching to a longer-acting insulin administered once a day or administering NPH or lente insulin in the morning and regular insulin at bedtime (i.e., 16 to 18 hours after the morning insulin injection) can be tried. When using different types of insulin in the

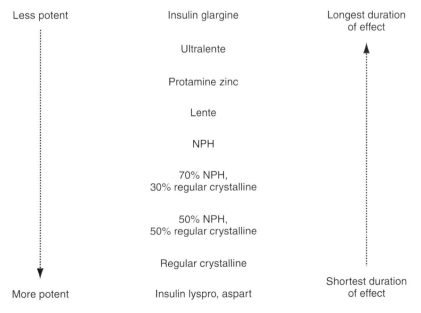

FIGURE 11-19. Categorization of types of commercial insulin based on the potency and duration of effect. Notice the inverse relationship between the potency and duration of effect. (From Nelson RW, Couto CG: Small Animal Internal Medicine, 3rd ed. St Louis, Mosby Inc, 2003, p 747.)

same 24-hour period, the goal is to have the combined duration of effect of the insulins equal 24 hours. For example, if the duration of effect of lente insulin is approximately 16 hours and regular insulin is 6 to 8 hours, the combination of the two insulins is approximately 22 to 24 hours. Differences in potency of intermediate- and long-acting insulins versus regular insulin often necessitates use of different dosages for the morning and evening insulin injection; regular insulin is more potent, and less of it is required to get the same glycemic effect, compared with lente, NPH, and ultralente insulin.

Inadequate Insulin Absorption

Slow or inadequate absorption of subcutaneously deposited insulin is an uncommon problem in diabetic

dogs treated with NPH or lente insulin but is a potential concern with ultralente and insulin glargine. See page 571 for information on inadequate absorption of longer-acting insulins.

Circulating Anti-Insulin Antibodies

Although all species of commercial insulin are effective in diabetic dogs, insulin immunogenicity and production of insulin antibodies can enhance and prolong the pharmacodynamic action of insulin by serving as a carrier, or they can reduce insulin action by neutralization (Bolli et al, 1984; Marshall et al, 1988; Lahtela et al, 1997). Antibodies may also have no apparent clinical effect on insulin dosage or status of glycemic control (Lindholm et al, 2002). In our experience, anti-insulin antibody production in diabetic dogs

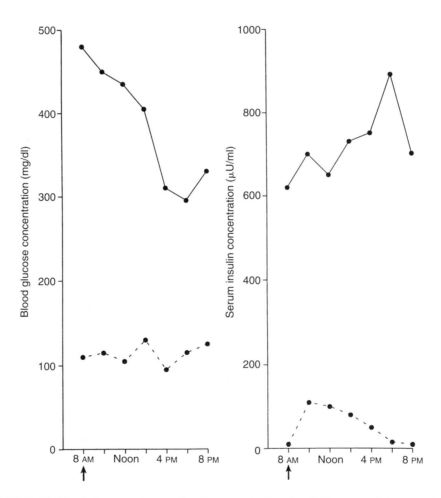

FIGURE 11-20. Blood glucose and serum insulin concentrations in a 7.6-kg, spayed dog receiving 1.1 U/kg beef/pork source lente insulin *(solid line)* SC. The dog had severe polyuria, polydipsia, and weight loss. A baseline serum insulin concentration was greater than 1000 μU/ml 48 hours after discontinuing insulin therapy. Interference from anti-insulin antibodies was suspected, and the source of insulin was changed to recombinant human insulin. Clinical signs improved within 2 weeks and a blood glucose curve obtained 4 weeks later, with the dog receiving 0.9 U/kg recombinant human lente insulin *(broken line),* showed excellent glycemic control. Presumably, loss of anti-insulin antibody interference with the insulin radioimmunoassay allowed a more accurate assessment of changes in the serum insulin concentration after recombinant human insulin administration. ↑ = insulin injection and food.

can have a deleterious impact on insulin effectiveness, hamper the ability to maintain control of glycemia, and in extreme cases, cause severe insulin resistance (Fig. 11-20). Insulin antibodies can also cause erratic fluctuations in the blood glucose concentration, with no correlation between the timing of insulin administration and changes in blood glucose concentration (Fig. 11-21). Presumably, fluctuations in blood glucose concentration result from erratic and unpredictable changes in the circulating free (i.e., non–antibody-bound) insulin concentration (Bolli et al, 1984). This phenomenon causes inappropriate and potentially life-threatening hypoglycemia at unexpected times in humans with diabetes. We have observed a similar syndrome in diabetic dogs treated with beef/pork insulin.

Insulin antibodies result from repeated injections of a foreign protein (i.e., insulin). The structure and amino acid sequence of the injected insulin relative to the native endogenous insulin influences the development of anti-insulin antibodies. Conformational insulin epitopes are believed to be more important in the development of anti-insulin antibodies than differences in the linear subunits of the insulin molecule, per se (Thomas et al, 1985; Thomas et al, 1988; Nell and Thomas, 1989; Davison et al, 2001). Nevertheless, the more divergent the insulin molecule being administered from the species being treated, the greater the likelihood that significant or worrisome amounts of insulin antibodies will be formed. The amino acid sequence of canine, porcine, and recombinant human insulin are similar, suggesting that recombinant human insulin should not be strongly antigenic when administered to diabetic dogs (Feldman et al, 1983; Ganong, 1991). Studies using an ELISA to detect insulin antibodies in serum of insulin-treated diabetic dogs identified serum insulin antibodies in approximately 5% of dogs treated with recombinant human insulin (Harb-Hauser et al, 1998). In contrast, the amino acid sequences of canine and beef insulin differ, and serum insulin antibodies have been identified in approximately 40% and 50% of dogs treated with beef/pork-source insulin (which is 90% beef insulin) (Haines, 1986; Harb-Hauser et al, 1998) and 65% of dogs treated with bovine insulin (Davison et al, 2003). In our experience, the presence of serum insulin antibodies in these dogs was associated with erratic and often poor control of glycemia, an inability to maintain control of glycemia for extended periods of time, frequent adjustments in insulin dose and occasional development of severe insulin resistance (i.e., blood glucose concentrations consistently >400 mg/dl). Dogs treated with recombinant human insulin consistently had more stable control of glycemia for extended periods of time. In fact, ELISA titers reverted to negative and glycemic control improved by 4 to 6 weeks after changing from beef/pork to human recombinant insulin in insulin antibody–positive dogs. Recombinant human-source insulin should be used in diabetic dogs to avoid problems with insulin effectiveness presumably caused by circulating insulin antibodies.

Although uncommon, insulin antibody formation should be suspected in poorly controlled diabetic dogs treated with recombinant human insulin in which another cause for the poor glycemic control cannot be identified. Documentation of serum insulin–binding antibodies should use assays that have been validated in diabetic dogs, assays that are currently not readily available commercially. However, circulating insulin antibodies may interfere with some RIA techniques used to measure serum insulin concentration in a manner similar to the effects of thyroid hormone antibodies on RIA techniques for serum T_3 and T_4 concentrations (see Fig. 3-14, page 112). This interference can be used to raise the clinician's index of suspicion for insulin-binding antibodies as a cause for insulin resistance. A single-phase separation system using antibody-coated tubes is used in our laboratory to measure serum insulin concentration. The presence of insulin antibodies in the serum sample causes spuriously high insulin values using this RIA. The

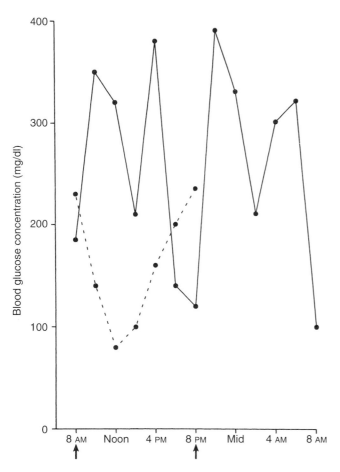

FIGURE 11-21. Blood glucose curve in a 50-kg male dog receiving 0.7 U/kg beef/pork source lente insulin *(solid line)* SC. Note the erratic fluctuations in the blood glucose concentration. The dog had polyuria, polydipsia, and weight loss and was blind from cataract formation. A baseline serum insulin concentration was 825 µU/ml 24 hours after discontinuing insulin therapy. Interference from anti-insulin antibodies was suspected, and the source of insulin was changed to recombinant human insulin. Clinical signs improved within 1 month and a blood glucose curve obtained 8 weeks later, with the dog receiving 0.5 U/kg recombinant human lente insulin *(broken line),* showed excellent glycemic control and loss of erratic fluctuations in the blood glucose concentration.

serum insulin concentration is typically less than 50 µU/ml 24 hours after insulin administration in diabetic dogs and cats without antibodies causing interference with the RIA. In contrast, serum insulin concentrations are typically greater than 400 µU/ml and may be greater than 1000 µU/ml 24 hours after insulin administration when insulin antibodies interfere with the RIA results; insulin values are erroneously increased because of the antibodies (see Fig. 11-20). A switch to purified porcine insulin, a switch to a purer form of insulin (i.e., regular crystalline insulin), or both, should be considered if insulin antibodies are identified in a diabetic dog being treated with recombinant human insulin. Because regular crystalline insulin has a duration of effect of approximately 6 to 8 hours when injected subcutaneously, it should be administered every 8 hours when used to treat diabetic dogs or cats at home.

Allergic Reactions to Insulin

Significant allergic reactions to insulin occur in up to 5% of human diabetics treated with insulin and include erythema, pruritus, induration at the injection site, and uncommonly, systemic manifestations characterized by urticaria, angioneurotic edema, or frank anaphylaxis (Unger and Foster, 1998). Atrophy or hypertrophy of subcutaneous tissue (i.e., lipoatrophy and lipodystrophy) may also occur at the insulin injection site. Many humans with insulin allergy have histories of sensitivity to other drugs as well. Allergic reactions to insulin have been poorly documented in diabetic dogs and cats. Pain on injection of insulin is usually caused by inappropriate injection technique or site of injection and not an adverse reaction to insulin, per se. Chronic injection of insulin in the same area of the body may cause inflammation and thickening of the skin and subcutaneous tissues and may be caused by an immune reaction to insulin or some other protein (e.g., protamine) in the insulin bottle. Inflammation and thickening of the skin and subcutaneous tissues may impair insulin absorption, resulting in recurrence of clinical signs of diabetes. Rotation of the injection site will help prevent this problem. Rarely, diabetic dogs and cats will develop focal subcutaneous edema and swelling at the site of insulin injection. Insulin allergy is suspected in these animals. Treatment includes switching to a more homologous insulin (purified porcine insulin for dogs, purified beef insulin for cats) and to a more purified insulin preparation (e.g., regular crystalline insulin) in the hopes of minimizing a potential immune reaction to the species of insulin or some contaminant in the insulin preparation. We have not yet confirmed systemic allergic reactions to insulin in dogs or cats.

Concurrent Disorders Causing Insulin Resistance

Insulin resistance is a condition in which a normal amount of insulin produces a subnormal biologic response. Insulin resistance may result from problems occurring before the interaction of insulin with its receptor (i.e., prereceptor), at the receptor, or at steps distal to the interaction of insulin and its receptor (i.e., postreceptor) (Ihle and Nelson, 1991). Prereceptor problems reduce free metabolically active insulin concentration and include increased insulin degradation and insulin-binding antibodies. Receptor problems include alterations in insulin-receptor binding affinity and concentration and insulin-receptor antibodies. Postreceptor problems are difficult to differentiate clinically from receptor problems, and both often coexist. In dogs and cats, receptor and postreceptor abnormalities are usually attributable to obesity or a disorder causing excessive secretion of an insulin-antagonistic hormone, such as cortisol, glucagon, epinephrine, growth hormone, progesterone, or thyroid hormone.

No insulin dose clearly defines insulin resistance. When insulin effectiveness in a diabetic dog is being assessed, the insulin dose relative to body weight and adequacy of glycemic control should be evaluated simultaneously. For most diabetic dogs, good glycemic control (i.e., blood glucose concentration between 100 and 250 mg/dl) can be achieved with less than 1.0 U of intermediate or long-acting insulin per kilogram of body weight given twice daily. Insulin resistance should be suspected if control of glycemia is poor despite an insulin dosage in excess of 1.5 U/kg, when excessive amounts of insulin (i.e., insulin dosage >1.5 U/kg) are necessary to maintain the blood glucose concentration below 300 mg/dl (Fig. 11-22), and when control of glycemia is erratic and insulin requirements are constantly changing every few weeks in an attempt to maintain control of glycemia (Fig. 11-23). Failure of the blood glucose concentration to decrease below 300 mg/dl during a serial blood glucose curve is suggestive of, but not definitive for, the presence of insulin resistance. An insulin resistance–type blood glucose curve can also result from stress-induced hyperglycemia, the Somogyi phenomenon, and other problems with insulin therapy (Table 11-16), and a

TABLE 11-16   RECOGNIZED CAUSES OF INSULIN INEFFECTIVENESS OR INSULIN RESISTANCE IN DIABETIC DOGS AND CATS

Caused by Insulin Therapy	Caused by Concurrent Disorder
Inactive insulin	Diabetogenic drugs
Diluted insulin	Hyperadrenocorticism
Improper administration technique	Diestrus (bitch)
	Acromegaly (cat)
Inadequate dose	Infection, especially of oral cavity and urinary tract
Somogyi effect	
Inadequate frequency of insulin administration	Hypothyroidism (dog)
	Hyperthyroidism (cat)
Impaired insulin absorption, especially ultralente insulin	Renal insufficiency
	Liver insufficiency
Anti-insulin antibody excess	Cardiac insufficiency
	Glucagonoma (dog)
	Pheochromocytoma
	Chronic inflammation, especially pancreatitis
	Pancreatic exocrine insufficiency
	Severe obesity
	Hyperlipidemia
	Neoplasia

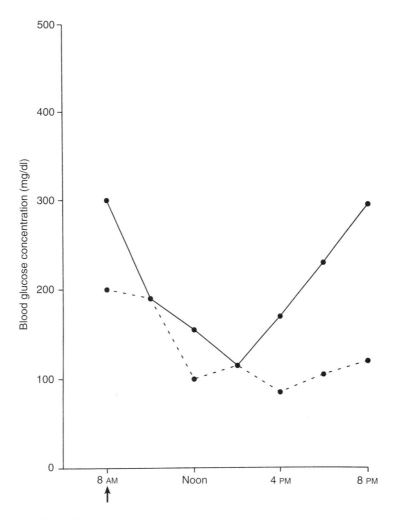

FIGURE 11-22. Blood glucose curve in a 12-kg male diabetic dog with untreated hypothyroidism receiving 2.2 U/kg recombinant human lente insulin *(solid line)*. The large amount of insulin required to lower the blood glucose concentration suggests insulin resistance. Glycemic control was improved and the insulin dosage decreased to 0.9 U/kg after sodium levothyroxine therapy was initiated *(broken line)*. ↑ = SC insulin injection and food.

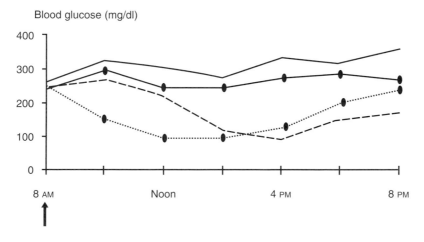

FIGURE 11-23. Blood glucose curves in a 9-year-old diabetic cat with recurring clinical signs of chronic pancreatitis. The cat developed lethargy, inappetence, polyuria, polydipsia, and weight loss, and blood glucose concentrations were increased *(solid lines)* when pancreatitis was symptomatic. Clinical signs were absent and blood glucose concentrations were in an acceptable range *(broken lines)* when pancreatitis was quiescent. Blood glucose curves were obtained when the cat was receiving 4 units ultralente insulin *(solid and broken lines - no circles)* SC twice a day and 3 units lente insulin *(solid and broken lines - solid circles)* SC twice a day. Note the negative impact of pancreatitis on glycemic control. ↑ = SC insulin injection and food.

decrease in the blood glucose concentration below 300 mg/dl can occur with disorders causing relatively mild insulin resistance. Serum fructosamine concentrations are typically greater than 500 µmol/L in animals with insulin resistance and can exceed 700 µmol/L if insulin resistance is persistent and severe. Unfortunately, an increased serum fructosamine concentration is merely indicative of poor glycemic control not insulin resistance, per se.

The severity of insulin resistance is dependent, in part, on the underlying etiology. Insulin resistance may be mild and easily overcome by increasing the dosage of insulin or may be severe, causing marked hyperglycemia regardless of the type and dosage of insulin administered. Some causes of insulin resistance are readily apparent at the time diabetes is diagnosed, such as obesity and the administration of insulin-antagonistic drugs (e.g., glucocorticoids, megestrol acetate). Other causes of insulin resistance are not readily apparent and require an extensive diagnostic evaluation to be identified. In general, any concurrent inflammatory, infectious, hormonal, or neoplastic disorder can cause insulin resistance and interfere with the effectiveness of insulin therapy (see Table 11-16). In our experience, the most common concurrent disorders interfering with insulin effectiveness in dogs include diabetogenic drugs (glucocorticoids), severe obesity, hyperadrenocorticism, diestrus, chronic pancreatitis, renal insufficiency, oral, skin, and urinary tract infections, hyperlipidemia, and anti-insulin antibodies in dogs receiving beef insulin. Obtaining a complete history and performing a thorough physical examination is the most important step in identifying these concurrent disorders. Is the dog severely obese? Is the dog taking any medications that may have insulin-antagonistic properties? Has the female diabetic dog been spayed, and if not, when was the last estrus observed? Has the owner noticed any clinical signs that may suggest concurrent infection (e.g., hematuria, vaginal discharge)? Abnormalities identified on a thorough physical examination may suggest a concurrent insulin-antagonistic disorder or infectious process, which will give the clinician direction in the diagnostic evaluation of the animal. If the history and physical examination are unremarkable, a CBC, serum biochemical analysis, serum progesterone concentration (intact female dog), abdominal ultrasound, and urinalysis with bacterial culture should be obtained to further screen for concurrent illness. Additional tests will be dependent on the results of the initial screening tests (Table 11-17).

OBESITY. Obesity causes a reversible insulin resistance secondary to obesity-induced downregulation of insulin receptors, reduced insulin-receptor binding affinity, and intracellular, postreceptor defects in glucose metabolism (Truglia et al, 1985). Weight reduction improves tissue responsiveness to insulin, presumably via improvement in obesity-induced insulin resistance. Whenever possible, correction of obesity through dietary modifications (see page 501) and exercise should be attempted. Glycemic control may improve if persistent hyperglycemia is caused by

TABLE 11-17 DIAGNOSTIC TESTS TO CONSIDER FOR THE EVALUATION OF INSULIN RESISTANCE IN DIABETIC DOGS AND CATS

CBC, serum biochemistry panel, urinalysis
Bacterial culture of the urine
Serum lipase and amylase activities (pancreatitis)
Serum trypsin-like immunoreactivity (exocrine pancreatic insufficiency, pancreatitis)
Adrenocortical function tests
  ACTH stimulation test (spontaneous or iatrogenic hyperadrenocorticism)
  Low-dose dexamethasone suppression test (spontaneous hyperadrenocorticism)
Thyroid function tests
  Baseline serum total and free thyroxine (hypothyroidism or hyperthyroidism)
  Endogenous TSH (hypothyroidism)
  Thyroid-stimulating hormone stimulation test (hypothyroidism)
  Thyroid-releasing hormone stimulation test (hypothyroidism or hyperthyroidism)
  Triiodothyronine suppression test (hyperthyroidism)
Serum progesterone concentration (diestrus in intact female dog)
Plasma growth hormone or serum insulin-like growth factor I concentration (acromegaly)
Serum insulin concentration 24 hours after discontinuation of insulin therapy (insulin antibodies)
Serum triglyceride concentration (hyperlipidemia)
Abdominal ultrasonography (adrenomegaly, adrenal mass, pancreatitis, pancreatic mass)
Thoracic radiography (cardiomegaly, neoplasia)
Computed tomography or magnetic resonance imaging (pituitary mass)

a combination of obesity, inappropriate diet, and problems with insulin therapy. However, improvement in blood glucose concentrations is unlikely if insulin resistance is caused by concurrent inflammatory, infectious, neoplastic, or hormonal disorders.

PROGESTOGENS. Insulin resistance induced by diestrus should *always* be suspected in any newly diagnosed or poorly controlled intact diabetic female dog, regardless of the history concerning estrus activity. The diestrual increase in blood progesterone concentration has a direct insulin-antagonistic effect and also stimulates secretion of growth hormone. Progesterone reduces insulin binding and glucose transport in tissues (Ryan and Enns, 1988). The insulin-antagonistic effects of growth hormone result from a decrease in the number of insulin receptors and inhibition of glucose transport, possibly through effects on the expression of glucose-transporter genes (Moller and Flier, 1991). Administration of progestogens (e.g., medroxyprogesterone acetate) in the dog also stimulates growth hormone secretion (Eigenmann and Rijnberk, 1981; Eigenmann et al, 1983).

Diestrus-induced insulin resistance quickly becomes severe as plasma growth hormone concentrations increase in response to progesterone secretion from the corpora lutea. Insulin quickly becomes ineffective in lowering the blood glucose concentration, despite the administration of insulin dosages well in excess of 2.2 U/kg/injection. Life-threatening diabetic ketoacidosis can develop. Rapid identification of increased serum progesterone concentration followed by ovario-

TABLE 11-18 FREQUENCY OF OCCURRENCE OF CAUSES OF INSULIN RESISTANCE IN 65 DIABETIC DOGS AND 54 DIABETIC CATS RANDOMLY EVALUATED FROM UC DAVIS RECORDS BETWEEN 1990 AND 1995

Cause	Diabetic Dogs	Diabetic Cats
Hyperadrenocorticism	38%	17%
Acromegaly	–	19%
Bacterial infection	16%	9%
Diestrus	8%	–
Renal, hepatic, cardiac insufficiency	6%	15%
Hypothyroidism	9%	–
Hyperthyroidism	–	9%
Diabetogenic drugs	3%	9%
Chronic pancreatitis	5%	6%
Exocrine pancreatic insufficiency	5%	4%
Anti-insulin antibodies	5%	2%
Glucagonoma	4%	–
Pheochromocytoma	2%	–
Miscellaneous neoplasia	–	9%

hysterectomy is strongly recommended, especially if diabetic ketoacidosis is present. For most commercial endocrine laboratories, a serum progesterone concentration greater than 2 ng/ml is consistent with diestrus. The stimulus for growth hormone secretion declines once the blood progesterone concentration returns to anestrus levels, following either spontaneous regression of the corpora lutea, ovariohysterectomy, or withdrawal of progestogen therapy. Improvement in insulin effectiveness typically occurs within 7 days after ovariohysterectomy or withdrawal of progestogens. Carbohydrate intolerance may resolve in bitches with adequate numbers of functional beta cells once growth hormone returns to normal baseline concentration (see Secondary Diabetes in Dogs, page 490).

HYPERADRENOCORTICISM. Hyperadrenocorticism, whether naturally occurring or due to exogenous glucocorticoid administration, is the most common cause of severe insulin resistance in diabetic dogs (Table 11-18). Glucocorticoids antagonize the actions of insulin in both hepatic and peripheral cells. Glucocorticoids may induce insulin resistance directly by reducing the number or efficacy of glucose transporters and indirectly by increasing the circulating levels of glucagon and free fatty acids (Moller and Flier, 1991). The decreased cellular use of glucose induced by glucocorticoids does not involve changes at the level of the insulin receptor.

Naturally occurring hyperadrenocorticism and diabetes mellitus are common concurrent diseases in the dog. The question is often raised: which disorder came first? Although the answer to this question is not known, we suspect that hyperadrenocorticism develops initially and subclinical diabetes mellitus becomes clinically apparent as a result of the insulin resistance caused by the hyperadrenal state. Invariably diabetes mellitus is diagnosed first, in part because the initial diagnostic evaluation for polyuria and polydipsia includes evaluation of a CBC, serum biochemistry panel, and urinalysis. Hyperglycemia and glycosuria are readily apparent in the results. Physical findings suggestive of hyperadrenocorticism, such as endocrine alopecia, thin skin, and abdominal enlargement, are usually not apparent at the time diabetes is diagnosed but often become apparent weeks later as the severity of hyperadrenocorticism progresses. In addition, hepatomegaly, hypercholesterolemia, and hepatic enzyme alterations are quickly ascribed to the diabetic state. Early indicators for possible hyperadrenocorticism in diabetic dogs include a serum alkaline phosphatase activity greater than 500 IU/L, urine specific gravity less than 1.020 (especially in the presence of glycosuria), and adrenomegaly on abdominal ultrasound. Glycemic control in diabetic dogs with untreated hyperadrenocorticism is variable and dependent, in part, on the severity and duration of hypercortisolemia. Diabetic dogs presumably in the early stages of hyperadrenocorticism may be responsive to insulin and initially well-controlled with typical doses of insulin. However, during the ensuing months, control of glycemia becomes progressively more difficult, and eventually severe insulin resistance develops. Hyperadrenocorticism should always be considered in any poorly controlled diabetic dog in which problems with the insulin treatment regimen are not readily apparent, regardless of the findings on physical examination and routine diagnostic tests.

When interpreting results of tests of the pituitary-adrenocortical axis (e.g., ACTH stimulation test, low-dose dexamethasone suppression test, urine cortisol: creatinine ratio), the influence of poorly regulated diabetes mellitus on adrenocortical function and results of these diagnostic tests should be considered. Although one study found normal adrenal function test results in 15 well-regulated diabetic dogs (Zerbe et al, 1988), many of our poorly regulated diabetic dogs have had one or more adrenal function test results suggestive of hyperadrenocorticism despite normal pituitary and adrenal glands at necropsy. A mildly exaggerated response to ACTH administration (i.e., post-ACTH cortisol, 18 to 24 μg/dl), an increased urine cortisol: creatinine ratio, and less commonly, failure of plasma cortisol to suppress to less than 1.5 μg/dl during low-dose dexamethasone suppression testing can occur in poorly regulated (and occasionally well-regulated) diabetic dogs. Presumably, the chronic "stress" related to poorly regulated diabetes mellitus and its associated problems is responsible for these results. Because of the potential interplay between the stress of poorly regulated diabetes mellitus and results of tests of the pituitary-adrenocortical axis, the diagnosis of hyperadrenocorticism should always be based on a combination of history, findings on physical examination, clinical pathologic abnormalities, results of tests of the pituitary-adrenocortical axis, ultrasound evaluation of adrenal size, and clinical suspicion for the disorder. The decision to treat should be based on the etiology (pituitary- versus adrenal-dependent disease), severity of clinical signs and insulin resistance, and status of glycemic control. Treatment may not be indicated at the time pituitary-dependent hyperadrenocorticism is diagnosed, especially if clinical signs are absent, insulin resistance is not apparent, and control of glycemia is good. The reader is referred to Chapter 6 for a complete discussion on the diagnosis and treatment of hyperadrenocorticism in dogs.

BACTERIAL INFECTIONS. The detrimental impact of diabetes on the risk for infection-related morbidity and mortality is well recognized in humans (Bertoni et al, 2001). Infections are also commonly identified in diabetic dogs and cats, suggesting that diabetes causes a similar increased susceptibility of infection in these species (Hess et al, 2000b; Peikes et al, 2001). Proposed mechanisms for the increased susceptibility to infections in diabetics include decreased blood supply secondary to the associated microangiopathy and atherosclerosis, resulting in decreased delivery of oxygen, phagocytes, and antibodies to the site of infection; impaired humoral immunity, resulting in decreased antibody production; abnormal chemotaxis of neutrophils; defects in the phagocytosis and intracellular killing of organisms; and impaired cell-mediated immunity (Possilli and Leslie, 1994; McMahon and Abistrian, 1995; Joshi et al, 1999). Many of these host defense abnormalities improve, at least partially, with better glycemic control.

Sustained hyperglucagonemia and insulin resistance have been documented in diabetic humans with bacterial infections (Nelson, 1989). The anti-insulin effects of glucagon are confined largely to the liver (i.e., stimulation of hepatic gluconeogenesis, glycogenolysis, and ketogenesis), although impaired glucose transport has also been described in peripheral tissues (Moller and Flier, 1991). The clinical significance of glucagon in insulin resistance in the diabetic dog and cat remains to be clarified. Clinically, correction of concurrent severe bacterial infection (most notably affecting the urinary tract, skin, and oral cavity) has improved glycemic control.

Bacterial infections are usually identified during the physical examination or following evaluation of the CBC, urinalysis, urine culture, and rarely, blood cultures. Because of the relatively high incidence of bacterial infections in diabetic dogs and cats, evaluation of the effect of trial antibiotic therapy on improving glycemic control should be considered when a cause for insulin resistance is not identified. Under these circumstances, a broad-spectrum, bactericidal antibiotic (e.g., amoxicillin-clavulanate) should be administered for 10 to 14 days and glycemic control reevaluated before antibiotic therapy is discontinued.

RENAL INSUFFICIENCY. Renal insufficiency and diabetes mellitus are common geriatric diseases and often occur concurrently, especially in older cats. Abnormal renal function may result from the deleterious effects of the diabetic state (i.e., diabetic nephropathy; see page 532) or may be an independent problem that has developed in conjunction with diabetes in the geriatric pet. As renal function declines, human diabetics with concurrent nephropathy are at increased risk for severe hypoglycemia as a result of decreased renal clearance of insulin and decreased renal glucose production by gluconeogenesis (see page 617) (Stumvoll et al, 1997; Rave et al, 2001). Tissue responsiveness to insulin (i.e., insulin sensitivity) is also attenuated, resulting in poorer metabolic control of the diabetic state (Eidemak et al, 1995). Prolonged duration of insulin effect, insulin resistance, and less commonly, hypoglycemia are recognized problems in diabetic dogs and cats with concurrent renal insufficiency. The interplay between progression and severity of renal insufficiency, severity of insulin resistance, and impairment of insulin clearance creates unpredictable fluctuations in control of glycemia and insulin requirements and frustration for the owner and veterinarian. In addition, reliance on an important indicator of diabetic control (i.e., severity of polyuria and polydipsia) is no longer reliable because of the concurrent renal insufficiency. In most cases, treatment for renal insufficiency and failure takes priority and insulin therapy is modified, as needed, to attain the best possible control of the diabetic state while trying to avoid hypoglycemia, recognizing that attainment of good control will be difficult and polyuria and polydipsia will persist regardless of the status of glycemic control.

CHRONIC PANCREATITIS. Chronic inflammatory disorders can deleteriously affect glycemic control. The most significant inflammatory disorder in the diabetic dog and cat is pancreatitis. Chronic pancreatitis is identified at necropsy in approximately 35% of diabetic dogs and 50% of diabetic cats (Alejandro et al, 1988; Goosens et al, 1995). Most of these animals have a similar history, characterized by poorly controlled diabetes, fluctuating insulin requirements, blood glucose concentrations often greater than 300 mg/dl, intermittent lethargy and inappetence, and owner concerns that their pet is "just not doing well" (see Fig. 11-23). An inability to correct these problems ultimately leads to euthanasia for many dogs and cats. Documentation of chronic pancreatitis can be difficult and must rely on a combination of clinical signs, physical examination findings, serum lipase concentration, serum trypsin–like immunoreactivity, ultrasound evaluation of the pancreas, and clinical suspicion for the disorder (see Pancreatic Enzymes, page 495). A successful response to therapy, including intravenous fluids, dietary modifications, and anti-inflammatory doses of prednisone, can be difficult to attain, and many of these dogs and cats continue to do poorly

EXOCRINE PANCREATIC INSUFFICIENCY. Exocrine pancreatic insufficiency (EPI) is an uncommon complication of diabetes mellitus, presumably developing as a sequela of chronic pancreatitis. In our experience, most diabetic dogs with EPI are difficult to regulate with insulin; have persistent weight loss despite a ravenous appetite, ultimately becoming emaciated; and defecate increased amounts of soft stools, not the voluminous, rancid stools considered classic for EPI. Mild diffuse thickening of the small intestine may be evident during abdominal palpation. Diagnosis of EPI in the diabetic dog requires evaluation of serum trypsin–like immunoreactivity (TLI), which is low (i.e., <2.5 μg/L)

(Widberg et al, 1999; Widberg and Westermarck, 2002). Treatment with pancreatic enzyme replacement therapy, metronidazole, and if necessary, a highly digestible, low-fat diet has resulted in improvement in clinical signs and glycemic control, often with a reduction in daily insulin requirements.

HYPOTHYROIDISM. Insulin resistance has been documented in diabetic dogs with hypothyroidism, which resolved following correction of the thyroid hormone deficiency (Ford et al, 1993). The mechanisms of carbohydrate intolerance in states of thyroid hormone deficiency are controversial. Most studies agree that a postreceptor defect in insulin-mediated glucose transport and metabolism exists (Arner et al, 1984; Pedersen et al, 1988). The effect of thyroid hormone deficiency on insulin secretion and on insulin receptors is less clear. Depending on the study, insulin secretion may be increased or decreased and insulin receptor concentration and binding affinity may be increased, decreased, or unaffected (Czech et al, 1980; Arner et al, 1984; Pedersen et al, 1988). Other factors associated with hypothyroidism and diabetes mellitus may also contribute to insulin resistance, most notably obesity and hyperlipidemia (see below).

Interpretation of serum thyroxine (T_4) concentrations must take into consideration the status of glycemic control of the dog, the severity of concurrent illness, and the effects these factors may have on thyroid gland function (i.e., euthyroid sick syndrome; see Serum Thyroxine Concentration, page 112). A low serum thyroxine concentration does not, by itself, confirm hypothyroidism in the dog. If hypothyroidism is strongly suspected after evaluation of the history, findings on physical examination, and results of routine blood work and serum T_4 concentration, we evaluate serum free T_4 and thyrotropin (TSH) concentrations before initiating levothyroxine sodium treatment. Refer to Chapter 3 for a more detailed discussion of the effects of concurrent illness and drug therapy on serum thyroid hormone concentrations and the tests used to diagnose hypothyroidism in dogs.

If levothyroxine sodium is administered, a concurrent reduction in insulin dosage should be considered, and glycemic control monitored weekly during the first month of administration (see Fig. 11-22). Further reductions in insulin dosage may be required if hypoglycemia develops as the hypothyroid-induced insulin resistance resolves. In one report on diabetic, hypothyroid dogs, insulin requirements decreased 50% to 60% within 2 weeks after initiating levothyroxine sodium therapy (Ford et al, 1993).

PHEOCHROMOCYTOMA, GLUCAGONOMA, AND OTHER NEOPLASIA. Neoplasia not causing hyperadrenocorticism was believed to contribute to insulin resistance in 5% to 10% of our diabetic dogs (see Table 11-18). Insulin resistance in diabetic dogs with glucagonoma and pheochromocytoma could be explained by excess secretion of the diabetogenic hormones glucagon and catecholamines, respectively. The effects of glucagon on glycemic control and insulin action are discussed in the bacterial infection section above and in Chapter 15.

Catecholamines have both direct and indirect effects to stimulate hepatic glycogenolysis and hepatic and renal gluconeogenesis; provide muscle tissue with an alternative source of fuel by mobilizing muscle glycogen and stimulating lipolysis; mobilize gluconeogenic precursors (e.g., lactate, alanine, and glycerol); and inhibit glucose use by insulin-sensitive tissues such as skeletal muscle (Moller and Flier, 1991; Cryer, 1993; Karam, 2001).

The carbohydrate intolerance that develops in humans with pheochromocytoma is usually mild and does not require therapy, in part because excessive catecholamine secretion is usually episodic, not sustained. Although pheochromocytoma may interfere with the effectiveness of insulin in diabetic dogs, development of severe insulin resistance is uncommon, presumably for the same reasons as in humans, that is, excess catecholamine secretion is usually episodic, not sustained. Identification of a pancreatic or adrenal mass with abdominal ultrasonography should raise suspicion for glucagonoma and pheochromocytoma, respectively, especially if other tests do not support hyperadrenocorticism. Additional diagnostic tests for pheochromocytoma and glucagonoma are discussed in Chapters 9 and 15, respectively.

Lymphoma and mast cell tumor are the most common nonendocrine tumors identified in diabetic dogs and cats with insulin resistance. The mechanisms involved with poor glycemic control of diabetics with nonendocrine tumors are poorly characterized but undoubtedly relate to effects on diabetogenic hormone secretion, hepatic function, lipid metabolism and/or tissue responsiveness to insulin (Vail et al, 1990; Ogilvie et al, 1997).

HYPERTRIGLYCERIDEMIA. Fasting lipemia is common in dogs with diabetes mellitus. Lipemia is caused by hypertriglyceridemia, which has been associated with insulin resistance and carbohydrate intolerance in humans and dogs. Hypertriglyceridemia may impair insulin receptor–binding affinity, promote downregulation of insulin receptors, and cause a postreceptor defect in insulin action (Bieger et al, 1984; Berlinger et al, 1984). Hyperlipidemia-induced increase in hepatic glucose secretion, in conjunction with insulin resistance, worsens carbohydrate intolerance. The insulin resistance caused by hypertriglyceridemia is most commonly appreciated in diabetic dogs that develop hypothyroidism and in diabetic Miniature Schnauzers with idiopathic hyperlipoproteinemia but should be considered in any poorly controlled diabetic dog with persistent lipemia.

Hypertriglyceridemia can be confirmed by measuring serum triglyceride concentration, preferably from a blood sample obtained after a 24-hour fast. In our laboratory, the upper limit of normal for serum triglyceride concentration is 150 mg/dl in healthy dogs. Hypertriglyceridemia may be secondary to other disorders or may be a primary idiopathic hyperlipidemia disorder (see Table 3-10, page 107).

Unfortunately, hypertriglyceridemia is common in poorly regulated diabetic dogs, and the differentiation between hypertriglyceridemia caused by poorly controlled diabetes and hypertriglyceridemia that has developed independent of the diabetic state can be difficult. As a general rule, serum triglyceride concentrations in poorly controlled diabetics are usually less than 500 mg/dl. Serum triglyceride concentrations in excess of 500 mg/dl, especially 800 mg/dl, should raise suspicion for a concurrent disorder causing the hypertriglyceridemia, most notably pancreatitis, hypothyroidism, and primary hyperlipidemic disorders. However, a serum triglyceride concentration less than 800 mg/dl does not rule out a concurrent disorder causing hyperlipidemia (Armstrong and Ford, 1989).

Restriction of dietary fat is the cornerstone of therapy for hypertriglyceridemia. The dietary history should be reviewed and the diet altered to one that contains less than 20% fat on a metabolic energy basis. Treatment with drugs, all of which have the potential for toxicity, should be undertaken with particular care. In general, drugs should not be used in dogs whose serum triglyceride concentration is less than 500 mg/dl. Several classes of drugs are used to treat hypertriglyceridemia in humans, however; there are few reports of their use in dogs. Niacin (100 mg/day) reduces serum triglyceride concentrations by decreasing fatty acid release from adipocytes and reducing the production of VLDL particles. Adverse effects are frequent and include vomiting, diarrhea, erythema, pruritus, and abnormalities in liver function tests. Fibric acid derivatives (clofibrate, bezafibrate, gemfibrozil, ciprofibrate, fenofibrate) lower plasma triglyceride concentrations by stimulating lipoprotein lipase activity, in addition to reducing the free fatty acid concentration, which decreases the substrate for VLDL synthesis (Garg, 1994; Haffner, 1998). In humans, the fibrates generally lower plasma triglyceride concentrations by 20% to 40%. Gemfibrozil has been used in the dog (200 mg/day) (Elliott, 2003). Reported adverse effects include abdominal pain, vomiting, diarrhea, and abnormal liver function tests. The statins (lovastatin, simvastatin, pravastatin, fluvastatin, cerivastatin, atorvastatin) are hydroxymethylglutaryl coenzyme A (HMG-CoA) reductase inhibitors and therefore primarily suppress cholesterol metabolism (Garg and Grundy, 1988; Haffner, 1998). However, in humans, the statins can lower triglyceride concentrations by 10% to 15%. Adverse effects include lethargy, diarrhea, muscle pain, and hepatotoxicity.

INTRINSIC RECEPTOR AND POSTRECEPTOR DEFECTS. Two categories of genetic syndromes causing severe insulin resistance have been described in humans with diabetes. The Type A syndrome of insulin resistance is characterized by marked endogenous hyperinsulinemia, acanthosis nigricans, and (in affected postpubertal women) ovarian hyperandrogenism (Moller and Flier, 1991). Insulin resistance of Type A syndrome is caused by insulin-receptor mutations or other target-cell defects in insulin action. The Type B syndrome of insulin resistance is caused by autoantibodies to the insulin receptor. Typically, humans with this syndrome have uncontrolled diabetes, acanthosis nigricans, and

(in premenopausal women) ovarian hyperandrogenism. Given that antireceptor antibodies can behave as agonists and antagonists, affected humans may have fasting hypoglycemia with or without postprandial hyperglycemia or may alternate among insulin-resistant diabetes, remission, and hypoglycemia (Moller and Flier, 1991). Most patients with the Type B syndrome have clinical or laboratory evidence of systemic autoimmune disease.

Primary insulin receptor and postreceptor defects have yet to be documented in diabetic dogs and cats. Problems in this area should be suspected when all other causes of insulin resistance have been ruled out, insulin absorption following subcutaneous administration has been documented, and minimal improvement in glycemic control has occurred with the use of less antigenic insulin preparations. Therapy is frustrating and usually involves a progressive increase in the insulin dosage to obtain some semblance of glycemic control.

CHRONIC COMPLICATIONS OF DIABETES MELLITUS

Complications resulting from the diabetes (e.g., cataracts) or the therapy (e.g., insulin-induced hypoglycemia) are common in diabetic dogs (see Table 11-7). The most common complications in the dog are blindness and anterior uveitis resulting from cataract formation, chronic pancreatitis, recurring infections, hypoglycemia, and ketoacidosis.

Many owners are hesitant to treat their newly diagnosed diabetic dog because of knowledge regarding chronic complications experienced in human diabetics and concern that a similar fate awaits their pet. The devastating chronic complications of human diabetes (e.g., nephropathy, vasculopathy, coronary artery disease) require 10 to 20 years or longer to develop and therefore are uncommon in diabetic dogs. Diabetes mellitus is a disease of older dogs, and most do not live beyond 5 years from the time of diagnosis. In our experience, owners are usually willing to "tackle" the care of a diabetic pet once the fears related to chronic complications seen in human diabetics are alleviated.

In humans, postulated pathogenetic mechanisms for development of long-term complications (e.g., retinopathy, nephropathy, neuropathy, coronary artery disease) are typically grouped into the following three categories: (1) glucose-related, including abnormalities in polyol (e.g., sorbitol) metabolism and excessive glycation of circulating and membrane-bound proteins; (2) vascular mechanisms, including abnormalities in the endothelium and supporting cells, such as pericytes in the retina and mesangial cells in the glomerulus, as well as hyperfiltration and intrarenal hypertension in the kidney; and (3) other mechanisms, including abnormalities in platelet function and growth factor, as well as genetic influences (Nathan, 1993). Some of the proposed pathogenetic mechanisms apply to only one complication or one stage of a complication. The pathophysiologic mechanisms for chronic complications in diabetic dogs and cats have been poorly characterized but are assumed to be comparable to those in diabetic humans.

Cataracts

Cataract formation is the most common and one of the most important long-term complications of diabetes mellitus in the dog (see Fig. 11-3). Cataracts are highly prevalent in diabetic dogs, in part because many of these animals have significant hyperglycemia despite insulin therapy. A retrospective-cohort study on the development of cataracts in 132 diabetic dogs referred to a university referral hospital found cataract formation in 14% of dogs at the time diabetes was diagnosed; additionally, 25%, 50%, 75% and 80% of the study population developed cataracts within 60, 170, 370, and 470 days of diagnosis, respectively (Beam et al, 1999). In contrast, diabetes-induced cataract formation is rare in cats. Differences in the prevalence of diabetic cataracts between dogs and cats are presumably related to the pathogenesis of diabetic cataract formation, which is thought to be related to altered osmotic relationships in the lens. The lens of the eye is freely permeable to glucose, which enters the lens from the aqueous humor by facilitated transport. Glucose is normally converted to lactic acid via the anaerobic glycolytic pathway; however, with elevated glucose concentrations, the glycolytic enzymes become saturated. Glucose is then metabolized through the polyol pathway to sorbitol and fructose (Feldman and Nelson, 1987). The polyol pathway consists of two consecutive reactions, with glucose first being reduced to sorbitol by aldose reductase and sorbitol subsequently oxidized to fructose by sorbitol dehydrogenase. High glucose concentration in the lens increases the activity of aldose reductase, which enhances glucose metabolism via the polyol pathway (Muirhead and Hothersall, 1995). Because sorbitol and fructose are not freely permeable to the cell membrane, they act as potent hydrophilic agents, causing an influx of water into the lens, leading to swelling and rupture of the lens fibers and the development of cataracts. In vitro studies identified similar glucose uptake by lenses from dogs and cats regardless of age but significantly lower aldose reductase activity in lenses of older cats, compared with lenses of dogs and young cats (Richter et al, 2002). Decreased aldose reductase activity and the high prevalence of diabetes in old cats may explain, in part, why diabetic cataracts are rare in cats.

Cataract formation is an irreversible process once it begins, and it can occur quite rapidly. Clinically, dogs may progress from having normal vision to being blind over a period of days, months, or years. Diabetic dogs that are poorly controlled and have problems with wide fluctuations in the blood glucose concentration seem especially at risk for rapid development of cataracts. Good glycemic control and minimal fluctuation in the blood glucose concentration delays the onset of cataract formation. Once blindness occurs as a result of cataract formation, the need for stringent blood glucose control is reduced.

Blindness may be eliminated by removing the abnormal lens. Vision is restored in approximately 75% to 80% of diabetic dogs that undergo cataract removal. Factors that affect the success of surgery include the degree of glycemic control, the presence of retinal disease, and the presence of lens-induced uveitis. Ideally, glycemic control should be the best possible before surgery, and retinal function should be normal. Acquired retinal degeneration affecting vision is more of a concern in older diabetic dogs than is diabetic retinopathy (see below). Fortunately, acquired retinal degeneration is unlikely in an older diabetic dog with vision immediately before cataract formation. If available, electroretinography should be performed before surgery to evaluate retinal function.

Although a study comparing the postoperative results and complications of phacoemulsification in dogs with and without diabetes mellitus did not find any clinical differences between the two groups (Bagley and Lavach, 1994), we have observed a higher prevalence of postoperative ulcerative keratitis in diabetic versus nondiabetic dogs. Several corneal ulcers were either recurrent or slow to heal. Diabetes mellitus has been associated with pathologic changes in the corneas of dogs, which are directly related to the degree of diabetic control (Yee et al, 1985), and a significant reduction in corneal sensitivity in all regions of the cornea has been documented in diabetic dogs, compared with nondiabetic normoglycemic dogs (Good et al, 2003). Corneal nerves are critical for eliciting and regulating corneal protection via their role in the mediation of tear production and eyelid closure and regulation of corneal collagen expression and epithelial cell function and integrity (Baker et al, 1993; Marfurt, 2000). Corneal sensory deficits are thought to be a component of the diffuse neuropathy affecting the peripheral sensorimotor nervous system of diabetic humans and animals (see page 576) and may have important implications regarding corneal healing and the development of recurrent or nonhealing corneal ulcers in diabetic dogs.

Lens-Induced Uveitis

During embryogenesis, the lens is formed within its own capsule, and its structural proteins are not exposed to the immune system. Therefore immune tolerance to the crystalline proteins does not develop (van der Woerdt et al, 1992). During cataract formation and reabsorption, lens proteins are exposed to local ocular immune systems, resulting in inflammation and uveitis. Uveitis that occurs in association with a reabsorbing, hypermature cataract may decrease the success of cataract surgery and must be controlled before surgery (Bagley and Lavach, 1994). The treatment of lens-induced uveitis focuses on decreasing the inflammation and preventing further intraocular damage. Topical ophthalmic corticosteroids are the most commonly used drug for the control of ocular inflammation. However, systemic absorption of topically applied corticosteroids may cause insulin antagonism and interfere with glycemic control of the diabetic state, especially in toy and miniature breeds. An alternative is the topical administration of nonsteroidal anti-inflammatory agents (e.g., 0.03% flurbiprofen [Ocufen, Allergan Pharmaceuticals, Irvine, CA]) or cyclosporine. Nonsteroidal anti-inflammatory drugs, although not as potent as corticosteroids, do not interfere with glycemic control.

Diabetic Retinopathy

Diabetic retinopathy is an uncommon clinical complication in the dog and cat. There is a close correlation between diabetic retinopathy and suboptimal glycemic control (Engerman and Kern, 1987). Microaneurysms, hemorrhages, and varicose and shunt capillaries may be observed with an ophthalmoscope (Herrtage et al, 1985; Ono et al, 1986). Histologic changes include an increased thickness of the capillary basement membrane, loss of pericytes, capillary shunts, and microaneurysms. The histologic changes are believed to result from retinal ischemia. Factors leading to decreased blood flow in the retina include increased blood viscosity, red blood cell sludging and aggregation, increased levels of fibrinogen, and diminished fibrinolysis (Unger and Foster, 1998). Involvement of polyol pathway activity is controversial, although studies in diabetic dogs suggest that the development of retinopathy is not critically dependent on excessive polyol production or accumulation (Engerman and Kern, 1993). Unfortunately, the rapid development of cataracts often inhibits the ability to evaluate the retina in the dog with diabetes mellitus. Because of the high incidence of cataract formation, the retinas should always be evaluated in the newly diagnosed diabetic pet to ensure normal function and lack of grossly visible disease, should cataract formation and subsequent lens removal become necessary in the future. Lens removal would be unwarranted in a diabetic dog with retinal changes sufficiently severe to result in blindness itself. An electroretinogram can also be used to evaluate the function of the retina prior to cataract surgery.

Diabetic Neuropathy

Although a common complication in the diabetic cat, diabetic neuropathy is infrequently recognized in the diabetic dog (Braund and Steiss, 1982; Katherman and Braund, 1983; Johnson et al, 1983). Subclinical neuropathy is probably more common than severe neuropathy resulting in clinical signs. In our experience, clinical signs consistent with diabetic neuropathy are most commonly recognized in dogs that have been diabetic for a long period of time (i.e., 5 years or longer).

Clinical signs and physical examination findings supportive of a coexistent neuropathy in the diabetic dog include weakness, knuckling, abnormal gait, muscle atrophy, depressed limb reflexes, and deficits in postural reaction testing. Diabetic neuropathy in the dog is primarily a distal polyneuropathy, characterized by segmental demyelination and remyelination and axonal degeneration and regeneration. Electrophysiologic testing may reveal fibrillation potentials and positive sharp waves, suggesting denervated muscle, and occasionally fasciculation potentials and bizarre high-frequency discharges (Steiss et al, 1981). Motor and sensory nerve conduction velocities are also decreased. There is no treatment, per se. See Chapter 12, page 576, for more information on diabetic neuropathy.

Diabetic Nephropathy

Although diabetic nephropathy has occasionally been reported in the dog, its clinical recognition appears to be low. In contrast, renal insufficiency occurs commonly in diabetic cats, being identified in 10 (19%) of 54 cats in one study (Goossens et al, 1995). Histologic evaluation of the kidney revealed glomerulosclerosis in most of these cats. Histopathologic findings in diabetic nephropathy depend on the duration of the disease prior to evaluation of the dog or cat and on the degree of glycemic control. Histologic findings consistent with diabetic nephropathy include membranous glomerulonephropathy with fusion of the foot processes, glomerular and tubular basement membrane thickening, an increase in the mesangial matrix material, the presence of subendothelial deposits, glomerular fibrosis, and glomerulosclerosis (Steffes et al, 1982; Jeraj et al, 1984). The pathogenic mechanism of diabetic nephropathy is unknown, but it probably results from several causes. The initial abnormality may be chronic intraglomerular hypertension and renal hyperperfusion induced by chronic hyperglycemia (Clark and Lee, 1995). Increased glomerular pressure results in the deposition of protein in the mesangium. Glomerular basement membrane thickening has also been ascribed to a rapid increase in membrane production (Unger and Foster, 1998). Mesangial expansion ultimately encroaches on the subendothelial space and the glomerular capillary lumen, causing a decline in glomerular blood flow and filtration and ultimately leading to glomerulosclerosis and renal failure.

Clinical signs depend on the severity of the glomerulosclerosis and the functional ability of the kidney to excrete metabolic wastes. Initially, diabetic nephropathy is manifested as severe proteinuria, primarily albuminuria, as a result of the glomerular dysfunction. As the glomerular changes progress, glomerular filtration becomes progressively impaired, resulting in the development of azotemia and eventually uremia. With severe fibrosis of the glomeruli, oliguric and then anuric renal failure develops. There is no specific treatment of diabetic nephropathy apart from meticulous metabolic control of the diabetic state, conservative medical management of the renal insufficiency, and control of systemic hypertension. The progression of the glomerulosclerosis is related to the degree of glycemic control. There appears to be a definite decrease in the incidence of glomerular microvascular changes with improved glycemic control (Nyberg et al, 1987; Wiseman et al, 1985).

Systemic Hypertension

Diabetes mellitus and hypertension commonly coexist in people. Together, these disorders double the risk for development of life-threatening cardiovascular disease (Sowers and Zemel, 1990). Estimates of the incidence of hypertension in diabetic people range from 40% to 80% and prevalence correlates with duration of diabetes. Control of glycemia appears to influence severity of hypertension; systolic blood pressures are higher in diabetic people with a history of poor control of blood glucose concentration. In a recent study, the prevalence of hypertension was 46% in 50 insulin-treated diabetic dogs, where hypertension was defined as systolic, diastolic, or mean blood pressure greater than 160, 100, and 120 mmHg, respectively (Struble et al, 1998). Hypertension was associated with duration of diabetes and an increased albumin-to-creatinine ratio in the urine. Diastolic and mean blood pressure were higher in dogs with longer duration of disease. A correlation between control of glycemia and blood pressure was not identified.

The mechanisms of hypertension in people with diabetes mellitus is not clear. Hypertension and diabetes-induced alterations, such as sodium retention, vasculopathies, and nephropathy, are thought to increase blood pressure (Weidman et al, 1993). However, it is unclear whether hypertension is the result of existing subclinical renal disease or whether those people with hypertension are more likely to develop nephropathy and microalbuminuria. Possible mechanisms associated with hypertension in diabetic dogs include disturbed lipid metabolism, leading to reduced vascular compliance and generalized glomerular hyperfiltration or an immune-mediated microangiopathy affecting basement membranes (Dukes, 1992).

PANCREATIC ISLET TRANSPLANTATION

Although the life expectancy of humans with IDDM has considerably improved since the availability of exogenous insulin in the 1920s, subcutaneously administered insulin exhibits nonphysiologic pharmacokinetics and fails to reproduce the stimulus-coupled pulsatile secretory responses of normal beta cells. The consequence is an altered state of metabolism that contributes to the chronic complications associated with the disease. During the last decade, remarkable advances have been made in islet cell transplantation. Increasing experimental evidence has shown that transplantation of the endocrine pancreas can normalize blood glucose levels and result in physiologic insulin secretion (Sutherland et al, 1984). The problem of rejection remains the biggest obstacle to successful transplantation. Current research efforts are centered on the prevention of rejection by immunomodulation of the graft and the recipient or by isolation of allografted islets from the host immune system and therapeutic strategies to prevent recurrence of the autoimmune process in the transplanted islet tissue.

Because the major goal of transplantation is prevention or reduction of long-term complications, the value of transplantation in pets must be questioned. Diabetic dogs and cats do not live long enough, even surviving past normal life expectancy, to develop the long-term complications known to occur in humans with IDDM. The reasons for transplantation in pets are, therefore, far less critical in terms of need than they are in humans. However, as the technology improves, application to pets remains a possibility.

WHOLE PANCREAS TRANSPLANTATION. The first human pancreatic transplantation was performed by Kelly and Lillehei in 1966, and since 1980, there has been a dramatic and steady increase in the number of these procedures performed. One of the most common techniques uses a duodenal segment of pancreas anastomosed to the urinary bladder (University of Michigan, 1988; Sutherland et al, 1989; Palmer, 1990). The bladder-drained pancreatic transplant provides a mechanism for eliminating pancreatic exocrine secretions. Urinary amylase concentrations can then be monitored, and a decrease in these concentrations can be found to be a sensitive and early marker of graft rejection. Because of the short-term operative risks, the long-term risks of immunosuppressive therapy, and the inability to accurately predict the 30% to 40% of diabetic patients in whom severe end-organ complications will develop, most physicians restrict pancreas transplantation to patients with end-stage diabetic nephropathy who need a kidney transplant.

Whole pancreas transplantation has been successfully performed in dogs with graft survival of more than 1 year (Alejandro et al, 1988). This procedure has been used exclusively in research, with the pancreatic ducts either surgically drained into the urinary bladder or the exocrine secretions allowed to flow freely into the peritoneal cavity. Owing to a lack of demand by the public, insufficient expertise within the veterinary profession, ethical questions regarding suitable donors, and the significant expense for these procedures (currently approximately $80,000 per transplant in humans), this method of treatment has not been used in clinical veterinary medicine.

PANCREATIC ISLET TRANSPLANTATION. Transplantation of pure islets of Langerhans is an attractive alternative to whole pancreas transplantation for the reversal of diabetes. Islets can be transplanted with little risk to the recipient; the immunogenicity of donor tissue might be altered to reduce immunosuppression requirements, cost can be moderated, and a greater number of individuals can be treated. In the past decade, methods of islet separation from whole pancreas have been described that have improved the yield from each donor pancreas. Islet transplantation to resolve diabetes has been successful in several small laboratory-animal species, in dogs, and in a limited number of humans (Soon-Shiong et al, 1993).

Pancreatic islets are potent antigenic stimuli and without recipient immunosuppression, rejection of this tissue typically occurs within 5 to 12 days of transplantation (Alejandro et al, 1988). Furthermore, the amount of immunosuppression required to prevent rejection correlates directly with the number of donors contributing to the graft. In other words, if cells from one donor are implanted, that recipient requires less immunosuppression to prevent rejection than a recipient receiving tissue from three donors. To complicate matters, numerous studies demonstrated that duration of graft survival may be correlated with the number of islets transplanted (Alejandro et al, 1988; Dafae and Uinik, 1990). The more islets transplanted, the better the short- and long-term control of the blood glucose concentration. Transplanting an "ideal" number of islets, however, often requires transplantation of islets collected from at least three to five donors (Alejandro et al, 1988; Tattersall, 1989).

Although tissue from several donors allows better control of diabetes mellitus, use of several donors increases the need for levels of immunosuppression that might harm the recipient. Also, the need for multiple donors creates the ethical question of multiple dog lives being sacrificed in order to treat one dog that could be treated with exogenous insulin. Adding to the confusion, immunosuppression with drugs such as cyclosporine is not benign. Dogs receiving long-term cyclosporine develop a number of problems directly due to the effects of the drug—weight loss, papillomatosis, anemia, hypoalbuminemia, and polyclonal gammopathies (Feldman and Alejandro, 1988). Finally, to further complicate an already complicated situation, blood concentrations of cyclosporine required to prevent pancreatic islet rejection are actually harmful to those very islets being "protected" (Alejandro et al, 1989).

IMMUNOPROTECTED ISLET TRANSPLANTATION. Many techniques have been used to circumvent the problems of immune rejection and/or to avoid the need for immunosuppression. One approach to this problem has been to use a technology called *microencapsulation*. The first report on microencapsulation appeared in *Science* in 1980. This novel approach to the previously mentioned rejection problems completely encloses each viable islet within a semipermeable membrane. The microcapsular membrane, composed of cross-linked alginate, a nontoxic polysaccharide, is permeable to small molecules such as glucose or insulin but totally impermeable to large molecules such as immunoglobulins (Soon-Shiong et al, 1992). Tissue transplanted within such membranes is essentially invisible to a recipient's immune system. Results in a group of natu-

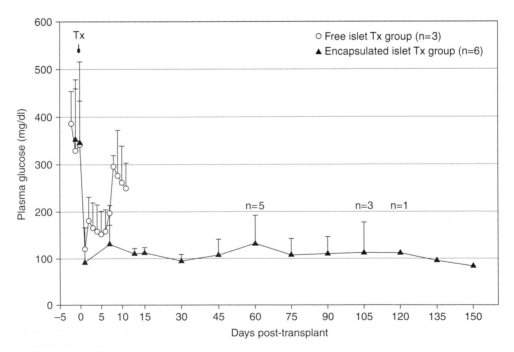

FIGURE 11-24. Fasting plasma glucose (mg/dl) monitored daily following an intraperitoneal injection of either free islet allografts (n = 3) or encapsulated islets (n = 6) in spontaneous diabetic dogs. Rejection occurred rapidly in the recipients receiving free islets, with recurrence of hyperglycemia 5.7 ± 3.7 days following implantation. In contrast, the dogs receiving encapsulated islets remained euglycemic, free of insulin requirements, for a median of 105 days. (From Soon-Shiong P, et al: Successful reversal of spontaneous diabetes in dogs by intraperitoneal microencapsulated islets. Transplantation 54:769, 1992, with permission.)

rally occurring type I diabetic dogs have reinforced the potential value of microencapsulation (Soon-Shiong et al, 1992). To date, transplantation has involved allografts (within species). A group of 12 pet dogs with naturally occurring diabetes mellitus received micro-encapsulated canine islets, transplanted free into the peritoneal cavity. Blood glucose concentrations fell to or below normal levels within 8 to 12 hours. These dogs remained euglycemic for 1 to 6 months, with a mean of 3.5 months (Fig. 11-24). Five of these dogs received second transplants following recurrence of insulin dependence. Success following the second transplant was equivalent to that observed after the first.

Transplantation of microencapsulated islets has been valuable in gathering information, but each donor must undergo extremely sophisticated surgery or be killed to allow harvesting of the pancreas. Allografting of islets, therefore, has limited potential in humans and would not be used in dogs. However, if such technology can be developed to use pig pancreas in harvesting islets of Langerhans, one can visualize a large resource for this novel treatment of diabetes mellitus. If such a tool is developed for humans, it will likely become available for diabetic dogs and cats as well.

PROGNOSIS

The prognosis for dogs diagnosed with diabetes mellitus depends, in part, on owner commitment to treating the disorder, ease of glycemic regulation, presence and reversibility of concurrent disorders (e.g., pancreatitis), and avoidance of chronic complications associated with the diabetic state (see Table 11-7). The mean survival time in diabetic dogs is approximately 3 years from time of diagnosis. This survival time is somewhat skewed because dogs are usually 7 to 10 years old at the time of diagnosis and there is a relatively high mortality rate during the first 6 months because of concurrent life-threatening or uncontrollable disease (e.g., ketoacidosis, acute pancreatitis, renal failure). Diabetic dogs that survive the first 6 months can easily live longer than 5 years with the disease and with proper care by the owners, timely evaluations by the veterinarian, and good client-veterinarian communication, most diabetic dogs can live relatively normal lives.

In general, death shortly after a diagnosis of diabetes is usually due to severe ketoacidosis, concurrent illness (e.g., severe pancreatitis or renal failure), or owner unwillingness to treat the disease. Death weeks to months after therapy is initiated for diabetes is usually caused by an inability to establish glycemic control with resultant persistence of clinical signs, development of chronic complications of diabetes (e.g., blindness due to cataracts), or unrelated problems. Inability to establish glycemic control is usually due to problems with insulin therapy or insulin resistance caused by concurrent insulin-antagonistic disorders. The latter may not be evident until weeks or months after diagnosing diabetes.

REFERENCES

Abraham AS, et al: The effects of chromium supplementation on serum glucose and lipids in patients with and without non-insulin-dependent diabetes. Metabolism 41:768, 1992.

Alejandro R, et al: Advances in canine diabetes mellitus research: Etiopathology and results of islet transplantation. JAVMA 193:1050, 1988.

Alejandro J, et al: Effects of cyclosporin on insulin and C-peptide secretion in healthy Beagles. Diabetes 38:698, 1989.

Anderson JW, Akanji AO: Dietary fiber— An overview. Diabetes Care 14:1126, 1991.

Anderson JW, et al: Metabolic effects of high carbohydrate, high fiber diets for insulin dependent diabetic individuals. Am J Clin Nutr 54:930, 1991.

Anderson RA: Chromium, glucose tolerance, and diabetes. Biol Trace Element Res 32:19, 1992.

Anderson RA, et al: Elevated intakes of supplemental chromium improve glucose and insulin variables in individuals with type 2 diabetes. Diabetes 46:1786, 1997.

Appleton DJ, et al: Insulin sensitivity decreases with obesity, and lean cats with low insulin sensitivity are at greatest risk of glucose intolerance with weight gain. J Feline Med Surg 3:211, 2001.

Armstrong PJ, Ford RB: Hyperlipidemia. In Kirk RW (ed): Current Veterinary Therapy X. Philadelphia, WB Saunders Co, 1989, p 1046.

Arner P, et al: Influence of thyroid hormone level on insulin action in human adipose tissue. Diabetes 33:369, 1984.

Atkins CE, et al: Morphologic and immunocytochemical study of young dogs with diabetes mellitus associated with pancreatic islet hypoplasia. Am J Vet Res 49:1577, 1988.

Atkinson MA, et al: Lack of bovine responsiveness to bovine serum albumin in insulin-dependent diabetes. N Engl J Med 329:1853, 1993.

Bagley LH, Lavach JD: Comparison of postoperative phacoemulsification results in dogs with and without diabetes mellitus: 153 cases (1991–1992). J Am Vet Med Assoc 205:1165, 1994.

Baker JR, et al: Use of protein-based standards in automated colorimetric determinations of fructosamine in serum. Clin Chem 31:1550, 1985.

Balfour JA, McTavish D: Acarbose: An update of its pharmacology and therapeutic use in diabetes mellitus. Drugs 46:1025, 1993.

Baker KS, et al: Trigeminal ganglion neurons affect corneal epithelial phenotype. Influence of type VII collagen expression in vitro. Invest Ophthalmol Vis Sci 34:137, 1993.

Beam S, et al: A retrospective-cohort study on the development of cataracts in dogs with diabetes mellitus: 200 cases. Vet Ophthalmology 2:169, 1999.

Bergman RN, Mittleman SD: Central role of the adipocyte in insulin resistance. J Basic Clin Physiol Pharmacol 9:205, 1998.

Berlinger JA, et al: Lipoprotein-induced insulin resistance in aortic endothelium. Diabetes 33:1039, 1984.

Bertoni AG, et al: Diabetes and the risk of infection-related mortality in the U.S. Diabetes Care 24:1044, 2001.

Bieger WP, et al: Diminished insulin receptors on monocytes and erythrocytes in hypertriglyceridemia. Metabolism 33:982, 1984.

Bolli GB, et al: Abnormal glucose counterregulation after subcutaneous insulin in insulin-dependent diabetes mellitus. N Engl J Med 310:1706, 1984.

Brange J, et al: Monomeric insulins obtained by protein engineering and their medical implications. Nature 333:679, 1988.

Braund KG, Steiss JE: Distal neuropathy in spontaneous diabetes mellitus in the dog. Acta Neuropathol (Berl) 57:263, 1982.

Brenner BM, et al: Dietary protein intake and the progressive nature of kidney disease: The role of hemodynamically mediated glomerular injury in the pathogenesis of progressive glomerular sclerosis in aging, renal ablation and intrinsic renal disease. N Engl J Med 307:652, 1982.

Briggs C, et al: Reliability of history and physical examination findings for assessing control of glycemia in dogs with diabetes mellitus: 53 cases (1995–1998). J Am Vet Med Assoc 217:48, 2000.

Clark CM, Lee DA: Prevention and treatment of the complications of diabetes mellitus. N Engl J Med 332:1210, 1995.

Cohn LA, et al: Effects of chromium supplementation on glucose tolerance in obese and nonobese cats. Am J Vet Res 60:1360, 1999.

Cohn LA, et al: Assessment of five portable blood glucose meters, a point-of-care analyzer, and color test strips for measuring blood glucose concentration in dogs. J Am Vet Med Assoc 216:198, 2000.

Coniff RF, et al: Reduction of glycosylated hemoglobin and postprandial hyperglycemia by acarbose in patients with NIDDM. A placebo-controlled dose-comparison study. Diabetes Care 18:817, 1995.

Crenshaw KL, et al: Serum fructosamine concentration as an index of glycemia in cats with diabetes mellitus and stress hyperglycemia. J Vet Intern Med 10:360, 1996.

Cryer PE: Catecholamines, pheochromocytoma and diabetes. Diabetes Rev 1:309, 1993.

Cryer PE, Polonsky KS: Glucose homeostasis and hypoglycemia. In Wilson JD, Foster DW, Kronenberg HM, Larsen PR (eds): Williams Textbook of Endocrinology, 9th ed. Philadelphia, WB Saunders Co, 1998, p 939.

Czech MP, et al: Effect of thyroid status on insulin action in rat adipocytes in skeletal muscle. J Clin Invest Med 66:574, 1980.

Dafae DA, Uinik AI: Is pancreas transplantation for insulin-dependent diabetes mellitus worthwhile? N Engl J Med 322:1608, 1990.

Davidson JK, et al: Insulin therapy. *In* Davidson JK (ed): Clinical Diabetes Mellitus: A Problem Oriented Approach. New York, Thieme Medical Publishers, 1991, p 266.

Davison LJ, et al: Anti-insulin antibodies in dogs with naturally occurring diabetes mellitus. J Immunol Immunopathol 91:53, 2003.

DeBowes LJ: Lipid metabolism and hyperlipoproteinemia in dogs. Comp Cont Ed 9:727, 1987.

DeFronzo RA: Pathogenesis of type 2 diabetes: Metabolic and molecular implications for identifying diabetes genes. Diabetes Rev 5:177, 1997.

DeFronzo RA: Pharmacologic therapy for type 2 diabetes mellitus. Ann Intern Med 131:281, 1999.

DeFronzo RA, et al: Fasting hyperglycemia in non-insulin dependent diabetes mellitus: Contributions of excessive hepatic glucose production and impaired tissue glucose uptake. Metabolism 38:387, 1989.

Devaux C, et al: What role does dietary protein restriction play in the management of chronic renal failure in dogs? Vet Clin North Am 26:1247, 1996.

Duesberg C, et al: Impaired counterregulatory response to insulin-induced hypoglycemia in diabetic dogs [abstract]. J Vet Intern Med 9:181, 1995.

Dukes J: Hypertension: A review of the mechanisms, manifestations and management. J Small Anim Pract 33:119, 1992.

Dutta SK, Hlasko J: Dietary fiber in pancreatic disease: Effect of high fiber diet on fat malabsorption in pancreatic insufficiency and in vitro study of the interaction of dietary fibers with pancreatic enzymes. Am J Clin Nutr 41:517, 1985.

Eckel RH: Lipoprotein lipase. A multifunctional enzyme relevant to common metabolic diseases. N Engl J Med 320:1060, 1989.

Eidemak I, et al: Insulin resistance and hyperinsulinaemia in mild to moderate progressive chronic renal failure and its association with aerobic work capacity. Diabetologia 38:565, 1995.

Eigenmann JE, Rijnberk A: Influence of medroxyprogesterone acetate (Provera) on plasma growth hormone levels and on carbohydrate metabolism. I. Studies in the ovariohysterectomized bitch. Acta Endocrinol 98:599, 1981.

Eigenmann JE, et al: Progesterone-controlled growth hormone overproduction and naturally occurring canine diabetes and acromegaly. Acta Endocrinol 104:167, 1983.

Eisenbarth GS: Type I diabetes mellitus. A chronic autoimmune disease. N Engl J Med 314:1360, 1986.

Elliott DA: Disorders of metabolism. *In* Nelson RW, Couto CG (eds): Small Animal Internal Medicine, 3rd ed. St Louis, Mosby, 2003, p 816.

Elliott DA, et al: Glycosylated hemoglobin concentrations in the blood of healthy dogs and dogs with naturally developing diabetes mellitus, pancreatic b-cell neoplasia, hyperadrenocorticism, and anemia. J Am Vet Med Assoc 211:723, 1997.

Elliott DA, et al: Comparison of serum fructosamine and blood glycosylated hemoglobin concentrations for assessment of glycemic control in cats with diabetes mellitus. J Am Vet Med Assoc 214:1794, 1999.

Engerman RL, Kern TS: Progression of incipient diabetic retinopathy during good glycemic control. Diabetes 36:808, 1987.

Engerman RL, Kern TS: Aldose reductase inhibition fails to prevent retinopathy in diabetic and galactosemic dogs. Diabetes 42:820, 1993.

Evans GW: The effect of chromium picolinate on insulin controlled parameters in humans. Internat J Biosoc Med Res 11:163, 1989.

Feldman EC, et al: Reduced immunogenicity of pork insulin in dogs with spontaneous insulin-dependent diabetes mellitus [abstract]. Diabetes 32(Suppl 1):153A, 1983.

Feldman EC, Alejandro R: Red blood cell and serum biochemical alterations in dogs receiving long term cyclosporin (CsA) therapy. Transplantation 45:837, 1988.

Feldman EC, Nelson RW: Insulin-induced hyperglycemia in diabetic dogs. JAVMA 180:1432, 1982.

Feldman EC, Nelson RW: Canine and Feline Endocrinology and Reproduction. Philadelphia, WB Saunders Co, 1987.

Fernqvist E, et al: Effects of physical exercise on insulin absorption in insulin-dependent diabetics: A comparison between human and porcine insulin. Clin Physiol 6:489, 1986.

Fluckiger R, et al: Evaluation of the fructosamine test for the measurement of plasma protein glycation. Diabetologia 30:648, 1987.

Ford SL, et al: Insulin resistance in three dogs with hypothyroidism and diabetes mellitus. JAVMA 202:1478, 1993.

Friedman EA: Diabetic nephropathy: Strategies in prevention and management. Kidney Int 21:780, 1982.

Galante P, et al: Acute hyperglycemia provides an insulin-independent inducer for GLUT4 translocation in C_2C_{12} myotubes and rat skeletal muscle. Diabetes 44:646, 1995.

Galloway JA: Chemistry and clinical use of insulin. *In* Galloway JA, et al (eds): Diabetes Mellitus. Indianapolis, Eli Lilly, 1988, p 105.

Ganong WF: Review of Medical Physiology, 15th ed. San Mateo, CA, Appleton & Lange, 1991.

Garg A: Management of dyslipidemia in IDDM patients. Diabetes Care 17:224, 1994.

Garg A, Grundy SM: Lovastatin for lowering cholesterol levels in non–insulin-dependent diabetes mellitus. N Engl J Med 318:81, 1988.

Garg A, Grundy SM: Management of dyslipidemia in NIDDM. Diabetes Care 13:153, 1990.

Gerstein HC: Cow's milk exposure and type 1 diabetes mellitus. Diabetes Care 17:13, 1994.

Good KL, et al: Corneal sensitivity in dogs with diabetes mellitus. Am J Vet Res 64:7, 2003.

Goossens M, et al: Response to therapy and survival in diabetic cats [abstract]. J Vet Intern Med 9:181, 1995.

Gorus FK, et al: IA-2-auto-antibodies complement GAD-65-autoantibodies in new-onset IDDM patients and help predict impending diabetes in their siblings. Diabetologia 40:95, 1997.

Graham PA, et al: Canned high fiber diet and postprandial glycemia in dogs with naturally occurring diabetes mellitus. J Nutri 124:2712S, 1994.

Graham PA, et al: Pharmacokinetics of a porcine insulin zinc suspension in diabetic dogs. J Small Anim Pract 38:434, 1997.

Groop LC, et al: Glucose and free fatty acid metabolism in non-insulin-dependent diabetes mellitus. Evidence for multiple sites of insulin resistance. J Clin Invest 84:205, 1989.

Gross KL, et al: Dietary chromium and carnitine supplementation does not affect glucose tolerance in obese dogs. JVIM 14:345, 2000 (abstr).

Guptill L et al: Is canine diabetes on the increase? *In* Recent Advances in Clinical Management of Diabetes Mellitus, Iams Company, Dayton, Ohio, 1999, p 24-27.

Hagopian WA, et al: Glutamate decarboxylase-, insulin-, and islet cell-antibodies and HL typing to detect diabetes in a general population-based study of Swedish children. J Clin Invest 95:1505, 1995.

Haines DM: A re-examination of islet cell cytoplasmic antibodies in diabetic dogs. Vet Immunol Immunopathol 11:225, 1986.

Haffner SM: Management of dyslipidemia in adults with diabetes. Diabetes Care 21:160, 1998.

Hallden G, et al: Characterization of cat insulin. Arch Biochem Biophys 247:20, 1986.

Harb-Hauser M, et al: Prevalence of insulin antibodies in diabetic dogs. J Vet Intern Med 12:213, 1998 (abstr).

Harte J, et al: Dietary management of naturally occurring chronic renal failure in cats. J Nutr 124:2660S, 1994.

Hasegawa S, et al: Glycated hemoglobin fractions in normal and diabetic dogs measured by high performance liquid chromatography. J Vet Med Sci 53:65, 1991.

Hasegawa S, et al: Glycated hemoglobin fractions in normal and diabetic cats measured by high performance liquid chromatography. J Vet Med Sci 54:789, 1992.

Henry RR: Protein content of the diabetic diet. Diabetes Care 17:1502, 1994.

Herrtage ME, et al: Diabetic retinopathy in a cat with megestrol acetate–induced diabetes. J Small Anim Pract 38:595, 1985.

Hess RS, Ward CR: Effect of insulin dosage on glycemic response in dogs with diabetes mellitus: 221 cases (1993-1998). J Am Vet Med Assoc 216:217, 2000.

Hess RS, et al: Clinical, clinicopathologic, radiographic, and ultrasonographic abnormalities in dogs with fatal acute pancreatitis: 70 cases (1986–1995). J Am Vet Med Assoc 213:665, 1998.

Hess RS, et al: Breed distribution of dogs with diabetes mellitus admitted to a tertiary care facility. J Am Vet Med Assoc 216:1414, 2000a.

Hess RS, et al: Concurrent disorders in dogs with diabetes mellitus: 221 cases (1993–1998). J Am Vet Med Assoc 217:1166, 2000b.

Hess RS, et al: Association between hypothyroidism, diabetes mellitus, and hyperadrenocorticism and development of atherosclerosis in dogs (abstr). J Vet Intern Med 16:360, 2002.

Hoenig M, Dawe DL: A qualitative assay for beta cell antibodies. Preliminary results in dogs with diabetes mellitus. Vet Immunol Immunopathol 32:195, 1992.

Holste LC, et al: Effect of dry, soft moist, and canned dog foods on postprandial blood glucose and insulin concentrations in healthy dogs. Am J Vet Res 50:984, 1989.

Home PD, et al: Comparative pharmacokinetics of the novel rapid-acting insulin analogue, insulin aspart, in healthy volunteers. Eur J Clin Pharmacol 55:199, 1999.

Hostetter TH, et al: The case for intrarenal hypertension in the initiation and progression of diabetic and other glomerulopathies. Am J Med 72:375, 1982.

Howard BV, et al: Integrated study of low density lipoprotein metabolism and very low density lipoprotein metabolism in non–insulin-dependent diabetes. Metabolism 36:870, 1987.

Howey DC, et al: Lys(B28)Pro(B29)-human insulin: A rapidly absorbed analog of human insulin. Diabetes 43:396, 1994.

Ihle SL, Nelson RW: Insulin resistance and diabetes mellitus. Comp Cont Educ 13:197, 1991.

Jacobs MA, et al: Metabolic efficacy of preprandial administration of Lys(B28),Pro(B29) human insulin analog in IDDM patients. A comparison with human regular insulin during a three-meal test period. Diabetes Care 20:1279, 1997.

Jain NC: Erythrocyte physiology and changes in disease. *In* Jain NC (ed): Essentials of veterinary hematology. Philadelphia: WB Saunders Co, 1993;133.

Jensen AL: Serum fructosamine in canine diabetes mellitus. An initial study. Vet Res Commun 16:1, 1992.

Jeraj K, et al: Immunofluorescence studies of renal basement membranes in dogs with spontaneous diabetes. Am J Vet Res 45:1162, 1984.

Johnson CA, et al: Peripheral neuropathy and hypotension in a diabetic dog. JAVMA 183:1007, 1983.

Johnson RN, et al: Relationship between albumin and fructosamine concenration in diabetic and non-diabetic sera. Clin Chim Acta 164:151, 1987.

Joshi N, et al: Infections in patients with diabetes mellitus. N Engl J Med 341:1906, 1999.

Kaiyala KJ, et al: Reduced β-cell function contributes to impaired glucose tolerance in dogs made obese by high-fat feeding. Am J Physiol 277(Endocrinol Metab 40):E659-E667, 1999.

Karam JH: Hypoglycemic disorders. In Greenspan FS, Gardner DG (eds): Basic and Clinical Endocrinology, 6th ed. New York, Lange Medical Books/McGraw-Hill, 2001, p 699.

Karjalainen J, et al: A bovine albumin peptide as a possible trigger of insulin-dependent diabetes mellitus. N Engl J Med 327:302, 1992.

Katherman AE, Braund KG: Polyneuropathy associated with diabetes mellitus in a dog. JAVMA 182:522, 1983.

Kawamoto M, et al: Relation of fructosamine to serum protein, albumin, and glucose concentrations in healthy and diabetic dogs. Am J Vet Res 53:851, 1992.

Kelley DE, et al: Efficacy and safety of acarbose in insulin-treated patients with type 2 diabetes. Diabetes Care 21:2056, 1998.

Kirk CA, et al: Diagnosis of naturally acquired type-I and type-II diabetes mellitus in cats. Am J Vet Res 54:463, 1993.

Krezowski PA, et al: The effect of protein ingestion on the metabolic response to oral glucose in normal individuals. Am J Clin Nutr 44:847, 1986.

Lahtela JT, et al: Severe antibody-mediated human insulin resistance: Successful treatment with the insulin analog lispro. Diabetes Care 20:71, 1997.

Leahy JL: Natural history of β-cell dysfunction in NIDDM. Diabetes Care 13:992, 1990.

Lembcke B, et al: Effect of 1-desoxynojirimycin derivatives on small intestinal disaccharidase activities and on active transport in vitro. Digestion 31:120, 1985.

Lewis L, et al: Small Animal Clinical Nutrition, 3rd ed. Topeka, KS, Mark Morris Associates, 1987.

Lindholm A, et al: Improved postprandial glycemic control with insulin aspart. A randomized double-blind cross-over trial in type 1 diabetes. Diabetes Care 22:801, 1999.

Lindholm A, et al: Immune responses to insulin aspart and biphasic insulin aspart in people with type 1 and type 2 diabetes. Diabetes Care 25:876, 2002.

Loste A, Marca MC: Study of the effect of total serum protein and albumin concentrations on canine fructosamine concentration. Can J Vet Res 63:138, 1999.

Lutz TA, et al: Fructosamine concentrations in hyperglycemic cats. Can Vet J 36:155, 1995.

Mahaffey EA, Cornelius LM: Evaluation of a commercial kit for measurement of glycosylated hemoglobin in canine blood. Vet Clin Path 10:21, 1981.

Mahaffey EA, Cornelius LM: Glycosylated hemoglobin in diabetic and non-diabetic dogs. JAVMA 180:635, 1982.

Malik RL, Jaspan JB: Role of protein in diabetes control. Diabetes Care 12:39, 1989.

Marca MC, Loste A: Glycosylated haemoglobin in dogs: Study of critical difference value. Res Vet Sci 71:115, 2001.

Marca MC, et al: Blood glycated hemoglobin evaluation in sick dogs. Can J Vet Res 64:141, 2000.

Marfurt C: Nervous control of the cornea. In Burnstock G, Sillito AM (eds): Nervous control of the eye. Amsterdam: Harwood Academic Publishers, 2000, p 41.

Marshall MO, et al: Development of insulin antibodies, metabolic control and β-cell function in newly diagnosed insulin dependent diabetic children treated with monocomponent human insulin or monocomponent porcine insulin. Diabetes Res 9:169, 1988.

Marshall RD, Rand JS: Comparison of the pharmacokinetics and pharmacodynamics of glargine, protamine zinc and porcine lente insulins in normal cats [abstr]. J Vet Intern Med 16:358, 2002.

Martin BC, et al: Role of glucose and insulin resistance in development of type 2 diabetes mellitus: Results of a 25-year follow-up study. Lancet 340:925, 1992.

Massillon D, et al: Induction of hepatic glucose-6-phosphatase gene expression by lipid infusion. Diabetes 46:153, 1997.

Mattheeuws D, et al: Diabetes mellitus in dogs: Relationship of obesity to glucose tolerance and insulin response. Am J Vet Res 45:98, 1984.

McGuire NC, et al: Detection of occult urinary tract infections in dogs with diabetes mellitus. J Am Anim Hosp Assoc 38:541, 2002.

McMahon MM, Bistrian BR: Host defenses and susceptibility to infection in patients with diabetes mellitus. Infect Dis Clin North Am 9:1, 1995.

Meyer JH, et al: Intragastric versus intraintestinal viscous polymers and glucose tolerance after liquid meals of glucose. Am J Clin Nutr 48:260, 1988.

Mitrakou A, et al: Contribution of abnormal muscle and liver glucose metabolism to post-prandial hyperglycemia in NIDDM. Diabetes 39:1381, 1990.

Moller DE, Flier JS: Insulin resistance. Mechanisms, syndromes, and implications. N Engl J Med 325:938, 1991.

Mossop RT: Effects of chromium (III) on fasting glucose, cholesterol, and cholesterol HDL levels in diabetics. Cent Afr J Med 29:80, 1983.

Muirhead RP, Hothersall JS: The effect of phenazine methosulphate on intermediary pathways of glucose metabolism in the lens at different glycaemic levels. Exp Eye Res 61; 619, 1995.

Nathan DM: Long-term complications of diabetes mellitus. N Engl J Med 328:1676, 1993.

Nell LJ, Thomas JW: Human insulin autoantibody fine specificity and H and L chain use. J Immunol 142:3063, 1989.

Nelson RW: Disorders of the endocrine pancreas. In Ettinger SJ (ed): Textbook of Veterinary Internal Medicine, 3rd ed. Philadelphia, WB Saunders Co, 1989, p 1676.

Nelson RW, Lewis LD: Nutritional management of diabetes mellitus. Semin Vet Med Surg 5:178, 1990.

Nelson RW, et al: Effects of dietary fiber supplementation on glycemic control in dogs with alloxan-induced diabetes mellitus. Am J Vet Res 52:2060, 1991.

Nelson RW, et al: Effect of an orally administered sulfonylurea, glipizide, for treatment of diabetes mellitus in dogs. JAVMA 203:821, 1993.

Nelson RW, et al: Transient clinical diabetes mellitus in cats: 10 cases (1989–1991). J Vet Intern Med 13:28, 1998a.

Nelson RW, et al: Effect of dietary insoluble fiber on control of glycemia in dogs with naturally acquired diabetes mellitus. JAVMA 212:380, 1998b.

Nelson RW, et al: Effect of the β-glucosidase inhibitor acarbose on control of glycemia in dogs with naturally acquired diabetes mellitus. JAVMA 216:1265, 2000.

Nerup J: On the pathogenesis of IDDM. Diabetologia 37(suppl 2):S82, 1994.

Nishida Y, et al: Effect of mild exercise training on glucose effectiveness in healthy men. Diabetes Care 24:1008, 2001.

Nuttall FQ: Dietary fiber in the management of diabetes. Diabetes 42:503, 1993.

Nyberg G, et al: Impact of metabolic control in progression of clinical diabetic nephropathy. Diabetologia 30:82, 1987.

Ogilvie GK, et al: Alterations in carbohydrate metabolism in dogs with nonhematopoietic malignancies. Am J Vet Res 58:277, 1997.

Ono K, et al: Fluorescein angiogram in diabetic dogs. Jpn J Vet Sci 48:1257, 1986.

Owens DR, et al: Pharmacokinetics of ^{125}I-labeled insulin glargine (HOE901) in healthy men-comparison with NPH insulin and the influence of different subcutaneous injection sites. Diabetes Care 23:813, 2000.

Palmer JP: Current management of Type I diabetes: Insulin, transplantation and immunotherapy. 42nd Postgraduate Assembly, The Endocrine Society 1, 1990.

Palmer JP, McCulloch DK: Prediction and prevention of IDDM-1991. Diabetes 40:943, 1991.

Panciera DL, et al: Epizootiologic patterns of diabetes mellitus in cats: 333 cases (1980–1986). JAVMA 197:1504, 1990.

Pastors JG, et al: Psyllium fiber reduces rise in postprandial glucose and insulin concentrations in patients with non-insulin-dependent diabetes. Am J Clin Nutr 53:1431, 1991.

Pedersen O, et al: Characterization of the insulin resistance of glucose utilization in adipocytes from patients with hyper- and hypothyroidism. Acta Endocrinol 119:228, 1988.

Peikes H, et al: Dermatologic disorders in dogs with diabetes mellitus: 45 cases (1986–2000). J Am Vet Med Assoc 219:203, 2001.

Phillips SM, et al: Increments in skeletal muscle GLUT-1 and GLUT-4 after endurance training in humans. Am J Physiol 270:E456, 1996.

Pieber TR, et al: Efficacy and safety of HOE 901 versus NPH insulin in patients with type 1 diabetes. Diabetes Care 23:157, 2000.

Polonsky KS: Lilly Lecture 1994. The β-cell in diabetes: From molecular genetics to clinical research. Diabetes 44:705, 1995.

Possilli P, Leslie RDG: Infection and diabetes: Mechanisms and prospects for prevention. Diabet Med 11:935, 1994.

Rabinowitz MB, et al: Effects of chromium and yeast supplements on carbohydrate and lipid metabolism in diabetic men. Diabetes Care 6:319, 1983.

Rave K, et al: Impact of diabetic nephropathy on pharmacodynamic and pharmacokinetic properties of insulin in type 1 diabetic patients. Diabetes Care 24:886, 2001.

Reaven GM: Role of insulin resistance in human disease. Diabetes 37:1595, 1988.

Remillard RL: Nutritional management of diabetic dogs. Compend Contin Educ Pract Vet 21:699, 1999.

Reusch CE: Fructosamine: A new parameter for diagnosis and metabolic control in diabetic dogs and cats. J Vet Int Med 7:177, 1993.

Reusch CE, Haberer B: Evaluation of fructosamine in dogs and cats with hypo- or hyperproteinaemia, azotaemia, hyperlipidaemia and hyperbilirubinaemia. Vet Rec 148:370, 2001.

Richter M, et al: Aldose reductase activity and glucose-related opacities in incubated lenses from dogs and cats. Am J Vet Res 63:1591, 2002.

Rios MS: Acarbose and insulin therapy in type I diabetes mellitus. Eur J Clin Invest 24:36, 1994.

Robertson J, et al: Effects of the β-glucosidase inhibitor acarbose on postprandial serum glucose and insulin concentrations in healthy dogs. AJVR 60:541, 1999.

Rosenstock J, et al: Basal insulin glargine (HOE901) versus NPH insulin in patients with type 1 diabetes on multiple daily insulin regimens. Diabetes Care 23:1137, 2000.

Rosenstock J, et al: Basal insulin therapy in type 2 diabetes: 28-week comparison of insulin glargine (HOE901) and NPH insulin. Diabetes Care 24:631, 2001.

Rossetti L, et al: Glucose toxicity. Diabetes Care 13:610, 1990.

Roszler J: Herbs, supplements and vitamins: What to try, what to buy. Diabetes Interviews August, 2001, p 45.

Ryan EA, Enns L: Role of gestational hormones in the induction of insulin resistance. J Clin Endocrinol Metab 67:341, 1988.

Saad MF, et al: Sequential changes in serum insulin concentration during development of non-insulin-dependent diabetes. Lancet 1:1356, 1989.

Savilahti E, et al: Increased levels of cow's milk and β-lactoglobulin antibodies in young children with newly diagnosed IDDM. Diabetes Care 16:984, 1993.

Scarlett JM, Donoghue S: Associations between body condition and disease in cats. J Am Vet Med Assoc 212:1725, 1998.

Schachter S, et al: Oral chromium picolinate and control of glycemia in insulin-treated diabetic dogs. J Vet Intern Med 15:379, 2001.

Schatz D, et al: Islet cell antibodies predict insulin-dependent diabetes in United States school children as powerfully as in unaffected relatives. J Clin Invest 93:2403, 1994.

Soon-Shiong P, et al: Successful reversal of spontaneous diabetes in dogs by intraperitoneal microencapsulated islets. Transplantation 54:769, 1992.

Soon-Shiong P, et al: Long-term reversal of diabetes by the injection of immunoprotected islet cells. Proceed Natl Acad Sci 90:5843, 1993.

Spears JW, et al: Influence of chromium on glucose metabolism and insulin sensitivity. In Reinhart GA, Carey DP (eds): Recent Advances in Canine and Feline Nutrition, Vol II. Wilmington, Ohio, Orange Frazer Press, 1998, p 97.

Spiller GA, et al: Effect of protein dose on serum glucose and insulin response to sugars. Am J Clin Nutr 45:474, 1987.

Srikanta S, et al: Assay for islet cell antibodies: Protein A–monoclonal antibody method. Diabetes 34:300, 1985.

Steffes MW, et al: Diabetic nephropathy in the uninephrectomized dog: Microscopic lesions after one year. Kidney Int 21:721, 1982.

Steiss JE, et al: Electrodiagnostic analysis of peripheral neuropathy in dogs with diabetes mellitus. Am J Vet Res 42:2061, 1981.

Striffler JS, et al: Chromium improves insulin response to glucose in rats. Metabolism 44:1314, 1995.

Struble AL, et al: Systemic hypertension and proteinuria in dogs with naturally occurring diabetes mellitus. J Am Vet Med Assoc 213:822, 1998.

Stumvoll M, et al: Renal glucose production and utilization: New aspects in humans. Diabetologia 40:749, 1997.

Sutherland DER, et al: One hundred pancreas transplants at a single institution. Ann Surg 200:414, 1984.

Sutherland DER, et al: Results of pancreas-transplant registry. Diabetes 38(Suppl 1):46, 1989.

Tattersall R: Is pancreas transplantation for insulin-dependent diabetes mellitus worthwhile? N Engl J Med 321:112, 1989.

Thomas JW, et al: Heterogeneity and specificity of human anti-insulin antibodies determined by isoelectric focusing. J Immunol 134:1048, 1985.

Thomas JW, et al: Spectrotypic analysis of antibodies to insulin A and B chains. Mol Immunol 25:173, 1988.

Truglia JA, et al: Insulin resistance: Receptor and post-binding defects in human obesity and non–insulin-dependent diabetes mellitus. Am J Med 979(Suppl 2B):13, 1985.

Tuomilehto J, et al: Antibodies to glutamic acid decarboxylase as predictors of insulin-dependent diabetes mellitus before clinical onset. Lancet 343:1383, 1994.

Unger RH, Foster DW: Diabetes mellitus. In Wilson JD, Foster DW, Kronenberg HM, Larsen PR (eds): Williams Textbook of Endocrinology, 9th ed. Philadelphia, WB Saunders Co, 1998, p 973.

University of Michigan Pancreas Transplant Evaluation Committee: Pancreatic transplantation as treatment for IDDM. Diabetes Care 11:669, 1988.

Vail DM, et al: Alterations in carbohydrate metabolism in canine lymphoma. J Vet Intern Med 4:8, 1990.

Verge CF, et al: Prediction of type 1 diabetes in first-degree relatives using a combination of insulin, GAD and ICA512bcd/IA-2 autoantibodies. Diabetes 45:926, 1996.

Villaume C et al: Long-term evolution of the effect of bran ingestion on meal-induced glucose and insulin responses in healthy men. Am J Clin Nutr 40:1023, 1984.

Vaaler S. Diabetic control is improved by guar gum and wheat bran supplementation. Diabetic Med 3:230, 1986.

van der Woerdt A et al: Lens-induced uveitis in dogs: 151 cases (1985-1990). J Am Vet Med Assoc 201:921, 1992.

Vuksan V, et al: American ginseng (Panax quinquefolius L) attenuates postprandial glycemia in a time-dependent but not dose-dependent manner in healthy individuals. Am J Clin Nutr 73:753, 2001.

Warram JH, et al: Slow glucose removal rate and hyperinsulinaemia precede the development of type II diabetes in the offspring of diabetic patients. Ann Intern Med 113:909, 1990.

Weidman P, et al: Pathogenesis and treatment of hypertension associated with diabetes mellitus. Am Heart J 125:1498, 1993.

Wess G, Reusch C: Evaluation of five portable blood glucose meters for use in dogs. J Am Vet Med Assoc 216:203, 2000a.

Wess G, Reusch C: Capillary blood sampling from the ear of dogs and cats and use of portable meters to measure glucose concentration. J Small Anim Pract 41:60, 2000b.

White NH, et al: Identification of type I diabetic patients at increased risk for hypoglycemia during intensive therapy. N Engl J Med 308:485, 1983.

Wiberg ME, et al: Serum trypsinlike immunoreactivity measurement for the diagnosis of subclinical exocrine pancreatic insufficiency. J Vet Intern Med 13:426, 1999.

Wiberg ME, Westermarck E: Subclinical exocrine pancreatic insufficiency in dogs. J Am Vet Med Assoc 220:1183, 2002.

Wiseman MJ, et al: Effect of blood glucose control on increased glomerular filtration rate and kidney size in insulin-dependent diabetes. N Engl J Med 312:617, 1985.

Witzum JL, et al: Nonenzymatic glucosylation of high-density lipoprotein accelerates its catabolism in guinea pigs. Diabetes 31:1029, 1982.

Wolfsheimer KJ, et al: The effects of caloric restriction on IV glucose tolerance tests in obese and non-obese beagle dogs. Proceedings of the American College of Veterinary Internal Medicine, Washington, DC, 1993, p 926.

Wood AW, Smith JE: Elevation rate of glycosylated hemoglobins in dogs after induction of experimental diabetes mellitus. Metab 31:906, 1982.

Wylie-Rosett J: Evaluation of protein in dietary management of diabetes mellitus. Diabetes Care 11:143, 1988.

Yee RW, et al: Corneal endothelial changes in diabetic dogs. Curr Eye Res 4:759, 1985.

Zerbe CA, et al: Adrenal function in 15 dogs with insulin-dependent diabetes mellitus. JAVMA 193:454, 1988.

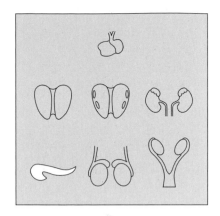

12

FELINE DIABETES MELLITUS

The incidence of diabetes mellitus is similar for the dog and cat, with a reported frequency varying from 1 in 100 to 1 in 500 (Panciera et al, 1990). Historically, veterinarians have taken a similar approach to the diagnosis and treatment of diabetes mellitus in dogs and cats. However, research and clinical experience over the past two decades have made it obvious that there are clinically important differences between diabetic dogs and diabetic cats, and failure to recognize these differences can lead to confusion and frustration for the owner and the veterinarian. For example, cats, unlike dogs, often have a significant population of residual functional beta cells, which allows some cats to oscillate between an insulin-dependent and a non–insulin-dependent state and provides opportunities for the use of oral hypoglycemic drugs in some cats. Cats, unlike dogs, are extremely "sympathoadrenal" animals; that is, they appear to have a rapid catecholamine response during times of stress, excitement, fear, or aggression. As a consequence, the traditional reliance on blood glucose concentrations to monitor therapy is often unreliable in cats because of problems with stress-induced hyperglycemia. Cats, more so than dogs, are prone to the development of hypoglycemia and the Somogyi phenomenon at dosages of insulin assumed to be safe for the treatment of diabetes—an assumption that leads to persistent poor control of the

diabetic state. Identifying an effective treatment regimen for diabetic cats can be challenging. Factors that affect the type and success of treatment include the severity of pancreatic beta cell loss, the responsiveness of tissues to insulin, the presence or absence of glucose toxicity, problems with absorption and duration of effect of exogenously administered insulin, and the presence of concurrent disease. This chapter focuses on specific aspects of diabetes as it relates to the cat. General information on various aspects of diabetes mellitus (e.g., classification of diabetes, overview of types of insulin) is provided in Chapter 11. Extensive cross-references have been provided in this chapter, where appropriate, to guide the reader to additional information on topics that are similar for the cat and dog.

CLASSIFICATION AND ETIOLOGY

Type 1 and type 2 diabetes mellitus

The etiologies of type 1 and type 2 diabetes mellitus are discussed on page 486. In humans, type 1 diabetes is characterized by a combination of genetic susceptibility and immunologic destruction of beta cells, with progressive and eventually complete insulin insufficiency. The presence of circulating autoantibodies against insulin, the beta cell, and/or glutamic acid decarboxylase (GAD) usually precedes the development of hyperglycemia or clinical signs. There is minimal evidence for the development of type 1 diabetes in cats. Lymphocytic infiltration of islets, in conjunction with islet amyloidosis and vacuolation, has been described in two diabetic cats (Nakayama et al, 1990), suggesting the possibility of immune-mediated insulitis. However, this histologic finding is very uncommon in diabetic cats. In addition, beta cell and insulin autoantibodies were not identified in 26 newly diagnosed, untreated diabetic cats (Hoenig et al, 2000a), findings that suggest that an immune-mediated process does not cause diabetes in most cats.

In humans, type 2 diabetes is characterized by insulin resistance and "dysfunctional" beta cells. Hepatic resistance to insulin results in excessive basal hepatic glucose production and fasting hyperglycemia, whereas muscle resistance to insulin impairs the ability of endogenously secreted insulin to augment muscle glucose uptake in response to a meal, resulting in an excessive postprandial increase in the blood glucose concentration. Impaired insulin secretion in response to an insulin secretagogue (e.g., glucose) creates an insulin deficiency state relative to the severity of insulin resistance and prevailing hyperglycemia. Humans with type 2 diabetes are typically not dependent on insulin to control the disease. Control of the diabetic state is usually possible through diet, exercise, and oral hypoglycemic drugs. However, insulin treatment may be necessary in some type 2 diabetics if insulin resistance and beta cell dysfunction are severe.

Insulin resistance and impaired insulin secretion have been identified in cats with obesity, and islet amyloid has been identified in insulin-dependent and non–insulin-dependent diabetes in cat (Yano et al, 1981a and 1981b; Nelson et al, 1990; Appleton et al, 2001); these findings are also associated with type 2 diabetes mellitus in humans. Low insulin sensitivity has also been identified in a group of lean cats subsequently identified to be at greater risk for developing impaired glucose tolerance with obesity, compared with lean cats with higher insulin sensitivity who subsequently developed obesity (Appleton et al, 2001). Although the role of genetics remains to be determined in cats, the findings of Appleton and colleagues suggest that similar etiologies exist for the development of type 2 diabetes in humans and in cats; that is, genetic predisposition, insulin resistance, impaired insulin secretion, islet amyloid, and environmental factors.

Just as in humans, diabetes is undoubtedly a multifactorial disease in cats. The severity of destruction of the pancreatic islets and the presence, severity, and reversibility of concurrent disorders that negatively affect insulin sensitivity are perhaps the two most important factors dictating the development of diabetes mellitus and the insulin dependency of the diabetic state in cats. Examples of concurrent insulin-resistant disorders include obesity, chronic pancreatitis and other chronic inflammatory diseases, and infection, and insulin-resistant diseases such as hyperthyroidism,

hyperadrenocorticism, and acromegaly. Identification and correction of concurrent problems that affect insulin sensitivity are critical to the successful treatment of diabetes in cats. Improvement in insulin sensitivity may promote a non–insulin-dependent or transient diabetic state in cats with partial loss of pancreatic beta cells (see Transient Diabetes in Cats). As such, it is more clinically relevant and perhaps more accurate to classify diabetes in cats as insulin-dependent diabetes mellitus (IDDM) or non–insulin-dependent diabetes mellitus (NIDDM) rather than as type 1 or type 2 for reasons discussed on page 488.

Classification of diabetic cats as IDDM or NIDDM based on their need for insulin treatment can be confusing, because some diabetic cats can initially appear to have NIDDM, which progresses to IDDM; or they may flip back and forth between IDDM and NIDDM as the severity of insulin resistance and impairment of beta cell function waxes and wanes. Apparent changes in the diabetic state (i.e., IDDM and NIDDM) are understandable when one realizes that islet pathology may be mild to severe and progressive or static; that the ability of the pancreas to secrete insulin depends on the severity of islet pathology and can decrease with time; that responsiveness of tissues to insulin varies, often in conjunction with the presence or absence of concurrent inflammatory, infectious, neoplastic, or hormonal disorders; and that all these variables affect the cat's need for insulin, the insulin dosage, and the ease of diabetic regulation.

Insulin-dependent diabetes in cats

The most common clinically recognized form of diabetes mellitus in the cat is IDDM. In our hospital, approximately 70% of cats have IDDM at the time diabetes mellitus is diagnosed. Cats with IDDM fail to respond to diet and oral hypoglycemic drugs and must be treated with exogenous insulin to obtain control of glycemia and prevent ketoacidosis. Common histologic abnormalities in cats with IDDM include islet-specific amyloidosis (see Non–insulin-dependent Diabetes in Cats), beta-cell vacuolation and degeneration, and chronic pancreatitis (Fig. 12-1) (O'Brien et al, 1986; Johnson et al, 1989; Goossens et al, 1998). The cause of beta-cell degeneration in cats is not yet known. Chronic pancreatitis occurs more commonly in diabetic cats than previously suspected. In one study, evidence of past or current pancreatitis was identified in 19 (51%) of 37 diabetic cats at necropsy (Goossens et al, 1998). Seemingly, pancreatitis may be responsible for islet destruction in some cats with IDDM. Still other diabetic cats do not have amyloidosis, inflammation, or degeneration of the pancreatic islets but have a reduction in the number of pancreatic islets and/or insulin-containing beta cells on immunohistochemical evaluation. This suggests that additional mechanisms are involved in the physiopathology of diabetes mellitus in cats. Immune-mediated destruction of the islets does not appear to play a significant role in the etiology of diabetes in cats (see discussion in previous

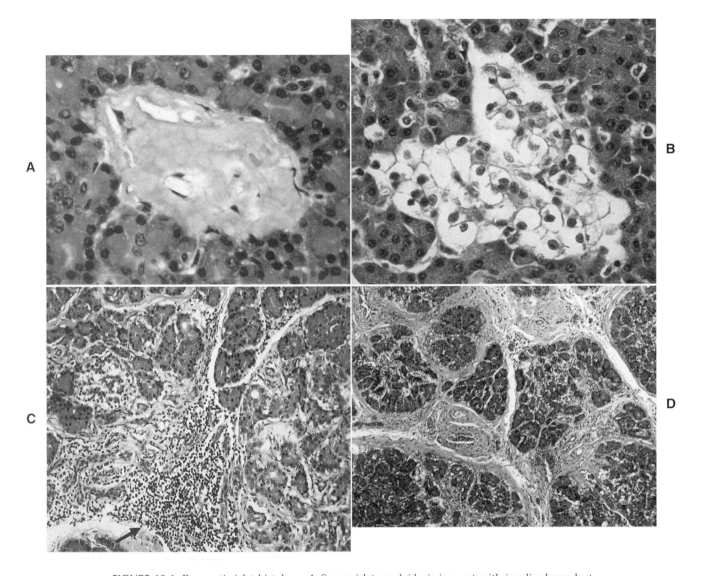

FIGURE 12-1. Pancreatic islet histology. *A,* Severe islet amyloidosis in a cat with insulin-dependent diabetes mellitus (IDDM). (H&E, ×100.) *B,* Severe vacuolar degeneration of islet cells. Pancreatic tissue was evaluated at necropsy 28 months after diabetes was diagnosed and 20 months after cat progressed from non–insulin-dependent diabetes mellitus (NIDDM) to IDDM. (H&E, ×500.) *C,* Chronic pancreatitis in a diabetic cat with IDDM. The inflammatory infiltrate *(arrow)* consists predominately of lymphocytes and plasma cells with a smaller number of neutrophils. (H&E, ×125.) *D,* Severe chronic pancreatitis with fibrosis in a diabetic cat with IDDM. The cat was euthanized because of persistent problems with lethargy, inappetence, and poorly controlled diabetes mellitus. (H&E, ×100.) (*D* from Nelson RW, Couto CG: Small Animal Internal Medicine, 3rd ed. St Louis, Mosby, 2003, p 749.)

section), and the role of genetics remains to be determined.

Insulin dependency may exist at the time hyperglycemia and clinical signs of diabetes are identified in the cat, presumably because of a relatively rapid destruction of beta cells. Alternatively, cats may gradually lose insulin secretion as beta cells are destroyed slowly. These cats may have an initial period when hyperglycemia and clinical signs of diabetes can be controlled with treatments other than insulin (i.e., NIDDM). However, if the underlying pathologic process causing destruction of beta cells is progressive, eventually insulin secretion is lost and IDDM develops.

The length of time between diagnosis of NIDDM and the development of IDDM is unpredictable and depends in part on the type and progression of islet pathology and the reversibility of concurrent insulin-resistant disease (see discussion in next section).

Non–insulin-dependent diabetes in cats

Clinical recognition of NIDDM is more frequent in the cat than the dog, accounting for approximately 30% of diabetic cats seen at our hospital. The etiopathogenesis of NIDDM is undoubtedly multifactorial. In humans, obesity, genetics, and islet amyloidosis are important

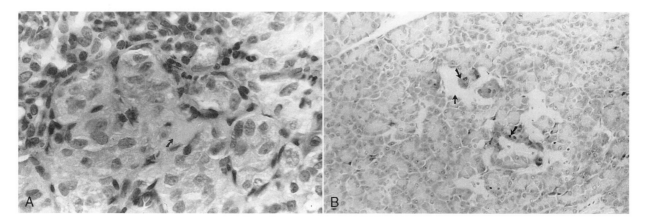

FIGURE 12-2. Pancreatic amyloidosis. *A,* Mild islet amyloidosis *(arrow)* and vacuolar degeneration in a cat with NIDDM treated with diet and glipizide (H&E, ×200). *B,* Severe islet amyloidosis *(straight arrow)* in a cat with initial NIDDM that progressed to IDDM. Pancreatic biopsy was obtained during IDDM state. Residual beta cells containing insulin *(curved arrows)* are also present (immunoperoxidase stain, ×100).

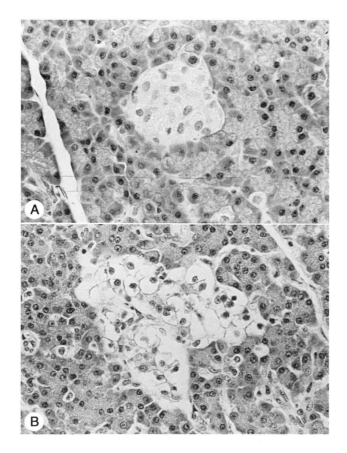

FIGURE 12-3. Pancreatic islet cell histology from a diabetic cat. Biopsies, which were obtained at different times during the course of the disease, illustrate the progressive degeneration of the islets. *A,* Mild vacuolar changes in the islet cells. Pancreatic biopsy was obtained 6 weeks after the cat was diagnosed with NIDDM and was responding well to diet and glipizide therapy (H&E, ×400). *B,* Severe vacuolar degeneration of islet cells. Pancreatic tissue was evaluated at necropsy 28 months after diabetes was diagnosed and 20 months after cat progressed from NIDDM to IDDM, requiring insulin to control blood glucose concentrations. The cat died from metastatic exocrine pancreatic adenocarcinoma (H&E, ×500).

factors in the development of NIDDM (Truglia et al, 1985; Johnson et al, 1989; Leahy, 1990). Similar factors appear to play a role in the development of diabetes mellitus in the cat. Our current understanding of the etiopathogenesis of diabetes in the cat suggests that the difference between IDDM and NIDDM is primarily a difference in the severity of loss of beta cells and the severity and reversibility of concurrent insulin resistance. Most cats with IDDM and NIDDM have islet amyloidosis, vacuolar degeneration of beta cells, or islet hypoplasia (Goossens et al, 1998; Nelson et al, 1998). The more severe the islet pathology, the more likely the cat will have IDDM, regardless of concurrent insulin resistance (Fig. 12-2). The less severe the islet pathology, the greater the role of concurrent insulin resistance in dictating whether the cat has IDDM or NIDDM. The more severe and the less reversible the cause of the insulin resistance, the more likely the cat with mild islet pathology will be insulin dependent, and vice versa. Fluctuations in the severity of insulin resistance, as occurs with chronic pancreatitis, can cause a cat with mild islet pathology to oscillate between IDDM and NIDDM as the severity of pancreatic inflammation waxes and wanes. Persistent insulin resistance can also worsen islet pathology and cause the diabetic cat to progress from NIDDM to IDDM as the progressive loss of beta cells leads to worsening insulin deficiency (see Fig. 12-2; Fig. 12-3) (Nelson et al, 1998; Hoenig et al, 2000b).

Amyloid is a common pathologic finding in the pancreatic islets of cats, with the severity of islet amyloid deposition increasing as the cat ages (Johnson et al, 1989; Lutz et al, 1994). Diabetic cats have significantly greater numbers of pancreatic islets with amyloid deposits and more extensive deposition of amyloid within islets than do nondiabetic cats, suggesting that diabetes mellitus and insular amyloid are causally related (Yano et al, 1981a and 1981b). Islet-amyloid polypeptide (IAPP), or amylin, is the principal constituent of amyloid isolated from the pancreatic tissue of humans with NIDDM and of adult cats with diabetes (Johnson et al, 1989). The amino acid sequences of human and feline IAPP are similar (Westermark et al, 1987a); immunoelectron microscopic studies have identified IAPP within beta-cell secretory granules in both cats and humans (Westermark et al, 1987b; Johnson et al, 1988); and amylin is co-secreted with insulin by the beta cell (Lutz and Rand, 1996). Stimulants of insulin secretion also stimulate the secretion of amylin. Amylin acts as a neuroendocrine hormone and has several glucoregulatory effects that collectively complement the actions of insulin in postprandial glucose control. These effects include a slowing of the rate at which nutrients are delivered from the stomach to the small intestine for absorption, suppression of nutrient-stimulated secretion of glucagon, and stimulation of satiety (Young et al, 1996; Gedulin et al, 1997). Although controversial, pharmacologic concentrations of amylin may induce insulin resistance (Johnson et al, 1990; Kassir et al, 1991). Chronic increased secretion of insulin and amylin, as occurs with obesity and other insulin-resistant states, results in aggregation and deposition of amylin in the islets as amyloid (see Fig. 12-2). IAPP-derived amyloid fibrils are cytotoxic and are associated with apoptotic cell death of islet cells and a resultant defect in insulin secretion (Lorenzo et al, 1994; O'Brien et al, 1995; Hiddinga and Eberhardt, 1999). If deposition of amyloid is progressive (e.g., persistent insulin-resistant states, such as obesity), islet cell destruction progresses and eventually leads to diabetes mellitus (Fig. 12-4). The severity of islet amyloidosis would determine in part whether the diabetic cat has IDDM or NIDDM (see Fig. 12-2, page 542). Total destruction of the islets results in IDDM and the need for insulin treatment for the rest of the cat's life. Partial destruction of the islets may or may not result in clinically evident diabetes, insulin treatment may or may not be required to control glycemia, and transient diabetes may or may not develop once treatment is initiated. If amyloid deposition is progressive, the cat will progress from a subclinical diabetic state to NIDDM and ultimately to IDDM.

The presence and severity of insulin resistance is an important variable that influences the clinical picture in cats with partial destruction of pancreatic islets. Insulin resistance increases the demand for insulin secretion, a demand that may not be met in some cats with partial destruction of islets. The more severe the insulin resistance and the more severe the loss of islets, the more likely hyperglycemia will develop. Persistent hyperglycemia in turn can suppress function of the remaining beta cells, causing hypoinsulinemia and worsening hyperglycemia (see Transient Diabetes in Cats). A sustained demand for insulin secretion in response to insulin resistance can also lead to worsening islet pathology and a further reduction in the population of beta cells. Any chronic insulin-resistant disorder can have a deleterious impact on the population and function of beta cells and can play a role in the development of NIDDM or IDDM. Examples in the cat include obesity, chronic pancreatitis, acromegaly, hyperadrenocorticism, and chronic administration of glucocorticoids or megestrol acetate. Obesity-induced carbohydrate intolerance is the classic insulin-resistant disorder affiliated with the development of NIDDM in humans and has been identified as a potential causative factor in the development of diabetes in cats as well (Panciera et al, 1990; Scarlett and Donoghue, 1998). Obesity causes a reversible insulin resistance that is a result of downregulation of insulin receptors, impaired receptor binding affinity for insulin, and post-receptor defects in insulin action (Truglia et al, 1985). Impaired glucose tolerance and an abnormal insulin secretory response have been documented in obese cats (Nelson et al, 1990; Appleton et al, 2001). This abnormal response is characterized by an initial delay in insulin secretion, followed by excessive insulin secretion (Fig. 12-5), results similar to those identified in humans with NIDDM. The abnormalities responsible for insulin resistance are reversible with correction of obesity, which is why correction and prevention of obesity is an important component of the treatment regimen for diabetes (Fig. 12-6) (Biourge et al, 1997; Fettman et al, 1998). With weight loss, insulin becomes more effective in controlling glycemia, and some diabetic cats revert to a non–insulin-dependent, subclinical diabetic state.

Leptin is an adipocyte-specific hormone that functions as an "adipostat" to sense and regulate body energy stores primarily by modulating the expression of hypothalamic neuropeptides known to regulate feeding behavior and body weight (Havel, 2001). A positive relationship between serum leptin immunoreactivity and body fat content has been identified in several species, including cats and dogs (Backus et al,

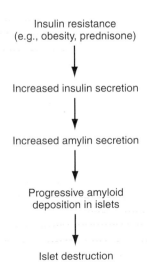

Insulin resistance
(e.g., obesity, prednisone)

↓

Increased insulin secretion

↓

Increased amylin secretion

↓

Progressive amyloid
deposition in islets

↓

Islet destruction

FIGURE 12-4. Schematic of the interplay between insulin resistance, amylin secretion, and amyloid deposition in the pancreatic islets. Insulin secretion increases to compensate for insulin resistance induced by environmental factors, insulin-antagonistic drugs, and concurrent illness. Because amylin and insulin are co-secreted, amylin secretion also increases in insulin-resistant states. If sustained, increased amylin secretion can lead to amylin aggregation and the formation of amyloid in the islets.

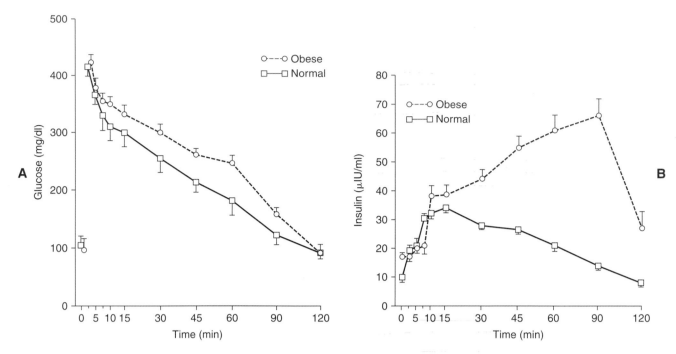

FIGURE 12-5. Serum glucose *(A)* and insulin *(B)* concentrations in normal-weight cats (n = 9) and obese cats (n=6) after IV administration of 0.5 g of glucose per kilogram of body weight. Results are expressed as mean ± SEM. * = P <0.05, comparing time in normal-weight cats versus obese cats . (From Nelson RW, et al: Glucose tolerance and insulin response in normal weight and obese cats. Am J Vet Res 51:1357, 1990.)

2000; Appleton et al, 2000; Sagawa et al, 2002). High leptin concentrations in the presence of obesity suggest that obese animals are resistant to leptin. A causal relationship between leptin and the insulin resistance of obesity has been suggested by some researchers (Segal et al, 1996; Zimmet et al, 1998). An inverse relationship between leptin concentrations and insulin sensitivity was recently reported in cats undergoing glucose tolerance testing before and after gaining weight, suggesting that increased leptin concentrations may contribute to the diminished insulin sensitivity observed in obese cats (Appleton et al, 2002a). However, insulin is an important stimulant for leptin production, and it is also possible that the compensatory hyperinsulinemia found with insulin resistance in obese cats stimulated leptin production (Havel, 2000).

Adiponectin is another adipocyte-specific hormone that has been proposed to be the link between obesity and insulin resistance. Adiponectin is believed to have an important role in the regulation of insulin action and energy homeostasis (Havel, 2002). Adiponectin decreases hepatic glucose production and increases glucose utilization by muscle (Berg et al, 2001; Fruebis et al, 2001). An inverse relationship between plasma adiponectin and leptin concentrations has been identified in normal-weight and obese humans, circulating concentrations of adiponectin are reduced in obese humans, and adiponectin is negatively correlated with fasting insulin concentrations and positively correlated with insulin sensitivity (Weyer et al, 2001). Finally, a decline in circulating adiponectin coincides

with the onset of decreased insulin sensitivity, insulin resistance, and onset of type 2 diabetes mellitus in monkeys (Hotta et al, 2001).

Transient diabetes in cats

Approximately 20% of diabetic cats become "transiently diabetic," usually within 4 to 6 weeks of establishment of the diagnosis of diabetes and initiation of treatment. In these cats, hyperglycemia, glycosuria, and clinical signs of diabetes resolve, and insulin treatment can be discontinued. Some diabetic cats may never require insulin treatment once the initial bout of clinical diabetes mellitus has dissipated, whereas others become permanently insulin dependent weeks to months after resolution of a prior diabetic state. Based on findings from a recent evaluation of a group of cats with transient diabetes mellitus, we theorize that cats with transient diabetes are in a subclinical diabetic state that becomes clinical when the pancreas is stressed by exposure to a concurrent insulin-antagonistic drug or disease, most notably glucocorticoids, megestrol acetate, and chronic pancreatitis (Fig. 12-7) (Nelson et al, 1998). Unlike healthy cats, those with transient diabetes mellitus have some abnormality of the islets (e.g., amyloidosis, vacuolar degeneration) and a significant reduction in the population of beta cells compared with healthy cats, which impairs their ability to compensate for concurrent insulin resistance and results in carbohydrate intolerance. Insulin secretion by beta cells becomes reversibly suppressed, most likely stemming from a worsening carbohydrate intolerance. Chronic

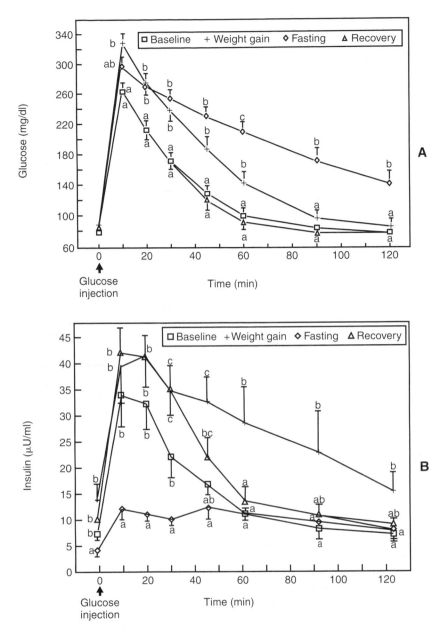

FIGURE 12-6. Mean serum glucose *(A)* and insulin *(B)* concentrations (± SEM) in 12 cats after IV administration of 0.5 g of glucose per kilogram of body weight at entry into the study (baseline), after 9 ± 2 months of weight gain, after a voluntary fast of 5 to 6 weeks (weight loss), and 5 weeks after the end of fasting (recovery). a-c: Points with a different letter are significantly different (p <0.05) among periods. Note the development of impaired glucose tolerance despite increased insulin secretion with weight gain and improvement in glucose tolerance and the exaggerated insulin secretory response with weight loss. (From Biourge V, et al: Effect of weight gain and subsequent weight loss on glucose tolerance and insulin response in healthy cats. J Vet Intern Med 11:86, 1997.)

hyperglycemia impairs insulin secretion by beta cells and induces peripheral insulin resistance by promoting the downregulation of glucose transport systems and causing a defect in posttransport insulin action; this phenomenon is referred to as glucose toxicity (Unger and Grundy, 1985; Rossetti et al, 1990). Beta cells have an impaired response to stimulation by insulin secretagogues, thereby mimicking IDDM (Fig. 12-8). The effects of glucose toxicity are potentially reversible upon correction of the hyperglycemic state. The clinician makes a correct diagnosis of diabetes and initiates appropriate treatment for diabetes and identifiable insulin-antagonistic disorders. Treatment improves hyperglycemia and insulin resistance, the suppressive effects of hyperglycemia decrease, beta-cell function improves, insulin secretion returns, and an apparent IDDM state resolves (see Figs. 12-7 and 12-8). The future requirement for insulin treatment depends on the underlying abnormality in the islets. If the islet pathology is progressive (e.g., amyloidosis), eventually enough beta cells are destroyed that permanent IDDM results.

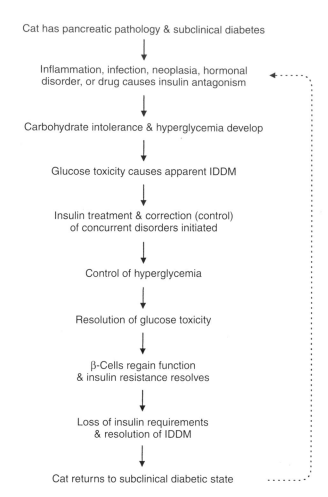

Cat has pancreatic pathology & subclinical diabetes

↓

Inflammation, infection, neoplasia, hormonal disorder, or drug causes insulin antagonism

↓

Carbohydrate intolerance & hyperglycemia develop

↓

Glucose toxicity causes apparent IDDM

↓

Insulin treatment & correction (control) of concurrent disorders initiated

↓

Control of hyperglycemia

↓

Resolution of glucose toxicity

↓

β-Cells regain function & insulin resistance resolves

↓

Loss of insulin requirements & resolution of IDDM

↓

Cat returns to subclinical diabetic state

FIGURE 12-7. Sequence of events in the development and resolution of an insulin-requiring diabetic episode in cats with transient diabetes.

Secondary diabetes in cats

See Secondary Diabetes in Dogs, page 490.

Diagnosis of IDDM versus NIDDM

Cats do not typically present to the clinician until clinical signs of diabetes become obvious and worrisome to an owner. Therefore at the time of diagnosis, all diabetic cats have fasting hyperglycemia and glycosuria, regardless of the type of diabetes mellitus present. Once the diagnosis of diabetes has been established, the clinician must consider the possibility of NIDDM. The significant incidence of NIDDM and transient diabetes in cats raises interesting questions concerning the need for insulin treatment. Glycemic control can be maintained in some diabetic cats with dietary changes and/or oral hypoglycemic drugs. Obviously, it would be advantageous to be able to prospectively differentiate IDDM from NIDDM. Insulin secretagogue tests have been used in humans for this purpose (Table 12-1). Unfortunately, measurements of the serum insulin concentration at baseline and after administration of an insulin secretagogue have not been consistent aids in differentiating IDDM and NIDDM in the cat (Nelson

TABLE 12-1 PROTOCOLS FOR INSULIN SECRETORY RESPONSE TESTS

Intravenous Glucose Tolerance Test (IVGTT)

1. Hospitalize 24 hours prior to testing.
2. Place indwelling catheter into jugular or medial saphenous vein to minimize stress with multiple blood samplings. Allow 24-hour recovery before performing the IVGTT.
3. Withhold all nonessential drugs for 24 to 48 hours prior to testing.
4. Withhold food overnight.
5. Collect baseline blood samples for blood glucose and insulin concentration 5 to 15 minutes before and immediately prior to glucose administration.
6. Administer 0.5 g (dog) or 1.0 g (cat) of 50% dextrose per kilogram of body weight IV over 30 seconds. Do not use the same catheter for glucose administration and blood sampling.
7. Collect blood samples for glucose and insulin determination 1, 5, 10, 15, 30, 45, 60, 90, and 120 minutes after glucose administration.

Intravenous Glucagon Tolerance Test

Steps 1 to 5: As in IVGTT.
6. Administer 0.5 mg (cat) or 1 mg (dog) glucagon IV over 30 seconds.
7. Collect blood samples for glucose and insulin determination 5, 10, 20, 30, 45, and 60 minutes after glucagon administration.

Oral Glucose Tolerance Test

Steps 1 to 5: As in IVGTT.
6. Administer 50 g dextrose (100 ml of 50% dextrose) diluted in water PO via stomach tube.
7. Collect blood samples for glucose and insulin determination 15, 30, 60, 90, and 120 minutes after glucose administration.

Intravenous Arginine Tolerance Test

Steps 1 to 5: As in IVGTT.
6. Administer 0.1 g of L-arginine hydrochloride per kilogram of body weight (cat) IV over 30 seconds.
7. Collect blood samples for glucose and insulin determination 2, 4, 6, 8, 10, 20, and 30 minutes after arginine administration.

et al, 1993; Kirk et al, 1993). A fasting serum insulin concentration or any postsecretagogue insulin concentration greater than one standard deviation above the reference mean (>18 μU/ml in our laboratory) suggests the existence of functional beta cells and the possibility of NIDDM. Unfortunately, cats subsequently identified as having IDDM and many of those with NIDDM have a low baseline serum insulin concentration and do not respond to a glucose or glucagon challenge (Nelson et al, 1993; Kirk et al, 1993; Nelson et al, 1998). This apparent insulin deficiency in cats subsequently identified with NIDDM is presumably the result of concurrent glucose toxicity (see Transient Diabetes in Cats). Because of problems with insulin-secretagogue tests in identifying beta-cell function, the ultimate differentiation between IDDM and NIDDM often is made retrospectively, after the clinician has had several weeks to assess the cat's response to therapy and to determine the animal's need for insulin. The initial decision between insulin treatment and oral hypoglycemic drugs is based on the severity of clinical signs, the presence or absence of ketoacidosis, the cat's general health, and the owner's wishes.

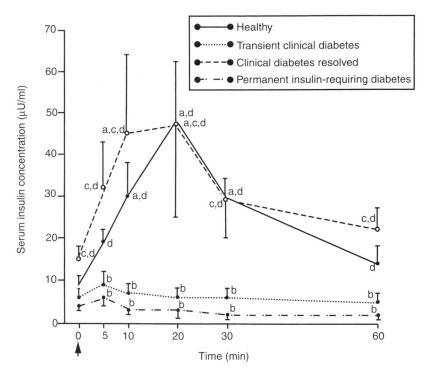

FIGURE 12-8. Mean (± SD) serum insulin concentrations before and after IV administration of 0.5 mg of glucagon per cat in 10 healthy cats, 10 cats with transient clinical diabetes at the time clinical diabetes was diagnosed and after clinical diabetes resolved, and 6 cats with permanent insulin-requiring diabetes at the time diabetes was diagnosed. *a,* Significantly (p <0.05) different compared with baseline value. *b,* Significantly (p <0.05) different compared with corresponding time in healthy cats. *c,* Significantly (p <0.05) different compared with corresponding time when clinical diabetes was diagnosed. *d,* Significantly (p <0.05) different compared with corresponding time in cats with permanent insulin-requiring diabetes. Arrow indicates glucagon administration. (From Nelson RW, et al: Transient clinical diabetes mellitus in cats: 10 cases [1989-1991]. J Vet Intern Med 13:28, 1998.)

PATHOPHYSIOLOGY

The pathophysiology of diabetes mellitus is similar for the dog and cat and is discussed in Chapter 11. The only significant difference between dogs and cats appears to be a greater variability in the renal tubular threshold for excretion of glucose in the urine in cats. Spillage of glucose into the urine occurs when the blood glucose concentration exceeds 180 to 220 mg/dl in the dog. The reported mean threshold for healthy cats is 290 mg/dl. Subjectively, diabetic cats appear to have thresholds for glucose ranging from 200 to 300 mg/dl. As such, the correlation between the blood glucose concentration and the onset of clinical signs is more variable in cats than dogs; that is, some cats are asymptomatic at blood glucose concentrations that would cause clinical signs in dogs.

SIGNALMENT

Although diabetes mellitus may be diagnosed in cats of any age, most diabetic cats are older than 6 years of age (mean, 10 years) at the time of diagnosis. Diabetes mellitus occurs predominantly in neutered male cats,

and there is no apparent breed predisposition, although Burmese cats may be overrepresented in Australia (Panciera et al, 1990; Rand et al, 1997).

ANAMNESIS

The history in diabetic dogs and cats is similar and is discussed in Chapter 11. A common complaint of cat owners is the constant need to change the litter and an increase in the size of the "kitty litter clumps," problems that reflect the polyuria associated with diabetes mellitus. Additional clinical signs include lethargy; decreased interaction with family members; lack of grooming behavior and the development of a dry, lusterless, unkempt or matted haircoat; and decreased jumping ability, rear limb weakness, or the development of a plantigrade posture (Fig. 12-9). If the clinical signs associated with uncomplicated diabetes are not observed by the owner, a diabetic cat may be at risk for the development of systemic signs of illness as progressive ketonemia and metabolic acidosis develop (see Chapter 13, page 584). The time sequence from the onset of initial clinical signs to the development of diabetic ketoacidosis (DKA) is unpredictable.

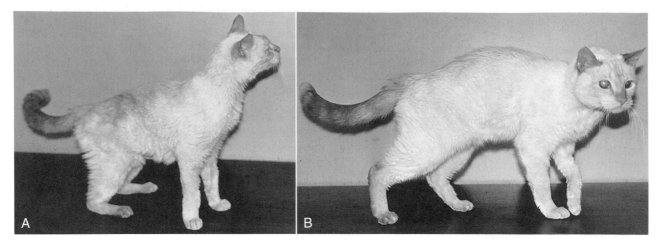

FIGURE 12-9. *A,* Plantigrade posture in a cat with diabetes mellitus and exocrine pancreatic insufficiency. *B,* Resolution of hindlimb weakness and plantigrade posture after glycemic control was improved by adjusting insulin therapy and initiating pancreatic enzyme replacement therapy.

PHYSICAL EXAMINATION

The physical examination findings depend on whether DKA is present and its severity and on the nature of any other concurrent disorder. The nonketotic diabetic cat has no classic physical examination findings. Many diabetic cats are obese but are otherwise in good physical condition. Cats with prolonged untreated diabetes may have lost weight but are rarely emaciated unless concurrent disease (e.g., hyperthyroidism) is present. Newly diagnosed and poorly controlled diabetic cats often stop grooming and develop a dry, lusterless haircoat. Diabetes-induced hepatic lipidosis may cause hepatomegaly. Impaired ability to jump, weakness in the rear limbs, ataxia, or a plantigrade posture (i.e., the hocks touch the ground when the cat walks) may be evident if the cat has developed diabetic neuropathy. Distal muscles of the rear limbs may feel hard on digital palpation, and cats may object to palpation or manipulation of the rear limbs or feet, presumably because of pain associated with the neuropathy. Additional abnormalities may be identified in the ketoacidotic diabetic cat (see Chapter 13, page 584).

ESTABLISHING THE DIAGNOSIS OF DIABETES MELLITUS

Establishment of the diagnosis of diabetes mellitus is similar for cats and dogs and is based on identification of appropriate clinical signs, hyperglycemia, and glycosuria (see page 493). Transient, stress-induced hyperglycemia is a common problem in cats and can cause the blood glucose concentration to increase above 300 mg/dl (see page 567). Unfortunately, stress is a subjective state that cannot be accurately measured, it is not always easily recognized, and it may evoke inconsistent responses among individual cats. Glycosuria usually does not develop in cats with stress hyper-

glycemia because the transient increase in the blood glucose concentration prevents glucose from accumulating in urine to a detectable concentration. For this reason, the clinician should always document persistent hyperglycemia and glycosuria when establishing a diagnosis of diabetes mellitus in cats. If the practitioner is in doubt, the "stressed" cat can be sent home with instructions for the owner to monitor the urine glucose concentration with the cat in the nonstressed home environment. Alternatively, a serum fructosamine concentration can be measured (see page 562). Documentation of an increase in the serum fructosamine concentration supports the presence of sustained hyperglycemia; however, a serum fructosamine concentration in the upper range of normal can occur in symptomatic diabetic cats if the diabetes developed shortly before presentation of the cat to the veterinarian (Elliott et al, 1999). Once the diagnosis of diabetes mellitus has been established, differentiation between NIDDM and IDDM can be considered (see Diagnosis of IDDM versus NIDDM).

CLINICAL PATHOLOGIC ABNORMALITIES

Information used to establish the diagnosis of diabetes mellitus does not provide information on the status of pancreatic islet health, the presence of glucose toxicity, the cat's ability to secrete insulin, or the severity and reversibility of concurrent insulin resistance. Identification of a serum insulin concentration greater than 18 µU/ml in a newly diagnosed, untreated diabetic cat supports the presence of functional beta cells and partial destruction of the islets; however, low or undetectable serum insulin concentrations do not rule out partial islet cell loss because of the suppressive effects of hyperglycemia on circulating insulin concentrations (Kirk et al, 1993; Nelson et al, 1998). Simply establishing the diagnosis of diabetes does not provide the whole picture; a thorough evaluation for concurrent disorders that may affect insulin sensitivity of tissues and evaluation of response to treatment are important pieces of the puzzle when trying to determine if the diabetic cat has IDDM, NIDDM, or transient diabetes mellitus. The minimum laboratory evaluation in any diabetic cat should include a complete blood count (CBC), serum biochemical panel, serum thyroxine concentration, and urinalysis with bacterial culture. If available, abdominal ultrasound should be a routine part of the diagnostic evaluation because of the high prevalence of chronic pancreatitis in diabetic cats. Measurement of the baseline serum insulin concentration or an insulin response test is not routinely done in cats because of the problems encountered with glucose toxicity. Additional tests may be warranted after the clinician has obtained the history, performed the physical examination, or identified ketoacidosis.

Clinical pathologic abnormalities are similar for diabetic dogs and cats and are discussed on page 493 and listed in Table 11-5, page 494. Of special note in the cat is assessment of thyroid gland function, the health of the exocrine pancreas, and concerns regarding radioimmunoassays for measuring the serum insulin concentration.

Serum thyroxine concentration

The serum thyroxine (T_4) concentration should be evaluated in all geriatric diabetic cats, in part because hyperthyroidism is common in older cats, small thyroid nodules (usually nonfunctional) are often palpable in older diabetic cats, and hyperthyroidism can cause insulin resistance (Hoenig and Ferguson, 1988; Hoenig et al, 1992). When interpreting serum T_4 concentrations in diabetic cats, the veterinarian must consider the current status of glycemic control and the severity of any concurrent illnesses. Poorly regulated diabetic cats, especially those with concurrent disorders, typically have falsely lowered serum T_4 concentrations, presumably as a result of the euthyroid sick syndrome. As a general rule, increased serum T_4 concentrations (i.e., >4 μg/dl) support hyperthyroidism, and serum T_4 concentrations in the lower half of the normal range or below the normal range (i.e., <2.0 μg/dl) support euthyroidism or the euthyroid sick syndrome, respectively. Serum T_4 concentrations in the upper half of the normal range (i.e., 2.0 to 4.0 μg/dl) are difficult to interpret because of the potentially suppressive effects of the uncontrolled diabetic state on the pituitary-thyroid axis. Serum T_4 results in this range are consistent with euthyroidism or mild hyperthyroidism with concurrent suppression of serum T_4 concentration into the upper normal range. Additional diagnostic tests (e.g., serum free T_4 concentration, sodium pertechnetate thyroid scan) may be warranted to determine the functional status of the thyroid gland. Chapter 4 presents a more detailed discussion of the interpretation of serum T_4 concentrations in cats suspected of having hyperthyroidism.

Pancreatic enzymes

Acute and especially chronic pancreatitis are common concurrent disorders in diabetic cats. Blood tests used to assess for the presence of pancreatitis should always be considered in the newly diagnosed diabetic cat, especially if abdominal ultrasound is not available. Measurement of the serum lipase concentration and serum feline trypsin-like immunoreactivity (fTLI) are most commonly recommended. In theory, cats with concomitant active pancreatitis should have an increase in the serum lipase concentration and serum fTLI. Unfortunately, serum lipase concentrations and serum fTLI do not always correlate accurately with the presence or absence of pancreatitis, especially when the inflammatory process is chronic and mild (Swift et al, 2000; Gerhardt et al, 2001). Interpretation of serum lipase and fTLI results should always be done in context with the history, physical examination findings, and additional findings on the laboratory tests. In our hospital and using sophisticated ultrasonographic equipment, abdominal ultrasound is the single best diagnostic test for identifying pancreatitis in the cat (Fig. 12-10). As such, abdominal ultrasound is part of the routine diagnostic evaluation of any newly diagnosed or poorly controlled diabetic cat. The concomitant presence of acute pancreatitis in a newly diagnosed diabetic cat may necessitate the instigation of intensive fluid therapy and modifications in the diet that may otherwise not have been done. Identification of chronic pancreatitis also has important prognostic implications regarding the success of establishing and maintaining control of glycemia and of long-term survival (see page 528).

Measurement of serum fTLI is also used to diagnose exocrine pancreatic insufficiency, an uncommon complication of diabetes mellitus that presumably develops as a sequela of chronic pancreatitis (Steiner and Williams, 2000). Exocrine pancreatic insufficiency should be suspected in diabetic cats that are difficult to regulate with insulin and are thin or emaciated despite polyphagia (see page 528).

Serum insulin concentration

Measurement of the serum insulin concentration, either baseline or after the administration of an insulin secretagogue, is not a routine part of our diagnostic evaluation of the newly diagnosed diabetic cat. In theory, identification of increased endogenous serum insulin concentrations (i.e., >18 μU/ml) in a newly diagnosed diabetic cat would suggest a likely response to administration of oral hypoglycemic drugs and the possibility for transient diabetes mellitus, especially if an underlying insulin antagonistic disorder can be identified and treated. Unfortunately, the suppressive effects of hyperglycemia on beta-cell function (i.e., glucose toxicity) often cause low serum insulin concentrations in animals subsequently identified as having NIDDM (see Transient Diabetes in Cats) (Nelson et al, 1998). Although increased serum insulin concentrations suggest the existence of functional beta cells, finding

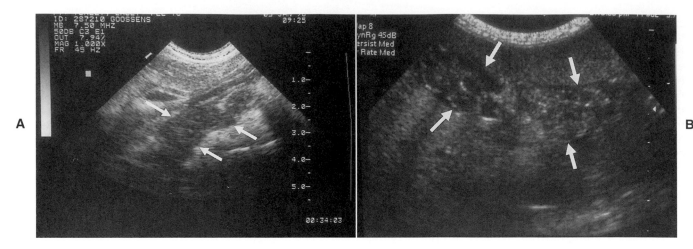

FIGURE 12-10. *A,* Abdominal ultrasound scan of a diabetic cat with acute pancreatitis, showing diffuse enlargement of the pancreas and a generalized hypoechoic pattern of the gland *(arrows),* suggestive of acute inflammation and edema. The cat presented for acute onset of lethargy, anorexia, and vomiting. Control of glycemia had been poor for several weeks prior to presentation. *B,* Abdominal ultrasound scan of a diabetic cat with chronic pancreatitis, showing diffuse enlargement of the pancreas and a mixed (hypoechoic and hyperechoic) echogenic pattern of the gland *(arrows),* suggestive of inflammation and fibrosis. The cat presented for mild lethargy, inappetence, and erratic control of glycemia.

low serum insulin concentrations (i.e., <12 μU/ml) does not rule out the existence of functional beta cells. Because the serum insulin concentration is low in most cats subsequently found to have NIDDM, routine measurement of the serum insulin concentration is not a cost-effective diagnostic procedure.

It is imperative that the radioimmunoassay (RIA) for insulin be validated for the cat. Commercial endocrine laboratories use RIAs designed for use in humans. Unfortunately, the amino acid sequences of human and cat insulins are different (see Table 11-6, page 496), and many RIAs designed for measurement of the serum insulin concentration in humans do not work in cats (Lutz and Rand, 1993). Interestingly, studies evaluating the pharmacokinetic properties of exogenously administered beef, pork, or recombinant human insulin in cats have used RIAs that do not detect cat insulin to ensure lack of interference of the cat's insulin in the results (Wallace et al, 1990).

TREATMENT OF NONKETOTIC DIABETES MELLITUS

Goals of Therapy

The goals of therapy are similar for the diabetic dog and cat; that is, elimination of owner-observed signs that occur secondary to hyperglycemia and glycosuria, maintenance of a "healthy" pet at a stable body weight, and avoidance of complications affiliated with diabetes mellitus and its treatment (see Table 11-7, page 496). These goals can usually be attained through proper insulin administration, diet, exercise, oral hypoglycemic medications, and/or the avoidance or control of concurrent inflammatory, infectious, neoplastic, and hormonal disorders. Which therapeutic regimen is ultimately successful depends in part on the number of functional beta cells remaining in the pancreas and individual variation of response to treatment.

Although attempting to normalize the blood glucose concentration is worthwhile, the veterinarian must also guard against the development of hypoglycemia, a serious and potentially fatal complication of therapy. Hypoglycemia is most likely to occur with overzealous insulin therapy. The veterinarian must balance the possible benefits of "tight" glucose control obtainable with insulin therapy against the risks of inducing hypoglycemia.

The significant incidence of NIDDM in cats raises interesting questions about the need for insulin treatment. Glycemic control can be maintained in some diabetic cats with dietary changes, oral hypoglycemic drugs, and control of current diseases. Obviously, it would be advantageous to be able to prospectively differentiate IDDM from NIDDM by assessing beta cell function. Unfortunately, measurement of the baseline serum insulin concentration or serum insulin concentrations after administration of an insulin secretagogue have not been consistent aids in differentiating IDDM from NIDDM in the cat. The ultimate differentiation between IDDM and NIDDM is often made retrospectively, after the clinician has had several weeks to assess the cat's response to therapy and to determine its need for insulin. The initial decision between insulin treatment and oral hypoglycemic drugs is based on the severity of clinical signs, the presence or absence of ketoacidosis, the cat's general health, and the owner's wishes.

Initial Insulin Therapy

The types and species of commercial insulin preparations are discussed in Chapter 11 (page 496). Diabetic cats are notoriously unpredictable in their response to exogenous insulin. No single type of insulin is routinely effective in maintaining control of glycemia, even with twice a day administration. Since the loss of protamine zinc insulin (PZI) a decade ago, neutral protamine Hagedorn (NPH), lente, and ultralente insulin of recombinant human origin have all been used to treat diabetic cats. Ultralente insulin is the longest acting but least potent of the commonly used commercial insulins (see Fig.11-19, page 521, and Fig. 12-11). Although considered a long-acting insulin, ultralente insulin has to be administered twice a day in most diabetic cats, and absorption of ultralente insulin is inadequate for controlling glycemia in approximately 25% of cats. Lente and NPH are more potent insulin preparations that are more consistently and rapidly absorbed after subcutaneous administration than is ultralente insulin. Unfortunately, the duration of effect of lente and especially NPH insulin can be considerably shorter than 12 hours in some diabetic cats, resulting in inadequate control of glycemia despite twice a day administration (see Table 11-8, page 497). Although the amino acid sequences of human and feline insulin differ, the prevalence of insulin antibodies causing problems with control of glycemia is uncommon in cats treated with recombinant human insulin (see page 572).

PZI of beef/pork origin at a concentration of 40 U/ml (i.e., U40) and produced using the same methods as the original manufacturer is now available (IDEXX, Westbrook, Maine). PZI is a longer acting insulin that is more consistently absorbed than ultralente insulin and has a more acceptable duration of effect than NPH insulin. However, the timing of the glucose nadir is quite variable and occurs within 9 hours of PZI administration in greater than 80% of treated diabetic cats (Nelson et al, 2001). We routinely administer PZI twice a day. In a recent study, PZI was very effective in significantly improving control of glycemia in newly diagnosed diabetic cats and poorly controlled diabetic cats previously treated with ultralente or NPH insulin (Fig. 12-12) (Nelson et al, 2001). Comparison of efficacy

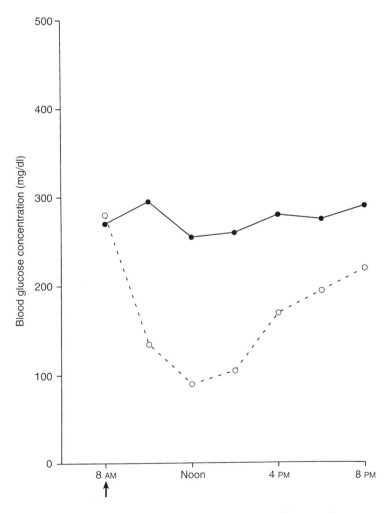

FIGURE 12-11. Blood glucose curve in a 5 kg male cat receiving 0.6 U/kg beef/pork source ultralente insulin *(solid line)* and 0.6 U/kg beef/pork source lente insulin *(broken line)* subcutaneously. At the same insulin dosage, lente insulin had a more "potent" glucose-lowering effect than ultralente insulin. ↑ = insulin injection and food.

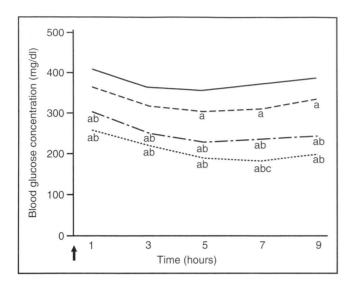

FIGURE 12-12. Mean blood glucose concentrations in 67 cats with insulin-dependent diabetes mellitus treated by administration of various dosages of protamine zinc insulin (PZI) twice daily for 45 days. Arrow indicates time of administration of insulin and consumption of half of daily caloric intake, which occurred 1 hour prior to first blood glucose measurement on each day of evaluation. Mean (± SD) daily insulin dosage was 0.4 ± 0.1 U/kg of body weight on day 7 *(solid line)*; 0.7 ± 0.2 U/kg on day 14 *(dashes)*; 0.8 ± 0.3 U/kg on day 30 *(dashes and dots)*; and 0.9 ± 0.4 U/kg on day 45 *(dots)*. [a]Value differs significantly (p <0.05) from value obtained on day 7. [b]Value differs significantly (p <0.05) from value obtained on day 14. [c]Value differs significantly (p <0.05) from value obtained on day 30. (From Nelson RW, et al: Efficacy of protamine zinc insulin for treatment of diabetes mellitus in cats. JAVMA 218:38, 2001.)

between PZI and lente has not been reported. PZI is not indicated for diabetic dogs because of the high probability of insulin antibody production directed against the bovine insulin in the product (see page 522). Insulin antibodies may interfere with insulin action, causing erratic and poor control of glycemia.

Insulin glargine (Lantus; Aventis Pharmaceuticals, Bridgewater, NJ) is a long-acting insulin analog that forms microprecipitates at the site of injection, from which small amounts of insulin glargine are slowly released (see page 498). In humans, the slow, sustained release of insulin glargine from these microprecipitates results in a relatively constant concentration/time profile over a 24-hour period with no pronounced peak in serum insulin. Insulin glargine is currently recommended as a basal insulin (i.e., sustained, long-acting insulin to inhibit hepatic glucose production) administered once a day at bedtime in human diabetics (Rosenstock et al, 2000 and 2001). In a preliminary study involving healthy cats, most of the pharmacokinetic and pharmacodynamic properties (i.e., onset of action, glucose nadir, time for blood glucose concentration to return to baseline, mean daily blood glucose concentration, and area under the 24-hour blood glucose curve) were similar for insulin glargine and PZI (Marshall and Rand, 2002). Similar studies in diabetic cats have yet to be reported. In our experience, insulin glargine has a duration of effect ranging from 10 to 16 hours in most diabetic cats. We have not yet

encountered problems with inadequate absorption of insulin glargine, as is described with ultralente insulin, although it seems likely that this problem will be encountered as we gain more experience with this insulin analog. Currently, we consider using insulin glargine in diabetic cats with problems of short duration of effect from NPH, lente, and PZI (see page 570). Based on our current experiences, we do not consider insulin glargine a first-choice insulin for the treatment of diabetes in cats.

It is impossible to predict which type of insulin will work best in individual diabetic cats. The initial insulin of choice ultimately is based on personal preference and experience. Currently, we recommend either lente insulin of recombinant human origin or PZI of beef/pork origin at a dosage of 1 U per cat administered twice daily. Dietary therapy is initiated concurrently (see below). Because greater than 80% to 90% of diabetic cats require recombinant human lente or beef/pork PZI twice a day, we prefer to start with twice a day insulin therapy. Establishing control of glycemia is easier and problems with hypoglycemia and the Somogyi effect (see page 569) are less likely when twice daily insulin therapy is initiated while the insulin dose is low; that is, when insulin treatment is started.

Dietary Therapy

The general principles for dietary therapy are discussed on page 499 (Table 12-2). Obesity, feeding practices, and content of the diet warrant discussion in diabetic cats.

Obesity

Obesity is common in diabetic cats and results from excessive caloric intake, typically caused by free-choice feeding of dry cat food. Obesity causes reversible insulin resistance, which resolves as obesity is corrected (see Fig. 12-6) (see page 545) (Nelson et al, 1990; Biourge et al, 1997). Control of glycemia often improves and some diabetic cats may revert to a subclinical diabetic state with weight reduction. The general principles for correcting obesity are similar for dogs and cats and are discussed on page 501. Correction of obesity is difficult in cats because it requires restriction of daily caloric intake with a minimal corresponding increase in caloric expenditure (i.e., exercise). The optimum body weight for cats is generally 3.5 to 5 kg. It is very important to set realistic and obtainable goals for weight loss in order to maintain client compliance. If the ideal body weight is below 15% of the current body weight, it is crucial to use a stepwise process to gradually achieve ideal body weight. The pet's initial goal should be set at 15% body weight loss. Once this goal has been achieved, a new target body weight can be selected until the pet has reached an ideal body weight. To achieve 15% body weight loss, cats can be fed 30 × (initial body weight in kg) kcal per day (Elliott, 2003). When fed at this level, cats achieve 15% body weight

TABLE 12-2 RECOMMENDATIONS FOR DIETARY TREATMENT OF DIABETES MELLITUS IN CATS

I. Dietary Composition (See Table 12-3)

Option 1: Moderate carbohydrate and fat, high fiber content
Option 2: High protein, low carbohydrate, low fiber content
Option 3: High fat, low carbohydrate, low fiber content
Diet options can be used interchangeably.
Which diet composition will improve glycemic control the most is unpredictable.

II. Feeding Recommendations

Feed canned and/or dry kibble foods.
Avoid diets containing monosaccharides, disaccharides, and propylene glycol.

III. Caloric Intake and Obesity

Average daily caloric intake for a geriatric pet should be 30 to 50 kcal/kg.
Adjust daily caloric intake on an individual basis.
Eliminate obesity, if present, by:
    Decreasing daily caloric intake
    Feeding diets designed for weight loss

IV. Feeding Schedule

Maintain consistent caloric content of the meals.
Maintain consistent timing of feeding.
Feed within time frame of insulin action.
Feed one half the total daily caloric intake at time of each insulin injection.
Let "nibbler" cats continue to nibble throughout day and night.

---

loss in 18 weeks. If the calculated amount of calories to achieve 15% body weight loss is actually less than the current daily caloric intake, the dietary history should be reevaluated to search for additional calories. If no additional daily calories are identified, the daily caloric intake of the pet should be reduced by 15% to 20%. Although several diets specifically formulated for weight reduction in cats are available, diets containing increased amounts of fiber or protein should be used in the diabetic cat for reasons discussed below.

Multicat households in which one cat is obese but the others are normal body weight or lean can present some management problems. Ideally cats should be fed in separate rooms, but this is not always possible. In general, fat cats cannot jump. Hence, it may be useful to place the healthy cat's food on an elevated bench so that healthy cats can jump up to consume their meals. Alternatively, a large cardboard box can be obtained. A small cat hole is cut into the box that will allow the normal body weight cats to fit but that restricts the entry of the fat cat. The normal weight cats are then fed in the box (Elliott, 2003).

Cats on a weight reduction program should be reevaluated every 2 weeks. The body weight and body condition score should be recorded, and the dietary history should be reviewed. Ideally, cats should achieve about 1% body weight loss per week. More rapid weight loss in cats increases the risk of hepatic lipidosis. If the rate of weight loss exceeds 2% body weight loss per week, the amount of calories fed should

be increased by 10% to 15%. If no weight loss has occurred, the dietary history should be reevaluated for additional calories. If none are found, the daily caloric intake should be further reduced by 10% to 15%.

Feeding schedule

The eating habits of cats vary considerably, from those that eat everything at the time it is offered to those that graze throughout the day and night. The primary goal of dietary therapy is to minimize the impact of a meal on postprandial blood glucose concentrations (see Feeding Schedule, page 502). Consuming the same amount of calories in multiple small amounts throughout a 12-hour period should have less impact than consuming the calories at a single large meal. Half of the cat's total daily caloric intake should be offered at the time of each insulin injection and should remain available to the cat to consume when it wishes. Attempts to force a "grazing" cat to eat the entire meal at one time usually fail and are not warranted as long as the cat has access to the food during the ensuing 12 hours. A similar approach is taken for diabetic dogs that are finicky eaters.

Dietary carbohydrate, protein, and fiber content

During the past decade, high fiber, moderately fat restricted diets (e.g., Prescription Diet w/d, Hill's Pet Products, Topeka, Kansas) have been recommended for diabetic cats based on studies that documented a significant improvement in glycemic control when diabetic cats consumed a canned insoluble-fiber (cellulose) diet containing 12% insoluble fiber on a dry matter basis, compared with a canned low-fiber diet (Fig. 12-13) (Nelson et al, 2000). A corresponding significant decrease in daily insulin dosages was seen when cats consumed the high-fiber diet compared with the low-fiber diet. As with diabetic dogs, increased frequency of defecation, inappetence caused by poor palatability, constipation, and obstipation are common when diabetic cats are fed diets containing large amounts of insoluble fiber.

Recently, dietary recommendations for diabetic cats have come under scrutiny, in part because of the seemingly increasing prevalence of obesity, chronic pancreatitis, and inflammatory bowel disease in cats during the past decade. Cats are carnivores and as such have higher dietary protein requirements than omnivores such as humans and dogs (Morris, 2002). The activity of hepatic enzymes responsible for the phosphorylation of glucose for subsequent storage or oxidation (glucokinase, hexokinase) and the conversion of glucose to glycogen for storage in the liver (glycogen synthetase) are lower in cats compared with that for carnivores with omnivorous dietary habits (Zoran, 2002). The low activity of these hepatic enzymes suggests that cats primarily use gluconeogenic amino acids and fat, rather than starch, in their diet for energy and suggests that diabetic cats may be predisposed to developing higher postprandial blood glucose concen-

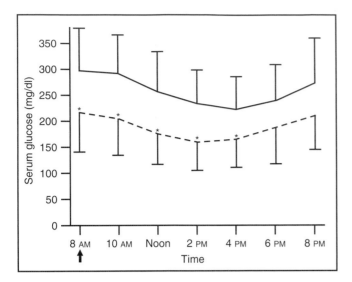

FIGURE 12-13. Mean (± SD) serum concentration of glucose in samples obtained from 16 cats with naturally acquired diabetes mellitus prior to feeding (8 AM) and obtained for 12 hours after insulin administration and concurrent consumption of a meal high in insoluble fiber *(dashed line)* or low in fiber *(solid line).* The mean serum concentration of glucose is the mean of all corresponding serum glucose values obtained during the 12-hour blood glucose–sampling period for each cat at 6, 12, 18, and 24 weeks after initiation of each diet. *Arrow* indicates time of administration of insulin and consumption of half of daily caloric intake. *Values differ significantly (p <0.05) from those for the low-fiber diet. (From Nelson RW, et al: Effect of dietary insoluble fiber on control of glycemia in cats with naturally acquired diabetes mellitus. J Am Vet Med Assoc 216:1082, 2000.)

trations after consumption of diets containing a high carbohydrate load, and vice versa. Two carbohydrate-restricted diets that have been recommended for diabetic cats are Purina DM (Ralston Purina, St. Louis, MO) and Science Diet Feline Growth (Hill's Pet Products, Topeka, KS). Purina DM is a high-protein, low-carbohydrate, low-fiber diet, and Science Diet Growth is a high-fat, low-carbohydrate, low-fiber diet (Table 12-3). In one study, consumption of the high-protein, low-carbohydrate diet was effective in improving control of glycemia, with a corresponding decrease in the daily insulin requirements in four of 9 diabetic cats; insulin was discontinued in one of the four cats (Frank et al, 2001). Although insulin was discontinued in two additional cats by the end of the study, the serum fructosamine concentration increased to 811 and 635 µmol/L (reference range, 175 to 400 µmol/L), and the average blood glucose concentration over 6 to 8 hours increased to 485 and 458 mg/dl in these cats. Improvement in clinical signs, the fasting blood glucose concentration, and the serum fructosamine concentration has been reported in diabetic cats fed the high-fat, low-carbohydrate diet, and insulin treatment was successfully discontinued in four of the 13 cats (Bennett et al, 2001). Improvement in control of glycemia also has been reported in diabetic cats fed the high-fat, low-carbohydrate diet and treated with the α-glucosidase inhibitor, acarbose (see page 504) (Mazzaferro et al, 2000). Interestingly, in retrospect, the high-fiber diet critically evaluated by Nelson and colleagues (2000) also contained 7% less carbohydrate and 5% more protein on a metabolizable energy basis than the low-fiber diet used in the study; differences that may have contributed to the beneficial glycemic effect of the high-fiber diet.

The central theme in all of these studies is restriction of carbohydrate absorption by the gastrointestinal tract, either by inhibiting starch digestion (acarbose), inhibiting intestinal glucose absorption (fiber), or decreasing carbohydrate ingestion (low-carbohydrate diets). Intuitively, the most effective means to minimize gastrointestinal absorption of carbohydrates in the diabetic cat is to feed diets that contain minimal amounts of carbohydrate. The beneficial role, if any, of the high protein or high fat content of these diets on the control of glycemia is not known at this time. It also is not known what effect, if any, a high-protein intake may have on the development of ketosis or diabetic nephropathy, the induction of satiety, or maintenance of a stable body weight. Similarly, it is not known what effect, if any, a high-fat intake may have on the development of obesity, hepatic lipidosis, and chronic pancreatitis or induction of insulin resistance and increased hepatic glucose production secondary

TABLE 12-3   APPROXIMATE NUTRIENT CONTENT OF SOME COMMERCIALLY AVAILABLE DIETS USED FOR THE TREATMENT OF DIABETES MELLITUS IN CATS

Diet	Crude Fiber*	Carbohydrates[†]	Fat[†]	Protein[†] (Can/Cup)	Calories[‡]
Prescription Diet w/d					
Canned	13	22	39	39	148
Dry	9	37	23	40	246
Purina DM					
Canned	4	7	44	49	194
Dry	1	11	37	52	592
Science Diet Feline Growth					
Canned	1	7	60	33	230
Dry	1	21	50	29	510

*Expressed as a percent of the diet dry matter.
[†]Expressed as percent metabolizable energy derived from carbohydrates, fat, or protein.
[‡]Expressed as kilocalories of metabolizable energy per can (5.5 oz.) or for the dry diets per standard (8 oz. volume) measuring cup full.

TABLE 12-4 INDICATIONS, EFFICACY, AND ADVERSE EFFECTS WITH ORAL HYPOGLYCEMIC DRUGS IN DIABETIC CATS AND DOGS

Drug Classification	Mechanism of Action	Indications	Efficacy	Adverse Effects	Prevalence of Adverse Effects
Sulfonylureas (e.g., glipizide, glyburide)	Stimulate insulin secretion	Cats with non–insulin-dependent diabetes mellitus (NIDDM); not indicated in dogs	~25% of cats respond	Cats: Vomiting, icterus, increased liver enzymes, hypoglycemia	<15% of treated cats
Meglitinides (e.g., Repaglinide)	Stimulate insulin secretion	Possibly cats with NIDDM	Unknown	Unknown	Unknown
Biguanides (e.g., metformin)	Insulin sensitizer	Possibly cats with NIDDM	Cats: <25% respond Dogs: Unknown	Cats: Inappetence, vomiting, weight loss	Cats: Common at dosages >75 mg Dogs: Unknown
Thiazolidinediones (e.g., rosiglitazone, pioglitazone)	Insulin sensitizer	Unknown	Unknown	Unknown	Unknown
α-Glucosidase inhibitors (e.g., acarbose)	Slows intestinal glucose absorption	Adjunct treatment in dogs and possibly cats	Cats: Unknown Dogs: Dose dependent	Cats: Unknown Dogs: Diarrhea, weight loss	Cats: Unknown Dogs: 35% of treated dogs

to the generation of nonesterified fatty acids, beta-hydroxybutyric acid, and hypertriglyceridemia, especially in older cats that may have decreased lipoprotein and hepatic lipase activity (Roden et al, 1996; Massillon et al, 1997; Butterwick et al, 2001). For now, all three diets listed in Table 12-3 are considered viable choices for the management of diabetes in cats. Which diet will be most beneficial in improving control of glycemia in any given diabetic cat is unpredictable. As such, the initial diet of choice is based on personal preferences and experience. If palatability or adverse effects become an issue or if poor control of glycemia persists despite adjustments in insulin therapy, a switch to one of the other diets should be considered.

Identification and Control of Concurrent Problems

In general, any concurrent inflammatory, infectious, hormonal, or neoplastic disorder can cause insulin resistance and can interfere with the effectiveness of insulin therapy (see page 506). Identification and treatment of concurrent disease play an integral role in successful management of the diabetic cat. A thorough history, a physical examination, and complete diagnostic evaluation (including CBC, serum biochemistry panel, serum T_4, urinalysis, and abdominal ultrasound scan) are indicated in any newly diagnosed diabetic cat to identify concurrent problems that may interfere with the success of treatment.

Oral Hypoglycemic Drugs

Oral hypoglycemic drugs are primarily used for the treatment of NIDDM, a form of diabetes that is uncommon in dogs but common in cats (see Etiology, page 541). In the United States, five classes of oral

hypoglycemic drugs have been approved for the treatment of NIDDM in human beings: sulfonylureas, meglitinides, biguanides, thiazolidinediones, and α-glucosidase inhibitors (Table 12-4). These drugs work by stimulating pancreatic insulin secretion, enhancing tissue sensitivity to insulin, or slowing postprandial intestinal glucose absorption. In addition, chromium and vanadium are trace minerals that may also enhance tissue sensitivity to insulin. Sulfonylureas have been the most extensively evaluated of the oral hypoglycemic drugs in diabetic cats.

Sulfonylureas

Sulfonylurea drugs (e.g., glipizide, glyburide) are the most commonly used oral hypoglycemic drugs for the treatment of diabetes mellitus in cats (Table 12-5) (DeFronzo, 1999). The primary effect of sulfonylureas is direct stimulation of insulin secretion by the beta cells of the pancreas (Fig. 12-14) (Gerich, 1989; Miller et al, 1992). Some endogenous pancreatic insulin secretory capacity must exist for sulfonylureas to be effective in improving glycemic control. Extrapancreatic effects include improvement of tissue sensitivity to circulating

TABLE 12-5 ORAL SULFONYLUREA DRUGS AVAILABLE IN THE UNITED STATES

Generic Name	Trade Name	Relative Potency
First Generation		
Tolbutamide	Ornase	1
Acetohexamide	Dymelor	2.5
Tolazamide	Tolinase	5
Chlorpropamide	Diabinese	6
Second Generation		
Glipizide	Glucotrol	100
Glyburide	Micronase, DiaBeta	150

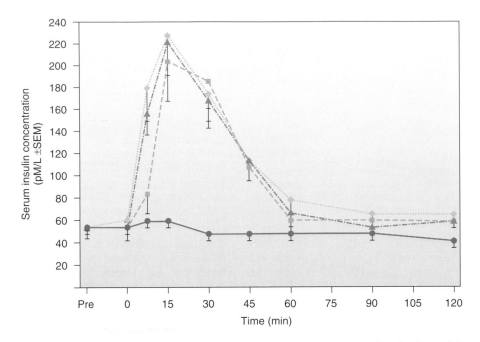

FIGURE 12-14. Mean serum insulin concentrations after oral administration of a placebo and three doses of glipizide (2.5, 5.0, and 10 mg) to 10 healthy cats. Placebo: Solid line; 2.5 mg: dashes-squares; 5.0 mg: dash-dot-triangle; 10 mg: dots-diamonds. (From Miller AB, et al: Effect of glipizide on serum insulin and glucose concentrations in healthy cats. Res Vet Sci 52:177, 1992.)

insulin, either through increased insulin receptor binding or improved postbinding action, inhibition of hepatic glycogenolysis, increased hepatic glucose utilization, and decreased hepatic insulin extraction (Gerich, 1989; Jaber et al, 1990; DeFronzo, 1999). These extrapancreatic effects may be the result of a direct action of the drug itself or may occur secondary to the resultant stimulation of insulin secretion.

GLIPIZIDE. The sulfonylurea drug glipizide (Glucotrol; Pfizer, New York, NY) has been used successfully as an alternative to insulin therapy in healthy, newly diagnosed diabetic cats (Nelson et al, 1993; Feldman et al, 1997). Clinical response is variable, ranging from excellent (i.e., blood glucose concentrations decreasing to less than 200 mg/dl) to partial response (i.e., clinical improvement but failure to resolve hyperglycemia) to no response. Presumably, the population of functioning beta cells varies from none (severe IDDM) to near normal (mild NIDDM) in treated cats, resulting in a response range from none to excellent. Cats with a partial response to glipizide have some functioning beta cells but not enough to decrease the blood glucose concentration to less than 200 mg/dl. These cats may have severe NIDDM or the early stages of IDDM. In our experience, glipizide treatment is effective in improving clinical signs and severity of hyperglycemia in approximately 30% of our diabetic cats in which it is used.

Selection Criteria. No consistent parameters allow the clinician to prospectively identify cats that will respond to glipizide therapy. Identification of a high preprandial serum insulin concentration or an increase in the serum insulin concentration during an insulin secretagogue test supports the diagnosis of NIDDM and the probability of a beneficial response to glipizide treatment; however, failure to identify these changes does not rule out NIDDM or the potential for a beneficial response to glipizide (Nelson et al, 1993). Selection of diabetic cats for treatment with glipizide must rely heavily on the veterinarian's assessment of the cat's health, the severity of clinical signs, the presence or absence of ketoacidosis and other diabetic complications (e.g., neuropathy), and the owner's desires.

Three sets of diabetic cats are obvious candidates for oral hypoglycemic drug therapy. The first group includes diabetic cats whose owners absolutely refuse to give injections. The second group includes cats that vacillate in and out of an insulin-requiring diabetic state (i.e., transiently diabetic). The third group includes cats that require insulin to control their diabetes but are very sensitive to the actions of insulin, have recurring problems with hypoglycemia, and require extremely low doses of insulin (i.e., <1 U/dose given once or twice daily). Conversely, oral hypoglycemic drugs are ineffective in improving glycemic control in poorly regulated diabetic cats with insulin resistance.

Adverse Reactions. Adverse reactions that have been identified with glipizide treatment in cats include hypoglycemia, vomiting shortly after administration of the drug, increases in serum hepatic enzyme activities, and icterus (Nelson et al, 1993; Feldman et al, 1997). The incidence of adverse reactions is less than 15% and can be significantly reduced by use of small initial doses. Hypoglycemia, hepatic enzyme alterations, and icterus resolve after discontinuation of glipizide. It is not known whether the increased serum hepatic enzyme activities are a result of hepatocellular damage and leakage or cellular death. In cats with hepatic reactions, glipizide treatment can be tried again, using a lower dosage, once hepatic enzyme abnormalities or icterus has resolved. In some cats the hepatic abnormalities do not recur, but in others hepatic abnormalities recur regardless of the glipizide dosage.

One theoretical adverse reaction of chronic glipizide therapy is accelerated loss of pancreatic beta-cell function caused by glipizide-induced stimulation of amylin secretion and worsening islet amyloidosis (see Fig. 12-4) (see Non–insulin-dependent Diabetes Mellitus). The effect of chronic sulfonylurea therapy on insulin secretion in human diabetics is controversial. In human diabetics treated with sulfonylureas, secondary failures (i.e., initial successful response for at least 6 months followed by subsequent failure to have an adequate response) range from 5% to 35% (Lebovitz, 1990). Secondary failure may be caused by patient-related factors (e.g., poor diet, stress), therapy-related factors (e.g., inadequate dose, impaired intestinal absorption), or disease-related factors (e.g., progression of islet pathology, insulin resistance) (Groop, 1992). What role sulfonylureas played in promoting disease-related factors is not known. Most studies have reported unchanged or decreased plasma levels of immunoreactive insulin after chronic administration (months to years) of sulfonylureas (Gerich, 1989; Groop, 1992). Other studies have reported continuously augmented insulin secretion with chronic sulfonylurea therapy (Lebovitz, 1990; Fajans and Brown, 1993).

Secondary failures also occur in diabetic cats treated with glipizide (Nelson et al, 1993). What role glipizide plays in accelerating secondary failures in cats is not known. In a recent study using an induced model of diabetes in cats (partial [~50%] pancreatectomy followed by 4 months of daily growth hormone injections and oral dexamethasone), mild to moderate islet amyloid deposition and moderate to severe islet vacuolar change were identified in three and one of four cats, respectively, that were treated with glipizide for 18 months, and in one and three of four cats, respectively, that were treated with recombinant human NPH insulin for 18 months (Hoenig et al, 2000b). The results suggested that glipizide treatment could cause progressive amyloid deposition as a result of glipizide-induced insulin and amylin secretion. Does this mean that glipizide should not be used for the treatment of diabetes in cats? To answer this question, one has to look at the underlying reason for using this drug. Glipizide has no advantage over insulin therapy with regard to cost of treatment, time required to treat, efficacy of treatment, or frequency of reevaluations by the veterinarian. However, glipizide gives many owners an initially more palatable option (i.e., pills versus injections) for the treatment of their newly diagnosed diabetic cat. Most owners who are unwilling to give insulin injections would euthanize their cat. Many of these people are willing to try oral medication. During the ensuing weeks, many of these owners become willing to try insulin injections if glipizide therapy fails. In our opinion, the real advantage of glipizide is in keeping more diabetic cats alive by giving the owner treatment options in lieu of insulin injections and not forcing a quick life-or-death decision at the time diabetes is diagnosed.

Treatment Protocol. Glipizide is initially administered at a dose of 2.5 mg per os two times a day in conjunction with a meal to diabetic cats that are nonketotic and relatively healthy on physical examination (Fig. 12-15). Each cat is examined weekly during the first month of glipizide therapy. The history, physical examination findings, body weight, urine glucose and ketone measurement, and blood glucose concentration are evaluated at each examination. If adverse reactions (Table 12-6) have not occurred after 2 weeks of treatment, the glipizide dosage is increased to 5.0 mg two times per day. Therapy is continued as long as the cat is stable, the owners are satisfied with the treatment, and the blood glucose and serum fructosamine concentrations are acceptable (i.e., average blood glucose concentration less than 300 mg/dl, serum fructosamine concentration less than 500 μmol/L). If euglycemia or hypoglycemia develops, the glipizide dosage may be tapered or discontinued and the blood glucose concentrations reevaluated 1 week later to assess the need for the drug. If hyperglycemia recurs, the dosage is increased or glipizide is reinitiated, with a reduction in dosage in cats that previously developed hypoglycemia. Glipizide is discontinued and insulin therapy is initiated if clinical signs continue to worsen; if the cat becomes ill or develops ketoacidosis or peripheral neuropathy;

TABLE 12-6 ADVERSE REACTIONS TO GLIPIZIDE TREATMENT IN DIABETIC CATS

Adverse Reaction	Recommendation
Vomiting within 1 hour of administration	Vomiting usually subsides after 2 to 5 days of glipizide therapy; decrease dose or frequency of administration if vomiting is severe; discontinue if vomiting persists longer than 1 week.
Increased serum hepatic enzyme activities	Continue treatment and monitor enzymes every 1 to 2 weeks initially; discontinue glipizide if cat becomes ill (lethargy, inappetence, vomiting) or the alanine transaminase activity exceeds 500 IU/L.
Icterus	Discontinue glipizide treatment; reinstitute glipizide therapy at lower dose and frequency of administration once icterus has resolved (usually within 2 weeks); discontinue treatment permanently if icterus recurs.
Hypoglycemia	Discontinue glipizide treatment; recheck blood glucose concentration in 1 week; reinstitute glipizide therapy at lower dose or frequency of administration if hyperglycemia recurs.

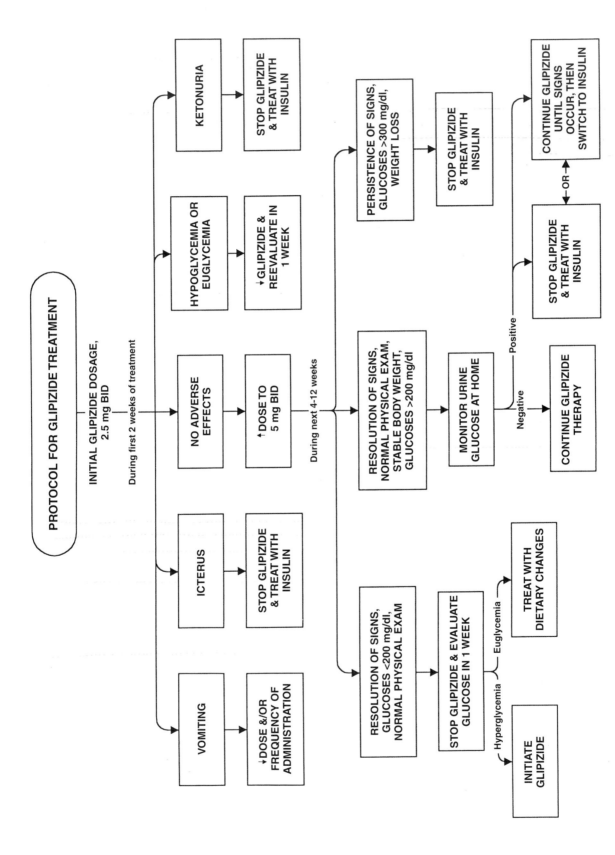

PROTOCOL FOR GLIPIZIDE TREATMENT

INITIAL GLIPIZIDE DOSAGE, 2.5 mg BID

During first 2 weeks of treatment

VOMITING → ↓DOSE &/OR FREQUENCY OF ADMINISTRATION

ICTERUS → STOP GLIPIZIDE & TREAT WITH INSULIN

NO ADVERSE EFFECTS → ↑DOSE TO 5 mg BID

HYPOGLYCEMIA OR EUGLYCEMIA → ↓GLIPIZIDE & REEVALUATE IN 1 WEEK

KETONURIA → STOP GLIPIZIDE & TREAT WITH INSULIN

During next 4-12 weeks

RESOLUTION OF SIGNS, GLUCOSES <200 mg/dl, NORMAL PHYSICAL EXAM → STOP GLIPIZIDE & EVALUATE GLUCOSE IN 1 WEEK

— Hyperglycemia → INITIATE GLIPIZIDE

— Euglycemia → TREAT WITH DIETARY CHANGES

RESOLUTION OF SIGNS, NORMAL PHYSICAL EXAM, STABLE BODY WEIGHT, GLUCOSES >200 mg/dl → MONITOR URINE GLUCOSE AT HOME

— Negative → CONTINUE GLIPIZIDE THERAPY

— Positive → STOP GLIPIZIDE & TREAT WITH INSULIN

PERSISTENCE OF SIGNS, GLUCOSES >300 mg/dl, WEIGHT LOSS → STOP GLIPIZIDE & TREAT WITH INSULIN

— OR — CONTINUE GLIPIZIDE UNTIL SIGNS OCCUR, THEN SWITCH TO INSULIN

FIGURE 12-15. Algorithm for treating diabetic cats with the oral sulfonylurea drug glipizide.

if the blood glucose or serum fructosamine concentration remains greater than 300 mg/dl and 500 μmol/L, respectively, after 1 to 2 months of therapy; or if the owners become dissatisfied with the treatment. In some cats, glipizide becomes ineffective weeks to months later, and exogenous insulin ultimately is required to control the diabetic state. Presumably the need to be switched from glipizide to insulin treatment results from the progression of the underlying pathophysiologic condition (e.g., islet-specific amyloid deposition). The more rapid the progression, the shorter the beneficial response to glipizide.

Potential Outcomes to Therapy. Several outcomes are possible using this therapeutic approach. The most common is failure to control hyperglycemia or the clinical signs of diabetes mellitus. For these cats, glipizide therapy is discontinued and insulin is used to control the blood glucose concentration. Human diabetics who do not achieve adequate glycemic control with sulfonylureas may achieve better glycemic control with combination therapy (i.e., insulin and sulfonylurea) than with insulin alone (Lebovitz and Pasmantier, 1990; Bailey and Mezitis, 1990). Some patients subsequently become responsive to sulfonylureas as the sole treatment, presumably as a consequence of insulin therapy correcting glucose toxicity. Unfortunately, we have not had similar experiences in our diabetic cats that failed to respond to glipizide. Concurrent administration of glipizide and insulin did not appear to affect insulin requirements or ease of glycemic regulation. Interestingly, the need for insulin therapy may dissipate in a small percentage of cats that fail to respond to glipizide.

Less commonly, the blood glucose concentration and clinical signs are controlled without the use of exogenous insulin. Cats that improve are usually classified as "partial" or "complete" responders. Complete responders have near-normal blood glucose concentrations and no glycosuria and are clinically well. Approximately 15% of the diabetic cats we have treated are either complete responders that require oral therapy to prevent hyperglycemia, or they eventually require no therapy and remain euglycemic.

Another 15% to 20% of the diabetic cats we have treated are partial responders. These cats are stable in body weight or gain weight, they are neither polydipsic or polyuric, and they appear well to their owners. The bothersome finding in these cats is their mean blood glucose concentration of 200 to 300 mg/dl. However, as a group, their pretreatment mean blood glucose concentration is typically greater than 400 mg/dl. Decreasing the blood glucose concentration below 300 mg/dl for much of each day appears to drop the blood glucose concentration below *their* renal threshold for spillage of glucose in urine, thereby eliminating or minimizing clinical signs of diabetes. We have successfully treated both "complete" and "partial" responders for longer than 7 years without the development of severe weight loss or peripheral neuropathy.

For some complete and partial responder cats, glipizide becomes ineffective and exogenous insulin is ultimately required to control the diabetic state. For these cats, the time from initiation of glipizide therapy to initiation of insulin therapy is unpredictable and quite variable, ranging from a few weeks to more than 3 years. Most cats remain on insulin for life once this form of therapy has been instituted. Rarely, insulin requirements continue to wax and wane. Presumably, the transition from NIDDM to IDDM is the result of progression of the underlying pathophysiologic mechanisms (e.g., islet-specific amyloid deposition) responsible for the development of diabetes in the cat (Nelson et al, 1998). The more rapid the rate of progression, the shorter the beneficial response to glipizide.

GLYBURIDE. Glyburide (DiaBeta, Hoechst-Roussel, Somerville, NJ; Micronase, Upjohn, Kalamazoo, MI) is another sulfonylurea with similar actions as glipizide (DeFronzo, 1999). Glyburide has a longer duration of action than glipizide and is usually administered once a day rather than the twice a day required for glipizide. Most studies in human diabetics have reported similar responses in comparisons of glyburide and glipizide (Groop, 1992; Birkeland et al, 1994). We have had minimal experience with glyburide for the treatment of diabetes in cats. However, in countries where glipizide is not available, treatment with glyburide should be considered at an initial dosage of 0.625 mg (one half of a 1.25 mg tablet) per cat once daily. The response to therapy and adverse reactions to glyburide are similar to those described for glipizide.

Meglitinides

Repaglinide (Prandin; Novo Nordisk), the only commercially available meglitinide, is a nonsulfonylurea drug that works by stimulating insulin secretion (DeFronzo, 1999). Improvement in the control of glycemia in humans with NIDDM is similar for Repaglinide and the sulfonylureas (Wolffenbuttel and Landgraf, 1999). Adverse effects in diabetic humans include hypoglycemia and weight gain. The prevalence of hypoglycemic reactions is less with Repaglinide than with the sulfonylureas (Damsbo et al, 1999). Repaglinide is used as monotherapy or in conjunction with metformin for the treatment of NIDDM in humans (Moses et al, 1999). Studies evaluating the efficacy of Repaglinide in diabetic cats have not yet been reported.

Biguanides

The most commonly used drug in this class of oral hypoglycemic agents is metformin (Glucophage; Bristol-Myers Squibb, Princeton, NJ). Metformin's mechanism of action is distinct from the sulfonylureas. Metformin has no direct effect on beta cell function but improves glycemic control in an insulin-dependent manner primarily by enhancing the sensitivity of both hepatic and peripheral tissues to insulin (Bailey and Turner, 1996; DeFronzo, 1999). Metformin inhibits hepatic gluconeogenesis and glycogenolysis; the decline in basal hepatic glucose production is closely correlated with the reduction in fasting blood glucose concentrations. Metformin also increases muscle glucose metabolism by enhancing muscle insulin sensitivity. The net effect of these actions is to lower blood glucose concentrations without causing hypoglycemia. The most common adverse effects are gastrointestinal in origin and include abdominal discomfort, inappetence, vomiting, and diarrhea (DeFronzo and Goodman, 1995). Although the development of severe lactic acidosis is a worrisome complication with metformin treatment in diabetic humans, its prevalence is now recognized to be low (Bailey and Turner, 1996). Metformin can be used as an initial therapeutic agent in human beings with NIDDM or in combination with sulfonylureas or insulin.

In human beings, therapeutic metformin concentrations in plasma range from 0.5 to 2.0 µg/ml (Sheen, 1996; Sambol et al, 1996). In cats, plasma metformin concentrations fall within the therapeutic range for humans at dosages of 25 to 50 mg/cat and are near baseline 12 hours after metformin administration (Fig. 12-16) (Michels et al, 1999; Nelson et al, in press). Lethargy and vomiting typically occur 1 to 4 hours after administration of doses exceeding 75 mg/cat. In one study, the results of routine blood work were unremarkable and lactic acidosis did not occur in healthy cats given 25 and 50 mg of metformin twice a day for 3 weeks (Nelson et al, in press). However, all cats experienced intermittent inappetence and vomiting during the 3-week drug trial, and most had lost weight by the end of the trial. Metformin was ineffective as a sole therapeutic agent in a small number of newly diagnosed diabetic cats and was discontinued in most cases because of progressively worsening clinical signs or the development of ketoacidosis (Nelson et al, in press). The only cat that responded to metformin had a fasting serum insulin

concentration greater than 20 µU/ml before initiating treatment. The serum insulin concentration was less than 5 µU/ml in all cats that failed to respond to the drug. These findings are consistent with the concept that metformin as an insulin-sensitizing drug is only effective in the presence of adequate blood concentrations of insulin. Diabetic cats with decreased serum insulin concentrations caused by loss of beta cells or suppression of beta cell function from concurrent glucose toxicity (see page 544) should not respond to metformin.

Unfortunately, the results of initial studies evaluating metformin in healthy and diabetic cats have not been encouraging, and the role, if any, for metformin in the treatment of diabetic cats remains to be clarified. Metformin is currently marketed in the United States as 500 mg tablets; administration of metformin to cats requires compounding the tablets to capsules, each containing 25 or 50 mg. Studies evaluating the usefulness of metformin as adjunct therapy in poorly controlled, insulin-treated diabetic cats or dogs have not been reported.

Thiazolidinediones

Thiazolidinediones are a new class of antidiabetic drugs that increases the sensitivity of target tissues to the action of insulin without directly stimulating insulin secretion from pancreatic beta cells. Thiazolidinediones bind to a novel receptor called the peroxisome proliferator-activated receptor-γ, leading to increased glucose transporter expression (Berger et al, 1996; Plosker and Faulds, 1999). Thiazolidinediones enhance insulin sensitivity in hepatic, muscle, and adipose tissue, thereby inhibiting hepatic glucose production, stimulating muscle glucose metabolism, and reducing circulating free fatty acid concentrations (DeFronzo, 1999). Troglitazone (Rezulin; Parke-Davis, Morris Plains, NJ) was the first commercially available thiazolidinedione in the United States and was used as monotherapy or in combination with sulfonylureas, metformin, or insulin to treat humans with NIDDM (Plosker and Faulds, 1999). Although often touted as a revolutionary new drug for treating NIDDM, several clinical studies found troglitazone monotherapy to be less effective than either sulfonylureas or metformin for treating humans with NIDDM (DeFronzo, 1999). The most serious adverse effect of troglitazone is death caused by hepatic failure (Gitlin et al, 1998), which has been reported in a large enough percentage of human diabetics that the U.S. Food and Drug Administration (FDA) withdrew troglitazone from the commercial market in the United States. Pioglitazone (Actos; Takeda Pharmaceuticals America, Lincolnshire, IL) and rosiglitazone (Avandia; SmithKline Beecham, Philadelphia, PA) are thiazolidinediones that have recently become available in the United States. Their hypoglycemic potency is at least equal to that of troglitazone (Patel et al, 1997; Grossman and Lessem, 1997). Rosiglitazone has been approved as monotherapy and for combination with metformin, and

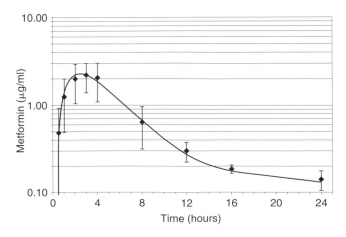

FIGURE 12-16. Mean (± SD) plasma concentration of metformin at various times following oral administration of 50 mg of metformin to five healthy cats. The therapeutic range of plasma metformin concentrations in human diabetics is 0.5 to 2.0 µg/ml. (From Nelson RW, et al: Evaluation of the oral antihyperglycemic drug metformin in normal and diabetic cats. J Vet Intern Med [in press].)

pioglitazone has been approved as monotherapy and for combination with sulfonylureas, metformin, and insulin.

The pharmacokinetics of intravenously and orally administered troglitazone have been reported in healthy cats (Michels et al, 2000). The general disposition pattern of troglitazone was similar to that reported for humans; however, the steady-state volume of distribution was lower in cats, and the oral bioavailability of troglitazone was low (7 ± 3%). Based on troglitazone pharmacokinetics in healthy cats, a dosage of 20 to 40 mg/kg administered orally once or twice a day should produce plasma concentrations of the insulin-sensitizing agent that has been documented to be effective in humans. Pharmacokinetic studies have not been reported in dogs. The role, if any, of thiazolidinediones in the treatment of diabetes in cats and dogs remains to be determined.

Chromium

Chromium is a ubiquitous trace element that exerts insulin-like effects in vitro. The exact mechanism of action is not known, but the overall effect of chromium is to increase insulin sensitivity, presumably through a postreceptor mechanism of action (Anderson, 1992; Striffler et al, 1995). Chromium is an essential cofactor for insulin function, and chromium deficiency results in insulin resistance. The effect of chromium tripicolinate supplementation on glucose tolerance has been controversial in cats, ranging from no effect in obese and nonobese healthy cats to a small but significant dose-dependent improvement in glucose tolerance in nonobese healthy cats (Cohn et al, 1999; Appleton et al, 2002b). Oral chromium tripicolinate supplementation did not improve glycemic control in a group of dogs with IDDM (Schachter et al, 2001). The effect of oral chromium tripicolinate supplementation in diabetic cats has not been reported. Chapter 11 presents more information on chromium (page 504).

Vanadium

Vanadium is another ubiquitous trace element that exerts insulin-like effects in vitro (Brichard et al, 1989). The mechanism of action is not known, but research suggests that vanadium acts at a post-receptor site to stimulate glucose metabolism (Brichard and Henquin, 1995; Goldfine et al, 1995). Vanadium does not increase serum insulin concentrations. Although the efficacy of vanadium is controversial, studies have identified decreased insulin requirements in humans with IDDM and improved control of glycemia in humans with NIDDM treated with vanadium (Goldfine et al, 1995; Cohen et al, 1995). Preliminary unpublished studies in cats performed by Dr. Greco and her colleagues have identified the following: 4 weeks of oral orthovanadate administered in the drinking water resulted in a significant reduction in mean daily water consumption and occasional vomiting and diarrhea, but therapy was otherwise well tolerated in healthy cats; blood glucose concentrations decreased and clinical signs of diabetes resolved in one diabetic cat treated with orthovanadate in the drinking water for 4 weeks; and control of glycemia appeared improved in a group of diabetic cats treated with PZI and oral vanadium dipicolinate compared with a group of cats treated with PZI alone (Plotnick et al, 1995; Fondacaro et al, 1999; Greco, 2000). The results of these studies suggest that vanadium may be a viable treatment option for cats with early NIDDM. The recommended dose is 0.2 mg/kg/day administered once a day in food or water. Adverse effects in cats include anorexia and vomiting. Long-term toxicity is related to the accumulation of the metal in organs such as bone, liver, and kidney. Acute renal failure occurred in one cat treated with vanadium for 1 year; the renal failure was reversible after discontinuation of the vanadium treatment (Greco, 2000).

Acarbose

Acarbose competitively inhibits pancreatic α-amylase and α-glucosidases in the brush border of the small intestinal mucosa, which delays digestion of complex carbohydrates and disaccharides and slows absorption of glucose from the intestinal tract (see page 504). Feeding of carbohydrate-restricted diets (see Table 12-3) is recommended in lieu of acarbose treatment in diabetic cats.

Herbs, supplements, and vitamins

See page 505.

Initial Adjustments in Insulin Therapy

The approach to initially adjusting insulin therapy is similar for the diabetic dog and cat and is discussed on page 507. The initial goal of insulin therapy is to improve the clinical signs of diabetes mellitus while avoiding hypoglycemia. Diabetic cats are typically evaluated every 7 to 14 days until an effective insulin treatment protocol is identified. At each evaluation, the owners' subjective opinion of water intake, urine output, and the overall health of their cat is discussed; a complete physical examination is performed; any change in body weight is noted; and serial blood glucose measurements between 7 to 9 AM and 4 to 6 PM are assessed. Adjustments in insulin therapy are based on this information, the pet is sent home, and an appointment is scheduled in 1 to 2 weeks to reevaluate the response to any change in therapy. Glycemic control is attained when clinical signs of diabetes have resolved, the pet is healthy and interactive in the home, its body weight is stable, the owner is satisfied with the progress of therapy and, if possible, the blood glucose concentrations range between 100 and 300 mg/dl throughout the day. Because the Somogyi phenomenon (see page 569) can occur at relatively small doses of insulin (2 to 3 U/injection) in diabetic cats, we prefer to have the owner administer a fixed dose of insulin once control of glycemia has been attained. Owners are discouraged from adjusting the insulin dose at home without first consulting their veterinarian.

TECHNIQUES FOR MONITORING DIABETIC CONTROL

Overview

The basic objective of insulin therapy is to eliminate the clinical signs of diabetes mellitus while avoiding the common complications associated with the disease. Common complications in cats include weakness, ataxia and a plantigrade stance caused by peripheral neuropathy, weight loss, poor haircoat from lack of grooming, hypoglycemia, recurring ketosis, and poor control of glycemia secondary to concurrent infection, inflammation, neoplasia, or hormonal disorders. The devastating chronic complications of human diabetes (e.g., nephropathy, vasculopathy, coronary artery disease) require several decades to develop and are uncommon in diabetic cats. As such, the need to establish near-normal blood glucose concentrations is not necessary in diabetic cats. Most owners are happy and most cats are healthy and relatively asymptomatic if most blood glucose concentrations are kept between 100 mg/dl and 300 mg/dl.

The techniques for monitoring diabetic control are similar for diabetic dogs and cats and have been discussed on page 508. One important factor that affects monitoring of diabetic cats is the propensity of cats to develop stress-induced hyperglycemia caused by frequent visits to the veterinary hospital for blood samplings (see page 567). Once stress-induced hyperglycemia develops, it is a perpetual problem and blood glucose measurements can no longer be considered accurate. Veterinarians must remain wary of stress hyperglycemia in diabetic cats and should take steps to avoid its development. Micromanaging diabetic cats should be avoided, and serial blood glucose curves should be done only when there is a perceived need to change insulin therapy. The determination of good versus poor control of glycemia should be based on the owner's subjective opinion of the presence and severity of clinical signs and the overall health of the pet, the cat's ability to jump, its grooming behavior, the findings on physical examination, and the stability of body weight. Generation of a serial blood glucose curve should be reserved for newly diagnosed and poorly controlled diabetic cats unless stress-induced hyperglycemia is suspected. If suspected, a switch from reliance on serial blood glucose curves generated in the veterinary hospital to reliance on blood glucose results generated by the owner in the less-stressful home environment (e.g., the marginal ear vein prick technique) or evaluation of sequential serum fructosamine concentrations should be done, in addition to the history and physical examination findings.

History and Physical Examination

The most important initial parameters to assess when evaluating control of glycemia are the owner's subjective opinion of the severity of clinical signs and the overall health of the pet, the findings on the physical examination, and the stability of body weight. If the owner is happy with the results of treatment, the physical examination is supportive of good glycemic control, and the body weight is stable, the diabetic cat is usually adequately controlled. Measurement of the serum fructosamine concentration can add further objective evidence for the status of glycemic control (see below).

Poor control of glycemia should be suspected and additional diagnostics (i.e., serial blood glucose curve, serum fructosamine concentration, tests for concurrent disorders) or a change in insulin therapy should be considered if the owner reports clinical signs suggestive of hyperglycemia or hypoglycemia (i.e., polyuria, polydipsia, lethargy, weakness, ataxia) or peripheral neuropathy (changes in jumping ability, weakness, ataxia, plantigrade stance); if the physical examination identifies problems consistent with poor control of glycemia (e.g., thin or emaciated appearance, poor haircoat); or if the cat is losing weight.

Serum Fructosamine Concentration

Fructosamines are glycated proteins found in blood that are used to monitor control of glycemia in diabetic dogs and cats (Reusch et al, 1993; Crenshaw et al, 1996; Elliott et al, 1999). Fructosamines result from an irreversible, nonenzymatic, insulin-independent binding of glucose to serum proteins. Serum fructosamine concentrations are a marker of the mean blood glucose concentration during the circulating life span of the protein, which varies from 1 to 3 weeks, depending on the protein (Kawamoto et al, 1991). The extent of glycosylation of serum proteins is directly related to the blood glucose concentration: the higher the average blood glucose concentration during the preceding 2 to 3 weeks, the higher the serum fructosamine concentration, and vice versa. The serum fructosamine concentration is not affected by acute increases in the blood glucose concentration, as occurs with stress or excitement-induced hyperglycemia (Lutz et al, 1995; Crenshaw et al, 1996; Plier et al, 1998; Elliott et al, 1999). Serum fructosamine concentrations can be measured during the routine evaluation of glycemic control performed every 3 to 6 months; to clarify the effect of stress or excitement on blood glucose concentrations; to clarify discrepancies between the history, physical examination findings, and serial blood glucose concentrations; and to assess the effectiveness of changes in insulin therapy (see page 567). Serum fructosamine concentrations increase when glycemic control of the diabetic cat worsens and decrease when glycemic control improves (Fig. 12-17).

Information on blood sample handling and the fructosamine assay are discussed on page 509. In our

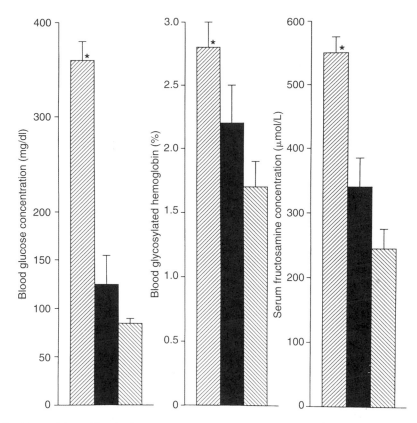

FIGURE 12-17. Mean blood glucose concentration per 12 hours after subcutaneous insulin administration, mean blood glycosylated hemoglobin concentration, and mean serum fructosamine concentration in 12 poorly regulated diabetic cats prior to (▨) and 6.5 ± 2.4 weeks after improving glycemic control (■) and in 20 healthy cats (▧) * = P <0.01 compared with value obtained after improving glycemic control.

laboratory, the normal reference range for serum fructosamine in cats is 190 to 365 µmol/L, a range determined in healthy cats with persistently normal blood glucose concentrations. The serum fructosamine concentration in newly diagnosed diabetic cats ranged from 350 to 730 µmol/L (Elliott et al, 1999). The normal serum fructosamine concentration in a few diabetic cats suggests that hyperglycemia severe enough to cause clinical signs had been present only for a short time prior to diagnosis. Interpretation of the serum fructosamine concentration is similar for the diabetic dog and cat and is discussed on page 509 (Table 12-7). Hypoproteinemia (total protein <5.5 g/dl) and hypoalbuminemia (albumin <2.5 g/dl) can decrease the serum fructosamine concentration below the reference range in healthy cats and presumably diabetic cats as well (Reusch and Haberer, 2001). In contrast, the presence of hyperproteinemia, hyperlipidemia, azotemia, and hyperbilirubinemia have no detectable effect on serum fructosamine results in healthy cats.

Blood Glycated Hemoglobin Concentration

Glycated hemoglobin (Gly Hb) is a glycated protein that results from an irreversible, nonenzymatic, insulin-independent binding of glucose to hemoglobin in red

TABLE 12-7 SAMPLE HANDLING, METHODOLOGY, AND NORMAL VALUES FOR SERUM FRUCTOSAMINE CONCENTRATIONS MEASURED IN OUR LABORATORY IN CATS

Parameter	Pertinent Information
Blood sample	1 to 2 ml; allow to clot, obtain serum
Sample handling	Freeze until assayed
Methodology	Automated colorimetric assay using nitroblue tetrazolium chloride
Factors affecting results	Hypoproteinemia and hypoalbuminemia (decreased), storage at room temperature (decreased)
Normal range	190 to 365 µmol/L
Interpretation in diabetic cats	
Excellent control	350 to 400 µmol/L
Good control	400 to 450 µmol/L
Fair control	450 to 500 µmol/L
Poor control	>500 µmol/L
Prolonged hypoglycemia	<300 µmol/L

blood cells. Blood Gly Hb is a marker of the mean blood glucose concentration during the circulating life span of the red blood cell, which is approximately 70 days in the cat (Jain, 1993). The extent of glycosylation of hemoglobin is directly related to the blood glucose concentration: the higher the average blood glucose concentration during the preceding 2 to 3 months, the higher the blood Gly Hb, and vice versa (Elliott et al, 1997; Hoenig and Ferguson, 1999). Gly Hb rather than fructosamine is used to monitor the long-term effectiveness of treatment in human diabetics, in part because diabetic humans self-monitor their blood glucose and adjust their insulin dose daily, and Gly Hb assesses a longer treatment interval than fructosamine (i.e., 3 to 4 months versus 2 to 3 weeks). In contrast, measurement of serum fructosamine is used more commonly to assess control of glycemia in diabetic cats, in part because the assay is readily available commercially and is better for assessing the impact of changes in insulin therapy on the control of glycemia in fractious or stressed cats because concentrations of fructosamine change more quickly than Gly Hb (i.e., 2 to 3 weeks versus 2 to 3 months).

Information on the fractions of Gly Hb, blood sample handling, and Gly Hb assays is presented on page 510. In our laboratory, the normal reference range for total Gly Hb as measured by affinity chromatography in cats is 0.9% to 2.5%, a range determined in healthy cats with persistently normal blood glucose concentrations. Blood total Gly Hb in newly diagnosed diabetic cats ranged from 1.2% to 4.7% (Elliott et al, 1997). The normal total Gly Hb in some diabetic cats suggests that diabetes had been present only for a short time prior to diagnosis. The reason for lower total Gly Hb percentages in cats versus dogs is not known but may be the result of a shorter life of the feline red blood cells; differences in amino acid composition or the conformation of the hemoglobin chain, which may reduce the number of binding sites for glucose; or differences in red blood cell membrane permeability to glucose (Hasegawa et al, 1992; Christopher et al, 1995; Elliott et al, 1997). Interpretation of the blood total Gly Hb is similar for the diabetic dog and cat and is discussed on page 511 (Table 12-8).

Urine Glucose Monitoring

Occasional monitoring of urine for glycosuria and ketonuria in the home environment is helpful in diabetic cats that have problems with recurring ketosis, to determine if ketonuria is present; in cats that have reverted to a non-insulin-requiring diabetic state, to determine if glycosuria has recurred; in cats treated with oral hypoglycemic drugs, to determine if glycosuria has improved or worsened; and in cats suspected of having stress-induced hyperglycemia, to differentiate transient from persistent hyperglycemia. In all of these situations, the time of day the urine sample is obtained is not critical to the interpretation of the results. A small amount of urine can be obtained by decreasing the amount of kitty litter in the pan or temporarily replacing the kitty litter with nonabsorbable material, such as aquarium gravel, or by assessing the change in color of urine glucose test squares

TABLE 12-8 SAMPLE HANDLING, METHODOLOGY, AND NORMAL VALUES FOR BLOOD TOTAL GLYCOSYLATED HEMOGLOBIN CONCENTRATIONS MEASURED IN OUR LABORATORY IN CATS

Parameter	Pertinent Information
Blood sample	1 to 2 ml whole blood in EDTA
Sample handling	Refrigerate until assayed
Methodology	Affinity chromatography and hemolysates derived from feline red blood cells
Factors affecting results	Storage at room temperature (decreased), storage at 4º C for longer than 7 days (decreased); anemia (Hct <35%) (decreased)
Normal range	0.9 to 2.5%
Interpretation in diabetic cats	
Excellent control	1.0 to 2.0%
Good control	2.0 to 2.5%
Fair control	2.5 to 3.0%
Poor control	>3.0%
Prolonged hypoglycemia	<1.0%

EDTA, Ethylenediamine tetra-acetic acid; *Hct,* hematocrit.

(Glucotest Feline Urinary Glucose Detection System; Ralston Purina, St. Louis, MO) that have been mixed into the kitty litter. Persistent glycosuria suggests inadequate control of the diabetic state and the need for a more complete evaluation of diabetic control using techniques discussed in this section. We never have owners adjust daily insulin dosages based on urine glucose measurements in diabetic cats.

Serial Blood Glucose Curve

If an adjustment in insulin therapy is deemed necessary after a review of the history, physical examination findings, changes in body weight, and serum fructosamine concentration, a serial blood glucose curve should be generated to provide guidance in making the adjustment unless blood glucose measurements are unreliable because of stress, aggression, or excitement (see page 567). The serial blood glucose curve provides guidelines for making rational adjustments in insulin therapy. Evaluation of a serial blood glucose curve is mandatory during the initial regulation of the diabetic cat and is necessary to reestablish glycemic control in the cat in which clinical manifestations of hyperglycemia or hypoglycemia have developed. Reliance on the history, physical examination findings, body weight, and serum fructosamine concentration to determine when a serial blood glucose curve is needed help reduce the frequency of serial blood glucose curves, reduce the number of venipunctures, and shorten the time the cat spends in the hospital, thereby minimizing the cat's aversion (and stress) to these evaluations and improving the chances of obtaining meaningful blood glucose results when a serial blood glucose curve is needed.

Protocol for generating the serial blood glucose curve in the hospital

The protocol for generating the serial blood glucose curve in the hospital is similar for the diabetic dog and cat and is discussed on page 512. In diabetic cats, we prefer to obtain blood for glucose determination using the marginal ear vein prick technique (see below). In our experience, cats are much more tolerant of frequent blood samplings using the marginal ear vein prick technique than repeated venipuncture, which minimizes problems with stress-induced hyperglycemia.

Protocol for generating the serial blood glucose curve at home

An alternative to hospital-generated blood glucose curves is to have the owner generate the blood glucose curve at home using the marginal ear vein prick technique and a portable home blood glucose monitoring device that allows the owner to touch the drop of blood on the ear with the end of the glucose-test strip (e.g., Glucometer Elite XL portable blood glucose meter, Bayer Diagnostics, Bayer Corp, Elkhart, IN) (Fig. 12-18). The marginal ear vein prick technique decreases the need for physical restraint during sample collection, thereby minimizing the cat's discomfort and stress. The accuracy of blood glucose results is similar when blood for glucose determination is obtained by ear prick and venipuncture (Wess and Reusch, 2000a; Thompson et al, 2002). However, blood glucose results obtained by portable blood glucose monitoring devices may overestimate or, more commonly, underestimate the actual blood glucose values obtained with reference methods (see page 513) (Wess and Reusch, 2000b). This inherent error must be considered when interpreting blood glucose results obtained by a portable home blood glucose monitoring device. Several web sites on the Internet (e.g., www.sugarcats.net/sites/harry/) explain in detail the marginal ear vein prick technique in layman's terms and provide information on owner experiences with the technique and with different portable home blood glucose meters. At the time diabetes is diagnosed, we provide a web site to the client and ask them to visit the web site and see if they would be interested in monitoring blood glucose concentrations at home. We spend time teaching the technique to those individuals willing to give it a try, advise them on how often to perform a blood glucose curve (ideally no more frequently than one day every 2 to 4 weeks), and how often to measure the blood glucose concentration on the day of the curve (typically at the time of insulin administration and 3, 6, 9, and 12 hours later). We have had excellent results using the marginal ear vein prick technique in cats (Fig. 12-19). Stress has been significantly reduced, and reliability of the blood glucose results has improved immensely. The biggest problem has been overzealous owners who start monitoring blood glucose concentrations too frequently. A similar approach can be used in diabetic dogs, using either the ear or lip prick technique. However, we do not push home glucose monitoring in dogs as much as cats, primarily because stress-induced hyperglycemia is not as big a problem in diabetic dogs.

When the marginal ear vein prick technique is performed, the cat is allowed to remain in sternal recumbency with restraint only as needed to keep the animal stationary. The marginal ear vein is identified, and a damp cloth or gauze sponge previously warmed in water is applied to the vein for 15 to 30 seconds to increase perfusion. A thin film of petrolatum is placed over the sampling site to allow a drop of blood to form without dissipating into the fur, the pinna is immobilized with a digit, an automatic lancing device (e.g., Microlet automatic lancing device; Bayer Diagnostics, Bayer Corp, Elkhart, Ind.) is placed over the vein, the ejected needle is used to nick the ear vein and, if necessary, the pinna in the region of the nick site is gently squeezed to promote formation of a drop of blood. A glucose-test strip previously inserted into the blood glucose meter is applied to the drop of blood to measure the blood glucose concentration (see Fig. 12-18). Digital pressure is then applied at the marginal ear vein prick site until bleeding stops. The skin puncture is rarely painful, and the puncture sites are barely visible even after numerous blood collections. Application of a thin film of petrolatum is critical for formation of the drop of blood. A small amount of padding (e.g., cotton ball, gauze sponge) between the pinna and the digit used to stabilize the pinna helps prevent inadvertent pricking of the finger if the lancet goes through the pinna. Finally, dehydration can interfere with the ability to obtain a drop of blood, a problem that occurs in some poorly controlled cats with marked hyperglycemia and severe polyuria and polydipsia. Administration of subcutaneous fluids may improve circulation to the ear. Only portable home blood glucose monitoring devices that allow the end of the glucose-test strip to touch the drop of blood formed on the pinna while the strip is in the glucose monitoring device are used.

Interpreting the serial blood glucose curve

The principles for interpreting the serial blood glucose curve are similar for diabetic dogs and cats and are discussed on page 514. Ideally, all blood glucose concentrations should range between 100 and 300 mg/dl during the period between insulin injections. Insulin effectiveness, the glucose nadir, and the duration of insulin effect are the critical determinations from the serial blood glucose curve. If the insulin is not effective in lowering the blood glucose concentration, the clinician must consider insulin underdosage, stress-induced hyperglycemia, and the differentials for insulin ineffectiveness and resistance (see Recurrence or Persistence of Clinical Signs, page 518). In general, insulin underdosage should be considered if the insulin dosage is less than 1.0 U/kg/injection in the diabetic cat, and insulin ineffectiveness and resistance should be considered if the insulin dosage exceeds these guidelines. However, the veterinarian should

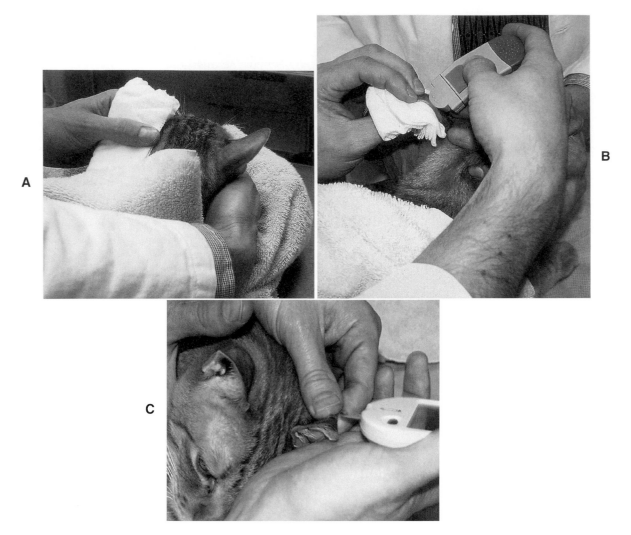

FIGURE 12-18. Marginal ear vein prick technique for measuring blood glucose concentration. *A,* A hot washcloth is applied to the pinna for 2 to 3 minutes to increase circulation to the ear. *B,* The marginal ear vein is identified on the periphery of the outer side of the pinna. A light coating of petrolatum jelly is applied over a spot on the vein, and the spot is pricked with the lancet device supplied with the portable blood glucose meter. Gauze should be placed between the pinna and the digit holding the pinna to prevent pricking of the finger if the blade of the lancet accidentally passes through the pinna. Petrolatum jelly is applied to help the blood form into a ball on the pinna as it seeps from the site that has been lanced. *C,* Digital pressure is applied in the area of the lanced skin to promote bleeding. The glucose test strip is touched to the drop of capillary blood that forms and is removed once enough blood has been drawn into the test strip to activate the meter. (From Nelson RW, Couto CG: Small Animal Internal Medicine, 3rd ed. St Louis, Mosby, 2003, p 759.)

always be wary of the development of the Somogyi phenomenon (see page 570).

If insulin is effective in lowering the blood glucose concentration, the lowest blood glucose concentration (i.e., glucose nadir) should ideally fall between 100 and 125 mg/dl. If the glucose nadir is greater than 150 mg/dl, the insulin dosage may need to be increased, and if the nadir is less than 80 mg/dl, the insulin dosage should be decreased. In the latter case, the reduction in insulin dosage depends on the amount of insulin given at the time the glucose curve is generated. If the diabetic cat is receiving an "acceptable" dose of insulin (i.e., <1.0 U/kg/injection), the insulin dosage should be decreased approximately 10% to 25%. If

the cat is receiving a large amount of insulin (e.g., >1.5 U/kg/injection), glycemic regulation should be started over again using the insulin dose recommended for the initial regulation of the diabetic cat (see page 499). Control of glycemia should be reevaluated 7 to 14 days after initiation of the new dose of insulin and adjustments in the insulin dose made accordingly.

The duration of the insulin effect can be assessed if the glucose nadir is greater than 80 mg/dl and there has not been a rapid decrease in the blood glucose concentration after insulin administration. The duration of effect is roughly defined as the time from the insulin injection, through the lowest glucose concentration, until the blood glucose concentration exceeds 250 mg/dl

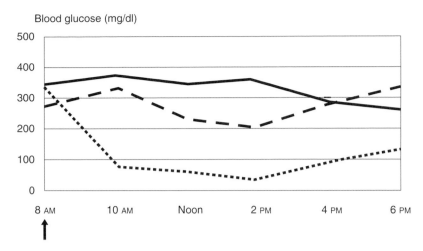

FIGURE 12-19. Initial regulation of insulin-dependent diabetes mellitus in a 6.5 kg Maine Coon cat using blood glucose measurements determined by the owner at home and using the marginal ear vein prick technique described in Figure 12-18. The cat initially was treated with 2 U of PZI administered twice daily. The cat remained symptomatic, and the blood glucose concentrations were still too high at 3 U *(solid line)* and 5 U *(dashed line)* of PZI twice daily. Clinical signs resolved and control of glycemia was attained with 6 U *(dotted line)* of PZI administered twice daily. The arrow indicates insulin administration and fed half of total daily caloric intake.

(see Fig. 11-15, page 515). Cats are usually symptomatic for diabetes if the duration of insulin effect is less than 10 hours (see page 570); they may develop hypoglycemia or the Somogyi phenomenon if the duration of insulin effect is greater than 14 hours and the insulin is being administered twice a day (see Fig. 11-16, page 516). A change in the type of insulin or the frequency of administration is usually necessary when the duration of insulin effect is too short or too long. Alterations in the dosage of insulin are often necessary at the same time as alterations in the type of insulin. The reader is referred to page 515 for guidelines on changing the insulin dosage when the type of insulin is changed.

Reproducibility of the serial blood glucose curve

See page 515.

Role of Serum Fructosamine in Stressed Diabetic Cats

Use of serum fructosamine concentrations for assessing control of glycemia has been discussed on page 562. Serum fructosamine concentrations are not affected by acute transient increases in blood glucose concentration (Lutz et al, 1995; Crenshaw et al, 1996). Unlike with blood glucose measurements, evaluation of the serum fructosamine concentration in fractious or stressed diabetic cats provides reliable, objective information on the status of glycemic control during the previous 2 to 3 weeks. In fractious or stressed cats, the clinician must make an educated guess as to where the problem lies (e.g., wrong type of insulin, low insulin dose), make an adjustment in therapy, and rely on changes

in the serum fructosamine concentration to assess the benefit of the change in treatment. Because serum proteins have a relatively short half-life, the serum fructosamine concentration changes relatively quickly (i.e., 2 to 3 weeks) in response to a change in glycemic control. This short period for change in the serum fructosamine concentration is advantageous for detecting improvement or deterioration of glycemic control quickly in fractious, stressed, or scared cats in which blood glucose concentrations are unreliable. As such, serum fructosamine concentrations can be measured prior to and 2 to 3 weeks after changes in insulin therapy to assess the effectiveness of the change. If a change in insulin therapy improved control of glycemia, a decrease in the serum fructosamine concentration should occur (see Fig. 12-17). If the serum fructosamine concentration is the same or has increased, the change was ineffective in improving glycemic control, another change in therapy based on an educated guess should be done, and the serum fructosamine concentration measured again 2 to 3 weeks later.

INSULIN THERAPY DURING SURGERY

The approach to managing the diabetic cat and dog during surgery is similar and is discussed on page 516.

COMPLICATIONS OF INSULIN THERAPY

Overview

Complications of insulin therapy are similar for diabetic dogs and cats and are discussed on page 517. Complications of insulin therapy result in poor control of glycemia. Poor control is defined as an inability to meet the goals for treating diabetes; that is, resolving clinical signs, maintaining a healthy pet, and avoiding complications caused by diabetes and its treatment. In diabetic cats, poor control is characterized by persistence or recurrence of polyuria, polydipsia, and polyphagia; lethargy and decreased interaction with family members; progressive weight loss, leading to a thin or emaciated body condition (the exception is acromegaly); lack of grooming behavior, leading to a poor, unkempt haircoat; peripheral neuropathy, causing weakness, inability to jump, a plantigrade stance, and ataxia; or clinical signs of hypoglycemia.

Poor control usually results from one of two basic problems: an inability to resolve hyperglycemia or an inability to avoid hypoglycemia. The most common complications of insulin therapy in the diabetic cat are recurring hypoglycemia; insulin overdosage, resulting in the Somogyi phenomenon; incorrect assessment of glycemic control caused by stress-induced hyperglycemia; inadequate absorption of longer acting insulin preparations; short duration of effect of intermediate acting insulin preparations; and insulin resistance caused by concurrent inflammatory and hormonal disorders, most notably chronic pancreatitis. Although the etiologies, clinical presentations, diagnostic approach, and treatment are different for these basic problems, the end result is the same—a frustrated, unhappy owner and a symptomatic diabetic cat.

Stress Hyperglycemia

Transient hyperglycemia is a well-recognized problem in fractious, scared, or otherwise stressed cats. Hyperglycemia develops as a result of an increase in catecholamines and, in struggling cats, lactate concentrations and presumably increased hepatic glucose production (Feldhahn et al, 1999; Rand et al, 2002). Blood glucose concentrations typically exceed 200 mg/dl in these cats, and values in excess of 300 mg/dl are common. Diabetes mellitus may be inadvertently diagnosed in these cats if the diagnosis is based solely on the blood glucose concentration. Because stress hyperglycemia is transient, clinical signs caused by hyperglycemia do not occur and urine testing for glucose is usually negative, findings inconsistent with a diagnosis of diabetes mellitus.

Stress hyperglycemia can significantly increase blood glucose concentrations in diabetic cats despite the administration of insulin, an effect that has serious consequences on the clinician's ability to accurately judge the effectiveness of the insulin injection. Unfortunately, the frequent blood samples required for the generation of a serial blood glucose curve can become very stressful, especially if serial blood glucose curves are performed frequently, as occurs during the initial month of treatment in newly diagnosed diabetic cats and in poorly regulated diabetic cats. Most diabetic cats do not tolerate frequent venipunctures and eventually develop a change in temperament, typically toward

aggression, and stress hyperglycemia. Induction of stress hyperglycemia is variable but usually starts during a venipuncture procedure and begins earlier and earlier on subsequent visits to the veterinarian, until eventually stress hyperglycemia is induced by hospitalization and ultimately by the car ride to the veterinary hospital. Blood glucose concentrations can remain greater than 400 mg/dl throughout the day when stress hyperglycemia develops prior to the first venipuncture of the day, despite administration of insulin (Fig. 12-20). Failure to recognize the effect of stress on the blood glucose results may lead to the erroneous perception that the diabetic cat is poorly controlled. Insulin therapy is invariably adjusted, often by increasing the insulin dosage, and another blood glucose curve recommended 1 to 2 weeks later. A vicious cycle ensues, which eventually culminates in the Somogyi phenomenon, clinically apparent hypoglycemia, or referral for evaluation of insulin resistance. Failure to identify the presence of stress hyperglycemia and its impact on interpretation of blood glucose measurements is one of the most important reasons for misinterpretation of the status of glycemic control in diabetic cats.

Stress hyperglycemia should be suspected if the cat is visibly upset, aggressive, or struggles during restraint and the venipuncture process. However, stress hyperglycemia can also be present in diabetic cats that are easily removed from the cage and do not resist the blood sampling procedure. These cats are scared, but rather than become aggressive, they remain crouched in the back of the cage, often have dilated pupils, and usually are flaccid when handled. Stress hyperglycemia should also be suspected when there is disparity between the assessment of glycemic control based on the results of the history and physical examination and the stability of body weight, and the assessment of glycemic control based on the results of blood glucose measurements, or when the initial blood glucose concentration measured in the morning is in an acceptable range (i.e., 150 to 250 mg/dl) but subsequent blood glucose concentrations increase steadily throughout the day (see Fig. 12-20). Once stress hyperglycemia develops, it is a perpetual problem and blood glucose measurements can no longer be considered accurate. If stress hyperglycemia is suspected, a switch from reliance on serial blood glucose curves generated in the veterinary hospital to reliance on blood glucose results generated by the owner in the less stressful home environment (see page 565) or evaluation of sequential serum fructosamine concentrations (see page 567) should be done, in addition to the history and physical examination.

Hypoglycemia

Hypoglycemia is a common complication of insulin therapy and is discussed on page 517. In diabetic cats, symptomatic hypoglycemia is most apt to occur after sudden large increases in the insulin dose, after sudden

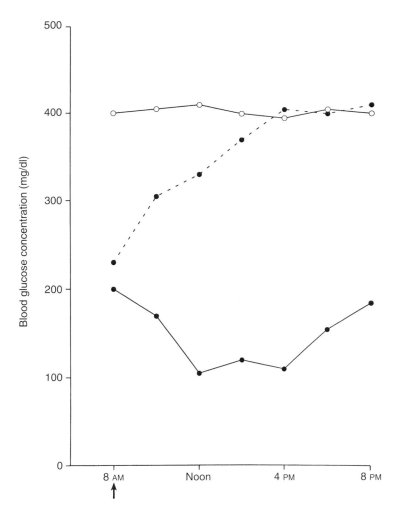

FIGURE 12-20. Blood glucose curves in a 5.3 kg male cat receiving 2 U recombinant human ultralente insulin *(solid line-solid circles)* 2 weeks after initiation of insulin therapy; 2 U recombinant human ultralente insulin *(broken line)* 2 months later; and 6 U recombinant human ultralente insulin *(solid line-open circles)* 4 months later. The insulin dosage had been gradually increased based on the results of the blood glucose curves. The owner reported minimal clinical signs regardless of the insulin dosage, the cat had maintained its body weight, and a blood glycosylated hemoglobin concentration was 2.2% at the 4-month recheck. The cat became progressively more fractious during each hospitalization, supporting stress-induced hyperglycemia as the reason for the discrepancy between blood glucose values and other parameters used to evaluate glycemic control. ↑ = Subcutaneous insulin injection and food.

improvement in concurrent insulin resistance, with excessive overlap of insulin action in cats receiving insulin twice a day, after prolonged inappetence, and in insulin-treated cats that have reverted to a non–insulin-dependent state. In these situations, severe hypoglycemia may occur before the diabetogenic hormones (i.e., glucagon, cortisol, epinephrine, and growth hormone) are able to compensate for and reverse low blood glucose concentrations. The initial treatment approach for hypoglycemia is to discontinue insulin until hyperglycemia recurs and then reduce the ensuing insulin dosage 25% to 50%. If hypoglycemia remains a reoccurring problem despite reductions in the insulin dose, prolonged duration of insulin effect or reversion to a non–insulin-dependent diabetic state should be considered. Hypoglycemia caused by prolonged duration of insulin effect results from twice a day administration of an insulin preparation with a duration of effect considerably longer than 12 hours, a problem that may occur with twice a day administration of ultralente, PZI, and insulin glargine but usually not with NPH or lente insulin (see page 571).

Reversion to a non–insulin-dependent diabetic state should be suspected if hypoglycemia remains a persistent problem despite administration of small doses of insulin (i.e., 1 U or less per injection) and administration of insulin once a day, if blood glucose concentrations are consistently below 150 mg/dl prior to insulin administration, if the serum fructosamine concentration is less than 350 µmol/L (reference range, 190 to 365 µmol/L), or if urine glucose test strips are consistently negative. Maintaining blood glucose concentrations below 150 mg/dl is very difficult with once or twice a day injection of intermediate or long acting insulin. All of the scenarios listed above suggest the presence of endogenously derived circulating insulin, the existence of partial rather than complete destruction of pancreatic islets, and probably the presence of glucose toxicity at the time diabetes was initially diagnosed (see page 544) (Nelson et al, 1998). Correction of concurrent disorders identified around the time diabetes was diagnosed may have also improved tissue sensitivity to insulin. Insulin therapy should be discontinued and diet modified to help minimize the recurrence of hyperglycemia (see Dietary Therapy, page 552). Treatment with the oral sulfonylurea drug glipizide may also be considered if clinically relevant hyperglycemia waxes and wanes (see Sulfonylureas, page 555).

Insulin Overdosing and Glucose Counterregulation (Somogyi Phenomenon)

The Somogyi phenomenon is discussed on page 519. A similar phenomenon characterized by wide fluctuations in the blood glucose concentration followed by several days of persistent hyperglycemia is recognized clinically in diabetic cats (Fig. 12-21) (McMillan and Feldman, 1986), although the exact role of the counterregulatory hormones remains to be clarified. Insulin overdosage inducing glucose counterregulation is one of the most common causes of insulin resistance and poor glycemic control in cats. Glucose counterregulation can be induced with insulin doses of 2 to 3 U/injection and can result in cats receiving 10 to 15 U of insulin per injection as veterinarians react to the persistence of clinical signs and increased blood glucose and serum fructosamine concentrations. A cyclic history of 1 or 2 days of good glycemic control followed by several days of poor control should raise suspicion for insulin resistance caused by glucose counterregulation. Serum fructosamine concentrations are unpredictable but are usually increased (>500 μmol/L), results that confirm poor glycemic control but do not identify the underlying cause. Establishing the diagnosis may require several days of hospitalization and serial blood glucose curves, an approach that eventually leads to problems with stress-induced hyperglycemia. An alternative approach, which we prefer, is to arbitrarily reduce the insulin dose 1 to 2 U and have the owner evaluate the cat's clinical response over the ensuing 2 to 5 days.

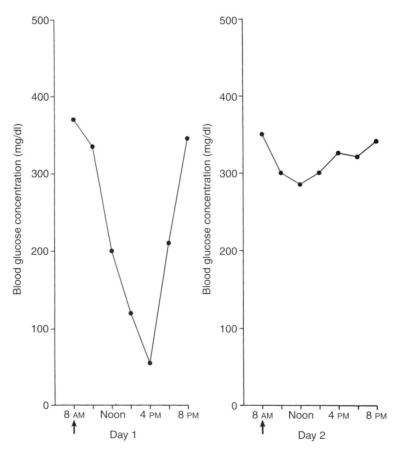

FIGURE 12-21. Blood glucose curves on 2 consecutive days in a 5.2 kg male cat receiving 4 U beef/pork source PZI subcutaneously. Results of the blood glucose curve on day 1 are consistent with the Somogyi phenomenon, whereas results on day 2 suggest insulin underdosage or insulin resistance. Presumably, release of diabetogenic hormones during the hypoglycemic period on day 1 deleteriously affected insulin's effectiveness on day 2. ↑ = Insulin injection and food.

If clinical signs of diabetes worsen after a small reduction in the insulin dose, another cause for the insulin resistance should be pursued. However, if the owner reports no change or improvement in clinical signs, continued gradual reduction of the insulin dose should be pursued. Alternatively, glycemic regulation of the diabetic cat could be started over, using an insulin dose of 1 U/cat given twice daily.

Insulin Underdosage

Control of glycemia can be established in most diabetic cats using 1 U or less of insulin per kilogram of body weight administered twice each day. An inadequate dose of insulin in conjunction with once a day insulin therapy is a common cause of persistence of clinical signs. In general, insulin underdosage should be considered if the insulin dosage is less than 1 U/kg/injection and the cat is receiving insulin twice a day. If insulin underdosage is suspected, the dose of insulin should be gradually increased by 0.5 to 1 U per injection per week. The effectiveness of the change in therapy should be evaluated by client perception of clinical response and measurement of the serum fructosamine or serial blood glucose concentrations. Before considering increasing the insulin dose above 1 U/kg/injection, the clinician should rule out other causes of insulin ineffectiveness and resistance, most notably the Somogyi phenomenon and chronic pancreatitis.

Short Duration of Insulin Effect

Short duration of insulin effect (i.e., less than 10 hours) is a common problem in diabetic cats despite twice a day insulin administration (see page 520) (Moise and Reimers, 1983; Wallace et al, 1990). Short duration of effect is most common with NPH and, to a lesser extent, lente insulin. In some diabetic cats the duration of effect of NPH and lente insulin is less than 8 hours (see Table 11-8, page 497). As a result, significant hyperglycemia (>300 mg/dl) occurs for several hours each day, and the owners of these pets usually mention continuing problems with polyuria and polydipsia, or weight loss or the development of weakness caused by the development of peripheral neuropathy. A diagnosis of short duration of insulin effect is made by demonstrating hyperglycemia (>250 mg/dl) within 6 to 10 hours of the insulin injection, whereas the lowest blood glucose concentration is maintained above 80 mg/dl (see Fig. 11-16, page 516). Treatment involves changing the type of insulin (e.g., switching to PZI, ultralente, or insulin glargine) or the frequency of insulin administration (e.g., initiating three times a day therapy) if the duration of effect of the insulin preparation is less than 8 hours. Glycemic control should be evaluated 1 to 2 weeks after a change in insulin therapy, and further adjustments in the insulin dose are made accordingly.

Prolonged Duration of Insulin Effect

Prolonged duration of insulin effect is discussed on page 521. Problems with prolonged duration of insulin effect result from twice a day administration of an insulin preparation with a duration of effect considerably longer than 12 hours, a problem that may occur with twice a day administration of ultralente, PZI, and insulin glargine but usually not with NPH or lente insulin. The excessive overlap in insulin action eventually leads to symptomatic hypoglycemia or, more commonly, the Somogyi phenomenon. Prolonged duration of insulin effect is an uncommon problem in cats, occurring in fewer than 10% of insulin-treated diabetic cats that we have evaluated for poor control of glycemia. Indications of excessive overlap include a glucose nadir that occurs 10 hours or later after insulin administration or gradually decreasing blood glucose concentrations measured at the time of sequential insulin injections (see Fig. 11-16, page 516). If prolonged duration of insulin effect is suspected as the cause of poor glycemic control, a decrease in the frequency of insulin administration to once a day (PZI, ultralente, insulin glargine) or a switch to a shorter acting insulin (e.g., lente, NPH) administered twice a day can be tried.

Inadequate or Impaired Insulin Absorption

Slow or inadequate absorption of subcutaneously deposited insulin is most commonly observed in diabetic cats receiving ultralente insulin, a long-acting insulin that has a slow onset and prolonged duration of effect (Broussard and Peterson, 1994; Bertoy et al, 1995). In approximately 25% of cats evaluated at our hospital, ultralente insulin is absorbed from the subcutaneous site of deposition too slowly for it to be effective in maintaining acceptable glycemic control. In these cats, the blood glucose concentration may not decrease until 6 to 10 hours after the injection or, more commonly, it decreases minimally despite insulin doses of 8 to 12 U/cat given every 12 hours. As a consequence, the blood glucose concentration remains greater than 300 mg/dl for most of the day. We have had success in these cats by switching from ultralente to lente or PZI given twice a day (Fig. 12-22) (Bertoy et al, 1995). When switching the type of insulin, the insulin dose is decreased (usually to amounts initially used to regulate the diabetic cat) to avoid hypoglycemia. The duration of effect of the insulin becomes shorter as the potency of the insulin increases, which may create problems with short duration of insulin effect (see Fig. 11-19, page 521). We have not yet identified similar problems with insulin glargine in diabetic cats, although our experience with insulin glargine is limited at this time.

Impaired absorption of insulin may also occur as a result of thickening of the skin and inflammation of the subcutaneous tissues caused by chronic injection of insulin in the same area of the body (see Allergic Reactions to Insulin, page 524). Rotation of the injection

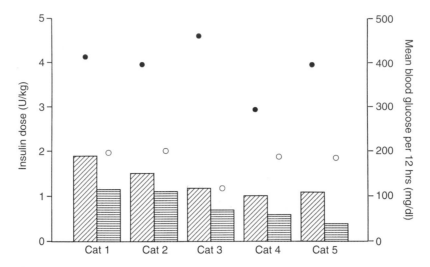

FIGURE 12-22. Insulin dosage *(bars)* and mean blood glucose concentration per 12 hours after subcutaneous insulin administration *(circles)* in five cats receiving beef/pork source ultralente insulin *(diagonal-hatched bars, closed circles)* and beef/pork source lente insulin *(horizontal-hatched bars, open circles)*. Note the improved glycemic control at a lower insulin dosage with lente versus ultralente insulin.

site helps prevent this problem. A rare cause of insulin inactivity in humans with diabetes mellitus is excess degradation of insulin at the site of subcutaneous deposition (Schade and Duckworth, 1986). Proteases at the site of insulin deposition are believed to degrade the insulin prior to absorption. As a result, the blood insulin concentration remains at basal levels after administration of large amounts of insulin. Documentation of the subcutaneous insulin resistance syndrome has relied on the following: (1) resistance to the hypoglycemic action of subcutaneously injected insulin but normal sensitivity to insulin administered intravenously, (2) a lack of increase in the serum free insulin concentration after injection of large doses of insulin subcutaneously, and (3) increased insulin-degrading activity in the subcutaneous tissue. Treatment is aimed at the use of an alternative route of insulin delivery or the use of additives to prevent enzymatic degradation of the insulin or to increase subcutaneous blood flow, or both (Freidenberg et al, 1981).

Circulating Antiinsulin Antibodies

The impact of antiinsulin antibodies on the control of glycemia was discussed on page 522. Fortunately, antiinsulin antibody formation is not common in diabetic cats treated with exogenous human insulin despite differences in the amino acid sequence of human and feline insulin (see Table 11-6, page 496) (Hallden et al, 1986). Surprisingly, two studies identified an approximately equal frequency of positive serum antiinsulin antibody titers in diabetic cats treated with beef insulin, compared with recombinant human insulin (Harb-Hauser et al, 1998; Hoenig et al, 2000a); these results suggest that conformational insulin epitopes may be more important than linear subunits of the insulin

molecule in the induction of antiinsulin antibodies (Thomas et al, 1985 and 1988; Nell and Thomas, 1989). Fortunately, antiinsulin antibody titers were weakly positive in most cats, the prevalence of persistent titers was low, and the presence of serum antiinsulin antibodies did not appear to affect control of glycemia (Harb-Hauser et al, 1998). These results suggest that the prevalence of antiinsulin antibodies causing problems with control of glycemia similar to those identified in dogs (see page 522) is uncommon in cats treated with recombinant human insulin. In our experience, overt insulin resistance caused by antiinsulin antibody formation occurs in fewer than 5% of diabetic cats with insulin resistance that are being treated with recombinant human insulin. Switching from the recombinant human insulin preparation to beef/pork-source PZI may improve control of glycemia if circulating antiinsulin antibodies are the cause of the insulin ineffectiveness.

Concurrent Disorders Causing Insulin Resistance

The definition and etiology of insulin resistance were discussed on page 524. No insulin dose clearly defines insulin resistance in the cat. For most diabetic cats, control of glycemia can usually be attained using 1.0 U or less of intermediate- or long-acting insulin per kilogram of body weight given twice daily. Insulin resistance should be suspected if control of glycemia is poor despite an insulin dosage in excess of 1.5 U/kg, when excessive amounts of insulin (i.e., insulin dosage greater than 1.5 U/kg) are necessary to maintain the blood glucose concentration below 300 mg/dl, and when control of glycemia is erratic and insulin dosages are changed every few weeks in an attempt to maintain control of glycemia (see Fig. 11-23, page 525). Failure of the blood glucose concentration to decrease below 300 mg/dl during a serial blood glucose curve is suggestive of but not definitive for the presence of insulin resistance. An insulin resistance–type blood glucose curve can also result from stress-induced hyperglycemia and problems with insulin therapy (see Problems with Insulin Treatment Regimen, page 518, and Table 11-16, page 524), and a decrease in the blood glucose concentration below 300 mg/dl can occur with disorders that cause relatively mild insulin resistance. Serum fructosamine concentrations are typically greater than 500 µmol/L in cats with insulin resistance and can exceed 700 µmol/L if insulin resistance is severe. Unfortunately, an increased serum fructosamine concentration is merely indicative of poor glycemic control, not of insulin resistance per se.

Many disorders can interfere with insulin action in cats (see Table 11-16, page 524). In our experience, the most common concurrent disorders interfering with insulin effectiveness in cats are severe obesity, chronic pancreatitis, renal insufficiency, hyperthyroidism, oral infections, acromegaly, and hyperadrenocorticism. The severity of insulin resistance depends in part on the underlying etiology. Insulin resistance may be mild and easily overcome by increasing the dosage of insulin (e.g., obesity, renal insufficiency); it may be severe and cause sustained hyperglycemia in excess of 400 mg/dl regardless of the type and dosage of insulin administered (e.g., acromegaly, hyperadrenocorticism); or it may fluctuate with time and cause erratic control of glycemia (e.g., chronic pancreatitis). Some causes of insulin resistance are readily apparent at the time diabetes is diagnosed, such as obesity and the administration of insulin-antagonistic drugs (e.g., glucocorticoids, megestrol acetate). Other causes of insulin resistance are not readily apparent and require an extensive diagnostic evaluation to be identified. Obtaining a complete history and performing a thorough physical examination are the most important steps in identifying these concurrent disorders. Abnormalities identified on a thorough physical examination may suggest a concurrent insulin-antagonistic disorder or infectious process, which gives the clinician direction in the diagnostic evaluation of the patient. If the history and physical examination are unremarkable, a CBC, serum biochemical analysis, serum thyroxine concentration, abdominal ultrasound scan, and urinalysis with bacterial culture should be obtained to further screen for concurrent illness. Additional tests depend on the results of the initial screening tests (see Table 11-17, page 526).

Many of the causes of insulin resistance in diabetic dogs and cats are similar and are discussed on page 524. Disorders worthy of emphasis in cats are discussed below.

Obesity

Obesity is a common cause of insulin resistance in diabetic cats. The interplay between obesity, insulin resistance, and development of diabetes mellitus is discussed on page 543. Obesity causes relatively mild insulin resistance, and improvement in control of glycemia can often be attained by increasing the dosage of insulin. Fortunately obesity-induced insulin resistance is reversible with weight loss, and in some cats, insulin-requiring diabetes mellitus may resolve with correction of the obese state. Treatment of obesity is discussed on page 552.

Chronic pancreatitis

See page 528.

Renal insufficiency

See page 528.

Bacterial infections

See page 527.

Hyperthyroidism

Insulin resistance has been documented in diabetic cats with hyperthyroidism. In these cats, insulin resistance resolved after correction of the hyperthyroid state. Several mechanisms for the carbohydrate intolerance of hyperthyroidism have been proposed, including decreased insulin synthesis and secretion, insulin resistance caused by impaired insulin receptor binding affinity or postreceptor defect, and a disproportionate increase in proinsulin secretion by the pancreatic beta cells (Pedersen et al, 1988; Hoenig and Ferguson, 1988; Hoenig et al, 1992). The diagnosis of hyperthyroidism should be based on a combination of the history, the physical examination findings, the serum thyroxine concentration, the clinician's index of suspicion for the disease and, if necessary, the serum free thyroxine concentration or a sodium pertechnetate scan (see Chapter 4). Interpretation of serum thyroxine concentrations must take into consideration the status of glycemic control of the cat, the severity of other concurrent illness, and the suppressive effects these factors may have on thyroid gland function, especially if hyperthyroidism is mild. A normal serum thyroxine concentration, especially a value in the upper range of normal, does not by itself rule out hyperthyroidism. We have documented insulin resistance in several diabetic cats with mild hyperthyroidism and serum total thyroxine concentrations between 2.5 and 3.5 µg/dl (reference range, 1.0 to 4.0 µg/dl).

Methimazole is the initial treatment of choice, especially if the diagnosis of hyperthyroidism is debatable (e.g., minimal clinical signs, palpable thyroid nodule, serum total thyroxine concentration between 2.5 and 3.5 µg/dl) but suspected as a potential cause for poor glycemic control. If methimazole is administered, a concurrent reduction in insulin dosage should be considered and the blood glucose concentration monitored weekly during the first month of administration to avoid hypoglycemia (Fig. 12-23). Further

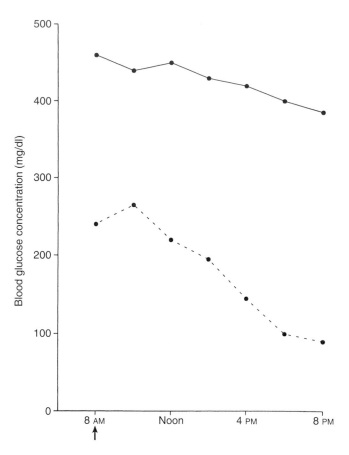

FIGURE 12-23. Blood glucose curve in a 7.4 kg male diabetic cat with untreated mild hyperthyroidism receiving 7 U beef/pork source lente insulin *(solid line)*. Glycemic control was improved and the insulin dosage decreased to 5 U after methimazole therapy was initiated *(broken line)*. ↑ = Subcutaneous insulin injection and food.

reductions in the insulin dosage may be required if hypoglycemia develops as the hyperthyroid-induced insulin resistance resolves.

Progestogens

Chronic administration of progestogens (e.g., megestrol acetate) and progesterone-secreting adrenocortical tumors can cause insulin resistance and the development of diabetes mellitus (Boord and Griffin, 1999; Rossmeisl et al, 2000). The development of carbohydrate intolerance is believed to result from the intrinsic insulin-antagonistic activity of progesterone. Unlike in the dog, progesterone does not stimulate growth hormone secretion in the cat (Peterson, 1987). Progesterone can also cause the feline fragile skin syndrome, which is characterized by progressively worsening dermal and epidermal atrophy, patchy endocrine alopecia, and easily torn skin (see Fig. 7-3, page 364). The clinical features of excess progesterone mimic feline hyperadrenocorticism, which is the primary differential diagnosis (see Chapter 7). The results of tests of the pituitary-adrenocortical axis are normal to suppressed in cats with progesterone-secreting adrenal tumors, and the contralateral adrenal

gland is normal in size and shape on abdominal ultrasound scans. Diagnosis requires documentation of an increased plasma progesterone concentration. For most commercial endocrine laboratories, a serum progesterone concentration greater than 2 ng/ml is consistent with a progesterone-secreting adrenocortical tumor. Adrenalectomy or withdrawal of progestogen therapy decreases the blood progesterone concentration, corrects insulin resistance, and improves diabetic control. Insulin-requiring diabetes may resolve in cats with adequate numbers of functional beta cells once the serum progesterone concentration decreases below 1 ng/ml and the severity of hyperglycemia improves.

For cats treated with progestogens, it is difficult to predict which cats are susceptible to the development of diabetes, when diabetes will occur, and whether diabetes will resolve after discontinuation of progestogen therapy. Many cats that develop diabetes are believed to have islet pathology, a decreased population of beta cells, and subclinical diabetes prior to progestogen administration. The development of clinical diabetes mellitus and the reversibility of the diabetic state are determined in part by the severity of islet pathology at the time progestogens are administered, the dosage of progestogen, and the duration of treatment. We recommend that owners periodically check their cat's urine for glucose whenever progestogens are administered and that they discontinue progestogens if glycosuria occurs.

Hyperadrenocorticism

Hyperadrenocorticism is an uncommon disorder that occurs in older cats; it has a strong association with diabetes mellitus; it can cause severe insulin resistance; and it is often associated with a pituitary macrotumor (Elliot et al, 2000). Clinical signs related to poorly controlled diabetes mellitus are common in cats with hyperadrenocorticism. The severity of insulin resistance is variable and depends on the severity of the hyperadrenal state. In the early stages of the disease, the diabetic cat may be responsive to insulin, although higher than anticipated dosages of insulin are required to maintain control of glycemia (Duesberg et al, 1995). Eventually severe insulin resistance develops. Acromegaly is the primary differential diagnosis when severe insulin resistance is identified. Unlike acromegaly, hyperadrenocorticism is a debilitating disease that results in progressive weight loss, leading to cachexia, and dermal and epidermal atrophy, leading to extremely fragile, thin, easily torn, and ulcerated skin (i.e., feline fragile skin syndrome) (see Fig. 7-4, page 365). Most of the abnormalities identified on routine blood and urine tests are caused by the concurrent poorly controlled diabetes mellitus. The usual markers for hyperadrenocorticism commonly identified in the dog (e.g., increased alkaline phosphatase activity, isosthenuric urine) are not present in diabetic cats with hyperadrenocorticism. Depending on the etiology, abdominal ultrasound may reveal bilateral adrenomegaly or an adrenal mass. Definitive diagnosis relies on tests of the pituitary-adrenocortical axis, most notably the urine cortisol:creatinine ratio and the dexamethasone suppression test. Adrenalectomy is currently the treatment of choice. Insulin requirements decrease and glycemic control is improved after the hyperadrenal state has been corrected. In one study, clinical signs and physical examination abnormalities resolved 2 to 4 months after adrenalectomy, and four of six diabetic cats reverted to a non–insulin-dependent diabetic state 2 to 8 months after surgery (Duesberg et al, 1995). Chapter 7 presents more detailed information on feline hyperadrenocorticism.

Acromegaly

Acromegaly is an uncommon disorder that occurs in older cats; it has a strong association with diabetes mellitus; it can cause severe insulin resistance; and it is often associated with a pituitary macrotumor (Peterson et al, 1990; Elliot et al, 2000). Initially, clinical signs related to poorly controlled diabetes mellitus dominate the clinical picture in cats with acromegaly. Conformational alterations (see Table 2-14, page 72) are insidious in onset and often not noted by owners or veterinarians initially. However, with time the conformational changes caused by the anabolic actions of chronic insulin-like growth factor-I (IGF-I) secretion come to dominate the clinical picture in acromegaly, most notably an increase in body size, prognathia inferior, and weight gain despite poorly regulated diabetes mellitus. Severe insulin resistance develops, but unlike in hyperadrenocorticism, the feline fragile skin syndrome and progressive weight loss do not occur with acromegaly. Most of the abnormalities identified on routine blood and urine tests are caused by the concurrent poorly controlled diabetes mellitus. Although the definitive diagnosis of acromegaly requires documentation of an increased baseline serum growth hormone (GH) concentration, a commercial GH assay is not available for cats. For most cats, the diagnosis is ultimately based on (1) the identification of conformational alterations (e.g., increased body size, large head, prognathia inferior, organomegaly) in a cat with insulin-resistant diabetes mellitus; (2) a persistent increase rather than decrease in the body weight of a cat with poorly controlled diabetes mellitus; (3) an increase in the serum IGF-I concentration in an insulin-resistant cat with clinical manifestations consistent with acromegaly; and (4) the documentation of a pituitary mass using contrast-enhanced computerized tomography or magnetic resonance imaging. The latter finding would support acromegaly in the cat with normal pituitary-adrenocortical axis test results.

The current treatment of choice for acromegaly is cobalt teletherapy. The response to cobalt teletherapy is unpredictable and ranges from no response, to a partial decrease in pituitary tumor size and/or serum GH concentration and increased responsiveness to insulin, to a dramatic response, characterized by significant shrinkage of the tumor, elimination of hypersomatotropism, resolution of insulin resistance and, in some cats, reversion to a subclinical diabetic state. Chapter 2 presents more detailed information on feline acromegaly.

Fluctuating Insulin Requirements

One of the most frustrating problems encountered with insulin treatment is the sudden inability to maintain control of glycemia in a previously well-controlled cat with IDDM. Typically, the diabetic cat has been well controlled with a consistent dose of insulin for weeks to months and then suddenly becomes symptomatic (e.g., polyuria, polydipsia, weight loss, lethargy). Concurrent problems are not readily apparent, and an increase in the insulin dose improves clinical signs for a short time (days to weeks), only to have clinical signs recur and often improve with a further increase in the insulin dose. If this routine continues, the insulin dose may eventually exceed 1.5 to 2.0 U/kg/injection with variable but inconsistent improvement in clinical signs. Control of glycemia often remains erratic and unpredictable, and the insulin dose is changed frequently in an attempt to reestablish consistent control of glycemia. Hypoglycemia (blood glucose <60 mg/dl) may suddenly be identified despite weeks to months of poor control and consistently high blood glucose concentrations. In many cats the increased frequency of visits to the veterinary hospital and of blood glucose measurements ultimately leads to stress-induced hyperglycemia, and the frustration of the veterinarian and owner intensifies.

In our experience, the most common explanation for sudden loss of glycemic control in a previously stable diabetic cat is the development of a concurrent disorder causing insulin resistance. The insulin resistance is usually mild, and it is either spontaneously reversible or it oscillates in severity over time. Inflammatory disorders, such as mild chronic pancreatitis, are the most common culprits, and they typically go unrecognized by the owner and veterinarian. In a diabetic cat receiving a fixed dose of insulin, the development of insulin resistance results in hyperglycemia and recurrence of clinical signs. An increase in the insulin dose improves control of glycemia because the insulin resistance is relatively mild. If the insulin resistance worsens, further increases in the insulin dose are required to maintain control of glycemia. However, if and when insulin resistance improves or resolves, the cat is suddenly at risk for developing symptomatic hypoglycemia or, more commonly, the Somogyi phenomenon. The Somogyi phenomenon can then perpetuate poor control of the diabetic state. In essence, what started out as an insulin resistance problem causing loss of glycemic control may evolve into perpetual loss of glycemic control because of the Somogyi phenomenon, which develops from an insulin overdosage created when the inflammatory process subsides and the insulin resistance improves. A thorough history and physical examination, evaluation of a serial blood glucose curve and, if indicated, diagnostic evaluation for disorders known to cause insulin resistance in the diabetic cat (see Table 11-16, page 524) should be undertaken whenever a previously well-controlled diabetic cat suddenly becomes symptomatic for the disease. The Somogyi phenomenon should always be considered if a reason for the sudden deterioration in glycemic control is not evident after a thorough evaluation of the cat, especially if the insulin dose has been arbitrarily increased prior to the evaluation.

CHRONIC COMPLICATIONS OF DIABETES MELLITUS

Complications resulting from the diabetic state (e.g., peripheral neuropathy) or its treatment (e.g., insulin-induced hypoglycemia) are common in diabetic cats (see Table 11-7, page 496). The most common complications in the cat are hypoglycemia; chronic pancreatitis; weight loss; poor grooming behavior, resulting in a dry, lusterless, and unkempt haircoat; and peripheral neuropathy of the hindlimbs, causing weakness, inability to jump, a plantigrade stance, and ataxia. Diabetic cats are also at risk for ketoacidosis. Most of the devastating chronic complications of human diabetes (e.g., nephropathy, vasculopathy, coronary artery disease) require 10 to 20 years or longer to develop and therefore are uncommon in diabetic cats. Diabetes mellitus is a disease of older cats, and most do not live beyond 5 years from the time of diagnosis (Goossens et al, 1998). In our experience, owners are usually willing to "tackle" the care of a diabetic pet once the fears related to chronic complications seen in human diabetics are alleviated. Postulated pathogenetic mechanisms for the development of long-term complications are discussed on page 530.

Many of the chronic complications in diabetic dogs and cats are similar and are discussed on page 530. Diabetic neuropathy is worthy of emphasis in cats and is discussed below.

Diabetic Neuropathy

Diabetic neuropathy is one of the most common chronic complications of diabetes in cats, with a prevalence of approximately 10% of cats with IDDM. Clinical signs of a coexistent neuropathy in the diabetic cat include hindlimb weakness; impaired ability to jump; a plantigrade posture, with the cat's hocks touching the ground when it walks (see Fig. 12-9), muscle atrophy, especially of the distal pelvic limb; depressed limb reflexes; deficits in postural reaction testing; and irritability on manipulation of the hindlimbs and feet (Kramek et al, 1984; Mizisin et al, 2002). Clinical signs may progress to include the thoracic limbs. Abnormalities on electrophysiologic testing are consistent with demyelination at all levels of the motor and sensory peripheral nerves and include decreased motor and sensory nerve conduction velocities in the pelvic and thoracic limbs and decreased muscle action potential amplitudes (Mizisin et al, 1998 and 2002). The more severe the clinical neuropathy, the more severe the decrease in motor and sensory nerve conduction and muscle action potential amplitudes. Sensory nerve conduction is not as severely affected as motor nerve conduction, and the thoracic limb tends to be less severely affected than the pelvic limb. Electromyographic abnormalities are usually absent and when identified are consistent with denervation. The most striking abnormality detected on histologic examination of nerve biopsies from affected cats is Schwann cell injury, characterized by myelin splitting, ballooning, and subsequent demyelination (Mizisin et al, 2002). Demyelination is presumed to be distributed along the whole length of the motor and sensory peripheral neuraxis and is responsible for the early signs of diabetic neuropathy. Axonal degeneration is identified in the most severely affected cats and is characterized by a decrease in average myelin nerve fiber density, morphologic evidence of fiber loss in nerve biopsies, and moderate denervation in muscle biopsies. Presumably, the early signs of diabetic neuropathy caused by Schwann cell injury and demyelination (e.g., weakness, decreased jumping ability) precede the more severe signs (e.g., full plantigrade stance when walking) derived from axonal pathology.

The cause of diabetic neuropathy is not known. Vascular, axonal, and metabolic hypotheses have been proposed in human diabetics (Unger and Foster, 1998). The vascular hypothesis proposes that a reduction in nerve blood flow may be an early defect leading to nerve ischemia and hypoxia (Asbury, 1988; Stevens et al, 1995; Ward, 1995). The axonal hypothesis supposes early functional changes, such as slow axonal transport, followed by structural degeneration. Potential metabolic derangements leading to neuropathy include altered polyol pathway activity, with accumulation of sorbitol and fructose and a corresponding decrease in myoinositol content in Schwann cells and axons (Winegard, 1986; Greene et al, 1988a); glycosylation of structural proteins in myelin and tubulin, with resultant formation of advanced glycosylation end products (Unger and Foster, 1998); decreases in Na^+-K^+ ATP'ase activity (Scarpini et al, 1993); oxidative stress resulting from enhanced free-radical formation and/or defects in antioxidant defense (Low et al, 1997); and induced growth factor deficiencies (Thomas, 1994; Zhuang et al, 1996).

An alteration in polyol pathway activity may play a role in the generation of diabetic neuropathy in cats. The polyol pathway consists of two consecutive reactions: glucose first is reduced to sorbitol by aldose reductase, and sorbitol subsequently is oxidized to fructose by sorbitol dehydrogenase. Aldose reductase is present in the retina, lens, Schwann cell, and renal papillae, and accumulation of polyols (e.g., sorbitol) has been implicated in the pathogenesis of cataracts (see page 530), retinopathy, nephropathy, and neuropathy (Greene et al, 1988b; Unger and Foster, 1998). In a recent study in cats with diabetic neuropathy, regression analysis suggested that the severity of clinical signs and the electrophysiologic abnormalities were best related to the blood glucose concentration, that nerve water content was significantly elevated in diabetic versus healthy cats, and that nerve glucose and fructose contents were increased eightfold and twelvefold in diabetic versus healthy cats, respectively (Mizisin et al, 2002). Sorbitol was not detected in the nerves of healthy cats, and only small amounts were detected in six of the 19 diabetic cats studied. Nerve myoinositol content in diabetic cats was reduced to 80% of the levels in healthy cats. These findings suggest an increase in the polyol pathway flux. Finding increased nerve glucose and fructose but not sorbitol content in cats with diabetic neuropathy suggests increased sorbitol dehydrogenase activity in diabetic cats and supports the idea that consequences of flux through the pathway, and not polyol accumulation itself, precipitate nerve disorders in diabetic cats (Mizisin et al, 2002). Activation of this polyol pathway by hyperglycemia results in depletion of myoinositol, a precursor of the polyphosphoinositides, which are important constituents of plasma membranes (Fig. 12-24) (Winegrad, 1986; Greene et al, 1988a and 1988b). Myoinositol is a key element in many nerve cellular functions, and myoinositol depletion correlates with reduced nerve conduction velocity in diabetic nerves (Forcier et al, 1991; Mizisin and Calcutt, 1991). The role, if any, of other metabolic derangements, such as glycosylation of myelin, in the pathogenesis of diabetic neuropathy in cats remains to be determined.

Currently, there is no specific therapy for diabetic neuropathy in cats. Intensive blood glucose control decreases the risk and improves the clinical manifestations of neuropathy in human diabetics (Diabetes Control and Complications Trial Research Group, 1993). Aggressive glucoregulation with insulin may also improve nerve conduction and reverse the posterior weakness and plantigrade posture in diabetic cats (see Fig. 12-9) (Kennedy et al, 1990). However, the response to therapy is variable, and the risks of hypoglycemia increase with aggressive insulin treatment. Generally, the longer the neuropathy has been present and the more severe the neuropathy, the less likely improving glycemic control is to reverse the clinical signs of neuropathy. Recent findings by Mizisin and colleagues (2002) suggest that treatment with aldose reductase inhibitors may be beneficial in diabetic cats and may warrant investigation.

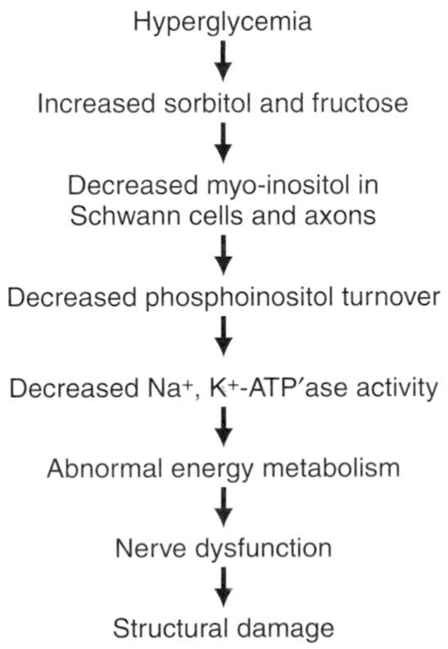

PROGNOSIS

The prognosis for diabetic cats depends in part on owner commitment to treating the disease, ease of glycemic regulation, the presence and nature of concurrent disorders (e.g., pancreatitis, acromegaly), and avoidance of chronic complications associated with the diabetic state (see Table 11-7, page 496). In general, diabetes mellitus carries a guarded long-term prognosis in the cat. In one retrospective study, 53 of 92 diabetic cats died 0 to 84 months after diabetes was diagnosed (Goossens et al, 1998). The mean and median survival times for these 53 cats were 25 and 17 months, respectively. Eleven cats died during the initial hospitalization as a result of severe ketoacidosis or concurrent illness (e.g., renal failure). Thirty-nine cats were alive and had survived a mean of 23 months (range, 2 to 66 months) after diagnosis of diabetes. Survival time can be somewhat misleading because cats are usually older (8 to 12 years) at the time of diagnosis, and the mortality rate during the first 6 months is high because of concurrent life-threatening or uncontrollable disease (e.g., ketoacidosis, acute pancreatitis, renal failure, hyperadrenocorticism). In our experience, diabetic cats that survive the first 6 months can easily maintain a good quality of life for more than 5 years with the disease.

Hyperglycemia
↓
Increased sorbitol and fructose
↓
Decreased myo-inositol in
Schwann cells and axons
↓
Decreased phosphoinositol turnover
↓
Decreased Na+, K+-ATP'ase activity
↓
Abnormal energy metabolism
↓
Nerve dysfunction
↓
Structural damage

FIGURE 12-24. Possible mechanism for the development of peripheral neuropathy in diabetic cats that involves stimulation of polyol pathway activity by hyperglycemia. The increased polyol pathway flux leads to a decrease in nerve myoinositol content, nerve dysfunction, and ultimately structural damage to the nerve.

REFERENCES

Anderson RW: Chromium, glucose tolerance, and diabetes. Biol Tr Elem Res 32:19, 1992.

Appleton DJ, et al: Plasma leptin concentrations in cats: reference range, effect of weight gain and relationship with adiposity as measured by dual energy x-ray absorptiometry. J Fel Med Surg 2:191, 2000.

Appleton DJ, et al: Insulin sensitivity decreases with obesity, and lean cats with low insulin sensitivity are at greatest risk of glucose intolerance with weight gain. J Fel Med Surg 3:211, 2001.

Appleton DJ, et al: Plasma leptin concentrations are independently associated with insulin sensitivity in lean and overweight cats. J Fel Med Surg 4:83, 2002a.

Appleton DJ, et al: Dietary chromium tripicolinate supplementation reduces glucose concentrations and improves glucose tolerance in normal-weight cats. J Fel Med Surg 4:13, 2002b.

Asbury AK: Understanding diabetic neuropathy. N Engl J Med 319:577, 1988.

Backus RC: Relationship between serum leptin immunoreactivity and body fat mass as estimated by use of a novel gas-phase Fourier transform infrared spectroscopy deuterium dilution method in cats. Am J Vet Res 61:796, 2000.

Bailey CJ, Turner RC: Metformin. N Engl J Med 334:574, 1996.

Bailey TS, Mezitis NHE: Combination therapy with insulin and sulfonylureas for type 2 diabetes. Diabetes Care 13:687, 1990.

Bennett N, et al: Comparison of a low carbohydrate versus high fiber diet in cats with diabetes mellitus. J Vet Intern Med 15:297, 2001 (abstract).

Berg AH, et al: The adipocyte-secreted protein Acrp30 enhances hepatic insulin action. Nat Med 7:947, 2001.

Berger J, et al: Thiazolidinediones produce a conformational change in paroxysmal proliferator-activated receptor-δ binding and activation correlated with antidiabetic actions in db/db mice. Endocrinology 137:4189, 1996.

Bertoy EH, et al: Treatment of diabetes mellitus with Lente insulin in 12 cats. J Am Vet Med Assoc 206:1729, 1995.

Biourge V, et al: Effect of weight gain and subsequent weight loss on glucose tolerance and insulin response in healthy cats. J Vet Intern Med 11:86, 1997.

Birkeland KI, et al: Long-term, randomized, placebo-controlled, double-blind therapeutic comparison of glipizide and glyburide. Diabetes Care 17:45, 1994.

Boord M, Griffin C: Progesterone secreting adrenal mass in a cat with clinical signs of hyperadrenocorticism. J Am Vet Med Assoc 214:666, 1999.

Brichard SM, Henquin J: The role of vanadium in the management of diabetes. Trends Pharmacol Sci 16:265, 1995.

Brichard SM, et al: Long-term improvement of glucose homeostasis by vanadate in obese hyperinsulinemic fa/fa rats. Endocrinology 125:2510, 1989.

Broussard JD, Peterson ME: Comparison of two Ultralente insulin preparations with protamine zinc insulin in clinically normal cats. Am J Vet Res 55:127, 1994.

Butterwick RF, et al: Influence of age and sex on plasma lipid and lipoprotein concentrations and associated enzyme activities in cats. Am J Vet Res 62:331, 2001.

Christopher MM, et al: Heinz body formation associated with ketoacidosis in diabetic cats. J Vet Intern Med 9:24, 1995.

Cohn LA, et al: Effects of chromium supplementation on glucose tolerance in obese and nonobese cats. Am J Vet Res 60:1360, 1999.

Cohen N, et al: Oral vanadyl sulfate improves hepatic and peripheral insulin sensitivity in patients with non–insulin-dependent diabetes mellitus. J Clin Invest 95:2501, 1995.

Crenshaw KL, et al: Serum fructosamine concentration as an index of glycemia in cats with diabetes mellitus and stress hyperglycemia. J Vet Intern Med 10:360, 1996.

Damsbo P, et al: A double-blind, randomized comparison of meal-related glycemic control by Repaglinide and glyburide in well-controlled type 2 diabetic patients. Diabetes Care 22:789, 1999.

DeFronzo RA: Pharmacologic therapy for type 2 diabetes mellitus. Ann Intern Med 131:281, 1999.

DeFronzo RA, Goodman AM: Efficacy of metformin in patients with non–insulin-dependent diabetes mellitus. The Multicenter Metformin Study Group. N Engl J Med 333:541, 1995.

Diabetes Control and Complications Trial Research Group: The effect of intensive treatment of diabetes on the development and progression of long-term complications in insulin-dependent diabetes mellitus. N Engl J Med 329:977, 1993.

Duesberg CA, et al: Adrenalectomy for treatment of hyperadrenocorticism in cats: ten cases (1988-1992). J Am Vet Med Assoc 207:1066, 1995.

Elliott DA: Disorders of metabolism. In Nelson RW, Couto CG (eds): Small Animal Internal Medicine, 3rd ed. St Louis, Mosby, 2003, p 816.

Elliott DA, et al: Glycosylated hemoglobin concentration for assessment of glycemic control in diabetic cats. J Vet Intern Med 11:161, 1997.

Elliott DA, et al: Comparison of serum fructosamine and blood glycosylated hemoglobin concentrations for assessment of glycemic control in cats with diabetes mellitus. J Am Vet Med Assoc 214:1794, 1999.

Elliott DA, et al: Prevalence of pituitary tumors among diabetic cats with insulin resistance. J Am Vet Med Assoc 216:1765, 2000.

Fajans SS, Brown MB: Administration of sulfonylureas can increase glucose-induced insulin secretion for decades in patients with maturity-onset diabetes of the young. Diabetes Care 16:1254, 1993.

Feldhahn JR, et al: The effect of interday variation and a short-term stressor on insulin sensitivity in clinically normal cats. J Fel Med Surg 1:233, 1999.

Feldman EC, et al: Intensive 50-week evaluation of glipizide administration in 50 cats with previously untreated diabetes mellitus. J Am Vet Med Assoc 210:772, 1997.

Fettman MJ, et al: Effects of weight gain and loss on metabolic rate, glucose tolerance, and serum lipids in domestic cats. Res Vet Sci 64:11, 1998.

Fondacaro JV, et al: Treatment of feline diabetes mellitus with protamine zinc analine insulin (PZI) alone compared with PZI and oral vanadium dipicolinate. J Vet Intern Med 13:244, 1999 (abstract).

Forcier NJ, et al: Cellular pathology of the nerve microenvironment in galactose intoxication. J Neuropathol Exp Neurol 50:235, 1991.

Frank G, et al: Use of a high-protein diet in the management of feline diabetes mellitus. Vet Therapeutics 2:238, 2001.

Freidenberg GR, et al: Diabetes responsive to intravenous but not subcutaneous insulin: effectiveness of aprotinin. N Engl J Med 305:363, 1981.

Fruebis J, et al: Proteolytic cleavage product of 30 kDa adipocyte complement-related protein increases fatty acid oxidation in muscle and causes weight loss in mice. Proc Natl Acad Sci USA 98:2005, 2001.

Gedulin BR, et al: Dose-response for glucagonostatic effect of amylin in rats. Metabolism 46:67, 1997.

Gerhardt A, et al: Comparison of the sensitivity of different diagnostic tests for pancreatitis in cats. J Vet Intern Med 15:329, 2001.

Gerich JE: Oral hypoglycemic agents. N Engl J Med 321:1231, 1989.

Gitlin N, et al: Two cases of severe clinical and histologic hepatotoxicity associated with troglitazone. Ann Intern Med 129:36, 1998.

Goldfine AB, et al: In vivo and in vitro studies of vanadate in human and rodent diabetes mellitus. Mol Cell Biochem 153:217, 1995.

Goossens MMC, et al: Response to insulin treatment and survival in 104 cats with diabetes mellitus (1985-1995). J Vet Intern Med 12:1, 1998.

Greco DS: Treatment of non–insulin-dependent diabetes mellitus in cats using oral hypoglycemic agents. In Bonagura JD (ed): Kirk's Current Veterinary Therapy XIII. Philadelphia, WB Saunders, 2000, p 350.

Greene DA, et al: Pathogenesis and prevention of diabetic neuropathy. Diabetes Metab Rev 4:201, 1988a.

Greene DA, et al: Are disturbances of sorbitol, phosphoinositide, and Na+-K+-ATPase regulation involved in pathogenesis of diabetic neuropathy? Diabetes 37:688, 1988b.

Groop LC: Sulfonylureas in NIDDM. Diabetes Care 15:737, 1992.

Grossman S, Lessem J: Mechanisms and clinical effects of thiazolidinediones. Exp Opin Invest Drugs 6:1025, 1997.

Hallden G, et al: Characterization of cat insulin. Arch Biochem Biophys 247:20, 1986.

Harb-Hauser M, et al: Prevalence of insulin antibodies in diabetic cats. J Vet Intern Med 12:245, 1998 (abstract).

Hasegawa S, et al: Glycated hemoglobin fractions in normal and diabetic cats measured by high-performance liquid chromatography. J Vet Med Sci 54:789, 1992.

Havel PJ: Role of adipose tissue in body weight regulation: mechanisms regulating leptin production and energy balance. Proc Nutri Soc 59:359, 2000.

Havel PJ: Peripheral signals conveying metabolic information to the brain: short-term and long-term regulation of food intake and energy homeostasis. Exp Biol Med 226:963, 2001.

Havel PJ: Control of energy homeostasis and insulin action by adipocyte hormones: leptin, acylation stimulating protein, and adiponectin. Curr Opin Lipidol 13:51, 2002.

Hiddinga HJ, Eberhardt NL: Intracellular amyloidogenesis by human islet amyloid polypeptide induces apoptosis in COS-1 cells. Am J Pathol 154:1077, 1999.

Hoenig M, Ferguson DC: Impairment of glucose tolerance in hyperthyroid cats. J Endocrinol 121:249, 1988.

Hoenig M, Ferguson DC: Diagnostic utility of glycosylated hemoglobin concentrations in the cat. Domest Anim Endocrinol 16:11, 1999.

Hoenig M, et al: Glucose tolerance and insulin secretion in spontaneously hyperthyroid cats. Res Vet Sci 53:338, 1992.

Hoenig M, et al: Beta cell and insulin antibodies in treated and untreated diabetic cats. Vet Immunol Immunopathol 77:93, 2000a.

Hoenig M, et al: A feline model of experimentally induced islet amyloidosis. Am J Pathol 157:2143, 2000b.

Hotta K, et al: Circulating concentrations of the adipocyte protein adiponectin are decreased in parallel with reduced insulin sensitivity during the progression to type 2 diabetes in rhesus monkeys. Diabetes 50:1126, 2001.

Jaber LA, et al: An evaluation of the therapeutic effects and dosage equivalents of glyburide and glipizide. J Clin Pharmacol 30:181, 1990.

Jain NC: Erythrocyte physiology and changes in disease. In Jain NC (ed): Essentials of Veterinary Hematology. Philadelphia, WB Saunders, 1993, p 133.

Johnson KH, et al: Immunolocalization of islet amyloid polypeptide (IAPP) in pancreatic beta cells using peroxidase antiperoxidase (PAP) and protein A gold techniques. Am J Pathol 130:1, 1988.

Johnson KH, et al: Islet amyloid, islet amyloid polypeptide, and diabetes mellitus. N Engl J Med 321:513, 1989.

Johnson KH, et al: The putative hormone islet amyloid polypeptide (IAPP) induces impaired glucose tolerance in cats. Biochem Biophys Res Commun 167:507, 1990.

Kassir AA, et al: Lack of effect of islet amyloid polypeptide in causing insulin resistance in conscious dogs during euglycemic clamp studies. Diabetes 40:998, 1991.

Kawamoto M, et al: Relation of fructosamine to serum protein, albumin, and glucose concentrations in healthy and diabetic dogs. Am J Vet Res 53:851, 1992.

Kennedy WR, et al: Effects of pancreatic transplantation on diabetic neuropathy. N Engl J Med 322:1031, 1990.

Kirk CA, et al: Diagnosis of naturally acquired type 1 and type 2 diabetes mellitus in cats. Am J Vet Res 54:463, 1993.

Kramek BA, et al: Neuropathy associated with diabetes mellitus in the cat. J Am Vet Med Assoc 184:42, 1984.

Leahy JL: Natural history of B-cell dysfunction in NIDDM. Diabetes Care 13:992, 1990.

Lebovitz HE: Oral hypoglycemic agents. In Rifkin H, Porte D (eds): Ellenberg and Rifkin's Diabetes Mellitus: Theory and Practice, 4th ed. New York, Elsevier, 1990, p 554.

Lebovitz HE, Pasmantier RM: Combination insulin-sulfonylurea therapy. Diabetes Care 13:667, 1990.

Lorenzo A, et al: Pancreatic islet cell toxicity of amylin associated with type 2 diabetes mellitus. Nature 368:756, 1994.

Low PA, et al: The roles of oxidative stress and antioxidant treatment in experimental diabetic neuropathy. Diabetes 46(suppl 2):S38, 1997.

Lutz TA, Rand JS: Comparison of five commercial radioimmunoassay kits for the measurement of feline insulin. Res Vet Sci 55:64, 1993.

Lutz TA, Rand JS: Plasma amylin and insulin concentrations in normoglycemic and hyperglycemic cats. Can Vet J 37:27, 1996.

Lutz TA, et al: Frequency of pancreatic amyloid deposition in cats from southeastern Queensland. Aust Vet J 71:254, 1994.

Lutz TA, et al: Fructosamine concentrations in hyperglycemic cats. Can Vet J 36:155, 1995.

Marshall RD, Rand JS: Comparison of the pharmacokinetics and pharmacodynamics of glargine, protamine zinc, and porcine Lente insulins in normal cats. J Vet Intern Med 16:358, 2002 (abstract).

Massillon D, et al: Induction of hepatic glucose-6-phosphatase gene expression by lipid infusion. Diabetes 46:153, 1997.

Mazzaferro EM: Treatment of feline diabetes mellitus with a high protein diet and acarbose. J Vet Intern Med 14:345, 2000 (abstract).

McMillan FD, Feldman EC: Rebound hyperglycemia following overdosing of insulin in cats with diabetes mellitus. J Am Vet Med Assoc 188:1426, 1986.

Michels GM, et al: Pharmacokinetics of the antihyperglycemic agent metformin in cats. Am J Vet Res 60:738, 1999.

Michels GM, et al: Pharmacokinetics of the insulin-sensitizing agent troglitazone in cats. Am J Vet Res 61:775, 2000.

Miller AB, et al: Effect of glipizide on serum insulin and glucose concentrations in healthy cats. Res Vet Sci 52:177, 1992.

Mizisin AP, Calcutt NA: Dose-dependent alterations in nerve polyols and (Na^+-K^+)-ATP'ase activity in galactose intoxication. Clin Exp Metab 40:1207, 1991.

Mizisin AP, et al: Myelin splitting, Schwann cell injury, and demyelination in feline diabetic neuropathy. Acta Neuropathol 95:171, 1998.

Mizisin AP, et al: Neurological complications associated with spontaneously occurring feline diabetes mellitus. J Neuropathol Exp Neurol 61:872, 2002.

Moise NS, Reimers TJ: Insulin therapy in cats with diabetes mellitus. J Am Vet Med Assoc 182:158, 1983.

Morris JG: Idiosyncratic nutrient requirements of cats appear to be diet-induced evolutionary adaptations. Nutr Res Rev 15:153, 2002.

Moses R, et al: Effect of Repaglinide addition to metformin monotherapy on glycemic control in patients with type 2 diabetes. Diabetes Care 22:119, 1999.

Nakayama H, et al: Pathological observations in six cases of feline diabetes mellitus. Jpn J Vet Sci 52:819, 1990.

Nell LJ, Thomas JW: Human insulin autoantibody fine specificity and H and L chain use. J Immunol 142:3063, 1989.

Nelson RW, et al: Glucose tolerance and insulin response in normal weight and obese cats. Am J Vet Res 51:1357, 1990.

Nelson RW, et al: Effect of an orally administered sulfonylurea, glipizide, for treatment of diabetes mellitus in cats. J Am Vet Med Assoc 203:821, 1993.

Nelson RW, et al: Transient clinical diabetes mellitus in cats: 10 cases (1989-1991). J Vet Intern Med 13:28, 1998.

Nelson RW, et al: Effect of dietary insoluble fiber on control of glycemia in cats with naturally acquired diabetes mellitus. J Am Vet Med Assoc 216:1082, 2000.

Nelson RW, et al: Efficacy of protamine zinc insulin for treatment of diabetes mellitus in cats. J Am Vet Med Assoc 218:38, 2001.

Nelson RW, et al: Evaluation of the oral antihyperglycemic drug metformin in normal and diabetic cats. J Vet Intern Med (in press).

O'Brien TD, et al: Immunohistochemical morphometry of pancreatic endocrine cells in diabetic, normoglycaemic, glucose-intolerant, and normal cats. J Comp Pathol 96:357, 1986.

O'Brien TD, et al: Intracellular amyloid associated with cytotoxicity in COS-1 cells expressing human islet amyloid polypeptide. Am J Pathol 147:609, 1995.

Panciera DL, et al: Epizootiologic patterns of diabetes mellitus in cats: 333 cases (1980-1986). J Am Vet Med Assoc 197:1504, 1990.

Patel J, et al: BRL 49653 (a thiazolidinedione) improves glycemic control in NIDDM patients. Diabetes 46:150A, 1997 (abstract).

Pedersen O, et al: Characterization of the insulin resistance of glucose utilization in adipocytes from patients with hyper- and hypothyroidism. Acta Endocrinol 119:228, 1988.

Peterson ME: Effects of megestrol acetate on glucose tolerance and growth hormone secretion in the cat. Res Vet Sci 42:354, 1987.

Peterson ME, et al: Acromegaly in 14 cats. J Vet Intern Med 4:192, 1990.

Plier ML, et al: Serum fructosamine concentration in nondiabetic and diabetic cats. Vet Clin Pathol 27:34, 1998.

Plosker GL, Faulds D: Troglitazone: a review of its use in the management of type 2 diabetes mellitus. Drugs 57:409, 1999.

Plotnick AN, et al: Oral vanadium compounds: preliminary studies on toxicity in normal cats and hypoglycemic potential in diabetic cats. J Vet Intern Med 9:181, 1995 (abstract).

Rand JS, et al: Overrepresentation of Burmese cats with diabetes mellitus. Aust Vet J 75:402, 1997.

Rand JS, et al: Acute stress hyperglycemia in cats is associated with struggling and increased concentrations of lactate and norepinephrine. J Vet Intern Med 16:1213, 2002.

Reusch CE, Haberer B: Evaluation of fructosamine in dogs and cats with hypo- or hyperproteinaemia, azotaemia, hyperlipidaemia, and hyperbilirubinaemia. Vet Rec 148:370, 2001.

Reusch CE, et al: Fructosamine: a new parameter for diagnosis and metabolic control in diabetic dogs and cats. J Vet Intern Med 7:177, 1993.

Roden M, et al: Mechanism of free fatty acid–induced insulin resistance in humans. J Clin Invest 97:2859, 1996.

Rosenstock J, et al: Basal insulin glargine (HOE901) versus NPH insulin in patients with type 1 diabetes on multiple daily insulin regimens. Diabetes Care 23:1137, 2000.

Rosenstock J, et al: Basal insulin therapy in type 2 diabetes: 28-week comparison of insulin glargine (HOE901) and NPH insulin. Diabetes Care 24:631, 2001.

Rossetti L, et al: Glucose toxicity. Diabetes Care 13:610, 1990.

Rossmeisl JH, et al: Hyperadrenocorticism and hyperprogesteronemia in a cat with an adrenocortical adenocarcinoma. J Am Anim Hosp Assoc 36:512, 2000.

Sagawa MM, et al: Correlation between plasma leptin concentration and body fat content in dogs. Am J Vet Res 63:7, 2002.

Sambol NC, et al: Pharmacokinetics and pharmacodynamics of metformin in healthy subjects and patients with non–insulin-dependent diabetes mellitus. J Clin Pharmacol 36:1012, 1996.

Scarlett JM, Donoghue S: Associations between body condition and disease in cats. J Am Vet Med Assoc 212:1725, 1998.

Scarpini E, et al: Decrease of nerve Na^+,K^+-ATPase activity in the pathogenesis of human diabetic neuropathy. J Neurol Sci 120:159, 1993.

Schachter S, et al: Oral chromium picolinate and control of glycemia in insulin-treated diabetic dogs. J Vet Intern Med 15:379, 2001.

Schade DS, Duckworth WC: In search of the subcutaneous insulin resistance syndrome. N Engl J Med 315:147, 1986.

Segal KR, et al: Relationship between insulin sensitivity and plasma leptin concentration in lean and obese men. Diabetes 45:988, 1996.

Sheen AJ: Clinical pharmacokinetics of metformin. Clin Pharmacol 30:359, 1996.

Steiner JM, Williams DA: Serum feline trypsin-like immunoreactivity in cats with exocrine pancreatic insufficiency. J Vet Intern Med 14:627, 2000.

Stevens MJ, et al: The aetiology of diabetic neuropathy: the combined roles of metabolic and vascular defects. Diabet Med 12:566, 1995.

Striffler JS, et al: Chromium improves insulin response to glucose in rats. Metabolism 44:1314, 1995.

Swift NC, et al: Evaluation of serum feline trypsin-like immunoreactivity for the diagnosis of pancreatitis in cats. J Am Vet Med Assoc 217:37, 2000.

Thomas JW, et al: Heterogeneity and specificity of human anti-insulin antibodies determined by isoelectric focusing. J Immunol 134:1048, 1985.

Thomas JW, et al: Spectrotypic analysis of antibodies to insulin A and B chains. Mol Immunol 25:173, 1988.

Thomas PK: Growth factors and diabetic neuropathy. Diabet Med 11:732, 1994.

Thompson MD, et al: Comparison of glucose concentrations in blood samples obtained with a marginal ear vein nick technique versus from a peripheral vein in healthy cats and cats with diabetes mellitus. J Am Vet Med Assoc 221:389, 2002.

Truglia JA, et al: Insulin resistance: receptor and postbinding defects in human obesity and non–insulin-dependent diabetes mellitus. Am J Med 979(suppl 2B):13, 1985.

Unger RH, Foster DW: Diabetes mellitus. In Wilson JD, et al (eds): Williams Textbook of Endocrinology, 9th ed. Philadelphia, WB Saunders, 1998, p 973.

Unger RH, Grundy S: Hyperglycemia as an inducer as well as a consequence of impaired islet cell function and insulin resistance: implications for the management of diabetes. Diabetologia 28:119, 1985.

Wallace MS, et al: Absorption kinetics of regular, isophane, and protamine zinc insulin in normal cats. Domest Anim Endocrinol 7:509, 1990.

Ward JD: Biochemical and vascular factors in the pathogenesis of diabetic neuropathy. Clin Invest Med 18:267, 1995.

Wess G, Reusch C: Capillary blood sampling from the ear of dogs and cats and use of portable meters to measure glucose concentration. J Small Anim Pract 41:60, 2000a.

Wess G, Reusch C: Assessment of five portable blood glucose meters for use in cats. Am J Vet Res 61:1587, 2000b.

Westermark P, et al: Islet amyloid in type 2 human diabetes mellitus and adult diabetic cats is composed of a novel putative polypeptide hormone. Am J Pathol 127:414, 1987a.

Westermark P, et al: Islet amyloid polypeptide–like immunoreactivity in the islet B cells of type 2 (non–insulin-dependent) diabetic and nondiabetic individuals. Diabetologia 30:887, 1987b.

Weyer C, et al: Hypoadiponectinemia in obesity and type 2 diabetes: close association with insulin resistance and hyperinsulinemia. J Clin Endocrinol Metab 86:1930, 2001.

Winegrad AI: Does a common mechanism induce the diverse complications of diabetes? Banting Lecture, 1986. Diabetes 36:396, 1986.

Wolffenbuttel BHR, Landgraf R: A 1-year, multicenter, randomized, double-blind comparison of Repaglinide and glyburide for the treatment of type 2 diabetes. Diabetes Care 22:463, 1999.

Yano BL, et al: Feline insular amyloid: incidence in adult cats with no clinicopathologic evidence of overt diabetes mellitus. Vet Pathol 18:310, 1981a.

Yano BL, et al: Feline insular amyloid: association with diabetes mellitus. Vet Pathol 18:621, 1981b.

Young AA, et al: Dose-responses for the slowing of gastric emptying in a rodent model by glucagon-like peptide (7-36)NH2, amylin, cholecystokinin, and other possible regulators of nutrient uptake. Metabolism 45:1, 1996.

Zhuang HX, et al: Insulin-like growth factors reverse or arrest diabetic neuropathy: effects on hyperalgesia and impaired nerve regeneration in rats. Exp Neurol 140:198, 1996.

Zimmet PZ, et al: Is there a relationship between leptin and insulin sensitivity independent of obesity? A population-based study in the Indian Ocean nation of Mauritius. Int J Obesity 22:171, 1998.

Zoran DL: The carnivore connection to nutrition in cats. J Am Vet Med Assoc 221:1559, 2002.

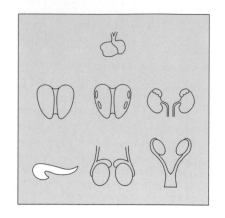

13

DIABETIC KETOACIDOSIS

Diabetic ketoacidosis (DKA) is a serious complication of diabetes mellitus. Before the availability of insulin in the 1920s, DKA was a uniformly fatal disorder. Even after the discovery of insulin, DKA continued to carry a grave prognosis, with a reported mortality rate in humans ranging from 10% to 30%. Despite expanding knowledge regarding the pathophysiology of DKA and the application of new treatment techniques for the complications of DKA, the mortality rate for this disorder remains at 5% to 10% in humans (Wagner et al, 1999; Masharani and Karam, 2001). DKA is a challenging disorder to treat, in part because of the deleterious impact of DKA on multiple organ systems and the common occurrence of concurrent, often serious, disorders that are primarily responsible for the high mortality rate of DKA. In humans, the incidence of DKA has not decreased, appropriate therapy remains controversial, and patients continue to succumb to this complication of diabetes mellitus. This chapter summarizes current concepts regarding the pathophysiology and management of DKA in dogs and cats.

PATHOGENESIS AND PATHOPHYSIOLOGY

GENERATION OF KETONE BODIES. Ketone bodies are derived from oxidation of nonesterified or free fatty acids (FFA) by the liver and are used as an energy source by many tissues during periods of glucose deficiency. FFAs released from adipose tissue are assimilated by the liver at a rate dependent on their plasma concentration. Within the liver, FFAs can be incorporated into triglycerides, can be metabolized via the tricarboxylic acid (TCA) cycle to CO_2 and water, or can be converted to ketone bodies (Fig. 13-1) (Hood and Tannen, 1994; Kitabchi et al, 2001). Oxidation of

FFAs leads to the production of acetoacetate. In the presence of NADH, acetoacetate is reduced to β-hydroxybutyrate. Acetone is formed by spontaneous decarboxylation of acetoacetate (Fig. 13-1). These ketone bodies—acetoacetate, β-hydroxybutyrate, and acetone—are substrates for energy metabolism by most tissues in addition to fulfilling a biosynthetic role in the brain of the neonate (Zammit, 1994). The metabolism of ketone bodies is integrated with that of other substrates of energy metabolism, both in peripheral tissues and in the liver. However, excessive production of ketone bodies, as occurs in uncontrolled diabetes, results in their accumulation in the circulation and development of the ketosis and acidosis of ketoacidosis.

ROLE OF INSULIN DEFICIENCY. The most important regulators of ketone body production are FFA availability and the ketogenic capacity of the liver (McGarry et al, 1989; Zammit, 1994). For the synthesis of ketone bodies to be enhanced, there must be two major alterations in intermediary metabolism: (1) enhanced mobilization of FFAs from triglycerides stored in adipose tissue and (2) a shift in hepatic metabolism from fat synthesis to fat oxidation and ketogenesis (Hood and Tannen, 1994; Kitabchi et al, 2001). Insulin is a powerful inhibitor of lipolysis and FFA oxidation (Groop et al, 1989). A relative or absolute deficiency of insulin "allows" lipolysis to increase, thus increasing the availability of FFAs to the liver and in turn promoting ketogenesis. Virtually all dogs and cats with DKA have a relative or absolute deficiency of insulin. In established diabetic animals in whom insulin is discontinued and in newly diagnosed diabetic animals who are diagnosed with ketoacidosis on initial examination, circulating insulin levels are low or undetectable. Some dogs and cats have serum insulin concentrations similar to those observed in

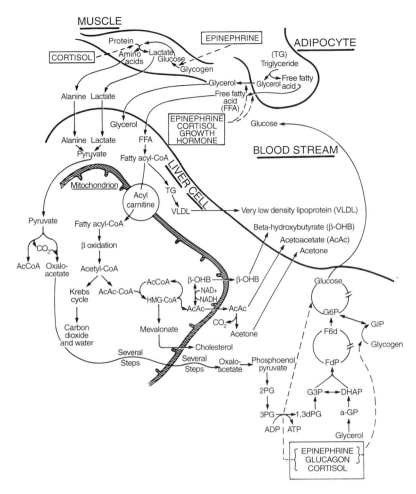

FIGURE 13–1. In response to a wide variety of stress situations, such as sepsis, heart failure, and pancreatitis, the body increases its production of the glucoregulatory hormones—insulin, glucagon, epinephrine, cortisol, and growth hormone. In diabetes, the lack of insulin allows the glucogenic effects of the stress hormones to be unopposed in liver, muscle, and adipose tissue. This results in excess ketone formation, fat and muscle breakdown, and a classic catabolic state.

normal, fasted nondiabetics (i.e., 5 to 20 µU/ml). However, such insulin concentrations are inappropriately low ("relative" insulin deficiency) for the severity of hyperglycemia encountered.

Some diabetic dogs and cats develop ketoacidosis despite receiving daily injections of insulin, and circulating insulin concentrations may even be increased. Insulin deficiency per se cannot be the sole physiologic cause for the development of DKA. In this group, a "relative" insulin deficiency is present. Presumably these dogs and cats have insulin resistance resulting from an increase in circulating glucose counterregulatory hormones (i.e., epinephrine, glucagon, cortisol, growth hormone) and an altered metabolic milieu (e.g., increased plasma FFAs and amino acids, metabolic acidosis). The ability to maintain normal glucose homeostasis represents a balance between the body's sensitivity to insulin and the amount of insulin secreted by the beta cell or injected exogenously. With the development of insulin resistance, the need for insulin may exceed the daily injected insulin dose, and

this leads to a predisposition for the development of DKA (Fig. 13-2).

ROLE OF GLUCOSE COUNTERREGULATORY HORMONES. Circulating levels of epinephrine, norepinephrine, glucagon, cortisol, and growth hormone are typically markedly increased in humans with DKA, as are plasma FFA and amino acid concentrations (Fig. 13-3; Luzi et al, 1988). Increased circulating concentrations of these counterregulatory hormones cause insulin resistance, stimulate lipolysis and the generation of FFAs in the circulation, and shift hepatic metabolism of FFAs from fat synthesis to fat oxidation and ketogenesis (Fig. 13-3) (McGarry et al, 1989; Zammit, 1994). Glucagon is considered the most influential ketogenic hormone. Increased concentrations accompany ketotic states, and low concentrations blunt ketogenesis in ketogenic conditions (Hood and Tannen, 1994). Glucagon can directly influence hepatic ketogenesis. However, its effects still depend on substrate availability, and ketogenesis can occur in the absence of glucagon. Catecholamines are also impor-

PATHOGENESIS OF DKA

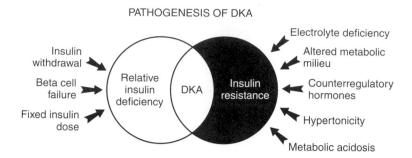

FIGURE 13–2. The pathogenesis of DKA, illustrating the interaction of insulin deficiency and insulin resistance necessary in the development of the ketoacidotic state.

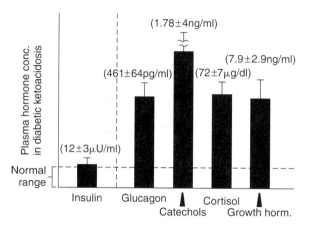

FIGURE 13–3. Plasma insulin and counterregulatory hormone concentrations in DKA (mean ± SEM). DKA is characterized by relative insulin deficiency and stress hormone excess. Plasma cortisol concentration is characteristically elevated in all animals admitted to the hospital in severe DKA. Although the mean growth hormone concentration also tends to be elevated in ketoacidosis, in many animals this hormone does not become elevated until therapy is begun with insulin and fluids. (Reprinted from Schade DS, et al: Diabetic ketoacidosis: Pathogenesis, prevention, and therapy. *In* Schade DS, et al (eds): Diabetic Coma. Albuquerque, University of New Mexico Press, 1981, p 84.)

tant modulators of ketogenesis, primarily through stimulation of lipolysis. Both epinephrine and glucagon contribute to insulin resistance by inhibiting insulin-mediated glucose uptake in muscle and by stimulating hepatic glucose production through an augmentation of both glycogenolysis and gluconeogenesis (Cherrington et al, 1987; Cryer, 1993). Cortisol and growth hormone enhance lipolysis in the presence of a relative or absolute deficiency of insulin (see Fig. 13-1), block insulin action in peripheral tissues (Bratusch-Marrain, et al, 1982; Boyle, 1993), and potentiate the stimulating effect of epinephrine and glucagon on hepatic glucose output (Sherwin et al, 1980). An elevation in plasma FFA concentration and FFA oxidation inhibits insulin-mediated glucose uptake in muscle and stimulates hepatic gluconeogenesis (Thiebaud et al, 1982; Ferrannini et al, 1983). The combination of insulin deficiency and excesses in counterregulatory hormones also stimulates protein catabolism. Increased plasma amino acid concen-

trations impair insulin action in muscle and provide substrate to drive gluconeogenesis (Tessari et al, 1985). The net effect of these hormonal disturbances is accentuation of insulin deficiency through the development of insulin resistance, stimulation of lipolysis leading to ketogenesis, and stimulation of gluconeogenesis, which worsens hyperglycemia. All these factors lead to the eventual onset of clinical manifestations associated with DKA.

The body increases its production of the glucose counterregulatory hormones in response to a wide variety of diseases and stress situations. Although this response is usually beneficial, in DKA the activity of these hormones as insulin antagonists usually worsens hyperglycemia and ketonemia, provoking acidosis, fluid depletion, and hypotension. This condition progresses in a self-perpetuating spiral of metabolic decompensation (Fig. 13-4). It is rare for the dog or cat with DKA not to have some coexisting disorder, such as pancreatitis, infection, renal insufficiency, or concurrent hormonal disorder. These disorders have the potential for increasing glucose counterregulatory hormone secretion. For example, infection causes a marked increase in the secretion of cortisol and glucagon, heart failure and trauma result in increased circulating levels of glucagon and catecholamines, and fever induces secretion of glucagon, growth hormone, catecholamines, and cortisol (Kandel and Aberman, 1983; Feldman and Nelson, 1987). The recognition and treatment of disorders that coexist with DKA are critically important for successful management of DKA (see Fig. 13-2).

PHYSIOLOGIC CONSEQUENCES OF ENHANCED KETONE BODY PRODUCTION. The physiologic derangements that accompany DKA are a direct result of relative or absolute insulin deficiency, hyperketonemia, and hyperglycemia (Table 13-1). In a short-term situation, the conversion of FFAs to ketone bodies is actually a positive metabolic development. Diabetes mellitus is interpreted physiologically as a state of starvation. With glucose deficiency, ketone bodies can be used as an energy source by many tissues. However, increasing plasma glucose and ketone concentrations eventually surpass the renal tubular threshold for complete reabsorption and spill into the urine, inducing an osmotic diuresis. During the development of DKA in

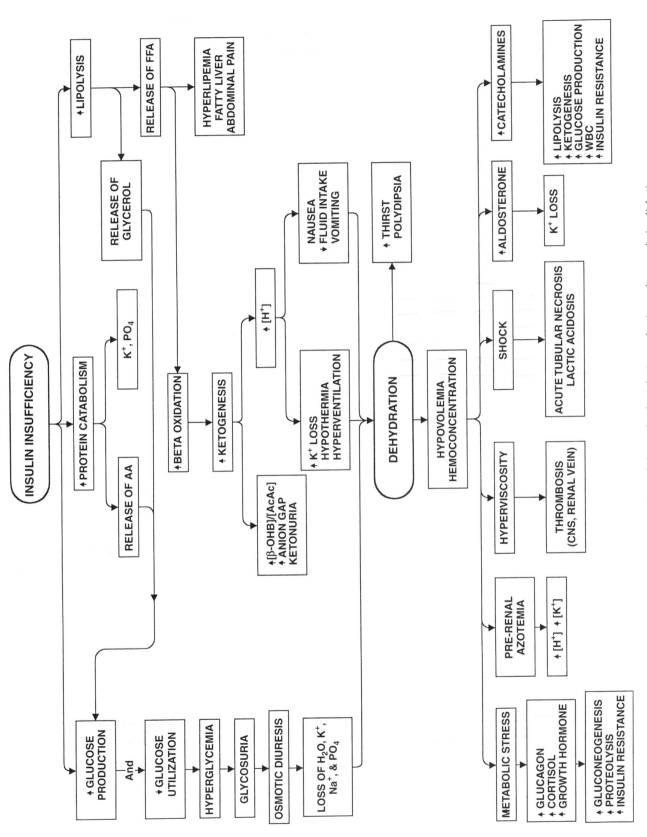

FIGURE 13-4. The interrelationship of the pathophysiologic mechanisms that result in diabetic ketoacidosis (DKA). *AA* = Amino acids; *FFA* = free fatty acids; *K* = potassium; *AcAc* = acetoacetate; β-*OHB* = β-hydroxybutyrate.

TABLE 13–1 PATHOPHYSIOLOGIC DERANGEMENTS IN DIABETIC KETOACIDOSIS

Hyperglycemia	Hyperketonemia	Insulin Deficiency
Osmotic diuresis	Osmotic diuresis	Electrolyte and fluid
Sodium	Sodium	losses
Potassium	Potassium	Sodium
Water	Water	Water
Calcium	Calcium	Phosphate
Phosphate	Phosphate	Negative nitrogen
Intracellular	Metabolic acidosis	balance
dehydration		

humans, the daily urinary losses of glucose can be as much as 150 to 200 g, and ketone excretion rates average 20 to 30 g (Luzi et al, 1988; Ennis et al, 1994). Each gram of glucose excreted via the kidneys adds a solute load of approximately 6 mOsm. The lower molecular weight of ketones accounts for a greater osmotic load per gram, and excretion of ketones is responsible for one-third to one-half of the osmotic diuresis in humans with DKA (DeFronzo et al, 1994; Kitabchi et al, 2001). Moreover, the anionic charge on the ketones, even at a maximally acid urine pH, obligates the excretion of positively charged ions, such as sodium, potassium, calcium, and magnesium, to maintain electrical neutrality. The total urinary osmolar load from glucose and ketones alone can amount to 1500 to 2000 mOsm, an amount that is two- to three-fold greater than the normal daily urinary osmolar losses (DeFronzo et al, 1994). This increased solute excretion impairs the reabsorption of water throughout the proximal tubule and loop of Henle, lowering the concentration of sodium and chloride in the tubular lumen, causing an increased concentration gradient for their reabsorption, and thereby inhibiting their transport from lumen to blood. The result is an excessive loss of electrolytes and water, leading to volume contraction and underperfusion of tissues.

Insulin deficiency per se also contributes to the excessive renal losses of water and electrolytes. Physiologic increases in plasma insulin concentration augment salt and water reabsorption in both the proximal and distal portions of the nephron and enhance proximal tubular phosphate reabsorption (DeFronzo et al, 1994). Conversely, insulin deficiency leads to enhanced water and electrolyte excretion; it also leads to an accelerated rate of proteolysis, impaired protein synthesis, and negative nitrogen balance (DeFronzo and Ferrannini, 1992). The composition of the urine in a person undergoing an osmotic diuresis is similar to that of half-normal saline. Consequently, water losses typically exceed sodium losses. Significant losses of potassium and phosphorus also occur and may complicate therapy. Although increased urinary calcium and magnesium losses occur, they usually do not present a problem during management of DKA.

The formation of ketones by the liver is associated with the production of an equivalent number of hydrogen ions, which titrate the plasma bicarbonate concentration. As ketones continue to accumulate in the blood, the body's buffering system becomes overwhelmed, causing an increase in arterial hydrogen ion concentration, a decrease in serum bicarbonate, and development of metabolic acidosis. Further loss of water and electrolytes occurs as a result of repeated bouts of vomiting or diarrhea combined with a lack of fluid intake, problems that often develop as the metabolic acidosis worsens (see Fig. 13-4). The excessive loss of electrolytes and water leads to further volume contraction, underperfusion of tissues, decline in the glomerular filtration rate (GFR), and worsening prerenal azotemia and dehydration. Hyperglycemic dogs and cats with reduced GFR lose the ability to excrete glucose and, to a lesser degree, hydrogen ions. Glucose and ketones then accumulate in the vascular space at a more rapid rate. The result is increasing hyperglycemia and ketonemia and worsening metabolic acidosis (see Fig. 13-4). The rise in the blood glucose concentration raises the plasma osmolality, and the resulting osmotic diuresis further aggravates the rise in plasma osmolality by causing water losses in excess of the salt loss. The increase in plasma osmolality causes water to be shifted out of cells, leading to cellular dehydration and the eventual development of obtundation and coma. The severe metabolic consequences of DKA, which include severe acidosis, hyperosmolality, obligatory osmotic diuresis, dehydration, and electrolyte derangements, ultimately become life-threatening.

SIGNALMENT

DKA is a serious complication of diabetes mellitus that occurs most commonly in dogs and cats with previously undiagnosed diabetes. Less commonly, DKA develops in an insulin-treated diabetic dog or cat that is receiving an inadequate dosage of insulin, often in conjunction with a concurrent infectious, inflammatory, or hormonal disorder. Because of the close association between DKA and newly diagnosed diabetes mellitus, the signalment for DKA in dogs and cats is similar to that for nonketotic diabetics (see Chapter 11, page 547 and Chapter 12, page 547). For the most part, DKA appears to be a disease of middle-aged and older dogs and cats, although DKA can be diagnosed at any age. In dogs DKA is diagnosed more commonly in females, whereas in cats it is more common in males. Any breed of dog or cat can develop DKA.

HISTORY AND PHYSICAL EXAMINATION

The history and findings on physical examination are variable, in part because of the progressive nature of the disorder and the variable time between DKA onset and owner recognition of a problem. The spectrum ranges from ketonuric dogs and cats that are otherwise healthy, are eating, and have not yet developed metabolic acidosis (i.e., diabetic ketosis [DK]) to ketonuric dogs and cats that have developed severe metabolic acidosis (i.e., DKA), have severe signs of illness, and are moribund.

The classic clinical signs of uncomplicated diabetes (i.e., polyuria, polydipsia, polyphagia, and weight loss) develop initially but either go unnoticed or are considered insignificant by the owner. Systemic signs of illness (i.e., lethargy, anorexia, vomiting) ensue as progressive ketonemia and metabolic acidosis develop, the severity of systemic signs being directly related to the severity of the metabolic acidosis and the nature of concurrent disorders (e.g., pancreatitis, infection) that are often present. The time sequence from the onset of initial clinical signs of diabetes to development of systemic signs due to DKA is unpredictable. We have seen diagnosed diabetic dogs and cats continue rather normal existences for longer than 6 months without therapy. Once ketonemia, ketonuria, and metabolic acidosis begin to develop, however, severe illness typically occurs within a week.

When a severely ill animal is brought to a veterinarian, the owner may not mention signs that were present prior to those most obvious and worrisome at the moment. If the owner is questioned closely with regard to the past history, the changes noted before severe illness include the classic history for diabetes mellitus (i.e., polydipsia, polyuria, polyphagia, and weight loss). It requires a careful historian to obtain this information from a distressed owner. Because of the increased incidence of concurrent diseases, it is imperative that the clinician spend ample time obtaining a careful history concerning all organ systems. Some of these diseases (e.g., pyometra, renal failure, hyperadrenocorticism) have historical signs resembling DKA and can initiate the metabolic derangements leading to DKA in a previously unidentified or insulin-regulated diabetic.

A complete and careful physical examination is critically important in any ketoacidotic animal (see Fig. 13-2). The initial physical examination should focus on an evaluation of the status of hydration, on the extent of central nervous system (CNS) depression, and on a careful search for any initiating cause for diabetic decompensation and ultimate ketoacidosis. Diabetic dogs and cats frequently suffer from concurrent infections, pyometra, pancreatitis, cholangiohepatitis, renal insufficiency, cardiac disease, or other insulin-antagonistic disorders (Bruskiewicz et al, 1997). A careful history, physical examination, and judicious use of laboratory tests can, in most circumstances, identify underlying concurrent disorders, lead to appropriate treatment, and increase the likelihood of successful therapy.

Common physical findings include dehydration, depression, weakness, tachypnea, vomiting, and sometimes a strong odor of acetone on the breath. With severe metabolic acidosis, slow, deep breathing (i.e., Kussmaul respiration) may be observed. Gastrointestinal signs of vomiting, abdominal pain, and distention may be identified and must be differentiated

from similar signs associated with pancreatitis, peritonitis, or other intra-abdominal disorders. The vomiting and abdominal pain that accompany DKA are usually acute in onset, beginning after diabetes mellitus is well established. Conversely, a history of intermittent abdominal pain or vomiting occurring over a period of days or weeks before examination should raise suspicion for a separate abdominal problem, especially chronic pancreatitis. Additional physical examination findings associated with uncomplicated diabetes mellitus (e.g., cataracts, peripheral neuropathy) may also be identified in the dog or cat with DKA (see Chapter 11, page 492, and Chapter 12, page 547).

ESTABLISHING THE DIAGNOSIS OF DIABETIC KETOSIS AND KETOACIDOSIS

A diagnosis of diabetes mellitus requires the presence of appropriate clinical signs (i.e., polyuria, polydipsia, polyphagia, weight loss) and documentation of persistent fasting hyperglycemia and glycosuria. Measurement of the blood glucose concentration using a portable blood glucose monitoring device (see page 512) and testing for the presence of glycosuria using urine reagent test strips (e.g., KetoDiastix; Ames Division, Miles Laboratories Inc., Elkhart, IN) allows the rapid confirmation of diabetes mellitus. The concurrent documentation of ketonuria establishes a diagnosis of diabetic ketosis or ketoacidosis. The subsequent documentation of metabolic acidosis differentiates DKA from DK. Urine reagent test strips for ketonuria measure acetoacetate and acetone. If ketonuria is not present but DK or DKA is suspected, blood can be tested for the presence of acetoacetate and acetone with Acetest tablets (Ames Division, Miles Laboratories, Inc, Elkhart, IN) or the presence of β-hydroxybutyrate using a bench-top chemistry analyzer. The nitroprusside reagents used for the rapid identification of ketoacidemia and ketoaciduria (Acetest and Ketostix) detect only ketone (–C=O) groups (i.e., acetoacetate, acetone). In humans, the predominate ketone body produced during DKA is β-hydroxybutyrate. The β-hydroxybutyrate:acetoacetate ratio can range from 3:1 to 20:1 depending on the severity of hypovolemia, tissue hypoxia, and lactic acidosis (Li et al, 1980; Goldstein, 1995). In the presence of circulatory collapse, an increase in lactic acid can shift the redox state to increase β-hydroxybutyrate at the expense of the readily detectable acetoacetate. In theory, severe hyperketonemia could be underestimated or even undetected if urine reagent test strips or blood tests using the nitroprusside reagent are used to identify DK or DKA. In one study, differences in the serum concentration of β-hydroxybutyrate were identified between dogs with nonketotic diabetes mellitus, DK and DKA, suggesting that measurement of serum β-hydroxybutyrate could be of value in diagnosing and monitoring ketosis and ketoacidosis in diabetic dogs (Fig. 13-5; Duarte et al, 2002).

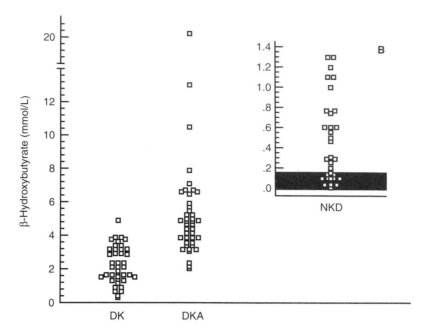

FIGURE 13–5. Serum β-hydroxybutyrate (β-OHB) concentrations from dogs with diabetic ketoacidosis (DKA) and diabetic ketosis (DK). The small plot *(B)* is a graphic depiction of serum β-OHB concentrations from dogs with nonketotic diabetes mellitus (NKD) compared with the reference interval *(shaded area)*. (From Duarte R, et al: Accuracy of serum β-hydroxybutyrate measurements for the diagnosis of diabetic ketoacidosis in 116 dogs. J Vet Intern Med 16:411, 2002.)

The aggressiveness of the diagnostic evaluation and treatment of a dog or cat with DKA is dictated primarily by results of the history and physical examination. A diagnosis of severe DKA is indicated in dogs and cats with systemic signs of illness (i.e., lethargy, anorexia, vomiting), a physical examination revealing dehydration, depression, weakness, and/or Kussmaul respiration; blood glucose concentration greater than 500 mg/dl; or severe metabolic acidosis as diagnosed by a total venous CO_2 or arterial bicarbonate concentration less than 12 mEq/L. History and physical examination findings are subjective, however, and a veterinarian may not be able to obtain quick acid-base information. Therefore a diagnosis of severe DKA is often initially based on having an ill dog or cat with glucose and ketones in the urine. Further diagnostic tests are necessary to care for these animals properly, but therapy can and should proceed while remaining tests are pending.

A tentative diagnosis of DK is reserved for diabetic dogs and cats that are apparently healthy but have both glucose and ketones present in the urine. Systemic signs of illness are absent or mild, serious abnormalities are not readily identifiable on physical examination, and metabolic acidosis has not yet developed or is mild (i.e., total venous CO_2 or arterial bicarbonate concentration greater than 16 mEq/L). Dogs and cats with DK are not in need of immediate aggressive therapy and must be distinguished from the pet with a critical metabolic emergency. The apparently healthy ketotic diabetic animal can be managed conservatively, usually without fluid therapy, whereas the animal with severe DKA requires a much more intensive therapeutic plan involving treatments with a variety of contingency alternatives based on numerous assessments of related parameters.

IN-HOSPITAL DIAGNOSTIC EVALUATION

OVERVIEW. The laboratory evaluation of "healthy" ketotic diabetic dogs and cats is similar to that for nonketotic diabetics (see Chapter 11, page 493 and Chapter 12, page 548). The healthy ketotic diabetic can usually be managed conservatively, as contrasted with the needs of an extremely ill DKA pet. To aid in the formulation of a treatment protocol, the clinician must perform a group of critically important studies in the ill ketoacidotic diabetic. Without these evaluations, an animal's metabolic status cannot be adequately assessed and the clinician cannot have sufficient knowledge of the specific abnormalities that require correction. The minimum required tests include urinalysis, hematocrit, total plasma protein concentration, blood glucose, venous total carbon dioxide or arterial acid-base evaluation, blood urea nitrogen (BUN) or serum creatinine, and serum electrolytes (Na, K, Ca, PO_4).

These studies are needed for the immediate assessment and intensive care of the animal. Knowing the results of these tests allows for proper choice of fluid therapy as well as for corrections that must be made with respect to electrolyte alterations, acidosis, and renal function. Other data, such as diagnostic imaging, electrocardiogram, or additional laboratory studies, may be needed for a complete medical assessment. However, the "ketoacidosis profile" provides the information necessary to begin proper emergency therapy.

Urinalysis and urine culture

The urinalysis can serve several purposes simultaneously. The most obvious reason for obtaining a urine sample is to identify glycosuria and ketonuria. A diagnosis of severe DKA should be made in the dehydrated, ill dog or cat with glycosuria and ketonuria. Fluid therapy should be initiated (see page 597) while confirmatory blood glucose and acid-base studies and determination of serum electrolyte concentrations are performed.

Urinary tract infection is a common and important contributing factor in DKA. The presence of bacteriuria, hematuria, and pyuria on urinalysis supports the diagnosis of urinary tract infection and the need for culture of a urine sample. If possible, urine should be obtained by cystocentesis. Because of the high incidence of urinary tract infections in our cats and especially dogs with DKA, we routinely culture urine, regardless of findings on urinalysis. Proteinuria may be the result of urinary tract infection or glomerular damage secondary to disruption of the basement membrane. Evaluation of a urine protein:creatinine ratio performed on a urine sample void of infection or inflammation can help determine whether the proteinuria is significant.

Azotemia is also common in DKA, and evaluation of urine specific gravity from a sample of urine obtained before initiation of fluid therapy is helpful in differentiating prerenal azotemia from primary renal failure. Urine specific gravity must be assessed with the severity of glycosuria and the hydration status of the dog or cat kept in mind. If the animal is clinically dehydrated and has normal renal function, its urine specific gravity should be greater than 1.030. Urine specific gravities that are less than 1.020 are suggestive of primary renal disease or concurrent disease causing secondary nephrogenic diabetes insipidus (e.g., hyperadrenocorticism). Glycosuria will increase the urine specific gravity measured by refractometers. As a general rule of thumb, 2% or 4+ glycosuria as measured on urine reagent test strips will increase the urine specific gravity 0.008 to 0.010 when urine specific gravity is measured by refractometry.

Oliguric and anuric renal failure is an infrequent but grave complication of DKA. Severe hyperglycemia (>500 mg/dl) is not likely to occur without a significant reduction in the GFR due to primary renal disease or severe dehydration and poor renal perfusion. It is critical that urine production be closely monitored in the severely ill DKA animal. Although diabetic animals are prone to develop infection, it is still strongly recommended that the animal with severe DKA have an indwelling urinary catheter secured in the bladder and attached to a closed collection system. The urine volume produced over the initial 12 hours of therapy can be assessed and anuric or oliguric renal failure quickly recognized. Rapid institution of appropriate measures to improve GFR and urine production can then be initiated. Urine production should increase once dehydration is corrected and normovolemia restored in the dog or cat with severe prerenal azotemia and decreased GFR. Once adequate urine production is confirmed, the indwelling urinary catheter can be removed.

The minimum data base (ketoacidosis profile)

BLOOD GLUCOSE. Although the average blood glucose concentration in dogs and cats with DKA is approximately 500 mg/dl, values can range from close to 200 mg/dl to concentrations that are characteristic of hyperosmolar coma (i.e., >1000 mg/dl; Fig. 13-6). Because hepatic production of glucose is excessive in dogs and cats with DKA and relative or absolute deficiencies of insulin always exist, it is likely that the degree of hyperglycemia is determined primarily by the severity of dehydration and corresponding decrease in GFR (Foster and McGarry, 1983). Evidence suggests that blood glucose concentrations become extremely elevated (i.e., >500 mg/dl) only when the extracellular fluid (ECF) volume has decreased to the point that urine flow and the capacity to excrete glucose are impaired. Studies have shown a marked reduction in the blood glucose concentration when humans with DKA were treated solely with fluids (i.e., no insulin; Owen et al, 1981), findings also seen clinically in diabetic dogs and cats (Fig. 13-7). An association has

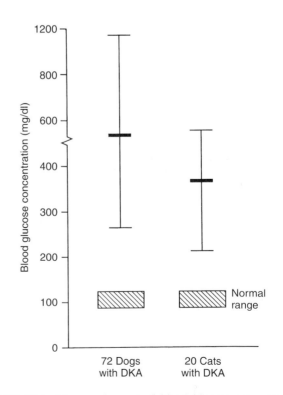

FIGURE 13–6. Mean and range of blood glucose concentration determined at the time diabetic ketoacidosis was diagnosed in 72 dogs and 20 cats.

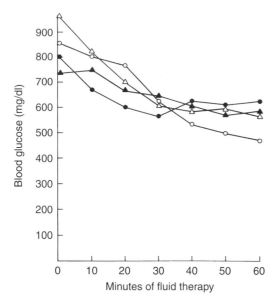

FIGURE 13–7. The effect of fluid therapy on four severely diabetic ketoacidotic dogs over a period of 1 hour, without insulin administration.

been made in humans with diabetes between the maximum attainable blood glucose concentration and the severity of reduction in GFR (Table 13-2; Kandel and Aberman, 1983).

The initial blood glucose concentration dictates, in part, how aggressive the initial fluid and insulin therapy should be and when glucose-containing fluids will be needed. The higher the blood glucose concentration, the higher the plasma osmolality, the more at-risk the animal is for developing cerebral edema following a sudden decrease in plasma osmolality, and therefore the slower the rate of blood glucose decline needs to be during the initial hours of treatment. Dextrose must be added to the IV fluids when the blood glucose concentration approaches 250 mg/dl to prevent hypoglycemia with continued insulin therapy. The closer the pretreatment blood glucose concentration is to 250 mg/dl, the sooner glucose-containing fluids are needed after initiating fluid and especially insulin therapy. When the pretreatment blood glucose concentration is 500 mg/dl or higher,

TABLE 13–2   MAXIMUM SERUM GLUCOSE CONCENTRATIONS IN DIABETIC HUMANS FOR GIVEN GLOMERULAR FILTRATION RATES

Glomerular Filtration Rate (ml/min)	Serum Glucose Concentration (mg/dl)
108	400
72	600
54	800
36	1200
27	1600

From Kandel G, Aberman A: Selected developments in the understanding of diabetic ketoacidosis. Can Med Assoc J 128:392, 1983.

glucose-containing fluids are usually not needed until several hours after initiating fluid and insulin therapy.

ACID-BASE STATUS.   Metabolic acidosis is one of the hallmark clinical pathologic changes in DKA and is the direct result of an excess accumulation of ketone bodies in the blood. Excessive serum ketones can overwhelm the body's buffering system, causing an increase in arterial hydrogen ion concentration, a decrease in serum bicarbonate, and a progressively worsening metabolic acidosis (Fig. 13-8).

Failure of the kidneys to compensate adequately for the acid load in DKA is partly the result of the physicochemical properties of β-hydroxybutyrate and acetoacetate. The renal threshold for these acids is low, and appreciable excretion occurs at plasma concentrations only slightly above normal. Thus the renal tubules are easily overwhelmed when these acids are synthesized in excessive quantities by the liver. This creates a situation in which the amount of acid present surpasses the renal capacity for urine acidification. Furthermore, β-hydroxybutyrate and acetoacetate are relatively strong acids (pKa 4.70 and 3.58, respectively). Even at the lowest urinary pH, they are excreted mostly as sodium and potassium salts, resulting in the concomitant loss of bicarbonate.

Recognition of acidosis is usually straightforward with the use of arterial blood gas or venous total CO_2 determinations (Table 13-3). In DKA, the severity of changes in arterial blood gas or venous total CO_2 depends on the duration and severity of hyper-

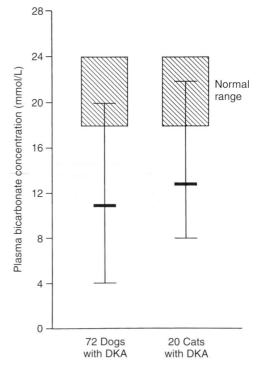

FIGURE 13–8. Mean and range of plasma bicarbonate concentration determined at the time diabetic ketoacidosis was diagnosed in 72 dogs and 20 cats.

TABLE 13–3 ARTERIAL PH, PCO$_2$, AND [HCO$_3^-$] IN SIMPLE ACUTE ACID-BASE DISORDERS

Condition	pH	Arterial PCO$_2$	Total Venous CO$_2$ = [HCO$_3^-$]*
Acidosis			
Respiratory	↓	↑↑	↑
Metabolic	↓	↓	↓↓
Alkalosis			
Respiratory	↑	↓↓	↓
Metabolic	↑	↑	↑↑

*The total venous CO$_2$ concentration is equal to the arterial bicarbonate concentration.
Double arrows indicate primary change.

ketonemia at the time of presentation to the veterinarian. Arterial pH can range from 7.2 to as low as 6.6. Dogs and cats with arterial blood pH values less than 7.0 have life-threatening DKA and are difficult to treat successfully. A tremendous amount of controversy surrounds therapy directed specifically at the acidosis component of DKA. A discussion on the pros and cons of bicarbonate therapy for animals with severe DKA is found on page 602.

SERUM SODIUM CONCENTRATION. The serum sodium concentration is a reflection of the relative amounts of water and sodium present in the body. With rare exception, dogs and cats with DKA have significant deficits in total body sodium, regardless of the measured serum concentration. In 72 dogs with DKA, 62% were hyponatremic and only 7% were hypernatremic (Fig. 13-9). Similarly, in 42 cats with DKA, 80% were hyponatremic and only 5% were hypernatremic (Bruskiewicz et al,1997).

Hyponatremia results from excessive urinary sodium loss caused by the osmotic diuresis induced by glycosuria and ketonuria. Because insulin enhances renal sodium reabsorption in the distal portion of the nephron, its absence results in sodium wasting. Hyperglucagonemia, vomiting, and diarrhea also contribute to the sodium loss in DKA (Foster and McGarry, 1983). Severe hypertriglyceridemia may occasionally cause factitious hyponatremia. Severe hypertriglyceridemia can be recognized by the presence of lipemia retinalis on ophthalmoscopic examination or by the presence of gross lipemia on visual inspection of serum or plasma. Saline and Ringer's solutions have adequate sodium quantities for replacement of severe sodium deficiencies and are recommended as the initial fluids of choice for the treatment of severe DKA (see page 597).

It is important to consider the severity of hyperglycemia when assessing the severity of hyponatremia in the dog or cat with DKA. Because glucose penetrates cells poorly in the absence of insulin, an increase in ECF glucose concentration creates a transcellular osmotic gradient that results in the movement of water out of the cells and a corresponding reduction in the plasma sodium concentration. In general, for each 100 mg/dl increment in serum glucose above the normal range, the plasma sodium concentration decreases by approximately 1.6 mEq/L (DiBartola, 2000). Conversely, as insulin therapy drives glucose into the cells, water will follow and the plasma sodium concentration will increase.

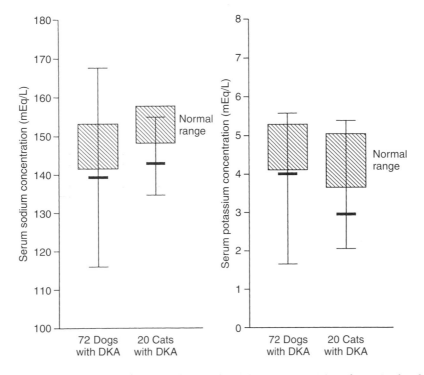

FIGURE 13–9. Mean and range of serum sodium and potassium concentrations determined at the time diabetic ketoacidosis was diagnosed in 72 dogs and 20 cats.

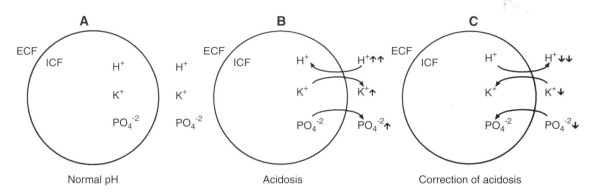

FIGURE 13–10. Redistribution of extracellular fluid (ECF) and intracellular fluid (ICF) hydrogen, potassium, and phosphate ions in response to a decrease in ECF pH (i.e., acidosis), an increase in ECF glucose and osmolality, and the translocation of water from the ICF to the ECF compartment and subsequent correction of acidosis and the intracellular shift of glucose and electrolytes with insulin treatment. *A,* Normal ECF pH. *B,* ECF H^+ concentration increases during acidosis, causing H^+ to move into cells and down its concentration gradient. Increase in ECF glucose and osmolality causes extracellular shift of water, K^+, and PO_4^{+2}. *C,* ECF H^+ concentration decreases during correction of acidosis, causing H^+ to move out of cells. Insulin administration and correction of acidemia cause an intracellular shift of glucose, K^+, and PO_4^{+2}, decreasing ECF K^+ and PO_4^{+2} concentration.

SERUM POTASSIUM CONCENTRATION. During DKA, intracellular dehydration occurs as hyperglycemia and water loss lead to increased plasma and ECF tonicity and a shift of water out of cells. This shift of water is also associated with a shift of potassium into the extracellular space (Fig. 13-10; Kitabchi et al, 2001). Potassium shifts are further enhanced by the presence of acidosis and the breakdown of intracellular protein secondary to insulin deficiency. Entry of potassium into cells is also impaired in the presence of insulinopenia. The osmotic diuresis induced by glycosuria and ketonuria causes marked urinary losses of potassium. Secondary hyperaldosteronism induced by plasma volume contraction, gastrointestinal losses, and decreased dietary intake augment the potassium deficiency (Kitabchi et al, 2001). As a consequence, most dogs and cats with DKA have a net deficit of total body potassium. Serum potassium concentrations can be decreased, normal, or increased, depending on the duration of illness, renal function, and previous nutritional state of the dog or cat. Most dogs and cats with DKA have either normal or decreased serum potassium concentrations on pretreatment testing (see Fig. 13-9). In 72 dogs and 42 cats with DKA, 43% and 67% were hypokalemic and 10% and 7% were hyperkalemic, respectively, at the time DKA was diagnosed (Bruskiewicz et al, 1997).

Knowing the serum potassium concentration and status of renal function is critical when deciding on the aggressiveness of potassium supplementation in the IV fluids. Polyuric DKA animals are predisposed to severe hypokalemia, and oliguric/anuric animals are predisposed to severe hyperkalemia. Insulin treatment causes a marked translocation of potassium from the ECF to the intracellular fluid (ICF) compartment, which when combined with continuing renal and gastrointestinal loss, can cause severe hypokalemia during the initial 24 to 48 hours of treatment. DKA dogs and cats that are hypokalemic on initial evaluation require aggressive potassium supplementation to their intravenous fluids to replace deficits and to prevent worsening hypokalemia (see page 600).

BLOOD UREA NITROGEN AND CREATININE. The BUN and serum creatinine concentrations are commonly elevated in DKA (Fig. 13-11) and are useful indicators of the severity of volume depletion. When evaluated in conjunction with the urine specific gravity and serum calcium:phosphorus ratio, they can also help to identify concurrent primary renal failure versus prerenal azotemia. In addition, the initial BUN or creatinine concentration can serve as a measure of the success of fluid therapy. A rapidly falling BUN is consistent with proper fluid therapy, good urine output, and a dog or cat that has prerenal azotemia. The increased BUN that is slowly declining or static suggests inadequate fluid therapy or primary renal failure.

Increased serum creatinine concentrations may be spurious, resulting from interference by acetoacetate (one of the ketone bodies). At serum acetoacetate concentrations of 8 to 10 mmol/L, the serum creatinine concentration is falsely elevated 3 to 4 mg/dl by the Beckman autoanalyzer method and 1 to 2 mg/dl by the Technicon autoanalyzer method. If the serum creatinine concentration is determined manually, elevated serum ketone levels do not interfere (Molitch et al, 1980; Nanji and Campbell, 1981).

SERUM OSMOLALITY. Hyperosmolality is a potentially serious development in DKA, one that can have profound effects on CNS function and consciousness. Of all the factors related to stupor or altered consciousness, including the serum levels of glucose, ketones, or arterial pH, the serum osmolality correlates best with the level of consciousness in humans with DKA. "Clouded consciousness" is an extremely subjective finding in humans, making recognition of such a problem guesswork in dogs or cats. Nevertheless, veterinarians and owners can usually recognize

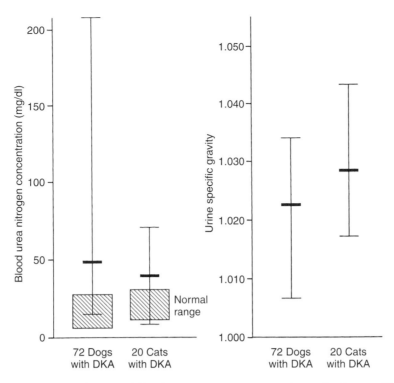

FIGURE 13–11. Mean and range of blood urea nitrogen concentration and urine specific gravity determined at the time diabetic ketoacidosis was diagnosed in 72 dogs and 20 cats.

"depression" in the dog and cat, and in our experience, the severity of this sign roughly correlates with the severity of hyperosmolality.

Fortunately, severe hyperosmolality (>350 to 400 mOsm/kg) occurs infrequently in dogs and cats with DKA, in part because of the concurrent prevalence of hyponatremia (see Fig. 13-9). Serum sodium concentration and, to a lesser extent, potassium and glucose are the primary determinants of effective serum osmolality. Hyperosmolality, if present, usually resolves with intravenous isotonic fluid and insulin therapy, although correction of the hyperosmolar state must be done slowly to minimize the shift of water from the extracellular to the intracellular compartment.

Many veterinary hospitals, especially those with a large emergency case load, have the necessary equipment to measure serum or plasma osmolality directly. One can calculate the approximate serum osmolality indirectly via related parameters and use the final determination as an aid in choosing proper fluid and insulin therapy. The effective osmolality of serum or plasma can be estimated from the following formula:

$$\text{Osmolality} = 2(Na^+ + K^+) + 0.05(\text{glucose})$$
$$(\text{mOsm/kg}) \quad (\text{mEq/L}) \quad \quad (\text{mg/dl})$$

In an insulin-deficient state, the intracellular movement of glucose in insulin-dependent tissues is impaired and the increase in extracellular glucose creates an osmotic gradient between the ECF and ICF compartments. For this reason, glucose is included in calculations of effective osmolality. In contrast, urea remains freely permeable across cell membranes regardless of insulin concentrations and therefore is not included in calculations of effective serum osmolality. The normal range for effective serum osmolality in the dog and cat is typically 280 to 300 mOsm/kg.

ANION GAP. The metabolic acidosis stemming from hyperketonemia is an anion gap acidosis, which must be differentiated from other causes of anion gap acidosis (e.g., lactic acidosis, renal failure, ethylene glycol intoxication) and from hyperchloremic acidosis (Narins et al, 1994). The anion gap is calculated by subtracting the negatively charged anions, chloride and bicarbonate, from the most important positively charged cations, sodium and potassium. The normal anion gap for dogs and cats is 12 to 16 mEq/L (Feldman and Rosenberg, 1981). Anything greater than 16 mEq/L indicates the presence of an anion gap acidosis. The unmeasured anions that comprise the normal anion gap include albumin and other circulating proteins, sulfate, phosphate, and a variety of organic acids.

The typical diabetic dog or cat in ketoacidosis has an anion gap that ranges from 20 to 35 mEq/L, and the increment in the anion gap above baseline approximates the decrement in serum bicarbonate concentration (Adrogué et al, 1982). A number of factors can disrupt the normal stoichiometry between acid retention, increment in the anion gap, and decrease in serum bicarbonate concentration (Table 13-4). Such disruption is common in DKA because urinary

TABLE 13–4 INFLUENCES OF COMMON METABOLIC DISORDERS ON THE CALCULATED ANION GAP*

Increased Anion Gap

Diabetic ketoacidosis
Lactic acidosis
   Tissue ischemia and/or hypoxemia
   Sepsis
   Malignancy
   Drugs
   Idiopathic causes
Chronic renal failure
Drugs
   Salicylates
   Ethylene glycol
   Others

Normal Anion Gap

Diarrhea
Renal tubular acidosis
Hyperchloremic acidosis
Hydrochloric acid or its precursors (i.e., ammonium chloride and
   others)

*These disorders are frequently associated with metabolic acidosis.

loss of ketoanions causes a disproportionately greater decrease in serum bicarbonate concentration compared with the increment in anion gap. In these cases, chloride replaces the missing ketoanion, and a component of hyperchloremic acidosis commonly accompanies the anion gap acidosis (Table 13-5; Adrogué et al, 1982; 1984). Dogs and cats that are volume-contracted tend to have a pure anion gap acidosis because the decrease in GFR and tubular avidity for sodium reabsorption limits the urinary loss of ketone bodies. Conversely, animals with DKA able to maintain salt and water intake avoid severe volume depletion. These animals have variable degrees of hyperchloremic acidosis because of the urinary excretion of ketone salts and a concomitant retention of chloride (Table 13-5).

Completing the data base

COMPLETE BLOOD COUNT. The complete blood count (CBC) in uncomplicated DKA usually reveals a leukocytosis without evidence of toxic neutrophils (Bruskiewicz et al,1997). The leukocytosis may occur secondary to the release of "stress" hormones or severe inflammation, especially if an underlying pancreatitis is present. White blood cell counts greater than 30,000/μl, the presence of toxic or degenerative neutrophils, or a significant left shift toward immaturity of the cells supports the presence of a severe inflammatory and/or infectious process as the cause of the leukocytosis. The red blood cell count and hematocrit should be consistent with hemoconcentration secondary to dehydration. A hematocrit below 35% in these typically volume-contracted animals should arouse suspicion that blood loss has occurred or that significant bone marrow suppression or another problem has resulted in anemia.

LIVER ENZYMES AND TOTAL BILIRUBIN. Clinical pathologic abnormalities associated with the liver are common in dogs and cats with DKA and are usually caused by hepatic lipidosis, pancreatitis, severe acidosis, hypovolemia, hypoxia, sepsis, and, less commonly, extrahepatic biliary obstruction caused by acute severe pancreatitis, chronic hepatitis, and cholangiohepatitis (see page 608). Aspartate transaminase (AST), alanine transaminase (ALT), and serum alkaline phosphatase (SAP) concentrations are usually increased (see page 493). Less commonly, fasting serum bile acid concentrations and serum total bilirubin concentrations may be increased, although icterus is not common. In some dogs and cats, a specific cause for the abnormal liver enzyme patterns cannot be identified. No significant correlation exists between the serum level of hepatic enzymes and the presence or severity of the hepatopathy.

PANCREATIC ENZYMES. Because acute and chronic pancreatitis is so common in dogs and cats with DKA, a diagnostic evaluation for its existence is always warranted (Bruskiewicz et al,1997). In our experience, abdominal ultrasound is the single best diagnostic test for identifying pancreatitis in the dog or cat with DKA (see Fig. 12-10, page 549). Measurement of serum lipase concentration and trypsin-like immunoreactivity (TLI) are also commonly recommended. In theory, dogs and cats with active inflammation of the pancreas should have an increase in serum lipase and TLI. Unfortunately, serum lipase concentrations and serum TLI do not always correlate accurately with the presence or absence of pancreatitis (Hess et al, 1998; Swift et al, 2000; Gerhardt et al, 2001). Pancreatic enzyme concentrations can be increased in dogs and cats with a histologically confirmed normal pancreas and normal in dogs and cats with histologically confirmed inflam-

TABLE 13–5 EXAMPLES OF SERUM ELECTROLYTE CONCENTRATIONS AND THEIR ASSOCIATED ANION GAPS IN ACIDOSIS

	Sodium (mEq/L)	Potassium (mEq/L)	Chloride (mEq/L)	Bicarbonate (mEq/L)	Anion Gap (mEq/L)
Normal	142	4	108	22	12
Hyperchloremic acidosis	142	4	118	12	12
Anion gap acidosis	142	4	108	12	22

Anion gap = Na – (Cl + bicarbonate).
The normal anion gap is 12 to 16 mEq/L.

mation of the pancreas, especially when the inflammatory process is chronic and mild. For these reasons, interpretation of serum lipase and TLI results should always be done in context with the history, physical examination findings, and additional findings on the laboratory tests. Recognition of concurrent pancreatitis in the dog or cat with DKA has important implications regarding initial fluid therapy, subsequent dietary therapy, and prognosis. Fortunately, aggressive fluid therapy is the cornerstone of treatment for both DKA and pancreatitis. In most cases, treating one disease also treats the other.

CALCIUM AND PHOSPHORUS. The serum calcium and phosphorus concentrations are usually normal in the diabetic dog or cat with "uncomplicated" DKA. If concurrent primary renal failure is present, the serum calcium concentration is typically normal, whereas the serum phosphorus concentration is increased. In pancreatitis, mild hypocalcemia may occur secondary to an acute shift of calcium into soft tissues such as muscle as a result of altered membrane integrity, alterations in thyrocalcitonin secretion or tissue responsiveness to parathyroid hormone, hypomagnesemia, hypoproteinemia, and deposition of calcium in plaques of saponified fat. Hypercalcemia supports the existence of concurrent disease, including chronic renal failure (see Chapter 16).

Attention has been directed to serum phosphorus concentrations in animals with DKA, especially during the initial 24 hours of treatment. Phosphate, along with potassium, shifts from the intracellular to the extracellular compartment in response to hyperglycemia and hyperosmolality (see Fig. 13-10; Kitabchi et al, 2001). Osmotic diuresis subsequently leads to enhanced urinary phosphate losses. Serum phosphorus concentrations can be decreased, normal, or increased, depending on the duration of illness and renal function. Most dogs and cats with DKA have either normal or decreased serum phosphorus concentrations on pretreatment testing. Hypophosphatemia (<3.0 mg/dl) was identified at initial presentation in 24% of 72 dogs and 48% of 42 cats with DKA (Bruskiewicz et al,1997). In contrast, hyperphosphatemia (>6.0 mg/dl) was identified in 14% and 26% of DKA dogs and cats, respectively, and usually occurred in conjunction with renal failure. Insulin treatment causes a marked translocation of phosphorus from the ECF to the ICF compartment. Within 24 hours of initiating treatment for DKA, serum phosphorus concentration can decline to severe levels (i.e., <1 mg/dl) as a result of the dilutional effects of fluid therapy, the intracellular shift of phosphorus following the initiation of insulin therapy, and continuing renal and gastrointestinal loss (Willard et al, 1987). Clinical signs may develop when the serum phosphorus concentration is less than 1.5 mg/dl, although signs are quite variable and severe hypophosphatemia is clinically silent in many animals. Hypophosphatemia primarily affects the hematologic and neuromuscular systems in the dog and cat (Forrester and Moreland, 1989). Hemolytic anemia is the most common and serious

sequela to hypophosphatemia. Hypophosphatemia may decrease erythrocyte concentration of ATP and/or alter red blood cell membrane lipids, which increases erythrocyte fragility, leading to hemolysis (Shilo et al, 1985; Adams et al, 1993). Hemolysis is usually not identified until the serum phosphorus concentration is 1 mg/dl or less. Hemolytic anemia can be life-threatening if not recognized and treated. Neuromuscular signs include weakness, ataxia, and seizures, as well as anorexia and vomiting secondary to intestinal ileus. Phosphate therapy is indicated if clinical signs of hemolysis are identified or if the serum phosphorus concentration is less than 1.5 mg/dl (see page 601).

MAGNESIUM. The osmotic diuresis of DKA may cause significant urinary losses of magnesium and the development of hypomagnesemia (serum total magnesium concentration <1.75 mg/dl; serum ionized magnesium concentration measured by ion-selective electrode <1.0 mg/dl) (Norris et al, 1999). In addition, the nature of the translocation of magnesium between the ICF and ECF compartments is similar to potassium in that factors which promote a shift of potassium into the ICF compartment (e.g., alkalosis, insulin, glucose infusion) promote a similar shift in magnesium. During therapy for DKA, the serum total and ionized magnesium concentration can decline to severely low levels (i.e., less than 1 mg/dl and 0.5 mg/dl, respectively) as a result of the dilutional effects of fluid therapy and the intracellular shift of magnesium after the initiation of insulin therapy (Norris et al, 1999). Clinical signs of hypomagnesemia do not usually occur until the serum total magnesium concentration is less than 1.0 mg/dl, and even at these low levels, many animals remain asymptomatic. A magnesium deficiency can result in several nonspecific clinical signs, including lethargy, anorexia, muscle weakness (including dysphagia and dyspnea), muscle fasciculations, seizures, ataxia, and coma (Martin et al, 1993; Abbott and Rude, 1993; Dhupa and Proulx, 1998). Concurrent hypokalemia, hyponatremia, and hypocalcemia occur in animals with hypomagnesemia, although the prevalence of these electrolyte abnormalities may differ between species. These electrolyte abnormalities may also contribute to the development of clinical signs. Magnesium is a cofactor for all enzyme reactions that involve ATP, most notably the sodium-potassium ATPase pump. Deficiencies in magnesium can lead to potassium wastage from the body and the resultant hypokalemia may be refractory to appropriate potassium replacement therapy. Magnesium deficiency inhibits PTH secretion from the parathyroid gland, resulting in hypocalcemia (Bush et al, 2001). Magnesium deficiency causes the resting membrane potential of myocardial cells to be decreased and leads to increased Purkinje fiber excitability, with the consequent generation of arrhythmias (Abbott and Rude, 1993). ECG changes include a prolonged PR interval, widened QRS complex, depressed ST segment, and peaked T waves. Cardiac arrhythmias associated with magnesium deficiency include atrial fibrillation, supraventricular tachycardia, ventricular tachycardia, and ventricular fibrillation. Hypomagnesemia also predisposes animals to digitalis-induced arrhythmias.

Unfortunately, assessing an animal's magnesium status is problematic because there is no simple, rapid, and accurate laboratory test to gauge the total body magnesium status. Approximately 1% of total body magnesium is present in serum; as a result, serum magnesium concentrations do not always reflect the total body magnesium status. A normal serum magnesium concentration may exist despite an intracellular magnesium deficiency. However, a low serum magnesium concentration does support the presence of a total body magnesium deficiency. Magnesium exists in three distinct forms in serum: an ionized fraction, an anion-complexed fraction, and a protein-bound fraction. A serum ionized magnesium concentration determined by using an ion-selective electrode is more accurate in assessing total body magnesium content and is recommended over measurement of serum total magnesium (Norris et al, 1999b). Fortunately, hypomagnesemia is not usually a clinically recognizable problem during management of DKA and magnesium supplementation is not recommended unless hypomagnesemia is documented in dogs and cats with complications that have been associated with hypomagnesemia (e.g., persistent lethargy and anorexia; refractory hypokalemia).

CHOLESTEROL AND TRIGLYCERIDES. Hyperlipidemia and obvious lipemia are common in untreated diabetic dogs and cats with DKA. Hypertriglyceridemia is responsible for lipemia. The mechanisms responsible for hyperlipidemia are discussed in Chapter 11, page 494. Most lipid derangements can be improved with aggressive insulin and dietary therapy.

Depending on the methodology used by the laboratory, hypertriglyceridemia causing lipemia may interfere with the results of several routine biochemistry tests (Table 13-6). Lipemia may also induce hemolysis, which in turn can interfere with some biochemical tests. These potential alterations in bio-chemical data must be considered when interpreting results in a dog or cat with DKA and hyperlipidemia.

DIAGNOSTIC IMAGING. Concurrent disorders such as acute or chronic pancreatitis, pyometra, cholangiohepatitis, heart failure, and bacterial pneumonia are common in dogs and cats with DKA. Many of these disorders actually perpetuate the metabolic derangements of DKA. Successful treatment of DKA requires recognition and treatment of these concurrent disorders. Abdominal and thoracic radiographs, as well as abdominal ultrasonography, are invaluable in confirming problems suspected after a review of the history and physical examination and in identifying problems previously unsuspected. In our hospital, thoracic radiography and abdominal ultrasonography are routine components of the diagnostic evaluation of any ill dog or cat with DKA. However, radiographs and ultrasound scans are not usually obtained until more critical laboratory data (i.e., the ketoacidotic profile) have been analyzed and appropriate treatment for DKA has been initiated.

ELECTROCARDIOGRAM. The electrocardiogram (ECG) remains one of the least expensive, simplest, and most valuable tools for identification of cardiac arrhythmias and for monitoring changes in serum potassium concentration during treatment of DKA. Use of the ECG is especially helpful for recognizing severe hypokalemia or hyperkalemia in hospitals where frequent monitoring of the serum potassium concentration is difficult because of lack of a point-of-care chemistry analyzer or because of economic constraints. If an animal with DKA is admitted to the hospital, blood should be obtained for pretreatment analysis of the serum potassium concentration, and a complete ECG with a good lead II "rhythm strip" should be performed. This rhythm strip with the documented serum potassium concentration serves as the "reference" ECG. Thereafter, all "unknown" rhythm strips can be compared with the one "reference" sample and educated estimates of the serum potassium concentration made.

The primary concern before and during treatment of DKA is hypokalemia. A complete description of the

TABLE 13–6 EFFECT OF LIPEMIA ON CLINICAL CHEMISTRY ANALYTES* IN CANINE AND FELINE SERA

FALSE INCREASE IN VALUES		FALSE DECREASE IN VALUES	
Canine Sera	Feline Sera	Canine Sera	Feline Sera
Total bilirubin	Total bilirubin	Creatinine	Creatinine
Conjugated bilirubin	Conjugated bilirubin	Total CO_2	Total CO_2
Phosphorus	Phosphorus	Cholesterol	ALT
Alkaline phosphatase[+]	Alkaline phosphatase[+]	Urea nitrogen	
Glucose[+]	Glucose[+]		
Total protein**	Total protein**		
Lipase			
ALT			

Adapted from Jacobs RM, et al: Effects of bilirubinemia, hemolysis, and lipemia on clinical chemistry analytes in bovine, canine, equine, and feline sera. Can Vet J 33:605, 1992.
*Analytes were measured using Coulter DACOS (Coulter Diagnostics, Hialeah, FL).
[+]Interference only occurs at very high concentrations of lipid.
**When measured using refractometer.
ALT, alanine aminotransferase.

ECG findings in hyperkalemia is provided in Chapter 8. It must be emphasized that hypokalemia usually causes subtle changes in the ECG, especially when the serum potassium concentration is above 3.0 mEq/L (Table 13-7; Fig. 13-12). Changes in the ECG are more obvious when the serum potassium concentration is between 2.5 and 3.0 mEq/L, and alterations invariably occur with serum potassium levels below 2.5 mEq/L.

The basic electrophysiologic alteration with hypokalemia is a gradual shift of the repolarization wave away from systole into diastole. The most consistent change on the ECG is prolongation of the Q-T interval. Additional findings include a progressive sagging of the S-T segment, a decreased amplitude of the T wave, and a repolarization wave occurring after the T wave (U wave). In advanced hypokalemia, the amplitude and duration of the QRS complex are increased. It is believed that the QRS complex widens diffusely secondary to a generalized slowing of conduction in the ventricular myocardium or Purkinje fibers. The amplitude and the duration of the P wave increase, and the P-R interval is slightly prolonged with hypokalemia. Atrial and ventricular premature contractions may also occur.

TABLE 13–7 ELECTROCARDIOGRAPHIC ALTERATIONS ASSOCIATED WITH HYPOKALEMIA AND HYPERKALEMIA IN THE DOG AND CAT

Hypokalemia

Depressed T-wave amplitude
Depressed S-T segment
Prolonged Q-T interval
Prominent U wave
Arrhythmias
   Supraventricular
   Ventricular

Hyperkalemia

Spiked T waves
Flattened P waves
Prolonged P-R interval
Prolonged QRS interval
Decreased R-wave amplitude
Bradycardia
Complete heart block
Ventricular arrhythmias
Cardiac arrest

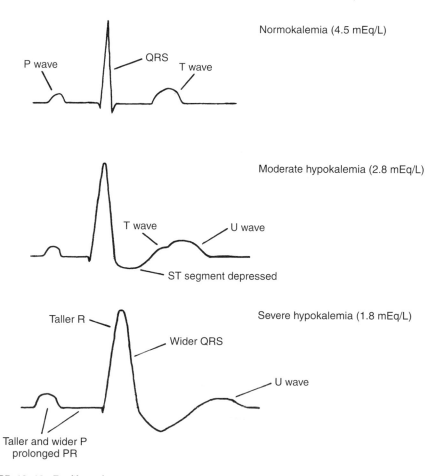

Normokalemia (4.5 mEq/L)

P wave — QRS — T wave

Moderate hypokalemia (2.8 mEq/L)

T wave — U wave
ST segment depressed

Severe hypokalemia (1.8 mEq/L)

Taller R — Wider QRS — U wave

Taller and wider P prolonged PR

FIGURE 13–12. Profiles of serum potassium are reflected in the electrocardiogram (ECG). These changes are exaggerated here for illustration purposes. In practice, these changes can be quite subtle, indicating the necessity of a baseline ECG with a simultaneous laboratory serum potassium.

TABLE 13–8 INITIAL MANAGEMENT OF THE DOG OR CAT WITH SEVERE DIABETIC KETOACIDOSIS

Fluid Therapy

Type: 0.9% saline solution initially
Rate: 60 to 100 ml/kg/24 hr initially; adjust based on hydration status, urine output, persistence of fluid losses.
Potassium supplement: based on serum K^+ concentration; if unknown, initially add 40 mEq KCl to each liter of fluids.
Phosphate supplement: administer if serum phosphorus concentration < 1.5 mg/dl or hemolytic anemia develops, initial IV infusion rate is 0.01 to 0.03 mmol/kg/hour in calcium-free fluids (e.g., 0.9% saline)
Dextrose supplement: not indicated until blood glucose concentration approaches 250 mg/dl, then begin 5% dextrose infusion.

Bicarbonate Therapy

Indication: administer if plasma bicarbonate concentration is less than 12 mEq/L or total venous CO_2 concentration is less than 12 mmol/L; if not known, do not administer unless animal is severely ill and then only once.
Amount: mEq HCO_3^- = body weight (kg) $\times$ 0.4 $\times$ (12 – animal's HCO_3^-) $\times$ 0.5; if animal's HCO_3^- or total CO_2 concentration is unknown, use 10 in place of (12 – animal's HCO_3^-).
Administration: add to IV fluids and give over 6 hours; do not give as bolus infusion.
Retreatment: only if plasma bicarbonate concentration remains less than 12 mEq/L after 6 hours of therapy.

Insulin Therapy

Type: regular crystalline insulin.
Administration technique: *Intermittent IM technique:* initial dose, 0.2 U/kg IM; then 0.1 U/kg IM hourly until blood glucose concentration approaches 250 mg/dl, then switch to SC regular insulin q 6 to 8 h. *Low-dose IV infusion technique:* initial rate, 0.05 to 0.1 U/kg/hr diluted in 0.9% NaCl and administered via infusion or syringe pump in a line separate from that used for fluid therapy; adjust infusion rate based on hourly blood glucose measurements; switch to SC regular insulin q 6 to 8 h once blood glucose approaches 250 mg/dl.
Decrease hourly IM insulin dose or IV insulin infusion rate for initial 2 to 3 hours of treatment if dog or cat is hypokalemic at time of diagnosis
Goal: gradual decline in blood glucose concentration, preferably around 75 mg/dl/hr until concentration is less than 250 mg/dl.

Ancillary Therapy

Concurrent pancreatitis is common in DKA; nothing per os and aggressive fluid therapy usually indicated.
Concurrent infections are common in DKA; use of broad-spectrum, parenteral antibiotics usually indicated.
Additional therapy may be needed, depending on nature of concurrent disorders.

Patient Monitoring

Blood glucose measurement every 1 to 2 hours initially; adjust insulin therapy and begin dextrose infusion when approaches 250 mg/dl.
Hydration status, respiration, pulse every 2 to 4 hours; adjust fluids accordingly.
Serum electrolyte and total venous CO_2 concentrations every 6 to 12 hours; adjust fluid and bicarbonate therapy accordingly.
Urine output, glycosuria, ketonuria every 2 to 4 hours; adjust fluid therapy accordingly.
Body weight, packed cell volume, temperature, and blood pressure daily.
Additional monitoring, depending on concurrent disease.

THERAPY OF THE "HEALTHY" DIABETIC KETOTIC ANIMAL

Diabetic dogs and cats that have ketonuria but not metabolic acidosis (i.e., diabetic ketosis) are often relatively healthy aside from the typical clinical signs of uncontrolled diabetes mellitus. Diabetic ketosis may be identified in newly diagnosed diabetic dogs and cats or diabetic dogs and cats that are being treated with insulin. Identification of ketonuria in insulin-treated diabetic dogs and cats indicates that insulin treatment has become ineffective, usually because of a problem with the insulin treatment regimen, development of a concurrent disorder causing insulin resistance, or both. We typically treat dogs and cats with diabetic ketosis and no systemic signs of illness (e.g., lethargy, inappetence, vomiting) with short-acting regular crystalline insulin (Eli Lilly and Co, Indianapolis, IN) administered sub-cutaneously every 8 hours until ketonuria resolves. Because regular crystalline insulin is a potent insulin, the initial dosage (0.1 to 0.2 U/kg/injection) is lower than that recommended for longer-acting insulin prep-arations. To minimize hypoglycemia, the owner should feed the dog or cat one-third of its daily caloric intake at the time of each insulin injection. Subsequent adjust-ments in the insulin dose are based on clinical response and results of blood glucose measurements (see pages 507 and 561). Urine ketone concentrations should also be monitored. If the blood glucose concentration is well controlled, blood and urine ketone concentrations fall. Although the time until resolution of ketonuria is quite variable, most dogs and cats are negative for urine ketones within 3 to 5 days of initiating three-times-a-day regular crystalline insulin therapy. However, some dogs and cats require several weeks of regular crystalline insulin treatment before excessive hepatic production of ketones resolves. Prolonged ketonuria or recurring ketonuria is suggestive of a concurrent illness causing insulin resistance, hyperglucagonemia, or both.

We always hospitalize ketotic diabetic dogs or cats when initiating three-times-a-day regular crystalline insulin treatment. Once the dose of regular crystalline insulin that provides acceptable control of glycemia has been identified, the dog or cat can be sent home for continuation of three-times-a-day insulin treatment by the owner, especially if ketonuria has not yet resolved. Once ketonuria has resolved, the dog or cat is stable, and control of glycemia is acceptable, a switch to a longer-acting insulin preparation administered twice a day can be tried (see Chapters 11 and 12). As a general rule of thumb, the initial dosage of the longer-acting insulin preparation is the same as the dosage of regular crys-talline insulin being administered at the time the switch in insulin is made, with subsequent adjustments in the dosage based on the animal's response to the insulin.

THERAPY OF THE ILL DIABETIC KETOACIDOTIC ANIMAL (TABLE 13-8)

The goals in the treatment of the severely ill ketoacidotic diabetic pet are (a) to provide adequate amounts of insulin to normalize intermediary metabolism, (b) to restore water and electrolyte losses, (c) to correct acidosis, (d) to identify precipitating factors for the present illness, and (e) to provide a carbohydrate substrate when required by the insulin treatment. Proper therapy does not imply forcing as rapid a return to normal as possible. Because osmotic and biochemical problems can be created by overly aggressive therapy as well as by the disease process itself, rapid changes in various vital parameters can be as harmful as, or more harmful than, no change. If all abnormal parameters can be slowly returned toward normal (i.e., over a period of 36 to 48 hours), there is a better likelihood of success in therapy.

Fluid Therapy (Fig. 13-13)

Initiation of appropriate fluid therapy should be the first step in the treatment of DKA. Replacement of fluid deficiencies and maintenance of normal fluid balance are critical to ensure adequate cardiac output,

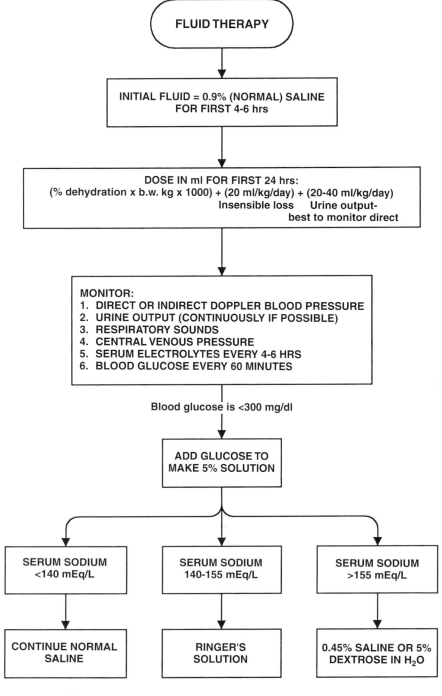

FIGURE 13–13. IV fluid treatment plans for the dog or cat in DKA.

blood pressure, and blood flow to all tissues. Improvement of renal blood flow is especially critical. In addition to the general beneficial aspects of fluid therapy in any dehydrated animal, fluid therapy can correct the deficiency in total body sodium and potassium, dampen the potassium-lowering effect of insulin treatment, and lower the blood glucose concentration in diabetics, even in the absence of insulin administration (see Fig. 13-7). Fluids enhance glucose excretion by increasing glomerular filtration and urine flow, and they decrease secretion of the diabetogenic hormones that stimulate hyperglycemia. The gradual decline in blood glucose combined with replacement of sodium for glucose in the ECF helps minimize the intracellular shift of water caused by a rapid decrease in ECF osmolality, thereby preventing cerebral edema (see page 611). Unfortunately, fluid therapy alone does not decrease the concentrations of acetoacetate and β-hydroxybutyrate, nor does it improve the severity of metabolic acidosis (Foster and McGarry, 1983; Lebovitz, 1995). For this reason, insulin is always required.

FLUID COMPOSITION AND RATE. The type of parenteral fluid initially used depends on the animal's electrolyte status, blood glucose concentration, and osmolality. With rare exceptions, all dogs and cats with DKA have significant deficits in total body sodium, regardless of the measured serum concentration (see page 589). Excessive urinary sodium loss is thought to result from the osmotic diuresis induced by glycosuria and ketonuria, as well as from the insulin deficiency. Insulin enhances renal sodium reabsorption in the distal portion of the nephron, and its absence results in sodium wasting. Hyperglucagonemia, vomiting, and diarrhea also contribute to sodium losses in DKA.

Unless serum electrolytes dictate otherwise, the initial intravenous fluid of choice is 0.9% (physiologic) saline with appropriate potassium supplementation (Fig. 13-14). Most dogs and cats with DKA have significant deficits in total body sodium that are best replaced with physiologic (0.9%) saline, even when the osmolality is greater than 350 mOsm/kg. Fortunately, most dogs and cats with severe DKA usually are sodium depleted and, therefore, do not suffer from dramatic hyperosmolality despite potentially remarkable elevations in the blood glucose concentration. Serum osmolality can be measured directly or can be estimated using the formula on page 591. Additional replacement crystalloid solutions may be used if physiologic (0.9%) saline is not available; these products include Ringer's solution, Ringer's lactated solution, Plasma-Lyte 148 (Baxter Healthcare Corporation, Deerfield, IL), and Normosol-R (Abbott Laboratories, Chicago, IL). Each of these solutions has a slightly different electrolyte composition; none contains as much sodium as 0.9% saline (Table 13-9).

Ringer's lactated solution contains lactate, and Plasma-Lyte and Normosol-R contain acetate. Lactate and acetate are metabolized to bicarbonate. A theoretical contraindication for the use of crystalloid solutions that contain lactate centers around the increase in serum lactate concentration that could occur with use of these fluids. Lactate is metabolized in the liver in a similar manner as ketones, and hyperketonemia could reduce hepatic lactate metabolism. As such, administration of fluids containing lactate could increase lactate concentrations in the circulation and, because lactate is a negatively charged ion, promote further sodium and potassium loss in the urine as lactate is excreted (Macintire, 1995). However, in our experience, use of Ringer's lactated solution has not had a recognizable deleterious impact on development of complications or resolution of DKA in dogs and cats. Ringer's lactated solution can be used in lieu of 0.9% saline to minimize the chloride load in animals that develop hyperchloremic acidosis during treatment of DKA.

Hypotonic fluids (e.g., 0.45% saline) are rarely indicated in dogs and cats with DKA, even when severe hyperosmolality is present. Hypotonic fluids do not provide adequate amounts of sodium to correct the sodium deficiency, restore normal fluid balance or stabilize blood pressure. In contrast, isotonic fluids are able to expand circulatory volume, enhance tissue perfusion, and improve renal GFR (Lebovitz, 1995; Kitabchi and Wall, 1995). Rapid administration of hypotonic fluids can also cause a rapid decrease in the osmolality of ECF. The rapid decrease in ECF

TABLE 13–9 ELECTROLYTE COMPOSITION OF COMMERCIALLY AVAILABLE FLUIDS

Fluid	Na⁺ (mEq/L)	Cl⁻ (mEq/L)	K⁺ (mEq/L)	Glucose (g/L)	Buffer* (mEq/L)	Osmolarity (mOsm/L)
0.9% saline[a]	154	154	0	0	0	308
0.45% saline[a]	77	77	0	0	0	154
Ringer's solution[a]	147	156	4	0	0	310
Ringer's lactated solution[a]	130	109	4	0	28 (L)	273
Plasma-Lyte 148[a]	140	98	5	0	27 (A) 23 (G)	294
Normosol-R[b]	140	98	5	0	27 (A) 23 (G)	294
5% dextrose in water[a]	0	0	0	50	0	252

* Buffers used: A, acetate; G, gluconate; L, lactate.
[a] Baxter Healthcare Corporation, Deerfield, Ill.
[b] Abbott laboratories, Chicago, Ill.

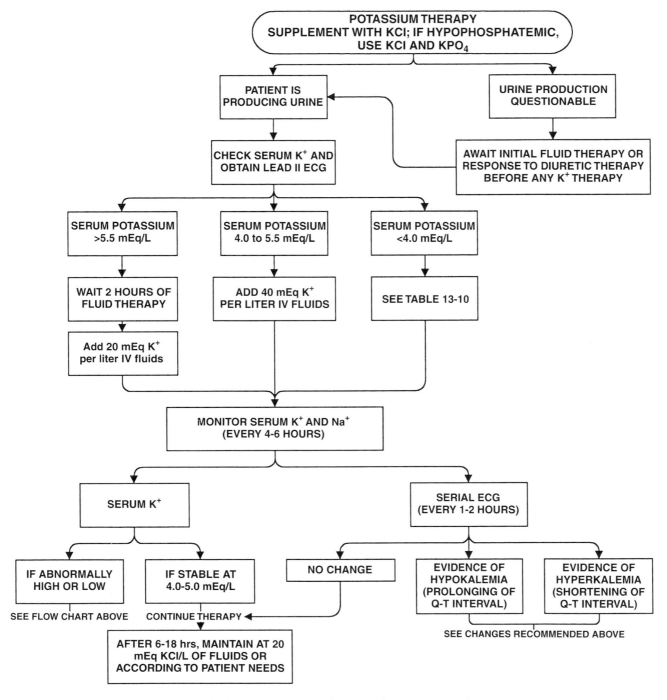

FIGURE 13–14. Potassium therapy in the management of DKA.

osmolality shifts water from the extracellular to the intracellular compartment, causing cerebral edema, deterioration in mentation, and eventually coma (see page 611). Hyperosmolality is best treated with isotonic fluids and the judicious administration of insulin.

RATE OF FLUID ADMINISTRATION. The initial volume and rate of fluid administration are determined by assessing the degree of shock, the dehydration deficit, the animal's maintenance requirements, plasma protein concentration, and presence or absence of cardiac disease. The typical dog or cat with DKA is 6% to 12%

dehydrated. Fluid administration should be directed at gradually replacing hydration deficits over 24 hours while also supplying maintenance fluid needs and matching ongoing losses. Rapid replacement of fluids is rarely indicated unless the dog or cat is in shock. Once out of this critical phase, fluid replacement should be decreased in an effort to correct the fluid imbalance in a slow but steady manner. As a general rule of thumb, a fluid rate of 1.5 to 2 times maintenance (i.e., 60 to 100 ml/kg/24 hr) is typically chosen initially, with subsequent adjustments based on frequent assessment of hydration status, urine output, severity of azotemia, and persistence of vomiting and diarrhea.

MONITORING FLUID THERAPY. The rate of fluid administration and its effects on the animal must be monitored. Overzealous fluid therapy can lead to overhydration, pulmonary edema, and other "third-space" fluid loss with potentially serious consequences. Inadequate fluid administration can result in prolonged tissue underperfusion, hypoxia, continuing pancreatitis (if present), persistent prerenal azotemia, and the potential for development of primary renal failure. Evaluation of fluid therapy should include subjective and objective assessments. Subjectively, the animal's alertness, heart rate, mucous membrane moisture, capillary refill time, pulse pressure, and skin turgor should be monitored and frequent pulmonary and cardiac auscultation performed. Objectively, serial evaluation of direct arterial or indirect Doppler blood pressure measurements, central venous pressure (CVP), urine output, body weight, and serum osmolality should be considered or completed. CVP should remain below 10 cm H_2O. The fasted dog or cat should also lose approximately 0.5 to 1.0% of its body weight daily.

Accurate assessment of urine output is extremely important in the severely ill ketoacidotic dog or cat. Diabetes-induced glomerular microangiopathy and/or the hemodynamic effects of ketoacidosis, concurrent necrotizing pancreatitis, or prolonged severe dehydration can lead to oliguric or anuric renal failure. Failure to produce urine within several hours of initiating fluid therapy is an alarming sign, one that demands rapid recognition and an aggressive course of action. If urine production is in doubt, an indwelling urinary catheter should be secured in the bladder and attached to a closed collection system. Palpation of the bladder is not an accurate method for assessing urine output. Frequent, accurate monitoring of urine production is imperative. A minimum of 1.0 to 2.0 ml of urine per kilogram of body weight per hour should be produced following the initial phase of fluid therapy. If urine production is minimal, the patency of the urinary catheter should be checked, the adequacy of fluid therapy should be evaluated (e.g., CVP, arterial blood pressure, subjective signs of excessive or inadequate fluids), and then attempts should be made to improve urine output (e.g., diuretics, dopamine infusion; see page 607).

An important aid in fluid therapy is the frequent assessment (ideally every 6 to 8 hours, initially) of serum sodium and potassium concentrations and total venous CO_2 or arterial blood gases. Measures taken to correct electrolyte imbalances are an integral part of fluid therapy. After the initial 6 to 8 hours of therapy, if the serum sodium concentration is between 140 and 155 mEq/L, the IV fluid solution should be changed to Ringer's or Ringer's lactated solution, both of which have less sodium than normal saline (see Table 13-9). If the serum sodium concentration is less than 140 mEq/L, the animal should be maintained on 0.9% saline. If the serum sodium concentration is greater than 155 mEq/L, 0.45% saline or a 50:50 mixture of 0.9% saline and 5% dextrose in water should be given. The IV infusion may need to be changed several times during the initial 24 hours of therapy.

POTASSIUM SUPPLEMENTATION (see Fig. 13-14). Most dogs and cats with DKA have a net deficit of total body potassium due primarily to the marked urinary losses caused by the osmotic diuresis of glycosuria and ketonuria. Most dogs and cats with DKA initially have either normal or decreased serum potassium concentrations (see Fig. 13-9; see page 589). Individual animals may have low, normal, or elevated potassium concentrations, depending on the duration of illness, renal function, and previous nutrition. During therapy for DKA the serum potassium concentration decreases because of rehydration (dilution), insulin-mediated cellular uptake of potassium (with glucose), continued urinary losses, and correction of acidemia (translocation of potassium into the ICF compartment). Dogs and cats with hypokalemia require aggressive potassium replacement therapy to replace deficits and to prevent worsening, life-threatening hypokalemia after initiation of insulin therapy. Normal saline does not contain potassium, and Ringer's solution contains 4 mEq of potassium per liter; thus supplementation of these fluids is required, especially with initially low or normal serum potassium concentrations. The exception to potassium supplementation of fluids is hyperkalemia associated with oliguric renal failure. Potassium supplementation should initially be withheld in these dogs and cats until glomerular filtration is restored, urine production increases, and hyperkalemia is resolving.

Ideally the amount of potassium required should be based on actual measurement of the serum potassium concentration (Table 13-10). If an accurate measurement of serum potassium is not available, 40 mEq of potassium should initially be added to each liter of intravenous fluids (36 mEq added to Ringer's solution). Subsequent adjustments in potassium supplementation should be based on measurement of serum potassium, preferably every 6 to 8 hours until

TABLE 13–10   GUIDELINES FOR POTASSIUM SUPPLEMENTATION IN IV FLUIDS

Serum K$^+$ (mEq/L)	TYPICAL GUIDELINES K$^+$ Supplement/ Liter of Fluids	GUIDELINES FOR DKA K$^+$ Supplement/ Liter of Fluids
> 5.0	Wait	Wait
4.0–5.5	10	20 to 30
3.5–4.0	20	30 to 40
3.0–3.5	30	40 to 50
2.5–3.0	40	50 to 60
2.0–2.5	60	60 to 80
< 2.0	80	80

Total hourly potassium administration should not exceed 0.5 mEq/kg body weight.

the dog or cat is stable and serum electrolytes are in the normal range. An alternative is to periodically evaluate an ECG for changes consistent with hyperkalemia or hypokalemia (see Table 13-7). If an ECG and a serum potassium determination are obtained before therapy, the ECG becomes an inexpensive and relatively reliable technique for detecting worrisome changes in the serum potassium concentration.

PHOSPHATE SUPPLEMENTATION. Serum phosphorus concentrations can be decreased, normal, or increased, depending on the duration of illness and renal function. Most dogs and cats with DKA have either normal or decreased serum phosphorus concentrations on pretreatment testing. Within 24 hours of initiating treatment for DKA, serum phosphorus concentration can decline to severe levels (i.e., <1 mg/dl) as a result of the dilutional effects of fluid therapy, the intracellular shift of phosphorus following the initiation of insulin therapy, and continuing renal and gastrointestinal loss (Willard et al, 1987). Hypophosphatemia affects primarily the hematologic and neuromuscular systems in dogs and cats (Forrester and Moreland, 1989). Hemolytic anemia is the most common problem and can be life-threatening if not recognized and treated (see page 612). Weakness, ataxia, and seizures may also be observed. Severe hypophosphatemia may be clinically silent in many animals.

Phosphate therapy is indicated if clinical signs or hemolysis are identified or if the serum phosphorus concentration decreases to less than 1.5 mg/dl. Phosphate is supplemented by intravenous infusion. Potassium and sodium phosphate solutions contain 3 mmol of phosphate and either 4.4 mEq of potassium or 4 mEq of sodium per milliliter. The recommended dosage for phosphate supplementation is 0.01 to 0.03 mmol of phosphate per kilogram of body weight per hour, preferably administered in calcium-free intravenous fluids (e.g., 0.9% sodium chloride) (Willard, 1987). In dogs and cats with severe hypophosphatemia, the dosage may need to be increased to 0.03 to 0.12 mmol/kg/hr (Nichols and Crenshaw, 1995). Because the dose of phosphate necessary to replete an animal and the animal's response to therapy cannot be predicted, it is important to monitor the serum phosphorus concentration initially every 8 to 12 hours and adjust the phosphate infusion accordingly. Adverse effects from overzealous phosphate administration include iatrogenic hypocalcemia and its associated neuromuscular signs, hypernatremia, hypotension, and metastatic calcification (Forrester and Moreland, 1989). Serum total or preferably ionized calcium concentration should be measured at the same time as serum phosphorus concentration and the rate of phosphate infusion decreased if hypocalcemia is identified. Phosphorus supplementation is not indicated in dogs and cats with hypercalcemia, hyperphosphatemia, oliguria, or suspected tissue necrosis. If renal function is in question, phosphorus supplementation should not be administered until the status of renal function and serum phosphorus concentration are known.

The routine supplementation of intravenous fluids with phosphorus during the initial 24 to 48 hours of treatment to prevent the development of severe hypophosphatemia is controversial and varies with the experiences of the veterinarian queried. Routine phosphate supplementation is seldom recommended in treating DKA in humans, in part because several studies have failed to identify any apparent clinical benefit from phosphate administration and overzealous phosphate administration may cause hypocalcemia with tetany (Becker et al, 1983; Fisher and Kitabchi, 1983; Masharani and Karam, 2001). The use of low-dose insulin treatment regimens, as described below, helps reduce the intracellular shift of phosphate, and the frequent monitoring of serum phosphorus concentrations during therapy ensures early recognition of worrisome changes in the serum phosphorus concentration. Arguments for routine phosphate administration, especially if the pretreatment phosphorus concentration is low, center around concerns with hemolytic anemia and the desire to avoid this serious complication. Studies documenting the impact, if any, of prophylactic phosphate supplementation on the prevalence of hemolytic anemia have not been reported in dogs and cats with DKA. If the decision is made to prophylactically administer phosphate, it can be administered separately using the dosages discussed above or can be included as a component of potassium replacement in the fluids. When the latter approach is used, 5 to 10 mEq of the potassium supplement added to the liter of fluids should be potassium phosphate and the remainder of the potassium supplemented as potassium chloride. The serum phosphorus concentration should be monitored every 8 to 12 hours and the phosphate supplement adjusted accordingly.

MAGNESIUM SUPPLEMENTATION. Hypomagnesemia is common in dogs and cats with DKA; it often worsens during the initial treatment of DKA but resolves without treatment as the DKA resolves (Norris et al, 1999). Clinical signs of hypomagnesemia do not usually occur unless the serum total and ionized magnesium concentration is less than 1.0 and 0.5 mg/dl, respectively, and even at these low levels, many dogs and cats remain asymptomatic (see page 593). What impact, if any, hypomagnesemia has on morbidity and response to treatment of DKA is not clear. To date there are no clinical studies that have yielded guidelines for magnesium replacement in dogs and cats; currently it is determined empirically. We do not routinely treat hypomagnesemia in dogs or cats with DKA unless problems with persistent lethargy, anorexia, weakness, or refractory hypokalemia or hypocalcemia are encountered after 24 to 48 hours of fluid and insulin therapy and another cause for the problem cannot be identified.

Parenteral solutions of magnesium sulfate (8.13 mEq of magnesium per gram) and magnesium chloride (9.25 mEq of magnesium per gram) salts are available; the initial IV dose for the first day is 0.75 to 1 mEq/kg, administered by continuous-rate infusion in 5%

dextrose in water (Dhupa, 1995; Hansen, 2000). Magnesium supplementation can be continued at half of the initial dose for an additional 3 to 5 days, if necessary. Renal function must be assessed before the administration of magnesium and the magnesium dose reduced by 50% to 75% in azotemic animals. The administration of magnesium to animals being treated with digitalis cardioglycosides may cause serious conduction disturbances. Magnesium is incompatible with solutions containing sodium bicarbonate, calcium, hydrocortisone, and dobutamine hydrochloride. Serum total or preferably ionized magnesium concentrations should be monitored every 12 to 24 hours and adjustments in the rate of magnesium infusion made accordingly. The goal of therapy is to return serum total and ionized magnesium concentrations to the normal range. The parenteral administration of magnesium sulfate may cause significant hypocalcemia such that calcium infusion may be necessary. Other adverse effects of magnesium therapy include hypotension, atrioventricular and bundle-branch blocks, and in the event of overdose, respiratory depression and cardiac arrest. Overdoses are treated with calcium gluconate (10 to 50 mg/kg IV).

Bicarbonate Therapy (Fig. 13-15)

Use of bicarbonate to aid in correcting the acidosis of DKA is controversial. Proponents of bicarbonate therapy argue that the deleterious effects of acidosis should be corrected. Severe acidosis interferes with insulin binding to receptors; impairs cardiac output and promotes arrhythmias; results in vasodilation with subsequent hypotension, CNS depression, and respiratory depression; causes renal and mesenteric vascular constriction, which predisposes the animal to acute renal tubular necrosis and ischemic bowel disease; enhances the development of hyperkalemia if renal function is impaired; decreases buffer reserve, and causes significant clinical signs (e.g., anorexia, nausea, vomiting; Whittaker et al, 1981; Feldman and Nelson, 1987). Decreasing buffer reserves are a major concern in the severely acidotic dog or cat with DKA because small changes in either PCO_2 or serum bicarbonate concentration can produce life-threatening changes in the blood pH.

Arguments for the use of bicarbonate therapy are countered by the potential deleterious consequences of bicarbonate administration. Administration of sodium bicarbonate may exacerbate hypokalemia,

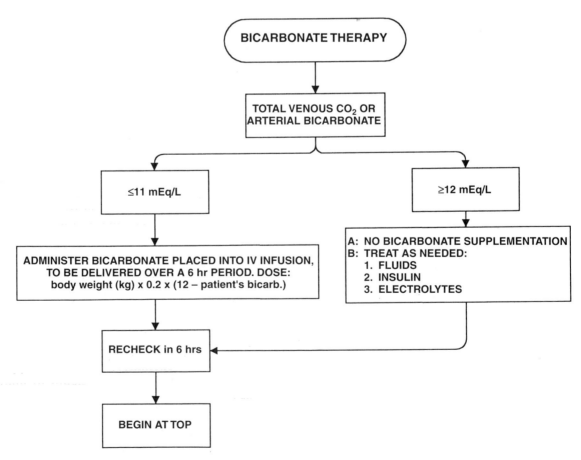

FIGURE 13–15. Bicarbonate treatment protocol for the management of DKA.

impair oxygen delivery to tissues by increasing hemoglobin affinity for oxygen, cause sodium overload and rebound alkalosis, promote an exaggerated decrease in the cerebrospinal fluid (CSF) pH with resultant worsening of CNS function, and delay the decrease in blood lactate and ketone-body concentrations (Hale et al, 1984; Hood and Tannen, 1994; Kitabchi et al, 2001). Adding to the controversy is the realization that pH can directly modify hepatic ketogenesis, with decreases in pH reducing hepatic output of β-hydroxybutyrate and acetoacetate (Okuda et al, 1986a; Farfournoux et al, 1987); treatment with insulin and fluids corrects the acidosis via oxidation of ketone bodies and excretion of hydrogen ions in the urine (Owen et al, 1980); and differences in the rates of recovery between animals and humans receiving bicarbonate therapy and animals and humans who did not receive such therapy have not been identified (Lever and Jaspan, 1983; Morris et al, 1986; Viallon et al, 1999). In one study, treatment with sodium bicarbonate actually delayed resolution of ketosis in humans with DKA (Okuda et al, 1996b).

The clinical presentation of the dog or cat, in conjunction with the plasma bicarbonate or total venous CO_2 concentration, should be used to determine the need for bicarbonate therapy. Bicarbonate supplementation is not recommended when plasma bicarbonate (or total venous CO_2) is 12 mEq/L or greater, especially if the animal is alert. An alert dog or cat probably has a normal or nearly normal pH in the CSF. The acidosis in these animals is corrected through insulin and fluid therapy. Improvement in renal perfusion enhances the urinary loss of ketoacids, and insulin therapy dramatically diminishes the production of ketoacids. Acetoacetate and β-hydroxybutyrate are also metabolically usable anions, and 1 mEq of bicarbonate is generated from each 1 mEq of ketoacid metabolized.

When the plasma bicarbonate concentration is 11 mEq/L or less (total venous CO_2 <12 mEq/L), bicarbonate therapy should be initiated. Many of these animals have severe depression that may be a result of concurrent severe CNS acidosis. These are difficult dogs and cats to treat, and the only safe therapeutic protocol involves correcting the metabolic acidosis slowly in the peripheral circulation via intravenous fluid supplementation, thereby avoiding major alterations in the pH of the CSF. As such, only a portion of the bicarbonate deficit is given initially over a 6-hour period of time.

The bicarbonate deficit (i.e., the milliequivalents of bicarbonate initially needed to correct acidosis to the critical level of 12 mEq/L over a period of 6 hours) is calculated as:

$$\text{mEq bicarbonate} = \text{body weight (kg)} \times 0.4 \times (12 - \text{animal's bicarbonate}) \times 0.5$$

or if the serum bicarbonate is not known:

$$\text{mEq bicarbonate} = \text{body weight (kg)} \times 2$$

The difference between the animal's serum bicarbonate concentration and the critical value of 12 mEq/L represents the treatable base deficit in DKA. If the animal's serum bicarbonate concentration is not known, the number 10 should be used for the treatable base deficit. The factor 0.4 corrects for the ECF space in which bicarbonate is distributed (40% of body weight). The factor 0.5 provides one-half of the required dose of bicarbonate in the IV infusion. In this manner, a conservative dose is given over a 6-hour period. Bicarbonate should never be given by bolus infusion (Ryder, 1984). After 6 hours of therapy, the acid-base status should be re-evaluated and a new dosage calculated. Once the plasma bicarbonate level is greater than 12 mEq/L, further bicarbonate supplementation is not needed.

Insulin Therapy

Insulin therapy is critical for the resolution of ketoacidosis. Insulin inhibits lipolysis and the mobilization of FFAs from triglycerides stored in adipose tissue, thereby decreasing the substrate necessary for ketone production; shifts hepatic metabolism from fat oxidation and ketogenesis to fat synthesis; suppresses hepatic gluconeogenesis; and promotes glucose and ketone metabolism by tissues (Hood and Tannen, 1994; DeFronzo et al, 1994). The net effect is decreased blood and urine glucose and ketone concentrations, decreased osmotic diuresis and electrolyte losses and correction of metabolic acidosis. Overzealous insulin treatment can cause severe hypokalemia, hypophosphatemia, and hypoglycemia during the first 24 hours of treatment; problems that can be minimized by appropriate fluid therapy, frequent monitoring of serum electrolytes and blood glucose concentrations, and modifying the initial insulin treatment protocol in those dogs and cats that are hypokalemic at the time DKA is diagnosed.

The decision on when to start insulin therapy varies with the experiences of the veterinarian queried. Initiating appropriate fluid therapy should always be the first step in the treatment of DKA (see page 597). Delaying insulin therapy allows the benefits of fluid therapy to begin to be realized before the glucose, potassium, and phosphorus-lowering effects of insulin therapy commence. The question is how long to delay insulin therapy. We typically delay insulin therapy for a minimum of 1 to 2 hours. Additional delays and decisions on the initial dosage of insulin administered are based on serum electrolyte results. If the serum potassium concentration is within the normal range, we begin insulin treatment as described below. If hypokalemia is identified, insulin therapy can be delayed an additional 1 to 2 hours to allow fluid therapy to replenish potassium, the initial insulin dose can be reduced to dampen the intracellular shift of potassium and phosphorus, or both can be done. The more severe the hypokalemia, the more inclined we are to delay insulin therapy and reduce the insulin dose initially. However, in our opinion, insulin therapy should always be started within 4 hours of initiating fluid therapy. If results of serum electrolyte tests will not be known for several hours, insulin therapy can be delayed for a couple of hours and the initial insulin dose reduced to help prevent severe hypokalemia.

Insulin therapy may not be as effective if a concurrent insulin-antagonistic disease is present, and it may be necessary to eliminate the disease while the animal is still ill to improve insulin effectiveness and resolve the ketoacidosis (e.g., female dog in diestrus [see page 609]). Regardless, insulin therapy is still indicated. The amount of insulin needed by an individual animal is difficult to predict. Therefore an insulin with a rapid onset of action and a brief duration of effect would be ideal for making rapid adjustments in the dose and frequency of administration to meet the needs of that particular dog or cat. Rapid-acting regular crystalline insulin meets these criteria (Nelson et al, 1990) and is recommended for the treatment of DKA.

Insulin protocols for the treatment of DKA include the hourly intramuscular technique (Chastain and Nichols, 1981), the continuous low-dose IV infusion technique (Macintire, 1993), and the intermittent intramuscular/subcutaneous technique (Feldman, 1980). All three routes (IV, IM, SC) of insulin administration are effective in decreasing plasma glucose and ketone concentrations (Fig. 13-16). Arguments abound regarding the most appropriate route for initial insulin administration. In our experience, the intermittent intramuscular regimen has worked well. This protocol is simple, reliable, and consistent and avoids the inherent difficulties of intravenous and subcutaneous regimens. Successful management of DKA does not depend on route of insulin administration. Rather, it depends on proper treatment of each disorder associated with DKA (see Table 13-8).

HOURLY INTRAMUSCULAR INSULIN TECHNIQUE. (FIG. 13-17). Dogs and cats with severe DKA should receive an initial regular insulin loading dose of 0.2 U/kg followed by 0.1 U/kg every 1 to 2 hours thereafter. The insulin dose can be reduced by 25% to 50% for the first 2 to 3 injections if hypokalemia is a concern. The insulin should be administered into the muscles of the rear legs to ensure that the injections are intramuscular and do not go into fat or subcutaneous tissue. Diluting regular insulin 1:10 with special diluents available from the insulin manufacturer and using 0.3 ml U100 insulin syringes are helpful when small doses of insulin are required.

By means of this insulin treatment regimen, the serum insulin concentration is typically increased to and maintained at approximately 100 μU/ml (Fig. 13-18), an insulin concentration that inhibits lipolysis, gluconeogenesis, and glycogenolysis and promotes utilization of glucose and ketones by tissues (Barrett and DeFronzo, 1984; Feldman and Nelson, 1987). The blood glucose concentration should be measured every hour using a point-of-care chemistry analyzer or portable blood glucose monitoring device, and the insulin dosage should be adjusted accordingly (see Fig. 13-17). The goal of initial insulin therapy is to slowly lower the blood glucose concentration to the range of 200 to 250 mg/dl, preferably over a 6- to 10-hour time period. An hourly decline of 50 mg/dl in the blood glucose concentration is ideal (Wagner et al, 1999). This provides a steady moderate decline, avoiding large shifts in osmolality. A declining blood glucose concentration also ensures that lipolysis and the supply of FFAs for ketone production have been effectively turned off. Glucose concentrations, however, decrease much more rapidly than do ketone levels (Barrett and DeFronzo, 1984; Yeates and Blaufuss, 1990). In general, hyperglycemia is corrected

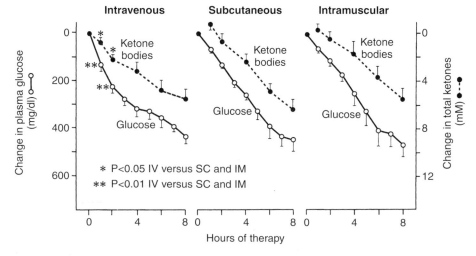

FIGURE 13–16. Effect of route of insulin therapy on reduction in plasma glucose and ketone concentrations in humans with DKA. Intravenous insulin was associated with a more rapid decline (initial 0–2 hr) in plasma glucose and ketone levels. Thereafter, no differences were noted between any of these groups. (From DeFronzo RA, et al: Diabetic ketoacidosis. A combined metabolic-nephrologic approach to therapy. Diabetes Rev 2:223, 1994; used with permission.)

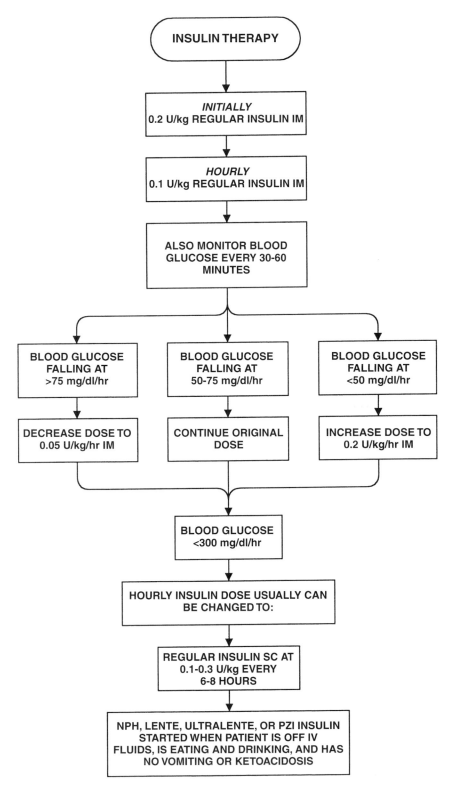

FIGURE 13–17. Insulin treatment protocol for the management of DKA.

within 12 hours, but ketosis often takes 48 to 72 hours to resolve.

Once the initial hourly insulin therapy brings the blood glucose concentration near 250 mg/dl, hourly administration of regular insulin should be dis-

continued and regular insulin given every 4 to 6 hours intramuscularly or, if hydration status is good, every 6 to 8 hours SC. The initial dose is usually 0.1 to 0.3 U/kg, with subsequent adjustments based on blood glucose concentrations. In addition, at this

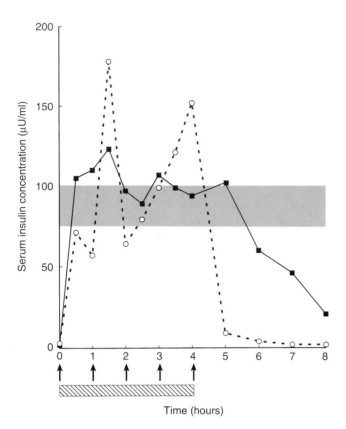

FIGURE 13–18. Mean serum insulin concentration in eight dogs with DKA before and after the administration of regular crystalline insulin, 0.2 U/kg of body weight IM (time 0), and then 0.1 U/kg IM hourly thereafter *(solid line)*, and in six dogs with DKA before and after continuous IV infusion of regular crystalline insulin *(dashed line)*, using a pediatric drip set. Insulin treatment was discontinued after the fourth hour in both groups of dogs. ↑, IM insulin administration; *hatched area*, IV insulin infusion; *shaded area*, ideal serum insulin concentration for treatment of DKA.

point, the intravenous infusion solution should have enough 50% dextrose added to create a 5% dextrose solution (100 ml of 50% dextrose added to each liter of fluids). The blood glucose concentration should be maintained between 150 and 300 mg/dl until the animal is stable and eating. Usually a 5% dextrose solution is adequate in maintaining the desired blood glucose concentration. If the blood glucose concentration dips below 150 mg/dl or rises above 300 mg/dl, the insulin dose can be lowered or raised accordingly. Dextrose helps minimize problems with hypoglycemia and allows insulin to be administered on schedule. Delaying the administration of insulin delays correction of the ketoacidotic state.

Longer-acting insulins (e.g., NPH, lente, PZI) should not be initiated until the dog or cat is stable, eating, maintaining fluid balance without any intravenous infusions, and no longer acidotic, azotemic, or electrolyte-deficient. The initial dose of these longer-acting insulins is similar to the regular insulin dose being used just before switching to the longer-acting insulins. Subsequent adjustments in the longer-acting insulin dosage should be based on clinical response

and measurement of blood glucose concentrations.

CONSTANT LOW-DOSE INSULIN INFUSION TECHNIQUE. Constant intravenous infusion of regular crystalline insulin is also effective in decreasing blood glucose concentrations. The decision to use the hourly intramuscular technique versus constant intravenous insulin infusion is based primarily on clinician preference and availability of technical support and infusion pumps. To prepare the infusion, regular crystalline insulin (2.2 U/kg for dogs; 1.1 U/kg for cats) is added to 250 ml of 0.9% saline and initially administered at a rate of 10 ml/hr in a line separate from that used for fluid therapy (Church, 1983; Macintire, 1993). This provides an insulin infusion of 0.05 (cat) and 0.1 (dog) U/kg/hr, an infusion rate that has been shown to produce plasma insulin concentrations between 100 and 200 µU/ml in dogs (Macintire, 1993). Because insulin adheres to glass and plastic surfaces, approximately 50 ml of the insulin-containing fluid should be run through the drip set before it is administered to the animal. The rate of insulin infusion can be reduced for the initial 2 to 3 hours if hypokalemia is a concern. Two separate catheters are recommended for treatment: a peripheral catheter for insulin administration and a central catheter for fluid administration and blood sampling. An infusion or syringe pump should be used to ensure a constant rate of insulin infusion. Insulin infusions using pediatric drip sets may not provide a constant insulin infusion rate, especially if frequent monitoring of fluid administration is not possible (see Fig. 13-18). The goal of therapy is identical to that described for the hourly intramuscular technique—to provide a continuous source of insulin at a dosage that causes a gradual decline in the blood glucose concentration. This goal is best attained with use of infusion or syringe pumps.

Adjustments in the infusion rate are based on hourly measurements of blood glucose concentration; an hourly decline of 50 mg/dl in the blood glucose concentration is ideal (Wagner et al, 1999). Once the blood glucose concentration approaches 250 mg/dl, the insulin infusion can be discontinued and regular insulin given every 4 to 6 hours intramuscularly or, if hydration status is good, every 6 to 8 hours subcutaneously, as discussed for the hourly IM protocol. Alternatively, the insulin infusion can be continued (at a decreased rate to prevent hypoglycemia) until the insulin preparation is exchanged for a longer-acting product. Dextrose should be added to the intravenous fluids once the blood glucose concentration approaches 250 mg/dl, as discussed in the section on hourly IM insulin technique.

INTERMITTENT INTRAMUSCULAR/SUBCUTANEOUS INSULIN TECHNIQUE. An intermittent intramuscular followed by intermittent subcutaneous insulin technique has been described (Feldman, 1980). Although we used this technique successfully for years, it has been replaced with the hourly IM and constant IV insulin techniques. The intermittent intramuscular technique is less labor-intensive than the other techniques for insulin administration, but the decrease in blood glucose can be rapid and the risk for hypoglycemia is greater with the intermittent IM technique. The initial regular crystalline insulin dose is 0.25 U/kg IM every 4 hours. Usually, insulin is administered intramuscularly only once or twice. Once the animal is rehydrated, subcutaneous administration is substituted for IM insulin administration and insulin is administered SC every 6 to 8 hours. Subcutaneous administration is not recommended initially, because of problems with insulin absorption from subcutaneous sites of deposition in a dehydrated dog or cat. The dosage of IM or SC insulin is adjusted according to blood glucose concentrations, which initially should be measured hourly beginning with the first IM injection. An hourly decline of 50 mg/dl in the blood glucose concentration is ideal (Wagner et al, 1999). Subsequent insulin dosages should be decreased by 25% to 50% if this goal is exceeded. Dextrose should be added to the IV fluids once the blood glucose concentration approaches 250 mg/dl, as discussed in the section on hourly IM insulin technique.

Concurrent Illness

Therapy for DKA frequently involves the management of concurrent, often serious illness. Common concurrent illness in the dog and cat with DKA include acute and chronic pancreatitis, bacterial infection, cholangiohepatitis, renal insufficiency, cardiac disease, and insulin antagonism induced by hormonal disorders, most notably iatrogenic or naturally developing hyperadrenocorticism and diestrus (Bruskiewicz et al,1997). Modifications in therapy for DKA (e.g., fluid therapy with concurrent heart failure) and/or additional therapy (e.g., antibiotics) may be required, depending on the concurrent illness. Insulin therapy, however, should never be delayed or discontinued. Resolution of ketoacidosis can be obtained only through insulin therapy. If nothing is to be given by mouth, insulin therapy should be continued and the blood glucose concentration maintained with intravenous dextrose infusions. If concurrent insulin-antagonistic disease is present, correction of the disease while the animal is still ill may be necessary to improve insulin effectiveness and resolve the ketoacidosis.

PANCREATITIS. Pancreatitis, acute or chronic, should always be assumed to be present in the dog or cat with DKA. The diagnosis should never be made solely on serum lipase concentrations, but on a combination of presence of appropriate clinical signs; physical examination findings; abnormalities on the CBC, serum biochemistry panel, urinalysis, and serum lipase; radiographic evidence of a loss of detail in the right cranial abdomen accompanied by gas-filled duodenal ileus; and ultrasonographic evidence of enlargement of the pancreas and a hypoechoic to mixed echogenic pattern with or without mild to severe blockage of the bile duct (see Fig. 12-10, page 549).

Fluid therapy is the cornerstone of treatment for both DKA and pancreatitis. In addition, most ill DKA dogs and cats are initially anorectic and food is not usually offered during the initial 24 to 72 hours of hospitalization; therapy that is also helpful for concurrent pancreatitis. Nutritional support by total or peripheral parenteral nutrition may be necessary in diabetic dogs and especially cats with protracted vomiting, in part to prevent development of hepatic lipidosis syndrome. Once the dog or cat is eating, the diet should be modified to meet the dietary principles established for the management of pancreatitis. Subsequent adjustments in the diet should be based on the clinical response of the dog or cat in the home environment. Acute severe necrotizing pancreatitis is a common cause of death during the initial days of treatment of DKA, and the inability to prevent recurring bouts of chronic pancreatitis is one reason owners eventually elect euthanasia of their pet (Goossens et al, 1998). Avoidance of recurrent bouts of pancreatitis is critical to the long-term survival of the diabetic dog and cat. In the dog, this is primarily accomplished through appropriate dietary therapy. To date, inciting factors for development of pancreatitis in the cat have been poorly characterized and the impact of diet, if any, on preventing recurrence of pancreatitis has not been determined.

BACTERIAL INFECTION/SEPSIS. The immunosuppressive effects of diabetes mellitus, in conjunction with the increased blood glucose concentration in body fluids, predisposes diabetic dogs and cats to bacterial infections (McMahon and Bistrian, 1995; Joshi et al, 1999). Urinary tract infections are most common, followed by infections of the oral cavity, skin, and pulmonary systems (Hess et al, 2000; Peikes et al, 2001). Life-threatening sepsis may develop in debilitated diabetics, those with severe concurrent illness (e.g., necrotizing pancreatitis), and those in which aseptic technique is not strictly followed during diagnostic and therapeutic procedures (e.g., placement of indwelling urinary or venous catheters). The clinician must always suspect infection in the DKA dog or cat. Urine cultures should be completed in all dogs and cats with DKA. Cultures of blood, joint fluid, CSF, or other tissues are usually dictated by the clinical signs and laboratory parameters. We routinely place all of our ill DKA animals on broad-spectrum, bactericidal antibiotics at the time of initial hospitalization. Subsequent changes in antibiotic therapy are based on results of culture and sensitivity testing.

RENAL FAILURE. Diabetes-induced glomerular microangiopathy causes progressive fibrosis of the glomeruli, with the ultimate development of glomerulosclerosis (see Chapter 11, page 532). Initially, diabetic nephropathy is characterized by proteinuria, which progresses to polyuric renal failure. As glomerular fibrosis and sclerosis worsen, end-stage oliguric to anuric renal failure develops. In our experience, a high incidence of oliguria is seen in ill dogs and cats diagnosed with both DKA and renal failure. This is due, in part, to the concurrent hemodynamic effects of ketoacidosis, concurrent necrotizing pancreatitis, or prolonged severe dehydration, in addition to diabetes-induced glomerular microangiopathy. Concurrent renal failure in the ill dog or cat with DKA carries a guarded to grave prognosis, depending on the status of urine production in the animal.

The clinician should always suspect oliguria when renal failure is diagnosed in an ill DKA animal. Accurate assessment of urine production during the initial 4 to 6 hours of therapy is imperative. Failure to produce urine within the first few hours of initiating fluid therapy or within 1 to 2 hours of establishing normal blood pressure is an alarming sign, one that demands rapid recognition and an aggressive course of action. If urine production is in doubt, an indwelling urinary catheter should be secured in the bladder and attached to a closed collection system. Palpation of the bladder is not an accurate method for assessing urine output. Frequent, accurate monitoring of urine production is imperative. A minimum of 1.0 to 2.0 ml of urine per kilogram of body weight per hour should be produced following rehydration of the animal. If urine production is minimal, the patency of the urinary catheter should be checked and the adequacy of fluid therapy evaluated (e.g., CVP, arterial blood pressure, subjective signs of excessive or inadequate fluids). If the animal is hypotensive, the CVP is very low (<1 to 2 cm H_2O), or questions concerning fluid volume remain, the rate of fluid administration should be increased for an additional 1 to 2 hours. Urine output, CVP, blood pressure, and signs of overzealous fluid administration should be carefully monitored during this time.

If fluid therapy is deemed adequate and anuria or severe oliguria persists, an attempt should be made to induce or increase the volume of urine produced with diuretics, mannitol, and/or dopamine. We prefer a slow bolus followed by a constant-rate infusion of mannitol initially. The dose for bolus injection is 0.5 g/kg administered IV over 10 to 20 minutes. Improvement in urine production should occur within 30 minutes. If diuresis improves, a constant-rate infusion of mannitol should be initiated at a dose of 1 mg/kg/min, preferably given by syringe or infusion pump in a separate IV line. Mannitol can be diluted to a 12.5% solution with 5% dextrose in water (i.e., 1:1 dilution of a 25% mannitol solution) to decrease the concentration and osmolality of the solution and increase the volume of fluid being administered. Mannitol precipitates if mixed with saline, potassium chloride, or blood products; these mixtures must be avoided (Dhupa and Shaffran, 1995).

If the intravenous bolus of mannitol does not improve urine production 30 minutes after its administration, a constant-rate infusion of furosemide and dopamine rather than mannitol should be initiated in the dog (furosemide in the cat). Dopamine (Intropin, Faulding, Elizabeth, NJ), a precursor of norepinephrine (see Fig. 9-1, page 441), is useful as a renal vasodilator in dogs and may work synergistically with furosemide to improve urine production. Cats are not believed to have dopamine receptors in the kidney. Dopamine is administered at an initial dose of 2 to 5 µg/kg/min. Dopamine needs to be diluted in saline or Ringer's solution and cannot be added to solutions containing sodium bicarbonate, because this inactivates the drug. For treatment, 50 mg of dopamine can be diluted in 500 ml of infusion solution to create 100 µg of dopamine per milliliter. The mixture should be used only for delivering dopamine; fluid therapy must be provided with a separate infusate. The dopamine solution is best administered with an infusion pump attached to a separate IV line. Furosemide can be added to the dopamine solution and administered concurrently. The initial dosage of furosemide for constant rate infusion is 0.1 mg/kg/hr, with a maximum dosage of 1 mg/kg/hr (Dhupa and Shaffran, 1995).

Improvement in urine production should be seen within 30 to 60 minutes. The dose of dopamine and furosemide can be increased if urine production still does not improve, but tachycardia and/or tachyarrhythmias may develop. Tachycardia or arrhythmias indicate that the dopamine dose is excessive and potentially dangerous. If significant diuresis develops, the dopamine/furosemide infusion should be slowly decreased over 12 to 24 hours until urine production is maintained with fluid therapy alone.

If the above therapy fails, peritoneal dialysis and hemodialysis are the only alternatives.

HEPATITIS AND CHOLANGIOHEPATITIS. Hepatic lipidosis is commonly identified in diabetic dogs and cats, does not usually cause clinical signs, and does not require specific treatment aside from that directed at the diabetic state. A more worrisome hepatopathy, most notably acute or chronic hepatitis and cholangiohepatitis, should be suspected when icterus, a marked increase in serum liver enzyme activities (higher than expected with hepatic lipidosis, see page 494), or abnormalities involving endogenous liver function tests (e.g., hypoalbuminemia, hypocholesterolemia, increased bile acids) are identified on the physical examination or routine diagnostic blood tests. Acute or chronic hepatitis and cholangiohepatitis should also be considered in diabetic dogs and cats with persistent lethargy and anorexia despite correction of the metabolic derangements associated with DKA. Hepatitis and cholangiohepatitis often occur in conjunction with pancreatitis. When appropriate, abdominal ultrasound scanning and histologic evaluation of a liver biopsy specimen may be indicated to establish concurrent liver disease. As with DKA and pancreatitis, fluid therapy is an important initial treatment for dogs and cats that are ill from acute and chronic hepatitis and cholangiohepatitis. Nonspecific therapy including dietary manipulations, antibiotics, and lactulose may be indicated, especially if hepatic encephalopathy is suspected. Nutritional support administered by forced feeding, nasogastric tube, or esophagostomy tube may be necessary in diabetic dogs and especially cats with persistent anorexia. Nutritional support by total or peripheral parenteral nutrition may be necessary in diabetic dogs and cats with protracted vomiting. Additional therapy will vary depending on the specific diagnosis (e.g., chronic active hepatitis, lymphocytic/plasmacytic cholangiohepatitis, etc).

HORMONAL DISORDERS CAUSING INSULIN RESISTANCE. Insulin resistance accompanies many of the concurrent disorders present in dogs and cats with DKA. The severity of insulin resistance is quite variable and depends on the underlying cause (see Chapter 11, page 524 and Chapter 12, page 572). Fortunately, most disorders cause mild insulin resistance; that is, the dog or cat remains responsive to insulin therapy even at the low insulin dosages often employed during the initial 24 to 72 hours of therapy, and ketoacidosis progressively resolves. Two major exceptions are diestrus-induced insulin resistance in the intact bitch and hyperadrenocorticism. Although acromegaly also causes severe insulin resistance in the cat, ketonuria is an infrequent finding and systemic illness from DKA is uncommon, despite an inability to establish any semblance of glycemic control with massive doses of insulin. Seemingly, insulin is able to inhibit lipolysis and the supply of FFAs for ketone production but unable to control hepatic glucose secretion and/or stimulate tissue glucose utilization to control hyperglycemia in these cats.

Diestrus. Increased progesterone secretion during the diestrual phase of the estrus cycle in the bitch directly antagonizes insulin action and stimulates growth hormone secretion which, in turn, causes severe insulin resistance and the potential for life-threatening DKA (see Chapter 11, page 526). Diestrus-induced insulin resistance can be difficult if not impossible to override, despite the administration of massive doses of regular crystalline insulin. As a consequence, the metabolic derangements associated with DKA progressively worsen, ultimately resulting in death of the bitch.

Intact bitches in DKA should always be assumed to be in diestrus and should be assumed to have a pyometra, regardless of owner statements regarding estrus activity. Once initial therapy for DKA is initiated, abdominal ultrasound scans or radiographs should be evaluated for pyometra and a blood progesterone concentration should be evaluated using an in-house ELISA that provides rapid results (see Chapter 20). A blood progesterone concentration greater than 2 ng/ml is diagnostic for ovarian luteal activity and supports the diagnosis of diestrus. The bitch should undergo ovariohysterectomy as soon as safely possible. Timing of surgery depends on the severity of clinical signs. Severely ill bitches with DKA should be stabilized as well as possible with IV fluids, regular crystalline insulin, and parenteral antibiotics for 6 to 24 hours before performing surgery. We rarely wait more than 24 hours from the time of diagnosis of pyometra or diestrus to ovariohysterectomy. Insulin resistance usually begins to resolve within a week of ovariohysterectomy. In some bitches, insulin-requiring diabetes mellitus may even resolve.

Diestrus-induced insulin resistance and its effect on responsiveness of DKA to insulin therapy are not commonly identified in queens, in part because progesterone does not stimulate growth hormone secretion in the cat (Peterson, 1987). Progesterone binds to glucocorticoid receptors and can cause insulin resistance, but the insulin resistance that develops during diestrus in the queen rarely causes significant problems, presumably because the insulin resistance is not severe and the increase in plasma progesterone is transient. In contrast, insulin resistance caused by chronic progesterone excess, as occurs with exogenous progestagen administration or a progesterone-secreting adrenocortical tumor, can cause diabetes mellitus and a clinical syndrome that mimics feline hyperadrenocorticism (see Chapter 7; Boord and Griffin, 1999; Rossmeisl et al, 2000).

Exogenous Glucocorticoids. Glucocorticoids facilitate lipolysis, promote protein catabolism and the conversion of amino acids to glucose by the liver and kidney, and limit glucose utilization by insulin-dependent tissues (Cryer and Polonsky, 1998). The limitation of glucose utilization may be due to alterations in insulin receptor binding sites on the cell membrane, postreceptor defects, and/or alterations in the number or efficacy of intracellular glucose transporters (Horner et al, 1987; Wolfsheimer and Peterson, 1991). The resultant insulin resistance can antagonize treatment for ketoacidosis. In general, glucocorticoids should not be given to dogs and cats with DKA and should be discontinued in previously undiagnosed diabetic ketoacidotic dogs and cats. This includes oral, ocular, aural, and skin preparations. The exceptions are those situations in which glucocorticoids are necessary to control life-threatening disorders (e.g., immune-mediated disease). In these situations, the lowest dosage of glucocorticoid needed to control the disorder should be administered and alternatives to glucocorticoids (e.g., azathioprine for immune-mediated diseases; nonsteroidal anti-inflammatory solution for uveitis [see Chapter 11, page 531]) should be sought. In addition, the clinician should be willing to compensate for the insulin-antagonistic effects of glucocorticoids by administering larger dosages of insulin than are typically required to control DKA.

Spontaneous Hyperadrenocorticism. Hyperadrenocorticism is a well-recognized disorder in dogs and cats with diabetes mellitus and is occasionally suspected in dogs and cats with newly diagnosed DK and DKA and insulin-treated dogs and cats with persistent ketonuria. Hyperadrenocorticism causes insulin resistance in a similar manner to exogenous glucocorticoids (see above). For these animals, appropriate diagnostic tests should be undertaken and appropriate treatment initiated once the diagnosis of hyperadrenocorticism is confirmed (see Chapter 6). Despite its impaired efficacy, insulin must continue to be administered to inhibit lipolysis, suppress ketone production, and prevent deterioration of the ketoacidotic state. Ketosis resolves once hyperadrenocorticism is controlled.

The approach to hyperadrenocorticism is tempered somewhat in the ill ketoacidotic dog or cat, in part because of concerns regarding accuracy of results when the diagnostic tests used to diagnose hyperadrenocorticism are performed in dogs and cats with severe illness (Kaplan et al, 1995). The primary goal is stabilization and, if possible, resolution of ketonemia and ketonuria through intravenous fluids and insulin therapy. This typically requires 24 to 72 hours. Diagnostic tests for hyperadrenocorticism are not performed until the dog or cat is stable and eating and electrolyte derangements and metabolic acidosis have resolved. We rely on results of the ACTH stimulation test, low-dose dexamethasone suppression test, and abdominal ultrasonography to help confirm the diagnosis. We do not rely on the urine cortisol:creatinine ratio because of the high prevalence of false positive results in sick dogs and cats. We do not use the high-dose dexamethasone suppression test because of the potential consequences of administering large doses of glucocorticoids to these fragile animals. We do not administer o,p'-DDD to ill DKA dogs with pituitary-dependent hyperadrenocorticism until the dog is stable and eating and dehydration, electrolyte derangements, and metabolic acidosis have resolved. Rarely, we administer ketoconazole to control hypercortisolemia and improve insulin resistance in ill dogs in which conventional therapy (i.e., fluids, insulin) has failed to improve the ketoacidotic state.

PULMONARY THROMBOEMBOLISM. Several concurrent diseases commonly identified in dogs and cats with DKA can predispose the animal to development of thromboembolism, including pancreatitis, hyperadrenocorticism, glomerulonephropathy, sepsis, cardiac disease, and neoplasia. Factors predisposing to thrombus formation include stasis of blood flow, damage to the vascular endothelium, alterations in platelet aggregation and clotting factors, and decreased concentrations of antithrombin III (LaRue and Murtaugh, 1990; Ewenstein, 1997; Jacoby et al, 2001). Pulmonary thromboembolism (PTE) occurs most commonly and is characterized by the acute onset of tachypnea and severe dyspnea. The primary differential diagnoses are bacterial and aspiration pneumonia, which can be readily identified with thoracic radiographs. The diagnosis of PTE is based on clinical signs, thoracic radiography, and arterial blood gas analysis. In many cases, the lungs appear normal on thoracic radiographs. Abnormalities identified on thoracic radiographs include blunted pulmonary arteries, typically in the caudal lung lobes, focal or diffuse interstitial or alveolar opacities, hyperlucent regions of lung where blood supply is absent, pleural effusion, and right-sided cardiac enlargement (Fluckiger and Gomez, 1984; Hawkins, 2003). Arterial blood gas studies typically reveal hypoxemia and hypocapnia (Burns et al, 1981). Confirmation of the diagnosis requires angiography or nuclear perfusion lung scan. Treatment of this acute life-threatening disorder involves keeping the animal quiet, providing an oxygen-rich environment, administering subcutaneous heparin and/or thrombolytic drugs, and tincture of time (see Chapter 6, page 293).

TABLE 13–11 COMMON COMPLICATIONS CAUSED BY TREATMENT OF DIABETIC KETOACIDOSIS IN DOGS AND CATS

Hypoglycemia from excessive use of insulin or inadequate administration of glucose
Hypokalemia from inadequate potassium supplementation
Hypophosphatemia and hemolytic anemia from inadequate phosphorus supplementation
Hypernatremia from excessive administration of physiologic saline or inadequate fluid intake
Persistent oliguria from inadequate or inappropriately slow administration of fluids
Persistent hypotension from inadequate or inappropriately slow administration of fluids
Cerebral edema and neurologic signs from too rapid decrease in blood glucose and/or osmolality
Paradoxical cerebral acidosis and neurologic signs from too rapid administration of bicarbonate

Complications of Therapy

Complications induced by treatment of DKA are common and usually result from overly aggressive therapy, inadequate animal monitoring, and failure to reevaluate biochemical parameters in a timely manner (Table 13-11). DKA is a complex disorder that carries a high mortality rate if improperly managed. To minimize the occurrence of therapeutic complications and improve the chances of successful response to therapy, all abnormal parameters should be slowly returned toward normal (i.e., over a period of 36 to 48 hours), the physical and mental status of the animal must be evaluated frequently (at least three to four times daily), and biochemical parameters (e.g., blood glucose, serum electrolytes, blood gases) must be evaluated in a timely fashion. During the initial 24 hours, blood glucose concentrations should be measured every 1 to 2 hours and serum electrolytes and blood gases every 6 to 8 hours. Fluid, insulin, and bicarbonate therapy typically require modification three or four times during the initial 24 hours of therapy. Failure to recognize changes in the status of DKA and to respond accordingly invariably leads to potentially serious complications. The more common complications are discussed below.

HYPOGLYCEMIA. Hypoglycemia is a common problem during the initial days of treatment, especially when the dog or cat is anorectic and unable to ingest a dietary source of glucose to counter the glucose-lowering effects of insulin. The goal of initial insulin therapy, regardless of how the insulin is administered, is to slowly lower the blood glucose concentration to the range of 200 to 250 mg/dl, preferably over an 8- to 10-hour time period. Unfortunately, this goal can be quite difficult to attain and the blood glucose concentration may drop precipitously. To avoid hypoglycemia, it is imperative that the blood glucose concentration be measured hourly with a point-of-care chemistry analyzer or portable blood glucose monitoring device. Whenever the blood glucose concentration approaches 250 mg/dl, 50% dextrose should be added to the intravenous infusion solution to create a 5% dextrose solution. If hypoglycemia occurs (i.e., blood glucose <80 mg/dl) or the dog or cat is symptomatic for hypoglycemia, 0.5- to 3-ml aliquots of 50% dextrose should be administered intravenously as needed until the 5% dextrose solution is able to maintain the blood glucose above 80 mg/dl. Insulin therapy should also be modified but not discontinued. Discontinuing insulin therapy interferes with resolution of the ketoacidosis.

CENTRAL NERVOUS SYSTEM SIGNS (CEREBRAL EDEMA). Cerebral edema may result from excessive free water accumulation in the intravascular space during therapy for DKA. This typically results from a rapid decrease in the blood glucose concentration or after infusion of large quantities of hypotonic solutions (e.g., 0.45% saline). With insulin deficiency, the movement of glucose from the ECF to the ICF compartment is impaired. Glucose accumulation in the ECF causes a significant increase in ECF osmolality. A rapid increase in ECF glucose can result in cellular dehydration as water moves from the ICF to the ECF compartment in response to the increase in ECF osmolality. Neurologic signs develop as a consequence of neuronal dehydration in the CNS. Neurons in the central nervous system produce osmotically active substances including lactate, sorbitol, myoinositol, and idiogenic osmoles to compensate for the increasing osmolality of the ECF and prevent cellular dehydration. These intracellular substances can cause water to diffuse into the cell if the osmolality within the cell exceeds that within the ECF space. Idiogenic osmols within the neurons of a severely hyperglycemic animal are not associated with an osmotic gradient because of the equilibrium between the hyperosmotic ECF space (induced by glucose) and the hyperosmotic intracellular space (induced by idiogenic osmols). However, with aggressive fluid therapy and exogenous insulin administration, rapid reduction in blood glucose concentration and improved renal perfusion may cause a rapid reduction in ECF osmolality. A relative excess in free water accumulates in the ECF space. This water can then diffuse into the idiogenic osmol-induced hyperosmotic brain cells. A rapid decline in blood glucose concentration can thus result in cerebral edema and worsening CNS function. For these reasons, the veterinarian must be aware of the CNS status of the animal before initiation of therapy. If the animal becomes depressed or obtunded during treatment, it may be the result of the relatively rapidly decreasing blood glucose concentration leading to cerebral edema.

Mannitol is the most effective treatment for cerebral edema (see page 608). Dexamethasone is usually recommended, but its efficacy has not been evaluated in diabetic animals. Passive hyperventilation to lower carbon dioxide pressure and diminish cerebral blood flow has also been recommended. Prophylactically avoiding cerebral edema through slow but progressive therapy is the critical lesson to be learned from the work of other investigators.

SEVERE HYPERNATREMIA AND HYPERCHLOREMIA. Occasionally, animals with DKA develop severe hypernatremia and hyperchloremia (see Fig. 13-9) as a result of water deprivation (i.e., inadequate fluid intake) in conjunction with urinary loss of large amounts of water in excess of electrolytes. Loss of water in excess of electrolytes creates hypertonic dehydration, a state of dehydration with few of the expected signs of severe fluid depletion (Edwards et al, 1983). Worsening hypernatremia, in combination with hyperglycemia, causes severe hyperosmolality (>400 mOsm/kg) and CNS dysfunction. The initial critical signs of hypernatremia include irritability, weakness, and ataxia, but as the hypernatremia worsens, stupor progresses to coma and seizures. The progression and severity of these signs depend on the rate of onset, degree, and duration of hypernatremia. Therapy should be designed to replace fluid deficits, match continuing fluid losses, and decrease those losses when possible. (See Chapter 1, page 31, for details on the treatment of hypernatremic, hypertonic dehydration.)

It is important to consider factors that can result in artifactual changes in serum sodium concentrations. Severe lipemia can appear to raise the serum sodium concentration because lipemia displaces sodium into the nonlipemic volume of serum, making a normal serum sodium concentration appear increased. Hyperglycemia can also alter the serum sodium concentration. For each 100 mg/dl increment of serum glucose above the normal range, the serum sodium concentration decreases approximately 1.6 mEq/L (i.e., a dog with a blood glucose concentration of 500 mg/dl and a laboratory serum sodium concentration of 135 mEq/L has a "corrected" serum sodium concentration of approximately 142 mEq/L) (DiBartola, 2000).

SEVERE HYPOKALEMIA. Dogs and cats with DKA are at risk for development of severe hypokalemia (<2.0 mEq/L) during the initial 48 hours of therapy for reasons discussed on page 600. The most common clinical sign of hypokalemia is generalized skeletal muscle weakness. In cats, ventroflexion of the neck, forelimb hypermetria, and a broad-based hindlimb stance may be observed. Cardiac consequences of hypokalemia include decreased myocardial contractility, decreased cardiac output, and disturbances in cardiac rhythm. Other metabolic effects of hypokalemia include hypokalemic nephropathy, which is characterized by chronic tubulointerstitial nephritis, impaired renal function, and azotemia and manifested clinically as polyuria, polydipsia, and impaired urine concentrating capability; hypokalemic polymyopathy, which is characterized by increased serum creatine kinase activity and electromyographic abnormalities; and paralytic ileus, manifested clinically as abdominal distention, anorexia, vomiting, and constipation (DiBartola and de Morais, 2000). Hypokalemic nephropathy and polymyopathy are most notable in cats. Cats seem more susceptible to the deleterious effects of hypokalemia than do dogs. In dogs, signs may not be evident until the serum potassium concentration is less than 2.5 mEq/L, whereas in cats signs can be seen with serum potassium concentrations between 3 and 3.5 mEq/L. Clinical signs of hypokalemia can be mistakenly ascribed to other commonly encountered concurrent disorders (e.g., pancreatitis), and hypokalemia may be overlooked as a possible cause. Initial aggressive potassium replacement therapy, frequent monitoring of serum electrolytes, and subsequent adjustments in potassium replacement therapy are necessary to identify and prevent hypokalemia.

HEMOLYTIC ANEMIA. Life-threatening hemolytic anemia may develop during the initial 72 hours of therapy as a consequence of hypophosphatemia (see page 601) (Willard et al, 1987; Adams et al, 1993; Bruskiewicz et al,1997). The mechanism of hypophosphatemia-induced hemolysis is not known, but hemolysis may occur secondary to depletion of erythrocyte adenosine triphosphate (ATP), which is necessary for maintenance of cell membrane integrity; malfunction of the sodium-potassium pump secondary to erythrocyte ATP depletion and subsequent osmotic lysis; or alterations in red blood cell membrane lipids (Shilo et al, 1985; Adams et al, 1993).

Hypophosphatemia-induced hemolytic anemia can be serious, with hematocrits less than 15% reported in dogs and cats (Willard et al, 1987; Adams et al, 1993). Additional findings on a CBC include spherocytes, Heinz bodies, and hemoglobinemia. Treatment involves the intravenous administration of phosphate (see page 601) and, if necessary, blood. Prevention of hypophosphatemia is the key to avoiding hemolytic anemia. Frequent monitoring of serum phosphorus concentration during the initial 24 to 48 hours of therapy for DKA and supplementation of the intravenous fluids with potassium or sodium phosphate when hypophosphatemia is identified are the cornerstones of prevention.

PROGNOSIS

DKA remains one of the most difficult metabolic therapeutic challenges in veterinary medicine. One must remain aware of all the complicating factors in treatment and remember that fluid therapy, insulin replacement, and potassium supplementation are the keys to successful management. Added to these factors are close supervision and monitoring of the animal, without which failure rates are high.

In humans, the mortality associated with DKA remains high (5% to 10%); however, diabetic humans rarely die of the metabolic complications of ketoacidosis (DeFronzo et al, 1994; Wagner et al, 1999). The persistently high mortality relates to the underlying medical disorders (e.g., infection, pancreatitis) that precipitate the DKA. Experiences in diabetic dogs and cats with DKA are similar (Macintire, 1993; Bruskiewicz et al, 1997). It is perhaps wise to reiterate that a careful search should always be made, at the time of initial history and physical examination and during therapy, for underlying problems that might have precipitated the episode of DKA. In particular, pneumonia, sepsis, pancreatitis, and hormonal diseases causing insulin resistance are often silent at the time of presentation.

Despite all precautions and diligent therapy, a fatal outcome cannot be avoided in some cases. In one study, 6 (29%) of 21 dogs with DKA died during initial therapy, primarily as a result of severe concurrent illness (Macintire, 1993). In our hospital, approximately 25% of cats and dogs presenting with severe DKA die or are euthanized during the initial hospitalization (Bruskiewicz et al, 1997). Death is usually the result of severe underlying illness (e.g., oliguric renal failure, necrotizing pancreatitis), severe metabolic acidosis (arterial pH <7), or development of complications (e.g., cerebral edema) during therapy. Nevertheless, with logical therapy and careful animal monitoring, the goal of therapy for diabetic ketoacidosis (i.e., achieving a healthy diabetic dog or cat) is attainable.

HYPEROSMOLAR NONKETOTIC DIABETES MELLITUS

Diabetic hyperosmolar nonketotic syndrome (DHNS) is an uncommon complication of diabetes mellitus in the dog and cat. This syndrome is characterized by severe hyperglycemia (blood glucose concentration >600 mg/dl), hyperosmolality (>350 mOsm/kg), and dehydration in the absence of significant ketosis. Progressively worsening lethargy ultimately leads to obtundation and coma as hyperosmolality becomes more severe. Underlying renal failure or congestive heart failure is common, and the presence of either worsens the prognosis. Additional precipitating disorders (e.g., sepsis, pancreatitis, glucocorticoids) contribute to the progression of this syndrome. DHNS is a remarkable diagnostic and therapeutic challenge because it is associated with a high fatality rate.

Pathogenesis

The pathogenesis of DHNS is similar to that of diabetic ketoacidosis—a partial or relative insulin deficiency reduces glucose utilization by muscle, fat, and the liver while at the same time inducing hyperglucagonemia and increasing hepatic glucose output. The result is hyperglycemia that leads to glycosuria and osmotic diuresis with obligatory water loss. In DHNS, a small population of functional beta cells exists and is capable of secreting insulin, albeit in insufficient amounts to prevent hyperglycemia. However, the presence of small amounts of insulin is believed to prevent the development of ketosis by inhibiting lipolysis (see page 580). Therefore, even though a low insulin: glucagon ratio promotes ketogenesis in the liver, the limited availability of precursor FFAs from the periphery restricts the rate at which ketones are formed

(Ennis et al, 1994). Hepatic resistance to glucagon may also play a role in the lack of ketosis with DHNS (Yen et al, 1980; Azain et al, 1985).

If a dog or cat is unable to maintain adequate fluid intake because of an associated acute or chronic illness (e.g., pancreatitis) or has suffered excessive fluid loss (e.g., diuretics for concurrent congestive heart failure), marked dehydration results. As plasma volume contracts, glomerular filtration is impaired, limiting renal glucose excretion and contributing markedly to the rise in blood glucose and plasma osmolality. As plasma osmolality increases, water is drawn out of cerebral neurons, resulting in mental obtundation and further impairment of water intake. A vicious cycle of worsening hyperosmolality, obtundation, inadequate fluid intake, and renal insufficiency ensues, ultimately resulting in coma and death.

The hyperglycemia of DHNS (600 to 1600 mg/dl) tends to be more severe than the hyperglycemia of DKA (300 to 800 mg/dl). The increase in blood glucose concentration in DHNS is, as in DKA, the result of increased production of glucose by the liver coupled with its diminished use by tissues. However, two additional factors in DHNS allow the hyperglycemia to become more severe. First, impaired urine output in DHNS diminishes excretion of glucose in urine (Foster and McGarry, 1989). Second, lack of ketosis in DHNS removes an important and early contributor to clinical signs. As a consequence, the hyperglycemia of DHNS progresses for a longer period of time, and it is not until signs of severe hyperosmolality (i.e., lethargy, obtundation) or signs related to concurrent problems become evident to the owner that veterinary care is sought.

Some dogs and cats with DHNS are acidotic despite low or undetectable concentrations of ketoacids in the plasma or urine. One cause for this disparity in expected versus real results is the fact that β-hydroxybutyrate (one of two major ketoacids) is not assayed by commonly used urine and plasma reagent strips or tablets. Unrecognized ketoacidosis appears to be a rare entity in dogs and cats. Another cause for acidosis in nonketotic diabetics is lactic acidosis. Lactic acid is the end product of anaerobic metabolism of glucose. The principal sources of this acid are erythrocytes (which lack the enzymes for aerobic oxidation), skeletal muscle, skin, and brain. Lactic acid is removed via hepatic, and to some degree renal, uptake with conversion first to pyruvate and eventually back to glucose, a process that requires oxygen. Lactic acidosis occurs when excess lactic acid accumulates in the blood. This can be the result of overproduction (tissue hypoxia), deficient removal (hepatic failure), or both (circulatory collapse). Like humans, dogs and cats with lactic acidosis are usually severely ill, with problems such as sepsis, anemia, pulmonary disease, liver disease, and renal failure.

Clinical Findings

CLINICAL SIGNS. The onset of DHNS may be insidious and preceded for days or weeks by the classic signs of diabetes mellitus (polydipsia, polyuria, polyphagia, and weight loss). Progressive weakness, anorexia, and lethargy develop, usually in conjunction with a reduction in water intake. Additional clinical signs depend on the underlying precipitating disorder(s). Physical examination often reveals the presence of profound dehydration. These pets are typically lethargic, extremely depressed, or actually comatose. There is a direct relationship between the severity of the hyperosmolality and the severity of neurologic signs. Hypothermia and slow capillary refill time are common. Kussmaul respirations are absent unless severe metabolic (lactic) acidosis is present.

LABORATORY FINDINGS. Severe hyperglycemia is present, with blood glucose concentrations ranging from 600 to as high as 1600 mg/dl. Virtually all of our animals with DHNS have had severe prerenal or renal azotemia. These animals all have considerably depleted body potassium stores, despite the fact that serum potassium concentrations can be high, normal, or low. Serum sodium concentrations are also variable. In mild cases, in which dehydration is less severe, dilutional hyponatremia as well as urinary sodium losses may reduce serum sodium concentrations to less than 130 mEq/L. This relative hyponatremia protects, to some extent, against extreme hyperosmolality. As dehydration progresses, however, the serum sodium concentration may exceed 145 mEq/L, producing serum osmolalities greater than 400 mOsm/L. Hyperosmolality is a consistent finding in DHNS. Plasma osmolality may be measured by determination of its freezing point with an osmometer or calculated using the formula given on page 591. The artifactual changes of severe hyperglycemia on serum sodium results should be considered when assessing serum sodium concentrations in dogs and cats with DHNS (see page 589).

Ketosis is usually absent. A small degree of ketosis is seen in humans who are fasting (Ennis et al, 1994), but this is uncommon in the dog or cat. Acidosis is not a part of the hyperglycemic hyperosmolar state, but it may be present (usually in the form of lactic acidosis) as a result of underlying conditions (see previous section on Pathogenesis). Lactic acidosis depresses plasma bicarbonate concentrations and the arterial pH. An anion gap is present (see page 591). Other causes of "anion gap" metabolic acidosis should be excluded (see Table 13-4). The diagnosis of lactic acidosis can be confirmed by measuring plasma lactate concentration.

Therapy

The goals of therapy for DHNS are similar to those for DKA, that is, to correct severe dehydration and restore electrolyte losses, to provide adequate amounts of insulin to normalize intermediary metabolism, to correct the hyperosmolar state, and to identify and treat precipitating factors. Restoring intravascular volume and lost electrolytes using isotonic fluids has the highest priority. Osmolality is returned to normal by lowering the blood glucose concentration and by replacing water deficits. Initially, fluid therapy is used to lower the blood glucose concentration; insulin should not be administered until intravascular volume is restored and blood pressure is stabilized. Careful and frequent monitoring of the dog's or cat's clinical and laboratory response to therapy is essential.

Fluid therapy is of paramount importance in treating DHNS and is the primary mode of therapy for the initial 4 to 6 hours. Total body water, sodium and potassium deficiencies, hyperglycemia, and hyperosmolality are usually severe, in part because the lack of ketoacidosis and associated systemic signs of illness allows DHNS to develop for a longer period of time before veterinary care is sought. Despite the severe hyperosmolality, the initial fluid of choice is isotonic (0.9%) saline with appropriate potassium supplementation. Isotonic saline will correct dehydration and improve blood flow to tissues, stabilize blood pressure, improve GFR and promote glycosuria, decrease blood glucose concentration, and replace sodium for glucose in the ECF space. The net effect is a slow reduction in ECF hyperosmolality, thereby minimizing development of cerebral edema (see page 611). Half of the estimated dehydration deficit plus maintenance requirements should be replaced in the first 12 hours and the remainder in the next 24 hours.

The principles of potassium and phosphorus supplementation are similar to those discussed for DKA (see pages 600 and 601). Most dogs and cats with DHNS are also in renal failure (often oliguric) and may have hyperkalemia, hyperphosphatemia, and/or impaired ability to excrete a potassium load. As such, potassium and phosphorus supplementation should be based on measurement of serum concentrations and awareness of the status of renal function and urine production. Usually, initial therapy consists of 20 mEq/L of potassium replacement (as potassium chloride) into the infusion fluids. Subsequent adjustments are based on measurements of serum electrolytes, which should be done frequently to quickly identify problems in serum electrolyte concentrations, should they arise.

Insulin therapy should be delayed (typically 4 to 6 hours) until the positive benefits of fluid therapy are documented, that is, correction of dehydration, stabilization of blood pressure, and improvement in urine production, hyperglycemia, hyperosmolality, and derangements in serum electrolyte concentrations. The need for insulin treatment is not as critical with DHNS as with DKA, in part because ketone production and its metabolic consequences are minimal to nonexistent with DHNS. Metabolic acidosis, if identified in DHNS, is more likely caused by lactic acidosis, which can be improved with fluid therapy. In addition, insulin can cause a rapid decrease in the blood glucose concentration and ECF osmolality, changes which promote cerebral edema (see page 611). The techniques for insulin administration are similar to those discussed for DKA (see page 603). However, the insulin dosage used for the hourly intramuscular technique or the insulin infusion rate used for the constant low-dose insulin infusion technique should be decreased by 50% initially to dampen the decrease in the blood glucose concentration and to avoid a rapid decrease in ECF osmolality. Subsequent adjustments in the amount of insulin being administered are based on the rate of decline in the blood glucose concentration. The goal is a decrease of 50 mg/dl/hr, although the rate of decrease is difficult to predict or control, in part because of differences in insulin sensitivity among animals. Once the blood glucose concentration approaches 250 mg/dl, dextrose should be added to the IV fluids to make a 5% dextrose solution.

Monitoring urine output, blood pressure, blood glucose, serum electrolytes, BUN, and urine glucose is imperative. As with ketoacidosis, the clinician must attempt to correct the hyperosmolality, hyperglycemia, and dehydration steadily (not precipitously) while stimulating diuresis to lower the BUN. These animals are critically ill and require close supervision.

The prognosis for recovery is poor to grave. The most common cause of death in our animals is renal failure.

REFERENCES

Abbott LG, Rude RK: Clinical manifestations of magnesium deficiency. Miner Electrolyte Metab 19:314, 1993.

Adams LG, et al: Hypophosphatemia and hemolytic anemia associated with diabetes mellitus and hepatic lipidosis in cats. J Vet Intern Med 7:266, 1993.

Adrogué HJ, et al: Plasma acid-base patterns in diabetic ketoacidosis. N Engl J Med 307:1603, 1982.

Adrogué HJ, et al: Diabetic ketoacidosis: Role of the kidney in acid-base homeostasis reevaluated. Kidney Int 25:591, 1984.

Azain MJ, et al: Contributions of fatty acid and sterol synthesis to triglyceride and cholesterol secretion by the perfused rat liver in genetic hyperlipemia and obesity. J Biol Chem 260:174, 1985.

Barrett EJ, DeFronzo RA: Diabetic ketoacidosis: Diagnosis and treatment. Hosp Pract 19:89, 1984.

Becker DJ, et al: Phosphate replacement during treatment of diabetic ketosis. Effects on calcium and phosphorus homeostasis. Am J Dis Child 137:241, 1983.

Boord M, Griffin C: Progesterone secreting adrenal mass in a cat with clinical signs of hyperadrenocorticism. J Am Vet Med Assoc 214:666, 1999.

Boyle PJ: Cushing's disease, glucocorticoid excess, glucocorticoid deficiency, and diabetes. Diabetes Rev 1:301, 1993.

Bratusch-Marrain PR, et al: The effect of growth hormone on glucose metabolism and insulin secretion in man. J Clin Endocrinol Metab 55:131, 1982.

Bruskiewicz KA, et al: Diabetic ketosis and ketoacidosis in cats: 42 cases (1980–1995). J Am Vet Med Assoc 211:188, 1997.

Burns MG, et al: Pulmonary artery thrombosis in three dogs with hyperadrenocorticism. JAVMA 178:388, 1981.

Bush WW, et al: Secondary hypoparathyroidism attributed to hypomagnesemia in a dog with protein-losing enteropathy. J Am Vet Med Assoc 219:1732, 2001.

Chastain CB, Nichols CS: Low-dose intramuscular insulin therapy for diabetic ketoacidosis in dogs. JAVMA 178:561, 1981.

Cherrington AD, et al: Insulin, glucagon, and glucose as regulators of hepatic glucose uptake and production in vivo. Diabetes Metab Rev 3:307, 1987.

Church DB: Diabetes mellitus. In Kirk RW (ed): Current Veterinary Therapy VIII. Philadelphia, WB Saunders Co, 1983, p 838.

Cryer PE: Catecholamines, pheochromocytoma, and diabetes. Diabetes Rev 1:309, 1993.

Cryer PE, Polonsky KS: Glucose homeostasis and hypoglycemia. In Wilson JD, Foster DW, Kronenberg HM, Larsen PR (eds): Williams Textbook of Endocrinology, 9th ed. Philadelphia, WB Saunders Co, 1998, p 939.

DeFronzo RA, et al: Diabetic ketoacidosis. A combined metabolic-nephrologic approach to therapy. Diabetes Rev 2:209, 1994.

DeFronzo RA, Ferrannini E: Insulin action in vivo: Protein metabolism. *In* Alberti KGMM, et al (eds): International Textbook of Diabetes Mellitus. Chichester, UK, Wiley, 1992, p 467.

Dhupa N: Magnesium therapy. *In* Bonagura JD (ed): Kirk's Current Veterinary Therapy XII. Philadelphia, WB Saunders Co, 1995, p. 132.

Dhupa N, Shaffran N: Continuous rate infusion formulas. *In* Ettinger SJ, Feldman EC (eds): Textbook of Veterinary Internal Medicine, 4th ed. Philadelphia, WB Saunders Co, 1995, p 2130.

Dhupa N, Proulx J: Hypocalcemia and hypomagnesemia. Vet Clin North Am Small Anim Pract 28:587, 1998.

DiBartola SP: Disorders of sodium and water. *In* DiBartola SP (ed): Fluid Therapy in Small Animal Practice, 2nd ed. Philadelphia, WB Saunders Co, 2000, p 45.

DiBartola SP, de Morais HA: Disorders of potassium. *In* DiBartola SP (ed): Fluid Therapy in Small Animal Practice, 2nd ed. Philadelphia, WB Saunders Co, 2000, p 83.

Duarte R, et al: Accuracy of serum β-hydroxybutyrate measurements for the diagnosis of diabetic ketoacidosis in 116 dogs. J Vet Intern Med 16:411, 2002.

Edwards DF, et al: Hypernatremic, hypertonic dehydration in the dog with diabetes insipidus and gastric dilatation-volvulus. JAVMA 182:973, 1983.

Ennis ED, et al: The hyperosmolar hyperglycemic syndrome. Diabetes Rev 2:115, 1994.

Ewensteim BM: Antithrombotic agents and thromboembolic disease. N Engl J Med 337:1383, 1997.

Farfournoux P, et al: Mechanisms involved in ketone body release by rat liver cells: Influence of pH and bicarbonate. Am J Physiol 252:G200, 1987.

Feldman BF, Rosenberg DP: Clinical use of anion and osmolal gaps in veterinary medicine. JAVMA 178:396, 1981.

Feldman EC: Diabetic ketoacidosis in dogs. Comp Cont Educ 11:456, 1980.

Feldman EC, Nelson RW: Canine and Feline Endocrinology and Reproduction. Philadelphia, WB Saunders Co, 1987.

Ferrannini E, et al: Effect of free fatty acids on glucose production and utilization in man. J Clin Invest 72:1737, 1983.

Fisher JN, Kitabchi AE: A randomized study of phosphate therapy in the treatment of diabetic ketoacidosis. J Clin Endocrinol Metab 57:177, 1983.

Fluckiger MA, Gomez JA: Radiographic findings in dogs with spontaneous pulmonary thromboembolism or embolism. Vet Radiol 25:124, 1984.

Forrester SD, Moreland KJ: Hypophosphatemia. Causes and clinical consequences. J Vet Intern Med 3:149, 1989.

Foster DW, McGarry JD: The metabolic derangements and treatment of diabetic ketoacidosis. N Engl J Med 309:159, 1983.

Foster DW, McGarry JD: Acute complications of diabetes: Ketoacidosis, hyperosmolar coma, lactic acidosis. *In* DeGroot LJ (ed): Endocrinology, 2nd ed. Philadelphia, WB Saunders Co, 1989, p 1439.

Gerhardt A, et al: Comparison of the sensitivity of different diagnostic tests for pancreatitis in cats. J Vet Intern Med 15:329, 2001.

Goldstein DE: Tests of glycemia in diabetes. Diabetes Care 18:896, 1995.

Goossens MMC, et al: Response to insulin treatment and survival in 104 cats with diabetes mellitus (1985-1995). J Vet Intern Med 12:1, 1998.

Groop LC, et al: Effect of insulin on oxidative and non-oxidative pathways of glucose and FFA metabolism in NIDDM. Evidence for multiple sites of insulin resistance. J Clin Invest 84:205, 1989.

Hale RJ, et al: Metabolic effects of bicarbonate in the treatment of diabetic ketoacidosis. Br Med J 289:1035, 1984.

Hansen B: Disorders of magnesium. *In* DiBartola SP (ed): Fluid Therapy in Small Animal Practice, 2nd ed. Philadelphia, WB Saunders Co, 2000, p. 175.

Hawkins EC: Disorders of the Pulmonary Parenchyma. *In* Nelson RW, Couto CG (eds): Small Animal Internal Medicine, 3rd ed. St Louis, Mosby Inc, 2003, p. 299.

Hess RS, et al: Clinical, clinicopathologic, radiographic, and ultrasonographic abnormalities in dogs with fatal acute pancreatitis: 70 cases (1986-1995). J Am Vet Med Assoc 213:665, 1998.

Hess RS, et al: Concurrent disorders in dogs with diabetes mellitus: 221 cases (1993-1998). J Am Vet Med Assoc 217:1166, 2000.

Hood VL, Tannen RL: Maintenance of acid-base homeostasis during ketoacidosis and lactic acidosis. Implications for therapy. Diabetes Rev 2:177, 1994.

Horner HC, et al: Dexamethasone causes translocation of glucose transporters from the plasma membrane to an intracellular site in human fibroblasts. J Biol Chem 262:17696, 1987.

Jacoby RC, et al: Biochemical basis for the hypercoagulable state seen in Cushing's syndrome. Arch Surg 136:1003, 2001.

Joshi N, et al: Infections in patients with diabetes mellitus. N Engl J Med 341:1906, 1999.

Kandel G, Aberman A: Selected developments in the understanding of diabetic ketoacidosis. Can Med Assoc J 128:392, 1983.

Kaplan AJ, et al: Effects of disease on the results of diagnostic tests for use in detecting hyperadrenocorticism in dogs. J Am Vet Med Assoc 207:445, 1995.

Kitabchi AE, Wall BM: Diabetic ketoacidosis. Med Clin North Am 79:9, 1995.

Kitabchi AE, et al: Management of hyperglycemic crises in patients with diabetes. Diabetes Care 24:131, 2001.

LaRue MJ, Murtaugh RJ: Pulmonary thromboembolism in dogs: 47 cases (1986–1987). J Am Vet Med Assoc 197:1368, 1990.

Lebovitz HE: Diabetic ketoacidosis. Lancet 345:767, 1995.

Lever N, Jaspan J: Sodium bicarbonate therapy in severe diabetic ketoacidosis. Am J Med 75:263, 1983.

Li PK, et al: Direct, fixed time kinetic assays for β-hydroxybutyrate and acetoacetate with a centrifugal analyzer or a computer-baked spectrophotometer. Clin Chem 26:1713, 1980.

Luzi L, et al: Metabolic effects of low-dose insulin therapy on glucose metabolism in diabetic ketoacidosis. Diabetes 37:1470, 1988.

Martin L, et al: Magnesium in the 1990's: Implications for veterinary critical care. J Vet Emerg Crit Care 3:105, 1993.

Masharani U, Karam JH: Pancreatic hormones and diabetes mellitus. *In* Greenspan FS, Gardner DG (eds): Basic and Clinical Endocrinology, 6th ed. New York, McGraw-Hill, 2001, p 623.

Macintire DK: Treatment of diabetic ketoacidosis in dogs by continuous low-dose intravenous infusion of insulin. JAVMA 202:1266, 1993.

Macintire DK: Emergency therapy of diabetic crises: Insulin overdose, diabetic ketoacidosis, and hyperosmolar coma. Vet Clin North Am Small Anim Pract 25:639, 1995.

McGarry JD, et al: Regulation of ketogenesis and the renaissance of carnitine palmitoyltransferase. Diabetes Metab Rev 5:271, 1989.

McMahon MM, Bistrian BR: Host defenses and susceptibility to infection in patients with diabetes mellitus. Infect Dis Clin North Am 9:1, 1995.

Molitch ME, et al: Spurious serum creatinine elevations in ketoacidosis. Ann Intern Med 93:290, 1980.

Morris LR, et al: Bicarbonate therapy in severe diabetic ketoacidosis. Ann Intern Med 105:836, 1986.

Nanji AA, Campbell DJ: Falsely elevated serum creatinine values in diabetic ketoacidosis—clinical implications. Clin Biochem 14:91, 1981.

Narins RG, et al: The metabolic acidoses. *In* Maxwell MH, Kleeman CR (eds): Clinical Disorders of Fluid and Electrolyte Metabolism. New York, McGraw-Hill, 1994, p 769.

Nelson RW, et al: Absorption kinetics of regular insulin in dogs with alloxan-induced diabetes mellitus. Am J Vet Res 51:1671, 1990.

Nichols R, Crenshaw KL: Complications and concurrent disease associated with diabetic ketoacidosis and other severe forms of diabetes mellitus. Vet Clin N Amer Small Anim Pract 25:617, 1995.

Norris CR, et al: Serum total and ionized magnesium concentrations and urinary fractional excretion of magnesium in cats with diabetes mellitus and diabetic ketoacidosis. J Am Vet Med Assoc 215:1455, 1999.

Norris CR, et al: Effect of a magnesium-deficient diet on serum and urine magnesium concentrations in healthy cats. Am J Vet Res 60:1159, 1999b.

Okuda Y, et al: Time course of ketone body production in the isolated perfused rat liver in response to various stimuli. Endocrinol Jpn 33:827, 1986a.

Okuda Y, et al: Counterproductive effects of sodium bicarbonate in diabetic ketoacidosis. J Clin Endocrinol Metab 81:314, 1996.

Owen OE, et al: Effects of therapy on the nature and quantity of fuels oxidized during diabetic ketoacidosis. Diabetes 29:365, 1980.

Owen OE, et al: Renal function and effects of partial rehydration during diabetic ketoacidosis. Diabetes 30:510, 1981.

Peikes H, et al: Dermatologic disorders in dogs with diabetes mellitus: 45 cases (1986-2000). J Am Vet Med Assoc 219:203, 2001.

Peterson ME: Effects of megestrol acetate on glucose tolerance and growth hormone secretion in the cat. Res Vet Sci 42:354, 1987.

Rossmeisl JH, et al: Hyperadrenocorticism and hyperprogesteronemia in a cat with an adrenocortical adenocarcinoma. J Am Anim Hosp Assoc 36:512, 2000.

Ryder RE: Lactic acidosis: High-dose or low-dose bicarbonate therapy? Diabetes Care 7:99, 1984.

Sherwin RS, et al: Epinephrine and the regulation of glucose metabolism. Effect of diabetes and hormonal interactions. Metabolism 29(Suppl 1):1146, 1980.

Shilo S, et al: Acute hemolytic anemia caused by severe hypophosphatemia in diabetic ketoacidosis. Acta Haematol 73:55, 1985.

Swift NC, et al: Evaluation of serum feline trypsin-like immunoreactivity for the diagnosis of pancreatitis in cats. J Am Vet Med Assoc 217:37, 2000.

Tessari P, et al: Hyperaminoacidemia reduces insulin-mediated glucose disposal in healthy man. Diabetologia 28:870, 1985.

Thiebaud D, et al: Effect of long chain triglyceride infusion on glucose metabolism in man. Metabolism 21:1128, 1982.

Viallon A, et al: Does bicarbonate therapy improve the management of severe diabetic ketoacidosis? Crit Care Med 27:2690, 1999.

Wagner A, et al: Therapy of severe diabetic ketoacidosis: zero-mortality under very-low-dose insulin application. Diabetes Care 22:674, 1999.

Whittaker J, et al: Impaired insulin binding in diabetic ketoacidosis. Diabetologia 21:563, 1981.

Willard MD, et al: Severe hypophosphatemia associated with diabetes mellitus in six dogs and one cat. JAVMA 190:1007, 1987.

Wolfsheimer KJ, Peterson ME: Erythrocyte insulin receptors in dogs with spontaneous hyperadrenocorticism. Am J Vet Res 52:917, 1991.

Yeates S, Blaufuss J: Managing the animal in diabetic ketoacidosis. Focus Crit Care 17:240, 1990.

Yen TT, et al: Hepatic insensitivity to glucagon in ob/ob mice. Res Commun Chem Pathol Pharmacol 30:29, 1980.

Zammit VA: Regulation of ketone body metabolism: A cellular perspective. Diabetes Rev 2:132, 1994.

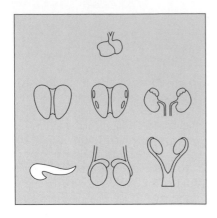

14

BETA-CELL NEOPLASIA: INSULINOMA

Insulin-secreting beta-cell tumors were first described in the dog by Slye and Wells in 1935. During the past 68 years, numerous publications have appeared in the veterinary literature addressing the clinical manifestations, diagnosis, treatment, and pathology of beta-cell tumors in dogs. Despite excellent documentation of this disease and well-established methods for determining the diagnosis, insulin-secreting beta-cell neoplasia remains an uncommon diagnosis in dogs and a rare entity in cats.

ETIOLOGY

Functional tumors arising from the beta cells of the pancreatic islets are malignant tumors that secrete insulin independent of the typically suppressive effects of hypoglycemia. Beta-cell tumors, however, are not completely autonomous, and they respond to provocative stimuli (e.g., glucose) by secreting insulin, often in excessive amounts. Immunohistochemical analysis of beta-cell tumors has revealed a high incidence of multihormonal production, including pancreatic polypeptide, somatostatin, glucagon, serotonin, and gastrin (Hawkins et al, 1987; O'Brien et al, 1987; Minkus et al, 1997). However, insulin has been the most common product demonstrated in the neoplastic cells, and the clinical signs in such animals are primarily those that result from a hyperinsulinemia-induced hypoglycemia.

MALIGNANT VERSUS BENIGN POTENTIAL. Beta-cell tumors are notorious for masking their malignant tendencies in the dog. Discrepancy is noted between the orderly arrangement of well-differentiated cells, the rarity of the mitotic figures seen in most islet cell tumors, and the frequent metastasis of beta-cell tumors (Kruth et al, 1982). Differentiation of malignant from benign neoplasia is usually based on identification of metastasis at surgery or necropsy, or the recurrence of hyperinsulinism weeks to months after surgical removal of a "solitary" pancreatic mass. Image analysis techniques applied to tumor tissue have also shown promise for differentiating between metastatic and nonmetastatic islet cell tumors (Minkus et al, 1997).

The malignant potential of beta-cell tumors is often underestimated in the dog. In our experience, virtually all beta-cell tumors in dogs are malignant, and most animals have microscopic or grossly visible metastatic lesions at the time of surgery. The most common sites of tumor spread are the regional lymphatics and lymph nodes (duodenal, mesenteric, hepatic, splenic), the liver, and the peripancreatic omentum. Pulmonary metastasis is rare. In most dogs, hypoglycemia recurs weeks to months after surgical excision of the tumor. The high incidence of metastasis at the time afflicted dogs are initially examined results in part from the typically protracted time for clinical signs to develop and become apparent to the owner and the interval between the time an owner initially observes signs and when assistance is sought from a veterinarian. Most dogs are symptomatic for 1 to 6 months before being brought to a veterinarian.

PATHOPHYSIOLOGY

The beta cells of the pancreatic islets are responsible for monitoring and controlling the blood glucose concentration. Unlike with most other cells, glucose enters beta cells independent of insulin. When the blood glucose concentration exceeds approximately 110 mg/dl, insulin is secreted and the blood glucose concentration declines into the normal physiologic range (i.e., 70 to 110 mg/dl). When the blood glucose concentration decreases below 60 mg/dl, normal insulin synthesis and secretion are inhibited, which limits tissue utilization of glucose and allows the blood glucose concentration to increase to the normal physiologic range. Minor fluctuations in insulin secretion maintain glucose concentrations in a narrower range.

Maintenance of euglycemia in the healthy dog

Cell metabolism and function depend on the delivery of energy sources via the circulation. Exogenously derived energy, in the form of ingested carbohydrate, fat, and protein, provides enough fuel for 4 to 8 hours of cell metabolism. After this postprandial period, fuel for cellular metabolism must be derived from endogenous sources, primarily through production of glucose by the liver (Fig. 14-1). The liver initially provides glucose by the breakdown of stored hepatic glycogen (glycogenolysis). Liver glycogen stores are exhausted slowly in dogs, requiring 2 to 3 days of fasting, compared with only 24 hours of fasting in humans (de Bruijne, 1982). Hepatic glucose production is augmented by gluconeogenesis as the postprandial period increases and hepatic glycogen stores become depleted (Rothman et al, 1991). Gluconeogenesis is the formation of glucose from precursors, including amino acids (especially alanine and glutamine), lactate, and glycerol. These substrates are delivered to the liver from peripheral stores. Muscle and other structural tissue supply amino acids, mainly alanine; blood cell elements supply lactate, the end product of glycolytic metabolism; and adipose tissue supplies glycerol from lipolysis of triglycerides (Karam, 2001). Oxidation of free fatty acids released from adipose cells during lipolysis supplies the energy required for gluconeogenesis and provides ketone bodies (i.e., acetoacetate, β-hydroxybutyrate), which can serve as alternative metabolic fuels for the central nervous system (CNS) during periods of prolonged fasting. Fatty acids are believed to be the major mediator of hepatic gluconeogenesis (Karam, 2001).

Hepatic glucose production depends on an adequate supply of substrates, including certain amino acids, glycerol, and free fatty acids mobilized from muscle and adipose tissue (Cryer and Polonsky, 1998). Other requirements include a normal hepatic circulation, functioning hepatocytes capable of removing substrates from the circulation, and a complete complement of hepatic enzymes capable of converting these noncarbohydrate precursors into glucose.

The renal cortex also has the requisite enzymes for the production and release of glucose into the circulation, albeit the contribution is only about 5% during fasting (Stumvoll et al, 1995; Gerich et al, 2001). However, renal glucose production is regulated, and under certain circumstances (e.g., glucose counterregulation, hepatic insufficiency), the contribution of glucose derived from renal gluconeogenesis can be as high as 40%. The kidney does not have glycogen stores and depends on gluconeogenesis as its only source of glucose production. Glutamine rather than alanine is the predominant amino acid substrate for renal gluconeogenesis. In addition to its contribution to glucose homeostasis during fasting, the kidney has been shown to be an important contributor to glucose counterregulation in the event of hypoglycemia. Although glucagon does not affect the kidney, the counterregulatory increase in epinephrine has been shown to stimulate gluconeogenesis in the renal cortex (Stumvall et al, 1995; Gerich et al, 2001).

A normally functioning endocrine system is also necessary to maintain glucose homeostasis and prevent hypoglycemia. Insulin is the dominant glucose-lowering hormone. It suppresses endogenous glucose production and stimulates glucose utilization. Glucose-raising or counterregulatory hormones include glucagon, epinephrine, growth hormone, and cortisol. These hormones increase hepatic glucose production by stimulating glycogenolysis and gluconeogenesis. They also inhibit glucose utilization by tissues (Cryer and Polonsky, 1998).

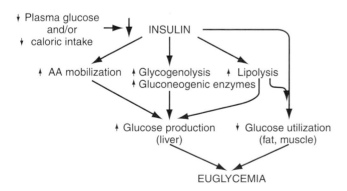

FIGURE 14-1. Hormonal and substrate changes by which euglycemia is maintained (and hypoglycemia is prevented) in normal subjects during a fast. The fall in the plasma insulin concentration is the key hormonal change resulting in increased glucose production and decreased glucose utilization. The decline in the plasma insulin concentration is, in turn, a result of a small decrease in the plasma glucose level (5 to 10 mg/dl) and/or a decrease in caloric intake.

Hypoglycemia and the counterregulatory response

Identification of a randomly obtained or fasting blood glucose concentration below 60 mg/dl is cause for concern in either dogs or cats. Although this finding is not always diagnostic of organic disease, "normal" dogs and cats have consistently been shown to not have blood glucose concentrations decline below this level. Therefore, once artifactual error has been eliminated as a possible cause, organic disease is a likely cause of persistent hypoglycemia (see page 623). Failure in any one of the steps involved in hepatic glucose production may result in hypoglycemia and its related clinical signs. Abnormalities affecting any of the key steps involved in the production and conservation of glucose may also cause hypoglycemia.

Under the usual metabolic conditions, the CNS is wholly dependent on plasma glucose and counteracts declining blood glucose concentrations with a carefully programmed neurogenic and hormonal response to mobilize storage depots of glycogen and fat and raise the plasma glucose concentration (Tables 14-1 and 14-2). Hepatic glycogen reserves and gluconeogenesis in the liver and kidney directly supply the CNS with glucose, and the mobilization of fatty acids from triglyceride depots provides energy for the large mass of skeletal and cardiac muscle, the renal cortex, the liver, and other tissues that use fatty acids as basic fuel; this spares glucose for use by tissues that remain dependent on glucose, including the CNS, erythrocytes, bone marrow, and renal medulla (Karam, 2001). The cascade of events leading to endogenous glucose production is initiated by a decreasing blood glucose concentration that eventually declines below a critical level (approximately 65 mg/dl). When this occurs, the autonomic nervous system and counterregulatory hormone response are stimulated to restore an adequate supply of glucose for cerebral function.

Hormones are the most important glucoregulatory factors, and glucose is the most important determinant of the secretion of glucoregulatory hormones. Insulin is the dominant glucose-lowering hormone. Hypo-

TABLE 14–1   AUTONOMIC NERVOUS SYSTEM RESPONSE TO HYPOGLYCEMIA

Alpha-Adrenergic Effects

Inhibition of endogenous insulin secretion
Stimulation of peripheral vasoconstriction causing increase in
  cerebral blood flow

Beta-Adrenergic Effects

Stimulation of hepatic and muscle glycogenolysis
Stimulation of plasma glucagon secretion
Stimulation of lipolysis generating free fatty acids
Impairment of glucose uptake by muscle
Increase in cardiac output causing increase in cerebral blood flow

Adrenomedullary Catecholamine Effects

Augmentation of alpha- and beta-adrenergic effects

Cholinergic Effects

Stimulation of pancreatic polypeptide secretion
Increase gastric motility
Produce hunger

Adapted from Karam JH: Hypoglycemic disorders. *In* Greenspan FS, Gardner DG (eds): Basic and Clinical Endocrinology, 6th ed. New York, Lange Medical Books/McGraw-Hill, 2001, p 702.

TABLE 14–2   INSULIN AND COUNTERREGULATORY HORMONAL RESPONSE TO HYPOGLYCEMIA

Insulin: Decreased Secretion

Reduced stimulation of beta cells by low glucose
Inhibition of insulin secretion by alpha-adrenergic nervous
  system and adrenomedullary catecholamines

Glucagon: Increased Secretion

Direct stimulation of alpha cells by low glucose
Stimulation of glucagon secretion by beta-adrenergic nervous
  system and adrenomedullary catecholamines

Catecholamines: Increased Secretion

Direct stimulation of sympathetic nervous system by low glucose
Direct secretion from the adrenal medulla in response to low
  glucose

ACTH and Cortisol: Increased Secretion

Direct stimulation of pituitary ACTH secretion in response to low
  glucose
Stimulation of pituitary-adrenocortical axis by the sympathetic
  nervous system

Growth Hormone: Increased Secretion

Direct stimulation of growth hormone in response to low glucose

glycemia suppresses insulin secretion, which facilitates the mobilization of energy from existing energy stores (glycogenolysis, lipolysis), promotes hepatic gluconeogenesis and ketogenesis, promotes renal gluconeogenesis, and decreases glucose utilization by insulin-dependent tissues (Cryer and Polonsky, 1998; Karam, 2001). Glucose-raising or counterregulatory hormones include glucagon, epinephrine, growth hormone, and cortisol (see Table 14-2). Insulin-induced hypoglycemia causes an increase in plasma glucagon, epinephrine, and norepinephrine concentrations at the onset of the glucose counterregulatory response, with increases in plasma growth hormone and cortisol occurring later. Glucagon is the key counterregulatory hormone affecting recovery from acute hypoglycemia, although its role in recovery from chronic hypoglycemia appears to be less influential (Cryer and Gerich, 1985). In response to falling plasma glucose levels, glucagon is secreted by the alpha cells of the pancreatic islets into the hepatic portal circulation; it acts exclusively on the liver to activate glycogenolysis and gluconeogenesis (Cryer and Polonsky, 1998). Hepatic glucose production increases within minutes.

The adrenergic-catecholamine response to hypoglycemia also plays a major role in recovery from hypoglycemia. Epinephrine has both direct and indirect effects, which stimulate hepatic glycogenolysis and hepatic and renal gluconeogenesis; provide muscle tissue with an alternative source of fuel by mobilizing muscle glycogen and stimulating lipolysis; mobilize gluconeogenic precursors (e.g., lactate, alanine, and glycerol); and inhibit glucose utilization by insulin-sensitive tissues (e.g., skeletal muscle) (Cryer, 1993; Karam, 2001). The role of cortisol and growth hormone in the acute response to hypoglycemia is probably minimal. Longer term elevation of cortisol facilitates lipolysis, promotes protein catabolism and the conversion of amino acids to glucose by the liver and kidney, and limits glucose utilization by insulin-dependent tissues. Similarly, growth hormone promotes lipolysis and antagonizes the action of insulin on glucose utilization in muscle cells. However, the hyperglycemic effects of cortisol and growth hormone do not appear for several hours after the hypoglycemic episode (Cryer and Polonsky, 1998). Cortisol and growth hormone play roles in the defense against prolonged hypoglycemia (Boyle and Cryer, 1991).

The adrenergic neurogenic response to hypoglycemia acts directly to raise the blood glucose concentration and to stimulate hormonal responses that augment the adrenergic mobilization of energy stores (see Table 14-1). In dogs, hepatic glucose autoregulation is also an important glucose counterregulatory factor (Cryer and Polonsky, 1998). That is, the rate of hepatic glucose production is an inverse function of the blood glucose concentration independent of hormonal and neural regulatory factors.

Regulation of insulin secretion in the healthy dog

The ratio between the blood insulin and glucose concentration appears to remain constant, even during a prolonged fast (de Bruijne et al, 1981). The beta cells of the pancreatic islets are primarily responsible for monitoring and controlling the blood glucose concentration. Unlike with most other cells, the entrance of glucose into beta cells occurs independent of insulin. When blood glucose concentrations exceed approximately 110 mg/dl, the insulin secretion rate increases and the blood glucose concentration declines. When blood glucose concentrations decrease below 60 mg/dl, insulin secretion is inhibited, which limits continued tissue utilization of glucose and increases the blood glucose concentration.

Insulin secretion in dogs with beta-cell neoplasia

In the dog or cat with an insulin-secreting tumor, neoplastic beta cells of the pancreas autonomously synthesize and release insulin despite hypoglycemia. As a result, tissue utilization of glucose continues, hypoglycemia progressively worsens, and signs eventually appear. The onset of clinical signs is related to both the degree of hypoglycemia achieved and the rate at which it occurs. For example, a blood glucose concentration that gradually drops to 35 mg/dl over an extended period (i.e., weeks) is much less likely to result in signs of hypoglycemia than is a blood glucose concentration of 35 mg/dl that develops rapidly over a few hours.

Failure of insulin secretion to decrease during periods of hypoglycemia predisposes a dog with a beta-cell tumor to the development of clinical signs of hypoglycemia during fasting and exercise. Insulin-secreting beta-cell tumors also remain responsive to many of the stimuli that promote insulin secretion in the healthy dog, but the secretory response is often exaggerated, resulting in severe hypoglycemia. For example, clinical signs of hypoglycemia often occur after consumption of food or intravenous administration of glucose to correct hypoglycemia (see page 621).

Mechanism for insulin-induced hypoglycemia

Insulin-secreting tumors and the associated hyper-insulinemia interfere with glucose homeostasis by decreasing the rate of glucose release from the liver and increasing the utilization of glucose by insulin-sensitive tissues (e.g., muscle, adipose tissue). Insulin interferes with mechanisms that promote hepatic glucose output by limiting circulating concentrations of substrates needed for gluconeogenesis. This effect is accomplished by inhibiting enzymes necessary for mobilizing amino acids from muscle and glycerol from adipose tissue. In addition, insulin decreases the activity of hepatic enzymes used in gluconeogenesis and glycogenolysis. Insulin also lowers blood glucose concentrations by stimulating glucose uptake and utilization in the liver, muscle, and adipose tissue. Thus insulin increases tissue utilization of glucose already present in the extracellular space while interfering with hepatic production of glucose. The net effect is decreasing blood glucose concentrations because of increased tissue utilization of glucose (see Feldman and Nelson, 1987 for references).

Origin of clinical signs

Glucose is the primary fuel used by the CNS. Carbohydrate reserves in neural tissue are limited, and function of these cells depends on a continuous supply of glucose from sources outside the CNS. If the blood glucose concentration drops below a critical level, nervous system dysfunction occurs. In mammals the cerebral cortex is the first area to be affected by a shortage of glucose. The metabolically slower vegetative centers in the brain stem have less demand for blood glucose and are affected after the cerebral cortex.

The entrance of glucose into the neurons of the CNS occurs primarily by diffusion and is not insulin dependent. Because cell membranes are impermeable to hydrophilic molecules such as glucose, all cells require carrier proteins to transport glucose across the lipid bilayers into the cytosol. All cells except those in the intestine and kidney have non-energy-dependent transporters that facilitate diffusion of glucose across cell membranes. At least five "facilitative glucose transporters" have been described in humans, and these are called GLUT 1 through GLUT 5, with the numbers designating the order of their identity (Table 14-3) (Masharani and Karam, 2001). GLUT 1 is present in all tissues, has a very high affinity for glucose, and appears to mediate basal glucose uptake. GLUT 1 is an important component of the brain vascular system (blood-brain barrier) that ensures adequate transport of plasma glucose into the CNS (Fig. 14-2). GLUT 3 is

TABLE 14–3   GLUCOSE TRANSPORTERS IDENTIFIED IN HUMANS

Name	Major Sites of Expression	Affinity for Glucose*
GLUT 1	Brain vasculature, red blood cells, all tissues	High (Km = 1 mmol/L)
GLUT 2	Liver, pancreatic B cells, serosal surfaces of gut and kidney	Low (Km = 15-20 mmol/L)
GLUT 3	Brain neurons, also found in all tissues	High (Km < 1 mmol/L)
GLUT 4	Muscle, fat cells	Medium (Km = 2.5 to 5 mmol/L)
GLUT 5	Jejunum, liver, spermatozoa	Medium (Km = 6 mmol/L)

From Masharani U, Karam JH: Pancreatic hormones and diabetes mellitus. *In* Greenspan FS, Gardner DG (eds): Basic and Clinical Endocrinology, 6th ed. New York, Lange Medical Books/McGraw-Hill, 2001, p 630.
*Km represents the level of blood glucose at which the transporter has reached one-half of its maximum capacity to transport glucose. It is inversely proportional to the affinity.

the major glucose transporter on the neuronal surface, has a very high affinity for glucose, and is responsible for transferring glucose from the cerebrospinal fluid into the neuronal cells.

Blood insulin concentrations do not affect neuronal glucose transport or utilization. However, if hyperinsulinemia results in an inadequate glucose supply for intracellular oxidative processes in neurons, a resultant decline occurs in energy-rich phosphorylated compounds (adenosine triphosphate [ATP]) in neurons. This in turn results in cellular changes typical of hypoxia, increased vascular permeability, vasospasm, vascular dilation, and edema. Neuron death from anoxia follows. In acute hypoglycemia, histologic alterations are most marked in the cerebral cortex, basal ganglia, hippocampus, and vasomotor centers (see Feldman and Nelson, 1987 for references). Although most of the damage from hypoglycemia occurs in the brain, peripheral nerve degeneration and demyelination are sometimes encountered (Braund et al, 1987). Other major organ systems, such as the heart, kidneys, and liver, also depend on glucose. However, an acute decrease in the blood glucose concentration results in clinical signs that involve the CNS before signs of any other major organ system dysfunction become apparent.

Prolonged, severe hypoglycemia may result in irreversible brain damage; however, it is uncommon for a dog to die during a hypoglycemic episode. Hypoglycemia is a potent stimulus for the release of the counterregulatory hormones that function to antagonize the effects of insulin and stimulate an increase in the blood glucose concentration (see Hypoglycemia and the Counterregulatory Response, page 617).

The clinical manifestations of hypoglycemia are believed to result from both a lack of glucose supply to the brain (neuroglycopenia) and stimulation of the sympathoadrenal system. The neuroglycopenic signs common to dogs include lethargy, weakness, ataxia, bizarre behavior, convulsions, and coma (Table 14-4).

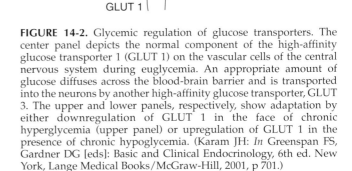

FIGURE 14-2. Glycemic regulation of glucose transporters. The center panel depicts the normal component of the high-affinity glucose transporter 1 (GLUT 1) on the vascular cells of the central nervous system during euglycemia. An appropriate amount of glucose diffuses across the blood-brain barrier and is transported into the neurons by another high-affinity glucose transporter, GLUT 3. The upper and lower panels, respectively, show adaptation by either downregulation of GLUT 1 in the face of chronic hyperglycemia (upper panel) or upregulation of GLUT 1 in the presence of chronic hypoglycemia. (Karam JH: *In* Greenspan FS, Gardner DG [eds]: Basic and Clinical Endocrinology, 6th ed. New York, Lange Medical Books/McGraw-Hill, 2001, p 701.)

Clinical signs resulting from stimulation of the sympathoadrenal system include muscle tremors, nervousness, restlessness, and hunger. In humans, the symptoms related to release of catecholamines often precede those of neuroglycopenia and act as an early warning sign of an impending hypoglycemic attack (Karam, 2001). This illustrates the rapid response of catecholamine secretion to hypoglycemia and partly explains why canine patients with insulin-secreting tumors do not always progress to generalized seizure activity during a fast.

Clinical manifestations depend on the duration and severity of hypoglycemia. Animals with chronic

TABLE 14–4 CLINICAL SIGNS ASSOCIATED WITH INSULIN-SECRETING TUMORS IN 91 DOGS

Clinical Sign	Number of Dogs	Percent
Seizures	51	56
Weakness	43	47
Collapse	27	30
Ataxia	17	19
Muscle fasciculations	16	18
Posterior weakness	15	16
Depression, lethargy	15	16
Bizarre behavior	11	12
Polyphagia	6	7
Polyuria, polydipsia	6	7
Weight gain	6	7
Diarrhea	4	4
Syncope	3	3
Nervousness	3	3
Head tilt	3	3
Anorexia	3	3
Urinary incontinence	2	2
Blindness	2	2
Panting	1	1

TABLE 14–5 BREED DISTRIBUTION OF 89 DOGS WITH ISLET CELL TUMORS

Breed	Number of Dogs	Percent
Labrador Retriever	12	13
Golden Retriever	10	11
German Shepherd	7	8
Irish Setter	6	7
Terriers (Fox, Kerry Blue, West Highland White, Norwich)	6	7
Poodle	6	7
Collie	5	6
Cocker Spaniel	5	6
Mixed-breeds	5	6
Doberman Pinscher	3	3
Boxer	3	3
Border Collie	3	3
Rottweiler	3	3
Samoyed	2	2
Other breeds (1 dog each)	13	15

and/or recurring fasting hypoglycemia appear to tolerate low blood glucose levels (i.e., 20 to 30 mg/dl) for prolonged periods without exhibiting clinical signs. In these dogs, slight reductions in the blood glucose level often produce symptomatic episodes. The "adaptation process" to chronic severe hypoglycemia is believed to involve "up-regulation" of the high-affinity glucose transporter GLUT 1 on the vascular cells forming the blood-brain barrier (see Fig. 14-2) (Karam, 2001).

CLINICAL FEATURES

Signalment

Insulin-secreting tumors typically occur in middle-aged or older dogs. The mean age at the time of diagnosis of an insulin-secreting tumor in 97 dogs in our series was 9.8 years, with a median age of 10 years and an age range of 3 to 14 years (Fig. 14-3). There is no gender predilection. A variety of breeds have been diagnosed with an insulin-secreting tumor at our hospital (Table 14-5). Labrador Retrievers, Golden Retrievers, and German Shepherd dogs are the breeds most commonly diagnosed with this disease, which is probably a reflection of breed popularity in our region rather than a breed predisposition per se. In general, insulin-secreting tumors occur more commonly in large breeds of dogs. However, the size of the dog should never preclude an investigation for an insulin-secreting tumor in a hypoglycemic dog. We have diagnosed insulin-secreting tumors in dogs as small as a Pomeranian.

History

Clinical signs of an insulin-secreting tumor may have been observed for more than a year or as briefly as 1 day before veterinary care is sought. Most dogs, however, are symptomatic for 1 to 6 months before being brought to a veterinarian. In our most recent 30 dogs with an insulin-secreting tumor, clinical signs had been observed by the owners for an average of 3 months (range, 2 days to 12 months) before veterinary care was sought.

The clinical signs of an insulin-secreting tumor typically are caused by neuroglycopenia (hypoglycemia) and an increase in circulating catecholamine concentrations; the signs include seizures, weakness, collapse, ataxia, muscle fasciculations, and bizarre behavior (see Table 14-4). One characteristic of hypoglycemic signs, regardless of the cause, is their episodic nature. Signs are generally observed intermittently for only a few seconds to minutes because of the compensatory counterregulatory mechanisms that usually increase the blood glucose concentration after the development of hypoglycemia. If these mechanisms are inadequate, seizures may occur as the blood glucose concentration

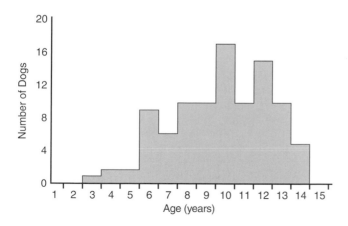

FIGURE 14-3. Age of 97 dogs at the time of initial diagnosis of an insulin-secreting islet cell tumor.

continues to decrease. Seizures are usually self-limiting, typically lasting from 30 seconds to 5 minutes. The seizure may stimulate further catecholamine secretion and other counterregulatory mechanisms that increase the blood glucose level above critical concentrations.

The severity of clinical signs depends on the duration and severity of the hypoglycemia. Dogs with chronic fasting hypoglycemia or with recurring episodes appear to tolerate low blood glucose concentrations (i.e., 20 to 30 mg/dl) for prolonged periods without clinical signs, and only small additional changes in the blood glucose concentration are then required to produce symptomatic episodes. As such, fasting, excitement, exercise, and eating may trigger the development of clinical signs. In the healthy, exercising dog, a balance between increased glucose utilization by muscle, decreased glucose utilization by other tissues, and increased glucose production by the liver maintains the circulating blood glucose concentration in the normal range, allowing the brain to continue to function. The exercising dog with an insulin-secreting tumor has continuing glucose utilization not just by muscle but by all tissues, owing to the autonomous and continuing secretion of insulin. In addition, hepatic release of glucose is impaired. The potential for severe hypoglycemia is great, and this fact is supported by the number of owners who associate symptoms in their pets with jogging, play, or long walks. A similar pathophysiology is thought to explain the development of symptoms during periods of excitement.

Insulin-secreting tumors are usually responsive to increases in the blood glucose concentration. Food consumption stimulates insulin secretion, which can be excessive and can result in postprandial hypoglycemia and the development of clinical signs 2 to 6 hours after consumption of food.

Physical Examination

Physical examination findings in dogs with an insulin-secreting tumor are often surprisingly unremarkable, especially if clinical signs of hypoglycemia have been present for several months prior to presentation. Most abnormalities identified on the physical examination are nonspecific and supportive of a diagnosis of hypoglycemia (Table 14-6). Weakness and lethargy, the most common findings, are identified in approximately 40% and 20% of our cases, respectively. Episodes of collapse and seizures may occur during the examination but are uncommon. Afflicted dogs are usually free of palpable abnormalities, aside from findings commonly associated with aging (e.g., lipomas). Weight gain is evident in some dogs and is probably a result of insulin's potent anabolic effects. Failure to identify abnormalities on the physical examination, especially in an older, large-breed dog, is an important finding supportive of an insulin-secreting tumor.

PERIPHERAL NEUROPATHY. Peripheral neuropathies have been reported in dogs with insulin-secreting

TABLE 14–6 PHYSICAL EXAMINATION FINDINGS ASSOCIATED WITH INSULIN-SECRETING TUMORS IN 52 DOGS

Physical Examination Finding	Number of Dogs	Percent
Weakness	22	42
Lethargy	10	19
Collapsing	6	12
Seizures	4	8
Tremors	4	8
Obtunded	4	8
Peripheral neuropathy	3	6
Obese	2	4
No abnormalities identified	24	46

tumors (Shahar et al, 1985; Braund et al, 1987; van Ham et al, 1997). Clinical signs and physical examination findings range from paraparesis to tetraparesis, facial paresis to paralysis, hyporeflexia to areflexia, hypotonia, and muscle atrophy of the appendicular, masticatory and/or facial muscles. Sensory nerves may also be affected. A subclinical polyneuropathy has also been reported (Braund et al, 1987). The onset of clinical signs may be acute (days) or insidious (weeks to months). Abnormalities identified on electrodiagnostic testing include abnormal spontaneous potentials (e.g., positive sharp waves, fibrillation potentials) and slowed motor nerve conduction velocities (Braund et al, 1987). Cerebrospinal fluid (CSF) analysis produces a normal result (van Ham et al, 1997). Histopathologic findings in motor and sensory nerves include moderate to severe axonal necrosis, nerve fiber loss, and variable demyelination-remyelination (Braund et al, 1987; Schrauwen et al, 1996; van Ham et al, 1997). Muscle changes reflect neurogenic atrophy. The pathogenesis of the polyneuropathy is not known. Proposed theories include metabolic derangements of the nerves induced by chronic and severe hypoglycemia or some other tumor-induced metabolic deficiency, an immune-mediated paraneoplastic syndrome resulting from shared antigens between tumor and nerves, or toxic factors produced by the tumor that deleteriously affect the nerves (Kudo and Noguchi, 1985; Das and Hochberg, 1999; Heckmann et al, 2000). Treatment is aimed at surgical removal of the beta-cell tumor (Jeffery et al, 1994). Prednisone therapy (initially 1 mg/kg daily) may also improve clinical signs (van Ham et al, 1997). Correction of hypoglycemia, by itself, may not improve clinical signs caused by the peripheral neuropathy (Bergman et al, 1994).

CLINICAL PATHOLOGIC ABNORMALITIES

Virtually all dogs with insulin-secreting tumors remain undiagnosed and often unsuspected of having such tumors after completion of the history and physical examination. Most afflicted dogs have in common the history of episodic weakness or seizures. These signs encompass a wide variety of organic disorders (Table 14-7). The minimum diagnostic evaluation for dogs with these signs should include a complete blood count (CBC), serum biochemical panel, and urinalysis in an effort to identify abnormalities supportive of one of the disorders outlined in Table 14-7. Therapy other than that required for an emergency situation should be withheld until a diagnosis has been made.

The results of the CBC and urinalysis in dogs with an insulin-secreting tumor are usually normal. The results of the serum biochemical profile, aside from the blood glucose level, are also usually normal. Hypoalbuminemia, hypophosphatemia, hypokalemia, and increased activity in alkaline phosphatase and alanine aminotransferase have been reported (Leifer et al, 1986), but these findings are considered nonspecific and not helpful in achieving a definitive diagnosis. A correlation has not been established between increased liver enzyme activity and obvious metastasis of pancreatic tumors to the liver.

The only consistent abnormality identified in serum biochemistry profiles is hypoglycemia. The mean initial blood glucose concentration in 97 of our dogs with an insulin-secreting tumor was 42 mg/dl, with a range of 15 to 78 mg/dl. The median blood glucose concentration was 38 mg/dl. Eighty-seven of the 97 dogs (90%) had a random blood glucose concentration less than 60 mg/dl. Dogs with insulin-secreting

TABLE 14–7 A PARTIAL LISTING OF THE NUMEROUS DISORDERS THAT MAY RESULT IN EPISODIC WEAKNESS (INCLUDES SEIZURES)

Neuromuscular Disorders

Infectious: viral encephalitis (canine distemper), cryptococcosis, toxoplasmosis
Congenital: hydrocephalus
Trauma
Acquired: myasthenia gravis, tetanus, discospondylitis, idiopathic polyradiculoneuritis (Coon Hound paralysis), polymyositis, polyarthritis
Neoplasia
Toxin: lead poisoning
Idiopathic epilepsy
Idiopathic polyneuropathy

Cardiovascular Disorders

Congenital: anatomic defects
Acquired: tachyarrhythmias or bradyarrhythmias, heartworm, bacterial endocarditis
Neoplasm: hemangiosarcoma
Coagulopathy (warfarin-induced)

Metabolic Disorders

Hepatic encephalopathy
Hypocalcemia
Polycythemia
Hypoadrenocorticism
Hyperviscosity syndrome
Pheochromocytoma
Hypoglycemia
Hypokalemia
Anemia

tumors may occasionally have a blood glucose concentration between 70 and 80 mg/dl on random testing. However, such a finding does not eliminate hypoglycemia as a cause of episodic weakness or seizure activity. Fasting, with hourly evaluation of the blood glucose level, should be done in dogs suspected of having hypoglycemia. A fast of 8 or fewer hours was successful in demonstrating hypoglycemia in 33 of 35 trials in 31 dogs with insulin-secreting tumor. Longer fasts have been reported to be needed in some dogs; however, it is rare that fasts beyond 12 hours fail to produce hypoglycemia in dogs with insulin-secreting tumors.

DIFFERENTIAL DIAGNOSES FOR FASTING HYPOGLYCEMIA

Hypoglycemia is defined as a blood glucose concentration less than 60 mg/dl. Hypoglycemia typically results from excessive glucose utilization by normal (e.g., with hyperinsulinism) or neoplastic cells, impaired hepatic gluconeogenesis and glycogenolysis (e.g., portal shunt), a deficiency in glucose counterregulatory hormones (e.g., cortisol or glucagon deficiency), inadequate dietary intake of glucose and other substrates required for hepatic gluconeogenesis (e.g., anorexia in the neonate or toy breeds), or a combination of these mechanisms (e.g., sepsis) (Table 14-8) (Service, 1995). Iatrogenic hypoglycemia is a common problem with overzealous insulin administration to diabetic animals.

Congenital hepatic disease

Portovascular anomalies are the most common congenital cause of hepatic-induced hypoglycemia. Hypoglycemia develops despite the proper reduction in the circulating insulin concentration because of insufficient hepatic glycogen stores and inadequate hepatocellular function to support gluconeogenesis. Dogs and cats with portovascular anomalies are typically younger than 3 years of age, are thin or cachectic, and may have any of the signs, aside from weight gain, outlined in Table 14-4. Ascites, icterus, hemorrhage, and additional neurologic signs induced by hepatic encephalopathy may also be present. Behavior abnormalities may be enhanced by eating protein and by the administration of drugs (anesthetics, tranquilizers, diuretics). Additional abnormalities suggestive of this disorder that are identified with a CBC, serum biochemistry panel, and urinalysis include microcytosis, hypoalbuminemia, hypocholesterolemia, decreased urea nitrogen, increased total bilirubin, ammonium biurate crystals in the urine, abnormal preprandial and postprandial bile acid concentrations, and small liver size on abdominal radiography or ultrasonography. Confirmatory tests include liver biopsy, angiography, nuclear scintigraphy, and identification of the shunt during abdominal ultrasound scanning or exploratory celiotomy.

TABLE 14–8 CLASSIFICATION OF FASTING HYPOGLYCEMIA

I. Endocrine
  A. Excess insulin or insulin-like factors
    1. Insulin-producing islet cell tumors
    2. Extrapancreatic tumors secreting insulin-like substances (e.g., IGF-II*)
    3. Iatrogenic-insulin overdose
  B. Growth hormone deficiency
    1. Pituitary hypoplasia
    2. Pituitary cyst
  C. Cortisol deficiency
    1. Secondary hypoadrenocorticism
    2. Primary hypoadrenocorticism
  D. Glucagon deficiency
    1. Chronic pancreatitis?
    2. Exocrine pancreatic adenocarcinoma?
II. Hepatic
  A. Congenital
    1. Vascular shunts
    2. Glycogen storage diseases
  B. Acquired
    1. Vascular shunts
    2. Chronic fibrosis (cirrhosis)
    3. Hepatic necrosis: toxins, infectious agents
    4. Primary or metastatic neoplasia
III. Substrate
  A. Extrapancreatic tumors (e.g., leiomyosarcoma)
  B. Endotoxic or sepsis-induced
  C. Fasting hypoglycemia of pregnancy
  D. Neonatal or juvenile hypoglycemia
  E. Uremia
  F. Severe malnutrition
  G. Severe polycythemia
IV. Miscellaneous
  A. Artifact
    1. Prolonged storage of whole blood
    2. Portable glucose monitoring devices
  B. Iatrogenic-insulin overdose

*IGF-II, Insulin-like growth factor II.

Glycogen storage diseases are rare congenital hepatic disorders in dogs in which hypoglycemia results from an inability to convert glycogen to glucose because of a congenital absolute or relative deficiency of one of the enzymes necessary for the catabolism of glycogen. Type III glycogen storage disease (Cori's disease), a deficiency in amylo-1,6-glucosidase, has been documented in puppies with clinical signs of massive hepatomegaly (caused by glycogen accumulation), failure to thrive, and muscle weakness (Fig. 14-4) (Hardy, 1989). Glycogen storage disease type Ia (GSD Ia) (von Gierke's disease) is a deficiency in glucose-6-phosphatase caused by a mutated, defective glucose-6-phosphatase gene. GSD Ia has been documented in the Maltese breed, and a canine model for GSD Ia has been established by crossbreeding Maltese and Beagle dogs (Brix et al, 1995; Kishnani et al, 2001). Affected puppies exhibited tremors, weakness, and neurologic signs when hypoglycemic. Biochemical abnormalities included fasting hypoglycemia, hyperlactacidemia, hypercholesterolemia, hypertriglyceridemia, and hyperuricemia. Affected puppies developed progressive hepatomegaly characterized histologically by diffuse, marked hepatocellular vacuolation. One screening test for glycogen storage disease is the glucagon tolerance test. Plasma glucose concentrations typically fail to increase after injection of glucagon in dogs with type Ia and type III glycogen storage diseases. Confirmatory tests include histologic evaluation of hepatic biopsies and specific hepatic enzyme assays that are rarely performed in veterinary medicine.

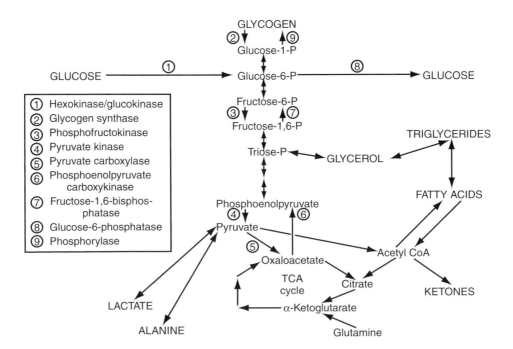

FIGURE 14-4. Schematic representation of glucose metabolism. (Cryer PE, Polonsky KS: *In* Wilson JD, et al [eds]: Williams Textbook of Endocrinology, 9th ed. Philadelphia, WB Saunders, 1998, p 940.)

Acquired hepatic dysfunction

Hypoglycemia may result from severe destruction of the liver by primary or metastatic neoplasia, bacterial infection, hepatotoxin (especially chronic administration of anticonvulsants), trauma or, more commonly, severe and chronic fibrosis (cirrhosis) of the liver and the development of *acquired* hepatic vascular shunts. There are numerous potential causes of chronic hepatic fibrosis in older dogs and cats. Hypoglycemia results from inadequate amounts of functional hepatic tissue for adequate storage of glycogen or for sufficient gluconeogenesis to sustain a normal blood glucose concentration during a fast. Serum insulin concentrations decline appropriately with worsening hypoglycemia, but this alone may be insufficient to prevent problems. Additional abnormalities identified on a CBC, serum biochemistry panel, and urinalysis suggestive of hepatic insufficiency include microcytosis, hypoalbuminemia, hypocholesterolemia, decreased urea nitrogen, increased total bilirubin, ammonium biurate crystals in the urine, abnormal preprandial and postprandial bile acid concentrations, abnormal liver size on abdominal radiography, or abnormal echotexture or liver size on ultrasonography. Liver biopsy is helpful in confirming severe fibrosis or cirrhosis and may even identify a cause (e.g., neoplasia). The etiology of the hepatic fibrosis and cirrhosis goes undiagnosed in most cases.

Adrenocortical insufficiency (Addison's disease)

Hypoglycemia in dogs with hypoadrenocorticism is caused by insufficient secretion of the glucocorticoids needed to stimulate hepatic mobilization and production of glucose (see Chapter 8). In this disorder, hypoglycemia occurs despite an appropriate reduction in the blood insulin concentration. Reduced insulin secretion must be accompanied by an increase in hepatic gluconeogenesis to correct hypoglycemia. The increasing glucose synthesis is normally stimulated by gluconeogenic hormones. Without secretion of these hormones, as observed in hypoadrenocorticism, hypoglycemia is possible (Sherwin and Felig, 1981). Hypoadrenocorticism is most common in young and middle-aged dogs, and there is a gender predisposition for the female. Abnormalities on screening tests supportive of this diagnosis include a relative increase in the eosinophil and lymphocyte counts, mild nonregenerative anemia, mild to severe prerenal azotemia, hyperkalemia, hyponatremia, and hypercalcemia. Radiographs of the thorax may reveal changes consistent with hypovolemia (e.g., microcardia), and an electrocardiogram may reveal abnormalities consistent with hyperkalemia. The diagnosis can be confirmed by abnormal results on adrenocorticotropic hormone (ACTH) stimulation tests.

Glucagon deficiency

Glucagon is the key counterregulatory hormone affecting recovery from acute hypoglycemia (Cryer and Gerich, 1985). In response to falling plasma glucose concentrations, glucagon is secreted by the alpha cells of the pancreatic islets into the hepatic portal circulation, and it acts exclusively on the liver to activate glycogenolysis and gluconeogenesis (Cryer and Polonsky, 1998). Hepatic glucose production is increased within minutes. Abnormalities in the production or secretion of glucagon prevent a normal counterregulatory response to decreasing blood glucose concentrations and predispose the animal to hypoglycemia. A classic example is hypoglycemia unawareness in diabetic humans, a syndrome caused by deficient glucagon and catecholamine secretion, resulting in defective counterregulation, severe hypoglycemia, and diabetic coma (Gerich et al, 1991; Mokan et al, 1994; Meyer et al, 1998). Isolated glucagon deficiency that causes hypoglycemia has been reported in humans but is rare (Cryer and Polonsky, 1998). Typically, glucagon deficiency occurs in conjunction with excess insulin secretion, deficient catecholamine secretion or increased tissue sensitivity to the actions of insulin, and this combination results in hypoglycemia. We have identified hypoglycemia in dogs and especially cats with pancreatitis and exocrine pancreatic adenocarcinoma and speculate that the destructive process associated with these disorders may cause glucagon deficiency, inappropriate insulin release, or both.

Hypopituitarism

Growth hormone and cortisol are important glucose counterregulatory hormones involved in hepatic glucose synthesis and secretion (see page 617). Failure of the pituitary gland to secrete ACTH, growth hormone, or both has a deleterious impact on maintenance of glucose homeostasis and predisposes the animal to hypoglycemia, especially in the fasting state. As in primary hypoadrenocorticism, insulin secretion diminishes appropriately for the degree of hypoglycemia, but this alone may not be sufficient to prevent signs. Growth hormone deficiency is a rare cause of hypoglycemia and is usually diagnosed in young German Shepherd dogs as a congenital defect or in dogs with acquired pituitary deficiency secondary to destruction by cancer, trauma, or inflammation. Growth hormone stimulation testing is used to establish a definitive diagnosis (see Chapter 2). Pituitary failure to secrete ACTH results in atrophy of the zona fasciculata of the adrenal cortex, impaired secretion of cortisol, and the development of secondary hypoadrenocorticism. No classic abnormalities are found on screening laboratory studies in animals with secondary hypoadrenocorticism. These dogs may have a mild nonregenerative anemia and fasting hypoglycemia, but serum electrolyte concentrations are usually normal. An ACTH stimulation test and determination of a baseline endogenous ACTH concentration are used to establish the diagnosis of secondary hypoadrenocorticism (see Chapter 8).

Non–beta-cell tumors

In humans, non–beta-cell tumors that cause hypoglycemia are usually of mesenchymal origin (e.g., leiomyosarcoma, fibrosarcoma); hypoglycemia is caused less often by tumors of epithelial origin (e.g., hepatoma, carcinoid tumors) and hematopoietic origin (e.g., lymphoma, multiple myeloma) (Cryer and Polonsky, 1998). A variety of tumor types has also been reported to cause hypoglycemia in the dog (Table 14-9). In our hospital, hepatocellular carcinoma, hepatoma, leiomyoma, leiomyosarcoma, and tumors with extensive hepatic metastasis are most commonly associated with hypoglycemia.

The pathogenesis of hypoglycemia associated with non–beta-cell tumors is poorly understood and undoubtedly multifactorial. Proposed mechanisms include excessive glucose utilization by the tumor, impaired hepatic glycogenolysis and gluconeogenesis as a result of tumor-induced hepatic destruction or inhibition of normal counterregulatory responses that prevent hypoglycemia, and secretion of an insulin-like molecule that lowers the blood glucose concentration by enhancing glucose utilization by normal cells (Cryer and Polonsky, 1998). In humans, excessive glucose utilization in conjunction with reduced or inappropriately low hepatic glucose production frequently plays a role in the development of hypoglycemia associated with a non–beta-cell tumor. Only rarely have nonpancreatic tumors been shown to produce insulin that can be assayed using conventional radioimmunoassays (Kahn, 1980). In most humans with nonpancreatic tumors and hypoglycemia, the serum insulin concentration is suppressed (Scully et al, 1983). Similarly, serum insulin concentrations are typically undetectable or in the low-normal range in dogs with non–beta-cell tumors, in contrast to the high-normal to increased serum insulin concentrations seen with hypoglycemia induced by a beta-cell tumor (Beaudry et al, 1995; Bagley et al, 1996; Bellah and Ginn, 1996).

Excessive production of insulin-like growth factor-II (IGF-II) is believed to be involved in the pathogenesis of hypoglycemia in many humans with mesenchymal tumors and with hepatocellular carcinoma (Merimee, 1986; LeRoith et al, 1992; Fukuda et al, 1994; Daughaday, 1995). Although the major organ responsible for circulating insulin-like growth factors is the liver, it has been demonstrated that these factors are produced ubiquitously, particularly by mesenchymal cells (D'Ercole et al, 1984; Barreca et al, 1992); this is in agreement with the finding that tumors resulting in hypoglycemia are usually of mesenchymal origin. However, unlike in healthy humans, the 150 kD complex (IGF-II, insulin-like growth factor binding protein 3 [IGFBP-3], and an acid-labile subunit) that normally transports most of the IGF-II in the circulation is greatly decreased in patients with tumor-induced hypoglycemia (see page 45 for information on IGFBP-3). As a result, most of the IGF-II is transported in a smaller complex that enters target tissues more readily, and serum free IGF-II concentrations are increased. IGF-II is structurally homologous to proinsulin, can bind to insulin receptors, and has direct insulin-like actions that result in hypoglycemia. In addition, IGF-II may suppress glucagon and growth hormone secretion, which may also contribute to hypoglycemia (Cryer and Polonsky, 1998).

A similar pathophysiologic mechanism for hypoglycemia was identified in a dog with gastric leiomyoma and hypoglycemia (Boari et al, 1995). In this dog, the serum IGF-II concentrations were increased prior to surgery, and the blood glucose concentration and serum IGF-II concentrations returned to the reference range after removal of the tumor. The results of immunohistochemical staining of tumor tissue were positive for IGF-II; the tumor tissue IGF-II concentration was higher than normal (5.7 nmol/kg tissue, compared with a range in normal gastric wall tissue of 1.1 to 3.7 nmol/kg); and in situ hybridization evidenced the expression of IGF-II messenger ribonucleic acid (mRNA) in tumor tissue. Evaluation of the molecular distribution of IGF-II in the circulation revealed immunoreactivity predominantly in the 50 kD region (versus the 150 kD region), which was reduced to normal after surgery. These findings suggest that the hypoglycemia in this dog was caused by overproduction of IGF-II circulating in a smaller than normal molecular form that could more easily cross the capillary wall and exert its insulin-like effects on target tissues.

In another study involving four dogs with hypoglycemia caused by smooth muscle tumors, the results of immunohistochemical staining for insulin were negative in the four tumors but positive for glucagon in three of the four tumors (Beaudry et al, 1995). The three smooth muscle tumors that stained positive for glucagon originated in either the stomach or jejunum, whereas the tumor that stained negative for glucagon

TABLE 14–9 HISTOLOGIC CLASSIFICATION OF NONPANCREATIC TUMORS ASSOCIATED WITH HYPOGLYCEMIA REPORTED IN THE VETERINARY LITERATURE SINCE 1974

Epithelial Origin	16 dogs
Hepatocellular carcinoma	11 dogs
Hepatoma	2 dogs
Metastatic mammary carcinoma	1 dog
Salivary adenocarcinoma	1 dog
Pulmonary carcinoma	1 dog
Mesenchymal Origin	22 dogs
Leiomyosarcoma	10 dogs
Hepatic	3 dogs
Gastric	3 dogs
Small intestine	2 dogs
Splenic	2 dogs
Leiomyoma	10 dogs
Gastric	6 dogs
Small intestine	4 dogs
Hemangiosarcoma	2 dogs
Splenic	1 dog
Hepatic	1 dog
Miscellaneous Tumors	3 dogs
Plasmacytoma	1 dog
Lymphocytic leukemia	1 dog
Metastatic melanoma	1 dog

originated in the spleen. Immunohistochemical staining for glucagon was negative in smooth muscle cells in normal adjacent tissue. The clinical relevance of this finding remains to be determined, especially considering that glucagon should increase, not decrease, the blood glucose concentration.

Dogs with hypoglycemia caused by a non–beta-cell tumor may be brought to the veterinarian with clinical signs of hypoglycemia, or hypoglycemia may be a serendipitous finding on a serum biochemistry panel. In most dogs, non–beta-cell tumors that cause hypoglycemia are located in the liver or abdomen. Identification of a non–beta-cell tumor requires a thorough physical examination of the dog or cat, thoracic and abdominal radiography, abdominal ultrasonography, and histopathologic evaluation of biopsy specimens from identifiable masses. The association between a non–beta-cell tumor and hypoglycemia requires resolution of hypoglycemia after surgical excision of the tumor.

Neonatal and juvenile hypoglycemia

The fetus receives a continuous source of glucose via the placenta and does not depend on its own gluconeogenic capabilities to maintain an adequate blood glucose concentration. In contrast, the neonate depends on glycogenolysis and gluconeogenesis to maintain euglycemia during fasts, even if brief. Limited hepatic glycogen stores, small muscle mass, lack of adipose tissue, and decreased use of free fatty acids as an alternative energy source place the neonate at risk for developing hypoglycemia within hours of fasting (Chastain, 1990). Impaired gluconeogenesis as a result of delayed induction of one or more of the rate-limiting gluconeogenic enzymes is suspected in neonatal hypoglycemia of human infants (Cryer and Polonsky, 1998) and may play a role in neonatal hypoglycemia of puppies and kittens as well.

Hypoglycemia often occurs in conjunction with hypothermia, sepsis, starvation, toxic milk syndrome, or a combination of these problems. The ill neonate should always be evaluated for hypoglycemia. Orally administered glucose (e.g., 0.01 ml of 5% to 10% solution per gram of body weight) and frequent nursing or bottle feeding help correct and prevent hypoglycemia in the neonate.

Hypoglycemia of toy and miniature breed dogs younger than 6 months of age is common. Alanine deficiency has been implicated in this syndrome, as it has in young children (Chew et al, 1982). In humans, the rate of alanine release from muscle determines the rate of gluconeogenesis during starvation. Puppies with juvenile hypoglycemia are usually under extreme stress. They frequently have a history of recently being purchased, with an associated change in environment and diet. Gastrointestinal upset (vomiting, diarrhea, anorexia) is typical and may or may not be associated with parasites. These puppies are quite fragile and are brought to veterinarians with signs that may include weakness, collapse, depression, ataxia, stupor, con-vulsions, hypothermia, and/or loose stools. Intravenous administration of glucose usually results in rapid clinical improvement. Frequent feedings prevent recurrences. This disorder virtually disappears with attainment of adult height and weight. If signs persist, a search for another disease that may be causing the hypoglycemia should be considered.

Endotoxic or sepsis-induced hypoglycemia

Endotoxic or sepsis-induced hypoglycemia is a relatively uncommon cause of hypoglycemia in the dog and cat (Breitschwerdt et al, 1981). The pathogenesis of sepsis-induced hypoglycemia is not well characterized but is believed to result from increased tissue utilization of glucose in conjunction with decreased hepatic glucose production (Naylor and Kronfeld, 1985; Hargrove et al, 1988a and 1988b). The factors responsible for increased glucose utilization and failure of glucose production are unclear. Proposed mechanisms for increased glucose utilization include sepsis-induced production of insulin-like substances, interleukin-1–enhanced insulin secretion by beta cells, cytokine-enhanced increase in glucose transport into cells, and increased glucose utilization by bacteria and neutrophils (Commens et al, 1987; del Ray and Besedovsky, 1987). Increased glucose use by macrophage-rich tissues such as the liver, spleen, and ileum is responsible for most of the glucose utilization (Meszaros et al, 1988), with skeletal muscle accounting for an additional 25% (Meszaros et al, 1987). Decreased hepatic glucose production may result from impaired hepatic oxidative metabolism, increased anaerobic glycolysis of liver glucose, hypoxic injury to hepatic cells, or sepsis-induced interference with substrate delivery to the liver (see Feldman and Nelson, 1987 for references). Endotoxin may also decrease glycogenolysis through depletion of hepatic and muscle glycogen stores, or it may impair hepatic gluconeogenesis.

In our hospital, sepsis-induced hypoglycemia is most commonly associated with parvovirus infection, prostatic or liver abscess, hemorrhagic gastroenteritis, pyothorax, pyometra, and gram-negative septicemia. Sepsis-induced hypoglycemia should be considered if a hypoglycemic animal is suffering from severe infection or significant leukocytosis (>30,000 cells/μl). A diagnosis of sepsis-induced hypoglycemia is based on identification of infection by means of a physical examination, CBC, radiography and ultrasonography, appropriate bacterial cultures, and resolution of hypoglycemia after initiation of appropriate antibiotic therapy. If severe infection is diagnosed in a dog or cat with hypoglycemia, pursuit of other causes of hypoglycemia is usually not warranted unless screening tests dictate otherwise or the hypoglycemia fails to resolve after initiation of appropriate antibiotic therapy.

Renal failure

The impact of renal failure on the blood glucose concentration is unpredictable in dogs and cats. The blood glucose concentration is usually normal. However, hyperglycemia may develop as a result of uremia-induced carbohydrate intolerance and insulin resistance in a dog or cat with impaired insulin secretion (see Chapter 11). Alternatively, renal failure may induce hypoglycemia, presumably because of uremia-induced alterations in carbohydrate metabolism, impaired glucose counterregulation, and decreased renal gluconeogenesis (Edwards et al, 1987; Gerich et al, 2001). Decreased renal glucose production, by itself, does not cause hypoglycemia because hepatic glucose production will maintain a normal blood glucose concentration (see page 617). Presumably, the development of hypoglycemia in renal failure centers on impaired glucose production by the liver as a consequence of defective hepatic glycogenolysis and gluconeogenesis, limited availability of glucogenic substrates, inadequate glucose counterregulatory responses, or a combination of these factors (Fischer et al, 1986). Decreased caloric intake and decreased renal degradation and/or excretion of insulin may also contribute to hypoglycemia.

Cardiac disease

Hypoglycemia may occur in humans with severe cardiac failure of diverse causes, but this is an unrecognized cause of hypoglycemia in the dog and cat. The pathogenesis of cardiac-induced hypoglycemia is not known. Suggested possibilities include hepatic congestion, cachexia, gluconeogenic substrate limitation, and hepatic hypoxia (Cryer and Polonsky, 1998).

Polycythemia

Severe polycythemia (hematocrit >65%) may cause hypoglycemia secondary to increased glucose utilization by the huge number of red blood cells. The utilization of glucose may deplete glycogen stores. Polycythemia may be primary (i.e., polycythemia vera), or it may occur secondary to disorders that cause chronic systemic hypoxia (e.g., congenital right-to-left shunting of blood in the heart), to chronic renal hypoxia (e.g., renal neoplasia), or to erythropoietin-producing tumors.

Artifactual hypoglycemia

Prolonged storage of blood before separation of serum or plasma can cause artifactual hypoglycemia. The glucose concentration decreases in a whole blood sample kept at room temperature because of the continuing metabolism of glucose by cells present in the blood. Decrements in the glucose concentration as high as 10 mg/dl/hr have been reported (Chew et al, 1982). Glucose metabolism by red and white blood cells becomes even more apparent in dogs and cats with erythrocytosis, leukocytosis, or sepsis. In addition, the concentration of glucose in blood refrigerated for 24 hours at 4° C may be reduced as much as 20 mg/dl. Therefore whole blood obtained for measurement of the glucose concentration should be centrifuged soon after collection (within 1 hour) and the serum or plasma harvested and refrigerated or frozen to minimize artifactual lowering of the blood glucose concentration. Glucose can be accurately measured from serum or plasma that has been refrigerated or frozen. Refrigerated samples should be assayed preferably less than 24 hours after collection, although reasonably accurate values can still be obtained after 48 hours.

Sodium fluoride–treated tubes have been advocated for collection of plasma and subsequent assessment of the plasma glucose concentration. The fluoride inhibits cellular utilization of glucose by acting as an enzyme inhibitor. Unfortunately, hemolysis is common when blood is collected in sodium fluoride–treated tubes, which can result in slight decrements in glucose values owing to methodological problems in the laboratory determination. For this reason, we do not use sodium fluoride–treated tubes.

It is a very common practice to measure glucose in whole blood immediately after it is collected, using a hand-held portable blood glucose monitoring device (e.g., Bayer Glucometer Elite-XL; Bayer, Elkhart, IN). It is very important to remember that blood glucose values determined by many portable blood glucose monitoring devices are lower than actual glucose values determined by bench-top methodologies (i.e., glucose oxidase and hexokinase methods) (see Fig. 11-12, page 513). Failure to consider this "error" could result in an incorrect diagnosis of hypoglycemia. Fortunately, for most portable blood glucose monitoring devices, the more severe the hypoglycemia, the more accurate the device becomes. In our experience, the actual blood glucose concentration is usually less than 60 mg/dl when most portable blood glucose monitoring devices report the concentration as less than 40 mg/dl; the actual blood glucose concentration is usually greater than 60 mg/dl and often greater than 70 mg/dl when the device reports the concentration as 50 to 60 mg/dl; and the actual blood glucose concentration may or may not be less than 60 mg/dl when the device reports the blood glucose level as 40 to 50 mg/dl.

Laboratory error may result in an incorrect value for any assay. Therefore it is wise to confirm a finding of hypoglycemia by means of evaluation of a second blood sample before more sophisticated and expensive studies are performed.

Iatrogenic hypoglycemia

Insulin and oral sulfonylurea drugs (e.g., glipizide, glyburide) are the only commonly available drugs that consistently lower the blood glucose concentration. Self-administration of insulin is an important cause of hypoglycemia in humans. In veterinary medicine, the diabetic animal receiving insulin always has the potential of becoming hypoglycemic. However, owners administering insulin to animals without the veterinarian's knowledge is not a realistic concern.

DIAGNOSTIC APPROACH TO HYPOGLYCEMIA: PRIORITIZING THE DIFFERENTIALS

A finding of hypoglycemia should always be confirmed before diagnostic studies are begun to identify the cause. Careful evaluation of the animal's history, the physical examination findings, and the results of routine blood tests (i.e., CBC, serum biochemistry panel, urinalysis) usually provide clues to the underlying cause (Fig. 14-5). Hypoglycemia in the puppy or kitten is usually caused by idiopathic hypoglycemia, starvation, liver insufficiency (i.e., portal shunt), or sepsis. In young adult dogs or cats, hypoglycemia is usually caused by liver insufficiency, hypoadrenocorticism, or sepsis. In older dogs or cats, liver insufficiency, beta-cell neoplasia, extrapancreatic neoplasia, hypoadrenocorticism, and sepsis are the most common causes.

Hypoglycemia tends to be mild (i.e., blood glucose concentration >45 mg/dl) and is often an incidental finding in dogs and cats with hypoadrenocorticism or liver insufficiency. Additional clinical pathologic alterations are usually present (e.g., hyponatremia and hyperkalemia in animals with Addison's disease or alterations in liver enzymes, hypocholesterolemia, hypoalbuminemia, and a low blood urea nitrogen [BUN] concentration in animals with liver insufficiency). An ACTH stimulation test or liver function test (i.e., preprandial and postprandial bile acids) may be required to confirm the diagnosis. Severe hypoglycemia (<40 mg/dl) may develop in neonates and juvenile kittens and puppies (especially toy breeds) and in animals with sepsis, beta-cell neoplasia, and extrapancreatic neoplasia, most notably hepatic adenocarcinoma and leiomyosarcoma. Sepsis is readily identified on the basis of physical examination findings and abnormal CBC findings, which include a neutrophilic leukocytosis (typically >30,000/μl), a shift toward immaturity, and signs of toxicity. Extrapancreatic neoplasia can usually be identified on the basis of the physical examination, abdominal or thoracic radiography, and abdominal ultrasonography. Dogs with beta-cell neoplasia typically have normal physical examination findings aside from findings suggestive of hypoglycemia (e.g., weakness) and no abnormalities other than hypoglycemia shown on routine blood and urine tests. Measurement of the baseline serum insulin concentration when the blood glucose is less than 60 mg/dl (preferably <50 mg/dl) is used to confirm the diagnosis of a beta-cell tumor.

CONFIRMING THE DIAGNOSIS OF AN INSULIN-SECRETING BETA-CELL TUMOR: SERUM INSULIN DETERMINATION

The diagnosis of an insulin-secreting tumor requires an initial confirmation of hypoglycemia followed by documentation of inappropriate insulin secretion and identification of a pancreatic mass using ultrasonography or exploratory celiotomy. Considering the potential differential diagnoses for hypoglycemia (see Table 14-8), a tentative diagnosis of insulin-secreting neoplasia can often be made on the basis of the history, physical examination findings, and an absence of abnormalities other than hypoglycemia shown by routine blood tests.

Whipple's Triad

In 1935 the report that established insulin-secreting tumors of the pancreas as a clinical entity included a discussion of the three criteria to be used in confirming the diagnosis (Whipple and Grantz, 1935). These standards, now referred to as Whipple's triad, are: (1) the symptoms occur after fasting or exercise; (2) at the time of symptoms, the serum glucose concentration is less than 50 mg/dl; and (3) the symptoms are relieved by administration of glucose. Unfortunately, this triad can result from numerous causes of hypoglycemia and as such is nonspecific.

Determination of Baseline Insulin and Glucose Concentrations

THEORY. The diagnosis of an insulin-secreting tumor is established by evaluating the blood insulin concentration at a time when hypoglycemia is present. Hypoglycemia suppresses insulin secretion in normal animals, with the degree of suppression directly related to the severity of the hypoglycemia. Hypoglycemia fails to have this same suppressive effect on insulin secretion if the insulin is synthesized and secreted from autonomous neoplastic cells, because tumor cells that produce and secrete insulin are less responsive to hypoglycemia than normal beta cells. Invariably the dog with an insulin-secreting tumor has inappropriate excesses in the blood insulin concentration relative to that needed for a particular blood glucose concentration. The relative excess of insulin is easiest to recognize when the blood glucose concentration is low, preferably less than 50 mg/dl. If the blood glucose concentration is low and the insulin concentration is in the upper half of the normal range or increased (typically >10 μU/ml), the animal has a relative or absolute excess of insulin that can be explained by the presence of an insulin-secreting tumor that is insensitive to hypoglycemia.

PROTOCOL. Most dogs with insulin-secreting neoplasia are persistently hypoglycemic. If the blood glucose concentration is less than 60 mg/dl (preferably less than 50 mg/dl), serum should be submitted to a commercial veterinary endocrine laboratory for determination of the glucose and insulin concentrations. If the dog's blood glucose concentration is greater than 60 mg/dl, a 4- to 12-hour fast may be necessary to induce hypoglycemia. Blood glucose concentrations should be evaluated hourly during the fast. Portable home blood glucose monitoring devices are typically used to monitor the

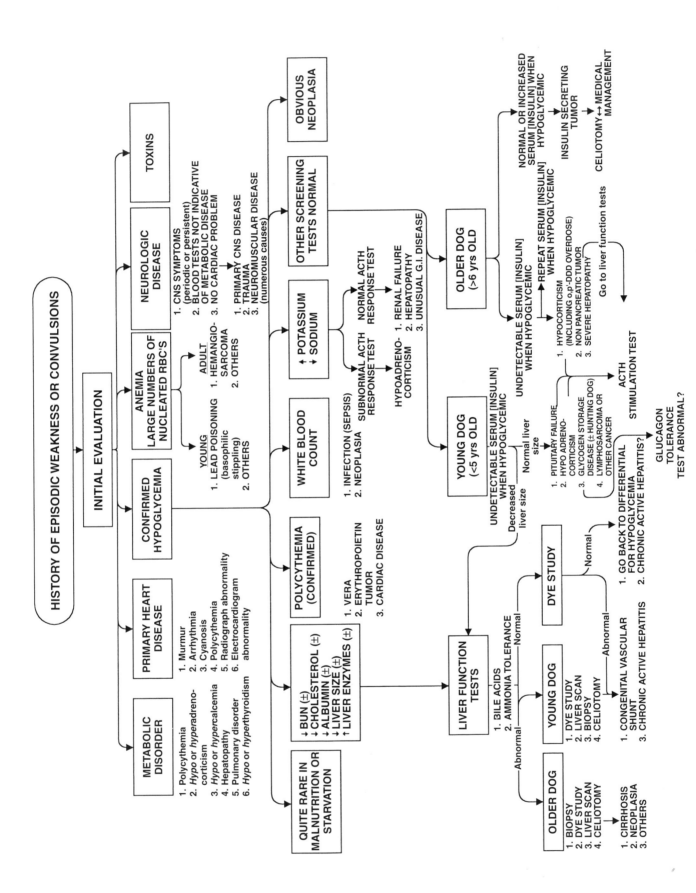

FIGURE 14-5. Flow chart for the diagnosis of episodic weakness and, more completely, hypoglycemia.

TABLE 14–10   INTERPRETATION OF BASELINE SERUM INSULIN CONCENTRATION IN DOGS WITH HYPOGLYCEMIA BELIEVED TO BE CAUSED BY INSULIN-SECRETING BETA CELL NEOPLASIA

Serum Insulin Concentration	Probability of Beta Cell Tumor*
> 20 μU/ml	High
10-20 μU/ml	Possible
5-10 μU/ml	Low
< 5 μU/ml	Ruled out

*Ideally, the blood glucose concentration determined by a bench-top methodology (i.e., glucose oxidase or hexokinase method) should be less than 50 mg/dl in the same blood sample submitted to the laboratory for insulin determination. Interpretation of serum insulin concentration is unreliable if the blood glucose concentration is greater than 60 mg/dl.

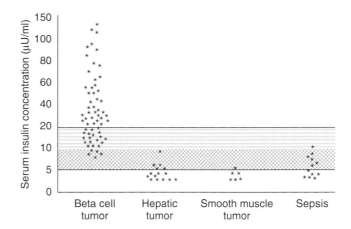

FIGURE 14-6. Serum insulin concentrations in dogs with hypoglycemia caused by an insulin-secreting beta-cell tumor, hepatoma or hepatocellular carcinoma, leiomyosarcoma, or sepsis. Although a serum insulin concentration in the high end of the normal range (i.e., >10 μU/ml) is consistent with a beta-cell tumor, a serum insulin concentration in the low end of the normal range (i.e., 5 to 10 μU/ml) is not diagnostic for a beta-cell tumor. Shaded regions represent the high (horizontal lines) and low (hatched area) ends of the normal range.

blood glucose concentration in most veterinary hospitals. Because blood glucose results obtained from many of these devices are erroneously low (Cohn et al, 2000; Wess and Reusch, 2000), a blood sample for submission to a commercial laboratory for glucose and insulin determinations should not be obtained until the blood glucose level measured on these devices is approximately 40 mg/dl or less. The dog can then be fed several small meals over the next 1 to 3 hours to prevent marked fluctuations in the blood glucose concentration and a potential postprandial reactive hypoglycemia.

INTERPRETATION.   The serum insulin concentration must be evaluated from the same blood sample as and in relation to the blood glucose concentration (Table 14-10). The serum insulin and glucose concentrations in a healthy fasted dog are usually between 5 and 20 μU/ml and 70 and 110 mg/dl, respectively. A serum insulin concentration that exceeds 20 μU/ml in a dog with a corresponding blood glucose concentration of less than 60 mg/dl (preferably less than 50 mg/dl), in combination with appropriate clinical signs and clinical pathologic findings, strongly supports the diagnosis of an insulin-secreting tumor. An insulin-secreting tumor is also possible if the serum insulin concentration is in the high-normal range (10 to 20 μU/ml). Insulin values in the low-normal range (5 to 10 μU/ml) may be found in animals with other causes of hypoglycemia, as well as in those with insulin-secreting tumors (Fig. 14-6). Careful assessment of the history, physical examination findings, and clinical pathologic and abdominal ultrasonographic findings, and possibly repeated serum glucose and insulin measurements, can usually identify the cause of the hypoglycemia. In 85 of our dogs with a histologically confirmed beta-cell tumor and a blood glucose concentration less than 60 mg/dl, the serum insulin concentration was greater than 20 μU/ml in 62 dogs (73%); 10 to 20 μU/ml in 18 dogs (21%); and 5 to 10 μU/ml in 5 dogs (6%). No dog had a serum insulin concentration less than 5 μU/ml. Any serum insulin concentration below the normal range (typically <5 μU/ml) is consistent with insulinopenia and does not indicate the presence of an insulin-secreting tumor. Confidence in identifying inappropriate hyper-

insulinemia depends on the severity of the hypoglycemia; the lower the blood glucose concentration, the more confident the clinician can be in identifying inappropriate hyperinsulinemia, especially when the serum insulin concentration falls in the normal range.

Insulin:Glucose Ratios

Several insulin:glucose ratios, including the insulin:glucose ratio, the glucose:insulin ratio, and the amended insulin:glucose ratio, have been recommended to evaluate the interrelationship between the blood glucose and insulin concentrations and to help establish the diagnosis of insulin-secreting tumor when the laboratory results are ambiguous (e.g., hypoglycemia is marginal and serum insulin concentrations remain in the normal range). Of these ratios, the amended insulin:glucose ratio is most commonly used. The amended insulin:glucose ratio is determined by entering the blood glucose and serum insulin concentrations in the following formula:

$$\frac{\text{Serum insulin (μU/ml)} \times 10}{\text{Blood glucose (mg/dl)} - 30}$$

The use of "– 30" in the formula is based on the theory that in normal humans, serum insulin concentrations are undetectable when the blood glucose concentration is less than 30 mg/dl. Whenever the blood glucose level is less than 30 mg/dl, the number 1 is used as the divisor. Extrapolating from the human literature, most authors have suggested that an amended insulin:glucose ratio greater than 30 is diagnostic of an insulin-secreting tumor. However, this test is not specific; that is, some dogs with other causes of hypoglycemia may have abnormal amended ratios (Leifer et al, 1986). The most common reason for lack of specificity is a detectable serum insulin concentration, albeit usually in the low-normal range, despite hypoglycemia. This occurs most commonly with hepatic tumors and sepsis. We do not rely on insulin:glucose ratios for interpretation of blood insulin and glucose results. Rather, we interpret the absolute serum insulin concentration during hypoglycemia (see Table 14-10) in conjunction with the history, physical findings, and results of clinical pathologic tests.

Provocative Testing

Several tests have been described that use agents that stimulate insulin secretion by normal and neoplastic beta cells; these include the glucagon tolerance test, the oral and intravenous glucose tolerance test, the tolbutamide tolerance test, and the epinephrine stimulation test. By evaluating the response of blood glucose and insulin concentrations for a period of time after administration of these agents, a differentiation between normal and neoplastic beta cells can potentially be made. We do not use any of these tests to establish the diagnosis of an insulin-secreting tumor, and they are not recommended. The reader is referred to the first edition of *Canine and Feline Endocrinology and Reproduction* for more information on the use of provocative testing in dogs suspected of having beta-cell neoplasia.

DIAGNOSTIC IMAGING

Radiography

Abdominal radiographs are not helpful in establishing the diagnosis of an insulin-secreting tumor, partly because of the location of the pancreas and the small size of most insulin-secreting tumors. Insulin-secreting tumors are typically less than 3 cm in diameter at the time the diagnosis is established. Displacement of viscera or a visible mass in the right cranial quadrant of the abdominal cavity is extremely rare. Thoracic radiographs are of limited help in documenting metastatic disease, primarily because beta-cell tumors rarely metastasize to the lungs until late in the course of the disease. The most common sites of early metastasis are the liver, regional lymph nodes, and peripancreatic omentum, which are regions where abdominal radiographs are also ineffective in identifying metastatic disease.

Beta-cell tumors do not spread to the lungs until late in the course of the disease. As such, thoracic radiographs are typically negative for metastatic disease when obtained at the time the diagnosis is established and surgery is contemplated.

Ultrasonography

Ultrasonic detection of a mass lesion in the region of the pancreas helps confirm the suspicion of beta-cell tumor in a dog with appropriate clinical signs and clinical pathologic abnormalities (Fig. 14-7). Identification of mass lesions in the hepatic parenchyma or peripancreatic tissue suggests metastatic disease. Occasionally only the metastatic sites are identified with ultrasound, and the tumor in the pancreas goes undetected. Failure to identify a mass lesion in the region of the pancreas or metastatic sites is common and does not rule out the presence of a beta-cell tumor. In our most recent 44 dogs with surgically and histologically confirmed beta-cell neoplasia, ultrasound evaluation of the abdomen prior to surgery identified a mass lesion in only 14 dogs (32%). Ultrasonography failed to identify diffuse infiltration of the pancreas by the tumor in one dog and a mass that was not grossly visible at the time of surgery in one dog. In the latter dog, a 2.3 × 1.3 cm pancreatic mass was identified 1 year after the initial exploratory surgery. Tumors in the left lobe of the pancreas were identified by ultrasound more often than those in the body or right lobe. Similarly, larger tumors were more likely to be identified with ultrasonography, but there was considerable overlap in tumor size. The mean size of excised tumors identified on ultrasonography was 2.7 × 2.4 cm (range, 1 × 1 cm to 5 × 4 cm), versus 1.7 × 1.5 cm (range, 0.4 × 0.4 cm to 5 × 2 cm) for excised tumors not identified on ultrasonography. Failure to identify a pancreatic mass in a dog suspected of having a beta-cell tumor is a further indication for exploratory surgery in the hopes of finding a small, excisable tumor.

Scintigraphy

Somatostatin receptor scintigraphy has been used to image pancreatic islet cell tumors in humans (Kvols et al, 1993; Lamberts et al, 1993). Positive and negative scan results have been correlated with the presence or absence of somatostatin receptors in tumor biopsy samples. In humans, detection of beta-cell tumors with somatostatin receptor scintigraphy is inconsistent, being only about 60% to 70% positive (Buetow et al, 1997). Ligand binding studies on beta-cell tumors in humans have identified different subtypes of somatostatin receptors, with variable binding capacities for somatostatin and somatostatin analogs, which may explain the variability of results (Lamberts et al, 1991; Bruns et al, 1994). Presumably, positive scintigraphic findings may also predict a positive response to treatment with the somatostatin analog octreotide (see page 640).

In the dog, only one somatostatin receptor that contains high-affinity binding sites for the somatostatin analog octreotide has been identified in insulin-secreting tumors (Robben et al, 1997). Recently, somatostatin receptor scintigraphy using radio-

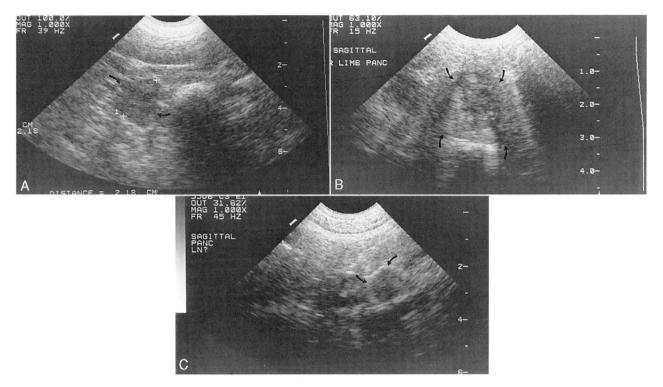

FIGURE 14-7. Ultrasonograms of the pancreas showing an islet beta-cell tumor (*arrows*) in a 13-year-old Borzoi (*A*) and a 14-year-old Miniature Poodle (*B*). *C*, Ultrasonogram of the peripancreatic tissue showing a metastatic beta-cell tumor (*arrows*) in a 5-year-old Golden Retriever.

labeled octreotide or indium (In-111) pentetreotide was used to identify beta-cell neoplasia in seven dogs with inconclusive findings on abdominal ultrasonography (Robben et al, 1997; Lester et al, 1999). Somatostatin receptor scintigraphy was effective in identifying the primary insulin-secreting tumor in five of seven dogs and larger metastases in the regional lymph nodes and liver in three of three dogs and two of three dogs, respectively. Small metastases in the liver were not detected in one dog. Although somatostatin receptor scintigraphy offers intriguing options for identifying insulin-secreting tumors and determining potential responsiveness of the tumor to octreotide therapy, the expense of the radiopharmaceutical and the need for specialized facilities will probably limit the role of scintigraphy in the diagnosis of beta-cell tumors in dogs for the foreseeable future.

TREATMENT OF BETA-CELL NEOPLASIA

Surgical versus Medical Therapy

Surgical exploration appears to be the best diagnostic, therapeutic, and prognostic tool in dogs with insulin-secreting tumors. Surgery offers a chance to cure dogs with a resectable solitary mass. In dogs with non-resectable tumors or with obvious metastatic lesions, removal or "debulking" of as much abnormal tissue as possible has frequently resulted in remission, or at

least alleviation, of clinical signs and an improved response to medical therapy lasting for weeks to months. Survival time is also longer in dogs that undergo surgical exploration and tumor debulking followed by medical therapy, compared with dogs only treated medically (Tobin et al, 1999). Despite these benefits, surgery remains a relatively aggressive mode of diagnosis and treatment, in part because of the high prevalence of metastatic disease, the older age of many dogs at the time beta-cell neoplasia is diagnosed, and the unpredictable response to surgery as it relates to improvement in hypoglycemia and clinical signs. As a general rule, we are less aggressive about recommending surgery in aged dogs (i.e., older than 12 years of age), dogs with extensive metastatic disease identified by ultrasonography, and dogs with concurrent disease that significantly enhances the anesthetic risk.

Medical management of chronic hypoglycemia should be initiated when an exploratory celiotomy is not performed or when metastatic or inoperable neoplasia results in recurrence of clinical signs. Medical therapy revolves around nonspecific antihormonal therapy designed to increase the blood glucose concentration and decrease the occurrence of clinical signs. Many dogs with metastatic disease can be managed medically for several months to more than a year. Medical therapy, however, has no potential for providing a "cure" or for preventing metastasis of malignant beta-cell neoplasia.

Surgical Therapy

The actual procedures involved in the surgical approach to the dog with an insulin-secreting tumor are not described here; the interested reader is referred to Nelson and Salisbury (2000). However, several general principles are discussed.

The intent of surgery should be to remove as much abnormal tissue as possible, including resectable sites of metastases. The success of surgery depends in part on providing appropriate fluid therapy, dextrose, and supportive care during the perioperative period to avoid severe hypoglycemia and postoperative pancreatitis and to improve the likelihood of an uneventful recovery. Euthanasia is not recommended regardless of the findings at surgery. Many dogs with metastatic disease can be managed medically for several months to more than a year.

PREOPERATIVE CONSIDERATIONS. Until surgery is performed, the dog with an insulin-secreting tumor must be protected from episodes of severe hypo-

TABLE 14–11   LONG-TERM MEDICAL THERAPY FOR DOGS WITH BETA-CELL TUMOR

Standard Treatments

1. Dietary Therapy
   a. Feed canned or dry food in three to six small meals daily
   b. Avoid foods containing monosaccharides, disaccharides or propylene glycol
2. Limit Exercise
3. Glucocorticoid Therapy
   a. Prednisone, 0.5 mg/kg divided bid initially
   b. Gradually increase dose and frequency of administration, as needed
   c. Goal is to control clinical signs, not to reestablish euglycemia
   d. Consider alternative treatments if signs of iatrogenic hypercortisolism become severe or glucocorticoids become ineffective

Additional Treatments

1. Diazoxide Therapy
   a. Continue standard treatment; reduce glucocorticoid dose to minimize adverse signs
   b. Diazoxide, 5 mg/kg bid initially
   c. Gradually increase dose as needed, not to exceed 60 mg/kg/day
   d. Goal is to control clinical signs, not to reestablish euglycemia
2. Somatostatin Therapy
   a. Continue standard treatment; reduce glucocorticoid dose to minimize adverse signs
   b. Octreotide (Novartis Pharmaceuticals), 10 to 50 µg/dog SC bid to tid
3. Streptozocin Therapy
   a. Continue standard treatment; reduce glucocorticoid dose to minimize adverse signs
   b. 0.9% saline diuresis for 3 hours, then streptozocin, 500 mg/m², in 0.9% saline and administered IV over 2 hours, then 0.9% saline diuresis for 2 additional hours
   c. Administer antiemetics immediately after streptozocin administration to minimize vomiting
   d. Repeat treatment every 3 weeks until hypoglycemia resolves or adverse reactions develop (e.g., pancreatitis, renal failure)

From Nelson RW, Couto CG: Small Animal Internal Medicine. St Louis, Mosby–Year Book, 2003, p. 772.

glycemia. This can usually be accomplished through frequent feeding of small meals and administration of glucocorticoids (Table 14-11). A continuous intravenous infusion of a balanced electrolyte solution containing 2.5% to 5% dextrose before, during, and immediately after surgery is important. Although this does not restore euglycemia, these solutions provide a substrate for adequate central nervous system function, thereby preventing CNS signs in most dogs and cats. Concentrations of dextrose in excess of 5% are extremely dangerous and *must* be avoided to prevent overstimulation of the pancreatic tumor and rebound, sometimes fatal, hypoglycemia. The intravenous dextrose infusion can be initiated the evening before surgery, at the time food and water are withheld, and continued throughout the perioperative period. Initiation of fluid therapy before surgery also helps ensure adequate circulation to the pancreas, thereby minimizing the risk of postoperative pancreatitis. The goal of the dextrose infusion is to prevent clinical signs of hypoglycemia and to maintain the blood glucose concentration at greater than 35 mg/dl. If the dextrose infusion is ineffective at preventing severe hypoglycemia during the perioperative period, a constant-rate infusion of glucagon should be considered (see Medical Therapy for an Acute Hypoglycemic Crisis, page 638).

INTRAOPERATIVE SURGICAL CONSIDERATIONS. During surgery, as much of the pancreas as possible should be examined visually. A complete, *gentle* digital inspection of this organ should then be undertaken. The importance of gentle handling of the pancreas cannot be overemphasized; failure to handle the organ gently may result in severe, potentially life-threatening pancreatitis. A thorough examination of the liver, surrounding lymph nodes, and omentum for metastatic sites should also be done.

Frequency of Tumor Identification. Most dogs with insulin-secreting tumors have masses that are easily visible to the surgeon inspecting the pancreas (Fig. 14-8). In a minority of dogs, the tumor is not visible but can be palpated during gentle but thorough digital examination of the pancreas. Multiple pancreatic masses may also occur. Seventy-eight (92%) of 85 dogs with insulin-secreting tumors in our practice had an obvious mass in the pancreas at the time of surgery.

Tumor Location. There is no predisposition for tumor location in the pancreas (Fig. 14-9). In our dogs, the mass was located in the right (duodenal) lobe of the pancreas in approximately 42%, in the left (splenic) lobe of the pancreas in 41%, and in the central region of the pancreas in 17%. In four of 85 dogs, a diffuse, microscopic islet cell carcinoma was recognized histologically in an arbitrarily resected portion of the right lobe of the pancreas. Diffuse thickening of the pancreas was evident on digital palpation of the pancreas at the time of surgery in two of these four dogs; the pancreas was visually and digitally normal in two dogs. In two of 85 dogs, there was no visible mass and no metastatic sites and the pancreas was normal on digital palpation. Histologic examination of a portion of the right limb of the pancreas failed to

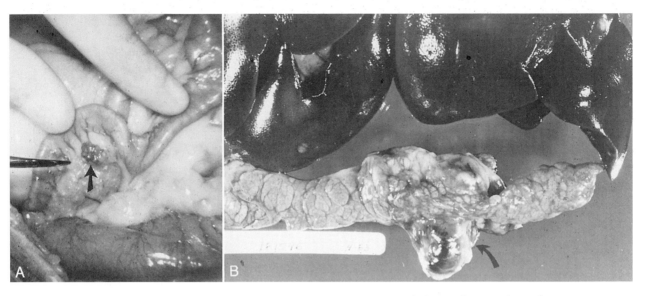

FIGURE 14-8. *A* and *B*, Photographs of pancreatic insulin-secreting islet beta-cell tumors (*arrows*).

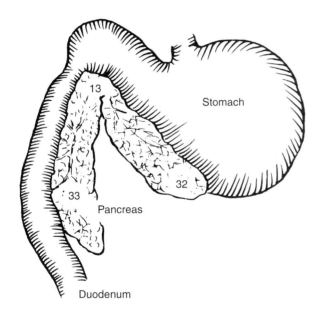

FIGURE 14-9. Diagram of tumor location in the pancreas in 78 dogs with an insulin-secreting islet beta-cell tumor.

identify an insulin-secreting tumor in either dog. A pancreatic mass was identified in one of these dogs 1 year after the initial surgery. The other dog was lost to follow-up at 18 months postsurgery; periodic evaluations of the dog identified persistent hypoglycemia and hyperinsulinemia but failed to identify a pancreatic mass. Enlargement of a mesenteric lymph node adjacent to the pancreas was evident in one dog, but a mass was not identified in the pancreas per se. Histologic examination of the excised lymph node confirmed metastatic beta-cell tumor. Hyperinsulinism and hypoglycemia persisted in this dog after surgery.

Tumor location has important ramifications for the success of surgery. In general, solitary tumors in the left or right limb of the pancreas are readily excisable with minimal damage to the pancreas and a low prevalence of postoperative pancreatitis. In contrast, tumors in the body of the pancreas are often intimately intertwined with the pancreatic ducts, blood vessels, and lymphatics. Surgical removal often requires extensive manipulation and dissection of the pancreas. Severe and potentially life-threatening pancreatitis that requires aggressive and often extended treatment is a common postoperative complication. In addition, complete excision of the tumor is almost impossible, and hypoglycemia typically recurs shortly after surgery. Prior to surgery we routinely discuss with the client the possible locations of the tumor and the implications that location has on attaining a successful outcome. We strongly recommend against tumor removal if the insulin-secreting tumor is located in the body of the pancreas because of the high probability of postoperative complications. We inform the client that there is a one in five chance of the dog having inoperable disease and that if such disease is found, we advise closing the abdomen and treating the dog medically rather than risk the development of severe pancreatitis by trying to remove the tumor.

Failure to Identify a Mass: Use of Methylene Blue. Intravenous methylene blue infusion has been advocated for intraoperative identification of a beta-cell tumor in the dog (Fingeroth and Smeak, 1988; Fingeroth et al, 1988). Methylene blue is an azodye that, when administered intravenously, is concentrated in the parathyroid glands and endocrine pancreas. Methylene blue intensely stains hyperfunctional, adenomatous, or carcinomatous areas of these organs. Normal pancreatic endocrine tissue is stained a dusky slate blue, whereas hyperfunctioning tissue is stained more intensely, often a reddish blue. In one dog, methylene blue also successfully identified an ectopic islet cell tumor and differentiated metastatic from nonmetastatic nodules in surrounding tissue (Smeak et al, 1988).

Methylene blue is administered as an intravenous infusion by mixing appropriate volumes of methylene blue in 250 ml of normal isotonic saline solution to obtain a total dose of 3 mg methylene blue per kilogram of body weight (Fingeroth and Smeak, 1988). The entire solution is given over a period of 30 to 40 minutes. Maximal staining of the endocrine pancreas occurs approximately 30 minutes after initiation of the infusion. Complications with methylene blue infusion include Heinz body hemolytic anemia, acute renal failure, pseudocyanosis (i.e., blue-appearing oral mucous membranes), green-tinged urine, and possibly pancreatitis. Hemolytic anemia is common, with the hematocrit declining to less than 25% 2 to 3 days after surgery.

We do not routinely use methylene blue because of its postoperative complications and because we have been able to grossly identify abnormal tissue in the vast majority of our dogs with beta-cell neoplasia. If our surgeon fails to recognize a mass and the diagnosis has been confirmed by glucose and insulin measurements, the recommendation is to remove the right or left limb of the pancreas in the hope of removing the portion that contains the tumor. In theory, 90% of the pancreas could be removed without causing overt diabetes mellitus or exocrine pancreatic insufficiency.

Sites of Metastasis. Little correlation appears to exist between tumor size or shape and its malignant potential. A complete inspection of the abdominal contents is imperative to identify unsuspected abnormalities as well as sites of metastasis. The most common sites of tumor spread include the regional lymphatics and lymph nodes (duodenal, mesenteric, hepatic, splenic), the liver, and the peripancreatic omentum. Failure to identify metastatic disease is common during surgery. A solitary pancreatic mass is commonly removed in toto, with the belief that the dog has been "cured," only to have clinical signs of hyperinsulinism recur months later. In our experience, almost all beta-cell tumors in the dog are malignant. Unfortunately, initial clinical signs are often vague and not worrisome to the owner; weeks to months may elapse between the onset of clinical signs and establishment of the diagnosis, and as a result, the likelihood of metastasis at the time of exploratory surgery is high.

Recommendations if Metastasis Is Identified. Ideally, all abnormal-appearing tissue should be removed, if possible, and submitted for histologic evaluation. When abnormal tissue cannot be entirely removed, debulking of the tumor mass may be beneficial. Biopsy of tumor tissue is the least a surgeon should accomplish. The surgeon must always weigh the potential gains obtained with aggressive tumor removal and debulking against the potential complications that may develop as a result of the surgical procedure. This is especially important when dealing with the pancreas, because life-threatening pancreatitis can develop after extensive manipulation and dissection of the gland. Because medical treatment is a viable option after surgery, euthanasia at the time of

surgery and heroic attempts to remove all abnormal tissue are not recommended in a dog with metastatic disease, especially if the latter course increases the risk of postoperative complications.

INTRAOPERATIVE MEDICAL THERAPY. Attention to the patient's blood glucose concentration and maintenance of adequate fluid therapy during surgery are imperative for the dog with beta-cell neoplasia. Monitoring of the blood glucose concentration every 30 to 60 minutes during surgery using a point-of-care or portable blood glucose monitoring device allows objective assessment of the dog's blood glucose status. The goal is to maintain the blood glucose concentration greater than 40 mg/dl, not to establish a normal blood glucose concentration per se. Moderate changes in the blood glucose concentration can be monitored and adjustments made in the rate of intravenous dextrose administration, as needed, to prevent the development of severe hypoglycemia (i.e., a blood glucose concentration <35 mg/dl). Fortunately, it is uncommon for a dog in stable condition with a beta-cell tumor to require more than a 5% dextrose solution given intravenously during surgery. This infusion usually maintains the blood glucose concentration above 35 mg/dl. If a 5% dextrose infusion is ineffective in preventing severe hypoglycemia during surgery, a constant-rate infusion of glucagon should be considered (see Medical Therapy for an Acute Hypoglycemic Crisis, page 638).

Adequate fluid therapy just prior to, during, and immediately after surgery is extremely important for minimizing the development of pancreatitis. Digital manipulation and dissection of the pancreas cause inflammation. The severity of inflammation depends on the gentleness of the palpation, circulation to the pancreas, and surgical procedures performed. Providing adequate fluid therapy prior to and during surgery ensures that every means of maintaining circulation through the microvasculature of the pancreas has been used and helps minimize the development of pancreatitis. We routinely administer fluids at a rate of 60 to 100 ml/kg/24 hr during surgery and for 24 to 72 hours after the procedure, unless concurrent problems (e.g., heart failure, hypoproteinemia) are present that may affect the dog's ability to handle intravenous fluids.

POSTOPERATIVE COMPLICATIONS. The most common postoperative complications are pancreatitis, hyperglycemia, and hypoglycemia. The development of these complications is directly related to the expertise of the surgeon in handling the pancreas and excising these tumors, the location of the tumor in the pancreas (i.e., peripheral lobe versus central region), the presence or absence of functional metastases, and the adequacy of fluid therapy during the perioperative period.

Pancreatitis. Intravenous administration of polyionic fluids with 2.5% to 5% dextrose (60 to 100 ml/kg/24 hr) and nothing per os just before and during and for 24 to 48 hours after surgery, followed by appropriate dietary therapy during the ensuing week, is helpful in minimizing the development of pancreatitis. Serum electrolytes and the blood glucose concentration should be measured twice a day during treatment with intravenous fluids, and appropriate adjustments should be made in the electrolyte or dextrose composition of the fluids. We rely on physical examination findings in determining when to initiate water and a bland diet. Circulating pancreatic enzyme concentrations (e.g., lipase and amylase) are rarely determined after surgery. Arbitrarily treating the dog for pancreatitis without determining the serum pancreatic enzyme concentrations beforehand has produced excellent results. Despite gentle handling of the pancreas during surgery, aggressive fluid therapy during the perioperative period, and appropriate dietary therapy during the postoperative period, 8 (12%) of 69 dogs undergoing surgery for beta-cell tumor still developed clinical signs of acute pancreatitis. Two of the eight dogs died as a result of pancreatitis; in both dogs, the tumor was located in the body of the pancreas and was difficult to excise.

Diabetes Mellitus. Occasionally dogs develop diabetes mellitus after surgical removal of an insulin-secreting tumor. Diabetes mellitus is believed to result from inadequate insulin secretion by atrophied normal beta cells. Removal of all or a majority of the neoplastic cells acutely deprives the animal of insulin. Until the atrophied normal cells regain their secretory capabilities, the animal is hypoinsulinemic and may require exogenous insulin injections to maintain euglycemia. It was once thought that postsurgical hyperglycemia and glucosuria were excellent prognostic signs indicating total removal of insulin-secreting neoplastic cells. However, most of our dogs have required exogenous insulin only transiently after surgery and ultimately have required medical management for an exacerbation of an insulin-secreting tumor several weeks to months after their need for insulin therapy dissipates.

Postsurgical insulin therapy is initiated only when hyperglycemia and glucosuria persist for longer than 2 or 3 days after the discontinuation of all dextrose-containing intravenous fluids. Initial insulin therapy should be conservative, that is, 0.25 U of NPH or lente insulin per kilogram of body weight given once daily. Subsequent adjustments in insulin therapy should be based on clinical response and serial blood glucose determinations (see Chapter 11, page 507).

Diabetes mellitus is usually transient, lasting from a few days to several months. Most of these dogs still have neoplastic beta cells in the pancreas, liver, lymph nodes, or peripancreatic tissues that multiply and eventually reach a population density capable of secreting enough insulin to cause hypoglycemic signs to recur. For these dogs, resolution of diabetes is followed by a variable period of euglycemia, which eventually progresses to hypoglycemia. Owner evaluation of the pet's urine glucose is helpful in identifying when insulin therapy is no longer needed. Persistently negative urine glucose in conjunction with cessation of polyuria and polydipsia is an indication to discontinue insulin therapy. If hyperglycemia and glucosuria recur,

insulin therapy can be reinstituted, but at a lower insulin dosage. The development of permanent insulin-requiring diabetes mellitus after surgical removal of a solitary insulin-secreting tumor is uncommon and implies additional abnormalities involving the beta cells (e.g., beta-cell degeneration, beta-cell hypoplasia; see Chapter 11). Permanent diabetes mellitus has developed in only one dog that underwent surgical removal of an insulin-secreting tumor at our hospital. The dog was lost to follow-up after 2.5 years, and at that time the dog was still receiving insulin injections twice a day to control hyperglycemia.

Persistent Hypoglycemia. Dogs that remain hypoglycemic after surgical removal of an insulin-secreting tumor are assumed to have functional metastases. Medical therapy should be initiated in dogs with persistent postoperative hypoglycemia. During the initial 48 to 72 postoperative hours, intravenous infusion of 2.5% to 5% dextrose should be continued. The goal is to prevent clinical signs of hypoglycemia (especially seizures), not to reestablish a normal blood glucose concentration. Additional therapy may be needed if hypoglycemic seizures occur (Table 14-12; also see Medical Therapy for an Acute Hypoglycemic Crisis, page 638). Small meals should be fed every 4 to 6 hours, beginning as soon after surgery as possible. A diet acceptable for the treatment of pancreatitis (e.g., boiled white rice and low-fat cottage cheese) should be fed initially. Additional therapy may be needed, depending on the efficacy of the frequent feedings in maintaining remission of clinical hypoglycemia (see

TABLE 14–12   MEDICAL THERAPY FOR HYPOGLYCEMIC SEIZURES CAUSED BY AN INSULIN-SECRETING BETA-CELL TUMOR

Seizures at Home

Step 1. Rub or pour sugar solution on pet's gums
Step 2. Once pet is sternal, feed a small meal
Step 3. Call the veterinarian

Seizures in Hospital

Step 1. Administer 1 to 5 ml of 50% dextrose IV *slowly* over 10 minutes
Step 2. Once animal is sternal, feed a small meal
Step 3. Initiate long-term medical therapy (see Table 14-11)

Intractable Seizures in Hospital

Step 1. Administer 2.5% to 5% dextrose in water IV at 1.5 to 2 times maintenance fluid rate
Step 2. Add 0.5 or 1 mg of dexamethasone/kg to IV fluids and administer over 6 hours; repeat every 12 to 24 hours, as necessary
Step 3. Administer glucagon USP (Eli Lilly Co.) IV by constant rate infusion at an initial dosage of 5 to 10 ng/kg/min
Step 4. Somatostatin analog (Octreotide, Novartis Pharmaceuticals), 10 to 50 μg SC bid to tid
Step 5. If above fails, anesthetize animal with pentobarbital for 4 to 8 hours while continuing above therapy; consider surgery to debulk functional tumor

From Nelson RW, Couto CG: Small Animal Internal Medicine. St Louis, Mosby–Year Book, 2003, p. 774.

Medical Therapy for Chronic Hypoglycemia, page 639). If a dog becomes symptomatic despite the frequent feedings, medical therapy should be attempted before euthanasia is recommended.

EVALUATING THE LONG-TERM SUCCESS OF SURGERY: IS THE DOG CURED? The long-term success of surgery can be difficult to predict in dogs with a "solitary" mass that is removed in toto. The most efficient and logical initial method for evaluating these patients for recurrence of beta-cell neoplasia is periodic measurement (i.e., every 1 to 3 months) of a fasting blood glucose concentration. Blood for glucose determination should be obtained after food has been withheld from the dog for 8 to 12 hours. The fasting blood glucose concentration should be consistently greater than 70 mg/dl if beta-cell neoplasia has not recurred. Recurrence of beta-cell neoplasia should be suspected if the blood glucose concentration is less than 70 mg/dl. Confirmation of recurrence requires measurement of the serum insulin concentration when the blood glucose concentration is less than 60 mg/dl (see Confirming an Insulin-Secreting Beta-Cell Tumor, page 629).

Medical Therapy for an Acute Hypoglycemic Crisis

The acute onset of clinical signs caused by hypoglycemia typically occurs at home after exercise, excitement, or eating; during the immediate postoperative period in the dog with functioning metastases or inoperable neoplasia; or as a result of inadvertently aggressive intravenous dextrose administration at the time hypoglycemia is initially identified. Therapy depends on the severity of clinical signs and the location of the dog (i.e., home versus hospital) and initially involves administration of glucose, either as food or sugar water by mouth or as an intravenous 50% dextrose solution.

If an owner contacts a veterinarian by telephone and reports that the pet is having a hypoglycemic seizure, we do not recommend transporting the dog to a veterinary hospital. Rather, the owner should be instructed to pour a sugar solution (e.g., Karo syrup) over the fingers and rub the syrup on the pet's buccal mucosa. Hypoglycemic dogs usually respond in 1 to 2 minutes. The owner should not place a hand or object into an animal's mouth during a seizure because the person might be bitten, and the sugar solution should not be poured directly into the animal's mouth because the animal may aspirate the liquid. If a dog responds to glucose administration, it should be fed a small, high-protein meal once it is sternal and cognizant of its surroundings. The dog should then be kept as quiet as possible, and veterinary attention can then be considered.

In the hospital, clinical signs of hypoglycemia can usually be alleviated with intravenous administration of 50% dextrose. It is imperative to avoid overstimulating the tumor when administering dextrose

intravenously. Overstimulation of the tumor can result in a massive release of insulin into the circulation and rebound, severe hypoglycemia. A vicious circle can result, with the clinician "chasing" the hypoglycemia with larger and larger amounts of 50% dextrose and the resultant rebound hypoglycemia becoming more and more severe. This cycle can result in persistent convulsions and death from cerebral edema. Persistent cycles of hypoglycemia and hyperglycemia require intensive medical therapy (see Table 14-12) and can be difficult to break.

Cycles of hyperglycemia and hypoglycemia can be avoided by minimizing rapid increases in the blood glucose concentration. Dextrose should be administered in small amounts slowly rather than in large boluses rapidly. The goal of therapy is to control the clinical signs, not correct hypoglycemia. Once the signs have been controlled with judicious intravenous administration of dextrose, frequent feedings and glucocorticoids can be initiated (see Table 14-11).

If the dextrose infusion is ineffective in preventing severe hypoglycemia or breaking the cycle of hypoglycemia and hyperglycemia, a constant-rate infusion of glucagon should be considered. Glucagon is a potent stimulant of hepatic glycogenolysis and gluconeogenesis and is effective in maintaining normal blood glucose concentrations in dogs with beta-cell neoplasia when administered by constant-rate infusion (Fig. 14-10) (Fischer et al, 2000). One milligram of lyophilized glucagon USP (Eli Lilly, Indianapolis, IN) is reconstituted with the diluent provided by the manufacturer, and the solution is added to 1 L of 0.9% saline, making a 1 µg/ml solution, which can be administered by syringe pump. The initial dosage is 5 to 10 ng per kilogram of body weight per minute. The dosage is adjusted as needed to maintain the blood glucose concentration between 50 and 100 mg/dl. When discontinuing glucagon, the

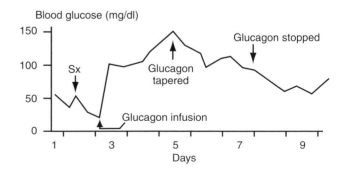

FIGURE 14-10. Blood glucose concentrations in a 13-year-old female spayed Pomeranian before and after surgical removal of an insulin-secreting islet beta-cell tumor. Pancreatitis and severe hypoglycemia developed postoperatively. The hypoglycemia resolved, and euglycemia was maintained after initiation of a constant-rate intravenous infusion of glucagon. The dosage of glucagon was gradually tapered beginning on day 5, feeding of small amounts of food was begun on day 7, and the intravenous glucagon infusion was stopped on day 8. Severe hypoglycemia did not recur.

dose should be gradually decreased over 1 to 2 days and the blood glucose level monitored for recurrence of severe hypoglycemia.

Occasionally, a hypoglycemic dog or cat with CNS signs fails to respond to glucose or glucagon administration. These signs could be the result of a disorder unrelated to hypoglycemia. However, irreversible cerebral lesions may result from long-term, severe hypoglycemia and the resultant cerebral hypoxia. Cerebral hypoxia predisposes the nervous tissue to edema, causing increased cerebrospinal fluid pressure and cell death. These animals have a guarded to grave prognosis. Therapy is directed at providing a continuous supply of glucose as a 5% solution given intravenously or by stimulating hepatic glucose production with a constant-rate infusion of glucagon. Simultaneously, seizure activity is controlled with diazepam or stronger anticonvulsant medication. Last, if cerebral edema is suspected, it may be treated with mannitol (1 g/kg body weight IV as a 20% solution administered at a rate of 2 ml/kg/min), furosemide (0.7 mg/kg as an IV bolus, repeated in 4 hours), and glucocorticoids (prednisone sodium succinate at 30 mg/kg IV followed by 0.1 mg/kg dexamethasone IV twice every 12 hours for 3 days) (Fenner, 1995).

Medical Therapy for Chronic Hypoglycemia (see Table 14-11)

BACKGROUND. Medical management for chronic hypoglycemia should be initiated when an exploratory celiotomy is not performed or when metastatic or inoperable neoplasia results in recurrence of clinical signs. The goals of medical therapy are to reduce the frequency and severity of clinical signs and to avoid an acute hypoglycemic crisis, not to establish euglycemia per se. Medical therapy typically involves nonspecific antihormonal therapy. Antihormonal therapy is palliative and should minimize hypoglycemia by providing a continuous source of glucose from the gastrointestinal tract, increasing hepatic glycogenolysis and gluconeogenesis, or inhibiting the synthesis, secretion, or peripheral cellular actions of insulin. Antihormonal therapy consists primarily of frequent feedings and glucocorticoids (see Table 14-11). Surgical debulking of functional masses may enhance the effectiveness of medical therapy. The best results are obtained when surgical debulking is performed shortly after the diagnosis of insulin-secreting tumor has been established, although we have had a few dogs benefit from surgical debulking after medical treatment has become ineffective in controlling clinical signs of hypoglycemia. One of our dogs underwent surgical debulking on three separate occasions; the dog survived 3 years before succumbing to metastatic disease involving the lungs.

Alloxan and streptozocin are drugs with specific toxicity directed at beta cells. The potential for serious adverse reactions has limited the use of these drugs for the treatment of insulin-secreting tumors in dogs. However, a viable treatment protocol using streptozocin was recently described, and studies are underway to determine its value in the treatment of insulin-secreting tumors (Moore et al, 2002).

FREQUENT FEEDINGS. Dogs with insulin-secreting tumors have a persistent absolute or relative excess of circulating insulin. If a constant source of calories is provided as a substrate for this insulin, hypoglycemic episodes can be reduced in frequency or prevented. Diets high in fat, complex carbohydrates, and fiber delay gastric emptying, slow intestinal glucose absorption, and help minimize a rapid increase in the portal blood glucose concentration that could stimulate excessive pancreatic insulin secretion. Simple sugars are rapidly absorbed, have a potent stimulatory effect on insulin secretion by neoplastic beta cells, and therefore should be avoided in the animal's diet. If dog food is used, a combination of canned and dry food, fed in three to six small meals daily, is recommended. Daily caloric intake should be controlled because hyperinsulinemia promotes obesity. Exercise should be limited to short walks on a leash.

GLUCOCORTICOID THERAPY. Glucocorticoid therapy should be initiated when dietary manipulations are no longer effective in preventing the signs of hypoglycemia. Glucocorticoids antagonize the effects of insulin at the cellular level, stimulate hepatic glycogenolysis, and indirectly provide the necessary substrates for hepatic gluconeogenesis. Prednisone, the glucocorticoid most often used, is given at an initial dosage of 0.5 mg/kg/day in divided oral doses twice daily. If this controls the signs of hypoglycemia, the medication is continued without dosage adjustment. If signs persist or recur, the dose of prednisone should be gradually increased until signs of hypoglycemia abate or signs of iatrogenic hyperadrenocorticism become unacceptable to the owner. For most owners, the severity of polydipsia, polyuria, polyphagia, weight gain, or panting eventually becomes unacceptable. When this occurs, the prednisone should be reduced (not stopped) to a dosage that minimizes signs of iatrogenic hyperadrenocorticism, and diazoxide or possibly streptozocin therapy should be considered.

DIAZOXIDE THERAPY. Diazoxide (Proglycem; Baker Norton Pharmaceuticals, Miami, FL) is a benzothiadiazide diuretic that inhibits insulin secretion, stimulates hepatic gluconeogenesis and glycogenolysis, and inhibits tissue use of glucose. The net effect is the development of hyperglycemia. Diazoxide does not inhibit insulin synthesis and does not have cytotoxic (antineoplastic) effects. Unfortunately, diazoxide is difficult to procure and expensive. The initial dosage is 10 mg/kg orally, divided into two doses daily. The dosage may gradually be increased as needed to control signs of hypoglycemia but should not exceed 60 mg/kg/day. Thiazide diuretics may potentiate the effects of diazoxide. The two drugs can be administered together to enhance hyperglycemic effects if diazoxide alone is not effective. The dosage of hydrochlorothiazide is 2 to 4 mg/kg/day orally, divided into two doses daily.

The goal of diazoxide therapy is to establish a dosage at which hypoglycemia and its clinical signs are reduced or absent. In addition, the dosage should be low enough to avoid hyperglycemia (blood glucose concentrations >180 mg/dl) and its associated clinical signs. Reports of diazoxide use have appeared in the veterinary literature only sporadically (Leifer et al, 1986; Feldman and Nelson, 1987). Thirteen of 17 dogs with an insulin-secreting tumor in our series had a good clinical response, lasting 6 weeks to 20 months. In another report, nine of 14 dogs had a good response to diazoxide therapy (Leifer et al, 1986).

The most common adverse reactions to diazoxide administration are anorexia and vomiting. Administering diazoxide with a meal or decreasing the dosage, at least temporarily, is usually effective in controlling adverse gastrointestinal signs. Other potential complications include diarrhea, tachycardia, bone marrow suppression, aplastic anemia, thrombocytopenia, pancreatitis, diabetes mellitus, cataracts, and sodium and fluid retention (Feldman and Nelson, 1987). Diazoxide is metabolized in the liver, and the metabolites are excreted via the kidneys and biliary system. Adverse reactions or complications may develop more rapidly or at a lower dosage of diazoxide in a dog with concurrent hepatic dysfunction.

SOMATOSTATIN THERAPY. Octreotide (Novartis Pharmaceuticals, East Hanover, NJ) is an analog of somatostatin that inhibits the synthesis and secretion of insulin by normal and neoplastic beta cells. Intravenous administration of octreotide can rapidly decrease the serum insulin concentration, causing a corresponding increase in the serum glucose concentration in dogs with insulin-secreting neoplasia (Fig. 14-11) (Robben et al, 1997). The inhibitory actions of octreotide on insulin secretion can be maintained for several hours with subcutaneous administration (Fig. 14-12). The responsiveness of insulin-secreting tumors to the suppressive effects of octreotide varies and depends on the presence of membrane receptors on the tumor cells that bind somatostatin (Lamberts et al, 1990; Simpson et al, 1995). To date, five subtypes of somatostatin receptors have been identified in humans (Kubota et al, 1994). These subtypes show a tissue-specific distribution and differences in affinity for somatostatin and its analogs (Bruns et al, 1994). In humans, some insulin-secreting tumors have receptor subtypes that do not or only minimally bind octreotide, resulting in minimal to no effect by the analog on the serum insulin and glucose concentrations (Lamberts et al, 1991 and 1996). Autoradiography performed in dogs with insulin-secreting neoplasia suggest the presence of only one type of somatostatin receptor in canine insulin-secreting tumors (Robben et al, 1997). The somatostatin receptor identified in canine insulin-secreting tumors contains high-affinity binding sites for octreotide. In that study, baseline plasma insulin concentrations, although varying widely, decreased significantly in all 10 dogs after octreotide administration. In our experience, somatostatin is beneficial in

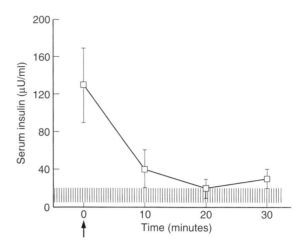

FIGURE 14-11. Mean (± SD) serum insulin concentration prior to and after intravenous administration of 100 μg of octreotide in six dogs with an insulin-secreting islet cell tumor. *Arrow,* Octreotide administration; *hatched area,* normal range for fasting serum insulin concentration.

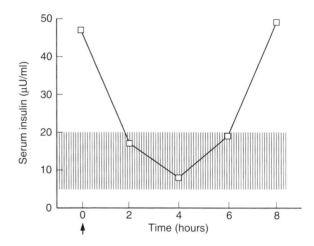

FIGURE 14-12. Serum insulin concentration prior to and after subcutaneous administration of 20 μg of octreotide to a dog with an insulin-secreting islet cell tumor. *Arrow,* Octreotide administration; *hatched area,* normal range for fasting serum insulin concentration.

alleviating hypoglycemia in approximately 40% to 50% of treated dogs. Unfortunately, some dogs become refractory to octreotide treatment (Lothrop, 1989). Nevertheless, octreotide (10 to 50 μg SC bid to tid) is well tolerated and can be used for the management of both acute and chronic hypoglycemia in some dogs with insulin-secreting neoplasia. Adverse reactions have not been reported at these dosages.

CHEMOTHERAPEUTIC DRUGS. Streptozocin and alloxan have been used for the treatment of human insulin-secreting tumors, but such use has appeared only sporadically in the veterinary literature. The potential for serious adverse reactions has limited the use of these drugs for the treatment of insulin-secreting tumors in dogs, although a viable treatment protocol using streptozocin was recently described (Moore et al, 2002).

Streptozocin. Streptozocin is a naturally occurring nitrosourea that selectively destroys pancreatic beta cells by depressing the pyridine nucleotides nicotinamide adenine dinucleotide (NAD) and reduced nicotinamide adenine dinucleotide (NADH). Streptozocin at a dosage of 500 mg/m^2 given intravenously for 5 consecutive days has proved effective at reducing tumor size and improving clinical signs of hyperinsulinism in humans with advanced beta-cell carcinoma (Moertel et al, 1980). The major toxicity associated with streptozocin treatment in humans is proximal renal tubular necrosis, which is dose related and cumulative and may lead to renal failure. Less common toxicities include nausea, vomiting, and increases in serum hepatic enzyme activity.

Two dogs with confirmed hyperinsulinism were treated with streptozocin by Meyer in the 1970s. The first dog developed nephrotoxicosis and was euthanized 3 weeks after a single treatment with streptozocin at a dosage of 1000 mg/kg body weight given intravenously over a 1-minute period. The second dog developed temporary remission of hypoglycemia that lasted approximately 50 days after two treatments with streptozocin at a dosage of 500 mg/m^2 given intravenously over a 30-second period. The treatments were given 1 week apart, and mannitol was infused for 20 minutes before and after each streptozocin treatment. The dog developed a nephropathy and hepatopathy after a third treatment administered at day 97 and was euthanized shortly thereafter. As a result of these clinical reports, streptozocin was not considered a viable treatment for insulin-secreting tumors in dogs.

Recently, Moore and colleagues (2002) described a fluid diuresis protocol that allows streptozocin to be administered to dogs with insulin-secreting tumors with a minimum of adverse reactions. Fluid diuresis has been reported to ameliorate the renal toxicity of streptozocin in humans, presumably as a result of less contact time between the drug and the renal tubular epithelium (Tobin et al, 1987; Kintzel, 2001). In Moore's study, diuresis with 0.9% sodium chloride at a rate of 18.3 ml/kg/hr administered through a peripherally located over-the-needle catheter was performed for 7 hours. Streptozocin (Zanosar; Upjohn, Kalamazoo, MI) was administered over a 2-hour period beginning 3 hours after initiation of the saline diuresis. The dose of streptozocin (500 mg/m^2) was diluted in an appropriate volume of 0.9% saline to maintain the same rate of fluid administration for 2 hours. Saline diuresis was continued at the same fluid rate for an additional 2 hours after completion of the streptozocin administration. Butorphanol (0.4 mg/kg IV) was given immediately after streptozocin administration as an antiemetic. Streptozocin treatments were repeated at 3-week intervals until there was evidence of tumor progression (i.e., increase in tumor size by greater than 50%), recurrence of hypoglycemia, or streptozocin-induced toxicity that required supportive treatment. Fifty-eight treatments were administered to 17 dogs with an insulin-secreting tumor at variable times after surgery (Moore et al, 2002). Sixteen of 17 dogs had metastatic disease. One dog developed azotemia, several dogs developed increases in serum alanine transaminase activity that appeared to resolve with cessation of treatment, and vomiting occurred in 18 (31%) of 58 streptozocin treatments and was occasionally severe. Two dogs developed diabetes mellitus after receiving five treatments; two of three dogs had rapid resolution of paraneoplastic peripheral neuropathy; and two dogs had a measurable reduction in tumor size. Although the median survival time was longer in dogs treated with streptozocin than in 15 control dogs with a similar stage of disease (163 versus 90 days, respectively), this difference was not statistically significant. The range for survival time was also similar between the two groups of dogs (streptozocin-treated dogs, 16 to 309 days; control dogs, 0 to 426 days). Based on the results of this study, it appears that streptozocin can be administered safely to dogs when combined with fluid diuresis, and streptozocin may be of benefit in some dogs with metastatic insulin-secreting tumors.

Alloxan. Alloxan is an unstable uric acid derivative that has a direct cytotoxic effect on the pancreatic beta cells, primarily by altering beta-cell membrane permeability (Dublin et al, 1983). The toxic effect of alloxan on beta cells appears to be dose related. In addition, alloxan enhances hepatic gluconeogenesis, possibly by enhancing glucagon secretion from pancreatic alpha cells (Dublin et al, 1983).

Alloxan has not been helpful in the management of beta-cell neoplasia in humans (Sherwin and Felig, 1981). We have had mixed results using the drug to treat eight dogs with metastatic beta-cell neoplasia. Alloxan (65 mg/kg IV) was given only once to each dog. Four dogs initially responded favorably, with hyperglycemia or euglycemia developing within 3 to 5 days of treatment and lasting for several months without other medical therapy except frequent feedings. Hypoglycemia eventually recurred in these four dogs. Hyperglycemia was transient in one dog, with hypoglycemia developing 3 weeks after alloxan administration. One dog died of acute renal failure, and two dogs died of acute respiratory distress syndrome within 24 hours of alloxan treatment.

Toxicities associated with alloxan therapy include renal tubular necrosis and resultant acute renal failure, acute respiratory distress syndrome with fulminate pulmonary edema, and hepatic necrosis. Renal toxicity is dose dependent and potentially reversible with appropriate fluid therapy and supportive care. At a dosage of 65 mg/kg given intravenously, alloxan can be used as a one-time injection to induce diabetes mellitus in healthy dogs. In our experience, problems with acute renal tubular necrosis and uremia, acute respiratory distress syndrome, or both develop in 10% to 20% of healthy dogs given intravenous alloxan. Alloxan has also been associated with hepatic central lobular necrosis and fatty infiltration when used at dosages greater than the diabetogenic dose.

OTHER DRUGS. Additional drugs that have been suggested to be helpful in decreasing the likelihood of hypoglycemic episodes include propranolol and phenytoin. These drugs have not been critically evaluated in dogs or cats with beta-cell neoplasia, and we rarely, if ever, use them.

Phenytoin. Phenytoin is an anticonvulsant that inhibits the release of insulin by the beta cells of the pancreas and that may also directly impair the effects of insulin on peripheral tissues (Haemers and Rottiers, 1981). Unfortunately, phenytoin is not usually successful in controlling clinical signs of hypoglycemia. Only 30% of human patients with hyperinsulinism showed any beneficial effects after phenytoin administration (Haemers and Rottiers, 1981). Concurrent diazoxide administration is not recommended, because it results in a decrease in blood concentrations of phenytoin.

Propranolol. Propranolol is a nonselective beta-adrenergic blocking drug that has no intrinsic sympathomimetic activity. Its potential usefulness in patients with beta-cell neoplasia probably involves its ability to block insulin secretion by beta cells. Insulin secretion is stimulated by the beta-adrenergic nervous system. However, propranolol may also induce hypoglycemia by impairing hepatic gluconeogenesis and glycogenolysis, normally induced by endogenous catecholamines.

PROGNOSIS

Owing to the extremely high likelihood of malignancy in any dog with an insulin-secreting tumor, the long-term prognosis is guarded to poor at best. Survival time depends partly on the owner's willingness to treat the disease. Tobin and colleagues (1999) reported a median survival time after diagnosis of only 74 days (range, 8 to 508 days) in dogs treated medically, compared with 381 days (range, 20 to 1758 days) in dogs that initially underwent surgery. The shorter survival time for dogs treated medically was partly due to a more severe stage of the disease at the time of diagnosis and the owners' feelings of hopelessness, which translated into early acceptance of euthanasia when clinical signs recurred.

The extent to which surgery can alter the prognosis depends on the clinical stage of the disease, most notably the extent of metastatic lesions. In one multiuniversity study, dogs with tumors confined to the pancreas (stage I) were normoglycemic for a median of 14 months after surgery, whereas dogs with metastasis to regional lymph nodes (stage II) or distant metastasis (stage III) were normoglycemic a median of approximately 1 month (Caywood et al, 1988). Dogs with stage I or stage II disease had a median survival time of approximately 18 months, whereas those with stage III disease had a median survival time of less than 6 months. Approximately 50% of dogs with metastases to the liver (the most common site) were dead by 6 months, and all were dead by 18 months from the time of diagnosis.

In our experience, approximately 10% to 15% of dogs undergoing surgery for an insulin-secreting tumor die or are euthanized at the time of or within 1 month of surgery because of severe metastatic disease, uncontrollable postoperative hypoglycemia, or complications related to pancreatitis. An additional 20% to 25% of dogs die or are euthanized within 6 months of surgery because of severe metastatic disease and recurrence of clinical hypoglycemia. The remaining 60% to 70% live beyond 6 months postoperatively, many beyond 1 year after surgery, before uncontrollable hypoglycemia develops, resulting in death or necessitating euthanasia. Additional surgery to debulk metastatic lesions may improve the animal's responsiveness to medical therapy and prolong the survival time in some dogs that become nonresponsive to medical treatment after the initial surgery. Some dogs with metastatic disease do remarkably well (i.e., survive longer than 2 years) after aggressive surgical debulking of the tumor and its metastases.

INSULIN-SECRETING BETA-CELL TUMORS IN CATS

Insulin-secreting beta-cell tumors are rare in cats. There are only three case reports of beta-cell neoplasia in cats in the literature (McMillan, 1985; O'Brien et al, 1990; Hawks et al, 1992) and one additional report in which the beta-cell tumor was an incidental finding at necropsy in a cat with ductal pancreatic adenocarcinoma (Carpenter et al, 1987). We have seen only two cats with beta-cell neoplasia during the past two decades, in contrast to more than 120 dogs with the disease during the same time interval.

The clinical characteristics of insulin-secreting beta-cell tumors in cats appear to be similar to those in dogs. To date, the disorder has affected aged cats, 12 to 17 years old. Interestingly, three of four cats have been Siamese. Immunohistochemical analysis of the beta-cell tumor in three cats revealed multihormonal productivity, with insulin being the most common peptide demonstrated in the neoplastic cells. Clinical signs appeared to result from the effects of hyperinsulinism and included seizures, weakness, ataxia, and muscle twitching. Hypoglycemia (blood glucose concentration <60 mg/dl) was documented in each cat, and an inappropriately increased blood insulin concentration was documented in two cats in which insulin was measured. A pancreatic mass was identified in three cats that underwent surgery, and hypoglycemia and clinical signs resolved in two of three cats after surgical excision of the mass. These three cats died 5 weeks, 18 months, and 2 years after surgery, and all cats were hypoglycemic at the time of death. Necropsy in one of these cats revealed metastasis to the liver and pancreatic lymph nodes.

Until more experience is gained with beta-cell neoplasia in cats, it seems prudent to approach this disorder in a manner similar to that used for dogs. Beta-cell neoplasia should be included in the list of differential diagnoses for persistent hypoglycemia in the older cat (see Table 14-8). The index of suspicion for beta-cell neoplasia should be heightened after a thorough review of the history, physical examination, and results of clinicopathologic tests and diagnostic imaging. The diagnosis should be confirmed by documentation of an inappropriate serum insulin concentration despite the presence of hypoglycemia (see Confirming an Insulin-Secreting Beta-Cell Tumor, page 629). Many commercially available radio-immunoassays for insulin work well in the dog but do not work in the cat (Lutz and Rand, 1993). It is imperative that the radioimmunoassay used to measure feline insulin be validated for cats.

Surgical exploration should be the initial treatment of choice for beta-cell neoplasia in the cat. However, the age of the cat, identification of metastatic disease using ultrasonography, or the existence of concurrent disease that increases the anesthetic risk may warrant a more conservative medical approach in some cats. Frequent feedings and glucocorticoid therapy have been effective in controlling clinical signs of hyperinsulinism (Hawks et al, 1992) and should be the mainstay of medical therapy for chronic hypoglycemia. The use of diazoxide has not been reported in the cat, therefore diazoxide should be used with caution until its safety is reported in cats. We have administered relatively large doses of the somatostatin analog octreotide (i.e., 200 µg SC) to cats with acromegaly with no adverse reactions. Dosages recommended for the treatment of beta-cell tumor in dogs should be safe in cats. However, the efficacy of octreotide for the treatment of feline beta-cell neoplasia remains to be reported.

REFERENCES

Bagley RS, et al: Hypoglycemia associated with intraabdominal leiomyoma and leiomyosarcoma in six dogs. J Am Vet Med Assoc 208:69, 1996.

Barreca A, et al: In vitro paracrine regulation of human keratinocyte growth by fibroblast-derived insulin-like growth factors. J Cell Physiol 151:262, 1992.

Beaudry D, et al: Hypoglycemia in four dogs with smooth muscle tumors. J Vet Intern Med 9:415, 1995.

Bellah JR, Ginn PE: Gastric leiomyosarcoma associated with hypoglycemia in a dog. J Am Anim Hosp Assoc 32:283, 1996.

Bergman PJ, et al: Canine clinical peripheral neuropathy associated with pancreatic islet cell carcinoma. Prog Vet Neurol 5:57, 1994.

Boari A, et al: Hypoglycemia in a dog with a leiomyoma of the gastric wall producing an insulin-like growth factor II–like peptide. Eur J Endocrinol 132:744, 1995.

Boyle PJ, Cryer PE: Growth hormone, cortisol, or both are involved in defense against but are not critical to recovery from prolonged hypoglycemia in humans. Am J Physiol 260:E395, 1991.

Braund KG, et al: Insulinoma and subclinical peripheral neuropathy in two dogs. J Vet Intern Med 1:86, 1987.

Breitschwerdt EB, et al: Hypoglycemia in four dogs with sepsis. J Am Vet Med Assoc 178:1072, 1981.

Brix A, et al: Glycogen storage disease type Ia in two littermate Maltese puppies. Vet Pathol 32:460, 1995.

Bruns C, et al: Molecular pharmacology of somatostatin receptor subtypes. Ann N Y Acad Sci 733:138, 1994.

Buetow PC, et al: Islet cell tumors of the pancreas: Clinical, radiological, and pathologic correlation in diagnosis and localization. Radiographics 17:453, 1997.

Carpenter JL, et al: Tumors and tumorlike lesions. In Holsworth J (ed): Diseases of the Cat: Medicine and Surgery. Philadelphia, WB Saunders, 1987, p 406.

Caywood DD, et al: Pancreatic insulin-secreting neoplasms: Clinical, diagnostic, and prognostic features in 73 dogs. J Am Anim Hosp Assoc 24:577, 1988.

Chastain CB: Endocrine and metabolic systems. In Hoskins JD (ed): Veterinary Pediatrics. Philadelphia, WB Saunders, 1990, p 249.

Chew DJ, et al: Hyperglycemia and hypoglycemia. In Klenner WR (ed): Quick Reference to Veterinary Medicine. Philadelphia, JB Lippincott, 1982, p 432.

Cohn LA, et al: Assessment of five portable blood glucose meters, a point-of-care analyzer, and color test strips for measuring blood glucose concentration in dogs. J Am Vet Med Assoc 216:198, 2000.

Commens PJ, et al: Interleukin-1 is a potent modulator of insulin secretion from isolated rat islets of Langerhans. Diabetes 36:963, 1987.

Cryer PE: Catecholamines, pheochromocytoma and diabetes. Diabetes Rev 1:309, 1993.

Cryer PE, Gerich JE: Glucose counterregulation, hypoglycemia, and intensive insulin therapy in diabetes mellitus. N Engl J Med 313:232, 1985.

Cryer PE, Polonsky KS: Glucose homeostasis and hypoglycemia. In Wilson JD, et al (eds): Williams Textbook of Endocrinology, 9th ed. Philadelphia, WB Saunders, 1998, p 939.

Das H, Hochberg FH: Metastatic neoplasms and paraneoplastic syndromes. In Goetz CG, Pappert EJ (eds): Textbook of Clinical Neurology. Philadelphia, WB Saunders, 1999, p 957.

Daughaday WH: The pathophysiology of IGF-II hypersecretion in non-islet tumor hypoglycemia. Diabetes Rev 3:62, 1995.

Daughaday WH, et al: Synthesis and secretion of insulin-like growth factor II by a leiomyosarcoma with associated hypoglycemia. N Engl J Med 319:1434, 1988.

D'Ercole AJ, et al: Tissue concentration of somatomedin-C: Further evidence for multiple sites of synthesis and paracrine or autocrine mechanisms of action. Proc Natl Acad Sci USA 81:935, 1984.

de Bruijne JJ: Ketone-body metabolism in fasting dogs. Doctoral thesis. University of Utrecht, 1982, The Netherlands.

de Bruijne JJ, et al: Fat mobilization and plasma hormone levels in fasted dogs. Metabolism 30:190, 1981.

del Ray A, Besedovsky H: Interleukin-1 affects glucose homeostasis. Am J Physiol 253:R794, 1987.

Dublin WE, et al: Experimental and spontaneous diabetes in animals. In Ellenberg M, Rifkin H (eds): Diabetes Mellitus, Theory and Practice, 3rd ed. New York, Medical Examination Publishing, 1983, p 361.

Edwards DF, et al: Hypoglycemia and chronic renal failure in a cat. J Am Vet Med Assoc 190:435, 1987.

Feldman EC, Nelson RW: Canine and Feline Endocrinology and Reproduction. Philadelphia, WB Saunders, 1987.

Fenner WR: Diseases of the brain. In Ettinger SJ, Feldman EC (eds): Textbook of Veterinary Internal Medicine, 4th ed. Philadelphia, WB Saunders, 1995, p 578.

Fingeroth JM, Smeak DD: Intravenous methylene blue infusion for intraoperative identification of pancreatic islet cell tumors in dogs. II. Clinical trials and results in four dogs. J Am Anim Hosp Assoc 24:175, 1988.

Fingeroth JM, et al: Intravenous methylene blue infusion for intraoperative identification of parathyroid gland and pancreatic islet cell tumors in dogs. I. Experimental determination of dose-related staining efficacy and toxicity. J Am Anim Hosp Assoc 24:165, 1988.

Fischer JR et al: Glucagon constant-rate infusion: A novel strategy for the management of hyperinsulinemic-hypoglycemic crisis in the dog. J Am Anim Hosp Assoc 36:27, 2000.

Fischer KF, et al: Hypoglycemia in hospitalized patients: Causes and outcomes. N Engl J Med 315:1245, 1986.

Fukuda I, et al: Circulating forms of insulin-like growth factor II (IGF-II) in patients with non-islet cell tumor hypoglycemia. Endocrinol Metab 1:89, 1994.

Gerich J, et al: Hypoglycemia unawareness. Endocr Rev 12:356, 1991.

Gerich JE, et al: Renal gluconeogenesis: Its importance in human glucose homeostasis. Diabetes Care 24:382, 2001.

Haemers S, Rottiers R: Medical treatment of insulinoma. Acta Clin Belg 36:199, 1981.

Hardy RM: Diseases of the liver and their treatment. In Ettinger SJ (ed): Textbook of Veterinary Internal Medicine, 3rd ed. Philadelphia, WB Saunders, 1989, p 1479.

Hargrove DM, et al: Adrenergic blockade does not abolish elevated glucose turnover during bacterial infection. Am J Physiol 254:E16, 1988a.

Hargrove DM, et al: Adrenergic blockade prevents endotoxin-induced increases in glucose metabolism. Am J Physiol 255:E629, 1988b.

Hawkins KL, et al: Immunocytochemistry of normal pancreatic islets and spontaneous islet cell tumors in dogs. Vet Pathol 24:170, 1987.

Hawks D, et al: Insulin-secreting pancreatic (islet cell) carcinoma in a cat. J Vet Intern Med 6:193, 1992.

Heckmann JG, et al: Hypoglycemic sensorimotor polyneuropathy associated with insulinoma. Muscle Nerve 23:1891, 2000.

Jeffery ND, et al: Letter to the editor. Prog Vet Neurol 5:135, 1994.

Kahn CR: The riddle of tumour hypoglycemia revisited. Clin Endocrinol Metab 9:335, 1980.

Karam JH: Hypoglycemic disorders. In Greenspan FS, Gardner DG (eds): Basic and Clinical Endocrinology, 6th ed. New York, Lange Medical Books/McGraw-Hill, 2001, p 699.

Kintzel PE: Anticancer drug–induced kidney disorders. Drug Safety 24:19, 2001.

Kishnani PS, et al: Canine model and genomic structural organization of glycogen storage disease type Ia (GSD Ia). Vet Pathol 38:83, 2001.

Kruth SA, et al: Insulin-secreting islet cell tumors: Establishing a diagnosis and the clinical course of 25 dogs. J Am Vet Med Assoc 181:54, 1982.

Kubota A, et al: Identification of somatostatin receptor subtypes and an implication for the efficacy of somatostatin analog SMS 201-995 for treatment of human endocrine tumors. J Clin Invest 93:1321, 1994.

Kudo M, Noguchi T: Immunoreactive myelin basic protein in tumor cells associated with carcinomatous neuropathy. Am J Clin Pathol 84:741, 1985.

Kvols LK, et al: Evaluation of a radio-labeled somatostatin analog (I-123 octreotide) in the detection and localization of carcinoid and islet cell tumors. Radiology 197:129, 1993.

Lamberts SJW, et al: Parallel in vivo and in vitro detection of functional somatostatin receptors in human endocrine pancreatic tumors: Consequences with regard to diagnosis, localization and therapy. J Clin Endocrinol Metab 71:566, 1990.

Lamberts SJW, et al: The role of somatostatin and its analogs in the diagnosis and treatment of tumors. Endocrinol Rev 12:450, 1991.

Lamberts SJW, et al: Octreotide and related somatostatin analogs in the diagnosis and treatment of pituitary disease and somatostatin receptor scintigraphy. Neuroendocrinology 14:27, 1993.

Lamberts SWJ, et al: Somatostatin analogs: Future directions. Metabolism 45:104, 1996.

Leifer CE, et al: Hypoglycemia associated with non-islet cell tumor in 13 dogs. J Am Vet Med Assoc 186:53, 1985.

Leifer CE, et al: Insulin-secreting tumor: Diagnosis and medical and surgical management in 55 dogs. J Am Vet Med Assoc 188:60, 1986.

LeRoith D, et al: Insulin-like growth factors in health and disease. Ann Intern Med 116:854, 1992.

Lester NV, et al: Scintigraphic diagnosis of insulinoma in a dog. Vet Radiol Ultrasound 40:174, 1999.

Lothrop CD: Medical treatment of neuroendocrine tumors of the gastroenteropancreatic system with somatostatin. In Kirk RW (ed): Current Veterinary Therapy X. Philadelphia, WB Saunders, 1989, p 1020.

Lutz TA, Rand JS: Comparison of five commercial radioimmunoassay kits for the measurement of feline insulin. Res Vet Sci 55:64, 1993.

Masharani U, Karam JH: Pancreatic hormones and diabetes mellitus. In Greenspan FS, Gardner DG (eds): Basic and Clinical Endocrinology, 6th ed. New York, Lange Medical Books/McGraw-Hill, 2001, p 623.

McMillan F: Functional pancreatic islet cell tumor in a cat. J Am Anim Hosp Assoc 21:741, 1985.

Merimee TJ: Insulin-like growth factors in patients with non-islet cell tumors and hypoglycemia. Metabolism 35:360, 1986.

Meszaros K, et al: Increased uptake and phosphorylation of 2-deoxyglucose by skeletal muscles in endotoxin-treated rats. Am J Physiol 253:E33, 1987.

Meszaros K, et al: In vivo glucose utilization by individual tissues during nonlethal hypermetabolic sepsis. FASEB J 2:3083, 1988.

Meyer C, et al: Effects of autonomic neuropathy on counterregulation and awareness of hypoglycemia in type 1 diabetic patients. Diabetes Care 21:1960, 1998.

Minkus G, et al: Canine neuroendocrine tumors of the pancreas: A study using image analysis techniques for the discrimination of metastatic versus nonmetastatic tumors. Vet Pathol 34:138, 1997.

Moertel CG, et al: Streptozotocin alone compared with streptozotocin plus fluorouracil in the treatment of advanced islet cell carcinoma. N Engl J Med 303:1189, 1980.

Mokan M, et al: Hypoglycemia unawareness in IDDM. Diabetes Care 17:1397, 1994.

Moore AS, et al: Streptozotocin for treatment of pancreatic islet cell tumors in dogs: 17 cases (1989-1999). J Am Vet Med Assoc 221:811, 2002.

Naylor JM, Kronfeld DS: In vivo studies of hypoglycemia and lactic acidosis in endotoxic shock. Am J Physiol 248:E309, 1985.

Nelson RW, Salisbury SK: Pancreatic beta-cell neoplasia. In Birchard SJ, Sherding RG (eds): Saunders Manual of Small Animal Practice, 2nd ed. Philadelphia, WB Saunders, 2000, p 288.

O'Brien TD, et al: Canine pancreatic endocrine tumors: Immunohistochemical analysis of hormone content and amyloid. Vet Pathol 24:308, 1987.

O'Brien TD, et al: Pancreatic endocrine tumor in a cat: Clinical, pathological, and immunohistochemical evaluation. J Am Anim Hosp Assoc 26:453, 1990.

Robben JH, et al: In vitro and in vivo detection of functional somatostatin receptors in canine insulinomas. J Nucl Med 38:1036, 1997.

Rothman DL, et al: Quantitation of hepatic glycogenolysis and gluconeogenesis in fasting humans with ^{13}C NMR. Science 254:573, 1991.

Schrauwen E, et al: Peripheral polyneuropathy associated with insulinoma in the dog: Clinical, pathological, and electrodiagnostic features. Prog Vet Neurol 7:16, 1996.

Scully RE, et al: Case records of the Massachusetts General Hospital. N Engl J Med 308:30, 1983.

Service FJ: Hypoglycemic disorders. N Engl J Med 332:1144, 1995.

Shahar R, et al: Peripheral neuropathy in a dog with functional islet B-cell tumor and widespread metastasis. J Am Vet Med Assoc 187:175, 1985.

Sherwin RS, Felig P: Hypoglycemia. In Felig P, et al (eds): Endocrinology and Metabolism. New York, McGraw-Hill, 1981, p 869.

Simpson KW, et al: Evaluation of the long-acting somatostatin analogue octreotide in the management of insulinoma in three dogs. J Small Anim Pract 36:161, 1995.

Slye M, Wells HG: Tumor of islet tissue with hyperinsulinism in a dog. Arch Pathol 19:537, 1935.

Smeak DD, et al: Intravenous methylene blue as a specific stain for primary and metastatic insulinoma in a dog. J Am Anim Hosp Assoc 24:478, 1988.

Stumvoll M, et al: Uptake and release of glucose by the human kidney. J Clin Invest 96:2528, 1995.

Tobin MV, et al: Forced diuresis to reduce nephrotoxicity of streptozocin in the treatment of advanced metastatic insulinoma. Br Med J 294:1128, 1987.

Tobin RL, et al: Outcome of surgical versus medical treatment of dogs with beta-cell neoplasia: 39 cases (1990-1997). J Am Vet Med Assoc 215:226, 1999.

van Ham L, et al: Treatment of a dog with an insulinoma-related peripheral polyneuropathy with corticosteroids. Vet Rec 141:98, 1997.

Wess G, Reusch C: Evaluation of five portable blood glucose meters for use in dogs. J Am Vet Med Assoc 216:203, 2000.

Whipple AO, Grantz VK: Adenoma of islet cells with hyperinsulinism. A review. Ann Surg 101:1299, 1935.

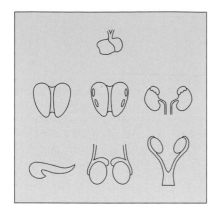

15

GASTRINOMA, GLUCAGONOMA, AND OTHER APUDomas

REGULATORY PEPTIDES OF THE GUT

CLASSIFICATION AND DISTRIBUTION OF GUT PEPTIDES. Throughout the gastrointestinal tract, from the esophagus to the rectum, is found a spectrum of specialized endocrine cells that secrete peptides involved with the normal physiologic functions of the gastrointestinal tract (Table 15-1). In addition to specialized endocrine cells, gut peptides are also located in neurons widely dispersed throughout the gastrointestinal tract (Table 15-2). In enteric neurons, gut peptides probably act as neurotransmitters or neurocrine agents (Mulvihill and Debas, 2001). The bodies of enteric neurons are located within the gut wall, usually in the submucosal or myenteric plexus, from which their pathways extend to cells of the mucosa, smooth muscle, blood vessels, and other endocrine cells. This enteric nervous system is considered a division of the autonomic nervous system.

PHYSIOLOGIC ACTIONS. Gastrointestinal peptides regulate gastrointestinal motility as well as secretion of fluid and digestive enzymes (see Table 15-1). Gastrointestinal peptides also have several trophic actions that regulate metabolism and growth of gastrointestinal tissues by stimulating protein, RNA, and DNA synthesis; minimizing protein catabolism; and enhancing cellular uptake of amino acids (Mulvihill and Debas, 2001). The interactions between these peptides are diverse and complex, encompassing not only stimulation or repression of each other's secretion but also potentiation or inhibition of each other's actions on target organs within the gastrointestinal tract. These complex interactions maintain an optimal environment for efficient digestion and absorption of nutrients. As such, gastrointestinal endocrine cells must be capable of monitoring and responding to changes within the environment of the gastrointestinal tract. These responses must occur in a coordinated fashion if optimal assimilation of ingested nutrients is to be maintained.

MODES OF GUT PEPTIDE DELIVERY. Gastrointestinal peptides are delivered to their sites of action in three main ways: some circulate in the bloodstream in order to reach the target cell (endocrine delivery); some are released into the interstitial fluid and affect nearby cells (paracrine delivery); and still others, within neurons, act as neurotransmitters or neuromodulators (neurocrine delivery; Fig. 15-1; Mulvihill and Debas, 2001). Some peptides have more than one delivery. Because of their various modes of delivery, it is preferable to refer to these substances as regulatory peptides rather than as hormones.

BRAIN-GUT AXIS. The discovery that many of these peptides are located in the central nervous system (CNS) and in enteric neurons—in addition to being found in specialized endocrine cells of the gastrointestinal tract—has led to the concept of the brain-gut axis. In the CNS, gut peptides are thought to be important in the regulation of bodily functions such as satiety. Furthermore, neurons of the CNS interact with those of the enteric nervous system to influence digestive processes. Many of these neurons are peptidergic. Neurons of the enteric nervous system exert local control over digestive processes, including absorption, secretion, motility, and blood flow. It is believed that some poorly understood conditions (e.g., irritable bowel syndrome in humans) are the result of abnormalities of regulation of gut function by the enteric nervous system and CNS.

THE APUD CONCEPT

All specialized peptide-secreting cells, including the gastrointestinal endocrine cells, have a number of ultrastructural and cytochemical features in common,

TABLE 15–1   GASTROINTESTINAL HORMONES

| | MODE OF DELIVERY | | | |
	Endocrine	Neurocrine	Paracrine	MAJOR ACTION
Gastrin	+	(+)	–	Gastric acid and pepsin secretion
Cholecystokinin	+	+	–	Pancreatic enzyme secretion; gallbladder contraction
Secretin	+	–	–	Pancreatic bicarbonate secretion
Gastric inhibitory polypeptide	+	–	–	Enhances glucose-mediated insulin release; inhibits gastric acid secretion
Vasoactive intestinal polypeptide	–	+	(+)	Smooth muscle relaxation; stimulates pancreatic bicarbonate secretion
Motilin	+	–	–	Initiates interdigestive intestinal motility
Somatostatin	+	+	+	Numerous inhibitory effects
Pancreatic polypeptide	+	–	(+)	Inhibits pancreatic bicarbonate and protein secretion
Enkephalins	–	+	(+)	Inhibition of gut motility
Substance P	–	+	(+)	Smooth muscle contractions
Gastrin-releasing peptide	–	+	(+)	Stimulates release of gastrin and cholecystokinin
Neurotensin	+	–	(+)	Vasodilation
Enteroglucagon	(+)	(+)	(+)	Incretin; mucosal mitogen
Peptide YY	+	–	(+)	Inhibits pancreatic bicarbonate and protein secretion
Neuropeptide Y	–	+	–	Inhibits pancreatic bicarbonate and protein secretion
Calcitonin gene-related peptide	–	+	–	Stimulates acid secretion and somatostatin release
Ghrelin	+	–	(+)	Stimulates appetite, gastric acid secretion, and gastric motility

From Mulvihill SJ, Debas HT: *In* Greenspan FS, Gardner DG (eds): Basic and Clinical Endocrinology, 6th ed. New York, Lange Medical Books/McGraw-Hill, 2001, p 604.
(   ) denotes inconclusive evidence

some of which reflect the ability of these cells to synthesize and metabolize biogenic amines (i.e., epinephrine, norepinephrine, dopamine, and serotonin). Two of these characteristic features (i.e., amine precursor uptake and decarboxylation) earned the cells the acronym APUD. Most of the cells possessing these characteristics are found in the gut or CNS (hypothalamus, pituitary gland), but they are also present in the thyroid (calcitonin cell), parathyroid, and placenta (Mulvihill and Debas, 2001). Despite their disparate locations, cells that exhibit these

properties have important developmental and functional characteristics in common, including the ability to secrete peptide hormones.

An APUDoma is a tumor arising from the APUD cells. This name was first applied by Szijj et al in 1969 to a medullary carcinoma of the thyroid C cells that was secreting ACTH. Since then, several different APUDomas have been described in both the human and the veterinary literature (Table 15-3). APUDomas are named after the endocrine product that they secrete.

TABLE 15–2   DISTRIBUTION OF GASTROINTESTINAL HORMONES*

	Endocrine Cell[†]	Localization	Localized in Gut Nerves
Gastrin	G	Gastric antrum, duodenum	No
Cholecystokinin	I	Duodenum, jejunum	Yes
Secretin	S	Duodenum, jejunum	No
Gastric inhibitory polypeptide	K	Small bowel	No
Vasoactive intestinal polypeptide	D_1	Pancreas	Yes
Motilin	EC_2	Small bowel	No
Substance P	EC_1	Entire gastrointestinal tract	Yes
Neurotensin	N	Ileum	No
Somatostatin	D	Stomach, duodenum, pancreas	Yes
Enkephalins	–	Stomach, duodenum, gallbladder	Yes
GRP	–	Stomach, duodenum	Yes
Pancreatic polypeptide	D_2F	Pancreas	No
Enteroglucagon	A	Pancreas	No
Enteroglucagon	L	Small intestine	No
Peptide YY	–	Small intestine, colon	No
Calcitonin gene-related peptide	–	Entire gastrointestinal tract	Yes
Neuropeptide Y	–	Small intestine	Yes
Ghrelin	–	Entire gastrointestinal tract, primarily stomach	Unknown

From Mulvihill SJ, Debas HT: *In* Greenspan FS, Gardner DG (eds): Basic and Clinical Endocrinology, 6th ed. New York, Lange Medical Books/McGraw-Hill, 2001, p 607.
*Note that several peptides are found both in nerves and in endocrine cells. VIP has been found only in nerves and is probably not present in endocrine cells.
†Endocrine cells identified with a specific hormone are identified by a letter. *EC* = Enterochromaffin cell. The cells containing enkephalins and PYY have yet to be named.

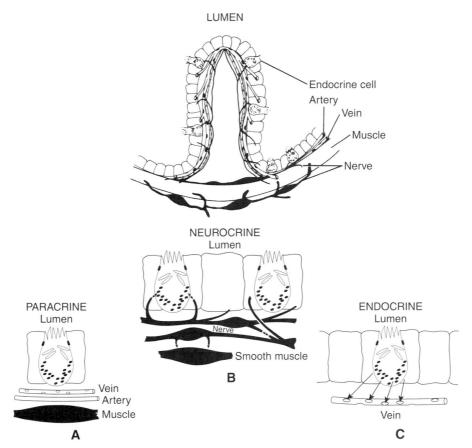

FIGURE 15-1. Schematic representation of the wall of the small intestine. Note the close proximity of endocrine cells and nerves to mucosal cells, blood vessels, and smooth muscle. Anatomically, local release of hormone by endocrine cells or nerves could affect secretion and absorption (mucosal cells), motility (muscle), and blood flow (blood vessels). *A,* Paracrine delivery—release of a messenger locally to affect adjacent cells. *B,* Neurocrine delivery—release of messenger by nerves to affect mucosal cells, other endocrine cells, or smooth muscle of both small intestine and blood vessels. *C,* Endocrine delivery—release of messenger into the blood to act as a circulating hormone. (From Mulvihill SJ, Debas HT: *In* Greenspan FS, Baxter JD (eds): Basic and Clinical Endocrinology, 4th ed. Norwalk, CT, Appleton & Lange, 1994, p 551.)

The cells composing an APUDoma usually possess the APUD characteristics with even greater clarity than the parent cells. Although it is relatively easy to distinguish one normal APUD cell from another by ultrastructural evaluation of the granules, it is difficult to predict the nature of the polypeptide synthesized or the cell of origin of an APUDoma based on evaluation of the tumor granules. In addition, one tumor may

secrete several hormones (Middleton and Watson, 1983).

APUDomas that secrete excessive quantities of the polypeptide or amine product typical for their cell of origin cause "orthoendocrine" syndromes. Those that secrete one or more polypeptides that are foreign to the presumed cell of origin, but are characteristic of other APUD cells, cause "paraendocrine" syndromes. Orthoendocrine syndromes are the most common entities in veterinary medicine, with insulinoma, pheochromocytoma, and gastrinoma accounting for the vast majority of APUDomas. However, as ultrastructural techniques and immunocytochemical evaluation of APUDomas in animals improve, paraendocrine syndromes with multiple hormone potential will undoubtedly become more frequently recognized.

TABLE 15–3   CLASSIFICATION OF GASTROINTESTINAL APUDomas AND PRINCIPAL HORMONE SECRETED

Tumor Type	Principal Hormone Secreted
Insulinoma	Insulin
Pheochromocytoma	Epinephrine, norepinephrine
Gastrinoma	Gastrin
VIPoma	Vasoactive intestinal polypeptide
Glucagonoma	Glucagon
Somatostatinoma	Somatostatin
Pancreatic polypeptide-oma	Pancreatic polypeptide
Carcinoid syndrome	Serotonin

INSULINOMA

Insulin-secreting islet cell tumors of the pancreas are the most commonly recognized APUDoma in the dog but are rare in the cat. Beta-cell tumors occur most frequently as a single entity. However, they may also represent part of the syndrome of multiple endocrine neoplasia (see Chapter 9). Refer to Chapter 14 for a complete discussion of beta-cell tumors.

PHEOCHROMOCYTOMA

Pheochromocytoma is the second most commonly recognized APUDoma in the dog but is rare in the cat. Pheochromocytoma is a catecholamine-producing tumor derived from chromaffin cells in the adrenal medulla. It occurs most frequently as a single entity but may also be part of the syndrome of multiple endocrine neoplasia. See Chapter 9 for a complete discussion of pheochromocytoma and multiple endocrine neoplasia syndrome.

GASTRINOMA: ZOLLINGER-ELLISON SYNDROME

ETIOLOGY. In 1955, Zollinger and Ellison described a clinical entity in two human patients consisting of gastric hypersecretion, multiple gastrointestinal ulcers, and a non–beta-cell tumor of the pancreas. It was subsequently shown that these tumors produce gastrin (Mulvihill and Debas, 2001) and the triad of hypergastrinemia, a neuroendocrine tumor, and gastrointestinal ulceration became known as the Zollinger-Ellison syndrome (Jensen and Fraker, 1994). The main actions of gastrin are stimulation of gastric acid secretion and parietal cell growth. Hypergastrinemia induces excessive gastric secretion of hydrochloric acid, which is responsible for the development of esophageal, gastric, and duodenal ulcers, the disruption of intestinal digestive and absorptive functions, and the development of clinical signs. The first reported case of a gastrinoma in veterinary medicine resembling the Zollinger-Ellison syndrome was by Jones et al in 1976. Although sporadic case reports in dogs and cats have since appeared in the literature (Happe et al, 1980; Drazner, 1981; Middleton and Watson, 1983; Breitschwerdt et al, 1986; English et al, 1988; Eng et al, 1992; Brooks and Watson, 1997; Altschul et al, 1997; Green and Gartrell, 1997), this syndrome is still considered a rare entity.

In humans, gastrin-producing tumors are found primarily in the pancreas, proximal duodenum, and gastric antrum, although other sites have been reported (Wolfe et al, 1982; Wolfe and Jensen, 1987). These tumors tend to be small, multiple, slow-growing, and malignant. They cause clinical signs primarily as a result of excessive secretion of gastrin. Occasionally, clinical signs are related to the malignant, space-occupying nature of the multiple metastatic masses. Metastasis is primarily to the liver, lymph nodes, and adjacent omentum. Gastrinomas may also be associated with tumors in other endocrine organs, a condition known as multiple endocrine neoplasia (MEN)

syndrome (see Chapter 9) (Pipeleers-Marichal et al, 1990).

Similar behavior patterns of gastrinoma are difficult to assess in dogs and cats, primarily because of the small number of affected animals that have been described to date. Nevertheless, of the 24 dogs and 4 cats with Zollinger-Ellison syndrome either reported in the literature or seen by us, 21 dogs and all cats with gastrinoma had a tumor arising from islet cells in the pancreas, with multiple pancreatic masses identified in 4 animals. The tumor was not identified in the pancreas but was identified in the regional lymph nodes in 2 dogs and at the root of the mesentery in 1 dog (Zerbe and Washabau, 2000; Brooks and Watson, 1997; Green and Gatrell, 1997). Metastatic disease involving the liver, adjacent lymph nodes, spleen, or mesentery was identified in 70% of the cases.

The cell of origin of the pancreatic gastrinoma is disputed. The normal pancreatic islets in the adult contain four cell types: A cells secrete glucagon, B cells secrete insulin, D cells secrete somatostatin, and F cells secrete pancreatic polypeptide. However, gastrin appears to be produced during fetal life by D cells. The most widely accepted current hypothesis is a reversion of D cell function back to fetal function, with subsequent secretion of gastrin instead of somatostatin (Krejs, 1998).

Gastrinomas may secrete other hormones (e.g., insulin, ACTH, pancreatic polypeptide) as well as gastrin, a phenomenon that has been documented in dogs and cats as well as in humans. A canine gastrinoma has been reported that produced gastrin and ACTH, while a gastrinoma in a cat produced gastrin, glucagon, and possibly cholecystokinin (Middleton and Watson, 1983; Feldman and Nelson, 1987). In humans, the clinical syndrome resulting from excessive hormone secretion by one of the cell types in multihormonal neoplasms may not be the result of the predominant cell type in the tumor. In addition, metastatic masses from multihormonal tumors are not necessarily composed of the cell type responsible for the clinical picture.

SIGNALMENT. Dogs and cats with confirmed gastrinomas were 3 to 12 years old, with a median age in dogs of approximately 8 years. There does not appear to be a gender or breed predisposition, although the number of reported confirmed cases is too small for definite conclusions to be drawn.

CLINICAL SIGNS. Almost all of the clinical signs are a result of severe gastric acid hypersecretion. The most common clinical signs are vomiting, weight loss, anorexia, and diarrhea (Table 15-4). Gastric hyperacidity eventually results in ulcer formation, most commonly involving the stomach and duodenum. Gastrointestinal ulceration was found during gastroduodenoscopy, surgery, or at necropsy in 20 (80%) of 25 dogs and cats with gastrinoma, with perforation of the ulcer identified in 4 animals (Zerbe and Washabau, 2000; Brooks and Watson, 1997; Altschul et al, 1997; Green and Gartrell, 1997). Ulcerations, in turn, may cause vomiting, hematemesis, hematochezia, melena,

TABLE 15–4   FREQUENCY OF OCCURRENCE OF CLINICAL SIGNS IN 24 DOGS AND 3 CATS WITH GASTRINOMA AND THE ZOLLINGER-ELLISON SYNDROME

Clinical Sign	Percent of Patients
Vomiting	93
Weight loss	89
Anorexia	75
Diarrhea	67
Lethargy, depression	56
Polydipsia	22
Melena	22
Fever	19
Abdominal pain	15
Hematemesis	15
Hematochezia	7
Tachycardia	7
Abdominal mass	4
Polyphagia	4
Obstipation (alternating with diarrhea)	4

inappetence, weight loss, depression, and abdominal pain. Esophageal reflux of acid gastric contents may lead to esophagitis and ulceration with worsening inappetence, regurgitation, and weight loss. Diarrhea with malabsorption and steatorrhea may develop following acidification of the intestinal contents, with subsequent inactivation of lipase, precipitation of bile salts, interference with chylomicron formation, and damage to intestinal mucosal cells. Hypergastrinemia may also alter intestinal absorption of water and electrolytes.

Acidification of the intestinal lumen is a stimulant for the secretion of secretin and cholecystokinin. Secretin has been shown to stimulate the secretion of gastrin from gastrinomas, so its endogenous release may contribute to the maintenance of hypergastrinemia. Thus a cycle may develop that perpetuates the hyperacidity and resultant pathology.

PHYSICAL EXAMINATION. Findings on the physical examination depend, in part, on the chronicity of the disorder, severity of hyperacidity and ulceration, and presence of a perforated ulcer. Findings of the physical examination can vary from relatively unremarkable to a dog or cat that is extremely sick. Animals with the Zollinger-Ellison syndrome may be lethargic, thin to emaciated, febrile, dehydrated, and in shock. Mucous membranes may appear pale as a result of anemia due to ulcer diathesis. Compensatory tachycardia and abdominal tenderness during palpation may also be present. One cat affected with gastrinoma had a palpable abdominal mass at the time of presentation (Zerbe and Washabau, 2000).

CLINICAL PATHOLOGY. Abnormalities in the complete blood count that have been associated with the Zollinger-Ellison syndrome in dogs and cats include a neutrophilic leukocytosis, hypoproteinemia, and regenerative anemia, presumably caused by gastrointestinal inflammation and blood loss. Abnormalities identified in the serum biochemistry panel include hypoproteinemia, hypoalbuminemia, hypocalcemia,

and mild increases in serum alanine aminotransferase and alkaline phosphatase activities. Hypocalcemia may be a result of concurrent hypoalbuminemia or secondary to gastrin-induced thyroid C-cell hyperplasia and increased calcitonin secretion. Hypokalemia, hypochloremia, and metabolic alkalosis may develop in those dogs and cats with frequent vomiting. Hyperglycemia and hypoglycemia have been reported in a few cases, the cause of which is unknown but may be related to tumor-associated secretion of other hormones (e.g., ACTH, insulin; Zerbe and Washabau, 2000). Results of the urinalysis are usually unremarkable. Evaluation of a fecal sample with Sudan stain may reveal steatorrhea due to both lipid and fatty acid accumulation. A positive occult blood reaction or overt melena is usually present.

DIAGNOSTIC IMAGING. Survey abdominal radiographs are usually normal. If an ulcer has perforated through the serosal surface, radiographic signs consistent with peritonitis may be present. Contrast radiographic studies may demonstrate gastric or duodenal ulcers; thickening of the gastric rugal folds, pyloric antrum, and/or intestine; and rapid intestinal transit of barium (Zerbe and Washabau, 2000). With concurrent severe esophagitis, a secondary megaesophagus or aberrant, nonperistaltic esophageal motility may be demonstrable fluoroscopically. Potential abnormalities identified with abdominal ultrasound include thickening of the gastric and intestinal wall, gastric ulcers, and a pancreatic mass or its metastases. However, gastrinomas vary tremendously in size and may be microscopic (Roche et al, 1982). Failure to identify a pancreatic mass with ultrasonography does not rule out gastrinoma. Because a high concentration of high affinity somatostatin receptors is present in greater than 90% of tissue from human gastrinomas, the use of radiolabeled somatostatin analogues has enabled successful imaging of many gastrinomas, including previously unsuspected metastases (Schirmer et al, 1995; Gibril et al, 1996). A positive scan can also suggest whether a patient will be likely to benefit from therapy with the long-acting somatostatin analogue octreotide, which decreases gastrin release (Ellison et al, 1986). [111]Indium-pentetreotide scintigraphy successfully detected gastrinoma and its metastases in a dog with metastatic gastrinoma, and octreotide treatment was beneficial in decreasing plasma gastrin concentrations (Altschul et al, 1997).

ENDOSCOPY. Gastroduodenoscopy in a dog or cat with the Zollinger-Ellison syndrome may reveal severe esophagitis and ulceration, especially in the vicinity of the cardia. Gastric rugal folds may be thickened and persist despite insufflation of the gastric lumen with air. Gastric and duodenal hyperemia, erosions, or ulceration is often visible (Fig. 15-2). Histologic evaluation of esophageal, gastric, and duodenal biopsies obtained during endoscopy may reveal mild to severe inflammation with infiltrates of lymphocytes, plasma cells, neutrophils and/or eosinophils, as well as gastric mucosal hypertrophy, fibrosis, and loss of the mucosal barrier.

DIAGNOSIS. Gastrinoma should be included in the differential diagnoses for any dog or cat presenting with severe gastrointestinal signs, especially vomiting with weight loss, melena or hematemesis, or any dog or cat in which severe gastric and duodenal ulceration is identified via gastroduodenoscopy. Identifying a pancreatic mass or metastasis with abdominal ultrasound followed by exploratory surgery, paying special attention to the pancreas and peripancreatic region, is perhaps the most cost-effective method to diagnose (and treat) gastrinoma in dogs and cats. Histologic and immunocytochemical evaluation of the mass excised at surgery confirms the diagnosis. Measurement of baseline serum gastrin concentration provides further evidence for or against gastrinoma and should be considered before surgery, especially if a mass is not identified with abdominal ultrasound. Unfortunately, gastrin-secreting tumors are often smaller than 1 cm and not discernible with routine imaging techniques, exploratory celiotomy is not typically considered unless a perforated gastric ulcer or peritonitis is suspected, and measurement of serum gastrin is not considered simply because gastrinoma is rare in dogs and cats. As such, most dogs and cats with gastrinoma are inadvertently treated for severe inflammatory bowel disease and gastroduodenal erosions/ulcers with inhibitors of gastric acid secretion, mucosal protectants, antibiotics, and diet. Presumably many of these dogs and cats respond to treatment and gastrinoma would be considered only if the dog or cat became recalcitrant to medical therapy directed at nonspecific inflammation and ulceration of the gastrointestinal tract or if clinical signs and gastrointestinal ulceration recurred after discontinuing antiulcer therapy.

Measurement of Fasting Serum Gastrin Concentration. Demonstration of persistent hypergastrinemia in a dog or cat with appropriate clinical signs adds further support for the diagnosis of gastrinoma. Multiple blood samples drawn after an overnight fast provide the most accurate means of establishing hypergastrinemia. Although the normal range for serum gastrin concentration varies among laboratories, the upper limit of the normal range using current radioimmunoassays is typically less than 100 pg/ml in dogs and cats (Altschul et al, 1997; Brooks and Watson, 1997). In dogs with the Zollinger-Ellison syndrome, serum gastrin concentrations have ranged from 72 to 2780 pg/ml, and in two cats it was 350 and 1000 pg/ml. To date, all but one dog and all cats with histologically confirmed gastrinoma had fasting serum gastrin concentrations greater than three times the upper normal value for the laboratory. Fasting serum gastrin concentration was 72 pg/ml (reference range, 10 to 40 pg/ml) in one dog with a 1-month history of vomiting and a neuroendocrine tumor identified at surgery (Green and Gartrell, 1997).

Serum gastrin concentrations may be normal in some humans with proven gastrinoma (Zimmer et al, 1995). Although not yet reported, normal serum gastrin concentrations also seem possible in dogs and

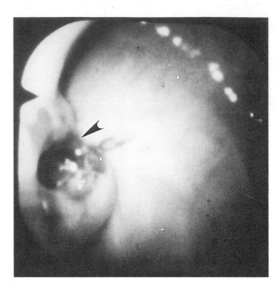

FIGURE 15-2. Endoscopic visualization of a hemorrhagic ulcer *(arrow)* in the body of the stomach in a dog with Zollinger-Ellison syndrome (gastrinoma).

cats, especially in the early stages of the disorder. High fasting serum gastrin concentrations are supportive of, but not pathognomonic for gastrinoma. Hypergastrinemia is found with many other disorders, including chronic renal failure, chronic gastritis, gastric outflow obstruction, liver disease, and achlorhydria, and following administration of H_2-receptor antagonists (Table 15-5; Breitschwerdt et al, 1986; Breitschwerdt et al, 1991; Goldstein et al, 1998). Fortunately, most of the conditions that cause hypergastrinemia in the dog and cat can be readily differentiated from the Zollinger-Ellison syndrome following evaluation of the initial data base and appropriate diagnostic imaging studies.

Gastrin Stimulation Tests. Several provocative stimulation tests have been used to confirm the diagnosis of gastrinoma in humans with borderline fasting serum gastrin concentrations whose acid secretion is in the range associated with ordinary

TABLE 15–5 FACTORS ASSOCIATED WITH HYPERGASTRINEMIA IN HUMANS AND IN DOGS AND CATS

Documented in Dogs and Cats	Documented in Humans
Gastrinoma	Gastrinoma
Renal failure	Renal failure
Gastric outflow obstruction	Gastric outflow obstruction
Achlorhydria/hypochlorhydria	Achlorhydria/hypochlorhydria
Atrophic gastritis	Atrophic gastritis
Gastric dilatation/volvulus	Antral gastrin-cell hyperplasia
Liver disease	Gastric carcinoma
Immunoproliferative enteropathy of Basenji dogs	Short bowel syndrome
Antacids	Peptic ulcer disease
H_2 receptor antagonists	Pheochromocytoma
Proton pump inhibitors	Vagotomy
Glucocorticoids	Antacids
	H_2 receptor antagonists
	Proton pump inhibitors

duodenal ulcer disease. These tests include the secretin stimulation test, the calcium stimulation test, the test meal, the bombesin test, and the glucagon test (Wolfe and Jensen, 1987).

SECRETIN STIMULATION TEST. The secretin stimulation test is the most reliable test and is preferred in humans suspected of having gastrinoma (Slaff et al, 1986). Exogenous secretin administration has an exaggerated effect on stimulating gastrin secretion in humans with gastrinoma compared with healthy humans (Brady et al, 1987). In humans, blood samples are obtained before and every 5 minutes for 30 minutes after the administration of secretin, 2 units/kg body weight as an IV bolus. An increase in serum gastrin concentration of 200 pg/ml within 15 minutes of secretin administration is diagnostic for gastrinoma (Wolfe and Jensen, 1987). In 80% of humans with the Zollinger-Ellison syndrome, serum gastrin concentrations increase within 5 to 10 minutes after secretin administration. In 20% of humans with gastrinoma, the secretin stimulation test is nondiagnostic. Measurement of the plasma level of progastrin, a high-molecular-weight precursor of gastrin, may also be useful in diagnosis of gastrinoma in humans (Bardram, 1990).

Experience with the secretin stimulation test in dogs with gastrinoma is limited, and its use in cats has not been reported. The currently recommended procedure in dogs and cats is to administer 2 units of secretin per kilogram of body weight IV and collect blood samples for gastrin determination before and 2, 5, 10, 15, and 30 minutes after secretin administration (Breitschwerdt et al, 1991). In three dogs with gastrinoma, there was a 1.4-fold (one dog) and greater than 2-fold (two dogs) increase in serum gastrin concentration within 5 minutes of secretin administration (Fig. 15-3; Zerbe and Washabau, 2000). In contrast, healthy dogs and Basenji dogs with immunoproliferative enteropathy had a gradual decrease in serum gastrin concentration immediately after secretin administration (Breitschwerdt et al, 1991).

CALCIUM CHALLENGE TEST. An alternative stimulation test is the calcium challenge test. As with secretin, calcium infusion stimulates an increase in serum gastrin concentration in humans with gastrinoma but not in nongastrinoma patients. The secretin test is preferred over the calcium challenge test in humans because the secretin stimulation test is shorter in duration, has fewer adverse effects, and yields fewer false-positive and false-negative results (McGuigan and Wolfe, 1980). However, expense and sporadic availability of secretin make the calcium challenge test appealing.

For the calcium challenge test, calcium gluconate is administered as a 1-minute IV bolus infusion (2 mg/kg) or as an IV continuous infusion for several hours (5 mg/kg/hr; Zerbe and Washabau, 2000). Blood samples are collected before and 15, 30, 60, 90, and 120 minutes after calcium administration. Maximum serum gastrin concentrations occurred 60 minutes after calcium bolus infusion in two dogs with gastrinoma (see Fig. 15-3). Both dogs had a

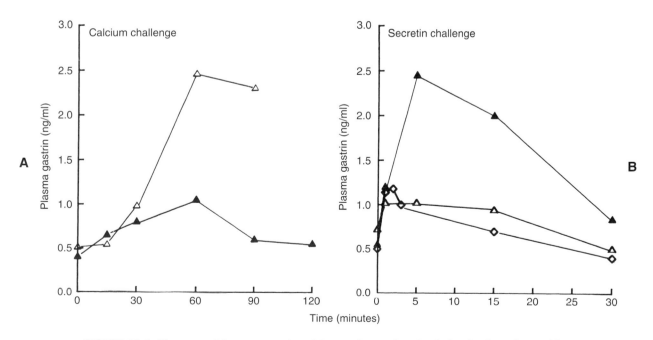

FIGURE 15-3. Plasma gastrin responses to calcium and secretin stimulation in three dogs with gastrinoma. *A,* Note the greater than twofold increase in gastrin concentrations at 60 minutes following calcium infusion. *B,* Note the greater than twofold increase in gastrin concentrations within minutes of secretin challenge. Identical line symbols represent results from testing the same dog. (From Zerbe CA, Washabau RJ: Gastrointestinal endocrine disease. *In* Ettinger SJ, Feldman EC (eds): Textbook of Veterinary Internal Medicine, 4th ed. Philadelphia, WB Saunders Co, 1995, p 1593.)

twofold increase in serum gastrin concentration in response to calcium infusion. In one dog, calcium stimulation, but not secretin stimulation, was diagnostic for gastrinoma (see Fig. 15-3). A combined secretin-calcium stimulation test has been shown to be superior to secretin stimulation in the diagnosis of gastrinoma in humans (Zerbe and Washabau, 2000). A 1-minute infusion of 2 mg/kg of calcium gluconate, together with an IV bolus of 2 U/kg of secretin, generally causes a twofold increase in gastrin in humans with gastrinoma.

Gastric Secretory Testing. Marked fasting acid hypersecretion occurs in most humans with gastrinoma. Collection of several 15-minute aliquots of gastric secretions through an orogastric tube and determination of gastric acid content may help identify hyperacidic secretory states. Basal acid output is usually negligible in the normal fasted dog. Fasting levels of 3 to 15 mEq of hydrogen ion per hour have been measured in dogs with gastrinomas (Happe et al, 1980). Unfortunately, gastric secretory testing is nonspecific. Documentation of gastric hypersecretion of hydrochloric acid is indicative of hypergastrinemia of any cause (see Table 15-5), as well as of increased blood concentrations of histamine (e.g., mast cell neoplasia), another potent stimulant of parietal cell function.

Measurement of maximal hydrochloric acid secretion following stimulation of the parietal cells with betazole or pentagastrin may help differentiate gastrinoma from other causes of gastric hyperacidity in the patient with excessive basal gastric acid output. Stimulation of maximal hydrochloric acid secretion in the normal dog using betazole or pentagastrin should result in an increase of 3 to 12 mEq of hydrogen ion per 15-minute period (Feldman and Nelson, 1987). In dogs with the Zollinger-Ellison syndrome, the gastric acid output is already nearly maximum, so stimulation causes minimal to no further increase in acid output.

TREATMENT. Treatment of gastrinoma patients is directed at surgical excision of the tumor and control of gastric acid hypersecretion. Gastrointestinal ulceration is common and can usually be successfully managed by reducing gastric hyperacidity (see below) and administering sucralfate (Carafate, Hoechst-Marion Roussel, Kansas City, MO) and misoprostol (Cytotec, Searle, St. Louis, MO). Surgical resection of an ulcer may be required, especially if the ulcer has perforated the bowel.

Surgical Excision of Primary Tumor. In the absence of known metastases, humans with gastrinoma are explored with the intent of curative excision of the tumor, an approach that has resulted in a 5-year survival rate of over 90% for completely resected tumors (Ellison, 1995; Weber et al, 1995; Cadiot et al, 1999). Unfortunately, surgical removal of the tumor may not be curative because of the high incidence of metastasis at the time gastrinoma is diagnosed (Jensen and Fraker, 1994). Tumor recurrence is reported in approximately 50% of humans with "completely resected tumors" in long-term studies. Before the

advent of the H_2-receptor antagonists (e.g., ranitidine, famotidine), total gastrectomy was used for managing Zollinger-Ellison syndrome in humans with metastatic disease. However, since the advent of the H_2-receptor antagonists and proton pump inhibitors, surgical therapy in humans with known metastatic disease is controversial and typically reserved for noncompliant humans with unresectable tumors (Landor, 1984; Hirschowitz, 1997). Because medical therapy has such a high degree of success in controlling the hypersecretory state associated with gastrinomas, little reason exists to operate on patients with a nonresectable neoplasm. Similar reasoning could be applied to dogs and cats, especially considering that 70% of reported cases already had metastatic disease at the time of the animal's initial examination. In addition to the malignant potential of these tumors, the possibility of ectopic sites of disease, the severity of clinical signs at the time of presentation, and the easy use of H_2-receptor blocking agents or proton pump inhibitors are further arguments against surgical intervention.

Nevertheless, strong arguments can also be made in support of surgical exploration in the dog or cat with suspected gastrinoma. We support surgical intervention in conjunction with concurrent medical management. Accurate preoperative localization of the tumor and the prediction of resectability are difficult in humans, even with the use of sophisticated diagnostic techniques such as ultrasonography, nuclear scintigraphy, computed tomography, and magnetic resonance imaging (Landor, 1984; Wolfe and Jensen, 1987; Norton, 1998). Surgery is perhaps the easiest and best method of establishing the diagnosis while offering a chance for cure in those few animals with solitary, nonmetastatic gastrinomas (Wolfe et al, 1982; Eng et al, 1992). Even if metastatic disease is present, tumor debulking may enhance the success of medical therapy. Dogs and cats with metastatic gastrinomas should not be euthanized because of metastatic disease. Humans with the Zollinger-Ellison syndrome and metastatic disease may live for years with appropriate medical therapy (Landor, 1984; Weber et al, 1995).

Surgery also offers a chance for excision of "deep" or perforated ulcers. The potential for perforation of a gastric or duodenal ulcer with subsequent development of peritonitis is a very real concern. Gastrointestinal ulceration was found in 20 (80%) of 25 dogs and cats with gastrinoma, with perforation of the ulcer identified in 5 animals (Table 15-6; Zerbe and Washabau, 2000). In the extremely ill animal, initial stabilization using IV fluids, antibiotics, and gastric acid-blocking drugs is necessary before considering surgery. Surgical exploration, however, should be undertaken quickly if a perforated ulcer and peritonitis are suspected.

Twenty-one of 24 dogs and all cats with gastrinoma had a tumor arising from islet cells in the pancreas, with multiple pancreatic masses identified in 4 animals. A tumor in the pancreas was not identified

TABLE 15–6 PREVALENCE OF GROSS PATHOLOGIC ALTERATIONS (SURGICAL OR NECROPSY) IN 21 DOGS AND 2 CATS WITH GASTRINOMA AND SIGNS CONSISTENT WITH THE ZOLLINGER-ELLISON SYNDROME

Pathology	Number of Animals	Percent of Animals
Tumor location		
Pancreas	21/22	95
Left lobe	1/16	6
Body	6/16	38
Right lobe	10/16	63
Liver	13/21	62
Lymph node	6/21	29
Other	5/21	24
Gastrointestinal ulceration	22/23	96
Esophagus	4/21	19
Stomach	10/22	45
Duodenum	14/19	74
Jejunum	1/18	6
Perforated ulcer	5/21	24
Gastric hypertrophy	14/19	74
Thyroid C-cell hyperplasia	4/9	44
Adrenocortical hyperplasia	2/9	22
Thyroid follicular cell carcinoma	1/9	11

From Zerbe CA, Washabau RJ: *In* Ettinger SJ, Feldman EC (eds): Textbook of Veterinary Internal Medicine, 5th ed. Philadelphia, WB Saunders Co, 2000, p 1505 and case accessions at the School of Veterinary Medicine, University of California, Davis.

at surgery in 3 dogs but was identified in the regional lymph nodes in 2 of the dogs and at the root of the mesentery in the third dog (Brooks and Watson, 1997; Green and Gatrell, 1997). Because gastrinomas can be small and the likelihood of metastasis high, the pancreas, regional lymph nodes, liver, and peripancreatic mesentery should be carefully inspected during surgery and any abnormalities removed or biopsied. Gastrin-secreting tumors occurred most commonly in the right lobe (10 animals) and body (6 animals) of the pancreas, with only one report of a tumor in the left lobe of the pancreas. A right lobe pancreatectomy should be performed if a specific tumor nodule cannot be located.

Gastric Hyperacidity. Current medical management is centered on blocking the hypersecretion of acid with histamine H_2-receptor antagonists and the $H^+–K^+$ ATPase inhibitor, omeprazole. Parietal cells have receptor sites that bind gastrin, histamine (H_2 receptors), and acetylcholine. All three receptor sites must be stimulated by the appropriate molecule for maximal hydrochloric acid secretion by the parietal cell. The occupation of H_2 receptors by the H_2 antagonist blocks gastrin's stimulatory effect on hydrochloric acid secretion because all three receptor sites are not occupied by their respective peptide. Serum gastrin concentrations are not altered by this mode of therapy (i.e., hypergastrinemia persists), nor is the gastrinoma. Treatment with H_2-receptor antagonists has been effective in reducing gastric acid hypersecretion, improving symptoms, and inducing ulcer healing in most humans with gastrinoma (McCarthy, 1980). Similar improvement in clinical signs has been documented in several dogs and one cat with gastrinoma (Drazner, 1981; Zerbe and Washabau, 2000). Histamine H_2-receptor antagonists include cimetidine (Tagamet, SmithKline-Beecham, Pittsburgh, PA; initial oral dosage, 10 mg/kg given every 6 to 8 hours), ranitidine (Zantac, Glaxo Wellcome, Research Triangle Park, NC; initial oral dosage, 2.2 mg/kg given every 12 hours), and famotidine (Pepcid, Merck, West Point, PA; initial oral dosage, 0.5 to 1.0 mg/kg given every 12 to 24 hours). Because the amount of medication required to suppress acid output is highly variable and, in humans, tends to increase with time (Jensen, 1984), the dosage of these medications must be individualized and periodically reevaluated. Dosages higher than those typically used for control of gastric acid secretion are usually required in humans with gastrinoma.

Omeprazole (Prilosec, AstraZenecka, Wilmington, DE) suppresses gastric acid secretion more effectively than H_2-receptor antagonists and is currently the preferred drug for inhibition of gastric acid secretion in humans with gastrinoma (Jensen and Fraker, 1994; Mulvihill and Debas, 2001). Omeprazole acts to inhibit parietal cell $H^+–K^+$ ATPase (i.e., proton pump inhibitor), which is the final common step in gastric acid secretion (Howden, 1991). Omeprazole inhibits gastric acid secretion stimulated by any of the secretagogues, whereas the H_2-receptor antagonists block only the actions of histamine. Omeprazole is a potent inhibitor of gastric acid secretion with a long duration of action (Larrson et al, 1983) and is effective in controlling clinical signs of gastrinoma in dogs (Brooks and Watson, 1997). The initial dosage in the dog is 0.7 to 1.0 mg/kg given every 24 hours.

The long-acting somatostatin analogue, octreotide, inhibits gastrin release, gastric acid secretion, and diarrhea in humans with gastrinoma (Kvols et al, 1987; Maton, 1989; Mulvihill and Debas, 2001). It is used occasionally in humans refractory to histamine H_2-receptor antagonists or omeprazole and was used in one dog with gastrinoma, in conjunction with cimetidine and sucralfate, for more than 10 months (Lothrop et al, 1989) and in one dog with metastatic gastrinoma, in conjunction with famotidine, sucralfate, and omeprazole, for 14 months (Altschul et al, 1997). The dosage is 5 to 20 μg subcutaneously every 8 hours.

PATHOLOGY. Twenty-five of 28 reported cases of Zollinger-Ellison syndrome in dogs and cats had the primary tumor in the pancreas, with the majority of tumors located in the right lobe or body of the pancreas (see Table 15-6; Zerbe and Washabau, 2000). Multiple pancreatic masses were found in 4 animals. A tumor in the pancreas was not identified at surgery in 3 dogs but was identified in the regional lymph nodes in 2 of the dogs and at the root of the mesentery in the third dog (Brooks and Watson, 1997; Green and Gatrell, 1997). A necropsy was not reported in these dogs. Metastatic disease involving the liver, adjacent lymph nodes, spleen, or mesentery was identified in

70% of the cases. Histologically, the tumor cells were arranged in sheets, cords, or acini with variable degrees of fibrosis interspersed within or encapsulating the mass (Happe et al, 1980; Middleton and Watson, 1983). Immunocytochemical analysis, when performed, revealed positive immunoreactivity to gastrin within the neoplastic cells, as well as to other hormones such as glucagon, ACTH, or somatostatin in a few of the tumors (Happe et al, 1980; Middleton and Watson, 1983). Pathologic alterations of other organ systems were also found and presumably resulted from hypergastrinemia and hypersecretion of gastric hydrochloric acid (see Table 15-6).

PROGNOSIS. Gastrinomas in dogs and cats are malignant tumors that carry a poor long-term prognosis. Evidence of metastasis was present in 70% of dogs and cats at the time gastrinoma was diagnosed (Zerbe and Washabau, 2000). Approximately one-third of reported affected animals died or were euthanized without the benefit of treatment. The diagnosis of gastrinoma was established at postmortem examination in these animals. Dogs and cats that were treated surgically and/or medically survived from 1 week to more than 2 years; most survived less than 8 months from the time of diagnosis (Zerbe, 1992). However, the prognosis has improved in recent years with the availability of drugs to reduce gastric hyperacidity (e.g., famotidine, omeprazole) and drugs that protect and promote healing of the ulcers (e.g., sucralfate, misoprostol).

GLUCAGONOMA (SUPERFICIAL NECROLYTIC DERMATITIS)

Glucagonomas arise from the A cells in the pancreatic islets and may occur as individual entities or as part of the multiple endocrine neoplasia syndrome. About 25% of glucagonomas in humans are benign and confined to the pancreas (Mulvihill and Debas, 2001). The remainder have metastasized by the time of diagnosis, most often to the liver, lymph nodes, adrenal glands, or vertebrae. Glucagon has been demonstrated by immunohistochemical analysis in canine islet cell tumors (Hawkins et al, 1987; O'Brien et al, 1987; Minkus et al, 1997) and solitary glucagonomas have been described in dogs (Gross et al, 1990; Torres et al, 1997a; Allenspach et al, 2000). Glucagonoma has not yet been described in cats.

Excessive secretion of glucagon causes a disorder in humans characterized by necrolytic migratory erythema, cheilosis, diabetes mellitus, normocytic normochromic anemia, venous thrombosis, weight loss, and neuropsychiatric manifestations (Krejs, 1998). The characteristic rash, necrolytic migratory erythema, is the primary clinical manifestation. Necrolytic migratory erythema commences as red patches that progress to form bullae and then break down and become encrusted, followed by healing and pigmentation. The lesions tend to coalesce, often with extensive skin involvement and secondary infection.

A similar syndrome, superficial necrolytic dermatitis, has been described in 7 dogs with glucagon-secreting pancreatic islet tumor and more than 40 dogs with advanced liver disease (Walton et al, 1986; Gross et al, 1990; 1993; Bond et al, 1995; Nyland et al, 1996; Torres et al, 1997a; Allenspach et al, 2000). Superficial necrolytic dermatitis has also been described in a cat with pancreatic adenocarcinoma (Patal et al, 1996). Superficial necrolytic dermatitis usually affects middle-aged to older dogs and is characterized by ulcerative, erythematous lesions of the footpads, mucocutaneous junctions, genital area, and at pressure points, such as the elbow and tarsus (Scott et al, 2001). The footpads are often extremely hyperkeratotic and may be fissured. Secondary infections are common. Histologically, epidermal parakeratotic hyperkeratosis and severe inter- and intracellular edema with subsequent clefts or subcorneal vesicles are identified in skin biopsies of affected areas. Histologic lesions of superficial necrolytic dermatitis are similar to those of human necrolytic migratory erythema.

Skin lesions are caused by degeneration of the keratinocytes, which results in laminar high-level epidermal edema and degeneration (Scott et al, 2001). The pathogenesis of necrolytic migratory erythema in humans and superficial necrolytic dermatitis in dogs is not known, although cellular starvation or some other nutritional imbalance is probably involved. Hyperglucagonemia, hypoaminoacidemia, and low essential fatty acid and zinc concentrations have been suggested to play a role in the pathogenesis of the skin lesions of necrolytic migratory erythema (Wood et al, 1983; Krejs, 1998) and are believed also to play a role in superficial necrolytic dermatitis. Hyperglucagonemia may play a direct or, more likely, an indirect role in the generation of the skin lesions. Glucagon is involved in the catabolism of amino acids to glucose, and increased concentrations of glucagon may create the decrease in amino acid concentrations that are consistently found in this syndrome. Low amino acid concentrations lead to epidermal protein depletion and subsequent keratinocyte necrolysis. In addition, increased glucagon levels may stimulate arachidonic acid synthesis in keratinocytes, causing increased arachidonic acid release and subsequent inflammation and necrosis (Walton et al, 1986; Gross et al, 1993). Hypoaminoacidemia has been documented in dogs with a glucagon-secreting tumor (Torres et al, 1997a; Allenspach et al, 2000) and was identified in eight dogs with superficial necrolytic dermatitis (Gross et al, 1993). In six of these eight dogs, marked improvement in cutaneous lesions was noted when egg yolks, a concentrated source of protein, were used to supplement the diet (Gross et al, 1993). Similarly, resolution of hyperglucagonemia, hypoaminoacidemia, and cutaneous lesions occurred following surgical excision of a pancreatic glucagonoma in a dog (Torres et al, 1997a).

Hyperglycemia or overt diabetes mellitus and small intestinal diarrhea are additional problems identified in dogs with glucagonoma (Walton et al, 1986). Diabetes mellitus results from the diabetogenic action of glucagon, which acts exclusively on the liver to activate glycogenolysis and gluconeogenesis (Cryer and Polonsky, 1998). Diarrhea is believed to result from the secretory effects of glucagon on the small bowel mucosa (reduction of absorption or enhancement of net secretion of water and electrolytes; Krejs, 1998).

A glucagon-producing pancreatic neuroendocrine tumor may be confirmed by documenting elevated plasma glucagon concentrations in the presence of a pancreatic tumor immunoreactive for glucagon. In humans, plasma glucagon concentrations are usually increased 5 to 10 times above normal (i.e., 300 to 1000 pg/ml; Misra and Baruh, 1983). Plasma glucagon concentration was increased 1.6 to 18-fold above the upper limit of the reference range in 5 dogs with histologically and immunohistochemically confirmed glucagon-producing neuroendocrine tumor in which plasma glucagon was measured (Allenspach et al, 2000). In contrast, most dogs with superficial necrolytic dermatitis associated with advanced liver disease have had normal concentrations of plasma glucagon (Nyland et al, 1996). Abdominal ultrasound may identify a pancreatic mass or metastases in the regional lymph nodes, liver, or peripancreatic tissue. However, failure to identify a pancreatic mass with abdominal ultrasound does not rule out a glucagon-secreting pancreatic tumor. A well-defined reticular or "honey-combed" pattern has been identified ultrasonographically in the liver of dogs with superficial necrolytic dermatitis caused by advanced liver disease but has not been reported in dogs with glucagon-producing neoplasia (Nyland et al, 1996).

The treatment of choice for glucagonoma is surgical excision of the tumor, which may be curative. Streptozocin, dacarbazine, and somatostatin analogues are effective palliative agents for unresectable lesions in humans (Maton, 1989; Nightingale et al, 1999; Mulvihill and Debas, 2001). Death in humans with nontreatable glucagon-secreting tumors usually occurs following extreme debilitation or thromboembolic complications. One dog had resolution of hyperglucagonemia, hypoaminoacidemia, and cutaneous lesions within 45 days of surgical excision of a metastatic pancreatic glucagonoma but cutaneous lesions recurred 9 months later and the dog was euthanized (Torres et al, 1997a), three dogs with pancreatic glucagonoma died shortly after surgery because of complications related to pancreatitis (Gross et al, 1990; Bond et al, 1995), and three dogs with pancreatic glucagonoma were euthanized 2, 4, and 6 weeks after establishing the diagnosis because of progression of the disease (Miller et al, 1991; Torres et al, 1997b; Allenspach et al, 2000). Palliative treatments for superficial necrolytic dermatitis caused by advanced liver disease have included the intravenous or oral administration of amino acid supplements (e.g., eggs; Prescription Diet a/d, Hill's Pet Products [Topeka, KS]; Aminosyn, Abbott Laboratories [Abbott Park, IL]), the subcutaneous administration of the somatostatin analogue octreotide (Sandostatin, Novartis Pharmaceuticals [East Hanover, NJ]), essen-

tial fatty acid supplements, topical astringents, hydrotherapy, and systemic antibiotics for secondary bacterial infections (Byrne, 1999). The prognosis for dogs with superficial necrolytic dermatitis associated with advanced liver disease is poor (Gross et al, 1993; Byrne, 1999). Mean survival time is approximately 5 months, with many dogs dying within 1 to 2 months of establishing the diagnosis.

VIPoma: VERNER-MORRISON SYNDROME

VIPoma was first described in humans by Verner and Morrison in 1958 and has not yet been described in dogs and cats. Clinical signs are caused by intestinal secretion of fluid and electrolytes in response to elevated circulating levels of vasoactive intestinal polypeptide (VIP), usually from an islet cell tumor of the pancreas (Smith et al, 1998; Soga and Yakuwa, 1998). Co-secretion of peptide histidine-methionine (PHM) occurs in humans with VIPomas, PHM concentrations are high in plasma, and both VIP and PHM are present in the same tumor cells (Bloom et al, 1983). PHM has effects on intestinal mucosa similar to VIP and may be responsible, in part, for the clinical signs.

VIPoma is characterized by profuse watery diarrhea, marked fecal loss of potassium and bicarbonate, hypokalemia, and low or absent gastric acid secretion. Severe metabolic acidosis may develop following excessive loss of bicarbonate in the stool (Smith et al, 1998; Soga and Yakuwa, 1998). Many humans are hypercalcemic, perhaps from secretion by the tumor of a parathyroid hormone–like substance. Abnormal glucose tolerance may result from hypokalemia and altered sensitivity to insulin. The average duration of symptoms prior to diagnosis is 3 years, with a range of 2 months to 4 years (Krejs, 1987).

The diagnosis of VIPoma is suspected by the clinical presentation of severe watery secretory diarrhea and hypokalemia. The diagnosis is confirmed by measurement of serum fasting VIP concentrations by radioimmunoassay and histologic confirmation of a non–beta-cell pancreatic tumor containing a high content of VIP (Krejs, 1987).

Surgical excision is the current treatment of choice. The prognosis is good, with remission achieved in 50% of patients when the tumor has not grown extensively or metastasized (Smith et al, 1998; Soga and Yakuwa, 1998). Metastasis is primarily to the liver and adjacent lymph nodes and is present in about one-third of humans at the time of diagnosis. Streptozocin plus fluorouracil have been used in patients with nonresectable or metastatic carcinoma (Nguyen et al, 1999). The long-acting somatostatin analogue octreotide has also been used to treat a patient resistant to all other modes of therapy (Maton et al, 1985; Maton, 1989). Somatostatin lowers plasma concentration of VIP in patients with VIPomas (Ruskone et al, 1982). Other agents that occasionally elicit a clinical response are corticosteroids and indomethacin (Deveney and Way, 1983).

SOMATOSTATINOMA

Somatostatinomas are rare tumors in humans and have not yet been described in dogs or cats. However, somatostatin has been documented by immunohistochemical analysis in canine islet cell tumors (Hawkins et al, 1987; O'Brien et al, 1987; Minkus et al, 1997). The syndrome results from secretion of somatostatin by an islet cell tumor arising from the D cells of the pancreas, which in most human cases is malignant and accompanied by hepatic metastasis (Mulvihill and Debas, 2001). Clinical features include glucose intolerance (mild diabetes mellitus), cholelithiasis, diarrhea, steatorrhea, hypochlorhydria, and weight loss (Krejs, 1998). In some individuals, hypoglycemia, flushing, and signs of hyperadrenocorticism may be present (Wright et al, 1980; Penman et al, 1980). Somatostatinomas frequently contain subpopulations of other endocrine cells, which may explain, in part, the variability of symptoms. Variability in symptoms and the fact that the cardinal manifestations (diabetes mellitus, cholelithiasis, diarrhea, steatorrhea) are common make antemortem recognition of somatostatinoma difficult.

The diagnosis is based on recognition of appropriate clinical features, documentation of increased serum concentrations of somatostatin, and histologic examination of a biopsied or excised tumor. Appropriate immunohistochemical evaluation of the tumor is necessary for definitive documentation. Pancreatic somatostatinomas tend to be slow-growing, with metastasis to the liver and adjacent lymph nodes often present at the time of the diagnosis (Misra and Baruh, 1983). Surgical excision is the recommended treatment, although chemotherapy with streptozocin has been tried.

Somatostatinomas have also been found in the gastrointestinal tract (Marcial et al, 1983). Gastrointestinal somatostatinomas appear to be histologically and clinically distinct from pancreatic somatostatinomas. Clinically, they tend to cause biliary tract or intestinal obstruction. Somatostatin is only rarely released by gastrointestinal somatostatinomas, so other signs associated with this syndrome are usually absent (Marcial et al, 1983).

PANCREATIC POLYPEPTIDE–PRODUCING TUMOR

Pancreatic polypeptide (PP) has been found in high concentrations in many types of pancreatic endocrine tumors, including gastrinomas, VIPomas, glucagonomas, and insulinomas (Adrian et al, 1986). PP is the second most common hormone identified by immunocytochemistry within canine pancreatic endocrine tumors (Zerbe et al, 1989). PP has been used as a marker for the diagnosis of pancreatic endocrine tumors in humans and for monitoring the response to treatment when initial plasma PP concentrations are elevated (Adrian et al, 1986; Krejs, 1998). Plasma PP concentrations have also been used to monitor humans at risk for and with a family history of multiple endocrine neoplasia (Tomita et al, 1983).

Several reports have been published describing humans with tumors secreting only PP (Tomita et al, 1983; Strodel et al, 1984). Humans with high circulating levels of PP do not display a characteristic clinical syndrome. The most common symptoms include watery diarrhea, abdominal pain, gastrointestinal bleeding, weight loss, and jaundice. An elevation in plasma PP concentrations and immunohistochemical documentation of PP production by the tumor were used to establish a definitive diagnosis. An increase in plasma PP levels is not necessarily diagnostic of a PP-producing tumor, because certain inflammatory diseases, duodenal ulcers, diabetes mellitus, pancreatic exocrine insufficiency, and renal dysfunction are also associated with increased plasma PP concentrations (Oberg et al, 1981; Whitehead, 1980). Ultrasonography or provocative testing, either stimulatory (e.g., tolbutamide, pentagastrin, secretin) or suppressive (e.g., atropine) may be necessary to identify PP–producing tumors presurgically (Strodel et al, 1984). Surgical excision is the recommended treatment. Sites of metastasis include the liver and adjacent lymph nodes.

Although PP has been demonstrated in canine islet cell tumors by immunohistochemical analysis (O'Brien et al, 1987), an islet cell tumor secreting only PP has not been documented in dogs or cats. Increased serum PP concentrations were documented in one dog with a pancreatic endocrine tumor that was positive for several hormones on immunocytochemical staining, including PP (Zerbe et al, 1989). Clinical signs in the affected dog were suggestive of gastrinoma (i.e., chronic vomiting, hypertrophic gastritis, duodenal ulceration), and basal serum insulin, gastrin, and PP concentrations were increased. However, results of secretin stimulation and calcium challenge tests (see page 651) were not consistent with gastrinoma, and immunocytochemical staining of the tumor for gastrin was negative. Because serum PP concentrations were extremely increased (637,000 pg/ml; normal <155 pg/ml) and the tumor and its metastasis were strongly positive for PP on immunocytochemical staining, the investigators proposed that high serum PP concentrations may have contributed to the dog's gastrointestinal ulceration and vomiting (Zerbe et al, 1989).

CARCINOIDS AND THE CARCINOID SYNDROME

Carcinoid tumors arise from enterochromaffin cells of the gastrointestinal tract. Carcinoids can be found anywhere in the gastrointestinal tract from the gastroesophageal junction to the anus. Extraintestinal sites such as the bronchus and ovary have also been described in humans (Mulvihill and Debas, 2001). Carcinoids in humans have been categorized as foregut (bronchus and stomach), midgut (small intestine and colon), or hindgut (rectum) tumors. Foregut carcinoids secrete 5-hydroxytryptophan, midgut tumors secrete 5-hydroxytryptamine (serotonin), and hindgut carcinoids synthesize no specific by-products.

Carcinoid syndrome is caused by the systemic release of substances from carcinoid tumors. Although 5-hydroxytryptamine (serotonin) is the primary mediator released from carcinoids, additional mediators also play a role in the development of the carcinoid syndrome, including bradykinin, prostaglandins, histamine, and substance P (Roberts and Oates, 1985). Because the humoral substances liberated by carcinoids are metabolized by the liver, the presence of the carcinoid syndrome implies either a primary lesion draining into the systemic circulation or hepatic metastasis from a gastrointestinal lesion (Misra and Baruh, 1983; Mulvihill and Debas, 2001).

The most common symptoms of the carcinoid syndrome in humans are paroxysmal flushing of the head and neck and diarrhea. Diarrhea is believed to be caused by serotonin secretion, whereas flushing is due to release of tachykinins from the tumor. Additional clinical features include abdominal cramping, bronchospasm, hyperventilation, and cardiac disease, with the potential for development of pulmonic stenosis and tricuspid valve insufficiency (Misra and Baruh, 1983; Roberts and Oates, 1985).

In dogs, carcinoid tumors have been reported in the intestine, lung, and liver (Patniak et al, 1980; 1981; Sykes and Cooper, 1982), whereas in the cat they have been found in the stomach and intestinal tract. In dogs and cats, carcinoid tumors affect primarily the aged animal; all reported cases involved animals at least 9 years old. The carcinoid tumors reported in dogs and cats have not resulted in the development of the "carcinoid syndrome." Instead, the signs have been related predominantly to the presence of a mass lesion causing gastrointestinal obstruction or signs associated with metastatic cancer (Table 15-7). Sites of metastasis in dogs and cats include regional lymph nodes, mesentery, peritoneal wall, lung, pancreas, liver, and local invasion (Patniak et al, 1980; 1981).

In humans, diagnosis of the carcinoid syndrome is based on clinical signs, documentation of large amounts of serotonin metabolites, especially 5-hydroxyindoleacetic acid (HIAA), in the urine, and histologic examination of a biopsied or excised tumor. In most laboratories, the urinary excretion of 5-HIAA in normal humans is below 10 mg/24 hr, whereas it ranges from 10 to 600 mg/24 hr in patients with the carcinoid syndrome (Roberts and Oates, 1985). Measurement of serotonin, histamine, prostaglandins, and bradykinin concentrations in blood is less reliable than measurement of urinary concentrations of serotonin metabolites (Mulvihill and Debas, 2001).

When feasible, localized carcinoids should be resected. If metastatic lesions are present, tumor debulking should still be considered, especially if clinical signs are present (Que et al, 1995; Krishnamurthy et al, 1996). In humans, palliation of the symptoms of carcinoid syndrome is best achieved with the long-acting analogue of somatostatin, octreotide (Kvols et al, 1986), which is successful in about 80% of humans. Cytotoxic chemotherapy is used in humans with rapidly progressive tumors and for those with carcinoid-induced valvular heart disease. The most widely used regimen consists of streptozocin plus fluorouracil (Roberts and Oates, 1985). The 5-year survival rate in humans with metastasis is 20%. If only regional lymph nodes are involved, the 5-year survival rate is 65%. If the tumor is locally invasive without lymph node involvement, the 5-year survival rate is 95% (Shebani, 1999). Death is usually a result of cardiac failure, electrolyte problems from severe diarrhea, or cachexia.

REFERENCES

Adrian TE, et al: Secretion of pancreatic polypeptide in patients with pancreatic endocrine tumors. N Engl J Med 315:287, 1986.

Allenspach K, et al: Glucagon-producing neuroendocrine tumour associated with hypoaminoacidemia and skin lesions. J Sm Anim Pract 41:402, 2000.

Altschul M, et al: Evaluation of somatostatin analogues for the detection and treatment of gastrinoma in a dog. J Sm Anim Pract 38:286, 1997.

Bardram L: Progastrin in serum from Zollinger-Ellison patients. Gastroenterology 98:1420, 1990.

Bloom SR, et al: Diarrhea in VIPoma patients associated with cosecretion of a second active peptide (peptide histidine isoleucine) explained by a single coding gene. Lancet 2:1163, 1983.

Bond R, et al: Metabolic epidermal necrosis in two dogs with different underlying diseases. Vet Rec 136:466, 1995.

Brady CE, et al: Secretin provocation in normal and duodenal ulcer subjects: Is the gastrin rise in Zollinger-Ellison syndrome paradoxic or exaggeration? Dig Dis Sci 32:232, 1987.

Breitschwerdt EB, et al: Hypergastrinemia in canine gastrointestinal disease. J Am Anim Hosp Assoc 22:585, 1986.

Breitschwerdt EB, et al: Gastric acid secretion in Basenji dogs with immunoproliferative enteropathy. J Vet Intern Med 5:34, 1991.

Brooks D, Watson GL: Omeprazole in a dog with gastrinoma. J Vet Intern Med 11:379, 1997.

Byrne KP: Metabolic epidermal necrosis-hepatocutaneous syndrome. Vet Clin N Amer (Sm Anim Pract) 29:1337, 1999.

Cadiot G, et al: Prognostic factors in patients with Zollinger-Ellison syndrome and multiple endocrine neoplasia type 1. Gastroenterology 116:286, 1999.

Cryer PE, Polonsky KS: Glucose homeostasis and hypoglycemia. In Wilson JD, Foster DW, Kronenberg HM, Larsen PR (eds): Williams Textbook of Endocrinology, 9th ed. Philadelphia, WB Saunders Co, 1998, p 939.

Deveney CW, Way LW: Regulatory peptides of the gut. In Greenspan FS, Forsham PH (eds): Basic and Clinical Endocrinology. Los Altos, CA, Lange Medical Publications, 1983, p 479.

Drazner FH: Canine gastrinoma: A condition analogous to the Zollinger-Ellison syndrome in man. Calif Vet 11:6, 1981.

Ellison EC: Forty-year appraisal of gastrinoma: Back to the future. Ann Surg 222:511, 1995.

TABLE 15–7 FREQUENCY OF OCCURRENCE OF CLINICAL SIGNS REPORTED IN 20 DOGS AND 1 CAT WITH CARCINOID TUMOR

Clinical Sign	Percent of Animals
Weight loss	52
Anorexia	38
Diarrhea	38
Ascites	29
Jaundice	24
Polyuria, polydipsia	24
Intestinal bleeding	10
Visible rectal mass	10
Vomiting	5

Ellison EC, et al: Characterization of the in vivo and in vitro inhibition of gastrin secretion from gastrinoma by a somatostatin analogue (SMS 201-995). Am J Med 81:56, 1986.

Eng J, et al: Cat gastrinoma and the sequence of cat gastrins. Reg Peptides 37:9, 1992.

English RV, et al: Zollinger-Ellison syndrome and myelofibrosis in a dog. JAVMA 192:1430, 1988.

Feldman EC, Nelson RW: Canine and Feline Endocrinology and Reproduction. Philadelphia, WB Saunders Co, 1987, p 375.

Gibril F, et al: Somatostatin receptor scintigraphy: Its sensitivity compared with that of other imaging methods in detecting primary and metastatic gastrinoma. Ann Intern Med 125:26, 1996.

Goldstein RE, et al: Gastrin concentrations in plasma of cats with chronic renal failure. J Am Vet Med Assoc 213:826, 1998.

Gorden P, et al: Somatostatin and somatostatin analogue (SMS 201-995) in treatment of hormone-secreting tumors of the pituitary and gastrointestinal tract and non-neoplastic diseases of the gut. Ann Intern Med 110:35, 1989.

Green RA, Gartrell CL: Gastrinoma: A retrospective study of four cases (1985-1995). J Am Anim Hosp Assoc 33:524, 1997.

Gross TL, et al: Glucagon-producing pancreatic endocrine tumors in two dogs with superficial necrolytic dermatitis. JAVMA 197:1619, 1990.

Gross TL, et al: Superficial necrolytic dermatitis (necrolytic migratory erythema) in dogs. Vet Pathol 30:75, 1993.

Happe RP, et al: Zollinger-Ellison syndrome in three dogs. Vet Pathol 17:177, 1980.

Hawkins KL, et al: Immunocytochemistry of normal pancreatic islets and spontaneous islet cell tumors in dogs. Vet Pathol 24:170, 1987.

Hirschowitz BI: Zollinger-Ellison syndrome: pathogenesis, diagnosis, and management. Am J Gastroenterol 92(4 suppl):44S, 1997.

Howden CW: Clinical pharmacology of omeprazole. Clin Pharmacokinet 20:38, 1991.

Jensen RT: Basis for failure of cimetidine in patients with Zollinger-Ellison syndrome. Dig Dis Sci 29:363, 1984.

Jensen RT, Fraker DL: Zollinger-Ellison syndrome: Advances in treatment of gastric hypersecretion and the gastrinoma. J Am Med Assoc 271:1429, 1994.

Krejs GJ: VIPoma syndrome. Am J Med 82(Suppl 5B):37, 1987.

Krejs GJ: Non–insulin-secreting tumors of the gastroenteropancreatic system. In Wilson JD, Foster DW, Kronenberg HM, Larsen PR (eds): Williams Textbook of Endocrinology, 9th ed. Philadelphia, WB Saunders Co, 1998, p 1663.

Krishnamurthy SC, et al: Primary carcinoid tumor of the liver: Report of four resected cases including one with gastrin production. J Surg Oncol 62:218, 1996

Kvols LK, et al: Treatment of the malignant carcinoid syndrome. Evaluation of a long-acting somatostatin analogue. N Engl J Med 315:663, 1986.

Kvols LK, et al: Treatment of metastatic islet cell carcinoma with somatostatin analogue (SMS 201-995). Ann Intern Med 107:162, 1987.

Landor JH: Control of the Zollinger-Ellison syndrome by excision of primary and metastatic tumor. Am J Surg 147:406, 1984.

Larrson H, et al: Inhibition of gastric acid secretion by omeprazole in the dog and rat. N Engl J Med 85:900, 1983.

Lothrop CD, et al: Medical treatment of neuroendocrine tumors of the gastroenteropancreatic system with somatostatin. In Kirk RW (ed): Current Veterinary Therapy X. Philadelphia, WB Saunders Co, 1989, p 1021.

Marcial MA, et al: Ampullary somatostatinoma: Psammomatous variant of gastrointestinal carcinoid tumor—An immunohistochemical and ultrastructural study. Report of a case and review of the literature. Am J Clin Pathol 80:755, 1983.

Maton PN, et al: Effect of a long-acting somatostatin analogue (SMS 201-995) in a patient with pancreatic cholera. N Engl J Med 312:17, 1985.

McCarthy DM: The place of surgery in the Zollinger-Ellison syndrome. N Engl J Med 302:1344, 1980.

McGuigan JE, Wolfe MM: Secretin injection test in the diagnosis of gastrinoma. Gastroenterology 79:1324, 1980.

Middleton DJ, Watson AD: Duodenal ulceration associated with gastrin-secreting pancreatic tumor in a cat. JAVMA 183:461, 1983.

Miller WH, et al: Necrolytic migratory erythema in a dog with a glucagon-secreting endocrine tumor. Vet Dermatol 2:179, 1991.

Minkus G, et al: Canine neuroendocrine tumors of the pancreas: A study using image analysis techniques for the discrimination of metastatic versus nonmetastatic tumors. Vet Pathol 34:138, 1997.

Misra P, Baruh S: Diagnostic and therapeutic applications of gastrointestinal hormones. In Essman WB (ed): Hormonal Actions in Non-Endocrine Systems. New York, Spectrum Publications, 1983, p 63.

Mulvihill SJ, Debas HT: Regulatory peptides of the gut. In Greenspan FS, Gardner DG (eds): Basic and Clinical Endocrinology, 6th ed. New York, Lange Medical Books/McGraw-Hill, 2001, p 603.

Nguyen HN, et al: Long-term survival after diagnosis of hepatic metastatic VIPoma: report of two cases with disparate courses and review of therapeutic options. Dig Dis Sci 44:1148, 1999.

Nightingale KJ, et al: Glucagonoma syndrome: survival 24 years following diagnosis. Dig Surg 16:68, 1999.

Norton JA: Gastrinoma: advances in localization and treatment. Surg Oncol Clin N Am 7:845, 1998.

Nyland TG, et al: Hepatic ultrasonographic and pathologic findings in dogs with canine superficial necrolytic dermatitis. Vet Radiol Ultra 37:200, 1996.

Oberg K, et al: Update on pancreatic polypeptide as a specific marker for endocrine tumors of the pancreas and gut. Acta Med Scand 210:145, 1981.

O'Brien TD, et al: Canine pancreatic endocrine tumors: Immunohistochemical analysis of hormone content and amyloid. Vet Pathol 24:308, 1987.

Patal A, et al: A case of metabolic epidermal necrosis in a cat. Vet Dermatol 7:221, 1996.

Patniak AK, et al: Canine intestinal adenocarcinoma and carcinoid. Vet Pathol 17:149, 1980.

Patniak AK, et al: Canine hepatic carcinoids. Vet Pathol 18:445, 1981.

Penman E, et al: Molecular forms of somatostatin in normal subjects and in patients with pancreatic somatostatinoma. Clin Endocrinol (Oxf) 12:611, 1980.

Pipeleers-Marichal M, et al: Gastrinomas in the duodenums of patients with multiple endocrine neoplasia type 1 and the Zollinger-Ellison syndrome. N Engl J Med 322:723, 1990.

Que FG, et al: Hepatic resection for metastatic neuroendocrine carcinomas. Am J Surg 169:36, 1995.

Roberts LJ, Oates JA: Disorders of vasodilator hormones: The carcinoid syndrome and mastocytosis. In Wilson JD, Foster DW (eds): Williams Textbook of Endocrinology, 7th ed. Philadelphia, WB Saunders Co, 1985, p 1363.

Roche A, et al: Pancreatic venous sampling and arteriography in localizing insulinomas and gastrinomas: Procedure and results in 55 cases. Radiology 145:621, 1982.

Ruskone A, et al: Effect of somatostatin on diarrhea and on small intestinal water and electrolyte transport in a patient with pancreatic cholera. Dig Dis Sci 27:459, 1982.

Schirmer WJ, et al: Indium-111-pentetreotide scanning versus conventional imaging techniques for the localization of gastrinoma. Surgery 118:1105, 1995.

Scott DW, Miller WH, Griffin CE (eds): Muller & Kirk's Small Animal Dermatology, 6th ed. Philadelphia, WB Saunders Co, 2001, p 780.

Shebani KO: Prognosis and survival in patients with gastrointestinal tract carcinoid tumors. Ann Surg 229:815, 1999.

Slaff JI, et al: Prospective assessment of provocative gastrin tests in 81 consecutive patients with Zollinger-Ellison syndrome (ZES) [abstract]. Gastroenterology 90:1637, 1986.

Smith SL, et al: Vasoactive intestinal polypeptide secreting islet cell tumors: A 15-year experience and review of the literature. Surgery 124:1050, 1998.

Soga J, Yakuwa Y: Vipoma/diarrheogenic syndrome: A statistical evaluation of 241 reported cases. J Exp Clin Cancer Res 17:389, 1998.

Strodel WE, et al: Pancreatic polypeptide–producing tumors. Arch Surg 119:508, 1984.

Sykes GP, Cooper BJ: Canine intestinal carcinoids. Vet Pathol 19:120, 1982.

Tomita T, et al: Pancreatic polypeptide–secreting islet cell tumors. A study of three cases. Am J Pathol 113:134, 1983.

Torres SMF, et al: Resolution of superficial necrolytic dermatitis following excision of a glucagon-secreting pancreatic neoplasm in a dog. J Am Anim Hosp Assoc 33:313, 1997a.

Torres S, et al: Superficial necrolytic dermatitis and a pancreatic endocrine tumour in a dog. J Sm Anim Pract 38:246, 1997b.

Walton DK, et al: Ulcerative dermatosis associated with diabetes mellitus in the dog: A report of four cases. JAAHA 22:79, 1986.

Weber HC, et al: Determinants of metastatic rate and survival in patients with Zollinger-Ellison syndrome: A prospective long-term study. Gastroenterology 108:1637, 1995.

Whitehead R: The APUD system—An update. Pathology 12:333, 1980.

Wolfe MM, et al: Extrapancreatic, extraintestinal gastrinoma: Effective treatment by surgery. N Engl J Med 306:1533, 1982.

Wolfe MM, Jensen RT: Zollinger-Ellison syndrome. Current concepts in diagnosis and management. N Engl J Med 317:1200, 1987.

Wood SM, et al: Glucagonoma syndrome. In Lefebore PJ (ed): Glucagon II. Hand Book of Experimental Pharmacology, Vol 66/II. Stuttgart, Springer-Verlag, 1983, p 411.

Wright J, et al: Pancreatic somatostatinoma presenting with hypoglycemia. Clin Endocrinol (Oxf) 12:603, 1980.

Zerbe CA: Islet cell tumors secreting insulin, pancreatic polypeptide, gastrin, or glucagon. In Kirk RW, Bonagura GD (eds): Current Veterinary Therapy XI. Philadelphia, WB Saunders Co, 1992, p 368.

Zerbe CA, et al: Pancreatic polypeptide and insulin-secreting tumor in a dog with duodenal ulcers and hypertrophic gastritis. J Vet Intern Med 3:178, 1989.

Zerbe CA, Washabau RJ: Gastrointestinal endocrine disease. In Ettinger SJ, Feldman EC (eds): Textbook of Veterinary Internal Medicine, 5th ed. Philadelphia, WB Saunders Co, 2000, p 1500.

Zimmer T, et al: A duodenal gastrinoma in a patient with diarrhea and normal serum gastrin concentrations. N Engl J Med 333:634, 1995.

PARATHYROID GLAND

16

HYPERCALCEMIA AND PRIMARY HYPERPARATHYROIDISM

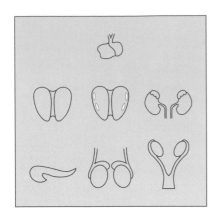

HYPERCALCEMIA

INTRODUCTION

Calcium is required for numerous vital intracellular and extracellular functions. For example, calcium is necessary for various enzymatic reactions, transport of substances across membranes and membrane stability, blood coagulation, nerve conduction, neuromuscular transmission, muscle contraction, smooth muscle tone, hormone secretion, bone formation, control of hepatic glycogen metabolism, and cell growth and division (Rosol et al, 2000). Calcium serves as an almost universal ionic messenger, conveying signals received at cell surfaces into cells (Rasmussen, 1989). In the extracellular fluid, calcium helps regulate the cellular function of various organs, including the parathyroid glands, kidneys, and thyroid C cells (Brown et al, 1995).

The concentration of serum ionized calcium (physiologically "active" calcium) is normally maintained within narrow limits by the action of parathyroid hormone (PTH) on bone resorption, renal calcium excretion, and metabolism of vitamin D (Table 16-1). PTH (primarily an 84–amino acid, single-chain polypeptide) is synthesized, stored, and secreted by chief cells in the four parathyroid glands. Secretion is regulated, in turn, by the serum calcium concentration: high concentrations inhibit secretion of PTH, and low concentrations stimulate it (Aurbach et al, 1985a; Brown et al, 1999). The amino acid sequence of PTH is

known for humans, dogs, cows, pigs, rats, chickens, and cats. Based on immunologic reactivities, most mammals appear to have similar amino-terminal portions of the molecule (Toribio et al, 2002). It is recognized that the amino terminal of PTH binds to cell membrane receptors. The carboxyl terminus is thought to serve only as a guide for PTH through the cellular secretory pathway (Orloff and Stewart, 1995). A synthetic 1-34 amino-terminal fragment is biologically active, but relatively minor modifications at the amino terminal (especially at the first two residues) can completely abolish its biologic activity (Marx, 2000). The effect of PTH on mineral metabolism is initiated by binding of PTH to type 1 receptors in target tissues, which results in regulation of large calcium fluxes across bone, kidneys, and intestines (Fig. 16-1).

Parathyroid hormone–related peptide (PTHrP) is a distant homologue of PTH and is not considered a true hormone. It is produced widely in the body and has numerous actions in the normal fetus and adult. However, this substance is best recognized as having a central role in the pathogenesis of humoral hypercalcemia of malignancy and is used as a "tumor marker." Since its discovery in the early 1980s, assay of PTHrP has been used in the evaluation of hypercalcemic patients in whom cancer is a possibility (Philbrick et al, 1996).

TABLE 16–1 NORMAL SERUM CONCENTRATIONS*

	Dog	Cat
Total Calcium		
(mg/dl)	9.0–11.7	8.0–10.5
(mmol/L)	2.2–3.9	2.0–2.6
Ionized Calcium		
(mg/dl)	4.6–5.6	4.5–5.5
(mmol/L)	1.12–1.42	1.1–1.4
Parathyroid Hormone		
(pmol/L)	2–13	0–4
Parathyroid Hormone-Related Protein (PTH-P)		
(pmol/L)	<2	<2
1,25-Dihydroxyvitamin D (Calcitriol)		
(pg/ml)		
Adults	20–50*	20–40*
10–12 wk old	60–120*	20–80*

*From Rosol, et al, 2000.

ETIOLOGY

The essential disorder in primary hyperparathyroidism (PHPTH) is the excessive synthesis and secretion of PTH by abnormal, autonomously functioning parathyroid "chief" cells. The cause of this hormonal excess is usually a solitary adenoma, but adenomatous hyperplasia of one or more parathyroid glands and parathyroid carcinomas have been identified in both dogs and cats. In contrast, other forms of hyperparathyroidism (e.g., renal secondary or nutritional secondary hyperparathyroidism) are usually the result of alterations in calcium and phosphorus homeostasis caused by nonendocrine disturbances. Such disturbances indirectly affect the parathyroid glands, causing diffuse parathyroid gland hyperplasia (see Differential Diagnosis of Hypercalcemia, page 669). Depending on the underlying cause, the serum calcium concentration in secondary disorders may range from low to normal to increased. *Primary* hyperparathyroidism is virtually always associated with hypercalcemia, as reflected by increases in circulating concentrations of the total or ionized calcium concentration or both.

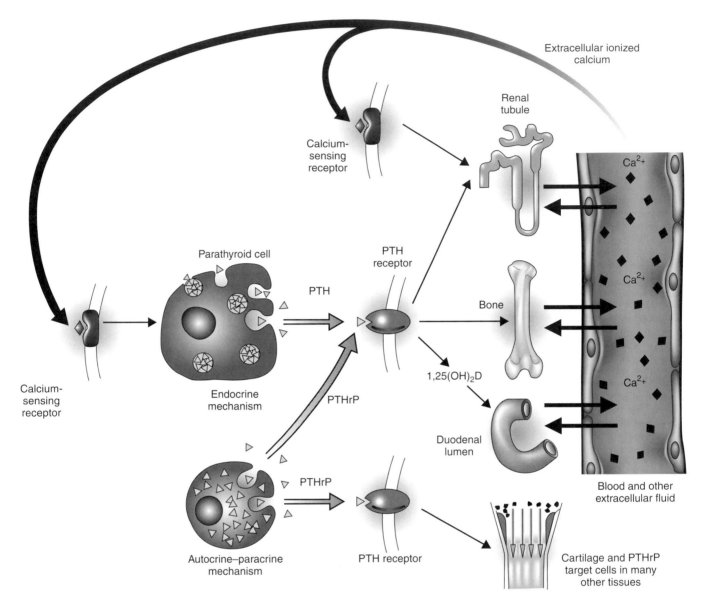

FIGURE 16–1. The parathyroid axis. The synthesis of parathyroid hormone (PTH) and parathyroid hormone–related peptide (PTHrP) is shown on the left and the target sites on the right. Both act by means of the same receptor (also called the type 1 receptor). Negative feedback of 1,25-dihydroxyvitamin D is not shown. (Modified from Marx SJ: N Engl J Med 343:1863, 2000.)

PATHOPHYSIOLOGY

Calcium–Parathyroid Hormone Feedback System

In primary hyperparathyroidism, normal negative-feedback homeostatic control is lost, and PTH secretion is increased either autonomously or as a result of a change in the set point. The autonomous secretion of PTH is not suppressible by the increased concentration of calcium perfusing the parathyroid glands. Conversely, the parathyroid glands in *secondary* hyperparathyroidism are normally suppressible by increased concentrations of calcium.

Severe Hypercalcemia, Bone Resorption, and the Kidneys

BONE. The process leading to severe hypercalcemia is initiated by accelerated bone resorption caused by the activation of osteoclasts in the skeleton (Attie, 1989). The activity of these cells, caused by PTH or PTHrP, is the foundation for virtually all cases of marked hypercalcemia. Excessive absorption of calcium from the gastrointestinal tract is not usually an important cause of hypercalcemia, although it is a contributor to the hypercalcemia resulting from vitamin D toxicosis. Hypercalcemia develops when the entry of calcium into the extracellular fluid (regardless of the source) overwhelms the mechanisms that maintain normocalcemia. One of these mechanisms is suppressed secretion of PTH, a process obviously negated when the cause of the hypercalcemia is the autonomous secretion of PTH. In cancer-associated hypercalcemia, the secretion of PTH is suppressed, but the humoral factor that activates osteoclasts is the autonomous secretion of PTHrP. PTHrP, as previously discussed, has biologic activity quite similar to that of PTH (Sleeboom and Bijvoet, 1982; Harinck et al, 1987). In the setting of accelerated bone resorption, the kidneys become the principal defense against hypercalcemia (Bilezikian, 1992a; Hruska and Teitelbaum, 1995).

Associated with accelerated osteocytic and osteoclastic bone resorption, mineral is removed and replaced by immature fibrous connective tissue. The bone lesion of fibrous osteodystrophy in afflicted dogs is reported to be generalized throughout the skeleton but accentuated in certain areas, such as the cancellous bone of the skull (Capen and Martin, 1983). Iliac crest bone biopsies from virtually all humans with primary hyperparathyroidism reveal histomorphometric evidence of the effects of excess PTH (Arnaud and Kolb, 1991; Hruska and Teitelbaum, 1995). These findings may include increased bone resorption surfaces, increased numbers of osteoclasts, osteocytic osteolysis, and marrow fibrosis. Bone histomorphometric findings in dogs with primary hyperparathyroidism were similar to those reported in humans (i.e., parallel increases in osteoblastic and osteoclastic activity). The increased rate of bone formation in these dogs was reflected in an increased rate of mineral apposition and a greater extent of tetracycline-labeled bone-forming surface (Meuten et al, 1983a; Weir et al, 1986).

KIDNEYS. When renal and endocrine functions are normal, any tendency for a rise in serum calcium is attenuated by increased urinary excretion of calcium. This process is inhibited by PTH excess, the foundation of primary hyperparathyroidism. *Severe* hypercalcemia (defined as a serum calcium concentration >14 mg/dl in humans and, arbitrarily, >15 mg/dl in dogs) is the result of humoral factors (PTH or PTHrP) that induce osteoclast-mediated bone resorption and stimulate intestinal absorption of calcium and renal tubular resorption of calcium (Mundy, 1988; Hruska and Teitelbaum, 1995). This impairs the kidneys' ability to excrete the increased filtered load of calcium. Thus animals with an excess of PTH lack the first lines of defense against hypercalcemia.

The hypercalcemic condition also interferes with renal mechanisms for resorption of sodium and water, leading to polyuria. This is due to an acquired inability to respond to antidiuretic hormone (ADH, vasopressin, AVP). This represents a reversible form of *nephrogenic diabetes insipidus*. Increased serum calcium concentrations reduce the concentration of cyclic adenosine monophosphate (cAMP) in the renal tubular cells that normally respond to ADH, either

through alteration of ADH receptors or through inactivation of adenylate cyclase, the enzyme necessary for the generation of intracellular cAMP. Compensation for the resultant polyuria by commensurate intake of fluid may not occur in people because of hypercalcemia-induced anorexia or nausea. Polyuria and resultant polydipsia are also recognized in hypercalcemic dogs and cats. Although hypercalcemia in dogs may cause "inappetence," it does not commonly result in anorexia or lack of water intake. Rather, most hypercalcemic dogs exhibit mild to moderate polydipsia and polyuria. A small number of hypercalcemic dogs have a urine specific gravity less than 1.007 and thus are arbitrarily classified as having "severe" polyuria.

Depletion of the extracellular fluid volume and a reduced glomerular filtration rate (GFR) as a result of dehydration may further increase the serum calcium concentration (Bilezikian, 1991). Hypercalcemia alters the GFR by causing (1) volume contraction of the extracellular fluid space secondary to fluid losses; (2) alterations in glomerular capillary permeability; and/or (3) sustained vasoconstriction that may result in ischemic injury to the kidneys, directly potentiating the toxic effects of hypercalcemia on renal tubular cells. Furthermore, mineralization of tissues may begin in the basement membrane of the ascending loop of Henle, the distal convoluted renal tubule, and the collecting ducts. This damages the basement membrane and impairs renal tubular repair. At the organelle level, mineralization of mitochondria occurs in renal tubular epithelial cells, potentially leading to disrupted cellular function, death, and sloughing of mineralized cell debris into renal tubular lumina. Casts composed of renal tubular cells may contribute to obstruction of urine flow along affected nephrons.

Early in the course of the hyperparathyroidism, when hypercalcemia is mild, urinary calcium excretion is relatively low. PTH action, at the renal level, enhances tubular resorption of calcium. When serum calcium concentrations are greater than 12 to 14 mg/dl, the renal tubular mechanism for reabsorbing calcium becomes overwhelmed. Here, the kidney's adaptive mechanism for correcting hypercalcemia becomes operative despite excessive concentrations of PTH. This hypercalciuria, however, is not sufficient to correct the hypercalcemia or the resultant nephrocalcinosis.

Nephrocalcinosis may be mild and reversible or severe and progressive, leading to continued renal damage and uremia. Severe mineralization of the kidneys is characteristically located subjacent to the corticomedullary junction and has the appearance of a white gritty band (Meuten, 1984). Histologic findings include interstitial infiltration of mononuclear cells, varying degrees of renal tubular atrophy, calcification, necrosis, and sloughing of the epithelium. In humans, renal failure may initially result from prerenal factors, but if hypercalcemia persists, the failure may be the result of acquired intrinsic renal lesions. It is extremely important to point out that this series of physiologic events described in humans seems to be much less worrisome in dogs with PHPTH. Almost all dogs with PHPTH have normal blood urea nitrogen (BUN) and serum creatinine concentrations. Furthermore, as we have monitored a considerable number of untreated dogs for periods longer than 12 to 18 months, it is safe to say that we have observed no evidence of progressive renal damage. To the contrary, the kidneys in dogs appear to be "protected" by PHPTH. As has been noticed in untreated humans, virtually no dramatic changes in serum biochemical profiles (aside from increasing calcium and decreasing phosphate concentrations) are noted over time (Silverberg et al, 1999).

Uroliths and Urinary Tract Infections

Hypercalciuria resulting from primary hyperparathyroidism may contribute to the urolithiasis and urinary tract infections that are "common" with this disorder. The incidence of urinary tract infection approaches 25% of afflicted dogs and may be related to reduction of the urine specific gravity. This is not known for certain, however, and other factors may contribute to the development of infection.

Reports on dogs with primary hyperparathyroidism (PHPTH) have also included a percentage of dogs (~30%) with urinary calculi (Berger and Feldman, 1987; Klausner et al, 1987). Hypercalciuria results from increased glomerular filtration of calcium, which we have always presumed to predispose these animals to urolithiasis. However, other hypercalcemic conditions have not been associated with urolithiasis. This discrepancy may be explained by the chronic nature of the hypercalcemia in dogs with PHPTH, because many tend to be asymptomatic or to have only mild signs, as opposed to the short-term nature of hypercalcemia in dogs with neoplasia, toxin exposure, and other such conditions. In these other conditions, dogs tend to develop obvious or severe clinical signs quickly and, therefore, do not have chronic hypercalcemia. Additional factors may play a role in urolith formation or urinary solute saturation, including pH, ionic strength, and crystal aggregation inhibitors. Calcium phosphate, for example, is markedly less soluble in alkaline urine than in acidic urine.

Vitamin D Excesses and Deficiencies

An adaptive mechanism to *increases* in the serum calcium concentration is a decrease in the circulating vitamin D concentration, assuming that the hypercalcemia is not a result of a primary renal or endocrine disorder. Decreases in the vitamin D concentration should result in reduced calcium absorption from the intestine. By contrast, the response to mild *decreases* in the serum calcium concentration is secretion of both PTH and vitamin D. PTH-stimulated bone resorption and vitamin D–stimulated intestinal absorption of both calcium and phosphorus then stimulate a rise in the serum calcium and phosphate concentrations (see Fig. 16-1). The renal tubular effects of PTH aid mineral homeostasis by stimulating synthesis and secretion of $1,25[OH]_2D_3$ (vitamin D). PTH also functions at the renal tubular level to increase phosphate excretion into the urine. This is important for preventing hyperphosphatemia after phosphate is removed from bone with calcium and/or absorbed from the intestine with calcium.

In primary hyperparathyroidism, hypercalcemia is aggravated by the *increased* production of vitamin D and by a decrease in the amount of serum phosphate available to form complexes with serum ionized calcium. The result is decreased tubular resorption of phosphate, hyperphosphaturia, and hypophosphatemia. These actions are responsible for the development of the biochemical triad classic for primary hyperparathyroidism: hypercalcemia, hypophosphatemia, and hyperphosphaturia.

Vitamin D deficiency, after chronic PTH-stimulated use of vitamin D stores, is a possible natural adaptive mechanism for coping with primary hyperparathyroidism. This process seems unlikely in dogs with PHPTH because humans with vitamin D deficiency caused by chronic hyperparathyroidism typically have severe osteomalacia, a problem not yet reported in animals (Meuten et al, 1983a; Weir et al, 1986). Furthermore, in a study that included four dogs with primary hyperparathyroidism, three had calcitriol concentrations that were mildly increased or in the high normal range (Rosol et al, 1992a). If the results in these three dogs accurately reflect the physiology of most dogs with PHPTH, osteomalacia would be uncommon, and the previously discussed physiologic triad is better understood.

Renal Effects of Hypercalcemia and Soft Tissue Mineralization

Several natural adaptive mechanisms are initiated in an attempt to control and possibly correct the hypercalcemia associated with primary hyperparathyroidism. One mechanism is the previously described hypercalciuria. Another occurs once the renal tubular transport of calcium is overwhelmed. When the solubility product of the serum calcium (Ca^{++}) and phosphate (PO_4) concentrations exceed 60 to 80 mg/dl, deposition of calcium in soft tissue ensues (Meuten et al, 1981). The result of this trade-off to lower the serum calcium concentration is the development of progressive organ dysfunction, especially in the kidneys as a result of nephrocalcinosis. Soft tissue calcification may occur in a variety of other organs or tissues (or both), but none is quite as worrisome as that which occurs in the kidneys.

As discussed previously, azotemia occurs commonly in dogs with hypercalcemia of malignancy, hypoadrenocorticism, chronic renal failure (CRF), and hypervitaminosis D (Kruger et al, 1996). Hypercalcemia can contribute to azotemia with any combination of the following: prerenal reduction in extracellular fluid volume (anorexia, hypodipsia, vomiting, and polyuria); renal vasoconstriction; decreased permeability coefficient of the glomerulus (K_f); acute tubular necrosis from the ischemic and toxic effects of hypercalcemia; and CRF caused by nephron loss, nephrocalcinosis, tubulointerstitial inflammation, and interstitial fibrosis (Rosol et al, 2000).

The frequency of azotemia was higher in dogs with malignancy (71%) than in those with PHPTH (11%) (Kruger et al, 1996). It is our impression, however, that CRF is almost never caused by PHPTH in dogs. The incidence of CRF in our series of dogs with PHPTH is approximately 4%. It is likely that a similar incidence of CRF would be identified in any population of dogs in which the average age is 10 to 11 years. The most common cause of CRF in hypercalcemic dogs would be related to a calcium × phosphorus product above 60 to 80 mg/dl. Such increases in this product would be extremely unusual in PHPTH because of the low-normal or low serum phosphorus concentrations caused by PTH-induced excesses in vitamin D. Therefore, although a typical normal dog has a total serum calcium (Ca) concentration of about 10.5 mg/dl, a serum phosphate of about 4.5 mg/dl, and a product of 47, the typical dog with PHPTH has a total serum Ca concentration of about 15 mg/dl, a serum phosphate of about 3.0 mg/dl, and a product of 45. This is in contrast to a dog with CRF or vitamin D toxicosis, with a total serum Ca concentration of about 10.5 mg/dl (or higher), a serum phosphate of about 10.0 mg/dl (or higher), and a product in excess of 100.

Rapid Metabolism of PTH

Stimulation, via hypercalcemia, of rapid tissue degradation of the biologically active forms of PTH by parathyroid and nonparathyroid cells may represent a physiologic mechanism to curtail worsening hypercalcemia in PHPTH (Arnaud and Kolb, 1991). Plasma calcium may regulate PTH secretion and also determine the circulating quantities of biologically active PTH molecules versus inactive hormone fragments. This phenomenon may be more theoretical than practical because the disappearance rate of PTH from serum after the removal of a parathyroid tumor is no different from that of dogs with nonparathyroid disease in which the parathyroids are surgically removed.

Calcitonin

Calcitonin, a 32–amino acid polypeptide hormone produced by parafollicular or "C cells" located in the thyroid, is secreted in response to increases in serum calcium (Mol et al, 1991). This hormone has the primary responsibility of limiting postprandial hypercalcemia in normal mammals. Calcitonin decreases bone resorption by reducing the size of osteoclast brush borders, the number of osteoclasts, and osteoclast motility. Calcitonin does not affect the kidney or intestine. It may, however, influence the satiety center, decreasing appetite. The role of calcitonin in dogs with hypercalcemia secondary to PHPTH is not known. Increased calcitonin secretion in response to hypercalcemia seems a reasonable physiologic response. Parafollicular cells are markedly hyperplastic and appear as small white foci in the thyroid gland of dogs with primary hyperparathyroidism (Capen and Martin, 1983). Hyperplastic parafollicular cells may displace colloid-containing follicles lined by thyroid follicular cells, implying the presence of an adaptive response by the parafollicular cells. Studies in humans suggest that this adaptive mechanism is inconsistent (Arnaud and Kolb, 1991).

ASSAYS OF SERUM PARATHYROID HORMONE

History

The development of an assay for serum PTH in 1963 by Berson and coworkers was a major breakthrough in the diagnosis of human parathyroid disorders. Indirect tests of parathyroid function, such as the renal clearance of calcium, phosphate, or cAMP, had not proved satisfactory for differentiating parathyroid from nonparathyroid causes of hypercalcemia or hypocalcemia. In the 1960s and 1970s it became clear that an immunoassay for PTH would provide much more consistent information but that development of such an assay presented far more complex problems than routine immunoassays established for other peptide hormones.

Complete (84–amino acid) molecules of PTH and numerous incomplete "pieces" of PTH are found in the circulation of all animals. These circulating PTH and partial-PTH peptides have different metabolic half-lives. The half-lives of intact PTH and the N-terminal fragments are measured in minutes, whereas the half-lives of middle and carboxyl (C)-terminal PTH fragments are tenfold to twentyfold longer. Bioactivity resides in the intact molecule, the major secretory product of the parathyroid glands. The intact molecule is present in relatively low serum concentrations in dogs and cats. The N-terminal fragment, a product of PTH metabolism by the liver and kidneys, contributes little or not at all to the circulating pool of immunoreactive PTH. The C-terminal and midmolecule fragments are biologically inactive but are present in rather large concentrations. These biologically inactive fragments are excreted primarily by the kidneys, and they accumulate in the serum of patients with renal failure.

PTH Assay Systems

Development of the "two-site" PTH assay system currently used by most human and veterinary laboratories depends on the production of two different polyclonal antibodies. The two-site immunoradiometric (IRMA) system for intact human PTH (Allegro Intact PTH; Nichols Institute, San Juan Capistrano, Calif.) has been demonstrated to be valid for measurement of dog and cat PTH (Torrance and Nachreiner, 1989a; Flanders and Reimers, 1991; Barber et al, 1993). One antibody binds only the midregion and C-terminal 39-84 amino acids of human PTH. The other antibody binds only the N-terminal 1-34 amino acids of human PTH. Samples being assayed are incubated simultaneously with both antibodies, with a "sandwich" created composed of the 1-34 antibody plus the patient's intact hormone plus the 39-84 antibody. Only these "sandwiches" are detected by the assay system, eliminating any interference by midregion or C-terminal fragments, even if present in large concentrations. Two-site immunochemi-luminometric assays for intact PTH in humans use antibodies similar to those in the intact PTH IRMA assays and have the same range of applicability to animal sera (Michelangeli et al, 1997).

Clinical Usefulness

BACKGROUND. Determination of the serum PTH concentration is a useful diagnostic aid in the evaluation of dogs and cats suspected of having parathyroid disease. As with any assay, the clinician must be certain that the assay used is valid for dogs or cats. Furthermore, laboratories must develop their own reference values for normal conditions, as well as values typical for most disease states. The need for development of independent reference ranges cannot be overstated, even when the assay system used has been validated elsewhere.

Experience with the new PTH two-site assays has been extremely positive. Samples obtained for this assay should be stored and shipped frozen to prevent degradation of intact PTH. Stability is best achieved in plasma collected with ethylenediamine tetra-acetic acid (EDTA), but serum is adequate if stored frozen after separation from red blood cells. Normal values for the serum PTH concentration are 2 to 13 pmol/L in dogs and 0 to 4 pmol/L in cats. Samples should be shipped to the appropriate laboratory with two or three frozen gel packs (Torrance and Nachreiner, 1989a and 1989b).

As with most hormone assays, evaluation of the serum hormone concentration "out of context" is not as consistently informative as evaluation in the proper context. With this in mind, the serum PTH concentration must be evaluated relative to the total and, ideally, ionized serum calcium concentrations. Decreases in the serum calcium concentration are normally associated with increases in the serum PTH concentration. Increases in the serum calcium concentration are normally associated with decreases in the PTH concentration (Fig. 16-2). As with any laboratory value, a single PTH result may not provide correct information. Therefore practitioners are encouraged to complete a thorough evaluation of hypercalcemic dogs or cats. If test results do not appear logical, some tests may need to be repeated, including measurement of serum hormone concentrations, which may fluctuate.

ASSAYS OF IONIZED SERUM CALCIUM CONCENTRATIONS

The biologically active form of calcium in the circulation is the ionized fraction. Measurement of the serum *ionized* calcium concentration has become widely available and cost-effective (normal or "reference" concentrations for our laboratory are 1.12 to 1.42 mmol/L; see Table 16-1). Although samples can be obtained routinely rather than according to the previously described anaerobic requirements, anaerobically obtained, handled, and stored serum is stable for a longer time and therefore preferred (Schenck et al, 1995). Anaerobic collection ensures that no increase in pH occurs as a result of loss of carbon dioxide (CO_2). An acidic pH favors dissociation of calcium from protein and increases the amount of ionized calcium in the sample. An alkaline pH occurs with loss of CO_2 and favors calcium binding to protein, thus reducing the amount of ionized calcium. Mixing of serum and air increases the pH, decreasing the ionized calcium concentration. Ionized calcium and pH are more stable in serum than in whole or heparinized blood. The analysis of serum eliminates potential interference by heparin and allows longer storage periods. Serum may be stored for subsequent ionized calcium analysis as long as it has been handled anaerobically. Silicone separator tubes should not be used. Measurement of ionized calcium in canine serum was stable after storage at 23° C for 72 hours and for 7 days at 4° C (Schenck et al, 1995).

The use of automated equipment with calcium ion–selective electrodes has resulted in easy and accurate measurement that minimizes interference caused by magnesium, potassium, protein, hemolysis, and other factors (Gouget et al, 1988). However, differences among analyzers exist, and it is recommended that each laboratory establish reference ranges for the analyzer they use (Hristova et al, 1995). Some instruments mathematically manipulate the ionized calcium concentration and actual pH value of the sample and yield an "adjusted" value. Formulas have also been developed to "adjust" results for samples exposed to air. These formulas have not been validated in animals, and their use is not recommended (Rosol et al, 2000).

The addition of this diagnostic tool can be valuable in the evaluation of hypercalcemia and hypocalcemia as well as renal insufficiency. An effect of aging has been observed in both dogs and cats: young dogs and cats (up to 2 years of age) have serum ionized calcium concentrations slightly higher than those reported in "adult" animals (Deniz and Mischke, 1995; Mischke et al, 1996).

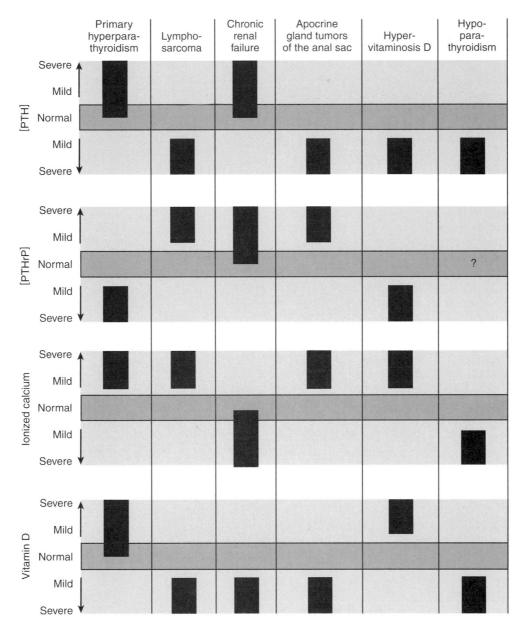

FIGURE 16–2. Graph showing the serum parathyroid hormone (PTH), parathyroid hormone–related peptide (PTHrP), ionized calcium, and vitamin D concentrations in the most common causes for hypercalcemia of dogs.

ASSAY OF VITAMIN D CONCENTRATIONS

Measurement of vitamin D metabolites, although not commonly used in veterinary medicine, would occasionally be helpful in the diagnosis of calcium disorders. 25[OH] vitamin D (calcidiol) and 1,25[OH]$_2$ vitamin D (calcitriol) are the metabolites of greatest clinical interest for detection of hypovitaminosis or hypervitaminosis D syndromes and in renal failure (Carothers et al, 1994). These metabolites are stable during refrigeration and freezing, but samples should not be exposed to light for any length of time. Both metabolites are chemically identical in all species, therefore receptor-binding assays or radioimmuno-

assays (RIAs) used for people are satisfactory for dogs and cats (Hollis et al, 1996). Young growing individuals have higher calcitriol concentrations than adults.

Calcitriol assays have demonstrated genetic errors of vitamin D metabolism and normal-to-increased concentrations in PHPTH, whereas patients with hypercalcemia of malignancy have levels that may be low, normal, or high. Dogs and cats with possible exposure to rat and mouse poisons containing vitamin D (e.g., Rat-B-Gone, Mouse-B-Gone, Rampage, Quintox) may present challenging diagnostic problems. Serum concentrations of vitamin D are increased in these toxicity states (Dougherty et al, 1990).

ASSAY OF PARATHYROID HORMONE–RELATED PROTEIN

Background

Parathyroid hormone–related protein (PTHrP) was identified in the 1980s as a tumor product that had the ability to activate PTH receptors and cause hypercalcemia. PTHrP resembles PTH not only in terms of its genetic sequence but also in terms of structure (Fig. 16-3), thus PTHrP is a second member of the PTH family of hormones (Broadus and Stewart, 1994). The first clues to the function of PTHrP came from studies of its expression in different tissues. In marked contrast to PTH, which is found only in the parathyroid glands, PTHrP is found in many tissues in both fetuses and adults, including epithelia, mesenchymal tissues, endocrine glands, and the central nervous system (Table 16-2). This widespread distribution suggests a diversity of roles for PTHrP (Fig. 16-4). Insights into these roles are now emerging from gene-knockout experiments and other approaches (Strewler, 2000). However, the key importance of this peptide is its central role in the development of humoral hypercalcemia of malignancy (HHM). It appears that the 1-36–amino acid peptide portion of PTHrP has an effect on cartilage, breast, and skin; the 38-94 midregion of PTHrP has an effect on placental calcium transport and perhaps on renal bicarbonate

transport; the 107-139–amino acid portion of the molecule has an effect on the brain and on bone resorption (Strewler, 2000).

PTHrP Assay Systems

Two-site IRMA and N-terminal RIAs are available for the measurement of human PTHrP, and these same assay systems have been validated for the dog because of the high degree of sequence homology between species (Brown et al, 1987; Burtis, 1992). PTHrP is susceptible to degradation by serum proteases, therefore these assays should be run from fresh or frozen plasma using EDTA as anticoagulant. The EDTA complexes with plasma calcium, limiting the action of most proteases. The addition of protease inhibitors, such as aprotinin, may provide further protection. Use of serum is not recommended (Rosol et al, 2000).

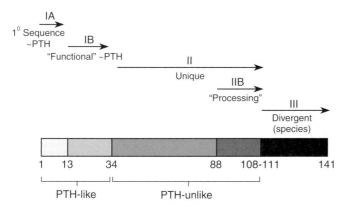

FIGURE 16–3. Structural and functional domains of parathyroid hormone–related protein (PTHrP). The 1-13 region of PTHrP is 70% homologous with the corresponding region of PTH and is believed to be involved in activation of adenylate cyclase and other second-messenger systems in target tissues. The 14-34 region shares no homology with the 14-34 region of PTH but has been shown to bind effectively to the PTH receptor. The 35-108 region of PTHrP is unique, sharing no homology with any other known peptide. This region is extraordinarily highly conserved among species, which suggests that it has a crucial but as yet unknown function or functions. The 88-108 region of the peptide is rich in potential proteolytic cleavage sites and contains several amidation signals and is therefore presumed to be the site of posttranslational processing, at least in some tissues. The 112-141 region of the peptide is poorly conserved among species. Preliminary evidence suggests that at least in some situations, C-terminal fragments derived from this region enter the circulation. The functional consequences of this are unknown. (Broadus AE, et al: N Engl J Med 319:556, 1988.)

TABLE 16–2   SITES AND PROPOSED ACTIONS OF PARATHYROID HORMONE-RELATED PROTEIN (PTHrP)

Site	Proposed Actions
Mesenchymal Tissues	
Cartilage	Promotes proliferation of chondrocytes; inhibits terminal differentiation and apoptosis of chondrocytes
Bone	Stimulates or inhibits bone resorption
Smooth muscle	Released in response to stretching; relaxes smooth muscle
Vascular system	
Myometrium	
Urinary bladder	
Cardiac muscle	Positive chronotropic stimulus; indirect positive inotropic stimulus
Skeletal muscle	Unknown
Epithelial Tissues	
Mammary	Induces branching morphogenesis; secreted in milk; possible roles in lactation
Epidermis	Unknown
Hair follicle	Inhibits anagen
Intestine	Unknown
Tooth enamel	Induces osteoclastic resorption of overlying bone
Endocrine Tissues	
Parathyroid glands	Stimulates placental transport of calcium?
Pancreatic islets	Stimulates insulin secretion and somatic growth
Pituitary	Unknown
Placenta	Calcium transport?
Central nervous system	Released from cerebellar granular neurons in response to activation of L-type calcium channels; receptors in cerebellum, hippocampus, hypothalamus

From Strewler, 2000.

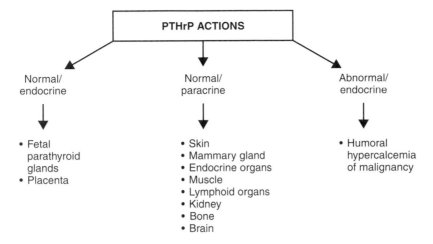

FIGURE 16–4. Actions of parathyroid hormone–related protein (PTHrP). (Rosol TJ, et al: *In* DiBartola SP [ed]: Fluid Therapy in Small Animal Practice, 2nd ed. Philadelphia, WB Saunders, 2000, pp 108-162.)

Clinical Usefulness

Simultaneous measurement of PTH and PTHrP in the plasma may be especially valuable when attempting to distinguish primary hyperparathyroidism (PHPTH) from hypercalcemia of malignancy (HHM) (Burtis et al, 1990). In several studies, the plasma PTHrP concentration was increased in most people with HHM, including those with metastatic disease. PTHrP has been detectable in only a small percentage of humans with primary hyperparathyroidism, this hypercalcemia being attributed to increased PTH concentrations. Impaired renal function is associated with increased immunoreactivity to PTHrP fragments (Budayr et al, 1989; Henderson et al, 1990).

There seems to be little doubt that valid assays for dog and cat PTHrP serve as an excellent *tumor marker*. In other words, simultaneous assaying for PTH and PTHrP in hypercalcemic dogs and cats has the potential to be a quick, reliable, noninvasive, and inexpensive means of distinguishing between malignant and nonmalignant hypercalcemia. However, animals with renal insufficiency may also have increased concentrations of PTHrP without malignancy (see Fig. 16-2).

DIFFERENTIAL DIAGNOSIS OF HYPERCALCEMIA

See Table 16-3.

Primary Hyperparathyroidism

See next section.

Hypercalcemia of Malignancy

GENERAL OVERVIEW. Malignancy-associated hypercalcemia is the most common cause of increased serum calcium concentrations in dogs and cats. Neoplasms can cause hypercalcemia by three recognized physiologic processes (Fig. 16-5): (1) humoral hypercalcemia of malignancy (HHM); (2) hematologic malignancies growing in the bone marrow; and (3) hypercalcemia induced by metastases of solid tumors to bone (Rosol et al, 2000). Dogs with lymphosarcoma, apocrine gland carcinomas of the anal sac, and multiple myeloma frequently have hypercalcemia. Some of the tumors less commonly associated with hypercalcemia include malignant mammary tumors, nasal adenocarcinomas, thyroid carcinoma, thymoma, squamous cell carcinoma of the gastrointestinal system or vagina, and melanoma.

TABLE 16–3 DIFFERENTIAL DIAGNOSES OF HYPERCALCEMIA

Common

Lymphosarcoma
Hypoadrenocorticism
Primary hyperparathyroidism
Chronic renal failure

Uncommon

Apocrine gland carcinoma of the anal sac
Multiple myeloma
Vitamin D toxicosis

Uncommon-to-Rare

Spurious
Hemoconcentration
Carcinomas:
    Lung, mammary, nasal, pancreas, testicle, thymus, thyroid,
      vagina
Melanoma
Acute renal failure
Hyperthyroidism
Nutritional secondary hyperparathyroidism
Granulomatous Disease
    blastomycosis, histoplasmosis, schistosomiasis

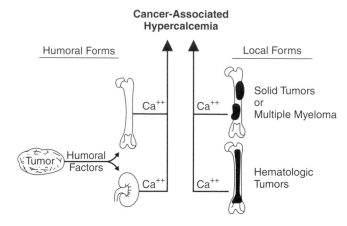

Cancer-Associated Hypercalcemia

FIGURE 16–5. Pathogenesis of cancer-associated hypercalcemia. Humoral and local forms of cancer-associated hypercalcemia increase circulating concentrations of calcium by stimulating osteoclastic bone resorption and increased renal tubular resorption of calcium. (Rosol TJ, et al: *In* DiBartola SP [ed]: Fluid Therapy in Small Animal Practice, 2nd ed. Philadelphia, WB Saunders, 2000, pp 108-162.)

HUMORAL HYPERCALCEMIA OF MALIGNANCY

Humoral "Factors." Tumor tissue at a site distant from bone may synthesize PTHrP, which is released into the circulation, stimulating bone resorption and causing hypercalcemia. Excessive secretion of biologically active PTHrP plays a central role in the pathogenesis of hypercalcemia in most forms of HHM. Cytokines, such as interleukin-1 (IL-1), tumor necrosis factor-α (TNF-α), transforming growth factor-α (TGF-α), transforming growth factor-β (TGF-β), or calcitriol, can have synergistic or cooperative actions with PTHrP (Fig. 16-6) (Rosol et al, 2000). PTHrP binds to the N-terminal PTH-PTHrP receptor in bone and kidney but does not cross-react immunologically with native PTH. The PTHrP stimulates osteoclastic bone resorption, increases renal tubular calcium resorption, and decreases renal tubular phosphate resorption. IL-1 and the transforming growth factors also have the potential to stimulate bone resorption (McCauley et al, 1991; Rosol et al, 2000). Not only does PTHrP provide the physiologic explanation for humoral hypercalcemia, it also explains why some tumors are not associated with hypercalcemia. Furthermore, assays for PTHrP are highly touted as tumor markers in that abnormal concentrations are obtained only from individuals with malignancies and renal failure (see Fig. 16-2).

Serum PTH concentrations in dogs with malignancy-associated hypercalcemia are typically low or undetectable. This should be seen as a normal response by the parathyroid glands to hypercalcemia. In an extremely small percentage of these dogs, PTH concentrations may be normal or increased. Obviously such results would be misleading, therefore it is important to evaluate each hypercalcemic dog or cat completely. Assay of PTH and PTHrP concentrations should not be viewed as a replacement for a complete physical examination, thoracic radiography, abdominal ultrasonography, or any other key parameter used to identify neoplasia. These assays complement other necessary components of an evaluation.

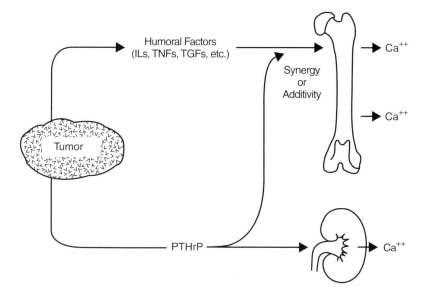

Humoral Factor and HHM

FIGURE 16–6. Humoral factors such as parathyroid hormone–related protein (PTHrP), interleukin-1, tumor necrosis factors (TNFs), and transforming growth factors (TGFs) produced by tumors induce humoral hypercalcemia of malignancy (HHM) by acting as systemic hormones and stimulating osteoclastic bone resorption or by increasing tubular resorption of calcium. (Rosol TJ, et al: *In* DiBartola SP [ed]: Fluid Therapy in Small Animal Practice, 2nd ed. Philadelphia, WB Saunders, 2000, pp 108-162.)

Hematopoietic Neoplasia. Lymphosarcoma is the most common hematopoietic tumor and the most common cause of hypercalcemia in dogs. It afflicts dogs of any age and either sex. Clinical signs may be subtle, moderate, or severe, or these dogs can be terminally ill. Approximately 20% to 40% of dogs with lymphosarcoma are hypercalcemic (Weller et al, 1982; Matus et al, 1986; Rosol et al, 2000). Hypercalcemia has been documented in cats with lymphosarcoma, but the incidence is much lower than in dogs. Studies on affected dogs have demonstrated parameters consistent with influence by PTHrP, including increased fractional excretion of phosphorus, increased nephrogenous cAMP, and increased osteoclastic bone resorption. PTHrP appears to differ from natural PTH in its inability to stimulate renal formation of 1,25 [OH]$_2$ vitamin D and its lack of cross-reactivity with specific, two-site, intact PTH assays. A significant percentage of these dogs have increased serum concentrations of PTHrP (Fig. 16-7) (Weir et al, 1988a, 1988b, and 1988c).

Lymphomas can synthesize both PTHrP and vitamin D, in which case the dog would not only have the expected increases in serum PTHrP but also would

have increased vitamin D concentrations (Seymour and Gagel, 1993). Some lymphocytes contain the 1α-hydroxylase (similar to that found in renal tubules) that converts 25-hydroxyvitamin D to the active metabolite, 1,25-[OH]$_2$ vitamin D (Rosol et al, 2000). Therefore lymphomas that retain this capability may synthesize excessive amounts of calcitriol, which would increase calcium absorption from the intestinal tract and exacerbate the hypercalcemia caused by PTHrP (see Fig. 16-2).

In contrast to the persistent hypercalcemia observed in dogs with PHPTH, dogs with malignancy-associated hypercalcemia may have fluctuating serum concentrations of calcium and sometimes are normocalcemic. Although the clinical signs associated with lymphoma are variable, it is safe to state that dogs with a combination of lymphoma and HHM, as a group, are considerably more ill than dogs with PHPTH. However, *until proven otherwise*, lymphoma must remain a possible explanation for hypercalcemia in any dog or cat. Lymphosarcoma may or may not be apparent to the veterinarian during the physical examination. At least 40% of dogs with both lymphoma and HHM do not have peripheral lymph node, liver,

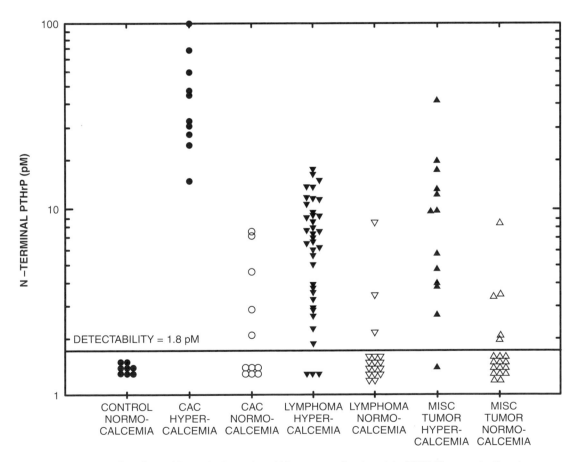

FIGURE 16–7. Circulating N-terminal parathyroid hormone–related protein (PTHrP) concentrations in normal dogs (control); dogs with hypercalcemia (>12 mg/dl) and anal sac adenocarcinoma (CAC), lymphoma, or miscellaneous tumors (MISC TUMOR); and dogs with normocalcemia (<12 mg/dl) and anal sac adenocarcinoma, lymphoma, or miscellaneous tumors. (Rosol TJ, et al: *In* DiBartola SP [ed]: Fluid Therapy in Small Animal Practice, 2nd ed. Philadelphia, WB Saunders, 2000, pp 108-162.)

spleen, or renal enlargement. Most of these dogs have an anterior mediastinal mass that is usually obvious on thoracic radiographs. The finding of an anterior mediastinal mass in a dog with hypercalcemia should suggest a diagnosis of lymphoma, although other forms of neoplasia (e.g., thymoma) may account for both the mass and the hypercalcemia (Foley et al, 2000).

Apocrine Gland Adenocarcinoma of the Anal Sac. Adenocarcinomas of the anal sac represent another classic example of a cancer commonly associated with hypercalcemia. Like lymphosarcoma, this neoplasm is known to synthesize PTHrP (Matus and Weir, 1989). This is a well-defined but relatively uncommon tumor, and the diagnosis is usually made in older dogs; the mean age at presentation is 10 to 11 years, but the range is 3 to 17 years (Bennett et al, 2002). Although early reports describe this neoplasia primarily in females, no obvious gender predilection was noted in recent studies. In a review of 238 dogs with this condition, numerous breeds were represented; in another report, mixed breed dogs were most commonly afflicted (Ross et al, 1991; Goldschmidt and Shofer, 1992; Bennett et al, 2002). Clinical signs associated with this condition include (among many owner observations): recognition of a mass near the rectum, tenesmus, poor appetite or anorexia, polyuria/polydipsia, and lethargy.

In dogs with polyuria/polydipsia, hypercalcemia was usually present. However, not all hypercalcemic dogs had evidence of polyuria/polydipsia (Bennett et al, 2002). The incidence of hypercalcemia has varied in different studies from about 25% of afflicted dogs to about 50% (Ross et al, 1991; Bennett et al, 2002). In one study, the serum calcium concentrations (upper reference value of 12.6 mg/dl) at the time of diagnosis ranged from 12.7 to 21.7 mg/dl (Bennett et al, 2002). Tumor resection results in normocalcemia. Local reappearance of the cancer or metastasis causes recurrence of hypercalcemia. Dogs afflicted with this form of cancer have increases in urinary cAMP and fractional phosphorus excretion. Serum PTH concentrations have been suppressed, and bone histomorphometry has revealed increased bone resorption with no compensatory increase in formation. These observations are consistent with the biologic actions of PTHrP (Meuten et al, 1983b). Apocrine gland adenocarcinoma cell lines established in mice have also demonstrated that of the potential factors responsible for HHM, only PTHrP is increased in the serum (Grone et al, 1998). Successful treatment of this neoplasia results in rapid normalization of serum calcium, phosphorus, calcitriol, and PTH concentrations (Rosol et al, 1992b).

With recognition of hypercalcemia in any dog, a rectal examination and careful palpation of the anal sac areas should be routine. In these dogs, the rectal examination commonly demonstrates a space-occupying mass that may be invasive and occasionally ulcerated. Careful digital rectal palpation is necessary to identify the presence of sublumbar lymph node enlargement.

Although radiography may also be used to evaluate the sublumbar area, abdominal ultrasonography has been our most sensitive diagnostic aid. Radiography of the thorax and abdomen can be used in searching for pulmonary metastases and/or bony metastases (lytic areas).

Other Nonneoplastic and Solid Tumors that May Synthesize PTHrP. Interstitial cell tumors of the testicle, squamous cell carcinoma, thymoma, melanoma, and thyroid adenocarcinoma are less commonly encountered solid tumors that cause hypercalcemia without bone metastasis (Grain and Walder, 1982; Meuten et al, 1983a; Pressler et al, 2002). This underscores the value of PTHrP assays in dogs with hypercalcemia. The remission of hypercalcemia after tumor excision and the return of hypercalcemia after tumor recurrence or growth of metastases support the presence of a hypercalcemic factor (PTHrP) secreted by these tumors, but studies are limited. In humans, other tumors that may produce PTHrP include bronchogenic non–small-cell carcinomas, breast cancer, squamous cell carcinoma of the esophagus, renal-cell carcinoma, and hepatoma (Harris et al, 2002). PTHrP has also been associated with hypercalcemia in nonneoplastic diseases, such as schistosomiasis (Fradkin et al, 2001).

HEMATOLOGIC MALIGNANCIES GROWING IN THE BONE MARROW: OSTEOLYTIC HYPERCALCEMIA

Background. Some types of hematologic malignancies in the bone marrow produce hypercalcemia by inducing bone resorption locally (Rosol et al, 2000). This condition is usually associated with lymphoma and multiple myeloma. In humans, metastatic breast cancer is another example, although this association is not common in dogs or cats. A number of paracrine factors, or cytokines, may be responsible for the stimulation of bone resorption in dogs with such tumors. The cytokines most often implicated in the pathogenesis of local bone resorption are IL-1 and IL-6, TNF-α and TNF-β, TGF-α and TGF-β, and PTHrP (Black and Mundy, 1994). Production of small amounts of PTHrP by a tumor in bone may stimulate local bone resorption without inducing a systemic response. Prostaglandins (especially prostaglandin E_2) may also contribute to local stimulation of bone resorption (Rosol et al, 2000). Together, these cytokines and prostaglandins comprise the *osteoclast-activating factors.*

Multiple Myeloma. Multiple myeloma is a tumor of the B-lymphocyte or plasma cell line that may be associated with the development of osteolytic bone lesions and, occasionally, hypercalcemia. The hypercalcemia develops secondary to production of osteoclast-activating factors. In addition, there is a correlation between the extent of bone destruction, the amount of tumor cell burden, and the amount of osteoclast-activating factor produced by myeloma cell cultures (Durie et al, 1981). Approximately 17% of dogs afflicted with this cancer are hypercalcemic (Matus et al, 1986), and 50% of dogs with multiple myeloma have radiographic evidence of bone lysis.

Bone pain is usually associated with the lytic areas. The initial database from these dogs often reveals abnormal increases in the total serum protein concentration as a result of a monoclonal spike in the globulin fraction. This monoclonal gammopathy can be demonstrated specifically with serum protein electrophoresis. Bone marrow aspiration confirms the diagnosis in most cases, demonstrating an infiltration of malignant plasma cells. Analysis of urine for light chains of myeloma protein (Bence Jones protein) has not been of much value.

HYPERCALCEMIA INDUCED BY METASTASES OF SOLID TUMORS TO BONE. Certain malignant neoplasms with osseous metastasis may cause hypercalcemia and hypercalciuria. Primary bone tumors, by contrast, do not commonly induce hypercalcemia. For example, hypercalcemia would be rare in a dog with osteosarcoma. In contrast, malignant mammary adenocarcinoma or squamous cell carcinoma is infrequently associated with both bone metastasis and hypercalcemia. Several different types of cells may be involved in the actual destruction of bone at sites of metastasis, including osteoclasts, tumor cells, lymphocytes, and monocytes. Lymphocytes and monocytes may accumulate as part of the cell-mediated immune response to a tumor (Mundy et al, 1984). Osteolysis is a result of the physical disruption of bone by proliferating neoplastic cells, but it also can be caused by secretion of cytokines or prostaglandins that stimulate local bone resorption (Garrett, 1993).

Epithelial tumors, especially squamous cell carcinomas, are the most likely neoplasms to metastasize to bone in dogs and cats (Quigley and Leedale, 1983). Common metastatic bone sites in the dog include the humerus, femur, and vertebrae, whereas in the cat, local invasion of bone rather than distant metastasis is more common. Although reported, these tumors are not commonly associated with hypercalcemia (Grain and Walder, 1982).

Hypervitaminosis D and Rodenticide Toxicosis

BACKGROUND. Vitamin D is cumulative in its action and may require 1 to 2 weeks before its maximum effects on mineral metabolism occur. However, acute toxicity after massive ingestion of cholecalciferol appears to be the more common experience when dealing with this problem in dogs. Hypercalcemia and hyperphosphatemia are the anticipated electrolyte abnormalities in animals with vitamin D toxicity, although normophosphatemia and transient periods of normocalcemia have been reported (Figs. 16-8 and 16-9) (Harrington and Page, 1983). Hypercalcemia begins as soon as 12 to 18 hours after ingestion, and peak concentrations are usually demonstrated by 48 to 72 hours, coinciding with increases in the BUN and creatinine (Rumbeiha, 2000). Increased resorption of bone, coupled with increased gastrointestinal absorption of calcium and phosphorus, is responsible for these abnormalities. Skeletal disease is usually not detectable radiographically, probably because of the acute nature of this form of toxicosis. The osteoclastic phase of bone resorption occurs early and is followed by osteoid deposition and hyperosteoidosis (Boyce and Weisbrode, 1983). Extensive soft tissue mineralization of the endocardium, blood vessels, tendons, kidney, and lung is frequently associated with vitamin D toxicity (Meuten, 1984).

RODENTICIDE TOXICOSIS. Hypercalcemia that develops secondary to cholecalciferol rodenticide toxicosis in dogs and cats is a recognized concern (Gunther et al, 1988; Moore et al, 1988; Fooshee and Forrester, 1990; Dougherty et al, 1990). Rat bait products containing cholecalciferol include Quintox, Rampage, and Muritan, among other proprietary names (Rumbeiha, 2000; Morrow, 2001). Dogs studied after being given this type of poison became weak, lethargic, and anorexic within 48 hours. Within 60 to 70 hours of consumption, all dogs became recumbent, exhibited hematemesis, and progressed into shock before dying or being euthanized (Gunther et al, 1988). Although the median lethal dose of cholecalciferol in dogs is widely reported to be 43 to 88 mg/kg, studies have shown that as little as 10 mg/kg given once orally can be lethal. Dogs that ingest as little as 4 to 6 mg/kg once become ill. Clinically healthy dogs that ingest single doses of 2 mg/kg develop hypercalcemia (Rumbeiha, 2000).

Most dogs and cats exposed to these toxins have had rapid increases in the serum calcium and phosphate concentrations (see Fig. 16-8). Diffuse hemorrhage in the stomach and small intestine was obvious. Histologic lesions consisting of hemorrhage or mineralization or both were identified in the gastrointestinal tract, kidneys, and myocardium and in the blood vessels of many organs (Gunther et al, 1988). The incidence of acute and/or severe renal failure was variable. Three exposed cats survived (Moore et al, 1988).

OTHER CAUSES OF VITAMIN D TOXICOSIS. Since 1997, perhaps the most common accidental cause of vitamin D toxicosis in pets has been ingestion of human psoriasis medications containing the vitamin D analogs calcipotriol or calcipotriene, and marketed as Davionex, Dovonex, or Psorcutan. Additional sources of vitamin D are dietary supplementation and overzealous administration of vitamin D by veterinarians to dogs or cats with hypoparathyroidism. This has become recognized as a problem in hyperthyroid cats as a result of the frequent use of surgery and the potential for iatrogenic disease. Removal of parathyroids is a concern during any major surgery involving the neck, especially when thyroid tissue is resected. *Cestrum diurnum* (day-blooming jessamine) is a popular houseplant that should be considered a possible source of vitamin D toxicity in pets because it contains the active metabolite of vitamin D. Jasmine, an indoor climbing plant without active vitamin D metabolites, should not be confused with day-blooming jessamine. Other plants containing glycosides of vitamin D include *Solanum malacoxylon* and *Trisetum flavescens*.

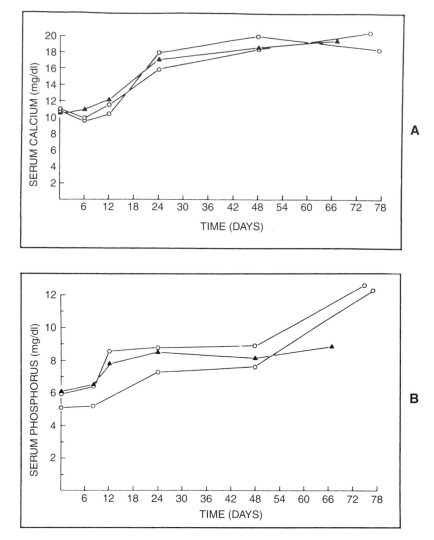

FIGURE 16–8. Serum calcium *(A)* and phosphorus *(B)* concentrations of dogs given vitamin D₃ at a dosage of 10 mg/kg *(circles)* and 20 mg/kg *(triangles)*. (Gunther R, et al: J Am Vet Med Assoc 193:211, 1988.)

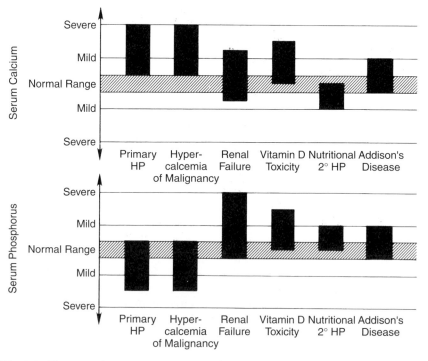

FIGURE 16–9. The range in serum calcium and phosphorus concentrations for the more common causes of hypercalcemia and/or hyperparathyroidism in the dog. *HP,* Hyperparathyroidism; *2° HP,* secondary hyperparathyroidism.

DIAGNOSIS. The diagnosis of vitamin D toxicosis is based on a history of exposure and the presence of dark, bloody feces, azotemia, oliguria or polyuria, proteinuria, and sometimes glucosuria. An additional clue to this diagnosis would be hyperphosphatemia in a hypercalcemic dog or cat. Most other causes of hypercalcemia are associated with hypophosphatemia or normal serum phosphate concentrations. Cholecalciferol-induced renal failure can be differentiated from ethylene glycol toxicosis or soluble oxalate toxicosis because those two conditions usually cause moderate hypocalcemia, as opposed to the severe hypercalcemia often associated with vitamin D toxicity. However, the history and signs of vitamin D toxicosis are strikingly similar to those seen in dogs with hypoadrenocorticism, acute renal failure, and chronic renal failure.

Hypoadrenocorticism

Hypoadrenocorticism (Addison's disease) is one of the more common causes of hypercalcemia in dogs, accounting for approximately 10% to 50% of cases (Uehlinger et al, 1998; Rosol et al, 2000). Serum calcium concentrations have been reported to be increased in as many as 33% of dogs with adrenocortical insufficiency (hypoadrenocorticism) (Peterson and Feinman, 1982; Peterson et al, 1996) as well as in a smaller percentage hypoadrenal cats (Johnessee et al, 1982; Peterson et al, 1989). In our series of hypoadrenal dogs, a correlation has been noted between the degree of hyperkalemia and the level of hypercalcemia (see Chapter 8). If the serum potassium concentration exceeds 6.0 to 6.5 mEq/L, a large percentage of these animals have serum calcium concentrations of 12 to 13.5 mg/dl. The hypercalcemia is not restricted to the extremely ill hypoadrenal dog. It is not common, however, for the serum calcium concentration to exceed 13.5 mg/dl, and it rarely exceeds 15 to 16 mg/dl. Despite the increased total serum calcium concentrations, serum ionized calcium levels usually remain in the reference range. Serum phosphate concentrations also correlate with serum calcium concentrations, with the hyperphosphatemic animal more likely to exhibit hypercalcemia (see Fig. 16-9).

Clinical signs and laboratory abnormalities associated with hypoaldosteronism (a primary component of Addison's disease) usually are striking and overshadow concerns related to hypercalcemia (see Chapter 8). Most dogs and cats with hypoadrenocorticism have hyperkalemia, hyponatremia, azotemia, hyperphosphatemia, and related problems. The only differential diagnoses for this combination of serum abnormalities are hypoadrenocorticism, renal failure, and vitamin D (rodenticide) toxicosis. Furthermore, the hypercalcemia rapidly resolves after treatment for the adrenal insufficiency, frequently within a few hours of initiation of saline resuscitation.

The pathogenesis of the hypercalcemia associated with hypoadrenocorticism is probably multifactorial. Any combination of the following may be involved:

(1) hyperproteinemia resulting from dehydration and hemoconcentration; (2) increased plasma protein–binding affinity for calcium; (3) increased concentrations of calcium-citrate complexes; and (4) increased renal tubular resorption of calcium (Peterson and Feinman, 1982).

Chronic Renal Failure

PATHOGENESIS OF HYPERCALCEMIA. The pathogenesis of hypercalcemia associated with chronic renal failure is complicated. Diffuse hyperplasia of the parathyroid glands is characteristic of chronic renal failure. Parathyroidectomy decreases the serum calcium and PTH concentrations in dogs with hypercalcemia and renal failure (Meuten and Armstrong, 1989). The development of hypercalcemia in experimentally nephrectomized dogs depends on the presence of the thyroparathyroid complex (Tuma and Mallette, 1983). The kidneys excrete PTH and its metabolic byproducts, a process impeded by renal failure. Additional possible mechanisms for hypercalcemia in renal failure include (1) decreased renal excretion of calcium due to a reduction in the GFR; (2) increased concentrations of PTH due to both excessive secretion and reduced renal tubular hormone degradation, which could enhance bone resorption; (3) renal failure or PTH-induced increased concentrations of organic cations (e.g., citrates), which would increase complexed calcium concentrations; (4) an exaggerated response to vitamin D, with increased intestinal absorption of calcium; and (5) autonomous parathyroid gland activity (tertiary hyperparathyroidism), causing enhanced secretion rates (Meuten and Armstrong, 1989). The actual presence or incidence of a syndrome involving "autonomously functioning" parathyroid glands that are the result of chronic stimulation due to the renal disease (i.e., tertiary hyperparathyroidism) is not known. *Tertiary* hyperparathyroidism is the name given to the syndrome of chronic renal *secondary* hyperparathyroidism, in which one or more of the parathyroid glands begin to *autonomously* secrete PTH ("tertiary" disease).

Transient hypercalcemia may develop after administration of oral phosphate-binding agents, presumably as a result of shifts in calcium from bone to extracellular fluid in response to the rapid lowering of the circulating phosphorus concentration (Capen and Martin, 1983).

PATHOGENESIS OF RENAL SECONDARY HYPERPARATHYROIDISM. The classic explanation for this syndrome involves the chronic, progressive inability of the kidneys to excrete phosphorus. Phosphate retention decreases extracellular calcium as a result of the mass law. The mass law simply suggests that the product of serum calcium and phosphate remains stable. Therefore, if calcium increases, phosphate decreases, and vice versa. The parathyroids become hyperplastic in response to chronic stimulation to maintain extracellular calcium concentrations in the normal range (renal secondary hyperparathyroidism) (Fig. 16-10;

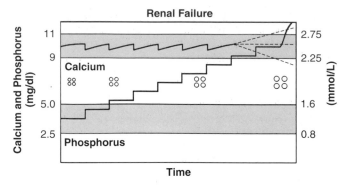

FIGURE 16–10. Diagrammatic illustration of progressive renal failure with time. Note the progressive loss in the ability to excrete phosphate, the small fluctuations in the serum calcium concentration until late in the disease, and the progressive enlargement of all four parathyroids secondary to the progressive renal failure (*open circles*, renal secondary hyperparathyroidism).

also see Figs. 16-2 and 16-9). Although this classic description has not been discounted, the "vitamin D trade-off" hypothesis has also been set forth. In this scenario, vitamin D deficits occur in chronic renal failure because of the decreasing population of proximal renal tubular cells that synthesize this "hormone." Decreases in extracellular calcium are the result of decreases in intestinal absorption of calcium, which is mediated by vitamin D. The decrease in vitamin D precedes the increase in serum phosphate in dogs and cats with chronic renal failure. Later in the course of chronic renal failure, hyperphosphatemia actually acts to further inhibit the synthesis of vitamin D. Vitamin D acts directly at the level of the parathyroid (negative feedback) to regulate PTH secretion. Decreases in vitamin D result in lack of negative feedback and subsequent excessive PTH secretion (renal secondary hyperparathyroidism) (Mattson et al, 1993).

Although the pathogenesis, diagnosis, and treatment of chronic renal failure are not the focus of this chapter, current theories regarding the management of renal failure are pertinent. The benefit of decreasing abnormal serum phosphate concentrations (low-phosphate diets, intestinal phosphate binders) in dogs or cats with renal failure cannot be disputed. The need for vitamin D therapy as a means of decreasing serum PTH concentrations is an area of clinical research. Administration of vitamin D is deemed important because PTH is considered a nephrotoxin that contributes to the relentless progression of most cases of chronic renal failure (Chew and Nagode, 1990). Research studies have also suggested that removal of the parathyroids (thereby removing all PTH) from dogs with induced renal failure was *not* beneficial in preventing progression of the disorder (Finco et al, 1994 and 1995). Thus the nephrotoxicity associated with excess serum PTH is an area of continuing study. Vitamin D (calcitriol, 1.5 to 3.5 ng/kg PO daily) has been recommended as a component of the treatment protocol for dogs and cats with chronic renal failure if the serum phosphate concentration is less than 6.0 mg/dl (usually as a result of diet or phosphate binders or both) and the calcium × phosphorus product is less than 60.

DIAGNOSTIC DILEMMAS. The finding of hypercalcemia and azotemia poses a diagnostic problem, because hypercalcemia can develop as a consequence of CRF or, it is claimed, hypercalcemia can cause azotemia. We do not believe that the hypercalcemia of PHPTH poses a threat of renal damage, except for such damage as may be caused by nephroliths or ureteroliths. However, this is an area of continuing research. It is fair to point out, therefore, that the serum PTH concentration should be within or above the reference range in PHPTH and CRF. However, two points should be made: (1) fewer than 4% of the 168 dogs in our series with PHPTH had azotemia, and (2) dogs with PHPTH have an increased serum ionized calcium concentration, whereas most dogs with CRF (>94%) have normal or decreased concentrations of ionized calcium (only 6% had increases in the serum ionized calcium concentration; see Figs. 16-2 and 16-9) (Rosol et al, 2000). As many as 10% to 20% of dogs and cats with CRF have mild to moderate increases in the total serum calcium concentration (usually values of 11.5 to 12.5 mg/dl) (Chew and Meuten, 1982; DiBartola et al, 1987). In one series of dogs with renal failure and hypercalcemia, most of the dogs that were hypercalcemic had normal or decreased ionized calcium concentrations (Chew and Nagode, 1990). Therefore low and normal ionized calcium concentrations in renal failure are more common than would be predicted from evaluation of the total serum calcium concentration, and hypercalcemia is actually relatively uncommon. However, because there is a rather large population of dogs and cats with renal failure, even if a small percentage of the total are hypercalcemic, they are periodically encountered.

CLINICAL SYNDROMES AND THE DECISION PROCESS. Dogs and cats with primary renal failure are azotemic and hyperphosphatemic and usually have isosthenuria. Their clinical signs typically include poor appetite to anorexia, weight loss, lethargy, polydipsia, and polyuria. Additional clinical problems include vomiting or diarrhea or both. The age, breed, and clinical signs of a dog with PHPTH may be similar, although we are continuously impressed that dogs with primary hyperparathyroidism have subtle to no signs, compared with the rather worrisome signs seen in pets with renal failure. The worse the clinical signs, the more likely that a dog (or cat) has primary renal disease. In addition, animals with hypercalcemia secondary to renal failure usually have serum calcium concentrations of 11.0 to 12.5 mg/dl, whereas those with PHPTH usually have serum calcium concentrations in excess of 13 mg/dl.

In summary, dogs or cats with no or minimal clinical signs, persistent hypercalcemia of a magnitude greater than 13.0 mg/dl, and a serum phosphate that is normal or low usually have PHPTH. Those with serum calcium concentrations less than 12.5 mg/dl and hyperphosphatemia are more likely to have primary renal failure. The dog or cat for which the diagnosis remains vague despite these guidelines may need further evaluation. Measurement of the serum ionized calcium concentration should help distinguish primary renal failure (normal or low) from a primary parathyroid problem (increased) (see Fig. 16-2). Cervical ultrasonography may aid in distinguishing enlargement of more than one gland (renal secondary hyperparathyroidism) from enlargement of one parathyroid (parathyroid adenoma). If the underlying disease process is still uncertain, the results of PTH and PTHrP assays would be helpful. Finally, surgery of the neck has the potential to be both diagnostic and therapeutic.

Acute Renal Failure

Dogs in which acute, severe hyperphosphatemia is a component of acute renal failure usually have normal or low serum calcium concentrations. Mild hypercalcemia occasionally is associated with acute renal failure, most commonly noted in dogs during the transition from the oliguric to the polyuric phase of recovery. As with chronic renal failure, the pathogenesis of hypercalcemia induced by acute renal failure is not certain. In the oliguric phase of acute renal failure, deposition of calcium and phosphorus in soft tissues may occur. During the polyuric phase, as renal function improves, this mineral may be mobilized, and hypercalcemia and hyperphosphatemia may develop (Llach et al, 1981). Alternatively, rapid improvement in both renal function and serum phosphate concentrations may lead to transient hypercalcemia as a result of changing mass law interactions.

Nutritional Secondary Hyperparathyroidism

The increased secretion of PTH in nutritional secondary hyperparathyroidism represents a normal compensatory response to nutritionally induced hypocalcemia. Dietary mineral imbalances capable of inducing this syndrome include diets low in calcium or vitamin D or diets containing excessive amounts of phosphorus with normal or low calcium levels (Crager and Nachreiner, 1993). Nutritional secondary hyperparathyroidism most commonly develops after the exclusive ingestion of all-meat diets, especially diets consisting of liver or beef hearts (Capen and Martin, 1983).

Subtle decreases in the serum calcium concentration (usually not below normal reference concentrations) develop in animals fed these diets. This subtle decrease in the serum calcium concentration stimulates the parathyroid glands to secrete PTH. With prolonged stimulation, chief cell hyperplasia and secondary hyperparathyroidism develop. Depletion of skeletal

calcium is the major disturbance in these animals. Because renal function is normal, hyperparathyroidism results in diminished renal tubular resorption of phosphate (hyperphosphaturia) and increased resorption of calcium. Therefore dogs and cats with this syndrome usually have a low-normal serum calcium concentration and a normal serum phosphorus concentration. Pathologic bone fractures are common, however, and are the reason many of these pets are brought to the veterinarian.

Septic Bone Disease, Sepsis, Schistosomiasis, and Systemic Mycoses

Bacterial or fungal osteomyelitis and primary or secondary tumors of bone are rare causes of hypercalcemia. Neonatal septicemia in puppies with septic emboli and lysis of bone is another rare cause of hypercalcemia. Hypercalcemia has been associated with blastomycosis, histoplasmosis, schistosomiasis, aspergillosis, and coccidioidomycosis in dogs without apparent bone involvement.* In one of these reports, increases in the PTHrP concentration was believed to cause hypercalcemia in two dogs with schistosomiasis (Fradkin et al, 2001). The pathogenesis for sepsis-induced hypercalcemia is not certain, but inflammation associated with sepsis may cause sufficient bone destruction and mobilization of calcium to cause hypercalcemia (Meuten, 1984). The production of bone-resorbing factors such as prostaglandins and cytokines comprise the osteoclast-activating factors produced by monocytes and lymphocytes that may be involved in the pathogenesis (Mundy et al, 1984). Viable macrophages have osteolytic capabi-lities that may be enhanced by endotoxin (McArthur et al, 1980). Abnormal metabolism of vitamin D may also be involved in the hypercalcemia associated with granulomatous disease (Lemann and Gray, 1984).

Disuse Osteoporosis/Tumors Metastasizing to Bone

Disuse osteoporosis is a rare cause of hypercalcemia seen in animals immobilized because of extensive musculoskeletal or neurologic injury. This form of hypercalcemia is mild and is associated with bone resorption and urinary hydroxyproline excretion, decreased bone production, hypercalciuria, and osteopenia (Chew and Meuten, 1982). Tumors that metastasize to bone are considered to be relatively common in dogs and cats. However, hypercalcemia is not usually associated with metastasis to bones in

---

*Legendre et al, 1981; Dow et al, 1986; Troy et al, 1987; Meuten and Armstrong, 1989; Rohrer et al, 2000; Fradkin et al, 2001; and Parker, 2001.

these animals. In contrast, hypercalcemia is common in humans with secondary bone tumors.

Hemoconcentration, Sodium Bicarbonate Infusion, and Plasma Transfusion

Hypercalcemia occasionally may develop in severely dehydrated animals, although it is a clinicopathologic problem we have not observed in our patients (hypoadrenocorticism may be an exception). The hypercalcemia is reported to be mild and is thought to result from fluid volume contraction and secondary hyperproteinemia. The hypercalcemia should resolve after fluid therapy. Sodium bicarbonate infusions have been demonstrated to decrease the total and ionized serum calcium concentrations (Chew et al, 1989). An increase in the serum total calcium concentration and a decrease in the ionized calcium concentration can occur transiently after plasma transfusion, presumably secondary to excesses in citrate–calcium ion complexes (Mischke, et al, 1996).

Hypothermia, Fetal Retention, and Endometritis

A dog and a cat have been described with severe, environmentally induced hypothermia and hypercalcemia (Ross and Goldstein, 1981). The hypercalcemia rapidly resolved after rewarming and fluid therapy. The pathogenesis is not known. Similarly, one dog with a retained fetus and concurrent endometritis had hypercalcemia (Hirt et al, 2000). It remains to be demonstrated that these conditions warrant being included in differential diagnosis lists for hypercalcemia.

Age

See Serum Total Calcium Concentration.

Laboratory Error

See Serum Total Calcium Concentration.

PRIMARY HYPERPARATHYROIDISM (PHPTH) IN DOGS

SIGNALMENT

Age

PHPTH is typically diagnosed in older dogs and appears to be much less common, or at least less frequently diagnosed, in cats. For the 168 dogs with PHPTH seen at our hospital during the past 20 years, the mean age was 11.2 years, and the range was 4 to 17 years (Fig. 16-11). Of the 168 dogs, 162 (96%) were 7 years of age or older. There is no apparent gender predilection; 94 of the dogs (56%) were male.

Breed

Reliable information about breed predisposition for any disorder requires sophisticated epidemiologic evaluation. To our knowledge, such an investigation has not been undertaken with respect to canine primary hyperparathyroidism. Regardless, it is reasonable to point out that Keeshonden are far removed from the most popular breeds seen at our hospital, as opposed to Poodles, German Shepherds, Retrievers,

and the like. Despite this relative lack of popularity, 44 of the 168 dogs in our series (26%) were Keeshonden. Although striking, the percentage of afflicted dogs that were Keeshonden is less than the 36% that we reported in the second edition of this text. Other breeds represented three or more times in our series were Labrador Retrievers, German Shepherds, Golden Retrievers, Shih Tzus, Poodles, Springer Spaniels, Australian Shepherds, Cocker Spaniels, Rhodesian Ridgebacks, Doberman Pinschers, and mixed breed dogs (Table 16-4). Several of these breeds, however, are simply popular. The question of whether breed predispositions exist awaits epidemiologic evaluation. However, two points should be made. First, the Keeshond is overrepresented, and second, dogs of any breed and any age from 4 years on can be afflicted by this condition.

Hereditary Disease

Hereditary neonatal primary hyperparathyroidism, with a possible autosomal recessive mode of inheritance, was reported in two German Shepherd dogs

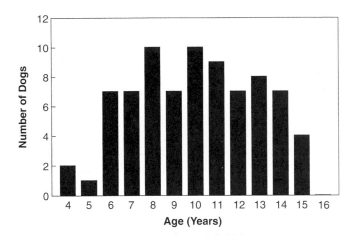

FIGURE 16–11. Age distribution of 78 dogs with primary hyperparathyroidism. The mean age at the time of diagnosis was 10.5 years.

TABLE 16–4 BREED DISTRIBUTION OF 187 DOGS WITH PRIMARY HYPERPARATHYROIDISM

Breed	Percentage
Keeshond	26
Labrador Retriever	10
German Shepherd dog	7
Cocker Spaniel	7
Golden Retriever	6
Springer Spaniel	5
Poodle	4
Shih Tzu	4
Australian Shepherd	4
Doberman Pinscher	3
Rhodesian Ridgeback	3
Breeds represented twice	11

(Thompson et al, 1984). The incidence of this syndrome in puppies and/or young dogs must be quite small, because no other report of neonatal disease has appeared in the literature. Our series of dogs with primary hyperparathyroidism did not include any less than 4 years of age.

ANAMNESIS: CLINICAL SIGNS

General

Clinical signs due solely to hypercalcemia are mild or absent in many dogs. The only condition in which hypercalcemia is the sole problem is PHPTH. The most common signs that we associate with PHPTH are polyuria, polydipsia, decreased appetite, decreased activity (muscle weakness?), and signs related to stones or infection in the urinary tract. Signs reported to be caused by hypercalcemia alone include the gastrointestinal signs of anorexia, vomiting, constipation and, in rare cases, pancreatitis. Renal signs include polyuria, polydipsia, and occasionally signs

related to urinary tract calculi. The central nervous system (CNS) signs include mental dullness, obtundation, and even coma. We have observed one dog with ataxia and circling in which those signs resolved after resolution of the PHPTH. Dogs with hypercalcemia that have worrisome signs almost always have a disease other than PHPTH. Worrisome signs are usually the result of the underlying cause for the hypercalcemia (e.g., cancer, renal failure, hypoadrenocorticism, toxin).

The mildest form of primary hyperparathyroidism may not be associated with any signs, and the hypercalcemia is identified serendipitously only after a standard biochemical panel has been obtained. This is certainly true in humans, in whom *occult* primary hyperparathyroidism is more prevalent than the symptomatic form of the disorder (Heath, 1989; Potts, 1990; Consensus Development Conference Panel, 1991; Silverberg et al, 1999). When clinical signs in dogs do develop, they initially tend to be mild, insidious, and nonspecific. Most owners are unaware of specific clinical signs. It is not until the pet has been treated for PHPTH that owners realize in retrospect that the dog had signs. It is this concept that resulted in an editorial in the *New England Journal of Medicine* suggesting that all people with PHPTH be treated (Utiger, 1999).

In our series of dogs with PHPTH, 35% had clinical signs related to primary hyperparathyroidism for more than 6 months and *all*, either retrospectively or prospectively, had signs for at least 1 month (Table 16-5). The clinical signs attributable to primary hyperparathyroidism and hypercalcemia usually involve one, two, or all three of the following: the renal, the gastrointestinal, and the neuromuscular organ systems (Table 16-6).

Renal: Kidneys, Bladder, and Urethra

POLYDIPSIA AND/OR POLYURIA. The most common clinical signs in dogs with PHPTH (136 of 168 dogs, or 81%) have been polyuria, polydipsia, and/or urinary incontinence (see Table 16-6). Signs develop as a result of impaired renal tubular response to ADH and impaired renal tubular resorption of sodium and chloride. Together, these alterations in normal physiologic mechanisms account for a significant increase in urine volume. The changes are a direct result of hypercalcemia or excessive concentrations of

TABLE 16–5 DURATION OF CLINICAL SIGNS IN 168 DOGS WITH NATURALLY OCCURRING PRIMARY HYPERPARATHYROIDISM

Duration (Months)	Percent of Dogs
<1	19
1–3	20
3–6	19
6–12	24
>12	18

TABLE 16–6 FREQUENCY OF CLINICAL SIGNS REPORTED PROSPECTIVELY OR RETROSPECTIVELY IN 168 DOGS WITH NATURALLY OCCURRING PRIMARY HYPERPARATHYROIDISM

Sign	Percent of Dogs
Polyuria/polydipsia	81
Listlessness	53
Incontinence	47
Weakness/exercise intolerance	47
Inappetence	37
Urinary tract signs (straining, blood, frequency)	29
Muscle wasting	17
Vomiting	12
Shivering	10
Constipation	6
Stiff gait	5

PTH, or both. The acquired and reversible form of nephrogenic diabetes insipidus causes the production of relatively dilute, solute-free urine. Compensatory polydipsia develops to maintain normovolemia. Surprisingly, the polydipsia and polyuria either are not observed or are thought to be mild by most owners, but they have seemed obvious to us on review of the routine database.

The specific gravity of initial urine samples obtained soon after hospital admission were much more dilute than we would have expected from owner comments. Of 168 dogs with PHPTH, 43 (26%) had a urine specific gravity of 1.001 to 1.007. In 65 dogs (39%), the urine specific gravity was in the isosthenuric range of 1.008 to 1.012. In 52 dogs (31%), the urine specific gravity was 1.013 to 1.020. Only four samples showed a value of 1.021 to 1.030, and in another four the value was greater than 1.030. Thus 96% of the dogs with PHPTH had a urine specific gravity less than or equal to 1.020 (Table 16-7).

URINARY TRACT CALCULI AND INFECTIONS. Another of the more common causes of owner concern regarding dogs with PHPTH was observation of clinical signs consistent with urinary tract infection or calculi or both (see page 687). These signs included frequency, urgency, incontinence, hematuria, stranguria, or apparent urinary obstruction. At some time in the year preceding diagnosis, 123 of 168 owners (73%) had seen at least one of these clinical signs in their dog. Of the 168 dogs with PHPTH in our series, 53 (32%) had uroliths (Fig. 16-12) and 41 (24%) had a urinary tract infection at the time of diagnosis.

Listlessness, Depression, and Decreased Activity

Listlessness or decreases in activity were observed in 89 (53%) of 168 dogs with PHPTH. Increased serum calcium concentrations depress the excitability of central and peripheral nervous tissue, which may be responsible for this clinical manifestation. Alternatively, these clinical signs may be a reflection of muscle weakness. Humans with this disorder may exhibit nonspecific neurologic abnormalities, which include impaired mentation, mental depression, hypoactive deep tendon reflexes, and loss of pain perception (Silverberg et al, 1999). Analogous abnormalities in dogs may explain the listlessness and/or depression associated with this disorder.

Weakness and Muscle Wasting

Weakness or exercise intolerance was observed in 79 (47%) of 168 dogs with PHPTH. Increased serum calcium concentrations decrease cell membrane permeability in nervous and muscular tissue, thereby depressing the excitability of these tissues. In addition, skeletal muscle weakness, primarily the proximal muscle groups, may result from a primary neuropathy that ultimately causes muscle atrophy. Muscle wasting and weight loss were observed in 28 (17%) of the 168 dogs in our series.

Inappetence

Owners observed some degree of reduced appetite in 62 (37%) of 168 dogs with PHPTH. In most of the dogs, this problem probably developed as a result of hypercalcemia-induced decreased excitability of gastrointestinal smooth muscle or from direct calcemic effects on the CNS (Chew and Capen, 1980; Parfitt and Kleerekoper, 1980). The development of gastric or

TABLE 16–7 SERUM BUN, CREATININE AND PHOSPHATE CONCENTRATIONS, AND URINE SPECIFIC GRAVITIES AT TIME OF DIAGNOSIS OF PRIMARY HYPERPARATHYROIDISM IN 168 DOGS

	BUN (mg/dl)	Serum Creatinine (mg/dl)	Serum Phosphate (mg/dl)	Urine Specific Gravity
Reference range	18–28	0.5–1.6	3.0–6.2	—
Mean (168 dogs)	17.1	1.0	2.8	1.011
	<10 = 6 (3%)	<0.5 = 0	<2 = 20 (12%)	<1.008 = 43 (26%)
	10–17 = 101 (60%)	0.6–0.9 = 76 (45%)	2.0–2.9 = 88 (53%)	1.008–1.012 = 65 (39%)
	18–22 = 37 (22%)	1.0–1.6 = 88 (52%)	3.0–3.9 = 47 (28%)	1.013–1.020 = 52 (31%)
	23–28 = 16 (10%)	1.7–2.0 = 3 (2%)	4.0–4.9 = 9 (5%)	1.021–1.030 = 4 (2%)
	29–47 = 7 (5%)	2.0–3.0 = 1	5.0–6.2 = 3 (2%)	1.030–1.039 = 4 (2%)
	>47 = 1	>3.0 = 0	>6.2 = 1	≥1.040 = 0

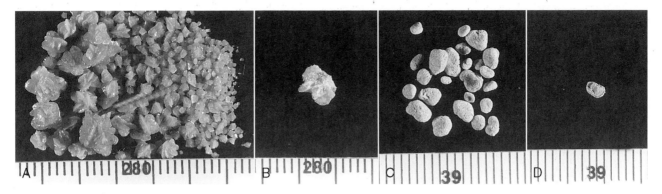

FIGURE 16–12. Calcium-containining cystic calculi from two dogs with primary hyperparathyroidism (*A* and *C*) and individual cracked calculi from each dog (*B* and *D*).

duodenal ulcers, as has been noted in hypercalcemic humans, has not yet been reported in dogs. In people, hypercalcemia causes an increase in the serum gastrin concentration and excess gastric acid secretion by the parietal cells of the stomach (Aurbach et al, 1985a).

One common assumption is that hypercalcemia-induced renal failure would cause inappetence in some dogs with PHPTH. However, only nine of 168 dogs (5%) in our series were azotemic, as defined by a BUN equal to or greater than 31 mg/dl. One of the 168 dogs had a BUN greater than 50 mg/dl. Four of the nine azotemic dogs had a serum creatinine concentration less than or equal to 1.4 mg/dl. Therefore renal problems, which could account for the inappetence, were not significant contributors in these dogs.

Shivering, Twitching, and Seizures

Shivering and muscle twitching have been observed in hypercalcemic dogs (Chew and Capen, 1980). Seizure activity has also been reported in a dog with primary hyperparathyroidism (Ihle et al, 1988). The mechanism for these problems is not well understood but may involve cerebral microthrombi, cerebral vasospasm, or interference with protective mechanisms in the brain that prevent the spread of a seizure impulse (Ihle et al, 1988). Neurologic signs may progress to stupor or coma as the hypercalcemia worsens, although this is extremely rare. Muscle twitching was not observed in any dog from our series; "shivering" was observed by the owners of 16 dogs in our series (10%); and one dog exhibited the previously mentioned circling and ataxia.

Miscellaneous (Uncommon) Signs

Other uncommon clinical signs that have been associated with PHPTH include vomiting, constipation, development of a stiff gait, and fractures (see Table 16-6). Vomiting and constipation are believed to result from hypercalcemia-induced decreased excitability of gastrointestinal smooth muscle (Chew and Capen,

1980; Parfitt and Kleerekoper, 1980). The development of pancreatitis, renal failure, or gastrointestinal ulcerations may also be responsible for vomiting in hypercalcemic dogs, but these must be considered quite rare. One dog in our series of 168 with PHPTH had concurrent pancreatitis.

Excessive osteoclastic resorption of bone induced by chronic hyperparathyroidism results in replacement of the bone matrix with fibrous tissue, thinning and weakening of cortical bone, and a predisposition to fractures from relatively minor physical trauma. Lameness may also develop with severe cortical thinning of the axial skeleton. Compression fractures of the vertebral bodies may result in peripheral motor dysfunction (Fig. 16-13). Nonspecific arthralgias are complications recognized in humans with primary hyperparathyroidism (Arnaud and Kolb, 1991). Metastatic calcification of tendons and joint capsules may contribute to stiffness and lameness. Apparent stiff gait was reported in 7 (4%) of our 168 dogs with PHPTH (see Table 16-6).

Summary

When present, the clinical signs of PHPTH in dogs are usually related to one of three systems: the renal system (polyuria, polydipsia, uroliths); the neuromuscular system (listlessness, generalized muscle weakness); and/or the gastrointestinal system (inappetence). The presence of any of these signs may raise suspicion of hypercalcemia, although this biochemical abnormality usually remains a serendipitous finding on review of a routine database obtained for nonspecific or unrelated concerns.

PHYSICAL EXAMINATION

General Observations

The physical examination is usually unremarkable in dogs with PHPTH. When abnormalities are found, they typically are related to the presence of uroliths or

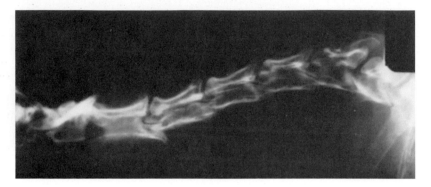

FIGURE 16–13. Lateral radiograph of the cervical spine from a dog with multiple myeloma and hypercalcemia. Note the severe osteolysis involving several vertebrae. These findings are consistent with a diagnosis of the hypercalcemia of malignancy syndrome.

to some concurrent and unrelated condition, or they are subtle and nonspecific. This concept is important, because the differential diagnoses for dogs with a serendipitous finding of hypercalcemia include diseases such as lymphosarcoma, chronic renal failure, apocrine gland carcinoma of the anal sac, hypoadrenocorticism, multiple myeloma, and vitamin D toxicosis. Dogs with any of these conditions are usually ill or quite ill. In other words, a relatively stable or apparently healthy older dog with hypercalcemia is more likely to have PHPTH than one of the serious conditions that cause secondary hypercalcemia.

Common Abnormalities

Potential physical examination findings in dogs with PHPTH, other than those caused by calculi in the urinary tract, include thin body condition, generalized muscle atrophy, and/or weakness. The severity of weakness is variable, but it usually is mild or undetectable. Bone deformities involving the mandible or maxilla and fractures of long bones have been reported (Capen and Martin, 1983), but such abnormalities were not identified in any of the 168 dogs from our series.

Ophthalmologic Changes

Infrequent ocular abnormalities in humans with PHPTH include "band keratopathy" and subconjunctival deposits of calcium (Aurbach et al, 1985a). Band keratopathy results from the deposition of calcium phosphate in the cornea. The condition is recognized as opaque material appearing as parallel lines in the limbus of the eye; these lines are best visualized on slitlamp examination.

Palpable Parathyroid Masses

It would be extremely unusual to palpate an enlarged parathyroid gland in dogs. We did not palpate any parathyroid mass in the 168 dogs we diagnosed and treated. Even with confirmed PHPTH, a nodule felt in the neck is much more likely to involve the thyroid or some other structure than a parathyroid. Parathyroid masses are not palpable because they are located dorsolateral to the trachea, they are usually 4 to 10 mm in diameter (a huge parathyroid tumor would be 20 mm in diameter), and they are covered by several muscle layers. Although an enlarged parathyroid gland was not palpable in any of our dogs, palpable tumors have been identified in four of eight cats with PHPTH.

Importance of a Thorough Physical Examination

A thorough physical examination is imperative in any animal with documented hypercalcemia. Physical examination results are usually normal in dogs with PHPTH. Abnormalities, when detected, are not related to this condition. Specific findings on physical examination may lead directly to a diagnosis. As previously discussed, the more common causes of hypercalcemia in dogs include such conditions as malignant cancers and chronic renal failure. The diagnostic approach to the dog with confirmed hypercalcemia is to rule out these differential diagnoses as completely as possible before pursuing the diagnosis of primary hyperparathyroidism.

Neoplasia may be suspected after careful palpation of peripheral lymph nodes, the mammary glands, or the perineal region. Rectal and vaginal examinations should always be included in the examination of a hypercalcemic patient. Lymphosarcoma, for example, can be extremely easy or extremely difficult to diagnose, and it is a condition that we do not remove from our differential diagnosis until an alternative diagnosis has been confirmed. In addition to hypercalcemia of malignancy, other causes of hypercalcemia may be suspected after a thorough physical examination. These include renal failure, in which the kidneys may be palpably abnormal, or there may be evidence of "rubber jaw." "Rubber jaw" is a soft mandible secondary to extensive bone resorption. Dogs with hypoadrenocorticism (Addison's disease) may have bradycardia, weak femoral pulses, melena, or a bloody rectal discharge.

CLINICAL PATHOLOGY

Hemogram

No typical hemogram abnormalities are found in dogs with PHPTH, whereas in humans a nonregenerative anemia and elevation in the erythrocyte sedimentation rate may be identified. In dogs with PHPTH, no specific changes in bone marrow aspirates or peripheral blood smears are seen.

Biochemical Profile

Owing to the various factors that can alter the serum calcium concentration (and keeping the differential diagnoses for hypercalcemia in mind), each parameter in a serum biochemistry profile has importance. Specifically, the serum calcium concentration should be evaluated relative to the serum albumin concentration and correlated with the phosphorus, BUN, and serum creatinine concentrations.

SERUM TOTAL CALCIUM CONCENTRATION

Results in Dogs and Humans. Hypercalcemia is the hallmark abnormality of primary hyperparathyroidism (PHPTH; see Figs. 16-2 and 16-9). In our series, the mean serum calcium concentration in 168 dogs with PHPTH was 14.3 mg/dl, with a range of 12.1 to 23.0 mg/dl (Table 16-8). This mean value could be arbitrarily inflated because the evaluation of hypercalcemia in our clinic is limited to animals with serum calcium concentrations greater than 12.0 mg/dl (the upper reference range limit is 11.7 mg/dl). In most of our dogs, hypercalcemia was initially identified by a referring veterinarian on at least two occasions and then rechecked several times at our hospital. Of 168 dogs with PHPTH, 92 (55%) had an initial total serum calcium concentration at our hospital of 12 to 14 mg/dl; 52 (31%) had an initial concentration of 14 to 16 mg/dl; 16 (9%) had an initial concentration of

16 to 18 mg/dl; and only 8 (5%) had an initial concentration greater than 18 mg/dl (range of 18 to 23 mg/dl). It is interesting that, among the eight dogs with severe hypercalcemia, the mean BUN concentration was 22 mg/dl, and only one dog had a BUN above the reference range limit of 28 mg/dl.

Although it is assumed that untreated PHPTH will result in progressively increasing serum calcium concentrations, this has not been the experience in all people with the same condition. A group of 60 people with PHPTH who were "asymptomatic" for the disease were not treated for 10 years. The mean total serum calcium concentration at the time of diagnosis was 10.5 mg/dl (reference range, 8.4 to 10.2 mg/dl); 5 years later it was 10.6 mg/dl, and a total of 10 years after diagnosis, it was 10.3 mg/dl (Silverberg et al, 1999). However, eight individuals developed uroliths during the decade, leaving 52 who remained asymptomatic. Two of the remaining 52 individuals developed "marked hypercalcemia" (defined as a serum calcium concentration greater than 12 mg/dl) during the study period, eight had significant hypercalciuria, and six had decreasing bone density. All 52, however, remained asymptomatic, and none developed uroliths. All dogs with PHPTH have persistent hypercalcemia. Our anecdotal experience suggests that hypercalcemia associated with PHPTH in dogs remains static or slowly increases with time, but studies on untreated, randomly selected dogs have not been completed.

FACTORS AFFECTING THE SERUM CALCIUM CONCENTRATION

Sample Error. Marked lipemia can falsely increase total calcium values determined by some automated analyzers. Severely lipemic blood samples may have calcium values ranging from normal to as high as 20 mg/dl or more as a result of interference caused by turbidity. Hemoconcentration (dehydration) can produce mild hypercalcemia (typically <13 mg/dl). Hemolysis can also falsely increase the total serum calcium concentration measured with an automated analyzer. Young animals may have mild increases in serum calcium concentration, and postprandial samples may, rarely, yield false increases. Excess use of oral

TABLE 16–8   SERUM TOTAL (168 DOGS) AND IONIZED (117 DOGS) CALCIUM CONCENTRACTIONS, SERUM PARATHYROID HORMONE (PTH) CONCENTRATIONS (121 DOGS), AND ULTRASONOGRAPHICALLY IDENTIFIED PARATHYROID MASSES (77 DOGS, 8 HAD 2 MASSES EACH) IN DOGS WITH PRIMARY HYPERPARATHYROIDISM (PHPTH)

	Total Calcium (mg/dl)	Ionized Calcium (mmol/L)	PTH (pmol/L)	Ultrasound Mass Size (mm)
Reference range	9.6–11.7	1.12–1.42	2–13	<4
Mean (PHPTH dogs)	14.3	1.72	11.9	7
Range (PHPTH dogs)	12.1–23.0	1.22–2.29	3.7–121	4–23
	12–14 = 92 (55%)	1.22–1.42 = 9 (8%)	3.7–7.9 = 54 (45%)	4–6 = 51 (60%
	14–16 = 52 (31%)	1.43–1.65 = 31 (26%)	8.0–13.0 = 34 (28%)	7–10 = 22 (26%)
	16–18 = 16 (9%)	1.66–1.90 = 57 (49%)	13.1–20.0 = 13 (11%)	11–15 = 7 (8%)
	≥18 = 8 (5%)	≥1.9 = 20 (17%)	≥20 = 20 (16%)	≥15 = 5 (6%)

phosphate binders may cause the serum calcium concentration to increase.

EDTA increases calcium values determined by atomic absorption spectrophotometry and decreases results obtained with other methods. Collection and storage of samples in glassware or plastic containers that have been washed with detergents may falsely increase or decrease calcium values. Samples handled in this manner usually have spurious values for other electrolytes as well (Meuten, 1984; Meuten and Armstrong, 1989). Simple prolonged storage may yield artifactual decreases in the calcium concentration, and contamination (chalk writing boards in the laboratory) may yield false increases. Confirmation of hypercalcemia with a fresh blood sample helps rule out sampling errors.

Plasma Protein Concentration. See Chapter 17, page 725 for a complete discussion of serum protein and albumin as they relate to the total and ionized calcium concentrations.

Acid-Base Status. Acidosis decreases plasma protein–binding affinity for calcium and increases ionic calcium concentrations, creating mild physiologic hypercalcemia. Alkalosis has the opposite effect, creating a physiologic hypocalcemia. The total serum calcium concentration appears to change with the acid-base status in a manner roughly parallel to the change in ionized calcium (Meuten, 1984). Acidosis, therefore, appears to increase both the ionized and the total serum calcium concentrations, whereas alkalosis has the opposite effect.

Age. Age should be considered when serum concentrations of calcium, phosphorus, and alkaline phosphatase are evaluated. Young dogs tend to have higher serum concentrations than adults (Meuten, 1984). Reference values for the total serum calcium in young dogs are approximately 11.1 ± 0.4 mg/dl (10.5 to 11.5 mg/dl), values above those observed in adults (8.8 to 11.0 mg/dl) (Meuten et al, 1982).

SERUM IONIZED CALCIUM CONCENTRATION. As previously discussed, the ionized fraction of the total circulating calcium concentration is the biologically active form. This fact, as well as the increasing availability of laboratories with valid assays for ionized calcium and the realization that dogs with chronic renal failure tend to have normal to low ionized concentrations versus the increased concentrations seen in most hypercalcemic conditions, has created a growing interest in the results of this parameter in hypercalcemic and hypocalcemic dogs (Figs. 16-14 and 16-15). The mean ionized calcium concentration in initial blood samples from 117 dogs with PHPTH was 1.72 mmol/L, with a range of 1.22 to 2.29 mmol/L (reference range, 1.12 to 1.42 mmol/L; see Table 16-8). Nine of the 117 dogs with PHPTH (8%) had a serum ionized calcium concentration in the reference range; 31 (26%) had a result between 1.43 and 1.65 mmol/L; 57 (49%) had concentrations of 1.66 to 1.9 mmol/L;

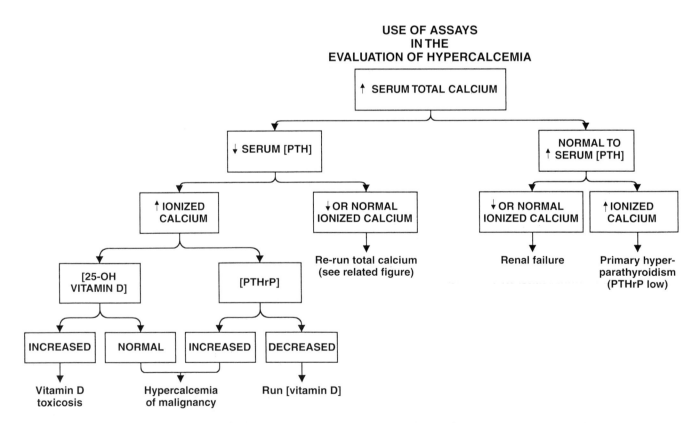

FIGURE 16–14. Algorithm showing the potential value and use of various new assays in the evaluation of hypercalcemic dogs.

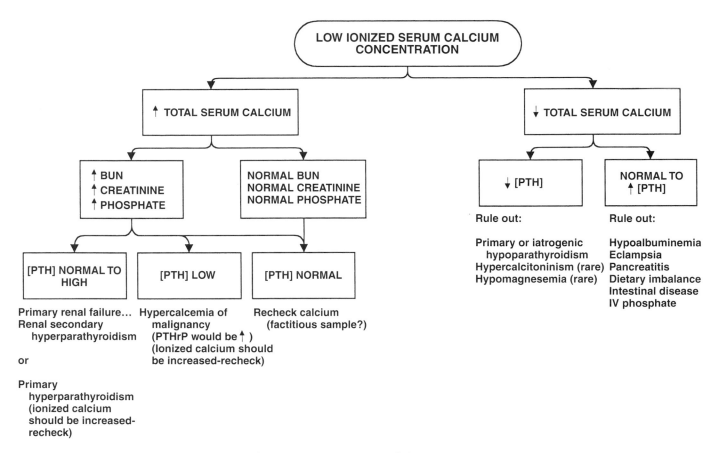

FIGURE 16–15. Algorithm for determining the cause of decreases in the ionized serum calcium concentration in dogs.

and 20 (17%) had concentrations greater than 1.9 mmol/L. In general, good correlation was seen between the serum total calcium and serum ionized calcium results. However, no dog had a total calcium concentration in the reference range, whereas 8% had ionized calcium concentrations in the reference range. It is our suspicion that these normal values may be the result of external factors (aerobic collection, pH) affecting the ionized result without altering the total calcium concentrations.

SERUM PHOSPHORUS CONCENTRATION. Low or low-normal serum phosphorus concentrations (<4.0 mg/dl) are typical of PHPTH (see Fig. 16-9). Hypophosphatemia develops after PTH-induced inhibition of renal tubular phosphorus resorption, resulting in excessive urinary losses of phosphate. In our series of 168 dogs with PHPTH, the mean serum phosphorus concentration was 2.8 mg/dl (less than the lower limit of the reference range), with a range of 1.5 to 6.8 mg/dl (reference range, 3.0 to 6.2 mg/dl; see Table 16-7). Twenty of our 168 dogs (12%) had serum phosphate concentrations less than 2.0 mg/dl; 88 (53%) had results of 2.0 to 2.9 mg/dl; 47 (28%) had results in the low-normal range of 3.0 to 3.9 mg/dl; 9 (5%) had values in the midnormal range of 4.0 to 4.9 mg/dl; and 4 (2%) had values greater than or equal to 5.0 mg/dl, with only 1 of those 4 having a serum phosphate

concentration above the reference limits (6.8 mg/dl). As a point of interest, 5 of the 168 dogs had BUN values above the reference limit of 28 mg/dl. The serum phosphate concentrations for those five dogs were 3.9, 3.9, 4.6, 4.8, and 6.8 mg/dl. As can be appreciated, the serum phosphate concentration is low to low normal in most dogs with PHPTH. Only 13 of 168 dogs with PHPTH had a serum phosphate concentration greater than or equal to 4.0 mg/dl (see Table 16-7).

The serum phosphorus concentration should always be evaluated relative to the serum calcium concentration and renal function. Hypophosphatemia, when dietary phosphate is adequate and oral phosphate-binding agents are not being given, is consistent with primary hyperparathyroidism and hypercalcemia of malignancy (see Fig. 16-9). Other causes of hypophosphatemia are less common (Table 16-9).

Hyperphosphatemia in the absence of azotemia suggests a nonparathyroid cause of hypercalcemia. When both hyperphosphatemia and azotemia are present, the clinician must rely on the history, physical examination, and other diagnostic tests to determine if the primary problem is hypercalcemia with secondary renal failure or renal failure with secondary hypercalcemia. The differentiation remains a difficult diagnostic dilemma. However, determination of the serum

TABLE 16–9 POTENTIAL CAUSES FOR HYPOPHOSPHATEMIA

Decreased Intestinal Absorption

Decreased dietary intake
Malabsorption/steatorrhea
Vomiting/diarrhea
Phosphate-binding antacids
Vitamin D deficiency

Increased Urinary Excretion

Primary hyperparathyroidism
Diabetes mellitus ± ketoacidosis
Hyperadrenocorticism (naturally occurring/iatrogenic)
Fanconi syndrome (renal tubular defects)
Diuretic or bicarbonate administration
Hypothermia recovery
Hyperaldosteronism
Aggressive parenteral fluid administration
Hypercalcemia of malignancy (early stages)

Transcellular Shifts

Insulin administration
Parenteral glucose administration
Hyperalimentation
Respiratory alkalosis

ionized calcium concentration can be of value. Dogs with renal failure and an increased total serum calcium concentration usually have normal results or a mild decrease in the ionized fraction, in contrast to dogs with PHPTH, in which both the total and the ionized fractions are increased.

Age should also be considered when evaluating the serum phosphorus concentration. Young dogs (<1 year old) tend to have a higher serum phosphorus concentration than adults. Puppies may have similar serum phosphorus and calcium concentrations (i.e., both approximately 10 mg/dl). However, the serum phosphorus concentration gradually declines during puppyhood, reaching normal adult concentrations by 9 to 12 months of age.

BLOOD UREA NITROGEN AND SERUM CREATININE. In dogs with uncomplicated primary hyperparathyroidism, serum renal parameters (BUN, creatinine) are usually normal (see Table 16-7). The mean BUN on the initial blood work from 168 dogs with PHPTH was 17.1 mg/dl (reference range, 18 to 28 mg/dl). Six dogs (3%) had BUN concentrations less than 10 mg/dl; 101 (60%) had concentrations of 10 to 17 mg/dl; 37 (22%) had concentrations of 18 to 22 mg/dl; 16 (10%) had results of 23 to 28 mg/dl; and 8 (5%) had values greater than or equal to 29 mg/dl. The range in BUN among the eight dogs with abnormally increased concentrations was 31 to 67 mg/dl.

No dog with a normal or decreased BUN concentration had an abnormal serum creatinine concentration. In addition, four of the eight dogs with an abnormal BUN concentration had a serum creatinine concentration in the reference range of 0.5 to 1.4 mg/dl. The highest serum creatinine concentration in the 168 dogs with PHPTH was 2.3 mg/dl. This is most impressive when the mean age of these dogs (11.2 years) is considered. The literature strongly suggests that hypercalcemia, especially when chronic, may damage kidneys. However, it is our impression that dogs with PHPTH are protected from renal damage. Whether this protective effect is the result of the low calcium × phosphate product in this population of dogs or some other factor, the BUN and serum creatinine values are striking.

The presence of azotemia in a hypercalcemic dog or cat that has a calcium × phosphate product in excess of 80 is an indication for medical intervention to reduce these concentrations and improve renal perfusion (see Acute Medical Therapy for the Hypercalcemic Patient, page 697). In addition, the combination of azotemia, hypercalcemia, and hyperphosphatemia represents a difficult diagnostic challenge because these abnormalities may be identified in dogs with primary renal failure (common) or primary hyperparathyroidism (quite uncommon). The availability of assays for ionized serum calcium and for PTH have made distinguishing between these disorders somewhat less difficult (see Figs. 16-14 and 16-15).

SERUM ALKALINE PHOSPHATASE (SAP). In humans, an increase in SAP is more common in hypercalcemia of malignancy than in primary hyperparathyroidism (Arnaud and Kolb, 1991). Serum increases of this parameter remain a nonspecific finding in veterinary medicine. In our series of dogs with PHPTH, only 19% had an increase in SAP. When present, increases were generally mild (twofold to sixfold), with a mean SAP of 176 IU/L (range, 52 to 866 IU/L). The increased activity of this enzyme, when present, is thought to result from a compensatory increase in osteoblastic activity in bone trabeculae as a response to mechanical stress in bone weakened by excessive resorption (Capen and Martin, 1983).

SERUM ALANINE AMINOTRANSFERASE (ALT). Serum ALT concentrations are usually normal in dogs with PHPTH. Mild increases are not worrisome and are nonspecific. The suggestion that mild increases may reflect hepatic ischemia after dehydration seems unlikely, because dehydration was virtually never a problem in our dogs. The alternative suggestion, that metastatic calcification of the liver results in ALT abnormalities, also seems unlikely in dogs with PHPTH, because metastatic calcification was seen rarely. A moderate to marked increase in ALT should raise suspicion of hypercalcemia of malignancy with concurrent liver involvement (e.g., lymphosarcoma).

SERUM CHLORIDE CONCENTRATION. In humans, excessive PTH secretion decreases the proximal renal tubular resorption of bicarbonate, leading to increased resorption of chloride and the production of a mild hyperchloremic renal tubular acidosis. Increased serum chloride concentrations in humans with hypercalcemia and hypophosphatemia and chloride: phosphate ratios greater than 33 are considered typical of PHPTH (Arnaud and Kolb, 1991). With the greater availability of reliable PTH and PTHrP assays, the increases in the serum chloride concentration are academic. However, hyperchloremia may aggravate existing hypercalcemia by impairing binding of calcium to albumin and by increasing the dissolution of bone mineral.

LIPASE. A serum lipase concentration could be evaluated to rule out the possibility of concurrent pancreatitis, although this test is not considered absolutely reliable. Chronic pancreatitis has been associated with primary hyperparathyroidism in humans (Aurbach et al, 1985b) but was identified in only one of the 168 dogs in our series.

Urinalysis

SPECIFIC GRAVITY. No abnormality on the routine urinalysis is considered pathognomonic for PHPTH in dogs. However, it is striking how many of these dogs have dilute urine. In our 168 dogs with PHPTH, the mean urine specific gravity was 1.011. Of the 168 dogs, 43 (26%) had a urine specific gravity less than 1.008 on initial evaluation at our hospital; 65 (39%) had a urine specific gravity of 1.008 to 1.012; 52 (31%) had a specific gravity of 1.013 to 1.020; 4 (2%) had a specific gravity of 1.021 to 1.030; and 4 had a specific gravity greater than 1.030 (see Table 16-7). These figures, as a group, are the result of hypercalcemia interfering with ADH action and renal concentrating ability. As previously discussed, hypercalcemia causes a reversible form of nephrogenic diabetes insipidus.

Isosthenuria (or hyposthenuria) may develop from *any* cause of hypercalcemia. Thus the combination of hypercalcemia and dilute urine is considered a cause-and-effect phenomenon, but it is not specific for any condition. However, confusion may arise because progressive renal failure is a differential diagnosis for isosthenuria. A thorough review of the serum chemistry profile and other parameters may be necessary to determine the cause of isosthenuria or hyposthenuria.

URINE SEDIMENT. Hematuria, pyuria, bacteriuria, and crystalluria are identified frequently on examination of the urine sediment of dogs with PHPTH. Of our 168 dogs with PHPTH, 53 (33%) either had a history of removal of uroliths by referring veterinarians in the 12 months prior to our examination, or uroliths were identified with radiographs or ultrasonography at the time of initial evaluation at our hospital. Urinary tract infection had been present or was present on initial examination at our hospital in 41 of 168 dogs with PHPTH (24%). Hypercalciuria, proximal renal tubular acidosis with impaired bicarbonate resorption, and the production of alkaline urine may predispose dogs to the development of bacterial cystitis and cystic or renal calculi. All uroliths have been composed of calcium phosphate, calcium oxalate, or mixtures of the two salts (see Fig. 16-12).

Blood Gas Analysis

Humans with primary hyperparathyroidism often have mild to moderate hyperchloremic metabolic acidosis as a result of impaired bicarbonate resorption by the proximal renal tubules. Urinary excretion of bicarbonate is increased, whereas excretion of hydrogen ions and chloride is decreased. The acidosis becomes even more severe as renal function deteriorates. Similar findings have not been reported in the dog.

ELECTROCARDIOGRAPHY

Experimentally induced hypercalcemia may increase myocardial contractility, shorten mechanical ventricular systole, and decrease myocardial automaticity. Potential electrocardiographic changes caused by hypercalcemia include a prolongation of the P-R interval and a shortening of the QT interval as a result of a shortened ST segment (Feldman, 1989). Theoretically, the decrease in myocardial conduction velocity and the shortened refractory period could predispose the heart to arrhythmias. However, in our dogs with primary hyperparathyroidism, severe hypercalcemia has not been associated with changes in the electrocardiogram aside from occasional ventricular premature contractions.

RADIOGRAPHY

General

Conventional radiography plays an integral role in the diagnostic evaluation of the hypercalcemic dog or cat (see Diagnostic Approach to the Hypercalcemic Patient, page 691). Thoracic and abdominal radiographs should be obtained in order to identify occult neoplasia not readily demonstrable on the physical examination. Abdominal ultrasonography may be more informative than radiography, although the two tests tend to complement each other. Lack of radiographic or ultrasonographic abnormalities in the hypercalcemic dog or cat would be consistent with PHPTH, but it is consistent with other differential diagnoses as well.

Thoracic Radiographs

The major purpose of evaluating radiographs in the hypercalcemic dog or cat is to identify abnormalities that would help establish a cause. The anterior mediastinum, perihilar, and sternal lymph nodes should be evaluated for a mass or lymphadenopathy. The classic finding in hypercalcemic dogs with lymphosarcoma is an anterior mediastinal mass (Fig. 16-16). The ribs, vertebrae, and any long bones included in the film can be evaluated for osteolytic areas arising from myeloma or other metastatic tumors. The lung fields should be carefully assessed for possible masses that might represent primary or metastatic lesions.

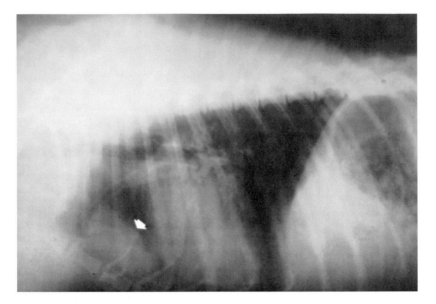

FIGURE 16–16. Lateral radiograph of the thorax of a dog with lymphosarcoma and hypercalcemia. Note the sternal lymphadenopathy *(arrow)*.

Abdomen and Skeleton

The sublumbar area and mesenteric lymph nodes can be evaluated for enlargements that would support a diagnosis of metastatic apocrine gland carcinoma of the anal sac or lymphoma (Fig. 16-17). The liver and spleen can be evaluated for enlargement or irregularities associated with lymphoma. Other than calculi in the urinary system, radiographic alterations associated with PHPTH are rare. As previously discussed, calculi in the urinary system, especially the bladder, are common; they are identified in approxi-mately one third of dogs with PHPTH. Calculi have also been detected in the kidneys, ureters, and urethra.

Osteitis fibrosa cystica, the classic bony abnormality of primary and secondary hyperparathyroidism in humans, is rarely seen in dogs. It is manifested radio-graphically as generalized osteopenia; increased bone resorption, especially at the subperiosteal surfaces; and the formation of cysts or cystlike areas in bone. In humans the phalanges and skull are usually involved. In severe cases, the long bones, patella, and ribs may become involved. The clinical manifestations of osteitis fibrosa cystica are bone pain, pathologic

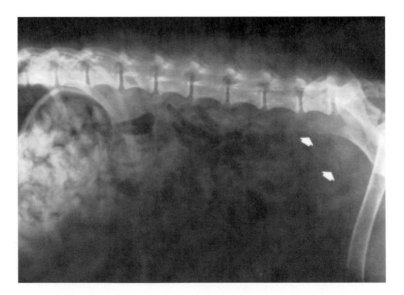

FIGURE 16–17. Lateral radiograph of the caudal abdomen of a dog with apocrine gland adenocarcinoma of the anal sac and hypercalcemia. Note the multiple masses in the sublumbar region and pelvic canal *(arrows)*, which are suggestive of sublumbar lymph nodes that have been invaded by the neoplasia.

fractures, bone cysts, and localized swelling of bone (Hruska and Teitelbaum, 1995). Other potential radiographic changes associated with PHPTH include loss of the lamina dura, fractures of the long bones and vertebrae, and soft tissue calcification. Such radiographic changes are neither common nor specific.

ULTRASONOGRAPHY

Neck

BACKGROUND. Parathyroid ultrasonography has been used extensively in humans as part of the evaluation process for hypercalcemia. Applications have included differentiation of primary and secondary hyperparathyroidism; confirmation of suspect lesions by ultrasound-guided, fine-needle aspiration biopsy; and presurgical localization of parathyroid adenomas. The sensitivity of ultrasonography in identifying one or more abnormal human parathyroid glands (69% to 88%) has been comparable to that of radioactive scintigraphy or angiography and slightly better than that of computed tomography (CT) or magnetic resonance imaging (MRI) (Attie et al, 1988; Krubsack et al, 1989). As ultrasound equipment has improved, the sensitivity of this tool has increased. Masses 2 or 3 mm in diameter or larger are usually easily visualized. The accuracy of ultrasound evaluation, more than with most other tools, is strongly operator dependent (Lloyd et al, 1990).

DOGS. In the past several years we have had the opportunity to use ultrasonography to examine the cervical area in numerous dogs with PHPTH, in normal dogs, and in dogs with secondary parathyroid hyperplasia (usually secondary to chronic renal failure). Normal parathyroid glands were not routinely visualized in early studies (Wisner et al, 1991). However, equipment sensitivity has improved, as has the experience of those performing ultrasonographic examinations, and normal parathyroid glands are now routinely visualized (Reusch et al, 2000).

Parathyroid masses (usually adenomas) from dogs with PHPTH have been as small as 2 mm in diameter and as large as 23 mm in diameter. Most adenomas are 4 to 10 mm in diameter and are easily visualized (Wisner et al, 1993; Wisner and Nyland, 1994). One recent study demonstrated a statistically significant difference in lesion size comparing hyperplastic parathyroid glands (2 to 6 mm, mean 2.9 mm) to parathyroid adenomas and adenocarcinomas (4 to 20 mm, mean 7.5 mm) (Wisner et al, 1997). Although this study is statistically sound, we are extremely reluctant to classify parathyroid tissue histologically based on an ultrasound examination. In part, our experience has not been similar. More important, pathologists do not always express confidence in classification of these masses when they can be carefully examined microscopically. Therefore the study results are interesting but, in our opinion, flawed. The choice of treatment should not be based on such observations.

In the most recent 77 dogs with PHPTH that we have studied, 51 parathyroid masses (60%) were 4 to 6 mm in diameter; 22 parathyroid masses (26%) were 7 to 10 mm in diameter; 7 parathyroid masses (8%) were 11 to 15 mm in diameter; and 5 parathyroid masses (6%) were 16 to 23 mm in diameter (see Table 16-8). Eight of the 77 dogs had two parathyroid nodules, thus 85 nodules were identified in the 77 dogs. In no dog were more than two parathyroid masses identified. Parathyroid masses are usually round or oval, well marginated, and hypoechoic to anechoic compared with surrounding thyroid gland parenchyma (Fig. 16-18). However, not every parathyroid nodule is obvious. We have had several dogs, especially those with large parathyroid masses, in which the radiologist was not certain about the

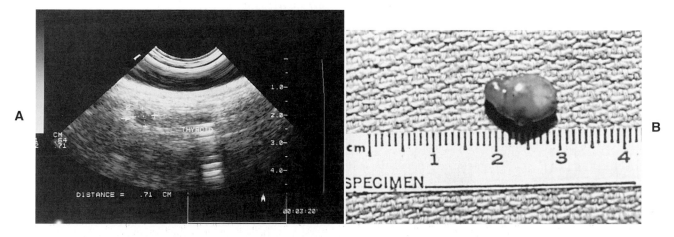

FIGURE 16–18. *A,* Cervical ultrasonogram of a dog with a functional parathyroid adenoma. Note the right thyroid lobe, in which a well-marginated, hypoechoic mass *(arrows)* is visible at the cranial pole of the thyroid. *B,* Solitary parathyroid adenoma removed from a dog with primary hyperparathyroidism (see Fig. 16-23, *C*). (*A* Courtesy Dr. Tom Nyland and Dr. Erik Wisner.)

tissue being examined. The most common confusion was whether a mass was thyroid tissue or parathyroid tissue. Another important issue that must be stressed is the subjective nature of this tool. In one of our studies, we demonstrated that experienced radiologists correctly identified a solitary parathyroid mass in 11 of 11 dogs and two parathyroid masses in another. However, less experienced radiologists identified a parathyroid mass in only four of seven dogs (Feldman et al, 1997). Ultrasound evaluation is only as reliable as the equipment and the experience of the individual performing the study allow.

The accuracy of cervical ultrasonography in dogs with PHPTH has been similar to that reported in humans: 90% to 95% of parathyroid adenomas and a smaller percentage of hyperplastic parathyroid glands can be visualized (Wisner and Nyland, 1998). It has been our experience that radiologists have identified parathyroid masses with ultrasonography more consistently than surgeons during a procedure. This observation can be explained by the occasional parathyroid mass located within a thyroid lobe that is neither visible nor palpable to the surgeon. Because of these encouraging results, we include cervical ultrasonography as a diagnostic aid strongly recommended for the evaluation of dogs with hypercalcemia. The experience of the operator and the sensitivity of the equipment must be considered. Also, a 10 MHz transducer is used for evaluating this area of the anatomy rather than the 7.5 MHz transducer used for abdominal scanning.

Abdomen

Ultrasonic scanning of the abdomen should also be a routine component of the diagnostic evaluation of hypercalcemic dogs and cats. If the liver, spleen, mesenteric lymph nodes, or other abdominal structures appear abnormal ultrasonographically, percutaneous biopsy of that structure should be strongly considered. Ultrasonography has proved an excellent tool for identifying uroliths as well. Most are found in the bladder, but renal, ureter, and urethral stones also have been seen.

ASSAYS: PTH, PTHrP, VITAMIN D (CALCITRIOL)

In dogs and cats with primary hyperparathyroidism, the serum PTH concentration is typically midnormal to exceedingly increased (Fig. 16-19; also see Fig. 16-2). In addition, PTHrP is usually undetectable, and calcitriol concentrations are expected to be normal to increased. The serum PTH concentration must *always* be evaluated relative to the serum calcium concentration. In normal animals, as the serum calcium concentration increases, the serum PTH concentration decreases. Relative to their hypercalcemia (using the total or, preferably, ionized calcium concentration), virtually all dogs and cats with PHPTH have excessive

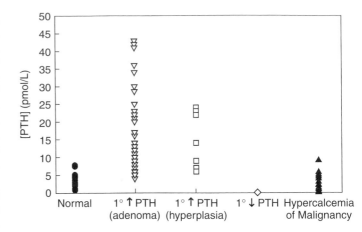

FIGURE 16–19. Serum PTH concentrations for normal dogs and those with various disorders of calcium homeostasis. Note that some overlap exists in test results and that the results as shown in Fig. 16-20 are easier to interpret.

concentrations of serum PTH (even though the PTH concentration may be within the "reference" range), which is consistent with a disease process associated with autonomous secretion of hormone (Fig. 16-20). To emphasize this concept, serum PTH concentrations in the reference range are inappropriate for individuals with concurrent hypercalcemia. Similarly, hypocalcemic animals with an abnormally decreased serum PTH concentration are most likely to be afflicted with primary hypoparathyroidism.

We have had considerable experience with the new "sandwich" assay for PTH, which was previously described, in our dogs with PHPTH. At least one serum PTH concentration was obtained from each of 121 dogs with PHPTH and assayed with the two-site IRMA system (see Table 16-8). Most laboratories have similar PTH reference ranges (2 to 13 pmol/L). Of the 121 results, 88 (73%) were within the reference range; 54 dogs (45%) had serum PTH concentrations of 3 to 7.9 pmol/L; 34 (28%) had values of 8 to 13 pmol/L; 13 (11%) had results of 13.1 to 20 pmol/L; and 20 (16%) had results greater than 20 pmol/L. Therefore, although almost 75% of the dogs with PHPTH had serum PTH concentrations in the reference range, those results should not be considered "normal," because all these dogs were hypercalcemic.

The availability of these relatively sensitive diagnostic tools has improved our ability to identify the specific problem causing hypercalcemia in most dogs and cats. These assays are accessible for practitioners. Fig. 16-2 reviews the expected results for these parameters with the various causes of hypercalcemia. A large majority of hypercalcemic dogs and cats have a disease that can be diagnosed without these sophisticated assays. However, all of us occasionally see patients that fail to yield a straightforward answer, even after the clinician follows a logical diagnostic plan. The results for any or all of these assays can only improve our ability to reach a correct diagnosis.

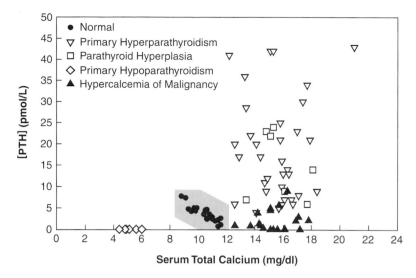

FIGURE 16–20. Serum PTH concentrations plotted against simultaneous serum calcium concentrations from normal dogs and those with abnormalities in calcium homeostasis. Note that the various groups are more distinguishable than would be the case if only the serum calcium or only the serum PTH concentrations were evaluated.

RADIONUCLIDE SCANS

Radionuclide procedures have been used for the detection and localization of parathyroid adenomas in humans (Fine, 1987). The most commonly used radionuclide imaging technique is a dual radioisotope procedure combining thallous chloride (^{201}Tl) with either pertechnetate (^{99m}Tc) or radioactive iodine (^{123}I) (Picard et al, 1987). Various problems with this methodology led to the use of one radionuclide: technetium-99m-sestamibi (^{99m}Tc-sestamibi) (O'Dougherty et al, 1992; Taillefer et al, 1992). The procedure and hospitalization time for radionuclide scans using ^{99m}Tc-sestamibi in humans are similar to those for ^{99m}Tc scans in cats. ^{99m}Tc-sestamibi radionuclide scans provide excellent results for localizing parathyroid adenomas in people (O'Dougherty et al, 1992; Taillefer et al, 1992).

Two reports suggested that this procedure might be helpful in localizing parathyroid adenomas in dogs with primary hyperparathyroidism (Wright et al, 1995; Matwichuk et al, 1996). In a subsequent study, double-phase parathyroid scintigraphy was evaluated in a group of hypercalcemic dogs. Only one of 10 dogs with PHPTH had a scan that correlated with surgery. The poor sensitivity and specificity of parathyroid gland scintigraphy led the authors to conclude that use of this tool could not be recommended (Matwichuk et al, 2000).

SELECTIVE VENOUS SAMPLING

An attempt was made to localize the correct side of the cervical area containing an autonomously functioning parathyroid mass using serum PTH assays. The hypothesis was that the vein draining the side of the mass would have greater amounts of PTH than the opposite side. Blood samples were obtained from each jugular vein prior to surgery from dogs with PHPTH caused by a solitary functioning adenoma. Unfortunately, a gradient between samples was identified in only one of 11 dogs. These disappointing results were most likely caused by sampling too high in the neck. Regardless, selective venous sampling was not reliable.

DIAGNOSTIC APPROACH TO THE HYPERCALCEMIC PATIENT

General Comments

The list of differential diagnoses for hypercalcemia is relatively short (Tables 16-3 and 16-10), allowing a logical approach to identification of its cause. Of these diagnoses, the most common cause in the dog and cat is *malignancy-associated hypercalcemia*. In an attempt to be practical, logical, and cost-effective, the veterinarian should design the diagnostic approach to first identify or rule out an underlying malignancy. Only after diagnostic tests have failed to identify a malignancy should primary hyperparathyroidism be considered.

Review of the History and Physical Examination

FIRST STEPS. The diagnostic approach to the hypercalcemic patient is usually relatively straightforward (see Table 16-3 and Fig. 16-21). The first step should always be to confirm the presence of hypercalcemia by submitting a *second* blood sample for calcium and phosphorus determinations, although the second sample virtually always has the same result as the first.

TABLE 16–10   DIFFERENTIAL DIAGNOSIS FOR HUMORAL HYPERCALCEMIA OF MALIGNANCY

Hematologic Cancers

Lymphosarcoma
Lymphocytic leukemia
Myeloproliferative disease
Myeloma

Solid Tumors with Bone Metastasis

Mammary adenocarcinoma
Nasal adenocarcinoma
Epithelial-derived tumors
Pancreatic adenocarcinoma
Lung carcinoma

Solid Tumors without Bone Metastasis

Apocrine gland adenocarcinoma of the anal sac
Interstitial cell tumor
Squamous cell carcinoma
Thyroid adenocarcinoma
Lung carcinoma
Pancreatic adenocarcinoma
Fibrosarcoma

In addition, the calcium concentration can be corrected for alterations in the serum protein and albumin concentrations (see Chapter 17 for a complete discussion). We agree that such formulas are inherently inaccurate. Therefore, whenever possible, veterinary practitioners would be well served to submit appropriate samples for the serum ionized calcium concentration. Such results, if increased appropriately, confirm hypercalcemia. If the ionized concentration is in or below the reference range in a dog with confirmed increases in the serum total calcium concentration, chronic renal failure or laboratory error should be considered.

Review of the signalment and a thorough history and physical examination often allow the clinician to identify the cause of the hypercalcemia or at least to develop a list of high-priority possibilities. Both the history and physical examination should be repeated with a serendipitous finding of hypercalcemia.

SIGNALMENT. Signalment (age, gender, breed) is emphasized in part because of the remarkable incidence of PHPTH in the Keeshond. Also, this condition is much more common in dogs 8 years of age or older. Renal failure can occur at any age, but certain breeds are predisposed to familial renal problems (e.g., Shih Tzu, Lhasa Apso, Doberman Pinscher). Young dogs are more likely to suffer from renal failure, malignancy (lymphosarcoma), or hypoadrenocorticism (especially females), whereas apocrine gland carcinoma of the anal sac, lymphoma, and other malignancies occur in older dogs.

HISTORY. The owner should be questioned about the pet's diet, vitamin-mineral supplementation, and exposure to rat or mouse poisons or houseplants that contain vitamin D analogs. An attempt can be made to determine whether the pet is in pain (lytic bone lesions). Responses to questions about the presence of polydipsia, polyuria, appetite, and activity, as well as any other information the owner may have, may be important. Generally, the more ill the pet appears, the less likely it is to have PHPTH and the more likely it is that a malignancy, renal failure, vitamin D toxicosis, granulomatous disease, or hypoadrenocorticism is the culprit.

PHYSICAL EXAMINATION. After assessment of the animal's hydration status and severity of illness, the physical examination should include careful palpation of peripheral lymph nodes and the mammary glands (lymphoma and mammary cancer). A thorough rectal and perirectal examination is imperative in the identification of neoplasia involving an apocrine gland of the anal sac. Anal sac tumors are frequently covered by haired skin and may not be identified unless rectal and perirectal examinations are performed. A digital vaginal examination should also be performed (vaginal tumor). The veterinarian should gently palpate as much of the skeleton as possible, searching for an area of focal bone pain, which then could be examined further with radiographs (multiple myeloma). The kidneys should be palpated in an attempt to assess size or irregularities.

Initial Database

BLOOD AND URINE. The initial database should include a hemogram (complete blood count [CBC]), serum biochemical profile, serum ionized calcium determination, urinalysis, and thoracic radiographs. The abdomen should be evaluated with ultrasonography or radiography or both. If the serum phosphorus concentration is normal or low, renal failure and rodenticide toxicosis are unlikely (see Fig. 16-21). Dogs with hypoadrenocorticism usually have hyperphosphatemia. The serum creatinine, sodium, potassium, and BUN concentrations are extremely valuable in this assessment as well. Evaluation of the sodium:potassium ratio should help rule out hypoadrenocorticism. A sodium:potassium ratio less than 27:1 is consistent with but not necessarily diagnostic of adrenal insufficiency. An adrenocorticotropic hormone (ACTH) stimulation test should be performed if this disease is considered likely or even possible. If the serum phosphorus concentration is increased and renal function is normal, bone osteolysis from metastatic disease should be considered. Low, low-normal, or normal serum phosphate concentrations are consistent with primary hyperparathyroidism and malignancy-associated hypercalcemia (see Fig. 16-9). A striking increase in the total protein concentration, specifically due to a monoclonal spike, is classic in multiple myeloma.

PRIMARY PARATHYROID DISEASE VERSUS PRIMARY RENAL DISEASE. A diagnostic dilemma exists when hyperphosphatemia and hypercalcemia coexist with azotemia. The clinician must determine whether the hypercalcemia is the cause or the consequence of renal disease. Other abnormalities in the initial database

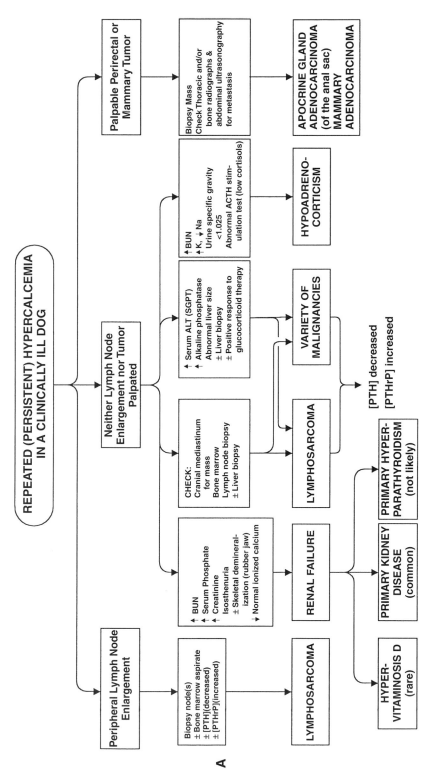

FIGURE 16–21. Algorithm for the clinical and diagnostic evaluation of dogs that are persistently hypercalcemic, including those that are ill (*A*) and those with mild clinical signs (*B*). *Continued*

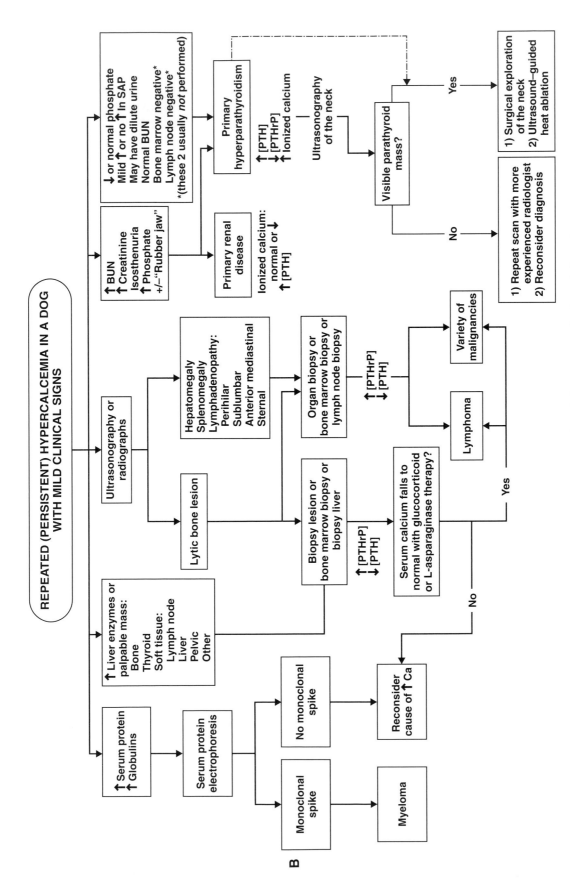

FIGURE 16–21.—cont'd. Algorithm for the clinical and diagnostic evaluation of dogs that are persistently hypercalcemic, including those that are ill (*A*) and those with mild clinical signs (*B*).

may support renal failure as the primary problem. These abnormalities include a marked increase in the serum phosphorus concentration, a low-normal or low serum ionized calcium concentration, a nonregenerative anemia, proteinuria, and/or palpably or radiographically small and irregular kidneys. The serum ionized calcium fraction in dogs with PHPTH is increased. If the hypercalcemia dissipates with aggressive fluid therapy and diuresis, PHPTH is less likely than primary renal failure. Furthermore, dogs with renal failure and hypercalcemia usually have a total serum calcium concentration less than 12.5 mg/dl. Dogs with PHPTH and secondary renal disease typically have a total serum calcium concentration greater than 13 mg/dl (see Figs. 16-2, 16-14, 16-15, and 16-21).

RADIOGRAPHY AND ULTRASONOGRAPHY. Radiographs of the thorax and ultrasonograms of the abdomen should be evaluated for soft tissue masses, soft tissue calcification, evidence of fungal disease, organomegaly, osteolysis, and/or osteoporosis. The goal is to identify an abnormal area that could be biopsied in the hope of providing a definitive explanation for hypercalcemia. An anterior mediastinal mass is demonstrable radiographically in as many as 40% of hypercalcemic dogs with lymphosarcoma (see Fig. 16-16) (Greenlee et al, 1990). If hepatomegaly or splenomegaly is identified, the histology of a biopsy (obtained percutaneously) taken from either of these organs should be evaluated to help establish a diagnosis.

Adenocarcinomas derived from the apocrine glands of the anal sac may appear radiographically as a mass in the pelvic canal. Sublumbar lymphadenopathy caused by tumor metastasis is also common (see Fig. 16-17) (Meuten et al, 1983b; Meuten, 1984). Soft tissue calcification is most frequently observed with hypervitaminosis D or chronic renal failure, although mineralization can be seen with any hypercalcemic disorder in association with hyperphosphatemia and a calcium × phosphorus product greater than 60 to 80.

Discrete lytic lesions in the vertebrae or long bones are suggestive of either myeloma or malignancy-associated hypercalcemia with bone metastasis (see Fig. 16-13). Radionuclide bone scans (Fig. 16-22) can be performed at specialty centers to identify or exclude focal bone lesions not detected with plain radiography. This is a routine procedure in people but not nearly as common in veterinary medicine (Chew et al, 1991). One of our dogs with PHPTH had lucent lesions in the long bones, but this is extremely uncommon. Concurrent hyperproteinemia is supportive of myeloma. Solid tumors with metastasis to bone are more likely if lytic bone lesions and normoproteinemia (especially a normal serum globulin concentration) are present. A core biopsy of a lytic lesion may be necessary to establish a definitive diagnosis of neoplasia, especially in a dog with occult neoplasia. Mild generalized osteoporosis is difficult to diagnose with plain survey radiographs. If present, however, it is suggestive of PHPTH or of hypercalcemia associated with hematologic neoplasia or solid tumors without bone metastasis (malignancy-associated hypercalcemia).

Ultrasonography of the cervical region has been reviewed. This tool is noninvasive and easily used (see Fig. 16-18). Identification of a solitary mass in or near one thyroid lobe supports the presence of an autonomously functioning parathyroid mass, if the dog is not in renal failure (Reusch et al, 2000). As mentioned, however, this tool requires the 10 MHz transducer and, most important, the results are subjective.

Lymph Node and Bone Marrow Evaluations

If the initial database has not established a diagnosis, the next diagnostic steps should include evaluation of lymph nodes or bone marrow or both. As has been mentioned repeatedly, lymphosarcoma is the most common neoplasm associated with hypercalcemia in the dog and cat. Involvement of the peripheral lymph nodes in lymphosarcoma can be present without enlargement of those nodes, although such a finding would be unusual. Ideally, the largest lymph node (*not* the submandibular node) should be assessed for histologic evaluation. Needle aspirates for cytology are occasionally acceptable, but pathologists may be hesitant to make a definitive diagnosis based on cytology alone. If any abnormalities are found on cytologic evaluation of an aspirate, histologic evaluation of a large biopsy sample or lymph node excision should be obtained to establish or rule out the diagnosis. As discussed, this step may be omitted in dogs that are relatively healthy based on an index of suspicion against the diagnosis of lymphosarcoma.

A bone marrow aspirate should also be considered in the hypercalcemic pet because the lymphosarcoma may be associated only with invasion of the marrow by neoplastic cells (Meuten et al, 1983b). As with the peripheral lymph node evaluation, the presence of a normal bone marrow aspirate does not definitively rule out lymphosarcoma. As with the lymph node aspirate or biopsy, we usually omit this diagnostic tool when a dog is clinically well and when a CBC is unremarkable.

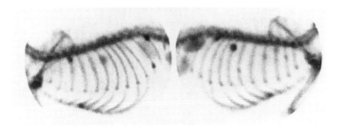

FIGURE 16–22. Bone scan from a dog with hypercalcemia caused by multiple myeloma. Note that the focal "black" areas are those of increased bone activity, as is typical for a metastatic lesion. (Courtesy Dr. William Hornof, Davis CA.)

Specific Assays: PTH, PTHrP, and Calcitriol

See previous discussions.

Cervical Surgery versus Chemotherapy (Trial Therapy)

PROBLEM. If a logical diagnostic evaluation fails to identify a cause of the hypercalcemia, the clinician is faced with a diagnostic decision. Most of the disorders that cause hypercalcemia are not "occult," but two diagnoses occasionally can be difficult to confirm or differentiate: PHPTH and malignancy-associated hypercalcemia (usually lymphosarcoma). However, because of the various assays and tools now available, especially a combination of cervical ultrasonography and PTH and PTHrP assays, this dilemma arises less often. Occasionally, the results of these assays are nebulous and the clinician must choose between chemotherapy and surgery. In dogs and cats with an "occult" cause of hypercalcemia, the clinician may choose between these two options to establish a diagnosis: (1) surgical exploration of the neck to look for a parathyroid tumor, or (2) trial therapy with a chemotherapeutic drug effective against lymphosarcoma to see if the hypercalcemia can be alleviated.

MEDICAL TREATMENT

Glucocorticoids. If hypercalcemia is caused by a lymphosarcoma (or other hematopoietic tumor), a rapid decline in the serum calcium concentration should be seen within 48 hours (sometimes overnight) of initiation of glucocorticoid therapy (Chew et al, 1991). The actions of glucocorticoids in inhibiting the growth of neoplastic lymphoid tissue and lymphocytolysis account for their rapid beneficial effect in most patients with hematologic cancers such as lymphoma and multiple myeloma (Goodwin et al, 1986). Glucocorticoids also counteract the effects of vitamin D, which accounts for their efficacy in animals with vitamin D toxicosis or granulomatous diseases (Sandler et al, 1984). In general, animals with nonhematologic cancers do not respond to glucocorticoids, nor do those with PHPTH (Bilezikian, 1992b). Therefore, if the serum calcium concentration fails to decline, PHPTH should be considered. Unfortunately, some of the effects of glucocorticoids on calcium homeostasis are nonspecific and may cause a mild transient decline in any hypercalcemic animal. If the serum calcium concentration decreases into the reference range after administration of a chemotherapeutic agent, lymphosarcoma should be suspected and further diagnostic tests implemented to confirm this diagnosis. However, confirmation of lymphosarcoma in dogs that have received glucocorticoids is extremely difficult. For this reason, we *strongly discourage* use of the "glucocorticoid response test," because it sometimes creates more problems than existed prior to the treatment.

L-ASPARAGINASE. Alternatives to glucocorticoid response in the diagnosis of malignancy-associated hypercalcemia include administration of L-asparaginase, diphosphonates, or mithramycin. Our experience has been restricted to the L-asparaginase trial, in which 20,000 IU/m² is administered intravenously. The serum calcium concentration should be measured prior to and every 12 to 24 hours after administration for as long as 72 hours. A decrease in the serum calcium concentration, especially into the reference range, is strongly suggestive of occult lymphosarcoma. Hypersensitivity reactions are an adverse side effect that has been reported with L-asparaginase; because these reactions are common, pretreatment with an antihistamine may be considered. Other adverse reactions include hepatopathy, nephropathy, coagulation abnormalities, and CNS dysfunction (Haemers and Rottiers, 1981; Haskell, 1981); fortunately, these reactions are not common. However, as with the use of glucocorticoids, using chemotherapy to establish a diagnosis must be considered crude compared with performing various assays (PTH, PTHrP, ionized calcium), which are more sensitive and specific.

SURGERY. Surgical exploration of the neck is an alternative for a dog with hypercalcemia of undetermined origin. The use of PTH, PTHrP, and ionized calcium assays plus cervical ultrasonography should improve patient selection. Ideally, one enlarged parathyroid gland is identified during surgery (Fig. 16-23). This surgery is straightforward, not difficult, and not associated with significant risk (see page 701). Therefore, in dogs over 7 years of age, cervical surgery is a viable diagnostic and therapeutic option. If an enlarged parathyroid gland is not found during surgery, one of two possibilities exists: the parathyroid mass exists in a site not evaluated, or the hypercalcemia is due to occult neoplasia. Further diagnostic tests, rather than trial therapy with glucocorticoids or L-asparaginase, are indicated once the patient has recovered from the surgery. We must emphasize, however, *confidence in a diagnosis prior to surgery or medical therapy is preferred over "exploratory" therapies.*

An ectopic location for a parathyroid mass is possible. Although reported in humans, ectopic parathyroid tumors have not been reported in dogs or cats. Localization of ectopic abnormal parathyroid tissue can be difficult. In humans, noninvasive procedures that can be used include esophagoscopy, CT, and radionuclide scans. Invasive procedures include thyroid arteriography, selective venous catheterization of the neck and mediastinal veins, and surgical exploration of the anterior mediastinum (Arnaud and Kolb, 1991).

SPONTANEOUS RESOLUTION OF PRIMARY HYPERPARATHYROIDISM. Acute hypocalcemia was diagnosed in two dogs with a history of chronic hypercalcemia. The acute hypocalcemia was interpreted in each dog to be caused by necrosis of a functional parathyroid gland adenoma after infarction. Hypocalcemia resulted because the remaining parathyroid glands were atrophied and unable to compensate for the loss of PTH (Rosol et al, 1988).

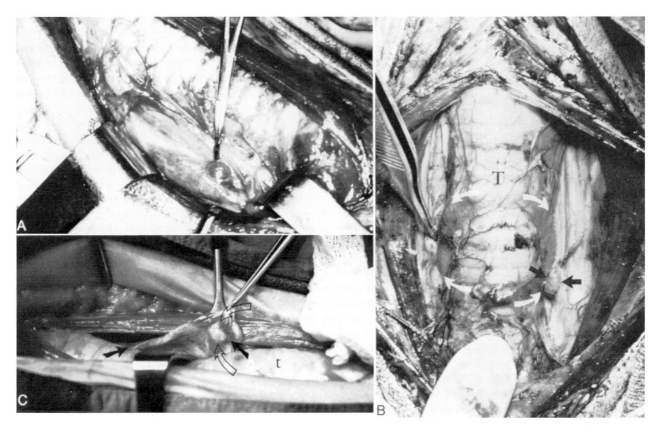

FIGURE 16–23. *A,* Surgical site during removal of a solitary parathyroid adenoma *(tip of forceps).* *B,* Surgical site during removal of a solitary parathyroid adenoma (*T,* trachea). White arrows delineate the cranial and caudal poles of the thyroid glands; black arrows point out the parathyroid adenoma. *C,* Surgical site during removal of an "internal" parathyroid adenoma (*t,* trachea). Solid arrows delineate the cranial and caudal poles of the thyroid, which is being retracted from the trachea to reveal the parathyroid adenoma *(open arrows)* on the dorsal surface of the thyroid.

ACUTE MEDICAL THERAPY FOR THE HYPERCALCEMIC PATIENT

Primary Hyperparathyroidism versus Other Disorders

PHPTH. The primary mode of therapy for severe hypercalcemia should be aimed at resolving the underlying cause. In dogs and cats with PHPTH, treatment involves surgical excision of abnormal parathyroid tissue. In these animals, however, the hypercalcemia is not an acute problem, and the calcium × phosphate product is usually well below 60. Therefore, although hypercalcemia can be damaging, primarily as a result of mineralization of nephrons, it is not a concern among a huge percentage of dogs with PHPTH.

RENAL FAILURE OR VITAMIN D TOXICOSIS. The severity of clinical signs and the degree of damage to tissues appear to depend most heavily on the serum phosphorus concentration. Renal damage induced by metastatic mineralization is thought to correlate with the product obtained by multiplying the serum total calcium concentration by the phosphate concentration. Products greater than 60 to 80 are likely to be associ-

ated with nephrotoxicity. Thus hypercalcemia associated with PHPTH is less worrisome and dangerous than the hypercalcemia associated with renal failure or hypervitaminosis D, two disorders that are almost always accompanied by hyperphosphatemia, a problem that amplifies the potential for soft tissue calcification (Table 16-11).

Indications

SOURCE OF ILLNESS VERSUS NEED FOR TREATMENT. Clinically, both to owners as well as on physical examination by veterinarians, dogs and cats with PHPTH are relatively healthy, and those that are ill usually have some concurrent problem. Despite a dramatic increase in the serum calcium concentration (mean serum calcium concentration >14 mg/dl), dogs and cats with PHPTH are typically stable and not in need of emergency therapy (see Table 16-11). In contrast, dogs with lymphosarcoma and hypercalcemia often exhibit extremely worrisome clinical signs that are caused by the malignancy rather than by the hypercalcemia. Treatment for cancer indirectly decreases the serum calcium concentration. Finally, dogs that have

TABLE 16–11 TYPICAL SERUM CALCIUM AND PHOSPHATE CONCENTRATIONS FOR VARIOUS CONDITIONS

	Typical Serum Calcium (mg/dl)	Typical Serum Phosphate (mg/dl)	Typical Calcium × Phosphate Product
Normal dog	10	4.5	45
Primary hyperparathyroidism	15	3.0	45
Lymphosarcoma	15	3.0	45
Apocrine cell carcinoma of the anal sac	15	3.0	45
Chronic renal failure	11.5	10	115
Vitamin D toxicosis	11.5	10	115

Note that aggressive therapy is recommended when the product of these two electrolytes exceeds 60 to 80. For most conditions causing hypercalcemia, emergency therapy is not necessary to reduce the serum calcium concentration.

mild hypercalcemia and renal failure typically have worrisome clinical signs and moderate to severe hyperphosphatemia. They are at risk for tissue mineralization, and they benefit from treatment directed specifically at decreasing the calcium × phosphorus product.

INDICATIONS FOR SYMPTOMATIC TREATMENT. Because of the deleterious effects of hypercalcemia, it may become necessary to treat a dog or cat symptomatically in an attempt to lower the blood calcium concentration while completing tests to establish a diagnosis or while waiting for surgery to remove an abnormal parathyroid gland or glands. The decision to implement symptomatic therapy should be based on the severity of the pet's clinical signs, the rapidity of progression of these signs, and the status of renal, cardiac, and neurologic function. *There is no specific serum calcium concentration above which therapy must be initiated.*

Symptomatic therapy for hypercalcemia is indicated when dehydration, azotemia, cardiac arrhythmia, severe neurologic dysfunction, or weakness exists (Bilezikian, 1992b). Death or encephalopathy directly attributable to hypercalcemia is not common, except after ingestion of large amounts of rat poison containing vitamin D. Symptomatic therapy (IV fluids with or without furosemide) may be indicated in the relatively stable patient in which progressive metastatic calcification of soft tissues is suspected. This can be assumed to be happening when the calcium × phosphorus product exceeds 60 to 80. With a product below 60, there is no urgent need to lower the serum calcium concentration in the stable patient, because the risk of soft tissue mineralization is not great (Chew and Meuten, 1982).

Several methods have been suggested for controlling acute or severe hypercalcemia (Tables 16-12 and 16-13). In the dog and cat, correction of fluid deficits, saline diuresis, diuretic therapy with furosemide or ethacrynic acid, and corticosteroids are the most commonly used modes of therapy. As a general rule, diuretic therapy and saline diuresis can be initiated without interfering with the diagnostic evaluation. Because the incidence of hypercalcemia associated with lymphosarcoma is great, glucocorticoids should not be administered unless a specific diagnosis has been confirmed.

TABLE 16–12 GENERAL TREATMENT OF HYPERCALCEMIA

Definitive
Remove underlying cause

Supportive

Initial considerations
  Fluid (0.9% sodium chloride)
  Furosemide
  Sodium bicarbonate
  Glucocorticosteroids
Secondary considerations
  Bisphosphonates
  Calcitonin
Tertiary considerations
  Mithramycin
  Ethylene diamine tetra-acetic acid (EDTA)
  Peritoneal dialysis
Future considerations
  Calcium channel blockers
  Somatostatin congeners
  Calcium receptor agonists
  Nonhypercalcemic calcitriol analogues

Fluid Therapy

CORRECTION OF FLUID DEFICITS. The primary indication for fluid therapy is dehydration. Decreases in fluid intake as a result of nausea and vomiting, plus an inability to concentrate urine, are common causes of dehydration, which in turn impairs calcium excretion by reducing the GFR and increasing renal tubular absorption of calcium (Parfitt and Kleerekoper, 1980). Dehydration also causes hemoconcentration, hyperproteinemia, and relative increases in the total and ionized serum calcium concentrations. Rehydration is an important initial step in treating severely hypercalcemic patients. Correction of fluid deficits should reduce the severity of the hypercalcemia, although it usually does not return the serum calcium concentration to normal except in dogs with hypoadrenocorticism or those that are not actually hypercalcemic. In humans, a rapid fall of 2 to 3 mg/dl in the total serum calcium concentration is typical after rehydration (Aurbach et al, 1985a).

SALINE DIURESIS. Once fluid deficits have been corrected, saline diuresis should promote continuing renal loss of calcium, and this is an effective short-term

TABLE 16–13   SPECIFIC TREATMENT OF HYPERCALCEMIA

Treatment	Dose	Indications	Comments
Volume Expansion			
SQ saline (0.9%)*	75–100 ml/kg/day	Mild hypercalcemia	Contraindicated if peripheral edema is present.
IV saline (0.9%)*	100–125 ml/kg/day	Moderate to severe hypercalcemia	Contraindicated in congestive heart failure and hypertension.
Diuretics			
Furosemide	2–4 mg/kg b.i.d. to t.i.d. IV, SQ, PO	Moderate to severe hypercalcemia	Volume expansion is necessary before use of this drug.
Alkalinizing Agent			
Sodium bicarbonate	1 mEq/kg IV slow bolus; may continue at 0.3 × base defcit × wt in kg/day	Severe hypercalcemia	Requires close monitoring.
Glucocorticoids			
Prednisone	1–2.2 mg/kg b.i.d. PO, SQ, IV	Moderate to severe hypercalcemia	Use of these drugs before identification of etiology may make definitive diagnosis difficult!
Dexamethasone	0.1–0.22 mg/kg b.i.d. IV, SQ		
Bone Resorption Inhibitors			
Calcitonin	4–6 IU/kg SQ b.i.d. to t.i.d.	Hypervitaminosis D	Response may be short-lived. Vomiting may occur.
Bisphosphonates			
EHDP-Didronel	15 mg/kg q24h to b.i.d.	Moderate to severe hypercalcemia	All are expensive and use in dogs is limited.
Clodronate	20–25 mg/kg in a 4-h IV infusion		
Pamidronate	1.3 mg/kg in 150 mL 0.9% saline in a 2-h IV infusion, can repeat in 1 wk		Clodronate is approved for use in humans in Europe; availability in United States may be limited.
Mithramycin	25 µg/kg IV in 5% dextrose over 2–4 h q2–4 wk	Severe hypercalcemia, refractory HHM	Limited use in dogs and cats. Nephrotoxicity, hepatotoxicity, thrombocytopenia.
Miscellaneous			
Sodium EDTA	25–75 mg/kg/h	Severe hypercalcemia	Nephrotoxicity.
Peritoneal dialysis	Low calcium dialysate	Severe hypercalcemia	Short duration of response. Use in hypercalcemia not reported.

*Potassium supplementation is necessary. Add 5–40 mEq KCl/L depending on serum potassium concentration.
Abbreviation: HHM, Humoral hypercalcemia of malignancy.

therapy for any cause of hypercalcemia. Physiologic saline promotes calciuresis because the large amount of filtered sodium competes with calcium for renal tubular resorption (Parfitt and Kleerekoper, 1980). Increased sodium excretion leads to increased calcium excretion. Normal saline given at two to three times the maintenance rate (120 to 180 ml/kg/day) is usually effective in promoting calciuresis. Potassium supplementation is often necessary to prevent hypokalemia. The pet should also be monitored carefully for adverse effects (e.g., pulmonary edema) resulting from the administration of large fluid volumes. Monitoring of body weight, urine output, and central venous pressure, as well as auscultation of the thorax, is recommended.

Diuretic Therapy (Furosemide)

The use of potent diuretics in conjunction with saline diuresis ensures maximal urinary sodium excretion and, in turn, calciuresis. Volume expansion must precede the administration of furosemide. Furosemide enhances the calciuric effects of volume expansion by inhibiting calcium resorption in the thick ascending limb of the loop of Henle. Furosemide also protects against significant volume overload (Bilezikian, 1992b). Recommended protocols typically suggest a 5 mg/kg intravenous bolus, followed by 2 to 4 mg/kg given twice or three times a day (Chew et al, 1991). Thiazide diuretics should not be used, because they decrease renal calcium excretion and may exacerbate hypercalcemia (Parfitt and Kleerekoper, 1980). Thiazides enhance distal tubular resorption of calcium (Bilezikian, 1992b).

Glucocorticoids

The beneficial effects of glucocorticoids in the symptomatic management of hypercalcemia have been discussed (see Diagnostic Approach to the Hypercalcemic Patient, page 691). These drugs reduce bone resorption of calcium, decrease intestinal calcium absorption, and increase renal calcium excretion. Glucocorticoids are cytotoxic to neoplastic lymphocytes, and they inhibit the growth of neoplastic tissue, which accounts for their beneficial effects in lymphoma and multiple myeloma (Bilezikian, 1992b). They counteract the effects of vitamin D in toxicosis (rat poison) or granulomatous diseases. In general, nonhematologic cancers do not respond to glucocorticoids (Percival et al, 1984), nor do animals with PHPTH.

Administration of glucocorticoids should be delayed until a definitive diagnosis has been established. Lymphosarcoma is the most common cause of hypercalcemia in the dog, and administration of glucocorticoids may interfere with the subsequent ability of the clinician and pathologist to confirm this diagnosis. Prednisone or prednisolone (1 to 2 mg/kg bid) or dexamethasone (0.1 to 0.2 mg/kg bid) can be used in the symptomatic management of hypercalcemia. These drugs can be given orally, subcutaneously, or intravenously.

Bisphosphonates

The bisphosphonates are compounds structurally related to pyrophosphate, a normal metabolic byproduct. The chief property of these compounds is their inhibitory effect on osteoclasts; not only can they inhibit osteoclast function, they also can decrease osteoclast viability (Fleisch, 1989). Gastrointestinal absorption is poor (<10%), but intravenous administration has been effective in the treatment of hypercalcemic humans (Bilezikian, 1992b). Considering the early occurrence of bone resorption and bone loss in humans with multiple myeloma, for example, the benefits bisphosphonates offer, even in patients who have no osteolytic lesions at the start of therapy, are impressive. These drugs not only have beneficial skeletal effects, they also slow tumor growth by inhibiting the production by osteoblasts of interleukin-6, a growth factor essential to myeloma cells (Bataille, 1996).

Three bisphosphonates (etidronate, clodronate, and pamidronate) have been approved in Western countries for the treatment of hypercalcemia in humans. The availability of other potent bisphosphonates (aminohexane bisphosphonate, risedronate, and alendronate) and other inhibitors of bone resorption (gallium nitrate, paclitaxel) open new avenues for more efficient treatment of hypercalcemia and bone disease. Clodronate was used successfully to treat lymphoma-induced hypercalcemia in one dog and vitamin D toxicosis in another dog (Petrie, 1996). Pamidronate has been used successfully to reverse vitamin D–induced toxicosis in dogs (Rumbeiha et al, 1999 and 2000).

Calcitonin

Calcitonin reduces both osteoclast activity and the formation of new osteoclasts. It may be effective at least temporarily in decreasing serum calcium levels in cases of hypercalcemia associated with excessive osteoclastic activity (Parfitt and Kleerekoper, 1980). In humans, calcitonin has not been uniformly effective in lowering the serum calcium concentration, either because the mechanisms of hypercalcemia induced by the disease are nonresponsive to calcitonin or because the patient becomes refractory to the effects of calcitonin (Aurbach et al, 1985a). The drug has been described as "weak," short-acting, and having few side effects (Bilezikian, 1992b).

Salmon calcitonin (Calcimar solution; USV Laboratories, Tarrytown, NY) is the most potent congener available. Dosages used in humans have been quite variable (Arnaud and Kolb, 1991). Reports in the veterinary literature support the use of this drug for the treatment of cholecalciferol rodenticide intoxication. Several dosages have been reported, but the number of dogs and cats in which the drug has been used is too small for recommendations regarding their effectiveness. Some reported doses in dogs include 4.5 U/kg given subcutaneously every 8 hours; 8 U/kg given subcutaneously every 24 hours; and 5 U/kg given subcutaneously every 12 hours (Dougherty et al, 1990; Fooshee and Forrester, 1990). In cats, a dosage of 4 U/kg given intramuscularly every 12 hours was used (Peterson et al, 1991). In each animal treated, the drug was effective in decreasing the serum calcium concentration.

Plicamycin (Mithramycin)

Plicamycin (previously called mithramycin) is a cytotoxic compound initially evaluated as a cancer chemotherapeutic agent. It is a potent inhibitor of RNA synthesis in osteoclasts and an effective treatment for hypercalcemia. The drug has caused significant toxicity, including thrombocytopenia, hepatic necrosis, renal damage, and hypocalcemia. Clinically significant toxicity was not observed in normal dogs after two intravenous treatments. Shivering was noted during the infusion, and osteoclastic activity was reduced (Rosol et al, 1992a and 1992b). Two dosages have been reported: 0.5 μg/kg and 0.25 μg/kg given intravenously once or twice weekly to control hypercalcemia (Finco, 1982). The effects of this drug on the serum total and ionized calcium concentrations were studied in nine dogs with hypercalcemia of malignancy, one dog with PHPTH, and one dog with vitamin D toxicosis. High-dose plicamycin (100 μg/kg) caused fatal acute hepatocellular necrosis in two dogs. A low dose of the drug (25 μg/kg) was effective in normalizing the total and ionized calcium concentrations within 24 to 48 hours in six of nine dogs, including the dog with vitamin D toxicosis. The effects were short-lived (1 to 3 days) in three dogs and lasted longer (~7 days) in three dogs. Side effects, which were mild in dogs treated with the low dose, included mild gastrointestinal signs in three dogs and reduction in platelet counts in three dogs. The low dose did not cause evidence of hepatic disease. The drug did not appear to reduce either tumor size or PTHrP concentrations (Rosol et al, 1994).

Ethylenediamine Tetra-Acetic Acid (EDTA)

Intravenous injection of sodium EDTA has been used to reduce the ionized calcium concentration immediately in humans with life-threatening hypercalcemia. Infused EDTA forms complexes with ionized calcium that are rapidly excreted by the kidney (Parfitt and Kleerekoper, 1980). A dosage of 25 to 75 mg/kg/hr has been suggested as a starting point for the treatment of hypercalcemia in the dog (Rosol et al, 2000). Unfortunately, EDTA is nephrotoxic, and acute renal failure may be a consequence of its infusion.

Bicarbonate

The ionized fraction of serum calcium is determined partly by the patient's acid-base status. Correcting the acidosis or creating a slight alkalosis with bicarbonate therapy shifts ionized calcium to the protein-bound fraction, rendering it less harmful (Chew and Meuten, 1982). A dosage of 1 to 4 mEq/kg has been recommended (Kruger et al, 1986). A single intravenous dose may last as long as 3 hours in normal cats (Chew et al, 1989). The effect of the drug is mild, and it may be helpful when administered with other treatments.

Dialysis

Hemodialysis and peritoneal dialysis with calcium-free dialysate solutions have been used effectively in humans to lower the serum calcium concentration when other methods have failed (Parfitt and Kleerekoper, 1980; Aurbach et al, 1985a). These techniques are particularly effective in patients with severe renal failure, because fluid and diuretic therapy depends on enhanced renal excretion of calcium. Significant amounts of phosphate may also be dialyzed from the blood. Because phosphate depletion may aggravate hypercalcemia, the serum phosphorus concentration should be monitored and phosphate supplements given as required.

Calcium Receptor Agonists

Medical therapy for PHPTH has been limited, although new approaches have followed discovery of a calcium-sensing receptor on parathyroid cells that downregulate the synthesis and secretion of PTH. Molecules that mimic the effect of extracellular calcium could also activate this receptor and inhibit parathyroid cell function. The phenylalkylamine (R)-N-(3-methoxy-α-phenylethyl)-3-(2-chlorophenyl)-1-propylamine, or R568, is one such calcimimetic compound. The drug did reduce serum PTH and ionized calcium concentrations in postmenopausal women with primary hyperparathyroidism (Silverberg et al, 1997).

Summary

In dogs, saline and furosemide are the most commonly used and recommended agents in the management of hypercalcemia. If these therapies fail, glucocorticoids may be given. In contrast to many other causes of hypercalcemia, primary hyperparathyroidism rarely requires medical management, except when concurrent renal failure is a factor.

SURGICAL THERAPY FOR PRIMARY HYPERPARATHYROIDISM

Number of Glands Involved

Surgical techniques for the thyroparathyroid complex have been adequately described (Bojrab, 1983; Slatter, 1985). It is important to identify and evaluate all four parathyroid glands before deciding on which gland or glands to remove. It is worth repeating that more than 90% of dogs with PHPTH have a solitary, autonomously functioning, parathyroid mass. Virtually all the remaining dogs have two abnormal glands. We would now be reluctant to send any dog with PHPTH to surgery if an abnormal mass or masses were not seen on cervical ultrasonography. Such findings support the diagnosis and indicate to the surgeon where abnormal tissue is located.

The process of evaluating parathyroid tissue at surgery without prior ultrasound evaluation can be extremely easy or quite difficult. The surgeon may easily visualize enlargement of one or more glands. However, it also has been our experience that no parathyroid tissue may be identified, or only one gland may be seen. Any enlarged and/or abnormal tissue should be removed and submitted for histologic evaluation, assuming that three or fewer parathyroids appear enlarged or discolored (or both). The remaining intact gland or glands should prevent permanent hypoparathyroidism, although transient hypocalcemia may develop shortly after surgery as a result of atrophy of normal glands after chronic suppression by the autonomously functioning abnormal gland or glands. An attempt must be made to ensure that at least one parathyroid gland remains intact to maintain calcium homeostasis and prevent permanent hypocalcemia. If none of the parathyroid glands appears enlarged or if all appear small, the diagnosis of primary hyperparathyroidism must be questioned. Uniform enlargement of all four glands should raise suspicion of secondary hyperparathyroidism.

Intravenous infusion of new methylene blue (3 mg/kg) has been described as a means of improving the surgeon's ability to recognize hyperfunctional glands. Three dogs with PHPTH were evaluated, and in each a tumor was identified after infusion with new methylene blue. Two of the three dogs developed anemia, Heinz bodies, and red blood cell "blistering" after the procedure (Fingeroth and Smeak, 1988). We have not needed to use this procedure.

Solitary Adenoma, Hyperplastic Nodule, or Carcinoma

Almost all dogs with PHPTH have a solitary, easily identified, parathyroid mass, usually an adenoma. Twelve of the 168 dogs with PHPTH in our series had parathyroid masses that at surgery appeared to be typical adenomas but histologically were diagnosed as carcinoma; another 11 dogs had parathyroid masses that were classified as hyperplasia. Approximately one half of the tumors in our series have been identified on the ventral surface of the thyroid glands. If the mass is not seen on the ventral surface, careful inspection of the dorsal surface of each thyroid lobe usually reveals it as a discrete structure on or within the adjacent thyroid tissue (see Fig. 16-23). "External" parathyroid adenomas have been easily removed without damage to surrounding tissue (see Figs. 16-18 and 16-23). In some dogs with an "internal" parathyroid adenoma, surgeons have chosen to remove the entire thyroid-parathyroid complex from the affected side. In about 5% of dogs, the surgeon was not able to identify abnormal tissue and removed the thyroid lobe that had been suggested by cervical ultrasonography as containing the parathyroid mass. In each case, that decision was correct. It should be emphasized that removal of a parathyroid mass is not difficult.

Enlargement of Multiple Parathyroid Glands

Only 13 of our 168 dogs with PHPTH (8%) had enlargement of more than one gland. Of these 13 dogs, 12 had two enlarged glands, and one had four enlarged glands. Three dogs had two "hyperplastic" parathyroids each; three dogs had two parathyroid adenomas each; three dogs had one adenoma and one hyperplastic gland each; two dogs had one hyperplastic gland and one carcinoma each; and one of the dogs with two masses had one adenoma and one carcinoma (histologic classification is discussed later in the chapter). One of the 168 dogs with PHPTH in our series had enlargement of all four glands (DeVries et al, 1993). Each of the four glands was classified histologically as primary parathyroid hyperplasia (i.e., no other cause for hyperplasia could be identified). Enlargement of all four glands suggests either multiple adenomas or, more likely, parathyroid hyperplasia.

When more than one enlarged gland is identified, the concern is primary versus secondary (renal or nutritional) hyperparathyroidism. The presurgical evaluation, as reviewed in this chapter, tends to eliminate secondary disease. If the clinician is convinced that primary disease is present, the decision to remove two glands is straightforward. However, if four glands are involved, the decision should be based on the patient's clinical status and renal function and the owner's ability to treat permanent hypoparathyroidism.

Recurrence of Primary Hyperparathyroidism

Fourteen of the 168 dogs with PHPTH in our series had a solitary parathyroid mass removed surgically, followed by resolution and then recurrence of the disease. In each case, resolution of the PHPTH persisted for at least 6 months, and in 12 of the 14 dogs, the PHPTH had resolved for 12 to 30 months. Each dog then had a recurrence of hypercalcemia caused by a second solitary, autonomously functioning parathyroid mass, which was surgically removed. The initial diagnosis in nine dogs was parathyroid adenoma; in three dogs it was parathyroid carcinoma; and in two dogs it was parathyroid hyperplasia. The histologic report after the second surgery was the same in eight dogs. However, two of the three dogs with carcinoma then had an adenoma removed; one dog with an adenoma initially had a carcinoma removed at the second surgery; and one dog with hyperplasia initially had an adenoma removed at the second surgery. The disorder, therefore, can recur, which suggests that periodic rechecks of the serum calcium concentration after stabilization would be warranted. Six of these 14 dogs were Keeshonden, and this breed may warrant more routine evaluations after initial treatment.

Absence of Parathyroid Mass at Surgery

If an enlarged parathyroid gland is not found after thorough inspection of both thyroid areas by an experienced surgeon, the most likely diagnoses include hypercalcemia due to occult neoplasia, PTH production by a parathyroid tumor located in the cranial mediastinum, or the presence of a non-parathyroid tumor producing PTH (i.e., ectopic hyperparathyroidism). The ventral neck should be carefully explored and any masses excised. New methylene blue infusion, as briefly described above, can also be considered (Fingeroth and Smeak, 1988). None of our surgeries have failed to resolve PHPTH.

We have no experience with surgical exploration of the cranial mediastinum for a parathyroid mass. Such surgeries have inherent technical difficulties. The poor likelihood of finding ectopic abnormal parathyroid tissue and the greater likelihood of dealing with an unidentified malignancy-associated hypercalcemia suggest that the decision to continue surgical exploration be carefully reconsidered. Further diagnostic tests should be undertaken to identify occult neoplasia.

NOVEL THERAPIES FOR PRIMARY HYPERPARATHYROIDISM IN DOGS

Percutaneous Ultrasound-Guided Ethanol Ablation

Ultrasonography is an excellent means of identifying parathyroid masses in dogs with hypercalcemia secondary to PHPTH. Based on our experience with this tool as a diagnostic aid and on studies performed on people with PHPTH (Bennedbaek et al, 1997), we elected to assess the efficacy of ethanol ablation as a treatment for this disorder (Long et al, 1999). Ethanol causes coagulation necrosis and vascular thrombosis in the parenchyma of exposed tissue.

PHPTH was diagnosed in 12 dogs. Their clinical and biochemical evaluation was typical for the disease. Each dog had a solitary, hypoechoic, round or oval mass near the thyroid gland on cervical ultrasonography. Parathyroid masses were identified on the right side of the neck in eight dogs and on the left side in the other four dogs. All the masses were 4 to 10 mm long; they were located at the cranial aspect of one thyroid lobe in six dogs, within the caudal pole of a thyroid lobe in three dogs, and in the midbody of the thyroid gland in three dogs. The calculated thyroid volume of the parathyroid masses ranged from 0.06 to 0.16 cm^3. It was assumed that each dog had an adenoma.

Each dog was placed under general anesthesia, and the ventral cervical region was clipped and aseptically prepared. The parathyroid mass was identified with ultrasound, and the tip of a 27-gauge needle, with arterial tubing attached, was inserted into the parathyroid under ultrasound guidance (Fig. 16-24). The approximate volume of the mass was matched with an equal volume of ethanol, which was placed in a syringe and attached to the tubing. Ethanol was slowly injected into the mass, and continuous ultrasound monitoring was used to ensure that it was injected into the target tissue. The goal of therapy was to inject enough ethanol to allow complete diffusion throughout the mass. The ablation (injection) procedure requires a high-resolution transducer (i.e., 10 MHz frequency) to allow assessment of the superficial tissues of the neck. Because parathyroid masses are small, considerable experience with ultrasound-guided needle placement is necessary. The parathyroid glands are also in close proximity to the carotid artery and vagosympathetic trunk, therefore absolute certainty about needle location is required prior to and during injection.

Because it is hyperechoic, the ethanol was easily seen using ultrasound (see Fig. 16-24). Each parathyroid mass was injected with 50% to 150% of the calculated parathyroid volume. No dog was under anesthesia for more than an hour, and the mean duration of anesthesia was 38 minutes. A single injection was administered to 11 of the 12 dogs. One dog was injected a second time 48 hours after the first dose failed to reduce the serum calcium concentration into the reference range. In all 12 dogs, the serum total calcium concentrations decreased into the reference range. In 11 dogs this decrease was documented within 48 hours of injection (10 after the first injection and one after the second injection). One dog remained hypercalcemic for 4 days, but the serum calcium concentration decreased into the reference range 5 days after treatment (Fig. 16-25). One dog had a recurrence of hypercalcemia 30 days after injection and was treated surgically. Each of the other 11 dogs remained normal for more than 18 months. The only adverse side effect was a transient change in the sound of the bark in two dogs. It is believed, retrospectively, that these two dogs suffered transient, unilateral laryngeal paralysis.

The conclusion of this study was that ultrasound-guided ethanol ablation was an efficacious mode of therapy for PHPTH in dogs. The cost of the procedure was considerably less than for surgery. Chemical ablation of parathyroid masses may be more effective in dogs than in humans because canine parathyroid masses are considerably smaller, thus requiring a smaller dose of ethanol for complete ablation. This procedure was excellent, and we abandoned the use of ethanol ablation only because the it was not consistently effective in the treatment of cats with hyperthyroidism. We therefore investigated another novel therapy for cats, once again using our dogs with PHPTH as animal models for treating hyperthyroid cats. Because the subsequent novel treatment (radio frequency heat ablation) was extremely successful, we have continued to use it rather than returning to the ethanol procedure.

Percutaneous Ultrasound-Guided Radio Frequency Heat Ablation

Ultrasonography is an excellent method of identifying parathyroid masses in dogs with hypercalcemia secondary to PHPTH. Based on our experience with this tool as a diagnostic aid, on studies performed on people, and on studies on dogs with PHPTH using ethanol ablation, we elected to assess the efficacy of percutaneous ultrasonographically guided radio frequency heat ablation as a treatment for this disorder (Pollard et al, 2001).

Radio frequency heat destroys tissue by causing thermal necrosis at the needle tip. This form of therapy has several advantages compared with ethanol

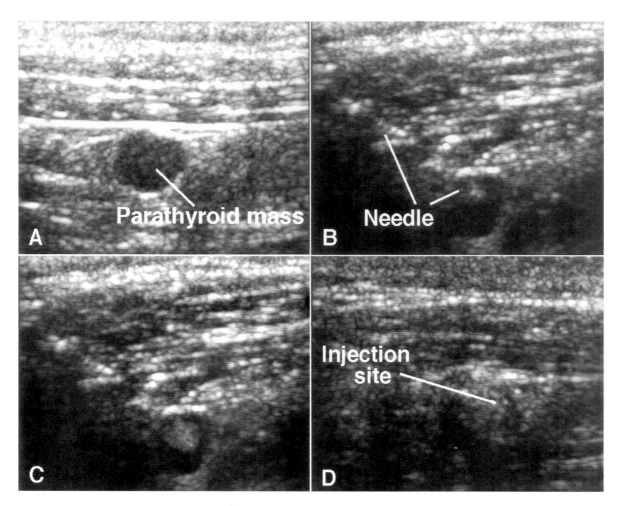

FIGURE 16–24. Ultrasonographic appearance of chemical ablation of a parathyroid mass in a dog. *A,* Sagittal view of the parathyroid mass prior to treatment. *B,* A 27-gauge needle is inserted into the mass. *C,* A test injection of 96% ethanol is used to confirm placement of the needle inside the mass. Note that the ethanol is hyperechoic in relation to the parenchyma of the mass. *D,* After injection of the target dose of ethanol, the entire mass has an echogenic appearance. (Long CD, et al: J Am Vet Med Assoc 215:217, 1999.)

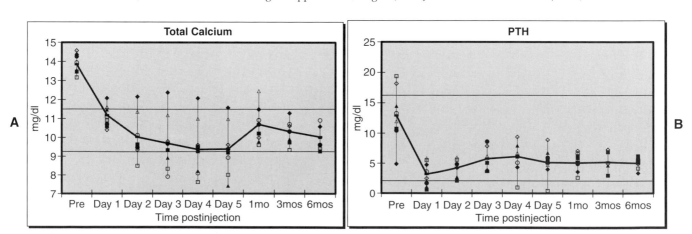

FIGURE 16–25. *A,* Serum total calcium concentration in eight dogs before (Pre) and after chemical ablation of a parathyroid mass. The horizontal black lines indicate the reference range. Dog 6 developed clinical signs of hypocalcemia 4 days after the ablation procedure. Dog 8 received two injections of ethanol (the data given represent values obtained after the second injection). Dog 7 underwent surgical removal of a parathyroid mass after the 1-month reevaluation. Dog 5 died of unrelated causes after the 3-month reevaluation. "Last" refers to the serum calcium concentration at the final follow-up evaluation (mean, 9 months after chemical ablation). *B,* Serum PTH concentrations in eight dogs before (Pre) and after chemical ablation of a parathyroid mass. The horizontal black lines indicate the reference range. (Long CD, et al: J Am Vet Med Assoc 215:217, 1999.)

ablation. First, radio frequency damages a discrete amount of tissue surrounding the uninsulated portion of the needle (there is no potential for "leakage," as there is with ethanol). Radio frequency offers the additional advantage of not damaging regional vasculature. Vascular blood flow disperses heat from vessel walls. In humans, this treatment modality has a higher success rate than ethanol for ablation of masses, and fewer treatments are required to achieve remission. Radio frequency heat ablation has been used in the treatment of multifocal hepatic masses, breast and nasal masses, and prostatic hypertrophy (Jiao et al, 1999; Livraghi et al, 1999). The disadvantage of the radio frequency technique is equipment cost.

Between September of 1999 and January of 2002, 27 dogs with PHPTH were treated with percutaneous heat ablation. Each dog had clinical and biochemical features typical of PHPTH. A solitary parathyroid nodule was identified through cervical ultrasonography in 22 dogs; five dogs had two nodules. In three of the five dogs, both nodules were on the left side of the neck; in two of the dogs, one nodule was associated with each thyroid lobe. The ultrasonic appearance of the 32 masses was similar. All masses were spherical or ovoid and hypoechoic to the surrounding thyroid parenchyma. Length of the masses varied from 3 to 15 mm.

Each dog with a solitary parathyroid mass was treated once. Each dog with two parathyroid nodules on the same side of the neck was treated once during the initial anesthesia. In the two dogs with one nodule on each side of the neck, each nodule was treated separately, 30 days apart. Each dog was placed under general anesthesia, and the ventral cervical region was clipped and aseptically prepared. The parathyroid mass was identified with ultrasound, and the tip of a 20-gauge, over-the-needle (insulated) catheter was directed into the parathyroid using ultrasound guidance. The needle hub was removed, allowing an area for connection of an insulated wire to the needle and to the radio frequency unit (Radiotherapeutics Inc., Redwood City, CA). Initially, 10 W of energy was applied to the tissue for 10 to 20 seconds. If echogenic bubbles were not seen sonographically at the needle tip during this time, the wattage was increased by 2 W every 5 to 10 seconds until echogenic foci became apparent (Fig. 16-26). Also, if a popping sound could be heard, the maximum heat application had been reached, and no additional increases in machine settings were made. The needle was arbitrarily redirected multiple times, if necessary, in an attempt to ablate the entire mass. Mean anesthesia time was 41 minutes, but it progressively decreased as experience with this procedure increased.

The procedure was uniformly successful in all 27 dogs. In 26 dogs, a dramatic reduction in the serum PTH concentration and normalization of both the total and ionized calcium concentrations occurred within days (Fig. 16-27). The serum calcium concentrations have remained in the reference range for more than a year. One dog improved for only 1 month and was treated surgically after hypercalcemia recurred. Immediately after heat ablation, one dog with a unilateral parathyroid mass developed a transient voice change, which resolved within 5 days. It is unclear whether this voice change occurred secondary to intubation or to the ablation procedure. Signs of pain, swelling, or respiratory distress were not detected in any of the dogs. Eleven of the 26 successfully treated dogs required vitamin D therapy for postablation hypocalcemia (see next section). This is currently our preferred mode of treating dogs with PHPTH that do not have cystic calculi.

During the time of this study, 18 additional dogs with PHPTH did not meet the criteria for inclusion. An attempt was made to treat two dogs

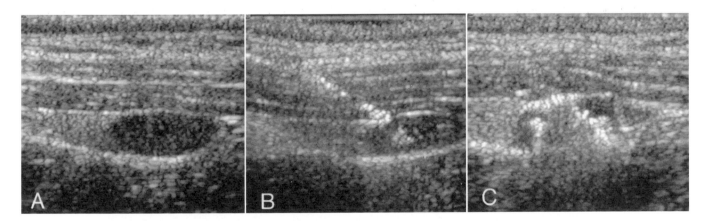

FIGURE 16–26. Left lateral sonographic images of an oval hypoechoic parathyroid nodule in a dog prior to heat ablation (A), with the insulated needle passing through the superficial soft tissues into the cranial aspect of the mass (B), and after heat ablation (C). Note the hyperechoic foci in the parenchyma of the gland in C. (Pollard RE, et al: J Am Vet Med Assoc 218:1106, 2001.)

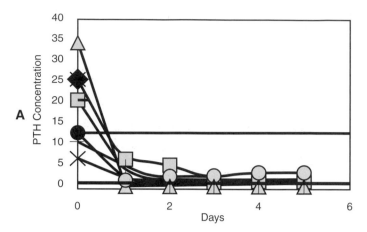
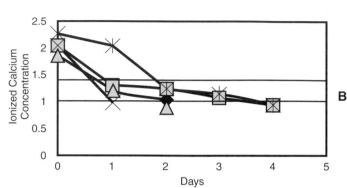

FIGURE 16–27. *A,* Serum PTH concentration (pmol/L: individual data points) of eight dogs that were successfully treated for primary hyperparathyroidism. The reference range is outlined. *B,* Serum ionized calcium concentrations (mmol/L; individual data points) in five dogs that were successfully treated for primary hyperparathyroidism on day 0 and eventually required vitamin D supplementation 1 to 4 days after treatment. The reference range is outlined. (Pollard RE, et al: J Am Vet Med Assoc 218:1106, 2001.)

early in the study period, but we were unable to penetrate the capsule of the mass with the needle, therefore percutaneous heat ablation was not pursued as the treatment method. Since then, we have used a sharper needle. In one dog, the parathyroid mass was too small for needle placement, and in four dogs the para thyroid mass was considered too close to the carotid artery for safe needle placement. Eleven dogs had cystic calculi, which required surgical removal. In each of these dogs, parathyroid surgery and abdominal surgery were performed at the same time.

POSTTREATMENT MANAGEMENT OF POTENTIAL HYPOCALCEMIA

A full discussion of vitamin D and calcium supplementation is presented in Chapter 17.

Background

Normal parathyroid glands atrophy if their function is suppressed for a prolonged period. Physiologically, the long-term response to autonomous secretion of PTH by a parathyroid adenoma, carcinoma, or primary hyperplasia is atrophy of normal glands. Surgical removal or percutaneous ablation of the autonomous source of PTH results in a rapid decline in the circulating PTH concentration (Fig. 16-28; also see Fig. 16-27) and a corresponding decline in the serum calcium concentration (see Figs. 16-25, 16-27, and 16-29). This process typically takes place over 1 to 7 days. There is little doubt that posttreatment hypocalcemia correlates with the duration and severity of hypercalcemia prior to surgery; that is, the higher the

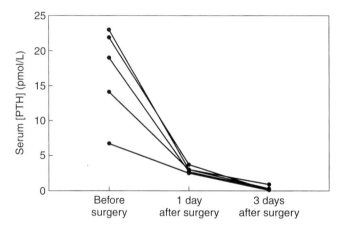

FIGURE 16–28. Serum PTH concentrations before and after surgery in eight dogs in which a solitary functional parathyroid adenoma was removed.

pretreatment calcium level and the longer a dog has been hypercalcemic, the greater the risk of hypocalcemia after resolution of the PHPTH.

Some veterinarians have suggested that it is imperative to document a decline in the serum calcium concentration after surgery. Although such a protocol allows further confirmation that PHPTH existed and that it was corrected by surgery, it places a dog at risk for pain and life-threatening hypocalcemia. The next two sections review the dogs for which no therapy or immediate therapy (posttreatment) is suggested. In our experience, beginning therapy immediately after surgery but before the serum calcium concentration has decreased has not prevented declines in the serum calcium concentration to or below the reference range.

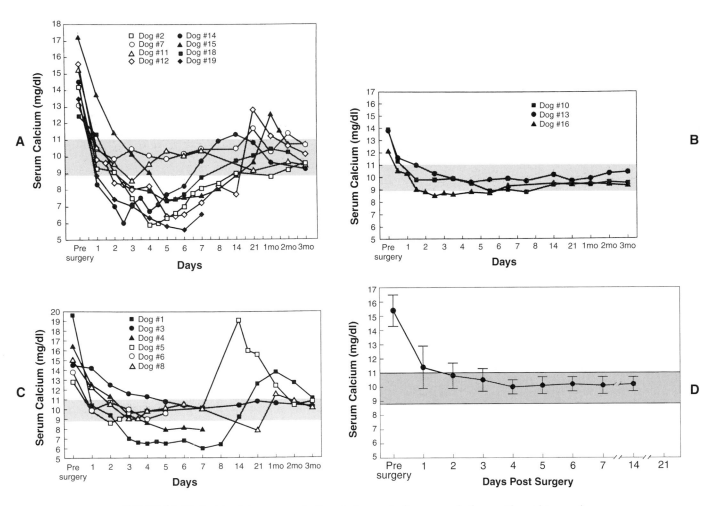

FIGURE 16–29. Serial calcium concentrations before and after removal of a parathyroid tumor from dogs with primary hyperparathyroidism. *A,* These eight dogs were placed on vitamin D_2 and calcium supplementation after hypocalcemia was identified. *B,* These three dogs had mild hypercalcemia prior to surgery, and they were not treated with vitamin D or calcium after surgery. *C,* These six dogs began receiving vitamin D_2 and calcium immediately after recovery from anesthesia. *D,* Serum calcium concentrations from 34 dogs that began receiving dihydrotachysterol immediately after recovery from anesthesia.

Presurgical Serum Calcium Level Less Than 14 mg/dl

If the serum calcium concentration prior to surgery is less than 14 mg/dl, the risk of postsurgical hypocalcemia is relatively small. The recommendation is to hospitalize the dog for at least 5 days after surgery to monitor the total serum calcium concentration once or twice daily. Hospitalization also reduces a dog's activity by maintaining it in a cage or run. The active hypocalcemic dog is at much greater risk of clinical tetany than one kept quiet. Exercise increases the risk of clinical tetany in any hypocalcemic patient. If the total serum calcium concentration remains above 8.5 mg/dl (assuming a lower reference limit of 9 to 10 mg/dl), treatment is not recommended. If the serum ionized calcium concentration remains above 0.8 mmol/L (assuming a lower reference limit of 1.12 mmol/L), treatment is not recommended. It should be noted, however, that these are general recommendations. It would be correct to begin vitamin D therapy if there is concern about the rate of decrease in the calcium concentration or if the clinician simply wants to be proactive.

If the serum calcium concentration declines below the limits suggested in the previous paragraph or if clinical signs of hypocalcemia are observed (Table 16-14), treatment with vitamin D (with or without calcium) is suggested. Chapter 17 presents a complete discussion of the acute and chronic management of hypocalcemia in the dog and cat.

Presurgical Serum Calcium Levels Greater Than 14 mg/dl

As previously discussed, the higher the presurgical serum calcium concentration and/or the more chronic the hypercalcemic condition, the more likely it is that a dog will become clinically hypocalcemic after resolution of PHPTH. Although the duration of the hypercalcemia is valuable information, it is usually unknown in veterinary patients. We assume that dogs with a serum calcium concentration persistently greater than 14 mg/dl due to PHPTH have been hypercalcemic chronically. The recommendation is to prophylactically attempt to avoid hypocalcemia after surgery by beginning vitamin D (Hytakerol or calcitriol) with or without calcium therapy the morning of surgery or immediately after recovery from anesthesia (see Chapter 17).

TABLE 16–14   CLINICAL SIGNS ASSOCIATED WITH THE ACUTE ONSET OF HYPOCALCEMIA

Panting	Stiff gait
Nervousness	Facial rubbing
Muscle trembling, twitching	Focal or generalized seizures
Leg cramping, pain	Biting of the feet
Ataxia	

In some cases we have begun vitamin D therapy 24 to 36 hours *before* surgery because of the known delay in the onset of vitamin D action. This becomes important in dogs severely hypercalcemic prior to surgery (>18 mg/dl). Initiation of these treatments has not prevented decreases in the serum calcium concentration to or below reference ranges after surgery. Each dog should be kept quiet in a cage or run for at least the 5 days after treatment. Postsurgical hypocalcemia has been seen in our dogs as early as 12 hours to as late as 20 days after the procedure. Most become hypocalcemic between the second and sixth days after surgery. Tetany, when it has occurred, most commonly is seen 4 to 7 days after treatment. The serum calcium concentration should be monitored once or twice daily.

The goal of calcium and vitamin D therapy is to maintain the serum calcium concentration in the low to low-normal range (i.e., 8 to 9.5 mg/dl). These serum calcium levels prevent clinical signs of hypocalcemia and minimize the risk of hypercalcemia, yet are low enough to stimulate recovery of function in atrophied parathyroid glands. Mid- to high-normal or greater serum calcium concentrations in dogs being given vitamin D should also be avoided. Such concentrations are typically associated with increases in the serum phosphate concentration, and they predispose the dog to tissue mineralization.

As the parathyroid glands regain control of calcium homeostasis, the calcium and vitamin D supplements can be gradually withdrawn. This process of returning parathyroid function in remaining glands is predictable, allowing the gradual withdrawal (tapering) of calcium and vitamin D supplements. Once the serum calcium concentration has stabilized and the dog has been returned to the owner, withdrawal of the supplements may be initiated. Vitamin D is usually withdrawn first by gradually extending the time between administration (e.g., twice daily to once daily for 2 weeks; to once every other day for 2 weeks; then once every third day for 2 weeks; then once every fourth day for 2 weeks; and finally, once weekly for 2 to 4 weeks). The serum calcium concentration should be checked prior to each adjustment in the dosing interval to prevent the development of occult hypocalcemia. If the serum calcium concentration drops below 8 mg/dl, reduction of the vitamin D supplementation should be delayed or the dose increased. The serum calcium concentration should remain above 8 mg/dl to minimize the risk of tetany. Once the vitamin D supplementation has been reduced to once weekly for 2 to 4 weeks, it may be discontinued. If the serum calcium concentration remains within the normal range, the calcium supplements can then be gradually withdrawn. The entire withdrawal process for vitamin D and calcium usually takes 3 to 4 months. It is important to remember that there is considerable individual variation in response to therapy; it is impossible, therefore, to check the serum calcium concentration too frequently.

Vitamin D Resistance/Time Until an Effect Is Documented

We have encountered dogs, but more often cats, that seem resistant to vitamin D in tablet form. This problem has been quickly resolved by using the liquid form. It is not common for the drug to begin to have an effect within the first 24 hours of therapy. Rather, vitamin D gradually takes effect during the first several days of therapy and almost always within 7 days of the first dose. However, we did have one dog with PHPTH and severe, persistent, vitamin D resistance. The dog had been diagnosed as having liver failure secondary to a portovascular anomaly 10 years earlier. In addition to hypercalcemia, this dog had all the biochemical features of severe liver insufficiency. Those hepatic features were present when she was 6 months of age and had not changed with time. After treatment for PHPTH, hypocalcemia developed. She did not respond to oral dihydrotachysterol. She did not respond to oral calcitriol. She did not respond to intravenous or subcutaneous calcitriol. This was an unusual combination of conditions, and we are not sure whether one affected the other.

PATHOLOGY

Subjectivity of Histologic Interpretation

Abnormal, autonomously functioning parathyroid glands from humans, dogs, and cats have been characterized histologically as adenoma, carcinoma, and hyperplasia. Unfortunately, controlled studies of histologic interpretations by pathologists have shown that it is difficult to consistently differentiate adenoma from hyperplasia and that nonmalignant parathyroid tissue in some cases may have many of the histologic features of malignancy (Aurbach et al, 1985a). Histologic classification of parathyroid disease, therefore, depends to some degree on gross features observed during surgery. The surgeon determines the number, size, and appearance of normal and abnormal glands. The pathologist then determines whether removed tissue is parathyroid.

Single-gland involvement (adenoma, carcinoma, or hyperplasia) occurs in about 80% of hyperparathyroid humans and multiple-gland involvement ("hyperplasia") in about 20% (Arnaud and Kolb, 1991). In dogs with PHPTH, it appears that single-gland involvement occurs in about 90% of cases and multiple-gland involvement (almost always two, but not more than two) in about 10% of cases. The diagnosis of carcinoma is based on a combination of gross appearance, histologic features and, ultimately, the biologic behavior of the lesion. Fewer than 2% of autonomously secreting parathyroid glands in humans are malignant. In dogs it seems that about 5% to 10% of our cases have been assigned the diagnosis of carcinoma, but we are not aware of any dog having distant metastases.

Solitary Parathyroid Mass

BACKGROUND. In humans, dogs, and cats, the most common cause of PHPTH is a functioning adenoma of the chief cells, resulting in the secretion of excessive amounts of PTH.* An adenoma is usually solitary (developing in an existing parathyroid gland), light brown-red in color, and located in the neck, closely apposed to the thyroid gland (see Figs. 16-18 and 16-23). Because of the difficulty involved in histologically classifying an enlarged parathyroid gland as an adenoma, carcinoma, or adenomatous hyperplasia, an "adenoma" is tentatively diagnosed during surgery when a single abnormally enlarged parathyroid gland is identified and the remaining glands are normal, atrophied, or not seen. The term *adenoma* is also arbitrary as applied to histologic evaluation of such tissue.

ADENOMA. Adenoma" is diagnosed when a single nodule greater than 5 mm in diameter is easily seen, is well demarcated, and compresses a rim of atrophied but otherwise normal parathyroid tissue (Capen and Martin, 1983; DeVries et al, 1993). Adenomas are generally composed of a diffuse pattern of parathyroid chief cells. In our series of dogs with this disease, about 85% had a solitary parathyroid adenoma found either during surgical exploration of the neck or during necropsy. Multiple adenomas have been reported in humans (Aurbach et al, 1985a) and were found in 3% to 5% of our dogs at the time of initial surgery.

In about 5% to 8% of our dogs with PHPTH, after removal of a solitary parathyroid adenoma, hypercalcemia recurred more than 12 months after successful surgery. Each of those dogs then had a second mass removed. In most cases the second mass was also an adenoma, but carcinoma and hyperplasia have been diagnosed. In none of these dogs were two masses present initially, demonstrated in part by complete, albeit transient, resolution of hypercalcemia for an extended period. Thorough exploration of the neck, initially, also failed to demonstrate two masses.

CARCINOMA. Chief cell carcinomas are identified in fewer than 3% to 4% of people with primary hyperparathyroidism (Shane and Bilezikian, 1982). In as many as 50% of these people, the malignant lesion may be palpable in the neck, and at surgery the mass is often firm and densely adherent to local structures (Aurbach et al, 1985a). Capsular and vascular invasion is a characteristic histologic finding. Parathyroid carcinomas tend to be locally invasive, with the potential to spread to regional lymph nodes, lung, liver, and bone.

Because chief cell carcinomas are rare in dogs and cats (Berger and Feldman, 1987), their biologic behavior is not well characterized. In our series of 168 dogs with PHPTH, seven (~4%) had carcinoma

---

*Aurbach et al, 1985a; Berger and Feldman, 1987; Feldman, 1989; Henderson et al, 1990; Shane, 1990; Bilezikian, 1991; Kallet et al, 1991; and Bruyette, 1992.

diagnosed histologically. At surgery, each of these masses had the appearance typical of adenomas. Local invasion or distant spread has not been recognized.

PRIMARY HYPERPLASIA. Hyperplasia implies an abnormality involving all parathyroid tissue and is frequently diagnosed when more than one parathyroid gland is grossly and microscopically abnormal. Gross enlargement of all four glands is not a prerequisite for a diagnosis of hyperplasia, because microscopic alterations may be present in a normal-sized gland (Aurbach et al, 1985a). Unfortunately, an accurate pathologic diagnosis requires clear criteria for distinguishing adenoma from hyperplasia and for distinguishing either of these from normal glands. Such criteria are not well established. As a result, a tentative differentiation often is based on the number of glands involved (i.e., one gland supports a diagnosis of adenoma and multiple glands a diagnosis of hyperplasia) (Verdonk and Edis, 1981).

We reported a group of six dogs with PHPTH (8% of the 72 in our series at the time) that had hyperplasia as determined by arbitrary criteria (DeVries et al, 1993). That percentage approximates our experience since completion of that study. The terms *nodular hyperplasia* and *adenomatous hyperplasia* were applied to parathyroids that contained multiple nodules less than 5 mm in diameter as opposed to adenomas, which were defined as parathyroid tumors consisting of solitary nodules greater than 5 mm in diameter.

Differentiation of hyperplasia and adenoma has important implications regarding surgery, medical therapy, and long-term prognosis. A dog or cat potentially can be cured after complete surgical removal of a solitary adenoma, with three normal parathyroid glands (albeit atrophied in the immediate postsurgical period) remaining to prevent permanent hypoparathyroidism. In contrast, parathyroid hyperplasia implies that if all abnormal parathyroid tissue is not removed, the chance for persistent or recurrent hyperparathyroidism is high. However, this has not consistently been observed in our series of dogs with PHPTH that have had less than all tissue removed. In three of the six dogs mentioned above, one parathyroid mass was removed, and in two dogs the disease resolved after more than one but less than four glands were extirpated, perhaps emphasizing the gap between histologic diagnosis and the biology of tissue involved. Only one of the six dogs required extirpation of all four glands (DeVries et al, 1993).

The cause of parathyroid hyperplasia in PHPTH is not known. A genetic factor may be involved in humans, because several families have been described in which the disease is inherited as an autosomal dominant trait (Arnaud and Kolb, 1991). This heritable nature of primary hyperparathyroidism is of interest because of the strikingly high incidence of PHPTH in the Keeshond. Other theories suggest that hyperplasia or adenomas in people may develop secondary to alterations in the response of chief cells to unusual secretagogues, such as glucagon, vasoactive intestinal polypeptide, and histamine (Brown, 1980 and 1982).

SUMMARY. In our series of dogs with PHPTH that have had surgery and that had a solitary mass, about 87% had a solitary parathyroid adenoma, about 8% had a diagnosis of solitary primary parathyroid hyperplasia, and 5% had a diagnosis of carcinoma. To our knowledge the histologic diagnosis is of academic interest. In each case, the long-term response to therapy was similar. Recurrences occur regardless of the initial histologic diagnosis. When recurrences occur (~10% of our dogs), the histologic diagnosis of tissue removed at second surgery is just as likely to be different from the initial diagnosis as it is to be similar. We have never seen distant metastasis from a solitary parathyroid carcinoma, nor have we seen local invasion. That is not to say that either scenario could not happen, but we do suggest that such problems would be extremely unusual.

It is also worth repeating that about 10% of dogs with PHPTH have two parathyroid nodules at the time of initial diagnosis. Again, the histologic classification of these masses is as likely to be different (e.g., one adenoma and one carcinoma or one hyperplasia and one adenoma) as they are to be the same. The recurrence rate in dogs with two masses at the time of diagnosis is actually 50% of the recurrence rate of dogs with a single solitary mass.

Mediastinal Parathyroid Tissue

Parathyroid tissue, displaced into the anterior mediastinum during the embryologic expansion of the thymus and often referred to as "ectopic" because its location is not associated with the thyroid, may also become neoplastic. In humans, this is an uncommon but recognized location for a solitary, autonomous, PTH-secreting adenoma causing primary hyperparathyroidism (Heath, 1989). Mediastinal parathyroid tissue that results in primary hyperparathyroidism has not been reported in the dog or cat, although a mediastinal parathyroid cyst was diagnosed in a normocalcemic cat (Swainson et al, 2000).

Multiple Endocrine Neoplasia

Multiple endocrine neoplasia (MEN) refers to a group of syndromes in humans (often familial) consisting of hyperplasia or neoplasia in two or more endocrine glands. Two patterns of MEN involve the parathyroid gland: MEN type I (parathyroid hyperplasia with pancreatic islet cell adenoma/carcinoma or adenoma/hyperplasia of the anterior pituitary) and MEN type IIa (medullary carcinoma of the thyroid with pheochromocytoma and/or parathyroid hyperplasia) (see Chapter 5). In both conditions, hyperplasia, not neoplasia, is the most common pathologic abnormality in the parathyroid. Although the clinical expression of the MEN components is variable, hyperparathyroidism usually predominates in MEN type I, whereas medullary thyroid carcinoma predominates in MEN type IIa (Leshin, 1985). Sporadic cases of dogs and cats with multiple endocrine disorders occasionally are encountered.

Hereditary Neonatal Primary Hyperparathyroidism

A rare form of hereditary neonatal primary hyperparathyroidism has been described in humans, associated with diffuse hyperplasia of the parathyroid chief cells. Primary parathyroid hyperplasia has also been reported in two German Shepherd pups from a litter of four females (Thompson et al, 1984). Clinical signs were apparent in these dogs by 2 weeks of age, including stunted growth, muscular weakness, and polyuria/polydipsia. An autosomal recessive mode of inheritance for the primary hyperparathyroidism was suggested, and analogies were drawn with the disease in children.

Breed Versus Histology of the Parathyroids

There is little doubt that the Keeshond is predisposed to primary hyperparathyroidism. Owing to this apparent familial tendency, we are always more suspicious of hyperplasia or recurrence in this breed. Forty percent of the dogs in our series with primary parathyroid hyperplasia were Keeshonden, as were 50% of the dogs with recurrence of the disease. Further studies likely will report the importance of breed in this disease.

PROGNOSIS

The prognosis for dogs with primary hyperparathyroidism is excellent. Hypocalcemia may occur after therapy but should be treatable with proper monitoring and appropriate supplementation and should not alter the prognosis. Only about 33% of the dogs we have treated developed clinically significant hypocalcemia. Routine use of vitamin D (dihydrotachysterol or calcitriol) and calcium supplementation has dramatically decreased the incidence of tetany. Care must be taken not to overdose vitamin D, because renal damage is much more likely in this situation than in dogs with PHPTH.

PRIMARY HYPERPARATHYROIDISM IN CATS

DIFFERENTIAL DIAGNOSIS FOR FELINE HYPERCALCEMIA

It is fair to state that, in general, the differential diagnoses for hypercalcemia in dogs apply to cats. In a study of 71 hypercalcemic cats, the mean age was about 9 years and the mean serum total calcium concentration was 12.2 mg/dl (lower than would likely be seen in hypercalcemic dogs). Anorexia and lethargy were the most common clinical signs (70%). Vomiting, diarrhea, and/or constipation was observed in 27% of the cats, polyuria and/or polydipsia was observed in 24%, and urinary signs were seen in 23%. Neurologic signs were observed in 14% of the cats (Savary et al, 2000).

Neoplasia was diagnosed in 30% of the cats. The most common cancers diagnosed included lymphoma and squamous cell carcinoma. Less common neoplasms included leukemia, osteosarcoma, fibrosarcoma, undifferentiated sarcoma, and bronchogenic carcinoma. The combination of bronchogenic carcinoma and hypercalcemia was also reported in a separate cat (Anderson et al, 2000). Renal failure was diagnosed in 25% of the cats, and half of those cats had urolithiasis. In a separate study, chronic renal failure in cats was usually associated with a total serum calcium concentration in the reference range and a low-normal to low serum ionized calcium concentration (Barber and Elliott, 1998). Of the cats with hypercalcemia, several had urolithiasis without renal failure. Four cats (6%) had PHPTH. One cat had hypoadrenocorticism. Several cats had hyperthyroidism or diabetes mellitus, but it would not seem likely that either of these endocrine problems would contribute to hypercalcemia. However, four cats (6%) had infectious or granulomatous disease (e.g., feline infectious peritonitis [FIP], toxoplasmosis, actinomycosis, or cryptococcosis). Thus the differential diagnosis for hypercalcemia in cats is not dramatically different from that in dogs (Mealey et al, 1999; Savary et al, 2000). Other differential diagnoses (e.g., vitamin D toxicosis, other neoplastic conditions,various granulomatous diseases) should also be considered.

IDIOPATHIC HYPERCALCEMIA OF CATS

Hypercalcemia is less common in cats than in dogs, but an increased frequency of hypercalcemia in cats has been observed in several geographically distinct veterinary centers since about 1990 (Barsanti, 1997; Refsal et al, 1998; Midkiff et al, 2000; Rosol et al, 2000). The striking feature of this hypercalcemia is that thus far, no explanation for it has been found. Veterinarians are seeing young, middle-age, and old cats with mild to moderate hypercalcemia and no identifiable cause. The serum total calcium concentration in some of these cats has been increased for years, often without clinical signs, but some of the cats have a poor appetite and weight loss and appear weak. The serum ionized calcium concentrations are also increased, sometimes out of proportion to the increase in the total calcium concentration (Rosol et al, 2000).

Nephrocalcinosis or uroliths may be observed on radiographs or on abdominal ultrasonography. It has been estimated that as many as 33% of cats with calcium oxalate urolithiasis have had hypercalcemia. Renal function parameters, based on the BUN and serum creatinine concentrations, initially are in reference ranges, but renal failure does develop in most cats. By definition these cats have no evidence of a neoplastic condition (including necropsy), and they test negative for feline leukemia virus (FeLV) and feline immuno-deficiency virus (FIV). Serum PTH concentrations have been normal or low, PTHrP has not been detectable, and vitamin D concentrations have been in reference ranges.

Chronic acidosis was thought to contribute to this condition, but venous blood gas analyses have not revealed significant abnormalities. It is not clear whether the pathophysiology of idiopathic hypercalcemia is different in cats with uroliths than in those without uroliths (Rosol et al, 2000).

Exploratory surgery of the cervical region has not identified any abnormalities, and subtotal para-thyroidectomy has failed to resolve the hypercalcemia. A change to high-fiber or nonacidifying diets has also failed to resolve the condition. Treatment with prednisone (usually 5 to 10 mg/cat/day) has resulted in long-term decreases in the serum calcium concentration in some cats. Regardless of its effect on the serum calcium concentration, prednisone has resulted in improved appetite and weight gain in some cats.

It is safe to state that almost all dogs with hypercalcemia have a specific diagnosis that explains this biochemical abnormality. It is also safe to state that a significant number of cats with hypercalcemia do not have an explanation for the condition. Some have suggested that the "problem" doesn't exist, that the profession should simply expand the reference range for feline calcium concentrations.

PRIMARY HYPERPARATHYROIDISM IN CATS

In addition to 10 cats in our series, we are aware of an additional nine cats with PHPTH having been reported. Thus we can comment on only 19 cats with

TABLE 16–15   CLINICAL, LABORATORY, AND HISTOLOGIC FINDINGS IN 10 CATS WITH PRIMARY, NATURALLY OCCURRING HYPERPARATHYROIDISM IN THE U.C. DAVIS SERIES

Signalment	Clinical Signs	Serum Ca (mg/dl)	Serum PO$_4$ (mg/dl)	BUN (mg/dl)	Serum Creatinine (mg/dl)	Urine Specific Gravity	Parathyroid Histology
15 y.o. M/N/, DLH	Anorexia Vomiting	14.6	3.4	35	1.8	1.011	Solitary adenoma
14 y.o. F/S, Siamese	Anorexia Vomiting Muscle fasciculation	22.8	6.6	70	3.2	1.013	Solitary adenoma
15 y.o. M/N, Siamese	None	13.5	3.3	21	2.2	1.031	Solitary adeboma
15 y.o. F/S, Siamese	Polydipsia Polyuria	13.3	2.2	31	2.7	1.010	Solitary adenoma
8 y.o. FlS, DSH	Anorexia Weight loss	13.8	1.8	15	1.0	1.015	Solitary adenoma
14 y.o. F/S, DSH	Polydipsia Polyuria Lethargy	15.4	2.5	30	1.2	1.010	Solitary adenoma
9 y.o. F/S, Siamese	Anorexia	17.1	6.2	63	2.6	1.026	Bilateral cystadenoma
9 y.o. M/N, DSH	Anorexia Vomiting Lethargy Dysuria	15.2	2.6	59	3.6	1.015	Solitary carcinoma
14 y.o. M/N, DSH	Constipation	13.4	3.7	41	2.2	1.022	Solitary adenoma
12 y.o. M/N, DSH	Weight loss Lethargy Constipation	14.1	3.2	27	1.4	1.018	Bilateral carcinomas
Reference values		8.8–11.4	2.4–6.1	10–30	0.8–2.0	—	—

y.o., years old; *M,* male; *N,* neutered; *F,* female; *S,* spay/ovariohysterectomy; *DLH,* Domestic Long-Haired; *DSH,* Domestic Short-Haired.

this condition, compared with a much larger number of similarly afflicted dogs. Of the 19 cats, 7 cats with hypercalcemia caused by primary hyperparathyroidism were described in one report, 4 in another, 2 in each of two, and 1 in another separate report (Kallet et al, 1991; Marquez et al, 1995; Den Hertog et al, 1997; Savary et al, 2000; Sueda and Stefanacci, 2000).

The mean age of these 19 cats was approximately 13 years (range, 8 to 20 years), and various breeds were represented. The most common clinical signs described by owners were anorexia, lethargy, and vomiting. Less common signs were constipation, polyuria, polydipsia, and weight loss. Other signs were uncommon. A parathyroid mass was palpable in at least 11 of the 19 cats. The presence of a palpable mass and the owners' observations contrast with our experience in dogs, in which none had a palpable cervical mass and polyuria, polydipsia, and muscle weakness are common.

The only consistent abnormality on CBC and serum biochemical profiles from as many of these cats as we were able to review, was hypercalcemia (Table 16-15). All afflicted cats had persistent increases in both the serum total calcium concentration and the ionized calcium concentration. Several cats had cystic calculi, and a large percentage had abnormalities in the BUN and serum creatinine concentrations, findings not typical of their canine counterparts. Cervical ultrasonography was described as normal in several cats, but others had visible masses that would be considered huge in a dog. On cervical ultrasonography, two cats each had a single parathyroid mass, one mass measuring $4.5 \times 2 \times 1$ cm and the other measuring $1.7 \times 1.1 \times 1$ cm (Sueda and Stefanacci, 2000). The serum PTH concentrations, when measured, ranged from within the reference range (0 to 4 pmol/L) to increased. In one cat, seven separate serum PTH samples were assayed; five results were in the reference range and two were increased. That would be a percentage of abnormally increased values that might apply to any series of cats.

Most of the 19 cats had surgery and showed resolution of the PHPTH after extirpation of the abnormal tissue. It seems that tetany has not been described in any cat treated with surgery, although several cats became hypocalcemic and were treated with vitamin D and calcium. Of the nine cats we followed after surgery, all lived well beyond 1 year from surgery, although at 1.5 years, one had recurrence of hypercalcemia and at necropsy was demonstrated to have had both a parathyroid adenoma and a parathyroid carcinoma. Histologic evaluation of tissue removed showed that 13 cats had had a parathyroid adenoma, three had had parathyroid carcinomas, two had had parathyroid hyperplasia (involving all four glands), and one had had bilateral cystadenomas.

REFERENCES

Anderson TE, et al: Probable hypercalcemia of malignancy in a cat with bronchogenic adenocarcinoma. J Am Anim Hosp Assoc 36:52, 2000.
Arnaud CD, Kolb FO: The calciotropic hormones and metabolic bone disease. In Greenspan FS (ed): Basic and Clinical Endocrinology. Los Altos, Calif, Lange Medical Publications, 1991, p 247.
Attie JN, et al: Preoperative localization of parathyroid adenomas. Am J Surg 156:323, 1988.
Attie MF: Treatment of hypercalcemia. Endocrinol Metab Clin North Am 18:807, 1989.
Aurbach GD, et al: Parathyroid hormone, calcitonin, and the calciferols. In Wilson JD, Foster DW (eds): Williams Textbook of Endocrinology, 7th ed. Philadelphia, WB Saunders, 1985a, p 1137.
Aurbach GD, et al: Metabolic bone disease. In Wilson JD, Foster DW (eds): Williams Textbook of Endocrinology, 7th ed. Philadelphia, WB Saunders, 1985b, p 1218.
Barber PJ, Elliott J: Feline chronic renal failure: Calcium homeostasis in 80 cases diagnosed between 1992 and 1995. J Small Anim Pract 39:108, 1998.
Barber PJ, et al: Measurement of feline intact parathyroid hormone: Assay validation and sample handling studies. J Small Anim Pract 34:614, 1993.
Barsanti JA: Hypercalcemia and urolithiasis in cats. Proc Am Coll Vet Intern Med Ann Forum 15:327, 1997.
Bataille R: Management of myeloma with bisphosphonates. N Engl J Med 334:529, 1996.
Bennedbaek FN, et al: Percutaneous ethanol injection therapy in the treatment of thyroid and parathyroid diseases. Eur J Endocrinol 136:240, 1997.
Bennett PF, et al: Canine anal sac adenocarcinomas: Clinical presentation and response to therapy. J Vet Intern Med 16:100, 2002.
Berger B, Feldman EC: Primary hyperparathyroidism in dogs. J Vet Med Assoc 191:350, 1987.
Bilezikian JP: Primary hyperparathyroidism. In Bardin CW (ed): Current Therapy in Endocrinology and Metabolism, 4th ed. Philadelphia, BC Decker, 1991, p 448.
Bilezikian JP: Hypercalcemic states. In Coe FL, et al (eds): Disorders of Bone and Mineral Metabolism. New York, Raven Press, 1992a, p 493.
Bilezikian JP: Management of acute hypercalcemia. N Engl J Med 326:1196, 1992b.
Black KS, Mundy GR: Other causes of hypercalcemia: Local and ectopic secretion syndromes. In Bilezikian JP, Marcus R, Levine MA (eds): The Parathyroids. New York, Raven Press, 1994, pp 341-358.
Bojrab MJ: Current Techniques in Small Animal Surgery, 2nd ed. Philadelphia, Lea & Febiger, 1983.
Boyce RA, Weisbrode SE: Effect of dietary calcium on the response of bone to 1,25(OH) vitamin D3. Lab Invest 48:683, 1983.
Broadus AE, Stewart AF: Parathyroid hormone–related protein: Structure, processing, and physiologic actions. In Bilezikian JP (ed): The Parathyroids: Basic and Clinical Concepts. New York, Raven Press, 1994, pp 259-294.
Brown EM: Histamine receptors on dispersed parathyroid cells from pathological human parathyroid tissue. J Clin Endocrinol 51:1325, 1980.
Brown EM: Parathyroid secretion in vivo and in vitro: Regulation by calcium and other secretagogues. Miner Electrolyte Metab 8:130, 1982.
Brown EM, et al: Calcium ion–sensing cell surface receptors. N Engl J Med 333:234, 1995.
Brown EM, et al: G-protein–coupled, extracellular Ca^{2+}–sensing receptor: A versatile regulator of diverse cellular functions. Vitam Horm 55:1, 1999.
Brown RC, et al: Circulating intact parathyroid hormone measured by a two-site immunochemiluminometric assay. J Clin Endocrinol Metab 65:407, 1987.
Bruyette D: Disorders of calcium metabolism. In Proceedings of the Tenth Annual Veterinary Medical Forum, 1992, p 161.
Budayr AA, et al: Increased serum levels of parathyroid hormone–like protein in malignancy-associated hypercalcemia. Ann Intern Med 111:807, 1989.
Burtis WJ: Parathyroid hormone–related protein: Structure, function, and measurement. Clin Chem 38:2171, 1992.
Burtis WJ, et al: Immunochemical characterization of circulating parathyroid hormone–related protein in patients with humoral hypercalcemia of cancer. N Engl J Med 322:1106, 1990.
Capen CC, Martin SL: Calcium-regulating hormones and diseases of the parathyroid glands. In Ettinger SJ (ed): Textbook of Veterinary Internal Medicine, 2nd ed. Philadelphia, WB Saunders, 1983, p 1550.
Carothers MA, et al: 25-OH-cholecalciferol intoxication in dogs. Proc Am Coll Vet Intern Med Forum 12:822, 1994.
Chew DJ, Capen CC: Hypercalcemic nephropathy and associated disorders. In Kirk RW (ed): Current Veterinary Therapy VII. Philadelphia, WB Saunders, 1980, p 1067.
Chew DJ, Meuten DJ: Disorders of calcium and phosphorus metabolism. Vet Clin North Am 12:411, 1982.
Chew DJ, Nagode LA: Renal secondary hyperparathyroidism. Proceedings of the Society for Comparative Endocrinology, 1990, p 17.
Chew DJ, et al: Effect of sodium bicarbonate infusions on ionized calcium and total calcium concentrations in serum of clinically normal cats. Am J Vet Res 50:145, 1989.

Chew DJ, et al: Hypercalcemia in dogs and cats: Overview of etiology, diagnostic approach, and therapy. Proceedings of the Waltham/OSU Symposium, 1991, p 35.

Consensus Development Conference Panel: Diagnosis and management of asymptomatic primary hyperparathyroidism. Ann Intern Med 114:593, 1991.

Crager CS, Nachreiner RF: Increased parathyroid hormone concentration in a Siamese kitten with nutritional secondary hyperparathyroidism. J Am Anim Hosp Assoc 29:331, 1993.

Den Hertog E, et al: Primary hyperparathyroidism in two cats. Vet Q 19:81, 1997.

Deniz A, Mischke R: Ionized calcium and total calcium in the cat. Berl Munch Teirarztl Wochenschr 108:105, 1995.

DeVries SE, et al: Primary parathyroid gland hyperplasia in dogs: Six cases (1982-1991). J Am Vet Med Assoc 202:1132, 1993.

DiBartola SP, et al: Clinicopathologic findings associated with chronic renal disease in cats: 74 cases (1973-1984). J Am Vet Med Assoc 190:1196, 1987.

Dougherty SA, et al: Salmon calcitonin as adjunct treatment for vitamin D toxicosis in a dog. J Am Vet Med Assoc 196:1269, 1990.

Dow SW, et al: Hypercalcemia associated with blastomycosis in dogs. J Am Vet Med Assoc 188:706, 1986.

Durie BGM, et al: Relation of osteoclast activating factor production to the extent of bone disease in multiple myeloma. Br J Haematol 47:21, 1981.

Feldman EC: Canine primary hyperparathyroidism. In Kirk RW, Bonagura JD (eds): Current Veterinary Therapy X. Philadelphia, WB Saunders, 1989, p 985.

Feldman EC, et al: Comparison of results of hormonal analysis of samples obtained from selected venous sites versus cervical ultrasonography for localizing parathyroid masses in dogs. J Am Vet Med Assoc 211:54, 1997.

Finco DR: Interpretations of serum calcium and phosphorus metabolism. Vet Clin North Am 12:411, 1982.

Finco DR, et al: Effects of parathyroid hormone depletion in dogs with induced renal failure. Am J Vet Res 55:867, 1994.

Finco DR, et al: Hypocalcemia has beneficial effects in dogs with induced renal failure. J Vet Intern Med 9:209, 1995 (abstract).

Fine EJ: Parathyroid imaging: Its current status and future role. Semin Nucl Med 17:350, 1987.

Fingeroth JM, Smeak DD: Intravenous methylene blue infusion for intraoperative identification of parathyroid gland tumors in dogs. III. Clinical trials and results in three dogs. J Am Anim Hosp Assoc 24:673, 1988.

Flanders JA, Reimers TJ: Radioimmunoassay of parathyroid hormone in cats. Am J Vet Res 52:422, 1991.

Fleisch H: Bisphosphonates: A new class of drug in diseases of bone and calcium metabolism. In Brunner KW, et al (eds): Bisphosphonates and Tumor Osteolysis. Berlin, Springer-Verlag, 1989, p 1.

Foley P, et al: Serum parathyroid hormone–related protein concentration in a dog with a thymoma and persistent hypercalcemia. Can Vet J 41:867, 2000.

Fooshee SK, Forrester SD: Hypercalcemia secondary to cholecalciferol rodenticide toxicosis in two dogs. J Am Vet Med Assoc 196:1265, 1990.

Fradkin JM, et al: Elevated parathyroid hormone–related protein and hypercalcemia in two dogs with schistosomiasis. J Am Anim Hosp Assoc 37:349, 2001.

Garrett IR: Bone destruction in cancer. Semin Oncol 20:4, 1993.

Goldschmidt MH, Shofer FS: Skin tumors of the Dog and Cat. Oxford, England, Pergamon Press; 1992, pp 103-108.

Goodwin JS, et al: Mechanism of action of glucocorticoids: Inhibition of T cell proliferation and interleukin-2 production by hydrocortisone is reversed by leukotriene B_4. J Clin Invest 77:1244, 1986.

Gouget B, et al: Ca^{2+} measurement with ion selective electrode. Ann Biol Chem 46:419, 1988.

Grain E, Walder EJ: Hypercalcemia associated with squamous cell carcinoma in a dog. J Am Vet Med Assoc 181:165, 1982.

Greenlee PG, et al: Lymphomas in dogs: A morphologic, immunologic and clinical study. Cancer 66:480, 1990.

Grone A, et al: Dependence of humoral hypercalcemia of malignancy on parathyroid hormone–related protein expression in the canine anal sac apocrine gland adenocarcinoma (CAC-8) nude mouse model. Vet Pathol 35:344, 1998.

Gunther R, et al: Toxicity of a vitamin D_3 rodenticide to dogs. J Am Vet Med Assoc 193:211, 1988.

Haemers S, Rottiers R: Medical treatment of insulinoma. Acta Clin Belg 36:199, 1981.

Harinck HIJ, et al: Role of bone and kidney in tumor-induced hypercalcemia and its treatment with bisphosphonate and sodium chloride. Am J Med 82:1133, 1987.

Harrington DD, Page EH: Acute vitamin D_2 (ergocalciferol) toxicosis in horses: Case report and experimental studies. J Am Vet Med Assoc 182:1358, 1983.

Harris NL, et al: Case records of the Massachusetts General Hospital. N Engl J Med 347:1952, 2002.

Haskell CM: L-Asparaginase: Human toxicology and single-agent activity in nonleukemic neoplasms. Cancer Treat Rep 65:57, 1981.

Heath DA: Primary hyperparathyroidism: Clinical presentation and factors influencing clinical management. Endocrinol Metab Clin North Am 18:631, 1989.

Henderson JE, et al: Circulating concentrations of parathyroid hormone–like peptide in malignancy and in hyperparathyroidism. J Bone Miner Res 5:105, 1990.

Hirt RA, et al: Severe hypercalcemia in a dog with a retained fetus and endometritis. J Am Vet Med Assoc 216:1423, 2000.

Hollis BW, et al: Quantification of circulating 1,25-dihydroxyvitamin D by radioimmunoassay with an ^{125}I-labeled tracer. Clin Chem 42:586, 1996.

Hristova EN, et al: Analyzer-dependent differences in results for ionized calcium, ionized magnesium, sodium and pH. Clin Chem 41:1649, 1995.

Hruska KA, Teitelbaum SL: Renal osteodystrophy. N Engl J Med 333:166, 1995.

Ihle SL, et al: Seizures as a manifestation of primary hyperparathyroidism in a dog. J Am Vet Med Assoc 192:71, 1988.

Jiao LR, et al: Clinical short-term results of radio frequency ablation in primary and secondary liver tumors. Am J Surg 177:303, 1999.

Johnessee JS, et al: Primary hypoadrenocorticism in a cat. J Am Vet Med Assoc 183:881, 1982.

Kallet AJ, et al: Primary hyperparathyroidism in cats: Seven cases (1984-1989). J Am Vet Med Assoc 199:1767, 1991.

Klausner JS, et al: Calcium urolithiasis in two dogs with parathyroid adenomas. J Am Vet Med Assoc 191:1423, 1987.

Krubsack AJ, et al: Prospective comparison of radionuclide, computed tomography, and sonographic and magnetic resonance localization of parathyroid tumors. Surgery 106:639, 1989.

Kruger JM, et al: Treatment of hypercalcemia. In Kirk RW (ed): Current Veterinary Therapy IX. Philadelphia, WB Saunders, 1986, p 75.

Kruger JM, et al: Hypercalcemia and renal failure: Etiology, pathophysiology, diagnosis, and treatment. Vet Clin North Am (Small Anim Pract) 26:1417, 1996.

Legendre AM, et al: Canine blastomycosis: A review of 47 clinical cases. J Am Vet Med Assoc 178:1163, 1981.

Lemann J, Gray RW: Calcitriol, calcium, and granulomatous disease. N Engl J Med 311:1115, 1984.

Leshin M: Multiple endocrine neoplasia. In Wilson JC, Foster DW (eds): Williams Textbook of Endocrinology, 7th ed. Philadelphia, WB Saunders, 1985, p 1274.

Livraghi T, et al: Small hepatocellular carcinoma: Treatment with radio frequency ablation versus ethanol ablation. Radiology 210:655, 1999.

Llach F, et al: The pathophysiology of altered calcium metabolism in rhabdomyolysis-induced acute renal failure. N Engl J Med 305:117, 1981.

Lloyd MNH, et al: Preoperative localization in primary hyperparathyroidism. Clin Radiol 41:239, 1990.

Long CD, et al: Percutaneous ultrasound–guided chemical parathyroid ablation for treatment of primary hyperparathyroidism in dogs. J Am Vet Med Assoc 215:217, 1999.

Marquez GA, et al: Calcium oxalate urolithiasis in a cat with a functional parathyroid adenocarcinoma. J Am Vet Med Assoc 206:817, 1995.

Martin TJ, Suva LJ: Parathyroid hormone–related protein in hypercalcemia of malignancy. Clin Endocrinol 31:631, 1989.

Marx SJ: Hyperparathyroid and hypoparathyroid disorders. N Engl J Med 343:1863, 2000.

Mattson A, et al: Renal secondary hyperparathyroidism in a cat. J Am Anim Hosp Assoc 29:345, 1993.

Matus RE, Weir EC: Hypercalcemia of malignancy. In Kirk RW, Bonagura JD (eds): Current Veterinary Therapy X. Philadelphia, WB Saunders, 1989, p 988.

Matus RE, et al: Prognostic factors for multiple myeloma in the dog. J Am Vet Med Assoc 188:1288, 1986.

Matwichuk C, et al: Use of ^{99m}Tc-sestamibi for detection of a parathyroid adenoma in a dog with primary hyperparathyroidism. J Am Vet Med Assoc 209:1733, 1996.

Matwichuk C, et al: Double-phase parathyroid scintigraphy in dogs using ^{99m}Tc-sestamibi. Vet Radiol Ultrasound 41:461, 2000.

McArthur W, et al: Bone solubilization by mononuclear cells. Lab Invest 42:452, 1980.

McCauley LK, et al: In vivo and in vitro effects of interleukin-1α and cyclosporin A on bone and lymphoid tissues in mice. Toxicol Pathol 19:1, 1991.

McClain HM, et al: Hypercalcemia and calcium oxalate urolithiasis in cats: A report of five cases. J Am Anim Hosp Assoc 25:297, 1999.

Mealey KL, et al: Hypercalcemia associated with granulomatous disease in a cat. J Am Vet Med Assoc 215:959, 1999.

Meuten DJ: Hypercalcemia. Vet Clin North Am (Small Anim Pract) 14:891, 1984.

Meuten DJ, Armstrong PJ: Parathyroid disease and calcium metabolism. In Ettinger SJ (ed): Textbook of Veterinary Internal Medicine: Diseases of the Dog and Cat, 3rd ed. Philadelphia, WB Saunders, 1989, p 1610.

Meuten DJ, et al: Hypercalcemia associated with an adenocarcinoma derived from the apocrine glands of the anal sac. Vet Pathol 18:454, 1981.

Meuten DJ, et al: Relationship of calcium to albumin and total proteins in dogs. J Am Vet Med Assoc 180:63, 1982.

Meuten DJ, et al: Hypercalcemia in dogs with lymphosarcoma: Biochemical, ultrastructural, and histomorphometric investigation. Lab Invest 49:553, 1983a.

Meuten DJ, et al: Hypercalcemia in dogs with adenocarcinoma derived from apocrine glands of the anal sacs: Biochemical and histomorphometric investigations. Lab Invest 48:428, 1983b.

Michelangeli VP, et al: Evaluation of a new, rapid, and automated immunochemiluminometric assay for the measurement of serum intact parathyroid hormone. Ann Clin Biochem 34:97, 1997.

Midkiff AM, et al: Idiopathic hypercalcemia in cats. J Vet Intern Med 14:619, 2000.

Mischke R, et al: The effect of the albumin concentration on the relation between the concentration of ionized calcium and total calcium in the blood of dogs. Dtsch Tierarztl Wochenschr 103:199, 1996.

Mol JA, et al: Elucidation of the sequence of canine (pro)-calcitonin: A molecular biological and protein chemical approach. Regul Pept 35:189, 1991.

Moore FM, et al: Hypercalcemia associated with rodenticide poisoning in three cats. J Am Vet Med Assoc 193:1099, 1988.

Morrow C: Cholecalciferol poisoning. Vet Med p. 905, 2001.

Mundy GR: Hypercalcemia of malignancy revisited. J Clin Invest 82:1, 1988.

Mundy GR, Martin TJ: Hypercalcemia of malignancy: Pathogenesis and management. Metabolism 31:1247, 1982.

Mundy GR, et al: The hypercalcemia of cancer: Clinical implications and pathogenic mechanisms. N Engl J Med 310:1718, 1984.

O'Dougherty MJ, et al: Parathyroid imaging with technetium-99m-sestamibi: Preoperative localization and tissue uptake studies. J Nucl Med 33:313, 1992.

Orloff JJ, Stewart AF: The carboxy-terminus of parathyroid hormone: Inert or invaluable. Endocrinology 136:4729, 1995.

Parfitt AM, Kleerekoper M: Clinical disorders of calcium, phosphorus, and magnesium metabolism. In Maxwell MH, Kellman CR (eds): Clinical Disorders of Fluid and Electrolyte Metabolism. New York, McGraw-Hill, 1980, p 947.

Parker, M: Personal communication, 2001.

Percival RC, et al: Role of glucocorticoids in the management of malignant hypercalcemia. Br Med J 289:287, 1984.

Peterson EN, et al: Cholecalciferol rodenticide intoxication in a cat. J Am Vet Med Assoc 199:904, 1991.

Peterson ME, Feinman JM: Hypercalcemia associated with hypo-adrenocorticism in sixteen dogs. J Am Vet Med Assoc 181:804, 1982.

Peterson ME: Primary hypoadrenocorticism in ten cats. J Vet Intern Med 3:55, 1989.

Peterson ME, et al: Pretreatment clinical and laboratory findings in dogs with hypoadrenocorticism: 225 cases (1979-1993). J Am Vet Med Assoc 208:85, 1996.

Petrie G: Management of hypercalcemia using dichloromethylene biphosphate (clodronate). Proceedings of the British Small Animal Veterinary Association Annual Congress, 1996, p. 80 (abstract).

Philbrick WM, et al: Defining the roles of parathyroid hormone–related protein in normal physiology. Physiol Rev 76:127, 1996.

Picard D, et al: Localization of abnormal parathyroid glands using ^{201}thallium/^{123}iodine subtraction scintigraphy in patients with primary hyperparathyroidism. Clin Nucl Med 12:61, 1987.

Pollard RE, et al: Percutaneous ultrasonographically guided radio frequency heat ablation for treatment of primary hyperparathyroidism in dogs. J Am Vet Med Assoc 218:1106, 2001.

Potts JT Jr: Management of asymptomatic hyperparathyroidism. J Clin Endocrinol Metab 70:1489, 1990.

Pressler BM, et al: Hypercalcemia and high parathyroid hormone–related protein concentration associated with malignant melanoma in a dog. J Am Vet Med Assoc 221:263, 2002.

Quigley PJ, Leedale AH: Tumors involving bone in domestic cats: A review of fifty-eight cases. Vet Pathol 20:670, 1983.

Rasmussen H: The cycling of calcium as an intracellular messenger. Sci Am 261:66, 1989.

Refsal KR, et al: Laboratory assessment of hypercalcemia. Proc Am Coll Vet Intern Med Forum 16:646, 1998.

Reusch CE, et al: Ultrasonography of the parathyroid glands as an aid in differentiation of acute and chronic renal failure in dogs. J Am Vet Med Assoc 217:1849, 2000.

Rohrer CR, et al: Hypercalcemia in a dog: A challenging case. J Am Anim Hosp Assoc 36:20, 2000.

Rosol TJ, et al: Acute hypocalcemia associated with infarction of parathyroid gland adenomas in two dogs. J Am Vet Med Assoc 192:212, 1988.

Rosol TJ, et al: Parathyroid hormone (PTH)–related protein, PTH, and 1,25-dihydroxyvitamin D in dogs with cancer-associated hypercalcemia. Endocrinology 131:1157, 1992a.

Rosol TJ, et al: Effects of mithramycin on calcium metabolism and bone in dogs. Vet Pathol 29:223, 1992b.

Rosol TJ, et al: Effect of mithramycin on hypercalcemia in dogs. J Am Anim Hosp Assoc 30:244, 1994.

Rosol TJ, et al: Disorders of calcium. In DiBartola SP (ed): Fluid Therapy in Small Animal Practice, 2nd ed. Philadelphia, WB Saunders, 2000, pp 108-162.

Ross LA, Goldstein M: Biochemical abnormalities associated with accidental hypothermia in a dog and in a cat. Proceedings of the Annual American College of Veterinary Internal Medicine Meeting, St Louis, 1981, p 66.

Ross JT, et al: Adenocarcinoma of the apocrine glands of the anal sac in dogs: A review of 32 cases. J Am Anim Hosp Assoc 27:349, 1991.

Rumbeiha WK: Nephrotoxins. In Bonagura JD (ed): Kirk's Current Veterinary Therapy XIII. Philadelphia, WB Saunders, 2000, pp 212-214.

Rumbeiha WK, et al: Use of pamidronate to reverse vitamin D_3–induced toxicosis in dogs. Am J Vet Res 60:1092, 1999.

Rumbeiha WK, et al: Use of pamidronate disodium to reduce cholecalciferol-induced toxicosis in dogs. Am J Vet Res 61:9, 2000.

Sandler LM, et al: Studies of the hypercalcemia of sarcoidosis: Effect of steroids and exogenous vitamin D_3 on the circulating concentration of 1,25-dihydroxy vitamin D_3. O J Med 53:165, 1984.

Savary KCM, et al: Hypercalcemia in cats: A retrospective study of 71 cases (1991-1997). J Vet Intern Med 14:184, 2000.

Schenck PA, et al: Effects of storage on serum ionized calcium and pH values in clinically normal dogs. Am J Vet Res 56:304, 1995.

Seymour JF, Gagel RF: Calcitriol: the major humoral mediator of hypercalcemia in Hodgkin's and non-Hodgkin's lymphomas. Blood 82:1383, 1993.

Shane E: Hypercalcemia: Differential diagnosis and management. In Savus MJ (ed): ASBMR Primer on Metabolic Bone Disease. Richmond, Va, William Byrd Press, 1990, p 107.

Shane E, Bilezikian JP: Parathyroid carcinoma: A review of 62 patients. Endocrinol Rev 3:218, 1982.

Silverberg SJ, et al: Short-term inhibition of parathyroid hormone secretion by a calcium receptor agonist in patients with primary hyperparathyroidism. N Engl J Med 337:1506, 1997.

Silverberg SJ, et al: A 10-year prospective study of primary hyperparathyroidism with or without parathyroid surgery. N Engl J Med 341:1249, 1999.

Slatter DH: Textbook of Small Animal Surgery. Philadelphia, WB Saunders, 1985.

Sleeboom HP, Bijvoet OL: Hypercalcemia due to malignancy: Role of the kidney and treatment. Contrib Nephrol 33:178, 1982.

Strewler GL: The physiology of parathyroid hormone–related protein. N Engl J Med 342:177, 2000.

Sueda MT, Stefanacci JD: Ultrasound evaluation of the parathyroid glands in two hypercalcemic cats. Vet Radiol Ultrasound 41:448, 2000.

Swainson SW, et al: Radiographic diagnosis: Mediastinal parathyroid cyst in a cat. Vet Radiol Ultrasound 41:41, 2000.

Taillefer R, et al: Detection and localization of parathyroid adenomas in patients with hyperparathyroidism using a single radionuclide imaging procedure with technetium-99m-sestamibi (double-phase study). J Nucl Med 33:1801, 1992.

Thompson KG, et al: Primary hyperparathyroidism in German Shepherd dogs: A disorder of probable genetic origin. Vet Pathol 21:370, 1984.

Toribio RE, et al: Cloning and sequence analysis of the complementary DNA for feline preproparathyroid hormone. Am J Vet Res 63:194, 2002.

Torrance AG, Nachreiner R: Human parathormone assay for use in dogs: Validation, sample handling studies, and parathyroid function testing. Am J Vet Res 50:1123, 1989a.

Torrance AG, Nachreiner R: Intact parathyroid hormone assay and total calcium concentration in the diagnosis of disorders of calcium metabolism in dogs. J Vet Intern Med 3:86, 1989b.

Troy GC, et al: Heterobilharzia americana infection and hypercalcemia in a dog: A case report. J Am Anim Hosp Assoc 23:35, 1987.

Tuma SN, Mallette LE: Hypercalcemia after nephrectomy in the dog: Role of the kidneys and parathyroid glands. J Lab Med 102:213, 1983.

Uehlinger P, et al: Differential diagnosis of hypercalcemia: A retrospective study of 46 dogs. Schweiz Arch Tierheilkd 140:188, 1998.

Utiger RD: Treatment of primary hyperparathyroidism. N Engl J Med 341:1301, 1999 (editorial).

Verdonk CA, Edis AJ: Parathyroid "double adenomas": Fact or fiction? Surgery 90:523, 1981.

Weir EC, et al: Primary hyperparathyroidism in a dog: Biochemical, bone histomorphometric, and pathologic findings. J Am Vet Med Assoc 189:1471, 1986.

Weir EC, et al: Humoral hypercalcemia of malignancy in canine lymphosarcoma. Endocrinology 122:602, 1988a.

Weir EC, et al: Adenyl cyclase stimulating, bone resorbing and β-TGF–like activities in canine apocrine cell adenocarcinoma of the anal sac. Calcif Tissue Int 43:359, 1988b.

Weir EC, et al: Isolation of 16,000-dalton parathyroid hormone–like proteins from two animal tumors causing humoral hypercalcemia of malignancy. Endocrinology 123:2744, 1988c.

Weller RE, et al: Chemotherapeutic responses in dogs with lymphosarcoma and hypercalcemia. J Am Vet Med Assoc 181:891, 1982.

Wisner ER, Nyland TG: Clinical vignette. J Vet Intern Med 8:244, 1994.

Wisner ER, Nyland TG: Ultrasonography of the thyroid and parathyroid glands. Vet Clin North Am (Small Anim Pract) 28:973, 1998.

Wisner ER, et al: Normal ultrasonographic anatomy of the canine neck. Vet Radiol 32:185, 1991.

Wisner ER, et al: Ultrasonographic evaluation of the parathyroid glands in hypercalcemic dogs. Vet Radiol Ultrasound 34:108, 1993.

Wisner ER, et al: High-resolution parathyroid sonography. Vet Radiol Ultrasound 38:462, 1997.

Wright KN, et al: Diagnostic and therapeutic considerations in a hypercalcemic dog with multiple endocrine neoplasia. J Am Anim Hosp Assoc 31:156, 1995.

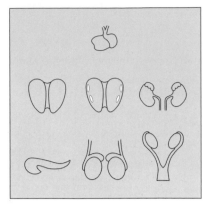

17

HYPOCALCEMIA AND PRIMARY HYPOPARATHYROIDISM

Several historical landmarks in the understanding of parathyroid physiology, maintenance of homeostasis, and calcium regulation are significant with respect to our knowledge of hypocalcemia. Rickets (hypovitaminosis D) was first described in 1645. More than 200 years later (1884), an association was made between thyroidectomy in dogs and cats and the development of clinical hypocalcemia (tetany). In 1891, Gley proved that the parathyroid glands must be removed with the thyroids to produce tetany. Shortly thereafter, administration of calcium salts following parathyroidectomy successfully prevented tetany. Almost a century later (1970), the amino acid sequence of parathyroid hormone (PTH) was determined (Tepperman, 1980). Almost 20 years later, the amino acid sequence of a parathyroid hormone–related peptide (PTHrP), produced by some cancers, was described in both humans and dogs (Weir, 1988; Broadus et al, 1988; Yates et al, 1988).

DEFINITION OF PRIMARY HYPOPARATHYROIDISM

A pair of parathyroid glands are located in close proximity to each thyroid lobe in normal individuals. Hypoparathyroidism, an uncommon endocrine disorder, develops as a result of an absolute or relative deficiency in secretion of PTH, the sole product of the four parathyroid glands. This deficiency causes various physiologic problems, with the final common pathway to clinical signs involving neurologic and neuromuscular disturbances resulting from hypocalcemia. The signs of hypocalcemia are similar, regardless of the cause (Table 17-1). Once identified, the clinician should attempt to determine the underlying pathogenesis (cause) for hypocalcemia, in order to formulate short- and long-term treatment strategies and a prognosis.

PATHOPHYSIOLOGY

Systemic Calcium Homeostasis

Maintenance of a normal serum calcium concentration

The parathyroid glands are exquisitely sensitive to small changes in the serum ionized calcium concentration. The integrated actions of PTH on calcium resorption from bone, distal renal tubular calcium reabsorption, and $1,25(OH)_2$ cholecalciferol (vitamin D; calcitriol)–mediated intestinal calcium absorption are responsible for the fine regulation of serum ionized calcium concentration. The precision in this integrated control is such that plasma ionized calcium

TABLE 17–1 SIGNS NOTED BY OWNERS OF DOGS WITH PRIMARY HYPOPARATHYROIDISM

Common

Muscle tremors, twitching, fasciculations
  (May be focal or diffuse)
  (Often worse with activity or excitement)
Facial rubbing (paresthesia?)
Generalized seizures (convulsions, "fits")
Rear leg muscle cramping or pain
Focal muscle fasciculations/twitching
Stiff gait
Behavior changes
  restless, nervous, "anxious"
  aggressive, biting
  hypersensitive (reluctant to be handled)
Poor appetite
Less active, listless
Intense biting or licking at paws (paresthesia?)

Uncommon

Weakness
Vomiting, diarrhea
Anorexia
Weight loss
Ataxia
Pyrexia
Prolapsed third eyelid (cats)
Ptyalism (cats)

Rare

None
Hypotension
Polydipsia or polyuria
Respiratory arrest or death

Note that almost all these signs are "episodic."

concentrations probably fluctuate day to day by no more than 0.1 mmol/L from their "set" normal value in healthy animals. The "acute" phases of bone resorption and distal renal tubular calcium reabsorption are major control sites in minute-to-minute calcium homeostasis. The effect of PTH on the distal renal tubule is quantitatively more important. Adjustments in the rate of intestinal calcium absorption via the calcium–PTH–vitamin D axis require approximately 24 to 48 hours to become maximal (Broadus, 1981).

Defense against hypocalcemia

THE CHALLENGES. The physiologic response to a hypocalcemic challenge can be characterized by several distinct categories of adjustment in mineral metabolism (Fig. 17-1). The classic challenges include (1) a minor, transient challenge, (2) a moderate challenge, and (3) a severe, prolonged challenge. Hypocalcemia elicits corrective homeostatic responses that are mediated by PTH and vitamin D. Acute effects occur in seconds to minutes, subacute or moderate effects occur over several hours and may last a few days, and chronic effects occur over days to weeks and longer (Rosol and Capen, 1997; Rosol et al, 2000).

MINOR, TRANSIENT CHALLENGE. A 12- to 15-hour fast (or consumption of a diet completely deficient in

calcium) in a normal mammal requires only subtle hormonal adjustments. The total quantity of calcium lost in the urine over this period is small. Negligible decreases in serum calcium concentration occur, causing a slight increase in PTH secretion. The dip in serum calcium concentration is corrected by this PTH-mediated increase in calcium reclamation efficiency from distal renal tubules and by rapid calcium resorptive responses from bone. Acute secretion of preformed PTH can maintain PTH concentrations for 1 to 1.5 hours during hypocalcemia. Hypocalcemia also decreases the proportion of PTH that is degraded in the parathyroid chief cells, making more hormone available for secretion. This effect typically occurs within 40 minutes. With increases in PTH secretion, renal calcium reabsorption and phosphorus excretion are enhanced within minutes, whereas bone mobilization of calcium and phosphate occurs over a period of 1 to 2 hours (Rosol et al, 2000). By 12 hours, only minor increases in $1,25(OH)_2$ vitamin D synthesis have occurred.

MODERATE CHALLENGE. An abrupt but significant reduction in dietary calcium intake (or other causes of hypocalcemia) initiates a series of adjustments in calcium metabolism, resulting in a new steady state of PTH secretion and vitamin D secretion. Several hours of persistent hypocalcemia increases PTH secretion, which in turn stimulates the synthesis and secretion of vitamin D (calcitriol). Calcitriol then increases intestinal transport of calcium and phosphorus into the vascular space, providing an external source of calcium that complements the internally mobilized calcium derived from bone. Hypocalcemia increases transcription of both the PTH gene and PTH mRNA, enhancing the ability of chief cells to produce PTH, a process that takes place within hours (Rosol et al, 2000).

Moderate increases in the secretion rate of PTH result in (1) increased calcium reabsorption from distal renal tubules, (2) increased mobilization of calcium and phosphorus from bone, and (3) increased synthesis of $1,25(OH)_2$ vitamin D (calcitriol), which participates with PTH in bone resorption and increases the efficiency of calcium and phosphorus absorption from the intestine (see Fig. 17-1). The increased concentrations of circulating PTH enhance renal excretion of phosphorus, thereby compensating for the increased amounts of phosphorus mobilized from bone and absorbed from the intestine. In this new steady state, the serum calcium concentration returns to normal, the serum phosphorus concentration is unchanged or slightly reduced, and a state of mild secondary hyperparathyroidism and enhanced intestinal mineral absorption efficiency exists. The initial requirement for calcium mobilization from the skeleton is largely replaced by the enhanced absorption of calcium from the intestine.

SEVERE, PROLONGED CHALLENGE. Significant lactation and chronic renal failure represent two examples of severe hypocalcemia-related challenges to calcium homeostasis that cannot be corrected by the processes

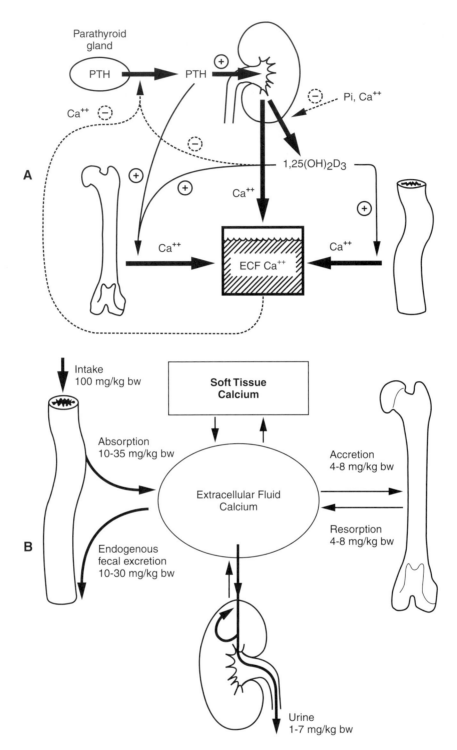

FIGURE 17-1. *A,* Regulation of extracellular fluid (ECF) calcium concentration by the effects of parathyroid hormone (PTH) and calcitriol (1,25-dihydroxyvitamin D$_3$) on gut, kidney, bone, and parathyroid gland. The principal effect of PTH is to increase the ECF calcium concentration by mobilizing calcium from bone, increasing tubular calcium reabsorption, and, indirectly on the gut, by increasing calcitriol synthesis. The principal effect of calcitriol is to increase intestinal absorption of calcium, but it also exerts negative regulatory control of PTH synthesis and further calcitriol synthesis. *B,* Normal calcium balance showing the major organs that supply or remove calcium from extracellular fluid: bone, gut, and kidney. Total calcium input into extracellular fluid equals total calcium leaving the extracellular space. (From Rosol et al, 2000.)

that are stimulated to occur within minutes or hours. Assuming that the four parathyroid glands are intact and functional, the previously described sequence of events resulting from "minor transient" and "moderate" challenges caused by hypocalcemia ensue. However, continuing losses of calcium into milk associated with lactation (for example) prevents complete compensation by the usual calcium–PTH–vitamin D absorption axis. Physiologic compensation in this setting includes (1) a maximal PTH secretion rate of approximately five times normal, (2) a maximal rate of $1,25(OH)_2$ vitamin D synthesis, and (3) initiation of maximal "rapid" and "late" phases of bone resorption in response to the combined effects of PTH and $1,25(OH)_2$ vitamin D.

Over days, weeks, or even longer periods of hypocalcemia, increases in PTH secretion, beyond those already described, are achieved largely via hypertrophy and hyperplasia of parathyroid gland chief cells (Roth and Capen, 1974; Rosol et al, 2000). Hypocalcemia directly stimulates the growth of parathyroid cells. This effect occurs regardless of vitamin D metabolite concentrations (Li et al, 1998; Malloy et al, 1999, Marx, 2000). With hyperplasia of parathyroid chief cells, PTH secretion rates approach 10 to 50 times normal. These circulating concentrations of PTH result in recruitment of an increasing osteoclast population and the incorporation of substantial bone surfaces into the resorption process. In the final steady state, serum calcium concentrations are maintained at the expense of the skeleton, and significant bone losses ensue. Thus the integrity of skeletal mineral homeostasis is sacrificed in an attempt to compensate for systemic mineral deficits (Broadus, 1981).

Hypoparathyroidism (Hypocalcemia)

Initial physiologic alterations

The pathologic and biochemical consequences of parathyroid gland removal (the most common cause of primary hypoparathyroidism) or loss of a critical number of parathyroid chief cells secondary to immune-mediated destruction (a less common phenomenon) can be appreciated by referring to the "butterfly" diagram (Fig. 17-2). In this condition, the right limbs of the three feedback loops predominate with (1) decreased bone resorption; (2) decreased renal phosphate excretion, increased serum phosphate, decreased calcitriol, and decreased intestinal absorption of calcium; and (3) increased renal excretion of calcium relative to the prevailing circulating concentrations of calcium. Typically, there is hypocalcemia and hyperphosphatemia, if dietary phosphate intake has been normal.

All of these changes can be explained by loss of PTH effects on various tissues. The processes that are not taking place include (1) mobilization of calcium and phosphate from bone, (2) retention of calcium and enhanced excretion of phosphate by kidneys, and (3) increased absorption of calcium and phosphate from intestine. An initial magnesium diuresis without significant change in plasma magnesium concentrations has also been observed in hypoparathyroidism. Urinary calcium is usually low unless eucalcemia has been restored with treatment. In the latter condition, urinary calcium is generally higher than it was before the development of hypoparathyroidism, and it occasionally reaches hypercalciuric levels (Arnaud, 1994).

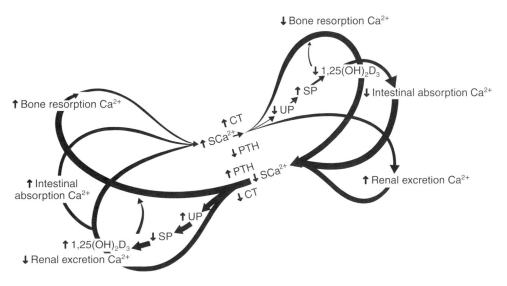

FIGURE 17-2. Regulation of calcium homeostasis. Three overlapping control loops interlock and relate to one another through the level of blood concentrations of ionic calcium, PTH, and CT. Each loop involves a calciotropic hormone target organ (bone, intestine, kidney). The limbs on the left depict physiologic events that increase the blood concentration of calcium (SCa^{2+}), and the limbs on the right, events that decrease this concentration. (*UP*, Urine phosphorus; *SP*, Serum phosphorus.) (Modified and reproduced with permission from Arnaud UD, 1994.)

In spite of dramatic changes in the concentration of plasma calcium and phosphate, bone mineralization is normal, bone resorption rates decline, and bone formation declines only slightly. Ultimately, bones are slightly more dense than normal in humans with hypoparathyroidism, and in long-standing cases, osteosclerosis may be seen. The major signs of hypoparathyroidism are directly attributable to decreases in circulating ionized calcium concentrations, which lead to increased neuromuscular excitability.

Neuromuscular activity

PERIPHERAL NEUROMUSCULAR DISORDERS. As discussed in Chapter 16, calcium ions are integral to the function of virtually all cells. However, although all cells in the body are affected by deficiencies in ionized calcium, clinical signs are most often associated with cells of the neuromuscular system simply because alteration in the function of these cells result in obvious visible abnormalities. Ionized calcium is involved in the release of acetylcholine during neuromuscular transmission. In addition, calcium is essential for muscle contractions and it stabilizes nerve cell membranes by decreasing their permeability to sodium. The role of calcium as a membrane stabilizer is most obvious during severe hypocalcemia, when insufficient stabilization exists.

When the extracellular fluid concentration of calcium ions declines below normal, the nervous system becomes progressively more excitable as a result of increases in neuronal membrane permeability. This increased excitability occurs both in the central nervous system (CNS) and in peripheral nerves, although the most obvious clinical signs are manifested peripherally. Nerve fibers may become so excitable that they begin to discharge spontaneously, initiating nerve impulses that pass to the peripheral skeletal muscles, where they elicit tetanic contraction ("cramps"). Consequently, hypocalcemia causes *tetany*, a random stiffening or tightening of various muscle groups. Nerve fibers seem particularly sensitive to decreases in calcium, in part because the signs are so acute, dramatic, and obvious. In fact, acute hypocalcemia usually results in death before effects in other major organ systems develop. Dogs with tetany that had previously undergone spinal cord transection at the thoracolumbar junction had classic signs of tetany above but not below the transection site (i.e., the rear legs were flaccid during the episodes of tetany). Thus tetany is initiated in the CNS, not peripherally (Arnaud, 1994).

Hypocalcemia is a relatively "common" laboratory abnormality, being observed on more than 13% of serum biochemical profiles in dogs in one report (Chew and Meuten, 1982). On the basis of *total* serum calcium concentration, hypocalcemia is usually defined as a concentration below 9.5 mg/dl in dogs and below 9 mg/dl in cats (Rosol et al, 2000). When serum ionized calcium concentration is used, hypocalcemia is generally defined as a concentration below 1.1 mmol/L in dogs and less than 1.0 mmol/L in cats. Clinical tetany, however, usually requires much lower serum calcium concentrations. For example, tetany can be assumed to exist whenever the serum total calcium concentration declines to or below 6 mg/dl or the serum ionized concentration to less than 0.7 mmol/L. These are values that are only 40% below normal. Total serum calcium concentrations below 4 mg/dl are frequently fatal.

Although dogs with untreated hypoparathyroidism consistently have abnormally decreased total serum calcium concentrations, the onset of *clinical* tetany is not entirely predictable. In studies on dogs undergoing total thyroparathyroidectomy, only approximately half developed tetany during a 96-hour period following the surgery. In each dog, however, the total serum calcium concentration decreased rapidly during the initial 24-hour postsurgical period. Why clinical tetany was not obvious in all the dogs was not understood. In our experience with dogs with primary *hyper*parathyroidism that have undergone surgical or alternative resolution of the condition, resulting in acute *hypo*parathyroidism, "clinical" signs of hypocalcemia have not always correlated with some absolute arbitrary serum calcium concentration. We tend to associate clinical signs with total calcium concentrations below 6 to 7 mg/dl and ionized serum calcium concentrations below 0.7 to 0.8 mmol/L. However, some dogs have had clinical signs with serum concentrations above these values, and others below our critical levels have had no signs. Without doubt, physical activity plays a role in development of clinical tetany. A quiet dog is much less likely than an active dog to exhibit signs at any low serum concentration of calcium. Individual variation, however, is the only consistent feature of this condition.

Calcium concentrations within cerebrospinal fluid (CSF) do not decrease as rapidly as serum concentrations in parathyroidectomized dogs. Although the serum total calcium concentration decreases as much as 27% (ionized calcium, 28%) within 24 hours of surgery, decreases in CSF total calcium concentration are less than 5% (ionized calcium, less than 10%). Rapid equilibrium does not occur between plasma and CSF ionic values. Thus the concentration of calcium ions in the CSF is relatively constant despite large fluctuations in plasma concentrations. However, relatively small changes in CSF calcium concentration may also result in dramatic changes in clinical appearance.

When serum calcium concentrations decline to abnormal levels, but not low enough to cause obvious clinical tetany, a physical state of "latent tetany" may exist. This condition is described as one in which an individual can progress from appearing clinically normal to becoming "tetanic" with minimal stimulation. Such a condition can be demonstrated to be present in people by weakly stimulating a nerve and observing an abnormal response (see Physical Examination, page 723). If a human with latent tetany hyperventilates, the resulting alkalinization of the body fluids can increase nerve irritability, causing overt signs of tetany. It is assumed that a similar situations develop in hypocalcemic dogs or cats.

In hypocalcemic pet dogs, latent tetany occurs, but the problem is less well documented. Owners mention that sudden excitement, activity, or petting may unpredictably cause muscle cramping, lameness, facial rubbing, pain, irritability, or aggressive behavior. These signs usually disappear quickly, only to recur sporadically. In addition, the nontetanic severely hypocalcemic pet is usually described by the owner as having a change in personality. These dogs are often observed to have poor appetites and to be irritable, nonplayful, and slow-moving. Frequently, owners report that the dogs "seem to be in pain." Such signs are vague, but after hypocalcemia is diagnosed, the clinical signs are consistent with those of an animal in latent tetany. The various disturbances are completely and quickly reversible with therapy.

THE HEART. In experimental animals, severe decreases in serum calcium concentration can result in marked dilatation of the heart, changes in cellular enzyme activities, and in increased membrane permeability in cells outside the nervous system. Calcium has both positive inotropic and chronotropic cardiac effects (Milnor, 1980). Hypocalcemia prolongs action potential duration in cardiac cells. This may result in decreased force of myocardial contraction (negative inotropic effect) and, in severe cases, bradycardia (negative chronotropic effect). An associated increase is seen electrocardiographically in the duration of the S-T and Q-T segments. The duration of the T wave itself is not altered with hypocalcemia. Although these disturbances in physical findings and the electrocardiogram (ECG) can be pronounced in humans, they are much less obvious in the hypocalcemic dog (Kornegay et al, 1980; Sherding et al, 1980). Rarely, hypocalcemia can cause a 2:1 heart block or heart failure requiring digitalis and diuretics in humans (Arnaud and Kolb, 1983).

Miscellaneous effects of hypocalcemia

Because calcium serves as a cofactor in both the intrinsic and extrinsic blood clotting systems, coagulopathies are theoretically possible in hypocalcemia. In hypocalcemic humans, disorders less common and less dramatic than tetany may be encountered, including (1) basal ganglia calcification and occasional extrapyramidal neurologic syndromes; (2) papilledema and increased intracranial pressure; (3) psychiatric disorders; (4) skin, hair, and fingernail abnormalities; (5) candidal infections; (6) inhibition of normal dental development; (7) lenticular cataracts; (8) intestinal malabsorption; and (9) increased serum concentrations of creatine phosphokinase and lactic dehydrogenase (Arnaud, 1994).

CLINICAL FEATURES OF NATURALLY OCCURRING HYPOPARATHYROIDISM IN DOGS

Signalment

Review of the records of 37 dogs we have seen with naturally occurring primary hypoparathyroidism (includes Bruyette and Feldman, 1988) and of reports

of an additional 13 dogs with hypoparathyroidism obtained from the veterinary literature (Table 17-2) reveals several characteristics of the syndrome. Hypoparathyroidism occurs at any age, the youngest dog being 6 weeks and the oldest being 13 years (Fig. 17-3). The average age was 4.8 years. Of the 50 dogs, 30 (60%) were female. The breeds most frequently identified as having primary hypoparathyroidism were Toy Poodles, Labrador Retrievers, Miniature Schnauzers, German Shepherds, and Terriers).

Anamnesis

DURATION OF ILLNESS. The clinical course in the 37 dogs of our series consisted of an abrupt onset of

TABLE 17–2 BREEDS IDENTIFIED AS HAVING PRIMARY, NATURALLY OCCURRING HYPOPARATHYROIDISM

Breed	Number of Dogs (Total = 50)*
Toy Poodle	10
Labrador Retriever	6
Miniature Schnauzer	5
German Shepherd dog	5
Terrier breeds	5
Beagle	2
Dachshund	2
Golden Retriever	2
English Pointer	1
Collie	1
Keeshond	1
Cocker Spaniel	1
Malamute	1
Irish Wolfhound	1
Siberian Husky	1
Mixed breed	6

*Includes 37 dogs from our series and 4 dogs from Kornegay et al, 1980; 6 dogs from Sherding et al, 1980; 1 dog from Meyer and Tyrrell, 1976; 1 dog from Burk and Schaubhut, 1975, and 1 dog from Crawford and Dunstan, 1985.

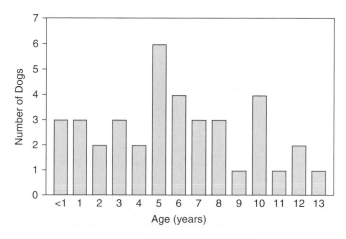

FIGURE 17-3. The ages of 38 dogs at the time of primary hypoparathyroidism diagnosis. These include 25 dogs in our series, as well as 4 dogs from Kornegay et al, 1980; 1 dog from Crawford and Dunstan, 1985; 6 dogs from Sherding et al, 1980; 1 dog from Meyer and Tyrrell, 1976; and 1 dog from Burk and Schaubhut, 1975.

intermittent neurologic or neuromuscular disturbances (see Table 17-1). In at least 20 dogs, owners noted that signs were initiated or worsened by excitement or exercise. The signs associated with hypocalcemia had been observed for periods of 1 day in some dogs to as long as 12 months in others. Only 8 of the 37 dogs had signs for longer than 14 days before the diagnosis was made and therapy initiated. The 8 dogs with prolonged illness had been symptomatic for 1 to 12 months and had been diagnosed and treated for nonspecific seizure disorders without the benefit of pretreatment laboratory testing. The dogs with signs for more than several days invariably had neuromuscular disturbances that became progressively more frequent and violent despite administration of anticonvulsant medication.

EARLY SIGNS. Most owners reported that one of their first observations (retrospectively) was that their pet appeared abnormally "tense," "nervous," or "anxious." Also retrospectively, owners noted that their dogs would intensely use their paws to rub their faces or the dog would use the ground for rubbing their faces (discussed below). Some owners noted their dogs intensely licking or chewing their paws. Although these signs were common, they were either not mentioned by owners until specifically questioned or were noted as having disappeared after treatment had been instituted.

The signs observed by owners that resulted in their seeking veterinary care were varied. The most common cause for seeking veterinary care was apparent grand mal convulsions (discussed in the next section). Owners also sought veterinary care after seeing apparent muscle cramping, tonic spasm of leg muscles, or pain in the legs. Focal muscle twitching, generalized tremors, fasciculations, or trembling was frequently observed. A stiff, stilted, hunched, or rigid gait was noted by most owners. Owners also commonly described their pets as having poor appetites or as being "slow," "less playful," or "not as friendly."

Nervousness is probably an expression of tetany exaggerated by adrenergic secretions. Aggressive behavior is assumed to be caused by the pain associated with muscle cramping. The muscle cramping could be elicited by petting, thus explaining why dogs that previously suffered acute pain from such a mild stimulus are reluctant to be handled. This accounts for the observations of dogs appearing to be less friendly or for their change in behavior or personality.

SEIZURES. Grand mal convulsions were observed by the owners in 32 of our 37 dogs with naturally occurring primary hypoparathyroidism. As previously reported, most of these dogs had typical grand mal convulsions. However, some seizures were atypical, in that the dogs either did not appear to lose consciousness or were not incontinent during the episode (Peterson, 1986). Of interest was the incidence of seizure activity seen by veterinarians. Of the 37 dogs, 32 were observed by a veterinarian to have seizures (often being suspected of having idiopathic epilepsy) or to be "in tetany." This represents a much higher

incidence of veterinarian-witnessed neuromuscular disorders than expected with idiopathic epilepsy. The neuromuscular problems became so severe that several dogs, although not having active obvious seizure activity, were not able to stand or walk. Also, as noted by other investigators (Sherding et al, 1980), the muscle tremors during some episodes began in one limb and gradually became generalized and progressively more violent, finally culminating in a generalized seizure. In some dogs, seizure episodes were as brief as 30 to 90 seconds; in others, they lasted for more than 30 minutes. Most, but not all, of the generalized seizures spontaneously abated.

MISCELLANEOUS SIGNS. As can be seen in Table 17-1, many owners observed overlapping neurologic and neuromuscular signs. It can be safely stated, retrospectively, that each dog suffered bouts of significant hypocalcemic tetany as a part of their initial signs. Some vague signs included panting, ataxia, episodic weakness, complete anorexia, vomiting, diarrhea, and weight loss. Veterinarians noted fever, a problem not observed by owners. Previously described signs of circling and/or disorientation (Sherding et al, 1980) were not observed in our group of 37 hypocalcemic dogs. All of our owners observed some clinical signs; failure to see any sign, reported by others, was not noted. Although hypocalcemia was almost always considered a serendipitous finding on laboratory testing, it remains an abnormality that "made sense" after being demonstrated. Death remains a potential sequela of untreated hypocalcemia but is quite uncommon.

FACIAL RUBBING. Of the 37 dogs in our series, 23 were observed to paw or rub violently at their muzzles, eyes, and ears and to rub their muzzles on the ground. Alternatively, owners noted their dogs intensely licking or chewing at their paws. These signs are thought to result from the pain associated with masseter and temporal muscle cramping caused by the hypocalcemia or as a result of the "tingling" sensation around the mouth or at the distal extremities. Classic signs of hypocalcemia in humans include "paresthesias," defined as numbness and tingling that often occur around the mouth, in the tips of fingers, and sometimes in the feet (Arnaud, 1994). Dogs, assuredly, suffer these same sensations, which may account for facial rubbing as well as biting of their feet (see Table 17-1).

HYPERVENTILATION. Because of the acute anxiety or pain associated with tetany, hypoparathyroid humans (and presumably dogs) may episodically hyperventilate and secrete increased amounts of epinephrine. Hyperventilation causes hypocapnia and alkalosis, which worsen hypocalcemia by causing increased binding of ionic calcium to plasma proteins. Prolonged hyperventilation in normal human subjects can cause a decrease in the serum ionic calcium concentration. It is almost impossible, however, for tetany to be caused solely by hyperventilation (Arnaud and Kolb, 1983).

EPISODIC NATURE OF THE ILLNESS. All neurologic and neuromuscular signs in our hypocalcemic dogs were episodic in nature. Episodes of apparent or confirmed hypocalcemic tetany were followed by asymptomatic periods. The periods of clinical well-being lasted minutes to days. Tetany was rather unpredictable, although retrospectively, these signs were much more frequent or inducible with exercise (even slow or short "leash" walks), excitement, petting ("latent tetany"?), or stress (being taken to the veterinarian).

All the dogs were persistently hypocalcemic but displayed tetany only episodically. This illustrates some adaptation in each dog to hypocalcemia and suggests that relatively minor alterations in these calcium concentrations would result in profound clinical signs. One dog in our series had been diagnosed as having primary hypoparathyroidism but remained untreated for almost a year because of owner reluctance to treat. This dog was persistently hypocalcemic but had only one or two clinically obvious hypocalcemic episodes monthly. In spite of this tragic history, the dog was relatively well, suffering primarily from a poor appetite and weight loss.

Physical Examination

GENERAL OBSERVATIONS. Other than signs related to hypocalcemia, dogs with primary hypoparathyroidism do not have other abnormalities on physical examination. Findings on physical examination performed on the 37 hypoparathyroid dogs varied (Table 17-3). Numerous dogs were in tetany on presentation. Most of the time this was an observation made after serum biochemical results were reviewed. Alternatively, 33 of the 37 dogs were referred for evaluation of hypocalcemia and the veterinarian who examined the dog initially (usually one of us) was "primed" to observe tetany. These observations (almost all of which are noted in Table 17-3), although impressive to the uninitiated, may not have been made had the history not alerted us to the underlying condition.

Five of the dogs appeared healthy, despite their previous history of neurologic or neuromuscular disorders. A few dogs were thin, and several growled when examined. Retrospectively, the growling dogs were in pain or were anticipating that handling would cause them pain, because after resolution of hypocalcemia, each became friendly. Cardiac abnormalities were apparent in 16 dogs on the initial examination. These abnormalities consisted of paroxysmal tachyarrhythmias suspected in 13 dogs and muffled heart sounds with weak pulses noted in 3 dogs.

SPONTANEOUS NEUROLOGIC AND NEUROMUSCULAR SIGNS. On initial examination, 32 of the 37 dogs with primary hypoparathyroidism had at least one abnormality that could be attributed to hypocalcemia. Most of these dogs (18) had convulsions. Others growled, were extremely tense or "rigid," or had "splinted" abdomens, stiff gaits, and/or muscle fasciculations. Virtually every time that a dog growled, the owner would comment that this was a "new behavior," one they had noticed at home as well. Retrospectively, these dogs were either in pain or they were anticipating pain from contact. Fever was noted in 26 of the 37 dogs.

Thirty-two of the 37 dogs had at least one convulsion during the initial 48 to 96 hours of hospitalization. Complete neurologic examinations were attempted on 30 dogs. These 30 examinations revealed a variety of problems. By far the most commonly reported disorder was that "the dog was too tense and nervous to complete a thorough evaluation." Retrospectively, these dogs were recognized to have been in tetany. Other findings included brisk reflexes, absent reflexes, clonus, and/or pain. Because these dogs were in latent or active tetany, their neurologic examinations were difficult to interpret until hypocalcemia was identified on laboratory testing.

INDUCED NEUROLOGIC OR NEUROMUSCULAR SIGNS. Two physical tests are used in humans as aids in diagnosing latent tetany (hypocalcemia). *Chvostek's sign* is elicited by tapping the facial nerve just anterior to the ear lobe. A positive sign is one of extensive facial muscle twitching or muscle contraction. *Trousseau's sign* is induced with a blood pressure cuff inflated above systolic blood pressure for at least 2 minutes. A positive response consists of carpal spasm, at least 5 to 10 seconds in duration, after release of the cuff or while the cuff is inflated (Arnaud, 1994; Meininger and Kendler, 2000). Although not well described in the dog, episodes of intense muscle spasm have been stimulated when testing reflexes in hypocalcemic dogs.

CATARACTS. Posterior lenticular cataract formation is the most common sequela of hypoparathyroidism in humans (Arnaud, 1994). Cataracts seen in hypoparathyroid human patients must be present and developing for 5 to 10 years before visual impairment occurs. Fully mature cataracts are confluent and produce total lens opacity. Successful treatment of hypocalcemia generally halts the progression of cataracts (Arnaud, 1994).

TABLE 17-3 INITIAL PHYSICAL EXAMINATION FINDINGS IN 37 DOGS WITH NATURALLY OCCURRING PRIMARY HYPOPARATHYROIDISM

Sign	Number of Dogs
Seizure or "in tetany"	
Initial examination	18
In first 4 days of hospitalization	32
Fever	26
Tense, splinted abdomen	24
Stiff gait	23
Thin	22
Generalized muscle fasciculations	21
Growling	21
Cardiac abnormalities	
Tachyarrhythmia	13
Muffled heart sounds/weak pulse	3
Neurologic examination difficult to complete and interpret	30/30
Cataracts	12
No abnormality	5

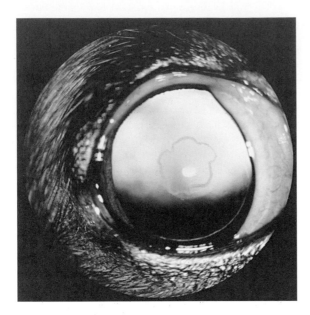

FIGURE 17-4. Lenticular cataract in the lens of a hypoparathyroid dog.

Cataracts were seen in 12 of the 37 dogs in our series and were first reported in 2 hypoparathyroid dogs in 1980 (Kornegay et al, 1980). Similar cataracts have been reported in several cats and were noted in 2 of the 5 cats with primary hypoparathyroidism in our series. These cataracts have been small punctate to linear white opacities in the anterior and posterior cortical subcapsular region. The opacities are randomly distributed along the lens fibers and are separated from the capsule by an intervening zone of normal thin cortex (Fig. 17-4). There has been no loss of vision. Other ocular signs not yet reported in dogs include papilledema, optic neuritis, conjunctivitis, keratitis, blepharospasm, loss of lashes, strabismus, nystagmus, and anisocoria.

CLINICAL FEATURES OF NATURALLY OCCURRING HYPOPARATHYROIDISM IN CATS

Nine cats with naturally occurring primary hypoparathyroidism have been reported in the veterinary literature, and we have seen five cats in our practice. Although this disease is not common, clinically and biochemically the syndrome is indistinguishable from iatrogenic destruction or removal of parathyroids in hyperthyroid cats undergoing surgery of the neck. Therefore this information is important, because an increasing number of veterinarians encounter hypoparathyroidism as an iatrogenic condition.

The clinical features of the 14 cats with naturally occurring hypoparathyroidism are much like those reported in humans and dogs except that a majority of the cats (9) have been male. The cats were 6 months to 7 years of age at the time of diagnosis and several breeds were represented. The clinical course of each cat was characterized by an abrupt or gradual onset of intermittent neurologic or neuromuscular disturbances, which included focal or generalized muscle tremors, seizures, ataxia, stilted gait, disorientation, and weakness. Other commonly observed abnormalities included lethargy, anorexia, panting, and raised nictitating membranes. Less commonly, dysphagia, pruritus, and ptyalism were observed by their owners. Physical examination findings included depression, weakness, fever, hypothermia, bradycardia, and mild to severe dehydration. Lenticular cataracts were detected in several of these cats (Forbes et al, 1990; Parker, 1991; Peterson et al, 1991; Bassett, 1998; Ruopp, 2001).

DIAGNOSTIC EVALUATION: ROUTINE STUDIES

Calcium

Hypocalcemia was a serendipitous finding in each of our 37 dogs with primary, naturally occurring hypoparathyroidism. Each dog had a history consistent with a behavioral, neurologic, muscular, or neuromuscular disorder. Therefore a database consisting of a complete blood count, urinalysis, and serum chemistry profile was deemed necessary in the evaluation of each dog. Each dog was severely and persistently hypocalcemic (Table 17-4). Since severe hypocalcemia (serum calcium concentration <6.5 mg/dl) is an unusual finding in our clinic population, this parameter was invariably rechecked with a separate blood sample. Then, because therapy for hypocalcemia was quickly instituted, each dog had its serum calcium concentration monitored three to five times during the first 72 hours of hospitalization. In no dog was the serum calcium concentration greater than 6.5 mg/dl until therapy began to have an effect. Since ionized plasma concentrations became routinely available, these values were also assessed. As can be noted from results reported in Table 17-4, each dog with primary hypoparathyroidism was profoundly deficient in the ionized fraction of calcium, as well as being deficient in the total fraction of calcium.

"Corrected" Calcium Values

Calcium in plasma or serum exists in three forms or fractions: ionized (free calcium), complexed or chelated (bound to phosphate, bicarbonate, sulfate, citrate, and lactate), and protein-bound (Fig. 17-5). In general, between 50% and 60% of total calcium is ionized in normal animals. In clinically normal dogs, protein-bound, complexed, and ionized calcium account for approximately 34%, 10%, and 56% of the total serum calcium, respectively (Schenck et al, 1996). Laboratories generally measure these components together and report them as a *total* calcium value.

TABLE 17–4 PERTINENT FINDINGS IN DOGS WITH PRIMARY HYPOPARATHYROIDISM

Dog	Age (Years)	Gender	Duration of Signs (Days)	Serum Calcium (mg/dl)	Serum Phosphorus (mg/dl)	Serum Magnesium (mg/dl)	BUN (mg/dl)	Plasma Ionized Ca (mmol/L)	PTH (pmol/L)	Parathyroid Histology
1	5	F/S	3	5.7	7.3	–	14	–	–	–
2	5	F/S	30	4.1	5.4	1.9	31	–	–	–
3	5	M	30	4.7	6.0	–	8	–	–	–
4	4	F	7	4.5	5.9	1.2	17	–	–	–
5	10	F/S	1	5.2	7.0	2.1	15	–	–	Lymphocytic parathyroiditis
6	11	F/S	3	5.6	8.9	–	4	–	–	–
7	1	F	14	4.2	9.8	–	20	–	–	–
8	5	M	180	5.7	10.2	–	12	–	–	–
9	10	F	3	5.5	7.2	1.9	9	–	–	–
10	1	M	1	5.2	7.8	–	19	–	–	–
11	10	M	11	4.9	5.9	1.8	10	–	1.0	Lymphocytic parathyroiditis
12	10	M	1	6.0	6.3	–	13	–	0.1	Lymphocytic parathyroiditis
13	4	F/S	14	3.9	4.9	1.9	16	–	0.1	–
14	7	F/S	10	6.0	8.3	2.3	12	–	1.0	Lymphocytic parathyroiditis
15	9	M	4	3.6	5.8	–	0	–	0.05	–
16	0.5	F/S	2	3.9	8.4	1.9	11	–	0.1	–
17	13	M	6	4.2	7.1	–	15	–	0.1	Lymphocytic parathyroiditis
18	1	F/S	7	5.1	8.7	1.2	14	–	0.1	Lymphocytic parathyroiditis
19	0.5	F/S	7	4.8	10.2	2.0	22	–	–	Lymphocytic parathyroiditis
20	2	M	45	4.4	7.4	2.1	16	–	0.1	–
21	3	F/S	9	5.1	6.8	–	25	–	0.5	–
22	6	M	360	5.1	8.8	2.2	23	0.4	0.1	Lymphocytic parathyroiditis
23	8	M	3	3.9	8.3	1.9	19	0.3	0.5	–
24	12	F/S	2	4.6	8.5	2.3	18	0.5	0.1	–
25	6	M	3	5.5	8.5	2.2	19	0.5	0.7	Fibrous tissue
26	5	M	2	5.6	7.6	–	23	0.5	1.1	Fibrous tissue
27	4	F	28	4.6	6.1	2.1	27	0.4	0.8	–
28	11	M	1	5.5	7.1	1.5	20	0.7	1.1	–
29	5	M	60	5.6	10.1	1.9	22	0.5	0.1	Lymphocytic parathyroiditis
30	1	M	1	5.1	7.3	–	19	0.4	–	–
31	10	M	9	5.9	6.1	2.0	26	0.5	0.1	Lymphocytic parathyroiditis
32	7	F/S	32	5.9	6.2	1.9	20	0.4	1.6	–
33	0.75	M	2	3.8	9.1	1.6	25	0.2	–	–
34	1	M	4	5.0	8.8	2.2	18	0.4	0.4	Fibrous tissue
35	2	M	5	4.3	7.9	–	26	0.4	1.0	–
36	6	M	320	5.0	9.0	2.2	17	0.3	1.7	–
37	12	F/S	3	4.5	8.1	–	27	0.3	1.2	–
Mean	6	–	30	4.8	7.6	1.9	15.6	0.3	0.4	–
Reference range	–	–	–	8.9–11.4	3.0–4.7	1.8–2.4	12–28	1.0–1.4	2–13	–

M, Male; *F*, female; *S*, spay/ovariohysterectomy.

Ionized calcium is the biologically active component, and the protein-bound calcium serves as a "reservoir" or storage pool for the ionized fraction. However, changes in serum concentration of albumin and globulins may alter the measured total serum calcium concentration without altering ionized calcium levels. Despite an alteration in the total amount of plasma calcium resulting from hyperproteinemia or hypoproteinemia, the biologically active ionized calcium concentration remains normal because of homeostatic mechanisms. Any dog or cat with hypocalcemia must be checked for hypoproteinemia and/or hypoalbuminemia (Chew and Meuten, 1983).

Two formulas were developed for use in dogs to account for changes in the reported serum calcium value attributed to changes in serum protein values (Meuten et al, 1982). The formulas were of significant value prior to routine availability of ionized calcium assays. These formulas are:

Corrected Total Ca (mg/dl) =
Measured Total Ca (mg/dl) – albumin (g/dl) + 3.5

Extracellular Calcium

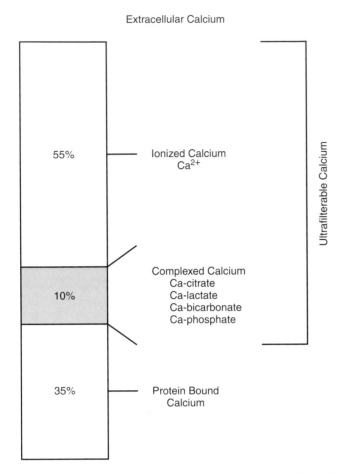

FIGURE 17-5. Serum total calcium concentration consists of ionized (free), complexed, and protein-bound fractions.

or

Corrected total Ca (mg/dl) =
  Measured total Ca (mg/dl) −
    [0.4 × total protein (g/dl)] + 3.3

Hypoalbuminemia is a common explanation for apparent hypocalcemia. However, it is the least important, causes no clinical signs, and is associated with only mild changes from reference ranges. While correction to normal limits implies that the ionized fraction is normal, the ionized fraction may yet be low. These formulas, developed more than 2 decades ago, were derived from serum albumin concentrations obtained with analytical methods no longer employed by modern automated analyzers. The normal range for serum albumin concentration reported then (Meuten et al, 1982) was considerably lower than those reported now. At the time, a positive correlation was noted, but only 33% of the variability in serum total calcium concentration could be attributed to serum albumin concentration and only 17% of the variability could be attributed to serum total protein. There was no association in cats between serum total protein and serum calcium concentrations, and only 18% of the

variability in total calcium concentration could be attributed to albumin concentration (Flanders et al, 1989). In another study, only 17% and 29% of the variability in total serum calcium concentration in dogs and cats, respectively, could be attributed to serum albumin concentration (Bienzle et al, 1993). For these reasons, use of these correction formulas are not recommended (Rosol et al, 2000).

Serum albumin concentrations (and total serum protein values) were normal in each of our 37 dogs with primary hypoparathyroidism. Using the formulas for correcting the serum calcium concentration did not alter the finding of severe hypocalcemia in any dog.

Serum Phosphorus

The diagnosis of hypoparathyroidism is strongly supported if both hypocalcemia and hyperphosphatemia are identified. As can be seen in Table 17-4, each dog with hypoparathyroidism in our series had a serum phosphorus concentration higher than its total calcium concentration, and all had a normal blood urea nitrogen (BUN). The absence of an absolute hyperphosphatemia in some of the dogs can be explained in part by the wide variation in what is considered "normal" by veterinary laboratories. Normal values usually include results from all ages, and young dogs usually have a relative hyperphosphatemia. Their serum phosphorus concentrations gradually decline until puberty, at which time the levels remain relatively constant. In addition, some hypoparathyroid dogs may be relatively phosphate-depleted because of dietary restriction or inappetence.

Remainder of the Chemistry Panel

The diagnosis of primary hypoparathyroidism in the dog is made "by exclusion." In other words, one must develop a complete differential diagnosis for hypocalcemia and then proceed to rule out the various causes of severe hypocalcemia. In this regard, a complete database is imperative when evaluating any nonlactating hypocalcemic animal. It has been suggested that hypoparathyroidism is the only possible diagnosis when one encounters a combination of low serum calcium concentration, increased serum phosphorous concentration, normal renal function, and a decreased (relative or absolute) serum PTH concentration (Rosol et al, 2000).

As will be discussed under Differential Diagnosis, there are three potential causes of hypoparathyroidism: suppressed secretion of PTH without parathyroid gland destruction (Dhupa and Proulx, 1998); sudden correction of chronic hypercalcemia in which the remaining parathyroid glands are severely atrophied; and absence or destruction of the parathyroid glands. In our experience, severe atrophy or destruction of the parathyroid glands is most common in dogs and cats. In reviewing the remaining routine laboratory tests performed on hypoparathyroid dogs, abnormalities were not seen. Therefore the only significant alterations were hypocalcemia in all patients and hyperphosphatemia in most.

Laboratory Testing of Cats

Laboratory testing in 14 cats (9 reported cases and 5 in our series) with naturally occurring primary hypoparathyroidism demonstrated severe hypocalcemia in each cat (range: 2.5 to 4.2 mg/dl). Serum phosphate concentrations were inappropriately increased in each cat (range: 5.2 to 19 mg/dl). Serum protein, albumin, urea nitrogen, creatinine, and magnesium concentrations were normal in each cat tested (Forbes et al, 1990; Parker, 1991; Peterson et al, 1991; Bassett, 1998; Ruopp, 2001).

Electrocardiogram

Hypocalcemia prolongs the duration of the action potential in cardiac cells, resulting in an increased duration of the S-T and Q-T segments. A good correlation exists between severity of hypocalcemia and duration of the S-T segment. Most of the hypocalcemic dogs in our series had no clinical evidence of cardiovascular disease. For this reason, only a few dogs were assessed electrocardiographically. The findings most consistent with hypocalcemia included (1) deep, wide T waves, (2) prolonged Q-T intervals, and (3) bradycardia. When the ECGs during hypocalcemia were compared with those taken following restoration of normal calcium concentrations, the R waves appeared taller during hypocalcemia (Fig. 17-6). No obvious ECG explanation could be found for the arrhythmias, weak pulses, or muffled heart sounds that were noted on several physical examinations.

Magnesium

Hypocalcemia, hyperphosphatemia, and a state of functional hypoparathyroidism and/or PTH resistance may be observed in humans with magnesium depletion and hypomagnesemia. Some individuals have low to undetectable serum PTH concentrations. In this setting, significant abnormalities in serum calcium and phosphorus concentrations are usually confined to patients with severe hypomagnesemia (serum magnesium concentration <1.2 mg/dl). Hypomagnesemia has a variety of well-recognized causes in humans (Table 17-5). The efficiency of renal tubular magnesium reabsorption is such that experimental magnesium depletion cannot be produced in humans by a deficient magnesium intake (Broadus, 1981). The magnesium depletion that has been described in severe protein-calorie malnutrition in children appears to result from multiple mechanisms. Excessive losses of magnesium-containing intestinal fluids, as occurs with prolonged diarrhea or nasogastric suction, may

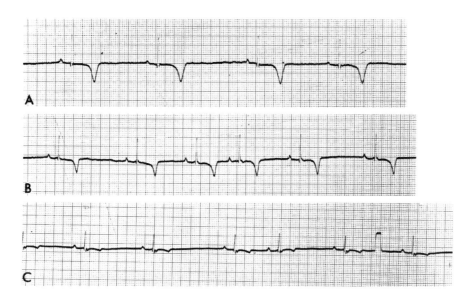

FIGURE 17-6. ECG illustrating various stages in the treatment of a dog with hypocalcemia secondary to primary hypoparathyroidism. *A,* The serum calcium level was 4.0 mg/dl. On this ECG, prolonged S-T and Q-T segments are obvious. The T wave itself is prolonged and deep. At this time the serum potassium (4.3 mEq/L), sodium (147 mEq/L), and chloride (103 mEq/L) levels were normal. The inorganic phosphorus level was 4.9 mg/dl. *B,* ECG taken when the serum calcium level was 6.2 mg/dl. The S-T, Q-T, and T wave durations are diminished, as is the T wave amplitude. *C,* ECG taken of the dog with a normal serum calcium level of 9.7 mg/dl. The S-T, Q-T, and T waves are normal. The three ECGs also suggest a diminishing R wave amplitude as the serum calcium level rises to normal.

TABLE 17–5 RECOGNIZED CAUSES OF HYPOMAGNESEMIA AND MAGNESIUM DEPLETION IN HUMANS

Decreased intake and/or absorption
  Protein-calorie malnutrition
  Magnesium-free fluid therapy
  Magnesium-free total parenteral nutrition
Gastrointestinal disorders
  Prolonged nasogastric suction
  Chronic diarrhea
  Malabsorption syndromes
  Extensive bowel resection, intestinal fistulas
Renal losses
  Chronic parenteral fluid therapy without magnesium
  Nonazotemic renal tubular dysfunction (see text)
  Loop and osmotic diuretics
  Hypercalcemia
  Hypokalemia
  Alcohol
Metabolic
  Hypercalcemia
  Hypophosphatemia
Endocrine
  Diabetes mellitus, insulin therapy
  Hyperthyroidism
  Primary hyperparathyroidism
  Primary and secondary hyperaldosteronism
  Hyperadrenocorticism
  Inappropriate secretion of antidiuretic hormone
Redistribution
  Pancreatitis
  Hyperadrenergic states
  Massive blood transfusion
  Hypothermia
  Acute respiratory alkalosis
  Sepsis
Other
  Burns
  Excessive lactation
  Excessive sweating

lead to magnesium depletion, particularly in patients receiving only parenteral fluids lacking magnesium supplements.

People with various intestinal disorders associated with small bowel malabsorption and/or steatorrhea may develop magnesium depletion. Responsible mechanisms include formation of magnesium soaps with unabsorbed fatty acids and losses of magnesium in intestinal fluids. Hypomagnesemia, with or without related symptoms, has been reported in as many as one-third of patients with malabsorption. Primary infantile hypomagnesemia is a rare autosomal recessive disorder that appears to be caused by a specific abnormality in intestinal magnesium absorption.

Decreased renal tubular magnesium reabsorption and hypomagnesemia have been reported in a minority of human patients during the diuretic phase of acute renal tubular necrosis and in patients with renal tubular acidosis, pyelonephritis, hydronephrosis, and other predominantly nonazotemic renal disorders. Impaired magnesium reabsorption and hypomagnesemia have also been observed as a component of gentamicin nephrotoxicity and following cisplatin chemotherapy. Virtually all diuretics increase magnesium excretion, but symptomatic hypomagnesemia also occurs in patients with primary hyperaldosteronism and those with various states of secondary hyperaldosteronism.

The osmotic diuresis associated with diabetic ketoacidosis (DKA) can be associated with significant urinary losses of magnesium. The time course for the development of hypomagnesemia in response to treatment of ketoacidosis is similar to that for decreasing serum potassium and phosphorus concentrations. Normal pretreatment magnesium concentrations may decrease to less than 1 mg/dl during the first 24 hours of insulin therapy. Treatment-associated hypomagnesemia occurs in approximately 50% of these people, and magnesium supplementation is now included in the routine management of DKA.

Hyperthyroidism is associated with negative magnesium balance and a tendency to develop hypomagnesemia. The responsible mechanisms are not entirely clear but appear to include bone resorption and altered distribution of magnesium into soft tissues.

Serum magnesium concentrations were determined in 23 of the 37 hypoparathyroid dogs listed in Table 17-4. In 19 dogs, the serum magnesium concentration was normal, with 4 dogs being hypomagnesemic. The significance of these four cases of hypomagnesemia is not known because specific magnesium therapy was not undertaken. However, hypocalcemia in people with concurrent hypomagnesemia is often refractory to calcium therapy unless magnesium is administered first (Hansen, 2000). In humans, symptoms of hypomagnesemia do not usually occur at serum levels of magnesium above 1.5 mg/dl. However, even at serum magnesium levels below 1.0 mg/dl, overt symptoms are not observed in all patients.

Poor quantitative relationships between testing and clinical relevance are the limitations created by having only 0.3% of total body magnesium stores in plasma or serum. Serum magnesium concentrations may be normal or high in the presence of intracellular depletion. Although serum concentrations routinely decrease during deficiency conditions, this test remains a weak predictor of magnesium status. While serum testing is least expensive and most convenient, most authorities recognize the inaccuracies associated with such assessments. Furthermore, interest in measuring serum ionized magnesium concentration has involved expensive equipment or facilities not widely available. In addition, the value and meaning of these assays, as compared with measurement of total magnesium concentration in animals is not known, nor are the various tissue assays (red cell, whole blood, bone, etc.) well understood (Hansen, 2000).

The definitive methods for measurement of serum magnesium concentration are "isotope dilution" and "mass spectrometry." The reference method established by the National Reference System for Clinical Laboratories of the National Committee for Clinical

Laboratory Standards is flame atomic absorption spectrometry (FAAS) (Elin, 1994). Most commercial laboratories utilize colorimetric assays, using primarily calmagite or methylthymol blue as a chromophore. Such assays are more susceptible to interference by other compounds (Hansen, 2000).

DIAGNOSTIC EVALUATION: PARATHYROID HORMONE (PTH) CONCENTRATIONS

Clinical usefulness

HUMANS. Measurement of serum PTH concentration is crucial to the correct diagnosis of potential parathyroid gland disorders in humans (Arnaud, 1994). Increased serum PTH concentrations, consistent with an appropriate physiologic response to hypocalcemia, rule out the diagnosis of hypoparathyroidism and suggest end-organ resistance to PTH (pseudohypoparathyroidism or vitamin D deficiency) or secondary hyperparathyroidism due to such disorders as dietary deficiency of calcium or intestinal malabsorption of calcium. Decreases in serum PTH concentration provide strong evidence for primary parathyroid gland failure.

DOGS AND CATS. Undetectable serum PTH concentrations in animals that are severely hypocalcemic confirm the diagnosis of primary hypoparathyroidism, assuming that the assay used is reliable and validated. Reliable and validated PTH assays are available for both cats and dogs via several veterinary laboratories. Serum PTH concentrations may be detectable or "low-normal" in some patients with hypoparathyroidism, if the assay employed is quite sensitive. However, a low-normal concentration, or even one within a provided reference range, may not be appropriate in a hypocalcemic individual that has healthy parathyroid glands (see Figs. 16-2, 16-19, and 16-20). Low to undetectable serum PTH concentrations were obtained from each of 24 dogs with primary hypoparathyroidism we tested (see Table 17-4; Fig. 16-19).

Response to therapy, coupled with review and ruling out of each of the various differential diagnoses for hypocalcemia, has served as a relatively reliable and logical method for supporting the diagnosis of primary hypoparathyroidism. This approach circumvents assessment of PTH concentrations and makes such assessments seem academic. However, because naturally occurring primary hypoparathyroidism is a permanent condition, assaying serum PTH concentrations is warranted and serves to aid both the veterinarian and client (Torrance, 1998). It is understood that the most important differential diagnoses for hypocalcemia are laboratory error, hypoalbuminemia, surgical removal of the parathyroids, use of phosphate enemas, acute or chronic renal failure, eclampsia, malabsorption, and severe pancreatitis. These problems can usually be identified by veterinary practitioners without sophisticated analyses, such as PTH assays. However, busy practices consistently encounter dogs or cats that present diagnostic dilemmas.

A review of earlier literature demonstrates that some hypocalcemic dogs have serum PTH concentrations consistent with a diagnosis of primary hypoparathyroidism (low or low-normal values) (Kornegay et al, 1980; Sherding et al, 1980; Feldman and Krutzik, 1981). One dog had elevated PTH concentrations, suggesting secretion of ineffective PTH or tissue unresponsiveness to PTH (see Differential Diagnosis of Hypocalcemia) (Kornegay et al, 1980), and one dog was hypomagnesemic but no serum PTH concentration was obtained (dog 4 in Table 17-4). However, these reports used assays no longer considered reliable. Reports based on the new "sandwich" intact PTH assays, in both dogs and cats, have been published. As expected, these assays have provided excellent results (Torrance and Nachreiner, 1989; Flanders and Reimers, 1991; Flanders et al, 1991; Barber et al, 1993; Chew et al, 1995).

DIFFERENTIAL DIAGNOSIS OF EPISODIC WEAKNESS

Because the clinical signs of hypocalcemia occur paroxysmally and episodically, the clinician may consider a variety of potential causes for recurrent apparent neurologic and/or neuromuscular disorders (Chapter 14 has a section on episodic weakness, because hypoglycemia results in somewhat similar problems). Several of the dogs in this series were initially believed to have idiopathic epilepsy. Toxins were also a commonly suspected problem (e.g., strychnine, metaldehyde, lead). Other tentative diagnoses after initial examination of hypocalcemic dogs included tetanus, trauma, cardiac disease, myasthenia gravis, hepatic disease, and hypoglycemia.

DIFFERENTIAL DIAGNOSIS OF HYPOCALCEMIA (TABLE 17-6; FIG. 17-7)

Parathyroid-Related

Primary Hypoparathyroidism: Causes

NATURALLY OCCURRING DISEASE—DOGS AND CATS. Naturally occurring hypoparathyroidism is a rare condition in dogs and cats. The onset of signs in these pets is typically abrupt and severe (tetany, seizures). Although the onset of signs almost always seems sudden to owners, the condition is likely insidious, with mild subclinical hypocalcemia present for prolonged periods. Surprisingly, some dogs and cats with naturally occurring disease have had signs for months at the time of diagnosis (one, in our series, for longer than a year) and survive without appropriate treatment.

Therefore dogs and cats have some capacity for "adapting" to hypocalcemia. Signs are not usually recognized until there has been a decline in the total serum calcium concentration below some critical level (<6.0–6.5 mg/dl?). At such serum calcium concentrations, relatively small decreases in calcium con-

TABLE 17–6 DIFFERENTIAL DIAGNOSIS OF HYPOCALCEMIA

Parathyroid-related hypocalcemia
  Primary hypoparathyroidism
    Destruction of glands
      Immune-mediated process
      Iatrogenic: surgical complication
      Any disease in neck causing damage
    Acute correction of chronic hypercalcemic condition
    Idiopathic atrophy (autoimmune process?)
  Pseudohypoparathyroidism
Chronic renal failure
Hypoalbuminemia
Acute pancreatitis
Puerperal tetany (eclampsia)
Intestinal malabsorption syndromes
Nutritional secondary hyperparathyroidism (rare)
Anticonvulsant therapy
Acute renal failure
Ethylene glycol toxicity
Phosphate-containing enemas
Hypomagnesemia
Miscellaneous diagnoses
  Laboratory error
  After bicarbonate administration
  Phosphate infusions
  Use of EDTA-coagulated blood
  Vitamin D deficiency
  Transfusion using citrated blood
  Soft tissue trauma
  Medullary carcinoma of the thyroid
  Primary and metastatic bone tumors
  Cancer chemotherapy

centration produce obvious clinical problems. For example, a serum calcium decline of 0.3 mg/dl in a dog or cat with a serum concentration of 10.5 mg/dl has no effect and is still considered normal, but the same decrease when the serum calcium concentration is 6.1 mg/dl could result in convulsions.

Diffuse lymphocytic "parathyroiditis" was described in 7 dogs with hypoparathyroidism (Kornegay, 1982). Our series includes an additional 10 dogs with similar histologic findings (see Table 17–4), and several had parathyroid tissue replaced by fibrous connective tissue. It is assumed that the fibrous tissue is an "end result" following lymphocytic/plasmacytic inflammation. Therefore the finding of either inflammatory infiltrates or scar tissue is most likely dependent on when tissue is obtained relative to the time course of the condition. Detection of antibodies against parathyroid tissue in human patients with idiopathic hypoparathyroidism has resulted in the understanding that many of these people have an autoimmune disease. An immune-mediated mechanism likely explains the condition in dogs and cats.

RARE DISORDERS IN HUMANS NOT REPORTED IN DOGS OR CATS. The DiGeorge syndrome in humans consists of parathyroid gland absence and thymic aplasia (Rasmussen, 1981; Marx, 2000). This disorder presumably results from abnormal development of the third pharyngeal pouch during embryogenesis. Parathyroid agenesis has also been reported in dogs (Meuten and Armstrong, 1989). Another form of idiopathic

hypoparathyroidism in humans is associated with an immune-mediated endocrine syndrome that includes hypofunction of the adrenal cortex, ovarian failure, pernicious anemia, thyroiditis, diabetes mellitus, candidiasis, and occasionally malabsorption (see Chapter 8). This is a familial disorder. Those patients who manifest disease before 6 months of age conform to an X-linked recessive inheritance pattern, and older individuals likely have an autosomal recessive inherited condition (Arnaud, 1994). Calcium-sensing receptor mutations have also been identified (Pearce et al, 1996).

SURGICALLY INDUCED. The most common cause for primary hypoparathyroidism in dogs, cats and people is surgical removal of or damage to (direct or indirect via damage to blood supply) these glands (Marx, 2000). Hypoparathyroidism can follow thyroid, parathyroid, or other surgeries of the neck. Because the incidence of hyperthyroidism in cats is high and because canine thyroid tumors have a high incidence of malignancy, thyroid surgery is common in both species.

One group estimated that as many as 10% of hyperthyroid cats undergoing surgery suffer from transient or permanent hypoparathyroidism (Peterson, 1986). Of 41 hyperthyroid cats that had bilateral thyroidectomy, postoperative hypocalcemia (not always associated with clinical signs) developed in 82% undergoing an extracapsular surgical technique, 36% with an intracapsular technique, and 11% with two separate thyroidectomies performed 3 to 4 weeks apart (Flanders et al, 1987). Of 106 cats studied in a subsequent report, postoperative hypocalcemia developed in 22%, 33%, and 23% of cats, depending on the surgical technique (Welches et al, 1989). Clinical signs related to hypocalcemia were observed only in severely hypocalcemic cats (<7.0 mg/dl). The incidence of permanent hypoparathyroidism is much lower today, because surgeons are more aware of this complication and because techniques have improved. Surgery remains the most common cause of hypoparathyroidism in dogs and cats (Henderson et al, 1991; Flanders, 1994; Graves, 1995; Klein et al, 1995). For this reason, autotransplantation of removed parathyroid tissue has been evaluated. This procedure has been successfully employed in humans and has excellent veterinary potential (Padgett et al, 1998).

The transient nature of hypoparathyroidism following surgery in many cats is not well understood. One group of cats had significantly reduced serum PTH concentrations after thyroparathyroidectomy. During the 12 weeks following surgery, serum PTH concentrations did not recover, but the serum calcium concentration did slowly increase. It was suggested that the most likely explanation for the increases in serum calcium concentration in these thyroparathyroidectomized cats was an "accommodation" of existing calcium-regulating systems that operate at suboptimal levels in the absence of PTH. One example of such an "accommodation" might involve changes in vitamin D metabolism to continue calcium absorption from the intestine despite a deficiency in PTH (Flanders et al,

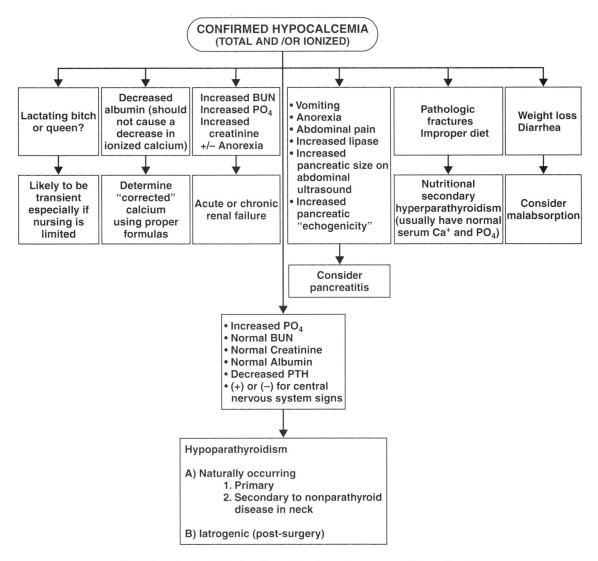

FIGURE 17-7. Algorithm for diagnosing the various causes of hypocalcemia.

1991). The onset of biochemical or clinical signs suggestive of parathyroid failure after neck surgery in dogs and cats can begin within days or take as long as several weeks. Other potential but rare destructive disorders of the parathyroids include neck injury, neoplastic conditions within the neck, thyroid irradiation, and aminoglycoside intoxication. We have not observed iodine[131]–induced parathyroid damage.

PSEUDOHYPOPARATHYROIDISM. Pseudohypoparathyroidism is a rare familial disorder in humans characterized by target tissue resistance to PTH. These individuals have hypocalcemia, increased serum concentrations of PTH, and a variety of congenital developmental growth and skeletal defects. Increases in serum PTH concentration represent an appropriate physiologic response to hypocalcemia. If the serum calcium concentration is transiently normalized by an infusion of calcium, the concentration of circulating PTH decreases. Therefore diagnosis of end-organ unresponsiveness involves (1) the inability of PTH to increase cyclic adenosine 3',5'-monophosphate

(cAMP) excretion, and (2) elevated circulating PTH concentrations. The hormone secreted by patients with pseudohypoparathyroidism is presumably normal in structure. Some of these patients have no developmental abnormalities (Arnaud, 1994). A deficiency in renal PTH-sensitive cAMP results in renal tubular resistance to PTH and diminished phosphaturia. Deficits in active vitamin D and/or bone cAMP have also been claimed to be the inciting factor leading to pseudohypoparathyroidism.

Dogs with this specific disease entity have not been recognized. However, one dog was reported that had apparent hypoparathyroidism, yet had elevations in serum PTH, urine cAMP, and plasma cAMP (Kornegay et al, 1980). Another dog had hypoparathyroidism. This dog had Fanconi's syndrome, which was thought to occur secondary to a 1,25–vitamin D deficiency (Freeman et al, 1994).

PSEUDOPSEUDOHYPOPARATHYROIDISM. Humans with this disorder have the typical developmental defects (growth and skeletal abnormalities) associated with pseudohypoparathyroidism. However, these individuals are not hypocalcemic or hyperphosphatemic, nor do they have abnormalities in serum PTH concentrations (Marx, 2000). This syndrome has not been recognized in cats or dogs.

HYPOMAGNESEMIA. Magnesium deficiency can result in hypocalcemia. Hypomagnesemia and hypocalcemia, as interrelated and distinct syndromes, have not been reported in dogs or cats. However, secondary hypoparathyroidism attributed to hypomagnesemia in dogs with protein-losing enteropathies and with eclampsia has been reported (Aroch et al, 1999; Kimmel et al, 2000; Bush et al, 2001). As seen in Table 17-4, four of our dogs with primary hypoparathyroidism were hypomagnesemic. The significance of these findings is inconclusive.

Chronic Renal Failure

Chronic renal failure (CRF) is an extremely common disorder in dogs and cats. The most common chemical feature of chronic renal failure is an increase in serum phosphate concentration with a normal serum calcium concentration. However, either hypocalcemia or hypercalcemia may occur in animals with chronic renal failure. Because renal failure is so common, it represents one of the most frequent explanations for hypocalcemia in dogs and cats. The clinical problems that are a direct result of renal failure (e.g., inappetence, vomiting, and weight loss) and the secondary bone disease are also of concern. Total serum calcium concentration was 8.0 mg/dl, or lower, in 10% of dogs with CRF, and the ionized calcium was below reference limits in 40% of these dogs. Approximately 15% of cats with CRF are hypocalcemic. Hypocalcemia, when it is noted, is a biochemical problem and rarely, if ever, clinically significant. The hypocalcemia is not severe (usually >8.0 mg/dl), and the accompanying metabolic acidosis usually associated with renal disease increases the ionized calcium concentration, further decreasing chance of tetany.

In the early stages of progressive CRF, a decrease in the number of functioning nephrons results in a decreased capacity to excrete phosphate. Transient hyperphosphatemia induces hypocalcemia. Hypocalcemia, in turn, stimulates an increase in PTH synthesis and secretion. This is the classically described genesis of renal secondary hyperparathyroidism (Fig. 17-8; see Fig. 16-10). Renal secondary hyperparathyroidism can cause skeletal osteocytic osteolysis, which in turn, reestablishes normal circulating concentrations of calcium and phosphorus. The hyperparathyroidism also augments phosphate excretion. As CRF continues to progress, however, secondary hyperparathyroidism can no longer compensate for the chemical abnormalities, and hyperphosphatemia develops with or without hypocalcemia (Chew and Nagode, 1990). Furthermore, normal kidneys convert inactive vitamin D to the active form. Progressive renal disease leads to reduced

capacity to form active vitamin D, limiting intestinal absorption of calcium and enhancing the potential for hypocalcemia. Additionally, increased urinary calcium excretion in the uremic state contributes to the hypocalcemia seen in chronic renal failure.

HYPOALBUMINEMIA. Reductions in total serum protein and/or albumin concentrations are encountered in a variety of disorders in veterinary medicine. These disorders include hepatopathies, glomerulopathies, malabsorption syndromes (such as lymphangiectasia), and blood loss to mention but a few. As previously described, reductions in circulating albumin concentration cause a decrease in the protein-bound fraction of circulating calcium. However, ionized calcium concentrations are typically normal. Therefore these animals rarely have clinical signs of hypocalcemia.

ACUTE PANCREATITIS. Hypocalcemia, when it occurs in dogs with acute pancreatitis, is usually mild and subclinical. Coexisting acidosis, which is commonly present, increases the ionized fraction of total calcium and further reduces the likelihood of clinical signs related to hypocalcemia (Hess et al, 1998). The incidence of hypocalcemia may be higher in cats with pancreatitis than in dogs. Results of one study suggest that low total and ionized calcium concentrations are common in cats with acute pancreatitis (41% and 61%, respectively). Furthermore, the cats with decreases in plasma ionized calcium concentration, even though

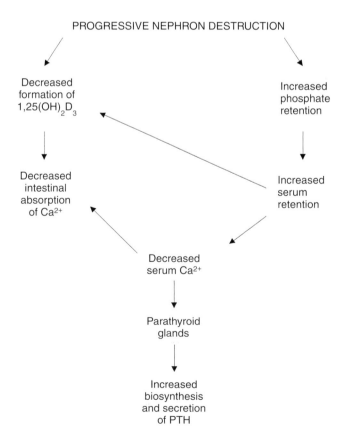

FIGURE 17-8. Pathogenesis of parathyroid hyperplasia during progressive destruction of nephrons.

none had clinical signs related to this complication, had a poorer prognosis than those with normal concentrations. A grave prognosis and aggressive medical therapy was recommended for cats with both acute pancreatitis and a plasma ionized calcium concentration <1.00 mmol/L (Kimmel et al, 2001).

The traditional theory for development of hypocalcemia in pancreatitis is that calcium is precipitated in the form of insoluble soaps via saponification of peripancreatic fatty acids formed subsequent to release of pancreatic lipase. Despite general agreement that this occurs, it is not clear whether it is sufficient to account completely for hypocalcemia in view of the large quantity of calcium that potentially can be mobilized from skeletal reserves. Other potential contributors to the hypocalcemia include hypomagnesemia, decreased secretion of PTH, hypoproteinemia, and glucagon-stimulated calcitonin secretion.

Diagnosis of pancreatitis has never been fool-proof. No test is totally reliable, and the diagnosis of pancreatitis in dogs is usually based on typical signalment (older, obese, small breed, female), typical signs (vomiting, anorexia, abdominal pain), and in-hospital testing (serum lipase concentration, ultrasonography). These dogs are not severely hypocalcemic, and their clinical signs are related to the gastrointestinal tract versus the severe hypocalcemia of hypoparathyroidism, in which signs are neuromuscular. In cats, the typical clinical signs include anorexia, lethargy, vomiting, abdominal pain, and icterus. Ultrasonographic findings considered consistent with a diagnosis of acute pancreatitis in cats include hypoechoic pancreatic parenchyma or hyperechoic peripancreatic mesentery (Kimmel et al, 2001).

Puerperal Tetany (Eclampsia)

Eclampsia is an acute life-threatening disease caused by extreme hypocalcemia in preparturient and lactating bitches and queens (Fascetti and Hickman, 1999; Drobatz and Casey, 2000). In most studies, dogs and cats with eclampsia are severely hypocalcemic (<6.5 mg/dl). Eclampsia is most common in small dogs and less common in cats and large dogs. Signs seen by veterinarians usually depend on how quickly the owner recognizes the problem and seeks professional care. Most bitches and queens are affected during the first 21 days of nursing a litter, although eclampsia has been diagnosed during the last 2 weeks of pregnancy and as long as 45 days after whelping (see Chapter 21).

The physiopathology of eclampsia is not well understood. The problem typically arises as a consequence of lactation, leading to excessive calcium loss, poor dietary use of calcium (sometimes the stress of nursing reduces a bitch's appetite or interferes with her ability to eat), and subsequent hypocalcemia. Other factors that may play a role in the development of hypocalcemia include parathyroid gland atrophy

caused by improper diet or dietary supplements, as well as calcium loss to the developing fetal skeletons. Additionally, in one study 44% of bitches with eclampsia had hypomagnesemia. Decreased magnesium-to-calcium ratios at the neuromuscular junctions can promote tetany. It was suggested that magnesium therapy may be beneficial in bitches with eclampsia (Aroch et al, 1999).

Regardless of the underlying physiology, hypocalcemia of eclampsia (if severe) causes the typical signs attributed to altered cell membrane potentials, spontaneous discharge of nerve fibers, and induction of tonic or tonoclonic contractions of skeletal muscle. The rate of fall in serum calcium concentration and the actual calcium level reached influence the onset and signs of tetany. Any factor increasing the protein-bound fraction of the serum calcium concentration favors the development of tetany, such as systemic alkalosis secondary to hyperventilation during dystocia. Hypoglycemia is another potential complication of eclampsia. The signs of hypoglycemia can be similar to those of hypocalcemia (see Chapter 14).

Diagnosis of eclampsia is usually based on the presence of neuromuscular signs in a lactating bitch or queen. In most situations, the diagnosis is so obvious that the serum calcium concentration is never checked. However, of four cats described with preparturient eclampsia, hypothermia was documented in three, and clinical signs included flaccid paralysis, rather than the more typical tonic-clonic muscle fasciculations noted in dogs (Fascetti and Hickman, 1999).

Malabsorption Syndromes

Malabsorption is a common cause of hypocalcemia in humans (Rasmussen, 1981) but is a rather uncommon cause for decreases in calcium concentrations in dogs. Canine hypocalcemia is usually thought to occur secondary to hypoalbuminemia. Two factors are important in the pathogenesis of hypocalcemia, their importance varying with the underlying disease. The first factor is an increase in fecal calcium excretion due to decreased absorption of dietary calcium, as well as decreased resorption of endogenous calcium secreted into the gastrointestinal tract in disorders such as lymphangiectasia. The degree of calcium malabsorption appears to correlate with the extent of small bowel disease. The second factor is the poor absorption of vitamin D in diseases that diffusely affect the small bowel.

Hypomagnesemia may also play an important role in producing hypocalcemia in people with malabsorption syndromes, and similar correlations have been made in dogs. In two studies, it was suggested that hypomagnesemia and hypocalcemia may have a related pathogenesis involving intestinal loss, malabsorption, and abnormalities of vitamin D and PTH metabolism. Supplementation with magnesium was demonstrated to normalize serum magnesium and PTH concentrations, improve plasma ionized calcium concentrations, and alleviate clinical signs of paresis (Kimmel et al, 2000; Bush et al, 2001).

Nutritional Secondary Hyperparathyroidism

Dogs and cats exclusively fed diets containing low calcium-to-phosphorus ratios, such as beef heart or liver, can develop severe mineral deficiencies. Dietary calcium deficiency results in transient decreases in circulating calcium concentrations, which induce increased PTH secretion, reduction in bone mass as calcium is removed from bone to replace that not taken in by diet, and diffuse skeletal disorders. These problems include bone pain and pathologic fractures. The skeletal disturbances are the result of an attempt to maintain *circulating* mineral homeostasis. Usually these animals have normal serum concentrations of both calcium and phosphorus. However, some cats may have mild to severe hypocalcemia (Tomsa et al, 1999). Treatment involves providing balanced diets and restricting activity until skeletal remodeling is complete. Diagnosis is based on recognizing skeletal disorders in a dog or cat receiving an improper diet. Neuromuscular problems (tetany) can be a major component of the history.

Acute Renal Failure and Ethylene Glycol Toxicity

Acute intrinsic renal failure, such as occurs with ethylene glycol poisoning, and postrenal failure, such as occurs with urethral obstruction, may result in abrupt and severe increases in serum phosphate concentration and a secondary reduction in serum calcium concentration. Hypocalcemia may be exaggerated in acute renal failure because the rapid onset of these disturbances blunts compensatory mechanisms. Dogs with acute intrinsic renal failure had a mean serum total calcium concentration of 9.8 mg/dl (Vaden et al, 1997). Ethylene glycol intoxication can cause severe renal failure, acidosis, and death. The metabolites of this toxin can chelate serum calcium ions and cause tetany. Hypocalcemia is one of several metabolic problems that can develop following ingestion of this toxin. Acute renal failure, with its associated blood urea nitrogen and serum creatinine abnormalities, is easily distinguished from primary hypoparathyroidism.

Urethral Obstruction

Male cats with long-standing (>12 to 24 hours) urethral obstruction and severe hyperphosphatemia often have associated hypocalcemia, hyperkalemia, azotemia, and sometimes experience seizures (Chew and Meuten, 1983). Hypocalcemia was diagnosed in 26% of male cats with urethral obstruction at initial presentation, based on total serum calcium assessment. On the basis of plasma ionized concentrations,

however, 75% were hypocalcemic. The hypocalcemia was defined as mild in 37.5%, moderate in 25%, and severe in 12.5% of affected cats. These abnormalities may contribute to cardiac dysfunction in severely affected cats. Although effects of IV administration of calcium were not evaluated, results in this study support their use in cats with urethral obstruction (Drobatz and Hughes, 1997).

Phosphate-Containing Enemas

Commercial phosphate-containing enemas may result in acute, marked hyperphosphatemia following colonic absorption of the enema solution, especially when administered to dehydrated cats with colonic atony and mucosal disruption. Colonic absorption of sodium and phosphate from the enema solution, as well as transfer of intravascular water to the colonic lumen (because of hypertonicity of the solution), causes hypernatremia and hyperphosphatemia. Acute increases in serum phosphate may cause reciprocal significant declines in serum calcium concentration (Atkins et al, 1985; Jorgensen et al, 1985). Therefore use of these enemas is not recommended in animals with severe obstipation, in animals with marginal renal function, or in those with abnormal serum calcium-to-phosphorus ratios. All these conditions predispose animals to hyperphosphatemia. Clinical signs of phosphate enema toxicosis (shock and neuromuscular irritability) result from hypocalcemia and hypernatremia. Treatment may require plasma volume expansion and calcium. Diagnosis is based on the history (Peterson, 1992).

Miscellaneous Causes

LABORATORY ERROR. Perhaps most important of the miscellaneous causes for hypocalcemia is laboratory error. Incorrect reporting of the serum calcium concentration can reflect a simple mistake or artifact due to samples submitted in tubes containing EDTA as an anticoagulant, because EDTA chelates calcium. Mixing of serum with air significantly decreases plasma ionized calcium concentrations. Freshly obtained plasma for ionized calcium determinations should be transported to reference laboratories with a cold pack. If a delay of more than 3 days is possible, plasma should be sent frozen (Schenck et al, 1995). Caution should be exercised in the interpretation of ionized calcium measured with portable analyzers, because results for dogs and cats are lower than those obtained with standard methodology. The use of dry heparin syringes for sample collection may negate this difference (Grosenbaugh et al, 1998). Whenever the reported serum calcium concentration is unexpectedly high or low, it should be rechecked.

ANTICONVULSANT THERAPY. Surveys of humans receiving long-term anticonvulsant therapy (principally phenobarbital and phenytoin) have shown a tendency to develop hypocalcemia, hypophosphatemia, and abnormal serum alkaline phosphatase activities. Studies in these subjects reveal a state similar to vitamin D deficiency. Bone biopsies and radiographs suggest osteomalacia without evidence of malabsorption or renal disease. Serum PTH concentrations are increased but remain normally suppressible with calcium infusions. Severity of the altered calcium metabolism is directly related to the dosage of medication (Arnaud, 1994).

Although this problem has not been recognized in the dog, it is described to remind practitioners that any drug has the potential to cause unexpected endocrine problems. Furthermore, several of our hypoparathyroid dogs were referred because of failure to respond to anticonvulsant therapy. The finding of hypocalcemia in dogs on relatively high doses of anticonvulsants may be mistakenly interpreted as iatrogenic.

HYPERTHYROID CATS. Cats with untreated hyperthyroidism have significantly lower serum ionized calcium concentrations than do control cats, although none had decreases in total calcium concentration and only 4 of 15 cats had ionized calcium concentrations below the reference range. Hyperthyroid cats also had significantly increased serum PTH concentrations. These changes are likely associated with the hyperphosphatemia often noted in hyperthyroid cats. The importance of these findings is not known (Barber and Elliott, 1996).

VITAMIN D DEFICIENCY. Vitamin D deficiency is an unlikely clinical cause of hypocalcemia (Henik et al, 1999).

CITRATED BLOOD. Blood for transfusion that contains citrates as an anticoagulant may induce hypocalcemia, particularly if the volume of donor blood is small compared with the volume of anticoagulant.

TRAUMA. Trauma, especially soft tissue trauma, has been reported as a cause of hypocalcemia (Chew and Meuten, 1983), but this is rare.

MEDULLARY CARCINOMA. Medullary carcinoma of the thyroid has been reported to cause severe hypocalcemia and tetany in one dog and represents an unusual cause of hypocalcemia in humans.

PRIMARY AND METASTATIC BONE TUMORS. Primary and metastatic bone tumors are common in small animal practice. Humans, dogs, and cats with tumors that have metastasized to bone usually have normal serum calcium concentrations. Hypercalcemia is the most common alteration of calcium metabolism induced by metastatic bone tumors. Occasionally in humans, however, hypocalcemia and hypophosphatemia occur. When osteoblastic metastases are present in humans, the incorporation of calcium into the lesions may be sufficient to result in measurable serum hypocalcemia and even clinical signs. This is not a reported problem in dogs or cats.

CHEMOTHERAPY. Tumor lysis syndrome occurs after acute release of intracellular contents during chemotherapy for highly sensitive neoplasms, such as lymphoid or bone marrow tumors (Persons et al, 1998). Among the multiple metabolic abnormalities that can occur in this setting is hypocalcemia due to mass law interactions related to acute and severe hyperphosphatemia (Calia et al, 1996; Piek and Teske, 1996). In addition to hypocalcemia, transient PTH deficiency may occur (Horn and Irwin, 2000). Transient hypocalcemia may also occur with sepsis and severe inflammatory conditions. One salicylate-intoxicated cat developed hypocalcemia associated with *sodium bicarbonate* therapy (Abrams, 1987).

THERAPY FOR HYPOPARATHYROIDISM AND HYPOCALCEMIA

General Approach

Eclampsia (puerperal tetany) is a classic condition of hypocalcemia in which specific and acute correction of the deficiency is necessary but chronic treatment is not. In contrast, hypoparathyroidism may be permanent, requiring acute and chronic management to alleviate or prevent clinical signs. No treatment is indicated for animals with hypocalcemia attributable entirely to hypoalbuminemia, assuming the ionized calcium fraction is normal.

Treatment of hypocalcemia virtually always requires a protocol tailored to the individual needs of a dog or cat. Management will be effected by the magnitude of the hypocalcemia and the rate of decline in calcium concentration. The trend in serum concentrations, either fluctuating, remaining stable, or quickly falling, will influence decision processes. Aggressive approaches are needed for dogs and cats with obvious clinical signs, for those with significant decreases in total or ionized calcium concentrations, or when severe hypocalcemia can be anticipated (such as with therapy for primary hyperparathyroid dogs and cats that have serum total calcium concentrations in excess of 14.5 to 15 mg/dl). Any suggestion that veterinarians should not treat for hypocalcemia until clinical signs are obvious must be questioned. Such an approach, at best, exposes the pet to an extremely painful condition. At worst, it places the pet at risk for developing a life-threatening event.

The goal of therapy—one that is difficult to achieve—is to increase serum calcium concentrations smoothly above the threshold responsible for clinical signs. That threshold is usually a total calcium concentration of 6.0 to 7.0 mg/dl, or above an ionized plasma calcium concentration of 0.6 to 0.7 mmol/L. Individual differences can be significant, however. Clinical signs typically improve with slight increases in measurable calcium. The veterinarian almost never needs to raise calcium concentrations within reference ranges; attempts to do so increase the risk for hypercalcemia, associated hyperphosphatemia, tissue mineralization, and stone formation. For anticipated or known postsurgical hypocalcemia that will be transient, as in pets with primary hyperparathyroidism, it is physiologically ideal to maintain calcium concentrations below established reference ranges since "below normal" values should enhance functional recovery of atrophied parathyroid glands.

Emergency Therapy for Tetany

DIAGNOSIS NOT APPARENT.   In the event that a practitioner is treating a seizuring animal without a specific diagnosis, diazepam is usually the initial drug of choice. This approach is usually beneficial, even in hypocalcemic pets. However, if treatment fails or if a diagnosis is still not obvious, blood should be drawn for glucose, calcium, and any other parameter that may lead to a diagnosis. In the meantime, intravenous glucose and/or calcium can be administered.

Hypocalcemic Tetany: IV Calcium

GENERAL.   Hypocalcemic tetany requires immediate replacement of calcium. 10% calcium gluconate should be administered by IV siowly, to effect. The dose is 0.5 to 1.5 ml/kg of body weight or 5 to 15 mg/kg, administered slowly over a 10- to 30-minute period. Calcium gluconate, as a 10% solution (Table 17-7), is recommended because this medication is readily available to veterinarians. More importantly, this solution is much less caustic than calcium chloride if any extravasates outside a vein. ECG monitoring is advisable; if bradycardia, premature ventricular complexes, and/or shortening of the Q-T interval are observed, the intravenous infusion should be slowed or briefly discontinued (Peterson, 1992). This emergency therapy is invariably successful. Cessation of seizures, for example, is usually noted within minutes of initiating the infusion. However, the final dose needed to control tetany is not predictable. Furthermore, some clinical signs may be slower to respond. Nervousness, panting, and behavioral changes may persist for as long as 30 to 60 minutes after return of eucalcemia, perhaps reflecting a lag in equilibrium between cerebrospinal fluid and circulating calcium. It is suggested that recommended doses be used as guidelines and patient response be the definitive factor in determining the volume administered.

The calcium content of different *salts* varies considerably. For example, both calcium gluconate and calcium chloride supplements are available as 10% solutions in 10-ml ampules, and each ampule provides 1 g of the parent compound. However, calcium chloride provides approximately 27 mg of calcium per milliliter, whereas calcium gluconate provides approximately 9 mg of calcium per milliliter. There is no difference in effectiveness of calcium administered intravenously to correct hypocalcemia when the dose is based on elemental calcium content. Thus the dose in *milligrams* is the same, regardless of the calcium solution chosen. Calcium chloride, when given outside a vein, can cause not only tremendous tissue death and sloughing but also calcinosis cutis (Schick et al, 1987). It is our opinion that calcium chloride should never be stocked by small animal practitioners, thus eliminating any possibility of its use.

Infusion of calcium-rich fluids should be performed with caution in a dog or cat with hyperphosphatemia. Hyperphosphatemia, however, is a common feature of hypocalcemia due to mass law effects. Therefore, although a concern, increases in circulating calcium should be accompanied by decreases in phosphate. However, in such conditions as renal failure, the combination of hyperphosphatemia and calcium administration could cause soft tissue mineralization. Therefore further damage to the kidneys may occur in animals with coexisting renal insufficiency or failure (Chew and Meuten, 1983).

FEVER.   Fever frequently accompanies tetany. It is common for a dog or cat in tetany to have a rectal temperature above 105° F. Veterinarians may be tempted to treat both hypocalcemia and fever (ice or

TABLE 17–7   SOME AVAILABLE CALCIUM PREPARATIONS

	Preparations Available		Approximate Calcium Content	Dose
Oral				
Calcium carbonate/gluconate	Chewable tablets: 700 mg		250 mg Ca/tablet	Cats: 0.5–1.0 g/day
Calcium gluconate	Tablets	325 mg	30 mg Ca/tablet	Dogs: 1.0–4.0 g/day
		500 mg	45 mg Ca/tablet	
		650 mg	60 mg Ca/tablet	
		1000 mg	90 mg Ca/tablet	
Calcium lactate	Tablets:	325 mg	42 mg Ca/tablet	
		650 mg	85 mg Ca/tablet	
Calcium carbonate	Capsules:	500 mg	145 mg Ca + 155 mg P/capsule	
		650 mg	190 mg Ca + 148 mg P/capsule	
Calcium glubionate	Tablets:	650 mg	190 mg Ca + 148 mg P/tablet	
		1000 mg	295 mg Ca + 228 mg P/tablet	
	Syrup:	360 mg/ml	20 mg/ml	
Injectable				
Calcium gluconate (IV, SQ)	10% solution, 10-ml ampule		9.3 mg Ca/ml	1.0–1.5 ml/kg; 5–15 mg/kg; slowly
Calcium chloride (IV)	10% solution, 10-ml ampule		27.2 mg/Ca/ml	Not recommended
Calcium gluceptate (IV, IM) (calcium glucoheptonate)	22% solution, 5-ml ampule		18 mg Ca/ml	–

Ca, Calcium; *P,* phosphate.

alcohol baths; parenteral drugs). However, with administration of calcium, the animal's fever should be monitored but not treated. Fever usually dissipates rapidly with control of tetany. Additional measures to lower body temperature may result in hypothermia and the development of shock. In fact, three of four cats recently reported to have had preparturient eclampsia were hypothermic (Fascetti and Hickman, 1999).

Subacute Management of Hypocalcemia (post-tetany maintenance)

THE PROBLEM. Once signs of hypocalcemic tetany are controlled with intravenous calcium, the effects of the infusion persist for 1 to 12 hours. Long-term maintenance therapy with oral vitamin D and oral calcium supplementation usually requires a minimum of 24 to 96 hours before an effect is achieved. Hypocalcemic animals require calcium support during the initial post-tetany period.

THE ALTERNATIVES. *Repeated Intravenous Boluses.* One method for managing hypocalcemia in the immediate post-tetany period is administration of repeated intravenous calcium boluses. This procedure is not recommended except in emergencies, because wide fluctuations in circulating calcium concentrations result.

Subcutaneous Calcium. Once tetany has been controlled with intravenous bolus calcium gluconate, administration of subcutaneous calcium has been effective, simple, and inexpensive. Continuous intravenous administration of fluids is expensive and usually demands hospitalization of the dog or cat. As an alternative, the veterinarian can determine the dose of calcium gluconate needed to control tetany originally and administer that dose subcutaneously every 6 to 8 hours. As a guide, a calcium dose of 60 to 90 mg/kg/day, divided, can be given. The calcium gluconate should be diluted as 1 part of calcium to 2, 3, or 4 parts of saline. This protocol has effectively supported serum calcium concentrations and has not caused inflammation or sloughing of skin over months in some of our canine patients. The subcutaneous regimen is an efficacious method of supporting circulating calcium while waiting for atrophied parathyroid glands to regain function, or while waiting for oral vitamin D and calcium to have effect. The procedure is easily taught to owners, further decreasing their expense.

Remember, calcium chloride cannot be administered subcutaneously, but calcium gluconate is usually safe. Two possible cases (1 dog and 1 cat) of calcinosis cutis following subcutaneous administration of calcium gluconate have been reported. The cat never had histologic confirmation of calcinosis cutis, bringing into question the diagnosis of this complication (Ruopp, 2001). In the dog, the subcutaneous calcium was not administered by the authors, leaving open the strong possibility that a more caustic form of calcium, rather than calcium gluconate, had been administered (Schaer et al, 2001). It is always possible

for an unexpected complication to follow any treatment. In our experience, however, subcutaneous calcium gluconate is efficacious.

After normal or near-normal serum calcium concentrations have been maintained for 48 hours, the frequency of subcutaneous calcium administration should be decreased from every 6 to every 8 hours. If serum calcium concentrations remain stable for the ensuing 48 to 72 hours, the subcutaneous calcium can be tapered to twice daily. This protocol is continued until parenteral calcium has been completely discontinued. Obviously, the tapering process in each patient may not be this smooth, because response to oral therapy is variable. Ideally, the total serum calcium concentration should be maintained above 8 mg/dl. Concentrations below 8 mg/dl indicate a need to increase the dose or frequency of parenteral calcium. Serum calcium concentrations of 8 to 9 mg/dl suggest maintaining the current parenteral dose. Concentrations greater than 9 mg/dl may indicate need for reducing the dose. The frequency and/or dosage of parenteral calcium are often increased before the therapy can be safely decreased and then discontinued. This is true regardless of the calcium supplementation protocol used.

Continuous Intravenous Infusion. Continuous infusion of calcium is recommended at 60 to 90 mg/kg/day elemental calcium (2.5 to 3.75 mg/kg/hr) until oral medications provide control of serum calcium concentration. Initial doses in the high end of this protocol are recommended for dogs and cats with severe hypocalcemia. The dose should be decreased according to the serum calcium concentration achieved and as oral calcium and vitamin D become effective.

Using 10% calcium gluconate solutions, 10 ml provides 93 mg of elemental calcium. A convenient method for infusing calcium can be used when intravenous fluids are administered at a typical maintenance rate of 60 ml/kg/day (2.5 ml/kg/hr). Approximately 1, 2, or 3 mg/kg/hr of elemental calcium is provided by adding 40, 80, or 120 ml of 10% calcium gluconate, respectively, to each liter of intravenous fluid solution. Calcium salts may precipitate if added to fluid solutions containing lactate, acetate, bicarbonate, or phosphates. Additionally, intravenous solutions containing sodium bicarbonate should be avoided because alkalinization can decrease ionized calcium and may precipitate clinical signs in dogs or cats with borderline hypocalcemia (Rosol et al, 2000).

Maintenance Therapy

The lack of commercially available PTH

Theoretically, the most appropriate therapy for hypoparathyroidism is the physiologic replacement of PTH. The practical limitation to this approach is the lack of suitable commercial PTH preparations. This has resulted in the use of vitamin D preparations as the primary means of treating hypoparathyroidism. Unfortunately, absence of endogenous PTH also causes a relative deficiency in the enzyme that converts inactive vitamin D (25[OH]D) to its active metabolite (1,25[OH]$_2$D). Thus hypoparathyroid patients are resistant to physiologic doses of vitamin D. Nevertheless, treatment with pharmacologic doses of vitamin D in combination with oral calcium administration has been the mainstay of managing hypoparathyroidism. Recurrent hypocalcemia and worrisome hypercalcemia represent potential complications of treatment if adequate calcium monitoring is neglected.

Vitamin D

GENERAL. Maintenance therapy for hypoparathyroidism consists of oral vitamin D and calcium supplementation. The need for vitamin D therapy is usually permanent in dogs and cats with primary, naturally occurring parathyroid gland failure. Calcium supplementation, however, can often be tapered and then stopped, because dietary calcium is sufficient for maintaining the needs of the animal. Conservative doses of supplemental calcium, however, ensure that vitamin D, which raises serum calcium by promoting its intestinal absorption, has substrate upon which to function. Iatrogenic hypoparathyroidism in dogs and cats following surgery is often transient and lifelong therapy is not always needed.

In contrast to tetany, for which the immediate goal of treatment is to avoid recurrence of neuromuscular signs, the aim of long-term therapy is to maintain serum calcium concentrations at mildly low to low-normal concentrations (8.0 to 9.5 mg/dl). Such calcium concentrations are above the level of risk for clinical hypocalcemia. Mild hypocalcemia should promote function of atrophied parathyroid glands and is below the level that might be associated with hypercalciuria (risk for calculi formation) or severe hypercalcemia and hyperphosphatemia (risk for nephrocalcinosis and renal failure).

VITAMIN D$_2$ (ERGOCALCIFEROL). Vitamin D$_2$ is a widely available, relatively inexpensive drug (40,000 USP U/mg; Table 17-8). Initially, large doses are required to induce normocalcemia. Dogs and cats can be given 4000 to 6000 U/kg once daily. These doses are needed to offset the decreased biologic potency of this product in hypoparathyroid patients. Additionally, large doses are required to saturate fat depots, important because vitamin D is a fat-soluble vitamin. Effect of the medication is usually obvious 5 to 14 days after beginning therapy. Parenteral calcium can usually be discontinued 1 to 5 days after starting oral treatment.

Dogs and cats receiving vitamin D$_2$ should be hospitalized until the total serum calcium concentration remains between 8 and 10 mg/dl without parenteral support. Once this goal is achieved, the pet can be returned to the owner and the vitamin D$_2$ is usually given every other day. Serum calcium concentrations should be monitored weekly, with vitamin D$_2$ doses adjusted to maintain a serum calcium concentration of 8 to 9.5 mg/dl. The aim of therapy is to avoid hypocalcemic tetany, but the most common problem with therapy is induction of hypercalcemia.

Even after a pet appears stable, monthly rechecks are strongly advised for 6 months and should be followed by rechecks every 2 to 3 months indefinitely. These animals cannot be rechecked too often. Drug-induced hypercalcemia can result in severe renal damage and renal failure, a problem that can be avoided or at least

TABLE 17-8   VITAMIN D PREPARATIONS

Preparation	Dosage Forms	Commercial Names (Manufacturer)	Daily Doses	Time Required for Maximal Effect	Time Required for Toxicity Relief
Vitamin D$_2$ (ergocalciferol)	Capsules 25,000 U 50,000 U	Calciferol (Rorer) Drisdol (Winthrop-Breon) Deltallin (Lilly)	Initial: 4000–6000 U/kg/day	5–21 days	1–18 weeks
	Oral syrup 8,000 U/ml IM injectable 50,000 U/ml	Drisdol (Winthrop-Breon) Calciferol (Rorer) Vitadee (Gotham)	Maintenance: 1000–2000 U/kg once daily–once weekly		
Dihydrotachysterol	Tablets 0.125 mg 0.2 mg 0.4 mg	Dihydrotachysterol (Philips-Roxane)	Initial: 0.02–0.03 mg/kg/day	1–7 days	1–3 week
	Capsules 0.125 mg Oral solution 0.25 mg/ml	Hytakerol (Winthrop-Breon) Hytakerol (Winthrop-Breon)	Maintenance: 0.01–0.02 mg/kg q24-48 hr		
Vitamin D$_3$ (calcitriol)	Capsules 0.25 µg 0.5 µg	Rocaltrol (Roche) (also generic)	Approximate: 0.03–0.06 µg/kg/day	1–4 days	24 hours–2 weeks
	Vitamin D$_3$ injectable 1.0 µg/ml	Calcijex (Abbott Laboratories)	Approximate: 0.02 µg/kg/day		1 to 7 days/week

minimized through proper monitoring. Vitamin D_2 has been used in cats and dogs with success and is relatively inexpensive. Some of our dogs and cats receive medication as infrequently as once weekly, whereas others require daily supplementation.

The drawbacks of vitamin D_2 include the previously described induction of hypercalcemia. Hypercalcemia, if it occurs, is not easily treated. Because of the fat-soluble nature of vitamin D_2, one may need to discontinue therapy for as long as 1 to 4 weeks before serum calcium concentrations decline. It is this physiologic condition that makes ergocalciferol the least attractive agent for treating hypocalcemia. Delays in correcting overdosage can certainly be life-threatening. Hypercalcemia should be aggressively treated with intravenous fluids and furosemide, especially if the product of the serum calcium multiplied by the serum phosphate is greater than 60 to 80. Some patients are further helped by corticosteroid therapy. We restrict use of ergocalciferol to owners with financial limitations that prevent use of DHT or calcitriol.

DIHYDROTACHYSTEROL (DHT). DHT is a synthetic vitamin D analogue. The advantages of DHT over vitamin D_2 are that it raises the serum calcium concentration more rapidly (1 to 7 days) and its effect dissipates faster when administration is discontinued. Veterinarians, therefore, have more control over therapy. DHT is readily available, more expensive than vitamin D_2, and more potent than vitamin D_2, 1.0 mg of DHT being equivalent to 120,000 U of vitamin D_2. The rapid onset of action and the increased effectiveness of DHT are a result of its stereochemistry; the A ring of the sterol structure is rotated 180 degrees so that the hydroxyl group in the 3 position serves as a pseudo-1-hydroxyl group (Fig. 17-9). Therefore, after hepatic 25-hydroxylation, DHT has biologic activity between that of 1,25-dihydroxyvitamin D and 25-hydroxyvitamin D (Peterson, 1982). The polarity and lower dose requirements of DHT limit its storage in fat compared with ergocalciferol.

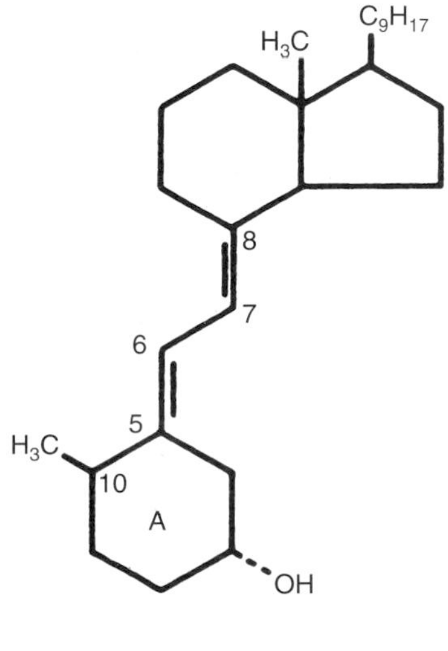

DHT has been our "drug of choice" for long-term management of hypocalcemia. The combination of ready availability, size of tablets, the alternative of a liquid form of the medication, reasonable cost, and effectiveness has made this an ideal therapy for a majority of our hypocalcemic dogs and cats. DHT is initially given at a dose of 0.03 mg/kg/day (divided and given twice a day) for 2 days or until effect is demonstrated, then 0.02 mg/kg/day for several days, and finally 0.01 mg/kg/day in divided dosages. As suggested with the less potent vitamin D, significant individual variation in dose requirements dictate that pets remain hospitalized until the serum calcium concentration remains stable between 8 and 9.5 mg/dl for several days. We have seen cats and dogs that appeared to be resistant to the tablet and capsule forms of this drug (0.125, 0.25, 0.4 mg) but which respond readily to the liquid (0.25 mg/ml). We have also seen dogs and cats fail to respond to any form of DHT but respond to calcitriol. Rechecks of the serum calcium concentration on a weekly basis allow dosage adjustment while avoiding prolonged hypercalcemia or hypocalcemia. As with vitamin D_2, long-term rechecks at least every 2 to 3 months are strongly encouraged.

High normal or increased circulating concentrations of calcium (>10.5 to 11.0 mg/dl) should be treated by lowering or discontinuing vitamin D therapy and, depending on the severity of the clinical signs and biochemistry abnormalities, possibly initiating intravenous fluids, furosemide, and/or corticosteroids (see Chapter 16). The lag period between stopping DHT and noting a fall in the serum calcium concentration has been 4 to 14 days, a much briefer period than with vitamin D_2.

ORAL 1,25-DIHYDROXYVITAMIN D; CALCITRIOL. Although we prefer DHT in managing our dogs with permanent or transient primary hypoparathyroidism, others consider calcitriol to be the "metabolite of choice." It is the most active known form of vitamin D_3 in stimulating intestinal calcium transport and osteoblastic activity in the skeleton, and it has the most rapid onset of maximal action and the shortest biologic half-life (Rosol et al, 2000; Chew and Nagode, 2000). It has been hypothesized that oral calcitriol has a direct effect on intestinal receptors, stimulating intestinal calcium absorption to a greater degree than other forms of vitamin D, including parenteral administration (Coburn, 1990).

The dose of calcitriol can be adjusted frequently because of its rapid onset of action and brief biologic effect. If hypercalcemia occurs, the effects of this drug abate quickly after stopping therapy or with dose reduction. The peak serum concentration of calcitriol is reached after 4 hours, the half-life is 4 to 6 hours, and the biologic half-life is 3 to 5 days. A loading dose of 20 to 40 ng/kg/day can be administered for 2 to 4 days

H_3C C_9H_{17}

8
7
6
5
H_3C
10
A
OH

Dihydrotachysterol$_2$

FIGURE 17-9. The chemical structure of dihydrotachysterol.

and then decreased to a maintenance dose of 10 to 20 ng/kg/day, divided and given twice daily (NOTE: This dose is in *nanograms*). The drug is available commercially in both original brand name and generic forms. Calcitriol is formulated for humans and may require reformulation for dogs and cats.

The concerns we have regarding calcitriol only relate to expense and the need for reformulation. Although reformulation should be reliable, inconsistencies occur among pharmacies. The reformulation by specialty pharmacies of calcitriol into liquid or into capsule sizes tailored to the need of specific pets will not likely provide the same "compound" and effectiveness to each patient. We have had experience with one dog that did not respond to oral calcitriol at any dose. This dog was known to have liver "insufficiency" since a diagnosis of vascular anomaly had been made 10 years earlier. Although calcitriol is "active," it is interesting to note lack of response in this setting.

PARENTERAL CALCITRIOL. In the event that oral medication cannot be administered or if oral calcitriol is ineffective, parenteral calcitriol can be given. Empirically, the same dose as that used for oral administration can be utilized (10 to 20 ng/kg/day). The drug is usually given intravenously to human dialysis patients, 3 times weekly, immediately after dialysis (Selgas et al, 1993; Rolla et al, 1993). The drug can be given subcutaneously and intraperitoneally, as well. We have used parenteral calcitriol successfully by administering it IV, TID, to effect and then progressively decreasing the dose. As with other forms of vitamin D, in-hospital monitoring is recommended until circulating calcium concentrations are stable. Owners can then administer the drug subcutaneously.

Calcium supplementation

INITIAL APPROACH TO ORAL CALCIUM. Dietary calcium must be adequate when treating hypoparathyroidism, because the primary mode of therapy depends on administration of vitamin D, which acts to increase absorption of calcium present in the intestinal lumen. Commercial pet food usually contains sufficient calcium to supply the needs of such dogs and cats. However, in order to avoid the catastrophic problems of hypocalcemia, especially early in the course of therapy, oral calcium supplementation is strongly recommended. Once tetany is controlled with bolus IV calcium, serum calcium levels should be maintained with a slow IV infusion or subcutaneous injections. At the same time, oral calcium and vitamin D therapy should be initiated. After 24 to 96 hours, the parenteral calcium administration can often be discontinued while oral therapy is maintained. In this manner, smooth continuous control is achieved.

CALCIUM SUPPLEMENTS. Supplements can be provided by administering calcium as the gluconate, lactate, chloride, or carbonate salt. Each has disadvantages. Calcium gluconate and lactate tablets contain relatively small quantities of elemental calcium, so relatively large numbers of tablets must be given. Calcium chloride tablets contain large quantities of calcium but tend to produce gastric irritation. Calcium carbonate tablets also contain large quantities of calcium but tend to produce alkalosis, which may aggravate hypocalcemia. Calcium carbonate is 40% calcium. One gram yields 20 mEq of calcium and gastric acid converts the calcium carbonate to calcium chloride. Calcium lactate is 13% calcium, and 1 g yields 6.5 mEq. Calcium gluconate contains 9% calcium, and 1 g yields 4.5 mEq.

Obviously, numerous calcium preparations are available (see Table 15-7). Calcium carbonate is the preparation of choice in treating hypoparathyroid humans because of its high percentage of calcium, low cost, lack of gastric irritation, and ready availability in drug stores in the form of antacids (Arnaud, 1994). No specific research to support recommendations for use of this drug is available for dogs and cats, although our success with calcium carbonate has been excellent.

TREATMENT PROTOCOL. In cats, the dosage of calcium is approximately 0.5 to 1.0 g/day in divided doses. In dogs, the dosage is usually 1.0 to 4.0 g/day in divided doses. These recommendations are approximate, and the primary therapy that determines stability of the serum calcium concentration is the use of vitamin D. As the vitamin D dose reaches a steady level, the dose of calcium can be gradually tapered over a period of 2 to 4 months. This method of treatment avoids unnecessary therapy, considering that dietary calcium should be sufficient to supply the needs of the pet and should decrease the demands of treatment placed on the owner. It must be emphasized that the ideal serum calcium concentration in these animals is 8 to 9.5 mg/dl. Concentrations above 10 are too high; they are unnecessary in avoiding tetany, and they increase the likelihood of unwanted hypercalcemia.

PARATHYROID HISTOLOGY IN HYPOPARATHYROIDISM

Animals have been classified as having idiopathic hypoparathyroidism when there is no evidence of trauma, malignant or surgical destruction, or other obvious damage to the neck or parathyroid glands. The glands are difficult to locate visually or via ultrasound and are microscopically atrophied. Approximately 60% to 80% of the glands are replaced by mature lymphocytes, occasional plasma cells, extensive degeneration of chief cells, and/or fibrous connective tissue. Chief cells are randomly isolated in multiple small areas or bands at the periphery. In the early stages of an immune-mediated attack, the gland is infiltrated with lymphocytes and plasma cells, with nodular regenerative hyperplasia of remaining chief cells. Later, the parathyroid gland is completely replaced by lymphocytes, fibroblasts, and neocapillaries, with only an occasional viable chief cell. The final interpretation is one of lymphocytic parathyroiditis (Capen and Marten, 1983; Sherding et al, 1980).

PROGNOSIS

The prognosis with primary hypoparathyroidism depends, for the most part, on the dedication of the owner and, to a lesser extent, on the experience of the veterinarian. With proper therapy, the prognosis is excellent. Thirty-three of our 37 dogs have lived more than 5 years from the time of diagnosis and treatment. However, proper management requires close monitoring of the serum calcium concentration, ideally every 1 to 3 months once the pet is stabilized. The more frequent the rechecks, the better chance the pet has of avoiding extremes in serum calcium concentrations. The chance for a normal life expectancy is excellent with proper care.

REFERENCES

Abrams KL: Hypocalcemia associated with administration of sodium bicarbonate for salicylate intoxication in a cat. JAVMA 191:235, 1987.

Arnaud CD: The calciotropic hormones and metabolic bone disease. In Greenspan FS, Baxter JD (eds): Basic and Clinical Endocrinology, 4th ed. Norwalk, Conn, Appleton & Lange, 1983, p 227.

Aroch I, et al: Serum electrolyte concentrations in bitches with eclampsia. Vet Rec 145:318, 1999.

Atkins CE, et al: Clinical, biochemical, acid-base, and electrolyte abnormalities in cats after hypertonic sodium phosphate enema administration. Am J Vet Res 46:980, 1985.

Barber PJ, Elliott J: Study of calcium homeostasis in feline hyperthyroidism. J Sm Anim Pract 37:575, 1996.

Barber PJ, et al: Measurement of feline parathyroid hormone: Assay validation and sample handling studies. J Small Anim Pract 34:614, 1993.

Bassett JR: Hypocalcemia and hyperphosphatemia due to primary hypoparathyroidism in a six-month-old kitten. J Am Anim Hosp Assoc 34:503, 1998.

Bienzle D, et al: Relationship of serum total calcium to serum albumin in dogs, cats, horses, and cattle. Can Vet J 34:360, 1993.

Broadus AE: Mineral metabolism. In Felig P, et al (eds): Endocrinology and Metabolism. New York, McGraw-Hill, 1981, p 1056.

Broadus AE, et al: Humoral hypercalcemia of cancer: identification of a novel parathyroid hormone-like peptide. N Engl J Med 319:556, 1988.

Bruyette DS, Feldman EC: Primary hypoparathyroidism in the dog: Report of 15 cases and review of 13 previously reported cases. J Vet Intern Med 2:7, 1988.

Burk RL, Schaubhut CW: Spontaneous primary hypoparathyroidism in a dog. J Am Anim Hosp Assoc 11:784, 1975.

Bush WW, et al: Secondary hypoparathyroidism attributed to hypomagnesemia in a dog with protein-losing enteropathy. JAVMA 219:1732, 2001.

Capen CC, Martin SL: Calcium-regulatory hormones and diseases of the parathyroid glands. In Ettinger SJ (ed): Textbook of Veterinary Internal Medicine. Philadelphia, WB Saunders Co, 1983, p 1581.

Chew DJ, Meuten DJ: Disorders of calcium and phosphorus metabolism. Vet Clin North Am 12:411, 1983.

Chew DJ, Nagode LA: Renal secondary hyperparathyroidism. Proceedings of the 4th Annual Meeting of The Society for Comparative Endocrinology, 1990, p 17.

Chew DJ, Nagode LA: Treatment of hypoparathyroidism. In Bonagura JD (ed): Kirk's Current Veterinary Therapy XIII. Philadelphia, WB Saunders Co, 2000, p 340.

Chew DJ, Meuten DJ: Disorders of calcium and phosphorus metabolism. Vet Clin North Am Small Anim Pract 12:411, 1982.

Chew DJ, et al: Utility of diagnostic assays in the evaluation of hypercalcemia and hypocalcemia: Parathyroid hormone, vitamin D metabolites, parathyroid hormone-related peptide, and ionized calcium. In Bonagura JD (ed): Kirk's Current Veterinary Therapy XII. Philadelphia, WB Saunders, 1995, p 378.

Coburn JW: Use of oral and parenteral calcitriol in the treatment of renal osteodystrophy. Kidney Int 38(Suppl):S54, 1990.

Crawford MA, Dunstan RW: Hypocalcemia secondary to primary hypoparathyroidism in a dog. Calif Vet, May/June, 1985, p 21.

Dhupa N, Proulx J: Hypocalcemia and hypomagnesemia. Vet Clin North Am Small Anim Pract 28:587, 1998.

Drobatz KJ, Casey KK: Eclampsia in dogs: 31 cases (1995-1998). JAVMA 217:216, 2000.

Drobatz KJ, Hughes D: Concentration of ionized calcium in plasma from cats with urethral obstruction. JAVMA 211:1392, 1997.

Elin RJ: Magnesium: The fifth but forgotten electrolyte. Clin Chem 102:616, 1994.

Fascetti AJ, Hickman MA: Preparturient hypocalcemia in four cats. JAVMA 215:1127, 1999.

Feldman EC, Krutzik S: Case reports of parathyroid hormone concentrations in spontaneous canine parathyroid disorders. JAAHA 17:393, 1981.

Flanders JA: Surgical therapy of the thyroid. Vet Clin N Am Small Anim Pract 24:607, 1994.

Flanders JA, et al: Feline thyroidectomy: A comparison of postoperative hypocalcemia associated with three different surgical techniques. Vet Surg 16:362, 1987.

Flanders JA, et al: Adjustment of total serum calcium concentration for binding to albumin and protein in cats: 291 cases (1986–1987). JAVMA 194:1609, 1989.

Flanders JA, et al: Functional analysis of ectopic parathyroid activity in cats. Am J Vet Res 52:1336, 1991.

Flanders JA, Reimers TJ: Radioimmunoassay of parathyroid hormone in cats. Am J Vet Res 52:422, 1991.

Forbes S, et al: Primary hypoparathyroidism in a cat. JAVMA 196:1285, 1990.

Freeman LM, et al: Fanconi's syndrome in a dog with primary hypoparathyroidism. J Vet Int Med 8:349, 1994.

Graves TK: Complications of treatment and concurrent illness associated with hyperthyroidism in cats. In Bonagura JD (ed): Kirk's Current Veterinary Therapy XII. Philadelphia, WB Saunders Co. 1995, p 369.

Grosenbaugh DA, et al: Evaluation of a portable clinical analyzer in a veterinary hospital setting. J Am Vet Med Assoc 213:691, 1998.

Hansen B: Disorders of Magnesium. In DiBartola SP (ed): Fluid Therapy in Small Animal Practice, 2nd ed. Philadelphia, WB Saunders Co. 2000, p 175.

Henderson RA, et al: Development of hypoparathyroidism after excision of laryngeal rhabdomyosarcoma in a dog. J Am Vet Med Assoc 198:639, 1991.

Henik RA, et al: Rickets caused by excessive renal phosphate loss and apparent abnormal vitamin D metabolism in a cat. JAVMA 215:1644, 1999.

Hess RS, et al: Clinical, clinicopathologic, radiologic, and ultrasonographic abnormalities in dogs with fatal acute pancreatitis: 70 cases (1986-1995). JAVMA 213:665, 1998.

Horn B, Irwin PJ: Transient hypoparathyroidism following successful treatment of hypercalcemia of malignancy in a dog. Aust Vet J 78:690, 2000.

Jorgensen LS, et al: Electrolyte abnormalities induced by hypertonic phosphate enemas in two cats. JAVMA 187:1367, 1985.

Kimmel SE, et al: Incidence and prognostic value of low plasma ionized calcium concentration in cats with acute pancreatitis: 46 cases (1996-1998). JAVMA 219:1105, 2001.

Kimmel SE, et al: Hypomagnesemia and hypocalcemia associated with protein-losing enteropathy in Yorkshire Terriers: five cases (1992-1998). JAVMA 217:703, 2000.

Klein MK, et al: Treatment of thyroid carcinoma in dogs by surgical resection alone: 20 cases (1981-1989). JAVMA 206:1007, 1995.

Kornegay JN: Hypocalcemia in dogs. Comp Cont Ed Small Anim Pract 4:103, 1982.

Kornegay JN, et al: Idiopathic hypocalcemia in four dogs. JAAHA 16:723, 1980.

Li YC, et al: Normalization of mineral ion homeostasis by dietary means prevents hyperparathyroidism, rickets, and osteomalacia, but not alopecia in vitamin D-receptor ablated mice. Endocrinol 139:4391, 1998.

Malloy PJ, et al: The vitamin D receptor and the syndrome of hereditary 1,25-dihydroxyvitamin D-resistant rickets. Endocr Rev 20:156, 1999.

Marx SJ: Hyperparathyroid and hypoparathyroid disorders. N Engl J Med: 343:1863, 2000.

Meininger ME, Kendler JS: Trousseau's Sign. N Engl J Med 343:1855, 2000.

Meuten DJ, Armstrong PJ: Parathyroid disease and calcium metabolism. In Ettinger SJ (ed): Textbook of Veterinary Internal Medicine. 3rd ed. Philadelphia, WB Saunders, 1989, p 1610.

Meuten DJ, et al: Relationship of serum total calcium to albumin and total protein in dogs. JAVMA 180:63, 1982.

Meyer DJ, Tyrrell TG: Idiopathic hypoparathyroidism in a dog. J Am Vet Med Assoc 168:858, 1976.

Milnor WR: Properties of cardiac tissues. In Mountcastle VB (ed): Medical Physiology. St Louis, CV Mosby Co, 1980, p 980.

Padgett SL, et al: Efficacy of parathyroid gland autotransplantation in maintaining serum calcium concentrations after bilateral thyroparathyroidectomy in cats. J Am Anim Hosp Assoc 34:219, 1998.

Parker JSL: A probable case of hypoparathyroidism in a cat. J Small Anim Pract 32:470, 1991.

Pearce SHS, et al: A familial syndrome of hypocalcemia with hypercalciuria due to mutations in the calcium-sensing receptor. N Engl J Med 335:1115, 1996.

Peterson ME: Treatment of canine and feline hypoparathyroidism. JAVMA 181:1434, 1982.

Peterson ME: Hypoparathyroidism: In Kirk RW (ed): Current Veterinary Therapy IX. Philadelphia, WB Saunders, 1986, p 1039.

Peterson ME: Hypoparathyroidism and other causes of hypocalcemia in cats. In Kirk RW, Bonagura JA (eds): Current Veterinary Therapy XI. Philadelphia, WB Saunders Co, 1992, p 376.

Peterson ME, et al: Idiopathic hypoparathyroidism in five cats. J Vet Intern Med 5:47, 1991.

Rasmussen H: Theoretical considerations in the treatment of osteoporosis. *In* De Luca HF (ed): Osteoporosis: Recent Advances in Pathogenesis and Treatment. Baltimore, University Park Press, 1981, p 383.

Rolla D, et al: Effects of subcutaneous calcitriol administration on plasma calcium and parathyroid hormone concentrations in continuous ambulatory peritoneal dialysis uremic patients. Peritoneal Dialysis Int 13:118, 1993.

Rosol TJ, Capen CC: Calcium-regulating hormones and diseases of abnormal mineral (calcium, phosphorus, magnesium) metabolism. *In* Kaneko JJ, Harvey JW, Bruss ML (eds): Clinical Biochemistry of Domestic Animals. San Diego, Academic Press, 1997, p 619.

Rosol TJ, et al: Disorders of Calcium. *In* DiBartola SP (ed): Fluid Therapy in Small Animal Practice, 2nd ed. Philadelphia, WB Saunders Co, 2000, p 108.

Ruopp JL: Primary hypoparathyroidism in a cat complicated by suspect iatrogenic calcinosis cutis. J Am Anim Hosp Assoc 37:370, 2001.

Schaer M, et al: Severe calcinosis cutis associated with treatment of hypoparathyroidism in a dog. J Am Anim Hosp Assoc 37:364, 2001.

Schenck PA, et al: Effects of storage on normal canine serum ionized calcium and pH. Am J Vet Res 56:304, 1995.

Schenck PA, et al: Effects of storage on serum ionized calcium and pH from horses with normal and abnormal ionized calcium concentrations. Vet Clin Pathol 25:118, 1996.

Schick MP, et al: Calcinosis cutis secondary to percutaneous penetration of calcium chloride in dogs. JAVMA 191:207, 1987.

Selgas R, et al: The pharmacokinetics of a single dose of calcitriol administered subcutaneously in continuous ambulatory peritoneal dialysis patients. Peritoneal Dialysis Int 13:122, 1993.

Sherding RG, et al: Primary hypoparathyroidism in the dog. JAVMA 176:439, 1980.

Tepperman J: Metabolic and Endocrine Physiology. Chicago, Year Book Medical Publishers, 1980, p 297.

Tomsa K, et al: Nutritional secondary hyperparathyroidism in six cats. J Sm Anim Pract 40:533, 1999.

Torrance AG: Disorders of Calcium Metabolism. *In* Torrance AG and Mooney CT (eds): Manual of Small Animal Endocrinology, 2nd ed. British Small Animal Veterinary Association, 1998, p 129.

Torrance AG, Nachreiner R: Intact parathyroid hormone assay and total calcium concentration in the diagnosis of disorders of calcium metabolism in dogs. J Vet Intern Med 3:86, 1989.

Vaden SL, et al: A retrospective case-control study of acute renal failure in 99 dogs. J Vet Intern Med 11:58, 1997.

Welches CD, et al: Occurrence of problems after three techniques of bilateral thyroidectomy in cats. Vet Surg 18:392, 1989.

Weir EC, et al: Isolation of 16,000-dalton parathyroid hormone like proteins from two animal tumors causing humoral hypercalcemia of malignancy. Endocrinol 123:2744, 1988.

Yates AJ, et al: Effects of a synthetic peptide of a parathyroid-related protein on calcium homeostasis, renal tubular calcium reabsorption and bone metabolism in vivo and in vitro in rodents. J Clin Invest 81:932, 1988.

RENAL HORMONES AND ATRIAL NATRIURETIC HORMONE

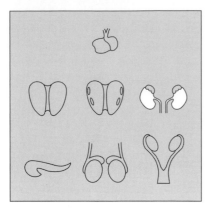

18

RENAL HORMONES AND ATRIAL NATRIURETIC HORMONE

THE KIDNEY

Hormones Synthesized by the Kidneys

The kidneys are involved in four major hormonal systems in the body. First, they secrete *renin*, a proteolytic enzyme that initiates a chain of events leading to production of the circulating peptide *angiotensin II*, which plays an important role in the regulation of salt and water metabolism, stimulates synthesis and secretion of *aldosterone*, and is a regulator of blood pressure. Second, the kidneys produce *kinins*, which are thought to enhance the effects of aldosterone and vasopressin in the kidneys. Kidney disease and renal hormones are frequently involved in the pathogenesis of hypertension. Third, the kidneys secrete *erythropoietin*, a glycoprotein that helps to control red cell production. Fourth, the final step in *activation of vitamin D* occurs in the kidneys. The kidneys remove 25-hydroxycholecalciferol from the bloodstream and hydroxylate it to *1,25-dihydroxycholecalciferol*. This agent increases the plasma calcium concentration by increasing its intestinal absorption, enhancing renal tubular resorption, and stimulating bone resorption. Vitamin D and its actions are discussed thoroughly in Chapters 16 and 17.

Erythropoietin

PHYSIOLOGY. It has long been realized that hypoxia is a potent stimulus to red cell production. In human subjects, within a few hours of exposure to hypoxia, the reticulocyte count increases, denoting the presence of new red blood cells in the circulation; this is followed by an increase in the circulating red cell mass. This response is the result of the increased production of a glycoprotein, erythropoietin. The kidney is the major source of this hormone, although it is also produced in the liver, particularly in fetuses. Day-to-day production of erythropoietin depends on the partial pressure of oxygen (PO_2) of blood perfusing the kidneys. The target cells for erythropoietin are the colony-forming units–erythroid (CFU-E) cells in the bone marrow. Erythropoietin reacts with receptors on CFU-E cells, leading to increased production of proerythroblasts and release of more erythrocytes into the circulation (Fig. 18-1) (Erslev, 1991).

Healthy adults continuously secrete erythropoietin. Because hypoxia is the most important stimulus to erythropoietin production, a number of pathologic conditions affecting the kidney, particularly those that reduce renal blood flow, may increase the rate of erythropoietin release and inevitably increase red blood cell production. A few cases of erythropoietin-releasing tumors have been described in dogs with severe polycythemia.

One of the explanations for the nonregenerative anemia in dogs and cats with chronic renal failure is a decreased capacity to synthesize erythropoietin because of underlying disease, which results in a loss of erythropoietin-producing cells. The suppressed rate of red blood cell formation caused by lack of renal production of erythropoietin is a major problem in the treatment of patients with severe renal failure. Renal transplantation not only restores renal function to individuals with severe renal failure but also restores normal erythropoiesis.

BENEFITS OF SYNTHETIC ERYTHROPOIETIN. Human erythropoietin has been cloned and represents one of the most successful products of recombinant deoxyribonucleic acid (DNA) technology. Recombinant human erythropoietin (rHuEPO; epoetin) is available for therapeutic use and has revolutionized the treatment of anemia in humans with chronic renal failure. Epoetin is virtually identical to human urinary erythropoietin; it has the same amino acid sequence but a slightly different glycosylation pattern. Most treated

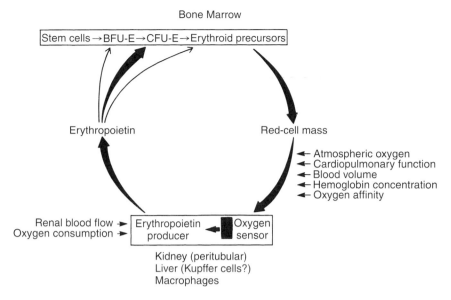

FIGURE 18-1. Feedback circuit that adjusts the rate of red cell production to the demand for oxygen. *BFU-E,* Burst-forming units–erythroid; *CFU-E,* colony-forming units–erythroid. (Erslev AJ: N Engl J Med 324:1339, 1991.)

humans have reported dramatic improvement in their quality of life and sense of well-being as a result of correction of anemia. The benefits of improved exercise tolerance, appetite, strength, and cognitive abilities without the need for blood transfusions outweigh some of the risks associated with the use of rHuEPO.

Most experience with the use of rHuEPO in animals has been with epoetin-α (Epogen). Epogen is suspended in human albumin to prevent adherence to glass and does not contain a preservative. The structure of erythropoietin is well conserved across species lines. Both dogs and cats respond appropriately to administration of this synthetic hormone. When given to dogs or cats with chronic renal failure, rHuEPO causes a dose-dependent increase in the hematocrit and corrects anemia (Cowgill, 1990, 1995). A transient, moderate reticulocytosis is initially observed within the first week of therapy in most animals. The bone marrow myeloid:erythroid ratio decreases, illustrating the increased erythropoietic response. Some animals have a transient thrombocytosis during therapy. This response may be seen in some human patients as well, and it is not known whether this is a direct effect of the rHuEPO on megakaryocytes or a secondary effect caused by iron deficiency (Polzin et al, 1995). Correction of the hematocrit to low normal takes about 2 to 8 weeks, depending on the measurement when treatment was initiated and the dose administered. Most clients observe improved clinical status in their pets as the hematocrit increases. These changes include improved appetite, body weight, energy, and sociability (Cowgill, 1990).

DOSAGE AND ROUTE OF rHuEPO ADMINISTRATION. Both intravenous and subcutaneous routes of administration of rHuEPO have been effective, and no difference has been seen in the percentage of patients that develop antibodies. Plasma concentrations persist

longer after subcutaneous administration, which allows lower total doses to be given. Definitive dosing schedules are continuing to evolve. Currently, starting doses of 50 to 150 U/kg given subcutaneously three times per week are recommended (Polzin et al, 1995). Weekly monitoring should continue until a target hematocrit is achieved; that is, a packed cell volume (PCV) of 33% to 40% in dogs and 30% to 35% in cats. If a dog or cat has severe anemia (PCV <14%) but does not require transfusion, daily therapy with 150 U/kg may be preferred for the first week. In hypertensive animals or if the anemia is not severe, 50 U/kg three times weekly may prevent progressive increases in blood pressure or iron-deficient erythropoiesis.

When a hematocrit at the low end of the target range has been achieved, the dosing interval should be decreased to twice weekly. Most animals require 50 to 100 U/kg two to three times weekly to maintain red blood cell counts and PCVs in the target range. The dosage required, however, varies significantly among treated individuals, therefore chronic monitoring of the PCV is necessary for proper adjustment of the dose or dosing interval or both. If a dosage exceeding 150 U/kg three times weekly is required, the animal may have erythropoietin resistance. Because of the time lag between dose adjustment and the effect on the PCV, patience must be exercised so that the dose is not adjusted too frequently, resulting in rather unpredictable changes in the PCV and inability to find a stable dose. Avoiding iatrogenic polycythemia is important.

Because of the high demand for iron associated with stimulated erythropoiesis, patients treated with rHuEPO are at risk of exhaustion of iron stores. Oral iron supplementation, therefore, is recommended for all patients treated with rHuEPO, even if the pretreatment transferrin concentrations are normal.

ADVERSE REACTIONS TO rHuEPO

Identified Adverse Reactions. A variety of adverse reactions to rHuEPO therapy have been identified, although a direct causal relationship between drug and side effect may not always be established. Adverse reactions include refractory anemia, polycythemia, vomiting, seizures, and discomfort at the site of injection. Transient cutaneous or mucocutaneous reactions with or without fever, hypertension, and cardiac complications have also been identified (Cowgill, 1992).

Neutralizing Antibodies. The problem of rHuEPO-related refractory anemia can be caused by the development of neutralizing anti-rHuEPO antibodies. The rHuEPO protein is antigenic in many dogs and cats, stimulating antibody titers as early as 4 weeks after treatment starts or many months later. Antibody titers decline after treatment stops, and attempts at immunosuppressive therapy to abrogate this response have not proved successful. It may be possible to test for antibody concentrations directly; as an alternative, bone marrow myeloid:erythroid ratios provide evidence of antibody formation. After rHuEPO is discontinued, pretreatment levels of erythropoiesis are attained (Polzin et al, 1995). However, such levels may not be sufficient to maintain adequate red cell numbers because severe anemia is present when rHuEPO is used.

Hypertension. It has been hypothesized that patients with chronic anemia (as occurs with chronic renal failure) have peripheral vasodilation. This vasodilation may be corrected with rHuEPO therapy, resulting in hypertension caused by increased peripheral vascular resistance. Hypertension has been identified as a complication of therapy and does not appear to be the result of a direct pressor effect of the rHuEPO (Nissenson et al, 1991; Cowgill, 1992).

Seizures and Allergic Reactions. Seizures have been observed after initiation of rHuEPO therapy in humans, dogs, and cats with chronic renal failure. Hypertensive and uremic encephalopathy are the most likely explanations in dogs and cats because the seizures have occurred in the animals with the most advanced renal disease. Allergic reactions, such as the cutaneous or mucocutaneous reactions observed in people, are not common in dogs or cats. Most lesions resolve within a few days of discontinuation of rHuEPO treatment, and some have not recurred if treatment is reinstated.

Serum Chemistries and Serum Iron. Abnormalities in serum chemistries have not been associated with rHuEPO therapy, although numerous alterations are attributed to the chronic renal failure. Decreases in serum iron and transferrin saturation are common. No evidence indicates that rHuEPO therapy has any effect on the progression of chronic renal failure.

Blunted Response to rHuEPO. Individual differences in response to rHuEPO are typical but not well understood. Several causes of blunted response or failure to resolve anemia have been identified in dogs and cats. These include antibodies to the rHuEPO in 20% to 30% of treated animals, functional or absolute iron deficiency, gastrointestinal loss of blood, hemolysis, and concurrent inflammatory or malignant diseases (Polzin et al, 1995).

WHEN TO INITIATE rHuEPO THERAPY. The prevalence of anti-rHuEPO antibodies in treated dogs and cats makes the decision process regarding when to initiate therapy quite important. Most recommend using the drug only when definitely necessary because once an animal develops the antibodies, the drug no longer has any value to that individual. When the hematocrit values are below 25% in dogs or 20% in cats, anemia probably contributes to the adverse clinical signs associated with chronic renal failure. These PCV guidelines usually can be used to judge the severity of anemia; however, the degree of azotemia, expected progression rate of chronic renal failure, appetite, willingness to eat therapeutic diets, and progression rate of the anemia should all be considered in the risk-benefit analysis of when to start therapy (Polzin et al, 1995). Because many pet owners consider quality of life of prime importance, the advantages and disadvantages of rHuEPO treatment should be discussed with owners when anemia appears to be contributing to the dog's or cat's deteriorating quality of life.

Kallikrein-Kinin System

The kidney contains all the elements of the kallikrein-kinin system. Renal kallikrein is a serine protease that is synthesized in distal tubule cells and is distinct from plasma kallikrein. Kallikrein is secreted into distal tubular fluid, where it reacts with filtered hepatic kininogen to form kinin. Kinin receptors are located in the cortical and medullary collecting tubules on both the luminal and peritubular surfaces. Kinins appear to increase the salt retention effects of aldosterone and the water excretion–inhibiting effects of vasopressin on the collecting tubular epithelium. The physiologic significance of the kallikrein-kinin system is not yet clear (Biglieri et al, 1994).

Renin and the Renin-Angiotensin System

BACKGROUND. In 1947, Goldblatt noted that a reduction in the flow of blood to the kidney in experimental animals was followed by an increase in blood pressure. This experiment implicated the kidney in the pathogenesis of hypertension. As the afferent arteriole enters the glomerulus (Fig. 18-2), the smooth muscle cells become modified to perform a secretory function. These *juxtaglomerular cells* produce and secrete renin, a proteolytic enzyme with a molecular weight of approximately 40,000. It is derived from the proteolysis of its precursor, prorenin. The kidney secretes both prorenin and renin into the bloodstream. Prorenin (previously called "inactive renin") can be present in the circulation at levels equal to or greater than those of renin. Prorenin can be converted into renin in vitro by a number of methods, but whether significant extra-

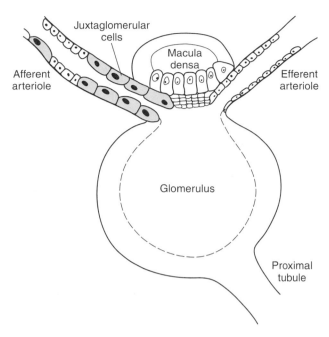

FIGURE 18-2. Diagram of a glomerulus, showing the juxtaglomerular apparatus and the macula densa. (Biglieri EG, et al: *In* Greenspan FS, Baxter JD [eds]: Basic and Clinical Endocrinology, 4th ed. Norwalk, Conn, Appleton & Lange, 1994, p 347.)

renal conversion of prorenin to renin occurs is not clear. In the bloodstream, renin acts on its substrate, angiotensinogen, to form a decapeptide, angiotensin I (Fig. 18-3), which is physiologically inert. Angiotensin I is converted to angiotensin II, the biologically active octapeptide, by the action of converting enzyme. The half-life of angiotensin II in plasma is less than 1 minute because of the action of multiple angiotensinases found in most tissues of the body (Biglieri et al, 1994).

ANGIOTENSINOGEN. Angiotensinogen (renin substrate) is an α_2-globulin secreted by the liver. It has a molecular weight of approximately 60,000 and is usually present in plasma at a concentration of 1 µmol/L. Although the rate of production of angiotensin II is normally determined by changes in the plasma renin

concentration, the concentration of angiotensinogen is below the V_{max} for the reaction. Thus, if the angiotensinogen concentration increases, the amount of angiotensin produced at the same plasma renin concentration also increases. Hepatic production of angiotensinogen is increased by both glucocorticoids and estrogens (Dzau et al, 1988; Kater et al, 1989; Biglieri, 1991).

In conditions such as sodium depletion, which involve a sustained increased concentration of circulating angiotensin II, the rate of breakdown of substrate by renin in the plasma is greatly increased. Because the plasma concentration of angiotensinogen remains constant in these situations, hepatic production must increase to match the increased rate of breakdown. The mechanism of this increase is not clear, although angiotensin II itself is a stimulus to substrate production (Biglieri et al, 1994).

CONVERTING ENZYME. Converting enzyme is found in most tissues and circulates in plasma. Thus, theoretically, the conversion of angiotensin I to angiotensin II could take place anywhere in the circulatory system. However, the activity of the enzyme in the lung is particularly high, such that on a single passage, 70% to 80% of angiotensin I is converted to angiotensin II.

Converting enzyme is a dipeptidyl carboxypeptidase, a glycoprotein of molecular weight 130,000 to 160,000 that cleaves dipeptides from a number of substrates. In addition to angiotensin I, these include bradykinin, enkephalins, and substance P. Inhibitors of converting enzyme are widely used to prevent the formation of angiotensin II in the circulation and thus block its biologic effects (see Fig. 18-3). Because converting enzyme acts on a number of substrates, blockage of the enzyme may not always exert its effects solely via the renin-angiotensin system (Biglieri et al, 1994).

PERIPHERAL EFFECTS OF ANGIOTENSIN II. Angiotensin II is a potent pressor agent that exerts its effects on peripheral arterioles, causing vasoconstriction and thereby increasing total peripheral resistance. Vasoconstriction occurs in all tissue beds, including the kidney, and has been implicated in the phenomenon of renal autoregulation. Angiotensin II may also increase

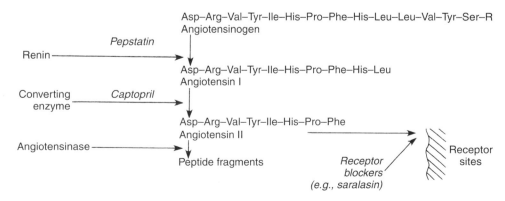

FIGURE 18-3. Sequence in the formation of angiotensin II. Drugs used in humans to block various steps are shown in italics. (Biglieri EG, et al: *In* Greenspan FS, Baxter JD [eds]: Basic and Clinical Endocrinology, 4th ed. Norwalk, Conn, Appleton & Lange, 1994, p 347.)

the rate and strength of cardiac contraction. The possible role of increased circulating levels of angiotensin II in the pathogenesis of hypertension is discussed below.

Angiotensin II acts directly on the adrenal cortex to stimulate aldosterone secretion, and in most situations it is the most important regulator of aldosterone secretion. Thus, it plays a central role in the regulation of sodium balance. For example, during dietary sodium depletion, extracellular fluid volume is reduced because of osmotic transfer of water to the intracellular fluid compartment. Subsequent stimulation of the renin-angiotensin system is important in two ways. Its vasoconstrictor actions help maintain blood pressure despite the reduced extracellular fluid volume, and its stimulation of aldosterone secretion and thus sodium retention allows volume to be conserved.

The intrarenal actions of angiotensin II also promote sodium retention. Angiotensin II preferentially constricts efferent arterioles, thus maintaining the glomerular filtration rate during hypovolemia and arterial hypotension. The subsequent fall in peritubular capillary hydrostatic pressure aids proximal tubular resorption of sodium and water. Angiotensin II also stimulates proximal tubular sodium resorption. Reduced loop of Henle flow—caused by a reduced glomerular filtration rate and increased proximal resorption—and reduced vasa recta flow aid countercurrent multiplication and urinary concentration mechanisms. Angiotensin II modulates activity at sympathetic nerve endings in peripheral blood vessels and in the heart. It increases sympathetic activity partly by facilitating adrenergic transmitter release and partly by increasing the responsiveness of smooth muscle to norepinephrine. Angiotensin II also stimulates the release of catecholamines from the adrenal medulla.

Blockade of the peripheral effects of angiotensin II is useful therapeutically. For example, in low-output congestive cardiac failure, plasma levels of angiotensin II are high. These high circulating levels promote salt and water retention and, by constricting arterioles, raise peripheral vascular resistance. Thus the increased angiotensin II concentration in heart failure enhances cardiac afterload. Treatment with converting enzyme inhibitors (e.g., captopril) results in peripheral vasodilation, which improves tissue perfusion and cardiac performance and aids renal elimination of salt and water (Ulick, 1991; Biglieri et al, 1994).

EXTRARENAL RENIN-ANGIOTENSIN SYSTEMS. Many tissues, including the brain, heart, ovary, adrenal, testis, and peripheral blood vessels, contain the components of the renin-angiotensin system. In some of these tissues, evidence indicates that angiotensin can be formed locally and that such formation may have physiologic functions. For example, production of angiotensin II in the brain has been implicated in several models of hypertension (Biglieri et al, 1994).

EFFECTS IN THE BRAIN AND CENTRAL NERVOUS SYSTEM. Many actions of angiotensin on the central nervous system have been described. Angiotensin II is a polar peptide that does not cross the blood-brain barrier.

Circulating angiotensin II, however, may affect the brain by acting through one or more of the circumventricular organs. These specialized regions in the brain lack a blood-brain barrier, so that receptive cells in these areas are sensitive to plasma composition. Of particular significance to the actions of angiotensin are the subfornical organ, the organum vasculosum of the lamina terminalis, and the area postrema.

Angiotensin II is a potent dipsogen when injected directly into the brain or administered systemically. The major receptors for the dipsogenic action of circulating angiotensin II are located in the subfornical organ. Angiotensin II also stimulates vasopressin secretion, particularly in association with increased plasma osmolality. As such, the renin-angiotensin system may have an important role in the control of water balance, particularly during hypovolemia.

Angiotensin also acts on the brain to increase blood pressure, although its effects at this site seem to be less potent than those exerted directly in the systemic circulation. In most animals, the receptors are located in the area postrema. Other central actions of angiotensin II include stimulation of adrenocorticotropic hormone (ACTH) secretion, suppression of plasma renin activity, and stimulation of sodium appetite, particularly in association with raised mineralocorticoid levels. The full implications of these (and other) central actions of angiotensin remain to be elucidated (Biglieri et al, 1994).

HYPERTENSION. Since the original observation that impaired renal perfusion leads to secretion of renin and an increase in blood pressure, renin has been implicated in the development of hypertension. For many years, the evidence linking renin to hypertension was inconclusive, and many investigators discounted the participation of the renin-angiotensin system in all but a few forms of hypertension. For example, rare renin-producing tumors can cause severe hypertension. Renal artery stenosis and coarctation of the aorta above the origin of the renal arteries are associated with renin-dependent hypertension. Similarly, malignant hypertension in end-stage renal disease is associated with increased plasma renin levels.

Essential Hypertension. Most hypertensive humans have "essential hypertension." This is not a single syndrome but a mixture of clinical entities. At one end of the spectrum are various causes of hypertension that have in common intense peripheral vasoconstriction ("dry hypertension"). Increased activity of any vasoconstrictor agent, such as angiotensin in renal vascular hypertension or catecholamines in pheochromocytomas, causes arteriolar vasoconstriction and an increase in total peripheral resistance, and therefore an increase in blood pressure. At the other end of the spectrum are increases in blood pressure caused by expansion of extracellular fluid volume ("wet hypertension"). Therefore any situation that leads to sodium or water retention can lead to an increase in blood pressure (Biglieri et al, 1994). As common as essential hypertension is in humans, it is not yet known how common this problem might be in dogs or cats.

Renovascular Hypertension. One recognized cause of renin-dependent hypertension in humans is renovascular hypertension. Various studies have reported it to be present in 1% to 4% of humans with hypertension. Renovascular hypertension is usually caused by either atherosclerosis or fibromuscular hyperplasia of the renal arteries. These disturbances result in decreased perfusion in the renal segment distal to the obstructed vessel, resulting in increased renin release and angiotensin II production. An increase in blood pressure and high levels of angiotensin II suppress renin release from the contralateral kidney. Consequently, total plasma renin activity may be only slightly elevated or even normal. Other anatomic lesions, such as renal infarction, solitary cysts, hydronephrosis, and other parenchymal lesions, also may cause hypertension (Krieger and Dzau, 1991; Pickering, 1990).

There is no reliable and simple single screening test for renovascular hypertension in humans. Because of this and because of the low incidence of the disorder, screening of all hypertensive individuals for renovascular hypertension is generally not recommended. Instead, most physicians look for indications that the hypertension is inappropriate before deciding to evaluate a person for renovascular hypertension. As a general guideline, any combination of severe hypertension, accelerated hypertension, onset of hypertension before age 20 or after age 50, presence of an abdominal bruit, or hypokalemia in a person without a family history of hypertension should lead to evaluation for this disorder (Biglieri et al, 1994). The incidence of this disorder in dogs and cats is not known.

ATRIAL NATRIURETIC PEPTIDE

Background

In 1981 DeBold and co-workers reported that intravenous administration of atrial extracts to rats induced profound natriuresis and diuresis. These effects were derived from a peptide synthesized and stored in atrial myocytes and thus termed atrial natriuretic peptide (ANP). In response to adequate stimuli, the biologically active ANP (99-125) is cleaved from the peptide's storage form, ANP (1-126), and is released into the circulation. The material is contained in densely staining granules of cardiocytes in the left and right atria of most mammalian species. Secretion of ANP is known to be stimulated by mechanical stretching of the atrial wall, and increases in the plasma concentration of ANP therefore have been associated with many cardiac disorders (Edwards et al, 1987). In instances of congestive heart failure, the ventricles may also be capable of synthesizing ANP (Laragh, 1985; Atlas and Maack, 1987; Genest and Cantin, 1988; Mantero et al, 1990; Melby, 1991).

A number of laboratories have sequenced and synthesized natriuretic peptides containing 22 to 28 amino acids. Rat and human atrial cDNA clones that encode atrial natriuretic peptides have been isolated and characterized. The 28–amino acid peptide is probably normally secreted into the bloodstream. In view of its natriuretic, diuretic, and vasodilative effects, as well as its inhibitory action on the release of renin, aldosterone, and vasopressin, this peptide was linked to the regulation of volume homeostasis (Cantin and Genest, 1985; Needleman et al, 1988).

Physiology

The primary effects of administration of atrial natriuretic peptide are natriuresis and a decrease in blood pressure. Although the peptide can cause relaxation of smooth muscle, the fall in blood pressure is caused primarily by reduction of venous return and depression of cardiac output in intact animals. In addition to its vasorelaxant properties, ANP has been documented to decrease intravascular volume. This effect not only is exerted by the natriuretic and aldosterone-inhibiting actions of the hormone but also is mediated by transportation of intravascular fluid to the interstitial space (DeBold et al, 1981; Atarashi et al, 1984; Sujimoto et al, 1989). The natriuresis is associated with a marked increase in filtration fraction without a sustained increase in renal blood flow, suggesting that the peptide may cause efferent arteriolar constriction. Observations suggest that glomerular membrane permeability may be increased and tubular resorption may be reduced by ANP. Evidence also suggests that baroreflex stimulation of the heart rate, as well as vasopressin and ACTH secretion, is inhibited by this peptide (Biglieri et al, 1994).

Assays

Recently, a number of radioimmunoassays for atrial natriuretic peptide have been developed. Although questions remain concerning the specificity of these assays, it is clear that measurable levels of the material are found in normal plasma. Maneuvers that expand plasma volume and experiments that increase atrial pressure are associated with increased levels of assayed peptide in plasma (Edwards et al, 1987; Goetz, 1988).

Atrial Natriuretic Peptide in Disease

Attention has subsequently been drawn to a possible involvement of ANP in the pathogenesis of diseases marked by volume overload, such as congestive heart failure, renal failure, and hypertension. Dogs with chronic renal failure were demonstrated to have a twofold increase in plasma ANP concentration (16 fmol/ml) over that in healthy dogs (8 fmol/ml) (Vollmar et al, 1991). This increase may be the result of expanded extracellular fluid typical of chronic renal failure. However, the kidneys are the major site of metabolism and degradation of ANP. Thus renal pathology and insufficiency may impair metabolism of ANP (Gerbes and Vollmar, 1990).

An even more distinct increase in the plasma ANP concentration (greater than sixfold) was observed in dogs with congestive heart failure (53 fmol/ml). Interestingly, in addition to ANP (99-126), all dogs with congestive heart failure had other molecular forms of ANP, including the ANP prohormone (1-126) (Vollmar et al, 1991). In congestive heart failure, the actions of ANP (which increase with increasing severity of heart failure) to promote sodium excretion and vasodilation may oppose those of the renin-angiotensin-aldosterone system, arginine vasopressin, and catechol-amines (Vollmar et al, 1994). In studies on congestive heart failure in the Cavalier King Charles Spaniel, it was concluded that plasma concentrations of ANP did not become markedly increased before decompensation of chronic mitral regurgitation associated with severe enlargement of the left atrium and ventricle (Haggstrom et al, 1994). Therefore increases in ANP may result from heart failure rather than represent a primary cause of the failure. However, ANP may have a role in maintaining diseases associated with impaired volume regulation. Increases in plasma ANP associated with congestive heart failure would be expected from experimental work because atrial distention is known to represent the principal stimulus for secretion (Dietz, 1984). Dehydrated dogs have decreased plasma ANP concentrations (Vollmar et al, 1994).

Dogs with hyperadrenocorticism did not show increases in the plasma ANP concentration (5.5 fmol/ml) despite the fact that a large percentage were hypertensive (Vollmar et al, 1991; Ortega et al, 1994). The observed polyuria in these dogs could indicate that they do not have volume overload, and the slight decrease in the ANP concentration might even indicate counterregulation to increased diuresis (Vollmar et al, 1991).

Qualitative and quantitative alterations of the plasma ANP concentration in dogs suggest that this peptide may be involved in the development and/or maintenance of diseases associated with impaired volume regulation (Vollmar et al, 1991).

REFERENCES

Atarashi K, et al: Inhibition of aldosterone production by an atrial extract. Science 224:992, 1984.

Atlas SA, Maack T: Effects of atrial natriuretic factor on the kidney and the renin-angiotensin-aldosterone system. Endocrinol Metab Clin North Am 16:107, 1987.

Biglieri EG: The spectrum of mineralocorticoid hypertension. Hypertension 18:251, 1991.

Biglieri EG, et al: Endocrine hypertension. In Greenspan FS, Baxter JD (eds): Basic and Clinical Endocrinology, 4th ed. Norwalk, Conn, Appleton & Lange, 1994, p 347.

Cantin M, Genest J: The heart and the atrial natriuretic factor. Endocrinol Rev 6:107, 1985.

Cowgill L: Efficacy of recombinant human erythropoietin for anemia in dogs and cats with renal failure. J Vet Intern Med 4:126, 1990 (abstract).

Cowgill L: Pathophysiology and management of anemia in chronic progressive renal failure. Semin Vet Med Surg 7:175, 1992.

Cowgill L: Medical management of the anemia of chronic renal failure. In Osborne C, Finco D (eds): Canine and Feline Nephrology and Urology. Philadelphia, Lea & Febiger, 1995.

DeBold AJ, et al: A rapid and potent natriuretic response to intravenous injection of atrial myocardial extract in rats. Life Sci 28:89, 1981.

Dietz JR: Release of atrial natriuretic factor from rat heart-lung preparation by atrial distension. Am J Physiol 247:R1093, 1984.

Dzau VJ, et al: Molecular biology of the renin-angiotensin system. Am J Physiol 255:F563, 1988.

Edwards BS, et al: Atrial natriuretic factor: Physiologic actions and implications in congestive heart failure. Cardiovasc Drugs Ther 1:89, 1987.

Erslev AJ: Erythropoietin. N Engl J Med 324:1339, 1991.

Genest J, Cantin M: The atrial natriuretic factor: Its physiology and biochemistry. Rev Physiol Biochem Pharm 110:1, 1988.

Gerbes AL, Vollmar AM: Degradation and clearance of atrial natriuretic factors. Life Sci 47:1173, 1990.

Goetz KL: Physiology and pathophysiology of atrial peptides. Am J Physiol 254:E1, 1988.

Haggstrom J, et al: Plasma concentration of atrial natriuretic peptide in relation to severity of mitral regurgitation in Cavalier King Charles Spaniels. Am J Vet Res 55:698, 1994.

Kater CE, et al: Stimulation and suppression of the mineralocorticoid hormones in normal subjects and adrenocortical disorders. Endocr Rev 11:149, 1989.

Krieger JE, Dzau VJ: Molecular biology of hypertension. Hypertension 18(Suppl):13, 1991.

Laragh JH: Atrial natriuretic hormone, the renin-aldosterone axis, and blood pressure: Electrolyte homeostasis. N Engl J Med 313:1330, 1985.

Mantero F, et al: New aspects of mineralocorticoid hypertension. Horm Res 34:175, 1990.

Melby JC: Diagnosis of hyperaldosteronism. Endocrinol Metab Clin North Am 20:247, 1991.

Needleman P, et al: The biochemical pharmacology of atrial peptides. Annu Rev Pharmacol Toxicol 29:23, 1988.

Nissenson A, et al: Recombinant human erythropoietin and renal anemia: Molecular biology, clinical efficacy, and nervous system effects. Ann Intern Med 114:402, 1991.

Ortega T, et al: Evaluation of arterial blood pressure and urine protein:creatinine ratio in dogs with hyperadrenocorticism. J Vet Intern Med 8:164, 1994 (abstract).

Pickering TG: Renovascular hypertension: Medical evaluation and nonsurgical treatment. In Laragh JH, Brenner BM (eds): Hypertension: Pathophysiology, Diagnosis, and Management. New York, Raven Press, 1990.

Polzin DJ, et al: Chronic renal failure. In Ettinger SJ, Feldman EC (eds): Textbook of Veterinary Internal Medicine. Philadelphia, WB Saunders, 1995, p 1734.

Sujimoto EKS, et al: Effect of ANP in circulating blood volume. Am J Physiol 257:R127, 1989.

Ulick S: Two uncommon causes of mineralocorticoid excess: Syndrome of apparent mineralocorticoid excess and glucocorticoid-remediable aldosteronism. Endocrinol Metab Clin North Am 20:269, 1991.

Vollmar AM, et al: Atrial natriuretic peptide concentration in dogs with congestive heart failure, chronic renal failure, and hyperadrenocorticism. Am J Vet Res 52:1831, 1991.

Vollmar AM, et al: Atrial natriuretic peptide and plasma volume of dogs suffering from heart failure or dehydration. J Am Vet Med Assoc 41:548, 1994.

CANINE FEMALE REPRODUCTION

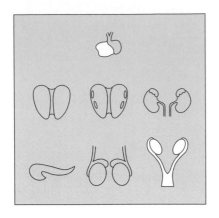

19

OVARIAN CYCLE AND VAGINAL CYTOLOGY

THE OVARIAN CYCLE

Onset of Puberty

Breed has a significant effect on the timing of a dog's first estrus. Generally, bitches exhibit their first cycle several months after they achieve adult height and body weight. There is, however, considerable variation within a breed as well as between different breeds. The Beagle, for example, usually exhibits her first proestrus between 7 and 10 months of age. Even in a controlled laboratory environment, the first proestrus may occur as early as 6 months of age or as late as 13 months (Concannon, 1987). Thus it is reasonable to advise owners that some small breeds enter their first heat between 6 and 10 months of age. Although a large-breed bitch may also begin her first proestrus before 1 year of age, some normal large-breed dogs may not begin to cycle until 18 to 24 months of age. A good deal of individual and breed variation is reported. This natural variability, coupled with cycles referred to as *silent heats,* adds to a veterinarian's or owner's inability to predict the timing of a first season (estrus) (Concannon, 1980; Evans and White, 1988; Johnston, et al, 2001).

Silent heat is simply one that goes unnoticed by the owner because little vulvar swelling, bleeding, attraction of males, or behavioral change may be associated with estrus in a young bitch. The owner's experience, hair length of the dog (vulvar bleeding is easier to see in a short-haired dog), cleanliness of the dog (one that licks a great deal is more apt to hide bleeding), and presence of a male dog in the home are just a few of the variables that determine the ease with which an owner may notice estrus (Concannon, 1980). We tend not to begin to evaluate a female dog clinically for failure to experience an ovarian cycle until she is at least 2 years

of age. (See Infertility, Chapter 24.) The ideal age for breeding is between 2 and 6 years. First breeding is recommended during the second or third estrus, *after* an owner has witnessed at least one complete normal ovarian cycle.

Seasonality of the Ovarian Cycle

Bitches experience ovarian cycles throughout the year. Breeding seasons depend on both genetic and management factors. The preference for late winter and early spring breedings may stem from an evolutionary advantage in whelping litters at a time when the food supply is beginning to increase in association with improving climatic conditions. Owner preferences may also play a role. Certainly, whelping puppies in October provides a breeder with puppies to sell for an upcoming Christmas season. For many breeders, a second choice for whelping is late winter, in order to have puppies for sale in the spring. Seasonal patterns to ovarian cycles of the bitch should be distinguished from owner preferences. Dogs experience ovarian cycle activity, breed, and whelp litters in all months of the year, but this process does tend to have subtle peaks in the late winter/early spring as well as in autumn months.

Intervals Between Ovarian Cycles

The "average" bitch begins proestrus approximately every 7 months. Thus, an ovarian cycle would begin at least once in every month of the year during a bitch's life if this schedule were maintained. There is a tendency to vary somewhat. The common *interestrus interval* (the period from the end of standing heat to the beginning of the following proestrus) is 5 to 11 months, with the normal interestrus interval as short as 3.5 months and as long as 13 months (Concannon, 1987). Interestrus intervals more frequent than every 4 months, however, are often associated with infertility, and those greater than every 12 months *may* be associated with sufertility or infertility. Breed and individual variability can be striking. The German Shepherd dog, for example, is one breed that often cycles every 4 to 4.5 months and yet maintains fertility. Rather than relying on knowledge concerning individual breeds, we use the 5- to 11-month interval as normal. It also appears that most dogs 2 to 6 years of age are relatively consistent in cycle length as well as in the duration of each phase. The obvious exceptions to the 7-month average normal interestrus interval are the African dog breeds such as the Basenji. These dogs cycle once yearly. Litters of this breed are typically whelped in December, with January and November following as likely months of births.

As dogs advance beyond the optimal breeding age (approximately 7 years), various changes are likely to occur, including progressive lengthening in the duration of the interestrus interval, reduction in litter size, increases in congenital birth defects, and problems at parturition. In one study, mean interestrus intervals increased from approximately 240 days to more than 330 for Beagle bitches after they reached 8 years of age, but healthy dogs continue to experience ovarian cycles throughout life (Anderson and Simpson, 1973).

Phases of the Ovarian Cycle

There are four phases of the canine ovarian cycle.

PROESTRUS. This is the period of heightened follicular activity preceding estrus when males are attracted to females but females refuse to breed.

ESTRUS. Estrus is the period during which the female allows the male to mount and breed. The term *estrus* is derived from the Greek word *oistros*, meaning "a vehement desire."

DIESTRUS. This is the period following mating. It is associated with corpora luteal activity. *Metestrus* refers to the period of corpora luteal activity as a distinct entity. In the dog, mating activity continues despite rising plasma progesterone concentrations. This progesterone is derived first from luteinized follicles and then from corpora lutea. Both estrus and diestrus are phases dominated by progesterone. In estrus the bitch breeds, whereas in diestrus she refuses to breed and is "physiologically pregnant." Thus, *diestrus* rather than *metestrus* is the term used as an aid in describing the unique sexual cycle of the bitch.

ANESTRUS. The time between the end of the luteal (progesterone) phase (diestrus) and the beginning of the following follicular phase (proestrus) is called *anestrus*. This has traditionally been described as a time of quiescence within the pituitary-ovarian axis. Clinically, this is a time of inactivity. Endocrinologically, hormonal activity continues.

Proestrus

DURATION. Proestrus is usually, and most reliably, defined as beginning when vaginal bleeding is first seen and ending when the bitch allows a male dog to mount and breed. Additional criteria used in defining the onset and completion of proestrus include changes in the appearance of the vaginal mucosa viewed endoscopically (Fig. 19-1) or changes seen on exfoliative cytology of vaginal epithelial cells (Fig. 19-2). Less reliable criteria used in describing the onset of proestrus include enlargement of the vulva, attraction of males, and changes in behavior toward males (Fig. 19-3).

The length of time from the onset of proestrus to the time of first breeding is usually 6 to 11 days, with an average of 9 days. However, variations within "normal" can be extreme (i.e., as brief as 2 or 3 days to as prolonged as 25 days) (Fig. 19-4). These extremes in normal duration of proestrus can be confusing, and their significance is discussed in greater detail in association with the evaluation of female infertility (Chapter 24).

CLINICAL SIGNS. Early proestrus behavior includes attraction of males, in part due to pheromone secretion (Goodwin et al, 1979). An increase in playful/teasing activity with discouragement of any mounting attempt by a male is common (Jeffcoate, 1998). This unwillingness to breed may involve antisexual growling, moving away, baring the teeth, and snapping. The bitch may also keep her tail tight against the perineum, between the rear legs and covering the vulva. This initial behavior pattern gradually changes as proestrus progresses. The female usually becomes more receptive, as demonstrated by actually seeking and playing with males. The response by the bitch to male mounting attempts progressively becomes more restrained, as she prevents mounting by retreating, crouching, or lying down. In late proestrus, the behavior of the bitch may be described as passive, and she may sit quietly when mounted, with or without intermittent displays of tail deviation and lordosis.

Proestrus is typically but not always associated with varying quantities of bloody vaginal discharge. Vaginal bleeding begins as diapedesis of erythrocytes through the endometrium and subepithelially as capillaries rupture within the endometrium. This blood seeps through a slightly relaxed cervix and enters the vaginal vault. Small numbers of erythrocytes may also originate from the vaginal mucosa, since erythrocytes have been observed in vaginal smears obtained from proestrus bitches that had been previously hysterectomized (Johnston et al, 2001). Rapid changes in thickness and development of the vaginal mucosa and the endometrium are responses to follicular estrogen secretion. The volume of bleeding and bloody vaginal discharge vary from bitch to bitch.

Bitches that keep themselves clean through licking may present a difficult challenge in detecting proestrus. Short-haired dogs without tails (e.g., German Short-Haired Pointers) can be contrasted with long-haired dogs with flowing tails (e.g., Newfoundlands). Obviously, vaginal bleeding associated with proestrus is easier

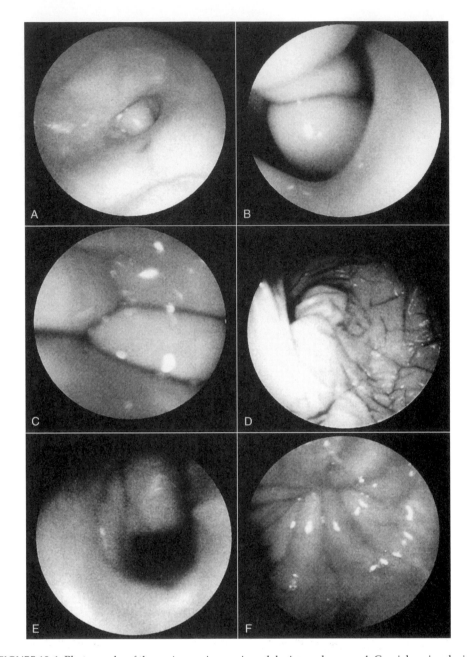

FIGURE 19-1. Photographs of the canine vagina as viewed during endoscopy. *A,* Cranial vagina during anestrus. In view is the round caudal tubercle of the dorsal median fold in center of field. *B,* Cranial vagina during early proestrus. Slightly oblique view of the dorsal median fold. Mucous membranes develop new folds and become edematous during proestrus. *C,* Cranial vagina during early proestrus. Note edematous folds of mucous membranes. *D,* Cranial vagina during late estrus (oblique view). Mucous membranes appear angulated during estrus. By the end of estrus, all folds are in their most shrunken and angular state. *E,* Cranial vagina as viewed on the first day of diestrus (first day of postestrus refusal). *F,* Cranial vagina showing the fully formed "rosette" that can be viewed with endoscopy during diestrus.

to detect in some breeds than in others. Occasionally, a grayish mucoid-like vaginal discharge is observed before actual bleeding or swelling of the vulva. Classically, dogs cease vaginal bleeding as proestrus proceeds into estrus. In these bitches the bloody discharge fades and becomes transparent to straw-colored. However, changes in color of the vaginal discharge are inconsistent, with some bitches showing bloody dis-

charge throughout proestrus, estrus, and into diestrus, whereas others bleed little or only at the beginning of proestrus.

THE VULVA. The vulva slowly enlarges throughout proestrus due to fluid accumulation. This edematous and turgid vulva impedes intromission by a male. As proestrus proceeds into estrus, however, the vulva softens dramatically, eliminating this obstacle.

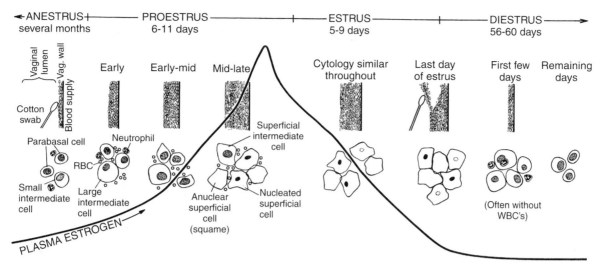

FIGURE 19-2. Illustration of the changes in vaginal wall thickness, vaginal cytology, and relative plasma estrogen concentrations in an average bitch experiencing an estrous cycle. Note that near the last day of estrus, rafts of vaginal cells are sloughed.

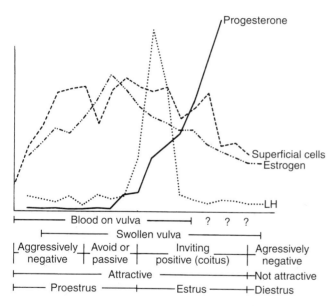

FIGURE 19-3. Diagrammatic illustration of the behavior changes, hormonal fluctuations, and vaginal cytology of a bitch experiencing proestrus and estrus.

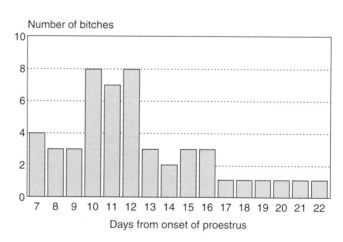

FIGURE 19-4. Predicted time of ovulation (or approximate onset of behavioral estrus) for 50 bitches, based on serum progesterone concentrations. More than 20 breeds were represented. (From Johnston SD, et al, 2001, with permission.)

HORMONAL CHANGES AND OVARIAN ANATOMY. The bitch in proestrus is under the influence of estrogen. This estrogen is synthesized and secreted by developing ovarian follicles. Proestrus is the phase of estrogen dominance in the bitch (see Fig. 19-2). FSH and LH pulses are released in concordance in late anestrus, and progression from anestrus into proestrus is associated with an increase in the secretion of FSH with a concomitant rise in LH secretion (Kooistra and Okkens, 2000). Follicles that develop at a time coinciding with gonadotropin stimulation mature and attain the capacity for estrogen synthesis and secretion. The secreted estrogen results in vaginal discharge, attraction of males, and uterine preparation for pregnancy.

The potent effects of estrogen can be demonstrated in the ovariohysterectomized female, which can easily be brought into a classic proestrus state (without vaginal bleeding) by administration of estrogens (Concannon, 1987). Estrogen alone usually does not result in breeding activity. Breeding in the dog is typically associated with a serum combination of decreasing estrogen and increasing progesterone concentrations. Estrogen alone usually does not cause behavioral estrus (Leedy, 1988).

The appearance of the ovaries has been monitored during proestrus with ultrasonography. Ovaries of bitches in anestrus can be visualized as structures with an echogenicity equal to or slightly greater than that of the renal cortex. Follicles appear as focal hypoechoic to anechoic rounded structures. Ovaries are easier to identify as follicular development progresses. Ovarian size increases throughout proestrus (England and Allen, 1989a, 1989b; Wallace et al, 1992).

The dramatically rising estrogen concentrations in venous plasma during proestrus correlate with dramatic changes in the uterus, the vaginal mucosa, and the vulva, as well as with follicular secretion and behavior patterns in the bitch. Circulating estrogen concentrations during anestrus are usually between 5 and 15 pg/ml. Proestrus is associated with an increase in estrogen (estradiol) concentration above 15 pg/ml. Early proestrus is usually associated with estradiol concentrations above 25 pg/ml, and late proestrus is associated with concentrations that may be in excess of 60 to 70 pg/ml. The peak in plasma estradiol concentration is achieved 24 to 48 hours *before* the termination of proestrus, that is, preceding estrus (standing heat).

Decreasing plasma estradiol concentrations stimulate the onset of estrus. During the subsequent 5 to 20 days, plasma estradiol concentrations taper progressively to basal levels. Therefore, proestrus is a phase of rising and then stable serum estrogen concentrations, and estrus is a phase of decreasing serum estrogen concentrations. "Basal" serum estrogen concentrations are observed in anestrus and in diestrus, although variations within individual dogs may be observed (Olson et al, 1982). Concentrations of testosterone increase in the serum of bitches during late proestrus, reaching concentrations of 0.3 to 1.0 ng/ml at the time of the LH surge that occurs in early estrus (Olson et al, 1984).

Progesterone concentrations throughout all but the last 24 to 72 hours of proestrus are low (basal: <0.5 ng/ml). The end of proestrus and the beginning of estrus are associated with a plasma progesterone concentration that rises above a critical plateau (1.0 ng/ml) while estrogen concentrations are decreasing. Serum progesterone concentrations of >1.0 ng/ml are required for induction of the behavior changes typical of estrus and maintenance of pregnancy. The progesterone is secreted by *follicles* progressively more *luteinized*, prior to ovulation and development of corpora lutea. Thus follicles begin to evolve from estrogen-producing "factories" in early and mid-proestrus to "factories" producing primarily estrogen and small amounts of progesterone in late proestrus. Progressively more progesterone and less estrogen are synthesized as the bitch progresses through estrus.

ANATOMY OF THE UTERUS, OVIDUCTS, AND MAMMARY GLANDS. Several "estrogen-target" tissues are affected by increases in serum estrogen concentrations during proestrus. These include growth of mammary gland ducts and tubules, proliferation of oviductal fimbria, thickening of oviducts, elongation of uterine horns, thickening of endometrium, increased myometrial sensitivity, enlargement of the cervix, elongation and edema of the vagina, proliferation of the vaginal wall, and synthesis of hepatic steroid-metabolizing enzymes (Concannon and DiGregorio, 1986; Concannon, 1987). The preparation for implantation in the endometrium includes a remarkable increase in

wall thickness and glandular activity, changes that are associated with bleeding. This uterine hemorrhage is the primary source of vaginal bleeding associated with proestrus and, in some bitches, estrus.

VAGINAL ANATOMY AND ENDOSCOPY. Increasing estrogen concentrations thicken the vaginal wall, which protects the bitch from the traumatic effects of breeding. The vaginal lining in anestrus is only a few cell layers thick and is relatively fragile. The basal or germinal cell layer is orderly, and the less orderly overlying cells are situated in rather close proximity to the blood supply present below the germinal layer. The increasing estrogen concentrations associated with proestrus cause rapid multiplication in the number of cell layers lining the vaginal vault, resulting in a wall 20 to 30 layers thick by the end of proestrus (Johnston et al, 2001). Thus intromission of the penis into the estrogen-primed vaginal vault is not harmful to the female.

This increased number of cell layers moves the cells lining the lumen further from their blood supply, causing the death of those cells. These dead cells function as a less sensitive and less fragile tissue. Fragility decreases not only because of increased cell layers, but also because of the development of keratin precursors within these cells. This nuclear material is similar to that found in fingernails. Thickening of the vaginal mucosa can be easily recognized with cytology (see Fig. 19-2).

Thickening in the vaginal mucosa, easily demonstrated with cytology, may also be detected with vaginoscopy. The procedure is simple and well tolerated by nonsedated bitches that have normal vaginovestibular anatomy, but does require some practice and experience. Before inserting any vaginoscope, one should first perform a digital examination of the vaginal vault to confirm that no stricture is present (see Chapter 25). The mid- to anterior vagina can be visualized using a rigid pediatric proctoscope or flexible endoscope. The less expensive proctoscope is an excellent tool for this purpose. Otoscopes are completely inadequate for viewing anything but the "vestibule" of the vagina. The vaginal mucosa is flat in anestrus because relatively few cell layers are present (see Fig. 19-1).

During proestrus, the mucosa appears markedly rounded, edematous, smooth, and shiny (Jeffcoate, 1988). Vaginal folds are pink and billow out into the lumen as a result of fluid retention, resulting in an inability to visualize the lumen (Goodman, 2001). The decreasing estrogen and increasing progesterone concentrations associated with the final 1 to 3 days of proestrus (or the first days of estrus in some bitches) cause edema in the vaginal mucosa to subside, and the stretched luminal surface becomes progressively wrinkled (see Fig. 19-1). This is referred to as *crenulation*. Initial vaginal crenulation, observed as this subtle wrinkling of the mucosa, appears within 24 hours of the preovulatory LH surge (Lindsay and Concannon, 1986; Concannon, 1987; Jeffcoate, 1998).

The LH surge, in turn, precedes the onset of ovulation by approximately 24 to 48 hours. Breeding should begin at this time. The mucosa becomes progressively more crenulated, the lumen more obvious, and the vaginal folds more flattened as the edema diminishes. This wrinkling is most obvious during the fertile period 4 to 7 days after the LH surge. By diestrus the mucosa is flat and variegated. Further, because the protective thickened layers of epithelium have disappeared, the mucosa once again becomes fragile and superficial hemorrhage may be associated with vaginoscopy (Goodman, 2001). With practice and observation of individual variation in this process, vaginoscopy becomes a useful adjunct when attempting to best time a breeding.

Classification of Vaginal Cells

GENERAL BACKGROUND. Changes in the vaginal mucosa due to increases in serum estrogen concentration during proestrus and estrus are reflected in the appearance of exfoliated vaginal epithelial cells. These alterations are believed to be due solely to increases in circulating estrogen concentrations. Therefore vaginal cytology can serve as a crude but reliable indirect estrogen assay.

Nomenclature of vaginal cells is based on cell morphology. Older literature refers to keratinized versus nonkeratinized cells and/or to cornified versus noncornified cells. Some species actually develop a hard keratin lining of the vaginal tract as a result of increasing circulating estrogen concentrations. The bitch, however, does not develop a "cornified" vaginal lining, which explains the different nomenclature used in describing alterations in canine vaginal cells due to estrogen influences. Different cell types represent stages of cell death. As healthy round vaginal cells die, they become larger and more irregular in shape. The nuclei within vaginal epithelial cells also undergo changes that reflect cell death: the nucleus becomes progressively smaller, then pyknotic, before eventually disintegrating, leaving a nuclear "ghost" and then an anuclear cell (see Fig. 19-2).

PARABASAL CELLS. Parabasal cells are the healthiest and smallest of the vaginal cells. They are round or slightly oval and have a large vesiculated nucleus and relatively small amounts of cytoplasm. They usually stain well with Wright-Giemsa stain or some of the rapid stains (Diff-Quik, American Scientific Products, McGraw, IL). These cells are exfoliated from near the germinal cell layer, close to the underlying blood supply (Fig. 19-5).

INTERMEDIATE CELLS. Intermediate cells vary in size from slightly larger than parabasal cells to twice their size. These cells have smooth, oval to rounded irregular borders and a nucleus that is vesiculated but generally smaller than those found in parabasal cells (Fig. 19-6). This change in morphology reflects the first step in cell death: cells appear larger, have relatively larger amounts of cytoplasm, and have smaller nuclei. For descriptive purposes they are classified as *small intermediate cells* and *large intermediate cells*.

SUPERFICIAL CELLS. Superficial cells are dead cells that line the vaginal lumen of bitches in estrus. They are the largest cells identified on vaginal cytology. These cells have sharp, flat, angular cytoplasmic borders and small, pyknotic, fading nuclei or no nuclei (Fig. 19-7).

SUPERFICIAL-INTERMEDIATE CELLS. These are vaginal cells that appear to have relatively healthy vesiculated nuclei but also have the angular, sharp, flat cytoplasmic border typical of superficial cells (Olson et al, 1984b; Olson, 1989) (Fig. 19-8). The superficial-intermediate cell provides evidence for potent estrogen effect on the vaginal lining, but not quite the full effect. Full estrogen effect is associated with superficial cells and *anuclear squames*. Vaginal exfoliative cytology may not progress beyond the presence of superficial-intermediate cells at the peak of estrogen effect. No study has demonstrated associations between failure to develop superficial cells on vaginal cytology and subsequent breeding or fertility problems.

ANUCLEAR SQUAMES. These large, dead, irregular vaginal cells with no nuclei represent the end of a process that began with healthy round parabasal cells. This cell death is caused by the thickened vaginal lining. As the vaginal wall thickens in response to increases in serum estrogen concentrations, from several cell layers to 20 to 30 cell layers, those cells lining the lumen become far removed from their blood supply and their death is inevitable (see Fig. 19-2). These cells are also called *anuclear superficial cells*. They are large cells with flat, angular borders (Fig. 19-9). These are the cells that have also been called "fully cornified" or "fully keratinized" cells.

METESTRUM CELLS. Metestrum cells are usually large intermediate vaginal cells that appear to have one or more neutrophils contained within their cytoplasm (Fig. 19-10). As described below, metestrum cells are usually seen in the vaginal smear from a bitch in early diestrus or one with vaginitis. Rarely, such cells are observed in early proestrus.

FOAM CELLS. Foam cells are parabasal and intermediate cells that have obvious cytoplasmic vacuoles. These cells may be associated with diestrus and anestrus.

Vaginal Cytology in Proestrus

EARLY PROESTRUS. The vaginal smear from a bitch in early proestrus is similar to that from a bitch in anestrus, with one difference: the presence of blood within the vagina derived primarily from a rapidly developing endometrium (see Fig. 19-2). In addition to varying numbers of red blood cells, the vaginal smear usually contains numerous parabasal, small, and large intermediate vaginal epithelial cells. Neutrophils are common in varying numbers, and bacteria may be present in small to large numbers (Fig. 19-11; Table 19-1). The background of these smears is often granular or "dirty" in appearance, owing to the presence of viscous cervical and vaginal secretions that appear to take a slight amount of stain.

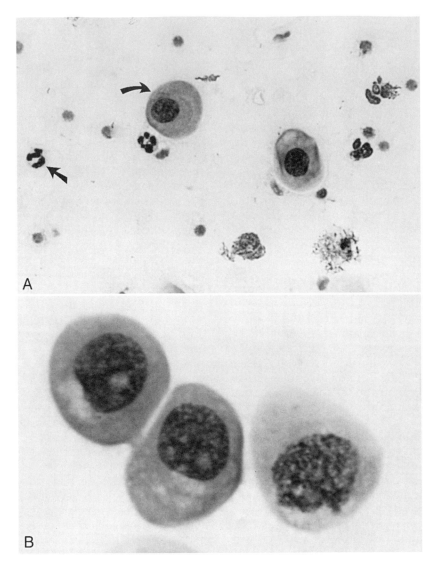

FIGURE 19-5. *A,* Parabasal cells *(curved arrow)* and neutrophils *(straight arrow)* on vaginal cytology. *B,* Parabasal/small intermediate cells on vaginal cytology.

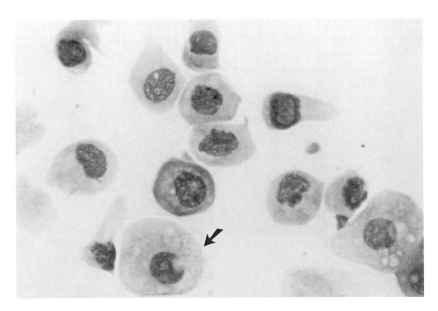

FIGURE 19-6. Intermediate cells on vaginal cytology; *arrow* points out one excellent example of a large intermediate cell.

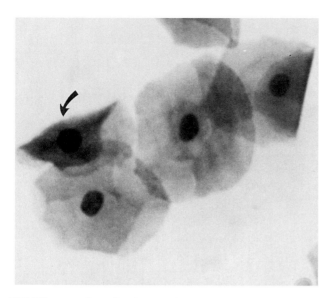

FIGURE 19-7. Superficial vaginal epithelial cells with angular perimeter borders and pyknotic nuclei. The variable density of the cell is caused by folding over *(arrow).*

MID-PROESTRUS. The first evidence of continued estrogen effect on the reproductive tract is visualized in the vaginal cytology. This includes (1) disappearance of neutrophils, (2) appearance of the red blood cells, and (3) progressively increasing percentage of superficial cells replacing the smaller parabasal and intermediate cells. White blood cells are believed to enter the vaginal lumen through the mucosal wall. With the dramatic thickening in the wall caused by estrogen, neutrophils are unable to penetrate this barrier and enter the lumen. Neutrophils are not normally visualized in vaginal smears from bitches between mid-proestrus and the start of diestrus Fig. 19-12).

LATE PROESTRUS. In late proestrus, the vaginal smear contains no neutrophils, the presence of red blood cells is variable, and the background is clear. It is important to remember that some bitches have a bloody vaginal discharge for only a few days into proestrus (if at all), most bleed throughout proestrus, some bleed throughout proestrus and estrus, and, finally, a small percentage exhibit vaginal bleeding in proestrus that continues into diestrus. Recognizing this variation in vaginal bleeding among healthy bitches prevents unnecessary worry.

More than 80% of exfoliated vaginal cells are "superficial," with either vesiculated nuclei, pyknotic nuclei, or no nucleus (anuclear superficial cells; Fig. 19-13). It is not possible to distinguish late proestrus from estrus with vaginal cytology. To the contrary, vaginal cytology from bitches in the final 1 to 8 days of proestrus is the same as that from bitches in estrus (see Table 19-1). In addition, variations in duration of proestrus (2 days to 3 weeks) in normal bitches may contribute to owner confusion when attempting to evaluate the ovarian cycle.

Estrus

The estrus phase encompasses the time during which the bitch allows a male to mount and breed. The first day that the female allows breeding (standing heat) is the start of estrus, and this phase ends when she no longer accepts the male. The other criterion defining the end to estrus is based on vaginal cytology (see page 764).

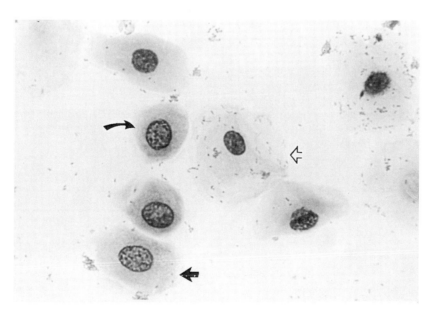

FIGURE 19-8. Vaginal cytology illustrating a small intermediate cell *(curved arrow)* and two different superficial-intermediate cells, one small *(closed arrow)* and one large *(open arrow).* Bacteria in background are not considered abnormal.

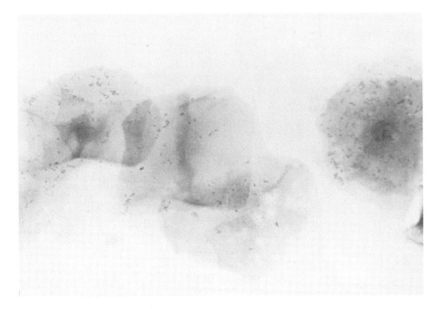

FIGURE 19-9. Vaginal cytology revealing anuclear superficial cells (squames). Note the angular perimeter to the cells and the light staining characteristics. Bacteria are often seen in normal bitches.

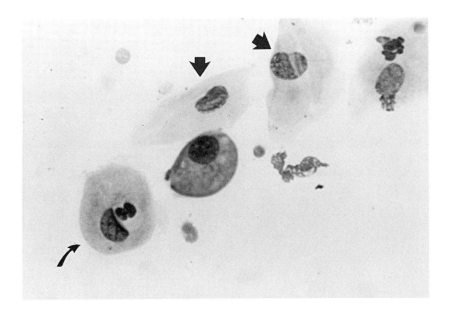

FIGURE 19-10. Vaginal cytology revealing one vaginal epithelial cell that contains a neutrophil within its cytoplasm (metestrum cell; *curved arrow*). Also note the superficial-intermediate cells *(straight arrows).*

TABLE 19–1 CYTOLOGIC STAGING OF ESTROUS CYCLE

Stage	Red Blood Cells	Neutrophils	Bacteria	Epithelial Cells
Early proestrus	Usually	Often	Many	Parabasal, intermediate, superficial intermediates, few superficial
Late proestrus	Usually	Few or none	Many	Superficial intermediates, superficial
Estrus	Present, may be decreased in number May be absent	None	Many	>80–90% superficial
Diestrus	Usually none	Few to many	May be clearing	Parabasal and intermediate predominate; dramatic decrease in superficial cells

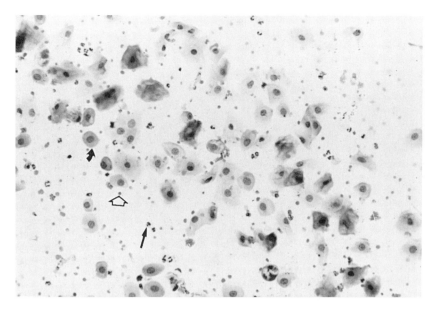

FIGURE 19-11. Vaginal cytology (at scanning microscope power) revealing neutrophils *(straight arrow)*, red blood cells *(open arrow)*, and vaginal epithelial cells that are primarily of the intermediate type *(curved arrow)*. This smear is typical of early proestrus.

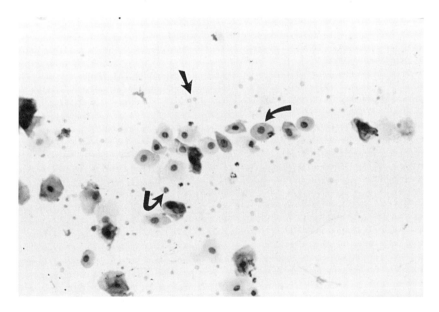

FIGURE 19-12. Vaginal cytology (at scanning microscope power) revealing red blood cells *(straight arrow)* and intermediate-type vaginal epithelial cells *(curved arrow)*. Presence of few neutrophils *(hairpin arrow)* makes this smear suggestive of mid-proestrus.

HORMONAL CHANGES. Serum estrogen concentrations peak 1 or 2 days *before* the onset of estrus (see Fig. 19-1). Typically, bitches usually begin to exhibit signs of standing heat only when circulating estrogen concentrations, that have progressively increased, begin to decrease. Decreasing serum estrogen concentrations reflect the final maturation process of ovarian follicles, several days before ovulation. Further demonstrating the importance of declining estrogen concentrations, ovariectomized bitches given estrogen parenterally exhibited behavioral signs of proestrus within 3 days, but not estrus. Of nine ovariectomized bitches given

estrogen for 9 days, three exhibited estrus behavior 1 to 2 days before the last estrogen injection, whereas the majority exhibited estrus only *after* the last injection; in other words, their behavior was enhanced by estrogen concentrations that were decreasing (Concannon, 1987).

Ovarian follicular cells begin synthesizing progesterone in excess of that required to serve as precursors for estrogen synthesis within days of beginning proestrus. In concert with declining estrogen levels, later in proestrus and immediately preceding the onset of estrus, additional follicular cells "luteinize" and secrete

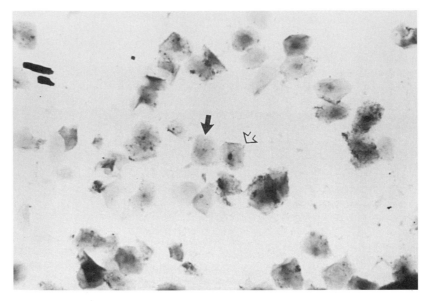

FIGURE 19-13. Vaginal cytology (at scanning microscope power) revealing both nucleated *(open arrow)* and anuclear *(closed arrow)* superficial cells. This smear is typical of late proestrus or estrus.

progressively greater amounts of progesterone. The combination of increasing serum progesterone concentrations and decreasing serum estrogen concentrations in the final days of proestrus stimulates two major events. The first is the change in behavior: the bitch that is passively resistant to breeding in late proestrus is transformed into one that actively seeks breeding in estrus. The second and equally important event stimulated by the decreasing serum estrogen and rising serum progesterone concentrations is the strong positive feedback to the hypothalamus and pituitary (Fig. 19-14), resulting in secretion of FSH and, most importantly, LH at the beginning of estrus.

Serum progesterone rises above basal concentrations *before* the LH surge. In other words, follicular cells capable of synthesizing and secreting progesterone are functioning before the development of corpora lutea. These cells cause the initial rise in progesterone concentration associated with the last day of proestrus and then the beginning of standing heat. This rise in progesterone concentration (see Fig. 19-3) enhances the intensity and duration of behavioral estrus. Ovariectomized bitches given progesterone-containing implants 6 hours following 9 days of estrogen injections had a 9-day mean duration of estrus behavior. In contrast, bitches that never received exogenous progesterone averaged only 5 days of estrus behavior following discontinuation of parenteral estrogen (Concannon, 1987). The combination of decreasing serum estrogen concentrations and increasing serum

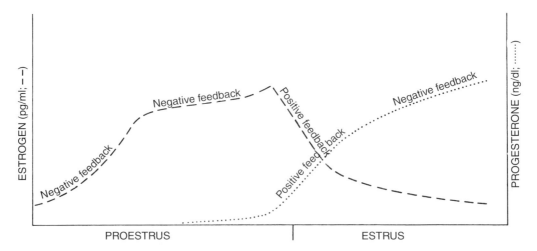

FIGURE 19-14. Diagrammatic illustration of the negative and positive feedback associated with estrogen and progesterone on the pituitary and hypothalamus by a normal bitch as she progresses through proestrus and estrus.

progesterone concentrations may be necessary for exhibition of maximal estrus behavior in most bitches (Olson et al, 1984c).

Declining estradiol concentrations with increasing progesterone concentrations are also thought to initiate the LH surge in the bitch (Concannon, 1987). The LH surge initiates ovulation within 24 to 48 hours, after which corpora lutea form. Progesterone concentrations steadily rise in the circulation during these first days of estrus. With the development of functioning corpora lutea, progesterone concentrations continue to increase further for a period of 1 to 3 weeks.

Thus, hormonally, estrus is a period of progressively decreasing estrogen concentrations, progressively increasing progesterone concentrations, and a brief (12- to 24-hour duration) burst of LH release (see Fig. 19-3). At the end of proestrus, the serum progesterone concentration usually rises to levels of 0.5 to 1.0 ng/ml from anestrus concentrations of less than 0.5 ng/ml. In contrast, approximately 24 to 48 hours before the preovulatory LH surge, the serum progesterone concentration rises above 1.0 ng/ml, reaching concentrations of 2 to 4 ng/ml. At the time of ovulation 2 days later, the serum progesterone concentration is typically in the range of 4 to 10 ng/ml. All this progesterone has been secreted *before* the development of corpora lutea, structures that are not identifiable until several days after ovulation.

Serum progesterone concentrations continue to increase throughout estrus and then several weeks into diestrus. Serum estrogen (estradiol) concentrations, which reach levels of 70 pg/ml and higher 1 to 3 days before the onset of estrus, progressively decrease throughout estrus. Estrogen concentrations greater than anestrus levels, even decreasing, maintain the various effects outlined in the description of proestrus. When the serum estrogen concentration decreases below basal levels of 15 pg/ml, estrus ends. This is reflected in the behavior of the bitch, vaginal cytology, vaginal wall thickness, vulvar size, and attraction of males.

Clinically, knowledge of plasma progesterone concentrations and how they change in a normal bitch progressing from proestrus into estrus can be extremely valuable. Several in-hospital ELISA kits are now available to estimate progesterone concentration as less than 1 ng/ml, 2 to 5 ng/ml, and greater than 5 ng/ml (Synbiotics Corp., San Diego, CA). Commercial laboratories are also beginning to provide results quickly (<24 hours) for this purpose. Establishing a plasma progesterone concentration less than 1 ng/ml in early-to-mid proestrus thereafter allows a veterinarian to obtain blood every 1 to 3 days in order to reliably detect the progesterone rise associated with the onset of estrus. The more frequent the sampling, the more precise the veterinarian can be in determining the day that progesterone begins to increase. From this knowledge, one can recommend breeding dates or predict whelping dates (Hegstad and Johnston, 1989; Cain, 1991; Manothaiudom et al, 1995).

It has been demonstrated that the normal bitch has increasing serum testosterone levels during proestrus.

Testosterone reaches maximal concentrations near the time of both the preovulatory surge of LH and behavioral receptivity. After this time, testosterone levels decline (Olson et al, 1984a). Whether testosterone contributes directly to behavioral estrus or to the surge of LH remains speculative. It is possible that testosterone is merely derived from progesterone during steroidogenesis. Aromatization of androgens to estrogens in the central nervous system (CNS) may be one contributory component initiating estrus behavior in the bitch (Olson et al, 1984a). CNS metabolism of androgens to estradiol could be one mechanism regulating the release of LH in the bitch, as has been postulated in the male (Worgul et al, 1981; Olson et al, 1984a).

OVARIES AND UTERUS. The hormonal changes described are reflected in the anatomic alterations that occur simultaneously within the ovary. Early estrus (standing heat) is associated with the final maturation process of developing follicles. Estrogen synthesis begins to wane and progesterone synthesis simultaneously increases. Ovulation, spontaneous in the bitch, occurs 24 to 72 hours following the LH surge. The number of ova released for future fertilization depends somewhat on the breed of the bitch. Smaller breeds, with their small litter size, ovulate fewer ova (2 to 10) than do larger breeds, which may ovulate 5 to 15 ova. Ovarian weight is greatest immediately before ovulation.

The enlarged ovaries with follicles may be visualized by means of abdominal ultrasonography. Apparent ovulation is characterized by a decrease in the number of follicles that can be visualized from one day to the next. The ovaries have an oval shape that becomes rounded after ovulation. At some time after ovulation, the ovaries have cystic, anechoic structures that are not distinguishable from follicles, demonstrating the value of a series of abdominal ultrasound studies. Structures identified after ovulation may represent nonovulatory follicles, corpora hemorrhagica, fluid-filled corpora lutea, or cystic luteinized follicles. Ovulation can be accurately identified using ultrasonography (England and Allen, 1989a, 1989b; Wallace et al, 1992).

All ovulatory follicles are thought to rupture within 12 to 96 hours (Jeffcoate, 1998). Because this process is not perfect, ova not released at precisely the same time are in similar stages of development, ensuring that embryonic development of all fetuses progresses similarly (Johnston et al, 1982) (see Chapter 20). This is an example of the exquisitely sensitive and synchronous nature of the delicate balance between falling estrogen concentrations, rising progesterone concentrations, the LH surge, and ovulation. Follicles that are not mature enough to ovulate following the LH surge undergo atresia, providing evidence against the possibility of ova being present for fertilization for more than 4 days.

Ruptured follicles luteinize rapidly. These rupture sites undergo reorganization, with development of mature corpora lutea capable of sustaining progesterone synthesis and secretion for 2 months and longer. The corpora lutea are bright salmon pink in color for approximately 10 days following ovulation and are easily recognized structures on the surface of the ovary.

The number of ova present in the ovaries of a newborn bitch has been estimated at 700,000. At puberty this number is reduced to 250,000; at 5 years of age, 30,000; and at 10 years, only a few hundred. Fertility appears to decline progressively once a bitch has reached 7 years of age or older. However, a corollary to the menopause of women is not typically seen in the bitch.

To review the timing of major events during the "average" standing heat, one must correlate changing hormone concentrations, follicular maturation, ovulation, corpora luteal development, and the behavior pattern of the bitch. Fig. 19-15 demonstrates that the "average" bitch first exhibits "standing" behavior as estrogen concentrations decline and progesterone concentrations rise (day 1). Day 2 is the day of the LH surge, and day 3 is associated with the final maturation process of the follicles and continued progesterone secretion by luteinized follicular cells. Days 4 through 7 are the time during which ovulation takes place. Days 5 to 9 include time for maturation of the primary oocytes to secondary oocytes, which can then be fertilized. Days 4 through 9 are the days of fertilization, and day 10 is the first day of diestrus.

Throughout this period, the uterus continues to prepare for implantation. Bleeding from the uterine microvasculature has usually but not always diminished or stopped, and glandular development with increased vascularity is nearing completion. The uterus may actually become palpable on a careful abdominal examination owing to its increase in size and thickness.

DURATION. The duration of estrus is usually 5 to 9 days. However, similar to proestrus, the length of this phase may vary dramatically among normal dogs. Estrus may be as brief as 1 to 2 days or as prolonged as 18 to 20 days. Individual bitches are usually consistent

from cycle to cycle within 2 to 6 years of age. However, variations within and among breeds make it difficult to predict the length of proestrus or estrus in any one dog.

CLINICAL SIGNS. The behavior changes in the female entering standing heat are those of reflexive receptivity to mounting and attempts at copulation by the male. These bitches may crouch and elevate the perineum toward the male. Any pressure placed on or near their lower back causes the tail to be held off to one side and an obvious tensing of the rear legs to support the weight of a mounting male. The bitch may attract males over long distances owing to the presence of potent pheromones. Typically, the vulva has progressed through the turgid phase associated with proestrus and becomes soft and flaccid, no longer the difficult barrier for a male to penetrate. The vaginal discharge is often a straw-colored or pink fluid. Less commonly, it continues to be obviously hemorrhagic.

Occasionally the vaginal discharge may contain enough glucose to register positive on urine test strips. This may be caused by rising progesterone concentrations that result in carbohydrate intolerance via insulin resistance (Ryan and Enns, 1988). The vaginal discharge during estrus is derived from uterine extracellular fluid, but such testing is not considered reliable.

The bitch in standing heat may be passive and accepting of a male or may actively approach a male as if to arouse his interest. It has been thought that the bitch breeds only with a dominant male and repels submissive males. This is a good reason to recommend delivery of the female to the home of the stud, where he is more likely to be comfortable and dominant. The female placed on the stud's territory is more likely to be submissive and receptive.

VAGINAL CYTOLOGY. Throughout standing heat the vaginal cytology remains relatively constant (see Fig. 19-2). No features on vaginal cytology identify the day

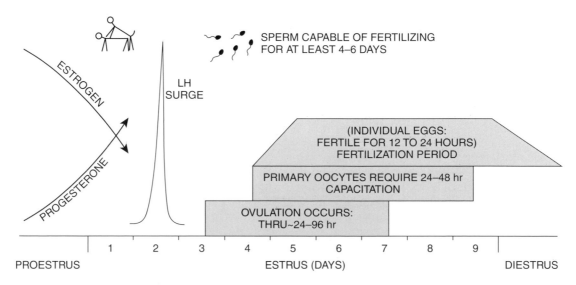

FIGURE 19-15. Illustration of the hormonal changes and sequence of events concerning the timing of ovulation and fertilization of ova in the average bitch.

of the LH peak, ovulation, or the timing of fertilization. Rather, the exfoliative vaginal cytology appears to be a reflection of serum estrogen concentrations, which continue to be greater than basal concentrations, even though they are declining toward basal levels. Superficial cells and anuclear squames account for greater than 80% of the total vaginal cells, often reaching 100%. No neutrophils are seen on cytology throughout this phase. Red blood cells may or may not be present. The background of the slide is clear of the granular material often seen in proestrus (Fig. 19-16).

The percentage of superficial vaginal epithelial cells has been described as progressively increasing throughout proestrus, with intermediate and parabasal cells simultaneously disappearing. With the onset of standing heat and the day of the LH surge, virtually 100% of the vaginal epithelial cells have been described as anuclear superficial cells (anuclear squames). These anuclear squames are then present for the duration of standing heat and continue to represent 100% of the vaginal epithelial cells.

Most researchers, however, have not found such a simple and predictable pattern to the vaginal exfoliative cytology in normal bitches. Vaginal epithelial cells at the beginning of proestrus are associated with 40% to 60% intermediate cells, and mid-proestrus with 40% to 60% superficial cells. Greater than 60% to 80% superficial cells (pyknotic nucleated and/or anuclear

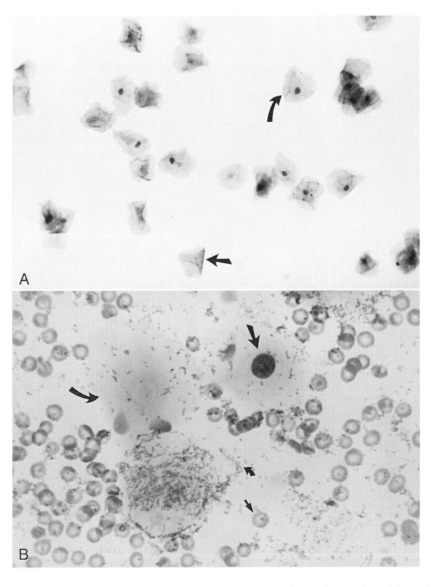

FIGURE 19-16. *A,* Vaginal cytology (at scanning microscope power) revealing nucleated *(curved arrow)* and anuclear superficial *(straight arrow)* vaginal cells, no red blood cells or neutrophils, and a clear background; this finding is classic for estrus in the bitch. *B,* Vaginal cytology at 40× revealing nucleated *(straight arrow)* and anuclear *(curved arrow)* superficial vaginal cells surrounded by large numbers of red blood cells *(small straight arrow)* and bacteria *(small curved arrow).* The Beagle bitch with this smear was also in estrus, bred on that day only, and had a litter of 11 healthy puppies.

squames) are consistently seen during the final 1 to 6 days of proestrus. More important, no further change in the percentage of superficial cells (with or without nuclei) is consistently noted from 3 to 4 days before the start of standing heat until the first day of diestrus (see Fig. 19-2). It is extremely valuable to remember that studies have demonstrated that the first day when 80% to 90% of vaginal epithelial cells are superficial in type ranged from 6 days before to 4 days after the LH surge (Olson, 1989).

Unpredictable but minor fluctuations are noted both in the percentage of superficial cells and in the presence of nuclei throughout estrus (see Table 19-1). Throughout the final days of proestrus and the entire period of standing heat the percentage of superficial cells typically does not fall below 60%, usually remaining between 90% and 100%. The presence or absence of pyknotic nuclei within these superficial cells fails to correlate consistently with alterations in plasma hormone concentrations or with the presence of follicles versus corpora lutea within the ovaries.

Vaginal cytology is a satisfactory means of estimating plasma estrogen concentrations. The effect of increased estrogen concentrations on vaginal wall thickness persists despite declining toward the basal levels typical of early diestrus. Perhaps the dramatic change in vaginal cytology noted on the first day of diestrus correlates best with the first or second day that plasma estrogen concentrations decrease to basal levels.

VAGINAL ENDOSCOPY. The switch from estrogen to progesterone secretion by pre-ovulatory follicles reduces vaginal mucosal vascularity and edema, reflected by a marked change in the appearance of the vaginal mucosa (Concannon, 1987). The luminal surface of the vagina then becomes progressively more wrinkled, or "crenulated." This effect is often visible to the trained individual within 24 hours of the surge in pituitary LH that is associated with the onset of estrus (see Fig. 19-1).

Maximal crenulation, seen as development of angulated folds of vaginal mucosa with sharp edges, is noted to occur in the interval between ovulation and oocyte maturation, 2 to 5 days later. This process translates into a time period beginning as early as 24 hours before the LH surge and continuing as long as 4 to 9 days after the surge. At the approximate time of the end of estrus, the vaginal mucosa again becomes flaccid with a patchy white and red surface (see Fig. 19-1). Thus vaginal endoscopy, as well as vaginal cytology, behavior of the bitch, and monitoring of plasma progesterone concentrations, can be a useful tool in determining breeding dates. This is especially true when only one or two breedings are allowed by the owner of the male or when using fresh extended or frozen semen (Lindsay and Concannon, 1986; Jeffcoate, 1998).

Diestrus

DEFINITION. *Diestrus* is defined as the phase of progesterone dominance following estrus. Diestrus begins with the cessation of standing heat (estrus) and ends when blood progesterone concentrations return to basal levels (<1.0 ng/ml). An alternative definition for the onset of diestrus is the day that a dramatic "shift" is observed on vaginal cytology: from a phase of 80% to 100% superficial cells (estrus) to one of 80% to 100% parabasal and intermediate cells (diestrus).

HORMONAL CHANGES. Progesterone concentrations in the plasma rise above basal concentrations (>0.5 ng/ml) at the end of proestrus to levels greater than 1.0 to 2.0 ng/ml at the onset of estrus. The progesterone rise contributing to the onset of estrus is derived from luteinized cells within follicles. After ovulation, corpora lutea develop on the ovaries within the ruptured follicular cavities, resulting in a cell population capable of synthesizing and secreting progesterone during the projected period of pregnancy. The zenith in progesterone synthesis from these corpora lutea is usually achieved 20 to 30 days after ovulation. This maximal rate of secretion occurs approximately 2 to 3 weeks after the beginning of diestrus (Johnston, 1980). A transient plateau in progesterone concentration persists for an additional 1 to 2 weeks. The progesterone concentrations at that time are dramatically higher than basal concentrations, usually in the range of 15 to 90 ng/ml (Concannon et al, 1989).

Statistically, pregnant bitches have higher progesterone concentrations than nonpregnant bitches, beginning several weeks after the onset of diestrus. Individual variation, however, precludes the use of progesterone assays for pregnancy diagnosis. This is extremely important. All nonpregnant healthy bitches that have progressed through standing heat (estrus) are "pseudopregnant" in the sense that they have functioning corpora lutea despite lack of pregnancy (i.e., a pregnancy recognition system does not exist in the bitch). Therefore corpora lutea function throughout a normal gestational period regardless of the presence or absence of a fetus (or fetuses). In fact, the corpora lutea of nonpregnant bitches have a longer functioning life expectancy than the corpora lutea of pregnant bitches (Johnston et al, 2001).

Once the plateau period in diestrual plasma progesterone concentration has passed, a prolonged decline in luteal function follows. The luteal phase ends abruptly in the pregnant bitch (approximately 65 days after fertilization) as part of the onset of parturition. However, the luteal phase slowly wanes in the nonpregnant bitch, often lasting 10 to 30 days longer than observed in pregnant bitches. The cause for the decline in luteal function, as well as its inevitable cessation in function, is not well understood. Corpora lutea represent functioning endocrine glands that have an inherent, rather brief lifespan. The function of declining corpora lutea is thought to cease abruptly with the initiation of parturition owing to the action of prostaglandins. The destructive effects of prostaglandins act on degenerated corpora lutea but fail to have a similar luteolytic effect in younger, healthier corpora lutea. Prostaglandins may be the sole luteolytic factor in nonpregnant as well as pregnant bitches.

Several studies have been completed in an effort to better understand the hormonal regulation of the cyclic corpus luteum in the dog. Since progesterone profiles are similar for pregnant, nonmated, and hysterectomized bitches during diestrus, it is unlikely that the uterus or uterine prostaglandins play a vital role in the physiologic maintenance or regression of corpora lutea (Olson et al, 1989; Jonhston et al, 2001). LH may be luteotrophic, and function of the canine corpus luteum may depend on basal LH secretion during the initial phase of the ovarian cycle (Concannon, 1980). Others believe that LH is not as important a factor in luteal function and that prolactin is the important luteotrophic factor for the second half of the luteal phase (Okkens et al, 1985a, 1985b, 1986, 1990; Concannon, 1987; Schaefers-Okkens, 1988).

It has been demonstrated that the pulsatile secretion pattern of growth hormone (GH) changes during the luteal phase, with higher serum basal concentrations and fewer pulses. It was hypothesized that this is caused by a partial suppression of pituitary GH release by progesterone-induced GH production in the mammary glands. This mammary GH may promote the physiological proliferation and differentiation of mammary gland tissue during the luteal phase of the bitch by local autocrine/paracrine effects. In addition, progesterone-induced mammary GH production may exert endocrine effects such as hyperplastic changes in the uterine epithelium and insulin resistance (Kooistra et al, 2000).

Estrogen concentrations early in diestrus are usually at basal levels (i.e., similar to anestrus concentrations). Corpora lutea initially synthesize only progesterone, but during the last week or two of gestation, estrogen concentrations have been shown to rise subtly (Concannon, 1987). Perhaps this slight increase in estrogen synthesis and secretion occurs in concert with falling progesterone concentrations as a component of the complex interactions that lead up to parturition. In any event, these small concentrations of estrogen do not cause attraction of males or any of the other obvious alterations associated with proestrus. It is not known whether the nonpregnant bitch experiences similar changes in estrogen concentration.

Secretion of LH and FSH from the pituitary during diestrus is thought to be episodic but of minimal importance. Mean LH concentrations are slightly increased during late diestrus, but the significance of this rise remains speculative. Prolactin is one of the key hormones of diestrus. Prolactin concentrations are low during anestrus, proestrus, and estrus. As progesterone concentrations decline in the latter half of diestrus, prolactin concentrations increase. An inverse relationship appears to exist between serum concentrations of progesterone and prolactin immediately prior to parturition as well as during pregnant and nonpregnant diestrus. Mammary enlargement and secretory activity during diestrus are presumed to be initiated and continued by prolactin (De Coster et al, 1983; Concannon, 1986).

Unlike concentrations of serum progesterone, which are similar among pregnant, nonmated, and hysterectomized bitches, serum immunoreactive relaxin concentrations differ between pregnant and nonpregnant dogs (Steinetz et al, 1989; Buff et al, 2000). Serum immunoreactive relaxin concentrations are <0.25 ng/ml in diestrus bitches that are not pregnant, but increase to maximum concentrations (>3.0 ng/ml) after about 6 to 7 weeks of gestation in pregnant bitches. While progesterone production is entirely of ovarian origin, relaxin production is primarily of placental origin (Tsutsui and Stewart, 1991).

OVARY AND UTERUS. Corpora lutea are located on the surface of the ovaries throughout diestrus. The uterus responds to increases in progesterone concentration by maintaining the glandular structure and vascularity required for pregnancy regardless of whether the bitch has mated. Maximum nonpregnant uterine size is seen 20 to 30 days following the onset of standing heat, a time coinciding with the highest progesterone concentrations. Earlier in diestrus, differences between the pregnant and nonpregnant uterus are insignificant. Once implantation occurs 17 to 21 days following fertilization, spherical fetal units become palpable.

With degeneration of corpora lutea and cessation of progesterone secretion, diestrus ends and the uterus undergoes a period of repair. This period of uterine involution requires 1 to 3 months in the bitch and may represent one of the factors that accounts for the relatively long interestrus period in normal bitches.

DURATION. Diestrus is the phase of progesterone dominance (increased plasma progesterone concentrations). The duration averages 56 to 58 days in pregnancy and 60 to 100 days in the nonpregnant bitch. Corpora lutea cease to function sooner in pregnancy than in nonpregnancy, presumably owing to the effects of prostaglandins. The fetus stimulates synthesis and secretion of prostaglandins, a process that has not been documented in nonpregnant bitches.

CLINICAL SIGNS. Diestrus begins when the "receptive" bitch abruptly refuses to breed. She may also no longer attract males. The vulva returns to a normal or anestrual size and is no longer enlarged or flaccid. Basically, no clinical difference is apparent between an anestrus bitch and one that is in diestrus and not pregnant. No obvious method has been found to distinguish a pregnant bitch early in diestrus (first 7 to 10 days) from one that is not pregnant.

VAGINAL CYTOLOGY. Vaginal cytology obtained from a bitch entering diestrus is *clearly different* from that of a bitch in early, mid-, or late estrus. The smears obtained during the final days of standing heat are no different on vaginal cytology from those obtained in early estrus (see Fig. 19-2). These smears contain more than 80% superficial cells, no neutrophils, and a clear background. Within a 24- to 48-hour period at the end of estrus, the percentage of superficial cells falls to approximately 20%, with the majority of cells being intermediate and/or parabasal cells (Fig. 19-17). This represents an abrupt and obvious change in the vaginal cytology (see Table 19-1).

Occasionally, sheets or rafts of vaginal epithelial cells are seen on vaginal cytologic smears, just preceding the onset of diestrus (see Fig. 19-17, B). This phenomenon

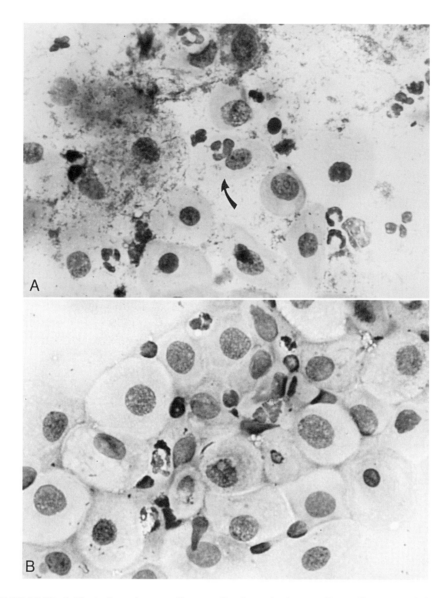

FIGURE 19-17. *A,* Vaginal cytology at 40× revealing bacteria, intermediate cells, neutrophils, and a metestrum cell *(arrow)* suggestive of diestrus. *B,* Vaginal cytology at 40× revealing sheets of large intermediate vaginal epithelial cells and a few neutrophils. Rafts of cells like this are sometimes seen on or around the first day of diestrus.

represents sloughing of large numbers of cells at once. Neutrophils may occasionally reappear, and the background may contain large amounts of debris. However, the dramatic change in the microscopic appearance of individual vaginal epithelial cells (from superficial cells to intermediate and parabasal cells) is usually the first indicator that diestrus has begun. The presence or absence of neutrophils is not a reliable criterion. The behavior of the stud or the bitch is even less reliable than the cytology (Olson, 1989).

Occasionally, specific "metestrum" cells associated with the diestrus phase are seen. These cells have been used as an aid in attempting to distinguish early proestrus from the beginning of diestrus. In examining the vaginal smear of a bitch with an unclear history, one may not be certain if the smear being examined represents early or mid-proestrus or represents a bitch that has just completed standing heat. "Metestrum" and "foam" cells are supposedly seen only in diestrus. Metestrum cells (see Fig. 19-10) are vaginal epithelial cells that contain one or two neutrophils within their cytoplasm. Unfortunately, we have identified these cells in other phases of the cycle whenever a large number of neutrophils are present. When there is doubt, a series of smears obtained every 2 or 3 days almost always identifies the correct stage of any cycle. The bitch in proestrus has a progressively increasing percentage of superficial cells on vaginal cytology and exhibits behavioral changes. The bitch in diestrus does not exhibit such changes.

Following the initial few days of diestrus, vaginal cytology smears from bitches in diestrus resemble those of anestrus. White blood cells may or may not be present, red blood cells are absent or present in small numbers, and the epithelial cells typically consist of small intermediate cells plus parabasal cells. Exfoliative vaginal cytology from the normal bitch is similar in comparing diestrus with anestrus. Smears from anestrus to proestrus and proestrus to estrus tend to change relatively slowly. However, the appearance of vaginal epithelial cells from estrus into diestrus change abruptly. In studying infertility patients and in attempting to identify whelping dates, recognizing the first day of diestrus becomes critically important (see Chapter 24).

MAMMARY GLANDS. The increasing progesterone concentrations of standing heat initiate glandular development in mammary tissue. These changes usually become obvious to the owner as the bitch reaches the final trimester of diestrus. Prolactin concentrations, which rise during the final weeks of gestation, cause overt lactation in preparation for the newborn.

Anestrus

DEFINITION. Anestrus is the phase of the female reproductive cycle in which the uterus involutes. Anestrus begins with whelping and ends with proestrus. The beginning of anestrus is not readily discernible in the nonpregnant bitch, in which no obvious demarcation between diestrus and anestrus is *clinically* detectable.

DURATION. Like the other phases of the ovarian cycle, anestrus varies in duration. This variation depends on breed, health, age, time of year, environment, and multiple other factors. The typical bitch begins proestrus every 7 months. Proestrus lasts 9 days; estrus, 7 to 9 days; diestrus, 58 days; and anestrus, 4.5 months. However, duration of these phases remains variable, in part because it is difficult to know when diestrus ends and anestrus begins in any nonpregnant bitch. The duration of diestrus progesterone secretion is likely to be the major factor determining the interval between nonfertile ovarian cycles. Shortening the luteal phase by either prostaglandin-induced luteolysis (Vickery and McRae, 1980) or prolonged administration of bromocriptine (Okkens et al, 1985b) reduced interestrus intervals by weeks to months (Concannon, 1987). In addition, the effect of pregnancy, the realization that interestrus periods are rarely totally constant, and other factors make predicting the onset of proestrus quite difficult.

CLINICAL SIGNS. No obvious clinical difference can be seen between the anestrus bitch and one that is not pregnant but in diestrus or one that has been ovariohysterectomized (spayed). In fact, sometimes one cannot tell whether a bitch has been spayed without assaying pituitary hormone (FSH and LH) concentrations. These gonadotrophs are dramatically elevated in the spayed bitch.

HORMONE CONCENTRATIONS. As with other species, sporadic bursts in LH secretion occur throughout anestrus in the dog. These transient abrupt increases in plasma LH appear to lead up to two major brief but potent secretory episodes. One LH peak immediately precedes the onset of proestrus, and one precedes or coincides with the onset of estrus and subsequent ovulation. Concentrations of serum FSH increase during anestrus, reaching levels in late anestrus that are as high as those present during the preovulatory FSH surge during estrus. It is hypothesized that these apparent paroxysmal pulses of pituitary secretion are not by chance. Rather, they likely represent a delicate mechanism necessary in recruiting follicles for the next cycle (Johnston et al, 2001). Once recruited into the preovulatory pool, these follicles selectively regulate pituitary gonadotroph secretion via negative feedback mechanisms, thereby affecting the subsequent cycle (see Fig. 19-3).

Estrogen concentrations fluctuate significantly throughout anestrus. Surges in estrogen concentration have been observed, and these are assumed to be derived from waves of follicle development that are subclinical in nature and probably short-lived. These follicles synthesize and secrete estrogen, causing minor increases in circulating estrogen concentrations. Because the follicles never fully mature, they regress, after brief periods of function, before ever developing luteinized cells that could synthesize progesterone. Serum estrogen concentrations decrease before the onset of proestrus (Olson et al, 1982). By contrast, progesterone remains at extremely low concentrations throughout anestrus.

It is not known what factor initiates proestrus and a new ovarian cycle. This is likely to be a result of complex interactions between environment, general health, ovarian status, uterine status, and age. This concept becomes clinically relevant in attempts to improve fertility through the parenteral administration of pituitary and/or ovarian hormones. The delicate coordination of events leading to ovulation is difficult to mimic.

THE UTERUS. The uterus during anestrus undergoes self-repair. It must reach a state of complete involution following the effects of pregnancy or pseudopregnancy (clinical or subclinical). Complete repair of the endometrium to a basal state requires approximately 120 days after serum progesterone concentrations return to basal levels in the nonpregnant cycle and after 140 days in a fertile cycle (Talwar et al, 1985; Johnston et al, 1985). Externally, the veterinarian detects little change in the palpable uterus once involution reduces the uterus to a size comparable with loops of bowel. At this point, further changes in uterine anatomy continue subclinically.

VAGINAL CYTOLOGY. The vaginal cytology of anestrus is relatively constant. One sees primarily parabasal and intermediate vaginal epithelial cells. Neutrophils may or may not be present, and red blood cells are absent. Bacteria may or may not be seen. When present, bacteria usually represent normal flora. The background appearance, after staining, may be clear or granular.

VAGINAL EXFOLIATIVE CYTOLOGY

Techniques or Methodology in Making Vaginal Smears

Various methods are recognized for obtaining exfoliated vaginal smears. All the techniques may succeed in providing necessary information. However, the criteria for choosing one method depends on several factors: the method (1) should be simple to perform and inexpensive, (2) should be applicable to dogs regardless of their size or temperament, (3) must not be painful, (4) should be successful regardless of the presence or absence of a vaginal discharge, and (5) should be able to be performed by owners after they have been given a brief lesson. A veterinarian should use and become familiar with one method for obtaining vaginal smears. The clinician can then become comfortable and confident in this one procedure. The cotton swab method described below is recommended because it best meets the suggested criteria.

Cotton Swab Technique

The lips of the vulva are gently separated with one hand. The other hand holds a sterile, cotton-tipped applicator, 5 to 7 inches long. We often use the cotton swab found within a culturette tube (Culturette; Marion Scientific, Kansas City, MO). The cotton-tipped end of this swab is passed into the dorsal commissure of the vulva.

Initially, the cotton tip is gently pressed against the caudodorsal surface of the vaginal vault to avoid the clitoral fossa and then advanced in a craniodorsal direction, toward the vertebral column, until it passes over the ischial arch (Fig. 19-18). The swab is inserted at least the distance needed to reach the pelvic canal. The applicator is then rotated a complete revolution in each direction and withdrawn. The entire procedure should take only seconds and is rarely painful. A bitch may appear uncomfortable if there is no vaginal discharge. Therefore the cotton should be moistened with two to three drops of sterile saline to act as a lubricant if a discharge is not obvious. The clitoral fossa must be avoided because this is a small blind pocket and attempts to advance the swab against this surface would be painful. In addition, the cells of the clitoral fossa may be confused with superficial vaginal epithelial cells (Olson, 1989).

Once the cotton swab is withdrawn, the cotton tip is *rolled* gently from one end of a glass microscope slide to the other. There should be space on the slide for two or

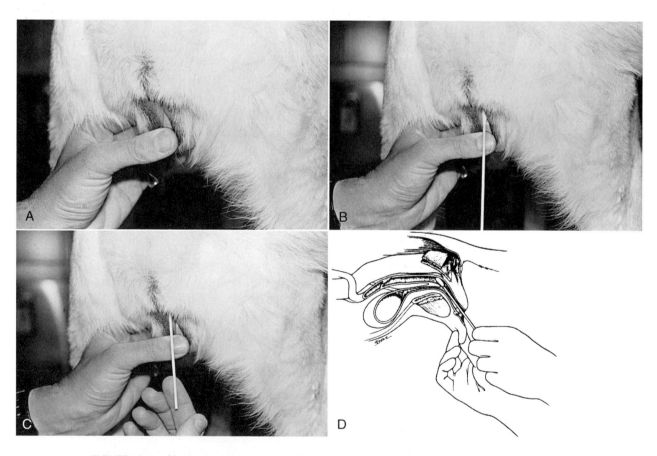

FIGURE 19-18. Obtaining a vaginal smear with a cotton swab. *A,* Spreading open the vulvar lips for insertion of the swab. *B,* The swab placed at the vulva, just before insertion into the vagina. *C,* The swab has been inserted into the vaginal vault. *D,* A diagram illustrating the location of the cotton-tipped swab. (*D* From Johnston SD: The Female. Vet Clin N Amer 11:543, 1981.)

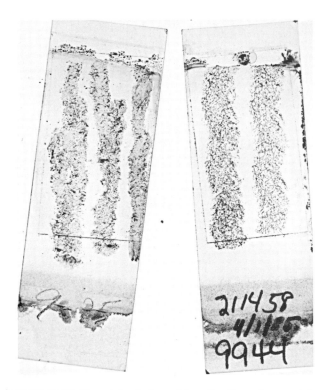

FIGURE 19-19. Two stained glass slides after the cotton swab has been rolled across the surface to make two or three columns containing vaginal smear material.

three separate linear impressions (Fig. 19-19). The swab should not be pressed firmly, and the cotton should not be rubbed or smeared against the glass, because the result of either mistake is nondiagnostic material. Usually two slides are prepared using one or two cotton swabs. The slides with the exfoliated cells can be quickly air dried and then dipped once or twice in 95% to 100% methanol to prevent cellular deterioration or distortion. Such slides can be stained immediately or stored and stained at a later date (Olson et al, 1984a).

Stains

CRITERIA FOR CHOOSING A STAIN. As with the techniques available for obtaining cells for vaginal exfoliative cytology, the staining of these smears is quite important. Several stains have been shown to be excellent. The stain chosen should be easy to use and inexpensive; it should also store well over a period of time and, ideally, provide a permanent slide that can be saved for years.

WRIGHT'S STAIN OR WRIGHT-GIEMSA STAIN. Wright's stain is methylene blue polychromated with sodium bicarbonate and heat, to which eosin is added. Giemsa stain consists of a combination of azure II dyes and eosin. Wright's stain is commonly used in staining peripheral blood smears. This stain is also used for vaginal cytology and provides easy-to-read slides with colors that are consistent, reproducible, and of excellent quality. The stain does require careful maintenance of

the solutions, and the clinician must carefully follow the instructions regarding their make-up.

DIFF-QUIK. Diff-Quik (American Scientific Products, McGraw, IL) is the stain we recommend for routine vaginal smears performed by veterinary practitioners. It is a modified Wright-Giemsa stain that is easy to use; it reliably stains both vaginal epithelial cells and red blood cells and is inexpensive. Slides must be immersed in methanol and two staining solutions. It has been recommended that vaginal smears be immersed in the two staining solutions longer than the period normally required for staining peripheral blood smears (Olson et al, 1984b). Diff-Quik–stained slides can be stored for several days if reference to a series of slides is desired. If a permanent coverslip is used, the slides can be stored indefinitely. This is a stain that all veterinary hospitals can use.

NEW METHYLENE BLUE. Vaginal smears are stained by placing a drop of the new methylene blue solution on the slide, followed by a coverslip. Slides can be viewed immediately. The stain is excellent for vaginal cell morphology but does not stain red blood cells. For a quick and simple stain, it is excellent. This is usually the stain we recommend for use by breeders, and it has also been chosen by a number of veterinarians.

PAP AND TRICHROME STAINING. The staining method most commonly used in human vaginal cytology is that of Papanicolaou (PAP). The PAP and trichrome methods are polychromatic staining reactions designed to display the many variations of cellular morphology, showing degrees of cellular maturity and metabolic activity. The major advantage of these techniques is provision of good differentiation of the exfoliated cells; keratinized cells stain orange-red, whereas nonkeratinized cells stain blue-green. Other advantages include definition of nuclear detail and cytoplasmic transparency. Despite the benefits, these staining methods are not recommended because they are labor-intensive, complicated, and impractical (Thomas, 1987).

Clinical Usefulness of Vaginal Cytology

MANAGEMENT OF NORMAL BREEDING. Vaginal cytology is one of the most commonly used diagnostic tools in clinical canine reproduction. This tool may be used in helping an owner to determine the proper time to breed a bitch. Observation of the behavior of a bitch with a stud is the most reliable method of learning when a bitch has entered standing heat (i.e., when the bitch is ready to breed, she will breed). However, numerous exceptions to this philosophy point out the value of vaginal cytology.

As described in the preceding section on phases of the ovarian cycle, vaginal cytology is an excellent aid in distinguishing between early proestrus, estrus, and diestrus. It is always wise to recommend that a minimum of two or three smears, taken over a period of 4 to 7 days, be examined. However, when the number of superficial cells makes up 80% or more of the vaginal epithelial cells, the bitch and stud should be brought together. If mating does not take place within 1 or 2 days, a second smear should be obtained. If it is similar to the first smear and not suggestive of diestrus, another breeding or artificial insemination should be pursued. The presence of 80% or more superficial cells often precedes estrus by as many as 3 to 6 days. Vaginal cytology becomes an extremely important diagnostic aid whenever an infertility problem or abnormality in behavior is believed to exist.

Vaginal cytology, behavior of a bitch, and monitoring of her serum progesterone concentrations are of real value in breeding management. Knowing the precise day of a cycle, beginning with the first day of vulvar swelling or vaginal bleeding, is helpful but should not be relied on as the sole criterion of when a bitch should be bred. Some bitches are in standing heat with 80% or more superficial cells without ever having had an obvious proestrus, whereas others begin estrus as long as 21 days after the apparent start of proestrus. Only the *average* dog enters standing heat on the tenth day after beginning proestrus. Some bitches never stand for a male (i.e., do not display behavioral estrus). Such dogs are often fertile, and correct use of vaginal cytology aids in determining dates for artificial insemination.

An attempt at breeding should be pursued, naturally or artificially, *throughout* the period when 80% or more superficial cells are seen on vaginal cytology. This advice is more reliable once the serum progesterone of the bitch has been documented to exceed 1.0 ng/ml. After the vaginal smear is suggestive of estrus, 3 to 6 days may pass before natural breeding commences, because of the overlap in vaginal cytology appearance seen at the end of proestrus and throughout estrus. However, once natural breeding begins, it should be allowed to continue until the bitch refuses to breed. *This is the most important advice we provide to owners.* We recommend breeding dogs every second, third, or fourth day of estrus. More frequent intervals are suggested if this is the first breeding or if the bitch is known to have an abbreviated estrus. Less frequent breedings are suggested if she is known to have been in standing heat for 9 days or longer in previous ovarian cycles.

SHIPPING OR RECEIVING A BITCH. Bitches may be sent long distances for breeding. Bitches should be shipped before finding 80% or more superficial cells on the vaginal smear. The duration of proestrus can be difficult to predict, and shipping early is recommended. When a bitch is received, her behavior status can be assessed. If she is not standing for the stud, a vaginal smear and a serum progesterone should be evaluated. Both parameters should be monitored serially.

UNUSUAL CYCLES. Any bitch that appears to have normal reproductive cycles but never stands for the stud may be hormonally normal and fertile. Some of these bitches apparently fail to stand for a male because they are not exposed to the stud during their standing heat (i.e., standing heat is often unrecognized because it does not occur between days 9 and 12 of the cycle). For various reasons, standing heat may not be recognized or may not occur. Bitches that refuse natural breeding can be artificially inseminated (AI). AI should begin the first day superficial cells reach or exceed 80% of the total vaginal cells. AI should be continued on an alternate-day basis throughout this phase. Insemination should be discontinued only when diestrus is definitively recognized on assessment of vaginal cytology.

PREDICTING WHELPING DATES. Vaginal cytology is a superb tool in predicting the approximate date of whelping. The prediction is based on the knowledge that whelping occurs near day 57 of diestrus (Olson et al, 1983; Linde and Karlsson, 1984). Obtaining a series of vaginal smears from a bitch on a daily basis readily allows recognition of the first day of diestrus. This method is considerably more reliable than using breeding dates.

INFERTILITY PROBLEMS. Vaginal cytology is a crude reflection of plasma estrogen concentrations and, as such, a test of ovarian follicular function. Infertility cases should be evaluated with vaginal cytology and serum progesterone concentrations to determine whether the problem is one of mismanagement (incorrect timing), inadequate estrogen (poor follicular development), or some less common disorder.

FOLLICULAR CYSTS. By definition, an ovarian follicular cyst is one that synthesizes and secretes estrogen. A bitch with a follicular cyst appears to have a prolonged proestrus and/or prolonged estrus. The first evidence that a bitch has a follicular cyst includes her behavior of prolonged proestrus and/or estrus and a persistent bloody vaginal discharge (> 2 to 3 weeks). With or without these parameters, the bitch should have persistent evidence of proestrus/estrus on vaginal cytology. The next diagnostic aid used in establishing a diagnosis is abdominal ultrasonography.

VAGINITIS. The vaginal smear from a bitch with vaginitis usually contains a large number of healthy to degenerated neutrophils. Neutrophils with engulfed bacteria may be observed if a bacterial vaginitis is present. Neutrophils and bacteria are often seen in smears from normal bitches as well, but large numbers of neutrophils may be abnormal. Early diestrus may be transiently associated with large numbers of bacteria and neutrophils within the vaginal cytology. Persistent significant neutrophilia seen on vaginal cytology may be consistent with vaginitis.

VAGINAL TUMORS. Not surprisingly, tumors invading the vaginal vault exfoliate cells that may then be recognized on vaginal cytology. The tumors most frequently identified with vaginal cytology include transmissible venereal tumor (Fig. 19-20) and transitional cell carcinomas of the bladder, which may extend into the vagina via the urethra.

PYOMETRA AND ACUTE METRITIS. These two disorders are serious problems that usually cause systemic illness. These conditions are often associated with fever, clinical signs, and abnormalities on blood, urine, radiographic, or ultrasonographic evaluations. Therefore vaginal cytology is not the most valuable or reliable diagnostic aid when a bitch is being evaluated for one of these disorders. Diagnosis of uterine disease should *not* be made with vaginal smears. However, animals with open-cervix pyometra or metritis may have large

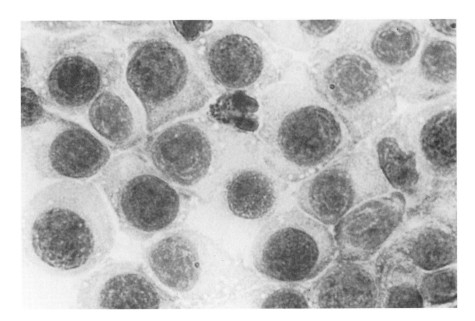

FIGURE 19-20. An impression smear obtained from a vaginal mass caused by a transmissible venereal tumor in a bitch.

numbers of degenerated neutrophils and, occasionally, vacuolated endometrial cells (Olson et al, 1984c).

DETERMINING WHETHER AN ABORTIFACIENT SHOULD BE ADMINISTERED TO A BITCH. An owner may not actually observe an unwanted breeding. However, if an unwanted breeding was likely, the finding of spermatozoa or the heads of spermatozoa on vaginal cytology confirms that breeding has occurred (Fig. 19-21). Lack of these findings does not eliminate the possibility that a breeding took place. In addition, if the vaginal smear is suggestive of proestrus, diestrus, or vaginitis, there is little reason for an owner to be concerned. (A complete discussion of mismating is presented in Chapter 22.)

Limitations of Vaginal Cytology

Vaginal cytology is an extremely useful tool in canine reproduction. Understanding the clinical applications of cytology increases the value of the procedure. It must be pointed out, however, that vaginal exfoliative cytology does not answer some common questions. Vaginal cytology cannot identify the day of ovulation or fertilization; therefore the "perfect" day for breeding cannot be determined from an evaluation of smears. Retrospectively, once the first day of diestrus is identified, ovulation can be assumed to have occurred approximately 6 days earlier. Vaginal cytology cannot be used for pregnancy diagnosis. Finally, vaginal cytology, although a valuable tool, is an imperfect substitute for owner observations of behavioral estrus. Observation of behavior plus a review of vaginal cytology is an excellent pairing of complementary assessments.

REFERENCES

Anderson AC, Simpson ME: The genital system during maturity and senescence. In The Ovary and Reproductive Cycle of the Dog (Beagle). Los Altos, CA, Geron-X, 1973, p 195.

Buff S, et al: Serum relaxin concentrations in pregnant and pseudopregnant bitches: evaluation of performances of a new enzyme-immunoassay for the determination of pregnancy. The Fourth International Symposium on Canine and Feline Reproduction, Norway, 2000, p 101.

Cain J: Timing ovulation in the bitch. Symposium on Canine Reproduction, Eastern States Veterinary Conference, 1991, p 1.

Concannon PW: Effects of hypophysectomy and of LH administration on the luteal phase plasma progesterone levels in the Beagle bitch. J Reprod Fertil 58:407, 1980.

Concannon PW: Canine pregnancy and parturition. Vet Clin North Am [Small Anim Pract] 16:453, 1986.

Concannon PW: The physiology of ovarian cycles, pregnancy and parturition in the domestic dog. Proceedings of the Society for Theriogenology, 1987, p 159.

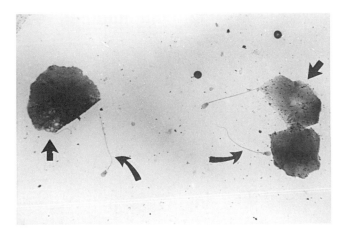

FIGURE 19-21. Vaginal smear from a bitch that had been bred to a normal male 12 hours earlier. Note the superficial vaginal epithelial cells (*straight arrows*) and the sperm (*curved arrows*).

Concannon PW, DiGregorio GB: Canine vaginal cytology. *In* Burke T (ed): Small Animal Reproduction and Infertility. Philadelphia, Lea & Febiger, 1986, p 96.

Concannon PW, et al: Biology and endocrinology of ovulation, pregnancy and parturition in the dog. J Reprod Fertil Suppl 39:3, 1989.

Concannon PW, et al: Suppression of luteal function in dogs by luteinizing hormone antiserum and by bromocriptine. J Reprod Fertil 81:175, 1987.

De Coster R, et al: A homologous radioimmunoassay for canine prolactin-plasma levels during the reproductive cycle. Acta Endocrinol 103:477, 1983.

England GCW, Allen WE: Ultrasonography and histological appearance of the canine ovary. Vet Rec 125:555, 1989a.

England GCW, Allen WE: Real-time ultrasonic imaging of the ovary and uterus of the dog. J Reprod Fertil 39(Suppl):91, 1989b.

Evans JM, White K: The Book of the Bitch: A Complete Guide to Understanding and Caring for Bitches. London, Henston Ltd, 1988.

Goodwin M, et al: Sex pheromone in the dog. Science 203:559, 1979.

Hegstad RL, Johnston SD: Use of a rapid, qualitative ELISA technique (Biometallics Inc) to determine serum progesterone concentrations in the bitch. Proceedings of the Society for Theriogenology, 1989, p 277.

Hoffman B, et al: Ovarian and pituitary function in dogs after hysterectomy. J Reprod Fertil 96:837, 1992.

Jeffcoate I: Physiology and endocrinology of the bitch. *In* Simpson G, editor: Manual of Small Animal Reproduction and Neonatology, London, British Small Animal Association, 1988, p 1.

Johnston SD: Diagnostic and therapeutic approach to infertility in the bitch. JAVMA 196:1335, 1980.

Johnston SD, Root Kustritz MV, Olson PNS: Canine and Feline Theriogenology. Philadelphia, Saunders, 2001.

Johnston SD, et al: Canine theriogenology. J Soc Theriogenol 11:1, 1982.

Johnston SD, et al: Cytoplasmic estrogen and progesterone receptors in canine endometrium during the estrous cycle. Am J Vet Res 46:1653, 1985.

Kooistra HS, Okkens AC: The role of follicle-stimulating hormone in the initiation of ovarian folliculogenesis in the bitch. The Fourth International Symposium on Canine and Feline Reproduction, Norway, 2000, p 44.

Kooistra HS, et al: Pulsatile secretion pattern of growth hormone during the luteal phase and mid-anoestrus in beagle bitches. The Fourth International Symposium on Canine and Feline Reproduction, Norway, 2000, p 46.

Leedy MG: Hormonal and neural control of sexual behavior in dogs and cats. *In* Sitsen JMA, editor: Handbook of Sexology. Vol. 6: The Pharmacology and Endocrinology of Sexual Function. Amsterdam, Elsevier, 1988, p 231.

Linde C, Karlsson I: The correlation between the cytology of the vaginal smear and the time of ovulation in the bitch. J Small Anim Pract 25:77, 1984.

Lindsay FEF: The normal endoscopic appearance of the caudal reproductive tract of the cyclic and non-cyclic bitch: post-uterine endoscopy. J Small Anim Pract 24:1, 1983.

Lindsay FEF, Concannon PW: Normal canine vaginoscopy. *In* Burke T (ed): Small Animal Reproduction and Infertility. Philadelphia, Lea & Febiger, 1986, p 112.

Manothaiudom K, et al: Evaluation of the ICAGEN-Target canine ovulation timing diagnostic test in detecting canine plasma progesterone concentrations. J Am Anim Hosp Assoc 31:57, 1995.

Okkens AC, et al: Evidence for the non-involvement of the uterus in the lifespan of the corpus luteum in the cyclic dog. Vet Q 7:169, 1985a.

Okkens AC, et al: Shortening of the interoestrous interval and the lifespan of the corpus luteum of the cyclic dog by bromocriptine treatment. Vet Q 7:193, 1985b.

Okkens AC, et al: Influence of hypophysectomy on the lifespan of the corpus luteum in the cyclic dog. J Reprod Fertil 77:187, 1986.

Okkens AC, et al: Evidence for prolactin as the main luteotrophic factor in the cyclic dogs. Vet Q 12:193, 1990.

Olson PN: Exfoliative cytology of the canine reproductive tract. Proceedings of the Society for Theriogenology, 1989, p 259.

Olson PN, et al: Concentrations of reproductive hormones in canine serum throughout late anestrus, proestrus, and estrus. Biol Reprod 27:1196, 1982.

Olson PN, et al: Infertility in the bitch. *In* Kirk RW (ed): Current Veterinary Therapy VIII. Philadelphia, WB Saunders Co, 1983, p 925.

Olson PN, et al: Concentrations of testosterone in canine serum during late anestrus, proestrus, estrus, and early diestrus. Am J Vet Res 45:145, 1984a.

Olson PN, et al: Vaginal cytology. Part I. A useful tool for staging the canine estrous cycle. Comp Cont Ed Pract Vet 6:288, 1984b.

Olson PN, et al: Vaginal cytology. Part II. Its use in diagnosing canine reproductive disorders. Comp Cont Ed Pract Vet 6:385, 1984c.

Olson PN, et al: Endocrine regulation of the corpus luteum of the bitch as a potential target for altering fertility. J Reprod Fertil Suppl 39:27, 1989.

Ryan EA, Enns L: Role of gestational hormones in the induction of insulin resistance. J Clin Endocrinol Metab 67:341, 1988.

Schaefers-Okkens AC: Hormonal regulation to the cyclic corpus luteum in the dog. Thesis, Utrecht, 1988.

Steinetz BG, et al: Serum relaxin and progesterone concentrations in pregnant, pseudopregnant, and ovariectomized, progestin-treated pregnant bitches: detection of relaxin as a marker of pregnancy. Am J Vet Res 50:68, 1989.

Talwar G, et al: Bioeffective monoclonal antibody against the gonadotropin releasing hormone: Reacting determinant and action on ovulation and estrus suppression. Proc Natl Acad Sci 82:1228, 1985.

Thomas TN: Staining techniques for vaginal cytology evaluation. Proceedings of the Society for Theriogenology, 1987, p 262.

Tsutsui T, Stewart DR: Determination of the source of relaxin immunoreactivity during pregnancy in the dog. J Vet Med Sci 53:1025, 1991.

Vickery B, McRae G: Effect of synthetic PG analogue on pregnancy in Beagle bitches. Biol Reprod 22:438, 1980.

Wallace SS, et al: Ultrasonic appearance of the ovaries of dogs during the follicular and luteal phases of the estrous cycle. Am J Vet Res 53:209, 1992.

Worgul TJ, et al: Evidence that brain aromatization regulates LH secretion in the male dog. Am J Physiol 241:E246, 1981.

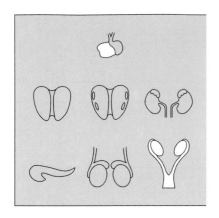

20

BREEDING, PREGNANCY, AND PARTURITION

SEXUAL BEHAVIOR

Breeding management of both the bitch and the stud involves a good deal of emphasis on normal "instincts" or normal "behavior." There is little doubt, however, that humans influence dogs and their behavior patterns. It can be difficult to understand and assess the effect of the interaction between owner influence and a variety of other environmental factors on pet dogs that do have strong instinctive behavior patterns.

Development of Sexual Behavior

Sexual behavior may be recognized in male puppies as young as 3 to 4 weeks of age. They are often observed to mount litter mates of either gender and display pelvic thrusting actions. This is normal behavior and should not be discouraged unless absolutely necessary (Farstad, 1998). Bitch puppies only occasionally show mounting behavior and, if mounted, they usually remain passive. This is considered normal play behavior. Dogs raised with exposure only to humans may respond incorrectly when placed in a breeding

situation. The past several decades have seen a trend toward selling puppies when they are quite young. With puppies arriving in their new homes at 5 to 7 weeks of age, it is possible that they are being deprived of some "sex education" they would have received had they remained with their litter mates for a longer time. However, the importance of mounting behavior during play and of interaction with other dogs for the development of normal adult sexual behavior remains speculative.

Courtship

Premating behavior is initiated by the male, and the female responds to these actions. The male is assumed to be sexually attracted to the female by means of pheromones. Most males are aggressive in their behavior, forcing positive or negative responses from the bitch. Courtship behavior includes the male sniffing at the bitch's nose, ear, neck, flank, and vulvar area while she sniffs the male in return. Licking of the vulvar area, chasing, wrestling, and urinating induce actions of a similar nature by the proestrual female. If

TABLE 20-1 BEHAVIORAL SCORING SYSTEM*

BEHAVIORAL CATEGORY	BEHAVIOR PATTERN LABELS AND POINT VALUES							
Male interest	Nil	= 0	Investigative	= 1	Mounting	= 2	Pelvic thrusting	= 3
Female interest	Hostile	= 0	Retreating	= 2	Passive	= 4	Presenting	= 6
Female stance	Retreat	= 0	Crouch	= 2	Stand poorly	= 4	Stand firmly	= 6
Female tail deviation	Nil	= 0	Minimal	= 2	Infrequent	= 4	Rapid and constant	= 6
Total possible score								= 21

*Adapted from Concannon PW, et al: LH release in ovariohysterectomized dogs in response to estrogen withdrawal and its facilitation by progesterone. Biol Reprod 20:523, 1979.

the female is in proestrus, further advances by the male, such as standing near her or placing his paw or head on her back, result in the bitch sitting, crouching, growling, snapping, or wheeling around.

Changes in Sexual Behavior in Proestrus and Estrus

In response to increases in plasma estrogen concentrations, the bitch is frequently observed to be more interested in interacting with other dogs, to be restless or nervous, to have an increase or decrease in appetite, to drink more, and/or to urinate more frequently (Farstad, 1998). The increase in urination may aid in dispersing pheromones present in the urine and vaginal secretions that attract male dogs. This pheromone has the chemical structure of methyl-hydroxybenzoate.

Using a scoring system to assess changes in the behavior of the bitch and the stud, an objective view of changing patterns can be appreciated (Tables 20-1 and 20-2) (Concannon et al, 1979). The female changes from being outwardly hostile to the male, to becoming passive but resistant, and finally to being actively receptive. Obviously, the key behavioral change during this series of events is the female becoming overtly receptive to males. The bitch in estrus stands still when approached by a male and deviates her tail to one side ("flagging"). Some females may present their vulva by elevating it when sniffed by a male. Often contractions may be observed in the perineal and rectal muscles. The bitch may assume a "lordosis" posture if a male places a paw on her back. If the male is timid, she may back up to him, poke him in the side with her nose, paw on his back, or even mount him. As estrus progresses,

the female may become less interested in mating. The behavior at the end of estrus is not marked by an abrupt alteration (Farstad, 1998).

Bitches tend to show a gradual decline in acceptance of males over 1 to 4 days. Behavior is definitely variable in late estrus and early diestrus when correlated with vaginal cytology. The female response to an aggressive or persistent male when she is in late estrus may be initial reluctance followed by acceptance of copulation. It should be pointed out that males, too, may show a relative or absolute lack of interest in bitches that have progressed to early diestrus.

Normal Mating

The six stages of normal mating are as follows (modified from Farstad, 1998):
1. Mounting
2. Pelvic thrusting and intromission
3. Erection (swelling of both penis and bulbus glandis) and release of the first fraction of the ejaculate (sperm free, clear, prostatic fluid)
4. Rotation (dismounting or "the turn") and ejaculation; release of the second fraction of the ejaculate (white, sperm-rich fraction)
5. Tie; release of the third fraction of the ejaculate (sperm free, clear, prostatic fluid)
6. Breaking of the tie

The Tie

Courtship behavior, as previously described, usually precedes copulation. Courtship may be prolonged by

TABLE 20–2 TYPICAL MAXIMUM SCORES OF EACH BEHAVIOR CATEGORY AND RANGE OF SCORES FOR EACH STAGE OF PROESTRUS AND ONSET OF ESTRUS*

BEHAVIOR CATEGORY	MAXIMUM POINTS			
	Onset of Proestrus	Mid-Proestrus	Late Proestrus	Onset of Estrus
Male interest	1	2	3	3
Female interest	0	2	4	6
Female stance	0	0	2–4	6
Female tail deviation	0	0	0–2	4–6
Range of total scores	0–1	2–4	5–12	16–21

*Adapted from Concannon PW, et al: LH release in ovariohysterectomized dogs in response to estrogen withdrawal and its facilitation by progesterone. Biol Reprod 20:523, 1979.

play or chasing activity, or it may consist of the male briefly licking the vulva prior to mounting. Any attempt at mounting by the male typically causes the bitch to stand firmly in place. Mounting (stage 1 of normal mating) consists of the male clasping the flanks of the female, with his forelegs anterior to the hip joints. Intromission appears to be achieved through tentative trial and error pelvic thrusting of the penis toward the vaginal opening (stage 2 of normal mating).

Intromission (stage 2 of mating; stage 1 of coitus; Fig. 20-1) can be accomplished without the male having an erection because the os penis provides rigidity. If the male had an erection prior to intromission, the enlarged bulbus glandis would actually prevent intromission. With normal breeding, intromission takes place, erection then begins (stage 3 of mating), and "stepping" movements of the male's rear legs are seen. Engorgement of the bulbus glandis takes place simultaneously with the stepping movements. The pelvic thrusting becomes more aggressive, and ejaculation of sperm-free prostatic fluid takes place during the initial 15 to 60 seconds of intromission.

After pelvic thrusting, the male typically dismounts (stage 4; see Fig. 20-1) by placing both front legs to one side of the bitch, lifting one hind leg over her back, and standing tail to tail with her (stage 4; see Fig. 20-1). Full

engorgement of the bulbus glandis makes withdrawal of the penis from the *relatively* small vaginal opening impossible. Thus the male and female are locked, or "tied," together (Fig. 20-2). This is described as an *inside tie*. If the male's erection precedes intromission, the relatively large bulbus glandis cannot enter the vagina, and the result is an *outside tie*. Dogs that have achieved an inside tie (normal mating) usually remain "locked" together for 5 to 60 minutes. They may actually drag each other around during this period. During the first 1 to 5 minutes of a tie, the male is ejaculating sperm-rich semen. The ejaculate throughout the remainder of a tie consists of sperm-free prostatic fluid.

Factors Affecting Sexual Behavior

ENVIRONMENT. Male dogs are more territorial than females, and it has been suggested that when a female is dominant to an individual male, he is not likely to succeed in breeding. Male dominance may be pronounced in his territory, therefore females are brought to the male for breeding (Farstad, 1998). Humans may also influence behavior. Some dogs respond positively or negatively to the presence of the owner, whereas others do not. Some dogs allow human assistance during breeding. Some males perform better if another male dog is in the area. Noise, lighting, flooring (traction), and numerous other environmental factors can also influence breeding.

EXPERIENCE. Young and inexperienced adult male dogs may become overexcited when near bitches "in estrus." They may attempt to mount the head, side, or flank before orienting correctly. Inexperience may result in failure to dismount the female until she literally throws the male off her back. Maiden bitches in estrus are reported to display longer play behavior prior to allowing copulation than do experienced females. Sexual behavior, therefore, is likely to reflect both innate and learned responses.

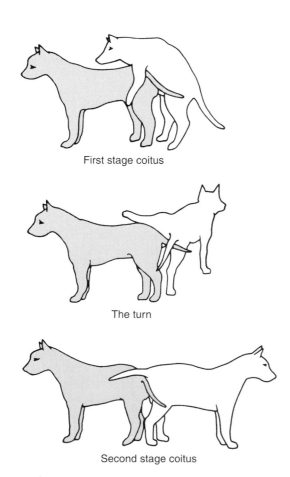

First stage coitus

The turn

Second stage coitus

FIGURE 20-1. Illustration of the three most obvious stages of breeding in dogs.

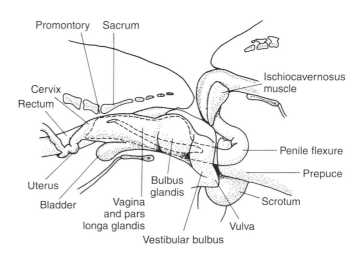

FIGURE 20-2. Illustration of the location of the penis in the vagina during normal breeding of dogs.

MATE PREFERENCE AND DOMINANCE. Studies have suggested that bitches show distinct preferences for particular males during mating by either accepting or actively rejecting one male. Preferences remain during several cycles and are unrelated to social affinity for males during anestrus. The role of dominance, although probably the most critical factor in mate selection, is difficult to assess. Males, however, are rarely particular if the female is receptive. The female, therefore, is likely to determine the success of copulation when a pair of dogs is chosen for mating.

ARTIFICIAL INSEMINATION (AI): GENERAL INFORMATION

Indications for Artificial Insemination

There are numerous reasons for an owner to choose AI over natural breeding, but the primary explanations are that the male and female live some distance from each other or there is a perceived inability for the male and female to breed. This inability may be the result of the presence of a vaginal stricture, which impedes intromission by the male and causes pain during breeding for the female (see Chapter 25). Additional reasons for failure to breed include orthopedic problems, such as disk disease, stifle problems, or muscle weakness.

AI may also be chosen because of a major size difference between the mates. Either the male or female may be inexperienced, or one dog may have a history of refusing to mate or to allow mating by the other. If the male or female has a history of attacking the other, the owner may simply want to avoid confrontation. Some bitches appear never to enter standing heat, refusing all breeding attempts by any male.

Less commonly, some owners wish to avoid venereal diseases resulting from contact between their dog and its mate. This seems uncalled for when working with *Brucella*-free animals. Any agent that could be transmitted from stud to bitch during natural mating is not avoided with AI. However, AI avoids transmission of any agent from the bitch to the stud. Some male dogs (particularly Doberman Pinschers) experience some prostatic bleeding after exposure to a bitch in heat (see Chapter 30). This may be associated with von Willebrand's disease. In this situation, AI can be performed without any contact between stud and bitch, occasionally avoiding this problem.

Fresh extended and frozen forms of semen are being used with increasing frequency. Obviously, shipped semen must be artificially inseminated into a bitch. Because semen collection is the "rate-limiting" factor in AI, insemination of extended or previously frozen semen remains a relatively simple procedure (Fontbonne et al, 2000).

Success Rates for Artificial Insemination

AI may be associated with lower conception rates and smaller litter sizes than would be achieved with natural breeding (Andersen, 1980). This is likely a result of several factors. During natural breeding, semen is pressure forced through the cervix into the uterus and oviducts (see Fig. 20-2), whereas in AI, the semen is placed posterior to the cervix. With natural breeding, uterine contractions aid in semen transport. This is an unlikely event in most AI situations. Also in natural breeding, the duration of the tie may contribute to improving conception rates.

A review of various reports shows that conception rates are less with every method of artificial insemination compared with natural breeding. Natural breeding has been reported to be associated with pregnancies at a rate of 80% to 100%; with fresh semen and artificial insemination, the rate is 62% to 100%; with chilled extended semen and intravaginal insemination, the rate is 60% to 80%; and with frozen semen and intravaginal insemination, the rate is 52% to 60% (Kustritz and Johnston, 2000b). Litter size also appears to be smaller with any insemination method compared with natural breeding (Linde-Forsberg and Forsberg, 1989, 1993; Fontbonne and Badinand, 1993; Silva, 1996).

It is our opinion that the above percentages, if incorrect, underestimate the success rates associated with each method of achieving conception. Experience and expertise have dramatically improved during the past decade, and each methodology has true attributes. There is little doubt that natural breeding, for numerous reasons, achieves the greatest conception rates. However, in various situations, natural breeding is not an option, therefore the various alternatives have potential to offer success. Nevertheless, we do not underestimate the value of experience with respect to relating conception rates to any "artificial" protocol.

ARTIFICIAL INSEMINATION (AI): INTRAVAGINAL TECHNIQUE

Collection of Semen

EQUIPMENT. Semen is usually collected in an artificial vagina. We cut off and use one end of a sterilized, soft rubber, cone-shaped bovine artificial vagina. To this is attached a 12 to 15 ml clear plastic tube (Fig. 20-3). The wide mouth end of the cone is folded over and sealed with rubber cement to make a smooth, nonabrasive edge. A small amount of nonspermicidal lubricating jelly is applied to the inner surface of the rubber cone. This is the only surface that makes penile contact. The only material reused is the bovine rubber cone artificial vagina. Although gas-sterilized equipment is claimed to harm sperm, there have been few problems with reused rubber cones. Perhaps this is because the cone is used primarily as a funnel, and the semen itself is held in the clear, new, disposable plastic tube (Johnston et al, 2001).

ENVIRONMENT. Most stud dogs can be collected in a clean, quiet room with a nonslippery floor and without any other dog present. However, having a bitch in heat can make collecting semen from a small percentage of males easier. It has been suggested that the presence

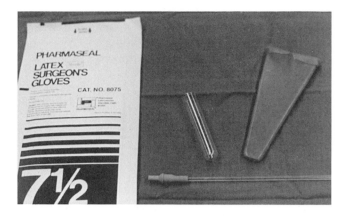

FIGURE 20-3. Artificial insemination equipment: sterile gloves, sterile soft rubber artificial vagina, sterile plastic tube that fits into the rubber vagina, and soft, flexible plastic catheter for insemination.

of a "teaser" bitch or use of the canine pheromone may improve the quality of semen collected (Kustritz and Johnston, 2000b). This concept has no scientific support.

PROTOCOL. With the owner holding the stud, to provide him with someone familiar and to protect the collector from being bitten, the penis and bulbus glandis are gently massaged within the penile sheath. When the bulbus glandis begins to enlarge, the sheath is slipped posteriorly, and the penis, including the

bulbus glandis, is exteriorized. Failure to exteriorize the penis and the bulbus glandis from the sheath usually results in an incomplete erection and failure to ejaculate, presumably due to pain.

Once the penis and bulbus glandis are extruded from the sheath, the collector firmly holds onto the base of the penis, *proximal* to the bulbus glandis. The thumb and index finger are used, providing both massaging movements and downward pressure around the base of the bulbus glandis (Fig. 20-4). During or immediately after achieving an erection, aggressive pelvic thrusting movements by the stud, which accompany the onset of ejaculation, may make it difficult to place the artificial vagina over the penis. However, the pelvic thrusting is typically short-lived (5 to 15 seconds) and, as previously described, the initial 5 to 30 seconds of ejaculate consists of sperm-free prostatic fluid. There is no need to collect this sperm-free fluid; therefore there should be no alarm if pelvic thrusting interferes with collection of the initial fluid of the ejaculate.

The sperm-rich second fraction of the ejaculate usually begins as the pelvic thrusting stops. At the same time, moreover, many males step over the collector's arm, as if dismounting the bitch. The collector should simply allow this instinctive movement by the male and bring the penis between the rear legs of the stud for continued collection (Fig. 20-4, B). Semen is usually collected for 2 to 5 minutes. The clear plastic tube should already have been connected to the rubber

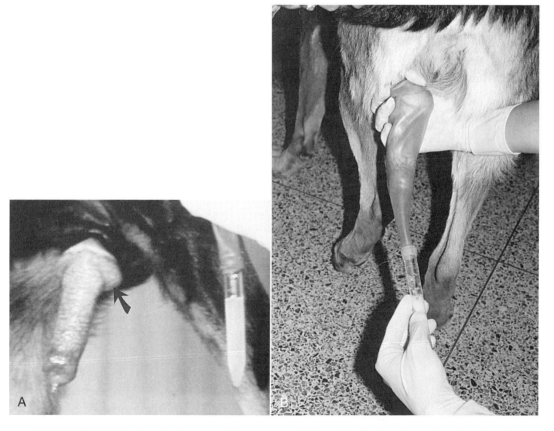

FIGURE 20-4. *A*, Erect penis of a dog with an engorged bulbus glandis (*curved arrow*) and a tube with normal ejaculate. *B*, Semen collection of a dog with the penis extended between the rear legs.

artificial vagina, and the apparatus can be held under the collector's arm during the initial stimulation period to provide some warmth. Canine semen is relatively resistant to cold shock, alleviating the need for warm water tanks or incubators for holding semen.

Use of a clear plastic collection tube allows visualization of the semen. We usually collect semen for approximately 2 to 4 minutes, keeping one hand over the plastic to avoid excessive exposure to light. As long as the ejaculate is obviously whitish or cloudy (normal and sperm rich), it continues to be collected. Whenever the ejaculate becomes clear (sperm free), collection can be discontinued. If the collector is not certain whether the male has stopped ejaculating the sperm-rich fraction, collection should be stopped after 3 to 4 minutes (Farstad, 1998). Continued collection only dilutes the sperm with the phase 3 clear, sperm-free prostatic fluid, resulting in cumbersome fluid volumes. Alternatively, the collection system containing sperm-rich semen can be exchanged for a clean system if there is any need to evaluate the prostatic fluid.

The most difficult task in AI is collection of semen from the male. Once this has been accomplished, the balance of the procedure is quite simple. The bitch should be inseminated within 10 to 15 minutes of collection of semen from the male. If the semen appears grossly normal, we inseminate the bitch immediately after collecting the semen, saving several drops for postinsemination microscopic evaluation. If there are any questions about the male or if the ejaculate is abnormal in color or consistency, it is evaluated prior to insemination. During any delay, the collector keeps the semen warm by holding the tube in the hand, which also keeps the semen out of potentially harmful ultraviolet rays.

Insemination Procedure

The male is taken out of the room to avoid any distractions. Wearing sterile gloves, the inseminator draws the semen into a sterile, new, 6 ml syringe. Every attempt should be made to stop semen collection as soon as sperm-free prostatic fluid is seen so as to avoid an excessive volume. The smaller the volume (less than 4 to 6 ml is excellent), the less leakage of semen from the vaginal vault of the bitch after AI. Once the semen is in the syringe with at least 1 to 2 ml of air, a new clean urethral catheter is attached (see Fig. 20-3). The owner is usually given the job of holding the bitch's head and keeping the bitch's tail to one side.

A gloved, nonlubricated index finger (except in very small dogs, in which case the little finger is used) is inserted into the vaginal vault, palm up. If lubricant is used, it must be nonspermicidal. Lubricant is often not needed, or only a tiny amount is necessary due to the normal vaginal discharge associated with estrus. The urethral catheter is then slid over the top of the finger and passed into the vaginal vault until resistance is met. Because of the unique anatomy of the canine cervix (Fig. 20-5), it is difficult at best to pass a catheter through the cervix and into the uterus (Roszel, 1992). Therefore the goal should be to pass the urethral

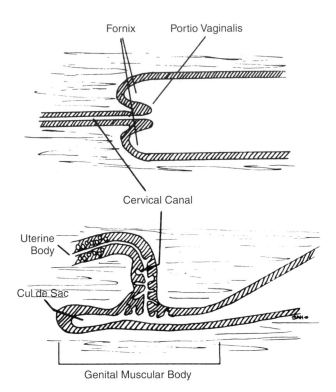

FIGURE 20-5. Schematic illustration of a longitudinal midline section through the cervical area in many species *(top)*. A 90-degree ventral rotation results in the appearance of the canine cervix *(bottom)* with loss of the dorsal fornical area and the dorsal portio vaginalis musculature continuous with the dorsal fold. The ventral fornical body forms a cul-de-sac (the cranial limit of the genital muscular body). The cervical canal (with epithelial invaginations) is at a right angle to the vaginal floor, and at a nearly right angle it joins the body of the uterus at the internal cervical opening. (From Roszel JF: Compend Contin Educ [Small Anim Pract] 14:751, 1992; used with permisson.)

catheter cranial to the "cervical os." Realistically, the inseminator passes the catheter as far cranially as possible, having first estimated the length of the catheter against the distance from the vulva to the cranial edge of the pelvic floor. The index finger aids in avoiding both the clitoral fossa and the urethra. The catheter follows the dorsal curvature of the vaginal vault. Semen is flushed into the vaginal vault and cleared with the air that was also in the syringe. Once this procedure has been completed, the catheter is removed.

The index finger can be used to stroke the roof of the vaginal vault or the clitoris, which sometimes causes obvious vaginal (uterine?) contractions. Once contractions have stopped, the index finger is withdrawn and the rear legs are raised so that the bitch is held in a "wheelbarrow" fashion. This helps the semen flow through the cervix. Usually we have the owners sit in a comfortable chair with a drape over their lap and have them hold the rear legs of the bitch up for at least 10 to 15 minutes. During this time the remaining semen is examined microscopically by the collector. The entire insemination procedure is rarely a problem for the bitch. There should not be any pain or discomfort associated with the procedure, making it rather simple and not time-consuming.

Intravaginal Insemination with Previously Frozen Semen

Experience has demonstrated that intravaginal insemination of previously frozen semen consistently fails, in part because this sperm loses the ability to migrate through the cervix. However, more recently, one study demonstrated success with intravaginal insemination of semen that had been frozen in Triladyl (Minitub, Germany) to which 0.5 ml of Equex STM paste was added. Prostatic fluid or TALP was also added to the thawed semen (Nothling et al, 2000).

ARTIFICIAL INSEMINATION (AI): TRANSCERVICAL INSEMINATION (TCI)

Background

HISTORY. Although the technology for freezing semen was developed long ago, use of this method has increased recently. Explanations for this include: an improved ability to "time" breedings; an understanding that the freezing process dramatically reduces the ability of sperm to migrate through the cervix; and the development of practical, nonsurgical, transcervical insemination techniques (Farstad and Anderson-Berg, 1989; Wilson, 2001). Direct surgical insemination into the uterus is possible, but such procedures are usually limited to one insemination, and many veterinarians are reluctant to become involved with a method with obvious surgical and anesthetic risks.

ANATOMY. Familiarity with canine anatomy is required to become competent with TCI. The vagina of the bitch is relatively long compared with other species. The total length of the vagina in the typical 11 kg female has been estimated to be 10 to 14 cm, and for large breed dogs it can be as long as 30 cm (Pineda et al, 1973). Visualization of the cervix is normally compromised by the dorsal median fold (Fig. 20-6), which extends caudally 2 to 4 cm from the cervix. The *paracervix* is the term used to identify this portion of the cranial vaginal vault (Lindsay, 1983). The caudal portion of the paracervix ends in a narrow "tubercle," which has the appearance of a cervix when viewed from the rear; this explains why some individuals incorrectly assume that they can routinely visualize the cervix with various scopes. Cranially, the paracervix ends in a fornix. The fornix is a slitlike space cranioventral to the true cervix and is a blind pouch (see Figs. 20-5 and 20-6).

The cervix lies diagonally across the uterovaginal junction and is directed craniodorsally, connecting the vagina with the uterus. Thus the external opening of the cervix faces the floor of the vagina and is located in the center of a rosette of furrows in most bitches. This angle, plus the small diameter of the cervical canal, creates natural obstacles to an attempt to pass a catheter from the vagina into the uterus (Wilson, 2001). Maiden bitches present a greater challenge because their cervical lumen is, on average, narrowest.

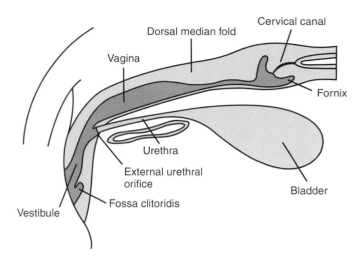

FIGURE 20-6. The anatomy of the paracervix, showing the dorsal median fold terminating caudally in the vagina, the vaginal portion of the cervix with the ventral-facing cervical os, and the fornix. (Courtesy Dr. Autumn Davidson, Davis, CA.)

"New Zealand" Endoscopic Technique

INTRODUCTION. The technique described here (Wilson, 1992, 2001) requires time, patience, and practice. A thorough knowledge of reproductive tract anatomy is indispensable. Practicing with a trained individual who can observe the endoscope and catheter via an attachable video camera is quite helpful. The equipment described in the next paragraph is easily cleaned and disinfected.

EQUIPMENT. The equipment used is a rigid, extended length cystourethroscope (Storz, Coleta, CA). This tool has a telescope with a 30-degree oblique viewing angle, a sheath, a bridge, and a cold light source. The working length of the assembled endoscope is 29 cm (Fig. 20-7). This tool can be used with virtually any breed, regardless of size. A nonessential video camera can be attached. Finally, the actual insemination is accomplished with a 6 or 8 French urinary catheter (the 6 French size is sometimes needed for small or maiden bitches). The best technique for this procedure also uses a specially designed hydraulic platform table that provides a tie point to the dog's collar and an abdominal band that prevents sitting or any sideways movement. The table can be placed at a level that gives the operator optimum positioning during the procedure (Fig. 20-8).

PROCEDURE. The endoscope is placed into the vagina and visually advanced through the vaginal folds. When a bitch is in proestrus or early estrus, the rounded vaginal folds (see Chapter 19) that tend to fill the vaginal lumen can impede placement of the endoscope. Dehydration of these folds, associated with continuing estrus, allows better visualization. The caudal tubercle of the dorsal median fold (DMF) is a prominent landmark (see Fig. 20-6). The lumen may be quite narrow in this region, sometimes requiring manipulation of the endoscope to the widest space and occasionally causing the endoscope to be pushed

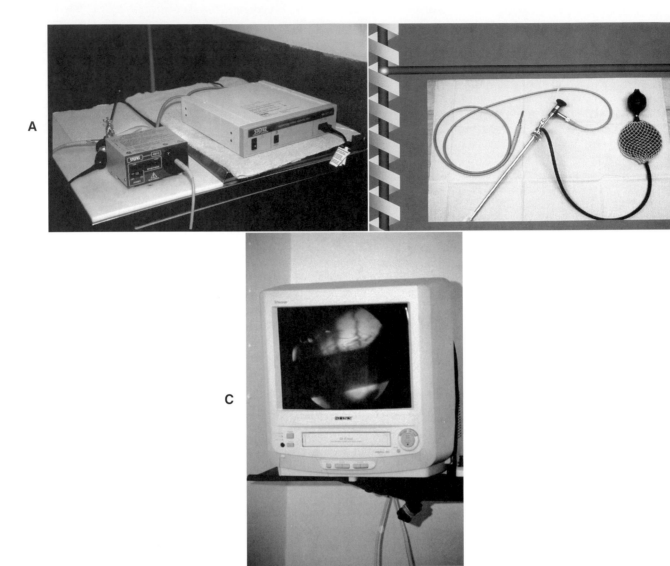

FIGURE 20-7. Endoscopic equipment for transcervical insemination consists of a light source and cable (A), a 30-degree, extended length cystourethroscope and sheath (B), and a video monitor to observe progress (C). (Courtesy, Dr. Autumn Davidson, Davis, CA.)

lateral to the DMF rather than being maintained in the more ideal midline. The vaginal cervix may not be obvious because it faces caudoventrally or ventrally. To locate the cervical os, the operator usually must advance the scope under the cervical tubercle. The os can be identified as being centered in the rosette of furrows or by observing the flow of serosanguineous uterine fluid through the cervix. The positioning of the os may appear to change during estrus as dehydration of vaginal folds progresses.

Most bitches in estrus tolerate transcervical insemination without anesthesia or sedation. The catheter should be advanced into the cervical os by careful manipulation of the endoscope and catheter. The rigidity of the endoscope allows the operator to move the cervical tubercle, line up the os, and change the canal angle. Air insufflation is not needed to visualize vaginal structures. Once the catheter tip has been introduced into the os, it can be steadily advanced with a twirling movement to aid passage through the cervical canal. The catheter is then advanced as far as possible, without force, for semen deposition. To ensure correct placement, it is important that the operator observe semen flow through the catheter and see no back flow. If back flow of semen does occur, the operator should stop the insemination and reposition the catheter, either inserting it farther in or withdrawing it slightly.

In some bitches, the amount of space in the paracervix is too small to accommodate the endoscope. This problem may be encountered in some small breed dogs and with some maiden bitches. Endoscopes with a smaller diameter may be used, although such scopes have a shorter length. The shorter length limits use of these scopes to small breeds. The longer scope may be difficult to manipulate in small breeds, sometimes requiring their sedation. Even when the scope can be positioned without difficulty, some bitches are not easily catheterized due to unusual anatomy, poor visibility

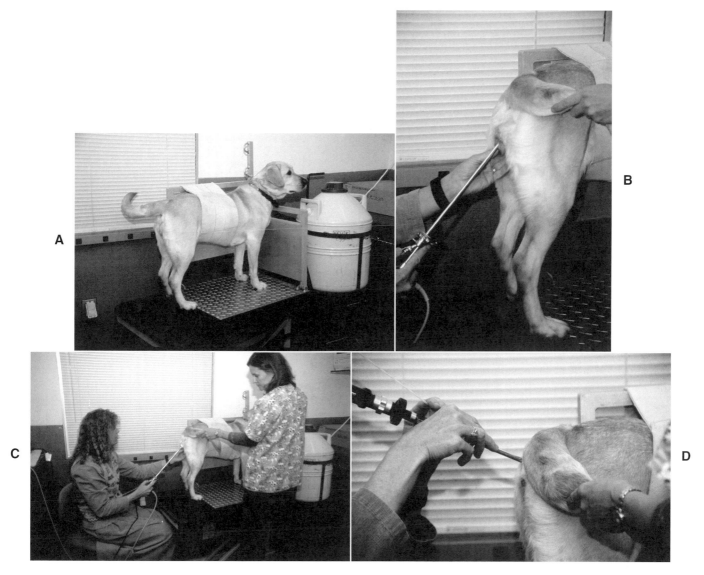

FIGURE 20-8. Endoscopic transcervical insemination. *A,* The bitch is restrained on a specially designed stand; the abdominal band limits sideways movement and attempts to sit. *B* and *C,* The operator advances the endoscope through the vaginal folds by observing the direction of the vaginal lumen. *D,* Catheterization of the cervical canal is achieved by manipulating the cervical tubercle, making use of the rigid endoscope and catheter. (Courtesy Dr. Autumn Davidson, Davis, CA.)

secondary to vaginal discharges, or lack of cooperation.

SAFETY. The procedure is safe. Trauma caused by the scope or catheter would be extremely unusual if a bitch is in estrus and would be most likely the result of abnormal preexisting problems in the vaginal tract or undo force on the equipment by the operator. Whenever the bitch shows discomfort, the procedure should be halted and the scope repositioned. Resistance to infection is heightened during estrus, and the likelihood of this procedure creating a greater risk of infection than natural breeding seems unwarranted (Watts et al, 1996). However, the equipment must be cleaned properly, and this discussion focuses on the bitch in estrus. Risk of infection is greater in the other phases of the estrous cycle.

RESULTS. The technique described here allows intra-uterine deposition of semen. It also allows repeated inseminations (unlike surgical semen placement). Conception depends on placement of the semen in the uterus, correct timing, quality of the semen, and fertility of the bitch. Conception rates in excess of 80% have been described (Sirivaidyapong et al, 2000; Wilson, 2001).

FERTILIZATION

The Egg

Understanding the temporal relationships between ovulation, fertilization, and breeding behavior of the bitch may aid in caring for dogs used in breeding programs, specifically dogs suspected of being infertile. In an "average" bitch, there is a consistent sequence of events leading to pregnancy as she progresses

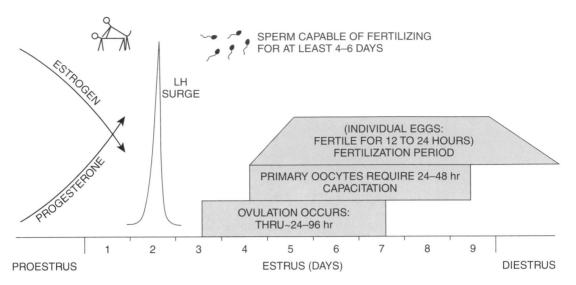

FIGURE 20-9. Hormonal changes and sequence of events in the timing of ovulation and fertilization of ova in the average bitch.

through proestrus and into estrus (standing heat). The luteinizing hormone (LH) peak occurs on the second day of standing heat (Concannon and Yeager, 1990). Twenty-four to 96 hours later, averaging the fourth day of standing heat, ovulation begins. Studies indicate that it takes 72 hours for approximately 75% of the follicles to rupture and 96 hours after the LH surge for more than 90% of the follicles to rupture (Wildt et al, 1978). The eggs released are "primary" oocytes that must undergo two meiotic divisions, requiring 48 to 72 hours, before they can be fertilized. Once mature, the fertile life of "secondary" oocytes may be as brief as 24 to 72 hours (Phemister et al, 1973). Fertilization, therefore, on average, takes place on day 7 of estrus (standing heat).

Eggs are fertilized in the average bitch from the middle of the fifth day of standing heat through the ninth day after the beginning of standing heat. Minimal fertility may persist for 1 or 2 days after the beginning of diestrus, as determined by vaginal cytology (Fig. 20-9). However, because most bitches are not precisely "average," predicting a precise day of fertilization is difficult (Concannon et al, 1989b), therefore no single day is optimal for a stud to breed the normal bitch. Conception usually occurs, however, with a single natural breeding (Figs. 20-9 and 20-10). When 21 bitches were bred twice, once 36 hours prior to ovulation and once 84 hours after ovulation, each time to a different male, only two of the bitches conceived pups from only the second male (Doak et al, 1967). This suggests that some advantage is gained by breeding early in estrus. The primary goal in breeding should be to obtain at least one mating every 2 to 4 days during standing heat. Embryonic cleavage between 2 and 16 cells occurs more rapidly after fertilization of more mature versus less mature oocytes, explaining in part why gestation length is similar whether mating occurs before or

after ovulation (Bysted et al, 2000; Concannon et al, 2000).

The Sperm

Knowing the potential life span of canine sperm in the uterus of the bitch is also helpful in understanding breeding management and conception. Sperm from a natural mating may reach the oviduct of the bitch within 25 seconds of ejaculation. More important, canine sperm has a relatively long survival period in the uterus. Undiminished concentrations of motile sperm have been found in the uterus 4 to 6 days after a single breeding. Breeding trials have suggested that canine sperm has a fertile intrauterine life span of 6 to 7 days after breeding (Doak et al, 1967; Concannon et al, 1983). Also, motile sperm have been observed in

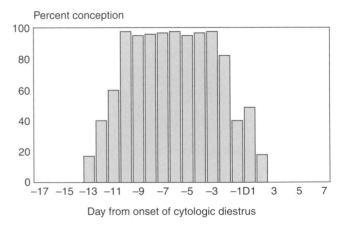

FIGURE 20-10. Conception rates relative to day of a single breeding (n = 267 Beagle bitches). (Holst PA, Phemister RD: Am J Vet Res 35:401, 1974; used with permission.)

bitches as late as 11 days after a single mating. Sperm requires 7 hours of capacitation in the uterus. Once this time period has passed, sperm can penetrate the zona pellucida. In vitro, sperm can enter the vitellus and undergo nuclear decondensation in immature (primary) oocytes (Mahi-Brown et al, 1982).

The length of time that *fertile* eggs (primary and secondary oocytes) remain in the oviducts (several days), coupled with the longevity of sperm capable of fertilization after a single mating, suggests that a single breeding is quite likely to result in conception (see Figs. 20-9 and 20-10). Single matings per bitch per cycle, beginning 2 days prior to the LH surge through 5 days after, have resulted in conception in 95% of healthy bitches. Maximum litter sizes have been observed among bitches bred once 4 to 10 days before the onset of diestrus. Conception rates fall to 80% if the single breeding takes place 6 days after the LH surge, and the percentage of successful conceptions continues to fall to virtually zero 10 days after the LH peak. Litter size also decreases. The average onset of diestrus was the eighth day after the LH surge. These various factors agree with the tentative scheme outlined in Fig. 20-9 and with the results of early research (see Fig. 20-10).

BREEDING MANAGEMENT OF THE BITCH

Most "Infertile" Dogs Are Healthy

The most common problem encountered by veterinarians working in canine reproduction is the "potentially" infertile bitch or stud. Owners bring these dogs to their veterinarian with the concern that the dog is failing to produce puppies. It is important to emphasize that a vast majority of these dogs are healthy fertile animals whose apparent infertility problems are related to misunderstanding of proper breeding management. It is wise to review proper breeding protocols versus those used by the client (owner or trainer) before embarking on an investigation of less common causes of infertility.

Age, Silent Heat, Split Heat, Inexperience, and Ovulation Failure

AGE. The bitch reaches sexual maturity and experiences her first ovarian cycle within 1 to 6 months of attaining adult height and weight. The average Miniature Poodle, therefore, begins her first proestrus at a younger age than the average Great Dane. However, the initial one or two ovarian cycles may be associated with irregularities that can be frustrating for an owner who wants to have a young dog bred. Several common problems include "silent heats," "split heats," behavior problems, and "infertile heats."

SILENT HEAT. A silent heat is simply a cycle that proceeds unseen by an owner. These bitches have little or no vaginal bleeding, or they are dogs that keep themselves clean or that are not in any contact with male dogs. Thus all but the most experienced owners fail to detect proestrus and estrus. Silent heats appear to be most common in the first and second heat cycles.

SPLIT HEAT. A split heat involves the bitch that has proestrual vaginal bleeding and vulvar swelling and that attracts males. The bitch experiencing a split heat may or may not exhibit standing heat (estrus) before proceeding into an apparent diestrus. However, these bitches begin proestrus again 2 to 10 weeks later. This may be repeated several times. Evidence indicates that each "apparent" proestrus is associated with follicular development and estrogen secretion. However, ovulation does not take place, and the follicles become atretic. A new group of follicles then develops, reexposing the bitch to increases in circulating estrogen concentrations and the signs of another proestrus (Okkens et al, 1992).

Once the follicles fully mature and ovulation does take place, the cycle is fertile and the expected interestrus interval, consisting of diestrus and anestrus, takes place. Split heats are frequently seen as a "behavior problem," and such dogs may be force bred or artificially inseminated. Without ovulation there is no chance of pregnancy. Split heats may occur at any age but are most commonly encountered in young bitches. Split heats are not associated with any major underlying problem.

INEXPERIENCE AND OVULATION FAILURE. It is not surprising that the young bitch, even one apparently in estrus, may not respond to a stud as would be expected. The inexperienced bitch and stud, controlled by inexperienced owners, may fail to achieve a tie, with one of two healthy dogs taking the blame. In addition, some bitches may proceed through an apparently normal cycle, including normal breeding, but fail to ovulate. The diagnosis of inexperience cannot be confirmed but is reserved for young bitches and dogs. The diagnosis of ovulation failure can be indirectly determined if estrus is not followed by a typical 60- to 90-day period of progesterone dominance (see Chapter 19).

SUMMARY. The problems of split heats, silent heats, inability to breed, and failure to ovulate are not worrisome in the young bitch less than 24 to 30 months of age. These problems are encountered with some frequency. Suggesting that an owner witness two cycles or wait until a bitch is older than 24 months of age before attempting the first breeding can reduce owner frustration and worry. This protocol also reduces the likelihood that simple immaturity will interfere with successful breeding.

Breeding Intervals per Estrus and When Breeding Should Begin

GOAL IN BREEDING. The simple goal in any breeding program is to have a sufficient number of sperm present in the uterus and oviducts to achieve the optimal chance for fertilization of mature eggs. Mature oocytes are typically fertilized during the 3 to 8 days after the LH surge, representing a period beginning 24 to 48 hours after ovulation of primary immature oocytes (see Fig. 20-9). Using reliable, clinically practical methods for estimating the day of the LH surge can be quite valuable. These criteria include behavior observation, vaginal cytology, vaginoscopy, and serial serum progesterone concentrations. None of these four criteria is considered perfect, but when used together, they enhance the chances of a bitch being inseminated at the proper times. Use of a direct LH assay is possible. Furthermore, normal sperm are known to survive and retain the capacity for fertilizing mature oocytes in the oviducts for at least 4 to 6 days and in some instances for as long as 11 days. Using this information, a breeding program can be offered to a client with reasonable confidence of success.

CRITERION 1: BEHAVIOR. Behavioral estrus (standing heat) is *the* factor in determining when breeding of the bitch should begin. In most bitches, estrus behavior is synonymous with fertility. Therefore observation of the bitch's response to a male is an inexpensive and reliable means of determining when to begin and end breedings. Occasionally it is advisable to have both the male and the female leashed, with one handler for each, in case of fighting. However, if possible, it is better to allow the male and female some freedom of movement, and if the female stands for the male, breeding should begin regardless of the color of the vaginal discharge, the vaginal exfoliative cytology interpretation, or the "day of the cycle."

On day 5 or 6 of proestrus, the bitch should be brought into contact with a male dog for approximately 10 to 20 minutes. This should be repeated every second or third day. Breeding should begin whenever the bitch is willing to breed (behavioral estrus) and should continue every other day (daily if AI is being used) until she is no longer willing to breed. The one variable that cannot be overstated is the inability to predict the number of days a bitch will be in estrus (will allow mating); the average is 7 to 9 days.

We recommend breeding the bitch every 2 to 4 days, beginning with the first day of acceptance and continuing *throughout* the acceptance period. If the period of standing heat for an individual bitch cannot be predicted, breeding every second or third day is an excellent routine. Based on observations from previous ovarian cycles in an individual bitch, an educated guess may be made regarding the duration of estrus, because a bitch 2 to 6 years of age tends to be similar from one cycle to the next. Bitches typically in standing heat for longer than 12 days should be bred every third or fourth day. Bitches typically in standing heat for only 3 or 4 days should be bred every 24 to 48 hours.

It is of paramount importance to recommend to owners that the male *continue breeding the bitch until the bitch refuses to breed or until the first day of diestrus is documented with vaginal cytology.* Fertilization of eggs is most likely occurring in the final 4 or 5 days of standing heat, regardless of the length of standing heat, or 4 to 5 days before the onset of diestrus.

CRITERION 2: VAGINAL CYTOLOGY. Vaginal exfoliative cytology provides a good reflection of rising plasma estrogen concentrations. Cytologically, full estrogen effect is seen as greater than 80% of epithelial cells being the superficial type, with no neutrophils present on the smear. This is a smear typical of standing heat. Whenever the number of superficial cells on vaginal cytology exceeds 60% to 80% of the exfoliated cells, the bitch should be brought to the male to see if she will allow breeding. This is also the time to begin AI. As described in Chapter 19, vaginal cytology is a simple, inexpensive, and reliable means of evaluating the bitch. The recommendation is to continue exposure to the male or breeding (or both) every other day (daily with AI) as long as the percentage of superficial cells remains above 80% and to discontinue breeding when the percentage of superficial cells decreases below 60%; that is, breeding is continued until diestrus is obvious on vaginal cytology. Vaginal smears should be monitored beginning with the second or third day of proestrus to avoid initiating contact with a male too late.

CRITERION 3: VAGINAL ENDOSCOPY. Vaginoscopy can be used to aid in staging the ovarian cycle of the bitch for timing natural breeding or AI. As reviewed in Chapter 19, the vaginal mucosa of the bitch in proestrus appears rounded and edematous. Subtle wrinkling (crenulation) of the mucosa is associated with the preovulatory LH surge. This is the time to begin breeding or AI. Breeding (assuming that the bitch is standing for the male) or AI should be continued through the phase of maximal mucosal crenulation, seen as angulated folds of vaginal mucosa with sharp profiles. Breedings or AIs should be discontinued when the vaginal mucosa again becomes flaccid and smooth, with a patchy red and white surface. This shift back to a smooth mucosal surface is typically observed 6 to 10 days after the LH surge (Lindsay and Concannon, 1986). In contrast to the other three primary criteria in determining breeding or AI dates, observation for crenulation in the vaginal mucosa is subjective, and experience in detecting subtle changes is beneficial.

CRITERION 4: SERUM PROGESTERONE CONCENTRATION. In-hospital test kits for determining the serum progesterone concentration are widely available, and reference laboratories are providing rapid turnaround of submitted samples, making progesterone a useful tool for timing ovulation. It is recommended that serum be assessed beginning 3 or 4 days after a bloody vaginal discharge is observed or within 1 or 2 days of detection of greater than 60% superficial cells on vaginal cytology. Ideally, the first sample documents plasma progesterone concentrations less than 1 ng/ml. The bitch should then be assessed daily or every other day until a distinct rise of greater than 1 ng/ml is noted, which suggests that the LH surge is occurring or has occurred (Eckersall and Harvey, 1987; England et al, 1989; Hegstad and Johnston, 1992; Manothaiudom et al, 1995; Goodman, 2001). Breeding or AI should then begin and continue every other day (or daily with AI) for 8 days or until another criterion (vaginal cytology or behavior) demonstrates that breeding should be discontinued.

The serum progesterone level begins to rise concurrently with the LH surge, reaching 1.0 to 1.9 ng/ml (3.1 to 5.9 nmol/L) on the day the surge takes place.

The day after the LH surge, 1 day before ovulation, the serum progesterone concentration is 2.0 to 3.9 ng/ml (6.2 to 12.1 nmol/L). On the day of ovulation, the serum progesterone concentration is 4.0 to 10.0 ng/ml (12.4 to 31.0 nmol/L). Several enzyme-linked immunosorbent assay (ELISA) kits for assessing the progesterone concentration are available for use in the veterinary hospital (i.e., PreMate, Camelot Farms, College Station, TX; Status-Pro, Synbiotics, Malvern, PA). Critical evaluation of these kits has demonstrated poor correlation with radioimmunoassay (RIA) systems, specifically in the 1.5 to 10.0 ng/ml range. This is the range of greatest importance for ovulation timing. Whenever possible, therefore, laboratory RIA testing should be used (Bouchard et al, 1993; Kustritz and Johnston, 2000a).

CRITERION 5: SERUM LH. Test kits are available for in-clinic LH measurement (e.g., Status LH, Synbiotics Corp., San Diego, CA). LH testing is considered the most accurate means of ovulation timing; however, the accuracy of these kits has not yet been critically evaluated (Kustritz and Johnston, 2000a, 2000b). Accurate identification of the LH surge is most important when chilled extended semen, frozen semen, historically infertile bitches, or a historically or known "subfertile" stud dog is used. Samples must be obtained daily, because the LH surge may be as brief as 24 hours in many bitches and may be missed if one day is skipped (Goodman, 2001). Such testing therefore may be impractical or too expensive for some owners.

CRITERIA THAT ARE NOT RELIABLE. A variety of unreliable criteria have been recommended for choosing the time to breed bitches. Included among these unreliable factors are the number of days since the onset of proestrus (onset of vaginal bleeding), the time that the color of a vaginal discharge changes from bloody to straw colored or clear, the behavior of the male, and the turgidity of the vulva.

Predetermined Dates. It is never recommended to breed the bitch routinely on days selected from the first observed day of proestrus. Initiating breeding around the tenth day assumes an *average* duration of proestrus (lasting 9 days) and an accurate detection of the first day of proestrus. The duration of proestrus in normal bitches is quite variable and may be as brief as a few days to as prolonged as 3 weeks. Furthermore, some bitches have an obvious bloody vaginal discharge, making detection of proestrus easy, whereas others bleed little or not at all, making detection of proestrus difficult or delayed. Thus breeding bitches on days 9 and 11, or days 10 and 13, is not as reliable or as likely to result in conception in all bitches as the criteria previously described as valuable.

Color of the Vaginal Discharge. It is often suggested that the optimal time to begin breeding is when the vaginal discharge changes from bloody to a translucent yellow, straw color, or clear. This can be misleading. Normal bitches have been observed never to have a bloody discharge, whereas others may bleed throughout standing heat (estrus). The color or consistency of the vaginal cytology should not determine breeding dates.

Turgidity of the Vulva. As the bitch progresses from proestrus into estrus, the swollen, turgid, enlarged vulva typical of proestrus becomes soft, flaccid, and pliable. Recognition of this change requires experience in dog management and is subjective. Because most owners seeking veterinary advice are not experienced, use of such a subjective criterion is not encouraged.

Glucose in Vaginal Secretions. The average bitch enters standing heat as plasma progesterone concentrations begin to increase. Rising progesterone concentrations may be associated with glucose intolerance due to insulin antagonism, resulting in an increasing extracellular glucose concentration (Ryan and Enns, 1988). Occasionally, vaginal secretions contain more glucose, as seen with test strips. However, this finding has been inconsistent and is not recommended for identifying breeding dates.

Behavior of the Male. The male dog is typically willing to breed any bitch in standing heat. Experienced studs have been described that breed the bitch only on the "correct" day. However, the bitch usually is the factor that determines when and if breeding occurs. When the bitch and stud are brought together, observation of the bitch's behavior is more informative than observation of the male.

Recommendations for Breeding Programs

A set of simple guidelines should be available for the conscientious breeder of an apparently healthy bitch. These guidelines cannot harm the animal and usually increase the success of any breeding program:
1. The first day of vulvar swelling, bloody vaginal discharge, and when males become obviously interested in the bitch should be recorded.
2. "Teasing" of the bitch with a male dog should begin on day 5 or 6 of proestrus and should be repeated every 2 or 3 days to determine the first day of standing heat. In cases of previous infertility, teasing is begun on the first day that proestrus is observed.
3. The bitch should be allowed to breed beginning on her first day of acceptance of the male, with breeding occurring every 2 to 4 days *throughout* the acceptance period.
4. In cases of infertility, as well as with bitches with short or prolonged standing heat, the owner should be taught how to obtain vaginal smears. Smears should be obtained once daily throughout apparent proestrus and estrus, as well as several days into diestrus. The veterinarian can stain and review slides as they are brought in, or the entire series of slides can be reviewed after estrus has apparently ended. The results of slide interpretation can be correlated with breeding dates and the conception rate. When possible, a series of serum progesterone measurements, with or without vaginoscopy, should be considered, as discussed previously.
5. Complete records should be kept on the dates of proestrus, breeding, and vaginal smears. Notes should be made on the presence or absence of ties,

the length of each tie, and the behavior of both the male and the female. The success of the male in siring litters with other bitches should be recorded. Records should also be kept on whelping dates, litter size, health of puppies, length of parturition, interval between births, and any other valuable information, including the reason for destroying any puppies.

Pups of Different Ages in Utero and Multiple Fathers

One reason some dog owners resist breeding a bitch and stud every 2 to 4 days is the fear of having fetuses developing that are distinctly different in age. However, eggs are fertilized over a short time (24 to 96 hours), and the age differences of developing fetuses are not significant. Furthermore, embryonic cleavage between 2 and 16 cells occurs more rapidly after fertilization of more mature oocytes compared with less mature oocytes. This is another explanation for similar gestation lengths regardless of whether mating occurs before or after ovulation (Bysted et al, 2000; Concannon et al, 2000).

Gross differences in the size, weight, and apparent maturity of newborn puppies are likely to be related to delayed implantation, the overall health of each pup, its placenta, the genetic background of the individual fetus, and the health of the area of the uterus in which each puppy develops. It is important to remember that sperm from more than one male can account for disparity in the size or color of puppies (i.e., one litter can have multiple fathers). Repeated breedings do not alter the synchronization of an LH surge.

Parasite Control and Vaccination Protocols

Parasite control and vaccinations should be current for the breeding bitch before she enters proestrus. If they are not, the bitch should be treated and vaccinated early in proestrus. Vaccination of any bitch that may be pregnant is not recommended. If vaccinations are demanded, killed vaccines should be used (rabies and parvovirus). *Toxocara canis* and *Ancylostoma caninum* can be treated with fenbendazole at a dosage of 50 mg/kg given orally from day 40 of gestation to day 14 after whelping. Pregnant bitches should be routinely tested for heartworm disease and maintained on heartworm preventative medication in at-risk areas. Both ivermectin and milbemycin oxime monthly preventatives are safe in pregnant bitches.

PREGNANCY

Litter Size

Generally, the larger the breed (not including adipose tissue), the larger the average litter size. Toy breeds usually have litters of one to four puppies, whereas larger breeds can average 8, 10, or even 12 puppies per litter. Litter size also correlates with the sperm count of the male (normal is 250 million to 800 million sperm per ejaculate), the timing of breeding, the health of the bitch, and the condition of her uterus, plus numerous other factors. Certainly the nutritional status of the bitch, the presence of concurrent endocrine problems, and exposure to various pharmaceuticals are additional variables that affect ultimate litter size. Maximal litter size correlates with successful breedings from 2 days prior until 5 days after the LH peak. Allowing the bitch and stud to breed every other day during the time that a bitch is receptive is the least expensive and most logical method of assuring maximal litter size. The additional criteria previously described (vaginal cytology, vaginal endoscopy, and serum progesterone measurements) should be considered tools that may be helpful but are not always needed.

Sequence of Events

Fertilization is completed in the oviducts. Embryos accumulate as morulae in the distal segments of the oviducts and develop into 32- to 64-cell blastocysts before they migrate to the uterus. Embryos have migrated into the uterus before day 16 to day 20 after the preovulatory LH surge. This is followed by a 3-day period in which blastocysts are free floating in their ipsilateral uterine horn, and then by another 3-day period when they freely migrate as 2 mm structures throughout the entire uterus. Focal areas of edema, which develop into equally spaced attachment sites in the endometrium, are formed 17 to 19 days after the LH surge, but blastocysts remain unattached as late as day 21 to 22. Attachment to the endometrium by placental trophectoderm invasion is noted as early as day 22 to as late as day 23. Attachment occurs only 1 to 2 days before heartbeats can be detected with ultrasonography (Concannon et al, 2000). There is no correlation between the number of eggs from one ovary or the number fertilized in one oviduct and the number of fetuses that implant in that horn of the uterus. Rather, the fetuses appear to become equally spaced throughout both uterine horns, regardless of the ovary of origin (Concannon and Yeager, 1990).

Uterine swellings, which are the implantation sites, are approximately 1 cm in diameter 20 days after the LH surge; they represent localized edema, expansion of embryonic membranes, and early placental development. The endothelium of the uterine vessels lies adjacent to the fetal chorion. Within this layer are the mesenchymal and endothelial tissues. Maternal blood and fetal blood are separated by four cell layers. The placentation is designated as *endotheliochorial*, describing its vascular nature. The placenta is anatomically *zonary* and *deciduate* (i.e., the placenta is shed at parturition, leaving a denuded endothelium).

The girdle of the fetal trophoblast develops marginal hematomas that contain stagnant maternal blood from which the future umbilical blood vessels absorb iron and other nutrients. The amnion, containing the fetus, floats free in the allantoic cavity, attached only by the umbilical stalk. By day 23 of gestation, these structural attachments between the uterus and the placental membranes are formed, and by day 30 the uterine swellings are approximately 3 cm in diameter. By day 35, canine body characteristics are recognizable. By day 40 the eyelids are closed with fused lids, each digit has its claw, hair and color markings are visible, and gender can be determined. Ossification of the skeleton can be seen radiographically after 42 to 45 days of gestation, and the remainder of in utero life is the maturation of fully formed fetuses (Concannon and Yeager, 1990).

The Bitch

Pregnancy results in alterations that may have clinical and routine biochemical importance. Body weight increases 20% to 50%; the average is 36% (Arthur et al, 1984). This increase is most dramatic in the second half of gestation. Between days 30 and 40 of gestation, the uterus may turn in on itself, resulting in some discomfort. The bitch may also develop mild leukocytosis (white blood cell count of 17,000 to 26,000 cells/mm^3). The hematocrit is usually less than 40% at day 35 and less than 35% at term. This is a normocytic, normochromic anemia thought to be due to an increase in plasma volume, which dilutes the red blood cell concentration. The fibrinogen concentration increases after day 20 of gestation, peaks at day 30, decreases prior to term, and rises again at parturition (Gentry and Liptrap, 1981; Concannon et al, 1996). A mild suppression in serum IgG concentrations has been described (Fisher and Fisher, 1981), and the uterus has been demonstrated to synthesize large quantities of prostacyclin, which may act as a circulating vasodepressor (Gerber et al, 1981). Pregnant bitches may also develop hypercholesterolemia and hyperproteinemia. Although no abnormal increases in prothrombin time or partial thromboplastin time are observed, pregnancy does result in increased activity of coagulation Factors VII, VIII, IX, and XI (Gentry and Liptrap, 1981).

Endocrinology

PITUITARY HORMONES. The role of the pituitary in maintaining pregnancy is not well defined in dogs. Circulating LH concentrations remain low throughout the latter half of estrus and the first half of gestation. LH release is pulsatile, as is release of other pituitary hormones, and it may increase slightly during the second half of the luteal phase (Fernandez et al, 1987). LH and prolactin are thought to be important luteotrophic hormones because pregnancy can be terminated at any time by hypophysectomy (Concannon, 1980). Follicle-stimulating hormone (FSH) concentrations have been reported to be increased in the latter half of pregnancy, and this may contribute to the mild increase in estrogen concentrations observed at that time (Concannon and Yeager, 1990).

Prolactin fluctuates at low concentrations during proestrus and estrus. Prolactin increases about tenfold during the last half of pregnancy, an amount significantly greater than that documented at the same diestrual stage in nonpregnant bitches (De Coster et al, 1983). This pregnancy-specific increase is presumably of pituitary origin, but some potential exists for placental or uterine secretion of a prolactin-like protein (Concannon and Yeager, 1990). The rise in serum prolactin concentrations during the second half of gestation culminates with a brief surge at the time that progesterone is acutely decreasing, immediately prior to parturition (Concannon and Yeager, 1990). After parturition, prolactin concentrations decrease for 1 to 2 days and then rise in response to suckling by puppies. Secretion of prolactin is suppressed by hypothalamic dopamine. Prolactin concentrations can be reduced by administration of the dopamine agonist bromocriptine (Concannon, 1981).

Progesterone

The ovaries, with their functioning corpora lutea, are essential for pregnancy. Ovariectomy performed after day 30 of gestation results in abortion within 24 to 72 hours. Plasma progesterone concentrations are typically greater than 0.5 ng/ml but less than 1.0 ng/ml in midproestrus, rising above 1.0 ng/ml prior to the onset of standing heat (before the LH peak), and continuing to increase for the next 15 to 25 days. By the first day of diestrus, serum progesterone concentrations are invariably above 5 ng/ml, and by day 10 to 15 of diestrus, the plasma progesterone concentration is usually above 25 ng/ml and in some bitches may reach levels of 50 to 90 ng/ml. Usually after progesterone concentrations peak, they plateau for 7 to 15 days before beginning to decrease slowly throughout the remainder of pregnancy. Progesterone concentrations less than 2 ng/ml can be consistently documented 36 to 48 hours prior to whelping. If the serum progesterone concentration is maintained above 2 ng/ml with implants, whelping can be completely inhibited.

Progesterone is thought to be necessary for endometrial glandular development, secretion of uterine fluids, endometrial growth, maintenance of placental attachments, inhibition of uterine motility, and elimination of leukocyte responsiveness in the uterus (Nelson et al, 1982). Numerous studies have demonstrated no significant difference in mean serum progesterone concentrations between pregnant and nonpregnant bitches in diestrus. Pregnancy-specific increases in progesterone in the second half of gestation are not obviously reflected in peripheral hormone measurements. Therefore measurement of serum concentrations cannot be used to diagnose pregnancy (Fig. 20-11).

Estrogen

Plasma estradiol (estrogen) concentrations are believed to be at basal (anestrus) concentrations (5 to 15 pg/ml)

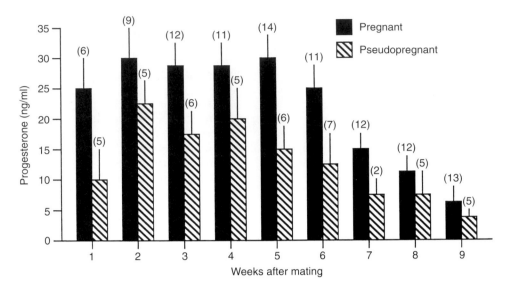

FIGURE 20-11. Serum progesterone concentrations in pregnant and pseudopregnant bitches (nonpregnant bitches in diestrus). Numbers in brackets are number of bitches. (Steinetz BG, et al: Am J Vet Res 50:68, 1989; used with permission.)

for the initial 5 or 6 weeks of gestation. Late in pregnancy, estradiol concentrations may increase slightly but remain below proestrual levels (<20 pg/ml). These increases persist until parturition, at which time plasma estrogen concentrations, like progesterone concentrations, decrease. Estrogen is thought to promote mammary development and perhaps aid in relaxing the cervix.

Thyroid and Adrenal Cortex

THYROID. Pregnancy alters the entire endocrine state of the bitch. In one study, concentrations of serum thyroxine (T_4) were demonstrated to be similar in diestrus regardless of pregnancy status. However, the T_4 concentrations (pre-TSH and post-TSH stimulation) were significantly lower when the bitch was in other phases of her cycle. Concentrations of triiodothyronine (T_3) were greater in the nonpregnant diestrual bitch than in pregnant dogs or those in any other phase of their cycle.

CORTISOL. Basal concentrations of plasma cortisol did not differ in different stages of a bitch's cycle. By contrast, cortisol concentrations after stimulation with adrenocorticotropic hormone (ACTH) did vary, with anestrus = diestrus > lactation = pregnancy > proestrus. The precise purpose of altered thyroid and/or adrenocortical function in pregnancy or diestrus is not understood. However, the stage of the cycle and the pregnancy status of the bitch must be taken into account when reviewing such hormone profiles (Reimers et al, 1984).

Glucose

The hormonal support of pregnancy may exacerbate a state of diabetes mellitus in a small number of bitches. These dogs have subclinical but definite carbohydrate intolerance prior to becoming pregnant. Insulin resistance becomes more pronounced throughout gestation (McCann and Concannon, 1983; McCann et al, 1988) and is probably due to the acute and chronic effects of increases in the plasma progesterone concentration (Ryan and Enns, 1988). Insulin resistance is a well-recognized problem in treated diabetic females that subsequently become pregnant.

Gestation Length and Prediction of the Whelping Date

Variation in the timing of ovulation, multiple breeding dates, and the inconsistent length of estrus make it difficult to identify the day of fertilization or the exact due date for a litter. The traditional 63 to 65 days from the time of first breeding is not a perfect formula (Figs. 20-12 and 20-13). A range of potential due dates, 55 to 72 days from the day of first breeding, is more correct. Knowing a precise due date can be critical when working with a bitch likely to require a cesarean section or for the owner who simply wants to know precise whelping dates. Vaginal cytology is the most consistent, inexpensive, and reliable means of predicting a whelping date. Smears should be obtained daily by the owner or veterinarian throughout standing heat and several days beyond the day of first refusal to breed. The whelping date is likely to be 56 to 58 days after the first day of diestrus, as determined from vaginal cytology. This is the first day that the percentage of superficial cells decreases from greater than 80% to less than 40%. Furthermore, after day 42 to 45 of gestation, radiographs of the abdomen can be reviewed and the number of fetuses counted. Larger litters tend to have shorter gestation lengths (55 to 56 days), whereas bitches with

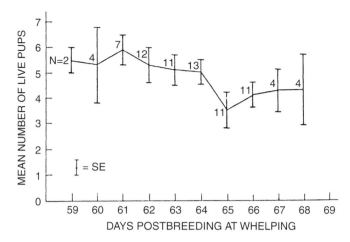

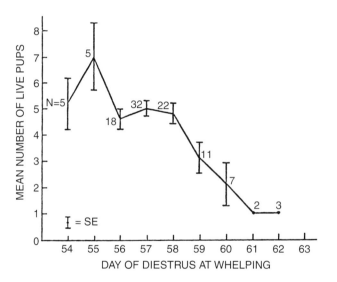

FIGURE 20-12. Litter size related to postbreeding gestation length. Only bitches bred on day 1 of estrus are included (*n* = 80). (Holst PA, Phemister RD: Am J Vet Res 35:401, 1974.; used with permission.)

FIGURE 20-13. Litter size relative to diestrus gestation length. Only bitches bred on day 1 or day 7 are included (*n* = 108). (Holst PA, Phemister RD: Am J Vet Res 35:401, 1974; used with permission.)

only one or two puppies tend to have longer gestation lengths (58 to 59 days).

Alternatives to using vaginal cytology to define the first day of diestrus in predicting whelping dates do exist. The two most popular alternatives are more expensive, require more time by both the veterinarian and the client, and require more expertise. For nearly all normal pregnancies, the time interval from the preovulatory LH surge to parturition is 64 to 66 days (Concannon et al, 1983). The date of the preovulatory LH surge can be estimated by determining serial serum progesterone concentrations and noting the date that they rise above 1 ng/ml, as previously described. Identification of the first day that the vaginal mucosa undergoes crenulation also has potential for noting the approximate day of the LH

surge. Finally, a drop in rectal temperature precedes whelping by 12 to 36 hours.

Pregnancy Diagnosis

PALPATION. Palpation of the abdomen is easy, inexpensive, and reliable for recognizing pregnancy. Between days 25 and 30 of gestation (or 20 to 30 days after first breeding if the progesterone level or vaginal cytology has not been monitored), uterine swelling at individual placental sites is usually palpable. Swellings are initially pear shaped and then become rounder with time. In a 20 kg bitch, the swellings average approximately 2 inches in length at days 28 to 30 of gestation (Johnston et al, 1982). It has been suggested that raising the forequarters of the bitch drops the uterus posteriorly and makes palpation somewhat easier. Palpation is always easier to describe than to perform. Differentiating a pregnant uterus from a stool-filled colon requires experience. Palpation of a lean, relaxed dog is not the same as palpation of one that is overweight or nervous.

As gestation proceeds beyond days 30 to 35, the uterus becomes diffusely enlarged and the horns drop to a more ventral position with the cranial ends pushed inside the rib cage. The uterus is enlarged and easier to palpate, but identification of individual fetal vesicles is more difficult. By day 35 the swellings are greater than 3 cm in diameter, elongated, nearly confluent, pliable rather than firm, and more difficult to palpate as distinct entities (Concannon, 1983). Beyond day 50 of gestation, individual fetuses can again be palpated because the uterus loses its diffusely swollen character.

RADIOGRAPHS. Radiographic evaluation of the abdomen is an excellent tool for diagnosing pregnancy and the most reliable aid for determining the number of developing fetuses. Between 21 and 42 days after mating, enlarged, fluid-filled horns may be seen. To recognize a fetus radiographically, radiopaque fetal skeletal development must be present (Fig. 20-14). Fetal skeletal elements may be first detected 20 to 21 days prior to parturition, which represents 42 to 52 days after mating or 44 to 47 days after the LH peak. An unequivocal diagnosis of pregnancy was made radiographically 17 to 20 days before parturition, which represented 46 to 49 days after the LH peak or 43 to 54 days after mating (Concannon and Rendano, 1983).

Fetal maturation during the last 2 weeks of gestation can be crudely estimated with radiographs. The fetal skull and spine become radiopaque 44 to 46 days after the LH peak. The fetal pelvis becomes detectable 53 to 57 days after the LH peak, and fetal teeth, 58 to 61 days after the peak. An elective cesarean section, for example, should be scheduled only after fetal teeth are readily detectable.

Usually radiographic evaluation is used not only to diagnose pregnancy but also to determine the number of fetuses and as a tool for predicting dystocia problems. The number of fetuses is best estimated by

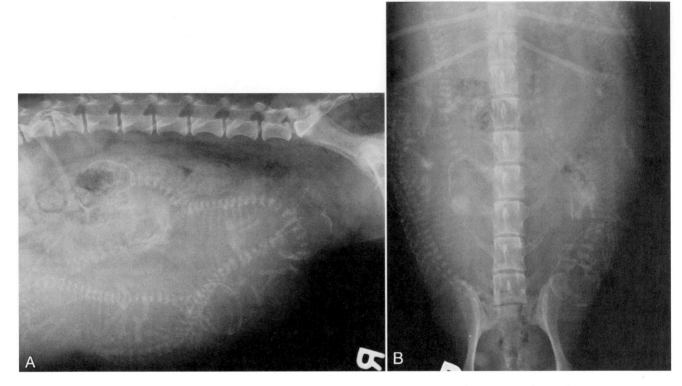

FIGURE 20-14. Lateral *(A)* and ventrodorsal *(B)* abdominal radiographs of a pregnant dog with a healthy litter on day 50 of diestrus. The easiest methods for estimating litter size are counting skulls or vertebral columns.

counting fetal skulls. This procedure is excellent in all situations except when a litter is exceptionally large or when the skeletal development is incomplete. Collapse of skeletal elements may suggest fetal death (Fig. 20-15). During normal parturition, the skull of a fetus barely squeezes through the birth canal (Fig. 20-16). Radiographic prediction of dystocia based on fetal skull versus maternal pelvic width is not reliable and is not recommended. It is impossible to predict the amount of pelvic relaxation that will occur during whelping.

ULTRASONOGRAPHY.   The use of ultrasonography for pregnancy diagnosis has been extremely rewarding, consistently allowing recognition of fetal vesicles in the uterus between days 18 and 20 of gestation, approximately 11 days after the first day of diestrus (Fig. 20-17). The stage of pregnancy can be estimated by measuring the biparietal diameter (longitudinal plane of the head aligned with the rest of the fetal body) and the trunk diameter (transverse plane at the level of the stomach) for one or more pups. Biparietal and trunk diameter correlate with fetal age (England et al, 1990). The times at which various structures can be detected have been studied and are reviewed in Table 20-3. Anticipated results of ultrasonography can be quite precise if the dates of the LH surge can be estimated but are not precise if dates of mating are used as the reference point. For example, 1 mm gestational sacs can be identified reliably 17 to 18 days after the LH surge but may be seen as early as 10 days or as late as 23 days after mating. Using ultra-

sonography, the chorionic cavity is identifiable on day 20, the embryo and heartbeat at days 23 to 25, and fetal movement at days 34 to 36 after the LH surge (Shille and Gontarek, 1985; Taverne et al, 1985; England et al, 1990; Yeager et al, 1992). Fetal well-being is often based on the heart rate, with normal reported as 200 to 225 beats per minute (Verstegen et al, 1993; Gradil et al, 2000).

The equipment for these procedures can be expensive but is becoming widely available. Differentiation of pregnancy from pyometra and early recognition of pregnancy can be accomplished quickly and safely with ultrasonography. Ultrasound Doppler units can be used in pregnancy diagnosis, although this is not recommended because of the limited usefulness of such a tool in clinical and practical settings.

BLOOD AND/OR URINE TESTS FOR PREGNANCY DIAGNOSIS. No routine blood or urine assays are available for the diagnosis of pregnancy in dogs. This reflects the fact that serum progesterone concentrations, although lower in pseudopregnant (nonpregnant) than in pregnant bitches, are not consistently different enough to identify pregnancy (see Fig. 20-11). This is true after implantation as well as before.

The hormone *relaxin* is detectable with immunoassays and is the only pregnancy-specific hormone in dogs. These assays are not yet commercially available (Steinetz et al, 2000). Unlike progesterone, serum relaxin concentrations increase during pregnancy but are not detectable at any time in pseudopregnant bitches

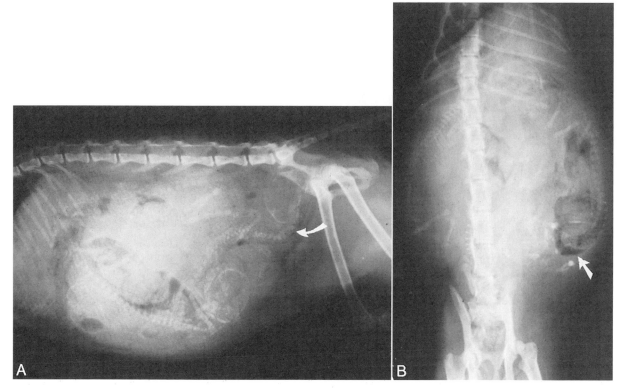

FIGURE 20-15. Lateral *(A)* and ventrodorsal *(B)* abdominal radiographs of a bitch with dead fetuses. Note the abnormal extension of the fetal neck *(arrow in A)* and the fetal gas best seen on the ventrodorsal view *(arrow in B)*.

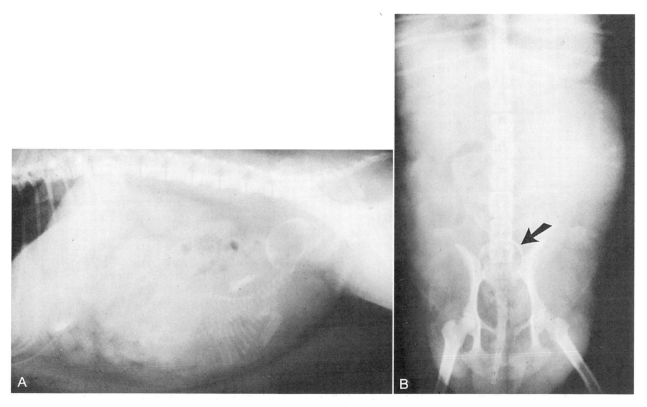

FIGURE 20-16. Lateral *(A)* and ventrodorsal *(B)* abdominal radiographs of a bitch with a single fetus. Notice the skull *(arrow)* width versus the pelvic width on the ventrodorsal view, which may possibly cause dystocia. Ligament relaxation can be difficult to predict. This fetus was delivered naturally with little apparent difficulty.

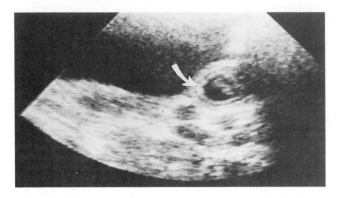

FIGURE 20-17. One fetal vesicle *(arrow)* on ultrasonography on day 20 after the LH surge in a bitch. (Courtesy Dr. Tom Nyland, Radiology Department, University of California, Davis.)

TABLE 20–3 GESTATIONAL AGE RANGE AT FIRST ULTRASONOGRAPHIC DETECTION OF SELECTED FEATURES IN PREGNANT BEAGLES

Pregnancy Feature	Days after the LH Surge	N*
Gestational sac	20	7
Uterine wall		
Echogenic at gestational sac	20–23	8
Placental layers	22–24	7
Zonary placenta	27–30	8
Embryo position		
Apposed to uterine wall	23–25	8
Dependent in chorionic cavity	29–33	8
Fetal membranes		
Yolk sac membrane	25–28	7
Allantoic membrane	27–31	7
Yolk sac tubular shape	27–31	8
Yolk sac folded cross-section	31–35	6
Embryo and fetus		
Heartbeat	23–25	8
Bipolar shape	25–28	8
Anechoic area in head	27–31	6
Choroid plexus	31–35	6
Limb buds	33–35	6
Fetal movement	34–36	5
Dorsal sagittal tube	30–39	6
Skeleton	33–39	4
Bladder	35–39	4
Stomach	36–39	4
Lung hyperechoic vs liver	38–42	4
Liver hypoechoic vs abdomen	39–47	4
Kidney	39–47	3
Eyes	39–47	4
Umbilical stalk	40–46	5
Intestine	57–63	4
Relative size relationships		
Body diameter 2 mm > head	38–42	4
Body diameter:chorionic cavity diameter >1:2	38–42	4
Crown-rump length > placenta	40–42	4
Body diameter:outer uterine diameter >1:2	46–48	5
Parturition	63–65	5

From Yeager AE, et al: Ultrasonographic appearance of the uterus, placenta, fetus, and fetal membranes throughout accurately timed pregnancy in Beagles. Am J Vet Res 53:342, 1992, with permission.
*N is the number of pregnancies examined.
LH, Luteinizing hormone.

(Steinetz et al, 1987, 1989). The amount of relaxin detected in pregnant bitches was significantly greater than in pregnant ovariectomized bitches. Both groups, however, had more relaxin than nonpregnant bitches (Figs. 20-18 and 20-19). Thus evidence suggests that relaxin is produced by the ovary and probably in smaller amounts by the placenta of pregnant bitches (Steinetz et al, 1989). Although apparently sensitive and reliable, serum relaxin concentrations are detectable as early as days 28 to 30 and reach peak concentrations at 40 to 50 days of gestation. Ultrasonography remains the tool that detects pregnancy earliest.

Commercially available pregnancy tests use "acute phase" protein concentrations. Whether such measurements include fibrinogen, C-reactive protein, or both, varies. Both of these proteins increase in the serum by approximately day 30, remain increased until day 50, then decrease near term (Gradil et al, 2000). False-positive test results are a concern because these proteins are increased in the serum of dogs with inflammatory conditions, such as pyometra. Currently, these tests are not recommended.

Therapeutic Considerations

The administration of drugs of any kind to a bitch known to be or suspected of being pregnant is always associated with some risk. The concern is well warranted because pregnant bitches may have an adverse reaction to medication that would not have occurred were they not pregnant. Some medications may result in rapid onset of abortion, whereas other drugs cause obvious congenital problems in a fetus or problems that may not be detected for months after whelping. Some drugs have reversible effects in the bitch and irreversible effects in developing embryos, and many drugs have not been studied in pregnant bitches or fetuses.

Ovarian function is controlled to varying degrees by the hypothalamus and pituitary. Therefore drugs that affect these higher centers can indirectly alter the function of the ovaries. In addition, the ovaries are perfused by a remarkable amount of blood. Blood flow to corpora lutea has been reported to reach levels of 20,000 ml/min/kg (Davis, 1983). The ovaries, therefore, can be exposed to high concentrations of any drug dispersed in the vascular space. The effects of most drugs on various ovarian functions are unknown, but the potential risks are still appreciated.

For decades it was believed that the placenta served as a barrier that protected the fetus from the adverse effects of drugs. The thalidomide disaster in women drastically changed this perception by demonstrating that fetal exposure to the drug during critical periods of development resulted in severe defects (Koren et al, 1998). Yet 40 years after recognition of the terrible consequences this drug can have in developing fetuses, fewer than 30 drugs have been proved teratogenic in humans when used in clinically effective doses (Table 20-4). Some commonly used drugs once thought

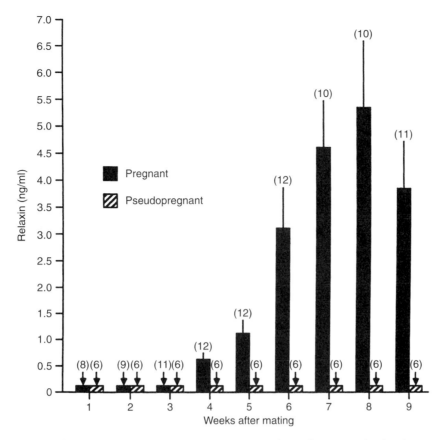

FIGURE 20-18. Serum relaxin concentrations in pregnant and pseudopregnant bitches (nonpregnant bitches in diestrus). Downward arrows represent less than the minimal detectable concentration (0.18 ng/ml). Numbers in brackets are the numbers of bitches studied. (Steinetz BG, et al: Am J Vet Res 50:68, 1989; used wth permission.)

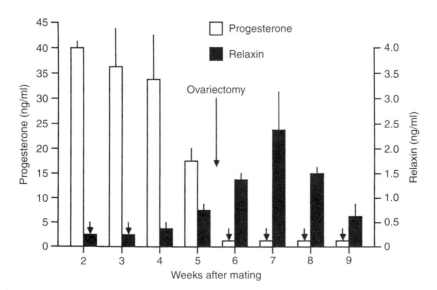

FIGURE 20-19. Serum relaxin and progesterone concentrations in ovariectomized, pregnant bitches in which gestation was maintained by daily administration of 17α-ethyl-19-nortestosterone at a dosage of 1 mg/kg body weight. Downward arrows indicate less than the minimal detectable concentration (progesterone, 0.5 ng/ml; relaxin, 0.25 ng/ml); n = 3. (Steinetz BG, et al: Am J Vet Res 50:68, 1989; used wth permission.)

TABLE 20-4   DRUGS WITH PROVEN TERATOGENIC EFFECTS IN HUMANS*

Drug	Teratogenic Effect
Aminopterin[†], methotrexate	CNS and limb malformations
Angiotensin-converting-enzyme inhibitors	Prolonged renal failure in neonates, decreased skull ossification, renal tubular dysgenesis
Anticholinergic drugs	Neonatal meconium ileus
Antithyroid drugs (propylthiouracil and methimazole)	Fetal and neonatal goiter and hypothyroidism, aplasia cutis (with methimazole)
Carbamazepine	Neural-tube defects
Cyclophosphamide	CNS malformations, secondary cancer
Danazol and other androgenic drugs	Masculinization of female fetuses
Diethylstilbestrol[†]	Vaginal carcinoma and other genitourinary defects in female and male offspring
Hypoglycemic drugs	Neonatal hypoglycemia
Lithium	Ebstein's anomaly
Misoprostol	Möbius sequence
Nonsteroidal anti-inflammatory drugs	Constriction of the ductus arteriosus[‡], necrotizing enterocolitis
Paramethadione[†]	Facial and CNS defects
Phenytoin	Growth retardation, CNS deficits
Psychoactive drugs (e.g., barbiturates, opioids, and benzodiazepines)	Neonatal withdrawal syndrome when drug is taken in late pregnancy
Systemic retinoids (isotretinoin and etretinate)	CNS, craniofacial, cardiovascular, and other defects
Tetracycline	Anomalies of teeth and bone
Thalidomide	Limb-shortening defects, internal-organ defects
Trimethadione[†]	Facial and CNS defects
Valproic acid	Neural-tube defects
Warfarin	Skeletal and CNS defects, Dandy-Walker syndrome

Koren et al, 1998 (used with permission)

*Only drugs that are teratogenic when used at clinically recommended doses are listed. The list includes all drugs proved to affect neonatal morphology or brain development and some of the toxic manifestations predicted on the basis of the pharmacologic actions of the drugs. CNS denotes central nervous system.

[†]The drug is not currently in clinical use.

[‡]Sulindac probably does not have this effect.

to be teratogenic have been shown safe in subsequent larger and better controlled studies (Table 20-5). Every drug since found to be teratogenic in humans has caused similar effects in animals except misoprostol, which causes a morphologic pattern known as the Möbius sequence in humans (Table 20-6). In at least one case, that of isotretinoin, the studies in animals probably prevented a disaster in humans (Koren et al, 1998). However, there are drugs that have a teratogenic effect in animals when administered in high doses (glucocorticoids, benzodiazepines, salicylates) that are not teratogenic in humans receiving clinically relevant doses.

The extent to which medications given to the bitch cross the placenta and reach the fetus is determined by a number of factors. Molecular size, lipid solubility, placental blood flow, protein-binding characteristics, and stage of gestation are some of the many factors that determine tissue concentrations of any drug. Some drugs are protein bound; others are rapidly metabolized or excreted by the bitch and never reach a fetus in significant quantities. Different drugs may reach high concentrations in the fetus and never reach those levels in the bitch. Generally the fetus is assumed to have limited ability to metabolize or excrete most drugs, and the fetus can be assumed to be exposed to substances circulating through the placenta (Davis, 1983).

The developing fetus is most likely to be harmed during the critical phases of organ development. Gestation represents a continuing process of precisely orchestrated events, which illustrates the point that no single critical time exists in development when drug therapy must be avoided. Potentially harmful drugs (any drug?) administered early in pregnancy (less than 20 days in the bitch and less than 16 days in the queen) are likely to result in embryotoxicity or abortion or both. Pregnancy may be quickly terminated if the blastocyst is exposed to drugs that inhibit implantation. Adverse effects of drugs administered in midgestation may cause internal or externally visible malformations. Lead, mercury, nicotine, and some pesticides are suggested to be most likely to cause morphologic changes during organogenesis but are less dangerous later in pregnancy (Davis, 1983).

Harmful drugs administered to a bitch in late gestation (after day 45) may cause problems in the

TABLE 20-5   COMMON DRUGS INITIALLY THOUGHT TO BE TERATOGENIC BUT SUBSEQUENTLY PROVED SAFE

Drug	Initial Evidence of Risk	Subsequent Evidence of Safety
Diazepam*	Oral clefts	No increase in risk in large cohort and case-control studies
Oral contraceptives	Birth defects involving the vertebrae, anus, heart, trachea, esophagus, kidney and limbs; masculinizing effects on female fetuses resulting in pseudohermaphroditism	No association between first-trimester exposure to oral contraceptives and malformations in general or external genital malformations in two meta-analyses
Spermicides	Limb defects, tumors, Down's syndrome, and hypospadias	No increase in risk in a meta-analysis
Salicylates	Cleft palate and congenital heart disease	No increase in risk in large cohort studies
Benedectin (doxylamine plus pyridoxine)	Cardiac and limb defects	No increase in risk in two meta-analyses

From Koren et al, 1998 (used with permission)

*Diazepam taken near term may cause the neonatal withdrawal syndrome or cardiorespiratory instability.

TABLE 20-6 TERATOGENIC EFFECTS OF DRUGS IN ANIMALS AND HUMANS*

Drug	Effects in Animals	Effects in Humans
Angiotensin-converting-enzyme inhibitors	Stillbirths and increased fetal loss in sheep and rabbits	Prolonged renal failure and hypotension in the newborn, decreased skull ossification, hypocalvaria, and renal tubular dysgenesis
Carbamazepine	Cleft palate, dilated cerebral ventricles, and growth retardation in mice	Neural-tube defects
Cocaine	Dose-dependent decrease in uterine blood flow, fetal hypoxemia, hypertension, and tachycardia in sheep; reduced fetal weight, fetal edema, and increased resorption in rats and mice	Growth retardation involving weight, length, and head circumference; placental abruption and uterine rupture
Ethanol	Microcephaly, growth deficiency, and limb anomalies in dogs, chickens, and mice	Fetal alcohol syndrome:prenatal and postnatal growth deficiency, CNS anomalies (microcephaly, behavioral abnormalities, and mental retardation), characteristic pattern of facial features (short palpebral fissures, hypoplastic philtrum, and flattened maxilla), and major organ-system malformations; with age, facial features may become less distinctive, but short stature, microcephaly, and behavioral abnormalities persist
Isotretinoin	CNS, head, limb, and cardiovascular defects in rats and rabbits	Retinoid embryopathy resulting in some or all of the following abnormalities; CNS defects (hydrocephalus, optic-nerve blindness, retinal defects, microphthalmia, posterior fossa defects, and cortical and cerebellar defects); craniofacial defects (microtia or anotia, low-set ears, hypertelorism, depressed nasal bridge, microcephaly, micrognathia, and agenesis or stenosis of external ear canals); cardiovascular defects (transportation of great vessels, tetralogy of Fallot, and ventricular or atrial septal defects); thymic defects (ectopia and hypoplasia or aplasia); miscellaneous defects (limb reduction, decreased muscle tone, spontaneous abortion, and behavioral abnormalities)
Lithium	Heart defects in rats	Ebstein's anomaly and other heart defects
Methyl mercury	CNS abnormalities in rats; growth retardation, motor disturbances, microencephaly, and brain lesions in rhesus monkeys	Fetal Minamata disease: diffuse neuronal disintegration with gliosis, cerebral palsy, microcephaly, strabismus, blindness, speech disorders, motor impairment, abnormal reflexes, and mental retardation
Phenytoin	Cleft palate, micromelia, renal defects, and hydrocephalus in rabbits, mice, and rats	Fetal hydantoin syndrome; prenatal and postnatal growth deficiency, motor or mental deficiency, short nose with broad nasal bridge, microcephaly, hypertelorism, strabismus, epicanthus, wide fontanelles, low-set or abnormally formed ears, positional deformities of limbs, hypoplasia of nails and distal phalanges, hypospadias, hernia, webbed neck, low hairline, impaired neurodevelopment and low performance scores on tests of intelligence
Thalidomide[†]	Limb-shortening defects in rabbits (most sensitive species)	Limb-shortening defects, loss of hearing, abducens paralysis, facial paralysis, anotia, microtia, renal malformations, congenital heart disease
Valproic acid	Exencephaly in hamsters and mice	Neural-tube defects
Warfarin[†]	Maxillonasal hypoplasia and skeletal anomalies in rats	Fetal warfarin syndrome: skeletal defects (nasal hypoplasia and stippled epiphyses), limb hypoplasia (particularly in distal digits), low birth weight (<10th percentile), hearing loss, and ophthalmic anomalies; CNS defects with exposure after first trimester; dorsal midline dysplasia (agenesis of corpus callosum and Dandy-Walker malformations) or ventral midline dysplasia (optic atrophy)

From Koren et al, 1998 (used with permission).
*CNS denotes central nervous system.
[†]Initial studies in animals failed to show teratogenicity; hence, documentation in humans preceded that in animals.

central nervous system or cardiovascular system or both. Drug-induced endocrine disorders may not be obvious until the dog is an adult, whereas nervous system damage may be quickly obvious or may cause only vague changes in behavior patterns. Drugs may alter the onset of parturition; delays may be dangerous or even fatal for the bitch, and early whelping can be harmful or fatal to the newborn (Papich, 1990). Table 20-7 presents a partial list of drugs that are probably safe, as well as those that should be avoided during pregnancy (Papich, 1990).

Drugs are not often administered during parturition. Anesthetics, the most commonly used agents during whelping, may depress the newborn. Inhalation

TABLE 20-7   SAFETY OF DRUGS IN PREGNANCY

Drug	Recommendation*	Comments
Antimicrobial Drugs		
Aminoglycosides (e.g., gentamicin, amikacin, tobramycin, kanamycin)	C	These drugs cross the placenta easily. They may cause renal toxicity or CN VIII nerve toxicity to the fetus.
Penicillins (e.g., penicillin G, ampicillin, amoxicillin)	A	The penicillins cross the placenta, but they are safe for the fetus.
Cephalosporins	A	Safe if used at therapeutic doses.
Chloramphenicol	C	This drug may adversely affect the bone marrow of the developing fetus.
Clindamycin (Antirobe)	A	Clindamycin and lincomycin cross the placenta but have not been shown to be harmful to the fetus.
Erythromycin	A	Erythromycin crosses the placenta, but problems in the fetus have not been documented.
Metronidazole (Flagyl)	C	This drug is teratogenic in laboratory animals, but there is no incidence of such effects in people, dogs, or cats.
Quinolones (e.g., enrofloxacin, ciprofloxacin)	D	Because quinolones have been shown to affect the developing cartilage in immature animals, their use is not recommended in pregnancy.
Sulfonamides	C	Sulfonamides cross the placenta and have produced malformations in developing mice and rats. In dogs they may adversely affect the thyroid.
Tetracyclines (e.g., doxycycline, oxytetracycline)	D	Tetracyclines cause bone and teeth malformations in the developing fetus and may be harmful to the mother.
Trimethoprimsulfonamides (e.g., Tribrissen, Bactrim)	C	Manufacturer states that it is safe, but there may be precautions regarding the sulfonamides (see above).
Antifungal Drugs		
Amphotericin B	C	There are no known teratogenic effects, but amphotericin is an extremely toxic antibiotic.
Griseofulvin	D	Malformations have been observed in cats and adverse effects have been seen in dogs.
Ketoconazole	C	Teratogenic in laboratory animals; decreases adrenocorticosteroid synthesis; may decrease testosterone in males and cause impotence; may cause dystocia.
Antiparasitic Drugs		
Amitraz (Mitaban)	C	According to manufacturer's label, no information is available.
Bunamide (Scoloban)	B	Slight interference in spermatogenesis is seen in male dogs. No effects on pregnancy in dogs or cats have been reported.
Diethylcarbamazine	A	Safe during all stages of pregnancy. The routine use has been reported to cause sterility in males. This is an individual idiosyncrasy rather than an expected reaction. Fertility is regained after daily use is stopped.
Diethazine iodide (Dizan)	C	No specific information is available, but iodides can cause congenital goiter.
Ivermectin	A	Reproduction studies in most species have not shown any adverse effects. Mice are the most sensitive laboratory animal, and it was teratogenic at 400 µg/kg.
Levamisole	C	No information available.
Mebendazole	A	Safe according to reproduction studies in dogs.
Organophosphates (e.g., dichlorvos, fenthion, trichlorfon)	C	These drugs can be harmful to puppies and kittens and should be avoided if possible in pregnant animals.
Piperazine	A	Safe.
Praziquantel	A	Safe when tested in dogs and cats.
Thiacetarsemide (Caparsolate sodium)	C	No specific studies have been performed, but it may be hepatotoxic. If possible, delay heartworm therapy until after parturition.
Anticancer Drugs		
Cyclophosphamide (Cytoxan)	C	This drug may decrease fertility. There is an increased risk of malformations, especially if used early in pregnancy.
Doxorubicin (Adriamycin)	C	Embryotoxic, teratogenic, and abortifacient. Avoid the use of doxorubicin, especially early in pregnancy.
Vincristine	C	There are no specific studies in dogs or cats, but it should be considered to be toxic to the fetus and may produce malformations.
Methotrexate (MTX)	C	Abortifacient; teratogenic; mutagenic.

TABLE 20-7   SAFETY OF DRUGS IN PREGNANCY—cont'd

Drug	Recommendation*	Comments
Analgesic and Antiinflammatory Drugs		
Aspirin, salicylates	C	Embryotoxicity and birth defects have been reported in laboratory animals, but not in dogs or cats. Pulmonary hypertension may occur if administered near term.
Acetaminophen (Tylenol)	C	Toxic in cats. Safety not established in dogs. Chronic toxicity has inhibited spermatogenesis.
Antihistamines (e.g., chlorpheniramine)	B	Studies in laboratory animals suggest that they are safe.
Dimethyl sulfoxide (DMSO)	D	Teratogenic in laboratory animals. Manufacturer states that it should not be administered to pregnant animals.
Flunixin meglumine (Banamine)	C	The safety in dogs and cats has not been established. Pulmonary hypertension is possible if administered near term. No adverse effects were seen in pregnant cows at six times the dose for 2 days.
Ibuprofen (Motrin, Advil)	C	Safety in dogs and cats has not been established.
Phenylbutazone	C	Safety in pregnancy has not been established. Long-term use may adversely affect the bone marrow.
Anesthetic and Preanesthetic Drugs		
Acepromazine, chlorpromazine, triflupromazine	C	Phenothiazine tranquilizers should be avoided near term because they may cause CNS depression. At high doses they may decrease spermatogenesis. There are reports of adverse effects in infants of women who received phenothiazines (nervous disorders and jaundice).
Atropine	C	Easily crosses the placenta; may cause fetal tachycardia. May inhibit gonadotropin secretion and ovulation.
Glycopyrrolate	B	Crosses the placenta readily. It may cause fetal tachycardia.
Opiates (e.g., morphine, butorphanol, codeine, oxymorphone)	B	These drugs are safe for short-term use during pregnancy, but if administered to the mother near term they may cause fetal depression. Fetal depression should be treated with naloxone.
Naloxone (Narcan)	A	Naloxone has been shown to be safe when administered to neonates within a few minutes of birth.
Halothane	C	Halothane should be avoided for C-sections. It may cause CNS depression and excessive uterine bleeding.
Isoflurane	B	Probably safe, although temporary depression has been seen in neonates following C-section.
Methoxyflurane	C	Neonatal depression has been seen following C-sections.
Ketamine	C	Probably safe, although neonatal depression may follow C-section. Ketamine increases uterine pressure, which may induce premature labor.
Local anesthetics (e.g., lidocaine, procaine)	A	All local anesthetics are probably safe if used in small doses for local infiltration.
Nitrous oxide	A	Probably safe. This drug has been used frequently for C-section without adverse effects.
Pentobarbital	D	This drug has a high incidence of fetal mortality.
Thiamylal, thiopental	C	The barbiturates cross the placenta and may cause fetal depression (especially respiratory depression at birth when they are used for C-section).
Xylazine (Rompun)	D	No information on teratogenicity, but it may induce early parturition or abortion.
Gastrointestinal Drugs		
Antacids (e.g., magnesium hydroxide, aluminum hydroxide)	A	These drugs are all safe if used in therapeutic doses.
Antiemetics	B	Probably safe because they are usually administered for just a short time.
Cimetidine, ranitidine	B	Safety has not been established. Administered to many pregnant women with no adverse effects.
Diphenoxylate (Lomotil)	C	Although studies in pregnant laboratory animals have shown some adverse effects, none has been reported in people, dogs, or cats.
Laxatives	B	All laxatives are probably safe, except castor oil, which may cause uterine contractions.
Loperamide (Imodium)	B	No adverse effects have been reported in laboratory animals, humans, dogs, or cats.
Metoclopramide (Reglan)	B	This drug was shown to be safe in laboratory animals, but information is not available for dogs and cats.
Misoprostol (Cytotec)	D	This is a prostaglandin analogue. It causes abortions.

(Continued)

TABLE 20-7   SAFETY OF DRUGS IN PREGNANCY—cont'd

Drug	Recommendation*	Comments
Omeprazole (Losec)	C	Studies in rats and rabbits have shown fetal toxicity when high doses were administered. No information is available for humans, dogs, or cats.
Sucralfate (Carafate, Sulcrate)	A	This drug is not absorbed systemically to any extent and is probably safe.
Sulfasalazine (Azulfidine)	B	The salicylate component is not absorbed sufficiently to cause adverse effects. The sulfonamide component is absorbed, however (see sulfonamides).
Cardiovascular Drugs		
ACE inhibitors, e.g., Captopril (Capoten), Enalapril (Vasotec)	C	These drugs have been shown to be embryotoxic in laboratory animals. They may produce decreased growth, hypotension, and decreased renal perfusion in the neonate.
Calcium-channel blocking drugs (e.g., verapamil, diltiazem)	C	High doses in laboratory animals caused embryotoxicity and fetal deaths.
Digoxin	A	Although it crosses the placenta, no adverse effects have been reported when it is administered in therapeutic doses. Advanced pregnancy may alter some of the pharmacokinetic characteristics.
Furosemide (Lasix)	A	No adverse effects have been reported.
Hydralazine (Apresoline)	B	Although this drug has produced adverse effects in laboratory animals, it has been administered to pregnant women safely.
Isoproterenol (Isuprel)	C	Beta-adrenergic drugs inhibit uterine contractions. This drug may produce fetal tachycardia.
Lidocaine (Xylocaine)	B	The use of lidocaine is accepted if the benefit outweighs the risk. Probably safe.
Procainamide (Pronestyl)	B	Probably safe.
Propranolol (Inderal)	C	May cause fetal cardiac depression and neonatal hypoglycemia; avoid its use near term.
Quinidine	C	Studies have not been done, but quinine, a related compound, has produced congenital abnormalities.
Theophylline, aminophylline	C	Crosses the placenta easily. Teratogenic in mice at high doses (30 × therapeutic dose), but there are no reported adverse effects in dogs or cats.
Anticonvulsant Drugs		
Diazepam (Valium)	C	Diazepam has been associated with congenital defects in mice, rats, and humans. The benefits of its use outweigh the risks when used for status epilepticus.
Phenobarbital	B	Phenobarbital has been associated with some congenital defects and bleeding tendencies in the newborn, but it is probably safer than other anticonvulsants.
Phenytoin (Dilantin)	D	Associated with fetal hydantoin syndrome. Teratogenic.
Primidone (Mylepsin)	B	Probably the same risks as phenobarbital.
Valproic acid	C	May cause congenital malformations.
Endocrine Drugs		
Anabolic steroids (e.g., stanozolol, testosterone, nandrolone deconate)	D	Do not administer to pregnant animals. These drugs may cause congenital malformations and masculinization of the female fetus.
Glucocorticoids (e.g., dexamethasone, prednisolone, prednisone)	C	Glucocorticoids have been associated with decreased birth weights, cleft palate, and other congenital malformations, but teratogenic effects have not been seen in dogs and cats. They may induce premature labor and abortion.
Diethylstilbestrol (DES)	D	Produces malformations of fetal reproductive organs.
Estradiol cypionate (ECP)	D	Produces malformations in the fetus and abortions.
Mitotane (o,p'-DDD)	D	Causes adrenocortical necrosis.
Thyroxine	B	Does not cross the placenta easily and has not been reported to produce problems in the fetus.

TABLE 20-7   SAFETY OF DRUGS IN PREGNANCY—cont'd

Drug	Recommendation*	Comments
Miscellaneous Drugs		
Ammonium chloride	B	May cause fetal acidosis; avoid its use during pregnancy.
Aspartame (NutraSweet)	A	Safe.
Caffeine	C	In laboratory animals caffeine produced skeletal abnormalities in the fetus at doses equivalent to 12 to 24 cups per day for a woman throughout pregnancy.
Ephedrine, pseudoephedrine	B	There are no studies in dogs and cats, but results in other species indicate that these drugs are probably safe.
Isotretinoin (Acutane)	D	This drug has caused major fetal abnormalities; do not use during pregnancy.

From Papich MG: Pharmacological considerations during pregnancy in small animals. Proceedings of the Society for Theriogenology, 1990, with permission.

*A: Probably safe. Although specific studies may not have proved the safety of all drugs in dogs and cats, there are no reports of adverse effects, and it has not been shown to be harmful in pregnant women or laboratory animals.

B: Safe if used cautiously. Studies in laboratory animals may have uncovered some risk, but specific problems have not been identified in dogs or cats. These drugs are safe if they are used for only a short course of therapy.

C: These drugs may have potential risks. Studies in laboratory animals have shown these drugs to have harmful effects, or scattered reports may have associated these drugs with adverse effects in women, dogs, or cats. These drugs should be used only as a last resort or when the benefits clearly outweigh the risks.

D: Do not use. These drugs definitely have been shown to be toxic to the fetus or pregnant mother. In most cases a suitable alternative can be used instead.

anesthetics are associated with the fewest problems. Ketamine may accumulate in the placenta and cause prolonged depression, whereas barbiturates require biotransformation, which could prolong their activity in the fetus. Opiates may cause respiratory depression but can be reversed with naloxone or nalorphine. The anticholinergic effects of meperidine may inhibit constriction of the ductus arteriosus, but the significance of this effect is not known. Adrenergic drugs do not enter the fetal circulation but still can do harm by causing vasoconstriction of placental vessels, resulting in fetal asphyxia. Severe weakness in puppies can result from the use of anticholinesterase agents, such as organophosphates, that cross the placental barrier. Tranquilizers, such as diazepam, chlordiazepoxide, and phenytoin, readily enter the fetus, potentially causing sedation. Chlorpromazine may cause prolonged sedation and retinopathy (Davis, 1983).

Corticosteroids are a real concern because they are used frequently by practitioners for various conditions. In the pregnant bitch, corticosteroids are contraindicated primarily because they induce abortion. This has been a consistent problem and one that owners and veterinarians should recognize. Corticosteroids are also known to cause cleft palates in mice, but mice may be more sensitive to these drugs than other species (Papich, 1990). Nonsteroidal antiinflammatory drugs have been associated with a wide variety of fetal effects; their use is controversial. The major problems with this class of drugs have been found in late gestation, when they may be associated with fetal pulmonary hypertension, prolonged gestation, or prolonged bleeding (Moise et al, 1988). Salicylates caused birth defects in laboratory animals, but no subsequent risk in humans was identified in large studies (see Table 20-5) (Koren et al, 1998).

Antibiotics must also be used cautiously in the pregnant bitch. The safest group of antibiotics are the β-lactam group: penicillins, aminopenicillins, and cephalosporins. Because their mechanism of action is on the cell wall, at therapeutic doses they are relatively safe (Papich, 1990). Tetracyclines may produce permanently abnormal teeth, and injectable tetracycline may cause a fulminating and usually fatal hepatitis in the bitch. Streptomycin may cause deafness in the neonate, and nitrofurantoin can cause hemolysis. Chloramphenicol is associated with fetal death, and long-acting sulfonamides may cause liver atrophy and hyperbilirubinemia (Davis, 1983). Quinolones may harmfully affect developing cartilage (Papich, 1990).

Nutrition and General Care during Pregnancy and Lactation

DIET. The diet for a breeding bitch or one in the first one half to two thirds of gestation should consist primarily or totally of good commercial "maintenance" dog food. These dogs should be fed normal amounts of food during the 4 weeks after standing heat. Increasing amounts of food should be offered beginning during the fifth to sixth week of gestation. An initial increase of 20% to 25% may progress to 50% by the eighth and ninth weeks of gestation and the first week after whelping. The last part of gestation and lactation should be nutritionally supported with a diet containing higher levels of protein, energy, and minerals.

Ideally, the label of the gestation/lactation diet should state that the food has passed the American Association of Feed Control Officers (AAFCO) trials (Ralston, 1990). The second and third weeks of lactation can be associated with the greatest stress to the bitch, and caloric requirements at these times may be twice that of anestrus. During the fourth week of lactation, the food allotment should begin to be tapered until a week after weaning, when caloric requirements should return to anestrus levels.

It is advisable to increase the number of meals offered to a bitch during the last few weeks of pregnancy. It is not unusual for dogs with large litters to have a limited capacity for food due solely to gastric compression by the fetuses. Offering small meals while keeping the bitch separated from other dogs is helpful. It is also important to allow the *lactating* bitch time to eat without being disturbed by her puppies. Some bitches lose significant amounts of weight while nursing a large litter because they have limited opportunity to eat.

SUPPLEMENTS. Some owners have a strong desire to supplement a pregnant or lactating bitch's diet. Multipurpose veterinary B-complex vitamins may be beneficial and should not be harmful. Vitamin D supplementation should always be discouraged. Bone meal or other calcium supplements should also be strongly discouraged. Commercial dog foods contain adequate amounts of calcium and the correct calcium:phosphorus ratio (1.2:1). Calcium requirements may be increased as much as threefold above maintenance in late gestation and/or early lactation. The bitch fed a properly balanced diet meets these needs via increased intake, which should also meet increasing energy requirements. Excess calcium supplementation in late gestation has been shown to be a factor in the predisposition of puppies to gastric dilation/volvulus; it also interferes with the absorption of zinc, manganese, and other essential divalent minerals, and it may predispose the bitch to dystocia. It is interesting that "raspberry tea," which is high in calcium, is a folk remedy for preventing dystocia. Calcium additives should be given only with the veterinarian's approval to bitches with a past history of eclampsia. Unfortunately, calcium supplementation may actually increase the chance of hypocalcemia by suppressing parathyroid hormone secretion. It remains to be determined when such medication is indicated and what the dosage or treatment strategy should be.

MIDGESTATION EXAMINATION. Many practitioners routinely recommend examining bitches at days 35 to 45 of gestation. This provides an opportunity to answer the owner's questions and to review the bitch's diet, supplements, exercise, wormings, and any other pertinent data. Ideally, the breeding bitch should have been vaccinated prior to breeding. It is preferable to vaccinate an unvaccinated pregnant bitch with killed vaccine than to risk peripartum or postpartum illness. A previously vaccinated bitch, even when overdue, is usually not vaccinated. The bitch should be tested for heartworm and fecal parasites prior to proestrus but can be tested if pregnant. Heartworm microfilaria can cross the placenta into the fetus. *A. caninum* (hookworms) and *T. canis* (roundworms) can be treated. Fenbendazole is an effective anthelmintic, reducing prenatal and lactogenic infections in pups, when treatment (50 mg/kg/day) extends from day 40 of pregnancy through postpartum day 14 (Burke and Robertson, 1983). Fenbendazole appears to be a safe drug that does not harm the bitch or her puppies.

Checking a complete blood count (CBC) and total protein concentration is not always warranted but remains simple and inexpensive. Mild anemia may be documented and is usually normal, as described earlier in this chapter (see page 789). The clinician may recommend abdominal radiography, after day 45, to confirm the pregnancy and to count fetuses and subjectively assess their health.

EXERCISE. Walking a bitch daily throughout gestation should be beneficial to the owner as well as the dog. Dogs accustomed to jogging may continue to do so for the initial 4 to 6 weeks of pregnancy. An owner must be careful not to overexert the pet, especially late in gestation.

BODY WEIGHT. The body weight of a pregnant bitch should not change much through the first 4 weeks of gestation. Noticeable weight gain after that time is expected. The ideal body weight of the bitch immediately after whelping is usually 10% to 15% above the prebreeding weight.

PARTURITION

Endocrinology of Parturition

INITIAL EVENTS. The bitch depends on progesterone secreted from the corpus luteum for the maintenance of pregnancy. The ovary appears to be the sole source of progesterone in the bitch (Concannon et al, 1990). The onset of parturition is timed primarily by the fetus via secretions of the fetal adrenal cortex. The fetal pituitary, secondary to some stress-related factor, secretes ACTH, which in turn causes glucocorticoid secretion by the fetal adrenal cortex. These fetal glucocorticoids probably boost the synthesis of estrogens in the placenta through induction of placental aromatizing enzymes, which cause secretion of prostaglandins.

PROSTAGLANDINS. Increased estrogen concentrations and cortisol concentrations and/or additional factors in the fetoplacental unit contribute to the synthesis and release of luteolytic amounts of prostaglandin $F_{2\alpha}$ ($PGF_{2\alpha}$), both in the placenta and subsequently in the myometrium (Concannon et al, 1989a). Prostaglandins (PGs) are a group of biologically active lipids that are synthesized in various forms by many tissues. They are essentially *locally acting hormones* that function at or near their site of synthesis. They are inactivated during one circulation through the lungs. In parturition, the endometrium is probably the most important site of $PGF_{2\alpha}$ synthesis. It is probable that the myometrium, cervix, placenta, and fetal membranes also synthesize PGs. The conceptus appears to inhibit PG production until late in gestation, when alterations in physiology promote PG synthesis and release.

PROSTAGLANDINS, PROGESTERONE, ESTROGEN, AND PARTURITION. Estrogens enhance PG synthesis, whereas progesterone antagonizes the effect. The increase in estrogen secretion near parturition, combined with a decreasing progesterone concentration, leads to increased PG synthesis. In addition, oxytocin stimulates the release of $PGF_{2\alpha}$ directly from the uterus. In sheep, estradiol has been shown to enhance this effect by increasing the number of oxytocin receptors in the endometrium, whereas progesterone has the reverse effect. This means that estradiol can directly promote PG synthesis and release and indirectly promote PG release via an oxytocin-dependent mechanism. Thus there are two routes to increased PG production at parturition, and both involve an increase in the estrogen:progesterone ratio.

$PGF_{2\alpha}$ causes corpora lutea to regress (i.e., it is luteolytic). Progesterone concentrations in the plasma plummet, removing the block on myometrial contractions, whereas $PGF_{2\alpha}$ synthesis and release are enhanced. $PGF_{2\alpha}$ also promotes myometrial contractions. Parturition can occur only after the plasma progesterone concentration sharply decreases. The increase in $PGF_{2\alpha}$ concentrations in the uterine vein precedes the final decline in the progesterone concentration by approximately 24 hours and precedes parturition by approximately 48 hours.

Parturition can be induced prematurely by injecting ACTH into the fetus. This is consistent with the known sequence of events. The consequent increased estrogen:progesterone ratio also facilitates oxytocin release from the posterior pituitary, a phenomenon reinforced by the positive feedback effects of uterine contractions and cervical dilation as parturition proceeds (Ferguson's reflex). The effects of oxytocin on myometrial activity also seem to be mediated largely by prostaglandins.

PROLACTIN. Prolactin concentrations begin to increase progressively in the plasma of pregnant bitches approximately 30 to 40 days prior to parturition, peaking 1 or 2 days before whelping. Prolactin then decreases for 1 or 2 days after parturition, before increasing to new peaks in response to suckling-induced reflex release. Concentrations remain high for 10 to 14 days, then slowly decline to basal levels 45 to 55 days after whelping (De Coster et al, 1983). Removal of suckling puppies from a bitch results in rapidly decreasing prolactin concentrations.

RELAXIN. Relaxin was first discovered in 1926 and is unique in that it is the only well-characterized *peptide* hormone produced by the ovary, specifically the follicle, and subsequently primarily by the placenta. During parturition, the classic role of relaxin is to elongate the collagenous interpubic ligament, allowing separation of the pubic bones. This separation is essential to fetal delivery, because neonatal puppies are relatively large and mature. Relaxin may be responsible for rendering the uterus quiescent, especially in the immediate prepartum period. Relaxin may have a role in priming the myometrium for subsequent responsiveness to oxytocin by inducing formation of oxytocin receptors. Relaxin has also been claimed to play a part in controlling uterine contractility before implantation, influencing blastocyst spacing (Bryant-Greenwood, 1982). Along with estrogen, progesterone, and prostaglandins, relaxin plays a major role in bringing about changes in cervical structural collagen. These alterations lead to increased distensibility of the cervix at parturition (Porter, 1980).

Care of the Bitch

WHELPING BOX. Providing a bitch with an area for whelping and nursing her pups can eliminate problems of the bitch choosing an undesirable location. Many breeders build a whelping box to meet certain criteria (Fig. 20-20). The box should be available to the bitch 7 to 14 days prior to her whelping date to allow ample opportunity for her to feel comfortable with the new environment. The box should be placed in relatively familiar surroundings that also provide some degree of privacy. It should be large enough for the bitch to stretch out comfortably and have room for a litter of puppies.

The sides should be high enough so that 4- to 6-week-old puppies cannot jump out, but the bitch

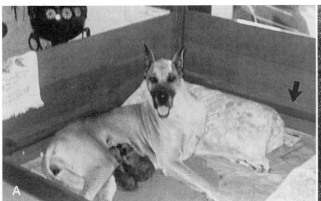 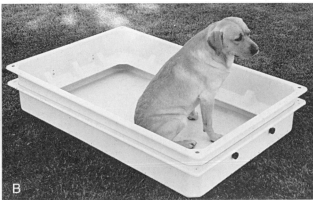

FIGURE 20-20. *A,* Great Dane bitch and her litter in a whelping box. Note the bedding and the ledge *(arrow),* which prevents the bitch from accidentally crushing a puppy between herself and the wall of the box. *B,* Yellow Labrador in a plastic whelping box. This prefabricated box is lightweight and easily cleaned.

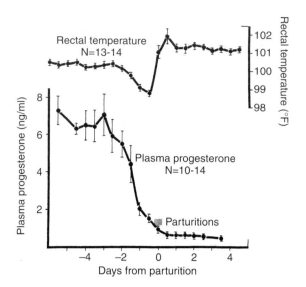

FIGURE 20-21. Peripartum changes in plasma progesterone and rectal temperature. (From Concannon PW, Yeager AE: Endocrine, ultrasonographic, radiographic and clinical changes during pregnancy, parturition, and lactation in dogs. Proceedings of the Society for Theriogenology, 1990, p 197; used with permission.)

must be able to escape her puppies. The wall of the box should have a ledge near the floor to prevent a bitch that is lying down from accidentally crushing a puppy between herself and the wall. The whelping box or area should be bedded down with towels to provide nesting material. Towels can be cleaned and reused countless times. Newspapers are not nearly as soft or warm, and newspaper print can discolor the puppies. The ideal temperature for the box floor is approximately 75° F, which can be attained with ordinary low-wattage light bulbs (care must be taken that the floor of the box is not *too* warm). Hot water bottles are cumbersome. During whelping, the owner should have some small towels available, as well as scissors, thread, tincture of iodine, and a rectal thermometer for monitoring the temperature of the bitch.

FINAL 30 HOURS. Eighteen to 30 hours before parturition, the plasma progesterone concentration declines below 2 ng/ml. Ten to 14 hours after this critical hormone change, the rectal temperature of the bitch falls below 100° F and often below 99° F (Fig. 20-21). If progesterone implants are administered, the rectal temperature does not decline, and parturition is delayed. The decrease in temperature usually precedes labor by 10 to 24 hours. The temperature decline is also seen prior to exogenous $PGF_{2\alpha}$-induced abortion (Concannon and Yeager, 1990).

Stages of Labor

STAGE I. This stage begins with the onset of uterine contractions and ends when the cervix is fully dilated. Contractions of the uterine musculature are usually *not* visible externally. These contractions occur at regular but progressively shorter intervals and result in strong intrauterine pressures. It is the longest stage of human labor, but the onset of this stage is usually not easily or confidently recognized in bitches. The shortening of each muscle cell during contraction is followed, during relaxation, by failure of the cell to regain its initial length. This phenomenon is referred to as *brachystasis* (Johnson and Everitt, 1980).

Stage I labor in the bitch averages 6 to 12 hours, but it may last 24 hours. During this time the bitch may appear restless, nervous, and anorectic and may be seen to shiver, pant, vomit, chew, scratch at the floor, or pace. Most of these dogs seek seclusion and/or exhibit nesting behavior (digging and/or tearing material to create a nest) during or near the end of this phase of labor. The owner can do little aside from providing the bitch with some privacy and an area for whelping.

STAGES II AND III. Stage II of labor begins with full dilation of the cervix and ends with complete expulsion of the fetus, and stage III begins after expulsion of the fetus and ends with expulsion of the placenta. The bitch with more than one puppy alternates between stages II and III. The length of these two stages is highly variable. Bitches may deliver pups over a period as short as a few hours to as long as 24 to 36 hours. Contractions are usually visible, and the bitch is either on her side or in a squatting position. With passage of each pup, either the chorioallantoic membrane ruptures or the bitch frees the pup by biting and/or licking the membrane away. The amniotic membranes, which the puppy is likely to still have at birth, must also be removed by the bitch.

The time between initiation of stage II labor and the birth of the first puppy varies. Commonly, it is only 10 to 30 minutes. Active straining for more than 30 minutes is worrisome, and a veterinarian should be consulted. The intervals between the births of subsequent puppies also vary. It is not unusual for a bitch to deliver several puppies, then rest for a time before beginning the delivery process again. In this situation, a lag of more than 4 to 6 hours is worrisome. However, a lag of 30 minutes to 1 hour *with straining* or abdominal contractions warrants veterinary consultation. A disturbed, frightened, or nervous bitch may actually interrupt whelping.

The placenta is usually passed within 5 to 15 minutes of the birth of each puppy. Occasionally, one or two placentas may follow the birth of two puppies that had no placentas (i.e., one puppy may be born from each uterine horn without placentas, but subsequent pups from either horn are typically preceded by the placenta associated with the previous birth).

The order of puppy delivery usually alternates between uterine horns. In a study of 14 bitches, one horn was never observed to empty completely before the other horn began expelling puppies. In six of eight bitches in which the uterine horns contained unequal numbers of fetuses, the first pup was born from the horn containing more pups. In almost 80% of the births, if one or more fetuses were left in each uterine horn, the next pup was produced by the horn with the greater number (van der Weyden et al, 1981).

Approximately 40% of puppies are born in a breech presentation. Breech presentation is normal and does not predispose the bitch to dystocia (Johnston et al, 1982).

The bitch may eat the placentas, although there is no known benefit, and this practice is not encouraged. Vomiting of the placental material is common. The bitch should lick each newborn vigorously to remove all membranes from the face and to promote respiration. If this does not occur within 1 to 3 minutes, the owner can intervene. All membranes should be removed by laying the puppy in a clean, soft towel and vigorously rubbing the puppy with the other end of the towel. Owners must be reminded that a large amount of fluid is associated with the birth of each neonate and that failure to use a new *dry* towel results in feeling as though one is attempting to hold onto a wet bar of soap. Fluids can be removed from the mouth by suction, usually using a soft, blunt-ended rubber air bulb. The owner can cup the puppy in the hands (with its head at the fingertips and its tail at the wrist) and

swing the arms in an up and down motion (as if chopping wood) to promote respiration and clean the respiratory tract.

The bitch severs the umbilical cord with her teeth. If she does not do this, the owner can use thread, tying two knots in the cord. The first knot should be at least 1 inch from the puppy, and the second is an additional $\frac{1}{4}$-inch away (Fig. 20-22). Clean scissors are used to cut between the knots, and the severed end is dipped into a mild antiseptic such as tincture of iodine or Betadine. The pups should definitely be left with the bitch, except in unusual circumstances, and handled as little as possible. Some bitches nurse newborn puppies while delivering subsequent puppies; others do not.

Normal Uterine Involution

After whelping, the uterus undergoes a period of repair called *involution*. Once involution is complete,

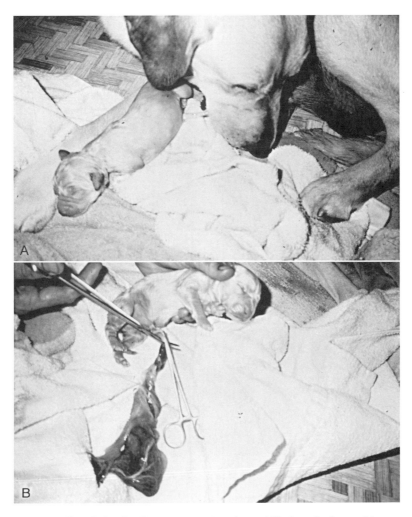

FIGURE 20-22. *A,* Yellow Labrador Retriever severing the umbilical cord of one of her puppies. *B,* If the bitch fails to sever the cord, it is cut distal to one hemostat. (Courtesy Dr. Autumn Davidson, Davis, CA.)

the uterus reaches an anestrus condition of small size and readiness for the upcoming proestrus. The major amount of involution occurs during the initial 4- to 6-week postpartum period. During this time the owner may notice an odorless green, dark red/brown, or obvious bloody vaginal discharge, called *lochia*. This discharge is a normal finding and varies from a rather significant amount immediately after parturition to quite small amounts 4 to 6 weeks later. The discharge is often licked clean by the bitch. The bitch should be normal in all respects during the period of uterine involution. The health of the bitch is important, because a healthy bitch with a vaginal discharge postpartum is considered normal, whereas an ill bitch with a vaginal discharge postpartum may have metritis. *It is important to realize that the 4- to 6-week postpartum period for vaginal discharge is approximate. Some normal bitches have a bloody discharge for as long as 8 to 12 weeks. As long as the bitch is healthy, not anemic, and not septic, the discharge is not likely to be worrisome.*

Copious amounts of bloody vaginal discharge can be worrisome. If the bitch is healthy, a wait-and-see attitude can be taken. However, continued bleeding may be consistent with a coagulopathy (inherited or acquired [e.g., toxin]), trauma in the birth canal, or continued bleeding from placental sites. Prostaglandin therapy using natural prostaglandin can be tried (0.25 mg/kg SC once daily for 2 to 3 days). Spaying the bitch may be necessary.

One week after parturition, the uterine horns should have significantly decreased in size, averaging 33.5 cm in thickness. Placental sites are 1.5 to 2 cm in diameter and are rough, granular, and covered with mucus and blood during the first postpartum week. By the fourth week, the placental sites have decreased in size and appear as nodular grayish tan areas with a clear mucous covering. At postpartum week 7, placental sites are light brown in color; by the ninth week they are narrow, light bands, and at 3 months the repair process is complete (AlBassam et al, 1981; Johnston et al, 1982). Histologically, during the first postpartum week, placental sites are covered by eosinophilic necrotic collagenous masses. These masses have sloughed by the ninth week (Wheeler, 1986).

The nonpregnant uterus also undergoes involution after diestrus. However, in the nonpregnant bitch, there is no vaginal discharge, and the period required for involution is approximately a month shorter.

REFERENCES

AlBassam MA, et al: Normal postpartum involution of the uterus in the dog. Can J Comp Med 45:217, 1981.

Andersen K: Artificial insemination and storage of canine semen. *In* Morrow DA (ed): Current Therapy in Theriogenology. Philadelphia, WB Saunders, 1980, p 661.

Arthur G, et al: Veterinary Reproduction and Obstetrics (Theriogenology), 5th ed. London, Bailliere Tindall, 1984.

Bouchard GF, et al: Determination of ovulation in the bitch with a qualitative progesterone enzyme immunoassay in serum, plasma, and whole blood. J Reprod Fertil Suppl 47:517, 1993.

Bryant-Greenwood GD: Relaxin as a new hormone. Endocrinology 3:62, 1982.

Burke TM, Robertson EL: Fenbendazole treatment of pregnant bitches to reduce prenatal and lactogenic infections of *Toxocara canis* and *Ancylostoma caninum* in pups. J Am Vet Med Assoc 183:987, 1983.

Bysted BV, et al: Embryonic development stages in relation to the LH peak in the bitch. *In* Farstad W, Steel C (eds): Proceedings, the Fourth International Symposium on Canine and Feline Reproduction, Oslo, Norway, 2000.

Concannon PW: Effects of hypophysectomy and of LH administration on luteal phase plasma progesterone levels in the Beagle bitch. J Reprod Fertil 58:407, 1980.

Concannon PW: Prolactin and LH: Two luteotrophic requirements in the dog. Program of the Annual Conference of the Society for the Study of Fertility, Edinburgh, 1981, p 19.

Concannon PW: Reproductive physiology and endocrine patterns of the bitch. *In* Kirk RW (ed): Current Veterinary Therapy VIII. Philadelphia, WB Saunders, 1983, p 886.

Concannon P, Rendano V: Radiographic diagnosis of canine pregnancy: Onset of fetal skeletal radiopacity in relation to times of breeding, preovulatory luteinizing hormone release, and parturition. Am J Vet Res 44:1506, 1983.

Concannon PW, Yeager AE: Endocrine, ultrasonographic, radiographic, and clinical changes during pregnancy, parturition, and lactation in dogs. Proceedings of the Society for Theriogenology, 1990, p 197.

Concannon PW, et al: LH release in ovariohysterectomized dogs in response to estrogen withdrawal and its facilitation by progesterone. Biol Reprod 20:523, 1979.

Concannon PW, et al: Canine gestation length: Variation related to time of mating and fertile life of sperm. Am J Vet Res 44:1819, 1983.

Concannon PW, et al: Elevated concentrations of 13,14-dihydro-15-keto-prostaglandin $F_{2\alpha}$ in maternal plasma during prepartum luteolysis and parturition in dogs (*Canis familiaris*). J Reprod Fertil 39:12, 1989a.

Concannon PW, et al: Biology and endocrinology of ovulation, pregnancy, and parturition in the dog. J Reprod Fertil 39:3, 1989b.

Concannon PW, et al: Termination of pregnancy and induction of premature luteolysis by the antiprogestagen, mifepristone, in dogs. J Reprod Fertil 88:99, 1990.

Concannon P, et al: Postimplantation increase in plasma fibrinogen concentration with increase in relaxin concentration in pregnant dogs. Am J Vet Res 57:1382, 1996.

Concannon PW, et al: Embryo development, hormonal requirements, and maternal responses during canine pregnancy. *In* Farstad W, Steel C (eds): Proceedings, the Fourth International Symposium on Canine and Feline Reproduction, Oslo, Norway, 2000.

Davis LE: Adverse effects of drugs on reproduction in dogs and cats. Mod Vet Pract 64:969, 1983.

De Coster R, et al: A homologous radioimmunoassay for canine prolactin plasma levels during the reproductive cycle. Acta Endocrinol 103:477, 1983.

Doak RL, et al: Longevity of spermatozoa in the reproductive tract of the bitch. J Reprod Fertil 13:51,1967.

Eckersall PD, Harvey MJA: The use of a bovine plasma progesterone ELISA kit to measure progesterone in equine, ovine, and canine plasmas. Vet Rec 120:5, 1987.

England GCW, et al: A comparison of radioimmunoassay with quantitative and qualitative enzyme-linked immunoassay for plasma progesterone detection in bitches. Vet Rec 125:107, 1989.

England GCW, et al: Studies on canine pregnancy using B-mode ultrasound: Development of the conceptus and determination of gestational age. J Small Anim Pract 31:324, 1990.

Farstad W: Mating and artificial insemination in the dog. *In* England GCW, Harvey M (eds): BSAVA Manual of Small Animal Reproduction and Neonatology. British Small Animal Association, Cheltenham, United Kingdom, 1998, p 95.

Farstad W, Anderson-Berg K: Factors influencing the success rate of artificial insemination with frozen semen in the dog. J Reprod Fertil Suppl 39:289, 1989.

Fernandez PA, et al: Luteal function in the bitch: Changes during diestrus in pituitary concentration of and the number of luteal receptors for luteinizing hormone and prolactin. Biol Reprod 37:804, 1987.

Fisher T, Fisher D: Serum assay for canine pregnancy testing. Mod Vet Pract 62:466, 1981.

Fontbonne A, Badinand F: Canine artificial insemination with frozen semen: Comparison of intravaginal and intrauterine deposition of semen. J Reprod Fertil Suppl 47:325, 1993.

Fontbonne A, et al: Artificial insemination with frozen semen in the bitch: Influence of progesterone level, inseminating dose, and number of inseminations performed in the same bitch. *In* Farstad W, Steel C (eds): Proceedings, the Fourth International Symposium on Canine and Feline Reproduction, Oslo, Norway, 2000.

Gentry PA, Liptrap RM: Influence of progesterone and pregnancy on canine fibrinogen values. J Small Anim Pract 22:185, 1981.

Gerber JG, et al: Prostacyclin produced by the pregnant uterus in the dog may act as a circulating vasodepressor substance. J Clin Invest 67:632, 1981.

Goodman M: Ovulation timing. Vet Clin North Am (Small Anim Pract) 31:219, 2001.

Gradil CM, et al: Pregnancy diagnosis in the bitch. *In* Bonagura JD (ed): Kirk's Current Veterinary Therapy XIII. Philadelphia, WB Saunders, 2000, p 918.

Hegstad RL, Johnston SD: Use of serum progesterone ELISA tests in canine breeding management. *In* Kirk RW, Bonagura JD (eds): Current Veterinary Therapy XI. Philadelphia, WB Saunders, 1992, p 943.

Johnson MH, Everitt BJ: Essential Reproduction. Oxford, UK, Blackwell Scientific Publications, 1980.

Johnston SD, Root Kustritz MV, Olson PNS: Canine and Feline Theriogenology. Philadelphia, WB Saunders, 2001, p 41.

Johnston SD, et al: Canine theriogenology. J Soc Theriogenol 11:1, 1982.

Koren G, et al: Drugs in pregnancy. N Engl J Med 338:1128, 1998.

Kustritz MVR, Johnston SD: Use of serum progesterone for ovulation timing in the bitch. *In* Bonagura JD (ed): Kirk's Current Veterinary Therapy XIII. Philadelphia, WB Saunders, 2000a, p 914.

Kustritz MVR, Johnston SD: Artificial insemination in the bitch. *In* Bonagura JD (ed): Kirk's Current Veterinary Therapy XIII. Philadelphia, WB Saunders, 2000b, p 916.

Linde-Forsberg C, Forsberg M: Fertility in dogs in relation to semen quality and time and site of insemination with fresh and frozen semen. J Reprod Fertil Suppl 39:299, 1989.

Linde-Forsberg C, Forsberg M: Results of 527 controlled artificial inseminations in dogs. J Reprod Fertil Suppl 47:313, 1993.

Lindsay FEF: The normal endoscopic appearance of the caudal reproductive tract of the cyclic and noncyclic bitch: Postuterine endoscopy. J Small Anim Pract 24:1, 1983.

Lindsay FEF, Concannon PW: Normal canine vaginoscopy. *In* Burke T (ed): Small Animal Reproduction and Infertility. Philadelphia, Lea & Febiger, 1986, p 112.

Mahi-Brown CA, et al: Infertility in bitches induced by active immunization with porcine zonae pellucidae. J Exp Zool 222:89, 1982.

Manothaiudom K, et al: Evaluation of the ICAGEN-Target canine ovulation timing diagnostic test in detecting canine plasma progesterone concentrations. J Am Anim Hosp Assoc 31:57, 1995.

McCann JP, Concannon PW: Effects of sex, ovarian cycles, pregnancy, and lactation on insulin and glucose response to exogenous glucose and glucagon in dogs. Biol Reprod 28:41, 1983.

McCann JP, et al: Pregnancy-specific alterations in the metabolic endocrinology of domestic dogs, including insulin resistance and modified regulation of growth hormone secretion. Proceedings of the Eleventh International Congress on Animal Reproduction, 1988.

Moise KJ, et al: Indomethacin in the treatment of premature labor. N Engl J Med 319:327, 1988.

Nelson RW, et al: Treatment of canine pyometra and endometritis with prostaglandin F$_{2\alpha}$. J Am Vet Med Assoc 181:899, 1982.

Nothling JO, et al: Intravaginal insemination of bitches with semen frozen in Triladyl with Equex STM paste to which prostatic fluid or modified TALP was added prior to insemination. *In* Farstad W, Steel C (eds): Proceedings, the Fourth International Symposium on Canine and Feline Reproduction, Oslo, Norway, 2000.

Okkens AC, et al: Fertility problems in the bitch. Anim Reprod Sci 28:379, 1992.

Papich MG: Pharmacological considerations during pregnancy in small animals. Proceedings of the Society for Theriogenology, 1990, p 224.

Phemister RD, et al: Time of ovulation in the Beagle bitch. Biol Reprod 8:74, 1973.

Pineda MH, et al: Dorsal median postcervical fold in the canine vagina. Am J Vet Res 34:1487, 1973.

Porter DG: Relaxin and cervical softening. *In* Anderson AM, Ellwood DA (eds): The Cervix in Pregnancy and Labour. Edinburgh, Churchill Livingstone, 1980.

Ralston SL: Feeding for breeding. Proceedings of the Society for Theriogenology, 1990, p 236.

Reimers TJ, et al: Effects of reproductive state on concentrations of thyroxine, 3,5,3N-triiodothyronine and cortisol in serum of dogs. Biol Reprod 31:148, 1984.

Roszel JF: Anatomy of the canine uterine cervix. Compend Contin Educ (Small Anim Pract) 14:751, 1992.

Ryan EA, Enns L: Role of gestational hormones in the induction of insulin resistance. J Clin Endocrinol Metab 67:341, 1988.

Shille VM, Gontarek J: The use of ultrasonography for pregnancy diagnosis in the bitch. J Am Vet Med Assoc 187:1021, 1985.

Silva LDM, et al: Comparison of intravaginal and intrauterine insemination of bitches with fresh and frozen semen. Vet Rec 138:154, 1996.

Sirivaidyapong S, et al: Successful pregnancy in bitches after transvaginal endoscope–guided intrauterine insemination. *In* Farstad W, Steel C (eds): Proceedings, the Fourth International Symposium on Canine and Feline Reproduction, Oslo, Norway, 2000.

Steinetz BG, et al: Plasma relaxin levels in pregnant and lactating dogs. Biol Reprod 37:719, 1987.

Steinetz BG, et al: Serum relaxin and progesterone concentrations in pregnant, pseudopregnant, and ovariectomized, progestin-treated pregnant bitches: Detection of relaxin as a marker of pregnancy. Am J Vet Res 50:68, 1989.

Steinetz BG, et al: Use of serum relaxin for pregnancy diagnosis in the bitch. *In* Bonagura JD (ed): Kirk's Current Veterinary Therapy XIII. Philadelphia, WB Saunders, 2000, p 924.

Taverne MA, et al: Pregnancy diagnosis in the dog: A comparison between abdominal palpation and linear array real-time echography. Vet Q 7:249, 1985.

van der Weyden GC, et al: Intrauterine position of canine fetuses and their sequence of expulsion at birth. J Small Anim Pract 22:503, 1981.

Verstegen J, et al: Echocardiographic study of heart rate in dog and cat fetuses in utero. J Reprod Fertil Suppl 47:175, 1993.

Watts JR, et al: Uterine, cervical, and vaginal microflora of the normal bitch throughout the reproductive cycle. J Small Anim Pract 37:54, 1996.

Wheeler SL: Subinvolution of placental sites in the bitch. *In* Morrow DA (ed): Current Therapy in Theriogenology 2. Philadelphia, WB Saunders, 1986, p 513.

Wildt DE, et al: Relationship of reproductive behavior, serum luteinizing hormone, and time of ovulation in the bitch. Biol Reprod 18:561, 1978.

Wilson MS: Some aspects of artificial insemination in the bitch using frozen semen. Master's thesis. Palmerston North, New Zealand, Massey University, 1992.

Wilson MS: Transcervical insemination techniques in the bitch. Vet Clin North Am (Small Anim Pract) 31:291, 2001.

Yeager AE, et al: Ultrasonographic appearance of the uterus, placenta, fetus, and fetal membranes throughout accurately timed pregnancy in Beagles. Am J Vet Res 53:342, 1992.

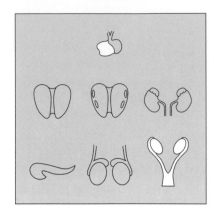

21

PERIPARTURIENT DISEASES

NORMAL PERIPARTURIENT CONDITION OF THE BITCH

Clinical

A variety of changes may be noted to occur in bitches before, at the time of, or soon after parturition. Some of these problems can be serious. Without doubt they are almost always unexpected and invariably of great concern. However, some apparent "problems" are, in fact, normal alterations associated with pregnancy in the bitch. For example, changes in personality may be observed. The bitch often has an increased appetite throughout gestation, but a decrease in stomach volume results in the need for frequent small meals late in gestation. Decreases in exercise and heat tolerance can be dramatic late in gestation.

Blood and Serum

Decreases in red blood cell numbers during pregnancy are expected, with hematocrits as low as 30% to 35%.

Serum cholesterol concentrations may increase during pregnancy whereas the total serum protein, albumin, and calcium concentrations decrease (Bebiak et al, 1987). Total serum thyroxine (T_4) concentrations increase during pregnancy (Reimers et al, 1984), as do the activities of coagulation factors VII, VIII, IX, and XI (Olson, 1988). Some breeds may have unique alterations. Knowing what is expected for bitches and their specific breeds can be important when determining whether a bitch is in need of medical assistance.

CLINICAL PSEUDOPREGNANCY (PSEUDOCYESIS)

Definition and Signs

All normal bitches enter a luteal phase (diestrus) of progesterone dominance following estrus (standing heat). Progesterone assays do not demonstrate any clear biochemical distinction between nonpregnant and pregnant bitches. Physiologically, all nonpregnant bitches in diestrus are pseudopregnant. However, this reference to a normal physiologic process needs to be differentiated from clinical pseudopregnancy, a syndrome recognized by breeders and veterinarians.

Signs of clinical pseudopregnancy are those commonly associated with pregnancy. They can be so convincing that owners have been known to insist that their bitch is pregnant, that she is about to whelp, or that she is suffering from dystocia. These clinical signs usually begin 6 to 12 weeks after estrus. They may be subtle, such as a change in appetite, weight gain, or abdominal enlargement. Sometimes the signs are suggestive of impending parturition: restlessness, decreased activity, nesting behavior, anorexia, vomiting, and/or mothering inanimate objects.

Less commonly, the signs may be quite overt and confusing, such as lactation or abdominal contractions. Certainly, some of these signs in a diestrual bitch would make an owner suspicious that his or her dog is pregnant. Bitches have been examined for delayed parturition, uterine inertia, or dystocia that have subsequently been demonstrated to be pseudopregnant! The phenomenon of nonpregnant bitches lactating could have had functional importance in evolution, when nonbred mature bitches (such as the wolf) have had to nurse and tend the litter of the pack-leading she-wolf (Voith, 1980).

Physiology

Because the physiology of diestrus in pregnant and nonpregnant bitches is quite similar, the physiology of clinical pseudopregnancy is thought to be an exaggerated response to the normal nonpregnant diestrual condition. The onset of clinical pseudopregnancy is most likely initiated by decreasing serum progesterone concentrations. The decreasing progesterone, in turn, stimulates synthesis and secretion of prolactin. Some nonpregnant bitches must be more sensitive than others to these normal endocrine events, resulting in the exhibition of obvious pseudopregnancy.

Lactating pseudopregnant bitches are definitely under the influence of prolactin. However, prolactin secretion has been demonstrated to rise in bitches that do not lactate, suggesting that excessive concentrations or an increased sensitivity to prolactin may explain the clinical condition (Harvey, 1998). Therefore, the physiologic process that causes clinical pseudopregnancy is a composite of exquisitely timed normal hormonal fluctuations. There has been a suggestion that restricted food intake may decrease the incidence of pseudopregnancy in dogs, but this observation may not have clinical implications (Lawler et al, 1999). It is most important that owners understand pseudopregnancy is an exaggeration of normal.

Diagnosis/Interpretation

The diagnosis of clinical pseudopregnancy is established in any bitch that exhibits the typical signs of this condition but is demonstrated not to be pregnant. Assuming abdominal radiography or ultrasonography is negative for pregnancy, no blood, urine, or other tests are required to confirm the diagnosis. It is not usually possible to determine whether a bitch was pregnant, subsequently aborted, or resorbed a litter only to later appear pseudopregnant. Although such a sequence of events is possible, uncomplicated clinical pseudopregnancy is much more common than a scenario involving abortion/resorption.

Perhaps the most important message that veterinarians are encouraged to discuss with owners is the concept that clinical pseudopregnancy is an exaggeration of normal and that the condition, left untreated, always resolves. A bitch that failed to ovulate, one with abnormal ovaries, or one with an abnormal pituitary would not be able to exhibit clinical pseudopregnancy. The condition can only occur in a bitch with normally functioning corpora lutea that begin to regress. Decreasing progesterone concentrations then stimulate prolactin secretion. Therefore the condition suggests that the bitch must also have ovulated in order to have developed corpora lutea. In this sense, clinical pseudopregnancy demonstrates that a bitch is normal.

One differential diagnosis for galactorrhea is hypothyroidism. It has been suggested that increases in thyrotrophin-releasing hormone (TRH) promotes prolactin secretion and then lactation. One dog has been described with hypothyroidism, increased serum prolactin concentration, and galactorrhea (Cortese et al, 1997).

Treatment

NO TREATMENT. Treatment may not be recommended for mild clinical pseudopregnancy, primarily because it is a self-limiting condition, typically lasting 1 to 3 weeks. The endocrine changes associated with the end of diestrus continue, and the signs of pseudopregnancy abate. The most worrisome clinical problems in pseudopregnancy are nesting behavior and lactation, because they bother the owner and may result in destruction or staining of household furnishings. Mammary enlargement and lactation may be uncomfortable for the bitch and represent a potential site of serious infection. When possible, no treatment is pursued. However, some bitches lactate for prolonged periods of time.

CONSERVATIVE THERAPY. Persistent lactation is a response to continuing stimuli for milk letdown. Some owners warm- or cold-pack the bitch's mammary glands or run water over the glands to relieve discomfort. However, most bitches stimulate themselves by licking, by mothering inanimate objects, or by having an unrelated litter of puppies in close proximity. Therefore measures by owners to create stimulation are discouraged. Placing an Elizabethan collar around the neck of the bitch and removing any objects she may be mothering should hasten the resolution of pseudopregnancy.

If these measures do not succeed or if a more aggressive strategy is deemed necessary, one or both of the following are helpful. We recommend that water be removed from the bitch for a 6- to 10-hour period each night for 3 to 7 nights. This water deprivation forces fluid conservation, and lactation quickly ceases. Alternatively, a bitch can be treated with furosemide (Lasix) at an oral dosage of 0.25 to 0.5 mg/kg TID until lactation ceases (usually less than 7 days). Water restriction should not be implemented if furosemide is used.

Light sedation with a tranquilizer for several days may be helpful. The use of phenothiazines has been discouraged in the management of pseudopregnancy because they may inhibit or antagonize dopamine, which is a prolactin-inhibiting factor; that is, they may stimulate synthesis and/or secretion of prolactin. Therefore other forms of sedative or tranquilization medication are recommended (Voith, 1983). An alternative to tranquilization is to exercise a bitch in an attempt to interrupt unwanted behavior.

AGGRESSIVE THERAPY. *Progesterone.* If conservative attempts at therapy are unsuccessful and lactation is persistent, alternatives may be considered. Progesterone administration (megestrol acetate, 2 mg/kg/day for 8 days) actually returns the bitch to a diestrus condition hormonally and usually alleviates signs of clinical pseudopregnancy. However, when progesterone administration is discontinued, there is a repetition of the same hormonal events that initially caused the signs. Thus lactation may recur as the effects of the progesterone dissipate and prolactin is secreted. This form of therapy is not recommended (Concannon and Lein, 1989).

Estrogen or Testosterone. Estrogen therapy (diethylstilbestrol [DES], 1 mg/day orally for 7 days) may alleviate pseudopregnancy but also may cause signs of proestrus or estrus. Testosterone can be administered at a dose of 1 to 2 mg/kg intramuscularly. The androgen mibolerone (Cheque) has been moderately successful in reducing the physical and psychologic signs of pseudopregnancy. The dose recommended is 0.016 mg/kg orally, once daily, for 5 days (Brown, 1984). However, fewer than 50% of the 63 dogs with physical evidence of pseudopregnancy responded. The response seen in bitches with psychologic problems associated with pseudopregnancy was better.

Prolactin Inhibitors. Ergot alkaloids (ergolines) and their derivatives have been identified as potent prolactin inhibitors (Krulich et al, 1981; Ferrari et al, 1982). They act via direct dopamine receptor stimulation at the level of the pituitary gland. Bromocriptine, an ergoline compound and dopamine agonist, inhibits pituitary secretion of prolactin. Bromocriptine, administered orally at 0.01 to 0.1 mg/kg/day in divided doses, does inhibit lactation and should be given until lactation ceases (Mialot et al, 1981, 1982; Janssens, 1986). Side effects to bromocriptine are common and include vomiting, anorexia, depression, and behavioral changes (Peterson and Drucker, 1981). Vomiting can be reduced by administering an antiemetic drug at the

time bromocriptine is given. This is our drug of choice if aggressive treatment of a bitch is necessary; however, we have never needed to use it.

An equally effective but better-tolerated ergoline compound (cabergoline) was identified and evaluated. Cabergoline, administered at a dose of 5 µg/kg once daily for 5 to 10 days, was effective at sharply dropping prolactin concentrations and suppressing lactation in more than 95% of the bitches treated (Di Salle et al, 1984; Jochle et al, 1987; Arbeiter et al 1988). Side effects were considered mild and included lethargy (25% of dogs), inappetence, and vomiting (<5% of dogs). Success was slightly lower (21 of 26 dogs) in a more recent study (Harvey et al, 1997). Furthermore, the conclusion of the most recent study was that cabergoline is effective in suppressing prolactin release from the pituitary gland, but that this suppression may only be transient.

The drug has also been used to induce abortion in the second half of pregnancy in the bitch (Post et al, 1988). In a comparison between cabergoline and bromocriptine use in women, cabergoline was more effective and better-tolerated when used for hyperprolactinemic amenorrhea (Webster et al, 1994).

Ovariohysterectomy. Ovariohysterectomy (OVH), also referred to as *spaying,* is the one therapy that should not be considered or recommended in any pseudopregnant dog. The procedure may exacerbate the syndrome by eliminating progesterone from the system and further stimulate prolactin secretion. On rare occasions, OVH may result in prolonged signs. In fact, because of this concern, some authors recommend avoiding OVH until a period of 4 to 5 months after the previous heat has passed (Harvey, 1998).

Pseudopregnancy-Induced Disorders and Incidence of Recurrence

No association appears to exist between clinical pseudopregnancy and the development of infertility, pyometra, poor mothering/nursing habits, or any other disorder. Clinical pseudopregnancy is simply an exaggeration of a normal state. If the owners of a bitch are distressed by repeated bouts of clinical pseudopregnancy, they should attempt to have the bitch become pregnant or consider ovariohysterectomy. (If repeated attempts at breeding have not been successful, consult the section Infertility of the Bitch and Associated Breeding Disorders.) Some dogs exhibit clinical pseudopregnancy after every heat. OVH should be strongly advised if breeding is not planned (Harvey, 1998).

EXTRAUTERINE FETUSES

Although extremely rare, it is possible for a dog to have fetuses develop outside the uterus. This could happen following a uterine tear that occurred during pregnancy, which would allow exteriorization of fetuses. The tear could be the result of external trauma to the uterus, or death of a fetus could cause local necrosis of the uterine wall. Clinical signs may be absent or a bitch may have vague signs of illness during pregnancy or following parturition. Definitive diagnosis would most likely be made with ultrasonography or at surgery (Shamir and Shahar, 1996).

SPONTANEOUS ABORTION AND RESORPTION OF FETUSES

Incidence

Premature expulsion of dead or living fetuses during late gestation (abortion) or resorption of a fetus or fetuses poses a difficult diagnostic dilemma for veterinarians. The incidence of abortion or resorption of canine fetuses is extremely difficult to assess, because no reliable method is available to confirm pregnancy during the first 3 weeks of gestation and because most bitches are never evaluated with abdominal ultrasonography or radiography until a problem develops. Many bitches thought to have aborted or resorbed a litter were likely never pregnant. Furthermore, bitches may consume or bury aborted fetuses, making it more difficult to confirm a diagnosis. However, a recent ultrasound study demonstrated that resorption of one or two conceptuses occurs in up to 10% of pregnancies (England, 1998).

Causes

GENERAL. A myriad of causes exists for any bitch to abort all or part of a litter. Even when aborted fetuses and/or placentas are evaluated histologically, the exact cause for pregnancy failure may not be understood. The causes of pregnancy failure can encompass congenital/hereditary defects; infectious causes; exposure to drugs, toxins, or trauma during pregnancy; uterine disease; hormonal abnormalities; severe malnutrition; and significant systemic illness. In general terms, these causes are categorized into fetal defects, abnormal maternal environment, and infectious agents (Table 21-1).

FETAL DEFECTS. Any defect in fetal development that is incompatible with life results in death and subsequent abortion or resorption. The defects include not only sperm, egg, or chromosomal abnormalities, but also major organ defects. Fetal resorption probably depends on its stage, with early fetal death resulting in resorption. Death later in gestation results in abortion.

ABNORMAL MATERNAL ENVIRONMENT. *Systemic Disease.* Any factor causing significant stress or damage to the uterus or fetus can cause fetal death. Included among these problems is any serious disease within or outside the reproductive tract. For example, a bitch that develops severe cardiac disease during pregnancy is likely to have a compromised uterine blood supply, leading to fetal death. Similar problems

can arise with any major organ disease. Hypothyroidism has been included as a potential cause for abortion. The veterinarian must remember that a bitch ill from any significant systemic illness may be euthyroid but have thyroid function test results consistent with hypothyroidism (euthyroid sick syndrome; see Chapter 3). Diabetes mellitus, perhaps the most common endocrine disease in dogs, is definitely associated with an inability to carry a litter to term and abortion. All female dogs with diabetes should undergo OVH.

Uterine Disease. Another broad subcategory includes the abnormal uterus that is unable to support pregnancy. Among these problems are cystic endometrial hyperplasia, chronic uterine infections, uterine neoplasia, and uterine adhesions.

Hypoluteoidism. Pregnancy is maintained by progesterone derived from ovarian corpora lutea. Failure to maintain progesterone concentrations above a critical level (1.0 to 2.0 ng/ml) is likely to result in expulsion of the fetus. A luteal phase defect has been associated with pregnancy failure in women, but the diagnosis is considered controversial (Meis et al, 2003). The syndrome has not been well documented in dogs (Olson, 1988), although one case has been described (Purswell, 1991). Progesterone insufficiency is possible, and progesterone concentrations may be low at the time of an abortion. The decreases, however, may be secondary to fetal death rather than representing the primary cause. It has been demonstrated that fetal death will result, within days, in subsequent decreases in serum progesterone concentration (Concannon et al, 1990). Furthermore, fetal distress secondary to virtually any cause may result in decreased serum progesterone concentrations (Johnston et al, 2001). Subnormal progesterone concentrations in a bitch that has already aborted is not proof of hypoluteoidism.

If progesterone is administered to a bitch with impending abortion, delivery may be interrupted even if the cause of the disorder is an infectious disease. Therefore it is advisable to educate owners regarding the potential adverse effects of preventing delivery: continued fetal growth and subsequent dystocia; and potential teratogenic effects, especially masculinization of female fetuses. Maintaining the inciting cause of abortion (e.g., infected fetus) could further harm or threaten the life of other fetuses or the bitch.

The diagnosis of hypoluteoidism is difficult, explaining the controversial nature of the diagnosis. It is imperative that pregnancy be confirmed with ultrasonography and closely monitored. Serum progesterone concentrations should be assessed at least twice weekly. If a known pregnant bitch aborts a litter following documented premature decreases in progesterone concentration in the serum, and no cause for the abortion is identified despite thorough necropsy, culture, and other testing of fetal and placental tissue, the diagnosis of hypoluteoidism can be considered.

It is accepted that serum progesterone concentrations must be in excess of 2 ng/ml for maintenance

TABLE 21–1   CAUSES AND METHODS OF DIAGNOSIS OF CANINE ABORTIONS

CAUSATIVE AGENTS	CLINICAL FINDINGS	NECROPSY FINDINGS	TESTS
Bacteria			
Brucella canis	Third-trimester abortion	Autolyzed fetuses	Culture (special media): vaginal discharge and blood Serology: RSAT, TAT, and AGID
B. abortus, B. suis, or *B. melitensis*	History of contact with infected livestock Third-trimester abortion	Autolyzed fetuses	Serology: specific for organism
Salmonella spp.	Systemic disease in bitch Purulent vaginal discharge	Fetal septicemia	Culture: vaginal discharge and fetal tissues
Campylobacter spp.	History of diarrhea in bitch or contact humans	Placentitis	Culture (special media): vaginal discharge and fetal tissues
Escherichia coli or *Streptococcus* spp.	Purulent vaginal discharge Systemic disease in bitch	Fetal septicemia	Culture: vaginal discharge and fetal tissues
Viruses			
Canine herpesvirus	Third-trimester abortion Bitch asymptomatic Vaginal vesicles Stillbirth Infertility	Fetal septicemia Multifocal petechiae and necrosis in fetal adrenal glands, kidney, liver, and lung	Serology in bitch: paired samples 2 weeks apart, run together
Canine distemper or canine adenovirus	Systemic involvement in bitch	Depends on virus involved	Depends on virus involved
Other Organisms			
Mycoplasmataceae (*Mycoplasma* or *Ureaplasma* spp.)	Asymptomatic bitch housed in overcrowded conditions Vaginal discharge Infertility	Fetal septicemia	Culture: vaginal discharge and fetal tissues
Toxoplasma gondii	May be asymptomatic bitch or have multisystemic involvement	Placentitis Multiorgan involvement in fetus	Serology: Paired samples 2 weeks apart, run together (fourfold increase significant)
Endocrine Causes			
Progesterone deficiency	Infectious causes ruled out	None	Serial progesterone assays during luteal phase
Hypothyroidism	Obesity Lethargy Symmetric hair loss	None	TSH-stimulation test

AGID, Agar gel immunodiffusion test; *RSAT,* rapid slide agglutination test; *TAT,* tube agglutination test; *TSH,* thyroid-stimulating hormone.

of pregnancy. However, such concentrations are at the detection limits of ELISA kits, which usually estimate concentrations as less than 1 ng/ml, 1 to 5 ng/ml, and greater than 5 ng/ml. Precise determination of progesterone concentration is critical in the diagnosis. The veterinarian cannot be completely confident using in-hospital assay systems. The bitch described in the Purswell report may not have had hypoluteoidism, because the laboratory progesterone value at the time of diagnosis with the kit was rechecked and documented to be 6.5 ng/ml (Purswell, 1991). One value should be considered inadequate to confirm a diagnosis. Laboratory progesterone concentrations should be used to confirm or deny borderline results. Does the syndrome exist? Possibly.

If treatment is attempted for hypoluteoidism, several strategies can be employed. It is important to know the first day of diestrus, as defined with vaginal cytology (see Chapter 19). Exogenous progesterone should be discontinued after 50 to 53 days of diestrus (whelping typically occurs 55 to 58 days into diestrus). A recent study demonstrated that 3 mg/kg of progesterone in oil, intramuscularly, once daily (Progesterone Injection; Steris Laboratories Inc, Phoenix, AZ) is adequate to maintain serum concentrations above 10 ng/ml. Serum progesterone concentrations decreased below 2 ng/ml 48 to 72 hours after the final injection (Scott-Moncrieff et al, 1990). As little as 2 mg/kg every 48 hours may be sufficient to maintain pregnancy (Eilts, 1992). Alternatively, synthetic progesterone (17α-ethyl-19-nor-testosterone [Steraloids Inc, Denville, NJ]), 1 mg/kg SC daily, has been used successfully in maintaining pregnancy in ovariectomized bitches (Steinetz et al, 1989). The use of Ovaban (Schering, Union City, NJ) for preventing hypoluteoidism has not been described, although undocumented reports of 5 mg/day until day 55 of diestrus have been suggested.

An oral progestogen, allytrenbolone (Regumate, Hoechst RA), has been evaluated for maintaining pregnancy in ovariectomized bitches. Bitches were treated following ovariectomy on day 30 to 32 of pregnancy. Treatment was continued through day 54 of cytologic diestrus. The use of 0.044 mg/kg daily maintained pregnancy in only two of six pregnant bitches. The use of 0.088 mg/kg (0.2 cc/10 pounds) resulted in three of three bitches carrying their litters to term, with parturition beginning on the expected date in each. However, although two bitches had normal parturition, one had dystocia and death of all puppies. None of the bitches receiving the Regumate at either dosage had optimal milk production. Several litters were said to have been nursed by untreated controls, one bitch was able to nurse most of her litter 3 days after whelping, and one was able to nurse her entire litter beginning 3 days after whelping. Prolactin secretion was assumed to be suppressed by the drug in all bitches. If use of the drug is contemplated, clients must be warned that milk supplementation may be needed. In addition, the drug should not be used unless whelping dates have been reliably estimated, with serial progesterone concentrations obtained during proestrus and early estrus or with vaginal smears used for identifying day one of diestrus (Eilts, 1992).

Trauma. Trauma is an extremely unlikely cause for abortion. However, any significant blow to the abdomen has the potential of causing damage to the uterus or fetus, which could lead to abortion.

Nutrition, Drugs, Vaccines. These factors are considered uncommon causes for abortion. Each is reviewed in Chapter 20.

INFECTIOUS AGENTS. Numerous agents have been implicated in causing uterine infection, fetal death, and resorption or expulsion of litters from the bitch (see Table 21-1). These agents include *Brucella, Escherichia coli, Streptococcus,* herpesvirus, canine parvovirus, distemper virus, mycoplasma, *Campylobacter* species, *Toxoplasma,* and others. In our experience, confirming that a litter has been lost and that the cause was an infectious agent is quite difficult. If infection is to be pursued, it is recommended that fetal/placental or neonatal tissue, stomach and stomach contents, and vaginal swabs of the bitch be submitted for culture. Infectious agents, such as *Campylobacter,* may require special handling (Bulgin et al, 1984).

Brucella canis *Infection.* See Chapter 26.

Canine Herpesvirus Infection. Canine herpesvirus (CHV) is fairly ubiquitous in dogs, with 80% to 100% of certain populations having been exposed. Dogs in contact with many other dogs, via shows or in kennels with a great deal of turnover, are at greatest risk. Lifelong states of latent infection can occur, and immune responses are characterized as minimal and/or short-lived. Therefore, any serum-neutralizing antibody titer is significant, especially if coupled with clinical signs. Recrudescent canine herpes with virus shedding may be stimulated by the stress of pregnancy and parturition.

CHV infection in neonatal pups is an acute fatal infectious disease characterized by generalized focal necrosis and hemorrhage. The disease in adult dogs is usually subclinical or mild, such as conjunctivitis, serous or mucopurulent ocular and/or nasal discharges, and vaginal/vestibular/vulvar lesions that are vesicular early in the course of the disease and later become circular and pock-like. Genital lesions usually disappear shortly after infection, but they may reappear with the onset of proestrus. Canine herpes virus infection can result in fetal resorption and/or mummification if the bitch is infected early in gestation, abortion if the bitch is infected in mid-gestation, or premature birth if infection occurs in late pregnancy (England, 1998). A bitch may have dead and/or mummified fetuses in the same litter with unaffected live pups. Abortion has occurred between 44 to 51 days of gestation following infection on day 30. It is also possible for an infected bitch to be infertile or to have litters that are small in number. The fetal placenta from a bitch with canine herpesvirus infection is typically underdeveloped and congested. Several grayish white foci ranging in size from miliary to "rice grain" in size can be observed in the placental labyrinth. Sometimes the lesions form zonal structures 2 to 3 mm wide. Typical changes are also seen histologically.

Transmission of herpesvirus can occur venereally, transplacentally, via fetal contact with virus-filled vesicles that rupture during birth, or through respiratory routes of infection. Diagnosis depends on viral isolation. Viral isolation requires fastidious sampling and culture techniques from refrigerated but not frozen tissue. A negative culture for this virus may be due to inadequate methodology. Separation of infected animals from noninfected animals is advisable, especially in the final 3 weeks of gestation and the first 3 weeks of life. Because no vaccine is available for prevention, veterinarians can only recommend careful physical examination and review of the history from dogs to be used in a breeding program (Hashimoto and Hirai, 1986; Evermann, 1989).

Toxoplasmosis. This is an uncommon cause of canine abortion; dogs are an intermediate host for *Toxoplasma* infection. Cats are the only definitive host. Routes of infection include congenital exposure, ingestion of oocysts in cat feces, or ingestion of infected meat. Diagnosis should be suspected when paired serum samples obtained 3 weeks apart demonstrate a greater than fourfold increase in titer. Previous exposure can produce increased titers. Prevention is accomplished by preventing exposure to cat litter or raw meat.

Mycoplasma *and* Ureaplasma *Infections.* These microorganisms are among the recognized normal flora in the canine vagina. *Mycoplasma* and *Ureaplasma* isolates have been implicated in infertility, early embryonic death/resorption, abortion, stillbirths, and neonatal morbidity and mortality. Dogs may be exposed to large concentrations of these organisms in crowded kennel conditions. Diagnosis is always tentative at best because positive vaginal cultures may simply include normal flora, and identifying the pathologic situation usually depends on demonstrating pure infection with one of these organisms in a bitch with metritis/vaginitis. *Mycoplasma-* or *Ureaplasma-*induced abortion is rare. Treatment involves the administration of chloramphenicol or tetracycline for 10 to 14 days. These antibiotics should not be given to neonates or to nursing bitches. The pregnant bitch can be treated with erythromycin, although this antibiotic is not as effective and it may result in gastrointestinal problems (Lein, 1986; Purswell, 1992).

Signs

Among the signs suggestive of impending abortion are anorexia, listlessness, vomiting, fever, abdominal pain, vaginal discharge, and abdominal contractions. The only certain external sign of abortion is seeing the premature expulsion of living or dead fetuses. Palpation of fetuses that do not materialize is subjective and should not be considered reliable. Owners or veterinarians may see abdominal contractions before day 55 of gestation, which is suggestive of imminent abortion. Vaginal discharges, especially fetid or off-colored, during pregnancy are abnormal and worrisome because such a finding is seen in bitches that resorb or abort their litters. Clear, odorless, egg white–like vaginal discharges may not be worrisome. However, bloody, black, dark green, or purulent and fetid vaginal discharges often precede abortion due to infection. Similar discharges can also occur with vaginitis, vaginal foreign bodies, urinary tract problems, and other disorders unrelated to the pregnancy (see Treatment, below). The pregnant bitch with a concurrent illness is always in danger of aborting the litter because of the illness, its therapy, or the effects of stressful diagnostic testing.

Bitches have the potential for aborting a portion of a litter and carrying the remainder of the fetuses to term. If owners see their bitch abort, they should remember that viable fetuses may still remain within the uterus.

Diagnosis (Fig. 21-1)

Abdominal ultrasonography is a highly sensitive and reliable means of diagnosing pregnancy (as early as 16 days of gestation) and detecting viable fetuses by recognition of functioning hearts (as early as 24 days of gestation). Confirmation of pregnancy early in gestation using ultrasonography allows a veterinarian the opportunity to recognize loss of a few fetuses or an entire litter.

Abdominal radiography can also serve as a tool in recognition of pregnancy and, therefore, of abortion or resorption. This tool is not as reliable as abdominal ultrasonography because pregnancy cannot be confirmed radiographically until skeletal development is complete; after 42 to 45 days of gestation. Thereafter, collapse or decalcification of the skeleton, intrafetal gas, or an abnormal fetal position can be helpful in assessing viability of fetuses (Fig. 21-2).

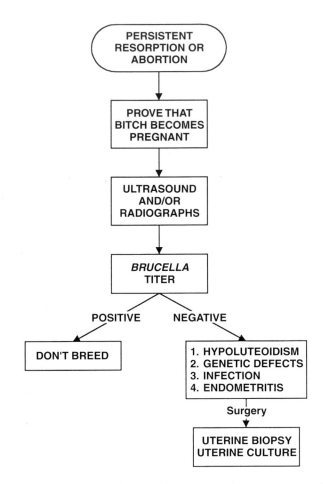

FIGURE 21–1. Algorithm on diagnosis and management of persistent resorption or abortion.

If a pregnant bitch is brought to the clinic exhibiting signs consistent with illness or abortion, the veterinarian must focus on completing a thorough history and physical examination. The reproductive history should include the results of previous matings and any previous problems possibly related to the reproductive tract. A careful accounting of this breeding and information regarding the male is imperative. Results of *Brucella* testing of the bitch and dog, as well as previous mates, are critical. Additional information to obtain includes vaccination and worming protocols; travel, contact, or exposure data; diets and supplements; environmental conditions; and medications (see Chapter 20). The physical examination should include careful and gentle abdominal palpation. Vaginal examination must be performed and culture and cytology obtained. Radiography and/or ultrasonography should be strongly considered. Blood and urine tests can be chosen as dictated by the history and physical examination. Titers for the various infectious agents may be diagnostic. Hormone assay for progesterone concentrations may be helpful in determining the likelihood of ovarian failure during the course of pregnancy. Low plasma progesterone concentrations (<2 ng/ml) indicate that corpora luteal

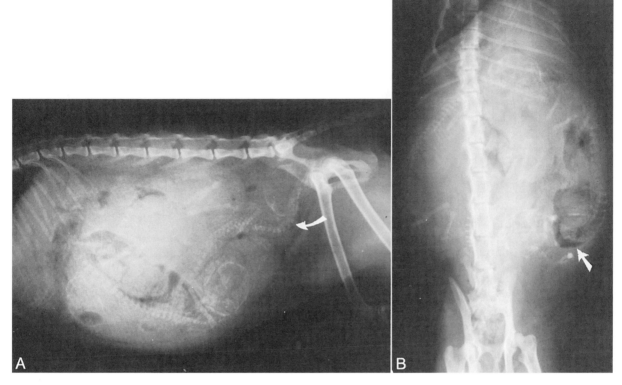

FIGURE 21–2. Lateral *(A)* and ventrodorsal *(B)* abdominal radiographs of a bitch with dead fetuses. Note the abnormal extension of the fetal neck *(arrow in A)* and the fetal gas best seen on the ventrodorsal view *(arrow in B)*.

function has failed as a primary defect or secondary to some other disorder.

If abortion/resorption is known to have taken place, a *Brucella* titer should be determined. Thorough necropsy of any fetus also may be informative. Bacterial or viral cultures of fetal and placental material are valuable, but results may be altered by contamination. The veterinarian must remember the long list of causes for abortion/resorption that cannot be detected using the few studies described here.

Any bitch undergoing cesarean section should also undergo complete inspection of her uterus and abdomen. Regardless of the number of ova released at ovulation or the ovary from which they arise, fetuses are normally implanted with equal and consistent spacing in both uterine horns. If obvious unequal spacing is recognized (i.e., four fetuses in one horn and one fetus in the other horn), the veterinarian should strongly suspect abortion or resorption of a portion of the litter during gestation. Close inspection with biopsy and culture of the uterus is strongly recommended in an effort to confirm suspicions of local or diffuse uterine abnormalities.

Treatment

PREVENTING ABORTION/RESORPTION. Therapy in the bitch with an impending abortion is surprisingly limited and is superficial at best (i.e., severely limiting exercise, administering antibiotics for obvious or suspected infection, and performing other diagnostic tests). One can obtain plasma for progesterone concentrations. Between days 15 and 50 of gestation, progesterone concentrations below 2 ng/ml may suggest hypoluteoidism (see discussion above); however, exogenous progesterone therapy must be used with caution even when the serum progesterone concentration is less than 1 ng/ml.

THE BITCH THAT HAS ABORTED A LITTER. The bitch that has a recent history of abortion and systemic illness should be evaluated for pyometra, retained or mummified fetuses, and/or retained placentas. Occasionally, palpation of the abdomen is sufficient to recognize these problems. The characteristics of any vaginal discharge may provide a clue in diagnosing ongoing uterine problems. A bitch with significant uterine infection rarely benefits from antibiotics alone. Prostaglandin therapy may be necessary if the owner wants to attempt future breeding (see pyometra, Chapter 23). Ovariohysterectomy may be considered if future breedings are not a priority.

The bitch that has aborted a litter but remains clinically healthy is easier to manage. A *Brucella* titer should be checked. If the bitch has aborted only once, she simply should be bred during the following estrus. If a bitch is *Brucella*-negative and has aborted several times, a different stud should be used. If that fails, monitoring plasma progesterone concentrations and ultrasonography of the fetuses during pregnancy may reveal a cause. Also, every attempt should be made to obtain a fetus or several fetuses immediately after they are aborted for necropsy and culture.

THE BITCH WITH RETAINED DEAD FETUSES. Rarely, a bitch is encountered that has dead fetuses in utero. This diagnosis can occasionally be made with abdominal radiography (see Fig. 21-2). The diagnosis is confirmed by using ultrasonography or surgery. Therapy involves ovariohysterectomy or uterotomy and removal of all fetuses. If the bitch has an open-cervix pyometra and the fetuses have undergone autolysis, prostaglandin therapy may be successful if fetal skeletal material is not present in utero. One bitch has been reported with severe hypercalcemia caused by retained fetus and endometritis (Hirt et al, 2000).

DYSTOCIA

Definition

Dystocia is defined as difficult birth or the inability to expel the conceptus from the uterus through the birth canal. Although dystocia is not a common problem in bitches, the condition occurs with enough frequency that veterinarians acquire some familiarity with the condition. However, management of dystocia is not always straightforward. Causes of dystocia are listed in Table 21-2 (Linde-Forsberg and Eneroth, 1998).

Practical Description

THE UTERUS. Uterine causes of dystocia include uterine weakness or insufficient uterine force to propel the conceptus through the birth canal. This is the type of dystocia most likely to respond to medical management.

THE PELVIS. If the birth canal is too small, dystocia results. This constriction may be the result of a congenitally small pelvic canal size or an acquired defect, such as the sequela to a pelvic fracture. Dystocia may also occur with various breeds that have a large head and a small pelvis (Bulldogs, Boston Terriers, etc.). These cases of dystocia usually require surgical intervention.

TABLE 21-2 CAUSES OF DYSTOCIA IN BITCHES AND QUEENS

Cause	Bitch (%)	Queen (%)
Maternal:	75.3	67.1
Primary complete inertia	48.9	36.8
Primary partial inertia	23.1	22.6
Birth canal too narrow	1.1	5.2
Uterine torsion	1.1	—
Uterine prolapse	—	0.6
Uterine strangulation	—	0.6
Hydrallantois	0.5	—
Vaginal septum formation	0.5	—
Fetal:	24.7	29.7
Malpresentations	15.4	15.5
Malformations	1.6	7.7
Fetal oversize	6.6	1.9
Fetal death	1.1	1.1

From Linde-Forsberg and Eneroth, 1998 (used with permission).

THE FETUS. Occasionally the fetus is too large for the birth canal. The most common explanation for fetal oversize is conception of a single fetus, potentially resulting in a fetus too large for the pelvic canal (Fig. 21-3). Normal "presentation" (posture of the fetus as it enters the pelvic canal) usually results in normal delivery (Fig 21-4, A, B). However, abnormal fetal presentation causes relative oversize. Examples of relative fetal oversize include headfirst presentation with retention of the forelegs, resulting in significantly increased shoulder width (Fig 21-4, C); breech presentation with retention of the rear legs (Fig 21-4, D); presentation of one foreleg and retention of the other; lateral or ventriflexion of the head (Fig 21-4, E, F); or transverse presentation (Fig 21-4, G; Johnston et al, 2001). These problems usually require surgical intervention. Fetal oversize typically does not result from breeding a large male to a small bitch. The bitch usually "dictates" the size of the newborn, whereas both bitch and stud determine adult size of their offspring.

THE VAGINAL VAULT. A bitch may be examined and found to have a puppy wedged in the vaginal vault. This may be caused by fetal oversize or an undersized pelvis. The vaginal vault itself may be too small, as occurs with a vaginal stricture (see Chapter 25 and Fig. 21-5) (Johnston et al, 2001). A vaginal stricture or band of tissue can obstruct fetal passage, resulting in the need for surgery or extensive manipulation. Vaginal strictures due to a band of tissue also usually prevent natural breeding. Such bands of tissue, however, do not prevent artificial insemination and may not be noted to be present.

Classic Description

PRIMARY UTERINE INERTIA. Failure of sufficient uterine contractions to expel the conceptus can be due to uterine inertia. In this situation, the bitch has a normal birth canal, normal-sized and normal presentation of fetuses, and fetuses that are small enough to pass through the birth canal. Despite these favorable factors, parturition may fail to proceed. *Complete inertia* indicates that no puppies are delivered because of apparent uterine muscle fatigue. *Incomplete inertia* occurs when there is normal delivery of a portion of the litter but the uterus fatigues before parturition is complete (Jones and Joshua, 1982).

Primary uterine inertia has been associated with an inherited breed predisposition in Terrier breeds, with overstretching of the uterus containing a large litter, with inadequate uterine stimulation in one- or two-pup litters, with systemic disease such as hypocalcemia or infection, and with inadequate nutrition, uterine torsion, and trauma (Johnston et al, 2001).

SECONDARY UTERINE INERTIA (FETAL OBSTRUCTION). With secondary uterine inertia, uterine contractions occur, but fatigue results from an unrelated cause. The fetus may be too large for the birth canal, as is seen with small bitches that have one fetus (Bennett, 1980). The fetus may simply grow beyond the limit of the

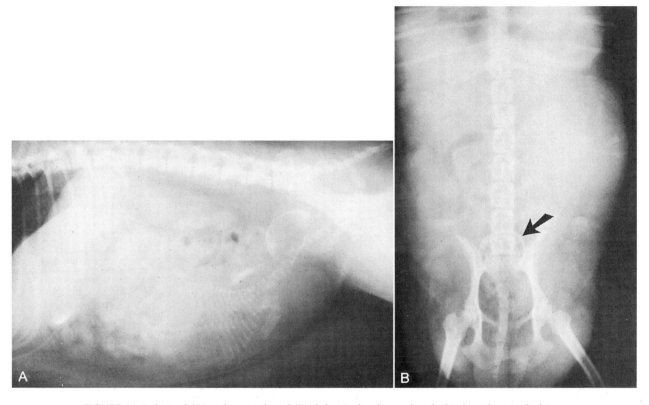

FIGURE 21–3. Lateral *(A)* and ventrodorsal *(B)* abdominal radiographs of a bitch with a single fetus. Notice the skull *(arrow)* width versus the pelvis width on the ventrodorsal view, which may possibly cause dystocia. Ligament relaxation can be difficult to predict. This fetus was delivered naturally with little apparent difficulty.

birth canal, as occurs with prolonged gestation. The fetus may be of normal size, but the birth canal may be too small for the conceptus. The small pelvic canal may be the result of previous pelvic fractures or other acquired anatomic defects. Congenitally, some breeds with a small pelvis and a large head can encounter dystocia problems. In addition, vaginal strictures, a vaginal mass, or insufficient dilation of the cervix can result in secondary inertia. Abnormal fetal positioning can also cause dystocia. One example here is the fetus with a head in one horn and rear quarters in the contralateral horn, resulting in presentation of the fetal trunk to the body of the uterus. Occasionally the head of the fetus is twisted, facing its tail, causing one shoulder to enter the uterine body. This position is typically larger than the dilated birth canal can accommodate (see previous discussion and Fig. 21-4). Fetal death can also cause abnormal positioning. Breech presentation is not included because it is normal and occurs in approximately 40% of deliveries.

MISCELLANEOUS CAUSES. The bitch that is nervous or frightened may actually inhibit her own uterine contractions (Shille, 1983). Such dogs should be provided with quiet, familiar surroundings. A veterinary hospital is often the least comfortable place for such an animal. Also, certain types of hernias (e.g., inguinal hernias) may entrap a fetus or an entire uterine horn. Uterine torsion has been reported, again making it impossible for normal whelping to proceed. Rarely, the obese bitch may have difficulty whelping (Donovan, 1980).

Breed Incidence

BRACHYCEPHALIC BREEDS. These breeds (Bulldogs, Pugs, Boston Terriers, Sealyham Terriers, Scottish Terriers, etc.) typically have a narrow or small pelvis with large heads and wide shoulders. These bitches are quite prone to secondary uterine inertia problems (Shille, 1983).

MINIATURE AND SMALL BREEDS. Not only are these dogs prone to small (1 or 2) litters, but subjectively, they are more often nervous and apprehensive. The psychologic state of the bitch can disrupt parturition and result in primary uterine inertia while a single fetus may be quite large, resulting in fetal obstruction.

LARGE BREEDS. As a group, large-breed bitches have a lower incidence of dystocia problems. However, occasionally, an extremely large litter of puppies is encountered. In this situation, incomplete uterine inertia may occur secondary to uterine fatigue or uterine over-stretching.

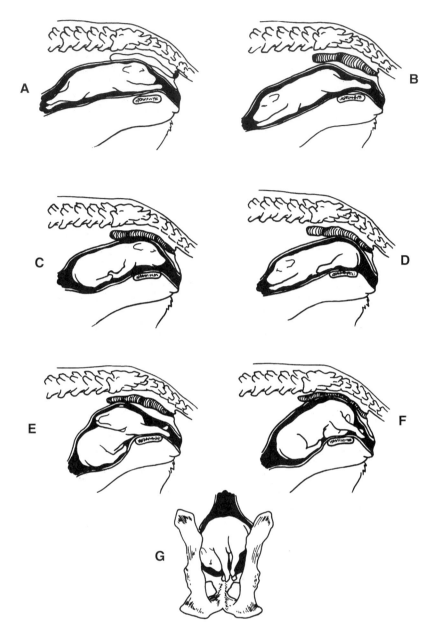

FIGURE 21–4. Fetal presentations, postures and positions. *A,* A normal cranial presentation. *B,* A normal caudal presentation. *C,* Front limbs are retained under the body. *D,* Rear limbs are retained under the body (breech posture). *E,* Lateral deviation of the neck. *F,* Ventral deviation of the neck. *G,* Transverse presentation. (From Johnston SD, Root Kustritz MV, Olson PNS. Canine and feline theriogenology. Philadelphia, WB Saunders Co, 2001, p 111; used with permission.)

Diagnosis (Fig. 21-6)

HISTORY. ***Definitions.*** The diagnosis of dystocia is usually based on owner observations. Dystocia is considered likely and veterinary consultation or examination is recommended when an owner reports one or more of the following: (1) 20 to 30 minutes of strong abdominal contractions without successful expelling of a puppy; (2) after delivering one or more puppies, more than 4 to 6 hours pass without another birth in a bitch known or suspected of having additional fetuses in utero; (3) a bitch fails to deliver pups 24 to 36 hours after the rectal temperature was noted to decrease below 100° F; (4) a bitch cries and licks or bites at the vulvar area during whelping; (5) a bitch fails to progress to stage II labor after 8 to 12 hours of apparent stage I labor; or (6) a bitch has prolonged gestation, lasting beyond a well-established due date, beyond 70 to 72 days from the first breeding, or beyond 60 days from the first day of diestrus (Schweizer and Meyers-Wallen, 1999).

General Considerations. Factors such as the bitch's age, reproductive history, and previous or current medical conditions may be more important than breed. Age, for example, is important because the 2-year-old bitch is less prone to primary uterine inertia

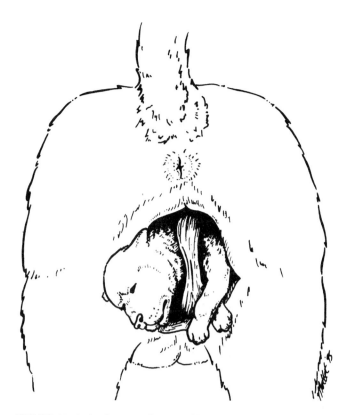

FIGURE 21–5. A schematic diagram illustrating how a dystocia can result from residual vaginal bands of tissue (hymen). (From Johnston SD, Root Kustritz MV, Olson PNS. Canine and feline theriogenology. Philadelphia, WB Saunders Co, 2001, p 114; used with permission.)

than is a 6- or 7-year-old. Heart problems, as another example, may become enhanced during the muscular exertion associated with labor.

Use of Breeding Dates. A thorough history can be valuable with any potential dystocia. It is helpful to be aware of any previous whelping difficulties or cesarean sections. If the first day of diestrus has been identified or the breeding dates are known, an approximate due date can be derived. The inexperienced owner may become concerned if day 63 of gestation passes without the bitch whelping. Owners need to be made aware that the average bitch does whelp on day 63 or 64, counting from the first breeding day. However, using the first day of breeding, whelping can occur in normal bitches at any time between days 56 and 72 of gestation.

Vaginal Cytology and/or Litter Size. Daily vaginal cytology can be used with excellent reliability to detect the first day of diestrus and, then, gestation length. Gestation lasts 56 to 58 diestrus days. With either vaginal cytology or breeding dates, litter size helps to further define likely whelping dates. Large litters have a shorter gestation length (56 diestrus days), and small litters experience longer gestation (58 diestrus days). For example, an owner worried because a 20-kg bitch with two fetuses has reached postbreeding day 64 without whelping may be informed that gestation

could be normal and may last 65 to 70 days. Often, a bitch thought to have primary uterine inertia, based on duration of gestation, has yet to enter stage I of labor.

Single Serum Progesterone. One serum progesterone concentration obtained during estrus can aid in determining whelping dates. Gestation length (from the day of obtaining a single serum progesterone concentration of 1.0 to 1.9 ng/ml during estrus) averages 65 days—64 days if the progesterone was between 2.0 and 3.9, and 62.4 days if 4.0 to 10.0 ng/ml (Johnston et al, 2001). These results, however, are not as reliable as recognizing the first day of diestrus with vaginal cytology (as previously discussed).

Owner Observations: Rectal Temperature. Most bitches exhibit a decrease in rectal temperature 12 to 24 hours (sometimes 48 hours) before onset of stage II labor. The temperature drop is usually 1° to 3° in magnitude and the temperature falls below 99° F. This temperature drop is associated with the abrupt and final drop in serum progesterone to basal levels.

Owner Observations: Labor. The timing of signs consistent with stage I labor (restlessness) or stage II labor (abdominal contractions) should be noted. Stage I signs can persist for 3 to 24 hours before actual abdominal contractions begin. Therefore, some owners simply need to be patient. However, 20 to 30 minutes of obvious abdominal contractions without delivery of a puppy is reason for concern. The frequency and intensity of expulsive efforts should be appraised, as well as the number of puppies delivered and their condition. Asking the owner about these events may help a veterinarian diagnose dystocia or determine how thoroughly an owner has observed the whelping. The time interval between delivery of each puppy is also an aid in recognizing dystocia.

Birth Rate. Puppies are delivered, on average, every 30 to 60 minutes. Several puppies may be born within a period of minutes. However, bitches may "rest" periodically during whelping for several hours. These rests are not associated with abdominal contractions and usually do not persist beyond 4 to 6 hours (Schweizer and Meyers-Wallen, 1999). The veterinarian needs to know the health of the bitch and whether any medications or other treatments have been attempted by the owner.

Size of the Stud. In general, the size of the stud dog is not helpful in the diagnosis of dystocia. Use of large males, relative to the height and weight of the bitch, does not result in an increased incidence of dystocia. The bitch and uterus are major determinants of fetal size in utero. The male does, however, affect the size of his adult offspring.

Uterine and Fetal Monitoring. The standard approach of guessing breeding dates, relying on subjective behavior observation of the bitch, measuring rectal temperature, and watching the progression of whelping through the eyes of the owner via a phone conversation is certainly far from ideal. The use of uterine and fetal monitors allows veterinarians to detect the onset of labor and to manage labor medically with greater accuracy. Recently, such systems for

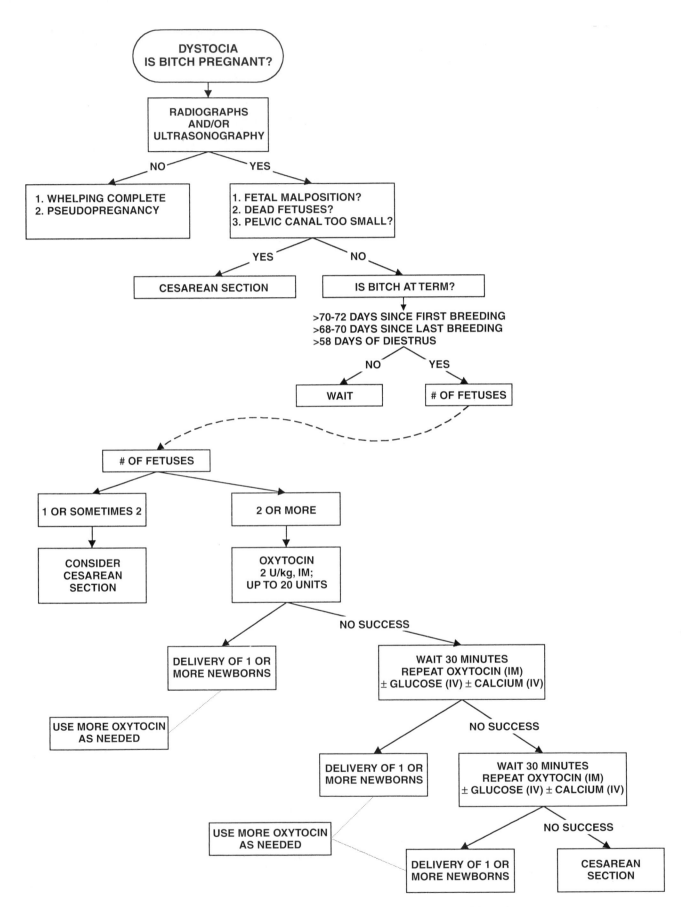

FIGURE 21–6. Algorithm on diagnosis and management of dystocia.

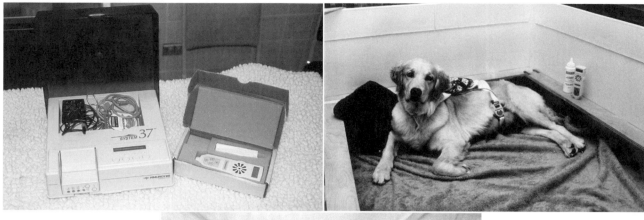

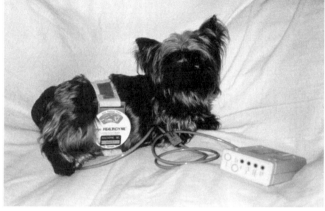

FIGURE 21–7. *A,* Whelping monitoring equipment includes a sensor, transducer, modem, and hand-held Doppler. This equipment can be used in large dogs *(B)* and small dogs or cats *(C)*. (From Dr. AP Davidson; used with permission.)

monitoring labor and delivery in the bitch have become commercially available (Davidson, 2000; Barber and Coley, 2000; Davidson, 2001). Commercially available services have been established by nurses trained in human obstetrical medicine.

Monitoring is recommended for inexperienced breeders, bitches with a history of whelping difficulty, bitches that are greater than 6 years of age (although we believe no bitch should be bred after 6 years of age), and bitches with unusually large or small litters. Radiographs should first be obtained after 45 days of gestation to determine litter size. Use of all fetal monitoring equipment (Fig. 21-7) is demonstrated by the veterinarian to the client well before the bitch is due to whelp. The hair coat of the bitch is lightly clipped over the gravid area of the lateral flanks to allow proper contact of the uterine sensor and fetal Doppler with acoustic gel.

The canine uterus exhibits characteristic patterns of activity during late gestation and labor, varying in strength and frequency. It is recommended that monitoring begin at least 1 week before predicted whelping dates, and is generally performed twice daily. Once a bitch enters stage I labor, the subsequent frequency of monitoring is based on recommendations of the nurse and the veterinarian. If problems are encountered and medication is deemed necessary, the

dog can be brought to the veterinarian. The uterine monitoring system consists of a tocodynamometer (sensor), a recorder, and a modem. The uterine sensor detects changes in intrauterine and intra-amniotic pressures. The sensor is maintained over the caudolateral abdomen with an elasticized strap. The recorder of the sensor is worn in a small backpack placed over the caudal shoulder area (Fig. 21-8). Bitches should be at rest in a whelping box crate during monitoring sessions. Fetal Doppler cardiac monitoring is performed with a hand-held unit on bitches in lateral recumbency. Directing the Doppler perpendicularly over a fetus causes a characteristic amplification of the fetal heart sounds, distinct from maternal arterial or cardiac sounds. After each session, data are transferred from the recorder via modem through the client's telephone to the nurse. The nurse then communicates acquired information and an interpretation to the veterinarian. The veterinarian, in turn, contacts the owner.

Generally, the two drugs most commonly recommended to treat uterine inertia, after fetal monitoring, are calcium and oxytocin. Administration of calcium gluconate increases strength of myometrial contractions, and oxytocin increases the frequency of contractions. Calcium is recommended when ineffective and weak uterine contractions are detected. Oxytocin is recommended when uterine contractions are less

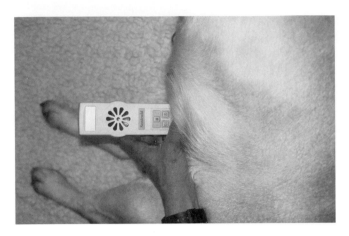

FIGURE 21–8. Uterine monitor placed over a lightly clipped region of the canine caudolateral abdomen, with the recorder in a harness worn over the scapulae. (From Dr. AP Davidson; used with permission.)

frequent than expected for the stage of labor and when fetal heart rates are normal. Uterine hyperstimulation with elevated baseline levels of contractility compromising placental blood supply, or a uterine obstructive pattern negate further use of calcium or oxytocin. Fetal distress is reflected by sustained deceleration of heart rates. Transient accelerations are noted with fetal movement. If fetal stress is evident and response to medication is poor, surgical intervention (cesarean section) may be indicated.

PHYSICAL EXAMINATION. Ideally, the bitch with suspected or known dystocia should undergo a complete physical examination before examination of the reproductive tract. However, initial examination of the vaginal area should take precedence to determine whether a fetus is present within the vaginal canal. If no fetus is visible or palpated in the vaginal canal, a quick but thorough physical examination should be completed to be certain that contributing problems (e.g., cardiac arrhythmias, dehydration, fever) are not missed. Sometimes, a concurrent problem is of greater concern than the dystocia, and occasionally, correction of an underlying problem such as hypoglycemia or hypocalcemia simultaneously treats the dystocia. If a bitch is nervous or trembling, the veterinarian must differentiate among anxiety, pain, and hypocalcemia.

The reproductive examination should include careful abdominal palpation, as well as digital examination and assessment of the vaginal vault. If no fetuses are identified in utero or in the vaginal vault, the bitch may have finished whelping or she could be in exaggerated clinical pseudopregnancy. If a fetus is palpated in the vaginal vault, its physical position and viability can be assessed. The vaginal vault can also be assessed for the presence of strictures, bands, or other defects.

The finding of significant amounts of fresh blood in the vaginal vault can be confusing. The presence of blood may be caused by normal events during whelping, but it can also be due to separation of placental sites, a condition that may be best managed with

surgery. Other causes of hemorrhage (coagulopathies, trauma to the vaginal lining, etc.) must always be considered.

RADIOGRAPHY AND/OR ULTRASONOGRAPHY. The most valuable tests that a veterinarian can perform on a bitch with possible dystocia are radiography and ultrasonography of the abdomen. Radiographs identify or dismiss the presence of pregnancy and are excellent for locating fetuses and identifying malpositioned fetuses that cannot be delivered vaginally. Ultrasonography is a superb means of assessing fetal viability. These studies should follow a thorough physical examination and review of the history.

The first condition established by the radiographs is the presence or absence of pregnancy. The nonpregnant bitch either has completed whelping or was only pseudopregnant. If pregnancy is confirmed, the veterinarian must ask the following: Are the fetuses viable? How many are present? Abdominal auscultation may answer the question of fetal viability if heart beats are heard, but not if heart beats cannot be auscultated. Ultrasonography definitively identifies contracting fetal hearts and is therefore a means of assessing viability. Ultrasonography also allows assessment of fetal heart rates. Heart rates of 150 to 200 bpm are normal, but rates below 150 bpm are cause for concern, especially when the rate is less than 100 bpm. If fetal movement does not result in upward rate excursions or if several minutes of observation do not reveal increases in heart rate, fetal distress is likely (Schweizer and Meyers-Wallen, 1999). If medical management is being considered, ultrasonography should be repeated every hour.

Fetal death is likely if the veterinarian finds on radiographs (1) evidence of collapse of the spinal column, (2) intrafetal gas patterns, (3) overlapping or misalignment of the bones that make up the skull, or (4) obviously abnormal fetal positioning (see Fig. 21-2). Radiographs also identify the presence of an obviously large single fetus with little chance of normal delivery. Radiographs may diagnose several normal fetuses that have not been delivered because of uterine inertia or because labor has not yet begun. Finally, radiographs allow an examination of the pelvic structure of the bitch, possibly identifying an obstruction (Rendano, 1983).

BLOOD AND/OR URINE STUDIES. Usually little time is available for laboratory assessment of the bitch with dystocia. However, the blood glucose, blood urea nitrogen, hematocrit, and urinalysis are all valuable diagnostic studies that can be evaluated in the hospital, using reagent sticks or simple centrifugation (packed cell volume). The serum calcium concentration is an important parameter to assess in bitches with dystocia, but most hospitals cannot quickly obtain this information.

Criteria for Diagnosis

Table 21-3 outlines the various criteria that are strongly suggestive of dystocia. If a bitch meets any of these

TABLE 21–3 CRITERIA FOR DIAGNOSIS OF DYSTOCIA

Prolonged gestation
>70–72 days from day of first breeding
>60 days of diestrus
Pelvic obstruction
Breed likelihood
Mass lesion or previous fracture
Strong contractions >45–60 min without expulsion of a puppy
Weak and infrequent contractions for >4–6 hr without expulsion of a puppy
Failure to enter labor 24–36 hr after the rectal temperature falls below 99°F
A bitch in obvious pain that is failing to expel a puppy
Obvious radiographic abnormalities
Malposition
Fetal gas suggestive of fetal death
Fetal oversize (single pup?)
Fetal death
Previous history of dystocia
An obviously ill or weak bitch

criteria, rapid institution of manual, medical, or surgical intervention is warranted.

Treatment

MANUAL THERAPY (FIG. 21-9). Palpation of the cervix is not possible in the bitch (see Chapter 19). Therefore, it is not possible to assess cervical dilation digitally or to determine whether a fetus is unable to pass through a narrowed cervix. These are rare problems in the bitch. Manual therapy is restricted solely to delivering a puppy lodged within the vaginal vault. For most situations, the fingers are the safest and most reliable tools available. Liberal use of lubricants and gentle traction on a living or dead fetus are the only therapies needed in some bitches. It is often difficult to know whether the newborn is alive, especially if it is weak. Use of gauze sponges helps to maintain a hold on a fetus. The bitch should be in a standing position to improve chances of delivery (Shille, 1983).

The vaginal vault is too small in most bitches to allow significant digital manipulation of the conceptus. Unfortunately, the veterinarian must then rely on lubrication and instrumentation. A spay hook, nonratcheted sponge forceps, and placental forceps are the instruments least likely to damage either the bitch or her newborn. Occasionally, turning the fetus to one side alleviates the obstruction. One finger must always be placed in the vaginal vault to direct the instrument. Gentle traction, avoiding the distal extremities, offers the best chance of successful delivery. Abdominal or rectal palpation may assist in placing instruments. The mouth of the newborn may be recognized by sucking action on the finger or by palpation of the ridges composing the hard palate.

The traction placed on a conceptus should be in a posterior and ventral direction, following the anatomy of the vaginal vault. Gentle shifting of the conceptus

from side to side may help release the obstruction. Although sterile technique is always recommended, it is nearly impossible to maintain.

Avoiding damage to the walls of the vaginal vault is imperative but quite difficult. Any bitch undergoing significant manipulation should be thoroughly examined for traumatic problems following the procedure, using vaginoscopy whenever possible. Before breeding in any subsequent estrus, a vaginal examination should again be performed to ensure that adhesions or other anatomic disturbances have not occurred. The decision to manage a dystocia with external manipulation must always be weighed against the ease of performing a cesarean section.

Throughout all fetal manipulations, several concepts should be remembered. First, the health of the bitch usually takes priority. Second, progress needs to be obvious. If no progress is being made in exteriorizing a fetus in 5 to 10 minutes, seriously consider cesarean section.

MEDICAL MANAGEMENT. *Uterine Inertia.* *General Approach.* If complete or incomplete uterine inertia has been diagnosed, medical management is usually successful. One must be certain that fetal or maternal obstructions are not present. Medical management consists of stimulating uterine contractions. If these contractions take place against an obstruction, uterine rupture and/or fetal death could result. Inducing uterine contraction against an obstruction may cause separation of placental sites, resulting in fetal hypoxia, anoxia, and/or possible fetal death.

Oxytocin. Oxytocin is the drug used to stimulate uterine contractions. An initial arbitrary dose of 5 to 20 units may be used. We recommend 2 units/kg, up to 20 units, intramuscularly (see Fig. 21-6). The bitch should be placed in a quiet, warm environment and should be observed by veterinary personnel. If no response is seen within 30 to 40 minutes, a second dose should be administered. This second injection of oxytocin should be preceded by the slow intravenous injection of 2 to 10 ml of 10% calcium gluconate. The infusion should be slowed or stopped if cardiac arrhythmias are detected. If an additional 30 to 40 minutes pass without passage of a puppy or at least some abdominal contractions, a third injection of oxytocin can be given. This oxytocin injection should be accompanied by administration of 5 to 10 ml of 50% dextrose in a slow intravenous infusion (see Fig. 21-6).

If the third injection of oxytocin does not result in expulsion of at least one fetus, a cesarean section is recommended. If oxytocin does cause delivery of a fetus, it is reasonable to wait 30 to 60 minutes to determine whether the bitch requires additional oxytocin. Oxytocin can be administered every hour, if needed and successful.

Oxytocin is also used in the induction of labor in pregnant women. In this situation, oxytocin is administered slowly in the form of a dilute intravenous solution containing approximately 10 units of oxytocin per liter of 5% dextrose. The rate of adminis-

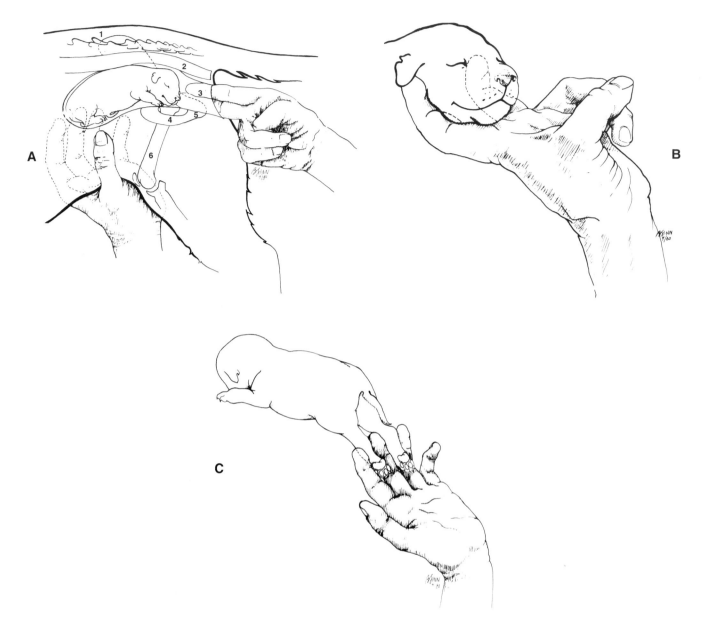

FIGURE 21–9. *A,* Determination of the fetal disposition when the head has entered the vaginal canal. The bitch should be standing for this procedure. (*1,* right wing of ilium; *2,* rectum; *3,* lumen of vaginal vestibule; *4,* right half of pubic symphysis; *5,* right wing of ischium; *6,* right femur.) *B,* The index and middle fingers are used to guide the head and to exert moderate traction in a cranial presentation. *C,* Manual traction as applied in a caudal presentation. The fingers should be positioned proximal to the hocks for best results. (From Shille VM: Diagnosis and management of dystocia in the bitch and queen. In Bojrab MJ (ed): Current Techniques in Small Animal Surgery. Philadelphia, Lea & Febiger, 1983, p 338; used with permission.)

tration can be gradually increased until effective contractions occur. If oxytocin is administered too rapidly or in too large a dose, intramuscularly or intravenously, tetanic contractions of the uterus occur. These contractions are of no value in expelling a fetus and may impair placental blood supply or cause a tear in the uterine wall.

We have had experience with both the intramuscular and intravenous administration protocols. Subjectively, the intravenous method appears more effective. Using a pediatric infusion set, the veterinarian can increase the initial slow infusion rate, at 15-minute intervals, until the desired response is achieved. This approach requires close patient monitoring.

Uterine tetany or tetanic contractions are not easily diagnosed. In the bitch, one sees extremely strong, intense contractions persisting for several minutes or longer. This recurs and resembles what would be seen in an obstructive dystocia (i.e., strong contractions without fetal expulsion). Uterine tetany is a poorly coordinated contraction that fails to propel the conceptus posteriorly. One must lower the oxytocin dose by at least 50% before successful coordinated contractions can be achieved.

TABLE 21-4 INDICATIONS FOR CESAREAN SECTION

Uterine inertia unresponsive to oxytocin
Pelvic obstruction
Fetal oversize
Vaginal obstruction that cannot be manipulated
In utero fetal death
Planned surgery

The Agitated or Nervous Bitch. Extreme excitement, fear, or nervousness (in the bitch or in the owner) can interfere with labor. If these traits are observed in the owner, he or she should be encouraged to leave the bitch to trained personnel. If these signs are observed in a bitch, it is occasionally helpful to lightly sedate her, helping her to relax so that whelping is allowed to proceed. Use of a conservative dose of acepromazine can be beneficial. In some cases, labor proceeds without any other manipulation or medication.

CESAREAN SECTION. *General.* Surgical removal of puppies from the uterus is a relatively safe, simple, and successful procedure. When other means of management fail (Table 21-4), cesarean section is well warranted. Numerous surgical and anesthetic review articles are available for current techniques (Probst and Webb, 1983; Gaudet and Kitchell, 1985; Funkquist et al, 1997). It is safe to state that mortality rates of bitches and puppies undergoing cesarean section in the United States and Canada are low. The most common methods for inducing and maintaining anesthesia are isoflurane alone or propofol for induction and isoflurane for maintenance. The most common breeds undergoing emergency surgery are the Bulldog, Labrador Retriever, Boxer, Corgi, and Chihuahua. Elective surgeries are most common in the Bulldog, Labrador Retriever, Mastiff, Golden Retriever, and Yorkshire Terrier (Moon et al, 1998). It should be pointed out that women who have had a cesarean section are at greater risk for uterine rupture during subsequent labors, especially if their labor is induced (Lydon-Rochelle et al, 2001). The need for repeat cesarean section in dogs and cats has not been evaluated.

Planning. Certain breeds are highly prone to dystocia. It is wise to be able to closely predict correct whelping due dates in order to avoid unnecessary surprises or emergencies. Such predictions are reliable and easy to achieve, allowing ready application to practical clinical situations (see Chapter 19). The owner of a bitch likely to require cesarean section can be taught how to obtain vaginal cytology smears. Each slide is dated. Smears should be obtained from the first day of standing heat until 7 days after the day of first refusal to breed. Each slide is air dried. The entire series of slides, unstained, can be delivered to the veterinarian for staining and review. The first day of diestrus is then identified (see Chapter 19).

Approximately 45 to 50 days into diestrus, abdominal radiographs should be obtained. The number of fetuses can then be counted. Small litters (one or two

puppies) should be assigned a due date of day 58 or 59 of diestrus. Large litters have shorter gestation duration and should have a due date of day 55 or 56 of diestrus. Average-sized litters should be delivered on day 57 of diestrus. Predictions are not perfect but do identify rather precise and logical whelping times for both the veterinarian and owner. Any bitch with a previous history of dystocia or from a breed prone to this problem should be evaluated using this simple procedure. Cesarean section should be scheduled 48 hours before the date that a bitch is due to whelp. In this manner, the surgery should precede labor but not take place at a time when the puppies would be too premature for survival.

Lack of Planning. Without accurate assessment of gestation duration based on vaginal cytology and/or serial progesterone determinations, cesarean section surgery always entails some risk. The risk is minimal if the bitch is an obvious dystocia patient. In this situation, the surgery is warranted and the primary risk is to the fetus(es) if the surgery is performed too late. Without an obvious set of signs confirming dystocia, the primary risk is that the surgery is performed too soon for neonatal survival. In this latter situation, it is always wise to be certain that the bitch is at least 57 days from her last breeding. One can use the criterion of 63 to 65 days after her first breeding, but this is the least reliable determinant.

PROLONGED GESTATION

Duration of gestation is quite variable if determined from date of first or last breeding. Based on breeding dates, whelping can begin as early as day 54 or as late as day 72. The inability to predict whelping dates more accurately, using breeding dates, is a reflection of the variation in duration of estrus (standing heat) of healthy bitches and the fact that canine spermatozoa are capable of fertilization for a period of 4 to 11 days from a single breeding. However, the duration of gestation can be reliably estimated if serial vaginal cytologic smears are obtained, serial serum progesterone concentrations are determined, or serial vaginal endoscopies are evaluated (see Chapter 19). Prolonged duration of pregnancy is of concern if it lasts beyond day 60 of confirmed diestrus (using vaginal cytology), beyond day 66 from the LH surge (using serial serum progesterones or vaginoscopy), or beyond day 68 from the date of first breeding.

The history should be evaluated to determine how whelping dates were determined. Abdominal radiography and/or ultrasonography must be evaluated, after a thorough physical examination is completed, to confirm that the bitch is pregnant as opposed to pseudopregnant. Ultrasonography is the preferred tool when fetal viability is to be assessed. If pregnant, the bitch may be healthy and nearing the end of a normal gestation. Radiographs can be used to assess approximate fetal age, by looking at their teeth for example (see Chapter 20). Fetal death can be associated with an apparent prolongation of gestation due to absence of fetal stress and the cascade of events culminating in parturition.

The bitch with a litter of dead fetuses usually requires surgery to remove the fetuses and to avoid infection. Gestation length may be abnormally prolonged with primary uterine inertia. In this situation, puppies cannot be delivered because of inadequate uterine contractions. Gestation may also be prolonged if a single fetus is present, presumably because a single fetus is less stressed in utero, delaying the onset of parturition. Severe hypocalcemia is uncommon in the prepartum bitch because she is not lactating or is lactating only small quantities of milk. However, mild hypocalcemia may decrease the number or strength of uterine contractions sufficient to create stage I or stage II labor.

The bitch with prolonged gestation is managed best following a thorough history and physical examination. As a general rule, if the bitch is healthy, if the fetuses are viable, and if gestation length is less than 70 days from the first day of breeding, the bitch should be returned home with the owner. The owner is instructed to monitor rectal temperature twice daily in order to help detect the onset of parturition. If stage II labor is not apparent within 48 hours after the drop in rectal temperature to less than 100° F or if gestation length exceeds 70 days from the first day of breeding, a cesarean section is recommended.

VULVAR DISCHARGE IN THE TERM BITCH

Green Discharge: Separation of Placental Sites

Lochia, or uteroverdin, is the green vulvar discharge observed following placental separation. Pigment originates at the margins of the zonary placenta. The uterus and the placenta surrounding the fetus must separate (placental separation) before the fetus can be born and the placenta passed. Thus a green vulvar discharge with or without small amounts of blood indicates that stage II labor will soon be seen and that puppies should quickly follow. If whelping does not begin within 2 hours of the time that lochia is observed, the bitch may be experiencing dystocia and veterinary attention is recommended.

Placental separation may occur days to weeks before parturition. This difficult problem should initially be assessed with a complete history and physical examination to determine whether the bitch has an unrelated problem, such as a coagulopathy or vaginal foreign body. The veterinarian can also determine whether there is any evidence of trauma. A complete blood count to assess for anemia and infection is warranted. Abdominal ultrasonography is recommended to determine viability of the fetus(es). Both tests are of great value in determining whether infection/metritis is a possibility and in determining whether surgical intervention is warranted. If no treatable problems are identified, all exercise involving the bitch should be discontinued and she should be kept as quiet as possible until the vaginal discharge is absent for several days or until after parturition. Remember that separation of placental sites can threaten the lives of the entire litter or only a portion of a litter, while the balance may remain quite healthy and be delivered at term (Olson, 1988).

Water-Like/Serous Vaginal Discharge

Water-like or "egg white–like" vulvar discharge in a term bitch often indicates that parturition is beginning. An owner may see a clear or water-filled bubble or balloon protruding from the vulva. This also could represent allantoic or amniotic fluid. If neonates are not delivered within 2 hours of these observations, the bitch should be examined for dystocia. Until a problem seems likely, however, the owner should be assured that his or her bitch is most likely normal and about to begin delivery of puppies.

Purulent Vaginal Discharge

Metritis may be present in the systemically ill bitch with a purulent vulvar discharge and a fever. If the bitch appears healthy, vaginitis (due to any cause) is more likely, although early stages of metritis may be present. As with many problems, the veterinarian must complete a thorough history and physical examination before pursuing diagnostic tests or reaching any conclusions. Complete blood counts and abdominal ultrasonography can be helpful in defining the location of the problem, in determining pregnancy, in assessing fetal viability, and in understanding the likelihood of infection.

Vaginal smears are usually not helpful or definitive, as degenerative neutrophils, free bacteria, and phagocytized bacteria are seen in smears from healthy bitches as well as those with metritis or vaginitis. Dogs with closed-cervix pyometra may not have bacteria in their vaginal cytologic smear. Skeletal muscle fibers are rarely observed in vaginal smears from bitches with metritis secondary to decomposing fetuses. It is possible, although quite rare, for a bitch to be pregnant with healthy fetuses in one uterine horn and to have a metritis/pyometra (open or closed cervix) in the other (Olson, 1988).

Blood: Hemorrhagic Vaginal Discharge

The normal vulvar discharge from the bitch, immediately preceding parturition, consists of small amounts of blood and/or greenish lochia. We occasionally receive phone calls regarding a term bitch with "large amounts of blood" from the vulva. Most of these calls are from concerned but inexperienced owners who overstate the situation. Most of these bitches are normal. However, a large amount of blood is worrisome, because it may be an indicator of dystocia, uterine/vaginal trauma, uterine torsion, coagulopathies, or excessive bleeding from placental sites of attachment. Uterine torsions result in a quickly deteriorating shock-like state associated with severe abdominal pain. If the decision is made to examine a pregnant bitch because of a bloody vaginal discharge, a history and complete physical examination are critically important. Vaginoscopy may be warranted to determine whether there has been any trauma to the vagina. The veterinarian is also obligated to at least assess her for anemia, fetal viability (via ultrasonography), and the location of any unborn fetuses that might be contributing to the blood.

SYSTEMIC ILLNESS IN THE TERM BITCH

The pregnant bitch with significant systemic illness represents a special challenge, because the owner and veterinarian want to help the bitch but not harm her litter. Unfortunately, this is not always possible. Close and honest communication with owners is imperative, because treatment directed at helping the bitch may harm or kill the litter. The veterinarian must initially establish what is wrong with the bitch (history and physical examination), determine whether she is pregnant, and evaluate the litter for viability. Uterine retention of dead fetuses is dangerous because of the potential for septicemia or toxemia.

Pregnancy toxemia is associated with inappetence/anorexia, lethargy, weakness, vomiting, and/or diarrhea. These bitches may have ketonuria without glycosuria, hypoglycemia, and abnormalities in serum liver enzymes or function test results. White blood cell numbers can be extremely depressed with a degenerative left shift. Alternatively, the white blood cell count may be dramatically increased owing to sepsis. Treatment consists of aggressive fluid therapy with dextrose-containing solutions and parenteral administration of appropriate antibiotics (ampicillin or Clavamox?). Cesarean section or ovariohysterectomy should be considered as soon as the bitch is deemed stable enough to withstand anesthesia. If glucocorticoids are administered for shock or to control severe immune-mediated disease, they may induce parturition, although this usually requires several days (Olson, 1988).

POSTWHELP OXYTOCIN INJECTION

Many veterinarians recommend administration of oxytocin at the end of parturition. This injection is thought to aid in expelling any retained placenta or fetuses, to hasten uterine involution, and to decrease postpartum hemorrhage. Other veterinarians have claimed that the injection does little good and is unnecessary. Subjectively, intramuscular oxytocin at 5 to 20 units or 2 units/kg, up to 20 units, has not been harmful. On request, injections are administered, although they are not strongly encouraged.

POSTPARTUM ENDOMETRITIS (ACUTE METRITIS)

Most normal bitches develop a mild fever (<104° F) without any related signs in the 24 to 48 hours immediately following parturition. However, if a bitch becomes clinically ill within 1 to 7 days of whelping, acute metritis should be considered. A similar disease entity may follow nonsterile artificial inseminations but rarely follows natural mating. Acute metritis in the postpartum period may be the result of dystocia, obstetric manipulations, the presence of devitalized uterine tissue, or retention of either a fetus or a placenta. Bacterial infection is usually the result of uterine invasion from the vaginal tract and overgrowth within the endometrium.

Signs seen by the owner usually consist of foul-smelling brownish or reddish brown vaginal discharge (remember that normal lochia is not foul smelling and is greenish in color), anorexia, listlessness, decreased or absent maternal instincts, fever, and decreased or absent milk production. Rarely, dogs may have concurrent septic polyarthritis. Counting placentas may aid in recognizing a retention problem. However, bitches are notorious for consuming a placenta when the owner's back is turned. On physical examination, the veterinarian should detect the vaginal discharge observed by the owner. An enlarged uterus or a "doughy" abdomen should be palpable. The bitch may appear stable or dehydrated, or she may be in shock and critically ill.

A complete blood count (CBC) usually reveals a leukocytosis with a left shift (leukopenia may occur in quite ill bitches). Vaginal cytology usually includes neutrophils (increased numbers and many degenerated), red blood cells, debris, mucus, bacteria (free and/or phagocytized), and perhaps endometrial cells (Olson et al, 1984). Chemistry abnormalities are related to dehydration and septicemia. Radiography reveals an enlarged uterus, which is of little help because all bitches have an enlarged uterus for the first few days after whelping. However, radiographs are helpful if a retained fetus is visualized. Ultrasonic evaluation of the uterus is extremely valuable because it can identify uterine enlargement, intrauterine fluid or pus accumulation, a retained fetus, and retained placentas. For most practitioners the diagnosis of acute metritis is based on the presence of the abnormal vaginal discharge and systemic illness within days of whelping.

Rapid institution of antibiotic therapy is imperative. It is helpful to obtain anterior vaginal swabs for aerobic and anaerobic cultures. Anaerobic testing may prove quite important. However, one should not await results before initiating oxacillin, ampicillin (20 mg/kg four times a day), or trimethoprimsulfonamide therapy. If puppies are nursing, oxacillin or ampicillin is relatively safe. Response to therapy, coupled with results of culture/sensitivity testing, can be used in determining any long-term treatment. Surgery may be necessary to remove retained placentas/fetuses. If all or a portion of the uterus is devitalized, ovario-hysterectomy may be warranted (Johnston et al, 2001).

Prognosis depends on owner recognition of a problem, how quickly the bitch is seen and treated by the veterinarian, and response by the bitch to the chosen antibiotic. Recommended therapy includes ovariohysterectomy, although initial stabilization of the bitch is required before anesthesia and surgery. $PGF_{2\alpha}$ (see Chapter 23, Medical Treatment of Pyometra [Prostaglandins]) has been extremely beneficial in several dogs when attempting to evacuate the uterus. The recommended dose of natural $PGF_{2\alpha}$ is 0.25 mg/kg subcutaneously once a day for 5 days. We have not had experience with oxytocin or ergonovine (given intra-muscularly at a dosage of 0.2 mg/15 kg three times daily for 2 to 3 days). Uterine rupture could follow this therapy but has not been reported (Magne, 1986).

SUBINVOLUTION OF PLACENTAL SITES (SIPS)

Uterine Involution

Normal postpartum uterine involution requires approximately 12 weeks (Al-Bassam et al, 1981a, 1981b). However, using ultrasonography, it appears that involution requires approximately 15 weeks to complete (Yeager and Concannon, 1990). After involution, the uterine horns should appear as uniform hypoechoic, tubular structures (0.3 to 0.6 cm in diameter). Normal reconstruction (involution) of the endometrium following parturition is typically associated with a serosanguinous vaginal discharge. This bloody vaginal discharge usually persists for 1 to 6 weeks, with only small to tiny amounts of discharge during the final few weeks.

In normal bitches, fetal trophoblasts or maternal decidual cells can be observed in the upper loose connective tissue of the lamina propria for the first 2 weeks after whelping. These trophoblasts, however, do not degenerate and continue to invade deep glandular layers of the endo- and myometrium in bitches with SIPS. This trophoblastic invasion with vascular damage is the proposed pathogenesis of SIPS (Johnston et al, 2001). Trophoblast-like cells may be present in the vaginal smears from affected bitches.

Definition/Clinical Signs

Some healthy bitches have a bloody discharge (without odor or off-color) lasting well beyond 6 weeks. Normal bitches have no fever or worrisome clinical signs other than the vulvar discharge. Furthermore, if such a dog is brought to a veterinarian by a concerned owner/handler, no treatment is recommended if the red and white blood cell counts are normal, the vaginal discharge has no purulent component, and abdominal ultrasonography fails to demonstrate significant fluid accumulation within the uterine lumen. The puppies from that litter have usually been weaned and distributed to their new owners before the healthy bitch is examined for persistent postpartum vaginal discharge. The bitches are usually less than 3 years of age, and the syndrome most commonly follows their first or second litter.

The vulva may be slightly enlarged and flaccid, but the vaginal mucosa is normal. Rarely, abdominal palpation reveals single or multiple discrete, firm, spheroid enlargements spaced along the length of the uterus. These palpable structures are the previously described trophoblastic/eosinophilic masses protruding into the uterine lumen. The lesions may be raw and ooze blood, explaining the vaginal discharge, but they do not result in red or white blood cell abnormalities in the peripheral blood. However, vaginal cytology may reveal syncytial trophoblast-like cells; this finding aids in confirming a clinical diagnosis (Wheeler, 1986).

Differential Diagnosis

The important differential diagnoses for prolonged vaginal bleeding postpartum include metritis, vaginitis, endometrial hyperplasia secondary to endogenous or exogenous estrogen excess, coagu-lopathies, proestrus, trauma, neoplasia, and cystitis (Wheeler, 1986). Brucellosis testing is advisable. Vaginoscopy has been recommended as a means of distinguishing vaginal bleeding from blood derived from the uterus (Reberg et al, 1992). Blood in the vagina, however, can be difficult to interpret, or the source of the blood may be difficult to identify. Blood interferes with interpretation of vaginoscopy unless an obvious mass, foreign body, or area of trauma and/or necrosis is visualized. Use of an otoscope is usually useless. Digital evaluation is helpful if a distal foreign body, mass, or area of trauma exists. Vaginal cultures, although recommended, often produce a mixed population of normal vaginal flora. Culture of large numbers of an individual organism, however, is as likely to be normal as it would be consistent with infection.

Treatment

Our approach is to monitor the bitch for the duration of the continuing discharge, specifically for evidence of infection or anemia. Examination once every 2 or 3 weeks is adequate. Treatment is usually unnecessary as long as the bitch remains healthy, and we are aware of no long-term problems. These dogs typically remain healthy and fertile, discounting the need for surgery. The prognosis for health and fertility is excellent.

Recommended therapies have included systemic antibiotics, curettage via hysterotomy, or ovario-hysterectomy. Antibiotics are helpful only if infection is present. Prostaglandins (natural prostaglandin, 0.25 mg/kg, once daily for 5 days) have been used in this setting, but beneficial effects have not been demonstrated. Medroxyprogesterone acetate was reported to be helpful but is not recommended. The injection of oxytocin to the bitch following whelping has been suggested as an aid in preventing subinvolution of placental sites, but this effect is not proven.

RETAINED PLACENTA

Retained placenta is an extremely uncommon postparturient problem in the bitch. Passage of the placenta usually occurs with the birth of each puppy or follows within approximately 15 minutes. The major problem is in diagnosing this syndrome. Owners who have attempted to count placentas realize that it is difficult. This is due, in part, to the confusion and excitement associated with observing a bitch whelp, as well as understanding how quickly a bitch can consume a placenta.

Failure to expel a placenta is reported to be most common in the toy breeds, but definitive diagnosis can be almost impossible without ultrasonography (even this is subjective) or exploratory celiotomy/hysterotomy. Therefore, if an owner is concerned about a retained placenta, a complete physical examination of the bitch is warranted, and an oxytocin injection should be considered. No other treatment or course of action is recommended unless the bitch becomes ill. If the bitch remains healthy, one should not be unduly concerned.

A bitch that becomes ill has clinical signs of postpartum endometritis, because retained tissue may represent a nidus for infection. Signs include a purulent, fetid vaginal discharge, fever, inappetence/anorexia, and listlessness. Ovariohysterectomy is the recommended treatment because other forms of therapy are not consistently successful when the uterus contains a great deal of solid material. However, $PGF_{2\alpha}$ therapy in conjunction with systemic antibiotics can be attempted.

PUERPERAL TETANY– ECLAMPSIA–HYPOCALCEMIA

Definition

Eclampsia is an acute, life-threatening condition caused by extremely decreased circulating serum calcium concentrations. It is seen most commonly in small to medium-sized bitches during early lactation after whelping and, rarely, in late pregnancy. Eclampsia has been demonstrated to be associated with relatively large litters (Drobatz and Casey, 2000).

Etiology

The physiopathology of eclampsia is not well understood. The problem arises as a consequence of hypocalcemia that alters cell membrane potentials and allows spontaneous discharge of nerve fibers to induce tonic or tonoclonic contractions of skeletal muscles. Both the rate of decline in the serum calcium concentration and the actual level to which the serum calcium concentration declines influence the onset and signs of tetany. The total serum calcium concentration is usually well below 7 mg/dl when signs are seen by the owner. Ionized calcium, rather than total calcium, is the active electrolyte. Bitches in tetany usually have ionized calcium concentrations less than 0.8 mmol/L (Drobatz and Casey, 2000).

The hypocalcemia is most likely due to calcium loss into lactated milk coupled with poor utilization of dietary calcium. In addition, the stresses of nursing a litter could reduce the bitch's appetite, further reducing calcium intake without affecting calcium loss into the milk. Other factors that may play a role in the development of hypocalcemia include parathyroid gland atrophy caused by improper diet or supplements and calcium loss to the developing fetal skeletons. In healthy animals, 50% of calcium is bound to protein, and the ionized fraction is free and biologically active. Any factor increasing the protein-bound fraction of the serum calcium theoretically favors the development of tetany, such as would occur with the systemic alkalosis secondary to hyperventilation during dystocia.

Hypoglycemia is a potential complication of hypocalcemia. In addition, the signs of hypoglycemia can be similar to those of hypocalcemia. Some authors suggest administering glucose intravenously whenever a dog or cat is being treated for hypocalcemia (Linde-Forsberg and Eneroth, 1998)

In a study of 27 dogs with naturally occurring eclampsia, all had decreases in both total and ionized serum calcium concentrations. Of interest, hypomagnesemia was observed in 12 of the 27 bitches (mean 0.7; range 0.3 to 1.0 mmol/L; reference range 0.7 to 1.1 mmol/L). The total magnesium-to-calcium ratio was significantly lower in bitches with eclampsia compared with the normal controls (0.32 versus 0.5 mmol/L, respectively). Of the 27 bitches with eclampsia, 8 had hypophosphatemia, 2 had hyperphosphatemia, and 14 had hyperkalemia (Aroch et al, 1999). It is not known whether any of these abnormalities require specific therapy.

Signs

Eclampsia is most common in small dogs and much less common in cats and large dogs. The signs seen by the veterinarian usually depend on how quickly the owner recognizes a problem and seeks professional care. Most bitches are affected during the first 21 days of nursing a litter, although eclampsia has been seen during the last 20 days of pregnancy and as long as 45 days postpartum.

The initial signs caused by hypocalcemia may be subtle and vague in a bitch, especially to the inexperienced owner. The behavior changes likely to be seen are similar to those alterations seen before whelping (i.e., restlessness, nervousness, pacing, panting, and whining). In addition, the bitch is likely to lose maternal responses to her puppies and begin to exhibit some of the early signs of hypocalcemic tetany: irritability, restlessness, increased salivation, stiffness of gait, ataxia, tremors, facial rubbing, biting at the feet, and pain.

Within minutes to several hours of manifesting early signs of hypocalcemia, a bitch may progress into a much more severe clinical state. Tetany can be expressed as tonic-clonic muscle spasms, twitching, obvious muscle fasciculations, facial rubbing, biting at the feet, or an inability to stand. These signs are usually associated with fever, tachycardia, and miosis. If untreated, the bitch may exhibit epileptiform-like seizures with preservation of consciousness. Auditory or tactile stimuli may initiate muscle spasms or seizure-like activity. Death can result from severe respiratory depression or from hyperthermia (heat prostration) and associated cerebral edema.

Diagnosis

The diagnosis is based on typical signs (neurologic signs or nervousness) in a lactating bitch. Although total serum calcium or ionized serum calcium determinations might confirm the suspicion of eclampsia, the clinician should treat these patients immediately. Do not wait for laboratory confirmation. Response to therapy is the most reliable diagnostic aid.

Acute Treatment

CALCIUM INFUSION. The immediate goal is to return the serum calcium concentration to normal by parenteral calcium therapy (Table 21-5). Usually, a 10% calcium solution (gluconate or gluceptate is preferred over chloride) is administered slowly by IV. A small bitch may require only 1 or 2 ml or as much as 10 to 15 ml. Calcium gluconate is recommended because it is less irritating than calcium chloride, should any of

the solution leak into the perivascular space. The use of gluconate solutions is important because the cephalic vein of a tetanic or seizuring dog is not an easy target. As previously discussed, the veterinarian should consider concurrent glucose administration with the calcium infusion. Also as previously mentioned, magnesium therapy may be of benefit in some dogs diagnosed as having eclampsia (Aroch et al, 1999).

CARDIAC MONITORING. During calcium administration, the heart should be monitored for bradycardia and/or arrhythmias. If cardiac problems are identified, calcium administration should be stopped. The infusion can again be given, if needed, at a slower rate once normal heart rate and rhythm return.

TEMPERATURE MONITORING. Occasionally, bitches with severe hyperthermia secondary to tetany are helped with an ice or alcohol bath. However, controlling tetany with calcium causes body temperature to decrease rapidly. If the animal is simultaneously cooled with ice or alcohol, close monitoring of rectal temperature is imperative because severe hypothermia may otherwise occur. The rectal temperature should be monitored until it is stable and the bitch is free of tetany signs. This may take 30 to 45 minutes or longer after the calcium has been injected. The temperature declines toward normal in this time period, and the bitch rarely requires any additional therapy (see Chapter 17 on hypocalcemia).

Long-Term Therapy

After resolution of the clinical signs, the bitch's serum calcium concentration may still require continued support. The volume of calcium gluconate (or gluceptate) administered intravenously to control the original signs should be tabulated. That same dose, mixed in an equal volume of saline, can be given subcutaneously, usually three times daily, to help prevent relapse. Calcium chloride can be administered only intravenously. Once a bitch is stable and no longer hyperthermic, she should be returned to the owner. The owner should be instructed to treat the

TABLE 21–5 CONCENTRATIONS OF CALCIUM IN VARIOUS COMMERCIAL PREPARATIONS

Form of Calcium	Concentration of Compound (g/100 ml)	Calcium in the Compound (%)	Elemental Calcium (mg/ml)	Calcium (mEq/ml)
Calcium gluconate*	23	9.3	21.4	1.07
	10		9.3	0.46
Calcium glycerophosphate*	1	19.07	1.87	0.09
Calcium lactate	Solution	18.37		
Calcium glycerophosphate‡	10	19.07	18.71	0.93
Calcium lactate	Suspension	18.37		
Calcium chloride†	5	27.2	13.6	0.68
(do *not* use)	10	27.2	27.2	1.36
Calcium gluceptate*	22	9.0	19.8	0.99
Calcium levulinate*	10	13.0	13.0	0.65

Concentration of compound (g/100 ml) × calcium in the compound (%) ÷ 10 = Elemental calcium (mg/ml).
*Can be given intravenously or intramuscularly.
†Can be given intravenously only.
‡Can be given intramuscularly only.

bitch with calcium replacement in tablet form. Calcium gluconate is available in generic tablets, and calcium carbonate tablets are also a commonly used form of medication. The average 40-kg bitch should receive one 500-mg tablet three times a day until the puppies have been weaned and lactation has ceased.

In addition to oral supplements, the owner should take further measures to prevent recurrence of eclampsia. Older puppies (>3 weeks) can be permanently removed from the bitch and hand-raised. Younger puppies can also be hand-raised, which reduces the likelihood of a relapse but requires a large amount of work by the owner. Alternatively, the puppies can be removed for 24 hours and then allowed to nurse. It would also be helpful to alternate nursing and bottle feeding daily for 10 days (i.e., hand-feed either one-half of the litter every day or the entire litter every other day). These approaches reduce milk production and thereby reduce the chances for a relapse. If a relapse occurs, all nursing by the puppies should be permanently discontinued. The mammary glands should not be hot-soaked or cold-soaked, because either of these measures may continue to stimulate lactation. The diet of any bitch that has had eclampsia should be a high-quality and balanced commercial dog food.

Acute Calcium Therapy Failure

If a bitch is thought to have eclampsia but fails to respond to intravenous calcium therapy, alternative medications should be available. Initially, intravenous glucose can be administered. Hypoglycemia and hypocalcemia can occur simultaneously, and each appears clinically similar. If the glucose administration also fails to bring about a reduction in nervous system signs, the acid-base status of the bitch should be evaluated because the hyperventilation of tetany may result in respiratory alkalosis. This results in a greater percentage of calcium being protein-bound and unavailable to the cells dependent on calcium for their function. Intravenous diazepam (Valium) and, if necessary, pentobarbital may need to be administered in the acute management of continued seizure activity. An alternative diagnosis or prolonged eclampsia with secondary cerebral edema must also be considered as possible causes for the signs.

Treating the Bitch That Has a History of Eclampsia

Bitches that have experienced eclampsia once may have a recurrence of hypocalcemia with subsequent litters. No study has demonstrated the effectiveness of preventing eclampsia with oral calcium therapy during the final week of gestation or throughout the period of lactation. High-quality, balanced commercial diets are recommended. These diets provide adequate but not excessive amounts of calcium. Because cattle are more prone to hypocalcemia after calving if they have received a high-calcium diet, it has been assumed that the same may be true of dogs. If so, owners should be warned of the dangers associated with high-calcium diets or calcium supplements given to bitches in the final few weeks of pregnancy or those nursing a litter. Owners should also be cautioned against feeding their pregnant bitches any diet high in legumes because they contain phytates that could bind dietary calcium and predispose to hypocalcemia (Olson, 1988).

It has been suggested that the ionic balance of foods may be important in controlling the postpartum hypocalcemia of cattle (Oetzel et al, 1988). Cattle fed ammonium chloride during late gestation may have a lower incidence of hypocalcemia. It is not known whether this would be of benefit to dogs (Olson, 1988). Bitches with large litters and a previous history of eclampsia benefit from limiting the number of nursing puppies per day, as previously described.

MASTITIS

Septic Mastitis

SIGNS. Bacterial mastitis is not a common problem in the lactating bitch. A bitch with mastitis may or may not be ill. The mammary gland involved is usually warm and painful, having areas within the tissue that feel firm or hard. Milk from these glands may be off-color, and the bitch is commonly febrile and listless and does not allow the puppies to nurse. She may or may not be inappetent. Usually the source of the infection is not found. Obvious potential causes include ascending infection via the nipples, penetrating wounds, and hematogenous spread of bacteria. Rarely, the puppies are ill, weak, and crying. Death of the bitch or puppies is possible.

DIAGNOSIS. The diagnosis is usually based on the history and physical examination. Before beginning therapy, the veterinarian may elect to obtain a milk sample for cytologic evaluation, as well as for culture and sensitivity testing. Alternatively, an attempt can be made to aspirate fluid from the affected gland, using a syringe and needle and culturing any material obtained. The cytologic examination of secretions from inflamed glands of bitches with septic mastitis frequently reveals bacteria and numerous degenerative neutrophils.

Quantitative bacteriology of the secretion from mastitic glands often shows dense bacterial growth. The bacteria most often isolated are *Escherichia coli*, beta-hemolytic streptococci, and staphylococci (Wheeler et al, 1984). In contrast, cytologic smears from normal-appearing mammary glands usually have fewer cells but may also contain bacteria (Olson and Olson, 1986; Olson, 1989).

TREATMENT. Regardless of the diagnostic procedures performed, antibiotics should be started. Ampicillin or oxacillin is the initial antibiotic of choice unless bacterial sensitivity test results indicate otherwise. These drugs are effective and are unlikely to harm the neonate. Chloramphenicol has also been recommended as the initial drug of choice (Olson and Olson, 1986). Because milk is slightly more acidic than normal plasma, weak bases achieve higher concentrations in milk than in plasma under normal circumstances (Olson, 1988; mastitis may not be a normal circumstance).

Antibiotics that are weak bases and might be used advantageously in the treatment of chronic mastitis include erythromycin, trimethoprim, clindamycin, and lincomycin (Olson, 1988). Although the aminoglycosides are weak bases, they fail to concentrate in acidic compartments because of poor lipid solubility. This group of drugs may also be nephrotoxic. Tetracyclines can be trapped in acidic or alkaline milk, but this drug can interfere with development of puppy teeth and should not be used if the bitch is allowed to nurse.

It is wise to keep the puppies nursing from the bitch in order to aid in draining the affected glands. Owners should work at being certain that puppies are nursing from the infected glands. Because the glands are painful, the bitch may stop her puppies from nursing. Careful consideration of the caloric intake of the puppies is important, especially with a bitch that is in pain and rejecting her puppies. Running warm water over the infected glands or packing them with hot compresses may aid in promoting drainage, but this is not remarkably effective.

Sometimes severely infected mammary glands become necrotic. In this situation, the puppies are removed from the bitch, and surgical debridement may be needed. If the gland is abscessed, it may require lancing, draining, and flushing with dilute (1%) povidone-iodine. It is possible to cannulate single orifices within a gland using a lacrimal duct cannula in order to facilitate infusion of antiseptics or antibiotics. Occasionally, removal of the entire gland may be the safest and most expedient means of treating the bitch.

Nonseptic Mastitis/Galactostasis

Swollen, enlarged, and painful mammary glands can result from milk stasis or noninfectious inflammation. This condition most commonly effects the most productive glands (the two most caudal pairs). The syndrome may follow acute weaning of puppies from an actively lactating bitch. These bitches are usually not as ill or feverish as those with septic mastitis. Bacteria are usually absent in milk or aspirate samples, although there might be increases in neutrophils, macrophages, and eosinophils. The leukograms fail to demonstrate leukocytosis. The inflammation may respond to warm or cool compresses and continued nursing by the puppies. If the mastitis is severe, the puppies can be hand-fed. The glands can be gently massaged and compressed with warm water to induce milk flow and relieve pressure.

Alternatively, it may be wise to stop lactation. Furosemide (1.0 mg/kg twice a day) and/or glucocorticoids can be administered to the bitch for 1 to 3 days. It may also be helpful to decrease food intake to no food for 24 hours, then 25% of normal for a day, 50% for a day, and 75% for a day, to aid in slowing milk flow. Cabergoline, a dopamine agonist, can be administered for 4 to 6 days using a dose of 2.5 to 5 microgram/kg. This reduces prolactin secretion and thereby lactation. The use of dopamine agonists should be restricted to bitches that have either lost their litter or have a litter old enough to be weaned (Linde-Forsberg and Eneroth, 1998).

AGALACTIA

Complete failure to lactate (agalactia) is rare in postpartum bitches. If present, it is likely the result of a congenital defect in the mammary glands. More commonly, young or nervous bitches may experience delays in milk letdown or are reluctant to allow their puppies to nurse. Slow and calm introduction of the puppies to the bitch by the owner usually resolves the situation, although some bitches may require tranquilization. Occasionally the bitch cannot be trusted with her litter because of previous cannibalism. Hand-rearing is the only alternative. Attempts at allowing the neonates to consume colostrum in the first 24 hours of life are worthwhile. Concerns regarding milk volume, especially in the first 1 or 2 days of nursing, are not often valid. Inadequately fed puppies continue to cry and remain restless after feeding, and hand-rearing must be considered.

PREGNANCY HYPOGLYCEMIA

Hypoglycemia and ketonemia have been described in the pregnant bitch (Jackson et al, 1980). This exceedingly rare syndrome was described in one bitch late in gestation. Under the influence of progesterone, the bitch is more likely to be hyperglycemic than hypoglycemic (see below). The syndrome of hypoglycemia in pregnancy was rapidly responsive to intravenous glucose and subsequent frequent feedings. Parturition or cesarean section alleviates the problem.

The differential diagnosis for pregnancy hypoglycemia includes the hypoglycemia associated with severe sepsis. In this situation the bitch is more likely to have pyometra, although there is also the rare syndrome of pregnancy in one uterine horn and pyometra in the other. The most valuable diagnostic aids include the leukogram and abdominal ultrasonography.

DIESTRUS ACROMEGALY

The elevations in plasma progesterone associated with diestrus may induce spontaneous and transient acromegaly in the bitch. We have observed this syndrome in a few bitches. It appears that progesterone stimulates excessive growth hormone (GH) secretion, which in turn causes growth of soft tissue in the

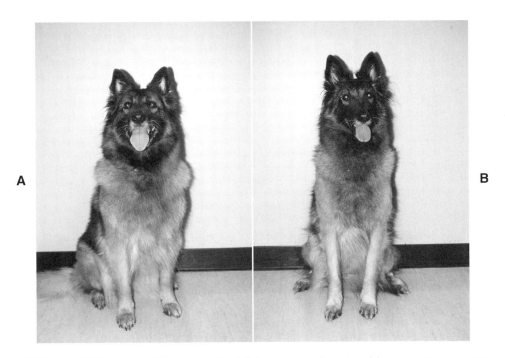

FIGURE 21–10. Litter-mates. The dog on the left has acromegaly induced by progesterone excess, which resolved following ovariohysterectomy. Although the clinical appearance did not seem remarkably different to the authors, the changes were dramatic to the owners.

orolingual/oropharyngeal/orolaryngeal regions. This can result in respiratory stridor as well. In addition, affected bitches are listless and have increased abdominal size, increased interdental spaces, polydipsia/ polyuria, weight gain, and excessive skin folds in the facial/neck areas. Many of the changes noted here may not be obvious to the veterinarian, but the alterations in facial appearance, personality, and respiratory rate, for example, may be quite obvious and worrisome to the owner (Fig. 21-10; Zimmerman et al, 2001).

The polydipsia and polyuria are usually due to secondary diabetes mellitus. Laboratory abnormalities in acromegaly may include elevation in the serum alkaline phosphatase, hyperglycemia, and mild depression in the packed cell volume (Eigenmann and Peterson, 1984). Therapy in these dogs is directed at decreasing plasma progesterone concentrations. Decreases naturally occur at the end of diestrus. If it is necessary to hasten reduction in serum progesterone concentrations, ovariohysterectomy or prostaglandin therapy must be considered. In one bitch, cystic endometrial hyperplasia was identified along with the expected multiple corpora lutea within the ovaries (Zimmerman et al, 2001).

DIABETES MELLITUS IN THE PREGNANT BITCH

Diabetes mellitus (DM) is a common endocrine disorder in the bitch. In the nonspayed diestrual bitch, DM can be difficult to treat by owner and veterinarian alike. Elevations in serum progesterone concentration during diestrus act as a potent insulin antagonist (see previous section on Acromegaly). A diabetic bitch in anestrus may have adequate carbohydrate control with insulin therapy. During diestrus (pregnancy), that same bitch may require large (sometimes huge) insulin doses, is likely to experience wide fluctuations in daily blood glucose concentrations, and may be prone to diabetic ketoacidosis.

Unfortunately, the problems in the diabetic bitch usually affect pregnancy as well. The pregnant diabetic bitch is prone to aborting her litter as a result of the effects of chronic hyperglycemia. Diabetes-related vascular changes can damage placental blood vessels, thus contributing to fetal death. Small, unthrifty puppies may also result from an abnormal placental blood supply. In contrast, some fetuses in a hyperglycemic environment experience an abnormally increased growth rate. Chronic hyperglycemia causes excess secretion of their insulin. These puppies tend to be large, often too large for natural delivery. Post-partum, the neonatal pancreas continues to secrete large amounts of insulin because of its previous hyperglycemic environment. These neonates are then prone to hypoglycemia for several weeks.

Most important, it is rare for a diabetic bitch to carry her litter to term. Most fetuses are aborted. The incidence of abortion and the additional serious potential health problems in the bitch with diabetes mellitus emphasize the importance of elective ovariohysterectomy. One must also consider the potential of contributing an inherited predisposition for diabetes mellitus to future offspring. Ovariohysterectomy is recommended for all such dogs once diabetes mellitus is recognized and adequately controlled.

REFERENCES

Al-Bassam MA, et al: Involution abnormalities in the postpartum uterus of the bitch. Vet Pathol 18:208, 1981a.

Al-Bassam MA, et al: Normal postpartum involution of the uterus in the dog. Can J Comp Med 45:217, 1981b.

Aroch I, et al: Serum electrolyte concentrations in bitches with eclampsia. Vet Rec 145:318, 1999.

Arbeiter K, et al: Treatment of pseudopregnancy in the bitch with cabergoline, an ergoline derivative. J Small Anim Pract 29:781, 1988.

Barber JA, Coley CJ. Labor monitoring in the bitch. Proceedings, 4th International Symposium on Canine and Feline Reproduction. Oslo, Norway, 84, 2000.

Bebiak DM, et al: Nutrition and management of the dog. Vet Clin North Am Small Anim Pract 16:495, 1986.

Brown J: Efficacy and dosage titration study of miboleone for treatment of pseudopregnancy in the bitch. JAVMA 184:1467, 1984.

Bulgin MS, et al: Abortion in the dog due to *Campylobacter* species. Am J Vet Res 45:555, 1984.

Concannon PW, et al: Termination of pregnancy and induction of premature luteolysis by the antiprogestagen, mifepristone, in dogs. J Reprod Fertil 88:99, 1990.

Concannon PW, Lein DH: Hormonal and clinical correlates of ovarian cycles, ovulation, pseudopregnancy, and pregnancy in dogs. In Kirk RW (ed): Current Veterinary Therapy X. Philadelphia, WB Saunders Co, 1989, p 1269.

Cortese L, et al: Hyperprolactinemia and galactorrhea associated with primary hypothyroidism in a bitch. J Am Anim Pract 38:572, 1997.

Davidson AP. Uterine and fetal monitoring in the bitch. Vet Clin N Amer 31:305, 2001.

Davidson AP. Uterine and fetal monitoring in the bitch. Proceedings, 4th International Symposium on Canine and Feline Reproduction. Oslo, Norway, 80, 2000.

Di Salle E, et al: Endocrine effects of the ergoline derivative FCE 21336, a new long lasting prolactin lowering drug [abstract 2777]. 7th International Congress of Endocrinology, Quebec City, Canada, 1984.

Donovan EF: Dystocia. In Kirk RE (ed): Current Veterinary Therapy VII. Philadelphia, WB Saunders Co, 1980, p 1212.

Drobatz KJ, Casey KK. Eclampsia in dogs: 31 cases (1995-1998). J Am Vet Med Assoc 217:216, 2000.

Eigenmann JE, Peterson ME: Diabetes mellitus associated with other endocrine disorders. Vet Clin North Am [Small Anim Pract] 14:837, 1984.

Eilts BE: Pregnancy maintenance in the bitch using Regumate. Proceedings of the Society for Theriogenology, 1992, p 144.

England GCW: Pregnancy diagnosis, abnormalities of pregnancy and pregnancy termination. In Simpson GM, England GCW, Harvey M (eds): BSAVA Manual of Small Animal Reproduction and Neonatology. Cheltenham, BSAVA, 1998, pp 113-125.

Evermann JF: Diagnosis of canine herpetic infections. In Kirk RW (ed): Current Veterinary Therapy X. Philadelphia, WB Saunders Co, 1989, p 1313.

Ferrari C, et al: Clinical application of prolactin lowering drugs. In Agarwal MK (ed): Hormone Agonist. New York, Walter de Gruyter & Co, 1982, p 503.

Funkquist PME, et al: Use of propofol-isoflurane as an anesthetic regimen for cesarean section in dogs. J Am Vet Med Assoc 211:313, 1997.

Gaudet DA, Kitchell BE: Canine dystocia. Comp Cont Ed Pract Vet 7:406, 1985.

Harvey M: Conditions of the non-pregnant female. In Simpson GM, England GCW, Harvey M (eds): BSAVA Manual of Small Animal Reproduction and Neonatology. Cheltenham, BSAVA, 1998, pp 35-51.

Harvey M, et al: Effect and mechanisms of the anti-prolactin drug cabergoline on pseudopregnancy in the bitch. J Am Anim Pract 38:336, 1997.

Hashimoto A, Hirai K: Canine herpesvirus infection. In Morrow DA (ed): Current Therapy in Theriogenology 2. Philadelphia, WB Saunders Co, 1986, p 516.

Hirt RA, et al: Severe hypercalcemia in a dog with a retained fetus and endometritis. J Am Vet Med Assoc 216:1423, 2000.

Jackson RF, et al: Hypoglycemiaketonemia in a pregnant bitch. J Am Vet Med Assoc 177:1123, 1980.

Janssens LAA: Treatment of pseudopregnancy with bromocriptine, an ergot alkaloid. Vet Rec 119:172, 1986.

Jochle W, et al: Inhibition of lactation in the Beagle bitch with the prolactin inhibitor cabergoline (FCE 21336): Dose response and aspects of long term safety. Theriogenology 27:799, 1987.

Johnston SD, Root Kustritz MV, Olson PNS. Canine and feline theriogenology. Philadelphia, WB Saunders Co, 2001.

Jones DE, Josuha JO: Reproductive Clinical Problems in the Dog. London, Wright PSG Co, 1982.

Krulich L, et al: On the mode of prolactin release inhibiting action of the serotonin receptor blockers metergoline, methysergide and cyproheptadine. Endocrinology 108:1115, 1981.

Lawler DF, et al: Influence of restricted food intake on estrous cycles and pseudopregnancies in dogs. Am J Vet Res 60:820, 1999.

Lein DH: Canine mycoplasma, ureaplasma, and bacterial infertility. In Kirk RW (ed): Current Veterinary Therapy IX. Philadelphia, WB Saunders Co, 1986, p 1240.

Linde-Forsberg C and Eneroth A: Parturition. In Simpson GM, England GCW, Harvey M (eds): BSAVA Manual of Small Animal Reproduction and Neonatology. Cheltenham, BSAVA, 1998, pp 127-142.

Lydon-Rochelle M, et al: Risk of uterine rupture during labor among women with a prior cesarean delivery. N Engl J Med 345:3, 2001.

Magne ML: Acute metritis in the bitch. In Morrow DA (ed): Current Therapy in Theriogenology 2. Philadelphia, WB Saunders Co, 1986, p 505.

Meis PJ, et al: Prevention of recurrent preterm delivery by 17 alpha-hydroxyprogesterone caproate. N Engl J Med 348:2379, 2003.

Moon PF, et al: Perioperative management and mortality rates of dogs undergoing cesarean section in the United States and Canada. J Am Vet Med Assoc 213:365, 1998.

Oetzel GR, et al: Ammonium chloride and ammonium sulfate for prevention of parturient paresis in dairy cows. J Dairy Sci 41:291, 1988.

Olson PN: Periparturient diseases of the bitch. Proceedings of the Society for Theriogenology, 1988, p 19.

Olson PN: Exfoliative cytology of the canine reproductive tract. Proceedings of the Society for Theriogenology, 1989, p 259.

Olson JD, Olson PN: Disorders of the canine pulmonary gland. In Morrow DA (ed): Current Therapy in Theriogenology 2. Philadelphia, WB Saunders Co, 1986, p 506.

Olson PN, et al: Vaginal cytology. Part II. Its use in diagnosing canine reproductive disorders. Comp Cont Ed Pract Vet 6:385, 1984.

Peterson ME, Drucker WD: Advances in the diagnosis and management of canine Cushing's syndrome. 31st Gaines Veterinary Symposium, Baton Rouge, LA, 1981, p 17.

Post K, et al: Effects of prolactin suppression with cabergoline on the pregnancy of the bitch. Theriogenology 29:1233, 1988.

Probst CW, Webb AI: Postural influence on systemic blood pressure, gas exchange, and acid/base status in the term pregnant bitch during general anesthesia. Am J Vet Res 44:1963, 1983.

Purswell BJ: Management of apparent luteal insufficiency in a bitch. JAVMA 199:902, 1991.

Purswell BJ: Differential diagnosis of canine abortion. In Kirk RW, Bonagura JD (eds): Current Veterinary Therapy XI. Philadelphia, WB Saunders Co, 1992, p 925.

Reberg SR, et al: Subinvolution of placental sites in dogs. Comp Cont Ed Pract Vet 14:789, 1992.

Reimers TJ, et al: Effects of reproductive state on concentrations of thyroxine, 3,5,3?-triiodothyronine and cortisol in serum of dogs. Biol Reprod 31:148, 1984.

Rendano VT Jr: Radiographic evaluation of fetal development in the bitch and fetal death in the bitch and queen. In Kirk RW (ed): Current Veterinary Therapy VIII. Philadelphia, WB Saunders Co, 1983, p 947.

Schweizer CM, Meyers-Wallen VN: Medical management of dystocia and indications for cesarean section in the bitch. In Bonagura J (ed): Current Veterinary Therapy XIII. Philadelphia, WB Saunders Co, 2000, p 933.

Scott-Moncrieff JC, et al: Serum disposition of exogenous progesterone after intramuscular administration in bitches. Am J Vet Res 51:893, 1990.

Shamir M, Shahar R: Extrauterine fetuses in an asymptomatic dog. Canine Practice 21:25, 1996.

Shille VM: Diagnosis and management of dystocia in the bitch and queen. In Bojrab MJ (ed): Current Techniques in Small Animal Surgery. Philadelphia, Lea & Febiger, 1983, p 338.

Steinetz BG, et al: Serum relaxin and progesterone concentrations in pregnant, pseudopregnant, and ovariectomized, progestin-treated pregnant bitches: Detection of relaxin as a marker of pregnancy. Am J Vet Res 50:68, 1989.

Voith VL: Functional significance of pseudocyesis. Mod Vet Pract 61:75, 1980.

Voith VL: Behavioral disorders. In Ettinger SJ (ed): Textbook of Veterinary Internal Medicine, 2nd ed. Philadelphia, WB Saunders Co, 1983, p 223.

Webster J, et al: A comparison of cabergoline and bromocriptine in the treatment of hyperprolactinemic amenorrhea. N Engl J Med 331:904, 1994.

Wheeler SL: Subinvolution of placental sites in the bitch. In Morrow DA (ed): Current Therapy in Theriogenology 2. Philadelphia, WB Saunders Co, 1986, p 513.

Wheeler SL, et al: Postpartum disorders in the bitch. Comp Cont Ed Pract Vet 6:493, 1984.

Yeager AE, Concannon PW: Serial ultrasonographic appearance of postpartum uterine involution in Beagle dogs. Theriogenology 34:523, 1990.

Zimmerman KL, et al: Challenging cases in internal medicine: What's your diagnosis? Veterinary Medicine 602, August, 2001.

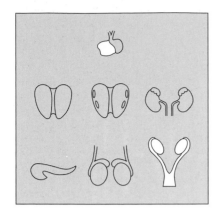

22

INDUCED ABORTION, PREGNANCY PREVENTION AND TERMINATION, AND MISMATING

THE PROBLEM: UNWANTED PREGNANCY

Unwanted pregnancies frequently occur in the bitch, and veterinarians may be asked by owners to terminate pregnancies early in gestation in an effort to avoid all the potential difficulties encountered with a pregnant bitch or an unwanted litter of puppies. The problem of an unwanted breeding may arise because dog owners are not aware that their pet is "in heat." Alternatively, the owner may be aware of estrus but may underestimate the will of a stud or bitch that wants to encounter the opposite sex. Even the best-educated and most careful owners may still find that their bitch has been or may have been bred (mismated, *misalliance*).

Reasons for having a bitch aborted vary, in addition to the obvious mating of two dogs not intended for breeding. This might be the bitch's first estrus; there may be pelvic abnormalities in the bitch that would prevent vaginal delivery of pups; or disproportionate size of the male and female may be a concern. The health of the bitch may be a factor, or an owner may simply not wish to have their bitch pregnant at this time.

Contraceptive medications are available that prevent a bitch from cycling by delaying the onset of proestrus. These drugs are approved for use in the bitch and are successful. However, such agents have limitations that prevent their widespread use in bitches. They are not to be used prior to the first estrus;

they cannot or should not be used for prolonged periods; they may change behavior or activity levels; and they are not recommended for use in brood bitches (Von Berky and Townsend, 1993).

INITIAL EVALUATION (FIG. 22-1)

A thorough history is valuable prior to treatment of the mismated bitch. Did the owner actually see a tie? What evidence is there of estrus? When was the dog last in heat? Is the bitch spayed? Although a tie is not necessary for conception, seeing a tie is the best evidence for realizing that the bitch is in standing heat. It is always possible that a bitch was not bred unless the owner actually saw the dog breeding.

A vaginal smear is the best diagnostic tool for evaluating mismated dogs. A large majority of bitches have sperm or sperm heads in the vaginal smears for 24 to 36 hours after breeding (Fig. 22-2). Forty-eight hours after breeding, 50% of bitches still have sperm or sperm heads on vaginal cytology (Olson, 1989). The presence of sperm or sperm heads confirms that breeding took place. However, lack of sperm does not prove that a fertile breeding did not occur.

The vaginal smear may also indicate the stage of the cycle. Bitches in diestrus, anestrus, or early to middle proestrus (majority of vaginal cells are parabasal and/or intermediate type) are unlikely to be fertile,

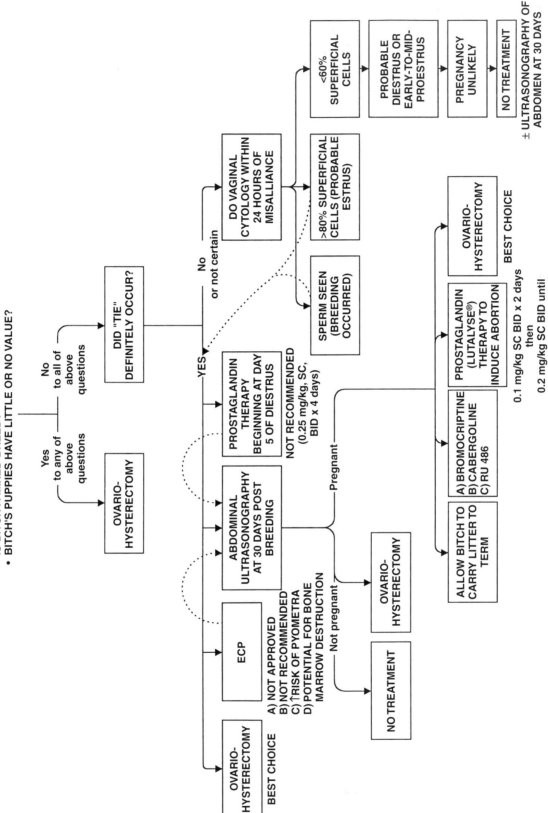

FIGURE 22–1. Algorithm outlining the differential diagnosis and management of bitches reported to have been "misbred." This assumes that the owner does not want the bitch to have this "potential" litter of puppies.

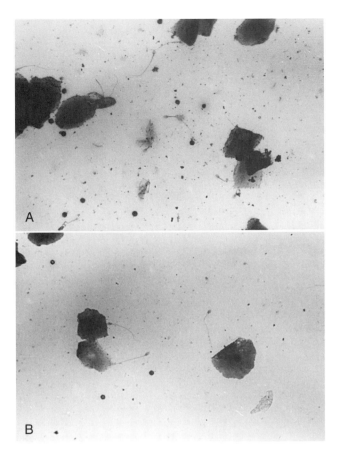

FIGURE 22–2. Vaginal smears (*A* and *B*) from a bitch that had been bred 8 hours earlier. Note the sperm present in the smears, confirming that breeding has taken place.

and the owners need not be concerned about an unwanted pregnancy. However, if the bitch is in estrus, she must be assumed to be fertile and may have bred. Greater than 80% superficial cells on vaginal cytology is strong evidence of estrus (standing heat) with or without the presence of sperm. However, greater than 80% superficial cells with a concurrent plasma progesterone concentration less than 2 ng/ml would indicate that the bitch is most likely in late proestrus, not willing to breed, and not fertile.

TREATMENT OF BITCHES NOT INTENDED FOR BREEDING PROGRAMS

Ovariohysterectomy

Several treatment options can be recommended by veterinarians to the owner of a mismated bitch. Convincing an owner to consider ovariohysterectomy is difficult at times but worth the effort. Ovariohysterectomy is the treatment of choice for the mismated bitch that is not intended for breeding. This procedure permanently eliminates chances of an unwanted pregnancy. It is safe, inexpensive, and eliminates any chance of reproductive problems in the future.

TREATMENT OF BITCHES VALUABLE FOR BREEDING PURPOSES

Overview

The objectives when planning to abort a bitch should be (1) to induce abortion only if the bitch is confirmed to be pregnant; (2) to use a product that is safe in the short and long term for the animal's health and her future fertility; and (3) to use a drug that is reliable, easily administered, and under veterinary control. In the past 10 to 15 years, a variety of alternatives have been established that meet these criteria.

Pregnancy "Trimesters"

FIRST TRIMESTER. The first period of pregnancy begins at fertilization and ends a few days after implantation. During this time, pregnancy cannot be confirmed, and induction of abortion during this first period is difficult because of the refractory nature of corpora lutea to exogenous medications. Medications recommended for use in this early period include estrogens, prostaglandins, and inhibitors of progesterone secretion or action. Invariably, these therapeutic options are not recommended because of the inability to confirm pregnancy and the likelihood of treating an animal unnecessarily. Furthermore, the medications used in this period may have dangerous side effects or the drugs efficacious for this time of pregnancy may not yet be commercially available.

SECOND TRIMESTER. Pregnancy can be confirmed during this second period and abortion induced if necessary. Abortion induction can be associated with fetal resorption or expulsion (Fig. 22-3). Abortion can be induced with prostaglandins (natural or synthetic), antiprolactin agents (e.g., dopamine agonists, such as bromocriptine and cabergoline), or antiserotoninergic agents (methergoline); with a combination of prostaglandins and dopamine agonists; or with inhibitors of progesterone secretion (epostane) or progesterone action (mifepristone or aglepristone). Inducing abortion in a bitch known to be pregnant has obvious advantages over attempting to cause abortion when pregnancy has not been confirmed (Verstegen, 2000).

THIRD TRIMESTER. The last trimester is one that begins with calcification of fetal skeletal structures. Fetuses are well developed, and abortion is always associated with fetal expulsion. Due to the wide variation in duration of pregnancy (when calculated from breeding dates, for example), abortion might induce premature parturition with delivery of live pups. For this reason, we recommend initiation of abortion protocols in bitches between days 30 and 35 after the onset of diestrus or from the date of last breeding (see Fig. 22-1).

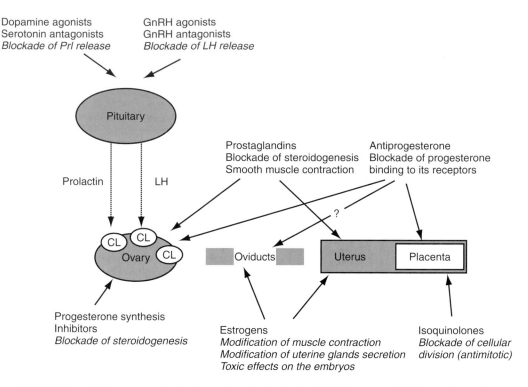

FIGURE 22–3. Mechanisms for induction of abortion in the bitch. *Prl,* Prolactin; *GnRH,* gonadotrophin-releasing hormone; *LH,* luteinizing hormone; *CL,* corpora lutea. (Verstegen JPL: *In* Bonagura J [ed)]: Current Veterinary Therapy XIII. Philadelphia, WB Saunders, 2000, p 947.)

Ovariohysterectomy

The bitch with potential value through the sale or use of her offspring is not usually a candidate for ovariohysterectomy because owners want to maintain her fertility. The age and reproductive history of such dogs should be considered. The bitch or dog may have conformation deficiencies that reduce the value of their offspring. Realistically, some bitches have little reproductive potential because of age, previous illness, or other factors. Discussion of these issues helps an owner to choose the appropriate therapy (Olson and Johnston, 1993).

Abortion Prior to Implantation: Estrogens (Not Recommended)

PHYSIOLOGY. Fertilization of eggs and the initial 6 to 10 days of canine embryonic development take place in the oviducts or fallopian tubes (Jackson and Johnston, 1980). Days later, the developing embryos migrate into the uterus and attach to the endometrium via a placenta for continued growth and nourishment. If embryos can be retained in the oviducts during the time they normally migrate and implant, degeneration and death occur. Large doses of estrogen can prolong the time the embryo is restricted to the oviduct, and this is the goal of therapy (Post, 1995).

Estrogens administered at the correct dose and time after an unwanted breeding have two potential

mechanisms of action. In one, estrogen tightens the uterotubular junction (the junction connecting the oviducts with the uterus), prolongs oviductal retention of embryos, and prevents migration of the developing embryo into the uterus, thereby ending pregnancy (Soderberg and Olson, 1983). In addition, estrogen may have direct degenerative effects on ova and may also alter the endometrium to prevent implantation (see Fig. 22-3). Several estrogen preparations have traditionally been used to prevent pregnancy in small animal practice.

DIETHYLSTILBESTROL (DES). Injection of DES (2 mg/kg body weight, up to 25 mg) once or twice within 5 days of mismating appeared to be quite successful in terminating pregnancy. However, injectable DES is no longer available to veterinarians. Oral DES has been recommended at a dosage of 1 to 2 mg/day for 7 days after mismating (Soderberg and Olson, 1983); or 75 μg/kg/day for 7 days (Bowen et al, 1985). However, oral DES has not been found to be a reliable therapy. Eleven of 12 bitches treated with DES during proestrus, estrus, or diestrus became pregnant (Olson et al, 1984; Bowen et al, 1985). Further, DES has been associated with potential side effects, which are discussed later.

ESTRADIOL CYPIONATE (ECP). Estradiol cypionate (estradiol 17β-cyclopentyl propionate) was an estrogen compound commonly used by veterinarians in the management of mismating (Jackson and Johnston, 1980). Several intramuscular dosage schedules were used and/or recommended. These protocols include one-time doses administered within 3 days of mismating: 0.25 to 1 mg total dose; 0.02 mg/kg, never to exceed 1 mg; and 0.04 mg/kg, never to exceed 1 mg (Burke, 1986). More so than DES, ECP has been associated with serious potential side effects. At 0.02 mg/kg, the drug was successful in preventing pregnancy in only 50% of bitches during proestrus or estrus and in 75% of bitches demonstrated to be in diestrus. The 0.04 mg/kg dose was 100% successful in preventing pregnancy in bitches receiving that dosage during estrus or diestrus (Olson et al, 1984; Bowen et al, 1985).

Despite the potentially favorable information on successful termination of pregnancy, ECP has major side effects that *limit or eliminate* its usefulness. Pyometra developed in two of eight dogs receiving ECP during diestrus (Bowen et al, 1985). Furthermore, ECP is well recognized as having the potential for causing permanent bone marrow suppression or destruction (or both) in dogs, resulting in severe anemia, leukopenia, thrombocytopenia, and death. This life-threatening syndrome may be caused even when ECP is given at proper dosages (Olson et al, 1984). Bone marrow suppression has been diagnosed 2 to 8 weeks after administration. For these reasons, *the manufacturer has not approved ECP for use in dogs for any purpose*, and we do *not* recommend its use.

ESTRADIOL BENZOATE, ESTRADIOL VALERATE, AND ESTRONE. Estradiol valerate has a long duration of action, and the recommended dosage is 3.0 to 7.0 mg administered once 4 to 10 days after mismating (Burke, 1986). Estradiol benzoate has a shorter duration of action, and the dosage recommendation is 5 to 10 µg/kg with a maximum of 1 mg per dog. This dose is divided into two or three subcutaneous injections, which are given at 48-hour intervals beginning on day 2 to day 4 after mating (Verstegen, 2000). Another protocol is 0.5 to 3.0 mg given every other day, for a total of three injections, beginning 4 to 10 days after misalliance (Burke, 1986). Estrone is also commercially available. The dose recommended is a single injection of 2.5 to 5.0 mg administered within 5 days of misalliance (Burke, 1986).

The efficacy of these drugs and of ethinyl estradiol and danazol has not been thoroughly evaluated in clinical trials. However, it must be remembered that potential harmful side effects are associated with the administration of estrogens to dogs. Alternatives to this mode of therapy, including allowing the bitch to become pregnant and carry the litter to term, are safer than estrogen-containing drugs. Use of estrogens, therefore, is not recommended, and most veterinary theriogenologists consider their use a form of malpractice.

ESTROGEN-INDUCED PYOMETRA. Estrogen preparations (DES and ECP) are thought to increase the incidence of pyometra. Estrogen predisposes bitches to pyometra by sensitizing progesterone receptors and enhancing the binding of progesterone to the endometrium (Niskanen and Thrusfield, 1998). There do appear to be two distinct pyometra syndromes in the dog. One is a uterine infection seen in older bitches that have an acquired uterine condition called *cystic endometrial hyperplasia* (CEH). Pyometra is a potential sequela to the chronic presence of CEH. The second, more common and more worrisome pyometra syndrome is uterine infection of young bitches secondary to estrogen administration. Pyometra, open or closed cervix, can occur 1 to 10 weeks after mismating therapy.

The pathogenesis of estrogen-induced pyometra is not well understood. The exogenous estrogen used in the management of misalliance is invariably administered when endogenous estrogen concentrations are decreasing (estrus) or low (diestrus). Thus the bitch is exposed to estrogen concentrations that are not physiologic and that are completely atypical for that phase of her ovarian cycle. Estrogens may stimulate synthesis of progesterone receptors in the endometrium, potentiating the effects of luteal progesterone. Chronic CEH is not a sequela of estrogen therapy.

Our continuing clinical trials provide evidence against long-term damage to the endometrium as a result of exogenous estrogen therapy. However, the exogenous estrogen causes transient uterine disease (pyometra); this condition is not only life threatening, it also is treated by ovariohysterectomy in most hospitals. Bitches with pyometra that are successfully treated with prostaglandins have an excellent prognosis for carrying pregnancies to term in subsequent cycles (Nelson et al, 1982). Thus a chronic endometrial disorder is not present. However, some bitches treated with estrogen do have recurrences of pyometra. Pyometra has been diagnosed in young bitches that never received estrogens at any time. However, pyometra as a naturally occurring disease in the young bitch (less than 6 years of age) is not nearly as common as it is in the estrogen-treated bitch. For these reasons (pyometra and bone marrow destruction), the use of estrogen compounds in the management of misalliance is strongly discouraged.

ESTROGEN-INDUCED BONE MARROW DESTRUCTION. Excesses in the serum estrogen concentration caused by exogenous estrogen treatment always have the potential to destroy the bone marrow in dogs (Verstegen et al, 1981). This bone marrow sensitivity to estrogen is not well understood. Bone marrow destruction may occur after exposure to abnormal increases in the serum estrogen concentration from endogenous sources (e.g., Sertoli and interstitial cell tumors in males) (Suess et al, 1992), as well as from exogenous sources. The most common and dangerous exogenous source of excess estrogen is administration of ECP.

Iatrogenic bone marrow destruction is frequently fatal. The pancytopenia results in immunosuppression, chronic bleeding, and anemia. Treatment traditionally has been supportive, with repeated transfusions to maintain life. This therapy usually provides transient improvement. Expense, time, frustration, and the bleak prognosis result in most owners having their pets euthanized.

Lithium carbonate (11 mg/kg PO bid for 6 weeks) has been reported as a possible treatment for estrogen-induced bone marrow hypoplasia (Hall, 1992). Lithium treatment, however, needs to be evaluated in a larger group of dogs to assess efficacy. Side effects of this drug include tremors, hypothyroidism, renal tubular nephropathy, edema, and cardiac "sick sinus" syndrome. Close patient monitoring, therefore, is critically important. Administration of recombinant canine granulocyte colony-stimulating factors may be more effective and safer than lithium therapy.

The iatrogenic syndrome is inexcusable and completely avoidable: *Do not administer ECP to any dog for any reason.*

ESTROGEN-INDUCED BEHAVIOR CHANGES. The least worrisome side effect of estrogen administration is induction or prolongation of estrus behavior (Jackson and Johnston, 1980). These bitches may continue attracting males for 7 to 10 days. Some have prolonged standing heat, and others reenter standing heat.

EXOGENOUS ESTROGEN AND FUTURE FERTILITY. Administration of estrogens may cause death of the bone marrow and open- or closed-cervix pyometra. Bitches that escape these problems may still become infertile. The incidence of estrogen-associated infertility is not well documented. The syndrome may be the result of estrogen-induced ovarian or uterine pathology.

Prostaglandins in General

BACKGROUND. Veterinarians in private practice need a safe, reliable, and cost-effective method of terminating an unwanted pregnancy in dogs. Unplanned and unwanted pregnancies in valuable bitches do occur, and owners appreciate an option other than surgery (spay) or pregnancy, or the use of estrogens, which could be deleterious to the uterus or bone marrow. The protocols described herein provide a reasonable treatment option until a more efficacious method is developed.

PHYSIOLOGY. Pregnancy in the bitch depends on progesterone secretion from corpora lutea. Ovariectomy (which would result in immediate loss of all progesterone) or inhibition of progesterone synthesis at any stage of gestation results in fetal resorption or abortion. Administration of prostaglandin $F_{2\alpha}$ ($PGF_{2\alpha}$) or its analogs has been repeatedly demonstrated by researchers to successfully terminate pregnancy in the bitch. Abortion with prostaglandins is induced through three different mechanisms: (1) by inducing vasoconstriction, reducing blood flow to the corpora lutea and causing cellular degeneration; (2) by interfering with progesterone synthesis through binding to specific receptors; and (3) by acting directly on the myometrium to cause smooth muscle contractions.* The myometrial contractions are associated with natural prostaglandins, not the synthetic analogs. Most of these studies have been performed on laboratory dogs using a variety of protocols. Several

clinical reports have also suggested that $PGF_{2\alpha}$ could be used by veterinary practitioners to terminate pregnancy in the bitch (Lein, 1983; Johnston, 1990; Feldman et al, 1993).

Currently, abortifacient therapy with prostaglandin has few limitations. As became apparent in our studies with bitches that have pyometra, canine corpora lutea may be relatively resistant to the luteolytic effects of prostaglandins during the first 14 to 28 days of pregnancy. Resistance after this time is still present but to a lesser degree. Thus the "mismated" bitch is not as consistently responsive to prostaglandin administration in the first few weeks of pregnancy as she is in the second half of gestation (beginning at approximately 30 days after breeding).

NATURAL VERSUS SYNTHETIC PROSTAGLANDINS. The natural prostaglandins (Lutalyse, Upjohn, Kalamazoo, MI; or Dinolytic, Upjohn, Europe) have a relatively short duration of action and side effects that may at times be worrisome. Therefore interest in synthetic analogs (e.g., cloprostenol) that are devoid of such side effects and that have a longer duration of action is logical.

The purpose of our ongoing clinical trials has been to evaluate the efficacy of $PGF_{2\alpha}$ as an abortifacient under conditions commonly encountered in veterinary practice; that is, privately owned pet dogs that become pregnant after an unplanned and unwanted mating. When initially examined, many of these bitches are in diestrus, therefore the precise date of onset of this phase can no longer be determined.

CRITERIA FOR SELECTION OF CASES. Since 1986 more than 120 privately owned pet bitches have been brought to our hospital for termination of pregnancy after an "observed," unplanned, and unwanted breeding. Each dog was examined 30 to 35 days after the breeding. To be considered for prostaglandin termination of pregnancy, bitches must be healthy and less than 7 years of age. When abdominal ultrasonography was used to confirm pregnancy, more than 60% of these bitches were not pregnant. Thus owner observation and/or veterinarian palpation is not considered sufficient reason to initiate administration of drugs to terminate pregnancy.

Natural Prostaglandins

RECOMMENDED TREATMENT PROTOCOL. Abdominal ultrasound is recommended approximately 30 days after the last (or unwanted) breeding or 30 days after the first day of diestrus as confirmed with vaginal cytology. After pregnancy has been confirmed, abortion should be discussed with the owner. In our opinion, the use of prostaglandins at this time of gestation is effective and safe. Treatment prior to day

---

*Vickery and McRae, 1980; Jackson et al, 1982; Oettle, 1982; Tsutsui et al, 1982; Paradis et al, 1983; Shille et al, 1984; Oettle et al, 1988; Lein et al, 1989; Romagnoli et al, 1991; Verstegen, 2000.

30 is not recommended. No evidence of straining or dystocia has been observed in any bitch. It is assumed, in part, that difficulty in delivery of fetuses is unlikely because each fetus is so small that it can be passed through the birth canal even if presented in an abnormal posture.

Commercially available $PGF_{2\alpha}$ is not licensed for use in dogs, and veterinarians may wish to obtain owner consent prior to its use. In our initial trials, three treatment protocols with $PGF_{2\alpha}$ were evaluated: (1) 0.1 mg/kg given subcutaneously every 8 hours; (2) 0.25 mg/kg given subcutaneously every 12 hours; and (3) 0.1 mg/kg given subcutaneously every 8 hours for 2 days, and then 0.2 mg/kg given subcutaneously every 8 hours thereafter. All the bitches in our studies were treated with natural $PGF_{2\alpha}$ daily until complete abortion was confirmed with abdominal ultrasonography. It is strongly recommended, as will be explained, that any bitch being treated with prostaglandins to induce abortion be hospitalized throughout the treatment period.

Our current recommendation is the protocol that acted most rapidly while resulting in the fewest and/or least severe side effects: natural $PGF_{2\alpha}$ at a dosage of 0.1 mg/kg given subcutaneously every 8 hours for 2 days, and then 0.2 mg/kg given subcutaneously every 8 hours daily until abortion has been completed, as confirmed by abdominal ultrasonography. This protocol resulted in the least severe side effects and the fewest number of days to complete the abortion process (Feldman et al, 1993).

MONITORING. Abdominal ultrasound was performed every 48 hours until abortion was completed. We now recommend that abdominal ultrasonography be performed within 6 to 12 hours and prior to the next scheduled administration of $PGF_{2\alpha}$ if abdominal contractions, fetuses, or bloody or dark vaginal discharge are observed. A physical examination, including abdominal palpation, should be performed at least twice daily. After each injection of $PGF_{2\alpha}$, the dog should be taken for a 20- to 30-minute walk, which allows close observation of the animal. The dog should be fed 1 to 2 hours *after* prostaglandin injection so as to avoid vomiting with feeding prior to treatment. The feeding period can also be used as an observation period (Feldman et al, 1993).

Amniotic vesicles are palpable in most 30- to 35-day pregnant bitches prior to therapy. Each dog we have treated has been demonstrated to have at least two viable fetuses on abdominal ultrasound examination, although exact litter size was not always known. It is important to emphasize that once $PGF_{2\alpha}$ treatment is initiated, abdominal palpation is no longer reliable in determining when abortion has begun or when and if it has been completed. Abdominal ultrasonography, however, is reliable in confirming whether abortion has been completed.

The need for repeated abdominal ultrasound examinations to confirm that abortion had been completed was disappointing because of the expense and the facilities required. However, ultrasonography has been the only reliable means of assessing pregnancy status in each bitch. The ultrasound examinations were easily performed, and the results were known immediately. Abdominal palpation was not considered reliable or acceptable as the sole means of determining which bitches were pregnant or when the abortion process was complete. Hospitalization is recommended to allow observation of the bitch and to spare owners from witnessing an abortion process they may not wish to see.

DURATION OF TREATMENT. All pregnant, prostaglandin-treated dogs aborted all fetuses within 9 days of beginning $PGF_{2\alpha}$ administration. One reason to strongly recommend hospitalization during the treatment period is the fact that owner response to observing aborted fetuses can be quite negative. In addition, one must dispose of any aborted fetuses not consumed by the bitch. The number of treatment days required to complete the abortions did not vary significantly with the treatment protocol used; the average was approximately 5 to 7 days, with all the bitches responding within 3 to 9 days.

COMPLETION OF PROSTAGLANDIN ADMINISTRATION. Several bitches were observed to abort one or more fetuses, only to have the subsequent abdominal ultrasound examination demonstrate live fetuses in utero. These dogs required 1 to 3 additional *days* of $PGF_{2\alpha}$ administration to complete the abortion process, a fact that demonstrates that monitoring any bitch being treated with prostaglandins without ultrasonography is not reliable. Furthermore, most of the bitches were not seen to abort any of their litters. In other words, many bitches quickly consume stillborn neonates. Most of the fetuses seen were expelled with membranes intact, and none survived longer than a few minutes. Fetal resorption, although possible, appears to be unlikely in bitches managed with prostaglandins because no in utero fetal material has been identified on ultrasonography performed on any of the bitches we have treated (Feldman et al, 1993).

SERUM PROGESTERONE CONCENTRATIONS. It has been suggested that plasma progesterone concentrations less than 2.0 ng/ml result in pregnancy termination in bitches (Olson et al, 1986). The pretreatment plasma progesterone concentrations were greater than 6.0 ng/ml in all bitches we treated. As shown in Fig. 22-4, the mean plasma progesterone concentration from all the bitches decreased after the start of $PGF_{2\alpha}$ administration. The plasma progesterone concentration decreased in all dogs approximately 50% from the pretreatment concentration after only 24 hours of $PGF_{2\alpha}$ treatment. After 72 hours and at each subsequent blood sampling time, all treated bitches had plasma progesterone concentrations less than 2.0 ng/ml. No bitch aborted any fetal material until at least 24 hours after the plasma progesterone concentration was less than 2.0 ng/ml (Feldman et al, 1993). Although monitoring of the plasma progesterone concentration is not necessary, these results demonstrate the physiologic effect of prostaglandin administration, as well as the speed with which it acts.

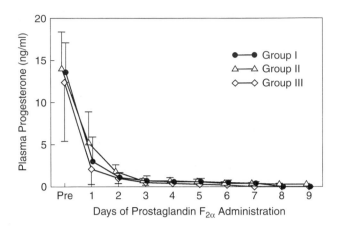

FIGURE 22–4. Mean (± SD) plasma progesterone concentrations for three treatment groups of bitches that were aborted with subcutaneous injections of prostaglandin $F_{2\alpha}$. Treatment was continued in each dog until abortion was confirmed to have been completed with abdominal ultrasonography. The values are from days 0, 1, 2, 3, 4, 5, 6, 7, 8, and 9 after initiation of treatment. Group I (●——●) was treated with 0.1 mg/kg every 8 hours; group II (△——△) was treated with 0.25 mg/kg every 12 hours; group III (◇——◇) was treated with 0.1 mg/kg every 8 hours for 2 days and 0.2 mg/kg every 8 hours thereafter. Each group was composed of six pregnant bitches. All bitches aborted all fetuses in 9 days or less.

SIDE EFFECTS. It would be quite unusual for a bitch not to demonstrate side effects after each of the first few doses of prostaglandins. All of the treated bitches exhibited at least one side effect after the initial injection of $PGF_{2\alpha}$. Side effects included panting, respiratory distress, excess salivation, vomiting, defecation, and stranguria and/or urination. Tachycardia greater than 180 beats per minute was noted in a few dogs. Side effects usually began within 30 seconds to 3 minutes after the subcutaneous injection and persisted for 4 to 55 minutes. Most often the side effects lasted 5 to 20 minutes.

Subjectively, the side effects were most obvious and severe in the dogs initially treated with the 0.25 mg/kg dosage. The bitches appeared to adapt to the $PGF_{2\alpha}$, with side effects diminishing after each subsequent injection (Nelson et al, 1982). After six to eight injections, side effects were minimal or absent in all the dogs regardless of the dosage protocol.

Within 24 to 48 hours preceding and after abortion, the bitches exhibited typical clinical signs of labor, including a mucoid vaginal discharge, dark red to black vaginal discharge, abdominal contractions, restlessness, nesting behavior, excessive grooming of the perineal area, a decrease in rectal temperature below 37.5° C, and trembling or muscle fasciculations. These side effects may be frightening to an owner or veterinarian but are rarely life threatening to a bitch. However, the salivation, diarrhea, vomiting, and respiratory distress may respond to atropine therapy (0.5 mg/kg IM) (Lein et al, 1989).

SHORT-TERM AND LONG-TERM RESULTS. No bitch treated with the protocols we have used aborted any fetal material after release from the hospital. All were hospitalized for at least 24 hours after ultrasound confirmation of pregnancy termination. Each bitch was considered healthy on a physical examination performed 2 weeks after treatment. In most of the dogs, no vaginal discharge was detected at that recheck, but a few had a slightly bloody vaginal discharge. The vaginal discharge in that small group cleared completely within 7 to 28 days. All the bitches observed for more than 8 months after completion of abortion have had normal ovarian cycles. All but four of the treated bitches bred after receiving prostaglandins whelped normal litters.

SUMMARY. Use of $PGF_{2\alpha}$ is a safe and consistent means of medically terminating pregnancy in the bitch. The physical side effects of $PGF_{2\alpha}$ are transient and not life threatening. It is recommended that pregnancy be confirmed prior to treatment. Abortion has required 3 to 9 days to be completed when this protocol is used in bitches bred 30 to 35 days earlier.

Combination prostaglandin and misoprostol

Induction of abortion in nine bitches using intravaginally administered misoprostol, a prostaglandin E_1 compound, and an injectable natural prostaglandin has been reported. Use of misoprostol as a component of combination protocols is gaining acceptance for early pregnancy termination in women (Spritz et al, 1998). Each of the nine bitches was beyond 30 days of gestation. The mean duration of therapy required to induce abortion was 5 days, compared with 7 days using prostaglandin alone (Davidson et al, 1998).

Prostaglandins: Immediate Postbreeding Administration (Not Recommended)

PROTOCOL. $PGF_{2\alpha}$ has been recommended for early diestrus luteolysis and, therefore, pregnancy termination in the bitch. It has been suggested that treatment be initiated as early as 5 days after the cytologic onset of diestrus. Different doses and treatment protocols have been reported in the literature, including a dosage of 0.25 mg/kg of the natural prostaglandin, administered subcutaneously twice daily for at least 4 days. This protocol should not be started earlier than the fifth day after cytologic diestrus (Romagnoli et al, 1991).

DRAWBACKS. This treatment protocol has several serious drawbacks. The most important problem is that it presumes that all "misbred" bitches are pregnant. In our series, however, fewer than 40% of "misbred" bitches were pregnant when examined with abdominal ultrasonography 30 to 35 days after breeding. It is likely that most bitches that naturally breed do become pregnant. However, most owners of "misbred" bitches simply assume that the dog has been bred, when in fact breeding was not witnessed and did not take place. Furthermore, because it is not currently possible to confirm pregnancy in a bitch within the first week of diestrus, immediate postbreeding protocols, such as this, result in unnecessary treatment of nonpregnant bitches.

The second drawback is that the treatment protocol requires knowledge of the first day of diestrus as determined by vaginal cytology. The owner phoning the veterinarian for advice is not likely to have access to this information. The bitch must be brought to the veterinarian for examination. If she is already in diestrus, that date can be assumed to be day 1, and treatment can begin 5 days later. However, if she is in estrus, vaginal smears must be obtained every 24 to 72 hours, stained, and interpreted to identify day 1 of diestrus.

The third drawback to this treatment regimen is the dose recommended; the 0.25 mg/kg dosage is relatively high. This is necessary because corpora lutea are resistant to prostaglandins early in diestrus. Lower doses can be used later in diestrus, when the corpora lutea are more sensitive to prostaglandins.

Finally, the authors of this protocol recommend that all treated bitches be examined with abdominal ultrasonography at approximately 30 days of gestation to determine if the prostaglandin protocol was successful. This seems to be a costly and inefficient method of managing misalliance. It is more logical to treat only bitches known to be pregnant (via ultrasonography 30 days after breeding) and then to continue treatment until the abortion process has been completed.

Prostaglandin Analogs

BACKGROUND. A good deal of work has been accomplished with prostaglandin analogs. Major improvements over natural $PGF_{2\alpha}$ appear to include greater luteolytic effectiveness at relatively low doses and decreases in the occurrence of myometrial contractions and the severity of side effects (Jackson et al, 1982). Side effects, which depend on the analog used, vary from mild (Jackson et al, 1982) to severe (Shille et al, 1984). Varying doses and routes of administration of fluprostenol and cloprostenol provided consistent abortifacient results when either drug was administered 25 days after the first breeding. These $PGF_{2\alpha}$ analogs were administered subcutaneously or via a plastic intravaginal device at single doses of 0.01 to 0.04 mg/kg. One dose of either fluprostenol or cloprostenol caused abortion by means of sustained luteolytic effects, resulting in suppressed luteal activity. Consistent and maintained depression of progesterone concentrations below 2.0 ng/ml appears to be the key in prostaglandin-induced abortion (Jackson et al, 1982). A transient drop in the progesterone concentration does not result in abortion (Shille et al, 1984). Intravaginally administered misoprostol has been reported to be effective for termination of second-trimester pregnancy in women (Jain and Mishell, 1994). Both fluprostenol and cloprostenol are marketed for use in large animals. They have not been approved for use in the dog or cat.

PROTOCOL USING CLOPROSTENOL. A variety of protocols for the use of prostaglandin analogs have appeared in the veterinary literature. Cloprostenol has a duration of action 12 to 24 hours; also, it does not cause uterine contractions, and administration to dogs has caused relatively few of the other side effects associated with the myometrial contractions induced by natural prostaglandins. The recommended regimen for cloprostenol is 1 to 2 µg/kg given subcutaneously once daily for 5 to 7 days, beginning at least 30 days after breeding (Verstegen, 2000). In bitches treated with this protocol, the plasma progesterone concentration decreased to less than 2.0 ng/ml for more than 24 hours after each injection. One of the advantages of this and the combination treatments discussed below is that abortion is less common than fetal resorption. However, this advantage depends partly on therapy being started at the appropriate time.

α-PROSTOL. Use of this synthetic prostaglandin (Gabbrostim; Centralvet-Vetem, Italy) was recently reported. Dogs were treated with 20 µg/kg either once or twice daily for 5 days beginning with day 10 of diestrus, as determined with vaginal cytology (Romagnoli et al, 2000). The results were disappointing, however, perhaps because treatment was initiated too early in diestrus.

Antiprogestin Therapy

BACKGROUND. Administration of progesterone antagonists at effective doses prevents establishment of pregnancy or terminates pregnancy in various species if the drug is given before implantation. These drugs have been shown to bind to the progesterone receptor with high affinity and to prevent progesterone-induced changes in deoxyribonucleic acid (DNA) transcription. It also should be noted that these drugs are associated with shortened interestrous intervals (Galac et al, 2000).

MIFEPRISTONE (RU486). Mifepristone is a progesterone receptor antagonist that may prevent pregnancy and/or induce the onset of menses in women (Spitz et al, 1998). The drug is orally active and has been shown to be safe and effective in terminating pregnancy in dogs if administered after day 30 of gestation. The protocol used in testing was oral administration of 2.5 mg/kg given twice daily for 4 to 5 days starting at day 32 of carefully timed gestation (Concannon et al, 1990). Serum progesterone concentrations declined to less than 1.0 ng/ml by days 40 to 45 after the preovulatory luteinizing hormone (LH) peak. Pregnancy was terminated without side effects within 3 to 4 days after treatment was begun.

As with midgestational use of prostaglandins, bitches did abort and consume fetuses or the fetuses required disposal. All bitches aborted all fetuses before serum progesterone concentrations decreased below 2.0 ng/ml. This demonstrates that the drug acts as a progesterone *receptor* antagonist at the level of the uterus, independent of any additional effects on luteal function. Premature cessation of luteal function may have occurred secondary to the termination of pregnancy or may represent a luteolytic effect of treatment independent of pregnancy status. Doses that would be effective prior to implantation or earlier in pregnancy were not established (Concannon et al, 1990).

Use of a single subcutaneous dose of RU486 was evaluated in eight pregnant bitches that were 11 to 56 days into gestation. The dosages used were 10 to 22.7 mg/kg. Six of the eight dogs aborted. The two dogs that delivered live puppies received the lowest dosage (10 mg/kg) and were near term (day 56 of gestation). No adverse effects were documented in any of the eight dogs (Sankai et al, 1991). The concept of a single subcutaneous treatment to abort bitches is of interest. However, one of the problems associated with other therapies remains: inability to predict when abortion will occur. Hospitalization, therefore, still needs to be considered (Concannon and Meyers-Wallen, 1991).

AGLEPRISTONE (RU534). This relatively new antiprogesterone drug (Alizine; Hoechst Roussel Vet, France) has been marketed in several European countries for use in dogs (Verstegen, 2000). In three studies, the drug was administered at a dosage of 10 mg/kg given twice at 24-hour intervals. One study included 367 bitches from 0 to 45 days of gestation, and another included 124 bitches an average of 30 days into gestation. Treatment was effective in 95% of animals confirmed pregnant on the first day of treatment in both groups (Fieni et al, 2000a and 2000b; Verstegen, 2000). No general or local side effects were observed except for mammary development and lactation (Fieni, 1995; Galac et al, 2000). In another study, 0.15 mg/kg was given twice at 24-hour intervals to two groups of dogs (Fieni et al, 2000a and 2000b). The dogs in one group were in early pregnancy (average of 13 days postovulation), and those in the other group were in midgestation (average of 32 days postovulation). In the early gestation group, the fetuses were resorbed, and in the midgestation group, the fetuses were aborted. Whether this type of drug will be available in more countries is unknown. Given its efficacy, safety, and absence of side effects, it would be an excellent alternative for small animals.

EPOSTANE. Experimental inhibition of progesterone synthesis has been accomplished with the drug epostane. The drug is a competitive inhibitor of the hydroxysteroid dehydrogenase–isomerase enzyme system, which results in decreased production of progesterone. In most species the effect is more prominent in the ovaries than in the adrenal glands. Epostane has been demonstrated to terminate pregnancy in dogs at a dosage of 50 mg/day given orally for 7 days, starting on the first day of diestrus as determined with vaginal cytology (Keister et al, 1989). In the past few years, interest in marketing epostane as a treatment for mismating in dogs has been high. However, additional trials are needed to determine the safety, efficacy, and dose requirements in dogs of various sizes and breeds (Concannon and Meyers-Wallen, 1991).

Dopamine Agonist Agents

BACKGROUND. Because prolactin is the primary luteotropic hormone in dogs, inhibition of its synthesis and release causes functional luteal arrest and a decrease in progesterone secretion. If treatment is continued for a sufficient time during the second "trimester" of pregnancy in dogs, luteolysis occurs. Prolactin secretion is primarily controlled by direct inhibition at the pituitary level by dopamine and by indirect stimulatory tone at the hypothalamic level by serotonin. Serotonin inhibits dopamine secretion. During pregnancy in the bitch, prolactin has been demonstrated to significantly increase from days 25 to 30 after the LH surge. During this period, dopamine agonists can be given orally or parenterally to induce abortion. Both bromocriptine and cabergoline are dopamine agonists. They inhibit prolactin secretion by direct action on pituitary receptors. Methergoline is one of the serotonin antagonists that inhibit prolactin secretion by increasing dopamine-inhibiting tone at the level of the hypothalamus (Verstegen, 2000). Use of these drugs is typically associated with a shortened interestrous interval.

BROMOCRIPTINE. Bromocriptine (Parlodel) is an ergot alkaloid commercially available for use in humans, primarily in the treatment of hyperprolactinemia (Webster et al, 1994). It is not licensed for veterinary use except in Italy. Bromocriptine has been reported to be an effective abortifacient after day 35 of gestation but not prior to day 30. Various treatment protocols have been reported. In one protocol, 0.1 mg/kg/day is given orally for 6 consecutive days beginning on day 35 of gestation (Concannon et al, 1987); in another protocol, 0.03 mg/kg is given orally twice a day for 4 days beginning after day 30 of gestation. Bromocriptine commonly causes inappetence, anorexia, vomiting, and depression. Furthermore, it is not 100% effective in inducing abortion before day 40 of gestation. Also, because the side effects are more severe and persistent than those seen in bitches treated with prostaglandins, this drug has not been used extensively.

CABERGOLINE. Cabergoline (Dostinex; Pharmacia & Upjohn, Peapack, NJ), like bromocriptine, is a synthetic ergot derivative, long-acting dopamine receptor agonist, prolactin inhibitor. It is a highly potent oral or parenterally administered drug. It is available in tablet form (0.5 mg) but can be expensive. A dose of 5 µg/kg given once daily caused a sharp decrease in serum prolactin concentrations and resulted in abortion in dogs without causing obvious systemic side effects (Arbeiter et al, 1988; Post et al, 1988; Jochle et al, 1989). The drug has been promoted as more effective and better tolerated than bromocriptine in women treated for hyperprolactinemia (Webster et al, 1994). This dose has been demonstrated to induce abortion in 100% of bitches treated from 40 days after the LH surge, but it is effective in only 25% of bitches when given from day 30 (Verstegen et al, 1993). Subcutaneous injections of 1.65 µg/kg given on alternate days over 5 days were more effective, with abortions induced in 100%, 66%, and 25% of bitches when treatments were started at 40, 30, and 25 days after the LH surge, respectively (Onclin et al, 1995). However, the injectable form is not commercially available.

Combination Prostaglandin and Dopamine Agonist

BACKGROUND. Simultaneous administration of a prostaglandin and a dopamine agonist for induction of abortion has been described. The purpose of combining two drugs is to reduce plasma progesterone concentrations, thus losing pregnancy support by (1) the direct local effect of prostaglandins in inhibiting progesterone synthesis and (2) an indirect effect secondary to interruption of pituitary prolactin secretion. Lower doses of each drug can be used, which reduces the side effects associated with use of prostaglandins alone.

PROTOCOL AND RESULTS. It is recommended that therapy begin after day 25 from the LH surge or 25 to 28 days after first breeding. Cloprostenol is administered every other day at a dosage of 1.0 µg/kg given subcutaneously. Three doses are given. In addition, oral cabergoline (5 µg/kg) is given daily for 9 days. This protocol induced abortion in 100% of five Beagles so treated within 5 to 8 days (Onclin and Verstegen, 1996). Pregnancy termination always took place by resorption of fetuses. No side effects were observed, although some sanguinous vaginal discharge was noted in each dog. Termination of pregnancy was accompanied in each case by a decline in the plasma progesterone level to less than 1.0 ng/ml within 72 hours of the start of treatment. If treatment is started after day 40, fetal expulsion rather than resorption occurs. Treatment before day 25 is not as effective (Verstegen, 2000).

Glucocorticoids

Occasionally a pregnant bitch develops a disease that requires glucocorticoid treatment. These disorders include immune-mediated diseases such as thrombocytopenia, hemolytic anemia, polyarthritis, systemic lupus erythematosus, and others. In these situations, the well-being of the fetuses may be of lesser priority than the health of the bitch. A regimen of 10 days of dexamethasone (5 mg IM bid) has been reported to cause intrauterine death and fetal resorption when started on day 30 of gestation and to cause abortion if administration is begun on day 45 (Jackson and Johnston, 1980). It is recommended that glucocorticoids be avoided whenever possible in the pregnant bitch. However, awareness of the side effects does allow for complete communication with owners prior to initiation of any therapy.

Dexamethasone may be used to terminate a pregnancy. In Beagles, a dosage of approximately 0.5 mg/kg given intramuscularly twice a day for 10 days terminated pregnancy (Shille, 1985). In Labrador Retrievers, the regimen to terminate pregnancy was approximately 0.15 mg/kg given intramuscularly once a day for 10 days. Currently, the use of glucocorticoids to terminate pregnancy is not recommended because of these drugs' immunosuppressive effects and because abortions, when they occur, are less predictable than with prostaglandin administration.

Gonadotropin-Releasing Hormone Antagonists

Antagonists of gonadotropin-releasing hormone (GnRH) act by rapidly suppressing the secretion of pituitary LH and follicle-stimulating hormone (FSH). The expected result is a decrease in ovarian steroid synthesis and secretion. A single injection of a GnRH antagonist did result in suppressed luteal function and termination of pregnancy in midgestational bitches (Vickery et al, 1989). Efficacy was reduced when the drug was administered earlier in gestation. If the drug was administered on the second day of diestrus in concert with a prostaglandin analog, as a single injection, the result was protracted luteolysis and better efficacy in terminating pregnancy. These drugs are classified as experimental, have not been thoroughly evaluated, and are not yet recommended for use (Concannon, 1991).

Tamoxifen Citrate

Tamoxifen citrate, an isomer of triphenylethylene, acts as an antiestrogen in premenopausal women but has estrogenic activity in dogs. It may interfere with zygote transport or implantation or both. The drug was effective in preventing or terminating pregnancy if administration began during proestrus or estrus or on day 2 of diestrus (Bowen et al 1988). Efficacy was much poorer if the treatment commenced on day 15 or day 30 of diestrus; in these two groups, 50% of the treated bitches remained normally pregnant. All bitches received 1 mg/kg orally twice a day for 10 days. Of the 20 bitches given tamoxifen citrate, five developed endometritis with or without pyometra, and four of these had ovarian cysts. Although tamoxifen citrate may have potential for preventing or terminating pregnancy in the bitch, the regimen used in the study reviewed was associated with an unacceptable frequency of pathologic abnormalities in the reproductive tract (England, 1998).

Management of the Bitch after Misalliance

As outlined in Fig. 22-1, the clinical approach to management of the mismated bitch must be practical and logical. If contacted within 24 to 36 hours of the unwanted breeding, the veterinarian can recommend an examination. This allows the veterinarian to complete a vaginal cytologic evaluation to determine (1) the phase of the ovarian cycle and (2) whether sperm are present in the vaginal smear. If sperm are in the smear or if the smear confirms that the bitch was in estrus, she is likely to be pregnant, and an abdominal ultrasound evaluation should be scheduled for 30 days hence. If no sperm are identified and if the vaginal smear is most consistent with early to midproestrus or with diestrus, pregnancy is not likely. Abdominal ultrasonography may be scheduled but probably will be negative.

If abdominal ultrasonography 30 days after breeding shows that the bitch is pregnant, the options of ovariohysterectomy, allowing the bitch to continue the pregnancy, and therapy directed at abortion can be explained to the client. The specific medication chosen for aborting the bitch should be based on the experience of the veterinarian and drug availability.

If prostaglandin therapy is selected, the bitch should be hospitalized until the abortion process has been completed. Natural $PGF_{2\alpha}$ is administered at a dosage of 0.1 mg/kg subcutaneously three times a day for 2 days, then 0.2 mg/kg subcutaneously twice a day until abortion is complete. Remember that fetuses not consumed by the bitch must be disposed of. Ultrasonography of the abdomen should be done at least every 48 hours until the abortion process is confirmed to have been completed (usually 4 to 9 days). The veterinarian may wish to perform abdominal ultrasonography prior to the scheduled time if signs of abortion have been observed (fetuses, straining, nesting behavior, bloody or greenish vaginal discharge). An attempt should always be made to administer only enough prostaglandin to complete the process.

The bitch should be walked for 30 to 60 minutes after each injection so that side effects can be observed and intervention provided needed (e.g., for shock or severe tachycardia). If necessary, atropine can be administered for excess panting, respiratory distress, vomiting, or diarrhea (0.5 mg/kg IM). If the bitch appears to go into shock (which was observed in only two of more than 120 bitches treated with prostaglandins for pyometra and not in any bitch treated for misalliance), rapid institution of intravenous fluids may be necessary. If severe tachycardia or ventricular arrhythmias are present, appropriate medications can be used. It must be emphasized that side effects are common but rarely life threatening or worrisome enough to require medical intervention.

PREVENTION OF OVARIAN CYCLES

Several treatment options are available to owners for prevention of ovarian cycles in the bitch. For permanent sterility and complete prevention of cycles, ovariohysterectomy is the most obvious and most popular treatment. Reversible contraception by pharmacologic means is occasionally requested. Pharmacologic contraception is one method of preventing or delaying estrus without precluding future fertility. These drugs are usually used in hunting, field trial, and show dogs because an ill-timed estrus could interfere with performance or preclude participation. Owners in North America usually choose ovariohysterectomy because they would rather not deal with administering drugs to their pet.

Surgical Sterilization: Ovariohysterectomy

RECOMMENDED PROCEDURE. Ovariohysterectomy (OVH) is the recommended method of sterilization in the bitch. The surgery is performed commonly and has no drawbacks. It is a procedure with distinct advantages over tubal ligation, salpingectomy, and hysterectomy, which sterilize a bitch but allow her to continue to experience ovarian cycles, with the behavior alterations that accompany estrus. Furthermore, the ovaries remain in situ and could become a site for neoplasia, infection, or torsion. Ovariectomy leaves the uterus, which is a site for potential infection. Ovariectomy, as part of the OVH procedure, has the additional advantage of substantially reducing the risk of mammary neoplasia if the procedure is done before the first ovarian cycle (Schneider, 1990).

QUALITY SURGERY. The need for good surgical practices cannot be overstated. Although OVH is considered routine, it is a major surgical procedure. Infection, dehiscence, adhesions, and incomplete organ extirpation are among the problems that do occur. Among these complications are incomplete removal of ovarian tissue, possibly resulting in a bitch that continues to exhibit ovarian cycle activity (see Chapter 24). If the cervix and cranial vaginal vault are included in the OVH, postsurgical problems are quite uncommon. However, if the cervix and a small portion of the uterine body fail to be removed, this tissue becomes a potential area for infection (see Chapter 23). Careful ligature placement dorsal/proximal to the ovaries and inspection of removed tissue prior to suture placement reduce the incidence of complications.

POST-OVH LACTATION. Lactation after elective OVH is almost always an unexpected and unwanted nuisance as well as a potential nidus for infection. This problem is encountered more commonly in cats than in dogs. The average owner assumes that the veterinary surgeon has done something incorrectly when lactation is observed after OVH. However, this most likely represents a normal physiologic response to acute decreases in the serum progesterone concentration after removal of the ovaries in a bitch in diestrus. The decrease in progesterone is a stimulus to prolactin and oxytocin secretion, just as it would be at parturition. Management of this unfortunate but normal sequela to surgery is the same as that recommended for bitches exhibiting pseudopregnancy (see Chapter 21).

OVH IN PREPUBERTAL BITCHES. Veterinarian and related organizations have debated the age at which bitches should undergo ovariohysterectomy. Common advice, which suggests that a bitch not be neutered until 6 months of age or until she has experienced one or two ovarian cycles, is no longer considered wise. Conclusions from several studies are that skeletal, physical, and behavioral development is not different, comparing puppies (of both sexes) neutered at 7 weeks of age with those neutered at 7 months of age (Salmeri et al, 1991; Howe et al, 2001).

The primary reason to neuter a bitch (or male) earlier than 5 to 6 months of age is to decrease the number of unwanted puppies with which our society must deal (Theran, 1993). Millions of unwanted puppies and kittens are euthanized yearly. The prepubertal neutering of puppies does not eliminate the problem, but it may reduce numbers. Early neutering has not been demonstrated to be in any way harmful. The cost, emotionally and financially, of millions of euthanasias every year *is* harmful. Unless serious damage can be demonstrated to follow the neutering of 6- to 12-week-old puppies, the procedure should be applauded and supported by the veterinary profession. Early spaying and neutering has been endorsed by the American Animal Hospital Association, the British Veterinary Association, and the American College of Veterinary Theriogenologists (Johnston et al, 2001).

POST-OVH OBESITY. Ovariohysterectomy has been implicated as a causative factor for obesity in pets. Some studies have demonstrated that neutering tends to promote increased food intake and weight gain (Concannon and Meyers-Wallen, 1991), whereas another study indicated that neutering did not influence these factors (Salmeri et al, 1991). It is wise to warn owners that some dogs are prone to gain weight after OVH and that this problem can be controlled with exercise and limited feeding. Reducing food intake alone may not resolve the tendency toward obesity in some bitches.

An owner may be concerned about depriving a bitch of the benefit derived from ovarian hormones. However, the estrogen and progesterone concentrations in a dog in anestrus are similar to those in a "spayed" bitch, therefore there is no obvious medical reason to avoid or delay ovariohysterectomy. Some bitches are susceptible to obesity after this surgery, but weight gain and activity can be controlled.

Laparoscopic Sterilization

Laparoscopic sterilization can be accomplished in the bitch. The uterine horns or the uterotubal junctions can be occluded using electrocoagulation or plastic clips. With either technique, the veterinarian must be certain that bilateral occlusion of the reproductive tract is complete. Laparoscopic sterilization is quick and safe, can be performed on young, prepubertal bitches, and could be used for mass sterilization (Wildt and Lawler, 1985). However, such dogs continue to cycle, breed, and attract males, therefore the disadvantages of continued ovarian activity must be considered.

Steroid Hormone Suppression of Ovarian Cycle Activity

BACKGROUND. A variety of natural and synthetic steroid hormones have been demonstrated to inhibit ovarian cycle activity in the bitch. Typically, this is a transient response that depends on continued exposure to the drug. When administration is discontinued and the effect of the drug dissipates, ovarian cycle activity usually but not always resumes. The effectiveness of steroids is due to negative feedback to the pituitary or hypothalamus or both, inhibiting gonadotropin synthesis and secretion.

It should be understood that these drugs can have side effects. Progestagens can promote the development of cystic endometrial hyperplasia with or without development of pyometra and/or mammary development with or without post-therapy lactation. Androgens can induce masculinization of behavior and appearance. Owners, therefore, must be completely informed about side effects. Attention to dose, timing of administration in ovarian cycles, and a review of the bitch's complete medical history and physical examination are always warranted.

MEGESTROL ACETATE

Drug Information. The progestin megestrol acetate is available in the United States as 5 mg and 20 mg tablets under the trade name Ovaban (Schering Corp., Kenilworth, NJ). The daily oral dose and treatment protocol depend on whether therapy begins during anestrus or proestrus (Table 22-1). The mechanism of action is not precisely known, although it is assumed that the drug suppresses gonadotropin hormone or releasing hormone secretion from the hypothalamus or pituitary or both. Megestrol acetate probably mimics the normal feedback action of endogenous ovarian steroids.

Contraindications. Several major contraindications are suggested for megestrol acetate, including avoiding use of the drug in dogs with any disease of the reproductive organs, mammary tumors, or mammary growth. It should not be administered to bitches that are or could be pregnant because of potential masculinization of female fetuses and because

TABLE 22–1 PERTINENT INFORMATION REGARDING THE USE OF MEGESTROL ACETATE* AS AN ESTRUS-PREVENTING CONTRACEPTIVE

Marketed as a canine contraceptive

Synthetic progestin; tablets; oral administration

Low daily dose for 1 month in anestrus will delay next cycle by 2–8 months, i.e., 0.55 mg/kg/day for 32 days

High dose for 8 days used in early proestrus to terminate current heat, i.e., 2.2 mg/kg/day for 8 days

Approved for up to two consecutive treatments only

Requires reproductive exam and vaginal smear to confirm anestrus or early proestrus, and absence of pregnancy

Potential problems: may promote uterine or mammary hyperplasia or disease; aggravation of diabetes or hepatobiliary diseases; fertile estrus can occur if started too late in proestrus

*Ovaban, Schering.

progestagens could delay parturition. This drug should not be used in dogs prior to or during the first ovarian cycle. If estrus occurs within 30 days of discontinuation of therapy, mating should be prevented. The drug should not be administered for more than two consecutive treatment periods because of the potential hazard of cystic endometrial hyperplasia. Megestrol acetate should not be administered to dogs known to have or suspected of having diabetes mellitus because of the insulin antagonistic effects of progestagens.

Side Effects. Side effects are not common with megestrol acetate administration. Occasionally the following transient progestational side effects have been noted in clinical studies: mammary enlargement, lactation, listlessness, increased appetite, and change in temperament. Long-term therapy may predispose a bitch to diabetes mellitus or acromegaly or both (Harding, 1981; Concannon and Meyers-Wallen, 1991). Veterinarians must follow the manufacturer's suggested doses. Pyometra develops in a rather small percentage of bitches (<1%). Megestrol acetate has been demonstrated to cause adrenocortical suppression in cats (see Chapter 8).

Anestrus Treatment. The recommended dose of megestrol acetate to postpone proestrus and estrus is 0.55 mg/kg body weight given orally once daily for 32 days. The return to estrus may occur at any time; in clinical trials, estrus activity began 1 to 7 months after discontinuation of treatment (average, 4 to 6 months). If a bitch is treated too early in anestrus, the effect of the drug may dissipate before any obvious postponement of the next cycle occurs. If the treatment is started too late, she may begin proestrus while receiving the drug or soon after, requiring a change in dosage to the proestrus protocol. Therefore, it is recommended that the time for beginning megestrol acetate therapy during anestrus be determined after a review of the bitch's past interestrous intervals. Treatment should begin 1 to 2 weeks prior to the next expected proestrus (Concannon, 1983).

Proestrus Treatment. Megestrol acetate can be administered to a bitch, beginning in the first 3 days of proestrus, to discontinue and postpone that cycle. The treatment protocol is based on the assumption that a bitch is progressing through an average proestrus. It has been suggested that a bitch that usually has a proestrus of less than 4 or greater than 20 days' duration not be considered a candidate for this therapy (Harding, 1981). Early proestrus should be confirmed with vaginal cytology before treatment is initiated.

The recommended dose of megestrol acetate for the proestrual bitch is 2.2 mg/kg body weight given orally once daily for 8 days. The bitch should be confined until the bloody vaginal discharge has stopped or for 1 to 2 weeks to avoid breeding and subsequent pregnancy in the event the treatment was initiated too late. Suppression of proestrus is seen within 3 to 8 days, and the cycle is typically delayed for 4 to 6 months. If treatment is initiated too soon, proestrus may begin shortly after the medication is stopped. If treatment

begins too late in proestrus, a fertile estrus may occur while the bitch is receiving the drug.

Additional protocols are available for the use of megestrol acetate in the United Kingdom (Evans, 1988).

MIBOLERONE

Drug Information. Mibolerone is useful for preventing estrus in adult female dogs not intended primarily for breeding purposes. Compared with methyltestosterone, this drug is 41 times more potent as an anabolic agent and 16 times more potent as an androgen. Mibolerone has no significant progestational nor estrogenic activity and is thought to block LH secretion. It is available as a liquid (100 mg/ml) that can be added to the food and is marketed under the trade name Cheque (Pharmacia & Upjohn, Peapack, NJ).

Side Effects. Mibolerone should not be used in pregnant bitches or female dogs with perianal adenoma, perianal adenocarcinoma, or other androgen-dependent neoplastic conditions. Other androgenic effects include clitoral enlargement, mounting behavior, and musky body odor. Approximately 10% of treated bitches develop a whitish, viscid vaginal discharge, and some have had small vaginal mucosal vesicles posterior to the urethral orifice.

Mibolerone is not recommended for any dog with a previous history of liver or kidney disease because it appears to be metabolized in the liver and excreted into the urine and feces. A few dogs have become icteric while receiving this agent, causing termination of treatment. Bitches treated for a prolonged period (longer than 8 months) should undergo periodic liver function testing. This medication is to be used with caution or not at all in bitches younger than 7 months of age because of the potential for induction of premature epiphyseal closure.

Drug Abuse. Several "side effects" caused by mibolerone actually encourage some owners to use this drug. Specifically, as a potent androgen, mibolerone appears to increase muscle strength, stamina, and aggressiveness in the bitch. These traits may be considered positive side effects for field trial bitches. Although this application is not recommended, it is recognized to occur.

Dosage and Administration. Administration of mibolerone should be initiated at least 30 days prior to the expected onset of proestrus. The dose depends on the breed and body weight (Table 22-2). The liquid is administered once daily in the food or placed in the mouth. The medication can be given for as long as 2 years, although longer periods of treatment (up to 5 years) have been successful (Concannon, 1983). After cessation of treatment, ovarian activity usually returns within 1 to 7 months. If the drug is started too late in anestrus, a treated bitch may begin proestrus within 30 days despite receiving the medication. If this happens, mibolerone should be discontinued.

DEPOT INJECTABLE PROGESTERONE.

A single intramuscular injection of medroxyprogesterone acetate maintains effective circulating levels of this progestagen for several months. The drug was marketed as a canine

TABLE 22–2 DOSE SCHEDULE OF MIBOLERONE RECOMMENDED FOR ESTRUS PREVENTION IN THE BITCH*

BODY WEIGHT OF DOG		MIBOLERONE DAILY DOSE	
lb	kg	ml	µg
1–25	0.5–12	0.3	30
26–50	13–23	0.6	60
51–100	24–45	1.2	120
100	>45	1.8	180
Any German Shepherd dog or German Shepherd mix any weight		1.8	180

*Medication begun during anestrus. Can be given orally once each day in the food or directly in the mouth.

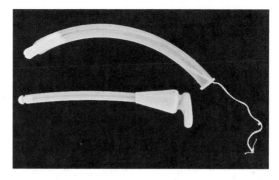

FIGURE 22–5. Two devices that have been proposed for intravaginal use in bitches to prevent breeding. No such device has been reported to have been used successfully in a group of privately owned bitches.

contraceptive (Promone) until 1969. Although successful in delaying heat cycles, the drug was not considered safe because it induced CEH and pyometra in a large number of bitches. Administered in midanestrus, the drug is reliable. However, the adverse effects were probably caused by overdosing and/or administration during stages of the cycle other than anestrus. High doses also contributed to mammary tumor development, adrenal suppression, and acromegaly (Concannon et al, 1980). The recommended dose is approximately 2 mg/kg every 3 months or 3 mg/kg every 4 months. The drug is *not recommended* for any use in the intact bitch because of an unacceptable incidence of uterine lesions (Von Berky and Townsend, 1993).

DepoProvera, another injectable form of medroxyprogesterone acetate, is available for use in the dog in Great Britain and Europe.

STEROID HORMONE IMPLANTS. Silastic capsules containing slow-release formulations of progestagens or androgens can result in long-term suppression of ovarian activity. However, because such implants require surgical placement, are not biodegradable, and are large, they have not gained acceptance in veterinary medicine. Smaller injectable implants of the progestin levonorgestrel have been developed for long-term contraception in women (Shoupe and Mishell, 1989). This has not been evaluated in dogs (Concannon and Meyers-Wallen, 1991).

TESTOSTERONE INJECTIONS. Weekly intramuscular injections of testosterone propionate (110 mg) and the use of oral androgens (25 mg of methyltestosterone) given weekly for as long as 5 years have been used to prevent ovarian activity in Greyhounds (Burke, 1982). Some believe the drug also enhances racing performance. Why such drug usage is allowed is not understood, nor is it considered acceptable.

PROLIGESTERONE. This progestin (14α,17α-propylidene dioxyprogesterone) is available as an injectable suspension for use as a canine contraceptive in the United Kingdom and Europe. It is administered subcutaneously (10 to 30 mg/kg), with injections subsequently given 3 months later, then after an additional 4 months, and finally every 5 months. In

clinical trials, this regimen did not cause development of uterine disease or mammary tumors. Furthermore, the investigators suggested little or no need to restrict usage according to the stage of the ovarian cycle. They have stated that this drug is safer than the use of other progestins as contraceptives in dogs (Evans and Sutton, 1989).

VAGINAL OR INTRAUTERINE DEVICES. Various vaginal devices have been marketed that are designed to block intromission by the male (Fig. 22-5). None has gained wide acceptance because of unacceptable failure rates, lack of practicality, problems with fitting, harm to the bitch, and owner dissatisfaction. Intrauterine devices cannot be used because of the difficulties associated with cannulating the canine cervix.

IMMUNIZATION. Immunization technology to provide reversible contraception in the bitch has been investigated and evaluated. One approach is immunization directed at antibody development against the zona pellucida of the egg. Such antibodies either prevent fertilization, destroy eggs prior to fertilization, or eventually deplete ovaries of fertile follicles (Shivers et al, 1981; Mahi-Brown et al, 1982, 1985, and 1988). However, the use of immunization has not yet undergone large-scale clinical trials, and its role in the future remains undetermined.

Immunization against endogenous LH may successfully result in contraceptive action in males and females. Evidence indicates that immunization against GnRH can have contraceptive activity in dogs. However, antibody titers obtained in one study were insufficient to prevent ovarian activity consistently (Gonzalez et al, 1989).

LONG-TERM GNRH AGONIST ADMINISTRATION. Continuous administration of large amounts of a GnRH agonist results in downregulation of pituitary GnRH receptors, subsequent decreases in the secretion of LH or FSH or both, and suppression of ovarian cycle activity (Concannon et al, 1988; Vickery et al, 1989). Such treatment requires surgical implantation of minipumps or some other method of maintaining chronic and continuous exposure to the drug. No clinical trials have been reported (Concannon and Meyers-Wallen, 1991).

REFERENCES

Arbeiter K, et al: Treatment of pseudopregnancy in the bitch with cabergoline, an ergoline derivative. J Small Anim Pract 29:781, 1988.

Bowen RA, et al: Efficacy and toxicity of estrogens commonly used to terminate canine pregnancy. J Am Vet Med Assoc 186:783, 1985.

Bowen RA, et al: Efficacy and toxicity of tamoxifen citrate for prevention and termination of pregnancy in bitches. Am J Vet Res 49:27, 1988.

Burke TJ: Pharmacologic control of estrus in the bitch and queen. Vet Clin North Am (Small Anim Pract) 12:79, 1982.

Burke TJ: Population control in the bitch. In Morrow DA (ed): Current Therapy in Theriogenology 2. Philadelphia, WB Saunders, 1986, p 528.

Concannon PW: Fertility regulation in the bitch: Contraception, sterilization, and pregnancy termination. In Kirk RW (ed): Current Veterinary Therapy VIII. Philadelphia, WB Saunders, 1983, p 901.

Concannon PW: New and proposed contraceptives for dogs. Proceedings of the Society for Theriogenology, 1991, p 221.

Concannon PW, Meyers-Wallen VN: Current and proposed methods for contraception and termination of pregnancy in dogs and cats. J Am Vet Med Assoc 198:1214, 1991.

Concannon PW, et al: Growth hormone, prolactin, and cortisol in dogs developing mammary nodules and an acromegaly-like appearance during treatment with medroxyprogesterone acetate. Endocrinology 106:1173, 1980.

Concannon PW, et al: Suppression of luteal function in dogs by luteinizing hormone antiserum and by bromocriptine. J Reprod Fertil 81:175, 1987.

Concannon PW, et al: Suppression of LH secretion by constant infusion of GnRH agonist in ovariectomized dogs and prolonged contraception of prepubertal bitches by constant subcutaneous administration of GnRH agonist. Proceedings of the Eleventh International Congress of Animal Reproduction and Artificial Insemination 4:427, 1988.

Concannon PW, et al: Termination of pregnancy and induction of premature luteolysis by the antiprogestagen, mifepristone, in dogs. J Reprod Fertil 88:99, 1990.

Davidson A: Induction of abortion in bitches with intravaginal misoprostol and parenteral PGF_{2alpha}. Proceedings of the Annual Meeting of the Society for Theriogenology, 1998, p 86.

England GCW: Pregnancy diagnosis, abnormalities of pregnancy, and pregnancy termination. In Simpson GM, England GCW, Harvey M (eds): BSAVA Manual of Small Animal Reproduction and Neonatology. United Kingdom, British Small Animal Veterinary Association, 1998, p 113.

Evans JM: Oestrus control in the bitch. J Small Anim Pract 29:535, 1988.

Evans JM, Sutton DJ: The use of hormones, especially progestagens, to control oestrus in bitches. J Reprod Fertil 39:163, 1989.

Feldman EC, et al: Prostaglandin induction of abortion in pregnant bitches after misalliance. J Am Vet Med Assoc 202:1855, 1993.

Fieni F: An original molecule to induce abortion in bitches: Aglepristone—A clinical study defining efficacy and absence of side effects. J Reprod Fertil Suppl 47:403, 1995.

Fieni F, et al: Midpregnancy termination in bitches with an antiprogestin: aglepristone (RU534). Proceedings: Advances in Dog, Cat and Exotic Carnivore Reproduction. Oslo, Norway, 2000a, p 111.

Fieni F, et al: Efficacy, safety, and hormonal kinetics in pregnancy termination in bitches with an antiprogestin: aglepristone (RU534). Proceedings: Advances in Dog, Cat and Exotic Carnivore Reproduction. Oslo, Norway, 2000b, p 81.

Galac S, et al: Pregnancy termination in bitches with aglepristone, a progesterone receptor antagonist. Proceedings: Advances in Dog, Cat and Exotic Carnivore Reproduction. Oslo, Norway, 2000, p 103.

Gonzalez A, et al: Immunological approaches to contraception in dogs. J Reprod Fertil Suppl 39:189, 1989.

Hall EJ: Use of lithium for treatment of estrogen-induced bone marrow hypoplasia in a dog. J Am Vet Med Assoc 200:814, 1992.

Harding RB: The use of megestrol acetate in oestrus control in dogs. Post Acak Onderstepoort 13:30, 1981.

Howe LM, et al: Long-term outcome of gonadectomy performed at an early age or traditional age in dogs. J Am Vet Med Assoc 218:217, 2001.

Jackson PS, et al: A preliminary study of pregnancy termination in the bitch with slow-release formulations of prostaglandin analogs. J Small Anim Pract 23:287, 1982.

Jackson W, Johnston S: Pregnancy prevention and termination. In Kirk RW (ed): Current Veterinary Therapy VII. Philadelphia, WB Saunders, 1980, p 1239.

Jain JK, Mishell DR: A comparison of intravaginal misoprostol with prostaglandin E_2 for termination of second-trimester pregnancy. N Engl J Med 331:290, 1994.

Jochle W, et al: Effects on pseudopregnancy and interoestrous intervals of pharmacological suppression of prolactin secretion in female dogs and cats. J Reprod Fertil Suppl 39:199, 1989.

Johnston SD: Canine pregnancy termination with prostaglandin $F_{2\alpha}$. Proceedings of the Annual Meeting of the Society of Theriogenology, 1990, p 264.

Johnston SD, Root Kustritz MV, Olson PNS: Canine and Feline Theriogenology. Philadelphia, WB Saunders, 2001, p 173.

Keister DM, et al: Efficacy of oral epostane administration to terminate pregnancy in mated laboratory bitches. J Reprod Fertil Suppl 39:241, 1989.

Lein DH: Prostaglandins in small animal reproduction. In Morrow DA (ed): Current Therapy in Theriogenology 2. Philadelphia, WB Saunders, 1983, p 481.

Lein DH, et al: Termination of pregnancy in bitches by administration of prostaglandin $F_{2\alpha}$. J Reprod Fertil Suppl 39:231, 1989.

Mahi-Brown CA, et al: Infertility in bitches induced by active immunization with porcine zonae pellucidae. J Exp Zool 222:89, 1982.

Mahi-Brown CA, et al: Fertility control in the bitch by active immunization with porcine zonae pellucidae: Use of different adjuvants and patterns of estradiol and progesterone level in estrous cycles. Biol Reprod 32:761, 1985.

Mahi-Brown CA, et al: Ovarian histology of bitches immunized with porcine zonae pellucidae. Am J Reprod Immunol Microbiol 18:94, 1988.

Nelson RW, et al: Treatment of canine pyometra and endometritis with prostaglandin $F_{2\alpha}$. J Am Vet Med Assoc 181:899, 1982.

Niskanen M, Thrusfield MV: Associations between age, parity, hormonal therapy, and breed, and pyometra in Finnish dogs. Vet Rec 143:493, 1998.

Oettle EE: Clinical experience with prostaglandin F_{2alpha} THAM as a luteolytic agent in pregnant and nonpregnant bitches. J S Afr Vet Assoc 53:239, 1982.

Oettle EE, et al: Luteolysis in early diestrous Beagle bitches. Theriogenology 29:757, 1988.

Olson PN: Exfoliative cytology of the canine reproductive tract. Proceedings of the Society for Theriogenology, 1989, p 259.

Olson PN, Johnston SD: New developments in small animal population control. J Am Vet Med Assoc 202:904, 1993.

Olson PN, et al: Evaluation of the efficacy and toxicity of estrogens used to terminate pregnancy in the bitch. Proceedings of the American College of Veterinary Internal Medicine, Washington, DC, 1984, p 35 (abstract).

Olson PN, et al: A need for sterilization, contraceptives, and abortifacients: Abandoned and unwanted pets. Part III. Abortifacients. Compend Contin Educ Prac Vet 8:235, 1986.

Onclin K, Verstegen JPL: Practical use of a combination of a dopamine agonist and a synthetic prostaglandin analogue to terminate unwanted pregnancy in dogs. J Small Anim Pract 37:211, 1996.

Onclin K et al: Termination of unwanted pregnancy in dogs with the dopamine agonist cabergoline in combination with synthetic analogue of either cloprostenol or alphaprostol. Theriogenology 43:813, 1995.

Paradis M, et al: Effects of prostaglandin $F_{2\alpha}$ on corpora lutea formation and function in mated bitches. Can Vet J 24:239, 1983.

Post K: Induced pregnancy termination in dogs. Theriogenology Handbook C2:1, 1995.

Post K, et al: Effects of prolactin suppression with cabergoline on the pregnancy of the bitch. Theriogenology 29:1233, 1988.

Romagnoli SE, et al: Use of prostaglandin $F_{2\alpha}$ for early pregnancy termination in the mismated bitch. Vet Clin North Am (Small Anim Pract) 21:487, 1991.

Romagnoli SE, et al: Clinical use of a-prostol (synthetic $PGF_{2\alpha}$ analogue) to induce early abortion in mismated bitches: Comparison between single vs bid treatment. Proceedings: Advances in Dog, Cat and Exotic Carnivore Reproduction. Oslo, Norway, 2000, p 108.

Salmeri KR, et al: Gonadectomy in immature dogs: Effects on skeletal, physical, and behavioral development. J Am Vet Med Assoc 198:1193, 1991.

Sankai T, et al: Antiprogesterone compound RU486 administration to terminate pregnancy in dogs and cats. J Vet Med Sci 53:1069, 1991.

Schneider R: Epidemiological aspects of mammary and genital neoplasia. In Morrow D (ed): Current Therapy in Theriogenology. Philadelphia, WB Saunders, 1990, p 636.

Shille VM: Mismating and termination of pregnancy. Vet Clin North Am 12:99, 1985.

Shille VM, et al: Induction of abortion in the bitch with a synthetic prostaglandin analogue. Am J Vet Res 45:1295, 1984.

Shivers CA, et al: Pregnancy prevention in the dog: Potential for a immunological approach. J Am Anim Hosp Assoc 17:823, 1981.

Shoupe D, Mishell DR: Norplant: Subdermal implant system for long-term contraception. Am J Obstet Gynecol 160:1286, 1989.

Soderberg SF, Olson PN: Abortifacients. In Kirk RW (ed): Current Veterinary Therapy VIII. Philadelphia, WB Saunders, 1983, p 945.

Spitz IM, et al. Early pregnancy termination with mifepristone and misoprostol in the United States. N Engl J Med 338:1241, 1998.

Suess RP, et al: Bone marrow hypoplasia in a feminized dog with an interstitial cell tumor. J Am Vet Med Assoc 200:1346, 1992.

Theran P: Early-age neutering of dogs and cats. J Am Vet Med Assoc 202:914, 1993.

Tsutsui T, et al: Effects of prostaglandin F_{2alpha} on implantation and maintenance of pregnancy in the dog. Jpn J Vet Sci 44:403, 1982.

Verstegen JPL: Overview of mismating regimens in the bitch. In Bonagura J (ed). Current Veterinary Therapy XIII. Philadelphia, WB Saunders, 2000, p 947.

Verstegen JPL, et al: Influence of estrogens on blood parameters in bitches. Ann Med Vet 125:397, 1981.

Verstegen JPL, et al: Abortion induction in queens and bitches using cabergoline, a specific dopamine agonist. Ann Med Vet 137:251, 1993.

Vickery B, McRae G: Effect of a synthetic prostaglandin analogue on pregnancy in Beagle bitches. Biol Reprod 22:438, 1980.

Vickery B, et al: Use of potent LHRH analogues for chronic contraception and pregnancy termination in dogs. J Reprod Fertil Suppl 39:175, 1989.

Von Berky AG, Townsend WL: The relationship between the prevalence of uterine lesions and the use of medroxyprogesterone acetate for canine population control. Aust Vet J 70:249, 1993.

Webster J, et al: A comparison of cabergoline and bromocriptine in the treatment of hyperprolactinemic amenorrhea. N Engl J Med 331:904, 1994.

Wildt DE, Lawler DF: Laparoscopic sterilization of the bitch and queen by uterine horn occlusion. Am J Vet Res 46:864, 1985.

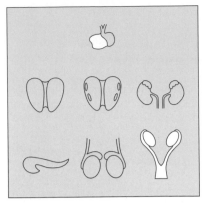

23

CYSTIC ENDOMETRIAL HYPERPLASIA/PYOMETRA COMPLEX

PATHOPHYSIOLOGY

Hormonal Influence (Progesterone)

CYSTIC ENDOMETRIAL HYPERPLASIA. Pyometra in the bitch is a hormonally mediated diestrual disorder. The disease is caused by a bacterial infection within the uterus and results in mild to severe and life-threatening bacteremia and toxemia. The uterus may have undergone a pathologic change that predisposed it to sepsis before development of infection; this underlying condition is called *cystic endometrial hyperplasia (CEH)*. CEH is assumed to be caused, in part, by an abnormal uterine response to chronic and repeated exposure to progesterone. However, other factors may have a role. A model of CEH has been developed by simply placing a silk suture in the uterine lumen of bitches during diestrus (Nomura, 1995). Estrogen may augment the effect of progesterone, enhancing development of CEH (Chen et al, 2000).

CEH DOES NOT ALWAYS PRECEDE PYOMETRA. Severe, life-threatening pyometra can occur in the absence of CEH. It is extremely rare, however, for pyometra to occur in a bitch that was not under the influence of progesterone at the time that infection began. On occasion, a bitch develops pyometra during diestrus (the progesterone-dominated phase of the ovarian cycle), but the syndrome progresses slowly, presumably because the infection is mild. In a small number of bitches, by the time the disease creates clinical signs or becomes severe enough for the owner to seek veterinary care for the dog, the ovarian cycle of the bitch may have progressed into anestrus. However, even in this situation, the disease began during diestrus.

PROGESTERONE CONCENTRATIONS. Plasma progesterone concentration in the anestrus bitch is low (basal; <0.5 ng/ml). Progesterone concentrations remain below 1.0 ng/ml during proestrus and then begin to rise at the onset of estrus, typically being greater than 2.0 ng/ml. Progesterone concentrations continue to increase throughout estrus and continues through the first several weeks of diestrus, followed by a plateau in serum concentrations and then a slow return toward basal concentrations. The return of concentrations less than 1.0 ng/ml marks the end of diestrus.

PROGESTERONE AND INFECTION. For approximately 9 to 12 weeks in normal bitches, following ovulation in each ovarian cycle, the plasma progesterone concentration is increased and often exceeds 40 ng/ml. During this phase, progesterone promotes or supports endometrial growth and glandular secretion while suppressing myometrial activity, allowing accumulation of uterine glandular secretions. These secretions provide an excellent environment for bacterial growth. Bacterial growth is further enhanced by inhibition of the leukocyte response to infection in the progesterone-primed uterus. Thus the uterus becomes a prime target for potential hostile takeover by bacteria. Bacterial infections associated with pyometra involve the same bacteria recognized as normal vaginal vault flora. These bacteria frequently cross the cervix and are found within the uterus during proestrus and estrus. However, there must be some combination of the ovarian (progesterone) phase of the estrous cycle and factors or changes in the uterine environment that allows overgrowth of bacteria normally isolated from this area of the anatomy.

Cystic Endometrial Hyperplasia

Progesterone-induced endometrial hyperplasia usually precedes the development of pyometra in bitches older than 6 years of age. Although pyometra is well recognized and commonly seen in bitches younger than 6 years of age, that population is less likely to have endometrial hyperplasia. Regardless of age, when pathologic hyperplasia is present and progressive, it becomes cystic, the result being cystic endometrial hyperplasia. Endometrial thickening is due to an increase in the size and number of endometrial glands, which may exhibit secretory activity. The mucosal epithelial cells are typically tortuous, with hypertrophic and clear cytoplasm. The stroma becomes edematous, and an inflammatory cell infiltrate is invariably present. CEH occasionally results in accumulation of thin or viscid fluid within the lumen of the uterus. This sterile, fluid-filled uterus is commonly referred to as *hydrometra* or *mucometra*, the degree of hydration of the mucin determining its description.

Pyometra is the most common problem associated with CEH. Much less frequently, CEH can cause infertility or chronic endometritis. Confirming the diagnosis of CEH is difficult because it is not usually associated with clinical signs unless the uterine contents become infected; this is referred to as *pyometra*. Confirmation of uninfected CEH requires uterine biopsy. No recognized therapy is available for CEH (Harvey, 1998).

Bacteria

Bacterial contamination of the uterus appears to be a normal phenomenon in the proestrual or estrual bitch, one that is naturally cleared before overgrowth becomes a problem. The most likely bacteria resulting in pathologic uterine infection are those known to inhabit the vaginal vault (Baba et al, 1983). These bacteria have the potential to, and commonly do, ascend through the relatively dilated cervix into the uterus during proestrus and estrus (Noakes et al, 2000). Biochemical fingerprinting of *Escherichia coli* (*E. coli*) cultured from the uterus of a bitch with pyometra showed that the organisms were identical or similar to those bacteria isolated from feces of these same dogs (Wadas et al, 1996).

Other bacterial sources for uterine infection have been suggested, including concomitant urinary tract infections and transient bacteremias. However, common vaginal flora is the logical source for uterine contamination. A predominance of *E. coli*, a common constituent of the normal vaginal flora, is recognized in uterine infections. *E. coli* may adhere via specific antigenic sites to receptors in the progesterone-stimulated endometrium and myometrium.

The presence of bacterial flora in the vaginal tract is constant. Cervical dilation is associated with proestrus and estrus, and it is assumed that bacterial contamination of the uterus occurs during these phases of the estrous cycle (Baba et al, 1983). However, uterine infection or pathology is rare, suggesting that the inevitable "contamination" is both controlled and rapidly cleared from the normal bitch. Intrauterine bacteria, therefore, cannot solely account for the pathogenesis of pyometra. Significant uterine disease or some other predisposing factor (progesterone or estrogen administration) predisposes bitches to pyometra. Part of the predisposition is the normal postovulation increase in plasma progesterone concentrations, because pyometra is seen only during or immediately following diestrus. Exogenous progesterone administration also increases the incidence of pyometra. Therefore, contributing factors to development of pyometra are CEH, bacteria, diestrus/elevation in serum progesterone concentrations, and exogenous progesterone or estrogen administration.

The bacterium usually associated with pyometra is *E. coli*. However, staphylococci, streptococci, *Klebsiella, Pseudomonas, Proteus, Haemophilus, Pasturella, Serratia,* and other bacteria have been isolated from the uteri of bitches with pyometra (Stone, 1985; Wheaton et al, 1989). These bacteria can be identified in the vaginal tracts of healthy normal bitches. The culture results from bitches with pyometra often demonstrate a pure growth of one bacterial species. However, some bitches with pyometra have two or more bacterial isolates cultured from the uterine contents (Memon and Mickelsen, 1993). Normal bitches can have vaginal bacterial flora composed of several bacterial species or a single isolate. It is uncommon for a bitch to have no growth (Bjurstrom and LindeForsberg, 1992).

E. coli is a gram-negative bacterium containing a chemically stable, biologically active lipopolysaccharide endotoxin in the cell membrane. The endotoxin is released as bacteria die and disintegrate. Clinical endotoxemia occurs when serum levels exceed ~0.05 ng/ml. Clinical signs of endotoxemia include hypothermia, disorientation, and signs of septic shock. The minimum lethal concentration of endotoxin in serum is approximately 0.7 ng/ml. In a review of 92 bitches with pyometra, 7 had endotoxemia. Furthermore, the release of endotoxin may be enhanced and clinical signs exacerbated by antibiotic treatment, since antibiotics should increase the rate at which bacteria die (Frannson et al, 1997; Johnston et al, 2001).

Estrogen

Exogenous estrogen, regardless of the specific chemical form used, enhances the stimulatory effect of progesterone on the uterus. This appears to be the result of estrogen sensitizing progesterone receptors and enhancing the binding of progesterone (Niskanen and Thrusfield, 1998). Supraphysiologic concentrations of estrogen resulting from exogenous administration (e.g., mismate injections) during estrus or diestrus dramatically increase the risk for developing pyometra. For this reason, estrogen injections to prevent pregnancy are strongly discouraged.

TWO DISTINCT PYOMETRA SYNDROMES: THE OLDER BITCH. The bitch that is older than 7 or 8 years of age is prone to CEH and subsequent pyometra. This appears to be an age-related phenomenon. The syndrome results from repeated exposure to progesterone during normal diestrus phases of the estrous cycle. After years of ovarian activity, the predisposition for and incidence of CEH increase. Therefore the risk for developing pyometra becomes exaggerated in the otherwise healthy older bitch.

TWO DISTINCT PYOMETRA SYNDROMES: THE YOUNGER BITCH. A significant number of young bitches (<6 years of age) have been diagnosed as having pyometra. It is unlikely that similar pathophysiologic processes account for uterine disease in old and young dogs. Chronic recurring exposure to progesterone cannot have occurred in these younger animals. However, a strong correlation exists between the incidence of pyometra in young dogs and estrogen administration by veterinarians attempting to prevent pregnancy (Bowen et al, 1985; Wheaton et al, 1989). Estrogen administration for accidental breedings is not recommended. If the misbred bitch is not valuable as a brood bitch, she should undergo ovariohysterectomy (be spayed). If she is of value, carrying the unwanted pregnancy to term or inducing an abortion (see Chapter 22) is preferable to estrogen therapy.

SIGNALMENT AND HISTORY

Traditional Description Versus Clinical Experience

Traditionally, pyometra has been described as a disorder of middle-aged bitches (>6 years of age). It theoretically develops after years of repetitive progesterone stimulation of the uterus, as part of each ovarian cycle. However, with the common use of estrogens for mismating in young bitches, we have seen open-cervix and closed-cervix pyometras develop in young dogs as well. This includes bitches less than 1 year of age, having just completed their first estrus. The mean age is 2.4 years in 192 bitches with open- and closed-cervix pyometra treated by the authors with $PGF_{2\alpha}$. A diagnosis of pyometra should be considered in any bitch with consistent clinical signs that appear during or immediately following diestrus, regardless of age.

TABLE 23-1 CLINICAL SIGNS COMMONLY SEEN IN BITCHES WITH PYOMETRA

Sign	Percent of Dogs
Vaginal discharge	85
Lethargy-depression	62
Inappetence/anorexia	42
Polyuria and/or polydipsia	28
Vomiting	15
Nocturia	5
Diarrhea	5
Abdominal enlargement	5

Pyometra occurs in dogs of any breed. There has been a report suggesting increased risk in rough-coated Collies, Rottweilers, Cavalier King Charles Spaniels, Golden Retrievers, Bernese Mountain Dogs, and English Cocker Spaniels compared with all other breeds, including mixed breed dogs. Breeds with a low risk for pyometra include Drevers, German Shepherds, Miniature and normal-sized Dachshunds, and Swedish Hounds (Egenvall et al, 2001).

Open-Cervix Pyometra

Owner-reported signs depend on the patency of the cervix (Table 23-1). An obvious sign seen in bitches with open-cervix pyometra is a sanguineous to muco-purulent discharge from the vagina. The discharge is usually first noticed 4 to 8 weeks after standing heat. Pyometra has been diagnosed as early as the end of standing heat and as late as 12 to 14 weeks after standing heat. Other common signs include lethargy, depression, inappetence/anorexia, polyuria, polydipsia, vomiting, and diarrhea (Wheaton et al, 1989). Open-cervix pyometra may be recognized quickly in some bitches by experienced owners. These bitches can be relatively healthy aside from the abnormal vaginal discharge. The overall health of the bitch with a pyometra depends primarily on how quickly the client recognizes the problem and seeks veterinary assistance.

Closed-Cervix Pyometra

The bitch with closed-cervix pyometra is often quite ill at the time of diagnosis compared with dogs that have open-cervix pyometra. This is due to the lack of an easily recognized, early sign of a serious problem. Specifically, dogs with closed-cervix pyometra do not have the purulent vaginal discharge seen with open-cervix infection. Instead, owners are more likely to notice insidious signs that usually include depression, lethargy, inappetence, polydipsia and/or polyuria, and weight loss. These signs, in conjunction with the vomiting and/or diarrhea associated with progressive septicemia and toxemia, can result in progressively worsening dehydration, shock, coma, and eventually death, unless owners realize that their pet is ill and seek attention.

Occasionally, owners report the observation of a vaginal discharge that lasted 1 or 2 days and occurred before the development of more serious systemic signs of illness. Because the discharge did not persist and because the bitch may have appeared healthy, veterinary consultation may have been delayed. Again, severity of illness at the time of examination depends to a large degree on the ability of the owner to recognize a problem and then seek veterinary care. A small number of bitches with closed-cervix pyometra have signs consistent with polyarthritis, secondary to bacteremia and joint infection.

PHYSICAL EXAMINATION

Abnormalities on physical examination consistent with pyometra include depression, dehydration, fever, palpable uterine enlargement, and a sanguineous to mucopurulent discharge from the vagina if the cervix is patent ("open"). The rectal temperature may be increased or within the normal range. Fever is associated with uterine inflammation and secondary bacterial infection, as well as septicemia or toxemia. With septicemia or toxemia, shock may ensue with tachycardia, prolonged capillary refill time, weak femoral pulses, and subnormal rectal temperature.

Uterine enlargement may be obvious. The uterus, however, could be difficult to palpate, especially if it is draining much of its content or if it is enlarged but flaccid. The size and weight of the dog plus the degree of abdominal relaxation also affect the ease of palpating uterine enlargement. Abdominal radiography can be used to confirm the diagnosis (one must remember that the pregnant bitch, prior to calcification of fetal skeletons, has uterine enlargement on radiographs, which could be confused with pyometra).

Overzealous palpation should be avoided to prevent uterine rupture. A palpable uterus is always considered an abnormal finding in the nonpregnant bitch in diestrus. Even if not palpable, the organ may still be massively inflamed and infected, causing obvious clinical signs.

CLINICAL PATHOLOGY

White Blood Cell Counts

The total white blood cell count in bitches with pyometra is variable. An absolute neutrophilia (usually >25,000 cells/μl) with variable degrees of cellular immaturity (presence of a "left shift," that is, >300 bands/μl) may be observed secondary to significant infection, inflammation, and septicemia. The infection, if severe and/or chronic, may cause a "degenerative left shift" with toxic neutrophils. Although increases in total white blood cell counts are identified in a slight majority of bitches with open-cervix pyometra (50% to 75%), normal or even decreased white blood cell counts may be docu-

mented. Some of these dogs do not exhibit evidence of the overwhelming infection seen in closed-cervix pyometra. Seventy-eight of the 163 (48%) bitches with open-cervix pyometra we have treated with PGF$_{2\alpha}$ had total white blood cell counts within the normal range before initiation of any therapy. Of those managed surgically, 20 of 80 (25%) had total white blood cell counts within the normal range (Wheaton et al, 1989).

The percentage of bitches with increased white blood cell counts that have closed-cervix pyometra is greater than those with increased white blood cell counts and open-cervix pyometra. Also, the percentage of bitches with abnormally decreased white blood cell counts and closed-cervix pyometra is greater than with open-cervix pyometra. In 42 closed-cervix pyometra dogs treated with prostaglandins at our clinic, 36 (86%) had abnormally increased white blood cell counts and 5 (12%) had decreased counts (<5000/μl).

Red Blood Cell Counts

Because pyometra is a chronic inflammatory disease, it is not surprising that a mild normocytic, normochromic, nonregenerative anemia (packed cell volume, 28% to 35%) often develops. The septicemia or toxemia associated with pyometra can suppress the bone marrow; this effect is most noticeable in the shift of neutrophils toward immaturity and the nonregenerative nature of the anemia. The anemia should resolve once the pyometra is corrected.

Serum Biochemistry Profile

Hyperproteinemia (total protein, 7.5 to 10.0 g/dl) and hyperglobulinemia commonly result from dehydration and/or chronic antigenic stimulation of the immune system. The BUN may be increased if dehydration and prerenal uremia are present. Occasionally, serum alanine aminotransferase (ALT) and alkaline phosphatase activities are mild to moderately increased as a result of hepatocellular damage caused by septicemia and/or diminished hepatic circulation and cellular hypoxia in the dehydrated bitch.

Urinalysis and Urine Culture

The urine specific gravity is unpredictable in bitches with pyometra because of the many variables that can affect the results. Early in the disease process, the urine specific gravity may be greater than 1.030 simply as a reflection of dehydration and the physiologic response to conserve fluids. With secondary bacterial infection, especially *E. coli*, toxemia develops and interferes with the resorption of sodium and chloride in the loop of Henle. This reduces renal medullary hypertonicity, impairing the ability of the renal collecting tubules to resorb free water. Polyuria and compensatory polydipsia result.

A renal tubular insensitivity to the action of antidiuretic hormone (ADH) can result in secondary nephrogenic diabetes insipidus. This represents a sequela to reversible renal tubular damage caused by *E. coli* endotoxins. This development may also contribute to a loss of concentrating ability. Renal tubular immune complex injury is another proposed mechanism for polydipsia/polyuria. Although not likely, prolonged polyuria and polydipsia may cause renal medullary solute washout, further impairing the kidney's ability to conserve water. Probably as a result of the reversible renal secondary diabetes insipidus, urine becomes progressively more dilute. Isosthenuria (urine specific gravity 1.008 to 1.015) or hyposthenuria (urine specific gravity <1.008) is well recognized in bitches with pyometra. Prerenal uremia may also be present if water consumption inadequately compensates for the polyuria.

Urinary tract infections may be suspected if pyuria, hematuria, and/or proteinuria are identified on urinalysis. However, urine obtained by a midstream collection is contaminated by the vaginal discharge. We do not recommend "blind" cystocentesis techniques on dogs with suspected or known pyometra because of the risk for puncturing an infected uterus and subsequent leakage of its contents into the abdomen. Cystocentesis using ultrasound guidance reduces the risk for penetrating the uterus. If an uncontaminated urine sample is considered important, it should be obtained only with ultrasound guidance. If ultrasonography is not available, one should not routinely culture the urine of dogs with pyometra.

Proteinuria without pyuria or hematuria may also be found with pyometra. Immune complex deposition in the glomeruli causes a mixed membranoproliferative glomerulonephropathy and leakage of plasma proteins into the glomerular filtrate. The proteinuria gradually resolves with correction of the pyometra.

RADIOLOGY

Pregnancy enhances uterine size and the ability to identify the uterus. It can be visualized radiographically beginning with the third to fourth week of gestation, continuing through pregnancy, and for 2 to 4 weeks after whelping. Radiographic visualization of the uterus at other times is abnormal. If a nonpregnant bitch is in diestrus and the uterus is easily identified, that would also be considered abnormal. Abdominal radiographs should be assessed in a bitch with suspected pyometra to confirm the diagnosis and to identify any unsuspected problems. With pyometra, a fluid-dense tubular structure that is larger in diameter than small-intestinal loops is typically seen in the ventral and caudal abdomen, displacing loops of intestine dorsally and cranially (Fig. 23-1, *A* and *B*).

Two additional concerns that might be seen radiographically in a dog with pyometra are the presence or absence of peritonitis from a uterine rupture and/or retained fetal tissue from a pregnancy occurring during the present cycle or a previous pregnancy (Fig. 23-1, *C*). Peritonitis should be suspected when there is a loss of normal contrast between abdominal structures. Abdominal compression may be of value, using a belly band or wooden spoon to displace the intestines away from the uterus. This procedure may enhance radiographic contrast and often allows improved visualization of the uterus. Inability to visualize the uterus radiographically does not rule out the presence of a relatively small pyometra with an open cervix and significant drainage.

ULTRASONOGRAPHY

Ultrasonography has greatly enhanced our ability to document the presence of pyometra and/or the success of medical treatment. The value of this diagnostic tool is emphasized when abdominal radiographs are inconclusive. Ultrasonography allows determination of uterine size, thickness of the uterine wall, and presence of fluid accumulation within the lumen. In some cases, the character of the fluid within the uterus (serous versus viscid) can be determined. More important, ultrasonography easily identifies fetal remnants or placental tissue within the uterus, factors that negatively impact potential success with prostaglandin therapy.

Endometritis and pyometra are readily distinguished from a gravid (pregnant) uterus with abdominal ultrasound, as the uterus is distended by fluid and no fetuses are present. The uterus takes on the appearance of an anechoic convoluted tubule with pyometra (Fig. 23-2). The tortuous convolutions may also appear as anechoic, circular structures when viewed in a transverse plane. Stump pyometras may be detected as a hypoechoic to mixed echo lesion located dorsal and caudal to the urinary bladder (Wrigley and Finn, 1989).

DIAGNOSIS AND COMPLICATIONS

Uncomplicated Pyometra

Pyometra can usually be easily recognized. Pyometra should be suspected in any ill bitch in diestrus. In fact, pyometra should be suspected in any ill, nonspayed, bitch. The diagnosis is confirmed when the appropriate clinical signs reported by the owner are present in conjunction with abnormalities on physical examination, laboratory studies, and radiographic or ultrasonographic evaluation. A definitive diagnosis becomes a challenge when the history is vague (especially regarding ovarian cycle activity), when a vulvar discharge is present yet the uterus feels normal, when no vaginal discharge is observed (Memon and Mickelsen, 1993), or when the dog has been previously spayed yet clinical signs and clinical pathology suggest pyometra.

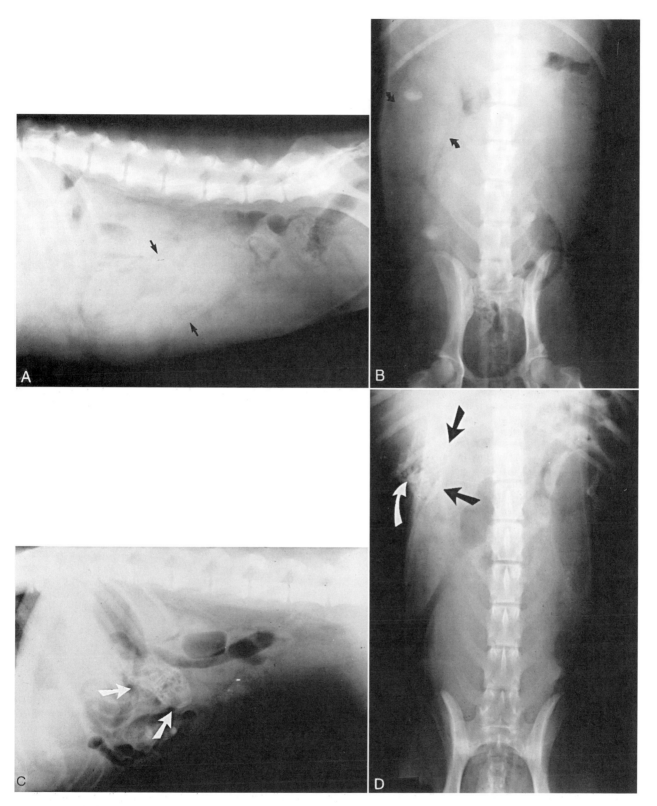

FIGURE 23-1. *A* and *B,* Lateral and ventrodorsal abdominal radiographs from a bitch with a large pyometra. The diameter of a single horn is illustrated by the *arrows. C* and *D,* Lateral and ventrodorsal abdominal radiographs from a bitch with a retained mummified fetus (*arrows*).

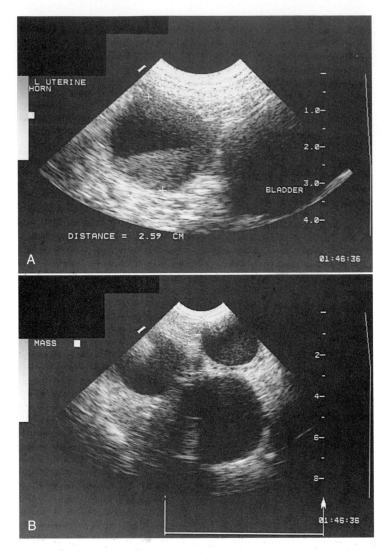

FIGURE 23-2. *A,* Ultrasonography of the abdomen of a bitch demonstrating a uterine "fluid line" consistent with pyometra. *B,* Ultrasonography of the abdomen of the same bitch with pyometra demonstrating three fluid-filled uterine cross-sections.

Polydipsia and Polyuria as the Sole Signs

Rarely, a bitch is brought to a veterinarian with a primary owner complaint of polyuria and polydipsia. There are numerous causes for polyuria and polydipsia in the dog (see Chapter 1). Evaluation of a hemogram, serum biochemistry panel, urinalysis, and abdominal radiographs may be necessary in differentiating these various disorders. However, pyometra must remain an important possible explanation for these signs in any intact bitch.

Renal Complications

It may be difficult to differentiate pyometra with concurrent renal failure from pyometra with prerenal uremia. If the urine specific gravity is less than 1.006, acquired secondary nephrogenic diabetes insipidus is likely. If the specific gravity is greater than 1.030,

prerenal uremia and not primary renal failure should be considered. If the urine specific gravity is 1.008 to 1.020 and dehydration is present, the clinician must rely on the history, presence or absence of other biochemical abnormalities (e.g., serum calcium and phosphorus concentrations), abdominal radiography and/or ultrasonography (evaluating uterus and kidneys), response to fluid therapy, and perhaps renal function tests to make an accurate diagnosis.

Use of Vaginal Cytology and Culture

The diagnosis of pyometra should neither be confirmed nor eliminated based on the results of vaginal cytology or vaginal cultures (Olsen et al, 1986). Results of either test are nonspecific and unreliable in the management of a bitch with pyometra. The presence of neutrophils and bacteria on vaginal cytologic smears can be seen in normal bitches as well as those

TABLE 23–2   AEROBIC BACTERIA RECOVERED FROM THE VAGINAS OF 59 HEALTHY BREEDING BITCHES*

Organism	Percent of Bitches
Pasturella multocida	98
β-Hemolytic streptococci	90
Escherichia coli	85
Unclassified gram-positive rods	90
Unclassified gram-negative rods	86
Mycoplasma spp.	60
Streptococcus spp. (α-hemolytic, nonhemolytic)	56
Pasturella spp.	68
Enterococci	44
Proteus mirabilis	25
Staphylococcus intermedius	34
Coryneforms	41
Coagulase-negative staphylococci	22
Pseudomonas spp.	10

Adapted from Bjurstrom L, Linde-Forsberg C: Long-term study of aerobic bacteria of the genital tract in breeding bitches. Am J Vet Res 53:665, 1992.
*All bitches had at least one positive culture; 826 vaginal swab specimens were obtained from these dogs.

with pyometra. That type of vaginal smear could also be associated with vaginitis from any cause. However, the vaginal smear from a bitch with an open-cervix pyometra often contains degenerated neutrophils. Differentiating distorted epithelial cells with ill-defined borders, vacuolated endometrial cells, macrophages, trophoblastic type cells, and vaginal epithelial cells undergoing cytolysis can be difficult.

Heavy bacterial growth from a vaginal culture can be due to almost any cause of vaginitis or to drainage from an open-cervix pyometra and may be observed in some apparently normal bitches. Bacteria commonly exist in the vaginal vault (Table 23-2). Bacterial growth from vaginal cultures does not prove that similar organisms are present in the uterus, even if the cervix is patent (almost an impossible diagnosis) and the culture is taken near the cervix with a guarded culture swab. It is usually impossible to be certain one is close to the cervix when obtaining a blind culture. Anterior vaginal cultures may be useful when medically treating a bitch with open-cervix pyometra, because results of antibiotic sensitivity testing can be considered in choosing appropriate antibiotic therapy. We do not routinely culture the anterior vagina of a bitch suspected of having or known to have an open-cervix or closed-cervix pyometra.

Lack of an Enlarged Uterus

A healthy bitch may have a copious vaginal discharge without uterine enlargement. The major differential diagnoses for such situations are significant vaginal inflammations with or without infection and pyometra that has drained sufficiently to avoid systemic toxemia. In an ovariohysterectomized bitch, a "stump pyometra" should also be considered. A carefully obtained history and results of a hemogram, vaginal examination, abdominal radiographs, and if possible, ultrasound examination of the uterus should be used to differentiate an open-cervix pyometra from a severe focal vaginal infection. The most valuable of these tests is abdominal ultrasonography.

Systemic signs of illness (i.e., lethargy, inappetence, bitch "does not seem right") may be subtle with an open-cervix pyometra. If present, however, these signs are more suggestive of uterine than vaginal disease. The bitch with an isolated vaginal infection rarely has systemic signs of illness. Likewise, fever, neutrophilic leukocytosis, and hyperproteinemia are suggestive of uterine disease, because these problems are not typical of an isolated vaginal infection.

Vaginoscopy, using a 15-cm proctoscope or a flexible endoscope, allows visualization of the vaginal mucosa for inflammation, infection, masses, foreign bodies, congenital abnormalities, and potential determination of the origin of the vulvar discharge. If the discharge appears to be coming from the anterior vaginal area, a uterine problem should be suspected. If doubt about the diagnosis still exists, the bitch is not severely ill, and the owners will not consider surgery, the bitch may be treated for vaginitis and reevaluated. However, abdominal ultrasonography is such an excellent diagnostic aid that the value of screening the abdomen with this tool should not be underestimated. If the reproductive potential of the dog is to be saved, medical therapy with $PGF_{2\alpha}$ can be started following documentation of the uterine source of the infection.

Stump Pyometra

Stump pyometra is an uncommon and difficult problem to diagnose. The condition involves inflammation and bacterial infection of a post-ovariohysterectomy remnant of the uterine body. If the cervix and a portion of the uterine body are left in situ during ovariohysterectomy, that area becomes a potential site for future infection. The stump of the uterus is located in an area favoring bacterial growth. An internal abscess could easily develop. If remnant ovarian tissue also remains following ovariohysterectomy, ovarian cycles, progesterone secretion, uterine stimulation, and inflammation could occur. These changes enhance the likelihood of future infection. However, stump pyometra due to an ascending infection from the vagina usually occurs without the presence of remnant ovarian tissue, because the site is one that can easily become infected.

The diagnosis can be extremely difficult if a vaginal discharge is not present. Clinical signs and laboratory abnormalities are those typically associated with pyometra—lethargy, inappetence, fever. Thus an isolated vaginal infection is less likely because such an infection does not usually cause systemic signs. Caudal abdominal radiographs with abdominal compression may demonstrate the diseased uterine stump. Ultrasonography is the most definitive noninvasive diagnostic tool for this disorder (Fig. 23-3).

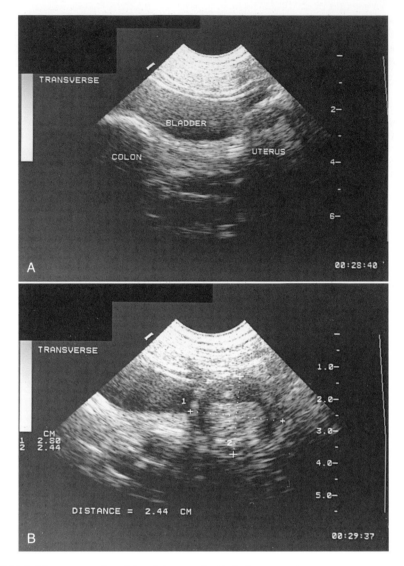

FIGURE 23-3. Ultrasonography of the abdomen of a bitch demonstrating a stump pyometra that had developed several years following ovariohysterectomy.

Many bitches require surgical exploration for a definitive diagnosis if ultrasonography is not available. A thorough exploratory evaluation of the abdomen to look for ovarian tissue is recommended if a uterine stump infection is removed at surgery.

SURGICAL TREATMENT

Ovariohysterectomy

Ovariohysterectomy is the preferred treatment for pyometra. The only reason for not performing surgery is an owner's adamant insistence on maintaining the reproductive potential of the bitch. Even then, the bitch must be 6 years of age or younger for the veterinarian to consider medical management rather than surgery. Relatively healthy bitches are usually excellent surgical candidates. Severely ill bitches should be vigorously treated with antibiotics and IV fluids. A recent study suggests that the combination of hypertonic saline and dextran 70 may be superior to isotonic saline in the management of septic shock secondary to pyometra in dogs (Fantoni et al, 1999). Bactericidal antibiotics effective against *E. coli* (Clavamox, trimethoprimsulfamethoxazole, cephalosporins) should be used and their effects closely monitored.

The bitch should undergo proper testing to identify abnormalities in serum electrolytes, acid-base status, cardiac rhythm, and fluid status. Any existing condition should be vigorously treated and veterinarians must remember that extremely ill dogs are not candidates for medical management of pyometra with prostaglandins. Complications associated with septicemia, toxemia, and uremia are common. One cannot always wait for "stabilization" of the animal before surgery is performed. In some dogs surgery may not be postponed more than a few hours. Septicemia originating from the diseased uterus is often responsible for the severe illness, and only surgical removal of that organ allows resolution of the septic state of the bitch to begin.

The injectable broad-spectrum antibiotics and IV fluids with appropriate electrolyte and bicarbonate supplementation should be initiated as quickly as possible in any bitch suspected of having pyometra. Rapid institution of these therapies improves the chances of surgical survival. Supportive therapy should be continued during and after surgery. Oral antibiotics should be continued for 7 to 10 days after removal of the infected uterus.

Surgical Drainage

Attempts have been made to treat pyometra surgically, while preserving the uterus and ovaries. Dogs and cats have been treated successfully with surgical drainage of the uterus (Vasseur and Feldman, 1982). Although we have used this aggressive approach in bitches and queens with retained uterine and extrauterine fetuses in the past, it is not recommended. Purulent material needs to be aspirated, and each uterine horn must be flushed with an antiseptic solution through indwelling tubes for several days after surgery (Fig. 23-4). Success with this procedure requires both skill and luck. Again, this procedure is not recommended.

Procedures have been described wherein the uterus was drained via catheters introduced through the vaginal vault and cervix, thereby avoiding surgery. Cannulation of the uterus was accomplished with the bitch under general anesthesia. Introduction of a rigid metal cannula was facilitated by continuous injection, with fluoroscopic observation, of a viscous contrast medium. Two radiopaque plastic catheters were inserted into the uterus through the cannula and the cannula was removed. The plastic catheters were left in place for several days and used for drainage and for instillation of antibiotics. The entire procedure involved multiple steps and various pieces of equipment (Lagerstedt et al, 1987). As with surgically placed catheters, this approach is impractical and may be life-threatening, and it is therefore not recommended.

MEDICAL TREATMENT (PROSTAGLANDINS)

Therapeutic Options

Results of medical therapy using estrogens, androgens, quinine, and oxytocin, have been inconsistent and rarely successful. In addition, systemic antibiotics are usually ineffective as the sole therapy for canine pyometra. However, results using $PGF_{2\alpha}$ have been extremely encouraging, and prostaglandins offer a consistently reliable medical alternative for therapy. Ovariohysterectomy remains the recommended therapy, but medical treatment in bitches or queens that are 6 years of age or younger can be rewarding.

Actions of Prostaglandins

$PGF_{2\alpha}$ has several physiologic effects on the female reproductive system, including contraction of the myometrium and reduction in circulating progesterone concentrations. The third and least consistent effect in the bitch or queen is relaxation of the cervix. Myometrial contractions result in expulsion of exudate from the uterus. Synthesis and secretion of progesterone are the primary functions of the corpora lutea. Lysis of the corpora lutea or transitory inhibition of

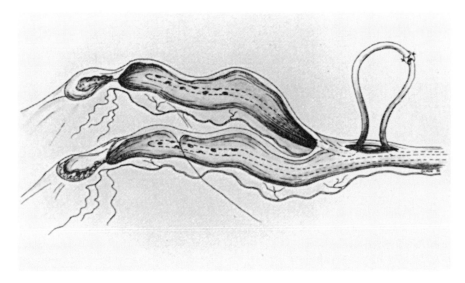

FIGURE 23-4. Schematic drawing showing the placement of intrauterine tubes in the surgical management of pyometra. (From Vasseur BB, Feldman EC: Pyometra associated with extrauterine pregnancy in a cat. JAAHA 18:872, 1982.)

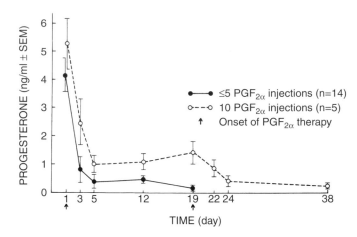

FIGURE 23-5. Illustration of the dramatic effect prostaglandin $F_{2\alpha}$ has on plasma progesterone concentrations in late diestrus of dogs with pyometra. The *solid line* reveals the changes seen in bitches requiring one 5-day course of injections. The *dashed line* reveals progesterone concentrations following onset of prostaglandin therapy earlier in diestrus and having an incomplete result until a second 5-day course of therapy is finished.

luteal steroidogenesis occurs with administration of $PGF_{2\alpha}$. These actions depend partially on the dosage, route, frequency of administration, and timing of $PGF_{2\alpha}$ therapy relative to when it is administered within the bitch's luteal cycle (i.e., the drug appears to be luteolytic late in diestrus but not early in diestrus). The resultant decreased plasma progesterone concentration reduces the stimulus for endometrial growth and glandular secretion (Fig. 23-5).

Clinical Use of Prostaglandins

GUIDELINES. When deciding whether to use $PGF_{2\alpha}$ the clinician should consider the age of the bitch, the owner's desire to save the animal's reproductive potential, the severity of illness at the time of examination, the presence or absence of other concurrent disease, and the patency of the cervix. Medical therapy using prostaglandins should be discouraged in older bitches (>6 years) or in bitches whose owners are unsure about, or not interested in, maintaining the reproductive capabilities of their dog. The drug should never be administered to dogs with known cardiac or respiratory disease. The drug should also never be administered to dogs that are critically ill. Ovariohysterectomy remains the treatment of choice in managing pyometra.

SEVERELY ILL BITCHES. Clinical response (reduction in uterine size and/or content) is not usually observed for at least 48 hours after beginning prostaglandin therapy. Therefore this drug is not ideal for use in severely ill animals that are poor anesthetic risks, in which some time would be desired to administer IV fluids and to "stabilize" a critically ill bitch before surgery. Although we have little experience in this setting, we believe that it is possible for the side effects

of the prostaglandins to cause significant morbidity and/or mortality in critically ill bitches. The drug should not be used in any critically ill dogs until studies demonstrating their effectiveness are published.

CLOSED-CERVIX PYOMETRA. $PGF_{2\alpha}$ should be used with caution in bitches with a closed-cervix pyometra because of relatively poor therapeutic response and the potential for failure of the cervix to dilate. Lack of cervical dilatation may result in uterine contents being expelled into the peritoneal cavity via the fallopian tubes or via a rupture in the uterine wall. In either situation, this exudate is likely to cause severe peritonitis. The use of estrogens to relax the cervix prior to $PGF_{2\alpha}$ therapy is not recommended because of potential enhancement of progesterone effects on the uterus.

DRUG LICENSING. $PGF_{2\alpha}$ is not licensed for use in the bitch, but it is available for use in the cow and mare. Owners should be informed that the use of $PGF_{2\alpha}$ for treating canine pyometra is an established therapy for the dog and cat and should be considered within the "standard care" of these pets.

INITIAL EVALUATION. The bitch to be treated with prostaglandins should first be screened for the presence of fetuses (living or dead) within the uterus using ultrasonography. Radiography is a relatively poor alternative. We have seen eleven bitches misdiagnosed as having pyometra, each of which was confirmed to be pregnant by ultrasonography. These bitches had been referred for $PGF_{2\alpha}$ therapy to resolve pyometra. Pyometra had been diagnosed based on copious mucopurulent vaginal discharges and "confirmed" with abdominal radiographs. It must be remembered that the pregnant bitch has a uniformly enlarged uterus that could be confused with pyometra before fetal skeletal calcification becomes obvious (Meyers-Wallen et al, 1986).

Each of these eleven dogs had severe vaginitis that responded to appropriate nitrofurazone (Furacin, Norden) or Betadine douche therapy, and each whelped healthy litters. Prostaglandin administration would have likely resulted in abortion of all fetuses in each bitch. The use of prostaglandins is also contraindicated in bitches with mummified fetuses and those with fetal skeletal material in utero, simply because our success rate in such bitches has been consistently nil.

Recommended Prostaglandin and Protocol

CHOICES. Only naturally occurring $PGF_{2\alpha}$ (Lutalyse and Prostin; Upjohn Co., Kalamazoo, MI 49006) should be used, at dosages recommended. Synthetic $PGF_{2\alpha}$ analogues (cloprostenol [Estrumate] and fluprostenol [Equimate], Haver-Lockhart, Cutter Laboratories, Inc, Shawnee, KS 66201; prostalene [Synchrocept], Diamond Laboratories, Inc, Des Moines, IA 50304) are more potent than natural $PGF_{2\alpha}$. Use of these synthetic products at our recommended dosage could result in shock and possibly death. The LD-50 for natural $PGF_{2\alpha}$ in the bitch is 5.13 mg/kg.

TABLE 23–3   PROTOCOL FOR PGF$_{2\alpha}$ THERAPY FOR CANINE OPEN-CERVIX PYOMETRA

1. Establish diagnosis definitively
   a. History and physical examination
   b. CBC, other blood tests
   c. Abdominal ultrasonography
   d. Radiography (not as good as ultrasonography)
2. Use natural prostaglandin (Lutalyse)
   a. Day 1: 0.1 mg/kg, SC, once
   b. Day 2: 0.2 mg/kg, SC, once
   c. Days 3–7: 0.25 mg/kg, SC, once daily
3. Antibiotics used during and for 14 days following prostaglandin treatment
4. Re-evaluate
   a. 7 days after completion of PGF$_{2\alpha}$
   b. 14 days after completion of PGF$_{2\alpha}$
5. Re-treat at 14 days if
   a. Purulent vaginal discharge persists
   b. Fever, increased WBC, and fluid-filled uterus persist

PROSTAGLANDIN THERAPY AND OBSERVATION PERIOD. The following protocol is recommended for the use of PGF$_{2\alpha}$ to treat pyometra (Table 23-3): day 1, 0.1 mg/kg subcutaneously once; day 2, 0.2 mg/kg subcutaneously once; days 3 through 7, 0.25 mg/kg of the natural prostaglandin salt (Lutalyse) subcutaneously once daily. All injections should be administered in the morning to allow observation of the bitch through the day. The low initial dose is used to minimize side effects, which tend to decrease in severity with continued use.

Seven days after the final day of prostaglandin administration, the bitch should be examined to be certain that she has not become clinically worse than she appeared before initiation of therapy. If she is worse, ovariohysterectomy should be strongly recommended. If she is stable, she should be evaluated again after 7 additional days (14 days after the final dose of prostaglandin).

An alternative protocol is administration of prostaglandin daily until vaginal discharges cease (Johnston et al, 2001). This appears to be inappropriate, in part because some bitches clean themselves so thoroughly that monitoring for any vaginal discharge can be difficult. In addition, most of our treated dogs continue to have a vaginal discharge for 2 weeks after therapy. This discharge progressively changes from purulent to clear before stopping. No evidence suggests that continuing therapy until the vaginal discharge stops has any advantage. Continuing therapy, however, carries the disadvantage of administering a potentially toxic drug to an animal that does not need it.

RETREATMENT? At the recheck scheduled 14 days after the seventh (and final) dose of prostaglandin, a decision regarding the need for a second course of therapy can be made based on clinical response and results of physical examination, CBC, and abdominal ultrasonography. If a sanguineous or mucopurulent vaginal discharge, fever, neutrophilia, or uterine enlargement is still present, treatment with PGF$_{2\alpha}$ should be reinstituted for an additional 7 days of injections, 0.25 mg/kg/day subcutaneously. The most important criterion regarding retreatment is presence of a purulent vaginal discharge; that is, if a purulent discharge continues to be present, the bitch should be retreated. If there are no worrisome clinical signs and if the discharge appears clear and serous, further treatment is not required. Only 7 bitches of the 192 with open- and closed-cervix pyometras treated with PGF$_{2\alpha}$ underwent three series of injections. Each of those bitches had a closed-cervix pyometra with marked uterine enlargement, did not respond to PGF$_{2\alpha}$ therapy, and eventually required an ovariohysterectomy.

DAILY MONITORING. During the initial 7-day course of treatment with prostaglandin, each bitch should be closely monitored with two or three thorough physical examinations per day. Management during each course of prostaglandin treatment should be the same: rectal temperature, abdominal palpation, hydration status, assessing the general well-being of the dog, and any other relevant parameter should be judged several times each day.

The side effects to prostaglandins, especially those witnessed after the first and second injections, can be striking and worrisome. As described in the next section, each bitch should be individually assessed regarding severity of side effects. It is suggested that each prostaglandin-treated bitch be walked outside from the time that the medication is administered until the post-injection side effects completely dissipate. Walking, just as for horses with colic, appears to minimize clinical signs. Most bitches recover within 20 minutes after injection, with a range of 5 to 60 minutes. They then appear well and can be fed. Do not feed within the 2 or 3 hours before prostaglandin administration, because all stomach contents will quickly be vomited.

It is strongly recommended that prostaglandins be administered in the morning for convenient observations throughout the day. The first injection *must* be administered in the morning. With this protocol, there is no reason that open-cervix pyometra bitches need to remain hospitalized at night. We encourage sending dogs or cats home each night, just as we encourage owners to allow us to keep their bitches for at least 4 hours after each injection. In this way, any unexpected drug-induced side effects can be observed and treated, if required. Bitches with closed-cervix pyometra should be hospitalized throughout the treatment period.

VAGINAL DISCHARGE. When treating a bitch with closed- or open-cervix pyometra, a prostaglandin-induced discharge from the vulva is not always obvious. Uterine response to prostaglandins appears to be slow and progressive, occurring over a period of days to weeks, not minutes to hours. As the uterine diameter slowly shrinks as a result of contraction, the contents are slowly discharged. The lack of a visible increase in the volume of discharge in many bitches is believed to be due to the small quantities of uterine contents discharged combined with the rapid response by the bitch to consume that material.

Peritonitis due to uterine rupture or fallopian tube leakage is always a worry when no discharge is obvious in a treated bitch. Ideally, if peritonitis is present, it can be identified through close observation and quickly treated. However, abdominal radiographs or ultrasound may need to be performed to ensure that peritonitis is not developing. Ultrasonography is far superior to radiology in assessing uterine content and size, presence of abdominal fluid or peritonitis, and response to prostaglandin treatment. Of the 192 bitches we have treated, none has developed peritonitis.

ANTIBIOTICS. Fifteen per cent of bitches with pyometra have had positive blood cultures before prostaglandin administration, supporting the need for antibiotic therapy (Nelson et al, 1982; Feldman and Nelson, 1989). Therefore broad-spectrum bactericidal antibiotics effective against *E. coli* should be administered for 7 days. Trimethoprimsulfamethoxazole and amoxicillin (Clavamox, Beecham, West Chester, PA) have proved to be reliable drugs.

Side Effects

Several reactions are usually observed after the subcutaneous injection of $PGF_{2\alpha}$ (Table 23-4). It is extremely rare to observe no side effects following the first dose. The first dose of a second course of therapy may not result in any reactions different from those of the initial response. Initially, the bitch may be restless and begin pacing. Hypersalivation and occasional panting then occur, followed by some or all of the following: abdominal pain or cramping, tachycardia, fever, vomiting, and defecation. These reactions disappear within 5 to 60 minutes of the injection. Generally, the side effects due to prostaglandin administration last for 20 to 30 minutes. Observance of uterine evacuation after an injection is variable.

Side effects typically diminish with each daily dose of prostaglandin. The bitch that exhibited alarming side effects after the first dose often appears to have no reaction or just mild reactions after the fifth to seventh dose. When present, side effects can be quite pronounced, causing dramatic signs of illness within 30 to 60 seconds of a subcutaneous injection. We have found that walking a dog continuously for 20 to 40 minutes following prostaglandin administration

TABLE 23-4 INCIDENCE OF REACTIONS IN 62 BITCHES RECEIVING SUBCUTANEOUS PROSTAGLANDIN THERAPY FOR PYOMETRA

Reaction	Percent of Dogs
Restlessness	85
Pacing	85
Hypersalivation	82
Panting	79
Vomiting	73
Abdominal pain or cramping	61
Tachycardia	55
Fever	33
Defecation	30
Uterine evacuation	30

not only minimizes the signs, but allows for close supervision by a veterinarian or trained technician.

The most worrisome reactions to the administration of prostaglandin have included a rapidly developing shock-like syndrome. This has been observed twice; the affected bitches became weak, pale, and tachycardic with poor pulse quality. Each was treated with IV fluids, and each recovered within 45 minutes of the initial signs. Two dogs have also been documented to suffer ventricular tachycardias within minutes of receiving prostaglandins. Their signs were similar to those described for the dogs that appeared to be in shock. These two dogs, however, were quickly managed with IV lidocaine infusions, and again recovery was noted in less than 60 minutes. Treatment was abandoned in one of these two bitches, and she underwent ovariohysterectomy. Two of the remaining three bitches had similar, but less severe, side effects after their second dosage. All three completed therapy without severe problems on the third or subsequent days of treatment. When worrisome side effects are observed, one may wish to lower the subsequent dose. Lower doses result in milder signs.

The use of atropine has been recommended to minimize the negative side effects of prostaglandin therapy (Lein et al, 1989). We have had no experience with this approach.

Need for Retreatment

In reviewing the records and test results from bitches treated for open-cervix pyometra with prostaglandin, those requiring two courses of medication before the pyometra resolved were compared with those requiring only one course of therapy. In both groups of bitches, resolution of pyometra correlated with serum progesterone concentrations decreasing below 1 ng/ml, 14 days after the fifth to seventh day of treatment. Bitches continuing to exhibit a purulent vaginal discharge had serum progesterone concentrations greater than 1 ng/ml. Furthermore, those bitches treated for pyometra less than 5 weeks after the end of estrus were less likely to respond to one course of therapy. Bitches whose previous estrus occurred more than 5 weeks previously usually responded to one course of treatment. It is obvious that most bitches treated with two series of prostaglandin injections began their first course of therapy relatively early in diestrus, whereas those requiring only one course of therapy began treatment later in diestrus. The implication is that corpora lutea become more sensitive to prostaglandin administration as diestrus progresses.

Corpora lutea of the bitch appear to become more sensitive to the "lytic" effects of prostaglandins as diestrus progresses (see Fig. 23-5). Therefore the bitch with pyometra treated more than 5 weeks after the end of estrus is more sensitive to prostaglandins than the bitch treated earlier in diestrus. Owners can be informed of the prognosis for response to one course of therapy based on the length of time the bitch has been in diestrus at the time treatment for pyometra begins.

Why serum progesterone concentrations must be reduced to anestrus levels before a response to prostaglandin therapy is obtained is not certain. Progesterone probably maintains endometrial glandular activity, which supports bacterial growth while suppressing leukocyte activity. The effects of progesterone enhance the continuation of pyometra. It is beneficial to eliminate progesterone as a means of improving the likelihood for resolving pyometra. However, in contrast to many authors, we do not recommend assaying plasma progesterone before or during therapy. This seems an academic pursuit, and results would not alter the recommended treatment protocol.

Results of Treatment

Indications of a successful response to $PGF_{2\alpha}$ therapy include loss of clinical signs, development of a serous vulvar discharge that then stops completely, decrease in the palpable uterine diameter, and a normal leukogram. After pyometra is surgically extirpated, the peripheral white blood cell count often increases dramatically. This is believed to be due to loss of the "sink" into which white cells flood, while the bone marrow continues to pour out cells. With medical management of pyometra, the sink remains but the infection clears. Thus, with this form of treatment the white blood cell count often quickly diminishes (Fig. 23-6).

Open-Cervix Pyometra

Of the 163 bitches with open-cervix pyometra treated by us, 153 (94%) had complete resolution of their uterine infection. Treatment was abandoned in eight dogs for various reasons: five bitches with fetal skeletal remnants in utero never demonstrated complete resolution of the pyometra, in spite of two courses of therapy; one dog had transient cerebellar signs as a result of treatment; one dog developed an acute cardiac tachyarrhythmia (ventricular tachycardia); and one dog was thought (incorrectly) to have developed peritonitis. Ovariohysterectomy was performed on each of these eight dogs.

Ninety-eight bitches (64%) responded to one series of injections, and 55 bitches (36%) required two series. Of the 153 bitches that responded favorably to treatment, 135 (88%) have whelped litters and 109 of these bitches have had more than one litter. Five bitches redeveloped pyometra after successfully carrying a litter to term on an earlier posttreatment heat.

Prostaglandin-treated bitches may begin their next estrous cycle early or late. No consistent pattern has been established, and owners are made aware that an early cycle is possible. We strongly recommend breeding the dog on the cycle immediately following

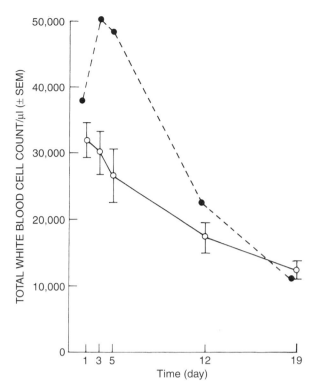

FIGURE 23-6. Illustration of the falling white blood cell count in bitches with pyometra treated successfully with prostaglandin $F_{2\alpha}$ (*solid line*) versus the initial increase in total white blood cell count in four dogs with pyometra that were successfully treated by ovariohysterectomy (*dashed line*).

therapy for several reasons: (1) these bitches may have an abnormal uterus, and recurrence of the pyometra is always possible; therefore an attempt should be made to obtain a litter while it is possible; (2) pregnant dogs may be less susceptible to infection than nonpregnant dogs; and (3) the bitch does not benefit from skipping a cycle.

A large number of successfully treated bitches have been spayed after whelping one or more litters. Histologic evaluations of the uteri from these bitches usually yield normal results. Failure to respond to prostaglandin therapy, however, may be associated with CEH. The fertility of the bitches that have responded to treatment, their ability to carry a litter to term, and their normal endometrial histology support the concept that pyometra in the young estrogen-treated bitch does not involve CEH.

Closed-Cervix Pyometra

RESULTS. The results of prostaglandin therapy in bitches with closed-cervix pyometra have not been as positive as with the open-cervix group. Fewer dogs have been treated because the syndrome is less common in our hospital population and because these bitches are often so ill that ovariohysterectomy is recommended with greater conviction. Fifty-three bitches with closed-cervix pyometra have been treated with prostaglandins, but only 16 (31%) have responded successfully. Of the 16 that had resolution of the pyometra, 12 dogs required two series of injections, whereas 4 required only the initial series of injections. These 16 dogs all subsequently whelped healthy litters.

Of the 37 failures, 4 dogs underwent one course of injections, 24 bitches had two series, and 9 were treated with three series of injections. Thirty-six bitches were spayed because of the lack of response to the prostaglandins. These bitches did not become more ill, nor did they seem to improve. Most simply remained static. One bitch died 6 hours after the initial injection. She was among the first 10 bitches ever treated, and she had completely recovered from the clinical side effects of the prostaglandins. She remains the only prostaglandin fatality among more than 200 dogs and cats treated at our institution. Necropsy did not identify the cause of death.

PROGNOSIS. A guarded prognosis with regard to resolving the pyometra should be given to owners of dogs with closed-cervix pyometra. Treatment failure is presumably due to an inability to evacuate the uterus because of the closed cervix. If a reliable method is developed for dilating the cervix, the ability to help these bitches will improve. We still attempt medical therapy in some bitches with closed-cervix pyometra despite the one reported death and the low percentage of successes. Medical therapy can be attempted and ovariohysterectomy maintained as an alternative if the prostaglandin injections fail to resolve the problem.

MONITORING. Careful monitoring is imperative during prostaglandin therapy for closed-cervix pyometra. In addition to physical examinations several times each day, monitoring should consist of abdominal ultrasonography performed before and every 2 or 3 days after beginning therapy. Ultrasonography should identify decreasing uterine size without evidence of peritonitis. Daily or every-other-day white blood cell counts should demonstrate decreasing counts as the infection clears. No decrease is expected in the first 2 or 3 days, but a progressive decline toward normal should then follow. From a clinical standpoint, these dogs should steadily improve, aside from the immediate and transient side effects associated with the prostaglandin injections. Appetite, attitude, and activity should quickly return toward normal. However, the clinical signs in many of these bitches persist for weeks without becoming worse or better. Uterine discharge, as a result of the injections, is not always obvious. Some fastidious bitches keep themselves extremely clean by licking. Thus constant licking may be the only evidence of an induced open cervix with vaginal discharge.

Long-Term Management

Once a bitch has been treated medically for pyometra with prostaglandin, it is assumed that a recurrence of pyometra is always possible. It is suggested that an owner objectively establish a realistic goal of the number of puppies to be obtained from that bitch. The bitch should be bred on each cycle until this goal is met. In addition to the goal of obtaining puppies while the chance exists, there is a medical reason for recommending that these bitches be bred: pregnancy may have a protective effect against development of pyometra (Niskanen and Thrusfield, 1998). The bitch should be spayed after whelping the last litter. Many owners have complied with these suggestions, and recurrences have perhaps been avoided.

MEDICAL TREATMENT (ALTERNATIVES TO USE OF NATURAL PROSTAGLANDINS)

Synthetic Prostaglandins

Cloprostenol, a prostaglandin analog, has been described for medical treatment of dogs with pyometra (Fazale et al, 1995; Valocky et al, 1997). We used doses of 10 µg/kg, subcutaneously, twice daily for 9 to 15 days. Only 60% of dogs responded completely to this regimen, and one dog died of shock. Side effects noted were similar to those observed with natural prostaglandins. Further investigation with synthetic prostaglandins is necessary before their use can be recommended.

Antiprogestagens

Use of the antiprogestagen aglepristone has been reported for the treatment of pyometra in dogs (Breitkopf et al, 1997; Fieni et al, 1999). Fieni et al treated 5 dogs once daily for 2 days at a dose of 10mg/kg, subcutaneously. Two of these five dogs developed disseminated intravascular coagulopathy (DIC) and were spayed; one dog did not improve and was treated successfully with natural prostaglandin; two dogs improved (Onclin and Verstegen, 2000). As with synthetic prostaglandin use, this mode of therapy needs further investigation before its use can be recommended.

POSTPARTUM ENDOMETRITIS

Although postpartum endometritis is a disease entity distinct from pyometra, it can be treated with prostaglandin. Nine of 11 bitches we have treated have responded well to therapy, with clearance of the uterine infection and subsequent successful pregnancy.

REFERENCES

Baba E, et al: Vaginal and uterine microflora of adult dogs. Am J Vet Res 44:606, 1983.
Bjurstrom L, LindeForsberg C: Long-term study of aerobic bacteria of the genital tract in breeding bitches. Am J Vet Res 53:665, 1992.

Bowen RA, et al: Efficacy and toxicity of estrogens commonly used to terminate canine pregnancy. JAVMA 186:783, 1985.

Breitkopf M, et al: Treatment of pyometra (cystic endometrial hyperplasia) in bitches with an antiprogestin. J Reprod Fert 51(Suppl):327, 1997.

Chen YMM, et al: A model for the study of cystic endometrial hyperplasia in the bitch. In Proceedings: Advances in dog, cat, and exotic carnivore reproduction. Oslo, Norway, 2000, p 30.

Egenvall A, et al: Breed risk of pyometra in insured dogs in Sweden. J Vet Intern Med 15:530, 2001.

Fantoni DT, et al: Intravenous administration of hypertonic sodium chloride solution with dextran or isotonic sodium chloride solution for treatment of septic shock secondary to pyometra in dogs. J Am Vet Med Assoc 215:1283, 1999.

Fazale A, et al: Comparative efficacy of hormonal and surgical treatment for pyometra in the dog. Int J Anim Sci 10:129, 1995.

Feldman EC, Nelson RW: Diagnosis and treatment alternatives for pyometra in dogs and cats. In Kirk RW (ed): Current Veterinary Therapy X. Philadelphia, WB Saunders Co, 1989, p 1305.

Fieni F, et al: Use of prostaglandins and antiprogestins in the treatment of metritis/pyometra in the bitch. In Proceedings: European Veterinary Society for Small Animal Reproduction. Lyons, France, 1999, Mondial Vet, p 63.

Frannson B, et al: Bacteriological findings, blood chemistry profile and plasma endotoxin levels in bitches with pyometra or other uterine diseases. J Vet Med Ser A 44:417, 1997.

Harvey M: Conditions of the non-pregnant female. In Simpson GM, England GCW, Harvey M (eds): BSAVA Manual of Small Animal Reproduction and Neonatology. United Kingdom, BSAVA, 1998, p 48.

Johnston SD, Root Kustritz MV, Olson PNS: Canine and Feline Theriogenology. Philadelphia, WB Saunders Co, 2001, p 210.

Lagerstedt AS, et al: Uterine drainage in the bitch for treatment of pyometra refractory to prostaglandin F_{2alpha}. J Small Anim Pract 28:215, 1987.

Lein DH, et al: Termination of pregnancy in bitches by administration of prostaglandin F_{2alpha}. J Reprod Fertil 39(Suppl):231, 1989.

Memon MA, Mickelsen WD: Diagnosis and treatment of closed-cervix pyometra in a bitch. JAVMA 203:509, 1993.

Meyers-Wallen VN, et al: Prostaglandin F_{2alpha} treatment of canine pyometra. JAVMA 189:1557, 1986.

Nelson RW, et al: Treatment of canine pyometra and endometritis with prostaglandin F_{2alpha}. JAVMA 181:899, 1982.

Niskanen M, Thrusfield MV: Associations between age, parity, hormonal therapy, and breed, and pyometra in Finnish dogs. Vet Rec 143:493, 1998.

Noakes DE, et al: Cystic endometrial hyperplasia/pyometra in the dog: A review of the causes and pathogenesis. In Proceedings: Advances in dog, cat, and exotic carnivore reproduction. Oslo, Norway, 2000, p 28.

Nomura K: Histological evaluation of the canine deciduoma induced by silk suture. J Vet Sci 57:9, 1995.

Olson PN, et al: The use and misuse of vaginal cultures in diagnosing reproductive disease in the bitch. In Morrow DA (ed): Current Therapy in Theriogenology 2. Philadelphia, WB Saunders Co, 1986, p 469.

Onclin K, Verstegen JP: Use of aglepristone (Alizine[R]) to treat pyometra in the canine and feline species. In Proceedings: Advances in dog, cat, and exotic carnivore reproduction. Oslo, Norway, 2000, p 114.

Stone EA: The uterus. In Slatter DH (ed): Textbook of Small Animal Surgery. Philadelphia, WB Saunders Co, 1985, p 1661.

Valocky I, et al: Experience with combined therapy with prostaglandin in bitches with the cystic endometrial/pyometra complex. Slovensky Vet Casopis 22:79, 1997.

Vasseur BB, Feldman EC: Pyometra associated with extrauterine pregnancy in a cat. JAAHA 18:872, 1982.

Wadas B, et al: Biochemical phenotypes of Escherichia coli in dogs: Comparison of isolates isolated from bitches suffering from pyometra and urinary tract infections with isolates from faeces of healthy dogs. Vet Microbiol 52:293, 1996.

Wheaton LG, et al: Results and complications of surgical treatment of pyometra: A review of 80 cases. JAAHA 25:563, 1989.

Wrigley RH, Finn ST: Ultrasonography of the canine uterus and ovary. In Kirk RW (ed): Current Veterinary Therapy X. Philadelphia, WB Saunders Co, 1989, p 1239.

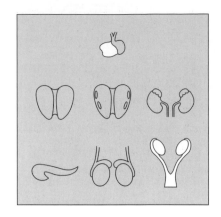

24

INFERTILITY, ASSOCIATED BREEDING DISORDERS, AND DISORDERS OF SEXUAL DEVELOPMENT

DEVELOPING THE PROBLEM LIST

Assessment of the Male

Before an investigation is begun into the potential causes of infertility in a bitch, the male should be assessed. The primary reason for evaluating the male before the female is that males are so much easier to study. The normal male is continuously fertile (i.e., continuously producing sperm). The female is usually fertile only 1 to 3 weeks per year. The easiest and usually most reliable method of establishing male fertility is a review of the male's previous breeding history. Any male that has sired one or more litters in the preceding 1 to 4 months usually can be assumed to be fertile. It is also helpful to know if the male sired any litters at the time the bitch in question was in heat and bred. However, even with positive responses to these inquiries, the fertility of the male should be demonstrated with a semen analysis.

All active stud dogs should be tested for brucellosis every 6 months. Less active studs should be checked yearly and immediately prior to use. A male that has not sired a litter or that has sired litters in the past but not in the preceding 6 to 12 months must be viewed with suspicion. Whenever the male's fertility is questionable, the owner of the bitch has three main alternatives: (1) have a semen analysis and *Brucella* titer performed on the male; (2) use an alternative, proven sire on the next heat; or (3) have the bitch evaluated, realizing that she may not be at fault.

A normal result on semen analysis is a major step toward ensuring that the male is not at fault. Abnormal semen or inability to obtain an ejaculate leaves suspicion directed at the male. Any normal male may have one or two abnormal semen analyses, but each abnormal study increases the likelihood of male infertility. In addition, males can have sperm that appear morphologically normal but that may not be capable of fertilization. Sophisticated studies on sperm function are not yet widely available in small animal reproduction. In any case, semen analysis is typically simple, safe, and inexpensive.

History (Anamnesis)

DEFINITION. Infertility or apparent infertility problems in the bitch are common. Veterinary advice is often sought if a bitch fails to conceive, if she fails to exhibit "normal" breeding behavior, when her cycles appear to be unusual, or for myriad other disturbances. "Infertility," therefore, is a huge category comprising a long list of anatomic, physiologic, and behavioral problems as well as a number of apparent husbandry misunderstandings. Also, if a bitch has earned a championship or other important title, a demand for puppies, as well as their value, are ensured before any attempt is made at breeding.

OBTAINING A "COMPLETE" HISTORY. Before the bitch is examined by the veterinarian, the various potential causes of infertility must be reduced to a workable number. In other words, the differential diagnosis for most infertility disorders is established by obtaining a thorough history from the owner. The initial history should include information about how well the owners know the bitch (e.g., does she live indoors with them, or 200 miles away at a hunt club?). Is she housed alone, with another bitch or bitches that recently completed ovarian cycles, with one or more ovariohysterectomized bitches, or with males? Is she of normal height and weight for her breed and her line? Is she receiving any medication, and is she well or ill?

To avoid the time-consuming chore of asking all the questions that help establish a problem list, differential diagnosis, and diagnostic plan, the veterinarian should have clients complete a questionnaire (Table 24-1). This list does not necessarily provide a complete background on every bitch, nor does it always provide the information needed to determine a diagnosis, but it does include the basic questions that must be answered to establish a foundation from which to work. Also, items can always be forgotten when reviewing a case history during a busy workday, and the question sheet helps avoid this problem.

AGE AND BREED. Small dogs reach sexual maturity at a younger age than large dogs. The onset of the pubertal (first) estrus in the bitch has been reported to occur at ages ranging from 6 to 23 months, with mean ages in different study populations of 9.6 to 13.9 months (Wildt et al, 1981; Johnston, 1991). Virtually all healthy bitches, therefore, begin ovarian cycles by 24 to 30 months of age.

Because first and second cycles may be irregular, unusual, short, or long (Wright and Watts, 1998), infertility evaluations are delayed in most dogs until 24 to 30 months of age. Just knowing the age and breed, therefore, can help the clinician decide how aggressive to be diagnostically. Toy Poodles may benefit from evaluation earlier in life than Bull Mastiffs. Each breed does have distinct average interestrous intervals, but the interval varies within a breed. As a general rule, almost all breeds cycle once every 4.5 to 10 months. The African breeds cycle once yearly. The remainder of the critical factors in an infertility evaluation are described under each major subheading.

Physical Examination

EXAMINE THE PROBLEM AREA LAST! As with any serious problem, the area of concern should be the last to be evaluated on physical examination. This approach ensures that each bitch receives a complete physical examination prior to an evaluation of the reproductive tract. The items specifically mentioned in this section involve the reproductive tract, but this should not suggest that a thorough examination be abbreviated in order to evaluate these areas.

VULVA. Examination of the reproductive tract usually begins with an external inspection of the vulva, which involves checking size and conformation and looking for any discharge. A small, immature vulva or one that is recessed under a fold of tissue, owing to body type or obesity, may impede normal breeding. An obese bitch is prone to perivulvar dermatitis. A swollen turgid vulva is suggestive of proestrus, and one that is swollen and flaccid may be consistent with dermatitis, estrus (standing heat), or approaching parturition.

VAGINAL DISCHARGES. The bitch in anestrus or diestrus usually has no vaginal discharge. A bloody discharge is most suggestive of proestrus, estrus, separation of the placental sites, or severe vaginitis. Greenish black or dark bloody vaginal discharges are associated with placental separation and postpartum "lochia." Reddish brown, yellowish, or grayish, thick, creamy, malodorous vaginal discharges are often seen in open-cervix pyometra, metritis, or severe vaginitis. Straw-colored vaginal discharges are sometimes seen when bitches are in estrus. Clear mucus can precede parturition and is rarely worrisome. A vaginal cytology specimen should be an integral part of any reproductive examination, because such specimens are easy to obtain, inexpensive, and informative. Vaginal cytology should be performed for any bitch with a vaginal discharge.

DIGITAL EXAMINATION OF THE VESTIBULE AND VAGINA. A digital examination of the vaginal vault should be

TABLE 24–1 CLIENT QUESTIONNAIRE—THE INFERTILE BITCH

A. Breed _____
   Age _____

B. General medical history (not including reproduction problems)
   1. Vaccinations current? _____
   2. Previous significant illness requiring hospitalization? If so, please briefly summarize:
      a. _____
      b. _____
   3. Does your dog:
      a. Have a vomiting problem?   Yes _____ No _____
      b. Have diarrhea?   Yes _____ No _____
      c. Drink excessively?   Yes _____ No _____
      d. Urinate excessively?   Yes _____ No _____
      e. Have normal ability to play and exercise?   Yes _____ No _____
      f. Appear to be of normal weight and height?   Yes _____ No _____
      g. Have a hair coat problem?   Yes _____ No _____
      h. Have any other problem? (If yes, please describe) Yes _____ No _____
   4. Has your dog ever had thyroid tests run?   Yes _____ No _____
   5. Has your dog received thyroid hormone?
      a. In the past?   No _____   Yes _____ Dose _____
      b. Now?   No _____   Yes _____ Dose _____
   6. Is your dog receiving any medication of any type?
      No _____ Yes _____ Drug and dose _____

   7. Has your dog ever received or is it now receiving medicine for fleas or scratching?
      No _____ Yes _____ Drug and dose _____

   8. Please list all foods and supplements presently being given to your dog:
      _____
      _____
      _____
      _____

C. Cycle history
   1. Is she cycling?   Yes _____ No _____
   2. Time interval between cycles _____
   3. Total number of cycles in her life _____
   4. How many days is a bloody discharge present (average in last 2 or 3 cycles)?
      _____
   5. How many days does she stand for the male (average in last 2 or 3 cycles)?
      _____
   6. Has a vaginal smear been checked by a veterinarian during a heat? _____
      _____
   7. Has a series of vaginal smears (several during one heat) ever been checked?
      _____
   8. Have any hormone assays been run?   No _____ Yes _____   Please describe
      _____
   9. Has your dog received any drug to cause a cycle (no _____ yes _____) or increase fertility?
      (no _____ yes _____) Please explain _____
      _____

D. Breeding history
   1. Does your bitch allow the male to mount and breed?   No _____ Yes _____
   2. How often is your dog bred in a cycle? _____
   3. How are breeding dates chosen? _____
   4. Has your bitch been bred to a male that has successfully sired litters
      within the last 6 months?   No _____ Yes _____
      1–2 years?   No _____ Yes _____
   5. Have you observed any ties?   No _____ Yes _____
   6. Duration of ties (average) _____
   7. Inside tie _____? Outside tie _____?
   8. Has the bitch been tranquilized prior to breeding or shipping? No _____ Yes _____
   9. Is the bitch bred locally or is she shipped for breeding? _____

TABLE 24–1   CLIENT QUESTIONNAIRE—THE INFERTILE BITCH—cont'd

E. Pregnancy history

   1. Has she had any litters?

      Dates: a. _____   Litter size a. _____

               b. _____   b. _____

               c. _____   c. _____

               d. _____   d. _____

   2. Any abortions? No _____ Yes _____ If so, how do you know she aborted?

   3. Any resorption of puppies?   No _____   Yes _____

      a. If so, how do you know she resorbed puppies?

        _____

      b. How was pregnancy proven? _____

      c. Was pregnancy examined at

        (1)   7 days _____

        (2) 14 days _____

        (3) 21 days _____

        (4) 28 days _____

        (5) 35 days _____

        (6) 45 days _____

   4. Has she ever been treated for mismating? _____

   5. Has she had a *Brucella* titer? _____

      Date of most recent check _____

   6. Has she ever had:

      Pyometra?   Yes _____   No _____

      Vaginitis?   Yes _____   No _____

   7. Has she ever had medication to prevent or delay a heat?

      No _____ Yes _____

      If yes, what drug? _____

      when given? _____

   8. Does she now or has she had an abnormal vaginal discharge?

      _____

F. Kennel history

   Do any other bitches in your kennel have reproductive disorders?

   No _____ Yes _____

G. Pedigree

   Do any other bitches in her line have reproductive disorders?

   No _____ Yes _____

performed routinely on any bitch examined for breeding soundness. If a culture or cytology specimen is needed, it should be obtained prior to the digital examination. Most bitches are easy to examine. A gloved, lubricated index finger should pass easily into the vaginal vault, allowing assessment of the lumen, the urethral opening, and the size and shape of the clitoris. Masses, foreign bodies, strictures, painful vaginitis, or abnormal tissue bands all prevent easy and painless examination.

If the digital examination result is abnormal but inconclusive, vaginoscopy can be performed for a more thorough evaluation. An otoscope or a vaginal speculum provides an extremely limited view of the vaginal vault and is of little value in most clinical situations. Pediatric proctoscopes are easy to use for vaginoscopy (Fig. 24-1), are relatively inexpensive, and can be used in all but the smallest of miniature breeds. An endoscope is a more expensive but smaller diameter alternative. In most breeds a small-diameter pediatric proctoscope can be used, which provides far better visualization of the area than an otoscope. If vaginoscopy is performed, the clinician must be knowledgeable about the changes in the appearance of the vaginal mucosa associated with each phase of the estrous cycle (Table 24-2).

MAMMARY GLANDS AND VENTRUM.   The mammary glands should be palpated. The primary concern is the presence of mammary tumors, although the glands can also be checked for evidence of lactation, mastitis, inverted teats, or benign nodules. The ventral midline can be checked for evidence of a surgical incision, which might suggest that the bitch has undergone ovariohysterectomy.

RECTAL EXAMINATION.   A rectal examination ensures that the pelvic canal has been assessed for previous

TABLE 24–2 CHANGES SEEN IN THE VAGINAL MUCOSA DURING THE ESTROUS CYCLE

ANESTRUS: Mucosa is flat and smooth.
PROESTRUS/ESTRUS PRIOR TO PREOVULATORY LH PEAK: Mucosa is edematous; vaginal folds are distended and rounded, causing obliteration of the vaginal canal.
PREOVULATORY LH PEAK ± 24 HOURS: Initial crenulation is a fine wrinkling in mucosa as vaginal edema begins to recede.
POST-LH PEAK/PERIOD OF FERTILITY: Crenulation continues with angulated appearance of mucosa with sharp-appearing profiles. Vaginal lumen easy to observe without insufflation.
DIESTRUS: Mucosa is irregularly flattened, blotchy red and white.

fractures or other unsuspected abnormalities. Compression of the pelvic canal is a potential cause of dystocia and, less commonly, inability to breed. An attempt can be made to palpate the vagina ventrally, although this organ would have to be extremely abnormal to reveal anything suspicious on palpation.

ABDOMINAL PALPATION. The abdomen should be palpated in an effort to identify and characterize the uterus. However, except in pregnancy and pyometra, the uterus almost never can be evaluated with confidence on abdominal palpation.

Owner Management Practices

DEFINITION. Improper management practices are the cause of a large majority of apparent infertility problems. A bitch that is bred or attempted to be bred at incorrect times may be completely normal. She may fail to conceive as a result of being brought to the male when she is not fertile.

COMMON MISTAKES. The following five major errors in breeding management are commonly encountered (negative results on *Brucella* tests are assumed).

1. Many people who own male dogs that are frequently in use allow only one breeding per cycle. (Although a single breeding can be associated with excellent conception rates, breeding several times per cycle helps eliminate the chance of a poorly timed or mistimed breeding and minimizes the risk of relying on one ejaculate.)
2. Many dog owners allow breeding only on certain predetermined days of the cycle, such as days 11 and 13 (first day of vaginal bleeding is day 1) or days 10 and 12, or one day only (such as day 14) may be chosen. (Predetermined dates are fine if they work, but what if the perfectly normal but not average bitch is in proestrus for 16 days or if proestrus lasts 4 days and estrus lasts 4 days?)
3. Breeding may be timed to begin only after the bloody vaginal discharge of proestrus becomes clear and/or straw-colored. (For some normal bitches this is a problem, because they may have a bloody vaginal discharge that begins with the onset of proestrus and ends several days after the onset of diestrus; that is, some bitches bleed throughout estrus. Others may discontinue bleeding *days* before the onset of estrus.)
4. Some owners allow the male dog to choose the breeding date. (Male response to a bitch is simply unreliable. Some males always want to breed, whereas others never want to breed because they may be submissive to a bitch. The male, therefore, is not reliable as a guide to breeding.)
5. It is always assumed that the male is fertile. (Any male may quickly become transiently or permanently infertile. Anytime the fertility of the male is in question, a semen analysis is warranted.)

These and similar practices do not consistently result in conception. They may work in a majority of bitches, but some normal bitches fail to conceive if bred according to such criteria.

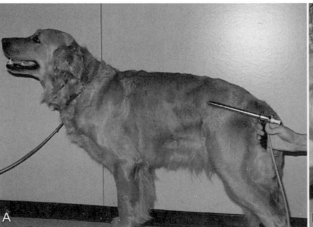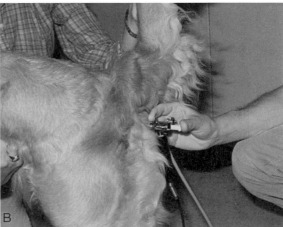

FIGURE 24-1. *A* and *B,* Vaginoscopy can be performed with a pediatric proctoscope. The instrument is easily passed into the vaginal vault for a thorough inspection. Despite its length, the pediatric proctoscope does not always allow visualization of the cervix, which illustrates the futility of using an otoscope for this procedure.

General Health of the Bitch

In the clinical evaluation of the infertile bitch, one underlying question is her overall health status. Some investigators have recommended complete blood counts, chemistry panels, urinalysis, and thyroid and adrenocortical function studies as initial steps in the evaluation of a potentially infertile bitch (Johnston, 1980; Johnston et al, 1982; Lein, 1983). Others have suggested that, "It is unethical and unprofessional to perform unnecessary tests without discussion with the owners as to the real value and cost of these investigations" (Wright and Watts, 1998).

We do not usually use extensive diagnostic testing unless the history or physical examination (or both) dictates that aggressive diagnostic testing is warranted. The bitch that appears healthy to an owner, that appears healthy on physical examination, and that has normal ovarian cycles does not have thyroid failure or adrenocortical disease and rarely has other significant organ disease. Therefore a complete blood count (CBC), a urinalysis, and a blood urea nitrogen (BUN) determination provide a sufficient database. Nonetheless, this approach depends on the completion of a thorough history and a competent physical examination. If abnormalities are identified through the history or physical examination, appropriate testing can then be done that may clarify the nature of the problem or specifically demonstrate the cause of infertility.

INFERTILITY IN THE *BRUCELLA*-NEGATIVE BITCH THAT HAS NORMAL OVARIAN CYCLES, NORMAL INTERESTROUS INTERVALS, AND THAT ALLOWS BREEDING (FIG. 24-2)

Initial Approach

COMMON STRATEGIES. Because the *average* proestrus lasts 9 days and the *average* estrus 7 to 9 days, commonly used management strategies succeed in the *average* bitch. The average bitch also has a clear, straw-colored vaginal discharge at the onset of estrus. However, if a "traditional" breeding protocol fails to result in conception, a new approach to breeding management may prove successful, and this is our initial approach to an "infertility problem."

BEHAVIOR OBSERVATION

Recommendation. As the initial approach to an apparently normal bitch that fails to conceive, the veterinarian should recommend that the owner adopt a reliable breeding schedule while simultaneously monitoring follicular function and the time of ovulation. In this manner, if the problem is management related, it is corrected. If the problem is physiologic, it may be identified and treated appropriately.

The proposed breeding schedule is aimed at better understanding the estrous cycle of the individual bitch in question. It is important to realize that in the "normal" bitch, proestrus can be as brief as 1 to 2 days

or as long as 25 days. Correct identification of day 1 of proestrus depends on an owner correctly detecting the first day of vaginal bleeding. Estrus (standing heat) can have a duration of 2 to 20 days. The recommendation, therefore, is to bring the bitch to a dominant male for evaluation of *her* behavior beginning on the second, third, or fourth day of proestrus and to continue to do so daily or every other day until *diestrus* is demonstrated both by *her* behavior and by vaginal cytology. If the male attempts to mount and the bitch is receptive, breeding should be allowed, regardless of the apparent timing in the ovarian cycle.

Handlers. It is wise to have someone hold the male and another person attend to the bitch. The dogs are allowed to interact for 5 to 15 minutes so that the bitch's response to the stud can be assessed. One is looking for evidence of standing heat. If the male is not the stud to be used in the actual breeding, the handlers must prevent mating. The handlers are also present to prevent fighting, which occasionally occurs.

Breeding Activity. Once the bitch displays standing heat, she should be bred on that day and every 2 to 4 days thereafter until she refuses to breed. In the context of this discussion, daily or every other day breeding is recommended because concern about infertility should not be complicated by uncertainty over whether breeding was occurring on appropriate days. Breeding is continued on this schedule, regardless of the duration of standing heat, the color of the vaginal discharge, the day of the cycle, or the interpretation of a vaginal cytology smear. This program ensures that viable sperm are present when eggs become available for fertilization. Bitches known to have a prolonged standing heat should be bred every 4 days until cytologic or behavioral diestrus is confirmed.

Predetermined Dates. If a bitch is bred only on specific predetermined days of her cycle (counting from the first day that vaginal bleeding is detected), several potential problems exist. The most common recipes are breeding on days 10 and 12, 11 and 13, or 11 and 15. If proestrus lasts 4 days and estrus 5 days, breeding will be attempted when the bitch is in diestrus and no longer likely to be receptive or, if receptive, no longer fertile (some healthy bitches allow breeding during the first 1 to 3 days of *diestrus* as defined by vaginal cytology).

If a bitch is in proestrus for 16 days and estrus for 10 days, ovulation is likely to begin on day 19 or 20 and fertilization on days 22 through 26. If she was bred (artificially inseminated because natural breeding would not have been allowed by the bitch) on days 10 and 12, few if any sperm would be alive when fertilization takes place (see Fig. 24-6). Forced mating or artificial insemination or both may be performed in an attempt to ensure that breeding occurs on the predetermined dates, only to have the bitch later appear infertile, with no consideration given to the fact that she was bred on the wrong dates. Forced breeding is never acceptable and should be a clue that errors in management are likely.

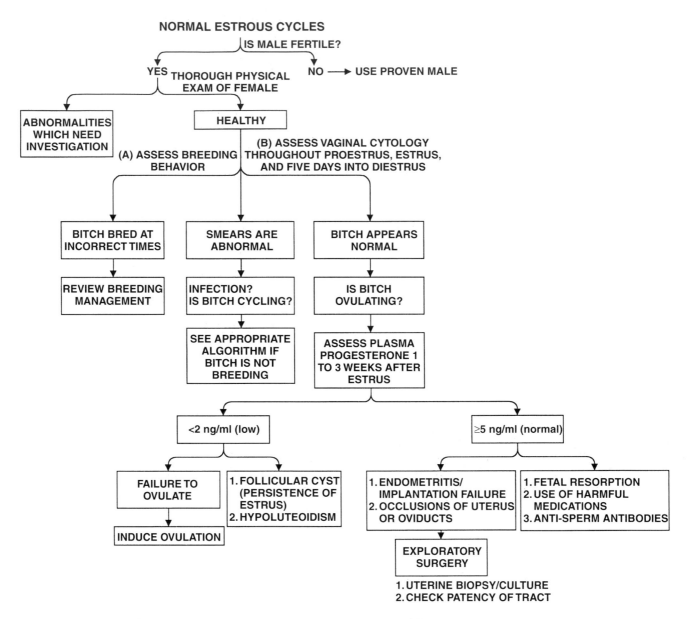

FIGURE 24-2. Algorithm for the evaluation of an infertile bitch that tests negative for *Brucella* infection but that has normal estrous cycle activity and apparent infertility.

Male Preference. Some bitches refuse a particular male or, less commonly, refuse mounting attempts by any male despite correct recognition of estrus. Preferences for particular mates have been documented in the bitch (Freshman, 1991). Three possible explanations for this frustrating dilemma are (1) the male has been brought to the bitch for mating, and she is dominant to him when she is at her home (the bitch does not allow submissive males to breed); (2) the male is submissive to the bitch in standing heat, regardless of the environment and regardless of the apparent relationship between these dogs at other times (Freshman, 1991); and (3) the bitch is housed with a bitch dominant to her and the other female may interfere with normal breeding behavior.

OVARIAN FUNCTION IN PROESTRUS AND ESTRUS. *Vaginal Cytology.* Like behavior, follicular function can be easily and inexpensively monitored. The owner should be taught how to obtain vaginal smears and then instructed to begin obtaining smears on the first day of proestrus, continuing daily until at least 4 to 5 days after the onset of behavioral or cytologic diestrus. Vaginal cytology is a reflection of peripheral estrogen concentrations, which in turn reflect follicular function. Vaginal smears identify the approximate days of estrus and can be used to definitively identify the beginning of diestrus (Olson et al, 1984). One can count back 6 days from day 1 of diestrus to the first likely day of ovulation and/or count back 1 through 4 days for the time of greatest fertility (see Chapter 19).

Recognizing that viable sperm can survive approximately 4 to 7 days in the uterus after breeding, the veterinarian can determine if the breeding dates were optimal for fertilization. If not, the bitch should be managed differently to better coordinate breeding with fertilization. If the breeding dates were optimal, management problems can be excluded from the list of causes of infertility.

Plasma Progesterone. The results of vaginal cytology can be reliable and helpful. However, to enhance evaluations, serial serum progesterone concentrations should be determined as the bitch progresses through proestrus and into estrus (see Chapter 19). Frequent serial progesterone assessments allow identification of the first day that the concentration rises above 2 ng/ml, which should coincide closely with the onset of behavioral estrus and the luteinizing hormone (LH) surge (Hegstad and Johnston, 1992). If an enzyme-linked immunosorbent assay (ELISA) in-hospital kit is used for the tests, the progesterone concentration usually is estimated as less than 1 ng/ml, greater than 1 to less than 5 ng/ml, and greater than 5 ng/ml (Manothaiudom et al, 1995). Breeding is recommended 4 days after the serum progesterone concentration is greater than 1 ng/ml as measured with these kits. Optimal breeding dates are 4 and 6 days after the rise in the serum progesterone concentration. Vaginal endoscopic evaluation of the bitch several times during proestrus and into estrus can also be informative (see Chapters 19 and 20) (Lindsay, 1990).

OVARIAN FUNCTION IN DIESTRUS: DETERMINING WHETHER OVULATION HAS OCCURRED. The question regarding ovulation cannot be answered with testing completed during proestrus or estrus. Vaginal cytologic identification of the first diestrual day offers an indirect method of determining an approximate ovulation date, as previously described. However, a more precise determination can be made by measuring the plasma progesterone concentration daily or on alternate days. Ovulation begins 2 to 4 days after the progesterone concentration rises above 2.0 ng/ml (see Fig. 19-15). Again, these values do not confirm that ovulation took place, because progesterone is initially derived from luteinized *follicles;* that is, the serum progesterone concentration increases *prior to* actual ovulation. The initial rise does not confirm that ovulation occurs.

If the veterinarian wishes to determine whether a bitch ovulates, daily vaginal cytology smears can be used to identify day 1 of diestrus, and that information can be coupled with measurement of the plasma progesterone concentration obtained between the 10th and 20th day of diestrus. During the initial few weeks of diestrus, the plasma progesterone concentration should be greater than 3 ng/ml and usually is 10 to 50 ng/ml. Concentrations into the ranges mentioned can be attained only by progesterone secretion from functioning corpora lutea (excluding exogenous sources), which exist as a result of previous ovulation. Normal diestrual progesterone concentrations, therefore, are consistent with ovulation and proper luteal function.

REVIEW OF SHIPPING PRACTICES: POSSIBLE STRESS. Breeding practices need to be reviewed as potential problem areas. For example, it is not known whether tranquilization or the stress of shipping can interfere with ovulation or early pregnancy (Wright and Watts, 1998). These factors could be a cause of "acquired infertility" and are worth avoiding during one cycle to see if the infertility problem can be resolved by keeping the bitch at home and having her bred locally.

Furthermore, if an owner never observes a breeding because the bitch is always being shipped to the male, only secondhand information about mating is available. The owner should be encouraged to have the bitch bred locally so that breedings can witnessed. This is the most reliable means of minimizing stress and ensuring that unsuspected problems are identified. For example, if outside ties persistently occur, an anatomic problem in the vaginal vault may be preventing penetration by the male but may not be observed or reported.

REVIEW OF MEDICATIONS. All previously or currently used medications should be noted. Previous use of gonadotropins may have long-term deleterious effects on pituitary function. Previous progesterone or estrogen administration may result in subclinical cystic endometrial hyperplasia (CEH), with infertility being the only outward effect seen by the owner or veterinarian.

HYPOTHYROIDISM. Most reviews concerning infertility in the bitch include discussion of hypothyroidism, a condition often described as common and as producing such signs as persistent anestrus, prolonged interestrous intervals, and prolonged proestrus, although some bitches demonstrate normal reproductive activity, pregnancy, and parturition (Johnston, 1980). However, only one bitch has been described in the veterinary literature since 1989 that had thyroid insufficiency and related ovarian disease (Johnston, 1989).

Hypothyroidism is an overdiagnosed endocrine disorder in veterinary practice. The diagnosis should always be viewed with suspicion, not because the disease does not exist but simply because many dogs treated for the disease are not so afflicted. If a bitch is being treated for hypothyroidism, the veterinarian must decide whether that diagnosis was correct and then whether thyroid replacement medication should be discontinued (see Chapter 3).

SUMMARY OF MANAGEMENT PROBLEMS. Management problems are the most common cause of *apparent* infertility in the bitch with a normal cycle (Johnston, 1980; Soderberg, 1989; Freshman, 1991). Veterinarians should remember to evaluate the male before embarking on the somewhat involved task of assessing the bitch. The entire question regarding proper management of an individual bitch can be answered through the relatively inexpensive approach of obtaining a thorough history, with corrections made, as needed, in past incorrect practices; behavior observation; review of vaginal cytology results; and monitoring of plasma progesterone concentrations. This approach answers the following questions: (1) how is the owner managing this bitch? (2) when does standing heat begin? (3) how long does standing heat persist? (4) what is the first day of true diestrus? (5) when is the bitch truly fertile? (6) what are her ideal breeding dates? (7) does she ovulate? (8) when does she ovulate? and (9) does she have the luteal function necessary to support pregnancy?

Brucella Infection

Brucella canis classically causes abortion late in gestation (see Chapter 26). In addition, the organism may render a bitch infertile or may cause resorption of fetuses early in gestation. *B. canis* infection can also result in ill or stillborn puppies (Olson et al, 1983). All bitches in active breeding programs should be repeatedly evaluated for canine brucellosis. The rapid slide agglutination test (Canine Brucellosis Diagnostic Test; Pitman-Moore, Washington Crossing, NJ) is an excellent screening test. False-negative results are unlikely, and a negative result can be trusted. Bitches that test seropositive should be retested with the tube agglutination method, because false-positive results do occur (Johnston, 1980).

Problems Arising from Infection

QUESTIONABLE VALUE OF A POSITIVE RESULT ON VAGINAL CULTURE. *Culture Technique.* Bacterial infections have been implicated as a cause of infertility in the bitch (Johnston, 1980; Lein, 1983). These infections are thought to be subclinical in the infertile bitch, only occasionally resulting in obvious vaginitis, metritis, pyometra, or systemic infection. It has been recommended that the anterior vagina of infertile bitches be cultured with a guarded swab (Accu-CulShure, from Accu-Med, Pleasantville, NY; Guarded Culture Instrument, from Kalayjian Industries, Long Beach, CA; and Tiegland Swab, HL 206400, from Haver-Lockhart Laboratories, Shawnee Mission, KS). Bacterial isolation and identification, as well as antimicrobial sensitivity, are suggested, after which the bitch can be given the appropriate antibiotics for 4 weeks (Johnston, 1980). However, it is difficult to establish the role of bacterial infections in canine infertility. Virtually all normal bitches have bacterial flora in the anterior vagina, and similar types of aerobic bacteria are present in the vaginal vaults of infertile bitches (Olson et al, 1983; Okkens et al, 1992). For these reasons, a request by stud owners that a vaginal culture be free of bacteria prior to mating is nonsensical (Watts et al, 1996; Wright and Watts, 1998).

Bacteria. Approximately 95% to 100% of normal bitches harbor aerobic bacteria in the vaginal tract (see Table 23-2; Bjurstrom and Linde-Forsberg, 1992a). A wide variety of bacteria have been isolated from normal canine vaginal tracts, and the numbers are often increased during proestrus and estrus. Merely isolating bacteria from the vagina does not constitute the basis for a diagnosis of disease; rather, it is likely to

confirm that a bitch is normal. Furthermore, the most worrisome organism, *B. canis,* may be difficult to isolate. A negative culture result, therefore, does not ensure that a bitch is free of an infectious disease.

The types of bacteria may vary with the age of the bitch; a higher percentage of prepubertal bitches have coagulase-positive staphylococci than do postpubertal dogs. The stage of the cycle did not alter the types of bacteria isolated in some studies, but other studies demonstrated increased numbers in proestrus and estrus (Allen and Dagnall, 1982; Baba et al, 1983). In a more recent study, the bacteria isolated did vary with the stage of the ovarian cycle (Fig. 24-3) (Bjurstrom and Linde-Forsberg, 1992a). The composition of the gram-positive and gram-negative organisms has been found to be unique to individual dogs.

Normal flora usually are recovered in mixed cultures of light to moderate growth (see Table 23-2; Bjurstrom and Linde-Forsberg, 1992a). If an organism is a significant pathogen, it usually produces clinical signs, is recovered in large numbers, and is present in a nearly pure culture because it gains advantage as a pathogen and overgrows the normal mixed flora (Allen and Dagnall, 1982; Allen, 1986; Olson et al, 1986). Of 826 vaginal swabs taken from 59 healthy, fertile bitches, cultures of only one organism were identified in 18%; mixed cultures were seen in 77%; and completely negative results occurred in only 5% (Fig. 24-4) (Bjurstrom and Linde-Forsberg, 1992a).

Some owners of stud dogs require a "negative" vaginal culture from the bitch to be used in breeding. However, most male dogs harbor microorganisms in the prepuce and urethra similar to those identified as normal vaginal flora (Bjurstrom and Linde-Forsberg, 1992b). There is no justification for refusing to breed a bitch to a stud dog because bacteria have been isolated from the vagina.

It should now be clear that it is unjustified to associate positive findings on vaginal cultures with infertility. Systemic antibiotics may have significant side effects. Heavy growth of one bacteria is more likely to be normal than abnormal. Treatment with vaginal douches for 2 to 3 weeks, with or without systemic antibiotics, may be beneficial, but such therapies should be reserved for bitches with obvious clinical signs of infection, such as a purulent vaginal discharge (Bjurstrom and Linde-Forsberg, 1992a and 1992b).

Finally, the canine uterus may contain small numbers of bacteria and still be normal (Baba et al, 1983). Obtaining a uterine culture requires laparotomy or transcervical uterine cannulation during proestrus, estrus, or diestrus. However, in normal fertile bitches these phases of the estrous cycle are associated with migration of bacteria from the vaginal vault into the uterus via the relaxed cervix (Watts and Wright, 1995). Without obvious vaginitis or pyometra, vaginal cultures are not believed to be of benefit in managing the infertile bitch.

MYCOPLASMA AND UREAPLASMA INFECTIONS. *Myco-plasma* and *Ureaplasma* are organisms commonly cultured from the vaginal tract of normal bitches. However, a syndrome of poor conception, early embryonic death,

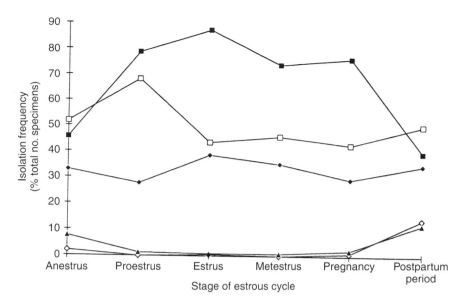

FIGURE 24-3. Variation in the frequency of isolation of five bacterial species from the vaginas of 59 bitches during various stages of the estrous cycle. (■———■), *Pasteurella multocida;* (□———□), β-Hemolytic streptococci; (◆———◆), *Escherichia coli;* (◇———◇), *Staphylococcus intermedius;* (▲———▲), Enterococci. (Bjurstrom L, Linde-Forsberg C: Am J Vet Res 53:665, 1992.)

embryonal or fetal resorption, abortion, stillborn pups, weak newborns, and neonatal death has been suggested to be caused by these smallest of free-living microorganisms. Currently, evidence regarding the pathogenesis of these disorders is circumstantial (Doig et al, 1981; Lein, 1989). As with bacterial culture results, if large numbers of these organisms are identified in pure or nearly pure growth from the vaginal vault of a breeding bitch with an infertility problem, these microorganisms may be at fault. However, in one study 59% of healthy, fertile bitches had *Mycoplasma* organisms recovered from vaginal swabs (Bjurstrom and Linde-Forsberg, 1992a). Management includes isolation of the animal and tetracycline or chloramphenicol therapy for 10 to 14 days (Lein, 1986).

VIRAL INFECTIONS. Viral infections, specifically herpesvirus (see Chapter 25), have been isolated in dogs that have had abortions and stillbirths. However, viral infections are not well documented as a cause of infertility. Moreover, viral cultures are not yet widely available to practitioners.

Chronic Endometritis: Cystic Endometrial Hyperplasia

BACKGROUND. The bitch with chronic endometrial disease is likely to be infertile. These dogs could experience normal ovarian cycles, ovulate, and have fertilized eggs but fail to support pregnancy because of the abnormal uterine environment that prevents implantation or that would result in fetal resorption (Allen and Dagnall, 1982). After evaluating the male and the owner's management practices, the clinician

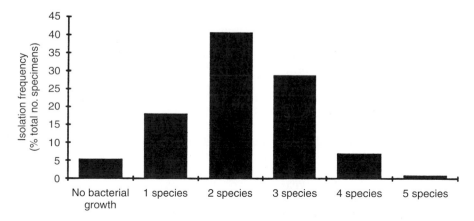

FIGURE 24-4. Frequency distribution of isolation of the number of bacterial species per vaginal swab specimen and per bitch. (Bjurstrom L, Linde-Forsberg C: Am J Vet Res 53:665, 1992.)

should be able to assess the likelihood of an ovarian problem. If the male is normal, ovarian function is normal, the bitch is free of brucellosis, and the timing of breeding is correct, an underlying endometrial problem is possible. CEH (sterile or infected) can be extremely difficult to confirm. The diagnosis is suspected if the nonpregnant uterus is thickened or abnormally large in anestrus or diestrus. Although a thickened uterine wall is a potentially palpable abnormality, it is difficult to be certain that one is palpating the uterus. Radiographically, the non-pregnant uterus is rarely visible. If the uterus is visible in a bitch with an infertility problem, endometrial disease is possible. Similarly, visualization of the nonpregnant uterus using abdominal ultrasonography may be a means of documenting the presence of a thickened endometrium or of intraluminal fluid. The diagnosis can be confirmed only by uterine biopsy.

TRANSCERVICAL UTERINE MICROBIOLOGY AND CYTOLOGY. Procedures for transcervical cannulation of the uterus are now feasible with injection and aspiration of sterile fluid for culture and cytology (see Chapter 20). Cells identified in normal aspirates include endometrial cells, leukocytes, erythrocytes, cervical cells, bacteria, and sperm. Endometrial cells appear degenerative in diestrus and anestrus. Neutrophils are the most common white cells present during proestrus and estrus (Watts et al, 1997 and 1998). This procedure can aid in the recognition of CEH and other endometrial disease.

Early Fetal Resorption

Early fetal resorption usually appears to both owner and veterinarian as primary infertility because early pregnancy is so difficult to confirm. Pregnancy cannot be recognized by palpation until after 21 days of gestation, and then the diagnosis is subjec-tive. Radiographically, pregnancy cannot be confirmed until 42 to 45 days of gestation. The earliest that pregnancy can confidently be identified is approximately 16 days after first breeding, using ultra-sonography. This imaging technique has been help-ful in the detection of early fetal resorption. Early fetal resorption suggests an endometrial disorder (infection or CEH), failure of corpora lutea to support pregnancy (hypoluteoidism), infectious disease (e.g., brucellosis), fetal defects (e.g., chromosomal anomalies), or some less common disorder. However, early embryonic loss has not been well investigated, and in most cases the diagnosis is speculative. Only definitive diagnosis of pregnancy through ultra-sonography with demonstration of fetal death and resorption is specific for recognition of this condition. With such a diagnosis, the management alternatives are to use a different male on the next cycle or to consider uterine culture and biopsy by means of surgery or transcervical cannulation (Wright and Watts, 1998).

Hypoluteoidism

Plasma progesterone concentrations begin to rise prior to the onset of standing heat and decline to basal levels immediately prior to parturition. The first 6 to 7 weeks of diestrus are usually associated with progesterone concentrations of 5 to 50 ng/ml. With any bitch diag-nosed as having an infertility problem, the plasma progesterone concentration should be evaluated 10 to 20 days after termination of standing heat and once or twice weekly thereafter. These studies should be completed in conjunction with evaluation by abdom-inal ultrasonography.

If the progesterone concentration is below 1.0 ng/ml when a bitch is timed to be in diestrus, either she never ovulated or the corpora lutea have failed to synthesize and/or secrete progesterone. Serum progesterone concentrations above 5 ng/ml should be sufficient to maintain pregnancy. If the progesterone concentration is 1.0 to 5.0 ng/ml, the amount of progesterone secreted may be insufficient to maintain pregnancy (hypoluteoidism), and abortion or fetal resorption may result. If fetuses are observed on abdominal ultrasonography early in gestation, abor-tion or fetal resorption should become demonstrable with repeated ultrasound examinations. (See Chapter 21 for a complete discussion of hypoluteoidism.)

To complicate matters, decreased progesterone concentrations in diestrus are not always a primary problem. Fetal factors, placentitis, or exogenous glucocorticoid therapy are a few of the many potential causes of premature luteal regression. In some situ-ations progesterone administration may be contra-indicated, but these conditions are not completely understood. Progesterone therapy should be recom-mended only with great caution.

Occlusion of the Uterus or Oviducts

It is impossible to evaluate the patency of the uterus and oviducts on a physical examination simply because these structures are too small. With bilateral segmental aplasia or other causes of obstruction of the uterine horns or with occlusion of the cervix or both oviducts, a bitch could cycle, ovulate, and breed normally but fail to conceive (Olson et al, 1983). Bilateral occlusion prevents sperm from ever reaching eggs. Diagnosing this rare anatomic defect is extremely difficult. The problem of diagnosis lies in the location of these tubular structures and in the physiology governing their accessibility.

Theoretically, it should be possible to pass radio-paque dye from the vagina through the cervix and uterus into both oviducts. Radiographs of the abdomen would then allow assessment of the reproductive tract for patency. However, even under a good deal of pressure, dye cannot easily be passed through the cervix except during proestrus and estrus, when the cervix is dilated. The uterotubular junction, how-ever, is tight (closed) under the influence of estrogen (i.e., during proestrus and perhaps early estrus).

Therefore this dye study (hysterosalpingography) is most likely to be successful only during estrus. Hysterosalpingography is an excellent theoretic tool but one that is difficult to use on a practical basis (Fig. 24-5) (Johnston, 1980; Buckrell and Johnson, 1988; Freshman, 1991). Rupture of the uterus rather than passage of dye through the oviducts has been reported in normal bitches (Freshman, 1991).

An alternative to the radiographic study is direct visualization. Laparoscopy is not a good tool because the oviducts are not visible with a laparoscope. Laparotomy is the only realistic remaining tool. The uterus can be closely studied and oviduct patency assessed by injecting saline into the uterus, occluding the uterus at the body, and watching the saline leak out of the oviducts. Other investigators have recommended using dye for the procedure, but in our experience this has not been necessary. Surgery also allows uterine biopsies and cultures to be obtained.

Little can be done if a bitch is diagnosed as having bilateral uterine or oviductal occlusion. Unilateral occlusion does not result in infertility. Opening of occluded uterine horns or oviducts has not been described, and such bitches are permanently infertile.

Miscellaneous Causes of Infertility

Among the recognized causes of infertility in species other than the dog, when the female has normal cycles and the male is fertile, are antisperm antibodies produced by the female and spermicidal substances in secretions of the cervix. Antisperm antibodies have been recognized in male dogs with *B. canis* (George and Carmichael, 1984). Antisperm antibodies have also been induced in dogs (Rosenthal et al, 1984). Studies on both systemic antibodies and cervical mucus may some day be part of the evaluation of the infertile bitch. However, such findings remain speculative. In addition, anti-egg zona pellucida antibodies have been developed in bitches through immunization procedures (Mahi-Brown et al, 1982). Such antibodies result in infertility. Spontaneous production of such antibodies may occur but has not yet been recognized.

THE BITCH WITH SHORTENED INTERESTROUS INTERVALS (LESS THAN 4.5 MONTHS) (FIG. 24-6)

Idiopathic Shortened Ovarian Cycles

PHYSIOPATHOLOGY. The "normal" bitch enters the proestrus phase of her ovarian cycle every 5 to 9 months. In some dogs, fertile cycles, culminating in a term pregnancy, occur every 4 to 4.5 months or as infrequently as every 10 to 12 months. The German Shepherd dog and the Rottweiler are breeds that reportedly have fertile cycles every 4.5 months. After the phase of progesterone dominance in which it is in

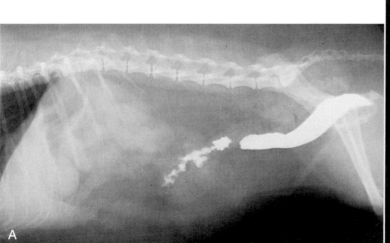

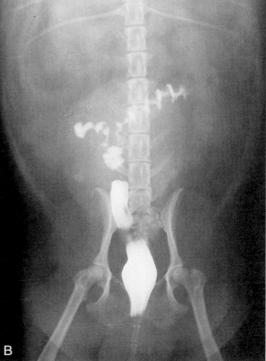

FIGURE 24-5. Lateral *(A)* and ventrodorsal *(B)* abdominal radiographs of a normal healthy bitch in which hysterosalpingography has been attempted by placing contrast material in the vaginal vault under pressure to identify the uterine horns and oviducts. One can appreciate how difficult it can be to identify oviducts with this procedure.

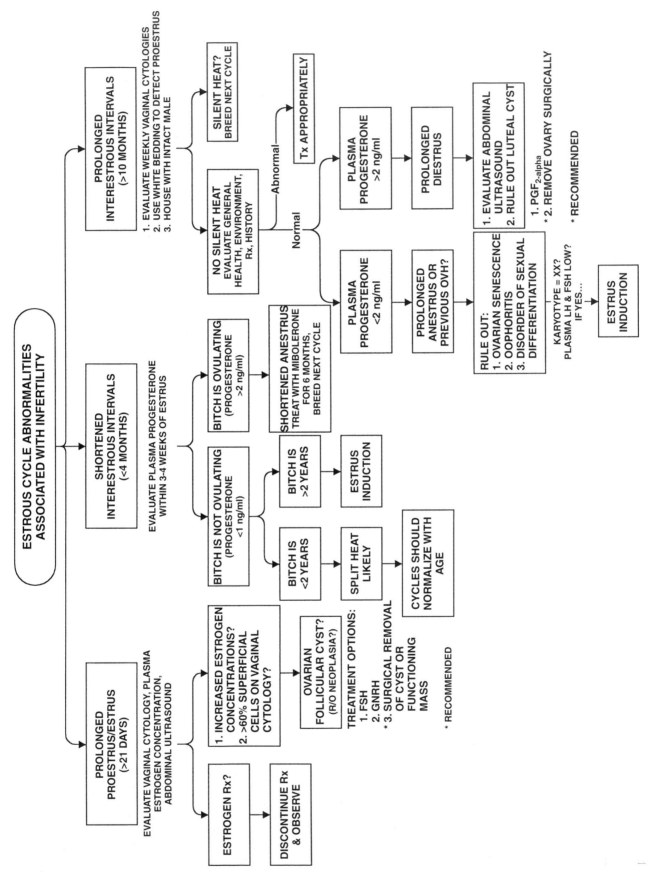

FIGURE 24-6. Algorithm for the evaluation of bitches with prolonged interestrous intervals, shortened interestrous intervals, or a prolonged proestrous or estrous phase of the estrous cycle.

a "pregnant" state, the uterus undergoes a period of breakdown and repair in preparation for the next cycle. This recovery period is thought to last 3 months (Al-Bassam et al, 1981; Shille et al, 1984b).

The 2 to 4 weeks needed for both proestrus and estrus, plus the 2 to 2.5 months of diestrus, and finally the 2 to 5 months of the uterine recovery phase (anestrus) account for the 4.5- to 8.5-month duration of a complete ovarian cycle. A bitch that enters proestrus prior to complete uterine repair may experience apparent infertility. Infertility could be the result of implantation failure caused by an abnormal endometrium that has not recovered from the previous effects of progesterone. Confirmation of these physiopathologic events is difficult. However, the presumptive diagnosis can be made from a careful review of the history.

OWNER MANAGEMENT PROBLEMS. Prior to making a diagnosis or instituting therapy, the clinician must obtain and study a complete history of the bitch. Ideally, specific dates for the onset of each proestrus are obtained. The goal here is to be certain that veterinarian and client are using the same terminology in describing a cycle and to rule out many of the more obvious causes of infertility. If any question arises regarding management practices or if the bitch has not been previously evaluated, it is prudent to study the bitch as she progresses through a cycle. In this manner, dates can be confirmed, vaginal cytology performed, progesterone data obtained, breedings confirmed, and postbreeding abdominal ultrasonography performed (3 to 5 weeks later), as suggested in the previous section on the infertile bitch with normal interestrous intervals. The bitch that cycles at less than 4-month intervals is typically normal in all respects and is infertile only as a result of incomplete uterine involution.

Changes in cycle length toward normal may be recognized as a bitch matures. Young bitches often have irregular, frequent, or silent ovarian cycles. These can be confusing to an owner attempting to predict when an upcoming cycle will begin. By the age of 2 to 3 years, a bitch's ovarian cycles should be consistent, and prediction of approximate dates for a future cycle is then possible. However, one must remain aware that some bitches mature more slowly than others. Normal ovarian cycle durations may not be appreciated until some bitches are older than 3 years of age.

It is recommended that no bitch be treated for shortened interestrous intervals until she is at least 2.5 to 3 years of age. In addition, a veterinarian should be allowed to observe and test the bitch through one cycle. By means of physical examination, vaginal cytology, and measurement of at least one diestrual plasma progesterone concentration (as described in the previous section), the nature of a cycle can be better understood. Most important, the presence of "split heats" must be ruled out.

TREATMENT. Treatment of the bitch older than 3 years that cycles too frequently involves medical induction of a normal anestrus period. This can usually be accomplished by treating the bitch with mibolerone drops (Cheque; Upjohn, Kalamazoo, MI) for 6 months. Medication is started 6 to 8 weeks after the end of the previous standing heat. The manufacturer provides the dosage with the medication; a separate schedule is used for German Shepherd dogs. The veterinarian must be certain that the bitch is not pregnant before beginning mibolerone therapy because this potent synthetic androgen causes urogenital defects in female fetuses (Johnston, 1980). The bitch also may undergo some virilization, but these signs are reversible and the drug is not thought to alter future reproductive performance. The bitch should be bred during the first estrus that follows therapy. This estrus can begin immediately after discontinuation of therapy or as long as 6 to 9 months later.

Follicular Cysts

Ovarian follicular cysts have been implicated as a cause of shortened interestrous intervals in the bitch (Freshman, 1991). This syndrome is not described here because it is not a problem that we have recognized. However, follicular cysts are well recognized in association with prolongation of proestrus or estrus or both. If this syndrome is among the differential diagnoses for shortened cycles, abdominal ultrasonography should be performed, because most cysts can be visualized. This is a simple, noninvasive, and reliable means of diagnosing an ovarian cyst (Fig. 24-7). Treatment involves surgical removal of the cyst or of the cyst and the ovary.

Uterine Disease

Uterine disease has been suggested as a cause of shortened interestrous intervals (Olson et al, 1988; Freshman, 1991). Like follicular cysts, this differential diagnosis has no physiologic basis and is not a syndrome we have recognized. It is presumed that a diagnosis would be based on histologic evaluation of submitted tissue, which requires uterine biopsy.

Split Heats

DEFINITION. Split heats occur most frequently in young pubertal bitches but can occur at any time in life. The initial phase of a split heat is associated with normal development of the ovarian follicles and their secretion of estrogen. Adequate estrogen is secreted to cause typical signs of proestrus; that is, vulvar swelling, vaginal bleeding, attraction of males, some behavior changes and, in rare cases, breeding. However, in the hypothalamic-pituitary-ovarian axis, the exquisitely timed coordination of endocrine events fails. The result is neither ovulation nor formation of corpora lutea. The owner observes vaginal bleeding

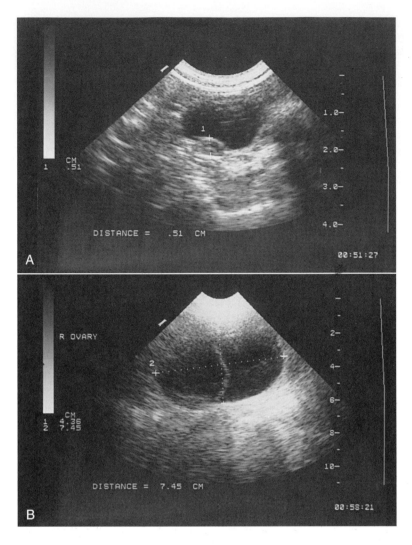

FIGURE 24-7. Abdominal ultrasonography of two bitches (*A* and *B*) with ovarian cysts that caused prolonged proestrus.

typical of a normal ovarian cycle, and the presumption is that all is well.

The follicles regress, and all signs of proestrus/estrus dissipate. Two to 10 weeks later, a new wave of follicles develops, secreting enough estrogen for signs of proestrus to reappear (Okkens et al, 1992). Now the owner sees vaginal bleeding once again, and the assumption is that a terrible problem exists. If the bitch proceeds through proestrus, ovulates, and continues through the cycle normally, she has undergone a typical split heat (i.e., follicular development is followed by signs of proestrus, which are followed by follicular regression; then several weeks pass, and a return of follicular development and a normal cycle occurs). The final or "true" heat is typically fertile. Breeding in the true cycle usually results in production of a normal litter.

OWNER OBSERVATIONS. This entire progression of events can be interpreted as two distinct cycles, and a bitch may be thought to have shortened interestrous

intervals. Also, she may simply be considered abnormal. Alternatively, the proestrual bleeding caused by the second follicular wave may be interpreted as the bleeding seen with abortion or resorption of fetuses. Split heats, therefore, can be confusing. Greater confusion can arise with split heats if several follicular waves occur prior to completion of a cycle (ovulation). In this situation, a bitch may be thought to be cycling every 2 or 3 months rather than having incomplete cycles. Two, three, or four independent follicular waves, with external signs of estrogen secretion, can take place before a complete cycle occurs.

DIAGNOSIS. Vaginal cytology can aid in confirmation of a diagnosis of split heat because each follicular wave is associated with estrogen secretion and typical estrogen-induced proestrual changes (see Figs. 19-2 and 19-3). The diagnosis may be further supported if serial serum progesterone values never exceed 2 ng/ml, which provides strong evidence that ovulation never took place. The progesterone concentration may rise during estrus (derived from follicles), but it then returns to basal levels. Such hormonal changes often result in estrous behavior, although the bitch has a split heat. Assessment of progesterone concentrations 1 to 3 weeks after breeding behavior dissipates or after diestrus is recognized (by means of vaginal cytology) demonstrates that ovulation never occurred.

CLINICAL INTERPRETATION. Split heats are not considered worrisome. They usually are seen in young bitches, not adults. No association exists between split heats and later infertility or between split heats and ovarian or uterine disorders. Recognition of split heats requires close supervision of the bitch and good communication between owner and veterinarian. The possibility of split heats is a reason for not treating any bitch for shortened interestrous intervals until she is at least 3 years of age. With maturity, split heats do not usually recur.

Ovulation Failure

Failure to ovulate may result in failure to form corpora lutea and failure to synthesize progesterone. The entire diestrus phase of the ovarian cycle is skipped, therefore the phase of uterine involution (anestrus) is also brief (Johnston, 1988). The diagnosis is based on serial serum progesterone determinations, as described in the previous section and in the section on hypoluteoidism. It is not known how this diagnosis differs from that of split heats. In the bitch less than 3 years of age, no treatment is recommended. In the bitch older than 3 years of age, an attempt to stimulate ovulation can be undertaken with LH or human chorionic gonadotropin (hCG; 500 IU/kg IM) administered the day before or the day after first breeding (Burke, 1986; Jones and Joshua, 1988).

Iatrogenic Causes of a Shortened Interestrous Interval

Administration of dopamine agonists, such as cabergoline or bromocriptine, have been associated with shortened interestrous intervals (Cinone et al, 2000). Similar effects are occasionally observed in bitches given prostaglandins. Use of progesterone receptor antagonists also may result in shortened interestrous intervals (Galac et al, 2000). From these early results, it would appear that subsequent cycles are normal and fertile.

THE BITCH WITH PROLONGED INTERESTROUS INTERVALS (GREATER THAN 10 MONTHS)

See Fig. 24-6.

Idiopathic Prolongation of the Interestrous Interval

OWNER MANAGEMENT PRACTICES AND HISTORY. As with other reproductive problems, a careful review of the history aids in avoiding unnecessary testing. Before asking any questions related directly to the reproductive past and present of the bitch, the veterinarian must first ask all questions necessary to be certain that the bitch is otherwise healthy. As a bitch becomes older, the interestrous interval increases (Olson et al, 1988). An interval of 10 to 12 months for a bitch older than 6 to 8 years of age is not worrisome. However, such prolonged intervals are not typical of the 2- to 6-year-old bitch.

It is important to know how the owner detects proestrus and estrus ("heat") and how closely the owner watches the dog. In some instances, a heat may simply be missed by the owner (called a *silent heat*). If no males are present and the owner does not specifically examine the vulva once or twice each week, heat cycles can be missed. If the veterinarian and owner are convinced that a bitch is cycling infrequently and that these are infertile cycles, further evaluation is warranted.

PHYSICAL EXAMINATION. Thorough and competent completion of a physical examination is outweighed in importance only by completion of a thorough history. The physical examination need not be time-consuming, but neither should it be omitted. The finding of a serious heart murmur, unsuspected organomegaly, a mass that was not expected, or a variety of other problems must be investigated to better treat the patient and to understand any potential cause for delay in an ovarian cycle.

BREED. Certain breeds experience ovarian cycles that normally have prolonged interestrous intervals. The classic examples are the Basenji and the wolf hybrid, both of which cycle once yearly (Barton, 1987). Individuals of any breed may have long interestrous intervals but remain fertile. The bitch that cycles less often than every 10 months and appears infertile is of greatest concern.

IN-HOSPITAL EVALUATION.

General Approach. Prolongation of the interval between ovarian cycles in the bitch can occur secondary to any underlying major medical disorder. This is an uncommon problem in the apparently healthy bitch, but a general screening panel to establish a database (i.e., CBC, serum chemistry profile, and urinalysis) is recommended. Any abnormality identified can then be pursued.

Hypothyroidism. The disorder most often associated with long interestrous periods is hypothyroidism. These dogs are usually slow, lethargic, inappetent, and dull and have poor hair coats or endocrine alopecia. Blood testing usually reveals a nonregenerative anemia and hypercholesterolemia. If the initial database is normal, thyroid testing can still be pursued. Test results are usually normal in apparently healthy bitches. However, it must be emphasized that no test of thyroid function is as reliable as the history and physical examination. It seems that occult hypothyroidism is not common and that the diagnosis of hypothyroidism is made far more frequently than the disorder is likely to occur.

A bitch diagnosed as having hypothyroidism can be appropriately treated with replacement hormones. These bitches usually cycle within 4 to 6 months of initiation of replacement thyroid hormone therapy. Initiation of normal cycles may follow successful management of any significant underlying disorder. If the bitch fails to cycle within 6 months of beginning thyroid treatment, the diagnosis may be incorrect, the treatment inadequate, or the diagnosis incomplete.

Silent Heat

See Failure to Cycle: Primary and Secondary Anestrus, next section.

Ovarian Cysts or Neoplasia

Ovarian cysts that secrete progesterone (luteal cysts) should cause prolonged interestrous intervals. Less commonly, neoplasia (e.g., granulosa-theca cell tumors) may secrete progesterone. Regardless of the source, progesterone causes strong negative feedback to the pituitary and hypothalamus, suppressing LH and follicle-stimulating hormone (FSH) secretion and thereby suppressing ovarian activity. In this physiologic environment, the bitch remains in prolonged "diestrus," which may not be associated with any clinical signs.

The diagnosis is based on demonstration of prolonged increases in the serum progesterone concentration (>9 to 10 weeks; >2 to 5 ng/ml) and the presence of a solitary cystic structure in one ovary on abdominal ultrasonography (see Fig. 24-7). More than one cyst in one ovary and one or more cysts in both ovaries are possible. Neoplasia may be palpable or may be seen on abdominal radiographs, but abdominal ultrasound is the most reliable tool for supporting this diagnosis. Ovarian cysts that do not appear to be functional (i.e., no increase in the serum estrogen or progesterone concentrations can be demonstrated, such as may occur with rete ovarii) may also result in a failure to cycle. In these cases also, abdominal ultrasound is a valuable diagnostic aid.

Treatment

If all test results are normal, a suspicion that silent heats are occurring is justified. In this situation, the owner can house the bitch with a normally cycling bitch, because this exposure may induce an earlier cycle. Alternatively, the bitch may be housed with a male. The owner may wish to obtain weekly vaginal smears, which can be evaluated for evidence of follicular function. The infrequent cycle can be closely monitored to verify that proper breeding dates are being chosen. Last, an ovarian cycle can be medically induced. Treatment of progesterone-secreting cysts may include administration of prostaglandins to induce regression of luteal tissue, but this mode of therapy has not been effective in our experience. Therefore the treatment for progesterone-secreting ovarian cysts, nonfunctional ovarian cysts, and possible ovarian tumors is surgical removal.

FAILURE TO CYCLE: PRIMARY AND SECONDARY ANESTRUS (FIG. 24-8)

Definition of the Problem

Rarely, veterinary advice is sought regarding a bitch that fails to cycle. *Primary anestrus* designates the condition of a bitch that has never had an ovarian cycle, and *secondary anestrus* describes the condition of a bitch that has had one or more ovarian cycles but subsequently fails to cycle. As with all reproductive disorders, the dog's age, breed, past history, current history, medications, and physical examination should be assessed before any major tests are undertaken. Some large-breed dogs experience the pubertal (first) estrus after 2 years of age, whereas small-breed dogs may have several silent heat cycles before exhibiting an obvious cycle. Failure to cycle, therefore, is a problem that we do not recommend pursuing until a bitch is older than 2 years of age. Evaluation of dogs with secondary anestrus should include all suggested approaches in the previous section on prolonged interestrous intervals.

Secondary anestrus can occur after the onset of thyroid, other endocrine, or nonendocrine disease. These bitches should be thoroughly evaluated with a history, physical examination, and laboratory testing (see Underlying Disease, page 887). If all tests results are normal, it is wise to wait at least 12 to 18 months from the previous cycle, in case one or two heat cycles were silent and therefore missed. The dog should be closely monitored during this time by the owner, and the veterinarian can recommend serial testing as outlined in the section on silent heat, below. As an alternative, an attempt at inducing estrus can be considered.

Previous Ovariohysterectomy

FOLLICLE-STIMULATING HORMONE AND LUTEINIZING HORMONE.   If the past history of a bitch is not known, a possible cause of failure to cycle that should be investigated is previous ovariohysterectomy. Examination of the ventral midline for an incision scar provides initial evidence of an earlier spay. Hair may need to be clipped from this area for a careful inspection. To confirm this finding, plasma can be submitted for LH and FSH determinations. An ovariohysterectomized female has a persistent elevation in LH and FSH concentrations. In one report, the

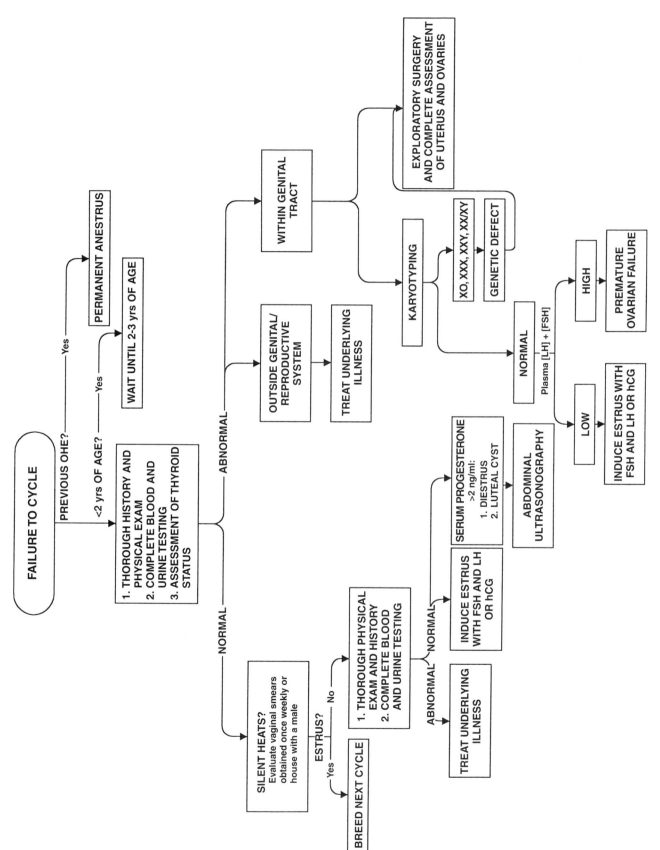

FIGURE 24-8. Algorithm for the evaluation of a bitch that apparently has no estrous cycle activity.

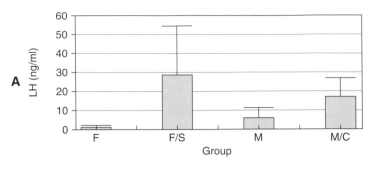

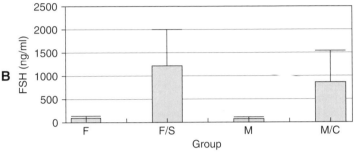

FIGURE 24-9. Plasma LH concentrations *(A)* and FSH concentrations *(B)* from intact and neutered dogs. The graphs demonstrate the potential value of these assays in distinguishing neutered from intact dogs. (Olson PN, et al: Am J Vet Res 53:762, 1992; used with permission.)

mean (± SD) serum LH concentration in intact bitches was 1.2 ± 0.9 ng/ml versus 28.7 ± 25.8 ng/ml in ovariohysterectomized dogs. The serum FSH concentration was 98 ± 49 ng/ml in intact bitches versus 1219 ± 763 ng/ml in spayed dogs (Fig. 24-9) (Olson et al, 1992). Assays for LH and FSH are not yet widely available but are likely to become so in the near future. A commercial test kit (ICG Status-LH canine ovulation timing test, Synbiotics Corp., San Diego, CA) has 98% sensitivity and 78% specificity in separating intact from ovariectomized bitches. A single low LH value indicated that a bitch was intact (Lofstedt and Van Leeuwen, 2002).

USE OF GONADOTROPIN-RELEASING HORMONE (GNRH) AGONISTS. Gonadotropin-releasing hormone controls FSH and LH synthesis. Intravenous administration of GnRH (0.01 µg/kg) in intact bitches produces a rise in LH with subsequent increases in the serum estrogen concentration. An increase in circulating estrogen would occur only in dogs with ovarian tissue (England, 1998). An alternative to administration of GnRH would be use of hCG or eCG (equine chorionic gonadotropin). One set of protocols (Jeffcoate et al, 2000) used hCG given intravenously at a dosage of 200 IU (for dogs that weigh 9 to 15 kg) or 300 IU (for dogs that weigh 15 to 20 kg). eCG was given intravenously at a dosage of 100 IU (for dogs weighing 9 to 15 kg) or 150 IU (for dogs weighing 15 to 20 kg). Plasma estradiol concentrations were measured before and 90 minutes after injection of either drug. Intact bitches either had basal estradiol concentrations that were increased and remained increased after

gonadotropin injection, or they had low basal values that increased significantly after injection. Spayed bitches had undetectable plasma estradiol concentrations before and after gonadotropin injection. Gonadotropin-induced stimulation of estrogen production, therefore, can be a useful method of determining whether a bitch is sexually intact or has been spayed.

Silent Heat

DEFINITION. Silent heat (defined as an ovarian cycle that was not detected by the owner) can be difficult to identify. Bitches in this condition may not have vulvar enlargement or a sanguineous vaginal discharge, or they may not attract males or allow breeding by males. Silent heats should be considered a possible cause of primary anestrus, especially if the owners of a bitch have little or no experience with an intact female, if the bitch is housed separately from any contact with a male dog, or if the bitch is not closely observed.

DIAGNOSIS AND MANAGEMENT. The plasma progesterone concentration can be assayed in any dog suspected of having a silent heat. A value greater than 2 ng/ml suggests that a previous heat has not taken place within the past 60 to 70 days. If the progesterone concentration is greater than 2 ng/ml, abdominal ultrasonography may reveal corpora lutea in the ovaries. If the progesterone level is less than 1 ng/ml, an owner may try bringing the bitch in question into contact with a male once weekly as an aid to recognizing estrus.

Close visual examination of the vulva once or twice weekly is an excellent method of detecting silent heat. Close observation allows the owner to develop some experience with the anestrus appearance of the vulva. Mild enlargement of the vulva or a slight bloody discharge is easier to see, and the owner is more comfortable identifying signs of early proestrus. More aggressive methods of evaluating bitches suspected of having silent heats include weekly reading of vaginal cytologic smears (looking for evidence of proestrus or estrus) or monthly serum progesterone assessments (looking for concentrations >2 to 5 ng/ml, which are consistent with ovulation).

Drug-Induced Anestrus

Anestrus may be induced by drugs specifically marketed for that purpose (see Chapter 22) and by drugs that result in anestrus as a side effect. Marketed drugs include androgens, which an owner interested in increasing the strength and/or endurance of a pet might use without realizing the effects on the hypothalamic-pituitary-ovarian axis. Progestogens are used in the treatment of a variety of maladies, with prolongation of anestrus (diestrus) as a side effect. Glucocorticoids can have negative feedback effects on the pituitary, suppressing gonadotropin activity and preventing ovarian cycles.

Underlying Disease

IMPORTANCE OF THE HISTORY AND PHYSICAL EXAMINATION. Any illness, mild or severe, has the potential to interfere with ovarian cycle activity in the bitch. For this reason, the importance of obtaining a thorough history and of performing a complete and competent physical examination cannot be overemphasized. Abnormalities identified through these evaluations must be pursued as possible explanations for infertility and to avoid the mistake of separating the reproductive tract from the rest of the animal.

IN-HOSPITAL EVALUATION. When silent heats, previous ovariohysterectomy, and owner error are considered unlikely explanations for apparent failure to cycle, blood and urine testing is advisable. It is recommended that a CBC, serum chemistry profile, and urinalysis be obtained. Another integral component of the screening of a bitch for unsuspected problems is abdominal ultrasonography. This is a noninvasive means of evaluating abdominal structures, especially the ovaries for a luteal (progesterone-secreting) cyst and the uterus for thickening and/or fluid (endometritis).

Hypothyroidism

Hypothyroidism has become a "popular" diagnosis for explaining why a bitch fails to cycle. Although the potential exists for a hypothyroid bitch to exhibit primary or secondary anestrus, such dogs should have signs of hypothyroidism (e.g., obesity, lethargy, poor appetite, poor hair coat, and bilaterally symmetric alopecia). An alert, active, vibrant bitch is not likely to be hypothyroid. As previously stated, we believe hypothyroidism is overdiagnosed by the profession and by breeders and trainers. However, subclinical hypothyroidism in women was associated with ovulatory dysfunction and infertility (Lincoln et al, 1999).

Hypothyroid dogs rapidly respond to thyroid replacement, becoming more alert, active, and responsive within days of initiation of therapy. The appetite quickly improves, and weight loss follows. Improvement in hair coat may take weeks. These dogs typically begin ovarian cycles within 3 to 6 months of initiation of therapy. If these responses are not observed, the thyroid hormone replacement dose is inadequate, a second medical problem exists, or the diagnosis is not correct.

Glucocorticoid Excess

Glucocorticoids are used in the treatment of numerous small animal conditions. However, they have negative feedback effects on pituitary adrenocorticotropin (ACTH), FSH, and LH secretion. A bitch receiving glucocorticoid therapy may not exhibit ovarian cycles unless the steroid dosages are kept to a minimum or administration is discontinued. Specific glucocorticoid doses capable of inhibiting ovarian cycles are variable. However, any bitch that has a blunted cortisol response to exogenous ACTH is likely to have sufficient negative feedback from the therapy to interfere with ovarian cycles (see Chapters 6 and 10).

Naturally occurring hyperadrenocorticism (Cushing's syndrome) is not usually a major consideration in the noncycling female because most bitches with Cushing's syndrome are older than 8 years of age. Therefore their failure to cycle is not recognized as a problem by the owners, whereas the other major signs of Cushing's syndrome are more obvious, dramatic, and worrisome.

Stress

Stress, heavy physical training, and poor nutrition are all potential causes of failing to cycle. Overcrowding, extreme temperatures, frequent exhibition at shows, and excess travel also could have negative effects on some bitches. These problems most likely would be revealed in a thorough history, and their correction would improve the likelihood of return of ovarian function.

Premature Ovarian Failure/Ovarian Aplasia

DEFINITION. A bitch that has never exhibited ovarian cycles (primary anestrus) may not have ovaries. Congenital absence or lack of development of one or both ovaries is extremely rare (Wright and Watts, 1998). Other causes of the aplasia may exist. Secondary hypoplasia simply suggests that one or more ovarian cycles preceded premature ovarian failure. The functional longevity of the ovaries of bitches is not known. On average, the ovaries are believed to decline in function gradually after the bitch has reached 7 to 10 years of age. However, the ovaries may cease functioning earlier (i.e., fail because of aplasia or hypoplasia). The result is a permanent anestrous state.

DIAGNOSIS. The diagnosis of ovarian failure may be suspected when all other differential diagnoses have been excluded and attempts to induce estrus fail. It is difficult to confirm this diagnosis, however. One method of confirmation is random evaluation of plasma FSH and LH concentrations. Premature ovarian failure is associated with extremely increased plasma FSH and LH concentrations, which develop in the absence of negative feedback to the pituitary and hypothalamus (see Fig. 24-9) (Olson et al, 1992). Alternatively, laparoscopy or exploratory surgery can be undertaken in order to inspect the reproductive tract and to biopsy the uterus and ovaries for confirmation of abnormalities. Finally, administration of hCG or GnRH would cause increases in the serum estrogen concentration if viable ovarian tissue is present. Protocols are discussed in this chapter under Previous Ovariohysterectomy (page 884) and Induction of Estrus (this page).

Progesterone-Secreting Ovarian Cyst

Progesterone-secreting ovarian cyst is a well-recognized but uncommon syndrome that results in persistent diestrus, although to the owner the dog usually appears to be persistently in anestrus. By definition, such a bitch must have had an ovarian cycle and would be classified as having *secondary* anestrus. However, if this follows a silent heat, the prolonged anestrus may appear to be *primary*. In either situation, abdominal ultrasonography and a plasma progesterone concentration greater than 2 ng/ml are diagnostic in most bitches (see Fig. 24-7). Treatment with prostaglandins to lyse these cysts is not usually successful, and surgical removal is recommended.

Immune-Mediated Oophoritis

Immune-mediated destruction of the ovaries has been described in one dog in the last 20 years (Johnston, 1989; 1991), a 5-year-old bitch with diffuse lymphocytic ovarian inflammation. Histology also revealed degenerating follicles, oocyte degeneration and necrosis, thickened zonae pellucidae, and absence of corpora lutea. The incidence of this syndrome is rare.

Surgical Diagnosis

Diagnostic evaluation of an adult bitch that has never exhibited ovarian cycle activity can be frustrating, because it involves the use of tests not commonly performed by veterinary practitioners. Many veterinarians view exploratory laparotomy as an expedient means of obtaining an answer, bypassing presurgical medical testing. During surgery the abdominal organs should be evaluated for normal versus abnormal appearance, and the veterinarian should be prepared to obtain biopsies of ovarian and uterine tissue, as well as cultures of the uterine lumen.

Although this method is expedient, it may not always be possible to distinguish normal from abnormal tissues externally. Furthermore, the veterinarian may not be able to answer the questions subsequently raised by an owner or breeder. The direct surgical approach, therefore, is tempered by the knowledge that a definitive diagnosis cannot always be made, even after visual inspection of the organs in question. We strongly recommend a thorough medical evaluation of the bitch, as previously discussed, before surgical exploration. If necessary, the bitch can be referred to an internist with the background and training necessary to provide definitive information about the individual and perhaps that entire line of dogs.

INDUCTION OF ESTRUS

Variable Rate of Success

Another approach to the problem of a bitch with prolonged interestrous intervals, primary anestrus, or secondary anestrus, besides exploring the use of diagnostic testing, is medical induction of estrus. This appears to be a potentially expedient diagnostic and therapeutic approach. However, most studies on induction of estrus in the bitch have been performed on healthy females, and success has been variable. When similar protocols are used on a bitch with a defect in the hypothalamic-pituitary-ovarian axis, great results should not be expected. Failure to induce ovarian cycle activity can be frustrating, because the lack of results may be a consequence either of an unsuccessful protocol or due to anatomic or physiologica defects that render the bitch incapable of responding.

Monitoring of the Treated Bitch

Regardless of the method chosen for estrus induction, vaginal cytology should be obtained on an alternate-day basis. It is recommended that natural breeding or artificial insemination begin when superficial cells compose 60% or more of the exfoliated vaginal epithelial cells and/or when plasma progesterone concentrations exceed 1 ng/ml. Insemination should continue on an alternate-day basis until diestrus is confirmed.

Drug Availability and Reliability

The gonadotropins FSH and LH are secreted by the anterior pituitary gland. FSH stimulates initial follicular development, and a surge in FSH contributes to ovulation. LH also contributes to follicular growth and is the trigger for ovulation. Neither FSH nor LH is commercially available for dogs. However, eCG (i.e., pregnant mare serum gonadotropin) and hCG are commercially available. eCG is produced in the mare during pregnancy and is mainly FSH-like in action, but it does have some LH effect. hCG is extracted from the urine of pregnant women and is primarily LH in effect (England, 1998).

Problems arise regarding the availability, quality, consistency, and dependability of the various hormone preparations used in the studies completed. This accounts to some degree for the different results seen with similar protocols used by separate research groups. Many of the agents used are not commercially available, and others vary significantly in potency, depending on where they are purchased and how they are prepared. The clinician is encouraged to maintain a wary attitude about these materials until assurances are made that the obvious problems recognized to date have been resolved.

Use of Pregnant Mare Serum Gonadotropin (PMSG) or Follicle-Stimulating Hormone

PREGNANT MARE SERUM GONADOTROPIN. A variety of protocols using PMSG (Gestyl, from Diosynth, Chicago, IL; Equinex, from Ayerst Laboratories, Montreal, Canada; and Folligon, from Intervet, Cambridge, UK) have been evaluated (Table 24-3). In one study, approximately 50% of bitches ovulated after 9 consecutive days of intramuscular or subcutaneous administration of PMSG, injected at a dosage of 44 IU/kg/day, followed by 500 IU of hCG given intramuscularly on day 10 (Archbald et al, 1980). The responding animals exhibited behavioral estrus 10 to 15 days after initiation of treatment, but this included only half of the dogs that ovulated.

In another study, pregnant mare serum (PMS) was administered subcutaneously to mature anestrus bitches for 10 consecutive days at dosages of 500 IU/day, 250 IU/day, or 20 IU/kg/day. This regimen was followed by a subcutaneous injection of 500 IU of hCG (Chorionic Gonadotropin for Injection, from Burns Biotech, Omaha, NE; Chorulon, from Intervet, Cambridge, UK) on day 10. These protocols resulted in abnormally high serum concentrations of estrogen, abnormal ovulations with shortened luteal phases, and toxic side effects attributed to the excess estrogen. Side effects included thrombocytopenia, uterine disease, and termination of pregnancy (Arnold et al, 1989).

If the PMSG (20 IU/kg) was administered subcutaneously for only 5 days before hCG adminis-

tration (25 IU/kg SQ once on day 5), the serum estrogen concentrations were more physiologic and the protocol resulted in a 50% conception rate (Arnold et al, 1989: England, 1998). This same protocol was evaluated in another study, in which excess concentrations of serum estrogen caused inhibition of implantation, bone marrow suppression, and death in some dogs (England and Allen, 1991). Differences in results may be partly due to differences in the potency of PMSG preparations used.

FSH WITH OR WITHOUT ESTROGEN PRIMING. Protocols using FSH (FSH-P; Schering, Kenilworth, NJ) as the sole stimulus of induction of estrus have not been as successful as those using PMSG (Olson et al, 1981; Shille et al, 1984a). Pretreatment of bitches with an "estrogen-priming" regimen of diethylstilbestrol (DES; Eli Lilly, Indianapolis, IN), at a dosage of 5 mg daily for 7 or more days, to produce signs of proestrus holds promise. Five days after induction of proestrus (vulvar enlargement/vaginal bleeding), 5 mg of LH was administered intramuscularly; 10 mg of FSH was administered intramuscularly 9 and 11 days after vaginal bleeding was observed. Each bitch so treated became pregnant (Moses and Shille, 1988). When hCG was substituted for the LH in a similar study performed by the same group, the data on onset of behavioral estrus and subsequent fertility were not nearly as promising as in the initial study (Shille et al, 1989).

A successful modification of the estrogen-FSH protocol included administration of DES (5 mg) daily for 4 to 10 days. DES administration was continued 3 days beyond the first day of induced proestrus (marked by bloody vaginal discharge and attraction of males). Counting from the first day that signs of induced proestrus were observed, 10 mg of FSH-P was given intramuscularly on days 5, 9, and 11. Estrus behavior was observed in 70%

TABLE 24–3 METHODS REPORTED FOR THE HORMONAL INDUCTION OF ESTRUS IN ANESTRUS BITCHES*

METHODS	ESTRUS (%)	OVULATION (%)	LITTER (%)	REFERENCES
Daily PMSG (2–50 IU/kg) for 9–14 days	50–100	50–100	0–20	Arnold et al, 1989 Archbald et al, 1980
Daily PMSG (20 IU/kg) for 5 days, then hCG	80–90	80–100	50	Arnold et al, 1989 England and Allen, 1991
Daily FSH (1–10 mg/day)	0–50	0–50	0	Olson et al, 1981 Shille et al, 1984a
Oral DES, then FSH, then hCG	90	30	—	Olson et al, 1984
Oral DES (5 mg/day) until proestrus induced, then				
a. LH, then FSH	100	100	100	Moses and Shille, 1988
b. hCG, then FSH	40	20	0	Shille et al, 1989
c. FSH (10 mg) q2–4d	70	50	30	Bouchard et al, 1991
GnRH, IV pulses q90 min	60–100	50–80	40–80	Cain et al, 1988 Vanderlip et al, 1987
GnRH agonist SC × 14 days	90	75	25–50	Concannon, 1989
GnRH agonist TID SC	80	80	80	Cain et al, 1990

*Adapted from Concannon PW: Methods for rapid induction of fertile estrus in dogs. *In* Kirk RW, Bonagura JD (eds): Current Veterinary Therapy XI. Philadelphia, WB Saunders Co, 1992, p 960.

DES, Diethylstilbestrol; *FSH,* follicle-stimulating hormone; *GnRH,* gonadotropin-releasing hormone; *hCG,* human chorionic gonadotropin; *IV,* intravenous; *LH,* luteinizing hormone; *PMSG,* pregnant mare serum gonadotropin; *SC,* subcutaneous; *TID,* three times a day.

of the bitches 5 to 10 days after the initial dose of DES. Subsequently, 46% ovulated, and 30% became pregnant, carrying litters to term (Bouchard et al, 1991).

Use of Gonadotropin-Releasing Hormone (GnRH) or a GnRH Agonist

REQUIREMENTS FOR SUCCESS. Use of GnRH or an agonist of that hormone induces a fertile ovarian cycle only if the pituitary-ovarian axis is normal. These drugs stimulate the secretion of pituitary gonadotropins, which should in turn stimulate the ovaries. Follicle development, estrogen secretion, behavioral estrus, and pituitary-stimulated ovulation depend on a normal physiologic response following "activation" of the system.

PROTOCOLS. One protocol used a surgically implanted infusion pump that administered a small dose of GnRH (40 to 400 ng/kg) every 90 minutes for 6 to 12 days. In the bitches treated, proestrus began in 3 to 6 days and fertile estrus in 7 to 14 days. The protocols were successful at inducing fertile cycles in 37% to 85% of bitches treated (Vanderlip et al, 1987; Cain et al, 1988). The cumbersome and impractical nature of expensive implanted infusion pumps that need to be removed makes this protocol interesting but unavailable to most practitioners.

Another protocol used a constant infusion of a GnRH agonist for 14 days. This approach resulted in rapid induction of proestrus and estrus, with fertility rates of 25% when the drug was administered immediately after lactation and 50% when it was given to anestrus bitches after a nonpregnant cycle (Concannon, 1989 and 1992). Although the results were promising, the agonist used is not commercially available. Also, the small, inexpensive osmotic pumps require minor surgery for subcutaneous placement and removal (Concannon, 1992).

A less stringent protocol used subcutaneous injections of a GnRH agonist (D-Trp-6 GnRH) at a dosage of 1 µg/kg three times daily for 11 days and then 0.5 µg/mg three times daily for 3 days. Estrus was observed within 9 to 11 days of initiation of treatment in 80% of the dogs, each of which became pregnant (Cain et al, 1990). Despite the inconvenience of a three times daily injection protocol, this method may present the best combination of efficacy and clinical utility among the various approaches involving GnRH (Concannon, 1992).

Use of Cabergoline

Six bitches with primary or secondary anestrus were treated with cabergoline (5 µg/kg, PO, daily) until 2 days after onset of proestrus. Five of the dogs had a normal proestrus and estrus. All 5 were bred naturally and whelped normal litters. No adverse effects were seen (Gobello et al, 2002).

PERSISTENT PROESTRUS AND/OR ESTRUS

See Fig. 24-6.

Definition

Persistent estrus is defined as a bitch willing to breed for longer than 21 to 28 consecutive days in any one ovarian cycle. Alternatively, and less directly, persistent estrus is defined as more than 21 to 28 consecutive days of greater than 80% to 90% superficial cells observed on vaginal cytology. Persistent presence of a large percentage of superficial cells on vaginal cytology is strong evidence of continued increases in the serum estrogen concentration.

Clinical Observations

Bitches with persistent proestrus have an enlarged vulva and persistent vaginal bleeding, attract males, and demonstrate estrogen effects on the reproductive tract. Although the causes for persistent proestrus/estrus may vary among bitches, the final common denominator is continued exposure to increases in the serum estrogen concentration.

Exogenous Estrogen Excess

Parenteral estrogen can be used in the bitch to prevent pregnancy (by preventing migration of embryos from the oviducts into the uterus) and in some bitches to prevent urinary incontinence. Estrogen administered during estrus to prevent pregnancy can prolong signs of estrus. In any bitch with prolonged proestrus/estrus, an investigation into the possible administration of estrogens for mismating should be considered. If estrogens were administered, the type and dosage should be ascertained. In addition to associations between exogenous estrogen and the development of pyometra or bone marrow aplasia, ovarian cysts are recognized sequelae to such medication (Olson et al, 1989b; Meyers-Wallen, 1992).

Endogenous Estrogen Excess

YOUNG BITCHES AND GONADOTROPIN-TREATED BITCHES. Rarely, the young bitch in her first or second ovarian cycle fails to ovulate and may exhibit prolonged proestrous or estrous activity as a result of continued follicular estrogen secretion. This appears to be a self-limiting problem that arises when the amounts of estrogen are inadequate to induce the LH surge or when LH fails to induce ovulation. One bitch began to demonstrate signs of proestrus at 7.5 months of age that persisted for more than 7 months. She was diagnosed as having X chromosomal monosomy (77,XO) (Lofstedt et al, 1992). Exogenous gonadotropins could have a similar physiologic and clinical effect (Meyers-Wallen, 1992).

FOLLICULAR CYSTS

Incidence. Little information is available in the veterinary literature on this disorder. Most follicular cysts have a granulosa cell lining, are anovulatory, and secrete significant amounts of estrogen. The cysts are usually solitary, occur in bitches less than 3 years of age, and measure 1 to 1.5 cm in diameter. A few are as large as 5 cm in diameter, and they typically contain a clear, watery fluid.

Clinical Signs and Diagnosis. The clinical signs in bitches with follicular cysts are those typical of estrogen dominance; that is, the bitch exhibits signs of proestrus and/or estrus. The most common reason owners seek veterinary care is vaginal bleeding that persists for weeks rather than the expected 7 to 10 days. Less commonly, owners may be concerned that the bitch appears to be in behavioral estrus (willing to breed) for weeks rather than the expected 6 to 10 days.

Cysts that secrete only progesterone are referred to as "luteinized cysts." They do not cause increases in the serum estrogen concentration, nor do they result in the clinical signs of proestrus and/or estrus. However, several of the bitches with follicular cysts that we have treated also have had mild increases in the serum progesterone concentration. Not surprisingly, bitches with cysts that produce only estrogen appear to exhibit prolonged *proestrus*. Those with cysts that produce both estrogen and small amounts of progesterone are most likely to exhibit persistent *estrus*.

The diagnosis of follicular cyst is based on observation of prolonged vaginal bleeding, persistent estrus behavior, continuous vaginal cytologic changes suggestive of late proestrus or estrus, and chronically increased plasma estrogen concentrations (>20 pg/ml). Vaginal cytology demonstrating greater than 80% to 90% superficial cells provides strong evidence of increased serum estrogen concentrations. Abdominal ultrasonography is one of the most important diagnostic aids. The finding of one or more anechoic cystic structures in the area of one or both ovaries in a bitch suspected of having a follicular cyst virtually confirms the diagnosis. Normal preovulatory follicles measure 4 to 9 mm in diameter (Meyers-Wallen, 1992), and functional cysts are usually larger and therefore easier to visualize (see Fig. 24-7).

Differential Diagnosis. There are few differential diagnoses for the bitch in persistent proestrus or estrus. The most common diagnosis is a *normal* bitch with longer than average proestrus or estrus. Proestrus may last as long as 3 to 4 weeks, although the duration is not usually longer than 14 days. Estrus, too, may persist for as long as 3 weeks, although durations of less than 2 weeks are most common. No treatment should be undertaken until it has been determined that the clinical signs are not those of a normal bitch. The signs, therefore, would have to persist well beyond 1 month before any treatment is recommended, especially in a pubertal bitch.

A split heat may be interpreted as or mistakenly thought by an owner to be a persistent proestrus or estrus. Similarly, the bitch with shortened interestrous intervals may be mistakenly thought to be persistently in proestrus or estrus. Any cause of persistent vaginal bleeding (e.g., foreign body, vaginal or urethral tumor) or of attraction of males (e.g., vaginitis, perivulvar dermatitis) could be interpreted as persistence in proestrus or estrus.

Bitches with ovarian tumors may have hormonal excesses. The evaluation of these bitches does not differ from that of bitches with ovarian cysts except that surgery is likely to be the only means of resolving the clinical signs. The diagnosis is first suspected with abdominal ultrasonography and then based on the histologic evaluation of removed tissue.

Treatment. In some bitches, treatment is not required because the follicular cyst or cysts may spontaneously undergo atresia or may completely luteinize. This can be monitored with abdominal ultrasonography, vaginal cytology, and measurement of serum progesterone concentrations. In either situation, the clinical signs rapidly dissipate.

PROGESTERONE. In bitches not intended for breeding, megestrol acetate (Ovaban; Schering, Kenilworth, NJ), at a dosage of 2 mg/kg given orally for 8 days, has been recommended to reduce clinical signs of estrus (Shille, 1986). Ovariohysterectomy is then considered mandatory because of the association between such therapy and the cystic endometrial hyperplasia/pyometra complex (Fayer-Hosken et al, 1992). This is not a treatment we have used, nor is it recommended.

GONADOTROPINS. In bitches whose offspring have potential value, several treatment protocols have been recommended to induce ovulation or to luteinize follicular cysts and thereby eliminate the clinical signs. A dosage of one to three injections of GnRH (Cystorelin; Sanofi, Overland Park, KS [50 to 100 µg IM q24-48h]) or a similar protocol using hCG (Follutein; Solvay Veterinary, Marietta, GA [22 U/kg IM q 24-48h]) has been suggested (Olson et al, 1989b). If serum estrogen concentrations decline and progesterone concentrations remain below 2 ng/ml, it is likely that the cyst has regressed and the bitch has progressed into anestrus. If the serum estrogen concentration decreases and the progesterone concentration increases, it is likely that the bitch has progressed into diestrus and will need to be monitored for pyometra.

It has been suggested that if either of these protocols fails to induce anestrus or diestrus (i.e., estrus persists), an ovarian tumor is likely (Olson et al, 1989b; Meyers-Wallen, 1992). Our experience has been different. Medical treatment has failed in most bitches with follicular cysts, and surgery has been curative and has maintained fertility because only one ovary has been removed; tumors have yet to be diagnosed.

SURGERY. As stated in the previous section, most of our bitches with follicular cysts that have not spontaneously regressed have been managed surgically. The plan has consistently been to attempt resection of the cyst without removing the ovary. Most often, however, the associated ovary could not be separated from the

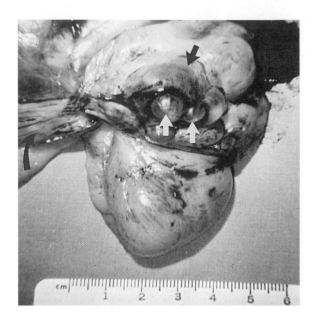

FIGURE 24-10. Ovary *(straight black arrow)* with two follicular cysts *(straight white arrows)* and uterus *(curved black arrow)* from a bitch with persistent proestrus.

cyst, and resection of both structures has been necessary (Fig. 24-10). These bitches have quickly responded to the surgery. The signs of proestrus and/or estrus dissipate within 1 to 4 days, and no long-term problems have developed. A large majority of these bitches have remained fertile and have whelped healthy litters after subsequent estrus cycles.

An alternative to surgical removal of ovarian cysts is surgical drainage of cysts. After drainage, one dog was treated with 22 IU/kg of hCG injected directly into the cyst (Brockus, 1998). Although successful in one case, this is a risky approach to management because treatment failure would dictate the need for a second major surgery, and the interval between the first and second surgery may allow the development of bone marrow suppression. For this reason, thorough owner education is imperative.

Histology. Histologic examination of removed tissue is mandatory. This examination should confirm the diagnosis and assure both veterinarian and owner that the syndrome was diagnosed correctly and should resolve. Most important, if the bitch had an ovarian tumor rather than a benign cyst, the tumor's malignant potential can be assessed. This information is of prime importance and must be made available to the owner.

OVARIAN TUMORS

Incidence

Ovarian tumors are quite uncommon. Such tumors may occur in bitches of any age, but the mean age is 8 to 10 years except for dogs with ovarian teratomas, for which the mean age was reported in one study to

be 4 years (Patnaik and Greenlee, 1987). Certainly the incidence is underestimated, owing to the fact that most female pet dogs are ovariohysterectomized by middle age.

Histology

Ovarian cystadenomas (serous or pseudomucinous) have been recognized more frequently than ovarian fibromas or adenocarcinomas. The most common primary ovarian tumors were, in order, epithelial, sex cord, and germ cell tumors. Granulosa cell and Sertoli-Leydig cell tumors are perhaps the most common sex cord ovarian neoplasms, whereas dysgerminomas and teratomas were the most common germ cell types (Patnaik and Greenlee, 1987). These tumors can be unilateral or bilateral and can range from small to large (Withrow and Susaneck, 1986).

Clinical Signs

Ovarian tumors have the potential to be functional and to cause syndromes of estrogen dominance, although this diagnosis has been extremely rare in our experience. Bitches with granulosa cell tumors may be brought to a veterinarian because of persistent proestrus/estrus or for cystic endometrial hyperplasia/pyometra. The ovarian tumor may mistakenly be believed to be an incidental finding in a bitch ovariohysterectomized for pyometra. Hematopoietic disorders may also result from the persistent estrogen secreted by functional tumors (Olson et al, 1989b).

OVARIAN REMNANT SYNDROME

Definition

Ovarian remnant syndrome is one of proestrus and/or estrus activity in a bitch or queen despite previous ovariohysterectomy. These animals not only exhibit the typical behavioral patterns consistent with either or both of these phases, they also have hormonal evidence of ovarian tissue.

Etiology

Three likely causes of ovarian remnant syndrome seem plausible. The most common explanation is improper surgical technique, resulting in incomplete resection of one or both ovaries. A second cause is dropping of some ovarian tissue into the peritoneal cavity after proper excision of all ovarian tissue. This tissue could revascularize and exhibit function at some later date; this has been demonstrated in cats, for which a prospective study was completed purposely creating this condition (DeNardo et al, 2001). The third possibility is ovarian "rest" tissue in a location other than the immediate ovarian area. This tissue can become functional at almost any time. We have identified such tissue in several bitches within the ovarian ligament at its junction with the abdominal wall.

Clinical Signs

The bitch with an ovarian remnant exhibits typical clinical signs of proestrus or estrus. The bitches with this syndrome seen in our hospital are usually brought to veterinarians because they are attracting males (some owners have described their homes as being surrounded by male dogs). Some of these people have had difficulty leaving home with their bitch because of the aggressive nature of the males and a similar interest in breeding by the female (flagging and standing). It should be understood that some remnant tissues function in cycles similar to normal cycles. Some of these bitches have had persistent estrus, but normal durations of proestrus and estrus are more typical.

These bitches also have vulvar enlargement. Typical changes consistent with increased serum estrogen concentrations are obvious in the examination of vaginal cytologic smears. Although bitches with ovarian remnant syndrome have been described with a sanguineous vaginal discharge (Wallace, 1992), those that we have treated do not have a discharge. Bloody vaginal discharge from a bitch without any uterine tissue is difficult to explain because the uterus is the source of blood. Thus bitches without a uterus are not expected to bleed. Those with uterine remnants in addition to ovarian remnants bleed as a result of the effects of estrogen on any endometrial tissue, and these dogs are predisposed to "stump pyometra."

Diagnosis

The diagnosis of ovarian remnant syndrome should be straightforward. Once exogenous estrogen administration has been ruled out, endogenous estrogen secretion can be demonstrated with vaginal cytology *obtained when the bitch is attracting males and is willing to breed*. The cytologic appearance of greater than 80% to 90% superficial cells is strong evidence for this diagnosis.

Because an ovarian remnant is unusual, we recommend supplementing the diagnosis with one or several serum estrogen determinations. Serum estradiol concentrations in excess of 15 pg/ml are abnormal and consistent with follicular activity. Some bitches with obvious signs of estrus also have mild increases in the serum progesterone concentration. Because these assays are readily available, one or several samples should be monitored for progesterone and estradiol. However, vaginal cytology may be more reliable than a solitary serum estradiol analysis and usually confirms the diagnosis.

Treatment

SURGERY. Exploratory laparotomy performed by a surgical specialist is strongly encouraged. Experience is the key to finding some ovarian remnants. It is wise to consider surgery when the bitch is in estrus or diestrus because the presence of follicles or corpora lutea enhances the chances of visualizing this tissue. The likely locations are the ovarian pedicles or anywhere within the ovarian ligaments. Any suspicious tissue should be removed and histologically examined by a veterinary pathologist. The tissue located at both ovarian pedicles should be completely resected, regardless of its appearance or the results of complete exploratory surgery. Elimination of signs, together with the histologic findings in the removed tissue, should confirm the diagnosis.

MEDICAL MANAGEMENT. Although not recommended, medical management may be necessary because the owners may refuse exploratory surgery or because one or more surgeries may have failed to resolve the syndrome. Use of megestrol acetate or mibolerone as directed (see Chapter 22) may be beneficial.

DISORDERS OF SEXUAL DEVELOPMENT

Normal Sexual Development

The sex chromosome composition of sperm determines the sex of mammals at fertilization. The embryo develops as a male if the fertilizing sperm has a Y chromosome. If the sperm contains an X chromosome, the embryo develops as a female. The genital system of early developing embryos is neither male nor female. Eventually, the embryo without a Y chromosome develops an ovary from the undifferentiated gonad, and the müllerian system persists as the fallopian tubes, uterus, and cranial vagina. The urogenital sinus and external genitalia develop in a female pattern.

In the presence of a Y chromosome, the indifferent gonad develops into a testis, which produces both testosterone and müllerian inhibiting substance (MIS). MIS, which is secreted by Sertoli cells, causes regression of the müllerian duct system. Testosterone, which is secreted by Leydig cells, stimulates formation of the epididymis and vas deferens from the wolffian duct system, as well as the male urethra, penis, prostate, and scrotum.

Normal sexual development occurs in three steps (Fig. 24-11). Step 1 is the establishment of chromosomal sex (XX versus XY). Development of gonadal sex follows as step 2 (ovaries versus testes). Assuming normal progression through these first two phases, the final step is development of phenotypic sex (the individual *looks* either like a female or a male). An error in any one of these steps can result in a disorder of sexual development, which may be occult or obvious to the owner or veterinarian (Table 24-4). Normal dogs have a total chromosome number of 78.

TABLE 24–4 OUTLINE OF DISORDERS OF SEXUAL DEVELOPMENT

Abnormalities of Chromosomal Sex
  Abnormalities of Chromosome Number
    XXY syndrome
    XO syndrome
    Triple-X syndrome
  Chimeras and Mosaics
    True hermaphrodite chimeras
    XX/XY chimeras with testes
    XY/XY chimeras with testes
Abnormalities of Gonadal Sex
  XX sex reversal
    XX true hermaphroditism
    XX male syndrome
Abnormalities of Phenotypic Sex
  Female pseudohermaphroditism
    Exogenous androgen exposure
    Endogenous androgen exposure
  Male pseudohermaphroditism
    Persistent müllerian duct syndrome
    Defects of androgen-dependent masculinization
      Hypospadias
      Androgen resistance
    Cryptorchidism

These 78 chromosomes include 38 pairs of non-sex chromosomes and two sex chromosomes. The sex chromosome constitution of females is XX and that of males is XY.

Abnormal Sexual Development

Dogs with obvious abnormalities in the external genitalia may be quickly recognized, but as the discussion in the previous section suggests, abnormalities may occur at any step in development. Many abnormalities in sexual development are subtle or occult with respect to what may be seen on physical examination. Definitive diagnosis of an abnormality in chromosomal sex may be derived from establishment of a karyotype. Chromosomal preparations from peripheral blood lymphocyte culture are most practical and are available at several veterinary schools (Meyers-Wallen and Patterson, 1986).

Intersex conditions include congenital malformations of the genital system such that the gender of the individual is ambiguous. "Intersex" is a generic term that encompasses numerous disorders. True

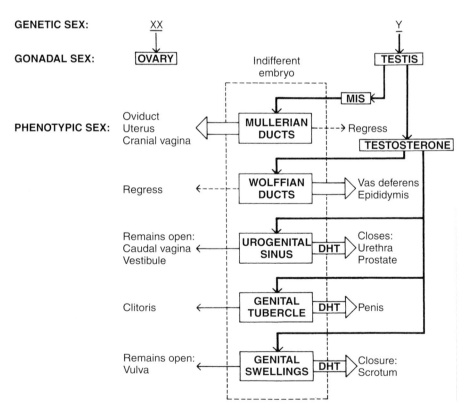

FIGURE 24-11. Normal sexual differentiation. *MIS*, Müllerian inhibiting substance; *DHT*, dihydrotestosterone. (Meyers-Wallen VN, Patterson DF: Disorders of sexual development in dogs and cats. *In* Kirk RW [ed]: Current Veterinary Therapy X. Philadelphia, WB Saunders, 1989, p 1261; used with permission.)

hermaphrodites are individuals with both testicular and ovarian tissue, either combined in one gonad (ovotestis) or existing as separate gonads. Pseudohermaphrodites have the gonads of one gender but have reproductive organs having characteristics of the opposite gender. Male pseudohermaphrodites have testes but have some female features, such as the presence of a uterus or external genitalia that are primarily female. Female pseudohermaphrodites have ovaries but are masculinized to some degree (Patterson, 1983).

Terminology needs to be defined. The *phenotype* is the external appearance (i.e., a phenotypic female is one that appears to be female). The *genotype* refers to the genetic makeup of an individual. In terms of gender, the genotype, or *chromosomal sex,* refers to XX, XY, XXY, XO, and the like. *Gonadal sex type* refers to the presence of ovaries or testicles.

Gonadal gender is best determined by histologic examination of the gonads. This may be accomplished with biopsy-obtained samples, although the entire gonad may need to be evaluated if conditions such as an ovotestis are to be recognized. Phenotypic sex can be established through review of a thorough description of both the internal and external genitalia. It is necessary to determine (1) whether the vulva or prepuce is appropriate in form and position; (2) whether a clitoris or penis is present; (3) the location of the urethral opening; and (4) whether the dog has a prostate or caudal vagina (Meyers-Wallen and Patterson, 1989).

Abnormalities of Chromosomal Sex

DEFINITION. Dogs and cats with abnormalities of chromosomal sex are normal-appearing males or females that have underdeveloped rather than ambiguous genitalia. Animals that are chimeras or mosaics may be exceptions to this rule. Most animals with chromosomal sex abnormalities are sterile, with no treatment advised (Meyers-Wallen and Patterson, 1989).

XXY SYNDROME. During the process of meiosis, the end result of which are gametes (sperm or eggs), abnormalities may occur. Among the abnormalities seen in the development of eggs or sperm is a condition called *nondisjunction.* If nondisjunction occurs in the development of an egg, one egg contains two X chromosomes and the other egg has no sex chromosomes. The two-X chromosome egg, fertilized by a Y chromosome sperm, develops into an XXY individual. The Y chromosome allows testicular development, which in turn results in production of MIS, testosterone, and the male phenotype (an individual with male external genitalia). However, the XX condition inhibits normal spermatogenesis, the result being an individual with testicular hypoplasia (Meyers-Wallen and Patterson, 1989). The XXY condition has been described in humans, mice, horses, cows, sheep, cats, and dogs (Patterson, 1983).

XO SYNDROME. As described above, an egg or sperm may contain no sex chromosome. If fertilization occurs by an X-containing gamete (egg or sperm), the result is an XO zygote. In humans, XO individuals develop as phenotypic females (an individual with female external genitalia), are short in stature, and have other developmental anomalies. The gonads develop as ovaries during fetal life, but they usually degenerate into fibrous streaks lacking germ cells. However, some dogs demonstrate prolonged proestrus and appear to have normal ovaries (Lofstedt et al, 1992). This condition should be considered in the differential diagnosis of bitches that fail to cycle within their first 2 to 4 years and in those with persistent proestrus. Females that are XO are also sex chromatin negative.

XXX SYNDROME. Fertile ovarian cycles have been observed in females of several species that were demonstrated to be chromosomally XXX. The cause is nondisjunction of the sex chromosomes, similar but opposite to the XXY syndrome. A bitch with primary anestrus has been described that had this unusual syndrome (Meyers-Wallen and Patterson, 1989). Among humans, the problem occurs in 1 in every 1000 women.

CHIMERAS AND MOSAICS. A *chimera* is an individual whose cells include two populations. Each set is derived from a different source; that is, if one source is an XX individual and the second source is an XY individual, the chimera is XX/XY. This individual, such as would result from the fusion of two zygotes, has an extra *pair* of chromosomes. A *mosaic* also has at least two cell populations, but the source of the extra chromosome or chromosomes is one individual. This defect is the result of mitotic nondisjunction, with four cell populations representing the result of such a process—YO, XXY, XO, XYY—and only one of these need survive with a normal cell population to create a mosaic such as XY/XXY, XY/XYY, or XY/XO. The end result, chimera or mosaic, is an individual composed of at least two cell populations having different chromosome constitutions (Meyers-Wallen and Patterson, 1989).

Gonadal sex in chimeras and mosaics depends on the distribution of cell populations in the tissue representing the embryonic gonad. If one population of cells has a Y chromosome and one has only X chromosomes, the result could be a combination of ovarian and testicular tissue that may end up looking like ovarian tissue, testicular tissue, or a combination. In any case, histologic examination should reveal both types of tissue (Meyers-Wallen and Patterson, 1989). The appearance of the individual (phenotype) depends on the *amount* of testicular tissue; the more testicular tissue, the more male it appears, and the more ovarian tissue, the more female it appears. The result could be an individual with normal-appearing external genitalia or "ambiguous" genitalia.

TRUE HERMAPHRODITES. An individual with both ovarian and testicular tissue is a true hermaphrodite. One gonad may be an ovary and the other a testicle, or both gonads may be a combination of the two (ovotestes). Most canine true hermaphrodites have an XX sex chromosome constitution and as such they represent examples of abnormalities in gonadal sex (see next section) rather than the much less commonly reported chimera or mosaic (Randolph et al, 1988; Olson et al, 1989a; Sommer and Meyers-Wallen, 1991). The chimeras have had either XX/XY or XX/XXY chromosome constitutions. Such dogs have been normal females in external appearance with an enlarged clitoris. Each had vulvar pruritus because of the protruding clitoral tissue, and each had failed to exhibit ovarian cycles (Meyers-Wallen and Patterson, 1986). The dog in Fig. 24-12 was demonstrated to be an XX/XY chimera with testes located near the kidneys, a fluid-filled enlarged uterus, a cranially displaced, vulvalike structure, and a hypoplastic penis in place of the clitoris. This penis was classified as such because the urethra was located within the structure and opened at its caudal (distal) pole.

Abnormalities of Gonadal Sex

XX SEX REVERSAL.   In this condition, chromosomal and gonadal sex do not agree. The individuals are referred to as *sex reversed*. Although XX sex reversal (a male-looking individual [phenotype] that is chromosomally [genotype] a female) is a well-described defect in the dog, XY sex reversal has not been described. In Cocker Spaniels, true hermaphroditism occurs as a familial, inherited, autosomal recessive trait, as does XX male syndrome. Sex reversal has also been described in Beagles, Chinese Pugs, Kerry Blue Terriers, Weimaraners, and German Short-Haired Pointers (Randolph et al, 1988; Olson et al, 1989a; Sommer and Meyers-Wallen, 1991).

XX TRUE HERMAPHRODITES.   The individual with this defect has both ovarian and testicular tissue. The most common combination is bilateral ovotestes (both tissues in one gonad). Dogs with one ovary and one ovotestis or one testis and one ovotestis have been described. If little testicular tissue is present, the dog appears to be a female externally, has uterine tissue, and is often (but not always) sterile.

If a significant amount of testicular tissue is present, the individual has epididymides, vasa deferentia, a uterus, and variable presence of oviducts. Externally, these dogs appear to be masculinized females or ambiguous, with obvious clitoral enlargement with or without abnormalities in the shape and location of the vulva (Fig. 24-13). Some XX true hermaphrodites have reproduced as normal females despite the testicular tissue and abnormal clitoris. All such offspring carry the trait, however.

Diagnosis of XX true hermaphroditism depends on suspicion gained from a careful physical examination,

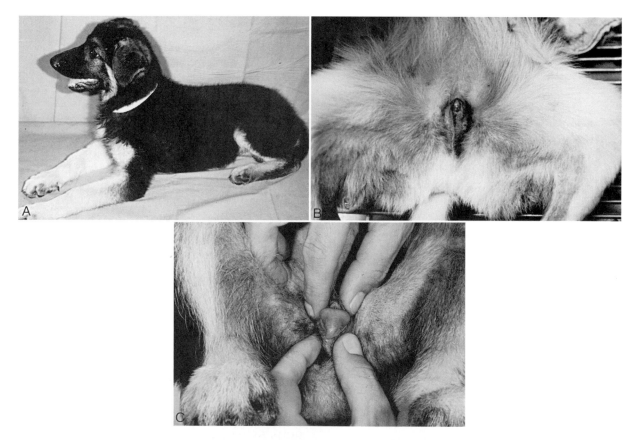

FIGURE 24-12. *A,* Healthy young German Shepherd dog with ambiguous genitalia. *B,* External genitalia of the dog in *A.* The genitalia are located midway between the normal location of the prepuce in males and the vulva in females. *C,* Small penile structure within the skin folds of the ambiguous genitalia.

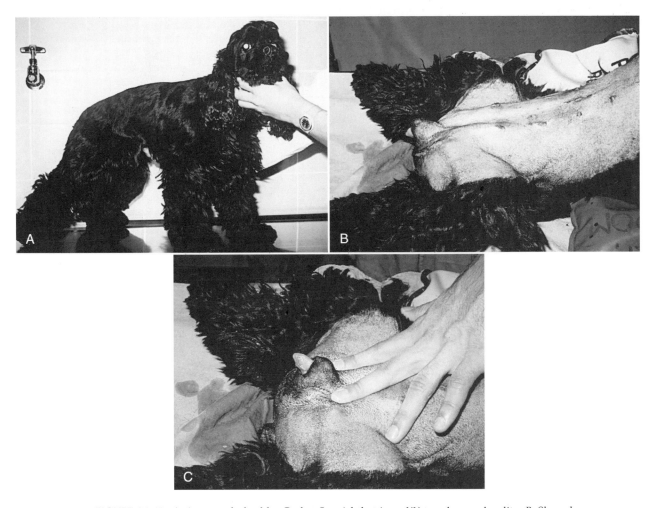

FIGURE 24-13. *A,* Apparently healthy Cocker Spaniel that is an XX true hermaphrodite. *B,* Shaved abdomen. *C,* Os clitoris extruded from the vulvar opening.

resulting in surgical exploration of the abdomen. Confirmation is based on histologic assessment of biopsied or completely extirpated tissue, demonstrating both ovarian and testicular tissue. Presurgical measurement of basal, post-LH, or post-GnRH serum testosterone concentrations may suggest the presence of testicular tissue in a dog that is phenotypically female, but a negative result does not rule it out. Karyotyping is necessary to prove that the individual is an XX hermaphrodite or an XX male (Meyers-Wallen et al, 1987).

XX MALE SYNDROME. An individual with a 78,XX cellular chromosome makeup, bilaterally undescended testicles, a prostate, and an entire wolffian duct system meets the criteria for an XX male. Externally, scrotal development is not evident, and the prepuce is present but abnormal in shape or position. These dogs typically have penile abnormalities that include *hypospadias* (an abnormality of the penis in which the urethra opens on the undersurface, usually proximal to the normal site in the glans penis), hypoplasia, or curvature (Fig. 24-14). They are sterile individuals without spermatogonia. Oviducts are absent, but a complete uterus is present. Oviduct regression is

proportional to the amount of MIS produced (see Fig. 24-11), but the continued presence of a uterus implies target organ insensitivity to this substance. Removal of the gonads and uterus is recommended to avoid problems with fluid accumulation in the uterus or the development of neoplasia in the gonads (Meyers-Wallen and Patterson, 1989).

Abnormalities of Phenotypic Sex: Pseudohermaphrodites

DEFINITION. Female and male pseudohermaphrodites have some degree of sexual ambiguity in the genitalia. Their chromosomal sex and gonadal sex agree, but their external appearance is reversed; that is, they are phenotypically abnormal.

FEMALE PSEUDOHERMAPHRODITES. An XX sex chromosome individual with ovaries that is masculinized in external appearance is a female pseudohermaphrodite. Such individuals may have mild to severe clitoral enlargement or nearly normal male external genitalia. If a penis is present, it is usually hypoplastic, and the prepuce resembles a vulva (see Fig. 24-12). These dogs do

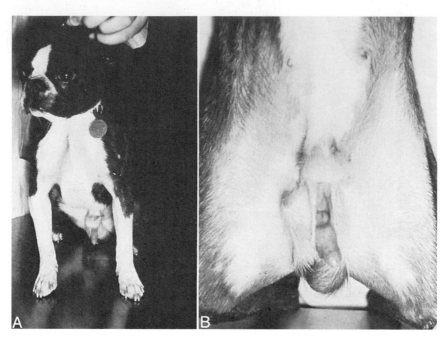

FIGURE 24-14. Puppy with hypospadias. Note the abnormal locations of the urethral openings.

have a cranial vagina and uterus. Such dogs may be mistaken for and raised as males, but they may periodically sexually attract other males because of the ovarian cycles. The underlying cause is not always recognized, but some cases are known to have occurred as a result of androgen administration to pregnant bitches, which alters the development of female fetuses. Sources of androgens include some vitamin-hormone combinations, progesterone, and androgenic preparations used to suppress estrus (Patterson, 1983). Management of these dogs includes ovariohysterectomy.

Human female pseudohermaphrodites may have genetic defects in adrenal steroid biosynthesis. Deficiencies in one of a number of enzymes in the pathway of glucocorticoid biosynthesis may result in low plasma cortisol concentrations. This causes lack of negative feedback to the pituitary and increased secretion of ACTH, stimulating production of steroid precursors from which androgens can be synthesized. The androgens alter the phenotypic appearance of the individual. The result in affected human infants is adrenal insufficiency as well as ambiguous genitalia. Defects of this type have not been documented in domestic animals (Patterson, 1983).

MALE PSEUDOHERMAPHRODITES. Male pseudohermaphrodites have a Y chromosome, testes, and female genitalia or varying degrees of penile and/or scrotal malformation. Various chromosomal defects have been documented. Affected individuals include those with both XX and XY cells (XX/XY chimerism) and those with XO and XY cells (XO/XY mosaicism). Some chromosomal male Miniature Schnauzers have persistent müllerian derivatives because of a deficiency in MIS or the presence of target cells that are refractory to MIS (Marshall et al, 1982). Affected dogs are usually cryptorchid and may develop Sertoli cell

tumors, pyometra, or mucometra. Those with one or both testicles descended may be fertile or subfertile. Treatment consists of surgical removal of the reproductive tissue (Patterson, 1983).

Other defects not yet reported in dogs include enzyme deficiencies in testosterone biosynthesis, which can result in incomplete masculinization of the external genitalia; low plasma testosterone concentrations; and glucocorticoid or mineralocorticoid insufficiencies. Also in this group are syndromes that result in an insensitivity of target tissues to androgens, resulting in female external genitalia, cryptorchid testicles, normal testosterone concentrations, and no uterus, fallopian tubes, or ovaries (testicular feminization).

HYPOSPADIAS. This condition (see Fig. 24-14) was defined in the previous section describing the XX male. Hypospadias may occur from a variety of causes, and the result is an incomplete fusion of the urethral folds in the formation of the male urethra. The common denominator may be inadequate production of fetal androgens (Wilson et al, 1983; Meyers-Wallen and Patterson, 1989). The Boston Terrier may have a familial predisposition to hypospadias. Cryptorchidism is the most common defect associated with hypospadias (Hayes and Wilson, 1986).

FAILURE TO PERMIT BREEDING (FIG. 24-15)

Mismanagement

The most common reason that bitches refuse a male's attempts at mounting is incorrect choice of breeding dates by the owner. For example, if it is predetermined that a bitch is to be bred on days 11 and 13 from the

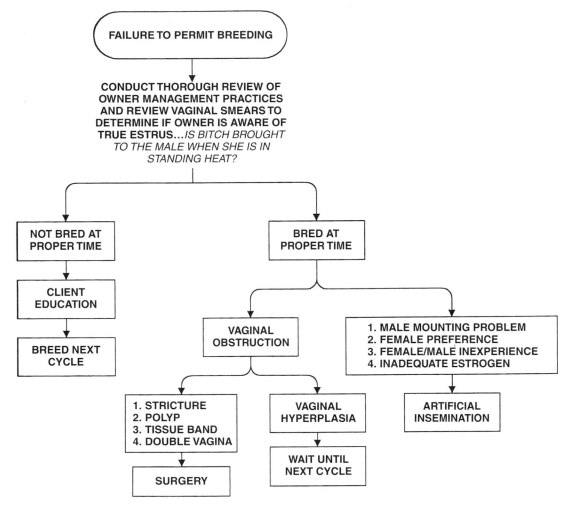

FIGURE 24-15. Algorithm for evaluation of a bitch that appears to be healthy but that refuses to allow breeding attempts by a male even when she is in the estrous phase of the ovarian cycle.

first day of proestrual vaginal bleeding and if proestrus lasted 5 days and estrus lasted 4 days, breeding will be attempted in diestrus, and the bitch will refuse to breed. Similarly, if proestrus was 14 days in duration, again she would not breed because attempts were being made during proestrus. Therefore bitches that fail to permit breeding are not always at fault. An owner who better understands the reproductive cycle of the bitch usually applies better management protocols and has better success. One potential cause of failing to permit breeding, however, is a vaginal defect (see Chapter 25).

Behavior

Bitches may be managed properly but still consistently refuse to breed with a particular male. Mate preference appears to be one potential cause for this problem. If no other cause is evident, the owner should attempt to breed the bitch to another, more dominant male before investigating unusual problems (see the section on sexual behavior in Chapter 20).

REFERENCES

Al-Bassam MA, et al: Normal postpartum involution of the uterus in the dog. Can J Comp Med 45:217, 1981.

Allen WE: Infertility in the bitch. In Practice 1:22, 1986.

Allen WE, Dagnall GJR: Some observations on the aerobic bacterial flora of the genital tract of the dog and bitch. J Small Anim Pract 23:325, 1982.

Archbald LF, et al: A surgical method for collecting canine embryos after induction of estrus and ovulation with exogenous gonadotropins. Vet Med Small Anim Clin 75:228, 1980.

Arnold S, et al: Effect of duration of PMSG treatment on induction of oestrus, pregnancy rates and the complications of hyperoestrogenism in dogs. J Reprod Fertil 39(Suppl):115, 1989.

Baba E, et al: Vaginal and uterine microflora of adult dogs. Am J Vet Res 44:606, 1983.

Barton CL: Infertility in the bitch. Proceedings of the Annual Meeting of the Society for Theriogenology, 1987, p 198.

Bjurstrom L, Linde-Forsberg C: Long-term study of aerobic bacteria of the genital tract in breeding bitches. Am J Vet Res 53:665, 1992a.

Bjurstrom L, Linde-Forsberg C: Long-term study of aerobic bacteria of the genital tract in stud dogs. Am J Vet Res 53:670, 1992b.

Bouchard G, et al: Estrus induction in the bitch using a combination of diethylstilbestrol and FSH-P. Theriogenology 36:51, 1991.

Brockus CW: Endogenous estrogen myelotoxicosis associated with functional cystic ovaries in a dog. Vet Clin Pathol 27:55, 1998.

Buckrell BC, Johnson WH: Infertility in the cyclic bitch. In Binnington AG, Cockshuti JR (eds): Decision Making in Small Animal Soft Tissue Surgery. Toronto, BC Decker, 1988, p 120.

Burke TJ: Causes of infertility. In Burke TJ (ed): Small Animal Reproduction and Infertility: A Clinical Approach to Diagnosis and Treatment. Philadelphia, Lea & Febiger, 1986, p 227.

Cain JL, et al: Use of pulsatile intravenous administration of gonadotropin-releasing hormone to induce fertile estrus in bitches. Am J Vet Res 49:1993, 1988.

Cain JL, et al: Induction of ovulation in bitches using subcutaneous injection of gonadotropin-releasing hormone analog. Scientific Proceedings of the American College of Veterinary Internal Medicine, 1990, p 1126.

Cinone M, et al: Termination of pregnancy in the bitch by means of PGF$_{2\alpha}$-gel and cabergoline administration. In Proceedings: Advances in Dog, Cat, and Exotic Carnivore Reproduction. Oslo, 2000, p 109.

Concannon PW: Induction of fertile oestrus in anoestrous dogs by constant infusion of GnRH agonist. J Reprod Fertil 39(Suppl):149, 1989.

Concannon PW: Methods for rapid induction of fertile estrus in dogs. In Kirk RW, Bonagura JD (eds): Current Veterinary Therapy XI. Philadelphia, WB Saunders, 1992, p 960.

DeNardo GA, et al: Ovarian remnant syndrome: Revascularization of free-floating ovarian tissue in the feline abdominal cavity. J Am Anim Hosp Assoc 37:290, 2001.

Doig PA, et al: The genital mycoplasma and ureaplasma flora of healthy and diseased dogs. Can J Comp Res 45:233, 1981.

England GCW, Allen WE: Repeatability of events during spontaneous and gonadotrophin-induced oestrus in bitches. J Reprod Fertil 93:443, 1991.

England GCW: Pharmacologic control of reproduction in the dog and bitch. In Simpson GM, England GWC, Harvey M (eds): BSAVA Manual of Small Animal Reproduction and Neonatology. United Kingdom, British Small Animal Veterinary Association, 1998, p 197.

Fayrer-Hosken RA, et al: Follicular cystic ovaries and cystic endometrial hyperplasia in a bitch. J Am Vet Med Assoc 201:107, 1992.

Freshman JL: Clinical approach to infertility in the cycling bitch. Vet Clin North Am (Small Anim Pract) 21:427, 1991.

Galac S: Pregnancy termination in bitches with aglepristone, a progesterone receptor antagonist. In Proceedings: Advances in Dog, Cat, and Exotic Carnivore Reproduction. Oslo, 2000, p 103.

George L, Carmichael L: Antisperm responses in male dogs with chronic Brucella canis infections. Am J Vet Res 45:274, 1984.

Gobello C, et al: Use of cabergoline to treat primary and secondary anestrus in dogs. J Am Vet Med Assoc 220:1653, 2002.

Hayes HM, Wilson GP: Hospital incidence of hypospadias in dogs in North America. Vet Rec 118:605, 1986.

Hegstad RL, Johnston SD: Use of serum progesterone ELISA tests in canine breeding management. In Kirk RW, Bonagura JD (eds): Current Veterinary Therapy XI. Philadelphia, WB Saunders, 1992, p 943.

Jeffcoate IA, et al: Measurement of plasma oestradiol after an injection of a gonadotrophin as a test for neutered bitches. Vet Rec 146:599, 2000.

Johnston SD: Diagnostic and therapeutic approach to infertility in the bitch. J Am Vet Med Assoc 176:1335, 1980.

Johnston SD: Noninfectious causes of infertility in the dog and cat. In Laing JA, et al (eds): Fertility and Infertility in Veterinary Practice. London, Bailliere Tindall, 1988, p 160.

Johnston SD: Premature gonadal failure in female dogs and cats. J Reprod Fertil 39(Suppl):65, 1989.

Johnston SD: Clinical approach to infertility in bitches with primary anestrus. Vet Clin North Am (Small Anim Pract) 21:421, 1991.

Johnston SD, et al: Canine theriogenology. J Soc Theriogenol 11:1, 1982.

Jones DE, Joshua JO: Infertility. In Reproductive Clinical Problems in the Dog, 2nd ed. London, Butterworths, 1988, p 187.

Lein DH: Examination of the bitch for breeding soundness. In Kirk RW (ed): Current Veterinary Therapy VIII. Philadelphia, WB Saunders, 1983, p 909.

Lein DH: Canine mycoplasma, ureaplasma, and bacterial infertility. In Kirk RW (ed): Current Veterinary Therapy IX. Philadelphia, WB Saunders, 1986, p 1240.

Lein DH: Mycoplasma infertility in the dog: Diagnosis and treatment. Proceedings of the Annual Meeting of the Society for Theriogenology, 1989, p 307.

Lincoln SR, et al: Value of screening infertile women for hypothyroidism. J Reprod Med 44:455, 1999.

Lindsay FEF: Postuterine endoscopy in the bitch. In Tams TR (ed): Small Animal Endoscopy. St Louis, Mosby, 1990, p 327.

Loftstedt RM, Van Leeuwen JA: Evaluation of a commercially available luteinizing hormone test for its ability to distinguish between ovariectomized and sexually intact bitches. J Am Vet Med Assoc 220:1331, 2002.

Lofstedt RM, et al: Prolonged proestrus in a bitch with X chromosomal monosomy (77, XO). J Am Vet Med Assoc 200:1104, 1992.

Mahi-Brown CA, et al: Infertility in bitches induced by active immunization with porcine zonae pellucidae. J Exp Zoo 222:89, 1982.

Manothaiudom K, et al: Evaluation of the ICAGEN-target canine ovulation timing diagnostic test in detecting canine plasma progesterone concentrations. J Am Anim Hosp Assoc 31:57, 1995.

Marshall LS, et al: Persistent müllerian duct syndrome in Miniature Schnauzers. J Am Vet Med Assoc 181:798, 1982.

Meyers-Wallen VN: Persistent estrus in the bitch. In Kirk RW, Bonagura JD (eds): Current Veterinary Therapy XI. Philadelphia, WB Saunders Co, 1992, p 963.

Meyers-Wallen VN, Patterson DF: Disorders of sexual development in the dog. In Morrow DA (ed): Current Therapy in Theriogenology, 2nd ed. Philadelphia, WB Saunders, 1986, p 567.

Meyers-Wallen VN, Patterson DF: Disorders of sexual development in dogs and cats. In Kirk RW (ed): Current Veterinary Therapy X. Philadelphia, WB Saunders, 1989, p 1261.

Meyers-Wallen VN, et al: Müllerian inhibiting substance in sex-reversed dogs. Biol Reprod 37:1015, 1987.

Moses DL, Shille VM: Induction of estrus in Greyhound bitches with prolonged idiopathic anestrus or with suppression of estrus after testosterone administration. J Am Vet Med Assoc 192:1541, 1988.

Okkens AC, et al: Fertility problems in the bitch. Anim Reprod Sci 28:379, 1992.

Olson PN, et al: Induction of estrus in the bitch. Proceedings of the American Veterinary Medical Association Annual Meeting, 1981, p 96.

Olson PN, et al: Infertility in the bitch. In Kirk RW (ed): Current Veterinary Therapy VIII. Philadelphia, WB Saunders, 1983, p 925.

Olson PN, et al: Vaginal cytology. I. A useful tool for staging the canine estrous cycle. Compend Contin Educ Pract Vet 6:288, 1984.

Olson PN, et al: The use and misuse of vaginal cultures in diagnosing reproductive diseases in the bitch. In Morrow DA (ed): Current Therapy in Theriogenology 2. Philadelphia, WB Saunders, 1986, p 469.

Olson PN, et al: Clinical evaluation of infertility in the bitch. In Ford RB (ed): Clinical Signs and Diagnosis in Small Animal Practice. New York, Churchill Livingstone, 1988, p 631.

Olson PN, et al: Female pseudohermaphrodism in three sibling Greyhounds. J Am Vet Med Assoc 194:1747, 1989a.

Olson PN, et al: Persistent estrus in the bitch. In Ettinger SJ (ed): Textbook of Veterinary Internal Medicine, 3rd ed. Philadelphia, WB Saunders, 1989b, p 1792.

Olson PN, et al: Concentrations of luteinizing hormone and follicle-stimulating hormone in the serum of sexually intact and neutered dogs. Am J Vet Res 53:762, 1992.

Patnaik AK, Greenlee PG: Canine ovarian neoplasms: A clinicopathologic study of 71 cases, including histology of 12 granulosa cell tumors. Vet Pathol 24:509, 1987.

Patterson DF: Disorders of sexual development. American Animal Hospital Association Scientific Proceedings, San Antonio, 1983, p 453.

Randolph JF, et al: H-Y antigen-positive XX true bilateral hermaphroditism in a German Short-haired Pointer. J Am Anim Hosp Assoc 24:417, 1988.

Rosenthal RC, et al: Detection of antisperm antibodies by indirect immunofluorescence and gelatin agglutination. Am J Vet Res 45:370, 1984.

Shille VM: Management of reproductive disorders in the bitch and queen. In Kirk RW (ed): Current Veterinary Therapy IX. Philadelphia, WB Saunders, 1986, p 1225.

Shille VM, et al: Efforts to induce estrus in the bitch using pituitary gonadotrophins. J Am Vet Med Assoc 184:1469, 1984a.

Shille VM, et al: Infertility in a bitch associated with short interestrous intervals and cystic follicles: A case report. J Am Anim Hosp Assoc 20:171, 1984b.

Shille VM, et al: Gonadotrophic control of follicular development and the use of exogenous gonadotrophins for induction of oestrus and ovulation in the bitch. J Reprod Fertil 39(Suppl):103, 1989.

Soderberg SF: Chronic vaginitis. Proceedings of the American College of Veterinary Internal Medicine Forum, 1989, p 182.

Sommer MM, Meyers-Wallen VN: XX true hermaphroditism in a dog. J Am Vet Med Assoc 198:435, 1991.

Vanderlip SL, et al: Ovulation induction in anestrous bitches by pulsatile administration of GnRH. Lab Anim Sci 27:459, 1987.

Wallace MS: Ovarian remnant syndrome. In Kirk RW, Bonagura JD (eds): Current Veterinary Therapy XI. Philadelphia, WB Saunders, 1992, p 966.

Watts JR, Wright PJ: Investigating uterine disease in the bitch: Uterine cannulation for cytology, microbiology, and hysteroscopy. J Small Anim Pract 36:201, 1995.

Watts JR, et al: The uterine, cervical and vaginal microflora of the normal bitch throughout the reproductive cycle. J Small Anim Pract 37:54, 1996.

Watts JR, et al: New techniques using transcervical uterine cannulation for the diagnosis of uterine disorders in the bitch. J Reprod Fertil (Suppl) 51:283, 1997.

Watts JR, et al: Endometrial cytology of the normal bitch throughout the reproductive cycle. J Small Anim Pract 39:2, 1998.

Wildt DE, et al: Behavioral, ovarian, and endocrine relationships in the pubertal bitch. J Anim Sci 53:182, 1981.

Wilson JD, et al: The androgen resistance syndromes: 5-α-reductase deficiency, testicular feminization, and related disorders. In Stanbury JB, et al (eds): The Metabolic Basis of Inherited Disease, 5th ed. New York, McGraw-Hill, 1983, p 1001.

Withrow SJ, Susaneck SJ: Tumors of the canine female reproductive tract. In Morrow DA (ed): Current Therapy in Theriogenology 2. Philadelphia, WB Saunders, 1986, p 52.

Wright PJ, Watts JR: The infertile female. In Simpson GM, England GWC, Harvey M (eds): BSAVA Manual of Small Animal Reproduction and Neonatology. United Kingdom, British Small Animal Veterinary Association.

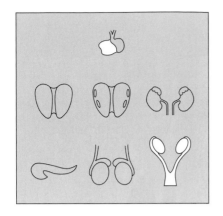

CONGENITAL ABNORMALITIES OF THE VAGINA AND VULVA

Embryonic Development

In the normal bitch, the external genitalia, the vestibule of the vagina, the urethra, and the urinary bladder are all derived from the embryonic urogenital sinus. The internal genitalia, including the anterior vagina, are derived from the pair of müllerian ducts. This distinct area of internal development is joined to the vestibule of the vagina with two epithelial linings sandwiching a thin layer of mesoderm. In the bitch, this hymen-like structure at the juncture of the internal and external genitalia often, but not always, disappears as a recognizable, palpable area before the bitch matures. Abnormalities, specifically *strictures*, involve this area immediately cranial (proximal) to the urethral opening into the vagina. These defects within the lumen of the vaginal vault and vestibule are one of the most common genital anomalies of the bitch.

Five major types of abnormalities in embryonic development of the vaginal vault have been reported in the dog, each resulting in a narrowing of the tract, called a "vaginal stricture" (Wykes and Soderberg, 1983). These five abnormalities include (1) a band of fibrous tissue crossing and narrowing the lumen of the vagina (Fig. 25-1); (2) an annular fibrous ring compressing the vaginal lumen (Fig. 25-2); (3) vulvar hypoplasia (immature vulva) that narrows the opening of the vulva; (4) incomplete fusion of the two müllerian ducts causing a "double" vagina (Fig. 25-3); and (5)

hypoplasia of the vaginal vault (as opposed to hypoplasia of the vulvar opening).

Of the five abnormalities described at the junction of the vagina and vestibule usually, two are quite common and either may result in an obstruction and cause clinical signs. These problems are almost always detected immediately proximal or cranial to the urethral opening into the vaginal vault, the site of embryonic external and internal genitalia fusion. One is a vertical septum or fibrous band of tissue that crosses the lumen of the vaginal vault (Root et al, 1995). Although not always vertical or central in location, most of these fibrous bands extend from the dorsal midline to the ventral midline, bisecting and compressing the lumen (Fig. 25-4). Vertical bands may represent persistence of a mesonephric duct (Harvey, 1998). The second most common obstruction is the presence of an annular fibrous structure in a similar area of the vaginal tract. This form of fibrous band usually involves the entire circumference of the lumen (Figs. 25-2 and 25-4). Occasionally, the veterinarian may identify an annular ring close to the entrance to the vestibule, located barely within the vulvar folds (Fig. 25-4). This latter obstruction may represent hypoplasia of the genital canal at the vaginal entrance. This defect has also been referred to as an *immature* or *infantile vulva* (Mathews, 2001). Regardless of the name, these defects both involve a narrowing of the lumen, although they each represent a different embryonic defect (Holt and Sayle, 1981).

In addition to these common defects, incomplete fusion of the two müllerian ducts can result in an elongated vertical vaginal band extending from the

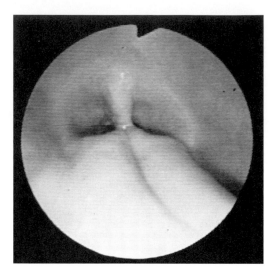

FIGURE 25-1. Endoscopic photograph of a vertical band (congenital defect) causing a vaginal stricture in a bitch.

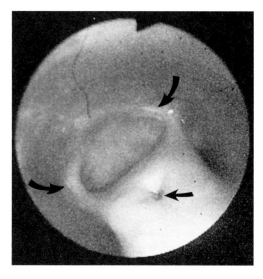

FIGURE 25-2. Endoscopic photograph of an annular fibrous band (congenital defect; *curved arrows*) causing a vaginal stricture in a bitch. The annular ring is located 1 to 2 mm proximal to the urethral opening *(straight arrow)*.

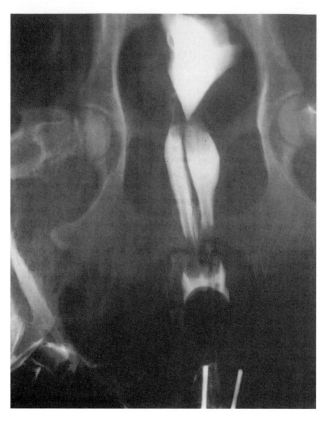

FIGURE 25-3. Ventrodorsal radiographic view with contrast material in the vaginal vault demonstrating a "double vagina" (congenital defect) in a bitch.

region of the urethral orifice cranially for variable distances. This septum may be short or long, bisecting the vagina, cervix, and uterine body (Figs. 25-3 and 25-4). This condition may be called a "double vagina" (Wykes and Soderberg, 1983; Root et al, 1995). The least common defect is hypoplasia of the vestibulovulvar junction, causing the lumen of the vaginal vault to narrow, perhaps as a result of imperfect joining of the genital folds and genital swellings (Fig. 25-4).

Clinical Signs

A large percentage of bitches with vaginal or vulvar strictures have no problems related to this defect at any time during their lives. Bitches with any of the above

defects that do have problems are usually brought to veterinarians for one, two, or all three of the following owner concerns: (1) vulvar discharge, (2) chronic vulvar licking, or (3) attracting male dogs. These three signs are the result of vaginitis, usually chronic and/or recurring, caused by the stricture. Inflammation of the vaginal mucosa results in increasing vaginal secretions (discharge), irritation causes the licking, and both of these problems, along with bacterial overgrowth, cause odors that attract males (Fig. 25-5). Additional common signs noted by owners include urinary incontinence and recurrent urinary tract infection (Kyles et al, 1996; Crawford and Adams, 2002).

Much less commonly, an owner seeks veterinary attention because a bitch is unwilling to breed, is unable to breed, or appears to be in pain when the male attempts or succeeds in breeding. Less common owner concerns include signs related to urination—dysuria and incontinence. Some owners have noted ambiguous genitalia. The least common owner concern, but perhaps most worrisome, is dystocia (Root et al, 1995).

Inability to breed is an uncommon reason for owners to seek veterinarian care, because most female dogs owned in this country have had an ovariohysterectomy and have never been bred. Therefore the defects described herein are diagnosed in our clinic far more often in spayed than in intact bitches. Lack of breeding may be important in the perceived incidence of these

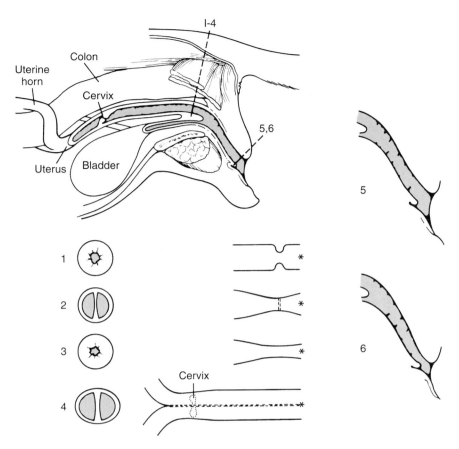

FIGURE 25-4. Various causes of vaginal obstructions in the bitch: *(1)* focal, circumferential stricture, on-end and lateral views; *(2)* band stricture, on-end and lateral views; *(3)* narrowing of the vaginal vault over a longer area, on-end and lateral views; *(4)* double vagina, or failure of the normal fusion of embryonic structures; *(5)* normal vaginal vestibule; *(6)* narrowed vestibule. The *asterisks* represent the urethral orifice.

defects in spayed bitches, because the male may break down some of these structures when penetrating the female.

The breeding bitch with a *vaginal stricture* usually exhibits a normal proestrus and a normal estrus with mating behavior, standing, and flagging the male. However, attempts at penetration by the male into the obstructed vaginal lumen are associated with the bitch showing signs of pain, moving away from the male, or biting at the stud dog and/or its handler. Attempts by the bitch to dissociate from the male can become quite violent. The male, too, may exhibit pain. Usually an "inside tie" cannot be accomplished if a bitch has such a defect. A bitch that associates standing heat with pain can become permanently afraid to breed. During estrus, these bitches can be shy, elusive, and irritable and may growl, even following surgical correction of the defect. This syndrome is a cause for an apparently normal bitch to refuse to permit breeding.

Chronic vaginitis or recurring urinary tract infections are potential sequelae to vaginal obstructions, sometimes causing the bitch to lick at the vulvar area excessively because of pain or discomfort. Vaginitis probably results from chronic retention of a small amount of normal vaginal secretions (±urine?) present in any bitch. If the defect prevents normal clearing of these secretions, they have the potential for serving as a medium for bacterial overgrowth. Therefore the problem is one of retained vaginal secretions followed by overgrowth of the normal bacterial flora and subsequent irritation of the vaginal lining or ascending urinary tract infection. These problems result in licking and increased volume of vaginal secretions. The vaginal secretions usually cause a vaginal discharge and attraction of males. These problems are typically self-limiting, perhaps due to eventual natural clearing of the overgrowth due to the volume of the secretions. Thus the irritation can naturally but transiently resolve, but the underlying cause remains (Fig. 25-5). Bacterial overgrowth within the vaginal tract is often implicated as causing ascending infection of the lower urinary tract.

The clinical signs of vaginitis caused by vaginal stricture typically wax and wane, being difficult to eliminate but rarely causing systemic illness. The entire described process usually repeats itself every few weeks or months, sometimes becoming more frequent or severe, causing owners to seek veterinary assistance. Rarely, an owner may believe that his or her bitch is experiencing an ovarian cycle because of the attraction

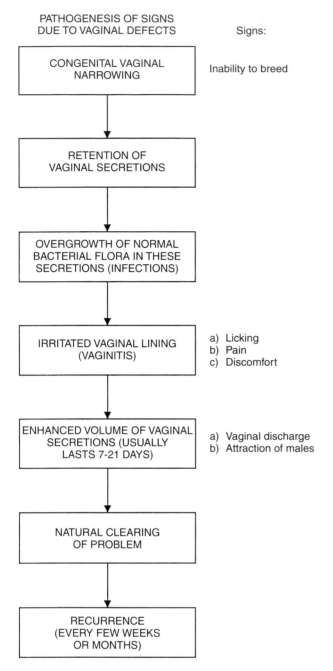

FIGURE 25-5. Flow chart illustrating a theoretic pathogenesis for clinical signs as a result of vaginal strictures in bitches.

of males. The odor created may cause this attraction, but the bitch does not allow the male to mount.

Diagnosis

THE OVARIOHYSTERECTOMIZED BITCH.   The diagnosis of any vaginal obstruction (vulvar stricture or vestibulovaginal stenosis) is best made with digital examination of the vaginal vault. Normally, a gloved and lubricated index finger can be passed into the vaginal vault, without pain or difficulty to the bitch,

in all but the most miniature breeds (Harvey, 1998). Remember that the veterinarian's finger is invariably smaller than the erection of the male of that breed. Therefore digital examination of the vaginal vault should be able to be completed without difficulty. If a stricture is suspected, one should proceed slowly and gently in order to avoid causing pain to the bitch. Sedation or anesthesia of the bitch is almost never used, being reserved for those dogs that become vicious when the vulvar area is examined.

USE OF OTOSCOPE OR VAGINAL SPECULUM.   Strictures are typically obvious and immediately evident on digital examination, blocking the normal cranial progress of the digit. Most important, any stricture is likely to be missed if the vaginal examination is performed with an otoscope or vaginal speculum, each of which is narrower and less sensitive than a finger. Such tools can easily bypass any one of these defects, and their use should be limited. It is possible, but rare, for a bitch to be so large that a vaginal stricture cannot be reached digitally or with one of these instruments.

THE ANESTRUAL OR VIRGIN PREPUBERTAL BITCH. There are two primary exceptions to a simple digital examination diagnosis. One is the virgin intact pubertal bitch that may not be easily palpated and can have remnants of a hymen that might be broken down during breeding or disappear following the relaxation of the vaginal vault. This relaxation can be dramatic when the bitch is under the influence of estrogen. Second, the vagina of an anestrual intact bitch can sometimes be small in diameter, nonpliable, difficult to palpate, or feel as if a stricture is present. In either situation, examination during a subsequent estrus is advised before recommending therapy. The veterinarian can also recommend at least one or two attempts at natural breeding and then repalpate if breeding is not achieved. Some bitches need to be muzzled for breeding or digital examination because of their pain or fear.

VAGINAL CYTOLOGY.   Vaginal cytology from the bitch with a vaginal stricture and an associated low-grade vaginitis usually contains mucoid debris, bacteria (in large or small numbers), and variable to large numbers of neutrophils engulfing bacteria. Large numbers of neutrophils may be seen, and degenerated neutrophils are common. The smears are usually easy to obtain. However, bacteria and neutrophils are seen in normal dogs as well as dogs with vaginitis. In either situation, the findings are nonspecific. If vaginitis is present, the causes are numerous and include common (strictures or foreign bodies, for example) and less common (neoplasia or polyps, for example) problems. Therefore any examination should include a digital evaluation before treatment is suggested or a diagnosis made.

VAGINOSCOPY.   Use of a fiberoptic pediatric procto-scope (see Fig. 25-1) can be an excellent diagnostic aid in visualizing a vaginal defect. Although these instruments are useful diagnostic tools, they are not as sensitive as the digital examination. Use of a vaginogram (radiographic dye study) has been recommended, especially when surgical correction of a vaginal defect is being considered and vaginoscopy is not available (Wykes and Soderberg, 1983; Root et al, 1995; Mathews, 2001; Crawford and Adams, 2002). This procedure has been beneficial diagnostically in some bitches because it has the potential of confirming a diagnosis, defining the location, and identifying a major defect such as a "double vagina" (Fig. 25-3) or a less extensive defect, such as an annular ring (Fig. 25-2).

RADIOLOGY. If vaginoscopy is not available, a radiographic dye study (vaginogram) is an alternative diagnostic aid. This tool is used in a bitch suspected of having a vaginal stricture not palpable because of its location (this is extremely unusual). We have used the vaginogram in bitches with *vulvar* hypoplasia because one cannot pass a finger or an instrument through the area of hypoplasia without causing pain or trauma to the bitch. Another indication for a vaginogram is a palpable stricture that prevents evaluation of the cranial vagina (Fig. 25-6). Before surgery or other therapy is considered, evaluation of the entire vagina may be warranted to rule out unsuspected abnormalities (polyp, tumor, foreign body, extensive congenital defect; see Figs. 25-3, 25-4, and 25-6). Furthermore, other congenital anomalies (e.g., urethral ectopia, pelvic bladder) should be ruled out. A urethral pressure profile should be considered (Mathews, 2001).

The bitch should be anesthetized for the vaginogram. A Foley catheter is placed in the vestibule of the vagina. The balloon is inflated, and a volume of dye is injected through the catheter into the vaginal vault. Radiographs can then be taken to determine whether enough dye has been injected to provide an adequate study. Determining the required volume of dye is a challenge, because it is difficult to predict what amount of dye will pass into the urinary bladder. One report describes a method of "grading" a vestibulovaginal stenosis (vaginal stricture). On review of radiographic cystourethrovaginograms, measurements were made. The dorsoventral height of the vagina was measured at its highest point, and the dorsoventral height of the vestibulovaginal junction was measured at its narrowest point on a lateral radiograph. The ratio of the height at the vestibulovaginal junction to the height of the vagina was calculated. A ratio >0.35 was suggested as normal. Ratios of 0.26 to 0.35 were classified as "mild," 0.20 to 0.25 as "moderate," and <0.2 as "severe" vestibulovaginal stenosis (Crawford and Adams, 2002).

Therapy

THE BREEDING BITCH. No treatment is recommended if the diagnosis of vaginal obstruction is made in a bitch without clinical signs. A bitch thought to have a vaginal obstruction may breed normally or be artificially inseminated. The artificially inseminated bitch requires close observation to be certain that a vaginal dystocia does not occur during whelping. The fibrous band defects are the easiest to correct because they can be isolated and incised without much difficulty or bleeding. Normal parturition may occur in the bitch with an annular ring if enough relaxation of the vaginal walls allows passage of the newborn through

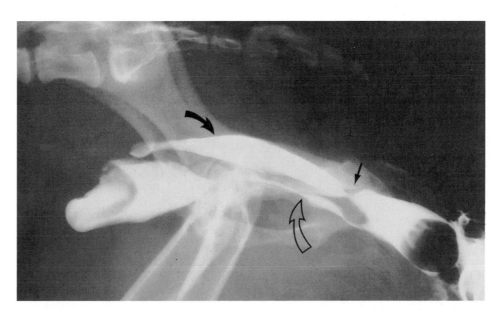

FIGURE 25-6. Lateral radiograph of the pelvic area from a bitch after the vaginal vault has been filled with radiographic contrast material. The contrast material, which was injected through a Foley catheter, demonstrates the vestibule of the vagina (cranial to the balloon of the catheter), the vaginal vault *(curved solid arrow)*, the stricture located at the juncture of the vestibule with the vault *(straight arrow)*, the urethra *(curved open arrow)*, and the bladder.

the narrowed area or if the obstruction is broken down during parturition. It is not known whether these defects are inherited, and some have suggested that their surgical correction would be unethical (Harvey, 1998).

Where indicated, correction of congenital vaginal ring obstructions can be accomplished surgically. In most cases, an episiotomy is necessary to provide adequate visualization of the defect. Postsurgical dilation of the vaginal vault may be required to prevent recurrence of vaginal strictures. In addition, correction of vaginal defects does not ensure that the bitch will subsequently allow breeding. (The interested reader should consult surgical references for the necessary procedures: Greene, 1983; Wykes and Soderberg, 1983; Mathews, 2001.) Antiseptic douches can be used as described in the following section.

THE OVARIOHYSTERECTOMIZED BITCH. Most bitches diagnosed with defects associated with their vaginal lumens have been previously spayed. Before making any treatment recommendation, the owner should be educated with a complete discussion and illustration, such as that in Fig. 25-4. In this manner the owner can understand the problem and can appreciate that no treatment except surgery will permanently resolve the signs. Many owners elect not to surgically treat their pet once they understand that the problem is self-limiting, that it almost never causes systemic illness, and that the signs, although likely to wax and wane throughout the dog's life, are not life-threatening and may not be as serious or dangerous as the surgery required to correct the defect. Reluctance to perform surgery on these defects stems from the knowledge that the surgical area is not easily reached and that recurrence of a vaginal stricture is always possible. Splitting a pelvis, for example, is considered extremely aggressive, and if the surgeon believes that such an approach would be needed, thorough owner education is advised. Similarly, because the surgery is often in the location of the urethra, iatrogenic incontinence problems would be catastrophic.

If treatment is deemed necessary, a less aggressive attempt at medical treatment is recommended before considering surgery. Treatment is indicated if the bitch is extremely uncomfortable and appears to be in significant pain or if the vaginal discharge is persistent and copious. In these dogs, the approach is to treat with a vaginal douche one to three times daily until the signs abate. We suggest that owners purchase several pediatric enema sets. The enema solution is discarded, but the bottle is a collapsible plastic container with a tapered tip, which is ideal for infusing an antiseptic solution into the vagina. The douche should be a "weak tea–colored" solution of Betadine. The bitch should be treated in an outside location that will not be discolored by the solution that invariably drips out. The bitch can be held up by her rear legs to ensure that the vaginal vault is thoroughly rinsed during or immediately after infusion. Use of antibiotic douche solutions is specifically contraindicated because resistant bacterial strains routinely develop.

VAGINAL HYPERPLASIA/VAGINAL PROLAPSE

Pathogenesis

A common cause of vaginal obstruction is the protrusion of edematous vaginal tissue into the vaginal lumen and often through the opening of the vulva (prolapse) in intact bitches during the proestrus or estrus phases of the ovarian cycle (Fig. 25-7). This is likely an exaggerated response by the vaginal lining to normal estrogen stimulation, although some of these dogs have had cystic follicles (Fig. 25-7, C through F). Frequently referred to as *vaginal hyperplasia* or *vaginal hypertrophy*, prolapsed vaginal membranes are histologically described as markedly edematous tissue.

Clinical Features (Table 25-1)

Excessive vaginal edema, with or without prolapse, is usually seen in younger (<2 to 3 years of age) large-breed bitches and usually precludes breeding if it is severe. A number of breeds have been identified as having this problem. In our experience, it is most common in the Boxer and the Mastiff breeds. Other breeds reported to have vaginal prolapse include St. Bernards, German Shepherd dogs, English Bulldogs, Labrador Retrievers, Walker Hounds, Chesapeake Bay Retrievers, Springer Spaniels, Weimaraners, and Airedale Terriers (Johnston, 1989). The frequent incidence in some breeds or lines suggests that this problem may be an inherited predisposition. Although the condition may occur in small-breed dogs, note that all those mentioned with any frequency are large.

Vaginal prolapse almost always is diagnosed when the bitch is in, or has just progressed through, proestrus or estrus (Table 25-1). The timing is consistent with a causal relationship between increases in serum estrogen concentration and the excessive edema. A few dogs have had excessive vaginal edema or prolapse near the end of diestrus, following the less dramatic but significant rise in serum estrogen concentrations that take place at this time in the normal ovarian cycle. These bitches often have had the problem in proestrus/estrus as well. Regression of the tissue mass usually begins in late estrus to early diestrus, as serum estrogen concentrations return to basal levels. This would explain the

TABLE 25–1 FEATURES OF VAGINAL EDEMA/HYPERPLASIA/PROLAPSE*

		NUMBER OF DOGS
Mean age	2.0 years	65
Age range	0.6-11 years	65
Stage of ovarian cycle		
Proestrus/estrus		57/66 dogs
Diestrus		4/66 dogs
Parturition/end of diestrus		5/66 dogs
Anestrus		0

*Adapted from Johnston SD: Vaginal prolapse. *In* Kirk RW (ed): Current Veterinary Therapy X. Philadelphia, WB Saunders Co, 1989, p 1302.

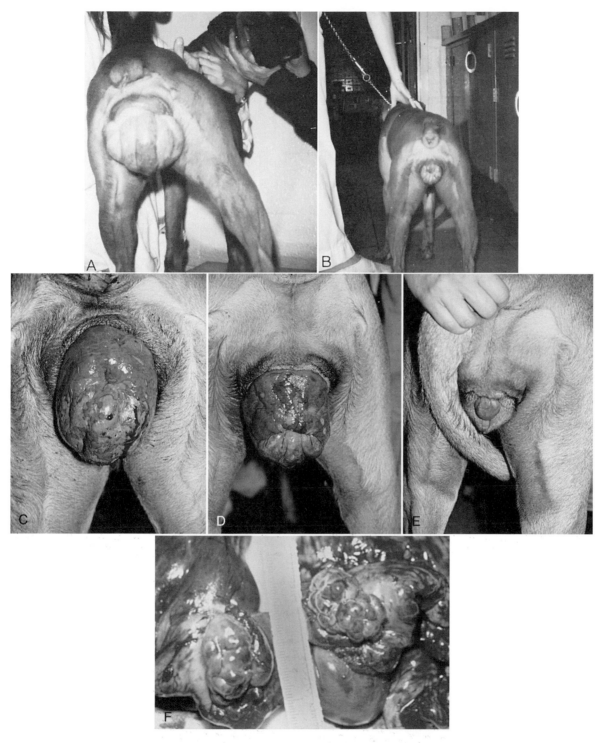

FIGURE 25-7. Severe vaginal hyperplasia in a young Boxer bitch before *(A)* and 1 week following *(B)* ovariohysterectomy. *C,* Photograph of a large, protruding vaginal hyperplasia in a 2-year-old Bull Mastiff at the time that the bitch underwent ovariohysterectomy. *D,* 4 days after surgery. *E,* 6 weeks after surgery. *F,* Photograph of the cystic follicles on both ovaries identified in the same 2-year-old Bull Mastiff.

response noted if the bitch is ovariohysterectomized as a treatment for this condition.

Presenting signs are usually reported by an owner who has noticed tissue protruding from the vulva. Although not common, it is possible for the owner to be concerned that the bitch cannot urinate or has difficulty urinating. Other owner concerns may include inability or unwillingness to breed or that the male appears unable to penetrate the bitch. Many bitches with vaginal prolapse lick the tissue, but only a small percentage of these have stranguria. No abnormalities are seen in serum chemistry values or hormonal profiles from afflicted bitches.

Some bitches develop a slight to severe vaginal hyperplasia in association with every proestrus. This problem is usually recognized in young bitches. Most bitches do not have severe problems once they have experienced their first few ovarian cycles. Ovariohysterectomy is the only definite means of permanent prevention. If an owner wants to breed a bitch with vaginal hyperplasia, artificial insemination is necessary. The hyperplasia is rarely present at the time of parturition.

Diagnosis

The diagnosis is straightforward because of the obvious mass protruding from the vulva (see Fig. 25-7) or a bulging perineum in a young bitch in proestrus or estrus. The major differential diagnoses include clitoral enlargement, a benign polyp, or a tumor such as leiomyoma, mast cell tumor, or transmissible venereal tumor. Clitoral enlargement is likely caused by the presence of an os clitoris (bone within the clitoris) and is palpable as a small, hard structure. Polyps are usually small and have a narrow pedicle or base (Fig. 25-8). Tumors are typically irregular in shape, occur in older females, and are not associated with the proestrus or estrus phases of the ovarian cycle. The exception to this rule is transmissible venereal tumor, which most often is identified in bitches that are young and sexually active.

Vaginal prolapsed tissue is usually relatively large and soft, often reducible, and associated with estrus. The tissue is in the form of a smooth, rounded mass with folds rising in a wide base from the floor of the vaginal vault (Fig. 25-7). The tissue usually arises cranial to the urethral opening. Less commonly, the vaginal prolapse is more severe and may include the entire circumference of the vaginal wall, in which case the tissue takes on the appearance of a large doughnut.

Treatment

Management of vaginal hyperplasia can be difficult. If the bitch can urinate despite the presence of the mass and no necrosis is present, the hyperplasia is not an emergency. If urination is not possible, an indwelling urethral catheter needs to be placed following identification of the urethral papilla. Virtually all vaginal prolapses shrink and disappear during diestrus, given enough time. Therefore most efforts are directed at keeping this tissue (1) clean with saline washes, (2) lubricated with appropriate jellies, and (3) non-traumatized. One can prevent trauma to exposed vaginal tissue by keeping the bitch indoors on smooth and padded surfaces and by placing an Elizabethan collar around the neck of the bitch to prevent her from causing any self-mutilation. "Diapers" can be rigged to minimize exposure of this tissue to the environment or to the dog herself.

Induction of ovulation using gonadotropin-releasing hormone (GnRH; Cystorelin, Abbott, North Chicago, IL; 2.2 µg/kg IM) or human chorionic gonadotropin (hCG; Pregnyl, Organon, West Orange, NJ; 1000 U, IM) has been recommended as a treatment for vaginal prolapse (Johnston, 1989). In theory, induction of ovulation shortens the phases of estrogen secretion (proestrus and estrus) and hastens regression of the edematous tissue. However, no study has demonstrated that such protocols result in ovulation, and even if ovulation were to occur, no evidence demonstrates that the duration of proestrus and estrus would be decreased.

Some of our clients have applied antihemorrhoidal creams to prolapsed tissue, claiming it causes shrinkage of the tissue. Necrotic tissue requires surgical debridement, and some eversions can be surgically reduced (Pettit, 1983; Mathews, 2001). One may elect to perform an ovariohysterectomy, which prevents recurrence but does not necessarily hasten shrinkage of the mass. Neither oral mibolerone nor megestrol acetate is recommended in treating this problem (Rushmer, 1980). Prostaglandin therapy is not indicated in the treatment of vaginal hyperplasia.

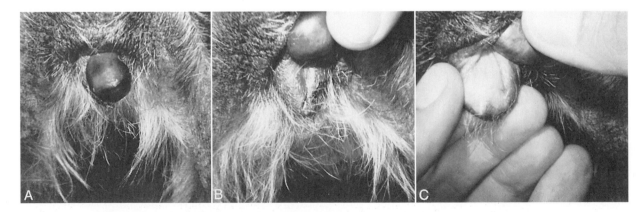

FIGURE 25-8. *A*, A vaginal polyp covering the surface of the vulva. *B*, The same polyp lifted up, revealing the vulva underneath. *C*, A close-up view of the same mass as in *A* and *B*, revealing the small pedicle connecting the vaginal polyp with the vaginal wall.

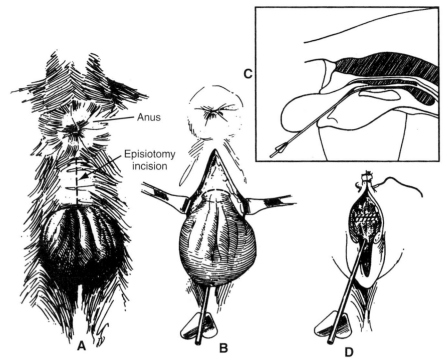

FIGURE 25-9. *A,* Edematous vaginal tissue protrudes (Type II vaginal prolapse) through the vulvar cleft. *B* and *C,* A urinary catheter is placed within the urethra ventral to the mass to prevent iatrogenic trauma to the urethral papilla during excision *(D).* (From Wykes and Olson, 1993; used with permission.)

For purebred bitches intended for breeding, some investigators have recommended surgical excision of the prolapsed tissue. Surgery should be considered only if the vaginal prolapse is associated with an inability to urinate, if it is large and likely to become infected, or if it has recurred in more than one cycle. Excision has been reported to prevent recurrence of prolapse (Johnston, 1989). Surgery is performed via episiotomy late in estrus or following induction of ovulation, when the mass is beginning to regress in size. After protecting the urethra by identifying it with placement of a catheter, an elliptic incision is made in the vaginal mucosa at the base of the mass. This is carefully dissected away and removed (Fig. 25-9). The vaginal mucosa is then closed with absorbable suture material (Johnston, 1989; Mathews, 2001). Surgery can be associated with a great deal of blood loss and can be complicated. It is performed in our hospital only if the vaginal tissue is extremely necrotic, if the bitch is unable to urinate, or if compromise of the vascular supply to that tissue, the uterus, or the bladder is suspected.

VULVAR DISCHARGES

Background

Vulvar discharges are usually quickly noticed by owners, who then may bring their pet to veterinarians if there is no ready explanation for the observation. The discharge may indicate a normal process (proestrus or whelping), but it may be the first clinical sign of a serious urogenital abnormality (pyometra, foreign body or neoplasia). As with any problem, a thorough history and physical examination should precede any testing. Most discussions of vulvar discharges are based on color and consistency. In this section, the age and clinical history serve as the basis for developing the differential diagnosis (Fig. 25-10, *A* to *C;* Table 25-2).

Perivulvar Dermatitis

Perhaps one of the most common causes of apparent vaginal discharge is perivulvar dermatitis. The most common problem in these dogs is a "recessed vulva" secondary to obesity. This is actually an example of the condition known as *skinfold pyoderma,* which can occur in various anatomic locations. Heat, moisture, and body excretions (in this case urine and/or vaginal secretions) accumulate within the folds, creating an environment conducive to skin maceration, bacterial overgrowth, and inflammation. Constant microtrauma to the skin created by the friction between opposing skin surfaces, in combination with maceration and inflammation, overwhelms normal skin defense mechanisms and allows secondary bacterial infections to develop.

Perivulvar dermatitis has been reported to develop in obese female dogs. It may also occur in dogs with infantile or atretic vulvas. It seems that this condition occurs in some dogs that are either not obese or do not have abnormally small vulvas. However, regardless of

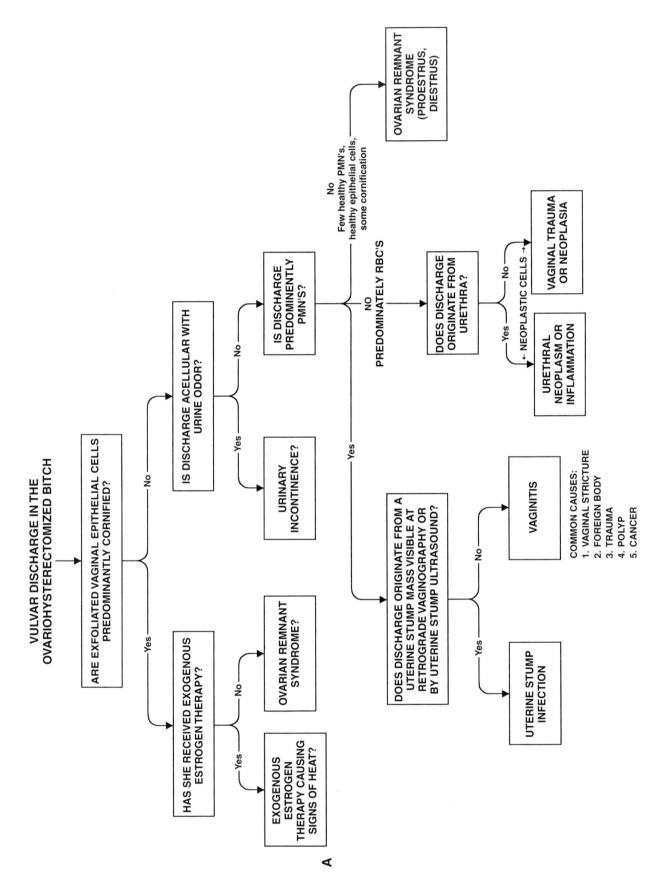

FIGURE 25-10. *A*, Algorithm for the diagnosis of vulvar discharges in ovariohysterectomized bitches.

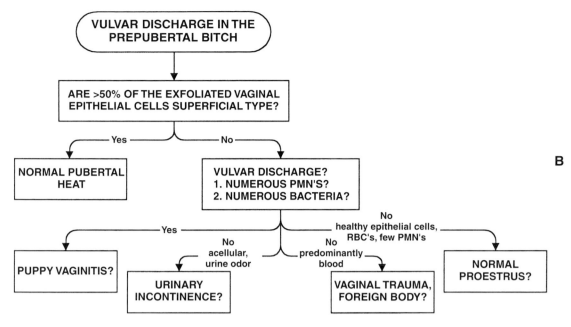

FIGURE 25-10. *B,* Algorithm for vulvar disharges in prepubertal intact bitches. *Continued*

TABLE 25–2 CAUSES OF ABNORMAL VULVAR DISCHARGE IN THE BITCH

Intact, Prepubertal Bitch

1. Normal pubertal estrous cycle
2. Puppy vaginitis
3. Urogenital trauma/neoplasia
4. Urinary incontinence

Intact, Postpubertal, Nonpregnant Bitch

1. Normal estrous cycle
2. Functional ovarian cyst/ovarian neoplasia
3. Pyometra
4. Vaginitis
5. Urogenital trauma/neoplasia
6. Urinary incontinence

Intact, Postpubertal, Pregnant, or Postpartum Bitch

1. Fetal loss (septic/nonseptic)
2. Normal placental fluid discharge at whelping
3. Lochia
4. Subinvolution of placental sites
5. Metritis
6. Urogenital trauma/neoplasia
7. Urinary incontinence

Ovariectomized Bitch

1. Exogenous estrogen therapy
2. Ovarian remnant syndrome
3. Vaginitis
4. Uterine stump infection
5. Urogenital trauma/neoplasia
6. Urinary incontinence

From Romagnoli SE: A diagnostic approach to vulvar discharge in the canine patient. Proceedings of the Society for Theriogenology, 1989, p 295; used with permission.

the cause, a "recessed" vulva predisposes that dog to perivulvar dermatitis. The superficial dermatitis can result in a foul odor and discharges from the skin. The dog may appear uncomfortable or in pain. Chronic vestibulitis, vaginitis, and cystitis have been reported to develop secondary to the perivulvar dermatitis.

Medical management of perivulvar dermatitis with administration of systemic antibiotics or topical treatments, such as antibiotic ointments, cleansing, drying agents, or lotions, is generally palliative and often unrewarding. Episioplasty, the surgical excision of the excessive perivulvar tissue, has been demonstrated to be an effective means of managing this chronic and sometimes frustrating condition. This surgical procedure is an effective low-morbidity treatment that can eliminate clinical signs, vaginitis, and chronic urinary tract infection (Lightner et al, 2001). However, resolution of recurring urinary tract infection or incontinence was not common following vulvoplasty for a recessed vulva if dogs also had a vestibulovaginal stenosis (Crawford and Adams, 2002).

The Healthy Bitch Less Than 6 Months of Age

The healthy immature bitch is most likely to have one of only a few causes for a vaginal discharge. If the discharge is purulent, "puppy vaginitis" (also called "prepubertal vaginitis") is likely. This is a self-limiting disorder that rarely requires therapy. It has been recommended that the puppy with vaginitis not be spayed until the problem resolves in order to avoid a chronic condition (Romagnoli, 1989). Such an approach usually means waiting until the dog has had her first estrous cycle. No proof (other than anecdotal comments) exists that delaying ovariohysterectomy is beneficial.

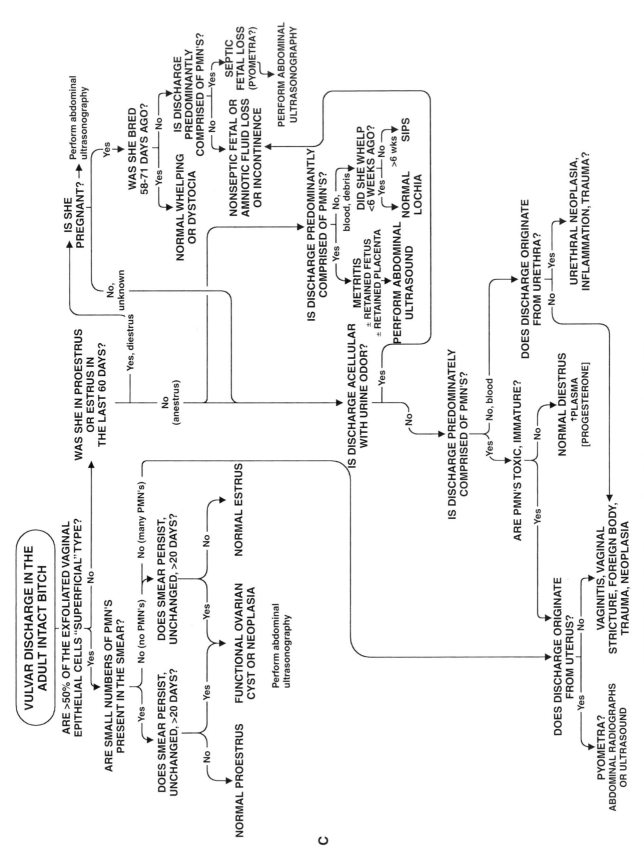

FIGURE 25-10. C, Algorithm for vulvar discharges in intact adult bitches.

We do not recommend delaying ovariohysterectomy because, in our experience, the puppy vaginitis will clear, regardless. If delay is recommended, the owner should be educated concerning an unwanted pregnancy. The major differential diagnoses for a purulent vaginal discharge in a puppy are presence of a foreign body and any of a variety of congenital disorders. Therefore, a careful digital examination and vaginoscopy may be warranted. Culture is rarely helpful (Harvey, 1998).

If the discharge is sanguineous (bloody), the bitch may be in proestrus, and vaginal cytology should support that diagnosis. The major differential diagnoses for bloody vaginal discharges are trauma, foreign bodies, and abnormalities in coagulation. The vaginal discharge may appear to be urine. If so, the differential diagnosis includes all causes of urinary incontinence. These include ectopic ureter(s), bladder problems, and urethral disease.

The Nonpregnant Bitch That Has Had at Least One Ovarian Cycle

SOON AFTER ESTRUS. If a bitch has recently cycled, a sanguineous (bloody) discharge noted within 1 to 8 weeks of estrus may be indicative of a *split heat*. This should be readily identified on vaginal cytologic examination, which would be consistent with proestrus or estrus (estrogen effect). The other possible diagnoses associated with a discharge in the 8 to 10 weeks following estrus are pyometra, which can cause a sanguineous, purulent, or mixed discharge; abortion or resorption; foreign bodies; trauma; tumors; or coagulopathies. It is wise to assume that all nonspayed dogs with a vaginal discharge, regardless of age, have a pyometra until proved otherwise.

PERSISTENT FOR WEEKS. Occasionally, a bloody vulvar discharge thought to be associated with proestrus becomes persistent over a period of weeks. Proestrus and estrus together can persist for as long as 7 weeks and still be considered normal. Thus, knowing the precise duration that the discharge has been observed is helpful. Abdominal ultrasonography may be useful if an estrogen-producing follicular cyst (less commonly a tumor) is under consideration because of persistent vaginal cytologic appearance of superficial cells.

PRESENCE OF BACTERIA. Vulvar discharges with large numbers of bacteria can be observed in healthy bitches recently beginning diestrus. Bacteria may be noted in normal bitches but without a vulvar discharge. The presence of a discharge containing large numbers of bacteria may be associated with metritis/pyometra or any cause of vaginitis (vaginal stricture, clitoral enlargement, mass, or foreign body). Vaginitis, a difficult diagnosis to confirm, is usually secondary to another problem.

The Bitch Bred Within the Last 30 to 70 Days

Vulvar discharge in a bitch that was recently bred is always of concern. A sanguineous discharge may be the only sign of a split heat. Vaginal cytology should indicate recurrence of estrogen effect (superficial cells in excess of 60% of cells seen). However, a vaginal discharge similar in appearance could be associated with a bitch aborting all or part of a litter. The vaginal cytologic examination if abortion is occurring would include blood and parabasal cells (i.e., no estrogen effect), with or without large numbers of bacteria. Abdominal ultrasonography is an important diagnostic aid. A purulent discharge suggests infection of uterine or vaginal origin as previously described.

If the bitch was bred 50 to 70 days earlier, a sanguineous discharge may be the first sign that the bitch is in labor and will soon begin to whelp. Some bitches have a vulvar discharge that appears to be clear mucus, serous to thick in consistency, immediately before whelping.

The Bitch That Has Recently Whelped

Sanguineous vulvar discharge in the first days after whelping is normal. This type of discharge may continue as long as 6 to 8 weeks and still be considered normal *lochia*. If the discharge persists beyond this amount of time, it is often referred to as *subinvolution of placental sites* (SIPS; see Chapter 21). Nevertheless, if the bitch appears healthy, is not anemic, does not have a leukocytosis, and does not have a fever, the discharge is probably not worrisome and no treatment is necessary.

Any time a vulvar discharge becomes purulent or the bitch becomes ill and/or stops mothering her litter, the problem is worrisome and she must be evaluated for postpartum metritis (see Chapter 21). This disorder may follow obstetric manipulation, abortion, or bacterial infection after normal whelping. Vaginal trauma related to whelping is a less common but possible consideration. Abdominal ultrasonography is an extremely important aid in determining whether a bitch has a retained fetus or placenta, pyometra, or some other disorder. Radiography, although useful, is not as valuable.

The Ovariohysterectomized Bitch

Purulent vulvar discharge in a spayed bitch is most commonly associated with vaginitis due to vaginal stricture (see Vaginitis/Vaginal Infections). Foreign bodies, polyps, neoplasia, perivulvar dermatitis, and stump pyometra are all possibilities that must be considered. These problems may cause sanguineous and/or purulent discharges. If vaginal cytology reveals superficial cells, exogenous administration of estrogen or the ovarian remnant syndrome is possible.

VAGINAL/VESTIBULAR MASSES

Differential Diagnosis

Various types of vaginal or vulvar masses have been recognized in bitches. Among the diagnoses are vaginal

TABLE 25–3 CLINICAL SIGNS IN 44 BITCHES WITH VAGINAL/VESTIBULAR MASSES

	Vaginal Prolapse (n = 18)	Clitoral Enlargement (n = 11)	NEOPLASIA Vaginal/Vestibular (n = 20)	Urethral (n = 5)	Total
Genital					
Vaginal prolapse	10		6	1	17
Vaginal mass/lump	3	1	6	1	11
Vaginal ulceration			1		1
Vulvar discharge	4	1	5	1	11
Vulvar bleeding			2	1	3
Licking at the vulva	1	1	3		5
Vulvar swelling	4			1	5
Urinary					
Hematuria				3	3
Inappropriate urination			1		1
Polyuria			1	1	2
Dysuria	4		5	4	13
Pollakiuria	1		4	2	7
Nocturia	1	1		2	4
Could not urinate	1				1
Gastrointestinal					
Vomiting			2	1	3
Diarrhea			1	1	2
Straining	1		3	1	5
Anorexia			4		4

From Manothaiudom K, Johnston SD: Clinical approach to vaginal/vestibular masses in the bitch. Vet Clin North Am Small Anim Pract 21:509, 1991. Used with permission.

prolapse, uterine prolapse, vaginal neoplasia, urethral neoplasia, clitoral hypertrophy, vaginal polyps, vaginal abscess, and hematomas. The history usually includes observation of tissue protruding from the vulva and various other owner concerns (Table 25-3).

Vaginal Neoplasia

Tumors of the vaginal tract are an uncommon cause of vaginal or vulvar obstructions. Tumors of the vagina and vulva account for 2% to 3% of neoplasms in dogs and are seen in older patients with a mean age of 10 years (Thacher and Bradley, 1983). Benign tumors commonly include fibromas, leiomyomas, polyps, and lipomas (Harvey, 1998). Malignant tumors include leiomyosarcomas, mast cell tumors, and transitional cell carcinomas that grow into the vagina from the urethra (Fig. 25-11; Thacher and Bradley, 1983; Herron, 1983). Benign tumors occur most frequently in sexually intact dogs, whereas malignant tumors occur more often in spayed dogs. Transmissible venereal tumor can be present as a genital mass lesion (see Chapter 26).

The most common clinical signs associated with vaginal neoplasia, in addition to a mass protruding from the vulva, are vaginal discharges, persistent licking of the area, and attraction of males. Less commonly, masses may result in mechanical interference with surrounding tissues, causing stranguria, tenesmus, dysuria, urinary or fecal incontinence, or perineal swelling (Weller and Park, 1983; Sahay et al, 1985; Withrow and Susaneck, 1986; Johnson, 1989b).

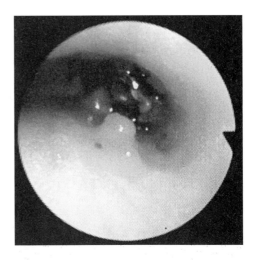

FIGURE 25-11. Vaginal endoscopy demonstrating a transitional cell carcinoma within the lumen of the vagina.

Diagnosis follows completion of a thorough history and physical examination. Invariably, an impression smear or biopsy of the mass is needed for determining cell type. In some cases surgical removal may precede identification of the mass, although this approach is strongly discouraged. Although surgery may be an expedient means of managing the bitch, it may be harmful in the long term. Understanding the nature of the mass, whether or not metastasis has occurred, and how it is best managed should precede surgery. Additional diagnostic information may be gained through vaginoscopy, abdominal ultrasonography, culture, vaginograms, and urethrocystograms.

Urethral Neoplasia

Canine urethral tumors are typically either epithelial (transitional cell carcinomas) or mesenchymal (leiomyoma) in origin. Most of these urethral tumors are malignant and locally invasive. Distant metastasis is less common. Females are more commonly afflicted than males. Afflicted dogs tend to be 8 to 10 years of age or older (Magne et al, 1985; Maxie, 1985; Davies and Read, 1990).

The most common tumors involving the distal urethra are transitional cell carcinoma and squamous cell carcinoma. The most common clinical signs associated with these tumors are stranguria, dysuria, and hematuria. Digital examination of the vagina and rectum, followed by subsequent cytology of the area, may be all that is needed to confirm the diagnosis. Occasionally, urine cytology is diagnostic and traumatic catheterization of the bladder may provide adequate cell numbers to confirm a diagnosis. Abdominal ultrasound or dye studies, however, may be warranted in determining the extent of a neoplastic process and whether any hope for surgical extirpation exists. Final diagnosis should be based on histology of biopsy material (Manothaiudom and Johnston, 1991).

Vaginal Polyps

Fibropapillomas (polyps) are relatively common in aging bitches. They are usually small, smooth, firm masses that may ulcerate following self-trauma. They rarely cause clinical problems and are usually attached by narrow pedicles (see Fig. 25-8). Surgical removal is typically straightforward and curative.

Uterine Prolapse

A rare complication of whelping is uterine prolapse. Prolapse has been most commonly observed to follow delivery of the last in a litter of puppies and may involve the cervix and one or both uterine horns. Partial or complete prolapse has been reported. Clinical signs include observation of a mass protruding from the vulva, vaginal discharge, straining, and licking (Wood, 1986; Johnson, 1989a). Diagnosis is based on the history of whelping and the appearance of the mass. Treatment options are surgical removal or manual reduction if the tissue appears viable and not traumatized (Manothaiudom and Johnston, 1991; Mathews, 2001).

Clitoral Enlargement

Normal-appearing bitches and male pseudohermaphrodites may have clitoral enlargement. Administration of androgens or anabolic steroids to pregnant bitches may result in development of an os clitoris in female offspring. Although it is not often recognized, bitches with hyperadrenocorticism may have clitoral hypertrophy as a result of virilization secondary to the excess steroid secretion.

Clinical signs include excessive licking of the area and observation of a mass protruding from the vulva. Less commonly, owners may observe vulvar discharge, attraction of males, or hematuria. The presence of a clitoral os results in protruding tissue, drying of the mucosa, and subsequent irritation, inflammation, and clinical signs. Diagnosis is straightforward and is made on digital examination of the vestibule of the vagina. The os clitoris is usually 1 to 1.5 inches in length and smaller in diameter than a pencil. It is readily palpated and is painful only if vaginitis is associated with the protruding or abnormal tissue. Some dogs have clitoral enlargement, tissue protrusion, and clinical signs without the presence of a bone within the clitoris.

Before any surgical procedure is considered, it is extremely important to identify the urethra. Surgical removal of the enlarged clitoris or the os clitoris is not difficult if the urethra is distinct from this defect. Removal of the bone or excessive tissue quickly resolves the clinical signs without complications. If the urethra passes through the os clitoris, however, a congenital chromosomal problem is quite likely. If the urethra is involved, surgical removal of the os is much more difficult.

VAGINITIS/VAGINAL INFECTIONS

Incidence

Vaginitis and vaginal infections are relatively common abnormalities in bitches of any age, regardless of whether or not they have undergone ovariohysterectomy. Primary, uncomplicated vaginitis seems not to be common. Naturally occurring bacterial overgrowth within an otherwise normal vaginal tract is not common. The significance or cause of *lymphoid-follicular* or *lymphocytic-plasmacytic* vaginitis is not known, but the condition is well recognized (Fig. 25-12).

Our experience indicates that vaginal infections are usually secondary to other problems, such as strictures. Less commonly, trauma, foreign bodies, or masses cause infection. The routine vaginal culture of a bitch before breeding, in order to prove that no infection is present before the male is allowed to breed, is a completely unfounded and highly questionable practice (Bjurstrom and Linde-Forsberg, 1992a). Culture of the vaginal tract in a bitch with a purulent vaginal discharge is completely unwarranted unless a digital examination has been performed and tests have been completed to rule out the presence of vaginal strictures, pyometra, foreign bodies, and os clitoris.

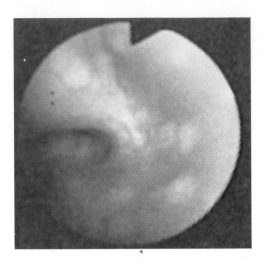

FIGURE 25-12. Vaginal endoscopy demonstrating lymphoid follicles in a bitch with vaginitis. Biopsy was interpreted as lymphocytic-plasmacytic vaginitis.

Clinical Signs and Diagnosis

Most bitches with vaginitis have a vaginal discharge that is mucous (cloudy), mucopurulent (cloudy white to yellow), or purulent (yellow to yellow-green) in appearance (Johnson, 1991). Much less commonly, the vulvar discharge is bloody or blood-tinged. Associated clinical signs are licking, attraction of males, and pollakiuria. If no discharge is present, the diagnosis is difficult to establish and is questionable. Additional findings on physical examination may include a variety of problems that caused the vaginitis, such as congenital abnormalities, tumors, and foreign bodies.

The diagnosis is supported by vaginal cytology and vaginoscopy. On vaginal cytology, vaginitis is usually associated with an inflammatory response—nonseptic, purulent, or septic with some or no red blood cells (Johnson, 1991). Neutrophils are the primary cell type identified, and the vaginal epithelial cells are expected to consist primarily of parabasal and intermediate cells. Vaginoscopy with a proctoscope (see Fig. 25-1) can be an excellent means of visualizing the underlying causes for vaginitis.

Complete blood counts and serum chemistry profiles do not demonstrate specific abnormalities that aid in the diagnosis of vaginitis. The only abnormality encountered with any frequency is the presence of eosinophilia in some of these bitches. Otherwise, these tests are used to rule out the presence of other problems. Urinalysis and urine cultures are warranted because infection or neoplasia of the urinary tract may appear initially as vaginitis. Contrast studies of the vagina and/or urinary tract may be indicated in some bitches.

Is a Positive Vaginal Culture Meaningful?
(See Chapter 24)

Bacterial infections have been implicated as a cause of infertility in the bitch and a source of disease for breeding males (Johnston, 1980; Lein, 1983). These infections have been thought to be subclinical in many infertile bitches, only occasionally resulting in obvious vaginitis, metritis, pyometra, or systemic infection. The recommendation has been made to culture the anterior vagina of infertile bitches with a guarded swab (AccuCulShure, AccuMed Co, Pleasantville, NY; Guarded Culture Instrument, Kalayjian Industries, Long Beach, CA; Tiegland Swab, HL 206400, Haver-Lockhart Laboratories, Shawnee Mission, KS). Bacterial isolation, identification, and antimicrobial sensitivity have been recommended, and the bitch can then be given appropriate antibiotics for 4 weeks (Johnston, 1980). However, it is difficult to establish the role of bacterial infections in canine infertility. Virtually all normal bitches have bacterial flora present in the anterior vagina, and similar types of aerobic bacteria are present in the vaginal vaults of infertile bitches (Olson et al, 1983; Bjurstrom and Linde-Forsberg, 1992a).

Bacteria

BACKGROUND. Virtually all normal bitches harbor aerobic bacteria in the vagina (Table 25-4; Bjurstrom and Linde-Forsberg, 1992a). Merely isolating bacteria from the vagina does not constitute the basis for a diagnosis of disease. Some organisms, such as *Brucella canis*, may be difficult to isolate. Thus a negative culture does not ensure that a bitch is free of an infectious disease.

TYPES OF BACTERIA. The types of bacteria may vary with the age of the bitch; a higher percentage of prepubertal bitches have coagulase-positive staphylococci than do postpubertal dogs. The stage of the cycle did not alter the types of bacteria isolated in some studies, but increased numbers were present in proestrus and estrus (Allen and Dagnall, 1982; Baba et al, 1983). In another study, the number and species of bacteria isolated did vary with the stage of the ovarian cycle (see Fig. 25-4; Bjurstrom and Linde-Forsberg, 1992a). Normal flora was usually recovered in mixed cultures of light to moderate growth (Table 25-4; Bjurstrom and Linde-Forsberg, 1992a). If an organism was a significant pathogen, it was believed that it would result in clinical signs, be recovered in large numbers, and be present in a nearly pure culture because it would have gained advantage as a pathogen and have overgrown the normal mixed flora (Allen and Dagnall, 1982; Allen, 1986; Olson et al, 1986). However, pure cultures of one organism were identified from 18% of vaginal swabs, mixed cultures were identified from 77%, and completely negative results were obtained from only 5% of 826 swab specimens from 59 healthy, fertile bitches. All the bitches had positive vaginal cultures at one time or another (see Fig. 25-5; Bjurstrom and Linde-Forsberg, 1992a).

Some owners of stud dogs require a "negative" vaginal culture from the bitch to be used in breeding. However, most male dogs harbor microorganisms in the prepuce and urethra that are similar to those

TABLE 25–4   AEROBIC BACTERIA ISOLATED FROM THE VAGINAS OF 59 BITCHES (826 VAGINAL SWAB SPECIMENS)

Organism	ISOLATES		BITCHES FROM WHICH ORGANISMS WERE ISOLATED	
	Number	Percent	Number	Percent
Pasteurella multocida	492	59.6	58	98.3
Beta-hemolytic streptococci	392	47.5	53	89.8
Escherichia coli	263	31.8	50	84.7
Gram-positive rods (unclassified)	141	17.1	53	89.8
Gram-negative rods (unclassified)	134	16.2	51	86.4
Mycoplasma spp.	73	8.8	35	59.3
Streptococcus spp. (alpha-hemolytic, nonhemolytic)	72	8.7	33	55.9
Pasteurella spp.	60	7.2	40	67.8
Enterococci	51	6.2	26	44.1
Proteus mirabilis	40	4.8	15	25.4
Staphylococcus intermedius	34	4.1	20	33.9
Coryneforms	25	3.0	24	40.7
Coagulase-negative staphylococci	17	2.1	13	22.0
Pseudomonas spp.	6	0.7	6	10.2
Total	1800	(2.3 isolates/bitch)		

From Bjurstrom L, Linde-Forsberg C: Long-term therapy of aerobic bacteria of the genital tract in breeding bitches. Am J Vet Res 53:665, 1992. Used with permission.

identified as normal vaginal flora (Bjurstrom and Linde-Forsberg, 1992b). It is unjustified to refuse to allow a stud dog to breed a particular bitch because bacteria have been isolated from her vagina (Olson et al, 1986).

It is also unjustified to associate all positive vaginal cultures with vaginitis or with infertility. Systemic antibiotics have been demonstrated to alter the bacterial flora of the vagina, but determining when antibiotics are warranted can be difficult. Heavy growth of one bacteria is more likely to be normal than abnormal.

The canine uterus may contain small numbers of bacteria and yet be normal (Baba et al, 1983). Obtaining a uterine culture requires laparotomy or training with transcervical endoscopy. The cervix "relaxes" in proestrus and estrus, suggesting that anterior vaginal cultures reflect uterine bacterial growth. Without obvious vaginitis or pyometra, vaginal cultures are not believed to be of benefit in managing the infertile bitch.

TREATMENT OF BACTERIA VAGINITIS.   As previously described in this chapter, treatment with vaginal douches for 2 to 3 weeks, with or without systemic antibiotics, may be beneficial. However, therapy should be reserved for bitches with obvious clinical signs of infection (Bjurstrom and Linde-Forsberg, 1992a and 1992b). We recommend using antiseptic douches (i.e., Betadine) because they can be quite effective and do not result in the development of bacterial resistances.

Mycoplasma and *Ureaplasma*

Mycoplasma and *Ureaplasma* are organisms commonly cultured from the vaginal tract of the normal bitch. However, a syndrome of vaginitis, poor conception, early embryonic death, embryonal or fetal resorption, abortion, stillborn pups, weak newborns, and/or neonatal death has been suggested to be caused by these smallest of free-living microorganisms. At present,

evidence regarding the pathogenesis of these disorders is circumstantial (Doig et al, 1981; Lein, 1989). As with bacterial culture results, if large numbers of these organisms are identified in pure or nearly pure growth from the vaginal vault of a breeding bitch with an infertility problem, these microorganisms may be at fault. However, 59% of healthy, fertile bitches had *Mycoplasma* recovered from vaginal swabs (Bjurstrom and Linde-Forsberg, 1992a). Management includes isolation of the animal and tetracycline or chloramphenicol therapy for 10 to 14 days (Lein, 1986).

Viral Infections

Viral infections, specifically herpesvirus (see Chapter 24), have been isolated in dogs with vaginitis, abortion, and stillbirths. However, viral infections as a cause of vaginitis are not well documented. Moreover, viral cultures are not yet widely available to practitioners. Thus the diagnosis of viral vaginitis remains difficult to prove, and its incidence is not yet appreciated.

REFERENCES

Allen WE: Infertility in the bitch. In Practice 1:22, 1986.
Allen WE, Dagnall GJR: Some observations on the aerobic bacterial flora of the genital tract of the dog and bitch. J Small Anim Pract 23:325, 1982.
Baba E, et al: Vaginal and uterine microflora of adult dogs. Am J Vet Res 44:606, 1983.
Bjurstrom L, Linde-Forsberg C: Long-term study of aerobic bacteria of the genital tract in breeding bitches. Am J Vet Res 53:665, 1992a.
Bjurstrom L, Linde-Forsberg C: Long-term study of aerobic bacteria of the genital tract in stud dogs. Am J Vet Res 53:670, 1992b.
Crawford JT, Adams WM: Influence of vestibulovaginal stenosis, pelvic bladder, and recessed vulva on response to treatment for clinical signs of lower urinary tract disease in dogs: 38 cases (1990-1999). J Am Vet Med Assoc 221:995, 2002.
Davies JV, Read HM: Urethral tumors in dogs. J Small Anim Pract 31:131, 1990.
Doig PA, et al: The genital mycoplasma and ureaplasma flora of healthy and diseased dogs. Can J Comp Med 45:233, 1981.
Greene JA: Episiotomy and episiostomy. In Bojrab MJ (ed): Current Techniques in Small Animal Surgery. Philadelphia, Lea & Febiger, 1983, p 357.

Harvey, M: Conditions of the non-pregnant female. *In* Simpson GM, England GCW, Harvey M (eds): BSAVA Manual of Small Animal Reproduction and Neonatology. United Kingdom, BSAVA, 1998, p 35.

Herron MA: Tumors of the canine genital system. JAAHA 19:981, 1983.

Holt PE, Sayle B: Congenital vestibulovaginal stenosis in the bitch. J Small Anim Pract 22:67, 1981.

Johnson CA: Uterine disease. *In* Ettinger SJ (ed): Textbook of Veterinary Internal Medicine, 2nd ed. Philadelphia, WB Saunders Co, 1989a, p 1801.

Johnson CA: Vaginal disorders. *In* Ettinger SJ (ed): Textbook of Veterinary Internal Medicine, 2nd ed. Philadelphia, WB Saunders Co, 1989b, p 1809.

Johnson CA: Diagnosis and treatment of chronic vaginitis in the bitch. Vet Clin North Am [Small Anim Pract] 21:523, 1991.

Johnston SD: Diagnostic and therapeutic approach to infertility in the bitch. JAVMA 176:1335, 1980.

Johnston SD: Vaginal prolapse. *In* Kirk RW (ed): Current Veterinary Therapy X. Philadelphia, WB Saunders Co, 1989, p 1302.

Kyles AE, et al: Vestibulovaginal stenosis in dogs: 18 cases (1987-1995). J Am Vet Med Assoc 209:1889, 1996.

Lein DH: Examination of the bitch for breeding soundness. *In* Kirk RW (ed): Current Veterinary Therapy VIII. Philadelphia, WB Saunders Co, 1983, p 909.

Lein DH: Canine mycoplasma, ureaplasma, and bacterial infertility. *In* Kirk RW (ed): Current Veterinary Therapy IX. Philadelphia, WB Saunders Co, 1986, p 1240.

Lein DH: Mycoplasma infertility in the dog: Diagnosis and treatment. Proceedings of the Annual Meeting of the Society for Theriogenology, 1989, p 307.

Lightner BA, et al: Episioplasty for the treatment of perivulvar dermatitis or recurrent urinary tract infections in dogs with excessive perivulvar skin folds: 31 cases (1983-2000). J Am Vet Med Assoc 219:1577, 2001.

Magne ML, et al: Urinary tract carcinoma involving the canine vagina and vestibule. JAVMA 21:767, 1985.

Manothaiudom K, Johnston SD: Clinical approach to vaginal/vestibular masses in the bitch. Vet Clin North Am [Small Anim Pract] 21:509, 1991.

Mathews KG: Surgery of the canine vagina and vulva. Vet Clin North Am (Small Anim Pract) 31: 271, 2001.

Maxie MG: The urinary system. *In* Jubb KVF, et al (eds): Pathology of Domestic Animals, 3rd ed. San Diego, Academic Press, 1985, p 398.

Olson PN, et al: Infertility in the bitch. *In* Kirk RW (ed): Current Veterinary Therapy VIII. Philadelphia, WB Saunders Co, 1983, p 925.

Olson PN, et al: The use and misuse of vaginal cultures in diagnosing reproductive diseases in the bitch. *In* Morrow DA (ed): Current Therapy in Theriogenology 2. Philadelphia, WB Saunders Co, 1986, p 469.

Pettit GD: Hyperplasia of the vaginal floor. *In* Bojrab MJ (ed): Current Techniques in Small Animal Surgery. Philadelphia, Lea & Febiger, 1983, p 352.

Romagnoli SE: A diagnostic approach to vulvar discharge in the canine patient. Proceedings of the Society for Theriogenology, 1989, p 295.

Root MV, et al: Vaginal septa in dogs: 15 cases (1983–1992). J Am Vet Med Assoc 206:56, 1995.

Rushmer RA: Vaginal hyperplasia and uterine prolapse. *In* Kirk RW (ed): Current Veterinary Therapy VII. Philadelphia, WB Saunders Co, 1980, p 1222.

Sahay PN, et al: Urinary incontinence in a bitch caused by vaginal fibroma. Vet Rec 116:76, 1985.

Thacher C, Bradley RL: Vulvar and vaginal tumors in the dog: A retrospective study. JAVMA 183:690, 1983.

Weller RE, Park JF: Vaginal leiomyoma and polyps in a Beagle dog. Calif Vet 37:6, 1983.

Withrow SJ, Susaneck SJ: Tumors of the canine female reproductive tract. *In* Morrow DA (ed): Current Therapy in Theriogenology 2. Philadelphia, WB Saunders Co, 1986, p 526.

Wood DS: Canine uterine prolapse. *In* Morrow DA (ed): Current Therapy in Theriogenology 2. Philadelphia, WB Saunders Co, 1986, p 510.

Wykes PM, Olson PN: Vagina, vestibule and vulva. *In* Slatter D (ed): Textbook of Small Animal Surgery, 2nd ed. Philadelphia, WB Saunders Co, 1993, pp 1308-1316.

Wykes PM, Soderberg SF: Congenital abnormalities of the canine vagina and vulva. JAAHA 19:995, 1983.

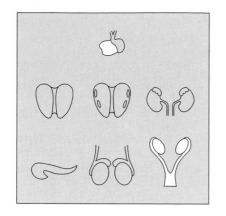

26

BRUCELLOSIS AND TRANSMISSIBLE VENEREAL TUMOR

BRUCELLOSIS

Infectious Agents

SPECIES. *Brucella canis* is one of six species of this nonmotile, gram-negative coccobacillus with a host range limited to domestic and wild canids. Of the six genus *Brucella* species that have been identified, dogs have been demonstrated to become infected by four: *B. melitensis, B. abortus, B. suis,* and *B. canis.* Dogs may occasionally be mechanical or biologic vectors for transmission to other animals or to humans. Except for *B. canis* infection, these infections are generally self-limiting.

INFECTION WITH *B. MELITENSIS, B. ABORTUS,* AND *B. SUIS.* These three species of *Brucella* have been reported to cause infections in the dog through either natural or experimental exposure. Natural infection occurs with ingestion of contaminated milk, meat, or aborted fetuses or the fetal membranes of infected livestock. Dogs appear to be relatively resistant to brucellosis because infection may result in no, few, or mild clinical signs. These infections may persist without clinical signs for varying periods after confirmation of the diagnosis (Pidgeon et al, 1987). Infected dogs usually show positive results on the conventional serologic tests used to diagnose brucellosis in livestock, such as the card or tube agglutination test (Barr et al, 1986; Nicoletti, 1989). Natural and experimentally induced infections have been transmitted to livestock (Kormendy and Nagy, 1982). Infected dogs therefore have the potential to infect not only cattle but also humans, and they pose a threat of longer duration of disease transmission in cattle than was once assumed (Johnston et al, 2001).

INFECTION WITH *B. CANIS.* Natural infection with *B. canis* appears to be limited to the Canidae family. Humans are accidental hosts, and infections are usually

relatively mild compared with the clinical signs in humans infected with other *Brucella* species. Livestock, primates, cats, and rabbits are quite resistant to experimental infection (Greene and George, 1984; Nicoletti, 1989).

Transmission of *Brucella canis*

TRANSMISSION BETWEEN DOGS. Infection can occur readily across mucous membranes, causing dogs to be infected by oronasal, conjunctival, or vaginal exposure. Transmission occurs readily when an uninfected bitch is mated with an infected male. Males can also acquire the disease from the female (Greene and George, 1984). Interestingly, in one study, when infected and uninfected dogs of the same gender were housed together for as long as 10 months, transmission did not occur (Hubbert et al, 1980). This suggests that urine and mucous membrane secretions are less important factors in the natural transmission of the bacteria. However, in a subsequent study, transmission between sexually mature male dogs was reported to occur after 4 to 6 months of cohabitation (Carmichael and Joubert, 1988).

Dogs without clinical signs can harbor *Brucella* organisms for prolonged periods. The time from exposure to bacteremia is usually 21 days (Meyer, 1983). After initiation of bacteremia, the organisms can become localized, causing continuous or recurrent bacteremia that lasts a few months to 3 to 4 years. Bacteria can be localized in the prostate or epididymis (or both) of an asymptomatic male. These focal infection sites can serve as a source of widespread dissemination if such a male is actively used in breeding. Venereal transmission probably occurs readily, even when low numbers of organisms are shed. Venereal transmission appears to occur most frequently when infected males are bred to susceptible females and somewhat less often when susceptible males are bred to infected females (Carmichael and Joubert, 1988).

In a kennel situation, a *Brucella*-infected aborting bitch is highly dangerous to *Brucella*-free dogs. Aborted placental tissues and fluids may contain huge numbers of organisms. Spread throughout a kennel is rapid, and persistent discharge of infected uterine secretions may continue for 4 to 6 weeks after a single abortion. Milk from infected bitches, which has been shown to contain abundant numbers of organisms, serves as an additional environmental contaminant. The effect on a breeding kennel can be devastating. With the potential for asymptomatic and prolonged bacteremia, blood transfusions also function as vectors for dissemination of brucellosis (Zoha and Walsh, 1982).

TRANSMISSION TO HUMANS. During the years since the initial isolation of *B. canis*, an extremely small number of cases have been reported in humans. Most of these individuals were laboratory personnel or kennel attendants who had repeated and/or massive exposure to the organism. However, a few people who had contact only with infected pets have contracted the organism. Therefore it is wise to advise but not frighten owners regarding the zoonotic potential of the disease (Johnston et al, 2001).

Clinical Signs of *Brucella canis*

NONSPECIFIC SIGNS. Dogs infected with *B. canis* are not always seriously ill. Deaths from such an infection have not been reported. Fever is an uncommon finding, presumably because the organism lacks endotoxin. Generalized lymph node enlargement, as a result of diffuse lymphoid and reticular cell hyperplasia, is common. The spleen may become enlarged, firm, and nodular. Inflammation of the liver may also occur.

Other systemic problems may be seen with *Brucella* infection. Discospondylitis of the thoracic and/or lumbar vertebrae has been reported (Smeak et al, 1987; Kerwin et al, 1992). Endophthalmitis and recurrent uveitis have been associated with brucellosis (Gwin et al, 1980; Johnson and Walker, 1992). A low-grade nonsuppurative meningitis (without clinical signs) was observed in dogs that were experimentally infected. Dogs with brucellosis can have arthritis or polyarthritis as the only clinical signs (Forbes, 1990). Most dogs show no clinical signs, or owners complain of subtle signs such as a poor hair coat, listlessness, and exercise intolerance (Gordon et al, 1985).

ABORTION AND VAGINAL DISCHARGE. The most common and obvious clinical sign of brucellosis in an otherwise healthy bitch is abortion between days 45 and 59 of gestation. The bitch may resorb fetuses and appear to be infertile because other clinical signs are absent. A bitch with brucellosis may abort puppies as early as day 30 of gestation or may carry pups nearly to term. A bitch with brucellosis also may deliver both living and dead fetuses. Surviving puppies are bacteremic for at least several months. Aborting bitches

may lose two or three litters in succession (Nicoletti, 1989).

Aborted puppies usually appear to be partly autolyzed. The vaginal discharge present in some bitches aborting their litters may be brown or greenish gray (Purswell, 1992). This discharge usually contains large numbers of organisms, and extreme caution should be taken to prevent humans or dogs from coming into contact with it. Prolonged vaginal discharge after abortion is characteristic of this condition. In addition to the infected vaginal discharge, mammary secretions, urine, saliva, nasal secretions, and semen may contain organisms and may cause transmission (Carmichael and Greene, 1990).

INFERTILITY. Apparent failure to conceive may be caused by canine brucellosis. In most cases bitches do conceive, but the fetuses are resorbed early or embryonic death and abortion go unnoticed by the owner. Upon examination, the placentas reveal focal coagulative necrosis of the chorionic villi, and numerous bacteria are present in the trophoblastic epithelial cells. Although none of the clinical signs of canine brucellosis is pathognomonic for the disease, it should always be considered in dogs examined for reproductive failure.

Diagnosis of *Brucella canis*

NONSPECIFIC FINDINGS. Hematologic and serum chemistry abnormalities in dogs with brucellosis are nonspecific, and the urinalysis results are usually unremarkable. Any inflammatory condition (involving the testes, intervertebral discs, joints, and the like) may be the result of brucellosis, but the disease is relatively uncommon. Even semen analyses and vaginal discharges from known diseased dogs show nonspecific changes, such as the head-to-head sperm agglutination with inflammatory cells described in the semen analyses from infected dogs (Greene and George, 1984).

SEROLOGIC TESTS

Background. Serologic tests for the presence of antibodies to cell wall and cytoplasmic antigens of *B. canis* are considered reliable, but such titers may not be detectable for 8 to 12 weeks. When bacteremia subsides after 30 to 60 weeks of infection, the serologic titer results may decline or become equivocal (Johnson et al, 1991). Therefore serologic titers, like many tests, are not perfect. Titers may fluctuate even with persistent bacteremia, and titer magnitudes do not reflect the stage of disease. Declining titers may not correctly reflect success of therapy (Table 26-1). Thus serologic testing may provide presumptive, but not definitive, diagnosis of canine brucellosis.

Two serologic tests are widely used in screening for the diagnosis of canine brucellosis: the slide agglutination test (SAT) and the tube agglutination test (TAT). Less commonly used tests are the agar gel immunodiffusion (AGID) test and the modified mercaptoethanol tube agglutination test. Direct culture of *Brucella* organisms is proof of infection, but bacteriologic confirmation is difficult.

TABLE 26–1   SEROLOGIC TESTS FOR *BRUCELLA CANIS*

Serologic Test	Antibody Affinity	Expected Positive	Comments
RSAT-ME	Cell wall	8–12 wk PI to 3 mn after abacteremic	Sensitive; common false +; few (1%) false negative; easy and fast
TAT	Cell wall	10–12 wk PI to 3 mn after abacteremic	False + as RSAT-ME semiquantitative
TAT-ME	Cell wall	As for TAT but longer to get positive result	More specific than TAT (somewhat)
AGID	Cell wall	12 wk PI up to 4 mn after abacteremic	More specific than RSAT, ME sensitive; complex
AGID	Cytoplasmic	12 wk PI up to 36 mn after abacteremic	Most specific, but not sensitive; detects chronic cases when other tests negative
ELISA	Cell wall	Unknown, expect similar to TAT	Specific, less sensitive than TAT, limited availability

From Johnson CA, et al: Diagnosis and control of *Brucella canis* in kennel situations. Proceedings of the Society for Theriogenology, 1991, p 236.
RSAT, Rapid slide agglutination test; *ME,* 2-mercaptoethanol test; *TAT,* tube agglutination test; *AGID,* agar gel immunodiffusion; *ELISA,* enzyme-linked immunosorbent assay; *mn,* month; *wk,* week; *PI,* postinfection; +, positive; –, negative.

Rapid Slide or Card Agglutination Tests (RSAT; RCAT). The RSAT (Canine Brucellosis Diagnosis Test Kit, made by Pitman-Moore, Washington Crossing, NJ; a version is also made by Synbiotics, San Diego, CA) is a rapid in-hospital presumptive screening test that can be used by practitioners to accurately identify *Brucella*-negative dogs. Because the test is widely available and practical, it is used much more often than culture protocols. The serum used for the test should be free of hemolysis. *B. ovis* is used as antigen because of its similarity to *B. canis.* The test is performed by mixing the patient's serum with a rose bengal–stained, heat-killed, *B. ovis* suspension on a glass slide. Agglutination of the bacteria is interpreted as suspicious for *B. canis* infection but is not by itself diagnostic (Greene and George, 1984).

The test is highly sensitive, and false-negative reactions are rare. However, when used according to the instructions, the kit identifies as many as 60% false-positive reactions. The false-positive results apparently are caused by cross-reactions between *B. ovis* antigen and antibodies to *Bordetella bronchiseptica, Pseudomonas* spp., a *Moraxella*-like organism, and other gram-negative bacteria (Greene and George, 1984). Therefore it may be stated with confidence that animals that do not show agglutination on the RSAT do not have brucellosis and that dogs that do show agglutination should be isolated and tested with the TAT.

A modification of the RSAT has been developed that uses 2-mercaptoethanol to reduce heterologous immunoglobulin M (IgM) agglutination (Badakhsh et al, 1982). This modification has been found to eliminate false-positive reactions (Nicoletti, 1989). However, the modified test could be falsely negative in the first few weeks after infection (Greene and George, 1984). An improved antigen was then described for the SAT; *B. ovis* antigen was replaced with *B. canis* (M–) cells, and the number of false-positive results declined (Carmichael and Joubert, 1987).

Tube Agglutination Test. The TAT is the most widely used serologic test for detecting antibodies to *B. canis* in dogs that have tested positive with the RSAT. In general, specific titers against *B. canis* are derived with this test. The TAT usually becomes positive by 2 to 4 weeks after exposure and concurrent bacteremia. The TAT is reliable, although test procedures may differ somewhat from laboratory to laboratory.

The test is performed by adding graded amounts of test serum to *B. canis* antigen solution to achieve different dilutions. The antigen solution is a suspension of heat-killed, washed *B. canis* organisms. A titer of 1:200 by the TAT is considered presumptive evidence of an active infection. Good correlations have been found between titers equal to or above 1:200 and recovery of the organism by blood cultures (Nicoletti and Chase, 1987b). A titer that is measurable but below 1:200 should be rechecked at least 2 weeks later.

The 2-mercaptoethanol tube agglutination test (2ME TAT) is similar to the TAT except for the addition of 2ME to the antigen solution. This is done in an attempt to increase test specificity. Obtaining positive titers with the TAT, after ME is added, may be delayed 1 to 2 weeks compared with the TAT, but there are fewer false-positive results (Greene and George, 1984; Nicoletti, 1989).

Although the SAT and TAT assess for the presence of agglutinating antibodies, the antibodies do not appear to protect the host producing them. Spontaneous recovery does occur after 1 to 3 years of infection, and these dogs are solidly immune to reinfection. Cell-mediated immunity does appear to be more important than humoral immunity. Agglutinating antibody titers decline to undetectable levels in recovered animals.

Specific antibiotic therapy may cause false-negative serologic results. For example, a 2-week regimen of tetracycline results in a period of abacteremia and a fall in antibody titer below significant levels. After therapy is stopped, bacteremia usually recurs and antibody titers rise.

Agar Gel Immunodiffusion Test. An AGID test using one or more antigens prepared by differing methods is available in some laboratories. The AGID test is recommended as an aid in confirming diagnoses suspected from RSAT, RCAT, or TAT results. The most specific but least sensitive AGID test used a protein antigen extracted from the cytoplasm of *B. canis* (Zoha and Carmichael, 1982). It was sensitive within 4 to 8 weeks of the onset of bacteremia and was positive for at least 12 months after the end of bacteremia, at times when other tests produced equivocal findings. The AGID test, however, may be negative in early infection when other tests would provide positive results (Nicoletti and Chase, 1987b). One advantage of the

AGID test is the rapid seroconversion from positive to negative that may be detected when a dog is successfully treated.

The test is not widely available because AGID antigens are not readily prepared free from cross-reacting lipopolysaccharides. Furthermore, immunodiffusion procedures are generally limited to laboratories with specialized facilities and specifically trained personnel (Nicoletti, 1989). In 1993 the American Association for Veterinary Diagnostic Laboratories agreed that the Cornell University Diagnostic Laboratory would serve as a *B. canis* reference laboratory. Therefore serum samples from dogs that test positive on the RSAT, RCAT, or TAT should be sent to this laboratory for further testing. The Cornell diagnostic laboratory reevaluates the serum with the AGID test using cytoplasmic protein antigens that are more unique and specific to *Brucella* species than cell wall antigens (Johnston et al, 2001). However, the AGID test result may be positive in dogs that have been exposed to *B. ovis*, *B. abortus*, or *B. suis* because some of these cytoplasmic antigens appear to be shared among the *Brucella* species (Johnson and Walker, 1992).

The disadvantage of the AGID test is that it is less sensitive than the RSAT, RCAT, and TAT in detecting early infections. The AGID test result may not become positive until 4 weeks after these other test results are positive. Blood cultures early in infection may test positive, but negative culture results should never be used to rule out brucellosis.

CULTURE. The definitive diagnosis of canine brucellosis is established by recovery of the organism from the animal. Although infected dogs may be bacteremic for 1 to 3 years, the number of organisms circulating is often small. Confirmation of infection with direct culture is difficult in living dogs with chronic disease because the organism may not be present in specimens obtained for culture. Nevertheless, isolation of organisms is not only proof of infection but valuable in kennel situations (Table 26-2).

Organisms can be recovered from a variety of tissues. Blood culture is the most practical test and it has the best chance of yielding positive growth from an infected dog. A bacteremia can first be demonstrated 2 to 4 weeks after oral exposure, and this condition may persist for as long as 2 years (Greene and George, 1984). Because the bacteria are located primarily in leukocytes, direct plating onto solid media is not reliable. Instead, it has been recommended that 5 ml of peripheral blood be added to 50 ml of tryptose broth and the mixture incubated at 37° C for approximately 9 days. Subcultures should be made onto tryptose agar on days 3, 6, and 9, and negative cultures should be discarded (Nicoletti, 1989). The organisms are usually identified by colonial morphology (rough or mucoid and translucent) and by agglutination using specific antiserum.

The organism has been isolated on solid media from milk, urine, vaginal discharges, semen, and placental and fetal tissue. It is usually necessary to use antibiotics to prevent overgrowth from contaminating organisms. The tissues most likely to be culture

TABLE 26–2 CONFIRMATION OF *BRUCELLA CANIS* INFECTION

Material To Culture	Time To Culture	Likely Results
Postabortion discharge	Whenever present	+++
Placenta	Whenever present	++
Abortus	Whenever present	May be negative
Semen	3–11 wk PI	+++
	12–60 wk PI	Lower numbers
	>60 wk PI	–
Blood	5–30 wk PI	"100%" +
	After 30 wk	Intermittent
	6–12 mn PI	>80% +
	28–48 mn PI	50–80% +
	48–58 mn PI	25–50% +
	>58 mn PI	<25% +
Epididymis	35–60 wk PI	50–100% +
	>100 wk PI	–
Urine	8–30 + wk PI	More organisms shed by male than female
Prostate	Up to 64 wk	Usually +
Lymph node, spleen, marrow	When bacteremic:	Usually +
	When abacteremic:	+/–
Eye	With uveitis	+++
Intervertebral disc	Discospondylitis	+/–

From Johnson CA, et al: Diagnosis and control of *Brucella canis* in kennel situations. Proceedings of the Society for Theriogenology, 1991, p 236. Used with permission.
PI, Postinfection; *wk*, weeks; *mn*, months; +, positive; –, negative.

positive on necropsy are lymph nodes and spleen. Other potential sites worth culturing are the prostate gland, testes, epididymides, bone marrow, and uterus. Specific infection sites, such as with discospondylitis or eye lesions, should be cultured. Negative culture results do not rule out the disease.

Treatment of *Brucella canis* Infection

BACKGROUND. The various investigators who have attempted to treat *B. canis* infections have reached similar conclusions. Although brucellosis may not in itself be life threatening, an infected dog should not be used as a breeding animal and does have the potential to be a source of infection for other dogs and other species, including humans. *B. canis* is susceptible to a variety of antibiotics, but therapy has resulted in failures or relapses in infection (Table 26-3). Treatment failure may occur because of the intracellular location of *Brucella* organisms and the inability of antibiotics to reach this site. For these reasons, veterinarians have not been optimistic about permanent cures. Aborting females may subsequently produce normal litters with or without treatment, but they may transmit the infection to their offspring. Treated males may have localized infection in the prostate gland and may continue to shed organisms (Greene and George, 1984). However, appropriate antibiotic regimens have led to successful results in many dogs, based on posttreatment serologic and/or bacteriologic results.

The owners of dogs infected with *Brucella* sp. have several options, including a commitment to repeated

TABLE 26–3   RESULTS OF SELECTED STUDIES ON CHEMOTHERAPY OF CANINE BRUCELLOSIS

Drug	Daily Dose	Route	Duration of Treatment	Success Ratio	Author
Tetracycline	10 mg/kg	Oral	14 days	0:5	Flores-Castro and Carmichael, 1981
Concurrent					
Tetracycline	10 mg/kg	Oral	14 days	0:6	Same
Sulfadimethoxine	23 mg/kg	Oral	14 days		
Concurrent					
Minocycline	10 mg/kg	Oral	14 days	15:18	Same
Streptomycin	4.5 mg/kg	IM	7 days		
Minocycline	10 mg/kg	Oral	14 days	3:11	Same
Concurrent					
Oxytetracycline	20 mg/kg	IM	4 inj over 3 wk	19:24	Zoha and Walsh, 1982
Streptomycin	30 mg/kg	IM	1st 7 days		
Successive					
Tetracycline	60 mg/kg	Oral	14 days		
Streptomycin	22 mg/kg	IM	14 days	0:6	Johnson et al, 1982
Trimethoprim- sulfadiazine	30 mg/kg	Oral	14 days		
Concurrent					
Tetracycline	10 mg/kg	Oral	30 days		Nicoletti and Chase, 1987a
Streptomycin	3.4 mg/kg	IM	days 1–7, 24–30	15:20	

courses of therapy, neutering, and euthanasia. Some investigators have consistently recommended euthanasia as the only safe alternative, whereas others are not that aggressive. Certainly the fact that immunocompromised people, pregnant women, and children should avoid exposure to such dogs limits treatment alternatives. However, most people who have become infected were laboratory workers exposed specifically to this bacteria. Symptoms in people include fever, sweats, weakness, weight loss, headache, lymphadenopathy, and splenomegaly. Agglutination tests that use only *B. abortus* antigen produce a negative result for humans infected with *B. canis* (Munford et al, 1975).

TETRACYCLINES AND AMINOGLYCOSIDES. Combination therapy with tetracyclines and aminoglycosides offers the best chance of eliminating infection. Aminoglycosides such as gentamicin are administered at a dosage of 2.2 mg/kg given intramuscularly once daily for the first week; doxycycline or minocycline is given at a high dosage (55 mg/kg bid) for 2 weeks. Less efficacy has been seen with the substitution of tetracycline or chloramphenicol, but such regimens are less expensive and therefore more practical.

ORAL TETRACYCLINE AND INJECTABLE STREPTOMYCIN. A treatment regimen used to control a *Brucella* outreak has been reviewed. The regimen consisted of tetracycline (10 mg/kg PO tid) for 30 days, with once-daily streptomycin (15 mg/kg IM) given on days 1 through 7 and days 24 through 30. Twenty of 28 dogs were treated, and 15 of the 20 were considered cured with one course of medication. Four of the five remaining dogs were retreated, and two of those four were also cured. The authors believed that there was justification for simultaneously treating seronegative and seropositive dogs when attempting to control an outbreak. Furthermore, serologic test results were considered useful for evaluating treatment, because titers decreased rapidly with successful responses but then became elevated again in dogs with relapsing infection (Nicoletti and Chase, 1987a; Nicoletti, 1989).

INJECTABLE TETRACYCLINE AND STREPTOMYCIN. In a study of 24 infected dogs, treatment consisted of four weekly intramuscular injections of oxytetracycline (Liquamycin La200; Pfizer, Irvine, CA) at a dosage of 20 mg/kg and daily intramuscular injections of streptomycin (15 mg/kg) for the first 7 days (Zoha and Walsh, 1982). Six months after completion of therapy, 19 of the 24 dogs had negative results on serologic and culture testing.

MINOCYCLINE. In extensive studies on 80 experimentally infected dogs, 13 different treatment regimens were evaluated in groups of three or more dogs each. The best results were documented after 14 days of administration of minocycline hydrochloride at a total daily dose of 10 mg/kg plus a total daily dose of streptomycin at 4.5 mg/kg, divided twice daily, for 7 days. On the basis of blood and tissue cultures at the time of euthanasia, 6 to 28 weeks after completing treatment, 83% of the dogs so treated were considered cured. Minocycline alone was not considered effective (Flores-Castro and Carmichael, 1981).

TETRACYCLINE, STREPTOMYCIN, AND TRIMETHOPRIMSULFADIAZINE. In one study, breeding bitches with spontaneous *B. canis* infection were treated with a combination of tetracycline, dihydrostreptomycin, and trimethoprim-sulfadiazine. Although the therapy did not eradicate the infection, it did prevent abortion (Johnson et al, 1982).

SUMMARY. Veterinarians must be candid when discussing this disease with the owners of infected dogs. Therapy, together with the necessary monitoring, may be expensive, and success is not predictable. Moreover, success or failure is difficult to confirm. The breeding bitch in a kennel situation should be permanently separated from other dogs to prevent spread of the bacteria. If euthanasia of a pet is unacceptable, spaying or castration should be recommended. Antibiotic therapy should also be strongly suggested in an attempt to protect other animals as well as the owners. However, a neutered and treated dog may still remain a source of infection to humans. Owners should be made aware of the zoonotic nature of brucellosis, the clinical signs of the disease in humans and dogs, and our lack of knowledge about how the disorder is passed to humans. They also should be urged to contact their physician if they think they have contracted the disease.

Prevention and Control of *Brucella canis*

Currently, there is no vaccine to provide protection against canine brucellosis. Prevention, therefore, depends on avoiding exposure to any infected dog. In a disease-free kennel all new additions should be isolated for at least 1 month. These dogs should have two negative *Brucella* titers 1 month apart before they are allowed into the kennel. Careful hygiene practices should be followed to avoid contamination in travel between facilities.

Breeding programs can involve dogs from a wide geographic area. It is important to instruct owners to use tested *Brucella*-free dogs. Dogs in active breeding programs should be tested at least every 6 months. Preferably, a dog is slide tested *before each breeding.* No *Brucella*-positive bitch should be bred, even with artificial insemination, because of the potential for spreading the disease via the vaginal discharge, milk, and living puppies.

If an infection is identified in a kennel situation, the dog demonstrated to have brucellosis may not be the source of infection to the colony. The *entire* colony must be evaluated, and all dogs with positive serologic test results should be isolated and retested after 1 month. Dogs should remain isolated until negative test results are obtained. Dogs that persistently test positive should be removed from the kennel. All modes of infection must be considered, because the organism readily penetrates any mucous membrane, allowing infection to follow oral, conjunctival, or venereal routes. The most important sources of infection are vaginal discharges, aborted material, semen, and urine. Transmission of aerosolized organisms can occur. *Brucella* organisms are reportedly killed by quaternary ammonium compounds and iodophors (Johnson et al, 1991).

It is important to remember that some tests do not become positive for weeks to months after infection, and testing must continue on a monthly basis until all animals with a positive result have been removed. The testing may need to continue indefinitely. All dogs in a colony must be subject to equal suspicion if the problem is to be eradicated.

TRANSMISSIBLE VENEREAL TUMOR

Definition

Transmissible venereal tumor (TVT) is a naturally occurring neoplastic disease in the dog that usually involves the external genitalia and is typically trans-

mitted at coitus (Cohen, 1985). There appears to be no heritable breed predisposition, and the disease is prevalent worldwide (Harmelin et al, 2001). Enzootic areas for TVT include the southern United States, southeastern Europe, Central and South America, Japan, the Far East, the Middle East, and parts of Africa. Stray dogs serve as the reservoir for this problem, which is seen most frequently in temperate climates and in large cities of the United States (Brown et al, 1981).

Etiology

The cell of origin of TVT is unknown, but the condition is assumed to be an undifferentiated round cell neoplasm of reticuloendothelial origin (Sandunsky et al, 1987; Mozos et al, 1996; Marchal et al, 1997). TVT is considered an example of a naturally occurring allograft (i.e., transplantation of cells between individuals of one species). Transmission is achieved by transplantation of viable tumor cells to a susceptible host. It is assumed that transmission is the result of exfoliated cells from the donor being "seeded" into the damaged genital mucosa of the recipient. A susceptible dog may contract TVT by licking the genitals of an infected dog and then licking its own genitals.

The first successful experimental transplantation of a tumor, in 1876, involved TVT, and transmission by coitus was reported in 1898. Homotransplantation of TVT using subcutaneous and intravenous routes has been widely reported. A viral cause has been suggested by some researchers, but other investigators have failed to demonstrate the presence of viral particles. A cell-free infiltrate of the tumor has not consistently resulted in transmission of the mass. Additional evidence against a viral cause is that host isoantigens cannot be demonstrated on TVT cell surfaces (Harmelin et al, 2001).

Molecular studies have revealed a consistent insertion of LINE transposable genetic element upstream to the *c-myc* oncogene, indicating that TVT in different geographic locations most likely developed from a common origin and has been continually transmitted by cell transplantation (Ameriglio et al, 1991). Other evidence supporting the allograft nature of transmission versus an oncogenic virus is the consistent number of chromosomes found in TVT cells. Cells infected with an oncogenic virus have varying numbers of chromosomes, whereas TVT cells consistently contain 50 chromosomes and similar quantities of DNA (Brown et al, 1981).

Signalment

TVT is most commonly diagnosed among free-roaming dogs. It therefore should not be surprising that most dogs described as having TVT in the United States have been large-breed dogs. In one study, 34 of 41 dogs weighed more than 20 kg, and in another study 26 of 29 dogs weighed more than 18 kg (Calvert

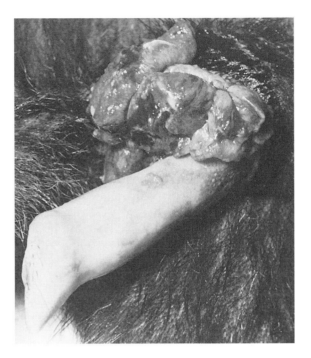

FIGURE 26-1. Large transmissible venereal tumor at the base of the penis. (Courtesy Dr. Jane Turrel, Davis, CA.)

et al, 1982; Rogers et al, 1998). The disease is most common in sexually intact dogs of either sex. The mean and median ages have been 4 to 5 years of age in each recent study (Brown et al, 1980; Calvert et al, 1982; Rogers et al, 1998).

Clinical Signs

TVTs are usually seen on the external genitalia of males and females (Figs. 26-1 and 26-2). The masses consist of solitary or multiple nodules that are irregular and friable and that may ulcerate. Because of the fragile nature of these tumors and their location, the most common clinical signs are bloody genital discharge, a visible mass, and deformation of external genitalia (Boscos, 1988; Rogers, 1997). In one study involving 29 dogs, of the genital lesions, 16 were found on the penis and prepuce and 11 involved the vagina and vulva (two dogs had lesions in the nasal cavity). It would be quite uncommon for TVT to cause urinary obstruction (Rogers et al, 1998).

In this group of dogs, because the nasal cavity was the primary site in two cases (in addition to the 27 cases in which the external genitalia was the primary site), additional signs included hemorrhagic discharge from the external nares and an abnormal "oral" odor. The mean time from the onset of clinical signs to diagnosis was 6.5 months, the median was 2 months, and the range was 2 weeks to 4 years (Rogers et al, 1998).

Such tumors may have a cauliflower-like shape, but they have also been reported to be pedunculated, nodular, papillary, or multilobulated. The tumor has been diagnosed in numerous extragenital locations with or without genital involvement. Some of these locations are the skin, face, nasal passages, and buccal cavities, as well as in and around the eyes. Metastasis is uncommon, and when it does occur, it is usually to the superficial inguinal and external iliac lymph nodes, although distant node involvement is possible. Metastases may also occur to the skin, subcutaneous sites, spleen, liver, brain, eyes, and lungs (Rogers et al, 1998; Ferreira et al, 2000). Metastasis to the eye or brain carries a poor prognosis.

In the bitch, TVT usually is recognized as a solitary mass on the vaginal wall. However, these masses have been seen to spread to the vestibule, vulva, labia, cervix, and uterus. The tumor may be gray or

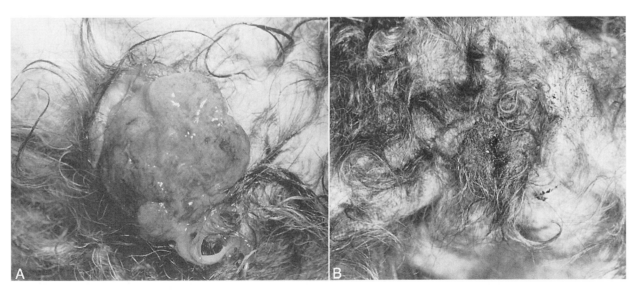

FIGURE 26-2. Large transmissible venereal tumor protruding from the vulva (A) and after radiation therapy (B). (Courtesy Dr. Jane Turrel, Davis, CA.)

pinkish gray. In males, in addition to the penis and prepuce, these tumors are also frequently identified in the oral or nasal cavities or both. The latter areas are involved as a result of prebreeding licking and/or smelling of the external genitalia of an infected bitch.

Diagnosis

The diagnosis of transmissible venereal tumor is initially suspected after a review of the history and physical examination. Examination of stained tissue impression smears is considered an accurate method of diagnosis, finding large, homogeneous sheets of large, round to oval cells with prominent nucleoli, scant cytoplasm, and multiple clear cytoplasmic vacuoles, often arranged in chains (Fig. 26-3). Microvilli are present, which interconnect the individual cells, making the cells adherent in sheets.

Tissue may be formalin fixed and then stained with hematoxylin and eosin. However, formalin fixation is said to distort the tumor cells and make the diagnosis difficult. The tumor can be histologically confused with histiocytoma, lymphoma, neuroblastoma, and reticulum cell sarcoma. Other methods of diagnosis are not commonly used. Tissue can be examined by electron microscopy, which reveals typical cell projections. Finally, an attempt could be made to transplant the tumor to susceptible dogs.

Treatment

RADIATION THERAPY. Radiation therapy is an effective modality if appropriate facilities are available. In one study, 18 of 18 dogs were successfully treated, and a single dose of radiation was effective in most dogs (Thrall, 1982). In a more recent report, 15 dogs were treated only with cobalt-60. Each received three fractions on a Monday-Wednesday-Friday schedule to an average minimum dose of 15 Gy (range, 10 to 18 Gy). Complete remission was obtained in each of these 15 dogs. No adverse reactions to the irradiation were noted. Response to therapy was observed as early as 48 hours after the first fraction was administered and was complete in all dogs within 1 month (Rogers et al, 1998). Radiation appeared to be effective for both genital and extragenital sites, even if the masses had been chemoresistant. Radiation was effective in the treatment of solitary tumors but was also curative at metastatic sites and for lesions resistant to vincristine and doxorubicin chemotherapy (Rogers et al, 1998).

A relatively low dose of radiation is needed to cure TVT. Possible explanations include interphase cell death, which does not require cell reproduction, as can be seen with lymphoid tissues. Another explanation for obvious sensitivity could be inherent radio-responsiveness as a result of the typical high mitotic index of TVTs. An average dose of 15 Gy was quite effective; however, the authors point out that lower doses may be adequate for some dogs (Rogers et al, 1998). The only disadvantage of using radiation as the "treatment of choice" would be access to facilities. However, such facilities are quickly becoming almost universally available in the United States.

SINGLE-DRUG THERAPY: VINCRISTINE SULFATE. Forty-one dogs with TVT were treated only with vincristine (0.025 mg/kg IV weekly to 1 mg maximum dose). Thirty-nine of the 41 dogs experienced complete response, one had greater than 90% reduction in tumor

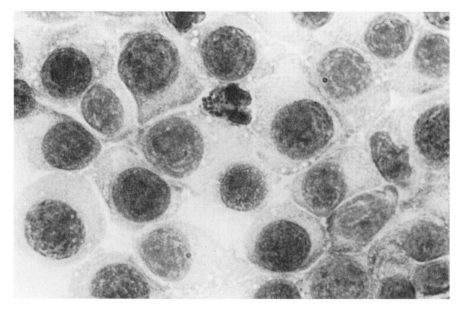

FIGURE 26-3. Impression smear obtained from a vaginal mass caused by a transmissible venereal tumor in a bitch.

volume, and one dog had a 25% reduction in volume of the TVT. In the 39 dogs experiencing a complete response, two to seven weekly injections (average, 3.3) were required. Nine dogs had transient side effects (Calvert et al, 1982).

In two subsequent studies, vincristine was administered intravenously (0.5 mg/m^2 body surface area [BSA]) weekly to a total of 25 dogs for 4 to 8 weeks or until a clinical response was noted. Complete remission was observed in 24 of the 25 dogs (Amber et al, 1990; Rogers et al, 1998). After a disease-free interval of 8 months, local recurrence of an intranasal TVT mass was diagnosed (Rogers et al, 1998). Vincristine appears to be an excellent mode of therapy and the medical treatment of choice (radiation is the overall treatment of choice). Chemotherapy is the treatment of choice for metastatic multifocal TVT.

Doxorubicin. If vincristine fails, the clinician should consider therapy with doxorubicin (30 mg/m^2 IV q3wk) until the tumor is gone. The average number of doxorubicin injections required is two.

SINGLE-DRUG THERAPY: CYCLOPHOSPHAMIDE AND METHOTREXATE. Forty-eight dogs with TVT were recently evaluated with a variety of treatment regimens. In four dogs, oral cyclophosphamide (50 mg/m^2 BSA) given 4 days per week for 6 weeks failed to elicit a response. Ten dogs received intravenous cyclophosphamide (50 mg/m^2 BSA) 4 days per week for 6 weeks. Two of the 10 dogs had a partial remission. Eight dogs were treated with oral methotrexate (2.5 mg/m^2 BSA) every other day for 6 weeks. No therapeutic response was observed in any of the eight dogs. Adverse reactions to the cyclophosphamide and methotrexate included anorexia, vomiting, diarrhea, and weight loss (Amber et al, 1990).

COMBINATION CHEMOTHERAPY. Various chemotherapy regimens have been used. In one report, 30 dogs with TVT were treated with combination chemotherapy consisting of vincristine (0.0125 or 0.025 mg/kg IV weekly), cyclophosphamide (1 mg/kg PO daily or 50 mg/m^2 PO on even-numbered days), and methotrexate (0.3 to 0.5 mg/kg IV weekly or 2.5 mg/m^2 PO on odd-numbered days). Four to six treatment periods consisting of 4 to 6 weeks each, on average, were needed to reach a point at which no evidence of disease remained. Of 30 dogs, 28 (93%) had a complete remission, 1 (3.5%) had a partial response, and 1 (3.3%) had a minimal response. Transient side effects of the treatment consisted of anorexia, vomiting, diarrhea, and neutropenia in six of the 30 dogs (Brown et al, 1980).

SURGERY. Small tumors can be surgically removed, but recurrence is common. Also, most tumors are non-resectable or would require extensive surgery at the time of diagnosis, and the risk of seeding surrounding tissue during surgery negates the chances of success. In a study of 35 dogs with naturally occurring TVT, the combined recurrence rate was 33% after attempts at surgical excision. However, some of the recurrences were at different sites, implying metastasis in at least some of the dogs (Amber and Henderson, 1982).

Surgery is not recommended (Boscos, 1988; Ogilvie and Moore, 1995).

SPONTANEOUS REMISSION. Before treatment is instituted, the clinician must realize that spontaneous regression of these tumor masses may occur naturally. In one report, 16% of dogs experimentally transplanted with TVT had spontaneous regression. Other dogs had alternate periods of progressive growth and regression. If complete regression occurs, regrowth is unlikely, and the dog is immune to all challenges with tumor cells except in exceedingly large volumes. The overall incidence of spontaneous TVT regression is not readily available from a review of the literature, although one recent report described no spontaneous remission in six dogs (Amber et al, 1990). However, because the veterinarian cannot rely on spontaneous regression of these tumor masses, therapy should be attempted.

REFERENCES

Amber EI, Henderson RA: Canine transmissible venereal tumor: Evaluation of surgical excision of primary and metastatic lesions in Zaria-Nigeria. J Am Anim Hosp Assoc 18:350, 1982.

Amber EI, et al: Single-drug chemotherapy of canine transmissible venereal tumor with cyclophosphamide, methotrexate, or vincristine. J Vet Intern Med 4:144, 1990.

Ameriglio EN, et al: Identity of rearranged LINE/c-MYC junction sequences specific for the canine transmissible venereal tumor. Proc Natl Acad Sci USA 88:8136, 1991.

Badakhsh FF, et al: Improved rapid slide agglutination test for presumptive diagnosis of canine brucellosis. J Clin Microbiol 15:286, 1982.

Barr SC, et al: *Brucella suis* biotype I infection in a dog. J Am Vet Med Assoc 189:686, 1986.

Boscos C: Canine transmissible venereal tumor: Clinical observations and treatment. Anim Familia 3:10, 1988.

Brown NO, et al: Chemotherapeutic management of transmissible venereal tumors in 30 dogs. J Am Vet Med Assoc 176:983, 1980.

Brown NO, et al: Transmissible venereal tumor in the dog. Calif Vet 3:6, 1981.

Calvert CA, et al: Vincristine for treatment of transmissible venereal tumor in the dog. J Am Vet Med Assoc 181:163, 1982.

Carmichael LE, Greene CE: Canine brucellosis. *In* Greene CE (ed): Infectious Disease of the Dog and Cat. Philadelphia, WB Saunders, 1990, p 573.

Carmichael LE, Joubert JC: A rapid slide agglutination test for the serodiagnosis of *Brucella canis* infection that employs a variant (M-) organism as antigen. Cornell Vet 77:3, 1987.

Carmichael LE, Joubert JC: Transmission of *Brucella canis* by contact exposure. Cornell Vet 78:63, 1988.

Cohen D: The canine transmissible venereal tumor: A unique result of tumor progression. Adv Cancer Res 43:75, 1985.

Ferreira AJA, et al: Brain and ocular metastases from a transmissible venereal tumour in a dog. J Small Anim Pract 41:165, 2000.

Flores-Castro R, Carmichael LE: *Brucella canis* infection in dogs. Rev Latinoam Microbiol 23:75, 1981.

Forbes LB: *Brucella abortus* infection in 14 farm dogs. J Am Vet Med Assoc 196:911, 1990.

Gordon JC, et al: Canine brucellosis in a household. J Am Vet Med Assoc 186:695, 1985.

Greene CE, George LW: Canine brucellosis. *In* Greene CE (ed): Clinical Microbiology and Infectious Diseases of the Dog and Cat. Philadelphia, WB Saunders, 1984, p 646.

Gwin RM, et al: Ocular lesions associated with *Brucella canis* infection in a dog. J Am Anim Hosp Assoc 16:607, 1980.

Harmelin A, et al: Use of a murine xenograft model for canine transmissible venereal tumor. Am J Vet Res 62:907, 2001.

Hubbert NL, et al: Canine brucellosis: Comparison of clinical manifestations with serologic test results. J Am Vet Med Assoc 177:168, 1980.

Johnson CA, Walker RD: Clinical signs and diagnosis of *Brucella canis* infection. Compend Contin Educ Pract Vet 14:763, 1992.

Johnson CA, et al: Effect of combined antibiotic therapy on fertility in brood bitches infected with *Brucella canis*. J Am Vet Med Assoc 180:1330, 1982.

Johnson CA, et al: Diagnosis and control of *Brucella canis* in kennel situations. Proceedings of the Society for Theriogenology, 1991, p 236.

Johnston SD, Root Kustritz MV, Olson PNS: Canine and Feline Theriogenology. Philadelphia, WB Saunders, 2001, p 88.

Kerwin SC, et al: Discospondylitis associated with *Brucella canis* infection in dogs: 14 cases (1980-1991). J Am Vet Med Assoc 201:1253, 1992.

Kormendy B, Nagy GY: The supposed involvement of dogs carrying *Brucella suis* in the spread of swine brucellosis. Acta Vet Acad Hung 30:3, 1982.

Marchal T, et al: Immunophenotype of the canine transmissible venereal tumor. Vet Immunol Immunopathol 57:1, 1997.

Meyer ME: Update on canine brucellosis. Mod Vet Pract 64:987, 1983.

Mozos E, et al: Immunohistochemical characterization of canine transmissible venereal tumor. Vet Pathol 33:257, 1996.

Munford RS, et al: Human disease caused by *Brucella canis*. Journal of the American Medical Association 231:1267, 1975.

Nicoletti P: Diagnosis and treatment of canine brucellosis. *In* Kirk RW (ed): Current Veterinary Therapy X. Philadelphia, WB Saunders, 1989, p 1317.

Nicoletti P, Chase A: The use of antibiotics to control canine brucellosis. Compend Contin Educ Pract Vet 9:1063, 1987a.

Nicoletti P, Chase A: An evaluation of methods to diagnose *Brucella canis* infection in dogs. Compend Contin Educ Pract Vet 9:1071, 1987b.

Ogilvie GK, Moore AS: Tumors of the reproductive system. *In* Ogilvie GK, Moore AS (eds): Managing the Veterinary Cancer Patient. Trenton, NJ, Veterinary Learning Systems, 1995, p 415.

Pidgeon GL, et al: Experimental infection of dogs with *Brucella abortus*. Cornell Vet 77:339, 1987.

Purswell BJ: Differential diagnosis of canine abortion. *In* Kirk RW, Bonagura JD (eds): Current Veterinary Therapy XI. Philadelphia, WB Saunders, 1992, p 925.

Rogers KS: Transmissible venereal tumor. Compend Contin Educ Pract Vet 19:1036, 1997.

Rogers KS, et al: Transmissible venereal tumor: A retrospective study of 29 cases. J Am Anim Hosp Assoc 34:463, 1998.

Sandunsky GE, et al: Diagnostic immunohistochemistry of canine round cell tumors. Vet Pathol 24:495, 1987.

Smeak DD, et al: *Brucella canis* osteomyelitis in two dogs with total hip replacements. J Am Vet Med Assoc 191:986, 1987.

Thrall DE: Orthovoltage radiotherapy of canine transmissible venereal tumors. Vet Radiol 23:217, 1982.

Zoha SJ, Carmichael LE: Serological responses of dogs to cell wall and internal antigens of *Brucella canis*. Vet Microbiol 17:35, 1982.

Zoha SJ, Walsh R: Effect of a two-stage antibiotic regimen on dogs naturally infected with *Brucella canis*. J Am Vet Med Assoc 180:1474, 1982.

CANINE MALE REPRODUCTION

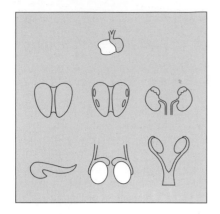

27

CLINICAL AND DIAGNOSTIC EVALUATION OF THE MALE REPRODUCTIVE TRACT

HISTORY

Regardless of an owner's primary concern with his or her pet's reproductive soundness, the veterinarian should always obtain a thorough and complete history with respect to all organ systems. Disorders of other organ systems may secondarily affect the reproductive tract through direct extension of infections or neoplasia or indirectly by altering the normal secretory patterns of testosterone, follicle-stimulating hormone (FSH), luteinizing hormone (LH), or gonadotropin-releasing hormone (GnRH). In addition, the exogenous administration of drugs (e.g., glucocorticoids), chronic stress, trauma, or previous systemic illness can affect the function of the reproductive tract. Failure to obtain a thorough history may allow these influencing factors to go unrecognized, potentially resulting in perpetuation of a disorder and ultimately causing frustration for the clinician and owner, as well as possibly harming the dog. After evaluation of all potential problem areas, a rational diagnostic and therapeutic plan can be formulated.

The types of historical questions about the reproductive system depend, in part, on the owner's reason for presenting the dog to the veterinarian and the results of the physical examination. For example, the line of questioning is different for the dog with suspected male feminizing syndrome due to Sertoli cell tumor than for the dog with suspected infertility. (See subsequent chapters for more information on the typical history associated with specific disorders of the male reproductive system.)

PHYSICAL EXAMINATION

A thorough physical examination is as important as a complete history. Recognition of underlying perpetuating problems of other organ systems is imperative for the successful management of any reproductive disorder. The reproductive tract should be thoroughly evaluated as part of a complete physical examination. Evaluation of the male reproductive tract is not as time-consuming as the balance of a thorough physical examination and should include the scrotum, testes, epididymis, penis, and prepuce and finish with rectal evaluation of the prostate gland.

SCROTUM. The scrotum in the normal dog should be sparsely covered with hair, feel relatively smooth and soft, have skin that is freely movable over the testes, be nonpainful to the touch, and have a uniform thickness. It should be assessed visually for signs of inflammation, trauma, or swelling by laying the dog comfortably on its side and gently lifting the upper leg. Chronic or severe scrotal inflammation may alter normal thermoregulatory processes, which in turn may alter spermatogenesis and/or spermatozoal storage in the epididymis. Palpation of the scrotum, separate from the testes, may reveal adhesions from previous or current inflammation. The presence of nodules may suggest granuloma or neoplasia development. Squamous cell carcinoma, melanoma, and mast cell tumors may involve the scrotum (Jones and Joshua, 1982). Scrotal thickening may result from inflammation, neoplasia, accumulation of fluid (e.g., lymphedema), testicular or epididymal enlargement, or inguinoscrotal hernia.

TESTES. In the dog, testicular descent is usually complete within 10 to 14 days of birth, and both testes should be readily palpable by 6 to 8 weeks of age. Failure to palpate both testes, especially in dogs older than 16 weeks of age, is supportive of cryptorchidism (see page 961). In younger dogs, however, temporary retraction of the testis into the inguinal canal or lateral to the penis may occur with nervousness or excitement. This should probably not be considered significant as long as the testis descends into the scrotum when the dog is quiet or relaxed.

The testes should be palpated for size, shape, and consistency. The left testis is usually caudal to the right. The size range for the dog testis is approximately 1 to 5 cm in length by 1 to 3 cm in diameter. Difference in breed sizes precludes an all-encompassing statement regarding normal size of the testis. In general, the size of the testes is roughly proportional to body size. Although evaluation of total scrotal width is an objective way to estimate testicular size, weight, and daily sperm production (Olar et al, 1983), such measurements are not usually made. Testicular asymmetry, bilaterally small testes, or symmetrical enlargement should be considered subjective information indicative of possible abnormalities. Potential causes for testicular enlargement include neoplasia, acute infection or inflammation, testicular torsion, and inguinoscrotal hernia. Potential causes for a decrease in testicular size include degeneration, chronic infection or inflammation, hypoplasia, or intersex states.

The paired testes should be oval in shape, with a smooth surface. They should be slightly thicker dorsoventrally than from side to side, with the scrotal covering freely movable. Palpation of an irregular surface, nodules, or scrotal adhesions suggests chronic inflammation, infection, or neoplasia. Pain on palpation of the testes suggests acute orchitis or torsion, especially if the testes are enlarged. The testes should feel firm but not hard, with soft, spongy, or doughy testes suggesting testicular degeneration and hard testes suggesting neoplasia or acute or chronic orchitis.

EPIDIDYMIS AND SPERMATIC CORD. The epididymis is attached to the dorsolateral surface of the testis, with the head and tail located at the cranial and caudal poles, respectively. The epididymis continues as the ductus deferens, located within the spermatic cord, originating at the tail of the epididymis, located medial and dorsal to each testis as it proceeds through the internal inguinal ring. The spermatic cord contains the ductus deferens, spermatic artery, pampiniform plexus of veins, lymphatics, nerves, and cremaster muscle. The epididymis and spermatic cord of each testis (although difficult to palpate) should be thoroughly palpated for areas of thickening or enlargement (suggestive of granuloma formation), epididymitis, adenomyosis of the epididymis, or an inguinal hernia. An apparent enlargement of the epididymis may also be caused by a decrease in the size of the testis. Aplasia of the epididymal duct or ductus deferens may be palpable. However, this disorder is most frequently associated with development of a sperm granuloma and/or testicular degeneration.

PENIS AND PREPUCE. Without an erection, the prepuce completely encloses the normal canine penis. Small quantities of preputial discharge are usually not clinically significant (i.e., mild balanoposthitis). Worrisome discharges include blood or large amounts of pus. "Normal" balanoposthitis is seen as a mild mucopurulent discharge covering the penile mucosa. The penis should be freely movable within the prepuce and easily exposed by pulling the prepuce caudally over the bulbus glandis. The prepuce can usually be retracted over the bulbus glandis. A narrow preputial opening (phimosis) or adhesions between the prepuce and penis should be suspected in a dog in which the penis cannot be fully exposed. The extruded penis should be thoroughly evaluated for the presence of inflammation, trauma, foreign bodies, or masses. Transmissible venereal tumors may be observed near the bulbus glandis and may be identified only following complete extrusion of the penis (Fig. 27-1). The

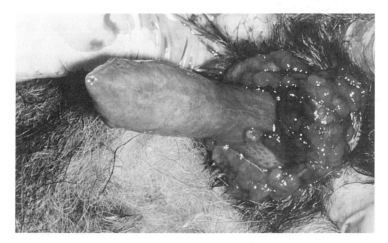

FIGURE 27-1. Transmissible venereal tumor involving the bulbus glandis. Note the cauliflower-like appearance and serosanguineous discharge associated with the tumor. (Courtesy of R.C. Richardson, Purdue University.)

penile mucosa should be pinkish white, smooth, and nonpainful to touch. Inflammation of the penile mucosa may result in lymphoid hyperplasia and the development of papular lesions.

The os penis should be thoroughly palpated for size and conformation. A congenitally deformed or fractured os penis may result in deviation of the penis and an inability to retract the penis fully into the preputial sheath. Likewise, a congenitally shortened os penis may result in excessive flaccidity of the penile tip and an impaired ability to copulate.

PROSTATE GLAND.   The prostate gland is the only accessory sex gland in the dog. It is normally located near the cranial rim of the pelvis, although cranial displacement into the abdomen may occur as the bladder distends with urine. The prostate gland encompasses the neck of the bladder, the proximal portion of the urethra, and the terminal portion of the ductus deferens. A median septum divides the gland into two equal-sized, smooth, firm lobes, which can usually be palpated per rectum. In large dogs, only the caudal pole of the prostate may be palpable. The size and weight of the prostate gland are variable and depend on the age, breed, and body weight of the dog. Because of the close association between the prostate and the ductus deferens, and thus the testis and epididymis, the prostate should always be evaluated by digital palpation per rectum. The presence of abnormal size, asymmetry between lobes, abnormal consistency, or pain supports the presence of prostatic dysfunction and dictates the need for a thorough diagnostic evaluation of the gland.

SEMEN EVALUATION

Semen analysis is integral to the evaluation of possible infertility or subfertility and should be performed as part of a routine prebreeding examination. Semen evaluation should be completed before artificial insemination or freezing (see Chapter 32). Culture of the semen is also indicated in dogs with suspected prostatitis, orchitis, or epididymitis (see Chapters 29 and 30). Because live sperm are normally present in the ejaculate, the clinician must carefully handle the semen to prevent death or artifactual changes in cell morphology or motility as a result of mishandling of the sample. Semen should be examined immediately after it is obtained; any delay may increase the number of dead sperm. Dramatic changes in environmental temperature should be avoided. Ideally, all equipment should be kept near 37° C to prevent temperature extremes. Glass slides and collection devices should be warm, clean, and free of alcohol, powder, or excessive lubricant.

The method of semen collection and the type and sequence of analytic techniques used for semen analysis should be kept consistent. Currently, most of the macroscopic and microscopic evaluation of semen is subjective and usually performed by a qualified technician. Automated sperm analyzer equipment is now commercially available and has become invaluable in the evaluation of semen from human, bovine, equine, and other species. Studies using computer-aided sperm analysis in dogs are beginning to appear in the literature (Smith and England, 2000; Verstegen et al, 2000). Use of techniques allowing objective assessment of spermatozoa function may help identify causes of infertility not previously appreciated (England and Plummer, 1993; Hewitt et al, 2000; Holst et al, 2000), although currently such techniques are not routinely performed. Regardless of the method used to evaluate semen, a standard semen analysis form (Fig. 27-2) should be completed and filed with the patient's medical records.

Techniques for Obtaining a Semen Sample

Collection of a semen sample can be accomplished by allowing the male to mount a bitch in heat, by use of a teaser bitch, or by masturbation. Electroejaculation requires general anesthesia and is not commonly used. Latex artificial vaginas (e.g., Canine Artificial Vagina; Synbiotics, San Diego, CA) that funnel semen into a plastic sterile test tube are ideal for collection of semen (Fig. 27-3). Although spermatozoal motility has been reported to be adversely affected by the warm latex lining, we have not recognized this as a clinically relevant problem. Scant amounts of lubricating jelly can be applied just inside the outer rim of the artificial vaginal device, avoiding contact with semen. Excessive lubrication can be deleterious to spermatozoal viability and should be avoided. Plastic (not glass) tubes should be used to prevent breakage of the collection device, which is most likely to occur when the male is exhibiting strong pelvic thrusting. Vinyl rather than latex gloves should be worn to minimize the detrimental effect of latex on spermatozoal motility (Althouse et al, 1991).

TEASER BITCH.   The easiest technique for obtaining a semen sample is to let the male mount a bitch in proestrus or estrus. A teaser bitch in anestrus may also be used, although the sexual interest of the male (thus the results) is less consistent. Application of a topical pheromone preparation (p-hydroxybenzoic acid methyl ester; Eau d'Estrus, Synbiotics, Malvern, PA) to the vulva and hindquarters of a bitch in anestrus to simulate estrus may help (Keenan, 1998). Unfortunately, we have only occasionally observed improvement in stimulating sexual excitement in the male when using pheromone preparations. Alternatively, vaginal secretions from a bitch in estrus can be collected on gauze pads or swabs, stored frozen, and when needed, thawed and held near or applied to the vulva of the teaser bitch for the dog to smell (Keenan, 1998; Freshman, 2001). Both the stud dog and the bitch should be kept on leashes and the bitch restrained to allow the male access to the rear quarters and vulva. The bitch may need to be muzzled (especially if she is not in standing heat) to prevent biting of the holder, collector, or male dog. If the collector is right-handed, he or she should be on the left side of the male dog, with the collection device

INFORMATION ON THE CANINE BREEDING SOUNDNESS EVALUATION CAN BE
FOUND ON PAGES 174-181 OF THE PROCEEDINGS OF THE
1992 ANNUAL CONFERENCE OF THE SOCIETY

Canine Breeding Soundness Evaluation

Guidelines Established by Society for Theriogenology
P.O. Box 2118, Hastings, NE 68902-2118
Phone (402)463-0392 Fax (402)461-4103

Case #_____ Date: _____
Client: _____ Address: _____
Dog's Name: _____ Breed and Color: _____
Date of Birth: _____ Registration Number: _____ Tattoo: _____

HISTORY
Reason for evaluation: _____ Date of last breeding: _____
Date of last litter: _____ Brucellosis tested: _____ Type of test: _____
Pedigree available: _____ Infertile relatives: _____

PHYSICAL EXAMINATION
Physical condition: _____ Weight: _____
Pertinent other health problems: _____
Penis/Prepuce: _____ Spermatic cord: _____
Scrotum: _____ Prostate: _____
Epididymides: (R) _____ (L) _____
Testes: Width (R) _____ (L) _____ Total: _____
        Consistency (hard/normal/soft): (R) _____ (L) _____
        Masses/fluid/pain/other: _____

SEMEN COLLECTION
Date last collected: _____ Libido/ease of collection: _____
Teaser bitch present: _____ Stage of cycle: _____ Pheromone used: _____
Equipment used (AV/other): _____

SEMEN EVALUATION

	Color	Volume	pH	Conc (sperm/ml)	Total Sperm Number (sperm/ejac)
Fraction 1	_____	_____	XXX*	XXXXXXXXXXXXX*	XXXXXXXXXXXXXX*
Fraction 2	_____	_____	XXX*	_____	_____
Fraction 3	_____	XXXXXXX*	____	XXXXXXXXXXXXX*	XXXXXXXXXXXXXX*

*Not applicable and/or necessary

MOTILITY:
    Total Motility (%): _____ Progressive Motility (%): _____
    Diluent (if used): _____ Speed: slow moderate fast

MORPHOLOGY:
    Method (Stain): _____ Phase Contrast (   )
    % Normal: _____ Total normal (% normal × sperm/ejac): _____
    Head abnormalities: _____
    Midpiece abnormalities: _____
    Tail abnormalities: _____
CYTOLOGY (0-4+) (RBC, WBC, Epith., Bact., Other):
    Fraction 1: _____ Fraction 2: _____ Fraction 3: _____

CONCLUSIONS:

Signed: _____ Clinic Name: _____
        Member–Society for Theriogenology

©Copyright 1992 Society for Theriogenology
FOR USE OF MEMBERS ONLY

FIGURE 27-2. Canine breeding soundness evaluation form distributed by the Society for Theriogenology.

in the left hand and the dog's prepuce/penis near the right. The dog is then lead up to the rear quarters of the bitch by an assistant. If the male is inexperienced, a period of foreplay and tentative mounting attempts should be allowed. The collector should gently massage the penis through the prepuce as the dog sniffs and licks the perineal region of the bitch. As sexual excitement increases in the male, he attempts mounting, pelvic thrusts begin, and the penis and bulbus glandis enlarge, all at about the same time. The collector must slide the prepuce back over the bulbus glandis before it becomes fully engorged. This must be done early during the erection process, or enlargement of the bulbus glandis exceeds the preputial opening and the handler is not able to exteriorize the penis and bulbus glandis. If full erection occurs before the bulbus glandis is exteriorized, the dog may experience discomfort or pain and lose the erection before ejaculation occurs or have an incomplete ejaculation. The collector should deviate the penis into the collection device as the male attempts to thrust the penis into the vulva. If an artificial vagina is used, it should be passed over the bulbus glandis and gentle digital pressure applied to the entire circumference of the penis just proximal to the bulbus

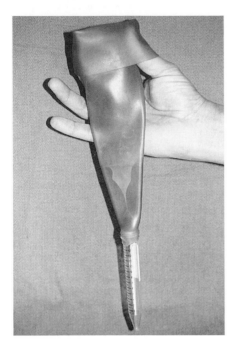

FIGURE 27-3. Latex artificial vagina and plastic sterile test tube used for collection of semen in dogs.

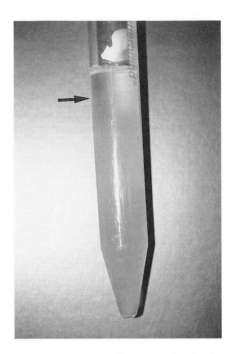

FIGURE 27-4. Semen from a dog, illustrating the cloudy, sperm-rich (second) fraction (below the *arrow*) and the clear prostatic (third) fraction (above the *arrow*).

glandis to maintain the erection. Rapid pelvic thrusting and ejaculation commence almost immediately. Care must be taken to prevent damage to the penis from forcing it too far into the artificial vagina. In addition, as ejaculation commences, the artificial vagina should be gradually withdrawn from the bulbus glandis (unless a soft distensible cone is used) to prevent trauma as the bulbus glandis continues to enlarge.

The first two ejaculate fractions (presperm, 5 to 20 seconds duration; sperm-rich, 30 seconds to 4 minutes duration) are ejaculated during and immediately following the pelvic thrusting phase of copulation, respectively. Once these fractions have been ejaculated, the dog usually dismounts and steps over the bitch and collector's arm with the hind leg so that the penis is rotated 180 degrees and directed caudally. Most dogs ejaculate prostatic fluid in spurts for several minutes, the volume ejaculated being dependent on the duration of the "tie." During manual collection, the application of constant pressure around the circumference of the penis proximal to the bulbus glandis maintains the erection and allows collection of prostatic fluid. The transition from a cloudy to a clear ejaculate indicates a transition from the sperm-rich fluid to prostatic fluid (Fig. 27-4). The collection device can be changed shortly after this transition from cloudy to clear fluid if only prostatic fluid is desired for culture and cytologic evaluation.

Collection of prostatic fluid is not necessary to evaluate spermatozoa for motility and morphology, nor is it needed for artificial insemination. The first two fractions of semen should be evaluated as soon as they are obtained to minimize artifacts that may result

during collection of prostatic fluid. If the semen is to be used for artificial insemination, enough prostatic fluid should be collected to increase the sample size to a volume that can be handled easily (usually 5 to 10 ml). Collection of excess prostatic fluid should be avoided because of potential deleterious effects on spermatozoal viability and motility.

Once a semen sample has been collected, the penis can be released by the collector, the artificial vagina carefully removed from the penis, and the bitch and dog separated, preferably into different rooms. With most dogs, the bitch can be removed as soon as ejaculation begins. The erection usually diminishes within a few minutes after withdrawal of digital pressure on the penis and bulbus glandis. The dog's penis and preputial sheath should always be examined before being released from the hospital to be certain the penis is completely inside the preputial sheath.

MASTURBATION.   Semen can be collected from most males without a teaser bitch. The general sequence of events is the same as outlined above; the difficulty is in initially obtaining an erection. The prepuce should be gently slid back and forth over the bulbus glandis and proximal penis until the erection begins. With initiation of an erection, the prepuce should be slid over the enlarging bulbus glandis and gentle digital pressure applied proximal to the bulbus glandis with the thumb and index finger. At the same time, the artificial vagina should be placed over the penis and bulbus glandis. Pelvic thrusts and ejaculation should begin. If the erection is lost during this sequence, the dog should be allowed to rest for a few minutes and the procedure attempted again.

Reasons for Failure to Obtain a Semen Sample

Although numerous reasons for failing to obtain an adequate semen sample exist, the most common include poor collection technique, an unusually nervous or agitated male, owner interference, and abnormalities in the male. Common technique errors include failure to expose the bulbus glandis, inappropriate timing of exteriorization of the penis, excessive force or pressure applied to the penis, use of cold collection devices, and premature touching of the penis. With practice, most of these technical problems can be resolved.

Another common reason for failure is placement of the male in an unfamiliar environment, such as a veterinary hospital. Males may show no sexual interest, even toward a bitch in estrus, when initially placed in a frightening environment. Leaving the dog in the new surroundings for a few hours often alleviates fear. When attempting to collect semen from a male, all possible distractions should be kept to a minimum. The collection room should be quiet and have proper flooring to provide the male with traction. Only those people absolutely necessary for the collection should be in the room. Crowds, excessive talking, laughter, and flash photography should be avoided. Removal of white lab coats may help alleviate fear or stress. The effect of owner presence on the ability to obtain a semen sample is variable. Some males refuse to perform unless a familiar person is present, and a few will perform only when at home. Others can be collected only by their owners, whereas a small number of dogs cannot be collected until their owner leaves the room. As a general rule of thumb, the owners of the male should be present during the initial attempts to obtain a semen sample and adjustments made if attempts at collecting semen are unsuccessful.

An underlying reproductive disorder may prevent collection of a semen sample. This is seen most commonly in dogs with poor libido, pain (e.g., acute orchitis or prostatitis, degenerative arthritis), or acquired behavioral abnormalities due to a previous negative sexual experience.

Macroscopic Evaluation of Semen

VOLUME. The volume of semen collected is highly variable and depends on the dog's age, size, frequency of service, and the amount of prostatic fluid collected. Normal volume may range from 1 to 40 ml per ejaculate. It is important to collect all of the sperm-rich (second) fraction when evaluating a dog's semen. The volume of this fraction varies between 0.5 and 12 ml and is cloudy. The third fraction (i.e., prostatic fluid) is translucent (Fig. 27-4). Once the ejaculate changes in appearance from cloudy to clear, the collector can assume that all of the second fraction has been obtained and the collection procedure can be discontinued. This usually occurs within 5 minutes following discontinuation of the pelvic thrusts. Volume does not correlate with fertility unless the animal fails to ejaculate.

COLOR. Dog semen is normally white to opalescent and opaque. The intensity of the opacity depends on the concentration of sperm. Clear and colorless semen suggests azoospermia. A yellow tint may be seen with urine or pus contamination. A green tint, with or without clumps, clots, or flakes, suggests pus and an infection in the reproductive tract. A red tint suggests blood, which usually originates from the prostate gland or from a traumatized, engorged penis. Hemorrhage does not necessarily imply pathology. Some males that experience prolonged sexual anticipation before being allowed to copulate may experience transient hemorrhage into the semen from the prostate gland. Normal semen may often be obtained if these dogs are isolated from the bitch in estrus for 12 to 24 hours and then recollected. Recurrence of any abnormality, however, is worrisome and suggests a need to investigate that problem.

In general, any abnormal color should alert the clinician that there may be a problem, and a careful evaluation of the reproductive tract should be considered. Any agent (i.e., urine, pus, blood) that produces discoloration can affect the concentration, motility, and viability of the sperm.

pH. The normal pH of canine semen ranges from 6.3 to 6.7 and depends, in part, on the amount of prostatic fluid collected. Prostatic fluid has a pH range of 6.0 to 7.4, with a normal mean of 6.8 (Nett and Olson, 1983). The alkaline nature of prostatic fluid is believed to increase sperm motility and help neutralize the acid environment in the vaginal vault during copulation (Jones and Joshua, 1982). An increase in the pH of semen is associated with incomplete ejaculation or inflammation of the testis, epididymis, or prostate gland.

Microscopic Evaluation of Semen

MOTILITY. Motility of individual spermatozoa should be assessed as quickly as possible after obtaining a semen sample. A drop of semen should be placed on a clean slide and microscopically examined at ×200 to ×400 for progressive forward motion of individual spermatozoa and presence of sperm agglutination. Canine spermatozoa are resistant to cold shock, so the slide need not be warmed (Johnston et al, 2001). Percentage of progressive spermatozoal motility has been demonstrated to decline less quickly in samples held at room temperature than in those held at body temperature. Motility will decline as the light from the microscope heats the drop of semen. Evaluation of spermatozoa under lower powers of magnification may give the false impression of forward motility, when in fact, abnormal side-to-side motion without forward motility is present. Evaluation of progressive forward motility may be difficult in heavily concentrated samples. Highly concentrated samples can be diluted with autologous prostatic fluid, phosphate-buffered saline, 2.9% sodium citrate solution, or a semen extender (Johnston et al, 2001).

Spermatozoal motility is assessed subjectively by visual appraisal; the percentage of motile sperm and the character of motility are evaluated. Progressive forward motility is considered normal movement for spermatozoa and is thought to reflect viability and ability to fertilize the ovum. A normal semen sample should have greater than 70% of the spermatozoa exhibiting vigorous forward motility. Individual spermatozoa should be carefully assessed for type of movement. Spermatozoa that are moving in small circles or that have side-to-side motion without forward progression are not normal. The percentage of actively motile spermatozoa may be altered by exposure of the semen to extremes in temperature, acidic diluents, water, urine, pus, blood, or lubricants. The first ejaculate from a dog following a prolonged period of sexual rest may contain a greater percentage of old and dead sperm that have been stored in the epididymis. This results in a decreased percentage of actively motile sperm. Semen samples obtained on subsequent days should be more normal. Rarely, hypomotile or nonmotile viable spermatozoa may also be seen with Kartagener's syndrome, an immotile cilia syndrome with an autosomal recessive mode of inheritance. In the dog, this syndrome is characterized by respiratory tract disease, male sterility, situs inversus, deafness, and hydrocephalus (Edwards et al, 1986).

A second semen sample should be evaluated whenever a large percentage of spermatozoa are immotile or dead. Special attention should be directed at collection and sample handling techniques to minimize or eliminate collection artifacts. Latex gloves may have a detrimental effect on spermatozoal motility (Althouse et al, 1991) and should be avoided when collecting a semen sample. Vinyl gloves have a minimal effect on motility. Persistent problems with sperm motility may reflect a problem in the testes, epididymides, or prostate gland (see page 999).

CONCENTRATION. The concentration or number of spermatozoa *per ejaculate* should be determined by multiplying the number of spermatozoa per milliliter of semen by the total volume (in milliliters) of semen collected. The total volume of semen depends, in part, on the volume of clear prostatic fluid (third ejaculate fraction) collected, thus becoming extremely variable. Evaluation of sperm concentration per milliliter is inaccurate and should not be done. Sperm can be counted using a calibrated spectrophotometer, Coulter counter, or hemacytometer. Use of the 1/100 Unopette (Becton-Dickinson and Co, Rutherford, NJ) white blood cell diluter kit and Neubauer hemacytometer is a relatively quick and inexpensive means of determining sperm concentration. The ejaculate should be mixed gently and the 20-μl Unopette capillary pipette filled with semen and dispensed into the reservoir chamber, which contains 2 ml of diluent. Diluted semen is then dispensed into both chambers of the Neubauer hemacytometer and the number of spermatozoa in the central square (Fig. 27-5) of the nine primary squares is counted on each side of the hemacytometer and the numbers averaged. The number of spermatozoa in the central square is the concentration, expressed in million spermatozoa per milliliter of semen. This value is then multiplied by the volume of the ejaculate to give the

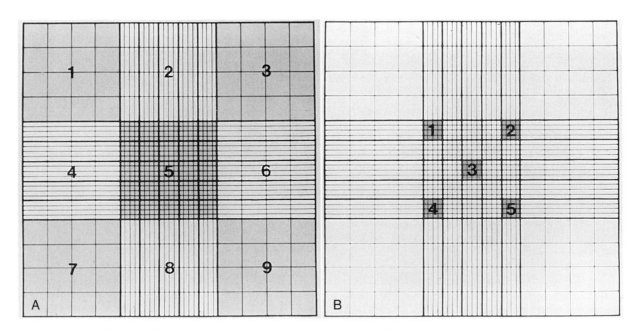

FIGURE 27-5. Schematic of a hemocytometer chamber as viewed through a microscope. There are nine 1 mm² primary squares *(A)* and 25 secondary squares within the central primary square *(B)*. For most dogs, to determine sperm count per milliliter of ejaculate, the total number of sperm in the central primary square (number 5 in *A*) is multiplied by 10⁶. If a large number of sperm are present, the total number of sperm in five of the secondary squares (numbers 1–5 in *B*) can be counted and multiplied by 10⁷ to determine the sperm count per milliliter of ejaculate.

total number of sperm per ejaculate. The total number of spermatozoa in the ejaculate of a normal adult dog ranges from 200 million to greater than a billion. The number of spermatozoa per ejaculate varies, depending in part on age, testicular weight, sexual activity, and perhaps, season of the year (see page 939). Larger breeds of dogs also have a higher number of total spermatozoa in the ejaculate than do smaller breeds (Amann, 1986).

MORPHOLOGY.   Smears of the undiluted ejaculate are examined microscopically for structural abnormalities of the spermatozoa. A small drop of fresh, undiluted semen can be placed on a slide and covered with a large coverslip. This spreads the fluid out into a thin film, allowing accurate evaluation of individual sperm without stains. This evaluation is best performed using phase contrast microscopy. Alternatively, semen can be smeared evenly on a glass slide in a manner similar to that of blood; the smear is then air-dried, fixed, and stained. Several stains are available. The rapid three-step Giemsa-Wright stain technique (e.g., Harleco Hemacolor, EM Diagnostic Systems, Gibbstown, NJ; Diff Quik, VWR International, West Chester, PA; Camco Stain Pack, Cambridge Diagnostic Products, Fort Lauderdale, FL) is quick, effective, and readily available in most practices. These stains do not stain the acrosomal area of sperm. India ink and eosin-nigrosin (e.g., Morphology stain, Society of Theriogenology, Lane Manufacturing, Denver, CO; Hancock, Lane Manufacturing, Denver, CO) are background stains that outline the sperm rather than stain the sperm directly. For the latter, a drop of eosin-nigrosin stain and a drop of semen are gently mixed on a warmed microscope slide before being smeared and allowed to air-dry. Spermac stain (Fertility Technologies Inc, Natick, MA) is a rapid stain that offers unique differential qualities. The sperm nucleus stains red; the acrosome, midpiece, and tail stain green; and the equatorial region of the acrosome stains pale green (Oettlé, 1995). Spermac stain can be used on extended semen, since constituents such as egg yolk, serum, and milk commonly included in extenders do not interfere with the staining. Leukocytes do not stain differentially with Spermac stain. Root Kustritz et al (1998) found the percentage of morphologically normal spermatozoa and the percentage of morphologic abnormalities differed depending on the staining technique, suggesting that staining or preparation technique may alter the morphology of canine spermatozoa artifactually. Results of this study emphasize the importance of consistency of preparation and staining technique when comparing sperm morphology within and between dogs.

Evaluation of sperm morphology should be completed microscopically using oil immersion. The normal spermatozoa consists of the acrosomal cap, head, neck, middle piece, and tail (Fig. 27-6). The acrosome is a cap-like structure covering slightly more than the anterior half of the head, and the middle piece is approximately 1.5 times the length of the head in normal spermatozoa. Individual spermatozoa should be evaluated for abnormalities arising in the head, middle piece,

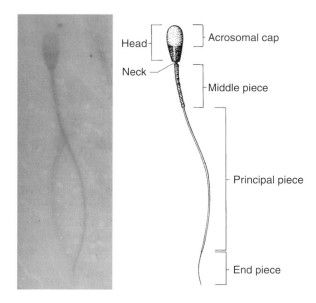

FIGURE 27-6. Normal canine spermatozoon (H&E stain ×1000).

and tail (Fig. 27-6). Commonly identified abnormalities include detached heads, knobbed acrosomes, detached acrosomes, proximal and distal cytoplasmic droplets, reflex (i.e., bent) midpiece, bent tails, tails tightly coiled over the midpiece, and proximally coiled tails (Root Kustritz et al, 1998). Abnormalities may be further classified into primary and secondary abnormalities (Table 27-1; Figs. 27-7 and 27-8). Primary abnormalities are believed to represent abnormalities in spermatogenesis (i.e., within the testes), whereas secondary abnormalities are nonspecific and may arise during transit through the duct system (i.e., within the epididymis), during handling of the semen or following infection, trauma, or fever (Johnston, 1991). A minimum of 200 spermatozoa should be counted and classified; only

TABLE 27-1 PRIMARY AND SECONDARY SPERMATOZOAL DEFECTS IN THE DOG

Primary Abnormalities

Head
  All deviations
Middle piece
  Abaxial attachments
  Double middle piece
  Frayed, thin middle piece
  Thickened middle piece
  Ruptured middle piece
  Kinked or bent middle piece
  Proximal cytoplasmic droplets (neck region)
Tail
  Coiled tail
  Multiple tails

Secondary Abnormalities

Detached normal heads, tails
Detached acrosome
Bent tail
Distal cytoplasmic droplet (distal midpiece)

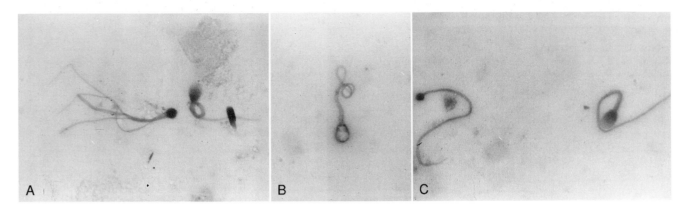

FIGURE 27-7. Examples of primary spermatozoal defects (H&E stain ×1000). *A,* Abnormal head with multiple tails; coiled tail. *B,* Coiled tail. *C,* Abnormal head; bent middle piece and tail of spermatozoon with normal head are secondary defects. (Courtesy of D.B. DeNicola, Purdue University.)

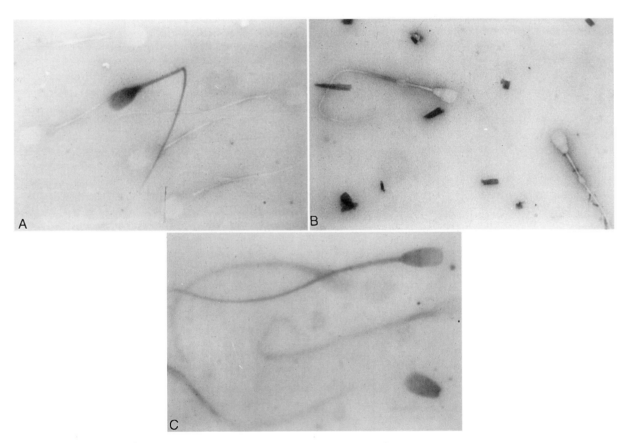

FIGURE 27-8. Examples of secondary spermatozoal defects (H&E stain ×1000). *A,* Bent tail. *B,* Distal cytoplasmic droplets; bent tail. *C,* Detached normal head; bent tail. (Courtesy of D.B. DeNicola, Purdue University.)

free heads should be counted, not free tails. The reader is referred to Oettlé (1995) for more information on classification of sperm abnormalities in the dog.

Historically, it has been suggested that normal males generally should have greater than 70% morphologically normal spermatozoa and that primary and secondary abnormalities should constitute less than 10% and 20% of the defective sperm, respectively. Positive correlations between percentage of morpho-

logically normal spermatozoa and fertility rate and total number of morphologically normal spermatozoa and pregnancy rate have been demonstrated in the dog (Oettlé, 1993; Mickelsen et al, 1993). Oettlé (1993) found that fertility of dogs was statistically reduced when the percentage of morphologically normal sperm fell below 60%. Using 60% normal sperm morphology as the cutoff point between normal and subnormal, fertility was 61% in a group of 23 normal dogs, compared with 13% in a group of 15 subnormal dogs. Mickelsen et al (1993) found that total numbers of morphologically normal and progressively motile spermatozoa per ejaculate was more important in predicting fertility. Artificial insemination with greater than 250×10^6 morphologically normal sperm resulted in a pregnancy rate of approximately 82% in 27 bitches evaluated. Obviously, total sperm per ejaculate and health of the spermatozoa (i.e., morphology, motility) are all critical in the assessment of fertility of the dog.

Although abnormal sperm morphology is associated with infertility in dogs, there are few descriptions of the effect of specific morphologic defects on fertility. Specific morphologic defects associated with infertility in the dog include abnormalities of midpiece attachment or ultrastructure, microcephalic spermatozoa, and proximal retained cytoplasmic droplets (Johnston et al, 2001).

CYTOLOGY. Smears of undiluted semen should also be stained with Wright's or new methylene blue stain and evaluated for the presence of inflammatory cells and bacteria. An occasional healthy inflammatory cell (i.e., neutrophil, macrophage, lymphocyte, plasma cell), red blood cell, or bacteria is common in the semen of a normal dog as a result of urethral contamination of the ejaculate. Epithelial cells are also commonly associated with urethral or preputial contamination of semen, especially after prolonged periods of sexual rest. Large numbers of inflammatory and red blood cells, however, should be considered abnormal. Intracellular bacteria or toxic changes in neutrophils support the presence of infection. However, their absence does not rule out infection. Large numbers of red blood cells imply hemorrhage, most commonly originating from the prostate gland or penis. Large numbers of mononuclear cells imply immune-mediated orchitis. In immune-mediated orchitis, neutrophils can

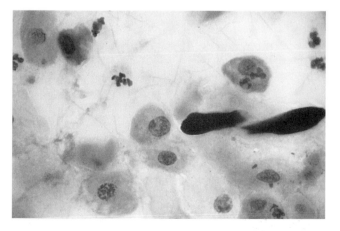

FIGURE 27-9. Cytologic smear of semen obtained from a 4-year-old Great Dane dog with infertility. Physical examination revealed small, "lumpy" testes; semen evaluation revealed oligospermia and inflammation; semen culture was negative; and testicular biopsy revealed lymphocytic orchitis. Note the mononuclear cells and neutrophils present on cytologic evaluation of the semen.

also be found in conjunction with mononuclear cells (Fig. 27-9).

Bacterial Culture

Bacterial culture of the semen should be a routine part of the semen evaluation. See page 941 for a detailed discussion on culture techniques and interpretation.

Factors Affecting Semen Characteristics

PUBERTY. The initial ejaculates from a dog after it reaches puberty often contain abnormal and dead spermatozoa. With subsequent ejaculations, the concentration of spermatozoa increases, the number of abnormal spermatozoa decreases, and the semen eventually contains normal numbers of mature spermatozoa (Taha et al, 1981b).

FREQUENCY OF EJACULATION. The frequency of ejaculation has a direct effect on semen volume and total number of spermatozoa in the ejaculate. A mild decrease in total spermatozoa count per ejaculate has been demonstrated when dogs are ejaculated once or twice daily, versus two and three times per week. This decrease is attributable to a reduction in the epididymal storage pool of sperm. When this storage pool is exhausted, the decline in spermatozoa count plateaus and subsequent counts represent the daily production rate within the testes, which is approximately 400×10^6 sperm for most dogs (Olar et al, 1983). Thus, although sperm count per ejaculate decreases with increased use, total sperm produced per week is relatively constant and may even increase with increased sexual use. The total sperm count per ejaculate may increase after a few days of sexual rest, presumably as the epididymal storage pool is replenished. Libido remains normal even when dogs are ejaculated daily.

This question frequently arises: How often can the stud dog be used without interfering with fertility? Recommendations concerning frequency of use must be tailored to the individual dog. What constitutes frequent use and what effect use has on libido and semen quality are quite variable from dog to dog. Sexual use of a healthy stud dog either once every 48 hours, daily for 3 days, then resting for 2 days; or twice in 1 day, then resting for 2 days, has been proposed as a guideline for use of the dog without affecting semen quality. Most healthy males can probably be used once daily for prolonged periods without causing oligospermia or subfertility. However, males with defective spermatogenesis may not be able to meet these demands, and oligospermia (sperm count <200 million per ejaculate) may result. A dog with frequent sexual usage, oligospermia, and subfertility may regain fertility when used sparingly to allow spermatozoa to accumulate in the epididymis (Olar et al, 1983).

SEASON OF YEAR. The season of the year may have some effect on the concentration of sperm per ejaculate, with an increased concentration occurring in spring/early summer and a lower concentration in late summer/fall (Taha et al, 1981a). Investigators have speculated that changes in sperm count may be related to photoperiod and/or environmental temperature. Although the concentration of sperm fluctuated, total numbers of sperm per ejaculate remained normal (i.e., $>200 \times 10^6$ per ejaculate) in most dogs. The normal dog can be assumed to be fertile, regardless of the season or environmental temperature.

PROSTATIC SIZE AND PATHOLOGY. A relationship between semen volume per ejaculate and prostatic size has been suggested in dogs with a normal prostate. The ejaculate volume of naturally collected semen increased in a linear manner with prostatic size and weight. In contrast, dogs with cystic hyperplasia of the prostate had a marked reduction in semen volume compared with dogs with comparable-sized normal prostate glands.

Brendler and colleagues (1983) evaluated prostatic size, histologic changes, semen volume, and plasma hormonal changes in a colony of Beagle dogs for several years. Their findings indicate that the prostate gland continues to enlarge during the first 6 years of life, but secretory function and therefore semen volume per ejaculate begin to decrease after 4 years of age. In addition, a close association was found between the onset of benign prostatic hyperplasia and a reduction in semen volume per ejaculate. A modest decrease occurred in plasma androgen concentration but not in plasma 17β-estradiol concentration with age in these dogs. It was speculated that changes in secretory function of the prostate gland may have been due to estrogen-induced blockade of prostatic fluid transport and/or to the pathologic changes within the gland. Although prostate secretory function decreases, fertility and total number of sperm per ejaculate are not deleteriously affected by benign prostatic hyperplasia. The influence of bacterial prostatitis or prostatic neoplasia on secretory function of the prostate has not been evaluated, although it is likely to be impaired. Prostatitis has a deleterious effect on sperm viability and motility (see page 977).

TESTICULAR SIZE. Testicular parenchymal weight, and thus testicular size, has been shown to correlate directly with daily production of spermatozoa (Olar et al, 1983; Amann, 1986). In a group of 11 normal dogs ejaculated daily for two 10-day intervals, daily sperm production averaged $11.7 \pm 0.5 \times 10^6$ spermatozoa per gram of testicular parenchyma. In another group of seven normal dogs ejaculated daily for two 20-day periods, daily sperm production averaged $16.7 \pm 1.4 \times 10^6$ spermatozoa per gram of testicular parenchyma. These findings suggest that as testicular weight (size) increases, daily sperm production and thus the number of sperm per ejaculate also increase. In general, small-breed dogs do not produce as much spermatozoa as large-breed dogs with larger testes.

Scrotal width (or circumference) may provide an objective index of testicular size and a method for detecting dogs with smaller than normal testes when scrotal width is corrected for body size (Woodall and Johnstone, 1988). However, scrotal width is not a precise measure. Considerable variation occurs in scrotal width for dogs of any particular body weight, in part because of breed differences. In addition, a "normal" scrotal width does not mean the dog is producing spermatozoa. Sequential evaluation of total scrotal width or circumference can be used to monitor a dog for decreasing testicular size, such as occurs with testicular degenerative processes. Sequential evaluation is more valuable than random determination of total scrotal width (or circumference) as an estimate of anticipated numbers of spermatozoa in an ejaculate.

Final Interpretation of the Semen Evaluation

Unfortunately, no single characteristic of a semen evaluation is, by itself, an accurate measure of fertility. The semen evaluation is just one of many factors to be considered in evaluating a male. The semen characteristics that appear to correlate most closely with fertility are total spermatozoa per ejaculate, percentage of progressive motility, and sperm morphology. For a male to be considered acceptable for breeding, his semen analysis should exceed the minimum criteria established for these three variables (Table 27-2). The male is not necessarily fertile, however, just because these criteria are met. Likewise, a male is not necessarily subfertile if these criteria are not met. Repeatable azoospermia (lack of sperm) or necrospermia (dead sperm) are the only characteristics that allow the clinician to declare a male sterile. Even then, it is important to remember that a single, random semen examination does not necessarily reflect what is occurring in the seminiferous tubules on that day. Transient disruptions in spermatogenesis may result in reversible, transient oligospermia or azoospermia. Reevaluation with several semen analyses should always be completed during the next 6 months before an apparently azoospermic dog is declared permanently sterile.

SEMINAL ALKALINE PHOSPHATASE

Measurement of seminal alkaline phosphatase should be assessed in dogs with azoospermia (see page 991). Alkaline phosphatase in semen is measured by the same

---

TABLE 27-2 CRITERIA FOR NORMAL SEMEN EVALUATION

Major Parameters for Assessing Fertility

Total spermatozoa per ejaculate: $>200 \times 10^6$/ejaculate
Spermatozoa motility: >70% with progressive forward motility
Spermatozoa morphology: >70% normal spermatozoa
   Primary defects: <10% of spermatozoa
   Secondary defects: <20% of spermatozoa

Additional Parameters

Volume of semen: variable, ranging from 1 to 40 ml/ejaculate
Color of semen: white to opalescent and opaque
Seminal pH: 6.3 to 6.7 (prostatic fluid, 6.0 to 7.4)
Seminal cytology: occasional epithelial cell, RBC, WBC, bacteria
Seminal alkaline phosphatase: >5000 U/L

methods as in serum. Seminal alkaline phosphatase originates from the epididymis in the dog (Frenette et al, 1986) and is a marker for the presence of epididymal fluid in the ejaculate. Seminal concentrations of alkaline phosphatase are typically greater than 5000 U/L in normospermic dogs (Johnston, 1991). Decreased concentrations suggest bilateral outflow obstruction of the vas deferentia or epididymides. The presperm fraction of semen originates from the prostate gland (England et al, 1990) and has a low concentration of alkaline phosphatase. As such, incomplete ejaculation can also result in low seminal alkaline phosphatase concentrations.

Seminal carnitine is believed to originate from the epididymis and can also be used as an epididymal marker in azoospermic dogs, in a manner similar to seminal alkaline phosphatase (Olson et al, 1987). Unfortunately, this test is not routinely available to veterinarians.

MICROBIOLOGIC ASSESSMENT OF THE REPRODUCTIVE TRACT

In the dog, bacterial culture of semen, urine obtained by antepubic cystocentesis, and prostatic fluid or tissue obtained by aspiration or biopsy of the prostate gland (see page 979) are used to identify infection of the reproductive tract. Urine cultures may provide a clue to the offending organism(s) and provide guidance for antibiotic selection in dogs with orchitis, epididymitis, or prostatitis. Culture of semen can be used to confirm infection of the testis and epididymis (culture of the second fraction of semen) or the prostate gland (culture of the third fraction of semen). Bacterial culture of semen should be a routine part of semen evaluation and is also indicated if inflammatory cells are identified on cytologic assessment of semen or if bacterial orchitis/epididymitis or prostatitis is suspected.

Bacterial cultures of the reproductive tract can be difficult to interpret, especially when obtained from healthy stud dogs and bitches. Cultures of the vagina, preputial cavity, and even semen are often positive for bacterial growth, even in healthy bitches and stud dogs. In the vast majority of bitches and stud dogs, positive bacterial growth represents the normal resident bacterial flora, which can include β-hemolytic streptococci and *Mycoplasma* (Bjurstrom and Linde-Forsberg, 1992a; 1992b). Many owners of stud dogs demand negative culture results from vaginal swabs as part of a prebreeding examination before they allow their dog to mate with the bitch. A less commonly employed practice is for owners of the bitch to demand negative culture results from the preputial cavity or semen before letting their bitch be bred by the male. There is no sound basis for these demands, especially if the dog is healthy. There should be some indication (i.e., clinical signs or other findings supportive of an infection) before recommending culturing the reproductive tract.

Before collection of the ejaculate, the clinician should take steps to minimize contamination of the semen sample and should decide what portion of the semen (i.e., second fraction, third fraction, entire sample) is to be cultured. The distal urethra and prepuce contain a normal bacterial flora (Table 27-3) that may contaminate the semen sample. The following steps should be taken to minimize contamination of the semen sample by this normal flora: the dog should be allowed to urinate before semen collection, preputial discharges should be removed, and the prepuce and penis should be cleansed with moistened sterile gauze sponges. A quantitative culture of the distal urethra can also be done. Finally, the few drops of the first fraction and the early part of the second fraction of the ejaculate can be discarded prior to collection of the remaining second and third fractions of semen. Aseptic technique and sterile collection devices should be used. Quantitative

TABLE 27-3   AEROBIC BACTERIA ISOLATED FROM PREPUTIAL CULTURES OF 15 HEALTHY STUD DOGS (232 SAMPLES)

Organism	ISOLATES		DOGS FROM WHICH ORGANISM WAS ISOLATED	
	Number	Percent	Number	Percent
Pasteurella multocida	123	55	15	100
β-Hemolytic streptococci	76	33	11	73
Escherichia coli	42	18	8	53
Coagulase-negative staphylococci	39	17	10	67
Mycoplasma spp.	25	11	12	80
Staphylococcus intermedius	22	10	9	60
Gram-negative rods (unclassified)	19	8	9	60
Gram-positive rods (unclassified)	11	5	7	40
Streptococcus spp. (α-hemolytic, nonhemolytic)	7	3	4	27
Pasteurella spp.	7	3	6	40
Coryneforms	4	2	3	20
Enterococci	4	2	4	27
Pseudomonas spp.	1	0.4	1	7
Proteus mirabilis	1	0.4	1	7
No bacterial growth	33	14		

From Bjurstrom L, Linde-Forsberg C: Long-term study of aerobic bacteria of the genital tract in stud dogs. Am J Vet Res 53:670, 1992.

TABLE 27-4   AEROBIC BACTERIA ISOLATED FROM THE SEMEN OF 15 STUD DOGS (232 SAMPLES)

	ISOLATES		DOGS FROM WHICH ORGANISM WAS ISOLATED	
Organism	Number	Percent	Number	Percent
Pasteurella multocida	44	19	10	67
β-Hemolytic streptococci	18	8	4	27
Escherichia coli	9	4	2	13
Mycoplasma spp.	8	3	4	27
Gram-positive rods (unclassified)	5	2	3	20
Gram-negative rods (unclassified)	5	2	4	27
Coagulase-negative staphylococci	4	2	3	20
Pasteurella spp.	1	0.4	1	7
Streptococcus spp. (α-hemolytic, nonhemolytic)	1	0.4	1	7
Staphylococcus intermedius	1	0.4	1	7
No bacterial growth	162	70		

From Bjurstrom L, Linde-Forsberg C: Long-term study of aerobic bacteria of the genital tract in stud dogs. Am J Vet Res 53:670, 1992.

cultures and cytologic assessment of the semen sample aid in differentiating simple contamination from serious infection.

Positive bacterial cultures may occur in normal dogs. In one study on normal dogs, 30% of semen cultures were positive for bacterial growth despite aseptic technique and precautions to prevent contamination of the semen sample (Bjurstrom and Linde-Forsberg, 1992b). In the normal dog, there should be less than 10^4 colony-forming units (CFUs) per milliliter of ejaculate (Table 27-4; Olson, 1984a). Most infections of the reproductive tract are caused by aerobic bacteria. As such, the clinician should always request aerobic culture of semen samples. Infection should be suspected if there are large numbers of CFUs (i.e., $>10^5$/ml), growth of a single organism, and inflammatory cells on cytologic assessment of the semen. Leukocytes by themselves do not necessarily indicate infection; they may be found in semen samples negative for bacterial growth and vice versa (Bjurstrom and Linde-Forsberg, 1992b). When interpreting results of semen culture, the clinician must always consider clinical signs, reasons for culturing the semen, technique used to obtain the semen sample, the cytology of the ejaculate, and the total numbers and variety of bacteria grown. If results are questionable, the clinician should repeat the culture.

The role of anaerobic bacteria remains to be clarified, but our experience, as well as that of others (Johnston, 1989), suggests that anaerobes are not commonly involved in reproductive tract infections in the dog, minimizing the need for anaerobic cultures. Anaerobic infections, however, should be suspected in the presence of necrotic, gangrenous tissue and if leukocytes and bacteria are identified on cytology but aerobic culture is negative for growth. Semen samples for anaerobic culture should be placed immediately into Anatrans tubes and transported immediately to the laboratory. The clinician should contact the microbiology laboratory for specific information concerning submission of anaerobic cultures.

The role of *Mycoplasma* and *Ureaplasma* in causing reproductive dysfunction remains to be clarified in the dog. *Mycoplasma* and *Ureaplasma* are members of the normal genital flora of the prepuce and distal urethra of dogs (Bjurstrom and Linde-Forsberg, 1992b; Doig et al, 1981), and few have been shown to be pathogenic. These organisms are commonly identified in preputial and, to a lesser extent, semen cultures of normal dogs. *Mycoplasma* and *Ureaplasma* have also been isolated from dogs with reproductive disorders, most notably balanoposthitis, orchiepididymitis, and infertility (Lein, 1989). The significance of positive *Mycoplasma/Ureaplasma* cultures is not certain. Culturing for these organisms may be indicated in dogs with infertility, orchitis, epididymitis, and prostatitis and dogs with inflammation identified in the semen.

Mycoplasma and *Ureaplasma* are fragile organisms and require special techniques for culturing. Semen samples should be collected in a sterile vial, avoiding the first fraction of the ejaculate to minimize contamination by bacteria colonizing the distal urethra (Linde-Forsberg and Bölske, 1995). It is also important to avoid any contact with the preputial mucous membrane. A sterile cotton culture swab (e.g., Culturette, Baxter Healthcare, McGaw Park, IL) is dipped into the semen sample and immediately transferred to a vial containing transport medium suitable for *Mycoplasma* and *Ureaplasma* (e.g., Amies Transport Media, Difco Laboratories, Detroit, MI; modified Stuarts medium, Baxter Healthcare, McGaw Park, IL). The vial should be sent overnight mail in a Styrofoam shipping box containing ice. Because *Mycoplasma* and *Ureaplasma* organisms have different growth requirements, the laboratory should be notified regarding which cultures are desired before obtaining the semen specimen.

Serology testing for *Mycoplasma* and *Ureaplasma* species is not routinely performed clinically because screening is limited to a few species, antibody titers are often low and slow to increase, and a positive titer may occur from normal flora. PCR testing for detection of *Mycoplasma* and *Ureaplasma* in semen, prostatic fluid and urine is also available (van Kuppeveld et al, 1994). See Linde-Forsberg and Bölske (1995) for more information on canine genital mycoplasmas and ureaplasmas.

BRUCELLA CANIS TESTING

Canine brucellosis is a cause of reproductive problems in both male and female dogs (see page 919). Brucellosis should be considered in any dog suspected of having infertility, orchitis, epididymitis, testicular atrophy, discospondylitis, generalized lymphadenopathy, or fever of unknown origin. Because infections are often subclinical, all males presented for reproductive failure should be screened for *B. canis*. Screening should also be a routine part of a prebreeding examination.

Serologic testing is the most frequently used screening diagnostic procedure for *B. canis* infection. Nonprotective antibodies are produced against cell wall antigens and cytoplasmic antigens of *B. canis*, become detectable 8 to 12 weeks after infection, and typically remain high (i.e., 1:400) as long as bacteremia persists (Carmichael et al, 1984; Carmichael and Greene, 1990). Serologic tests include the rapid slide agglutination test (RSAT; D-Tec CB, Pitman-Moore, Washington Crossing, NJ), the tube agglutination test (TAT), and the agar gel immunodiffusion (AGID) test. The latter two tests are available through most state diagnostic laboratories. The RSAT, TAT, and some of the AGID tests detect antibodies directed against cell wall antigens. Cell wall antigens are common to many of the *Brucella* species and to several other bacteria, including *Bordatella bronchiseptica, Pseudomonas aeruginosa,* and mucoid *Staphylococcus* species. Therefore test results are not specific for *Brucella*, and false-positive results are possible. Positive results using serologic tests that use cell wall antigens must be confirmed by other, more specific tests, such as AGID tests that use cytoplasmic antigen or isolation and identification of the organism by culture of blood or semen (see Chapter 26). Cytoplasmic or internal antigens of *B. canis* are unique to the genus *Brucella*.

False-negative serologic test results in dogs infected long enough to develop antibodies to cell wall antigens are rare. Antibodies to cell wall antigens are detectable 8 to 12 weeks after infection. Serologic tests are often negative in the first 4 to 8 weeks after infection. Recent infection may be missed by evaluation of a single test. All negative serology tests should be repeated after 30 days to decrease the possibility of false-negative results. When bacteremia becomes intermittent or subsides (e.g., during chronic infections exceeding 30 to 60 weeks or following antibiotic therapy), antibody titers decline and may become equivocal or negative, despite persistence of the organism in tissues (Carmichael et al, 1984).

HORMONAL EVALUATION

OVERVIEW. Spermatogenesis and steroidogenesis are closely related but performed by spatially distinct areas of the testis. Spermatogenesis occurs within the seminiferous tubule compartment, which consists of spermatogonia and Sertoli cells. Steroidogenesis occurs within the interstitial tissue compartment of the testis, which is composed of Leydig cells. Libido and sperm production are dependent on an intact hypothalamic-pituitary-testicular axis. Two hormonal systems exist in the male reproductive tract, one involving hypothalamic GnRH–pituitary LH–testicular testosterone and the other involving GnRH–pituitary FSH–testicular inhibin (Table 27-5; Fig. 27-10; Hewitt, 1998). The production of mature spermatozoa requires the presence of both FSH and male androgens, primarily testosterone and dihydrotestosterone, within the testes. Testosterone is converted to dihydrotestosterone by 5α-reductase. Dihydrotestosterone is approximately twice as potent as testosterone because of much greater binding affinity for and slower dissociation from intracellular androgen receptors (Wasmer and Rogers, 1996). Endogenous testosterone secretion from the interstitial (Leydig) cells bathes the seminiferous tubules and promotes spermatogenesis. Testosterone is also necessary for the maintenance of the secretory and absorptive activities of the efferent ducts, epididymis, and ductus deferens; for the growth and maintenance of the prostate gland; for maintaining libido; and for the development of secondary sexual characteristics.

GnRH stimulates the secretion of LH, which in turn, stimulates the secretion of testosterone. Prolactin may also act synergistically with LH in regulating testosterone production by the Leydig cells (Hewitt, 1998). GnRH is released into the hypophyseal portal system in discrete bursts (pulses; Kumar et al, 1980).

TABLE 27-5 ACTIONS OF REPRODUCTIVE HORMONES INVOLVED IN SPERMATOGENESIS AND STEROIDOGENESIS IN THE DOG

Hormone	Source	Primary Actions
GnRH	Hypothalamus	On anterior pituitary to stimulate LH and FSH secretion
LH	Anterior pituitary	On Leydig cells to stimulate steroidogenesis
FSH	Anterior pituitary	On Sertoli cells to stimulate spermatogenesis
Prolactin	Anterior pituitary	Synergistic action with LH to stimulate steroidogenesis by Leydig cells
Testosterone	Leydig cells	On Sertoli cells to stimulate spermatogenesis: On hypothalamus and anterior pituitary to inhibit GnRH, LH, and FSH secretion
Estradiol	Leydig cells?	Synergistic action with testosterone to inhibit GnRH, LH, and FSH secretion?
Inhibin	Sertoli cells	On anterior pituitary to inhibit FSH secretion
Activin?	Sertoli cells	On anterior pituitary to stimulate FSH secretion

Adapted from Hewitt D: Physiology and endocrinology of the male. *In* Simpson GM, England GCW, Harvey M (eds): BSAVA Manual of Small Animal Reproduction and Neonatology. Cheltenham, British Small Animal Veterinary Association, 1998, p 61.

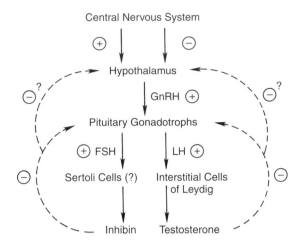

FIGURE 27-10. Proposed positive and negative feedback loops involved in the hormonal regulation of spermatogenesis and testosterone production.

TABLE 27-6   SERUM CONCENTRATIONS OF FSH, LH, AND TESTOSTERONE FROM DOGS WITH VARYING STAGES OF SEMINIFEROUS TUBULE DAMAGE AND IMPAIRED SPERMATOGENESIS

Grade	FSH (ng/ml ± SEM)	LH (ng/ml ± SEM)	Testosterone (ng/ml ± SEM)
I	73 ± 7	34 ± 9	3 ± 0.5
II	84 ± 9	85 ± 32	3 ± 0.6
III	236 ± 49	96 ± 18	3 ± 0.7
IV	321 ± 58	95 ± 26	3 ± 0.6

Grade I: All seminiferous tubules show active spermatogenesis
Grade II: Depression or arrest of spermatogenesis in some or all seminiferous tubules or diminished number of spermatogonia
Grade III: Some but not all seminiferous tubules have complete absence of spermatogonia
Grade IV: All seminiferous tubules have complete absence of spermatogonia

From Soderberg SF: PhD Thesis, Colorado State University, 1984; as reported by Olson PN: Clinical approach to infertility in the stud dog. Proceedings of the Annual Society for Theriogenology, 1984, p 33.

Consequently, LH and testosterone secretion is pulsatile and their serum concentrations fluctuate. Testosterone, possibly in conjunction with estradiol, inhibits GnRH and LH secretion (Kumar et al, 1980; Falvo et al, 1982). Estradiol is secreted by the testes or produced by local aromatization of testosterone.

FSH stimulates spermatogenesis indirectly by acting on Sertoli cells. FSH secretion is necessary to maintain germ cell differentiation and development of spermatozoa. FSH also facilitates the completion of spermatid maturation by stimulating Sertoli cell development, Sertoli cell function, and the synthesis of androgen-binding protein (Ganong, 2001). FSH secretion is stimulated by GnRH and inhibited by inhibin, a non-steroidal glycoprotein secreted by the Sertoli cells (de Kretser and Robertson, 1989) (Fig. 27-10). There may also be other products (activins) of the Sertoli cell that have the opposite effect and stimulate FSH secretion (Hewitt, 1998). Measurement of blood testosterone and gonadotropin concentrations provides information on the functional status of the hypothalamic-pituitary-gonadal axis. Indications for measurement of these hormones include oligospermia/azoospermia, poor libido, cryptorchidism, testicular neoplasia, and suspected intersex states.

TESTOSTERONE.   Canine blood contains testosterone and its precursors, including androstenedione, dehydroepiandrosterone, and 17-hydroxyprogesterone (Boulanger et al, 1982). Testosterone plays an important role in maintaining libido and spermatogenesis in the male. A deficiency in blood testosterone concentration can be safely predicted in most dogs with loss of libido. Dogs with normal libido and the ability to mate rarely have plasma testosterone concentrations below 0.4 ng/ml (400 pg/ml), regardless of fertility (Larsen and Johnston, 1980). In addition, testicular testosterone concentrations are 50 to 100 times greater than concentrations in blood, so blood levels may not reflect alterations in testicular testosterone nor be a useful diagnostic aid for evaluating spermatogenesis

(Table 27-6) (Olson, 1984b). For these reasons, we usually do not evaluate blood testosterone concentrations in dogs presented for infertility. Measurement of blood testosterone concentration, however, can be helpful in differentiating intact versus castrated versus bilaterally cryptorchid dogs (Table 27-7).

Determination of blood testosterone concentration by radioimmunoassay is offered by several commercial veterinary endocrine laboratories. The reported normal range is 0.4 to 10.0 ng/ml (Larsen and Johnston, 1980; Olson, 1984b), although our laboratory values are usually between 1 and 5 ng/ml. Dogs with retained testicles (cryptorchidism) usually have values of 0.10 to 2 ng/ml, whereas castrated males have concentrations less than 0.02 ng/ml (<20 pg/ml). A single baseline blood testosterone concentration is of limited value because of the wide and unpredictable fluctuation in blood testosterone concentration. It has been recommended that when using baseline testosterone concentration to assess Leydig cell function, three to six blood samples be obtained at 20-minute intervals and testosterone concentration be measured in each blood sample (Kamolpatana et al, 1998). Mean concentration of serum testosterone from the samples drawn should be greater than 2 ng/ml in normal, intact male dogs.

GnRH and human chorionic gonadotropin (hCG) stimulation tests can be used to assess Leydig cell function. The GnRH stimulation test is preferred. Dosage of GnRH, timing of blood sample collection and test results may differ depending on which GnRH analog is used (Purswell and Wilcke, 1993). It is important to follow the GnRH stimulation test protocol established by the laboratory performing the testosterone and LH assays. As a general rule, the intramuscular administration of GnRH elicits a peak in serum LH and testosterone concentration approximately 15 and 60 minutes after administration, respectively. For the GnRH stimulation test, 1.0 to 2.2 μg of GnRH per kilogram of body

TABLE 27-7 ALTERATIONS IN BASAL CONCENTRATIONS OF REPRODUCTIVE HORMONES SEEN IN ASSOCIATION WITH MORE COMMON DISORDERS OF THE TESTES

	Testosterone	Estrogen	FSH	LH
Normal dog	1–5 ng/ml	<15 pg/ml	N	N
Dog with 1 scrotal and 1 cryptorchid testis	1–5 ng/ml	<15 pg/ml	N	N
Dog with only cryptorchid testes	0.1–2 ng/ml (100–2000 pg/ml)	<15 pg/ml	N or ↑	N
Castrated dog	<20 pg/ml	<15 pg/ml	↑	↑
Dog with Sertoli cell tumor	0.1–2 ng/ml	10–200 pg/ml	N or ↓	N or ↓

N, Within normal range; ↑, increased; ↓, decreased

weight is administered IM, and blood for testosterone determination is obtained immediately before and 1 hour after GnRH administration. Blood for LH determination should be obtained before and 15 minutes after GnRH administration. In healthy dogs, serum testosterone concentration should increase after GnRH administration and post-GnRH serum testosterone concentration should be greater than 3 ng/ml (Meyers-Wallen, 1991). If serum testosterone concentration does not increase after GnRH administration, determination of serum LH concentrations will help localize the lesion to the pituitary gland or testes. In one study, mean serum LH and testosterone concentration increased by 947% (range, 433% to 2708%) and 189% (range, 53% to 518%) 15 and 60 minutes, respectively, after the intramuscular administration of 0.7 µg of GnRH (gonadorelin hydrochloride; Factrel, Fort Dodge, IA) per kilogram of body weight to eight healthy dogs (Purswell and Wilcke, 1993). Others have reported serum testosterone concentrations from 0.5 to 5 ng/ml and 3.7 to greater than 5 ng/ml before and 1 hour after the intramuscular administration of 1 µg of GnRH per kilogram of body weight, respectively, to healthy dogs (Schille and Olson, 1989).

For the hCG stimulation test, 40 IU of hCG (Chorionic gonadotropin, Rugby Laboratories, Long Island, NY) per kilogram of body weight is administered IM, and blood is obtained immediately before and 4 hours after hCG administration. In healthy dogs, serum testosterone concentration should increase after hCG administration, and post-hCG serum testosterone concentration should be greater than 4.5 ng/ml (Meyers-Wallen, 1991; Schille et al, 1991).

PITUITARY GONADOTROPINS (FSH, LH). Measurement of pituitary gonadotropins is used in the assessment of the hypothalamic-pituitary-gonadal axis in dogs with decreased libido or oligospermia/azoospermia and to determine neuter status. Normal baseline LH concentration is typically less than 20 ng/ml but can fluctuate to greater than 90 ng/ml during periods of episodic secretion (Amann, 1986). Normal baseline FSH concentration does not fluctuate to the same degree as LH and is typically less than 250 ng/ml (Schille and Olson, 1989). Loss of negative feedback inhibition following castration results in increased circulating concentrations of LH and FSH. In one study, mean (±SD) serum LH and FSH concentration was 6.0 ± 5.2 and 89 ± 28 ng/ml in intact dogs and 17.1 ± 9.9 and 858 ± 674 ng/ml in castrated dogs, respectively (Olson et al, 1992). Serum

LH values overlapped between intact and castrated dogs; however, no overlap was seen in serum FSH concentration. Serum FSH concentration was less than 150 ng/ml in intact dogs and greater than 150 ng/ml in castrated dogs. Overlap in serum LH concentration may be attributed to timing of blood sampling in relation to episodic bursts of LH secretion.

A similar increase in serum LH and FSH concentration may be found in some dogs with oligospermia/azoospermia and primary testicular dysfunction. Serum concentrations of FSH appear to correlate best with the severity of altered spermatogenesis (Table 27-6; Olson, 1984b). Infertile dogs with severe testicular dysfunction typically have serum FSH concentrations greater than 250 ng/ml (Soderberg, 1986). Plasma LH concentrations may also increase (Table 27-6), presumably as a result of increased GnRH secretion and/or testosterone deficiency from concomitant dysfunction of Leydig cells. In contrast, normal or low serum FSH and LH concentrations in oligospermic/azoospermic dogs suggest early degenerative changes in the testes, tubal obstruction within the duct system, retrograde ejaculation, or pituitary/hypothalamic dysfunction (e.g., hypogonadotropic hypogonadism). Interpretation of a single gonadotropin concentration must be done cautiously. Gonadotropins are secreted in an episodic manner, and serum concentrations can vary significantly in healthy dogs.

Pituitary response to GnRH administration may help differentiate hypothalamic/pituitary from primary testicular dysfunction (see prior discussion on testosterone) and help the clinician formulate a rational therapeutic plan for the oligospermic/azoospermic dog (see page 991). Falvo and colleagues (1982) showed a linear increase in LH response with increasing dosages of GnRH (5 to 250 ng/kg IV). An increase in plasma LH concentration occurred within 10 minutes, and peak response occurred within 30 minutes of GnRH administration. In six healthy dogs given 250 ng/kg GnRH IV, mean peak increase in plasma LH concentration was approximately 18 ng/ml. Concentrations of LH in serum obtained 10 minutes after administering 250 ng/kg GnRH IV to four intact Greyhounds ranged from 20.8 to 49.5 ng/ml (mean, 32 ± 11 ng/ml; Freshman et al, 1987), and in another study, mean serum LH concentration increased by 947% (range, 433% to 2708%) 15 minutes after the intramuscular administration of 0.7 µg/kg of GnRH to eight healthy dogs (Purswell and Wilcke, 1993). Failure of serum FSH and LH concentration to increase after GnRH administration suggests a hypothalamic/pituitary rather than primary testicular problem.

Because of poor cross-reactivity between species, only canine-specific assays should be used for measuring pituitary gonadotropins in the dog. Interpretation of results should also be based on normal values established by the endocrine laboratory being used. Unfortunately, canine-specific assays, especially for FSH, are not readily available commercially.

ESTRADIOL, PROGESTERONE. The primary indications for measuring blood estradiol and progesterone concentrations are in male dogs suspected of having steroid-secreting neoplasms, especially of the testes (see page 967), and in dogs with suspected intersexuality (see page 893).

THYROID HORMONE. The interplay between a deficiency of thyroid hormone and fertility in the dog is controversial. Historically, hypothyroidism has been cited as a cause of diminished libido, testicular degeneration, oligospermia, and subfertility. In humans, these abnormalities may result from decreased plasma FSH, LH, and testosterone concentrations secondary to thyroid hormone deficiency, but this relationship is not confirmed in dogs. Recently, reproductive function of Beagle dogs made hypothyroid by the administration of ^{131}iodine was compared with age- and breed-matched euthyroid dogs over a 2-year period (Johnson et al, 1999). Total scrotal width, daily sperm output, sperm motility, and sperm morphology did not change significantly in the hypothyroid dogs, compared with control dogs. Although libido was diminished, all dogs ejaculated readily. There was also no significant difference in serum concentrations of LH and testosterone before and after the administration of GnRH between the 2 groups of dogs. The consensus of academicians and researchers attending the International Symposium on Canine Hypothyroidism held at the University of California, Davis, in 1996 regarding the interplay between hypothyroidism and reproductive dysfunction in dogs was similar to results of Johnson's study—that is, hypothyroidism appears to be an uncommon cause of subfertility in dogs. Does this mean that thyroid gland function should not be assessed in a subfertile dog? Probably not, but it does suggest that if serum thyroid hormone concentrations are normal, other explanations for the subfertility should be sought rather than continuing to pursue hypothyroidism through trial therapy. When assessing thyroid gland function, we recommend measurement of serum total T_4, free T_4 by dialysis, endogenous cTSH, and thyroglobulin autoantibodies. (See Chapter 3, page 111, for a complete discussion on evaluation of thyroid gland function.)

CORTISOL. Elevations in plasma cortisol concentration are assumed to suppress the secretion of pituitary gonadotropins. As a result, plasma testosterone and FSH concentrations decline, resulting in testicular atrophy, loss of libido, oligospermia, and infertility. In one study, the mean morning plasma testosterone concentration as determined by radioimmunoassay in 11 healthy dogs was 4.7 ± 1.8 ng/ml. In 12 dogs with hyperadrenocorticism and testicular atrophy, the mean plasma testosterone concentration was 1.2 ± 0.7 ng/ml (Feldman and Tyrrell, 1982). The suppressive effect of cortisol can occur with prolonged oral, aural, ocular, or topical administration of glucocorticoids and with spontaneous hyperadrenocorticism. Dogs with spontaneous hyperadrenocorticism, however, are rarely presented to the veterinarian for a primary reproductive problem. (See Chapter 6, page 300, for a complete discussion on evaluation of the adrenal gland for hyperadrenocorticism.)

RADIOGRAPHY AND ULTRASONOGRAPHY

Radiographic assessment of the male reproductive tract is indicated in dogs with suspected prostatic disease, cryptorchid testis, or testicular tumor. Survey radiographs of the prostate gland may identify prostatomegaly, defined as prostatic dimensions exceeding 70% of the pubic brim-sacral promontory dimension in survey lateral radiographs (Feeney et al, 1987). Survey radiographs are also used to characterize prostatic margins (i.e., smooth versus irregular) and identify alterations in radiographic density of the prostate (e.g., uroliths, soft tissue mineralization, gas). In dogs with suspected prostatic adenocarcinoma, survey abdominal radiographs may identify metastatic lesions, such as lymphadenopathy or proliferative periosteal reaction of the ventral border of the lumbar vertebrae. Survey abdominal radiographs may also identify cryptorchid testes that have undergone malignant transformation and are enlarged, retroperitoneal lymphadenopathy of the iliac lymph nodes in dogs with metastatic testicular tumors, and discospondylitis or osteomyelitis in dogs with orchitis/epididymitis due to *Brucella canis* or other infectious agent. Positive contrast retrograde urethrocystography can be performed following survey radiography to assess the penile and prostatic urethra and the urinary bladder.

Ultrasonography is indicated in dogs with suspected disease of the prostate gland, testes, epididymis, or vas deferens. Ultrasonography allows examination of the internal structure of these organs and can also be used to obtain measurements of prostatic size and for directed aspiration or biopsy of identified lesions. The normal prostate should be symmetric with smooth borders, and a homogeneous parenchymal pattern with medium to fine texture. Echogenicity is variable, from hyperechoic to hypoechoic, although moderate echogenicity is most common (Fig. 27-11; Mattoon and Nyland, 1995). The prostatic urethra can often be imaged, appearing as a hypoechoic-to-anechoic round structure within the central-to-dorsal portion of the gland. Rarely, the ductus deferens can be seen as hypoechoic linear echoes coursing obliquely through the dorsal portion of the gland. Although one study found a good correlation between radiographic and ultrasonographic methods for assessing prostatic length but not depth when radiographic magnification was eliminated

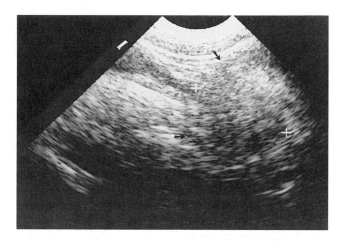

FIGURE 27-11. Ultrasonography of the normal prostate gland (*arrows* and *crosses*). Note the coarse, hyperechoic echotexture of the parenchyma.

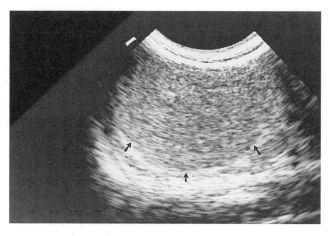

FIGURE 27-12. Ultrasonography of the normal testis (*arrows*). Note the homogeneous, coarse echogenicity of the parenchyma.

(Atalan et al, 1999), overall prostatic measurements from ultrasonographic images are considered more accurate and reliable because the contours of the prostate are better outlined, measurements are performed using integrated electronic calipers, and there is no magnification effect as occurs with abdominal radiographs. The size of the prostate gland in healthy dogs increases with size, body weight, and age, suggesting that assessment of prostate gland size should take into account the effect of body size and age (Table 27-8; Ruel et al, 1998).

The sonogram of the normal testes has a coarse homogeneous parenchyma with a linear hyperechoic mediastinum testis and well-defined hyperechoic capsule (the tunica albuginea; Fig. 27-12) (Pugh et al, 1990; Mattoon and Nyland, 1995). Visualization of the epididymis is variable. The tail of the epididymis is the most consistent structure seen with ultrasonography, is typically anechoic to hypoechoic relative to the testicular parenchyma, and is attached to the caudal pole of the testis. The head of the epididymis is smaller but has a similar ultrasonographic appearance. The ductus deferens is difficult to follow because it becomes quite small in size. It is rarely seen entering the prostate gland in the normal state. Alterations in echogenicity of tissue

parenchyma; sonographic shadowing; presence, size, shape, and location of cavitary lesions within the parenchyma; and irregularities in structure surface may provide clues to the underlying disease process (Tables 27-9 and 27-10; Johnston et al, 1991). In general, ultrasonography is of greater value than radiography when assessing the prostate gland and testes for disease and when attempting to identify intra-abdominal testes.

TESTICULAR ASPIRATION

Cytologic evaluation of a fine-needle aspirate of the testis is a quick, simple, inexpensive diagnostic aid in evaluating a discrete, focal testicular mass. This technique is especially helpful in differentiating testicular tumors (see page 964; Chapwanya et al, 2000). Fine-needle aspiration is less helpful as a diagnostic aid for oligospermia/azoospermia or degenerative changes in testicular parenchyma. The more severe the degenerative changes in the germinal epithelium, the more likely results of aspiration cytology are nondiagnostic. Fine-needle aspiration may identify inflammation (e.g., plasmacytic-lymphocytic or neutrophilic orchitis), an infectious agent, or the presence of spermatogenic cells (Figs. 27-13 and 27-14). Spermatogonia, spermatocytes, spermatids, spermatozoa, and Sertoli cells are identifiable; Leydig cells are difficult to identify on aspiration cytology (Dahlbom et al, 1997). The identification of active spermatogenesis on a testicular aspirate from an azoospermic dog suggests bilateral occlusion of the duct system or previous severe transient insult with regeneration of seminiferous tubule function. In contrast, failure to identify spermatogenic cells on a testicular aspirate from an azoospermic dog suggests severe arrest in spermatogenesis but provides no information on its reversibility. Condition of the basement membrane of the seminiferous tubule, architecture of the germinative epithelium, and status

TABLE 27-8 FORMULAS FOR CALCULATION OF THE PREDICTED MAXIMUM LENGTH (L), WIDTH (W), HEIGHT ON SAGITTAL IMAGES (H_{sag}), AND HEIGHT ON TRANSVERSE IMAGES (H_{tr}) (IN CENTIMETERS) OF THE PROSTATE GLAND IN HEALTHY DOGS, BASED ON BODY WEIGHT (BW) AND AGE (A) OF THE DOG

$$L = (0.055 \times BW) + (0.143 \times A) + 3.31$$
$$W = (0.047 \times BW) + (0.089 \times A) + 3.45$$
$$H_{sag} = (0.046 \times BW) + (0.069 \times A) + 2.68$$
$$H_{tr} = (0.044 \times BW) + (0.083 \times A) + 2.25$$

From Ruel Y, et al: Ultrasonographic evaluation of the prostate in healthy intact dogs. Vet Radiol Ultra 39: 212, 1998.

TABLE 27-9 GUIDELINES FOR INTERPRETATION OF ULTRASONOGRAPHIC FINDINGS IN THE CANINE PROSTATE GLAND

Prostatic Disorder	Ultrasonographic Findings
Normal prostate	Normal size; symmetrical shape; smooth borders; uniform homogeneous parenchymal pattern with medium to fine texture; variable echogenicity from hyperechoic to hypoechoic, moderate echogenicity most common
Benign hyperplasia	Normal to enlarged size; symmetric or asymmetric shape; usually smooth borders; echogenicity varies from hypoechoic to hyperechoic; texture may be smooth to coarse; scattered hyperechoic foci and intraparenchymal cysts may be present
Acute prostatitis	Normal to enlarged size; symmetric or asymmetric shape; smooth or irregular borders; heterogeneous pattern of mixed echogenicity with focal or multifocal areas of poorly marginated hypoechogenicity and focal irregular hyperechoic foci; hypoechoic or anechoic cavities with far enhancement if parenchymal cysts or abscesses present; sonographic shadowing if gas present
Chronic prostatitis	Variable size; symmetric or asymmetric shape; smooth or irregular borders; heterogenous pattern of mixed echogenicity with focal or diffuse increased parenchymal echogenicity; hypoechoic cavitating lesions with far enhancement if parenchymal cysts present; sonographic shadowing if mineralization or fibrosis present
Prostatic carcinoma	Enlarged size; asymmetric shape; irregular borders; heterogeneous echotexture; multiple, poorly defined hyperechoic foci that tend to coalesce; cavitary, cystlike lesions may be present; sonographic shadowing from mineralization possible; potential capsule disruption
Prostatic abscess	Normal to enlarged size; symmetric or asymmetric shape; smooth or irregular borders; hypoechoic or anechoic, poorly marginated cavitary lesions with variable far enhancement; normal to hyperechoic parenchyma
Prostatic cyst	Normal to enlarged size; symmetric or asymmetric shape; smooth or irregular borders; hypoechoic or anechoic foci with far enhancement; focal echogenicities may be present within cyst; normal to hyperechoic parenchyma

TABLE 27-10 GUIDELINES FOR INTERPRETATION OF ULTRASONOGRAPHIC FINDINGS OF THE TESTIS AND EPIDIDYMIS IN THE DOG

	Ultrasonographic Findings
Testicular Disorder	
Normal testis	Coarse, homogeneous parenchyma with linear hyperechoic mediastinum testis and well-defined hyperechoic capsule
Testicular tumor	Variable echogenicity depending on size of tumor and whether focal or diffuse distribution; often hypoechoic when small (<3 cm) and mixed echogenicity when large (>5 cm); hyperechoic, hypoechoic, or anechoic foci may develop within tumor
Testicular torsion	Testicular enlargement with uniform decrease in parenchymal echogenicity with concurrent enlargement of the epididymis and spermatic cord; absence of perfusion identified with color Doppler ultrasonography
Orchitis	*Acute:* Diffuse patchy hypoechoic parenchymal pattern; cavitating lesions (e.g., abscesses) may be present *Chronic:* Decrease in testicular size; diffuse hyperechoic or mixed echogenic parenchymal pattern
Abscess	Irregular, poorly defined internal wall marginations and variable internal echogenicity within cavitation; normal or hyperechoic testicular parenchyma
Cyst	Anechoic cavitations with smooth, well-defined walls
Extratesticular Disorder	
Normal epididymis	Anechoic to hypoechoic relative to testicular parenchyma
Epididymitis	Enlargement of epididymis with diffuse patchy hypoechoic to mixed echogenic parenchymal pattern
Epididymal cyst, spermatocele	Focal, anechoic cystic structures with sharp internal wall margins and far enhancement deep to the cyst
Hydrocele	Anechoic fluid accumulation around the testis with far enhancement
Scrotal hernia	Identifiable abdominal contents passing through inguinal canal into scrotum

of interstitial tissue of the testis cannot be determined from fine needle aspiration of the testis, and identification of stages of cellular differentiation of spermatogonia is difficult because normal cell-to-cell contact is lost.

The technique for fine-needle aspiration of the testis is similar to the technique used to aspirate other masses or lymph nodes. A 20- to 25-gauge needle on a 6-ml syringe should be used, depending on the size of the testis. Local anesthesia is not necessary, and sedation is usually needed only in the intractable dog. The epididymis should be avoided. The testicular material is gently smeared onto a clean glass slide, stained, and evaluated cytologically for the presence of spermatozoa, inflammatory cells, bacteria, and fungi (DeNicola et al, 1980). Aspiration of testicular

tissue causes minimal trauma and has not been found to have adverse effects on spermatogenesis (Dahlbom et al, 1997).

EPIDIDYMAL ASPIRATION

Cytologic evaluation of a fine-needle aspirate of the epididymis is indicated in dogs with palpably abnormal epididymides and in dogs with azoospermia (see page 991). The technique is similar to that described for testicular aspiration (see prior discussion). Aspirates of the caudal epididymis should be evaluated for the presence of live, motile sperm, inflammatory cells, and bacteria. In an azoospermic dog, the presence of spermatozoa from an epididymal aspirate implies

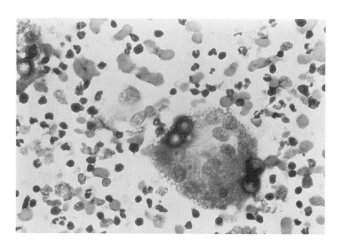

FIGURE 27-13. Testicular aspirate from a dog with swollen, painful testes, revealing a pyogranulomatous orchitis due to blastomycosis. Note the large, multinucleated giant cell containing a budding form of *Blastomyces dermatitides* (Wright's stain ×400). (From DeNicola DB, et al: Cytology of the Canine Urogenital Tract [brochure], copyright 1980. Reproduced by permission of Ralston Purina Company.)

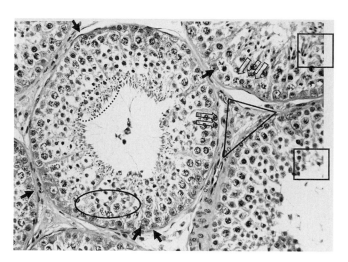

FIGURE 27-15. Histologic section of the testis from a healthy adult dog illustrating the cellular differentiation of the spermatogonia to spermatozoa. *Solid arrows,* Sertoli cells; *open arrows,* spermatogonia; *solid oval,* spermatocytes; *solid box,* round and elongated spermatids; *dashed oval;* spermatozoa; *solid triangle,* interstitial cells of Leydig (H&E ×400).

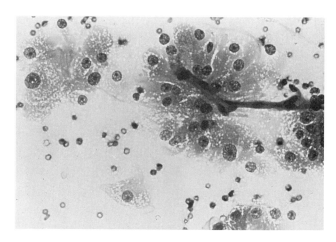

FIGURE 27-14. Aspirate of a small testicular mass, revealing an interstitial cell tumor. Note the cluster of variably sized polygonal cells surrounding an endothelium-lined capillary space (Diff Quik ×250). (From DeNicola DB, et al: Cytology of the Canine Urogenital Tract [brochure], copyright 1980. Reproduced by permission of Ralston Purina Company.)

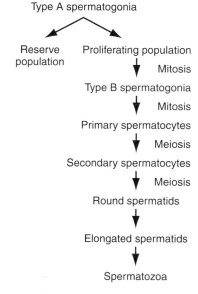

FIGURE 27-16. Schematic of spermatogenesis. In the dog, approximately 55 to 70 days are required for spermatozoa to develop from spermatogonia and appear in the ejaculate.

obstruction in the ductus deferens, whereas a lack of sperm implies duct obstruction or destruction of sperm proximal to the site of the aspirate or an arrest in spermatogenesis. Measurement of seminal alkaline phosphatase (see page 940) and evaluation of a testicular aspirate or biopsy help differentiate between the latter two diagnoses. The presence of inflammatory cells and bacteria is supportive of epididymitis. Depending on the amount of aspirate obtained, a portion can also be submitted for bacterial culture.

TESTICULAR BIOPSY

INDICATIONS. Biopsy of the testicular parenchyma allows evaluation of seminiferous tubule architecture, progression of spermatogenesis, interstitial and Sertoli cell numbers, and the presence or absence of inflammation or neoplasia (Figs. 27-15 and 27-16). Because tissue is obtained aseptically, a portion of the biopsy can also be submitted for bacterial and mycoplasmal culture. Testicular biopsy is indicated in the infertile dog with persistent oligospermia/azoospermia in which less invasive diagnostic tests have failed to identify the cause for the infertility. Testicular biopsy may also be considered in the dog with a discrete mass or diffuse change in consistency of the testis on digital palpation.

COMPLICATIONS. When considering a testicular biopsy, the clinician must always weigh the benefits gained against the potential risks of performing the

TABLE 27-11 POTENTIAL COMPLICATIONS RESULTING FROM TESTICULAR BIOPSY PROCEDURE

Hemorrhage
Inflammation
Infection
Scrotal, testicular hyperthermia
Immune-mediated orchitis
Scrotal swelling
Fibrosis
Scrotal-testicular adhesions
Duct obstruction
Sperm granuloma
Testicular atrophy
Transient or permanent decrease in sperm production

procedure. A number of potential complications may develop following testicular biopsy (Table 27-11). Fortunately, these complications are uncommon when care and aseptic technique are used. In studies evaluating serial percutaneous testicular biopsies, the only serious complication was the infrequent development of unilateral testicular atrophy. Nevertheless, a testicular biopsy should be performed only after other less invasive techniques have been explored and should never be performed on a valuable stud dog that has normal semen. There is obviously less to lose and more to gain from a testicular biopsy in an oligospermic or azoospermic dog.

FIXATIVES. Appropriate fixatives for testicular tissue include Bouin's, Zenker's, glutaraldehyde, and Karnovsky's fixative. The pathology laboratory should be contacted before obtaining the tissue sample to determine the clinician's preference of fixative. Tissues should not be fixed in formaldehyde. Fixation in buffered formaldehyde results in seminiferous tubule shrinkage, poor nuclear detail, and other artifacts that preclude meaningful interpretation (Amann, 1982). Tissues should be placed into the fixative immediately after they are obtained. If the excisional wedge biopsy technique is used, placement of both blade and specimen into the fixative without trying to separate the biopsy sample from the blade helps minimize tissue handling, artifacts, and cellular disruption. Hematoxylin and eosin, periodic acid–Schiff, or toluidine blue are suitable stains for analyzing testicular tissue.

TECHNIQUES. The percutaneous needle punch biopsy technique and the excisional wedge biopsy technique can be used to obtain testicular tissue for fixation and sectioning.

Percutaneous needle punch biopsy technique is a quick, simple, inexpensive technique. The dog should be placed under a short-acting general anesthetic (e.g., propofol) during the procedure. Ultrasound guidance is helpful during the biopsy procedure, especially if a focal lesion is present. Trauma to the inner parenchyma of the testis and the duct system is a risk with this procedure, and the tissue specimen may not be of sufficient size or quality for adequate histologic study. Heavy sedation or general anesthesia is required.

Several types of biopsy needles may be used, including the Bard Biopty-Cut, Franklin modified Vim-Silverman needle, Vim TruCut needle, Jamshidi

biopsy needle-syringe combination, and the Menghini needle. We prefer to biopsy the testes using the Bard Biopty-Cut needle (CR Bard, Inc, Covington, GA) and ultrasound guidance. An 18- to 22-gauge needle should be used, depending on the size of the testis and the needle size available. The testis should be immobilized, with one hand grasping the vas deferens tightly enough to compress the spermatic artery and a small skin incision made in the cranioventral scrotum. The needle should be directed posteriorly in the ventral portion of the testis so as not to penetrate the epididymis or efferent ductules. Ultrasound guidance is recommended, if available. Sutures at the biopsy site are not required. Hemostasis is obtained with local compression.

Excisional wedge biopsy technique is the preferred technique despite the potential for more gross and histologic lesions in the biopsied testis compared with the punch biopsy technique (Lopate, 1989). Testicular tissue removed through an incision in the tunica albuginea provides the best biopsy specimen for histologic interpretation. Using this technique, the clinician determines the size of the biopsy sample, artifacts from tissue handling are minimized, and avoidance of testicular vessels is maximized. Because the technique is aseptic, a portion of the biopsy specimen can be submitted for bacterial culture. Unfortunately, the excisional wedge biopsy technique requires general anesthesia, making it more time-consuming and expensive. However, the superior sample that is obtained for interpretive analysis by the pathologist warrants the extra time and expense required to obtain the specimen.

Although a biopsy can be obtained through a scrotal incision, it is preferable to incise the skin anterior to the scrotum (Fig. 27-17, *A*). This area is clipped and surgically prepared. The testis to be biopsied is moved forward, and an antescrotal midline incision is made. The testis is immobilized, and hemostasis is obtained by compression of the spermatic cord. The incision is extended through the subcutaneous tissue and tunica vaginalis on the medioventral surface of the testis. A thin scalpel blade is used to incise the white tunica albuginea. Testicular tissue then bulges into the incision site (Fig. 27-17, *B*). This bulging tissue can then be removed at its base by cutting it with a razor blade or fine Metzenbaum scissors. The tissue, either on the blade or following placement on cardboard, is immediately submerged into fixative. Cuts into the testicular parenchyma may be necessary to obtain a wedge of tissue for those testes in which the parenchyma fails to bulge following incision of the tunica albuginea. The tunicae may be closed with fine (5-0 or 6-0) absorbable nonreactive suture material (Fig. 27-17, *C*) and the skin closed with nonabsorbable material. The testis should resume its normal position within the scrotum. Inadvertent suturing of the testis to the tunicae should be suspected if the testis fails to return to its normal position.

KARYOTYPING

The determination of the chromosomal constitution aids in identifying abnormal sex chromosome patterns

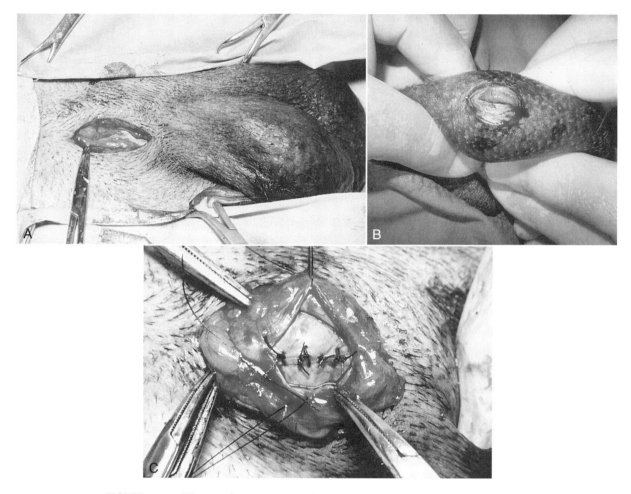

FIGURE 27-17. When performing a testicular biopsy, the skin just anterior to the scrotum is clipped and surgically prepared and an antescrotal midline incision made *(A)*. The testis to be biopsied is moved forward and immobilized, and the incision is extended through the subcutaneous tissue and tunica vaginalis on the medioventral surface of the testis. Testicular tissue bulges into the incision site following incision of the white tunica albuginea *(B)*. After biopsy is obtained, the tunicae may be closed with fine (5-0 or 6-0), absorbable, nonreactive suture material *(C)* and the skin closed with nonabsorbable material.

(e.g., XXY) in a congenitally infertile male dog or one with hypoplastic testes or penis. Unfortunately, only a limited number of institutions are currently involved with this diagnostic test. (See Chapter 24 for more information on karyotyping.)

REFERENCES

Althouse GC, et al: Effect of latex and vinyl examination gloves on canine spermatozoal motility. JAVMA 199:227, 1991.

Amann RP: Use of animal models for detecting specific alterations in reproduction. Fundam Appl Toxicol 2:13, 1982.

Amann RP: Reproductive physiology and endocrinology of the dog. *In* Morrow DA (ed): Current Therapy in Theriogenology, 2nd ed. Philadelphia, WB Saunders Co, 1986, p 532.

Atalan G, et al: Comparison of ultrasonographic and radiographic measurements of canine prostate dimensions. Vet Radiol Ultra 40: 408, 1999.

Bjurstrom L, Linde-Forsberg C: Long-term study of aerobic bacteria of the genital tract in breeding bitches. Am J Vet Res 53:665, 1992a.

Bjurstrom L, Linde-Forsberg C: Long-term study of aerobic bacteria of the genital tract in stud dogs. Am J Vet Res 53:670, 1992b.

Boulanger P, et al: Androgen levels in the liquid of the canine vas deferens and peripheral plasma. J Endocrinol 93:109, 1982.

Brendler CB, et al: Spontaneous benign prostatic hyperplasia in the Beagle: Age-associated changes in serum hormone levels, and the morphology and secretory function of the canine prostate. J Clin Invest 71:1114, 1983.

Carmichael LE, Greene CE: Canine brucellosis. *In* Greene CE (ed): Infectious Diseases of the Dog and Cat, 2nd ed. Philadelphia, WB Saunders Co, 1990, p 573.

Carmichael LE, et al: Problems with the serodiagnosis of canine brucellosis: Dog responses to cell-wall and internal antigens of *Brucella canis*. Dev Biol Standards 56:371, 1984.

Chapwanya A, et al: Diagnosing canine testicular neoplasia: Fine needle aspiration cytology and ultrasonography. Advances in Dog, Cat and Exotic Carnivore Reproduction—Book of Abstracts. The 4th International Symposium on Canine and Feline Reproduction and the 2nd Congress of the European Veterinary Society for Small Animal Reproduction. Oslo, Norway, June 29–July1, 2000, p 112.

Dahlbom M, et al: Testicular fine needle aspiration cytology as a diagnostic tool in dog infertility. J Sm Anim Pract 38: 506, 1997.

de Kretser DM, Robertson DM: The isolation and physiology of inhibin and related proteins. Biol Reprod 40:33, 1989.

DeNicola DB, et al: Cytology of the Canine Male Urogenital Tract. St. Louis, Ralston Purina Company, 1980.

Doig PA, et al: The genital *Mycoplasma* and *Ureaplasma* flora of healthy and diseased dogs. Can J Comp Med 45:233, 1981.

Edwards DF, et al: Immotile cilia syndrome—Primary cilia dyskinesia in the dog. Proceedings of the American College of Veterinary Internal Medicine, Washington, DC, 1986, p 1389.

England GCW, et al: An investigation into the origin of the first fraction of the canine ejaculate. Res Vet Sci 49:66, 1990.

England GCW, Plummer JM: Hypo-osmotic swelling of dog spermatozoa. J Reprod Fert Suppl 47:261, 1993.

Falvo RE, et al: Testosterone pretreatment and the response of pituitary LH to gonadotropin-releasing hormone (GnRH) in the male dog. J Androl 3:193, 1982.

Feldman EC, Tyrrell JB: Plasma testosterone, plasma glucose, and plasma insulin concentrations in spontaneous canine Cushing's syndrome. Proceedings of the American College of Veterinary Internal Medicine, Salt Lake City, 1982, p 81.

Feeney DA, et al: Canine prostatic disease—Comparison of radiographic appearance with morphologic and microbiologic findings: 30 cases (1981–1985). JAVMA 190:1018, 1987.

Frenette G, et al: Origin of alkaline phosphatase of canine seminal plasma. Arch Androl 16:235, 1986.

Freshman JL, et al: Effects of methyltestosterone on reproduction in male greyhounds. Proceedings of the American College of Veterinary Internal Medicine Fifth Annual Forum, San Diego, CA, 1987, p 917.

Freshman JL: Clinical management of the subfertile stud dog. Vet Clin North Am 31: 259, 2001.

Ganong WF: The gonads: Development and function of the reproductive system. In Ganong WF (ed): Review of Medical Physiology, 20th ed. New York, Lange Medical Books/McGraw Hill, 2001, p 398.

Hewitt D: Physiology and endocrinology of the male. In Simpson GM, England GCW, Harvey M (eds): BSAVA Manual of Small Animal Reproduction and Neonatology. Cheltenham, British Small Animal Veterinary Association, 1998, p 61.

Hewitt DA, et al: Test of canine sperm function in vitro using primary homologous oocytes and confocal microscopy. Advances in Dog, Cat and Exotic Carnivore Reproduction—Book of Abstracts. The 4th International Symposium on Canine and Feline Reproduction and the 2nd Congress of the European Veterinary Society for Small Animal Reproduction. Oslo, Norway, June 29–July1, 2000, p 69.

Holst BS, et al: Zona pellucida binding assay—A method for evaluation of canine spermatozoa. Advances in Dog, Cat and Exotic Carnivore Reproduction—Book of Abstracts. The 4th International Symposium on Canine and Feline Reproduction and the 2nd Congress of the European Veterinary Society for Small Animal Reproduction. Oslo, Norway, June 29–July1, 2000, p 67.

Johnson CA, et al: Effect of ^{131}I-induced hypothyroidism on indices of reproductive function in adult male dogs. J Vet Int Med 13:104, 1999.

Johnston GR, et al: Diagnostic imaging of the male canine reproductive organs. Vet Clin North Am 21:553, 1991.

Johnston SD: New canine semen evaluation techniques for the small animal practitioner. Proceedings of the Society for Theriogenology, Coeur d'Alene, ID, September 29–30, 1989, p 320.

Johnston SD: Performing a complete canine semen evaluation in a small animal hospital. Vet Clin North Am 21:545, 1991.

Johnston SD, Root Kustritz MV, Olson PNS: Semen collection, evaluation, and preservation. In Johnston SD, Root Kustritz MV, Olson PNS (eds): Canine and Feline Theriogenology. Philadelphia, WB Saunders Co, 2001, p 287.

Johnston SD, Root Kustritz MV, Olson PNS: Clinical approach to infertility in the male dog. In Johnston SD, Root Kustritz MV, Olson PNS (eds): Canine and Feline Theriogenology. Philadelphia, WB Saunders Co, 2001, p 371.

Jones DE, Joshua JO: Reproductive Clinical Problems in the Dog. Bristol, England, John Wright and Sons, 1982, p 49.

Keenan LRJ: The infertile male. In Simpson GM, England GCW, Harvey M (eds): BSAVA Manual of Small Animal Reproduction and Neonatology. Cheltenham, British Small Animal Veterinary Association, 1998, p 83.

Kumar MSA, et al: Distribution of luteinizing hormone releasing hormone in the canine hypothalamus: Effect of castration and exogenous gonadal steroids. Am J Vet Res 41:1304, 1980.

Larsen RE, Johnston SD: Management of canine infertility. In Kirk RW (ed): Current Veterinary Therapy VII. Philadelphia, WB Saunders Co, 1980, p 1226.

Lein DH: Mycoplasma infertility in the dog: Diagnosis and treatment. Proceedings of the Society for Theriogenology, Coeur d'Alene, ID, September 29–30, 1989, p 307.

Linde-Forsberg C, Bölske G: Canine genital mycoplasmas and ureaplasmas. In Bonagura JD, Kirk RW (eds): Kirk's Current Veterinary Therapy XII. Philadelphia, WB Saunders Co, 1995, p 1090.

Lopate C: Histopathologic and gross effects of testicular biopsy in the dog. Theriogenology 32: 585, 1989.

Mattoon JS, Nyland TG: Ultrasonography of the genital system. In Nyland TG, Mattoon JS (eds) Veterinary Diagnostic Ultrasound. Philadelphia, WB Saunders Co, 1995, p 141.

Mickelsen WD, et al: The relationship of semen quality to pregnancy rate and litter size following artificial insemination in the bitch. Theriogenology 39: 553, 1993.

Meyers-Wallen VN: Clinical approach to infertile male dogs with sperm in the ejaculate. Vet Clin North Amer 21: 609, 1991.

Nett TM, Olson PNS: Reproductive physiology of dogs and cats. In Ettinger SJ (ed): Textbook of Veterinary Internal Medicine, 2nd ed. Philadelphia, WB Saunders Co, 1983, p 1698.

Oettlé EE: Sperm morphology and fertility in the dog. J Reprod Fertil 47(Suppl):257, 1993.

Oettlé EE: Sperm abnormalities and fertility in the dog. In Bonagura JD, Kirk RW (eds): Kirk's Current Veterinary Therapy XII. Philadelphia, WB Saunders Co, 1995, p 1060.

Olar TT, et al: Relationships among testicular size, daily production and output of spermatozoa, and extragonadal spermatozoal reserves of the dog. Biol Reprod 29:1114, 1983.

Olson PN: Disorders of the canine prostate gland. Proceedings of the Annual Society for Theriogenology, Denver, CO, 1984a, p 46.

Olson PN: Clinical approach to infertility in the stud dog. Proceedings of the Annual Society for Theriogenology, Denver, CO, 1984b, p 33.

Olson PN, et al: Concentrations of carnitine in the seminal fluid of normospermic, vasectomized, and castrated dogs. Am J Vet Res 48:1211, 1987.

Olson PN, et al: Concentrations of luteinizing hormone and follicle-stimulating hormone in the serum of sexually intact and neutered dogs. Am J Vet Res 53:762, 1992.

Pugh CR, et al: Testicular ultrasound in the normal dog. Vet Radiol 31:195, 1990.

Purswell BJ, Wilcke JR: Response to gonadotrophin-releasing hormone by the intact male dog: Serum testosterone, luteinizing hormone and follicle-stimulating hormone. J Reprod Fert, 47(Suppl):335, 1993.

Root Kustritz MV, et al: The effects of stains and investigators on assessment of morphology of canine spermatozoa. J Am Anim Hosp Assoc 34: 348, 1998.

Ruel Y, et al: Ultrasonographic evaluation of the prostate in healthy intact dogs. Vet Radiol Ultra 39:212, 1998.

Smith SC, England GCW: Effect of technical settings and semen handling upon motility characteristics measured using computer-aided sperm analysis. Advances in Dog, Cat and Exotic Carnivore Reproduction—Book of Abstracts. The 4th International Symposium on Canine and Feline Reproduction and the 2nd Congress of the European Veterinary Society for Small Animal Reproduction. Oslo, Norway, June 29–July1, 2000, p 88.

Soderberg SF: Infertility in the male dog. In Morrow DA (ed): Current Therapy in Theriogenology, 2nd ed. Philadelphia, WB Saunders Co, 1986, p 544.

Taha MB, et al: The effect of season of the year on the characteristics and composition of dog semen. J Small Anim Pract 22:177, 1981a.

Taha MA, et al: Some aspects of reproductive function in the male Beagle at puberty. J Small Anim Pract 22:663, 1981b.

Van Kuppeveld, et al: Detection of mycoplasma contamination in cell cultures by a mycoplasma group-specific PCR. Appl Environ Micro 60: 149, 1994.

Verstegen J, et al: Objective evaluation of semen motility parameters in the dog: Comparison of Hamilton-Thorn Computer sperm assisted system and the Sperm quality analyser. Advances in Dog, Cat and Exotic Carnivore Reproduction—Book of Abstracts. The 4th International Symposium on Canine and Feline Reproduction and the 2nd Congress of the European Veterinary Society for Small Animal Reproduction. Oslo, Norway, June 29–July1, 2000, p 90.

Wasmer ML, Rogers KS: Pharmacologic androgen deprivation. Comp Cont Ed 18: 267, 1996.

Woodall PF, Johnstone IP: Scrotal width as an index of testicular size in dogs and its relationship to body size. J Small Anim Pract 29:543, 1988.

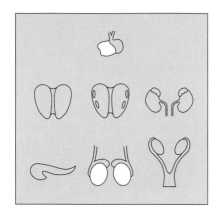

28

DISORDERS OF THE PENIS AND PREPUCE

CONGENITAL DISORDERS

Persistent Penile Frenulum

During fetal development, the epithelial surfaces of the penis and prepuce are attached by a single lamina of ectodermal cells that is incomplete ventrally. Here, a thin band of connective tissue, the frenulum, unites the penis and prepuce. Androgens secreted by the developing fetal testes cause the lamina to split, forming the preputial cavity. This normally occurs in the fetus or neonate, depending on the species. Androgens may cause thinning but not rupture of the frenulum; rupture of the frenulum is thought to result from mechanical stress early in life. Failure of the frenulum to rupture results in the persistence of a band of connective tissue extending from the ventral tip of the glans penis to either the prepuce or the ventral surface of the penis itself, causing a ventral or lateral deviation of the tip of the glans penis.

Persistent penile frenulum is usually identified during the physical examination of a puppy that has been brought in for its first vaccinations (Fig. 28-1). Owners may also complain that the puppy urinates on its back feet or in other unexpected directions, which may cause secondary dermatitis of the rear leg from urine scald. Additional clinical signs may include inability to extrude the penis from the prepuce during penile engorgement, discomfort or pain with penile engorgement, and repeated licking of the preputial area. If the problem is not identified, the dog may associate pain with sexual excitement and secondarily develop reduced libido and unwillingness to mate.

A diagnosis of persistent penile frenulum is made by identifying the abnormal band of tissue during visual examination of the penis and prepuce. The frenulum is usually avascular and can easily be transected with a scalpel blade after application of a topical anesthetic. Genetic implications for persistent penile frenulum are unknown, although Cocker Spaniels have been most commonly cited in the literature (Johnston et al, 2001).

Penile Hypoplasia

Penile hypoplasia is a rare disorder that has been reported in the Cocker Spaniel, Collie, Doberman Pinscher, and Great Dane (Johnston, 1989). Penile hypoplasia is a component of some intersex states (see page 893) and may be one of several reproductive abnormalities identified on physical examination. An abnormal karyotype has been identified in some animals with penile hypoplasia. A decrease in penile size may also occur in dogs castrated at an early age. Salmeri and colleagues (1991) found mixed breed dogs castrated at 7 weeks of age had immature genitalia, characterized by significantly smaller penile diameter, decreased size and radiodensity of the os penis, and immaturity of the prepuce, compared with male dogs castrated at 7 months of age or left intact. The mean penile diameter of the dogs castrated at 7 weeks of age was approximately half the penile diameter of the intact dogs; the penile diameter in dogs castrated at 7 months was intermediate between the other two groups.

Penile hypoplasia is usually asymptomatic and an incidental finding on physical examination. Urine pooling and infection inside the prepuce may develop if the dog also has a hypoplastic preputial opening (see page 954). The diagnosis of penile hypoplasia is based on physical examination. If it is identified, intersexuality should be suspected, and karyotyping (see page 893) may be indicated. No treatment is necessary in the asymptomatic dog. Enlargement of the preputial opening and surgical shortening of the prepuce may be necessary if urine pooling and infection are problems.

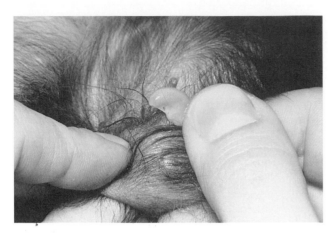

FIGURE 28-1. Persistent penile frenulum, causing deviation of the distal portion of the penis in a 3-month-old Lhasa Apso. The dog was presented for treatment for urinating in unexpected directions.

Hypospadias

Hypospadias is a congenital urogenital defect involving the external genitalia of males. It is characterized by an abnormal termination of the urethra ventral and posterior to the normal opening at the tip of the glans penis. Hypospadias is categorized as glandular, penile, scrotal, or perineal, depending on where the urethra opens (Hayes and Wilson, 1986). The perineal form is the most common and may represent a form of pseudohermaphroditism (see page 897). Hypospadias results from failure of fusion of the genital folds or genital swelling (or both) during fetal development, which may also cause abnormal development of the penis, prepuce, and/or scrotum. A short or deviated penis, malformed os penis, incomplete preputial closure, defects in the development of the scrotum, and other urogenital anomalies have been identified in dogs with hypospadias (see Fig. 24-14, page 898).

In addition to the visual abnormalities, clinical signs may include those related to urinary tract infection (e.g., dysuria, hematuria), urinary incontinence, and urine scalding. The diagnosis of hypospadias is made on visual inspection of the external genitalia and by catheterization of the urethra. The type of surgical correction required, if any, depends on the location and severity of the congenital defect. A thorough evaluation of the urogenital system should be completed before surgical correction is considered, because identification of additional abnormalities may alter the therapeutic plan. Penile amputation, ostectomy of the os penis, scrotal or perineal urethrostomy, or other reconstructive surgery may be necessary. Castration should always be performed because of the likely genetic implications of hypospadias, especially when the condition is present in conjunction with other developmental abnormalities (e.g., intersexuality, cryptorchidism). A familial occurrence in the Boston Terrier has been suggested (Hayes and Wilson, 1986).

Congenital Deformity of the Os Penis

Deformity of the os penis may result in deviation of the penis and, depending on the severity, inability to retract the penis fully into the preputial sheath. Some males are predisposed to urethral obstruction. Persistent exposure of a portion of the glans penis to the environment may result in desiccation, trauma, and necrosis of exposed tissue. Mild deformities of the os penis (e.g., bends or excessive shortness) may result in misdirected copulatory efforts, inability to achieve vaginal penetration, and apparent infertility.

Treatment depends on the severity of the deformity and the intended use of the dog. Severe deviations may require fracturing and straightening of the os penis. An excessively shortened or deviated os penis that impairs the dog's ability to copulate may necessitate the use of artificial insemination if breeding is desired. Therapy is probably not indicated if the dog is not intended for breeding and if paraphimosis or dysuria is not present.

Duplication of the Penis

Penile duplication (diphallia) is an extremely rare congenital anomaly that has been reported in a 5-month-old Pointer, a 6-month-old Poodle-cross, and a 5-month-old mixed breed dog with concurrent polymelia (Johnston, 1989; Zucker et al, 1993). All these dogs had multiple anomalies of the urogenital system (e.g., hydronephrosis, cryptorchidism, duplication of the urinary bladder and prostate gland). Diphallia may result from anomalous longitudinal duplication of the cloacal membrane, followed by ventral migration of primitive streak mesoderm around two cloacal membranes to form two genital tubercles. The diagnosis is made by visual inspection. There is no treatment.

ACQUIRED DISORDERS

Phimosis

Phimosis is the inability of the male dog to extrude the penis from the prepuce as a result of an abnormally small preputial orifice. Phimosis may be a congenital abnormality (i.e., congenital preputial stenosis, intersex dogs), or it may occur secondary to inflammation, edema, neoplasia, or scar tissue formation after trauma, chemical irritation, or infection.

The clinical signs depend on the severity of the defect. Complete congenital occlusion of the preputial orifice obstructs urinary outflow, resulting in neonatal death. Small openings may interfere with urination and cause accumulation of urine in the preputial cavity. Constant urine dribbling, an abnormal stream of urine during micturition, perpetual preputial swelling, and secondary bacterial infections and balanoposthitis may develop. More commonly, phimosis interferes with the extrusion of the penis during mating. Inability to copulate is quickly obvious. Pain may be associated with mating behavior, resulting in decreased libido.

The clinician can make the diagnosis relatively easily in severe cases by simply demonstrating that the flaccid penis cannot be extruded from the prepuce. Observation of the male during sexual excitement may be required to obtain a diagnosis if the phimosis interferes with extrusion of the penis only during periods of engorgement.

Any predisposing factors should be corrected in dogs with acquired phimosis. The need for surgical intervention to widen the preputial orifice depends on the severity of the phimosis and the intended use of the dog. Therapy is probably not indicated in an asymptomatic dog not intended for breeding. Surgical reconstruction of the preputial orifice is indicated if the phimosis interferes with urination or with extrusion of the engorged penis in a dog intended for breeding. Congenital preputial stenosis has been observed in a litter of mixed breed dogs and in multiple related Golden Retriever litters, which suggests that this condition may be heritable (Johnston, 1989).

Paraphimosis

Paraphimosis is the presence of an engorged or edematous penis that cannot be retracted into the preputial sheath (Fig. 28-2). Interference with venous drainage of the cavernous tissues during engorgement results in progressive enlargement of the glans penis, interference with circulation to the penis, exposure desiccation, ischemic necrosis, and eventually the development of urethral obstruction and gangrene. Paraphimosis is most commonly associated with coitus, in which preputial hairs become entangled around the base of the glans penis, forming a restrictive band, or the protruding penis becomes trapped as the preputial orifice adheres to the penis and is pulled into the preputial cavity when the erection subsides. Other causes of paraphimosis include mild phimosis, foreign objects (e.g., rubber bands), fracture of the os penis, chronic priapism (i.e., penile engorgement without associated sexual excitement), trauma, neoplasia, and chronic balanoposthitis (Greiner and Zolton, 1980).

Other conditions may result in chronic exposure of the glans penis and may be mistaken for paraphimosis. These include paralysis of the retractor penis muscle, congenital deformation of the os penis, an abnormally large preputial opening, or congenital shortening of the prepuce (Fig. 28-3). These conditions can be differentiated from paraphimosis by the lack of an engorged penis and the length of time the problem is observed (i.e., chronic condition).

Paraphimosis is an acute medical emergency. Failure or delay of treatment increases the risk of the development of urethral obstruction, ischemic necrosis, and gangrene of the penis. Amputation of the penis may be necessary when paraphimosis has been present for longer than 24 hours and no therapy has been provided (Burke, 1983). The goals of therapy are to reestablish venous drainage from the penis by removing any restrictive bands of tissue, hair, or foreign objects; to cleanse and debride necrotic areas of the penis; and to replace the penis in the prepuce. Tranquilizers (e.g., acepromazine) can be given to induce relaxation and hypotension, which allow detumescence and manual replacement (Verstegen, 1998). Lubricants and cold hypertonic dextrose solutions may be applied to the penis after cleansing in an attempt to reduce penile size. Surgical enlargement of the preputial orifice may be necessary in severe cases that do not respond to

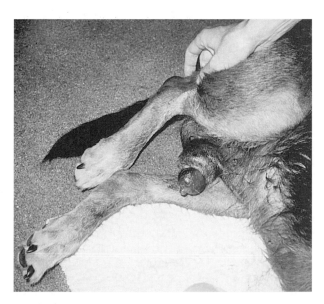

FIGURE 28-2. Postcoital paraphimosis in a 4-year-old German Shepherd dog. Paraphimosis developed after preputial hairs around the glans penis became entangled.

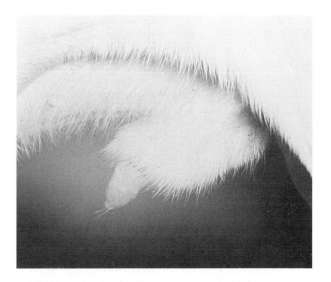

FIGURE 28-3. Congenitally shortened prepuce, resulting in persistent exposure of the glans penis. The lack of engorgement of the penis and the chronic nature of this problem help differentiate it from paraphimosis.

medical management. Placement of an indwelling soft rubber urinary catheter for 7 to 14 days helps prevent urethral strictures if the penis is severely traumatized and urethral involvement is suspected. Once the penis has been repositioned in the prepuce, daily penile extrusion and placement of antibiotic/steroid ointments in the preputial cavity for 1 to 2 weeks help prevent adhesions between the penis and prepuce. With severe necrosis or gangrene, penile amputation may be necessary.

Precautions taken prior to and after coitus can help prevent paraphimosis. Hairs around the preputial orifice should be clipped prior to breeding. After coitus, the penis and prepuce should be inspected frequently until the penis has completely retracted into the prepuce. The prepuce should move easily over the penis and should not be "turned in on itself." If reproductive function is not important, castration should be considered to minimize sexual excitement and recurrence of paraphimosis. Several surgical techniques have been described for the treatment of recurring paraphimosis, including narrowing of the preputial opening, preputial lengthening (preputioplasty), preputial muscle myorrhaphy, and creation of permanent adhesion between the surface of the penile shaft and the preputial mucosa (Fossum et al, 2002; Somerville and Anderson, 2001).

Priapism

Priapism is persistent penile engorgement without associated sexual excitement. Penile desiccation and ischemic necrosis may develop as a result of chronic external exposure of the penis and stagnation of blood in the penis. Penile erection results when parasympathetic stimuli via the pelvic nerve actively increase arterial blood flow to the corpus cavernosum penis and decrease venous outflow via contraction of smooth muscle fibers in the penis that surround the corpus cavernosum penis (Carati et al, 1988). Sympathetic stimuli reverse these effects. In humans, priapism usually occurs secondary either to neurologic dysfunction that causes prolonged or excessive parasympathetic stimulation or to decreased venous outflow from an occlusive thromboembolism or mass lesion (Winter and McDowell, 1988). Reported causes in the dog include trauma while mating, urinary tract infection, constipation, spinal cord lesions, chronic distemper encephalomyelitis, penile thromboembolism, and idiopathic (Guilford et al, 1990; Root Kustritz and Olson, 1999). Priapism has occurred in tomcats after castration and presumably from trauma after attempted mating with estrous queens (Orima et al, 1989; Swalec and Smeak, 1989; Gunn-Moore et al, 1995). The diagnosis of priapism is made by visual inspection. The primary differential diagnosis is paraphimosis, which is protrusion of the nonerect penis from the prepuce. Additional diagnostic tests are aimed at identifying the underlying etiology and should include routine blood work; thorough evaluation of the genitourinary system, including abdominal radiographs and ultrasound of the abdomen and external genitalia, as well as complete radiographic evaluation of the spinal cord; and cerebrospinal fluid analysis.

Although spontaneous recovery has been reported in some dogs, successful treatment of priapism usually requires identification and correction of the underlying etiology and symptomatic treatment to minimize desiccation and necrosis of the penis. Supportive care of the penis should include periodic cleansing, application of lubricants to prevent desiccation, and use of Elizabethan collars to prevent self-trauma from licking. Castration usually is not effective as a sole treatment (Root Kustritz, 2001). Orima and colleagues (1989) successfully treated priapism in a dog and cat by incising the penis over the bulbus glandis and pars longa glandis and through the tunica albuginea, after which pressure was applied to expel free blood and thrombi from the corpus cavernosum penis. The antihistamine and anticholinergic drugs benztropine mesylate (Cogentin; Merck & Co., West Point, PA) and diphenhydramine have been used successfully in two horses and in men with priapism, respectively, but treatment must be initiated within a few hours after the onset of priapism (Wilson et al, 1991). Terbutaline, a β-adrenergic agonist, has also been used successfully in the treatment of priapism in men (Shantha et al, 1989). Successful pharmacologic treatment of priapism has not been reported in the dog. Penile amputation and perineal urethrostomy may be necessary if the underlying cause cannot be corrected and the penis becomes irreparably damaged.

Failure to Achieve Erection

Achieving an erection depends in part on normal anatomy, circulation, and nerve supply in the penis and on adequate testosterone secretion from the interstitial Leydig cells. Failure to achieve erection may be caused by inadequate sexual stimulation, submissive behavior in the presence of a dominant or aggressive bitch, fear arising from pain encountered in a previous breeding as a result of joint or spinal inflammation or pain associated with ejaculation (e.g., prostatitis), androgen deficiency, pain associated with development of an erection (e.g., persistent penile frenulum), or intrapenile vascular shunts that prevent normal engorgement of the penis (Johnston, 1989). Androgen deficiency may be caused by testicular hypoplasia, abnormalities in sexual development (e.g., XXY syndrome), and disorders and drugs (e.g., glucocorticoids) that affect pituitary gonadotropin secretion. A decrease in libido often coincides with failure to achieve erection when the latter is caused by an androgen deficiency.

A thorough history and physical examination comprise the initial diagnostic approach. Questions concerning breeding management, drug therapy, and environment should be explored. During the physical examination, special attention should be paid to the size and consistency of the testes and prostate gland

and the size and conformation of the penis, with regard to any abnormalities that might suggest intersexuality or androgen deficiency. The musculoskeletal system should be evaluated for signs of arthritis, especially of the coxofemoral joints. Function of the Leydig cells can be assessed by measuring the testosterone concentration prior to and after the administration of gonadotropin-releasing hormone (GnRH) (see page 945). Karyotyping should be assessed if intersexuality is suspected. Finally, blood and urine tests (e.g., complete blood count [CBC], serum biochemical analysis, thyroid hormone panel, urinalysis) should be done to rule out endocrinopathies and other systemic disorders.

Identifiable abnormalities should be treated accordingly. The prognosis is usually grave in the presence of abnormal karyotype, low serum testosterone, or testicular hypoplasia unless concurrent drug therapy or a treatable endocrinopathy is identified. If diagnostic tests fail to identify a cause, attempts should be made to breed the male in his home environment with alternative estrous bitches. Application of a topical pheromone preparation (Eau d'Estrus; Synbiotics, Malvern, PA) or a swab from the vulva of a different estrous bitch to the vulva and hindquarters of the bitch in estrous can also be tried to induce sexual arousal in the dog.

Urethral Prolapse

Prolapse of the distal urethral mucosa is rare in the dog. The cause is not known, although excessive sexual excitement, self-stimulation from licking, and excessive straining to urinate after the development of genitourinary tract infections or calculi have been proposed. Urethral prolapse has been identified only in intact young males. After prolapse, the everted urethral mucosa becomes congested and edematous. Subsequent swelling results in a nonreducible, dark red to purplish mass at the tip of the penis (Fig. 28-4). Variable degrees of trauma may result from licking.

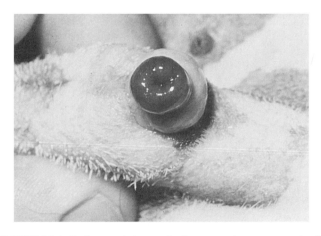

FIGURE 28-4. Prolapse of the urethral mucosa in a young mixed breed dog.

The most common clinical sign observed by the owner is intermittent bleeding from the penis (McDonald, 1989).

Surgical resection of the prolapsed tissue is the treatment of choice, especially if the prolapsed tissue is necrotic or severely traumatized. Dogs that respond well to surgical resection have been used successfully for breeding (Root Kustritz, 2001). Alternatively, medical therapy may be tried if the prolapsed tissue is reducible and viable. A temporary purse-string suture around the urethral orifice may be needed after reduction of the prolapsed tissue and should be maintained for 3 to 5 days to prevent recurrence of prolapse. Normal urination should be documented after placement of the purse-string suture. Tranquilizers may also be used during the initial healing period to minimize excitement and penile engorgement. Castration may be necessary if urethral prolapse is a recurrent problem associated with sexual excitement. The genetic implications of urethral prolapse are not known, although the English Bulldog is most commonly cited in the literature (Johnston et al, 2001).

Preputial Discharges

The normal dog should have no preputial discharge. Occasionally a small amount of yellow-white smegma, consisting of epithelial cells, inflammatory cells (primarily neutrophils), and bacteria, accumulates around the preputial orifice in an otherwise healthy dog; this is not clinically significant. Urine, blood, or significant amounts of purulent discharge from the prepuce should be considered abnormal.

URINE. Urine dribbling is uncommon in the male dog and is associated with urogenital anomalies (e.g., ectopic ureter), bacterial cystitis, urethral or cystic calculi, neurogenic incontinence, severe phimosis, and mass lesions that affect the urethral sphincter. Urine dribbling during sleep may also occur in dogs with polyuric/polydipsic disorders. A complete physical examination and evaluation of a CBC, serum biochemical analysis, urinalysis with bacterial culture, abdominal radiographs, and abdominal ultrasonography usually allow identification of the cause. Occasionally, radiographic contrast studies (e.g., intravenous pyelogram and positive contrast cystogram) and specialized neurogenic studies (e.g., cystometrogram, urethral pressure profile) may be required to establish the cause.

BLOOD. Blood dripping from the prepuce or penis is most commonly associated with acute or chronic prostatitis (see page 977). This sign is also associated with urethritis; urethral calculi; urethral prolapse; trauma to the penis, prepuce, or os penis; preputial, penile, or urethral neoplasia; foreign bodies lodged in the preputial cavity; or coagulopathies (e.g., clotting factor deficiencies, thrombocytopenia, and disseminated intravascular coagulation [DIC]). A complete physical examination, including examination of the extruded penis and rectal palpation of the prostate gland, CBC, urinalysis with bacterial culture, abdominal radiographs, abdominal ultrasonography, and blood clotting evaluation usually allow the clinician to localize the source and cause of hemorrhage.

Hematuria may be a sign of dysfunction in the genital or urinary system. Hematuria may be associated with a problem involving the kidney, bladder, prostate, urethra, penis, or prepuce. Occasionally the relationship between the onset of hematuria and the stage of micturition helps localize the site of the lesion. Hematuria that begins late in micturition suggests a bladder or prostate problem, whereas hematuria that occurs early in micturition suggests a problem involving the urethra, penis, or prepuce. Hematuria that is observed throughout micturition suggests a problem with the kidney, bladder, prostate or, in rare cases, the penis or prepuce.

MUCOPURULENT PREPUTIAL DISCHARGE. A mucopurulent preputial discharge is a common discharge in the male dog because of the predisposition to develop mild inflammation or infection in the preputial cavity. This type of discharge is usually associated with balanoposthitis, although neoplasia, preputial foreign bodies, and phimosis may also result in a mucopurulent discharge. Careful examination of the penis and prepuce usually reveals the underlying cause.

Balanoposthitis

Balanitis is inflammation of the glans penis, and posthitis is inflammation of the prepuce. Because inflammation in this area affects both, the term *balanoposthitis* is used. Balanoposthitis should be suspected whenever a dog is presented with the primary owner complaint of pus dripping from the preputial orifice.

The normal microflora of the preputial cavity includes *Escherichia coli*, *Streptococcus*, *Staphylococcus*, *Pseudomonas*, *Proteus*, *Klebsiella*, *Mycoplasma*, and *Ureaplasma* organisms (see Table 27-3, page 941) (Keenan, 1998). Balanoposthitis typically develops after a change in the ecosystem of the preputial cavity (e.g., foreign body, trauma) allows proliferation of the normal microflora and the subsequent development of infection. Viral causes of balanoposthitis include canine herpesvirus and calicivirus (Crandall, 1988; Anvik, 1991). Balanoposthitis may also be a component of atopic dermatitis or may occur secondary to self-trauma (Root Kustritz, 2001). *Mycoplasma canis* and *Ureaplasma* organisms have been incriminated as causes of balanoposthitis; however, there is no difference in the prevalence of these organisms between normal dogs and those with genital infections (Verstegen, 1998).

The history usually includes frequent licking, biting, and possibly self-mutilation of the penis and prepuce and a purulent or hemorrhagic preputial discharge. Mild balanoposthitis is common and usually clinically insignificant. Grossly visible inflammation of the mucosa of the glans penis and prepuce is usually not present, and culture is rarely indicated. Severe balanoposthitis may occur with infection of tissues in the glans penis or prepuce. Acute swelling, inflammation, copious purulent to sanguinopurulent preputial discharge, and pain develop. Abscess formation may occur, resulting in systemic signs of illness (e.g., lethargy, inappetence, fever). If the condition goes unrecognized and persists, local scarring and adhesions between the prepuce and penis may develop, which can lead to preputial stenosis, interference and pain with copulation, and reduced libido.

A thorough examination of the penis and prepuce should be performed on all dogs with balanoposthitis to ensure the absence of foreign bodies, lacerations, masses, and abscess formation. Follicular or papular lesions (composed of aggregates of lymphocytes), vesicles, or ulcerations may be found on the mucosa of the prepuce and bulbus glandis. The presence of small papules or vesicles can be related to herpesvirus infection; however, many vesicle-like lesions are not caused by herpesvirus (Verstegen, 1998). Depending on the severity of the balanoposthitis, exfoliative cytology of preputial smears, bacterial culture of infected tissue, determination of the *Brucella canis* titer and herpesvirus polymerase chain reaction (PCR) testing (see pages 813 and 920), and biopsy of unusual lesions may be indicated.

The treatment of balanoposthitis depends on its severity. Treatment of mild balanoposthitis is rarely required; when it is treated, topical antibiotics and antiseptic flushes provide only transient control. Treatment is indicated with the presence of visible signs of penile or preputial inflammation, necrosis, laceration, or abscess; systemic signs of illness; or owner insistence. Treatment involves removal of predisposing factors, cleansing of the preputial cavity and penis with mild antiseptic solutions (e.g., chlorhexidine, diluted Betadine) or sterile saline, and infusion of antibiotic ointments into the preputial cavity for 2 to 4 weeks. Abscesses should be lanced, drained, and flushed. Administration of oral broad-spectrum bactericidal antibiotics for 2 to 4 weeks should also be considered, especially if systemic signs of illness are present. Recurrence is common despite therapy, especially when a predisposing factor cannot be identified.

Penile Trauma

Any traumatic event that a dog experiences may cause penile damage, including mating, fights with other dogs, or impalement on a fence or other object during a jump. Laceration, contusion, puncture wounds, hematoma, a fractured os penis, urethral laceration, and obstruction may result. Clinical signs depend on the severity and type of trauma. Hemorrhage, swelling, and pain are common (Fig. 28-5). Urinary dysfunction (i.e., hematuria, dysuria, anuria) and signs caused by postrenal uremia may develop if urethral patency is compromised. Extravasation of urine into the subcutaneous tissues may occur if the urethra is ruptured, resulting in cellulitis, abscessation, and progressive edema of the ventral body wall.

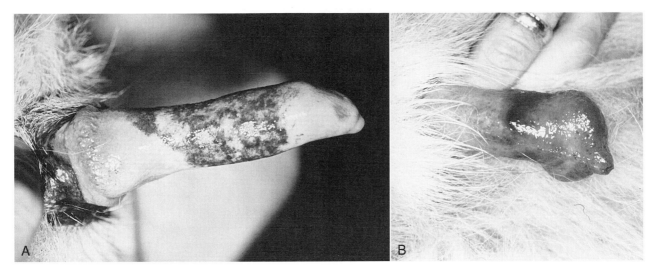

FIGURE 28-5. *A,* Penile hemorrhage secondary to trauma in a 5-year-old German Shepherd dog. *B,* Penile swelling and hemorrhage caused by trauma from self-licking in a 3-year-old mixed breed dog.

The first goal in the management of penile trauma is control of hemorrhage. The patency of the urethra and the status of the os penis should then be assessed by passage of a urinary catheter into the bladder, radiographic assessment of the os penis and, if necessary, retrograde urethrography. Wounds should be cleaned and debrided and severe lacerations sutured. An antibiotic cream should be applied to the penis twice daily until the lesions have healed. Fractures of the os penis may require surgical correction, especially if marked deviation of the os penis or impingement on urethral patency is present (Kelly and Clark, 1995). Perineal urethrostomy and penile amputation may be necessary with massive urethral trauma. During convalescence, the penis should be extruded twice a day to prevent adhesions. Topical antibiotic ointments can be applied at these times. Sexual excitement should be avoided.

Occasionally, excessive callus or fibrous tissue forms at the site of a previous os penis fracture, causing urethral obstruction or deviation of the penis (Bradley, 1985; Johnston et al, 2001). Clinical signs include dysuria, distention of the urinary bladder, and deviation of the penis. Postrenal azotemia may be present secondary to urinary tract obstruction. Definitive diagnosis requires radiographs of the penis and careful passage of a urinary catheter. Treatment involves surgical removal of excess bone and fibrous tissue and realignment and stabilization of the os penis (Bennett et al, 1986; Kelly and Clark, 1995). Alternatively, penile amputation can be considered.

Neoplasia of the Penis and Prepuce

The most common tumor involving the external genitalia of the male dog is the transmissible venereal tumor (see page 924; also see Fig. 27-1, page 931). Other tumors of the penis and prepuce include the mast cell tumor, squamous cell carcinoma, fibroma, lymphoma and papilloma. A mesenchymal chondrosarcoma of the os penis has also been reported (Patnaik et al, 1988). With the exception of transmissible venereal tumor, penile tumors typically occur in older dogs. Clinical signs may include swelling in the region of the prepuce, abnormal preputial discharge, excessive licking of the prepuce and penis, penile prolapse, hematuria, dysuria and, if urethral patency is affected, signs related to urethral obstruction and postrenal uremia (Michels et al, 2001). A definitive diagnosis requires histologic evaluation of a biopsy. The therapy and prognosis depend on the type of neoplasm.

REFERENCES

Anvik JO: Clinical considerations of canine herpesvirus infection. Vet Med 86:394, 1991.

Bennett D, et al: Wedge osteotomy of the os penis to correct penile deviation. J Small Anim Prac 27:379, 1986.

Bradley RL: Complete urethral obstruction secondary to fracture of the os penis. Compend Contin Educ Pract Vet 7:759, 1985.

Burke TJ: Reproductive disorders. *In* Ettinger SJ (ed): Textbook of Veterinary Internal Medicine, 2nd ed. Philadelphia, WB Saunders, 1983, p 1711.

Carati CJ, et al: Vascular changes during penile erection in the dog. J Physiol 400:75, 188.

Crandall RA: Isolation and characterization of caliciviruses from dogs with vesicular genital disease. Arch Virol 98:65, 1988.

Fossum TW, et al: Surgery of the Reproductive and Genital Systems. *In* Fossum TW, et al (eds): Small Animal Surgery. St Louis, Mosby, 2002, p 610.

Greiner TP, Zolton GM: Genital emergencies. *In* Morrow DA (ed): Current Therapy in Theriogenology: Diagnosis, Treatment, and Prevention of Reproductive Diseases in Animals. Philadelphia, WB Saunders, 1980, p 614.

Guilford WG, et al: Fecal incontinence, urinary incontinence and priapism associated with multifocal distemper encephalomyelitis in a dog. J Am Vet Med Assoc 197:90, 1990.

Gunn-Moore DA, et al: Priapism in seven cats. J Small Anim Pract 36:262, 1995.

Hayes HM, Wilson GP: Hospital incidence of hypospadias in dogs in North America. Vet Rec 118:605, 1986.

Johnston SD: Disorders of the external genitalia of the male. *In* Ettinger SJ (ed): Textbook of Veterinary Internal Medicine, 3rd ed. Philadelphia, WB Saunders, 1989, p 1881.

Johnston SD, Root Kustritz MV, Olson PNS: Disorders of the canine penis and prepuce. *In* Johnston SD, Root Kustritz MV, Olson PNS (eds): Canine and Feline Theriogenology. Philadelphia, WB Saunders, 2001, p. 356.

Keenan LRJ: The infertile male. *In* Simpson GM, England GCW, Harvey M (eds): BSAVA Manual of Small Animal Reproduction and Neonatology. Cheltenham, England, British Small Animal Veterinary Association, 1998, p 83.

Kelly SE, Clark WT: Surgical repair of fracture of the os penis in a dog. J Small Anim Pract 36:507, 1995.

McDonald RK: Urethral prolapse in a Yorkshire Terrier. Compend Contin Educ 11:682, 1989.

Michels GM, et al: Penile prolapse and urethral obstruction secondary to lymphosarcoma of the penis in a dog. J Am Anim Hosp Assoc 37:474, 2001.

Orima H, et al: Surgical treatment of priapism observed in a dog and a cat. Jpn J Vet Sci 51:1227, 1989.

Patnaik AK, et al: Two cases of canine penile neoplasms: Squamous cell carcinoma and mesenchymal chondrosarcoma. J Am Anim Hosp Assoc 24:403, 1988.

Root Kustritz MV: Disorders of the canine penis. Vet Clin North Am 31:247, 2001.

Root Kustritz MV, Olson PN: Theriogenology question of the month: Idiopathic priapism in a dog. J Am Vet Med Assoc 214:1483, 1999.

Salmeri KR, et al: Gonadectomy in immature dogs: Effects on skeletal, physical, and behavioral development. J Am Vet Med Assoc 198:1193, 1991.

Shantha TR, et al: Treatment of persistent penile erection and priapism using terbutaline. J Urol 141:1427, 1989.

Somerville ME, Anderson SM: Phallopexy for treatment of paraphimosis in the dog. J Am Anim Hosp Assoc 37:397, 2001.

Swalec KM, Smeak DD: Priapism after castration in a cat. J Am Vet Med Assoc 195:963, 1989.

Verstegen JP: Conditions of the male. *In* Simpson GM, England GCW, Harvey M (eds): BSAVA Manual of Small Animal Reproduction and Neonatology. Cheltenham, England, British Small Animal Veterinary Association, 1998, p 71.

Wilson DV, et al: Pharmacologic treatment of priapism in two horses. J Am Vet Med Assoc 199:1183, 1991.

Winter CC, McDowell G: Experience with 105 patients with priapism: Update review of all aspects. J Urol 140:980, 1988.

Zucker SA, et al: Diphallia and polymelia in a dog. Canine Pract 18:15, 1993.

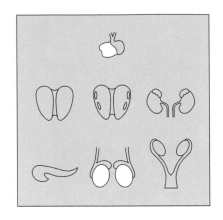

29

DISORDERS OF THE TESTES AND EPIDIDYMIDES

CONGENITAL DISORDERS

Cryptorchidism

NORMAL DESCENT. The first event in the sexual differentiation of the fetus is the differentiation and development of the gonads. The chromosomal sex normally determines gonadal sex. Testicular differentiation is controlled by the Y chromosome. The lack of a Y chromosome results in development of an ovary. The sex-determining region Y gene, SRY, is normally located on the Y chromosome. This gene encodes the testis-determining factor and is the genetic signal for initiating testis differentiation (Sinclair et al, 1990; Goodfellow and Lovell-Badge, 1993). SRY is distinctly different from the gene for H-Y antigen, which is no longer thought to have a role in testis induction (Koopman et al, 1991). Once differentiation has occurred and the gonad becomes a testis, it must migrate from its embryonic and fetal location near the caudal pole of the kidney into the scrotum to attain fertility. A mesenchymal structure, the gubernaculum testis, extends from the caudal pole of the testis through the inguinal canal to the genital tubercle and is responsible for guiding the testis into the scrotum. Shrinkage of the gubernaculum testis pulls the testis into the scrotum.

At the time of birth, the testes are usually within the abdomen, midway between the kidney and the inguinal ring (Baumans et al, 1981). Within 10 days, the testes move through the inguinal canal, and by 10 to 14 days of age, the testes are in the scrotum. Marked variability occurs in the time of descent of the testis into the scrotum, and scrotal positioning of the testis may not occur until 6 to 8 weeks of age. The inguinal rings of most dogs are closed by 6 months of age, precluding movement of testes from the abdomen to the inguinal canal if that has not already occurred (Johnston et al, 2001). Palpation of the testes in early life may be difficult because of small testicular size, small size of the neonate, poor scrotal development, variable amounts of scrotal fat, and involuntary withdrawal of the testes into the inguinal area. However, by 8 weeks of age, the testes should be palpable within the scrotum. Until 10 weeks of age, the testes of a few males may be periodically withdrawn into the inguinal region lateral to the penis following contracture of the cremaster muscle. These testes should move easily back into the scrotum with gentle digital pressure. The use of firm traction or failure to move the testicle into the scrotum should be viewed as a form of cryptorchidism.

DEFINITION. Cryptorchidism refers to failure of one or both testes to descend into the scrotum by 8 weeks of age. An underdeveloped or aberrant outgrowth of the gubernaculum and failure of the gubernaculum to regress and pull the testis into the scrotum results in cryptorchidism (Wensing, 1980). The most common location for the undescended testis is the abdomen, although it may also be present in the inguinal canal or lateral to the penis (Fig. 29-1). Failure of normal testicular descent may involve both testes (bilateral) or only one testis (unilateral), in which case the right testis is more commonly involved (Cox, 1986). Bilateral cryptorchidism can be associated with male pseudohermaphroditism and other intersex states (see page 893).

INCIDENCE AND GENETICS. Cryptorchidism is a common developmental defect. The incidence of cryptorchidism in the dog has been reported to range from 0.8% to 15% (Romagnoli, 1991; Ruble and Hird, 1993). Although nongenetic factors may be involved (e.g., relative size of testicle and the inguinal canal), genetics undoubtedly plays an important role in the development of cryptorchidism. The prevalence of cryptorchidism is higher in purebred dogs, in certain breeds of dogs (Table 29-1), and within certain families of a breed. Currently, cryptorchidism is believed to be a

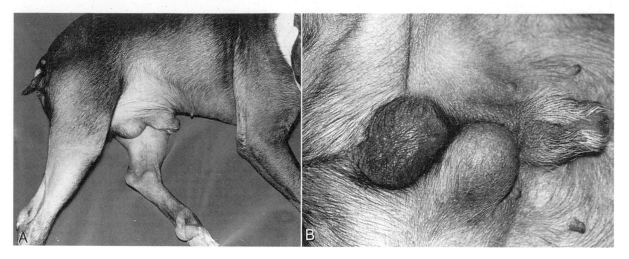

FIGURE 29-1. *A* and *B*, Unilateral cryptorchidism in an adult Boston Terrier. The left testis is located lateral to the penis, and the right testis is within the scrotum.

sex-limited autosomal recessive trait involving either a single gene locus or two gene loci. For the latter, one gene is believed to control internal testicular descent and organization of the epididymis and ductus deferens, and another gene controls external testicular descent.

Using the sex-limited autosomal recessive genetic model, both males and females carry the gene and can pass it on to their offspring. Only the homozygous males are phenotypically abnormal (i.e., cryptorchid) and readily identifiable. Heterozygous male and female and homozygous female puppies are phenotypically (clinically) normal. The genotype of the female and unaffected male can be determined only by progeny testing. Noncarrier status is difficult to prove because the absence of affected offspring is meaningless unless a large number of offspring are available for analysis. This fact is illustrated in a study in which the ratio of

TABLE 29–1 BREEDS OF DOGS AT HIGH AND LOW RISK FOR DEVELOPMENT OF CRYPTORCHIDISM

Increased Risk	Decreased Risk
Toy Poodle	Beagle
Pomeranian	Cocker Spaniel
Yorkshire Terrier	English Setter
Miniature Dachshund	Golden Retriever
Cairn Terrier	Great Dane
Chihuahua	Labrador Retriever
Maltese	Saint Bernard
Boxer	Mongrels
Pekinese	
English Bulldog	
Old English Sheepdog	
Miniature Poodle	
Miniature Schnauzer	
Shetland Sheepdog	
Siberian Husky	
Standard Poodle	

Data from Hayes HM, et al (1985), Hoskins and Taboada (1992) and Johnston SD, et al (2001).

cryptorchid to normal male offspring ranged from 1:1 to 1:20 among different carrier parents. In this case, more than 40 pups would have to be produced from a dam and survive to 6 months to establish noncarrier status. The occurrence of an occasional cryptorchid within a breed or breeding line may be attributed to chance or the presence of predisposing factors not necessarily related to genetics. As the incidence of such cases increases, however, the existence of a hereditary trait within the affected line becomes more likely.

DIAGNOSIS. The diagnosis of cryptorchidism is usually made on routine physical examination with the finding of only one or no scrotal testes. Occasionally, the veterinarian examines a dog obtained as an adult without scrotal testicles. Careful inspection of the scrotal and antepubic area for surgical scars may reveal evidence of previous surgery. Because retained testes are capable of steroidogenesis, digital palpation of the prostate gland may provide evidence for the presence or absence of circulating testosterone. The prostate gland in castrated dogs will be small on digital palpation, compared with the prostate gland in bilaterally cryptorchid dogs (Johnston et al, 2001). Sometimes a scar cannot be visualized, or the question of whether one retained testis is present still needs to be answered. Careful palpation and a thorough ultrasound examination of the abdomen and inguinal region usually identify a cryptorchid testicle. Abdominal radiography is usually ineffective because of the small size of the testicle and the inability to differentiate it from other soft tissue structures. If palpation and ultrasonography are inconclusive, a baseline plasma testosterone determination may distinguish dogs without testes from those with one or two retained testes (see Table 27-7). In our laboratory, castrated adult males typically have a random baseline plasma testosterone concentration of less than 20 pg/ml; those with only cryptorchid testes have a concentration of 100 to 2000 pg/ml (0.1 to 2 ng/ml); and adult males with one or two scrotal testes have plasma testosterone concentrations of 1 to

5 ng/ml. No difference in baseline plasma testosterone concentration is found in normal males and those with unilateral cryptorchidism (one retained and one scrotal testes), regardless of the location of the cryptorchid testis (Mattheeuws and Comhaire, 1989).

Monorchidism (only one testis) and anorchidism (no testes) are possible differential diagnoses but are extremely rare in dogs (Verstegen, 1998). For this reason, all cases of absence of one or both testes should be considered cryptorchidism until proved otherwise.

TREATMENT. Because of strong genetic implications and the increased potential for development of testicular neoplasia or torsion in cryptorchid testes, surgical removal of both testes is the treatment of choice. Genetic counseling aimed at reducing the prevalence of cryptorchidism in the family line should also be discussed with owners. Affected dogs should be removed from the breeding program. The father and mother as well as full siblings of affected dogs should be considered carriers and should also be removed from the breeding program.

Surgical therapy to place the retained testis into the scrotum is an unethical practice and should not be done. Medical therapy has been attempted, although results are quite variable and usually disappointing. Medical therapy for cryptorchidism has included the use of testosterone, human chorionic gonadotropin (hCG), or gonadotropin-releasing hormone (GnRH) injections. Testicular descent is believed to be under the influence of androgenic hormones secreted by the testes. Although testosterone production by the Leydig cells continues regardless of the location of the testes, plasma testosterone concentrations from cryptorchid dogs are usually less than that of normal males, suggesting that testosterone administration or administration of testosterone-stimulating hormones (i.e., hCG, GnRH) may promote testicular descent.

Historically, administration of testosterone or testosterone analogues has been ineffective in promoting testicular descent and is not recommended. The more commonly used medical therapy for cryptorchidism is serial injections of hCG, 100 to 1000 IU/dog intramuscularly four times over 2 weeks, or GnRH, 50 to 100 μg subcutaneously or intravenously twice at 7-day intervals. Results are variable and unpredictable and may be coincidental with spontaneous descent of mobile testes. Factors that affect success include location of the cryptorchid testis (inguinal canal versus intra-abdominal) and age of the dog. Success is more likely with mobile testes located in the inguinal canal and in dogs under 16 weeks of age. Dogs younger than 16 weeks of age have the best chance of responding to medical therapy. We have not successfully treated cryptorchid dogs older than 16 weeks of age. The ethics of medical management depend on the opinions of the veterinarian and the pet owner. However, it should be emphasized that the genes responsible for carrying the trait are still present and will be transmitted to offspring.

Fortunately, bilateral cryptorchid dogs are sterile as a result of destruction of the testicular germinal epithelium following prolonged exposure of the testes to normal intra-abdominal temperatures (i.e., body temperature). Most dogs with unilateral cryptorchidism are fertile, although total sperm per ejaculate may be decreased. Libido is typically normal in unilateral and bilateral cryptorchids because of continued testosterone secretion by interstitial Leydig cells.

Potential complications with cryptorchid testes include testicular torsion (see page 970), an increased incidence of testicular neoplasia (see page 964), male feminizing syndrome (see page 967), and blood dyscrasias. For these reasons, as well as the genetic implications, owners should be encouraged to have cryptorchid testes surgically removed once the dog has reached adulthood.

Testicular Hypoplasia

Testicular hypoplasia is a congenital, possibly hereditary disorder resulting from a lack of or marked reduction in the number of spermatogonia in the gonads. Testicular hypoplasia may result from inadequate primitive germ cell development in the yolk sac, failure of germ cells to migrate to the undifferentiated gonad, lack of an ability for these cells to multiply in the gonad, or early destruction of the cells during fetal development. Testicular hypoplasia may also be a component of some intersex states (see page 893). Because 50% to 70% of the volume of the testis is derived from the seminiferous tubules, a lack of germinal epithelial cells is associated with decreased testicular size. Testicular hypoplasia may be unilateral or bilateral. It is usually first noticed soon after puberty, which differentiates this condition from acquired testicular degeneration in the adult male (see page 974).

Testicular hypoplasia results in oligospermia or azoospermia and sterility. The interstitial Leydig cells are often present in normal numbers, maintaining testosterone secretion and libido. The severity of oligospermia depends on the amount of testicular tissue involved, with bilateral hypoplasia usually associated with azoospermia and sterility. Histologic evaluation of biopsies obtained from the involved testis reveals underdeveloped seminiferous tubules, lack of germinal epithelium, and variable numbers of Leydig cells.

A diagnosis of testicular hypoplasia should not be made until the dog is mature, that is, 1 to 2 years of age. There is no treatment. Injections of GnRH, FSH, or hCG are ineffective because no "receptors" (spermatogonia) are present to respond to these hormones. The prognosis for fertility depends on the severity of hypoplasia and oligospermia, although veterinarians tend to recognize only the most severe cases.

Aplasia of the Duct System

Failure of any part of the testicular duct system to develop results in impaired transportation of spermatozoa to the urethra, accumulation of sperm proximal to the obstruction, and possibly development of sperm granuloma and testicular degeneration (see pages 974 and 975). Although studies have not been done in the dog, aplasia of the duct system has been shown to be inherited in the bull, boar, and mink. Segmental aplasia is often unilateral, involving only one testis. Dogs with unilateral aplasia remain fertile, and the disorder is usually undiagnosed. If segmental aplasia is bilateral, the breeding dog is brought to the veterinarian with the primary complaint of infertility. Semen evaluation reveals azoospermia if bilateral aplasia is present. Seminal alkaline phosphatase concentration may be normal or decreased, depending on the site of aplasia (see page 940).

The aplastic portion of the duct may be palpable if the aplasia involves the epididymis or proximal portion of the vas deferens. The size of the testis and epididymis depends on the location of the aplasia. If the site of aplasia, and therefore obstruction, is distal to the head of the epididymis, seminiferous tubular secretions continue to be absorbed by the ductular epithelial cells in the head of the epididymis. Seminiferous fluid accumulation and secondary testicular degeneration are less likely to develop. If the site of aplasia involves the head of the epididymis, seminiferous tubule secretions are not absorbed and they accumulate, causing increased pressure and edema within the testis, seminiferous tubule degeneration, and testicular atrophy. The size of the testis is variable and may range from small through normal to slightly enlarged, depending on the age of the dog and the amount of fluid accumulation and testicular degeneration.

Results of testicular biopsy may reveal active spermatogenesis in an azoospermic dog, unless severe secondary testicular degeneration is present. A definitive diagnosis requires visual examination of the duct system during surgery, a step most veterinary surgeons would not recommend owing to the technical difficulty of such a procedure.

Because of the potential heredity involved with this disorder, bypass operations should be discouraged. The efficacy of these techniques has not been reported in the dog but is assumed to be extremely low. The probability of restoring fertility to an azoospermic dog with segmental aplasia is virtually nil.

ACQUIRED DISORDERS

Testicular Tumors

TYPES. Testicular neoplasia is common in the dog. The three most commonly recognized tumors are Sertoli cell, seminoma, and interstitial cell tumors. Embryonal carcinoma, granulosa cell tumor, hemangioma, fibrosarcoma, neurofibrosarcoma, and undifferentiated carcinoma and sarcoma have been reported but are rare.

Sertoli cell tumor. Sertoli cell tumors are derived from the Sertoli (nurse) cells of the seminiferous tubules. Sertoli cell tumors are usually slow-growing

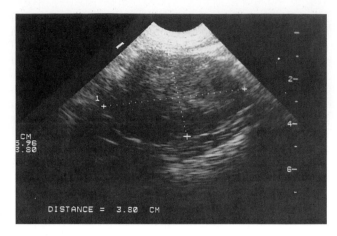

FIGURE 29-2. Ultrasonography of the caudal abdomen of a 16-year-old Coonhound dog with unilateral cryptorchidism, illustrating a 6 × 4 cm echogenic mass *(dotted lines)* located in the caudal right abdomen. Histologic evaluation of the mass revealed Sertoli cell tumor.

and noninvasive and typically range from 0.1 to 5 cm in diameter. Sertoli cell tumors may become quite large (i.e., 10 cm in diameter) when an intra-abdominal cryptorchid testis is involved (Fig. 29-2). These tumors feel firm and nodular on palpation. Approximately 10% to 20% are malignant, with metastasis occurring to the inguinal, iliac, and sublumbar lymph nodes and to the lungs, liver, spleen, kidneys, and pancreas (Crow, 1980). The male feminizing syndrome is most commonly caused by Sertoli cell tumors (see page 967).

Seminoma. Seminomas are derived from the spermatogenic cells of the seminiferous tubules and range in size from less than 1 cm to 10 cm in diameter. They feel soft on palpation. Seminomas are usually benign, although approximately 5% to 10% of seminomas are malignant (DeVico et al, 1994). Predisposing sites for metastasis are similar to those of malignant Sertoli cell tumors. Androgen secretion may be more common and male feminizing syndrome less common with seminoma versus Sertoli cell tumor.

Interstitial cell tumors. Interstitial cell tumors are derived from the Leydig cells. These tumors are usually small (0.1 to 2 cm in diameter), nonpalpable, discrete masses that are hormonally silent and most commonly identified as an incidental finding at necropsy (Crow, 1980). Only 25% of dogs with interstitial cell tumors evaluated in one study had enlargement of the testes as a result of the tumor. In the remaining 75%, the tumor was not detectable. Interstitial cell tumors are almost always benign, and they feel soft and nodular on palpation. Paraneoplastic syndromes are uncommon with interstitial cell tumors and result from hyperestrogenism or hyperandrogenism (Medleau, 1989; Suess et al, 1992).

INCIDENCE. Although individual reports of incidence vary, a review of the literature suggests an overall incidence of 44% for Sertoli cell tumor, 31% for seminoma, and 25% for interstitial cell tumor (Johnston et al, 2001). As many as 35% of dogs with testicular neoplasia have

TABLE 29-2 BREEDS OF DOGS AT HIGH AND LOW RISK FOR DEVELOPMENT OF TESTICULAR NEOPLASIA

Increased Risk	Decreased Risk
Boxer	Beagle
Chihuahua	Labrador Retriever
German Shepherd Dog	Mongrels
Pomeranian	
Miniature Poodle	
Standard Poodle	
Miniature Schnauzer	
Shetland Sheepdog	
Siberian Husky	
Yorkshire Terrier	

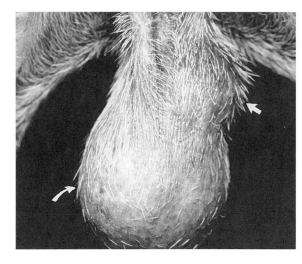

FIGURE 29-3. A 16-year-old German Short-Haired Pointer dog with marked asymmetry of the testes. Enlargement of the left testis was caused by a seminoma *(curved arrow)*. Note the atrophied right testis *(straight arrow)*.

two or all three tumor types present at one time. The mean age for development of testicular tumors is 10 years, with a range of 3 to 19 years. The age of onset is earlier when the involved testis is extrascrotal. Certain breeds appear to be at increased risk for development of testicular neoplasia (Table 29-2).

The incidence of testicular neoplasia is much greater in cryptorchid testes than in normally descended testes—approximately 10 times greater (Hayes et al, 1985). Because the right testis is more commonly cryptorchid, it has a higher frequency of neoplastic involvement. Sertoli cell tumor accounts for approximately 60% and seminoma for 40% of tumors in cryptorchid testes. The incidence of these tumors is greater in inguinal than in intra-abdominal testes. Interstitial cell tumors are almost always found in descended testicles. Differences in incidence of tumor type based on location of testis may be due to differences in parenchymal temperature when the testis is located in the abdomen versus the inguinal region and the effect of temperature on viability of spermatogonia, Sertoli cells, and Leydig cells (Wallace and Cox, 1980). Scrotally located testes are at the proper temperature to ensure viability and function of all three cell types, thereby accounting for the approximately equal incidence of all three tumor types in scrotal testes.

CLINICAL SIGNS. Clinical signs are variable and depend on the hormonal activity of the tumor. In general, clinical signs are caused by the space-occupying effect of the tumor itself or by its secretion of estrogens or androgens. Depending on the size of the tumor and the location of the involved testis, owners may bring their dog to the veterinarian with a complaint of scrotal or testicular enlargement, asymmetry in testicular size (Fig. 29-3), distended abdomen, or signs suggestive of a testicular torsion (see page 970). Rarely, stud dogs may be brought to a veterinarian for infertility. Infertility could result from pressure necrosis of normal testicular tissue by the tumor, a secondary immune-mediated reaction directed against spermatogonia following neoplasia-induced disruption of the blood-testis barrier, or hormonally induced testicular atrophy following secretion of estrogens or androgens by the neoplastic tissue. Peters et al (2000) documented a significant reduction in spermatogenesis in dogs with

testicular tumors. Grootenhuis et al (1990) reported that secretory products from Sertoli cell tumors in cryptorchid dogs suppressed pituitary gonadotropin secretion and decreased responsiveness of the pituitary gland to exogenously administered GnRH. Estrogen-secreting testicular tumors may cause the male feminizing syndrome (see page 967), whereas androgen secreting tumors may cause prostatic dysfunction.

ANDROGEN SECRETION AND ITS EFFECT ON THE PROSTATE. Testicular tumors may secrete androgens, a phenomenon believed to be responsible for the higher incidence of prostatic dysfunction and perianal tumors in dogs with testicular neoplasia. Androgens are thought to be essential for the development and maintenance of the canine prostate gland and are believed to play a role in the development of benign prostatic hypertrophy in humans. In addition, androgens have a direct stimulatory effect on the growth of perianal gland neoplasms. One study found a 33% incidence of prostatic disease and perineal neoplasia in dogs with either interstitial cell tumor or seminoma. This increased incidence is thought to be a result of preferential secretion of androgens by these tumors. In contrast, estrogens induce squamous metaplasia of the prostate gland, resulting in decreased size of the prostate, and they inhibit growth of perianal gland tumors. The low incidence of perianal gland tumors and prostatic hyperplasia in dogs with Sertoli cell tumors is believed to be a result of preferential secretion of estrogens.

Pathologic changes of the prostate gland that have been associated with testicular tumors include cysts, hyperplasia, abscesses, squamous metaplasia, inflammation, and atrophy. Clinical signs supportive of prostatic disease include blood dripping from the penis, dysuria, hematuria, constipation, rear limb weakness or gait abnormalities, and systemic signs of illness (i.e., fever, inappetence, weight loss, abdominal pain; see Chapter 30). In addition to prostatic disease, perianal

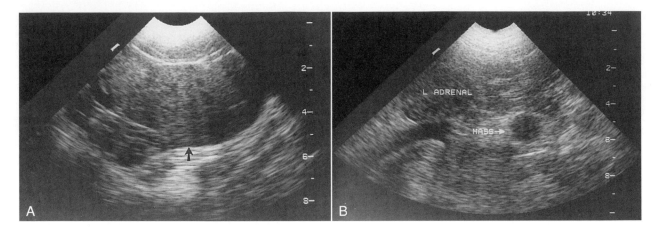

FIGURE 29-4. *A,* Ultrasonography of the right testis *(arrow)* of a 9-year-old Malamute dog with unilateral cryptorchidism. The right testis was enlarged and located in the right inguinal region. The testicular parenchyma appeared hypoechoic with multiple small cystic regions located throughout. *B,* Abdominal ultrasonography of dog in *A,* illustrating a hypoechoic mass *(arrow)* near the left adrenal gland. Hypoechoic masses were also visualized in the mesentery and sublumbar region. Histologic evaluation of the testis and several of the masses revealed metastatic seminoma.

adenoma, adenocarcinoma, and perineal hernias are associated with androgen-secreting testicular tumors.

DIAGNOSIS. The presence of a testicular tumor is usually suspected from a combination of clinical signs and physical examination findings. Signs typically caused by a testicular tumor include asymmetric testicular enlargement or the male feminizing syndrome. Testicular enlargement may be diffuse, or a discrete nodule may be palpable in the testis. It must be remembered that testicular tumors can be found within scrotal testes that are normal on digital palpation. Other less specific signs include prostatic dysfunction, perianal neoplasms, cryptorchidism, oligospermia, azoospermia, systemic signs of illness, or hemorrhage as a result of pancytopenia or prostatitis.

Abdominal radiography and ultrasonography can be used to identify and localize neoplastic intra-abdominal testes and to assess for metastases (Fig. 29-4). Testes smaller than twice the diameter of the small intestine, however, are difficult to identify radiographically. Ultrasonographic evaluation of scrotal testes by an experienced radiologist or internist is a helpful diagnostic aid for dogs in which neoplasia is suspected but not palpable. Testicular ultrasonography can localize the mass within the testis and provide guidance for subsequent biopsy. Testicular tumors have variable echotexture. Small discrete tumors (<3 cm) usually appear hypoechoic, whereas larger tumors, especially those greater than 5 cm, have mixed echogenicity (Fig. 29-5; Johnston et al, 1991; Pugh and Konde, 1991). Mixed echogenicity is caused by areas of hemorrhage, necrosis, infarction, and calcification within the tumor. It is difficult to predict the tumor type based on ultrasonographic appearance. In general, Sertoli cell tumors have a variable echogenic pattern, focal seminomas and interstitial cell tumors less than 3 cm in diameter tend to be hypoechoic, and focal seminomas and interstitial cell tumors greater than 3 cm in diameter have mixed echogenicity.

Occasionally, the clinician may elect to assay the plasma estrogen concentration in an effort to confirm a clinical suspicion of an estrogen-secreting testicular tumor. In our experience, dogs with Sertoli cell tumors have not consistently demonstrated increases in plasma estrogen (estradiol) concentration (see page 967). An alternative and perhaps more sensitive marker for Sertoli cell tumor is serum inhibin concentration. Inhibin is a glycoprotein hormone produced by Sertoli cells in the male (de Kretser and Robertson, 1989). The primary physiologic role of inhibin is the specific suppression of pituitary FSH secretion. Inhibin concentrations have been reported to be increased in dogs with Sertoli cell tumors versus healthy dogs (de Jong et al,

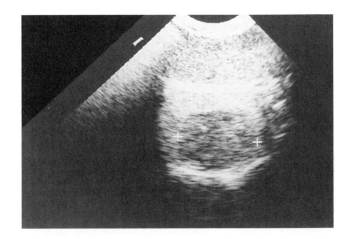

FIGURE 29-5. Ultrasonography of the left testis of a 9-year-old Miniature Poodle, illustrating a 1-cm diameter, hypoechoic nodule *(crosses)* within the parenchyma. Histology confirmed a seminoma.

1990; Grootenhuis et al, 1990). Exfoliative cytology of the preputial mucosa may also be useful in confirming the presence of hyperestrogenism. Preputial cytology of the normal dog yields noncornified epithelial cells, whereas cytology of dogs exposed to estrogen yields cornified epithelial cells with similar morphology to vaginal epithelial cells of estrous bitches (Johnston et al, 2001).

Definitive diagnosis of a testicular tumor requires cytologic evaluation of a fine-needle aspiration biopsy (see page 947) or histologic evaluation of a surgically excised testis.

THERAPY. Therapy for testicular neoplasia involves surgical excision of the involved testis. Before surgery, thoracic and abdominal radiographs and an abdominal sonogram should be evaluated for metastatic disease. Common metastatic sites include the sublumbar lymph nodes, liver, and spleen. If cryptorchidism is present, bilateral castration should always be performed. Scrotal testes are fertile; however, such dogs are not recommended for breeding.

Tumor-induced immune destruction of the testes rarely responds to selective removal of the neoplasm. Hormonally induced testicular atrophy, as a result of excessive estrogen secretion by a tumor, may be reversible once feedback inhibition on the hypothalamic-pituitary secretion of GnRH, LH, and FSH is removed. The presence of undetectable neoplasia in the "normal" testis or hormonally active metastatic masses may prevent return of fertility.

Chemotherapy or radiation therapy is indicated in those dogs with documented metastatic disease. Several chemotherapy protocols have been used. Combination chemotherapy using vinblastine, cyclophosphamide, and methotrexate has been reported to have some degree of efficacy in treating metastatic disease in dogs (Madewell and Theilen, 1987). Similar favorable results have been observed with cisplatin (Dhaliwal et al, 1999). Chemotherapy may reduce tumor volume and improve the dog's quality of life for several months, but chemotherapy does not induce a cure. The prognosis for metastatic testicular neoplasia is guarded to grave.

Seminomas are radiosensitive in humans and possibly dogs. Treatment with cesium-137 teleradiotherapy at a dose range of 17 to 40 gy given in 8 to 10 fractions, with 3 fractions given weekly, was effective treatment for seminoma with regional metastasis in four dogs (McDonald et al, 1988). The tumor and its metastases regressed in all dogs, and survival ranged from 6 to 57 months (mean, 36 months). All of the dogs died of non–tumor-related causes. No evidence of seminoma was found at necropsy.

Male Feminizing Syndrome

ETIOLOGY. The male feminizing syndrome is believed to result from either increased production of estrogens by testicular tumor cells, increased conversion of testosterone and androstenedione to estrogens by testicular cells or peripheral tissues (e.g., liver,

adipose tissue, hair follicles, neural tissue, muscle), or an abnormality in the balance of the sex hormones as a result of decreased androgen production concomitant with normal estrogen production. Conflicting information exists in the literature regarding the documentation of estrogen compounds as the cause of this syndrome. Some investigators have documented higher estrogen concentrations in peripheral blood, spermatic venous blood of the neoplastic testis, and urine in affected dogs compared with normal dogs, whereas others failed to document increased estrogen concentrations in plasma, urine, or neoplastic tissue. In our experience, dogs with Sertoli cell tumors have had normal to moderately increased plasma estrogen concentrations. Normal male dogs have plasma estrogen (estradiol) concentrations less than 15 pg/ml. Dogs with Sertoli cell tumors have had plasma estrogen concentrations of 10 to 150 pg/ml.

CELL TYPE. Sertoli cell tumors are most commonly associated with the male feminizing syndrome, although seminomas and interstitial cell tumors may also cause the syndrome. Approximately 25% of dogs with Sertoli cell tumors develop the male feminizing syndrome (Crow, 1980). A definite association exists between the syndrome and an extrascrotal location of the neoplastic testis. Approximately 70% of abdominally located testicular tumors are associated with the male feminizing syndrome, whereas 50% and 17% of dogs develop this syndrome when the testis is in the inguinal and scrotal position, respectively. Descended testes with no palpable abnormalities may contain a testicular tumor with or without causing signs of the male feminizing syndrome (Fig. 29-6).

CLINICAL SIGNS. The most obvious sign in dogs with the male feminizing syndrome is a nonpruritic, symmetric endocrine alopecia, which usually begins in the perineal and genital regions and spreads to the ventral abdomen, thorax, flanks, and neck (Fig. 29-6). Hyperpigmentation, gynecomastia, galactorrhea, a pendulous penile sheath, attraction of other males, and standing in a female posture to urinate are also commonly associated with this syndrome (Fig. 29-7). The negative feedback inhibition on hypothalamic-pituitary secretion of GnRH, LH, and/or FSH results in atrophy of the non-neoplastic testicular tissue, decreased libido, and oligospermia. Signs suggestive of prostatic dysfunction may develop as a result of prostatitis or prostatomegaly with squamous metaplasia of the epithelial cells of the gland.

BONE MARROW DYSFUNCTION. Severe bone marrow hypoplasia and pancytopenia may occur in some dogs with neoplastic testicular tumors and male feminizing syndrome. Bone marrow hypoplasia is believed to result from the effects of persistently increased plasma estrogen concentrations. This syndrome is identical to that resulting from estrogen injections administered to postcoital bitches as a treatment for preventing pregnancy or bitches with estrogen-secreting follicular ovarian cysts. Although the exact mechanisms are not completely understood, estrogens have been found to interfere with stem cell differentiation, alter iron

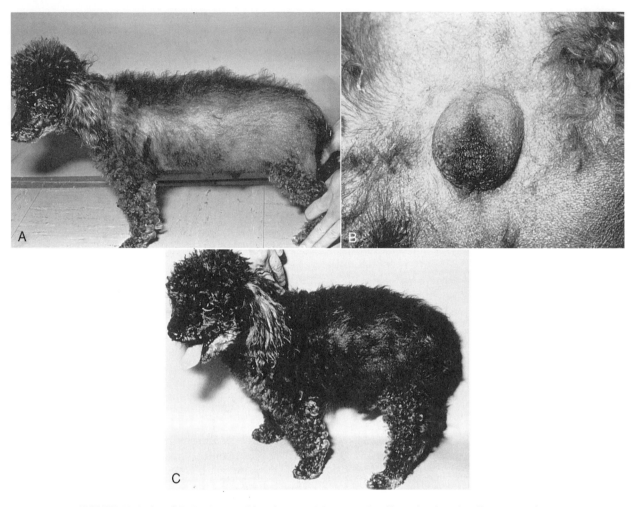

FIGURE 29-6. *A* and *B,* An 8-year-old male intact Miniature Poodle with a Sertoli cell tumor within a descended testis and with dermatologic signs of the feminizing syndrome. Note the characteristic symmetric alopecia involving the perineum, abdomen, chest, and neck. (Courtesy of J.C. Blakemore, Purdue University.) *C,* Same dog 2 months after castration.

utilization by erythrocyte precursors, and possibly inhibit the production of circulating erythrocyte-stimulating factor.

Estrogen-induced bone marrow toxicity initially results in a transient increase in granulocytopoiesis and a neutrophilic leukocytosis. This is followed by hypoplasia of all cell lines and eventual development of pancytopenia. Signs of bone marrow disease include listlessness, weakness, thrombocytopenic hemorrhage, petechiae, inappetence, fever, pallor, and vomiting. Evaluation of a complete blood count (CBC) reveals variable degrees of nonregenerative anemia, leukopenia with lymphocytosis, and thrombocytopenia. Bone marrow aspiration reveals hypoplasia with decreased numbers of leukocyte and erythrocyte precursors, as well as decreased megakaryocytes, suggesting complete maturation arrest of all three cell lines. Therapy is supportive (see below), and the condition is usually terminal.

DIAGNOSIS. The diagnosis of male feminizing syndrome is based on appropriate clinical signs in a dog with a testicular tumor, usually in a cryptorchid testis.

Identification of pancytopenia on a CBC, cornification of preputial mucosal cells or increased plasma estrogen concentration (i.e., >20 pg/ml) supports the diagnosis. Histologic confirmation of a testicular tumor and resolution of clinical signs following orchiectomy confirm the diagnosis.

Dogs with testicular tumor–associated male feminizing syndrome may be brought to the veterinarian with primary owner complaints of nonpruritic, bilaterally symmetric endocrine alopecia. If the testes are scrotal and are normal on palpation, diagnosis of a testicular tumor may not be readily apparent. Fortunately, the diagnostic approach to endocrine alopecia leads to the correct diagnosis (see Chapter 2, page 62).

THERAPY. Primary therapy for male feminizing syndrome is surgical removal of the testicular tumor. Before surgery, thoracic and abdominal radiographs and an abdominal sonogram should be evaluated for metastatic disease. Clinical signs of the male feminizing syndrome should begin to resolve 4 to 6 weeks following castration. If signs fail to resolve, the dog may have previously unidentified metastatic disease or there

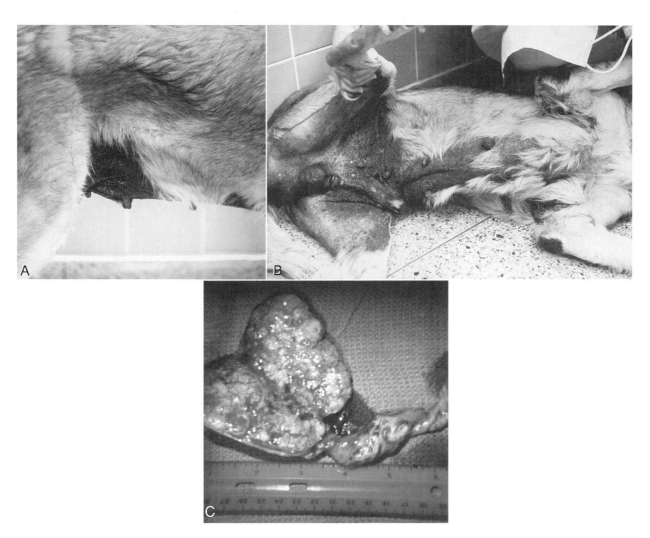

FIGURE 29-7. *A* and *B*, A 9-year-old German Shepherd cross with unilateral cryptorchidism, an intra-abdominal Sertoli cell tumor, and signs of the feminizing syndrome. Note the severe hyper-pigmentation and gynecomastia. *C*, A cross-sectional view of the Sertoli cell tumor removed from the abdomen of the dog shown in *A* and *B*.

may have been a misdiagnosis of the male feminizing syndrome. If metastatic disease is documented with radiography, ultrasonography, histologic findings, or continuing signs following castration, chemotherapy or radiation therapy should be considered (see page 967).

Dogs with pancytopenia often require intensive therapy for anemia, hemorrhage, and infection. Initial therapy depends on the severity of anemia and thrombocytopenia. Stabilization of these dogs often requires a combination of IV fluid therapy, fresh whole blood transfusions or platelet-rich plasma infusions, and broad-spectrum bactericidal antibiotics. Once the dog is stabilized and hemorrhage is controlled, castration should be performed to remove the source of estrogens that are causing the bone marrow toxicity. The use of hematinics, anabolic steroids (e.g., oxymetholone, nandrolone decanoate), and possibly glucocorticoids has been advocated for the treatment of estrogen-induced bone marrow toxicosis. However,

beneficial effects are not well documented, and the use of glucocorticoids is questionable in patients with concurrent infection and leukopenia.

Hematopoietic growth factors, specifically granulocyte colony-stimulating factor (G-CSF) and erythropoietin (EPO), offer interesting possibilities for the treatment of pancytopenia induced by estrogen. Recombinant G-CSF has been shown to accelerate bone marrow recovery after chemotherapy, to normalize neutrophil counts in humans with chronic idiopathic neutropenia, and to improve neutrophil counts in dogs with cyclic neutropenia (Obradovich et al, 1991; Ogilvie et al, 1992), whereas recombinant human EPO is routinely used to treat nonregenerative anemia of chronic renal failure in dogs and cats (Cowgill, 1992). Use of recombinant canine G-CSF has not been associated with clinically significant toxicosis (Obradovich et al, 1991); however, recombinant human G-CSF initially caused neutrophilia followed by a prolonged period of chronic neutropenia in healthy dogs (Hammond et al,

1991). Serum antibody to recombinant human G-CSF and endogenous canine G-CSF was responsible for the neutropenia. Serum antibody formation causing refractory anemia has also been documented in dogs treated with recombinant human EPO (Cowgill, 1992). Nevertheless, recombinant human EPO, 100 units/kg subcutaneously three times weekly, and recombinant G-CSF (preferably of canine origin), 5 μg/kg/day subcutaneously, should be considered for the treatment of pancytopenia in dogs with male feminizing syndrome (Ogilvie, 1995).

Repeated blood transfusions may be required during the course of therapy to support red blood cell, white blood cell, and platelet numbers until bone marrow activity returns. Periodic evaluation of a CBC, including reticulocyte and platelet count, is valuable in monitoring response to therapy and determining when additional blood transfusions are needed.

The prognosis for dogs with bone marrow hypoplasia is grave. Hypoplasia and progressively worsening pancytopenia usually persist despite removal of the testicular tumor. Affected dogs that respond to castration and supportive therapy usually show some signs of bone marrow regeneration within 3 to 6 weeks. Several months may be required before results of a CBC are normal in these dogs.

Testicular Torsion

CAUSE. Rotation of the testis on its horizontal axis results in torsion of the spermatic cord, occlusion of venous drainage from the testis, and subsequent testicular engorgement and necrosis. Testicular torsion is rare in the dog; it is most often diagnosed in dogs with an enlarged neoplastic abdominal testis (Fig. 29-8).

The presence of neoplasia is responsible for the abnormal amount of weight in a pendulous abdominal testis, predisposing that testis to rotation following physical activity or trauma.

A similar correlation between neoplasia and testicular torsion does not seem to exist for testes in an intrascrotal position. Intrascrotal testes that have undergone torsion are typically normal histologically. The cause of torsion of a scrotal testis remains unknown, although rupture of the scrotal ligament following trauma or excessive physical activity could predispose a testis to rotation.

CLINICAL SIGNS AND PHYSICAL EXAMINATION. Torsion of an intrascrotal testis causes acute pain, scrotal swelling, and a reluctance to stand or walk. Physical findings include an enlarged firm testis, scrotal edema, and pain on manipulation of the torsed testis. A thickened spermatic cord may be palpable.

An acute onset of abdominal pain and restlessness is typical in dogs with torsion of an intra-abdominal testis. Depending on the duration of torsion, lethargy, inappetence, vomiting, and shock may develop. Abdominal pain is the most consistent finding on physical examination. Additional findings may include abdominal distention, ascites, fever, and shock. A painful mass may be palpated in the mid- to caudal abdomen if ascites is not present. Other signs and physical findings may be related to the presence of a hormonally active testicular tumor (see pages 965 and 967).

DIFFERENTIAL DIAGNOSIS. Differential diagnoses include acute epididymitis and orchitis in swollen intrascrotal testes and pancreatitis, peritonitis, splenic torsion, or obstruction of the urinary tract or intestine in dogs with acute abdominal pain. Ultrasonography is quite valuable in confirming testicular torsion before surgery. Sonographic findings include testicular

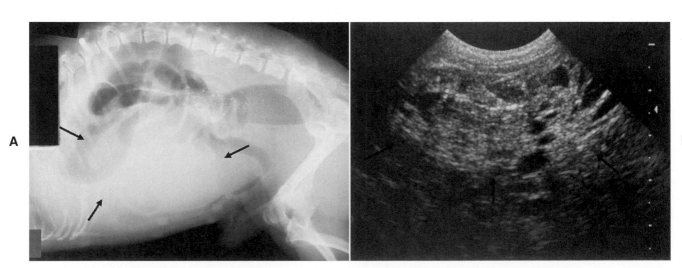

FIGURE 29-8. *A,* Abdominal radiograph of a 6-year-old male Pekinese with an acute onset of lethargy, vomiting, and abdominal pain, illustrating a mid-abdominal mass *(arrows). B,* Ultrasonography confirmed the presence of a large, multicameral mass with mixed echogenicity *(arrows).* Torsion of an intra-abdominal testicular mass was identified at surgery. Sertoli cell tumor was identified on histologic examination of the mass.

enlargement with a uniform decrease in parenchymal echogenicity, concurrent enlargement of the epididymis and spermatic cord, and cranial displacement of the tail of the epididymis (Mattoon and Nyland, 1995; Pinto et al, 2001). Color Doppler ultrasonography may identify lack of perfusion of the affected testis.

THERAPY. Testicular torsion is a medical emergency requiring surgical intervention. The treatment is orchiectomy and supportive care for concurrent problems (e.g., shock). The prognosis is good unless a metastatic testicular tumor is present. Any excised tissue should be submitted for histologic evaluation because of the strong association between testicular tumors and testicular torsion.

Acute Infectious Orchitis/Epididymitis

Because the testis and epididymis are in close apposition and connected via the duct system, any inflammatory or infectious process involving one usually also involves the other, although on occasion isolated orchitis or epididymitis may be seen. Involvement of the spermatic cord may also be present.

ETIOLOGY. Orchiepididymitis is typically caused by bacteria, which gain access to the testes and epididymides through direct trauma (e.g., puncture wounds), retrograde passage of infected urine or prostatic secretions, bacteremia, or infected lymph. Commonly isolated organisms include *Staphylococcus*, *Streptococcus*, *Escherichia coli*, and *Proteus*. *Mycoplasma* has also been isolated in a few dogs with orchiepididymitis (Lein, 1989). Symptomatic *Brucella canis* infections typically cause acute testicular/epididymal swelling and pain in the dog. Dogs with *B. canis* infection can also be asymptomatic, leading to an insidious destruction of the epididymis and testis, with the development of nonsuppurative inflammation, fibrosis, and oligo/azoospermia. Distemper virus has been reported to cause nonsuppurative inflammation and fibrosis of the testis and epididymis (Dahlbom and Andersson, 2000). Distemper inclusion bodies may be found in the epididymal epithelium and Sertoli cells. Finally, disseminated systemic mycoses (e.g., blastomycosis, coccidioidomycosis), canine ehrlichiosis, and Rocky Mountain spotted fever can cause acute orchitis/epididymitis (see Fig. 27-13).

CLINICAL SIGNS. Acute orchiepididymitis causes acute pain, scrotal swelling, and a reluctance to stand or walk. Lethargy and anorexia may also develop. Because of pain, these dogs often resist examination. Tranquilization may be required in some cases to allow completion of an adequate physical examination. The physical examination reveals variable degrees of testicular and/or epididymal swelling (Fig. 29-9), hyperemia, local hyperthermia, and pain on manipulation of the testis. Unilateral involvement is more common than bilateral. Scrotal dermatitis may be present if the dog has been allowed to lick the affected area. Mucopurulent exudate may be present on the scrotum if a suppurative process with abscessation has occurred. Fever is commonly associated with acute orchiepididymitis. Rectal palpation of the prostate gland may reveal an enlarged, painful gland, which in conjunction with the appropriate clinical signs, supports a diagnosis of acute prostatitis.

DIAGNOSTIC EVALUATION. In dogs with acute pain and scrotal swelling, the primary differential diagnosis is testicular torsion. Sonographic evaluation of the scrotum helps differentiate testicular torsion from acute orchiepididymitis (see Table 27-8) and may identify testicular or epididymal abscessation (Fig. 29-10). Once acute orchiepididymitis is suspected, an attempt should be made to isolate the underlying etiologic

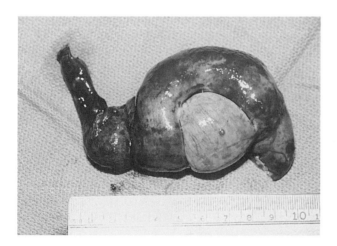

FIGURE 29-9. Unilateral suppurative epididymitis causing diffuse enlargement of the epididymis in a 7-year-old Rottweiler. The owner presented the dog for acute scrotal swelling and pain. The testis was normal.

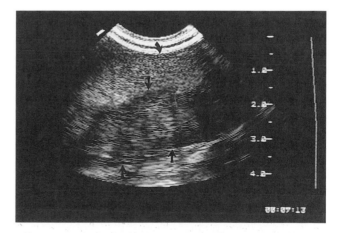

FIGURE 29-10. Ultrasonography of the right testis of a 7-year-old Rottweiler with a 3-day history of lethargy, inappetence, and a swollen, painful right testis, illustrating generalized enlargement of the epididymis *(straight arrows)*. The epididymal parenchyma appeared hypoechoic, and the testicular parenchyma *(curved arrow)* appeared unremarkable. Unilateral orchiectomy was performed (see Fig. 29-9). Histologic evaluation revealed severe suppurative epididymitis of undetermined cause and a normal testis. Aerobic and anaerobic cultures of epididymal tissue were negative.

agent through culture of blood, urine, and semen (see page 941). Draining scrotal tracts may also be cultured. Appropriate blood tests for *B. canis* should also be submitted to the laboratory (see page 920).

Semen collection may be difficult because of the pain associated with orchiepididymitis but should always be attempted. If an ejaculate is obtained, microscopic evaluation usually reveals inflammatory cells (primarily neutrophils), an increased percentage of primary and secondary morphologic defects in the spermatozoa, decreased numbers of spermatozoa, and possibly seminiferous epithelial cells. Head-to-head agglutination of spermatozoa is suggestive of *B. canis* infection.

Sonographic assessment of the prostate gland and prostatic aspiration, biopsy, or massage for cytologic evaluation and culture may be indicated if the initial prostatic examination is abnormal (see page 978). Samples for cytology and culture can also be obtained by fine-needle aspiration of the enlarged testes/epididymis (see page 947). Testicular biopsies are not performed routinely. If they are done, however, a portion of the biopsy specimen should be cultured for bacteria and *Mycoplasma*.

TREATMENT. Therapy should be initiated once appropriate bacterial cultures have been obtained. The therapeutic approach depends on the wishes of the owner. If fertility is of no concern, the dog should be stabilized with IV fluids, treated with broad-spectrum bactericidal antibiotics, and then castrated. Our initial antibiotics of choice are trimethoprim-sulfonamide, clavulanate-amoxicillin, or enrofloxacin. A more suitable antibiotic can be given once the antibiotic sensitivity of the organism is known.

If maintaining the reproductive potential of an individual dog is important to the owner, castration may not be an option unless the dog has an uncontrollable infection. Supportive care (i.e., IV fluids, antibiotics) should be initiated at once. In addition, cold compresses or water can be placed on the scrotum to help minimize thermal damage to the germinal epithelium of the seminiferous tubules. Prolonged exposure of the seminiferous epithelium to high temperatures created by the inflammation of acute orchitis may result in destruction of spermatogenic cells, azoospermia, and testicular atrophy. Anti-inflammatory agents (e.g., corticosteroids, aspirin) may be used to control inflammation, local hyperthermia, and exposure of the immune system to spermatozoal antigens following disruption of the blood-testis barrier.

Unilateral orchitis may damage the other testis as a result of heat liberated by the inflammatory process, immune-mediated destruction of spermatozoa following disruption of the blood-testis barrier, or extension of the infection to the unaffected testis. For these reasons, unilateral orchiectomy may be considered in a valuable stud dog in an attempt to salvage the normal testis. Dogs with one normal testis are fertile, although sperm numbers per ejaculate may be decreased. Owners should be aware that the American Kennel Club does not permit dogs with one testis to be shown.

PROGNOSIS. The prognosis for maintaining fertility in dogs following acute orchiepididymitis is guarded. Infertility may result from irreversible damage to the germinal basal epithelium during the inflammatory process, hyperthermia-induced tubular degeneration, and immune-mediated destruction of spermatocytes and spermatozoa following disruption of the blood-testis barrier or following duct obstruction by necrotic debris or fibrous tissue. Partial duct obstruction or the development of blind pockets as a result of destruction of some of the efferent ductules may result in development of spermatoceles and sperm granulomas (see page 975). Many of these sequelae may take several months to develop. Although semen evaluation and fertility may appear normal shortly after acute orchiepididymitis, oligospermia, azoospermia, and infertility may ultimately occur.

If the basal germinal epithelium remains intact and tubule obstruction does not occur, spermatogenesis and fertility may be restored several months following acute orchiepididymitis. It takes approximately 55 to 70 days for complete development and maturation of spermatozoa from primary (type A) spermatogonia. A dog should not be declared infertile based on semen evaluation until at least 3 months have elapsed following acute orchiepididymitis. The veterinarian should probably not prognosticate on fertility and spermatogenesis capabilities of a dog for at least 6 months from the time of the acute inflammatory process. Even then, the dog can be rechecked periodically to determine his status regarding sperm production.

Chronic Orchitis/Epididymitis

ETIOLOGY. Chronic orchitis and epididymitis may develop as a sequela of acute orchiepididymitis or be diagnosed with no previous history or owner awareness of an inflammatory testicular problem. The same agents cause acute and chronic orchiepididymitis. The most common source of infection is chronic subclinical bacterial prostatitis. Chronic orchiepididymitis is characterized by slowly progressive, low-grade, non-suppurative inflammation with fibrosis that eventually results in loss of seminiferous tubule function and sperm production in the affected testis.

CLINICAL SIGNS. The most common clinical sign is infertility in an otherwise asymptomatic dog. The dog may or may not have a prior history of acute orchitis, epididymitis, prostatitis, or recurring bacterial infection of the urinary system. Digital palpation of the testis may reveal atrophy, fibrosis, nodules, or fibrous attachments to the scrotum. Palpation of the epididymis may reveal indurations or enlargement, especially if a spermatocele or sperm granuloma has developed. A prostatic examination is important because chronic orchitis and prostatitis are often present concomitantly. In this instance, the prostate may feel irregular, soft or firm, asymmetric, possibly painful, and abnormal in size during rectal palpation.

DIAGNOSTIC EVALUATION. Chronic orchiepididymitis should be suspected in an infertile dog with nonpainful, palpably abnormal testes or epididymides. Diagnostic tests should confirm the diagnosis of chronic orchiepididymitis, identify the underlying etiologic agents, and assess the prostate gland (see page 978). Semen evaluation with culture, appropriate blood tests for identification of *B. canis*, and possible testicular biopsy should be considered for evaluation of the testis and epididymis. Morphologic and cytologic evaluation of a semen sample may identify azoospermia, oligospermia with abnormal sperm morphology, and leukocytes. Separate cultures of the second and third fractions of an ejaculate should be performed to localize infection to the testis and epididymis (second fraction) or prostate gland (third fraction). Findings on histologic evaluation of a testicular biopsy may include tubular degeneration, fibrosis, and atrophy in a testis with chronic inflammatory changes. A plasmacytic lymphocytic infiltrate may support immune-mediated destruction of the seminiferous tubules as a result of destruction of the blood-testis barrier (see Lymphocytic Orchitis). In an azoospermic dog, measurement of seminal alkaline phosphatase (see page 940) may help differentiate tubal obstruction with normal spermatogenesis from primary seminiferous tubular degeneration.

TREATMENT. Management of chronic orchiepididymitis is difficult because the underlying cause usually goes undiagnosed and severe, irreversible changes (i.e., fibrosis) are present. If bacterial cultures are positive, appropriate antibiotics should be administered for a minimum of 3 weeks. Semen should be recultured 7 to 14 days and 3 months after discontinuing antibiotics to ensure continued control of the infection. If a plasmacytic lymphocytic infiltration is identified histologically, treatment with immunosuppressive drugs may be tried (see Lymphocytic Orchitis).

PROGNOSIS. The prognosis for return of fertility in a dog with chronic orchiepididymitis is guarded to poor. Fibrotic changes and loss of tubular germinal epithelial cells are permanent. The ability to control immune-mediated destruction of the seminiferous tubules without inducing tubular atrophy is difficult. Eventual obstruction of the duct system is common, for which there is no reliable treatment. As a general rule, azoospermic dogs remain azoospermic.

Lymphocytic Orchitis

Lymphocytic orchitis is considered an immune-mediated disorder characterized by lymphocytic and plasmacytic inflammation in the testes. The blood-testes barrier is formed by Sertoli cell tight junctions, which isolate maturing germ cells in the seminiferous tubules from the immune system (Amann, 1989). The immune-mediated attack may be triggered following damage to the blood-testis barrier from trauma, infection, inflammation, and the like; may be a component of a more widespread, possibly genetic-based, autoimmune disorder affecting several endocrine glands (see page 91); or the underlying cause may not be evident. Disruption of the blood-testis barrier exposes the dog's immune system to spermatozoal antigens, which are not recognized as "self" antigens. If the damage to the barrier is severe or exposure to these antigens is prolonged, an immune-mediated orchitis may develop. Immune-mediated orchitis is characterized by an influx of plasma cells and lymphocytes into the testicular parenchyma, deposition of immunoglobulins within seminiferous tubules, seminiferous tubule destruction, loss of Leydig cells, and development of antisperm antibodies (Fig. 29-11; Olson et al, 1992). Clinically, oligospermia progressing to azoospermia with variable loss of libido develops. The involved testis is often small and soft on palpation. Biopsy demonstrates an immunocyte infiltration into the testicular parenchyma. Because of the progressive

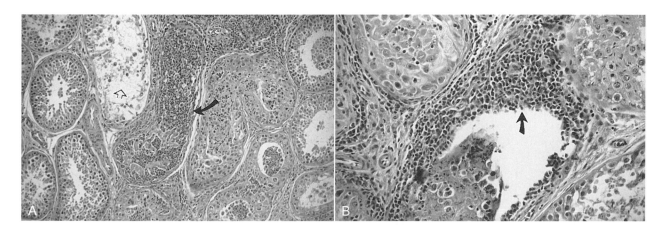

FIGURE 29-11. Histologic sections of a testicular biopsy from a 4-year-old Bearded Collie with azoospermia and normal libido. *A,* Moderate interstitial infiltration of plasma cells and lymphocytes *(curved arrow)* and marked diffuse tubular degeneration, with some seminiferous tubules *(open arrow)* containing only a single layer of primary spermatogonia and Sertoli cells (H&E ×100). *B,* Higher magnification illustrating lymphocytic infiltration in interstitium *(arrow)* (H&E ×450). The large white space is an artifact. The histologic diagnosis was lymphocytic orchitis and tubular degeneration.

TABLE 29–3 CHEMOTHERAPEUTIC DRUGS THAT AFFECT SPERMIOGENESIS IN HUMANS AND POSSIBLY DOGS

Busulfan
Chlorambucil
Cisplatin
Cyclophosphamide
Glucocorticoids
Methotrexate
Vinblastine
Vincristine

TABLE 29–4 POTENTIAL CAUSES OF TESTICULAR DEGENERATION

Thermal damage
Hormonally induced
  Hypothyroidism
  Hyperadrenocorticism
  Pituitary/hypothalamic dysfunction
  Exogenous hormones
  Testicular tumors
Trauma
Infections
Old age (>10 yr)
Testicular neoplasia
Chemicals, toxins, drugs
Nutrition
Vascular lesions, infarction
Irradiation
Duct obstruction
Idiopathic

nature of this condition, the prognosis for return of fertility is poor.

Therapy may be attempted using immunosuppressive dosages of glucocorticoids (e.g., prednisone, 2 to 4 mg/kg/day, divided twice a day initially) to control the immune reaction. Unfortunately, prolonged or excessive dosages of glucocorticoids, which are frequently required for the management of this disorder, adversely affect spermatogenesis and lead to infertility. Therefore, the clinician must attempt to control the immune reaction by using the least amount of glucocorticoid given as infrequently as possible to minimize the adverse effects of the therapy. This is rarely possible because controlling the immune-mediated orchitis usually requires large dosages of glucocorticoids, which in turn promotes infertility. Chemotherapeutic drugs, several of which are used for immunosuppression, can also affect fertility and may cause testicular degeneration (Table 29-3). The effectiveness of immunosuppressive drugs (e.g., azathioprine, 2 mg/kg/day) that may not adversely affect the reproductive tract has yet to be critically evaluated.

Lymphocytic orchitis may also occur spontaneously, often in conjunction with immunocytic destruction of other endocrine glands. For example, lymphocytic orchitis with concurrent lymphocytic thyroiditis has been reported to be an inherited disorder in Beagles. We have also observed testicular failure in dogs with primary hypoadrenocorticism, presumably as a result of immune-mediated destruction of the adrenal gland and testes. Testicular failure is also a component of polyglandular autoimmune syndrome type I in men (Neufeld et al, 1981) (see page 91). Lymphocytic orchitis should be suspected when testicular failure is identified in dogs with concurrent endocrine disorders (i.e., hypothyroidism, hypoadrenocorticism, diabetes mellitus). As previously discussed, therapy is difficult and, because of the genetic implications in these dogs, is probably not indicated.

Testicular Degeneration/Atrophy

Testicular degeneration occurs following damage to the cells within or surrounding the seminiferous tubules (i.e., spermatogonia, Sertoli cells, interstitial cells). Testicular degeneration may develop secondary to inflammatory or noninflammatory insults (Table 29-4).

Testicular degeneration may also be idiopathic, with no identifiable underlying cause. Idiopathic testicular degeneration is a noninflammatory form of degeneration that usually develops in dogs between 3 and 6 years of age. It is a progressive degeneration that ultimately results in testicular atrophy and sterility. There is no known treatment.

The clinical signs and physical findings with testicular degeneration depend on the progressive nature of the underlying cause, the cell lines that are damaged, and the severity of the degenerative process at the time the dog is initially examined. Testicular degeneration is typically characterized by damage to the spermatogonia, with the development of oligo/azoospermia, abnormal sperm morphology, and impaired motility of sperm cells. The primary owner complaint in these dogs is infertility. Affected testes may palpate normal to soft in consistency and normal to small in size, unless neoplasia or obstruction of the duct system is the cause of the degeneration. With chronic degeneration induced by inflammation, dystrophic calcification and fibrosis become more prominent, resulting in small, firm, "lumpy" testes that lack elasticity. With chronic degeneration induced by noninflammatory insults and with idiopathic degeneration, the testes become progressively softer and smaller and eventually atrophy. With severe atrophy (e.g., with end-stage idiopathic degeneration), only the epididymides remain palpable in the scrotum.

With most forms of testicular degeneration, an adequate population of functioning interstitial cells is maintained and libido is not initially affected. The exception is secondary testicular degeneration induced by concurrent endocrinopathies. Maintenance of libido often creates confusion for the owner, who frequently equates fertility with libido and cannot understand how his or her valuable stud dog can be sterile yet have normal libido.

Testicular degeneration should be suspected in the infertile dog with changes in the consistency and size of the testes. Semen evaluation usually confirms a testicular problem. The diagnostic approach should try to determine whether the degenerative process has been induced by an inflammatory or noninflammatory insult and then try to rule out potential secondary causes. The diagnostic evaluation is similar to that for the infertile dog with oligospermia or azoospermia and is described on page 991.

The treatment and prognosis for return to fertility depend on the cause, severity of damage to the primary tubular epithelial and Sertoli cells, and extent of fibrosis present within the testes. If the primary (type A) spermatogonia and Sertoli cells are destroyed, irreversible infertility results. If more differentiated cells in the spermatogenesis process are damaged but the primary spermatogonia and Sertoli cells are left intact and the inciting cause is transient or treatable, infertility may be transient. Likewise, if the Leydig cells remain functional, testosterone secretion and libido remain intact.

It takes approximately 55 to 70 days for mature, ejaculated spermatozoa to develop from primary spermatogonia; therefore a diagnosis of irreversible azoospermia should not be made until at least 3 to 6 months have elapsed following identification of the problem and removal of the inciting cause.

Spermatocele, Sperm Granuloma

Spermatocele is a sequela of occlusion of the epididymis for a variety of reasons. Spermatocele is a cystic dilatation of the epididymis, with accumulation of inspissated sperm proximal to the occlusion. The accumulation of sperm eventually results in a chronic inflammatory process and the development of a nodule of granulation tissue—the sperm granuloma. Blind rudimentary tubules of the rete testis or efferent ductules may also allow spermatozoa to accumulate, resulting in spermatoceles and sperm granulomas.

Sperm granulomas may be unilateral or bilateral. Dogs with unilateral testicular involvement remain fertile and the disorder may go undiagnosed. If both testes are involved, the breeding dog is brought to the veterinarian with the primary complaint of infertility. Semen evaluation reveals azoospermia if bilateral sperm granulomas are present. Seminal alkaline phosphatase concentration may be normal or decreased, depending on the site of obstruction (see page 940). Sperm granulomas may occasionally be palpable during the physical examination; however, the ability to palpate a nodule is not always possible. Spermatoceles appear as extratesticular focal, anechoic cystic structures on a scrotal sonogram, with sharp internal wall margins and distant enhancement deep to the cyst. Histologic evaluation of a testicular biopsy may reveal active spermatogenesis or variable degrees of tubular degeneration, depending on the site of the obstruction and the ability of the head of the epididymis to absorb seminiferous tubule secretions. Ligation of the tail of the epididymis causes degeneration of the seminiferous tubules within 1 to 3 months (Larsen, 1980). The closer the site of the obstruction to the head of the epididymis, the more

severe the degenerative changes within the testicle. Obstruction of the duct should be suspected in an azoospermic dog with normal spermatogenesis on testicular biopsy.

No treatment is available for bilateral sperm granulomas, and the prognosis for correcting infertility and azoospermia is poor. Bypass operations have a low percentage of cures and are not routinely performed in veterinary medicine.

Adenomyosis of the Epididymis

Adenomyosis of the epididymis refers to the invasion of the epithelial lining cells into the muscular layers of the epididymis (Larsen, 1980). Blind pockets may develop. Spermatozoa may accumulate in these pockets, leading to the development of spermatoceles and sperm granulomas. Epididymal duct obstruction and oligo/azoospermia may result from adenomyosis of the epididymis. This phenomenon is usually associated with the excessive endogenous secretion or exogenous administration of estrogens.

Inguinoscrotal Hernia

Herniation of abdominal contents into the inguinal canal is more common in the female than the male dog. However, if herniation occurs in the male, abdominal contents may pass through the inguinal canal into the scrotum. Structural defects, especially involving the internal inguinal ring, predispose some animals to the development of inguinoscrotal hernias. Increased intra-abdominal pressure (e.g., obesity, trauma) may force abdominal contents into the inguinal canal and cause a hernia.

Dogs with inguinoscrotal hernias are usually seen by veterinarians for a primary owner complaint of scrotal enlargement. A soft, painless thickening of the spermatic cord is highly suggestive of an inguinal hernia. Less common complaints are scrotal pain following impingement of the vasculature in the spermatic cord, testicular atrophy, infertility, and vomiting from gastrointestinal obstruction. Inguinoscrotal hernias may also be found during routine physical examinations. If the hernia is clinically silent and impairs the circulation to the testes or the thermoregulatory function of the scrotum, variable degrees of testicular degeneration, atrophy, and oligospermia result.

Ultrasonography can be used to confirm the diagnosis. Surgical reduction along with partial closure of the internal inguinal ring is the treatment of choice. Care must be taken to avoid interference with the spermatic vessels when closing the internal ring. If circulation in the spermatic cord is impaired, acute scrotal and testicular swelling with pain may result, often necessitating castration. Castration should also be considered because of the possible hereditary basis for this disease, especially if an underlying predisposing factor (e.g., trauma) is not present in the history.

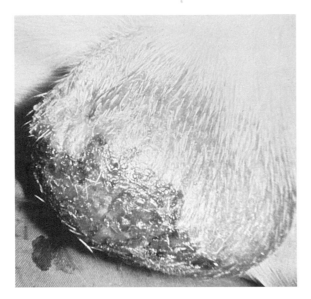

FIGURE 29-12. Scrotal dermatitis in a 2-year-old German Shepherd cross. The dermatitis developed secondary to self-trauma from licking, presumably as a result of a concurrent flea problem.

Disorders of the Scrotum

Primary scrotal dysfunction is relatively uncommon in dogs. Perhaps the biggest problem in dogs is scrotal dermatitis, the causes for which include chemical irritants, trauma, bacterial infections, parasites, and self-infliction from licking. The most common problem is flea allergy–induced scrotal dermatitis, primarily resulting from secondary self-trauma (Fig. 29-12). Appropriate therapy depends on the underlying cause and usually includes a combination of careful daily rinsing and cleaning of the scrotum, judicious use of topical ointments, systemic antibiotics, Elizabethan collars, and rarely, tranquilizers to prevent continued self-trauma to the area.

Neoplasia of the scrotum is rare. Squamous cell carcinoma, melanoma, and mast cell tumors have been reported. Scrotal melanomas are usually benign, and surgical removal is often curative.

REFERENCES

Amann RP: Structure and function of the normal testis and epididymis. J Am Coll Toxicol 8:457, 1989.

Baumans V, et al: Testicular descent in the dog. Zbl Vet Med C Anat Histol Embryol 10:97, 1981.

Cowgill L: Pathophysiology and management of anemia of chronic progressive renal failure. Semin Vet Med Surg 7:175, 1992.

Cox VS: Cryptorchidism in the dog. In Morrow DA (ed): Current Therapy in Theriogenology, 2nd ed. Philadelphia, WB Saunders Co, 1986, p 541.

Crow SE: Neoplasms of the reproductive organs and mammary glands of the dog. In Morrow DA (ed): Current Therapy in Theriogenology. Philadelphia, WB Saunders Co, 1980, p 640.

Dahlbom M, Andersson M: Long term effects of canine distemper on seminal characteristics and testicular tissue. Advances in Dog, Cat and Exotic Carnivore Reproduction—Book of Abstracts. The 4th International Symposium on Canine and Feline Reproduction and the 2nd Congress of the European Veterinary Society for Small Animal Reproduction. Oslo, Norway, June 29–July 1, 2000, p. 94.

de Jong FH, et al: Inhibin immunoreactivity in gonadal and non-gonadal tumors. J Steroid Biochem Molec Biol 37:863, 1990.

de Kretser DM, Robertson DM: The isolation and physiology of inhibin and related proteins. Biol Reprod 40:33, 1989.

DeVico G, et al: Number and size of silver stained nucleoli (AgNOR clusters) in canine seminomas: Correlation with histological features and tumour behavior. J Comp Pathol 110:267, 1994.

Dhaliwal RS, et al: Treatment of aggressive testicular tumors in four dogs. J Amer Anim Hosp Assoc 35: 311, 1999.

Goodfellow PN, Lovell-Badge R: SRY and sex determination in mammals. Annu Rev Genet 27:71-92, 1993.

Grootenhuis AJ, et al: Inhibin, gonadotrophins and sex steroids in dogs with Sertoli cell tumors. J Endocrinol 127:235, 1990.

Hammond WP, et al: Chronic neutropenia: A new canine model induced by human granulocyte colony-stimulating factor. J Clin Invest 87:704, 1991.

Hayes HM, et al: Canine cryptorchidism and subsequent testicular neoplasia: Case-control study with epidemiologic update. Teratology 32:51, 1985.

Johnston GR, et al: Ultrasonographic features of testicular neoplasia in dogs: 16 cases (1980–1988). JAVMA 198:1779, 1991.

Johnston SD, Root Kustritz MV, Olson PNS: Disorders of the canine testes and epididymes. In Johnston SD, Root Kustritz MV, Olson PNS (eds): Canine and Feline Theriogenology. Philadelphia, WB Saunders Co, 2001, p 312.

Koopman P, et al: Male development of chromosomally female mice transgenic for Sry. Nature (London) 351:117, 1991.

Larsen RE: Infertility in the male dog. In Morrow DA (ed): Current Therapy in Theriogenology. Philadelphia, WB Saunders Co, 1980, p 646.

Lein DH: Mycoplasma infertility in the dog: Diagnosis and treatment. Proceedings of the Society for Theriogenology, Coeur d'Alene, ID, September 29–30, 1989, p 307.

Madewell BR, Theilen GH: Tumors of the urogenital tract. In Theilen GH, Madewell BR (eds): Veterinary Cancer Medicine, 2nd ed. Philadelphia, Lea and Febiger, 1987, p 583.

Mattheeuws D, Comhaire FH: Concentrations of oestradiol and testosterone in peripheral and spermatic venous blood of dogs with unilateral cryptorchidism. Dom Anim Endocr 6:203, 1989.

Mattoon JS, Nyland TG: Ultrasonography of the genital system. In Nyland TG, Mattoon JS (eds) Veterinary Diagnostic Ultrasound. Philadelphia, WB Saunders Co, 1995, p 141.

McDonald RK, et al: Radiotherapy of metastatic seminoma in the dog. J Vet Intern Med 2:103, 1988.

Medleau L: Sex hormone-associated endocrine alopecias in dogs. J Am Anim Hosp Assoc 25:689, 1989.

Neufeld M, et al: Two types of autoimmune Addison's disease associated with different polyglandular autoimmune (PGA) syndromes. Medicine 60:355, 1981.

Obradovich JE, et al: Evaluation of recombinant canine granulocyte colony-stimulating factor as an inducer of granulopoiesis. J Vet Intern Med 5:75, 1991.

Ogilvie GK, et al: Use of recombinant canine granulocyte colony-stimulating factor to decrease myelosuppression associated with the administration of mitoxantrone in the dog. J Vet Intern Med 6:44, 1992.

Ogilvie GK: Hematopoietic growth factors: Frontiers for cure. Vet Clin North Am Small Anim Pract 25:1441, 1995.

Olson PN, et al: Clinical and laboratory findings associated with actual or suspected azoospermia in dogs: 18 cases (1979–1990). JAVMA 201:478, 1992.

Peters MAJ, et al: Spermatogenesis and testicular tumours in the ageing dog. Advances in Dog, Cat and Exotic Carnivore Reproduction—Book of Abstracts. The 4th International Symposium on Canine and Feline Reproduction and the 2nd Congress of the European Veterinary Society for Small Animal Reproduction. Oslo, Norway, June 29–July 1, 2000, p 35.

Pinto CRF, et al: Theriogenology question of the month. JAVMA 219:1343, 2001.

Pugh CR, Konde LJ: Sonographic evaluation of canine testicular and scrotal abnormalities: A review of 26 case histories. Vet Radiol 32:243, 1991.

Romagnoli SE: Canine cryptorchidism. Vet Clin North Am 21:533, 1991.

Ruble RP, Hird DW: Congenital abnormalities in immature dogs from a pet store: 253 cases (1987–1988). JAVMA 202:633, 1993.

Sinclair AH, et al: A gene from the human sex-determining region encodes a protein with homology to a conserved DNA-binding motif. Nature 346:240, 1990.

Suess RP, et al: Bone marrow hypoplasia in a feminized dog with an interstitial cell tumor. JAVMA 200:1346, 1992.

Verstegen JP: Conditions of the male. In Simpson GM, England GCW, Harvey M (eds): BSAVA Manual of Small Animal Reproduction and Neonatology. Cheltenham, British Small Animal Veterinary Association, 1998, p 71.

Wallace LJ, Cox VS: Canine cryptorchidism. In Kirk RW (ed): Current Veterinary Therapy VII. Philadelphia, WB Saunders Co, 1980, p 1244.

Wensing CJG: Developmental anomalies, including cryptorchidism. In Morrow DA (ed): Current Therapy in Theriogenology. Philadelphia, WB Saunders Co, 1980, p 583.

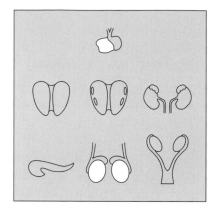

30
PROSTATITIS

The primary disorders affecting the prostate gland are benign hyperplasia with variable degrees of cyst formation, infection, abscessation, paraprostatic cysts, and neoplasia. Of these, bacterial prostatitis and benign prostatic hyperplasia are the most common prostatic disorders affecting the dog (Krawiec and Heflin, 1992) and the most likely disorders to affect fertility. Prostatic cysts and neoplasia are not commonly associated with reproductive dysfunction and are not discussed.

MECHANISMS OF PROSTATE-INDUCED INFERTILITY

Bacterial prostatitis is the most important prostatic disorder affecting fertility and should always be considered in any dog brought to a veterinarian for infertility. Bacterial prostatitis can affect fertility in a number of ways, including spread of infection to the epididymis and testis (Wallace, 1991). Prostatitis can cause fever-induced impairment of spermatogenesis, morphologic abnormalities and decreased motility of spermatozoa, decreased libido because of localized inflammation, pain, and systemic illness. It is also possible for prostatitis to result in mechanical obstruction of the ductus deferens as it courses through the inflamed, swollen prostate gland. Finally, prostatitis can cause hemorrhage into the ejaculate.

Spread of infection to the epididymis and testis is the most worrisome problem related to infertility. An infected prostate gland may serve as a source of infection to the epididymis and testis via the vas deferens or, less commonly, through hematogenous spread. Orchiepididymitis and immune-mediated orchitis can result. Bacterial prostatitis can affect semen without histologic abnormalities in the testis, presumably as a result of changes in seminal fluid. In one study of induced prostatic infection using *Escherichia coli*, two of six dogs had a marked decrease in the percentage of normal sperm (from >90% normal to <65%) and a marked increase in primary and secondary morphologic abnormalities despite histologically normal testes (Barsanti et al, 1986). Chronic *E. coli* prostatitis had no apparent effect on sperm concentration or motility; however, a deleterious effect on these parameters requires a large concentration of bacteria (>10^6/ml).

Benign prostatic hyperplasia is usually an insignificant finding in the dog but on occasion has been associated with infertility. The underlying cause of hyperplasia-induced infertility is not known, although hemorrhage into the ejaculate has been proposed as a possible reason. Blood is spermicidal and may cause infertility if consistently present in the ejaculate. The effect of benign prostatic hyperplasia on semen volume (see page 940) does not seem to be deleterious to fertility. Unlike in humans, benign prostatic hyperplasia does not usually cause occlusion of the urethral lumen in dogs.

ACUTE BACTERIAL PROSTATITIS

Etiology and Pathophysiology

The distal urethra of the dog has a normal microflora composed primarily of gram-positive bacteria (Barsanti and Finco, 1983). The prostate gland is the genital organ closest to the microflora of the distal urethra. Normally, the prostatic urethra and prostate gland are sterile. Migration of bacteria up the urethra to the prostate gland and bladder is prevented by various defense mechanisms, including the flushing action from unobstructed flow of urine and prostatic secretions, urethral peristalsis, the urethral high-pressure zone, surface characteristics of the urethral mucosa that trap bacteria, local IgA production, and prostatic antibacterial factor (Klausner and Osborne,

1983; Dorfman and Barsanti, 1995). Prostatic antibacterial factor is a low molecular weight zinc compound that inhibits bacterial growth, especially gram-negative enteric organisms. Alterations in any of these defense mechanisms may allow bacteria to ascend into, adhere to, and colonize the prostate gland.

Disorders that increase bacterial numbers in the prostatic urethra (e.g., bacterial cystitis, urethral calculi, neoplasia), compromise local immunity, or alter the architecture of the prostate (e.g., squamous metaplasia, hyperplasia) increase the risk of an infection of the prostate gland developing. Prostate growth is androgen dependent. The principal androgen regulating prostatic growth is 5α-dihydrotestosterone, which is formed from testosterone by the enzyme 5α-reductase (Rhodes, 1996). Estrogens induce squamous metaplasia and duct obstruction and reduce the conversion efficiency of testosterone to dihydrotestosterone by prostatic cells. Both estrogens and androgens must be present for significant hypertrophy and hyperplasia of the prostate gland to occur (Cochran et al, 1981; Winter and Liehr, 1996).

The bacteria that cause infection of the prostate are generally similar to those that cause urinary tract infection. It is likely that most cases of bacterial prostatitis occur secondary to infections with urinary tract bacterial pathogens that enter the prostate via the urinary tract. However, about one third of dogs in which prostatic infection is demonstrated do not have concurrent or historical urinary tract infections (Ling, 1995). *E. coli* is the most common cause of bacterial prostatitis in dogs. This infection is followed, in order of incidence, by infections with coagulase-positive staphylococci, streptococci, *Klebsiella* sp., *Proteus mirabilis*, *Enterobacter* sp., and *Pseudomonas aeruginosa* (Ling, 1995). A single organism is identified in approximately 70% of dogs with acute prostatitis (Dorfman and Barsanti, 1995). *Mycoplasma* sp. are identified in approximately 15% of dogs with bacterial prostatitis, compared with a prevalence of approximately 3% in dogs with urinary tract infections (Ling, 1995). *Brucella canis*, although an uncommon cause, can also give rise to acute and chronic prostatitis.

Clinical Signs

Clinical signs of acute prostatitis usually include lethargy, inappetence, urethral/preputial discharge (blood, pus), and abdominal pain. Additional clinical signs may develop, depending on the degree of involvement of the prostate gland, the presence or absence of abscessation, and involvement of the bladder, epididymis, and testis (Table 30-1). In one study, 26% of dogs diagnosed with prostatitis showed signs of urinary tract disease, 37% showed gastrointestinal signs, and 48% showed signs of systemic illness (Krawiec and Hefland, 1992).

Physical examination usually reveals fever and nonspecific or caudal abdominal pain. These dogs frequently have a painful prostate on rectal palpation.

TABLE 30–1 POTENTIAL CLINICAL SIGNS ASSOCIATED WITH ACUTE BACTERIAL PROSTATITIS

Preputial/urethral discharge
  Blood
  Pus
Lethargy, inappetence, vomiting, fever
Dysuria, hematuria, pyuria
Painful caudal abdomen
Tenesmus, constipation
Stilted gait
Weight loss
Painful, swollen testis, epididymis
Unwillingness to breed
Infertility

The prostate may be normal in size, shape, and symmetry or may be irregular in size and surface conformation. The median raphae may not be readily identifiable, and fluctuant areas may be present, especially if abscessation is present. In older dogs, benign prostatic hyperplasia and associated prostatic enlargement may be present in addition to prostatitis. If ascension to the testis and epididymis has occurred, findings suggestive of acute orchiepididymitis may also be present (see page 971).

Diagnostic Evaluation

A tentative diagnosis of acute prostatitis can usually be made from the history and physical findings. Results of a complete blood count (CBC) may reveal leukocytosis and neutrophilia with a variable shift toward immaturity and toxic changes. These alterations are exaggerated with prostatic abscessation (Barsanti and Finco, 1984). Measurement of serum concentrations of proteins of prostatic origin (i.e., acid phosphatase, prostate specific antigen, canine prostate specific esterase) is not helpful in differentiating dogs with bacterial prostatitis from healthy dogs or dogs with other prostate disorders (Bell et al, 1995). The results of a urinalysis may reveal hematuria, pyuria, and bacteriuria, although findings can be normal. Urine should be cultured if obtained by antepubic cystocentesis. The prostate is often assumed to be infected with the same organisms grown on urine culture (Black et al, 1998). However, mixed infections have been documented, in which the organism and its antibiotic sensitivity pattern differ between the bladder/urethra and the prostate (Ling et al, 1990). In these dogs, antibiotic therapy aimed at the organisms in the bladder may not control the prostate infection. For this reason, culture of prostatic fluid or tissue is recommended in dogs suspected of having prostatitis (see below).

Semen may be difficult to obtain and is usually not evaluated unless culture of the ejaculate is used to confirm bacterial prostatitis. The most common abnormalities identified on semen evaluation in acute bacterial prostatitis are neutrophils with variable degrees of toxicity, phagocytized bacteria, decreased sperm motility, and an increase in the number of spermatozoa with primary and secondary morphologic defects.

Radiographic evaluation of a dog suspected of having acute prostatitis is seldom informative. Normally, the prostate gland is located at the rim of the pelvis. However, the position of the prostate varies according to the degree of bladder distention. Radiographically, the normal prostate gland has a uniform soft tissue density and uniform, distinct margins. Radiographic alterations associated with acute prostatitis, if any, include an increase in size, mineralization, and indistinct margins (Feeney et al, 1987a). The presence of gas in the prostate gland may be iatrogenic from prior urinary bladder catheterization or may be indicative of an abscess. Reflux of contrast material into the stroma of the prostate gland and alterations in urethral diameter may be observed with positive-contrast urethrography, but these are nonspecific features of prostatic disease.

Ultrasonography provides the safest and most informative screening test of the prostate (see page 946). Ultrasonographic findings in dogs with acute prostatitis include normal to enlarged prostate gland size with symmetric or asymmetric shape and smooth or irregular borders. The prostatic parenchyma has a heterogeneous pattern of mixed echogenicity characterized by focal or multifocal areas of poorly marginated hypoechogenicity and focal irregular hyperechoic foci (Mattoon and Nyland, 1995). Hypoechoic to anechoic, fluid-filled parenchymal cavities may also be identified (Fig. 30-1) (Feeney et al, 1987b). The latter may be abscesses or cysts. Ultrasound-guided fine-needle aspiration (see below) of hypoechoic or anechoic areas provides prostatic fluid for culture and cytologic evaluation. Prostatic parenchyma can also be biopsied under ultrasound guidance.

PROSTATE SAMPLING TECHNIQUES. Attempts should be made to isolate, identify, and determine the antimicrobial susceptibility of the organism to confirm the diagnosis and to aid the selection of an appropriate antibiotic for therapy. This usually involves culturing of urine and prostatic fluid or tissue. Culture of prostatic fluid or tissue can and should be obtained initially in a dog suspected of having acute prostatitis and in dogs that fail to respond to antibiotic therapy selected from results of urine culture. Several methods have been described for obtaining prostatic fluid or tissue for cytologic evaluation and culture, including ultrasound-guided fine-needle aspiration, prostatic fluid sampling by ejaculation, and prostatic massage using a urinary catheter or urethral brush.

Regardless of the technique used, evaluation of results must take into account the number and type of organisms grown, their quantitative numbers, and the presence or absence of neutrophils and squamous cells containing bacteria in the sample (Barsanti et al, 1980). Contamination of the sample should be suspected with the following results: low numbers of neutrophils, growth of only gram-positive organisms or multiple organisms, or the presence of squamous cells containing bacteria (urethral origin). Infection should be suspected if large numbers of organisms ($>10^5$/ml) are grown, especially if they are gram-negative organisms or organisms grown in pure culture, or if large numbers of neutrophils are present (Ling, 1990).

SEMEN CULTURE. Culture of the third fraction of the ejaculate is an effective method of identifying organisms, especially when specimens from the urethra and bladder are obtained at the same time and are cultured simultaneously (Ling et al, 1983). Culture of the second fraction of the ejaculate can also be performed if concurrent orchitis/epididymitis is suspected or fractionation of the semen is difficult. Prostatic fluid is ejaculated into all three fractions of the semen

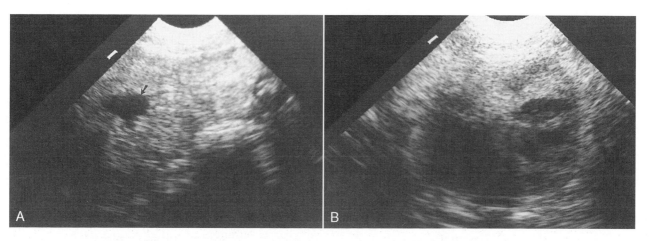

FIGURE 30-1. *A,* Ultrasonogram of the prostate gland of a 10-year-old Staffordshire Terrier with chronic prostatitis. Note the diffuse nodular increase in parenchymal echogenicity and the anechoic cyst in the prostatic parenchyma *(arrow). B,* Ultrasonogram of the prostate gland of a 12-year-old Rhodesian Ridgeback with prostatomegaly and acute prostatitis. Note the multiple anechoic cysts in the parenchyma.

(Johnston et al, 2001). Unfortunately, an ejaculate may be difficult to obtain from a dog with painful acute prostatitis. In addition, normal dogs have occasional white and red blood cells, and positive bacterial cultures of prostatic fluid obtained by ejaculation have been reported in 30% of healthy dogs (see Table 27-4, page 942) (Bjurstrom and Linde-Forsberg, 1992). Interpretation of culture results of an ejaculate may be made with confidence only if the urine, the urethral swab, and the ejaculate specimens are cultured quantitatively and the results compared. For a diagnosis of prostatitis, the number of bacteria in the ejaculate must be at least tenfold, and preferably 100-fold or more, greater than the number in the urethra for any single bacterial species (Ling, 1990). As a general rule, large numbers of bacteria ($>10^5$/ml) and high white blood cell numbers are indicative of infection. Interpretation becomes difficult if concurrent bacterial cystitis is present. Reculture after antimicrobial therapy has resolved bacterial cystitis and decreased the numbers of urethral bacteria aids in interpretation of ejaculate cultures.

FINE-NEEDLE ASPIRATION. Ultrasound-guided fine-needle aspiration is superior for obtaining specimens from the canine prostate for cytologic evaluation and culture. Dogs with bacterial prostatitis usually have one or more intraprostatic cysts, which can be as large as 4 cm in diameter (see Fig. 30-1) (Ling, 1990). The relationship between these cysts and bacterial prostatitis is not known; however, they provide a source of prostatic fluid for culture and cytologic evaluation and can be readily aspirated using ultrasound guidance. Cavitary prostatic parenchymal lesions greater than 0.75 cm in diameter can be aspirated transabdominally using aseptic technique and a sterile 22-gauge, 6 to 15 cm spinal needle with stylet. The needle is ultrasonographically directed to the desired location in the prostate (Fig. 30-2). Samples may be taken from cysts in the right or left lobe (or

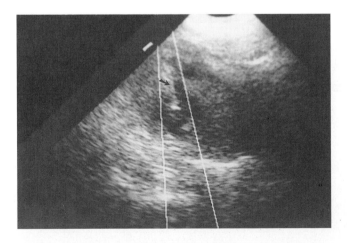

FIGURE 30-2. Ultrasound-guided fine-needle aspiration of a prostatic cyst in a 12-year-old Rhodesian Ridgeback with prostatomegaly, acute prostatitis, and multiple prostatic cysts. The prostatic cyst was aspirated transabdominally using aseptic technique and a sterile 22-gauge spinal needle (*arrow*).

both) of the prostate. Culture results of prostatic fluid obtained by this method accurately indicate the presence or absence of infection in the prostate (Ling, 1990; Black et al, 1998). Interpretation of culture results is simple. Any bacteria that are grown should be considered pathogens as long as contamination during collection and processing has not occurred. Failure to grow bacteria implies lack of prostate infection, sampling of a uninfected area, or infection by organisms requiring special culture techniques (e.g., *Mycoplasma* sp.).

Complications from prostatic aspiration are not common and include periprostatic hemorrhage, transient hematuria (usually lasting less than 48 hours), and inadvertent penetration of a prostatic abscess. Suspicion of an abscess is based primarily on the results of ultrasonography (see Table 27-9, page 948). The prostatic urethra should also be avoided to minimize the potential for peritonitis. Complications caused by spread of infection along the needle tract are uncommon and should not preclude the use of needle aspiration for obtaining a prostatic specimen.

PROSTATIC MASSAGE/WASH TECHNIQUE. Prostatic massage is an alternative technique for obtaining prostatic fluid and tissue for culture and cytologic evaluation. The prostatic massage/wash technique involves obtaining premassage and postmassage samples. The dog is allowed to urinate, and the bladder is then catheterized using aseptic technique. The bladder is emptied and then flushed with 5 to 10 ml of sterile physiologic saline, which is aspirated and saved for culture and cytologic evaluation. This is the premassage sample. The urinary catheter is then retracted distally to the prostate, as determined by rectal palpation, and the prostate is massaged digitally for 1 to 2 minutes (Fig. 30-3). Five to 10 ml of sterile physiologic saline is slowly infused through the catheter while the external urethral orifice is manually occluded. This is followed by gentle, continuous aspiration as the catheter is slowly advanced through the prostatic urethra and into the bladder. The fluid that is collected is saved and marked as the post-massage sample. The premassage and postmassage samples should be submitted for bacterial culture and cytologic evaluation.

Comparison of results from the premassage and postmassage samples should enable the clinician to determine the presence or absence of prostatic pathology. In normal dogs, the postmassage sample should be clear. Microscopically, only a few red blood, white blood, squamous, and transitional epithelial cells should be seen (Barsanti and Finco, 1995a). Cultures are usually negative or contain low numbers of organisms (<100/ml) consistent with urethral contamination associated with urethral catheterization. A cloudy or hemorrhagic postmassage sample, increased numbers of inflammatory cells, and greater quantities of bacterial growth in the postmassage sample support the diagnosis of prostatitis.

One problem with interpreting results of prostatic massage is the difficulty in detecting increases in

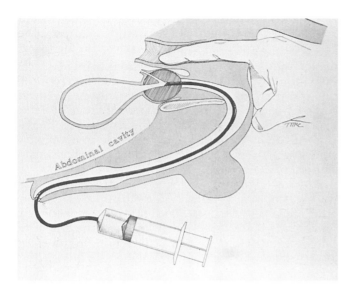

FIGURE 30-3. Schematic of the prostatic massage/wash technique for obtaining prostatic fluid for cytologic evaluation and culture. Digital massage of the prostate is done per rectum with the tip of the urinary catheter located in the prostatic urethra. Then, 5 to 10 ml of sterile physiologic saline is slowly infused through the catheter and collected for analysis.

bacterial numbers in the postmassage sample when urine is infected. If bacterial cystitis is suspected, this technique should not be used until the bladder infection has been resolved with appropriate antibiotics. An alternative is to administer an antibiotic that enters the urine but not the prostatic fluid (e.g., ampicillin) for 1 day prior to massage (Barsanti and Finco, 1995a). The samples obtained must be cultured immediately so that the antibiotic in the urine does not kill any bacteria in the prostatic fluid after collection.

The prostatic massage/wash technique does not ensure that prostatic fluid will be obtained in the post-massage sample. Failure to grow bacteria in the post-massage sample does not rule out chronic prostatitis. In one study, bacterial culture of prostatic fluid obtained by this technique failed to grow bacteria in nine of 11 dogs with confirmed chronic prostatitis (Barsanti and Finco, 1984).

PROSTATIC MASSAGE/BRUSH TECHNIQUE. Prostatic fluid sampling by urethral brush is similar to the prostatic massage/wash technique, except a guarded microbiology specimen brush (Fig. 30-4) is used instead of a urethral catheter for collection of the sample. The brush is used in an attempt to reduce urethral and bladder bacterial contamination of the prostatic fluid sample. This method is especially useful for obtaining specimens for cytologic evaluation.

For culture results to be meaningful, specimens from the urethra and bladder should be obtained immediately prior to obtaining the prostatic fluid sample. The guarded specimen brush is then advanced into the urethra and stopped with the tip of the device at the caudal pole of the prostate. The prostate is massaged for 1 minute per rectum, and the inner catheter then is advanced 1 cm into the prostatic urethra. The specimen brush is advanced about 1 cm into the prostatic urethra, retracted, and advanced again five or six times. A small amount of the prostatic fluid that is expelled into the urethra during the prostatic massage adheres to the brush. After collection of the specimen, the brush and the inner catheter are retracted into the outer catheter and the entire apparatus is withdrawn. Material in the inner catheter, that adhering to the brush, and urine and urethral samples are all submitted for culture and cytologic evaluation. Culture results of prostatic fluid obtained by this method accurately reflect the presence or absence of infection in the prostate, because there is little possibility of contamination of the sample with extraneous bacteria.

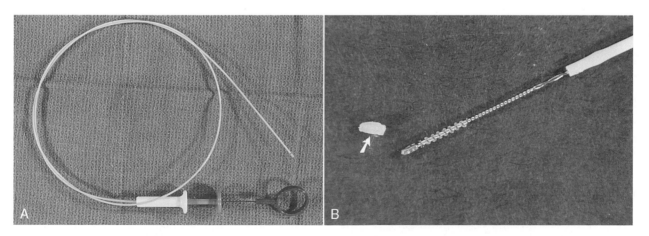

FIGURE 30-4. *A,* Guarded microbiology specimen brush for collection of prostatic fluid for cytologic evaluation and culture. *B,* Close-up of the specimen brush after it has been advanced out of the guarded sheath, displacing the catheter plug *(arrow).*

Therapy

The treatment of acute and chronic bacterial prostatitis is based on the administration of broad-spectrum bactericidal antibiotics. Additional therapy that has been proposed for the treatment of bacterial prostatitis includes castration, estrogen administration, 5α-reductase inhibitors, antiandrogens, and oral zinc supplementation.

ANTIBIOTIC THERAPY. The choice of antibiotic for treating acute prostatitis should be determined from results of bacterial culture and sensitivity. The blood-prostate fluid barrier is broken down with acute prostatitis and is not a major consideration in the choice of an antibiotic. If doubt exists, a nonionized, lipid-soluble, basic antibiotic should be administered (Klausner and Osborne, 1983). Chloramphenicol, trimethoprim-sulfonamide, erythromycin, tetracycline HCl, doxycycline, minocycline, and the fluoroquinolones (e.g., enrofloxacin, ciprofloxacin) are able to attain therapeutic concentrations in the canine prostate. The penicillins, cephalosporins, oxytetracycline, nitrofurantoin, most of the sulfonamides, and aminoglycosides have low lipid solubility and do not readily enter prostatic fluid in the healthy dog (Ling, 1995). These antibiotics should probably not be used for the treatment of prostatitis. The initial route of administration depends on the severity of systemic illness. In addition, appropriate supportive therapy should be provided until the dog is stable, drinking, and eating.

Antibiotics should be given until the prostatic fluid tests negative for bacterial growth. Antibiotics should be administered for at least 3 weeks. Dogs that respond favorably to treatment should be recultured after 3 weeks of antibiotic therapy and while still receiving antibiotics. Culture of prostatic fluid should be obtained sooner if clinical response to therapy is not observed, especially if prostatic fluid was not initially cultured. Prostatic fluid should be obtained by ejaculation or ultrasound-guided fine-needle aspiration. If these are not feasible, the urethral brush technique should be used to obtain fluid. If the infection is still present after 3 weeks of therapy, antibiotics should be continued and prostatic fluid cultured every 3 weeks until culture of the fluid is negative. This may take 6 to 9 weeks. Once prostatic fluid is negative for culture, antibiotics should be discontinued and prostatic fluid recultured 3 weeks later to ensure resolution of the infection. If the infection recurs after therapy is discontinued, the dog should be treated for chronic prostatitis (see page 984). If prostatic abscessation is suspected, surgical exploration with drainage or excision or both should be considered.

CASTRATION. Castration is an effective adjunct therapy for the management of bacterial prostatitis because it removes the source of androgens responsible for maintaining prostatic size, thereby reducing the amount of tissue available for infection. The prostatic zinc concentration also decreases after castration, but the loss of bactericidal properties of prostatic zinc does not appear to alter the beneficial effects of castration (Cowan et al, 1991a). In one study using induced prostatic infection with *E. coli*, castration 2 weeks after induction of infection reduced the duration of infection and resulted in fewer bacterial colony-forming units per milliliter of urine than with sham-operated controls (Cowan et al, 1991b). Unfortunately, castration is not feasible in a valuable stud dog whose reproductive potential is a primary concern of the owner.

ESTROGEN THERAPY. Exogenous estrogen administration impairs pituitary gonadotropin secretion, which results in decreased secretion of testosterone by the Leydig cells. Decreased testosterone and 5α-dihydrotestosterone cause a reduction in prostatic cellular mass and prostatic size; there may be no effect on intraparenchymal cysts. Estrogens may also cause growth of the fibromuscular stroma of the prostate, metaplasia of prostatic glandular epithelium, and secretory stasis; in the infected gland, estrogens may predispose the dog to the development of abscessation (Klausner and Osborne, 1983; Barsanti and Finco, 1995b). Estrogen therapy may also cause aplastic anemia. For these reasons, estrogen therapy is not recommended in the management of prostatitis.

5α-REDUCTASE INHIBITORS. Type 2 5α-reductase catalyzes the conversion of testosterone to dihydrotestosterone in most androgen-sensitive tissues, including the prostate. All 5α-reductase inhibitors (i.e., azasteroids) suppress the conversion of testosterone to dihydrotestosterone, thereby decreasing the actions of androgens in their target tissue. In the prostate, the result is a decrease in prostatic hyperplasia and volume (Gormley et al, 1992). Finasteride (Proscar; Merck & Co., Rahway, NJ) was the first 5α-reductase inhibitor to be approved by the U.S. Food and Drug Administration (FDA) for treatment of benign prostatic hyperplasia in humans. At dosages of 0.1 to 0.5 mg/kg/day, finasteride caused a significant decrease in prostatic diameter, prostatic volume, and serum dihydrotestosterone concentration, as well as a decrease in semen volume, without affecting semen quality or serum testosterone concentrations in sexually intact adult male dogs (Kamolpatana et al, 1998; Sirinarumitr et al, 2001). At dosages of 1 to 5 mg/kg/day, finasteride caused atrophy of the glandular compartment of the prostate and a decrease in prostate weight and volume in dogs with prostatic hyperplasia (Laroque et al, 1994 and 1995; Cohen et al, 1995). The decrease in prostatic volume was associated with decreases in volume occupied by both the glandular and stromal prostatic compartments. Maximum atrophy was noted after 6 to 9 weeks of therapy (Cohen et al, 1995; Iguer-Ouada and Verstegen, 1997). The prostate returned to pretreatment size within 8 weeks of cessation of therapy.

The current recommended dose is one 5 mg tablet per os daily for dogs weighing 5 to 50 kg (Kamolpatana et al, 1998). Optimum duration of treatment is not known. Adverse effects of finasteride treatment in humans include decreased libido and ejaculate volume and impotence (Gormley et al, 1992). Treatment with finasteride caused a reduction in prostatic secretions and ejaculate volume but did not have an effect on testicular weight, testicular histomorphology, daily sperm production, sperm motility, or libido in dogs. In one study, all bitches bred to males that had been treated with finasteride at a dosage of 1.0 mg/kg once daily for 21 weeks became pregnant (Iguer-Ouada and Verstegen, 1997). Finasteride can cause fetal anomalies in humans and is present in human semen (Medical Letter, 1992). Finasteride has not been evaluated for teratogenicity in dogs, but normal puppies have been born after its use (Iguer-Ouada and Verstegen, 1997). Although use of 5α-reductase inhibitors for treatment of benign prostatic hyperplasia shows promise, the role of these drugs, if any, as ancillary treatment for acute or chronic prostatitis has yet to be determined.

ANTIANDROGENS. Flutamide and hydroxyflutamide are antiandrogens that exert their effects by inhibiting androgen uptake and/or nuclear binding of androgens in target tissues (Neri, 1989). At oral dosages of 2.5 to 5.0 mg/kg/day, these drugs have been demonstrated to significantly decrease prostatic size within 6 weeks (Neri, 1989; Cartee et al, 1990). In one study, a significant decrease in prostatic size was detected by ultrasonography after 10 days of flutamide treatment in dogs (Cartee et al, 1990). No change in libido, overall sperm production, or fertility has been identified with use of these drugs, although a decrease in testicular diameter has been reported in 30% to 60% of treated dogs. The role of these drugs, if any, as ancillary treatment for acute or chronic prostatitis has yet to be determined.

ORAL ZINC THERAPY. Oral zinc supplementation has been recommended in the management of prostatic disease, although a beneficial effect in dogs has not been proven. Low zinc concentrations may impair or reduce the secretion of prostatic antibacterial factor in humans but not in dogs. Branam and colleagues (1984) found no statistical difference in prostatic fluid zinc concentrations between 36 dogs with bacterial prostatitis and 42 healthy dogs. In addition, oral zinc supplementation does not appear to increase the concentration of zinc in prostatic fluid (Barsanti and Finco, 1983).

EXTRACTS OF SERENOA REPENS. In Europe, one of the most commonly used natural compounds in the treatment of men with voiding symptoms secondary to prostatic hyperplasia is a liposterolic extract of the berry of the saw palmetto plant, *Serenoa repens* (Lowe and Fagelman, 1999). Active constituents are believed to be steroids chemically related to cholesterol, with sitosterols believed to be most important. The potential mechanism of action of this extract in prostatic hyperplasia is poorly understood but may result from inhibition of cytosolic androgenic receptors, inhibition of 5α-reductase, or an estrogenic effect (Barsanti et al, 2000). Beneficial or harmful effects of this plant extract have not been documented

in dogs with prostatic hyperplasia. At doses of 100 and 500 mg/dog administered every 8 hours for 91 days, treatment with an extract of *S. repens* did not significantly affect prostatic weight, volume, or histologic score, libido, semen characteristics, radiographs of the caudal portion of the abdomen, prostatic ultrasonographic findings, or serum testosterone concentrations in 12 dogs with prostatic hyperplasia (Barsanti et al, 2000). Adverse effects of treatment were not evident.

Sequelae of Acute Bacterial Prostatitis

Potential sequelae of acute prostatitis include the development of acute orchiepididymitis and chronic prostatitis, orchitis, and epididymitis. Recognition, appropriate antibacterial therapy, and especially reevaluation after discontinuation of antibiotics are important for preventing these sequelae.

CHRONIC BACTERIAL PROSTATITIS

Clinical Signs

Chronic prostatitis may develop as a sequela of treatment failure for acute prostatitis or may be an unexpected finding in a dog with no prior history of prostate disease. Chronic prostatitis is usually not associated with signs of systemic illness unless abscessation is present. The most common indicator of chronic prostatitis is recurrent urinary tract infections in an otherwise healthy intact male dog. Although nonspecific, blood or bloody fluid dripping from the prepuce/penis independent of urination, hematuria, abnormal gait in the rear limbs during walking, or discomfort when rising to a standing position are the most commonly encountered clinical signs (Ling, 1995). Orchiepididymitis and infertility are less common owner observations. However, as many as 35% of dogs with chronic prostatitis do not have any clinical signs of prostate infection, are afebrile, and do not have an increased white blood cell count in the blood.

The results of prostatic palpation vary and depend partly on the amount of concurrent hyperplasia and fibrosis present. Prostatic palpation may be normal or may reveal an asymmetric, firm, irregular gland. Fluctuant soft areas may be palpable if intraprostatic cysts or abscessation is present. The prostate gland is usually not painful on palpation.

Diagnostic Evaluation

The results of a clinical laboratory evaluation are variable and may be normal. The clinician must maintain a high index of suspicion for chronic prostatitis when appropriate clinical signs and physical findings are present. The most consistent findings on a CBC, serum biochemistry panel, and urinalysis are pyuria, hematuria, and bacteriuria. The results of a CBC are usually normal unless abscessation is present. With abscessation, a neutrophilic leukocytosis with variable shift toward immaturity and toxic changes may be found on the CBC (Barsanti and Finco, 1984).

Bacterial culture of urine obtained by antepubic cystocentesis is positive in more than 50% of dogs with chronic prostatitis (Barsanti and Finco, 1984). Identification of the inciting organism in dogs without a positive urine culture must rely on cytologic evaluation and culture of prostatic fluid, preferably obtained by ejaculation or ultrasound-guided fine-needle aspiration (see page 941).

The prostate gland is usually radiographically normal despite chronic infection. Prostatic mineralization may be present but is a nonspecific finding. With prostatic abscessation, the prostate may be enlarged and have irregular margins, and the prostatic urethra may be narrow (Feeney et al, 1987a). Similar changes may also be found with neoplasia and cystic hyperplasia. Ultrasonographic changes found with chronic prostatitis include a heterogeneous pattern of mixed echogenicity with a focal or diffuse increase in parenchymal echogenicity and hypoechoic to anechoic, fluid-filled parenchymal cavities (Feeney et al, 1987b; Mattoon and Nyland, 1995). The hypoechoic to anechoic fluid-filled cavities may be abscesses or cysts. Sonographic shadowing may be present if calcification, fibrosis, or gas is present.

The results of semen evaluation are quite variable and depend in part on the duration and severity of infection and the presence or absence of bacterial orchiepididymitis and immune-mediated orchitis. Typical findings in dogs with infertility induced by chronic bacterial prostatitis include neutrophils, macrophages, phagocytized bacteria, abnormal spermatozoal motility, increased numbers of spermatozoa with primary and secondary morphologic defects, and decreased total number of sperm per ejaculate. Azoospermia may occur in severe cases.

Therapy

The clinician should assume that the blood–prostate fluid barrier is intact in dogs with chronic bacterial prostatitis and should choose an antibiotic that is not only effective against the organism grown but also capable of penetrating the blood–prostate fluid barrier and gaining access to the prostatic fluid. The blood–prostate fluid barrier is based in part on the pH differences between blood (pH 7.4), the prostatic interstitium (pH 7.4), and prostatic fluid (pH 6.4); on the characteristics of the prostatic acinar epithelium; and on the plasma protein–binding characteristics of antibiotics (Klausner and Osborne, 1983; Branam et al, 1984). Effective antibiotics should have low protein binding in plasma (e.g., norfloxacin) and high lipid solubility. The prostatic epithelium's bilipid membrane serves as a structural and functional barrier that favors the passive diffusion of lipid-soluble antibiotics

(e.g., chloramphenicol, trimethoprim-sulfonamide, enrofloxacin) across the prostatic epithelium. Drugs with low lipid solubility (e.g., ampicillin, cephalosporins, oxytetracycline HCl, aminoglycosides) are unable to readily cross the prostatic epithelium.

A drug's lipid solubility depends on the pK_a of the drug and the pH of the body fluid in which the drug is present. The pK_a is the pH at which a drug exists equally in its ionized and unionized form. The unionized form of the drug crosses membranes readily, whereas the ionized form does not. Most dogs with prostatic infection have acidic prostatic fluid (Barsanti and Finco, 1995a). Ideally, antibiotics that are effective in crossing the blood–prostate fluid barrier should be basic with high pK_a values (e.g., trimethoprim-sulfonamide, erythromycin, clindamycin). With acidic prostatic fluid, basic antibiotics with high pK_a values ionize to a greater extent in prostatic fluid than in plasma, become trapped in prostatic fluid, and reach concentrations in prostatic fluid equal to or greater than those attained in plasma (Fig. 30-5) (Dorfman and Barsanti, 1995). Antibiotics that meet some or all of the criteria for crossing the blood-prostate barrier (i.e., high pK_a, high lipid solubility, low plasma protein binding) include chloramphenicol, trimethoprim-sulfonamide, erythromycin, clindamycin,

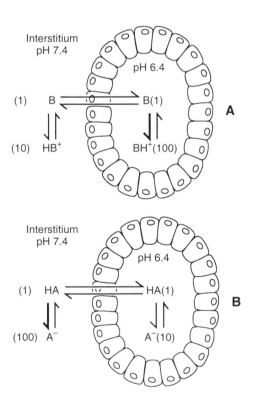

FIGURE 30-5. Effect of the pH difference between the prostatic interstitium and prostatic fluid on ion trapping of antibiotics. Basic antibiotics are present in larger concentrations in prostatic acini (*A*), whereas acidic antibiotics do not enter the acini (*B*). (From Barsanti JA, Finco DR: *In* Ettinger SJ, Feldman EC [eds]: Textbook of Veterinary Internal Medicine, 4th ed. Philadelphia, WB Saunders, 1995, p 1662.)

**TABLE 30–2 PHARMACOLOGIC CHARACTERISTICS
OF CERTAIN ANTIBIOTICS**

Antibiotic	Acid or Base	Lipid Soluble	pK$_a$	Diffusion into Prostate
Erythromycin	Base	Yes	8.8	Good
Oleandomycin	Base	Yes	8.5	Good
Polymyxin B	Base	No	8.0–9.0	Poor
Kanamycin	Base	No	7.2	Poor
Gentamicin	Base	No	7.9–8.2	Poor
Trimethoprim	Base	Yes	7.3	Good
Clindamycin*	Base	Yes	7.6	Good
Lincomycin	Base	Partly	7.6	Poor
Norfloxacin	Base	Yes	High	Good
Nalidixic acid*	Acid	Yes	6.7	Poor
Enrofloxacin	Acid	Yes	Zwitterion	Good
Ciprofloxacin	Acid	Yes	Zwitterion	Good
Penicillin G	Acid	No	2.7	Poor
Ampicillin	Acid	No	2.5	Poor
Cephalothin	Acid	No	2.5	Poor
Sulfisoxazole	Acid	Yes	Low	Poor
Sulfamethoxazole	Acid	Yes	Low	Poor
Oxytetracycline	Amphoteric	No	3.5, 7.6, 9.2	Poor
Tetracycline HCl	Amphoteric	Yes	3.3, 7.7, 9.7	Good
Chloramphenicol*	Not applicable	Yes	Not applicable	Good

Adapted from Barsanti JA, Finco DR: Vet Clin North Am 9:679, 1979.
*Highly protein-bound antibiotic.

and enrofloxacin (Table 30-2). Ciprofloxacin does not penetrate the prostate as well as enrofloxacin (Dorfman et al, 1995). The choice of antibiotic should also depend on results of culture and antibiotic sensitivity. As a general rule, if the causative organism is gram positive, trimethoprim-sulfonamide, chloramphenicol, tetracycline HCl, clindamycin, or erythromycin can be used pending antibiotic sensitivity results (Barsanti, 1990). If the causative organism is gram negative, trimethoprim-sulfonamide, chloramphenicol, tetracycline HCl, enrofloxacin, or ciprofloxacin is recommended.

Long-term antibiotic therapy is required for chronic prostatitis. Antibiotics should be administered for a minimum of 6 weeks. If a positive urine culture was found during the initial evaluation, urine should be recultured 7 to 10 days after initiation of antibiotic therapy to ensure negative growth and effectiveness of the antibiotic treatment. Prostatic fluid and urine should be recultured after 6 weeks of antibiotic treatment and while the dog is still being treated. If bacterial growth is still obtained, another 6-week cycle of appropriate antibiotics should be given and the prostatic fluid recultured. Once the culture results are negative, the antibiotic should be given for an additional 4 to 6 weeks. Reculture of the prostatic fluid 1 week and 1 to 2 months after discontinuation of the antibiotics should ensure successful therapy. If the infection recurs at this time, the entire cycle should be started again.

If the infection cannot be eliminated, antibiotics must be administered continuously for the rest of the dog's life to prevent infection of the urinary tract. Adverse reactions (e.g., keratoconjunctivitis sicca with chronic trimethoprim-sulfonamide therapy) must be considered when choosing an antibiotic for long-term therapy of recurring bacterial prostatitis. Chloramphenicol, tetracycline HCl, enrofloxacin, norfloxacin, and trimethoprim-sulfonamide have been recommended for long-term therapy of chronic prostatitis (Barsanti, 1990; Ling, 1995).

Castration should also be considered as adjunctive therapy to control chronic infection. In experimental chronic prostatitis in dogs, castration performed 2 weeks after induction of infection hastened spontaneous resolution of infection (Cowan et al, 1991b). Similar results in naturally occurring cases of chronic prostatitis have not been reported.

Sequelae of Chronic Bacterial Prostatitis

Possible sequelae of chronic prostatitis include orchitis, epididymitis, and infertility. Infertility may result from hyperthermia, immune-mediated destruction of spermatogenic cells with the development of orchitis, or sperm death from exposure to bacterial toxins.

REFERENCES

Barsanti JA: Male genital infections. In Greene CE (ed): Infectious Diseases of the Dog and Cat, 2nd ed. Philadelphia, WB Saunders, 1990, p 171.

Barsanti JA, Finco DR: Treatment of bacterial prostatitis. In Kirk RW (ed): Current Veterinary Therapy VIII. Philadelphia, WB Saunders, 1983, p 1101.

Barsanti JA, Finco DR: Evaluation of techniques for diagnosis of canine prostatic diseases. J Am Vet Med Assoc 185:198, 1984.

Barsanti JA, Finco DR: Prostatic diseases. In Ettinger SJ, Feldman EC (eds): Textbook of Veterinary Internal Medicine, 4th ed. Philadelphia, WB Saunders, 1995a, p 1662.

Barsanti JA, Finco D: Medical management of canine prostatic hyperplasia. In Bonagura J, Kirk R (eds): Current Veterinary Therapy XII. Philadelphia, WB Saunders, 1995b, p 1033.

Barsanti JA, et al: Evaluation of diagnostic techniques for canine prostatic diseases. J Am Vet Med Assoc 177:160, 1980.

Barsanti JA, et al: Effect of induced prostatic infection on semen quality in the dog. Am J Vet Res 47:709, 1986.

Barsanti JA, et al: Effects of an extract of *Serenoa repens* on dogs with hyperplasia of the prostate gland. Am J Vet Res 61:880, 2000.

Bell FW, et al: Evaluation of serum and seminal plasma markers in the diagnosis of canine prostatic disorders. J Vet Intern Med 9:149, 1995.

Bjurstrom L, Linde-Forsberg C: Long-term study of aerobic bacteria of the genital tract in study dogs. Am J Vet Res 53:670, 1992.

Black GM, et al: Prevalence of prostatic cysts in adult, large- breed dogs. J Am Anim Hosp Assoc 34:177, 1998.

Branam JE, et al: Selected physical and chemical characteristics of prostatic fluid collected by ejaculation from healthy dogs and from dogs with bacterial prostatitis. Am J Vet Res 45:825, 1984.

Cartee RE, et al: Evaluation of drug-induced prostatic involution in dogs by transabdominal B-mode ultrasonography. Am J Vet Res 51:1773, 1990.

Cochran RC, et al: Serum levels of follicle-stimulating hormone, luteinizing hormone, prolactin, testosterone, 5α-dihydrotestosterone, 5α-androstane-3α,17β-diol, and 17β-estradiol from male Beagles with spontaneously induced benign prostatic hyperplasia. Invest Urol 19:142, 1981.

Cohen S, et al: Comparison of the effects of new specific azasteroid inhibitors of steroid 5α-reductase on canine hyperplastic prostate: Suppression of prostatic dihydrotestosterone correlated with prostate regression. Prostate 26:55, 1995.

Cowan LA, et al: Effects of bacterial infection and castration on prostatic tissue zinc concentration in dogs. Am J Vet Res 52:1262, 1991a.

Cowan LA, et al: Effects of castration on chronic bacterial prostatitis in dogs. J Am Vet Med Assoc 199:346, 1991b.

Dorfman M, Barsanti J: CVT Update: Treatment of canine bacterial prostatitis. *In* Bonagura J, Kirk R (eds): Current Veterinary Therapy XII. Philadelphia, WB Saunders, 1995, p 1029.

Dorfman M et al: Enrofloxacin concentrations in dogs with normal prostates and dogs with chronic bacterial prostatitis. Am J Vet Res 56:386, 1995.

Feeney DA, et al: Canine prostatic disease: Comparison of radiographic appearance with morphologic and microbiologic findings: 30 cases (1981-1985). J Am Vet Med Assoc 190:1018, 1987a.

Feeney DA, et al: Canine prostatic disease: Comparison of ultrasonographic appearance with morphologic and microbiologic findings: 30 cases (1981-1985). J Am Vet Med Assoc 190:1027, 1987b.

Gormley GJ, et al: The effect of finasteride in men with benign prostatic hyperplasia. N Engl J Med 327:1185, 1992.

Iguer-Ouada M, Verstegen J: Effect of finasteride (Proscar MSD) on seminal composition, prostate function and fertility in male dogs. J Reprod Fertil Suppl 51:139, 1997.

Johnston SD, Root Kustritz MV, Olson PNS: Disorders of the canine prostate. *In*, Johnston SD, Root Kustritz MV, Olson PNS (eds): Canine and Feline Theriogenology. Philadelphia, WB Saunders, 2001, p 337.

Kamolpatana K, et al: Effect of finasteride on serum concentrations of dihydrotestosterone and testosterone in three clinically normal sexually intact adult male dogs. Am J Vet Res 59:762, 1998.

Klausner JS, Osborne CA: Management of canine bacterial prostatitis. J Am Vet Med Assoc 182:292, 1983.

Krawiec DR, Heflin D: Study of prostatic disease in dogs: 177 cases (1981-1986). J Am Vet Med Assoc 200:1119, 1992.

Laroque P, et al: Effects of chronic oral administration of a selective 5α-reductase inhibitor, finasteride, on the dog prostate. Prostate 24:93, 1994.

Laroque P, et al: Quantitative evaluation of glandular and stromal compartments in hyperplastic dog prostates: Effect of 5α-reductase inhibitors. Prostate 27:121, 1995.

Ling GV: Diagnosis and medical management of prostatic infections in dogs. Proceedings of the Society for Theriogenology, Toronto, Canada, 1990, p 254.

Ling GV: Disorders of the prostate. *In* Ling GV (ed): Lower Urinary Tract Diseases of Dogs and Cats: Diagnosis, Medical Management, Prognosis. St Louis, Mosby, 1995, p 129.

Ling GV, et al: Canine prostatic fluid: Techniques of collection, quantitative bacterial culture, and interpretation of results. Am J Vet Res 183:201, 1983.

Ling GV, et al: Comparison of two sample collection methods for quantitative bacteriologic culture of canine prostatic fluid. J Am Vet Med Assoc 196:1479, 1990.

Lowe FC, Fagelman E: Phytotherapy in the treatment of benign prostatic hyperplasia: An update. Urology 53:671, 1999.

Mattoon JS, Nyland TG: Ultrasonography of the genital system. *In* Nyland TG, Mattoon JS (eds): Veterinary Diagnostic Ultrasound. Philadelphia, WB Saunders, 1995, p 141.

Medical Letter: Finasteride for benign prostatic hypertrophy. Med Lett Drugs Ther 34:83, 1992.

Neri R: Pharmacology and pharmacokinetics of flutamide. Urology 34(suppl):19, 1989.

Rhodes L: The role of dihydrotestosterone in prostate physiology. *In* Proceedings of the Annual Meeting of the Society of Theriogenology, Kansas City, Mo, 1996, p 288.

Sirinarumitr K, et al: Effects of finasteride on size of the prostate gland and semen quality in dogs with benign prostatic hypertrophy. J Am Vet Med Assoc 218:1275, 2001.

Wallace MS: The diagnosis of infertility and subfertility secondary to prostatic disease in the dog. Proceedings of the Society for Theriogenology, San Diego, 1991, p 229.

Winter M, Liehr J: Possible mechanism of induction of benign prostatic hyperplasia by estradiol and dihydrotestosterone in dogs. Toxicol Appl Pharmacol 136:211, 1996.

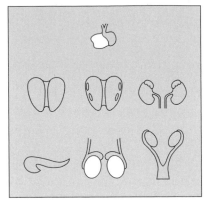

31

INFERTILITY

The diagnostic approach and therapeutic management of the infertile dog are perhaps the most difficult and least rewarding areas involving canine male reproduction. Unfortunately, the saying "an azoospermic dog remains azoospermic" is usually true. Nevertheless, a few disorders, if corrected, carry a good prognosis regarding return of fertility. A thorough, systematic diagnostic approach to the infertile dog offers the best chance of discovering the problem. Semen evaluation plays an integral role in the diagnostic evaluation of the infertile dog. It is important to remember that the characteristics of an ejaculate may vary from day to day; an abnormality should be consistently present in the semen before a definitive diagnosis is established. Therapy should be initiated only after a definitive diagnosis has been established. A definitive diagnosis enables the clinician to formulate a rational therapeutic plan and prognosis. The indiscriminate use of fertility drugs, androgens, and hormones is usually ineffective, potentially dangerous, and frequently confusing to both owner and veterinarian.

CLASSIFICATION

Developing a classification scheme for infertility based on information obtained from the history is a helpful aid in narrowing the list of differential diagnoses and providing insight into the initial diagnostic approach. Classifying infertility based on the dog's previous breeding history and current status of libido is easily done. Dogs have either acquired or congenital infertility and normal or decreased libido. The most common history we encounter is that of a proven stud dog with acquired infertility. Libido is typically normal but then wanes. Acquired infertility has many possible causes (Table 31-1). A dog that has never sired a litter despite numerous attempts should be considered congenitally

infertile until proved otherwise. Acquired infertility is possible in these dogs if the insult occurred before the onset of sexual use. In addition to acquired causes, the clinician must also consider congenital defects that would not be considered in the previously proven stud dog (Table 31-1).

Normal libido in an infertile dog implies dysfunction of the testis, epididymis, or prostate gland but normal Leydig cell function and plasma testosterone concentrations. Conversely, decreased libido in an infertile dog may result from destruction of the Leydig cells within the testes. Endocrinopathies, hormone-secreting testicular tumors, exogenous hormone administration, and psychologic problems resulting from trauma or pain during sexual arousal should also be considered.

DIAGNOSTIC APPROACH

Initial Evaluation

HISTORY. The differential diagnoses and diagnostic approach to potentially infertile dogs should be based on information obtained from the history and physical examination. A thorough history is extremely important in the evaluation of the infertile dog. The history should establish the previous fertility of the dog and the current status of libido. In addition, a complete reproductive history should be ascertained, as well as a knowledge of factors such as the dog's environment, use, previous illnesses, medications, and trauma (Table 31-2). Attention should be paid to the age of the animal, frequency of sexual use, breeding practices of the kennel, presence or absence of previous reproductive problems, and previous or current use of any hormones or other medications. Several drugs and exogenous hormones have been associated with infertility in the dog (Table 31-3). As a general rule, any

TABLE 31–1 CLASSIFICATION SCHEME FOR MALE INFERTILITY BASED ON HISTORICAL ABILITY TO SIRE A LITTER

Congenital Infertility	Acquired Infertility
Hormonal	Hormonal
Hypopituitarism	Hypopituitarism
Hypothyroidism	Hypothyroidism
Chromosomal aberration	Hyperadrenocorticism
Developmental	Metabolic
Cryptorchidism	Uremia
Penis, prepuce, os penis	Hepatic
anomaly	Neoplasia
Testicular hypoplasia,	Compression
aplasia	Hormonal secretion
Duct aplasia	Stress
Motility defect	Infection
Kartagener's syndrome	Fever
Retrograde ejaculation	Duct obstruction
	Immune-mediated orchitis
	Drugs, exogenous hormone
	therapy
	Retrograde ejaculation
	Idiopathic testicular degeneration
	Sexual overuse?
	Psychological?

drug therapy can potentially result in infertility. Genetic factors may also contribute to infertility and should be suspected if inbreeding, infertility in related dogs, or problems with other endocrine disorders (e.g., lymphocytic thyroiditis) are identified (Olson et al, 1992). Finally, a thorough review of breeding management practices and the fertility of bitches with which the dog has bred should be done. In many instances, the problem lies with inappropriate timing of the breedings, technical mistakes if artificial insemination was used, or fertility problems with the bitch rather than the dog.

PHYSICAL EXAMINATION. A complete physical examination is extremely important in the evaluation of the infertile dog. Abnormalities involving other organ systems besides the reproductive tract can interfere with spermatogenesis or libido. A thorough examination of the reproductive tract (see page 930) should be performed once all other organ systems have been examined. In the infertile dog, special attention should be given to the size, shape, and location of the os penis in relation to the tip of the glans penis; the preputial opening and the ability to extrude the penis; the size, shape, and consistency of the testes; the size and conformation of the epididymis and spermatic cord; and the size, symmetry, and consistency of the prostate gland. Any identified abnormalities should be evaluated as needed.

SUMMARY. A thorough evaluation of the overall health of the dog plays an integral role in the evaluation of infertility. Occasionally, the history or physical examination reveals what seems to be an unrelated abnormality that, when pursued, can be demonstrated to be the cause of infertility. After reviewing the reproductive history and findings on physical examination, the potentially infertile dog should be able to be placed into one of the following four categories: normal, decreased libido, acquired infertility with normal libido, and congenital infertility with normal libido.

Infertility and Decreased Libido

Decreased libido varies from complete lack of sexual interest and inability to mate, to slowness or delay in exhibiting libido or attaining an erection, to an increasing inability or disinterest in mounting the bitch and achieving intromission (Keenan, 1998). Decreased libido implies a reduction in the circulating concentration of testosterone or an acquired psychogenic problem resulting in loss of interest in mating (Fig. 31-1). Severe discipline for inappropriate mounting, exposure to aggressive or dominant bitches at the time of breeding, removal of the dog from his surroundings, or erratic behavior from the owner may deleteriously affect libido, especially if the negative influences occur early in life. Breeding at the incorrect time of estrus, sexual overuse, and painful orthopedic conditions can affect the performance of the dog. Some dogs also have pronounced mate preferences, resulting in inconsistent libido. Rarely, diminished olfactory function may inhibit libido by altering the dog's perception of pheromones (Freshman, 2001).

A reduction in circulating testosterone can result from either destruction of the Leydig cells within the testis or suppression of the pituitary–Leydig cell axis. The latter occurs most commonly with hypothyroidism, hyperadrenocorticism, exogenous drugs, most notably glucocorticoids, and hormone-secreting (estrogen-secreting) testicular tumors. Helpful in identifying these diagnoses are evaluations of thyroid gland function (i.e., serum thyroxine, free thyroxine and thyrotropin concentration), adrenocortical function (i.e., adrenocorticotropic hormone (ACTH) stimulation test), Leydig cell function (GnRH stimulation test), testicular ultrasonography, and aspiration cytology if a testicular mass is identified.

Most disorders causing acquired infertility with normal libido (see below) can also cause destruction of Leydig cells and loss of libido. The typical sequence is loss of fertility first, followed by loss of libido. The testes may be normal in size and consistency, soft but normal in size, or soft and decreased in size on palpation. Unfortunately, soft consistency or decreased testicular size may also be found with disorders affecting the pituitary–Leydig cell axis. Such a finding does not imply a primary testicular problem in the dog with decreased libido.

An ejaculate may be difficult to obtain in a dog with decreased libido, although obtaining a semen sample should be attempted. If an ejaculate can be obtained, a thorough evaluation and microbiologic culture should be performed (see pages 932 and 941). Results of these tests may provide clues to the underlying problem. If the semen evaluation and culture are inconclusive or an ejaculate cannot be obtained, cytologic evaluation of a testicular aspirate or histologic evaluation of a

TABLE 31–2 OWNER QUESTIONNAIRE—THE INFERTILE MALE

A. Age _____ Breed _____

B. General Medical History (not including reproductive problems)

   1. Vaccinations current? _____

   2. Previous significant illnesses requiring hospitalization: Yes _____ No _____ If yes, please summarize briefly:

     _____

     _____

   3. Previous trauma? Yes _____ No _____ If yes, please summarize briefly:

     _____

     _____

   4. Does your dog:

     a. Have a vomiting problem?   Yes _____ No _____

     b. Have diarrhea?   Yes _____ No _____

     c. Drink excessively?   Yes _____ No _____

     d. Urinate excessively?   Yes _____ No _____

     e. Have normal ability to play and exercise?   Yes _____ No _____

     f. Appear to be of normal weight and height?   Yes _____ No _____

     g. Have a hair coat problem?   Yes _____ No _____

     h. Have any other problem? (If yes, please describe)   Yes _____ No _____

     _____

     _____

   5. Has your dog ever had thyroid tests run?   Yes _____ No _____

   6. Has your dog received thyroid hormone?

     a. In the past?   No _____ Yes _____ Dose _____

     b. Now?   No _____ Yes _____ Dose _____

   7. Is your dog receiving any medication of any type?

     No _____ Yes _____ Drug and dose _____

   8. Has your dog undergone recent obedience or attack training?

     No _____ Yes _____ When _____

   9. Is your dog involved with the show circuit?

     No _____ Yes _____ If yes, please summarize frequency, method of travel, last showing:

     _____

     _____

   10. Please list all foods and supplements presently being given to your dog:

     _____

     _____

     _____

C. Reproductive History

   1. Is your dog a proven stud?

     No _____ Yes _____ If yes, date of last litter sired _____

   2. Does your dog show strong sexual desires in the presence of a female in estrus?

     No _____ Yes _____ If no, did he in the past? Yes _____ No _____ If so, when? _____

   3. Can your dog achieve:

     a. An erection   Yes _____ No _____

     b. Intromission   Yes _____ No _____

     c. A tie (If yes, duration of tie _____)   Yes _____ No _____

(Continued)

TABLE 31–2   OWNER QUESTIONNAIRE—THE INFERTILE MALE—cont'd

4. Does your dog ejaculate?   Yes _____ No _____

   If yes, does it occur before intromission?   Yes _____ No _____

5. Have you observed the semen?   Yes _____ No _____

   If yes, what is the color? _____

6. How frequently is your dog used for breeding? _____

7. When was your dog last used for breeding? _____

8. How do you determine when to mate your dog with the bitch?

   _____

   _____

9. How many times do you let your dog mate with the bitch?

   _____

10. Has your dog had a *Brucella* titer? Yes _____ No _____ Date of most recent check _____

11. Has your dog had a semen evaluation?   Yes _____ No _____

    If yes, date of most recent evaluation   _____

    Results of the evaluation:

    _____

    _____

12. Has your dog ever had a preputial discharge?   Yes _____ No _____

    If so, briefly describe what it was, when it occurred, and how it was treated:

    _____

    _____

    _____

    _____

13. Has your dog ever had scrotal:

    a. Swelling   Yes _____ No _____

    b. Pain   Yes _____ No _____

    c. Redness   Yes _____ No _____

    d. Dermatitis   Yes _____ No _____

14. Have you noticed any change in the size or consistency of your dog's testicles?   Yes _____ No _____

    If so, briefly describe:

    _____

    _____

    _____

D. Kennel History

   Do any other bitches or dogs in your kennel have reproductive disorders?   Yes _____ No _____

   If yes, briefly describe:

   _____

   _____

   _____

E. Pedigree

   Do any other bitches or dogs that are related to this dog have reproductive disorders?   Yes _____ No _____

   If yes, briefly describe:

   _____

   _____

   _____

TABLE 31–3 DRUGS AND EXOGENOUS HORMONES THAT AFFECT FERTILITY IN HUMANS AND POSSIBLY THE DOG

Chemotherapeutic drugs	Hormones
Busulfan	Anabolic steroids
Chlorambucil	Methyltestosterone*
Cisplatin	Testosterone esters*
Cyclophosphamide	Estrogens
Methotrexate	Estradiol 17β*
Vinblastine	Diethylstilbestrol*
Vincristine	KABI 1774*
	Progestogens
Miscellaneous drugs	Medroxyprogesterone acetate*
Amphotericin B*	Megestrol acetate*
Alloxan	Delmadinone acetate*
Cimetidine*	Glucocorticoids*
Clomipramine	Tamoxifen citrate*
Ketoconazole*	Gossypol*
Spironolactone	GnRH antagonists*
Sulfasalazine	GnRH agonists*

*Documented in the dog.

testicular biopsy should be considered to evaluate the condition of the seminiferous tubules and the Leydig cells (see pages 947 and 949). Secondary causes of decreased libido should be ruled out before performing a testicular biopsy. Blood luteinizing hormone (LH) concentrations are increased with loss of Leydig cells. Therefore assaying the blood LH concentration can be used to increase suspicion for a primary testicular problem (see page 945).

Acquired Infertility and Normal Libido

This is the most common cause for infertility in dogs. Normal libido suggests that the pituitary–Leydig cell axis is functional and that blood testosterone concentrations are adequate. Because of the large number of differential diagnoses (Table 31-4), an evaluation should be designed to progress from relatively easy and inexpensive to more difficult and time-consuming diagnostic tests. Three critical areas should be pursued in the history: (1) a thorough review of breeding practices,

TABLE 31–4 POTENTIAL CAUSES FOR ACQUIRED INFERTILITY AND NORMAL LIBIDO

Common Causes	Uncommon Causes
Normal dog	Sexual overuse
Breeding mismanagement	Testicular trauma
Problems with artificial	Testicular hyperthermia
insemination technique	Testicular neoplasia
Drugs, environmental insults	Retrograde ejaculation
Scrotal inflammation	Bilateral duct obstruction
Systemic illness	Chronic severe stress
(current or previous)	Kartagener's syndrome
Infectious orchitis	*Brucella canis*
Lymphocytic orchitis	Hemospermia
Idiopathic testicular degeneration	Asthenozoospermia
Old age	

focusing especially on the method by which the owner determines when a bitch is to be bred, the number of times the bitch is bred during estrus, the establishment of a tie, the fertility status of the bitch(es), the frequency of use of the dog, and the sexual experience of the dog; (2) a thorough review of medications currently or previously given to the dog; and (3) a thorough review of current and past illnesses, trauma, and stresses. Stress can inhibit reproductive function (Rivier and Rivest, 1991), and although the term *stress* is difficult to define, anything from serious illness to activity out of the expected ordinary routine for a dog should be considered. For example, frequent flying or participation in stressful activities (e.g., Schintzund training) can cause temporary infertility. Potential inciting factors identified in the history should be corrected, if possible.

Regardless of the historical findings, a thorough physical examination, *Brucella canis* test, and semen evaluation should be performed to rule out other possible problems. During the physical examination, the clinician should make special note of testicular size, symmetry, and consistency. The type of testicular abnormalities identified on palpation may provide clues to the underlying cause (see Physical Examination, page 930). Rectal palpation of the prostate should be performed to evaluate for changes consistent with chronic prostatitis. All dogs with an infertility problem should be evaluated for *B. canis*, using the rapid slide or tube agglutination test (see page 920).

A semen evaluation is critical in the diagnostic evaluation of the dog with acquired infertility and normal libido. (See page 932 for a complete discussion on obtaining and evaluating an ejaculate.) Abnormalities identified on evaluation of semen can provide clues to the underlying cause and dictate the next steps in the diagnostic evaluation of the dog. The diagnostic approach to some of the more common abnormalities identified on semen evaluation follows. The reader is referred to Chapter 27 for detailed information on the diagnostic tests discussed below.

Azoospermia (Fig. 31-2)

Azoospermia refers to a complete absence of spermatozoa in the ejaculate. Azoospermia is typically associated with normal seminal fluid. Identification of normal concentrations of seminal alkaline phosphatase confirms the presence of epididymal fluid in the ejaculate (see page 940). Identifiable abnormalities in seminal fluid can provide valuable insight into the possible underlying cause and should always be pursued (see below). In our experience, azoospermia is usually an acquired disorder that develops secondary to gonadal dysfunction, most notably idiopathic testicular degeneration (Table 31-5).

Azoospermia should always be confirmed with several ejaculates before embarking on an extensive evaluation for causes—and certainly before declaring a dog sterile. Incomplete ejaculation can result in "apparent" oligospermia and occasionally azoospermia,

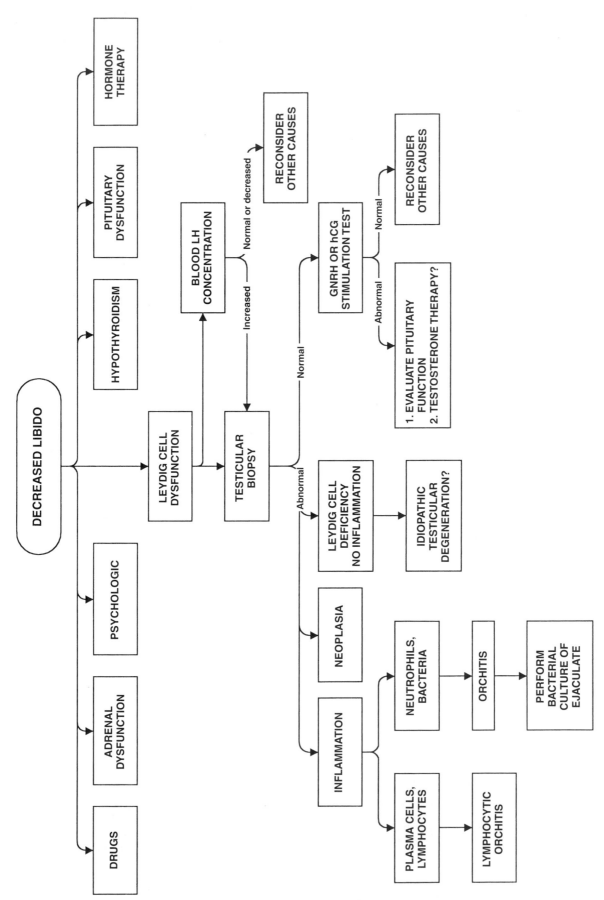

FIGURE 31-1. Diagnostic approach to decreased libido.

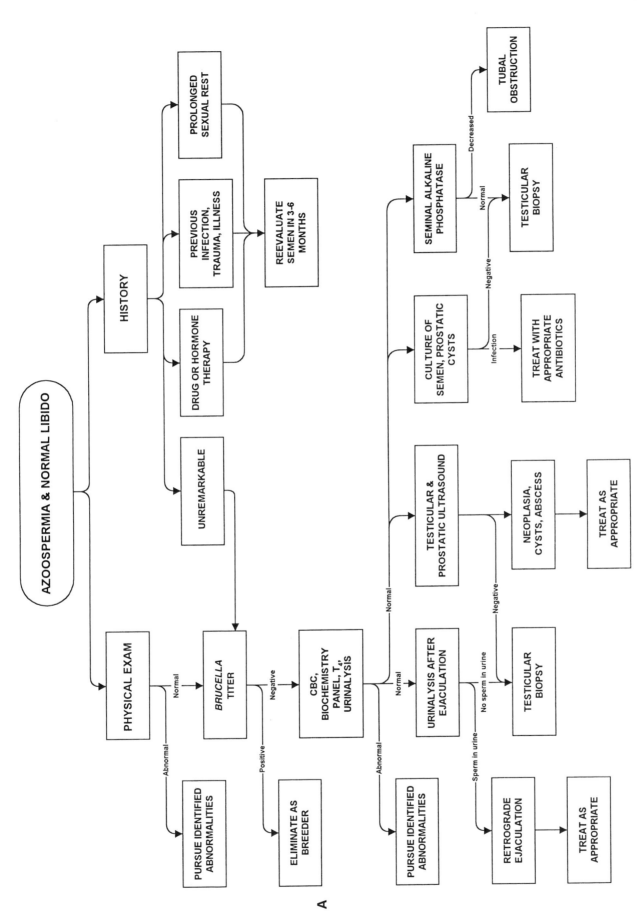

FIGURE 31-2. Diagnostic approach to azoospermia and normal libido. A, Initial approach prior to performing testicular biopsy or measuring pituitary gonadotropins. *Continued*

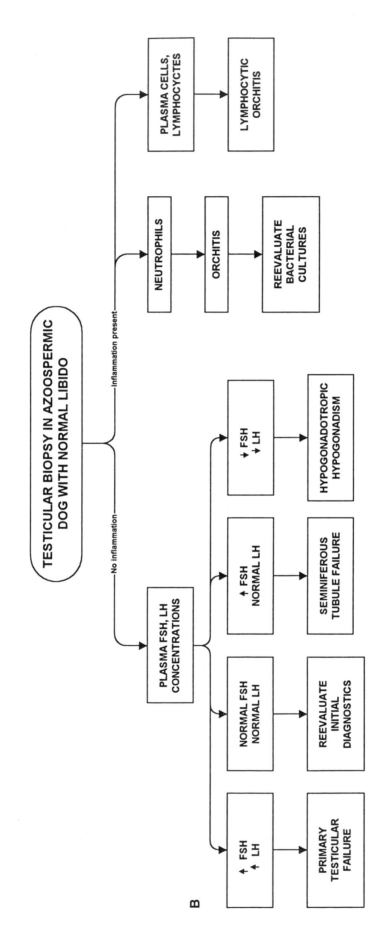

FIGURE 31-2.—cont'd *B,* Interpretation of results of testicular biopsy and measurement of pituitary gonadotropins in dogs for which initial diagnostic approach (*A*) failed to identify an etiology.

TABLE 31–5 POTENTIAL CAUSES FOR AZOOSPERMIA

Azoospermia May Be Transient	Azoospermia Usually Permanent
Drugs, hormones* (see Table 31–3)	Idiopathic testicular degeneration
Environmental insult	Lymphocytic orchitis
Systemic illness (current or previous)	*Brucella canis*
Testicular trauma, hyperthermia	Duct obstruction
Infectious orchitis, prostatitis	Bilateral testicular neoplasia
Retrograde ejaculation	Congenital defect
Hypothyroidism*	
Hypopituitarism*	
Hyperadrenocorticism*	
Estrogen-secreting Sertoli cell tumor*	

*Decreased libido often associated with these disorders.

especially in a young, timid male who is outside of his normal domain or in a dog experiencing pain during the collection procedure (e.g., failure to exteriorize the bulbus glandis). Evaluating several ejaculates and paying attention to careful and correct collection techniques usually allow identification of incomplete ejaculation.

Potential causes of azoospermia include drugs; environmental insults (e.g., exposure to heavy metals, mercurial compounds, and other toxins); systemic disease; bilateral obstruction of the vas deferens, epididymides, or ductulus deferens; retrograde ejaculation; gonadal dysfunction; and genetics (Olson, 1991). A thorough history concerning past and current drug therapy should always be obtained and reviewed (see Table 31–3). Information regarding the environment and potential for exposure to household and environmental chemicals and toxins should be pursued. Genetic factors may contribute to azoospermia and should be suspected if inbreeding, infertility in related dogs, or problems with endocrine disorders (e.g., lymphocytic thyroiditis) are identified (Olson et al, 1992). The following tests should be performed to screen for systemic disease that may be deleteriously affecting spermatogenesis: a complete blood count (CBC); serum biochemistry panel; thyroid panel, including total thyroxine, free thyroxine by modified equilibrium dialysis, and endogenous thyrotropin concentration; and urinalysis.

Obstruction of the duct system can result from inflammation, neoplasia, segmental aplasia, sperm granuloma, spermatocele, or prior vasectomy (Olson, 1991). A thorough palpation of the testes and epididymides may reveal pain, swelling, or mass lesions. An ultrasound examination of the testes, epididymides, vas deferens, and prostate gland may also reveal abnormalities in these structures. Patency of the duct system can be determined by measuring seminal alkaline phosphatase concentration (see page 940).

Retrograde ejaculation refers to the passage of semen into the urinary bladder during ejaculation. During normal antegrade ejaculation, sequential seminal emission, bladder neck closure and seminal expulsion through the penile urethra occur; these events are controlled primarily by the sympathetic portion of the autonomic nervous system (Root et al, 1994). Denervation or damage to the nerves or muscles in this system prevent this sequence of events. If there is inadequate closure of the bladder neck, semen will flow into the urinary bladder, because this is the path of least resistance (Frenette et al, 1986). Retrograde flow of some semen occurs during normal ejaculation in the dog (Dooley et al, 1990). Complete retrograde ejaculation is rare but should be considered a potential problem in the azoospermic dog. Partial retrograde ejaculation causing oligospermia can also occur. Documenting large numbers of spermatozoa in a urinalysis obtained after ejaculation versus one obtained before ejaculation establishes the diagnosis.

Congenital defects in testicular development and spermatogenesis should be considered in the young adult dog or in the dog that has never sired a litter despite multiple attempts. Intersex states (e.g., XXY syndrome) are the most common congenital causes for azoospermia (Nie et al, 1998). A thorough physical examination often reveals abnormalities (e.g., testicular hypoplasia) suggestive of a gonadal problem. Karyotyping should be done if intersexuality is suspected. Refer to Chapter 24 for information on intersexuality.

Acquired gonadal disorders that cause azoospermia in the dog with normal libido include idiopathic testicular degeneration, lymphocytic orchitis, infection, thermal insult, trauma, and neoplasia. Endocrine disorders, most sex hormones, and glucocorticoids typically affect libido as well as spermatogenesis; androgens are the exception (see page 1003). Most of these disorders typically cause oligospermia initially. With time, disorders causing acquired loss of spermatogenesis, most notably idiopathic testicular degeneration, may also decrease the dog's libido, as the Leydig cells also become affected. Acquired disorders often result in abnormalities identifiable on physical examination. Abnormalities (e.g., inflammatory cells, bacteria) in the seminal fluid may also be identified. Normal seminal fluid is common with idiopathic testicular degeneration and may also be found as an end-stage event with other disorders.

Dogs with suspected acquired gonadal dysfunction should have bacterial infection ruled out through cultures of the urine, semen, and, if identifiable with ultrasonography, prostatic cyst(s). An ultrasound examination of the testes and epididymides by an experienced ultrasonographer should be performed and any identifiable masses or cysts aspirated for cytology and culture. Cultures must be interpreted cautiously. Bacteria that are isolated may represent a primary infection causing infertility, may be secondary invaders and not the primary problem, or may be contaminants. In addition, bacteria isolated in semen may be different from those isolated from testicular tissue or prostatic cysts (Olson et al, 1992). Nevertheless, antibiotic therapy may be warranted in an azoospermic dog when bacterial cultures are positive.

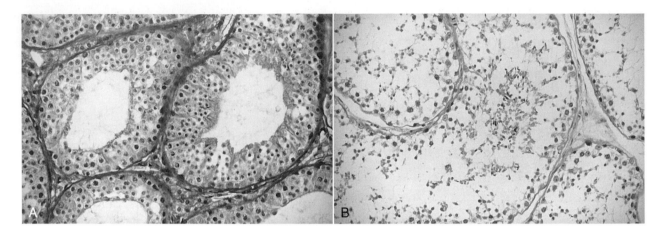

FIGURE 31-3. Histologic section of a testicular biopsy obtained from a 4-year-old Welsh Corgi at the time of the initial diagnostic evaluation for infertility *(A)* and 8 months later *(B)* (H&E ×250). Notice the marked degeneration of the seminiferous tubules and loss of interstitial Leydig cells with time. Libido was normal at the initial evaluation but gradually decreased with time. The diagnosis was idiopathic testicular degeneration.

If available, measurement of serum follicle-stimulating hormone (FSH) concentration can provide information on the health of the seminiferous tubules. The baseline serum FSH concentration is typically less than 130 ng/ml in healthy dogs. Infertile dogs with severe testicular dysfunction typically have serum FSH concentrations greater than 250 ng/ml (Soderberg, 1986). Increased concentration of FSH likely results from decreased production of inhibin by Sertoli cells in response to abnormal spermatogenesis and subsequent loss of feedback inhibition on pituitary FSH secretion. Conversely, normal or low serum FSH concentration in an azoospermic dog suggests bilateral tubal obstruction within the duct system, retrograde ejaculation, impaired pituitary FSH secretion (i.e., hypogonadotrophic hypogonadism), or sampling error (see page 945).

An epididymal aspirate or testicular biopsy should be considered if the diagnostics discussed above have failed to identify the cause of infertility. Aspirates of the caudal epididymis should be evaluated for the presence of live, motile sperm, inflammatory cells, and bacteria. In an azoospermic dog, the presence of spermatozoa from an epididymal aspirate implies an obstruction in the ductus deferens, whereas a lack of sperm implies duct obstruction or spermatozoa resorption proximal to the site of the aspirate, or an arrest in spermatogenesis.

Testicular biopsy provides concrete information on the underlying pathologic process (e.g., lymphocytic orchitis, seminiferous tubule degeneration), the state of the blood-testis barrier, the cellularity of the seminiferous tubules, and the potential for regeneration of spermatogenesis and may provide guidance regarding therapy (Olson et al, 1992). Aspirated testicular tissue can also be submitted for culture. When evaluating a testicular biopsy, it is important to remember that biopsied tissue represents a focal area of the testis and may not be representative of the disease process affecting the testis. In addition, it is often difficult to determine whether the seminiferous tubules are undergoing degeneration or regeneration based on a testicular biopsy obtained at one point in time, especially if inflammation is not present (Fig. 31-3).

An alternative to testicular biopsy is to wait for a period of time. If the cause of azoospermia is not identifiable, the dog should be sexually rested for a minimum of 2 months. During this time, any factors that could potentially affect spermatogenesis (e.g., drugs, dietary supplements, strenuous work) should be minimized or eliminated from the dog's routine. After 2 months, a complete physical examination should be performed, paying special attention to changes in the size, shape, and consistency of the testes. Semen analysis should also be performed. If azoospermia persists and the testes still feel normal, the dog should be evaluated again 2 and 4 months later. In our experience, the potential for regeneration of spermatogenesis can be determined in most dogs after 6 months of evaluation. Abnormal physical findings, especially regarding the testes, usually become evident during this time.

Oligospermia

Oligospermia refers to a decrease in the total number of spermatozoa per ejaculate, typically less than 100×10^6 spermatozoa per ejaculate. Sperm morphology may be normal or abnormal. Common causes of oligospermia include incomplete ejaculation, sexual overuse, and recent testicular insult. Most of the causes for azoospermia also cause oligospermia. The development of oligospermia versus azoospermia may depend on the severity of the disease process, the extent of the reproductive tract involvement (e.g., partial versus complete obstruction of the efferent ductules), and the timing of evaluation relative to the stage of the disorder (i.e., early versus late). With time, oligospermia may eventually lead to azoospermia.

The diagnostic evaluation for oligospermia is similar to that for azoospermia (see Fig. 31-2). Additional factors that must be considered in the dog with oligospermia include the age of the dog and the frequency of ejaculation. The frequency of ejaculation has a direct effect on spermatozoa concentration (see page 939). Total sperm count per ejaculate decreases with frequent use. This decrease is attributable to a reduction in the epididymal storage pool of sperm. When this storage pool is exhausted, the decline in spermatozoa count plateaus, and subsequent counts represent the production rate within the testes. Most healthy males can be used once daily for prolonged periods (months) without causing oligospermia or subfertility. However, males with defective spermatogenesis may not be able to meet these demands and oligospermia may result. This is more likely to be apparent in older dogs because of the potential for gradual reduction in daily sperm output associated with the aging process. A dog with frequent sexual usage, oligospermia, and subfertility may regain fertility when used sparingly to allow spermatozoa to accumulate in the epididymis (Olar et al, 1983).

Teratozoospermia (abnormal sperm morphology; Fig. 31-4)

Teratozoospermia refers to increased numbers of abnormal spermatozoa in the ejaculate. Total sperm count, sperm motility, and seminal fluid may be normal or abnormal, depending on the underlying cause. Morphologic defects of spermatozoa are classified as primary or secondary (see page 937). Primary abnormalities are believed to represent abnormalities in spermatogenesis (i.e., within the testes), whereas secondary abnormalities are nonspecific and may arise during transit through the duct system (i.e., within the epididymis), during handling of the semen or preparation of seminal smears, or following infection, trauma, or fever (Johnston, 1991). Normal males generally have greater than 70% morphologically normal spermatozoa. Primary abnormalities should constitute less than 10% and secondary abnormalities less than 20% of sperm in the normal dog. Positive correlations between percentage of morphologically normal spermatozoa and fertility rate and total number of morphologically normal spermatozoa and pregnancy rate have been demonstrated in the dog (Oettlé, 1993; Mickelsen et al, 1993). Using 60% normal sperm morphology as the cutoff point between normal and subnormal, fertility was 61% in a group of 23 normal dogs, compared with 13% in a group of 15 subnormal dogs (Oettlé, 1993). Based on these findings, morphologic defects affecting more than 40% of total spermatozoa should be considered a significant and worrisome finding, especially in an infertile dog. There are few descriptions of the effect of specific morphologic defects on fertility. Specific morphologic defects associated with infertility in the dog include abnormalities of midpiece attachment or ultrastructure, microcephalic spermatozoa,

and proximal retained cytoplasmic droplets (Johnston et al, 2001).

Morphologic defects may result from environmental insults, drugs, systemic illness, infectious or immune-mediated orchitis, epididymitis, prostatitis, and congenital defects in spermatogenesis. The only well-defined congenital cause is fucosidosis, a lysosomal storage disease affecting function of epididymal epithelial cells and causing a retention of cytoplasmic droplets (Taylor et al, 1989). Improper handling of the semen, abnormalities induced during preparation of the seminal smear, and sexual inactivity should be considered when a predominance of secondary morphologic defects are identified on semen analysis (Johnson et al, 1991). Several ejaculates should always be evaluated before embarking on an extensive diagnostic evaluation. If morphologic defects persist and there is nothing in the history or physical examination to suggest a cause, a CBC, serum biochemistry panel, and urinalysis should be performed to screen for systemic disorders. The testes, epididymides, and prostate gland should be evaluated with ultrasonography and any abnormalities pursued. Infection should be ruled out by culturing urine, semen, and, if present, prostatic cysts.

Although a testicular biopsy can be considered if the cause is still not identified, we prefer to sexually rest the dog and reevaluate in 2 months, hoping that teratozoospermia is transient. During this time, any factors that could potentially affect spermatogenesis should be minimized or eliminated from the dog's routine. If teratozoospermia has worsened at the 2-month reevaluation, a thorough review of the history and prior diagnostics should be done to identify diagnostics that may have been omitted in the previous evaluation and a complete physical examination performed to identify changes in the reproductive tract that may have occurred during the previous 2 months. If necessary, a testicular biopsy can be considered at this time. If the concentration of defective sperm has not worsened or is improving and no obvious changes in the reproductive tract are seen on physical examination, the dog should be reevaluated 2 and 4 months later.

Fertility of dogs with teratozoospermia depends on the type of morphologic defect and its effect on sperm function, the percentage of spermatozoa affected, and the total sperm count per ejaculate (Oettlé, 1993; Mickelsen et al, 1993). The dog may remain fertile despite morphologic defects if the number of healthy sperm per ejaculate is normal to high and good breeding management practices are followed (Wilson, 1993; Nöthling et al, 1995). Infertility is more likely if the morphologic defect interferes with sperm function, total sperm output is low, and good breeding practices are not used. A high incidence of a morphologic defect that deleteriously affects sperm function causes infertility regardless of the total sperm output per ejaculation (Plummer et al, 1987).

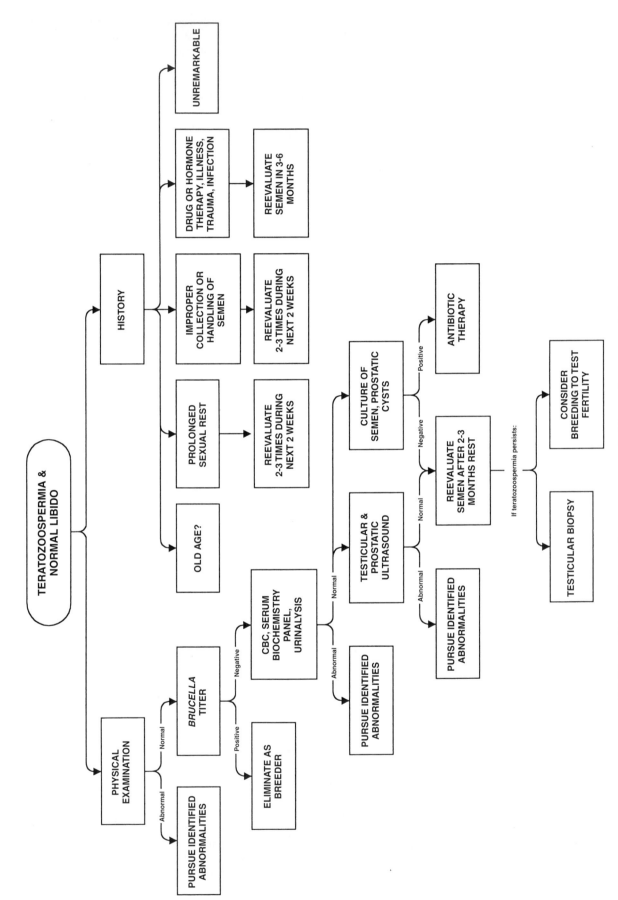

FIGURE 31-4. Diagnostic approach to teratozoospermia (abnormal sperm morphology).

Asthenozoospermia (decreased sperm motility; Fig. 31-5)

Asthenozoospermia refers to decreased motility of spermatozoa in an ejaculate. Progressive forward motility is considered normal movement for spermatozoa and is thought to reflect viability and ability to fertilize the ovum. A normal semen sample should have more than 70% of the spermatozoa exhibiting vigorous forward motility. Individual spermatozoa should be carefully assessed for type of movement. Spermatozoa that are moving in small circles or that have side-to-side motion without forward progression are not normal. It is unknown what percentage of sperm with abnormal motility results in canine infertility. Infertile men are categorized as having asthenozoospermia when normal sperm concentration is present but less than 25% of spermatozoa have normal motility (Meyers-

Wallen, 1991). It seems plausible that motility defects affecting more than 50% of total spermatozoa should be considered a significant finding, especially in an infertile dog.

Asthenozoospermia should be confirmed in several ejaculates before undertaking an extensive diagnostic evaluation. The first ejaculate from a dog following a prolonged period of sexual rest contains a greater percentage of old and dead sperm that has been stored in the epididymis. This results in a decreased percentage of actively motile sperm. Semen samples obtained on subsequent days should be closer to normal.

The most common cause for asthenozoospermia, especially when the remainder of the semen evaluation is unremarkable, is faulty semen collection technique or sample handling. The percentage of actively motile spermatozoa can be altered by exposure of the semen

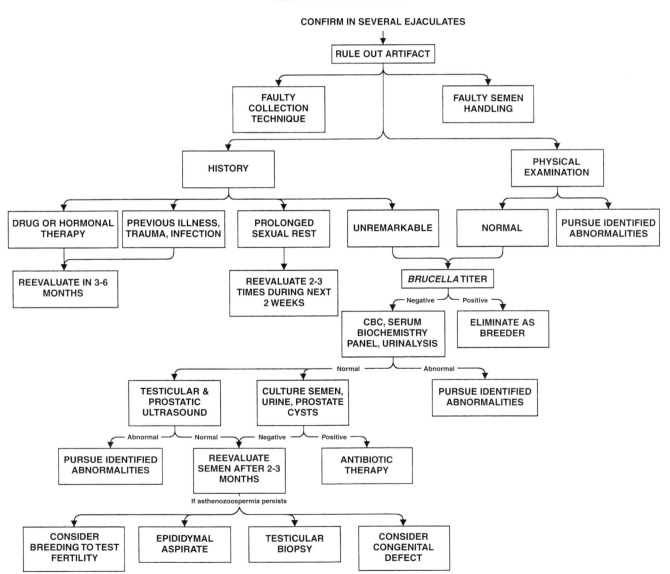

FIGURE 31-5. Diagnostic approach to asthenozoospermia (decreased sperm motility).

to latex artificial vagina liners, acidic diluents, water, urine, pus, blood, excessive lubricant, or extremes in temperature (<25° C and >40° C). The clinician must adhere to acceptable procedural techniques in the collection of semen to obtain reliable results (see page 932).

Persistent problems with sperm motility may reflect a problem in the testes, epididymides, or prostate. In general, causes for asthenozoospermia are similar to those for teratozoospermia. Asthenozoospermia may also result from primary sperm defects or enzyme deficiencies (Gagnon et al, 1982). The classic primary sperm defect is Kartagener's syndrome, an immotile cilia syndrome with an autosomal recessive mode of inheritance. In the dog, this syndrome is characterized by respiratory tract disease, male sterility, situs inversus, and hydrocephalus (Edwards et al, 1986). Spermatozoa are viable but immotile. The diagnosis of immotile cilia syndrome requires functional and ultra-structural analysis of cilia, including evaluation of tracheobronchial mucociliary clearance using nuclear scintigraphy, in vitro induction of ciliogenesis, and evaluation of cilia structure with transmission electron microscopy (Clercx et al, 2000).

Acquired disorders affecting sperm morphology (see above) can also affect sperm motility. Propulsion of spermatozoa requires normal function of the middle piece and tail. Defects in these structures affect motility. A decrease in sperm motility may be the first response to environmental insults, drugs, infection, inflammation, or any febrile disorder (Johnston, 1989). Abnormalities in sperm morphology or seminal fluid may provide clues to the cause. For example, head-to-head aggluti-nation of sperm may occur with *B. canis* infection (George and Carmichael, 1984), and this agglutination frequently results in abnormal motility. An abnor-mality affecting only the epididymis, however, can cause spermatozoal abnormalities without affecting other characteristics of semen (Amann, 1982).

If asthenozoospermia persists and nothing in the history, physical examination, or semen analysis suggests a cause, a CBC, serum biochemistry panel, and urinalysis should be performed to screen for systemic disorders. The testes, epididymides, and pro-state gland should be evaluated with ultrasonography and any abnormalities pursued. Infection should be ruled out by culturing urine, semen, and, if present, prostatic cysts.

If a cause is not identified, the dog should be sexually rested and reevaluated in 2 months. During this time, any factors that could affect sperm motility should be minimized or eliminated from the dog's routine. If asthenozoospermia has worsened at the 2-month reevaluation, a thorough review of the history and prior diagnostics, as well as a complete physical examination, should be done to identify anything that may have been omitted in the previous evaluation and to identify changes in the reproductive tract that may have occurred during the previous 2 months. If the severity of asthenozoospermia has not changed or is improving and no obvious changes in the repro-ductive tract are seen on physical examination, the dog should be reevaluated 2 and 4 months later. If asthenozoospermia remains mild and is the only abnormality identified on semen analysis, the dog may be able to sire litters provided good breeding management is practiced.

Abnormal seminal fluid

Abnormal seminal fluid may be grossly apparent at the time of semen collection or may become apparent during the microscopic examination. Gross abnor-malities in semen color and opacity are usually obvious. Dog semen is normally white to opalescent and opaque. Clear and colorless semen suggests azoo-spermia, which can be confirmed during the micro-scopic examination of the sample.

URINE.   Yellow discoloration is suggestive of conta-mination with urine. Occasional contamination prob-ably does not affect fertility, but persistent problems can affect fertility because urine is toxic to spermatozoa. A thorough evaluation of the lower urinary system, including urinalysis, urine culture, ultrasonography, contrast urethrocystography, and if possible, a urethral pressure profile study should be considered if urine contamination is a persistent problem. If dysfunction of the urethral sphincter is suspected, trial therapy with an alpha-adrenergic drug (e.g., phenylpropanolamine, pseudoephedrine) can be tried.

HEMOSPERMIA.   A red or brown tint in the semen suggests hemorrhage. Hemorrhage does not necessarily imply pathology, and mild hemospermia may not interfere with fertility. Hemospermia can occur in some males experiencing prolonged sexual anticipation before being allowed to copulate. In this condition, the blood is believed to arise from the prostate gland. Hemospermia can be prevented by minimizing expo-sure of the male to the bitch prior to breeding.

Persistent hemospermia may be caused by benign prostatic hyperplasia, prostatitis, prostatic neoplasia, coagulopathies, or lesions involving the urethra. The prostate gland should be evaluated digitally via the rectum and with ultrasonography. Abnormal tissue or prostatic cysts should be aspirated (see page 980) and samples submitted for cytology and culture. A CBC, urinalysis with culture, coagulation profile, and positive contrast urethrogram should also be considered. If available, visual inspection of the urethra can be done with a flexible urethroscope.

INFLAMMATION.   An occasional healthy inflamma-tory cell or bacteria are not uncommon in the semen of a healthy dog as a result of urethral contamination of the ejaculate. Large numbers of inflammatory cells or bacteria should always be considered worrisome, especially if they are a consistent finding. Grossly, the semen may appear normal or, with a severe inflam-matory process, may have a greenish tint, and clumps, clots, or flakes may be visible. Inflammation in the semen is usually a result of infectious prostatitis, infectious orchitis/epididymitis, or immune-mediated orchitis.

Infection should always be assumed, especially when the predominant inflammatory cell is the neutrophil. The diagnostic approach should be aimed at localizing the site of infection and isolating the offending organism(s). Appropriate serologic tests should be run for *B. canis.* The prostate gland, testes, and epididymides should be evaluated with ultrasonography, and identifiable prostatic cysts should be aspirated for cytology and culture. Urine and semen should also be submitted for culture. Culture for anaerobes, *Mycoplasma,* and *Ureaplasma* (see page 941) should be completed if an aerobic culture is negative. If all cultures are negative, trial therapy with a broad-spectrum bactericidal antibiotic may be considered and the dog reevaluated after 3 weeks of therapy. The possibility of immune-mediated orchitis/epididymitis should also be considered, especially if the predominant inflammatory cells identified in the semen are mononuclear. A diagnosis of immune-mediated orchitis is difficult to establish but should be suspected when a mononuclear inflammatory process is identified in the testis, cultures are consistently negative, and no improvement is seen after antibiotic therapy. A testicular biopsy for culture and histologic evaluation may be considered if the dog fails to respond to antibiotics and immune-mediated orchitis is suspected.

AGGLUTINATION. Agglutination of sperm is occasionally identified during the microscopic evaluation of semen. Agglutination of sperm is usually associated with infectious orchitis/epididymitis, most notably *B. canis* infection (George and Carmichael, 1984). Inflammation secondary to infection is believed to disrupt the blood-testis barrier, allowing spermatozoa to come in contact with the dog's immune system. Production of antisperm antibodies follows, and sperm agglutination results. In dogs infected with *B. canis,* seminal fluid containing primarily IgA had the highest sperm agglutination titers, but cytophilic factors causing adherence of sperm to macrophages also were present (George and Carmichael, 1984). Immune-mediated orchitis/epididymitis, as well as infections besides *B. canis,* should be considered when sperm agglutination is identified. In men, sperm agglutination can also be caused by amorphous material within semen and by proteins other than antibodies (Bronson et al, 1984).

Normal sperm count and seminal fluid

A dog labeled as infertile but with normal libido and normal semen analysis can be one of the more perplexing conditions to evaluate. In most cases, the dog is normal and the apparent infertility is a result of mistakes in breeding management or problems with the bitch. A thorough evaluation of breeding management and a critical assessment of the fertility of the bitch should be the first diagnostic steps. The reader is referred to Chapters 20 and 24 for detailed discussions of the more common breeding management problems and of assessment of fertility of the bitch, respectively.

Decreased spermatogenesis may occur with aging and keep the total sperm count per ejaculate consis-

tently around the lower end of the accepted normal range (i.e., 200×10^6 spermatozoa per ejaculate; see Oligospermia discussion above). Frequent ejaculation, especially in a dog with impaired spermatogenesis, can further reduce the sperm count. Subfertility may result. Improvement in fertility is possible with limited sexual use of such a dog to allow the epididymal storage pool of sperm to accumulate and with appropriate breeding management. Finally, ultrastructural or functional abnormalities of the sperm may exist that prevent fertilization of ova, despite viable and grossly normal-appearing sperm. Electron microscopy may identify ultrastructural abnormalities, but this is rarely performed. Tests to assess function of canine sperm are also not readily available, although these tests may become more accessible in the future (England and Plummer, 1993).

Congenital Infertility and Normal Libido

A dog that has never sired a litter despite numerous attempts should be considered congenitally infertile until proved otherwise. Acquired infertility is possible in these dogs if the insult occurred before the onset of sexual use. In addition to acquired causes, the clinician must also consider congenital defects that would not be considered in the previously proven stud dog with acquired infertility (see Table 31-1). The diagnostic approach to congenital infertility is similar to that for acquired infertility (see page 991), but with a greater concern for disorders of sexual development (e.g., XXY syndrome), anatomic defects (e.g., bilateral cryptorchidism, epididymal duct aplasia), and functional defects of spermatozoa (e.g., Kartagener's syndrome). A thorough history and physical examination are the cornerstones of a diagnostic evaluation for congenital infertility. The clinician should maintain a high index of suspicion for an intersex state. Chromosomal or developmental abnormalities of sexual differentiation that occur in phenotypically normal male dogs that are infertile include female pseudohermaphroditism and dogs with a 79, XXY karyotype or XX sex reversal (see page 893; Johnston et al, 2001). Subsequent diagnostics depend on the abnormalities identified during the initial evaluation of the dog. See the discussion on acquired infertility and normal libido for more detail.

TREATMENT OF INFERTILITY

Specific therapy depends on the underlying cause. Refer to the appropriate sections for management of such disorders as orchitis, epididymitis, prostatitis, and testicular neoplasia. It is important to remember that 55 to 70 days are required for spermatozoa to develop from spermatogonia and to appear in the ejaculate. Any therapy that is expected to increase the sperm count must be given for at least 3 months before its effectiveness can be critically evaluated. In addition, sexual rest becomes an important adjunct therapy for many infertility problems and may be all that is required following transient insults to the seminiferous tubules. Stress, sexual overuse, thermal damage, and some drugs are potentially transient problems, given enough time. Oligospermic and azoospermic dogs should always be reevaluated 3 to 6 months after initial examination before declaring a permanent spermatogenesis problem.

Idiopathic Testicular Degeneration

Idiopathic testicular degeneration is characterized by loss of function of the seminiferous tubules, with variable involvement of the Leydig cells (see page 974). Tubular cell degeneration is present with minimal inflammation. Libido may or may not be affected, although with time Leydig cells usually become sparse and libido decreases (see Fig. 31-3). Pituitary gland function is normal. Because of loss of the suppressive effects of inhibin, pituitary secretion of FSH is increased. Pituitary LH secretion may be normal or increased, depending on the status of the Leydig cells. Administration of gonadotropic hormones is ineffective in improving spermatogenesis because the target tissues (i.e., spermatogonia) are absent or nonresponsive. Administration of androgens is also ineffective in promoting spermatogenesis. Dogs with this problem do not respond to any known therapy. Sexual rest and reevaluation should be recommended to be sure a transient insult to the testes was not overlooked. The prognosis for return of fertility in these animals is grave.

Some oligospermic dogs have normal plasma FSH concentrations. This may represent an early stage of idiopathic testicular degeneration or a faulty feedback system between plasma inhibin and pituitary gonadotropin secretion. In theory, dogs with the latter problem may respond to GnRH injections or to antiestrogen agents that increase hypothalamic secretion of GnRH and therefore the pituitary secretion of LH and FSH, as well as the testicular production of testosterone. Examples of antiestrogenic agents used to treat oligospermia in humans include clomiphene citrate and tamoxifen (Howards, 1995). Although many uncontrolled studies report improvement in semen quality and pregnancy rate after use of antiestrogenic agents in humans, most controlled studies have found no evidence that treatment with these agents is effective in improving oligospermia or fertility (Sokol et al, 1988; WHO, 1992). Similar studies in the dog are lacking.

Testolactone is an aromatase inhibitor that prevents the conversion of testosterone to estradiol (Howards, 1995). Testolactone has been used to treat idiopathic oligospermia in men with variable results. Improvement in sperm concentration and fertility has been reported by some investigators (Vigersky and Glass, 1981), whereas others have found no effect of testolactone on semen quality or fertility (Clark and Sherins, 1989). Similar studies in the dog are lacking.

Mesterolone is a synthetic androgen used in Europe to treat idiopathic infertility in men. Unfortunately, a World Health Organization–sponsored double-blind study in men found no significant difference in pregnancy rates between placebo-treated and mesterolone-treated groups (WHO, 1989). Mesterolone has been shown to improve seminal characteristics in three healthy dogs and one dog with oligospermia (England and Allen, 1991). The three healthy dogs showed a significant increase in total sperm output beginning 3 weeks after 4 weeks of mesterolone administration (0.75 mg/kg q12h). When mesterolone (1.5 mg/kg q12h) was administered for 8 weeks to an oligospermic dog, a significant decrease in total sperm output but an increase in the percentage of live staining spermatozoa was seen. Unfortunately, drug therapy to improve spermatogenesis is usually ineffective; in those in which it is effective, it is unclear whether therapy or time played the major role in improving seminal characteristics.

Lymphocytic Orchitis

Lymphocytic orchitis is characterized by lymphocytic inflammation in the testes. The immune-mediated attack may be triggered following damage to the blood-testis barrier from trauma, infection, inflammation, and the like or may occur spontaneously in dogs with an underlying genetic predisposition (see page 973). Because of the progressive nature of this condition, the prognosis for return of fertility is poor. Because of the genetic implications in dogs with apparent spontaneous lymphocytic orchitis, attempts at therapy are probably not indicated.

Immunosuppressive dosages of glucocorticoids (e.g., prednisone, 2 to 4 mg/kg/day, divided BID initially) are used in an attempt to control the immune reaction. Unfortunately, prolonged or excessive dosages of glucocorticoids, which are frequently required for the management of this disorder, adversely affect spermatogenesis and lead to infertility. Therefore the clinician must attempt to control the immune reaction by using the smallest dose of glucocorticoid given as infrequently as possible to minimize the adverse effects of the therapy. This is rarely possible because controlling the immune-mediated orchitis usually requires large dosages of glucocorticoids, which in turn promote infertility. The effectiveness of other immunosuppressive agents (e.g., azathioprine, 2 mg/kg/day) that are less likely to adversely affect the reproductive tract has yet to be evaluated.

Retrograde Ejaculation

Small numbers of spermatozoa flow retrogradely into the urinary bladder during ejaculation in healthy dogs (Dooley et al, 1990). Failure of the internal urethral sphincter to contract fully during ejaculation may allow an excessive percentage of ejaculated spermatozoa to enter the bladder instead of exiting the penis (see page 995). This results in oligospermia or, less commonly, azoospermia in a dog with normal libido and mating behavior (Post et al, 1992; Root et al, 1994). This condition can be congenital or acquired. A diagnosis requires demonstrating the presence of large numbers of spermatozoa in the urinary bladder following ejaculation versus the number prior to ejaculation. Therapy for retrograde ejaculation involves the administration of alpha-agonist sympathomimetic drugs (e.g., pseudoephedrine, phenylpropanolamine) that contract the internal urethral sphincter and force antegrade ejaculation. Retrograde ejaculation was reversed in 1 dog following the administration of pseudoephedrine at a dosage of 4 mg/kg per os given 1 and 3 hours before semen collection and breeding; the inseminated bitch became pregnant and whelped 5 puppies (Post et al, 1994). The alpha-agonist sympathomimetic drug must be administered before every ejaculation to be effective in promoting antegrade flow of semen.

Leydig Cell Failure and Loss of Libido

Functional loss of the Leydig cells results in decreased serum testosterone concentrations, increased plasma LH concentrations, loss of libido, and variable degrees of impaired spermatogenesis. Suppression or loss of Leydig cells usually occurs in conjunction with disruption of spermatogenesis and is usually caused by a hormonal abnormality, infection, inflammation, neoplasia, or testicular degeneration. Primary testicular disorders affecting only the Leydig cells without affecting the seminiferous tubules are rare.

Treatment to improve libido must be done with caution because of the potential deleterious effects on spermatogenesis. Androgens have historically been used to improve libido. Normally, concentrations of testosterone are 50 to 100 times greater within the testes than in the plasma (Olson, 1984). To obtain these testicular concentrations, large doses of testosterone must be given. One protocol involves the oral administration of methyltestosterone, 0.1 mg/kg daily for 3 months, followed by reevaluation of a semen sample. Although administration of testosterone may improve libido, it is relatively ineffective in promoting spermatogenesis and may, in fact, have a significant deleterious impact on semen quality presumably secondary to its suppressive influence on GnRH and FSH secretion. In one study, a single subcutaneous injection of 5 mg of mixed testosterone esters per kg body weight to healthy dogs produced a significant decline in semen quality, including an increase in the number of primary sperm abnormalities 3 weeks after treatment; the abnormalities persisted for 3 months (England, 1997). Use of excessive dosages of androgens may also cause aggressive behavior and hepatopathy, as well as suppression of the hypothalamic-pituitary-testicular axis. In our experience, androgen therapy has been disappointing when overall fertility of the dog is considered.

Synthetic androgens that are capable of stimulating seminiferous tissue function without inhibiting the hypothalamic-pituitary-testicular axis have been used in human males with oligospermia, androgen deficiency, and infertility. Mesterolone lacks the hepatotoxic side effects commonly associated with other orally active androgens. An increase in sperm motility and concentration has been seen in approximately 30% of patients with oligospermia following administration of this androgen. In humans, the dose is 25 to 75 mg orally per day. One study in the dog used a dosage of 0.75 to 1.5 mg/kg q12h (see page 1002; England and Allen, 1991). Fluoxymesterone has also been successful in improving semen volume and sperm motility in a small percentage of oligospermic males. Currently no reports in the literature deal with the use of these synthetic androgens in dogs.

Hypogonadotropic Hypogonadism

In men, hypogonadotropic hypogonadism results from a congenital or acquired deficiency of GnRH. Acquired causes include defective biosynthesis or secretion of GnRH, infiltrative and space-occupying lesions, granulomatous disease, and lymphocytic hypophysitis (Nachtigall et al, 1997). Depending on the underlying etiology, treatment with GnRH may reverse the hypogonadism and restore fertility in affected men. GnRH deficiency causing infertility has not been reported in the dog. Anecdotal reports of pituitary disease causing impaired secretion of FSH and LH, decreased libido, impaired spermatogenesis, and testicular hypoplasia are found in the veterinary literature, but documentation is lacking. In theory, a congenital malformation of the pituitary gland can affect FSH and LH secretion. However, lack of other pituitary hormones (e.g., growth hormone, thyrotropin) play a more dominant role in the clinical presentation of affected dogs (see page 48). Similarly, acquired dysfunction of the pituitary secondary to trauma, infiltrative disease, or neoplasia can cause a deficiency of FSH and LH secretion, but clinical signs caused by an excess (e.g., ACTH) or deficiency (e.g., vasopressin) of other pituitary hormones or development of clinical signs caused by hypothalamic and thalamic dysfunction (see Pituitary Macrotumor Syndrome, page 296) dominate the clinical picture.

Infertility caused by loss of pituitary gonadotrophic cells should be suspected in dogs with decreased circulating concentrations of FSH, LH, and testosterone, decreased libido, testicular hypoplasia, and presence of Leydig cells, inactive seminiferous tubules, and minimal to no inflammation on biopsy of the testis. Drugs and concurrent disorders causing suppression of gonadotroph function (e.g., glucocorticoids, hypothyroidism) should be ruled out. Depending on the age of the dog, a developmental defect, trauma, or neoplasia involving the pituitary gland should be suspected (Olson et al, 1992). A complete diagnostic evaluation of the pituitary gland is warranted to identify the cause and formulate a therapeutic plan. The prognosis for the dog depends on the underlying cause.

Successful treatment of infertility caused by primary pituitary deficiency of FSH and LH has not been

documented in the dog. Recommendations for gonadotropin replacement therapy are in the veterinary literature, but documentation of their efficacy is lacking.
Therapy must be designed to stimulate libido and
spermatogenesis. Unfortunately, it is difficult to mimic
the normal pulsatile secretion of the pituitary gonadotropins with periodic injections of gonadotropins, and
the efficacy of such therapy is debatable. Administration of GnRH, 1 to 2 µg/kg SC, 2 to 3 hours prior to
attempted breeding may increase libido (Purswell, 1994).
Human chorionic gonadotropin, 500 IU biweekly SC,
may be given to stimulate Leydig cell function. Oral
methyltestosterone may be used to stimulate libido
but may prove ineffective in enhancing spermatogenesis for reasons discussed in the previous section.
The synthetic androgen mesterolone may prove more
reliable in stimulating libido and spermatogenesis.
Exogenous FSH injections at a dosage of 25 mg SC
once weekly (Larsen and Johnston, 1980) or 1 mg/kg
body weight IM every other day (Burke, 1983) have been
recommended to promote spermatogenesis. Equine
chorionic gonadotropin (eCG) has FSH properties
and has also been recommended for stimulation of
spermatogenesis. The recommended dosage is 20 IU/kg
body weight SC three times weekly. Use of GnRH injections should not be effective in stimulating endogenous
FSH and LH secretion in a dog with primary pituitary
deficiency of FSH and LH but may be effective if the
dysfunction is in the hypothalamus rather than the
pituitary gland. Hormonal therapy must be continued
for at least 3 months before an assessment of the effectiveness of these injections can be made. The prognosis
for return of fertility in these dogs is guarded.

REFERENCES

Amann RP: Use of animal models for detecting specific alterations in reproduction. Fund Appl Toxicol 2:13, 1982.
Bronson R, et al: Sperm antibodies: Their role in infertility. Fertil Steril 42:171, 1984.
Burke TJ: Reproductive disorders. In Ettinger SJ (ed): Textbook of Veterinary Internal Medicine, 2nd ed. Philadelphia, WB Saunders Co, 1983, p 1711.
Clark RV, Sherins RJ: Treatment of men with idiopathic oligozoospermic infertility using the aromatase inhibitor, testolactone: Results of a double-blinded, randomized, placebo-controlled trial with crossover. J Androl 10:240, 1989.
Clercx C, et al: Use of ciliogenesis in the diagnosis of primary ciliary dyskinesia in a dog. J Am Vet Med Assoc 217:1681, 2000.
Dooley MP, et al: Retrograde flow of spermatozoa into the urinary bladder of dogs during ejaculation or after sedation with xylazine. Am J Vet Res 51:1574, 1990.
Edwards DF, et al: Immotile cilia syndrome—Primary cilia dyskinesia in the dog. Proceedings of the American College of Veterinary Internal Medicine, Washington, DC, 1986, p 1389.
England GCW: Effect of progestogens and androgens upon spermatogenesis and steroidogenesis in dogs. J Repro Fertil Suppl 31:123, 1997.
England GCW, Allen WE: Effect of the synthetic androgen mesterolone upon seminal characteristics of dogs. J Small Anim Pract 32:271, 1991.
England GCW, Plummer JM: Hypo-osmotic swelling of dog spermatozoa. J Reprod Fert Suppl 47:261, 1993.
Frenette MD, et al: Effect of flushing the vasa deferentia at the time of vasectomy on the rate of clearance of spermatozoa from the ejaculate of dogs and cats. Am J Vet Res 47: 463, 1986.
Freshman JL: Clinical management of the subfertile stud dog. Vet Clin North Am 31:259, 2001.
Gagnon D, et al: Deficiency of protein carboxyl methylase in immotile spermatozoa of infertile men. N Engl J Med 306:821, 1982.
Ganong WF: The gonads: Development and function of the reproductive system. In Ganong WF (ed): Review of Medical Physiology, 10th ed. Los Altos, CA, Lange Medical Publications, 1981, p 331.
George L, Carmichael L: Antisperm responses in male dogs with chronic Brucella canis infections. Am J Vet Res 45:274, 1984.
Howards SS: Treatment of male infertility. N Engl J Med 332:312, 1995.
Johnson C, et al: Diagnosis and control of Brucella canis in kennel situations. Morphology-stain induced spermatozoal abnormalities. Proceedings of the Society for Theriogenology, San Diego, CA, August 16–17, 1991, p 236.
Johnston SD: New canine semen evaluation techniques for the small animal practitioner. Proceedings of the Society for Theriogenology, Coeur d'Alene, Idaho, September 29–30, 1989, p 320.
Johnston SD: Performing a complete canine semen evaluation in a small animal hospital. Vet Clin North Am 21:545, 1991.
Johnston SD, Root Kustritz MV, Olson PNS: Clinical approach to infertility in the male dog. In Johnston SD, Root Kustritz MV, Olson PNS (eds): Canine and Feline Theriogenology. Philadelphia, WB Saunders Co, 2001, p. 371.
Keenan LRJ: The infertile male. In Simpson GM, England GCW, Harvey M (eds): BSAVA Manual of Small Animal Reproduction and Neonatology. Cheltenham, British Small Animal Veterinary Association, 1998, p 83.
Larsen RE, Johnston SD: Management of canine infertility. In Kirk RW (ed): Current Veterinary Therapy VII. Philadelphia, WB Saunders Co, 1980, p 1226.
Meyers-Wallen VN: Clinical approach to infertile male dogs with sperm in the ejaculate. Vet Clin North Am 21:609, 1991.
Mickelsen WD: Maximizing fertility in stud dogs with poor semen quality. Proceedings of the Society for Theriogenology, San Diego, CA, August 16–17, 1991, p 244.
Mickelsen WD, et al: The relationship of semen quality to pregnancy rate and litter size following artificial insemination in the bitch. Theriogenology 39:553, 1993.
Nachtigall LB: Adult-onset idiopathic hypogonadotropic hypogonadism—A treatable form of male infertility. N Engl J Med 336:410, 1997.
Nie GJ, et al: Theriogenology question of the month. J Am Vet Med Assoc 212:1545, 1998.
Nöthling JO, et al: Success with intravaginal insemination of frozen-thawed dog semen—A retrospective study. J South African Vet Assoc 66:49, 1995.
Oettlé EE: Sperm morphology and fertility in the dog. J Reprod Fertil 47(Suppl):257, 1993.
Olar TT, et al: Relationships among testicular size, daily production and output of spermatozoa, and extragonadal spermatozoal reserves of the dog. Biol Reprod 29:1114, 1983.
Olson PN: Clinical approach to infertility in the stud dog. Proceedings of the Society for Theriogenology, Denver, CO, 1984, p 33.
Olson PN: Clinical approach for evaluating dogs with azoospermia or aspermia. Vet Clin North Am 21:591, 1991.
Olson PN, et al: Clinical and laboratory findings associated with actual or suspected azoospermia in dogs: 18 cases (1979–1990). JAVMA 201:478, 1992.
Plummer JM, et al: A spermatozoal midpiece abnormality associated with infertility in a Lhasa Apso dog. J Small Anim Pract 28:743, 1987.
Post K, et al: Retrograde ejaculation in a Shetland sheepdog. Can Vet J 33:53, 1992.
Purswell BJ: Pharmaceuticals used in canine reproduction. Semin Vet Med Surg 9: 54, 1994.
Rivier C, Rivest S: Effect of stress on the activity of the hypothalamic-pituitary-gonadal axis: Peripheral and central mechanisms. Biol Reprod 45:523, 1991.
Root MV, et al: Concurrent retrograde ejaculation and hypothyroidism in a dog: case report. Theriogenology 41:593, 1994.
Soderberg SF: Infertility in the male dog. In Morrow DA (ed): Current Therapy in Theriogenology, 2nd ed. Philadelphia, WB Saunders Co, 1986, p 544.
Sokol RZ, et al: A controlled comparison of the efficacy of clomiphene citrate in male infertility. Fertil Steril 49:865, 1988.
Taylor RM, et al: Reproduction abnormalities in canine fucosidosis. J Comp Pathol 100:369, 1989.
Vigersky RA, Glass AR: Effects of delta 1testolactone on the pituitary-testicular axis in oligospermic men. J Clin Endocrinol Metab 52:897, 1981.
Wilson MS: Non-surgical intrauterine artificial insemination in bitches using frozen semen. J Reprod Fert Suppl 47:307, 1993.
World Health Organization Task Force on the Diagnosis and Treatment of Infertility: Mesterolone and idiopathic male infertility: A double-blind study. Int J Androl 12:254, 1989.
World Health Organization: A double-blind trial of clomiphene citrate for the treatment of idiopathic male infertility. Int J Androl 15:299, 1992.

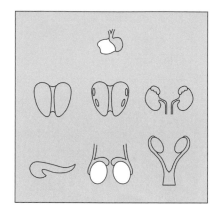

32

ARTIFICIAL INSEMINATION, FRESH EXTENDED SEMEN, AND FROZEN SEMEN

The manual collection and subsequent deposition of semen into the vaginal vault of a bitch in estrus (standing heat) is a common procedure used by breeders and veterinarians. As a result, artificial insemination (AI) is frequently requested by the dog owner or handler. Fresh undiluted semen, semen mixed with an extender, or frozen semen is used in dogs. The chances of success are enhanced if the veterinarian has a good understanding of the estrus cycle, semen collection, and AI techniques, as well as potential pitfalls.

INDICATIONS FOR ARTIFICIAL INSEMINATION

There are several situations in which AI may be used. The most obvious reason for AI is a perceived inability of the male and female to breed. For the bitch, this situation may involve problems such as vaginal strictures, conformational defects, rear leg weakness, psychological problems, and pain. AI is also used to ensure insemination early in estrus in a bitch with infertility of unknown cause. For the male, weakness, arthritis, back pain, premature ejaculation, and conformational defects that prevent intromission or a "tie" may prevent natural mating. AI may also be chosen because of a major size difference between the mates. Psychological problems (i.e., shyness, inexperience, dislike of the partner, previous breeding difficulties) may also result in the need for AI.

Some owners wish to use AI to avoid any possible venereal contact between their dog and its mate, thereby controlling the spread of potentially infectious diseases. This is not sound reasoning when the concern is the transmission of infectious agents from the dog to the bitch. Inseminating semen into the vagina still provides intimate contact between bitch and stud dog. Any infectious agent that could be transmitted from the dog to the bitch during natural

mating also has the potential to be transmitted during AI. However, AI does avoid transmission of infectious agents from the bitch to the stud dog. All breeding dogs and bitches should be free of *Brucella* infection, as determined by appropriate tests (see Chapter 26).

Some male dogs (particularly Doberman Pinschers) experience prostatic bleeding and hemospermia after exposure to a bitch "in heat" (estrus; see page 1000). The bleeding may be associated with von Willebrand's disease (VWD) but has also been observed in dogs not afflicted with VWD. Regardless, AI can be performed without any contact between stud dog and bitch, occasionally avoiding this problem.

Fresh extended and frozen forms of semen are being used with increasing frequency. Because semen collection is the difficult task, insemination of extended or previously frozen semen remains a relatively simple procedure. The shipment and use of fresh extended or frozen semen helps defray the cost and removes the hazards associated with shipping the female.

ARTIFICIAL INSEMINATION USING FRESH SEMEN

Collection of Semen

Semen is usually collected in an artificial vagina. We cut off and use one end of a sterilized, soft rubber, cone-shaped bovine artificial vagina. To this is attached a 12 to 15 ml plastic tube (Fig. 32-1; also see Fig. 27-3, page 934). The wide-mouth end of the cone is folded over and sealed with rubber cement to make a smooth, nonabrasive edge. A small amount of nonspermicidal lubricating jelly is applied to the inner surface of the rubber cone. This is the only surface that makes penile contact.

The most difficult task in AI is stimulating the male to ejaculate. Once this has been accomplished, the

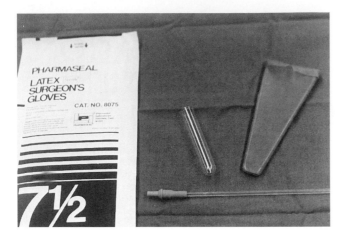

FIGURE 32-1. Artificial insemination equipment: sterile gloves, sterile soft rubber artificial vagina, sterile plastic tube that fits into the rubber vagina, and soft flexible plastic catheter for insemination.

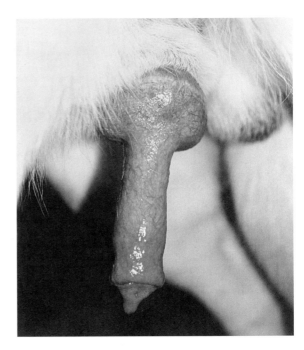

FIGURE 32-2. Erect penis of a dog with an engorged bulbus glandis and prepuce pulled posterior to the bulbus glandis.

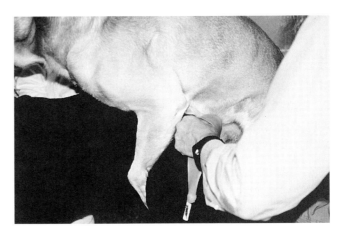

FIGURE 32-3. Collector holding erect penis during initial part of collection procedure.

balance of the procedure is quite simple. With most stud dogs, semen can be collected in a clean, quiet room with a nonslippery floor. A bitch is not often needed. However, for experienced males accustomed to natural breeding, a bitch in heat makes collecting semen easier and may improve the quality of the semen sample collected. Application of a topical pheromone preparation (Eau d'Estrus; Synbiotics, Malvern, PA) to a nonestrual bitch may also help. With the owner holding the stud dog to minimize movement and to protect the collector, the penis and bulbus glandis are gently massaged within the penile sheath. When the bulbus glandis begins to enlarge, the sheath is slipped posteriorly, and the penis with the bulbus glandis is exteriorized (Fig. 32-2). Failure to exteriorize both the penis and the bulbus glandis from the sheath usually results in an incomplete erection and failure to ejaculate or incomplete ejaculation, presumably due to pain.

Once the penis and bulbus glandis have been extruded from the sheath, the collector firmly holds onto the base of the penis, proximal to the bulbus glandis (Fig. 32-3). The thumb and index finger are used, providing both massaging movements and downward pressure around the base of the bulbus glandis. During or immediately after an erection has been achieved, aggressive pelvic thrusting movements by the stud dog, which accompany the onset of ejaculation, may make it difficult to place the artificial vagina over the penis. Fortunately, pelvic thrusting is typically short-lived (5 to 30 seconds), the initial phase of the ejaculate consists primarily of sperm-free prostatic fluid, and the sperm-rich second fraction of the ejaculate usually begins as the pelvic thrusting begins to subside. Therefore there should be no alarm over failure to collect ejaculate produced at the beginning of pelvic thrusting. Immediately after pelvic thrusting stops, many males try to "step over" the collector's arm, as if dismounting the bitch. The col-

lector should simply allow this movement by the male, which results in a 180-degree rotation of the engorged penis such that it is protruding caudally between the rear legs (Fig. 32-4). Digital pressure should be maintained on the bulbus glandis and collection continued until the ejaculate becomes clear (see Fig. 27-4, page 934).

Semen is usually collected for 2 to 5 minutes. This represents the typical duration of the second (sperm-rich) phase of ejaculation. The clear plastic tube should already have been connected to the rubber artificial vagina, and the apparatus can be held under the collector's arm during the initial stimulation period to provide some warmth. Canine semen is relatively resistant to cold shock, which alleviates the need for

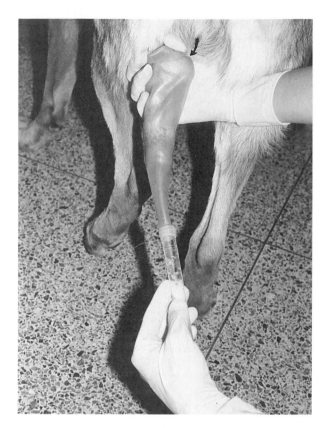

FIGURE 32-4. After completion of vigorous pelvic thrusting, the dog typically steps over the collector's arm, resulting in a 180-degree rotation of the penis such that the penis is now positioned caudally. Notice the collector's thumb and index finger, which continue to apply pressure to the proximal part of the engorged bulbus glandis to maintain the erection (*arrow*). (Courtesy A. Davidson, Davis, CA.)

warm water baths or incubators for holding semen. Use of a clear plastic collection tube allows visualization of the semen. One hand is kept over the plastic to avoid excessive light exposure. As long as the ejaculate is obviously whitish or creamy and cloudy (normal and sperm rich), the ejaculate continues to be collected. When the ejaculate becomes clear (sperm free), collection can be discontinued. If the collector is not certain when the male has stopped ejaculating the sperm-rich fraction, collection should be stopped after 5 minutes. Continued collection only dilutes the sperm with the third-phase clear, sperm-free prostatic fluid, resulting in cumbersome fluid volumes.

Collection of the third fraction of the ejaculate is not necessary for successful insemination. Enough of the third fraction should be collected to yield a final semen volume that is adequate for insemination. What constitutes adequate semen volume depends on the size of the bitch to be inseminated. The larger the bitch, the more semen is required for insemination. Adequate semen volume ranges from 2 to 10 ml, with bitches under 10 kg usually requiring 3 ml of semen or less and bitches over 20 kg requiring 5 ml of semen or more. The collection system containing sperm-rich

semen can be exchanged for a clean system if there is any need to evaluate the prostatic fluid.

The bitch should be inseminated within 5 to 10 minutes of collection of the semen. After collection, the male can be taken out of the room to avoid distractions. Prior to insemination, the color and consistency of the semen should be noted and a small drop placed on a warm glass slide. This semen can be quickly evaluated microscopically to ensure that a normal number of live, progressively motile spermatozoa are present. During this time, the semen is kept warm by holding the tube in one's hand, which also minimizes exposure of semen to potentially harmful ultraviolet rays. Alternatively, a drop of semen can be evaluated by a technician while the remainder of the semen is placed in the insemination device. Abnormal color or consistency, oligospermia, or dead sperm should be identified before insemination, because the breeder may wish to use a different stud dog. If these problems are not recognized until after insemination, another stud dog cannot be used if the litter is to be registered with the American Kennel Club (AKC).

Insemination Procedure

Vaginal and uterine insemination techniques have been described for the bitch. For vaginal insemination, semen is deposited into the cranial vagina near the cervix with a long insemination pipette. This technique is typically done with insemination of fresh and chilled semen. For uterine insemination, semen is deposited directly into the uterus. This technique results in a higher pregnancy rate and larger litter size than vaginal insemination, presumably because a greater percentage of inseminated spermatozoa reach the uterotubal junction (Thomassen et al, 2000). Uterine insemination techniques require specialized equipment or surgery. Uterine insemination is recommended with frozen-thawed semen because of the decreased viability of previously frozen spermatozoa.

VAGINAL INSEMINATION USING A URINARY CATHETER OR INSEMINATION PIPETTE. Although a variety of "tools" are available for vaginal insemination, we routinely use a 12 ml syringe, flexible disposable male urinary catheter or rigid plastic insemination pipette (Synbiotics; Malvern, PA), and surgical gloves. The catheter or insemination pipette should be long enough to reach the cranial vagina, which can be estimated as half the length from the vulvar lips to the costal arch (Root Kustritz and Johnston, 2000). These items should be sterile. After the gloves have been put on, the semen sample is drawn into the syringe, the sterile catheter is attached, and the syringe is filled with an additional 1 to 3 ml of air. The bitch's rear end is elevated above her head during and immediately after completion of the insemination. Usually we have owners sit in a chair and place a drape over the lap, and then hold the rear legs of the bitch in the lap (Fig. 32-5). With a technician holding the tail to the side, a gloved, nonlubricated index finger (except in very

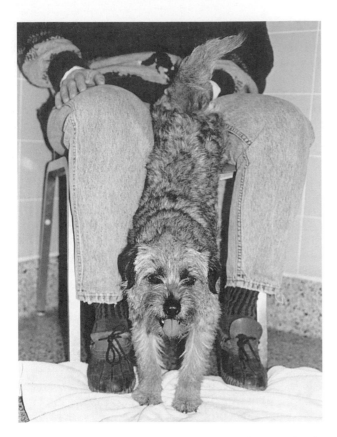

FIGURE 32-5. Owner sitting with rear quarters of bitch in her lap during insemination process to allow gravity to help move semen into uterus. The bitch is maintained in this position for 20 minutes after insemination.

small dogs) is placed into the vaginal vault, palm up. If a lubricant is used, it must be nonspermicidal. The catheter is slid over the top of the finger and passed into the vaginal vault, avoiding accidental catheterization of the urethra. Sliding the catheter over the index finger also aids in avoiding the clitoral fossa. The catheter follows the dorsal curvature of the vaginal vault. The catheter is inserted until resistance is met. The resistance indicates that the cranial end of the vaginal vault has been reached or that the catheter has simply become trapped within vaginal folds. The catheter should be gently advanced as far cranially as possible before the semen is deposited to ensure deposition of spermatozoa near the cervix. Blind cannulation of the cervix is difficult because of its relative inaccessibility and anatomy (Roszel, 1992).

When the syringe containing the semen has been emptied, it should be disconnected from the catheter, filled with a few more milliliters of air, reattached to the catheter, and emptied, thereby depositing any semen that may have remained in the catheter. Care should be taken to avoid injecting too much air into the vagina, as this may result in loss of semen out of the vulva once the procedure is complete.

Once the semen has been deposited, the catheter should be removed; the bitch's hindquarters should remain elevated above her head for a minimum of

20 minutes, aiding the movement of semen anteriorly in the reproductive tract and into the uterus. Insertion of a gloved finger and gentle stroking of the dorsal wall of the vagina (i.e., "feathering") during this time may stimulate muscular contractions within the reproductive tract, enhancing the movement of spermatozoa toward the ovaries. Unfortunately, no studies have evaluated the effectiveness or need for this procedure.

After the period for elevation of the hindquarters has been completed, the bitch should be kept quiet for an hour or so to minimize loss of semen out of the vagina. In addition, pressure should not be applied to the abdomen (e.g., lifting the dog up by the abdomen).

The entire insemination procedure is rarely a problem for the bitch; there should not be any pain or discomfort associated with it. The process is rather simple and is not time-consuming.

The only material reused is the rubber cone artificial vagina. Although gas-sterilized equipment is claimed to harm sperm, we have seen no problem with reused rubber cones. Perhaps this is because the cone is used primarily as a funnel and the semen is retained in the clear, new, disposable plastic tube.

VAGINAL INSEMINATION USING A SPECIAL BALLOON CATHETER. A specially designed balloon catheter (Osiris probe; I.M.V., l'Aigle, France) can be used to ensure movement of semen through the cervix and into the uterus. The catheter has two components, an outer sheath with the Foley bulb positioned at its tip and a second catheter with a side exit port that is inserted through the outer sheath. The catheter is inserted into the vagina up to the level of the cervix, and the bulb is inflated so that it forms a seal against the vaginal wall. The inner catheter is then advanced and the semen is deposited, after which the inner catheter is withdrawn inside the Foley catheter, thereby closing the side exit ports (England, 2000). The device is left in place for approximately 15 minutes to ensure that a pool of semen is located next to the cervix. During this time, the bitch's hindquarters should remain elevated above her head, which aids the movement of semen across the cervix and into the uterus. After the catheter has been removed and elevation of the hindquarters is complete, the bitch should be kept quiet for an hour or so to minimize loss of semen out of the vagina. In addition, pressure should not be applied to the abdomen (e.g., lifting the dog up by the abdomen).

TRANSCERVICAL UTERINE INSEMINATION. Transcervical catheterization and uterine insemination have been described. One method involves the use of a rigid catheter that is passed blindly through the vagina and cervix after digital fixation of the cervix through the abdominal wall (Andersen, 1980). A more commonly used method involves passage of a catheter through the cervix after endoscopic visualization of the external cervical os (see Fig. 32-7; Wilson, 1993). The endoscopic technique for transcervical uterine insemination is becoming increasingly popular, especially for insemination of frozen-thawed semen. A rigid or flexible endoscope, preferably with a mechanism for deflecting a catheter at the endoscope tip, is inserted into the vagina and advanced to the cervix. Inflation of the vagina improves identification of the cervical os. The insemination catheter is inserted through the endoscope, and the deflection device is used to direct the catheter into the cervical os. Sedation of the bitch may be required to minimize excessive movement during the procedure. After removal of the catheter and endoscope, the bitch's hindquarters should be elevated above her head for approximately 20 minutes to aid movement of semen toward the uterotubal junction and away from the cervix.

UTERINE INSEMINATION USING SURGERY. The body of the uterus is exposed through a caudal ventral midline incision into the abdominal cavity. A 22-gauge over-the-needle intravenous catheter is placed in the lumen of the uterine body, and the caudal portion of the uterine lumen is clamped to prevent semen from entering the vagina; the semen then is slowly infused into the uterine lumen and allowed to move proximally into the uterine horns. After removal of the catheter, digital pressure is applied to the site to promote hemostasis; sutures are not usually required (England, 2000). The abdominal incision is closed in a routine manner. The disadvantages of this technique include the need for general anesthesia, potential for morbidity secondary to the surgical technique, and the ethical limitation of only one insemination to try to establish a pregnancy. This technique should be considered only for insemination of frozen-thawed semen.

Success Rates for Artificial Insemination with Fresh Semen

The success of AI (i.e., pregnancy) depends on several variables, including the use of a fertile stud dog with normal semen, proper handling of the semen during collection and insemination, the fertility of the bitch, and the deposition of semen into the anterior vaginal vault of the bitch at the appropriate time of estrus. The importance of the timing factor cannot be over-emphasized. The determination of when to perform AI should always be based on a combination of the behavior of the bitch, sequential vaginal cytology, and plasma progesterone concentrations (using in-house enzyme-linked immunosorbent assay [ELISA] testing) and, if available, vaginal endoscopy (see Chapters 19 and 20). Evaluation of serial vaginal cytology and plasma progesterone concentrations, in conjunction with changes in the bitch's behavior, are easy, relatively inexpensive, and accurate methods for determining when the bitch should be inseminated.

Multiple inseminations, performed daily or every other day until diestrus is confirmed with vaginal cytology, should be done once the decision is made to perform AI. Because there is no way to predict exactly when ovulation has occurred, multiple inseminations increase the chance of conception by ensuring the presence of spermatozoa in the female tract both early and late in estrus.

Artificial insemination may be associated with lower conception rates and smaller litter sizes than would be achieved with natural breeding (Andersen, 1980; Linde-Forsberg and Forsberg, 1993). This is likely a result of several factors. During natural breeding, semen is pressure forced through the cervix into the uterus and oviducts, whereas in AI, the semen is placed posterior to the cervix. The erect penis virtually fills the vaginal vault, compressing the urethral opening, and the bulbus glandis prevents backward flow of semen. The large volume of ejaculate produced during the normally prolonged third phase is forced through the cervix because there is no other place for distribution. With natural breeding, uterine contractions may aid in semen transport. This is an unlikely event in most AI situations. Also in natural breeding, the duration of the tie may contribute to improved conception rates, because the male ejaculates during that entire period, producing a volume of semen too large for the vaginal vault.

Conception rates of 60% to 90% have been reported when AI with fresh semen is performed properly (Linde-Forsberg and Forsberg, 1993). Our results have been comparable with the vaginal technique described in depth above. Although deposition of fresh semen directly into the uterus may improve the conception rate, specialized equipment is required to ensure uterine placement of the semen. Placement of a catheter through the cervix is difficult because of its anatomic conformation. The conception rate was 76% in 17 bitches in which an intrauterine technique was used, comparable to results with vaginally deposited semen (Andersen, 1980). Use of an endoscope to assist with uterine insemination should improve conception rates, compared with older techniques, but the availability of this technique is currently limited.

ARTIFICIAL INSEMINATION WITH FRESH EXTENDED SEMEN

In 1986 the American Kennel Club began registering litters of puppies resulting from insemination with fresh extended semen. Semen that has been properly extended and chilled can be refrigerated for several days and still yield fertile sperm when warmed and inseminated. The extender helps keep the spermatozoal membranes from being harmed by changes in temperature or shaking during transport while also providing nutrients and stabilizing the pH, osmolality, and ionic strength of the medium (Linde-Forsberg, 1991). Common extenders for cold storage of fresh semen are outlined in Table 32-1 (Concannon and Battista, 1989; Johnston et al, 2001). After preparation, extender can be frozen in aliquots, with a shelf life of approximately 1 year (Held, 1997). In addition, proprietary canine semen extenders of unreported composition are available commercially (Synbiotics, San Diego, CA; International Canine Semen Bank,

TABLE 32–1 NAME AND COMPOSITION OF EXTENDERS REPORTED FOR 1 TO 4 DAYS' COLD STORAGE OF SPERM-RICH FRACTION OF CANINE SEMEN*

Citrate-bicarbonate–egg yolk extender
100 ml aqueous solution containing citric acid monohydrate (0.07 g), sodium bicarbonate (0.17 g), sodium citrate dihydrate (1.16 g), potassium chloride (0.03 g), glycine (0.75 g), glucose (0.24 g), egg yolk (20 ml); pH 6.8, 308 mOsm/kg (Province et al, 1984)

Citrate-dextrose-egg yolk extender
100 ml aqueous solution containing sodium citrate (1.45 g), dextrose (1.25 g) and egg yolk (250 ml) (Held, 1997)

Caprogen egg yolk extender
100 ml aqueous solution containing sodium citrate dihydrate (1.56 g), glycine (0.78 g), glucose (0.23 g), N-caproic acid (1.0 ml of 2.5% solution), catalase (1.0 ml of 45 mg/dl solution), egg yolk (20 ml); pH 7.0, 326 mOsm; bubbled with nitrogen gas immediately before use (Province et al, 1984)

TRIS-buffered egg yolk extender
100 ml aqueous solution containing 2.4 g TRIS base (THAM), 1.3 g citric acid monohydrate, 1 g fructose, 3.8 ml glycerol, 20% egg yolk (Gill et al, 1970)

Skim milk extender
Skim milk heated at 95° C for 10 min., then cooled; pH 6.5, 277 mOsm (Province et al, 1984)

Low-fat milk extender
Sterilized homogenized milk with 2% fat (Christiansen, 1984)

Cream–egg yolk extender
800 g cream (12% fat) and 200 g egg yolk (Linde-Forsberg, 1991)

Citrate–egg yolk extender
Sodium citrate, 2.9% solution (80%) and egg yolk (20%) (Christiansen, 1984)

From Concannon PW, Battista M: Canine semen freezing and artificial insemination. *In* Kirk RW (ed): Current Veterinary Therapy X. Philadelphia, WB Saunders Co, 1989, p 1248; Johnston SD, Root Kustritz MV, Olson PNS: Semen collection, evaluation, and preservation. *In*, Johnston SD, Root Kustritz MV, Olson PNS (eds): Canine and Feline Theriogenology. Philadelphia, WB Saunders Co, 2001, p. 287.
*Dilution rates used were 1 part semen to 3 to 10 parts extender at 23 to 35° C, with subsequent cooling to 5° C over a 2- to 3-hour period. Antibiotics typically added are 1000 IU penicillin and 1 mg dihydrostreptomycin per milliliter.

Sandy, OR; Camelot Farms, College Station, TX). Equine semen extenders may also be suitable for use in the dog (Paccamonti, 1997). Milk proteins protect against cold shock, and egg yolk protects acrosomal and mitochondrial membranes and protects against cold shock. A few drops of semen should be mixed with a small volume of the extender and evaluated for deleterious effects on sperm viability before the whole semen sample is mixed with the extender. Once extended, the semen is gradually cooled to 5° C over a period of 30 to 60 minutes and stored at this temperature. Rapid changes in temperature must be avoided. When prepared properly, chilled extended spermatozoa easily remain viable for 24 hours and, depending on the technique, may remain viable for as long as 5 days.

Short-term preservation of sperm allows overnight air delivery of freshly extended semen without the costs of frozen semen or shipment of the bitch. The ejaculate is extended, packaged in a small container, and shipped in a thermos-type container. The ejaculate should remain cold (approximately 5° C) during shipment and storage. Prior to insemination, the extended semen should be warmed slowly in a water bath at 37° C and once warmed, a sample should be evaluated under the microscope to ensure the presence of viable spermatozoa. The technique for insemination of the bitch with extended semen is as previously described for insemination with fresh semen. Vaginal insemination techniques are usually used, especially when the semen has been collected within 24 hours of insemination. Ideally, multiple inseminations beginning 3 to 4 days after the initial rise in the blood progesterone concentration should be completed to maximize the conception rate.

Conception rates for intravaginal insemination using fresh extended semen vary but generally average 50% to 80% (Farstad, 1984; Linde-Forsberg and Forsberg, 1989; Goodman and Cain, 1997; England, 2000). Conception rates for AI using fresh extended semen are higher than with frozen semen. With fresh extended semen, no damage to the sperm occurs from freezing, the cervix is less of a barrier, larger numbers of sperm are usually inseminated, fresh sperm live longer in the reproductive tract of the bitch, and the timing of inseminations is not as critical as with frozen semen.

ARTIFICIAL INSEMINATION WITH FROZEN SEMEN

Long-term preservation of semen using deep freezing techniques has been available for several years. The AKC approved the registration of litters resulting from insemination with frozen-thawed sperm in 1981. AKC approval is based on record-keeping practices as outlined in *Regulations Applying to the Registration of Litters Produced Through Artificial Insemination* (AKC form R198-1). Beginning in January 1999, the AKC required DNA identification of all male dogs from which semen is frozen. The DNA sample is retrieved from a cheek swab collected by the owner (Edwards et al, 1997). The number of freezing centers has increased considerably during the past decade, partly because of the emergence of proprietary companies (e.g., CLONE, Chester Springs, PA; International Canine Semen Bank, Sandy, OR; Synbiotics, San Diego, CA) that train and "license" semen freezers. Facilities that freeze canine semen must be approved by the AKC; this approval is not an indication of quality but instead verifies accurate record-keeping regarding semen collection and storage (Paccamonti, 1997).

The advantages of using frozen semen include wider dispersion of desirable genetic traits, disease prevention, decreased numbers of breeding males in a research colony, preservation of semen from dogs with diseases that are models of human disorders, and elimination of the need for shipping bitches. However, despite obvious advantages, AKC approval, and the relative access to necessary facilities, use of frozen semen has still not gained widespread use among breeders or veterinarians. This is partly because of the expense of shipping the male to the freezing facility, the expense of freezing and storing the semen, and the perceived low conception rate. Success in freezing, with resultant fertility, has been greatest with dairy cattle semen and worst with dog semen. Average pregnancy rates after AI with frozen semen in cattle and dogs have been 90% and 40% to 60%, respectively, of those obtained with natural breeding (Concannon and Battista, 1989; Linde-Forsberg and Forsberg, 1993). Differences among species in sperm shape, size, and biochemical makeup undoubtedly result in variability in the conditions required for successful freezing of sperm.

The techniques used in freezing semen have been reported (Smith, 1984; Concannon and Battista, 1989; England, 1993; Johnston et al, 2001). The steps involved in freezing semen for AI include semen collection, dilution in an extender, equilibration under refrigeration, freezing in convenient volumes, storage, thawing, and insemination of the bitch during the peak of her fertile period (Concannon and Battista, 1989). Semen extenders typically contain protective agents such as egg yolk, milk proteins, and bovine serum albumin that protect the sperm during cooling, freezing, and thawing and that control pH; cryoprotectants such as glycerol, ribose, and arabinose that reduce sperm cell damage during freezing and subsequent thawing; glycolyzable sugars such as glucose, fructose, and mannose for energy; and antibiotics to prevent growth of bacteria. A thorough semen evaluation should be performed on any dog whose semen is being considered for freezing (see page 932). Sperm are damaged during the cryopreservation process, and semen samples that are initially poor may be unusable after freeze/thawing. Freezing semen is an intricate process. Success is based on the viability of spermatozoa postthawing and requires a fine balance between the composition of the extender, the cooling rate, equilibration time, freezing rate, and thawing rate. The reader is referred to Smith (1987), Concannon and Battista (1989), and England (1993) for more details on semen cryoprecipitate techniques.

Semen can be frozen in pellets, glass ampules, or straws. Pellets are formed when cooled extended semen is deposited in 50 to 100 μl aliquots into depressions on solid dry ice and then stored in perforated nylon vials in liquid nitrogen (Concannon and Battista, 1989; Johnston et al, 2001). Polyvinylchloride (PVC) straws, 0.25 to 0.5 ml in volume, can be filled with cooled extended semen and an air bubble, plugged with cotton on one end and powdered PVC pyrrolidone on the other, and then frozen while suspended in liquid nitrogen vapor before the straw is plunged into the liquid nitrogen (Concannon and Battista, 1989; Held, 1997). The quality of canine semen samples after thawing may vary between those frozen as pellets and those frozen as straws (Battista et al, 1988). Variables such as the extender used also affect postthaw canine semen quality.

Frozen semen has been stored for as long as 9 years with little to no postthaw decrease in sperm motility. More than 4 years have been reported between semen collection and storage and thawing and conception. Thawing procedures and the number of straws or pellets used per insemination vary between facilities. Instructions in thawing usually accompany the semen and should be followed exactly. The thawing phase of the freeze-thaw process is as important to spermatozoa survival as the cooling process. At the time of insemination, a small drop of thawed semen should be evaluated microscopically for sperm viability and motility prior to the procedure.

The number of progressively motile spermatozoa at the time of insemination is the most important variable affecting the fertility rate (Nöthling et al, 1997). Maintenance of motility during incubation at 37° C after thawing is a major problem associated with canine sperm (Fig. 32-6). Motility can decline severely after only 30 to 60 minutes in the dog (Olar, 1984; Battista et al, 1988). In one study, motility was routinely less than 10% and often zero after 1 hour of incubation at 37° C (Olar, 1984). This may explain in part why depositing frozen-thawed semen in the cranial vagina generally results in a poorer conception rate than deposition of semen in the uterus (Linde-Forsberg and Forsberg, 1989; Fontbonne and Badinand, 1997).

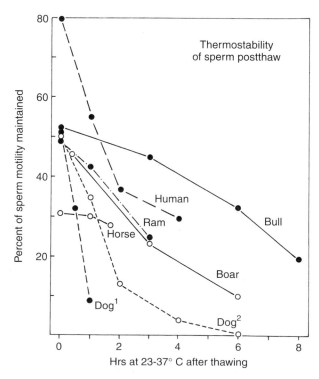

FIGURE 32-6. Typical sperm motility percentages for semen of several species, expressed as a percentage of total sperm after freezing and thawing, including semen from bulls, humans, rams, boars, and stallions during incubation at 37° C, and dog semen during incubation at (1) 37° C and (2) 23° C. (Adapted from Concannon PW, Battista M: In Kirk RW [ed]: Current Veterinary Therapy X. Philadelphia, WB Saunders, 1989, p 1247.)

The success rate for obtaining litters depends on the semen processing technique, the number of motile sperm per insemination, the site of insemination, the correct timing of the insemination, and the number of inseminations. The number of insemination doses of sperm in a single ejaculate varies with the quality of the semen and may range from one to 20 per ejaculate. The actual minimum insemination dose required to achieve pregnancy is not known. Historically, 100 to 200 × 10^6 sperm per insemination has been considered the minimum (Nöthling et al, 1997); however, pregnancy rates has high as 80% have been reported with multiple transcervical intrauterine inseminations of semen containing as little as 30 × 10^6 sperm per insemination (Wilson, 1993; Nöthling et al, 1995). Intrauterine insemination of spermatozoa requires fewer spermatozoa per insemination than intravaginal insemination.

Obtaining successful pregnancies and reasonable litter sizes with frozen-thawed semen depends greatly on inseminations being performed during the 2 to 3 days in which healthy, fertilizable ova reside in the oviducts of the bitch. In the bitch, the oocyte is ovulated in an immature state (primary oocyte) and cannot be fertilized immediately. Fertilization occurs after maturation of the primary oocyte, extrusion of the polar body, and completion of the first meiotic division. These events require at least 48 hours after ovulation. Fertilizable oocytes remain viable in the oviduct for a further 4 to 5 days. Fresh sperm can remain fertile in the bitch for at least 6 to 7 days. Frozen-thawed sperm die rapidly after being thawed and do not survive the long periods that fresh dog sperm do. As a consequence, AI with frozen-thawed semen should ideally be performed when all ova have been shed and are mature (i.e., 4 to 7 days after the luteinizing hormone [LH] peak). The initial increase in the serum progesterone concentration is often used as an estimate of the time of the LH peak when trying to determine the best time to inseminate the bitch. The fertile period is assumed to begin 4 days after the initial increase in the serum progesterone concentration. Once started, inseminations should be done every day or every other day for a minimum of three inseminations. Repeated inseminations with a moderate insemination dose results in a higher pregnancy rate than only one insemination with a large quantity of sperm (Fontbonne et al, 2000). The techniques for vaginal and uterine insemination of the bitch with frozen-thawed semen are as previously described for insemination with fresh semen.

In general, average pregnancy rates for fertile bitches intravaginally inseminated with frozen-thawed semen at the appropriate time is approximately 30% to 60%. Most commercial facilities claim a frozen semen fertility rate of 70% to 80% based on litters per bitch inseminated, or per bitch inseminated at the appropriate time and excluding mistimed inseminations performed primarily at the insistence of the owner (Concannon, 1991; Fontbonne et al, 2000; Thomassen et al, 2000). These high success rates are in contrast to published success rates of 0 to 60% when intravaginal insemination was used (Andersen, 1980; Smith, 1984; Fontbonne and Badinand, 1993). Properly timed intrauterine inseminations, using either surgical or transcervical deposition, have reported success rates of 45% to 85% (Smith, 1984; Farstad and Andersen-Berg, 1989; Linde-Forsberg and Forsberg, 1989 and 1993; Fontbonne and Badinand, 1993).

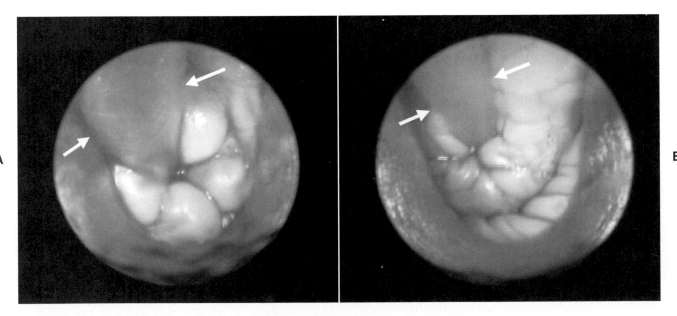

FIGURE 32-7. Transcervical insemination in a German Shepherd Dog (A) and a Labrador Retriever (B) utilizing a flexible catheter (*arrows*) and direct visualization of the cervix with a fiberoptic endoscope.

The poorer conception rates with intravaginal than with intrauterine insemination are probably related to the considerable decrease in spermatozoa motility and survival time after the freeze-thaw process, problems that probably impair sperm transport through the cervix. Insemination after cannulation of the cervix is preferable to deposition of the semen in the anterior vaginal vault. Cannulation of the cervix is difficult because of its relative inaccessibility (i.e., oblique orientation with the external cervical orifice directed toward the vaginal floor, occlusion of the anterior vagina by the prominent dorsal median vaginal fold, small vaginal lumen) and its anatomy (i.e., cervical folds; Fig. 32-7) (Concannon, 1991; Wilson, 1993). Nevertheless, cannulation can be accomplished with a flexible catheter under direct visualization with a fiberoptic endoscope or with a rigid cannula and fixation of the cervix by palpation per abdomen (Battista et al, 1988; Wilson, 1993).

REFERENCES

Andersen K: Artificial insemination and storage of canine semen. *In* Morrow DA (ed): Current Therapy in Theriogenology. Philadelphia, WB Saunders, 1980, p 661.

Battista M, et al: Canine sperm post-thaw survival following freezing in straws or pellets using pipes, lactose, tris or test extenders. Proceedings of the Eleventh International Congress on Animal Reproduction (Dublin) 3:229, 1988.

Concannon PW: Frozen semen artificial insemination in dogs. Proceedings, Society for Theriogenology, San Diego, 1991, p 247.

Concannon PW, Battista M: Canine semen freezing and artificial insemination. *In* Kirk RW (ed): Current Veterinary Therapy X. Philadelphia, WB Saunders, 1989, p 1247.

Edwards J, et al: DNA and the AKC. AKC Gazette 114:55, 1997.

England GCW: Cryopreservation of dog semen: A review. J Reprod Fertil Suppl 47:243, 1993.

England GCW: Semen evaluation, artificial insemination, and infertility in the male dog. *In* Ettinger SJ, Feldman EC (eds): Textbook of Veterinary Internal Medicine, 5th ed. Philadelphia, WB Saunders, 2000, p 1571.

Farstad W: Bitch fertility after natural mating and after artificial insemination with fresh or frozen semen. J Small Anim Pract 25:561, 1984.

Farstad W, Andersen-Berg K: Factors influencing the success rate of artificial insemination with frozen semen in the dog. J Reprod Fertil 39(Suppl):289, 1989.

Fontbonne A, Badinand F: Canine artificial insemination with frozen semen: Comparison of intravaginal and intrauterine deposition of semen. J Reprod Fertil Suppl 47:325, 1993.

Fontbonne A, et al: Artificial insemination with frozen semen in the bitch: Influence of progesterone level, inseminating dose and number of inseminations performed in the same bitch. Advances in Dog, Cat and Exotic Carnivore Reproduction: Book of Abstracts. The Fourth International Symposium on Canine and Feline Reproduction and the Second Congress of the European Veterinary Society for Small Animal Reproduction. Oslo, June 29-July 1, 2000, p 58.

Goodman MF, Cain JL: Retrospective evaluation of artificial insemination with chilled extended semen in the dog. J Reprod Fertil Suppl 51:554, 1997.

Held JJ: Critical evaluation of the success and role of chilled and frozen semen in today's veterinary practice. *In* Proceedings of the Canine Male Reproductive Symposium, Annual Meeting of the Society for Theriogenology, Montreal, September 17-20, 1997. Nashville, Society for Theriogenology, 1997, p 49.

Johnston SD, Root Kustritz MV, Olson PNS: Semen collection, evaluation, and preservation. *In* Johnston SD, Root Kustritz MV, Olson PNS (eds): Canine and Feline Theriogenology. Philadelphia, WB Saunders, 2001, p 287.

Linde-Forsberg C: Achieving canine pregnancy by using frozen or chilled extended semen. Vet Clin North Am 21:467, 1991.

Linde-Forsberg C, Forsberg M: Fertility in dogs in relation to semen quality and the time and site of insemination with fresh and frozen semen. J Reprod Fertil 39(Suppl):299, 1989.

Linde-Forsberg C, Forsberg M: Results of 527 controlled artificial inseminations in dogs. J Reprod Fertil Suppl 47:313, 1993.

Nöthling JO, et al: Success with intravaginal insemination of frozen-thawed dog semen: A retrospective study. J S Afr Vet Assoc 66:49, 1995.

Nöthling JO, et al: Semen quality after thawing: Correlation with fertility and fresh semen quality in dogs. J Reprod Fertil Suppl 51:109, 1997.

Olar TT: Cryopreservation of dog spermatozoa. Doctoral dissertation. Fort Collins, Colo, 1984, Colorado State University.

Paccamonti D: Technical aspects of using fresh cooled or frozen canine semen. *In* Proceedings of the Canine Male Reproductive Symposium, Annual Meeting of the Society for Theriogenology, Montreal, September 17-20, 1997. Nashville, Society for Theriogenology, 1997, p 81.

Root Kustritz MVR, Johnston SD: Artificial insemination in the bitch. *In* Bonagura JD (ed): Kirk's Current Veterinary Therapy XIII. Philadelphia, WB Saunders, 2000, p 916.

Roszel JF: Anatomy of the canine uterine cervix. Compend Contin Educ 14:751, 1992.

Smith FO: Update on freezing canine semen. Proceedings of the Annual Society for Theriogenology, Denver, 1984, p 61.

Smith FO: Cryopreservation of canine semen. Proceedings of the Society of Theriogenology, Austin, Texas, 1987, p 249.

Thomassen R, et al: Artificial insemination with frozen semen in the dog: Results from 1994 to 1998. Advances in Dog, Cat and Exotic Carnivore Reproduction: Book of Abstracts. The Fourth International Symposium on Canine and Feline Reproduction and the Second Congress of the European Veterinary Society for Small Animal Reproduction. Oslo, June 29-July 1, 2000, p 59.

Wilson MS: Nonsurgical intrauterine artificial insemination in bitches using frozen semen. J Reprod Fertil Suppl 47:307, 1993.

FELINE REPRODUCTION

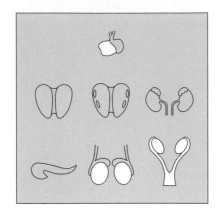

33

FELINE REPRODUCTION

THE QUEEN

ANATOMIC CONSIDERATIONS

The vulvar labia of the queen (female cat) are relatively nonresponsive to estrogen and thus remain small and covered with hair during proestrus and estrus, in contrast to the dramatic increase in size seen in bitches (female dogs). Also different from that in the bitch is the relatively straight horizontal anatomy of the vestibule of the vagina, the vagina, and the cervix of the queen. The vestibulovaginal junction is narrow and inelastic. Inspection of this area requires anesthesia and use of a rather small endoscope (3 mm) equipped with a device for insufflating the vaginal lumen (Shille and Sojka, 1995).

THE ESTROUS CYCLE

Onset of Puberty and Optimal Breeding Age

The domestic cat is generally thought to reach sexual puberty after she attains at least 80% of adult body weight (2.3 to 3.2 kg) and if the photoperiod is appropriate. In many cats puberty is observed by 6 to 9 months of age. The normal queen may go through puberty and experience her first estrus as early as 5 months of age and usually not later than 12 months. Subjectively, purebred cats are thought to reach puberty later than domestic or mixed-breed cats. Free-roaming cats may reach sexual maturity earlier than those kept constantly in the home.

The optimal breeding age for cats is between 1.5 and 7 years. Females older than 7 to 8 years tend to cycle irregularly, have smaller litters, and have more problems with abortions and congenital defects. Young cats (<1 year of age) may also have irregular cycles and be less predictable in their sexual behavior.

Seasonality of the Estrous Cycle

The adult queen is seasonally polyestrous. She typically cycles repeatedly throughout a breeding season unless the cycle is interrupted by pregnancy, pseudopregnancy, or illness. In temperate climate zones, the breeding season begins 1 to 2 months following the winter solstice and continues beyond the summer solstice. Although variation occurs between different latitudes and among various breeds, it is known that the hours of daylight have a major impact on the onset and duration of ovarian activity.

Inadequate intensity or duration of light is the major reason for prolonged anestrus in cats kept in apartments and indoor catteries. In the northern temperate zones, the breeding season usually begins in January or February. The highest incidence of estrus activity in cats is seen in February and March. The breeding season usually ends at any time between June and November. In the average queen, estrous cycles cease in September, and anestrus persists from October through late December.

Artificial light can alter the normal ovarian activity in cats. Those cats maintained with a minimum of 10 hours of artificial light (equivalent to a 100-watt bulb in a 4- × 4-meter room) may cycle throughout the year (Shille and Sojka, 1995). The effect of light on the estrous cycle of house cats can be quite complicated. Pet cats usually do not receive a consistent light pattern because of their exposure to both natural and artificial sources. The artificial lighting in a home may not always result in predictable ovarian cycles, although subjectively, most of these queens do not cycle in October, November, or December.

It has been suggested that the interestrous periods may lengthen during rather warm temperatures (Concannon and Lein, 1983). In our colony of cats, this has been true. However, the effect of heat and/or humidity on ovarian function remains subjective and depends, to some degree, on individual adaptation to extremes in the environment. Long-haired breeds seem to be more sensitive to the photoperiod than short-haired cats, with 90% and 40% showing winter anestrus, respectively (Banks, 1986; Shille and Sojka, 1995).

Phases of the Estrous Cycle

The queen and the bitch have four separate major phases in common that compose an estrous cycle: proestrus, estrus, diestrus, and anestrus. However, the combination of seasonally polyestrous cycles and induced ovulation makes the feline estrous cycle unlike that of the bitch. The normal queen also undergoes a fifth phase, called the nonestrous (interestrous) interval.

Proestrus

DEFINITION. Proestrus is usually defined as the period when males are attracted to nonreceptive females. This is the time of follicular function, estrogen synthesis and secretion, changes in vaginal exfoliative cytology, and preparation for both breeding and pregnancy. This phase ends when the female allows the male to mount and breed.

CLINICAL SIGNS AND DURATION. Proestrus is not observed regularly in queens. Rather, they typically proceed from an apparent anestrous or interestrous condition directly into estrus (standing heat). In one study, proestrus was noted in only 27 of 168 cycles (Shille and Sojka, 1995). The clinical signs associated with the onset of proestrus are changes in behavior consisting of continuous rubbing of the head and neck against any convenient object, constant vocalizing, lordosis posturing, and rolling.

The proestrual cat can be distinguished from one in estrus when she is placed with a male cat. During an observed proestrus, the queen may be less sexually demonstrative than is noted during the subsequent estrus; she does show estrus behavior but does not allow the male to mount. Recognition of proestrus is difficult because the signs may be subtle (affectionate behavior may be the only sign), and duration is only 0.5 to 2 days (Shille and Sojka, 1995). Many of the typical proestrual changes seen in the bitch are not observed in the queen (i.e., in the dog, proestrus has a duration of 5 to 9 days, vaginal bleeding, swelling of the vulva, and consistent changes in vaginal cytology).

HORMONAL CHANGES. Follicular growth consists of follicles enlarging from less than 1 mm in early proestrus to 1.5 mm at the start of estrus. The queen in the anestrous or interestrous period usually has plasma estrogen concentrations below 15 pg/ml. The follicular phase is associated with estrogen (17α-estradiol) concentrations exceeding 20 pg/ml. Proestrus, when seen, is associated with the abrupt rise in circulating estrogen concentrations, in association with rapid follicular growth and secretion. A two-fold increase in plasma estrogen concentration to values above 40 pg/ml is often observed in less than 24 to 48 hours. The abrupt nature of this initiation of follicular growth and the rapid onset of sexual receptivity in the cat can be contrasted with the more gradual sequence of changes typical of the bitch. The external genitalia of the queen are much less obvious than those of the bitch. This is another factor in explaining the brief or unseen proestrus period in the cat.

VAGINAL CYTOLOGY. *Technique.* Vaginal cytology is not a commonly used procedure in queens. This is primarily because the queen enters an obvious estrus abruptly and because the patterns seen on exfoliative vaginal cytology are not always clearly demarcated. Vaginal exfoliative cytology smears from the queen can be obtained as described for the bitch (see Chapter 19). The assistant usually grasps the queen by the scruff of her neck and holds her down on her elbows. The tail is held in the assistant's other hand, to raise the rear quarters slightly and allow visualization of the vulva. The veterinarian separates the lips of the vulva and can simultaneously raise the perineum slightly. A sterile cotton swab, moistened with saline, is placed into the vaginal vestibule and guided into the vaginal vault along the dorsal surface of the tract. The swab is gently rotated in both directions and smoothly withdrawn.

The entire procedure usually takes seconds and is rarely painful. Other methods have been described, as in the bitch, but the moistened cotton swab method is simple, quick, reliable, and inexpensive. The veterinarian must remember that the queen is an induced ovulator (i.e., coital contact induces ovulation). Therefore any method used in obtaining a vaginal smear may induce ovulation.

Once removed from the vaginal vault, the cotton swab is gently rolled across a glass slide two or three times and the slide is stained. Slides are usually air-dried or fixed with 90% methanol followed by air-drying. The slides can be stained with various solutions, as described for the bitch. Diff-Quik Stain (Harleco, Gibbstown, NJ) is recommended because it is reliable and easy to use.

Terminology. The stained slide is studied microscopically at low power to obtain an impression of the degree of "clearing" on the slide. Clearing is defined as the absence of noncellular debris and of eosinophilic

or basophilic strands of mucus, as well as a lack of coalescence of vaginal cells into sheetlike aggregates. Estrogen "liquefies" vaginal mucus in cats. Vaginal epithelial cells can be closely examined at higher magnification. These cells can be classified using the categories described in Chapter 19. These categories include parabasal, intermediate, superficial (cornified), and anuclear superficial cells.

Interpretation. It has been suggested that clearing of the background on a vaginal smear may be the most sensitive and consistent indicator of estrogen activity in the queen (Shille and Sojka, 1995) (Table 33-1). The vaginal epithelial cells become easier to visualize in association with the reduction and the absence of debris. Clearing of the vaginal smear is observed 2 days before the onset of the "follicular phase" in approximately 10% of queens. Clearing is observed in one-third of all estrous cycles before estrus behavior is noted and in more than 90% of estrous cycles during the follicular phase. If clearing is seen on vaginal cytology prior to the onset of estrus behavior, it is consistent with the occurrence of a brief proestrus period.

Cytologically and clinically, proestrus can be defined as starting with evidence of clearing on vaginal cytology smears and ending when the queen allows a tom (male cat) to mount and breed her. Progressive changes in the morphology of vaginal epithelial cells correspond with increasing follicular estrogen secretion rates. The proportion of anuclear superficial cells consistently increases above 10% on the first day of the follicular phase. The proportion of nucleated superficial

TABLE 33–1   VAGINAL CYTOLOGY DURING FOLLICULAR PHASE AND BEHAVIORAL ESTRUS IN A SERIES OF CATS*

DAYS OF FOLLICULAR PHASE	PERCENT OF QUEENS SHOWING BEHAVIORAL ESTRUS	CLEARING OF VAGINAL SMEAR (PERCENT)	EXFOLIATIVE VAGINAL EPITHELIAL CELLS					
			Parabasal	Intermediate	Superficial	Anuclear Superficial	RBC	WBC
−5	0	0	<10	40–50	40–60	<10	None	Few or more
−4	0	0	<10	40–50	40–60	<10	None	Few or more
−3	0	0	<10	40–50	40–60	<10	None	Few or more
−2	0	10–20	<10	40–50	40–60	<10	None	Few or more
−1	0	15–25	<5	30–40	40–60	<10	None	Few or more
F1	<10	30–50	<5	20–30	50–60	~10	Few or none	None
F2	30–40	60–80	<5	10–30	~60	10–15	Few or none	None
F3	40–60	80	<5	10–20	~60	15–35	None	None
F4	70–90	80	–	<10	~60	~40	None	None
F5	80–90	80	–	<10	~60	~40	None	None
F6	90–100	80	–	<10	~60	~40	None	None
F7	80–90	80	–	<10	~60	~40	None	None
I1	40–60	60–80	–	10–20	30–60	~40	None	Few or more
I2	30–50	40–60	<5	20–40	30–60	15–30	None	Few or more
I3	10–30	20–40	<5	20–40	30–60	10–20	None	Few or more
I4	<10	10–30	<5	30–60	30–60	~10	None	None
I5	<10	10–30	<5	30–60	30–60	~10	None	None

*Adapted from Shille VM, et al: Follicular function in the domestic cat as determined by estradiol-17α concentrations in plasma: Relation to estrous behavior and cornification of exfoliated vaginal epithelium. Biol Reprod 21:953, 1979.
F, Follicular phase; I, interestrous phase; RBC, red blood cells; WBC, white blood cells.

cells remains relatively constant whereas intermediate and parabasal cell numbers decline (see Table 33-1). Erythrocytes and leukocytes are not often seen in vaginal smears, the former occurring during the early follicular phase and the latter seen occasionally at the end of the follicular phase (Shille et al, 1979).

Estrus and the follicular phase

DEFINITION OF ESTRUS. Estrus in the queen is defined as the period of breeding. This phase, therefore, is recognized solely by the queen's behavioral response to the tomcat. Estrus begins when the queen allows the male to mount and breed and ends when this behavior ceases. Behavior changes from anestrus to estrus can be abrupt, usually occurring in less than 12 to 24 hours.

DEFINITION OF FOLLICULAR PHASE. Estrus behavior in the queen is associated with follicular estrogen synthesis and secretion. The ovaries become enlarged with 2- to 3-mm translucent follicles. Estrus is recognized, however, only by the sexual behavior of the queen, whereas the "follicular phase," or phase of active follicular function, is physiologic and recognized biochemically via plasma estrogen concentrations. Most queens either in anestrus or during an interestrous period have plasma estrogen concentrations below 12 to 15 pg/ml. Evidence of follicular activity is defined as plasma estrogen concentrations above 20 pg/ml.

The mean length of the follicular phase is approximately 7.5 days and ranges from 3 to 16 days. Coital contact, with or without induction of ovulation, does not alter the duration of the follicular phase. The follicular phase of queens that experience coitus and induced ovulation averages 7.0 days. Queens that experience coitus but do not ovulate have follicular phases that average 7.2 days, whereas those with no coital stimulation have an average follicular phase of 7.7 days (Shille et al, 1979).

During the follicular phase, the plasma estrogen concentration rapidly increases, remains elevated for 3 to 4 days, and abruptly begins to decline. The plasma estrogen concentration 1 day prior to the start of the follicular phase is below 12 to 15 pg/ml. The first day of the follicular phase is associated with estrogen concentrations of approximately 25 pg/ml, rising to approximately 45 pg/ml on day 3, slightly above 50 pg/ml on day 5, from 20 to 25 pg/ml on day 7, and usually back to 10 pg/ml on day 8. Because the mean estrogen concentration on day 8 is below 15 pg/ml, this actually represents the first day of the interestrous interval, assuming that ovulation was not induced. The mean peak follicular phase plasma estrogen concentration is slightly greater than 50 pg/ml, but it may range from levels near 25 pg/ml to those above 80 pg/ml (Shille et al, 1979).

Cessation of follicular function is characterized by an abrupt decline in plasma estrogen concentrations. These levels fall from peak concentrations to less than 20 pg/ml, usually within 2 to 3 days. Initiation of the decline in hormone concentrations is not altered by exposure to coitus or induction of ovulation.

POLYESTROUS CYCLES VERSUS FOLLICULAR PHASES. The queen has polyestrous breeding seasons. This means that the average queen repeatedly exhibits estrus behavior in a given season. These estrus periods are associated with recurring follicular phases, but not necessarily in a 1:1 ratio. Generally, each period of peak estrogen concentration is followed by a return to baseline concentrations (Fig. 33-1). Cats have repeating distinct waves of follicle development, maturation, and degeneration.

ESTRUS BEHAVIOR AND ITS RELATION TO THE FOLLICULAR PHASE. Estrus behavior in the queen can be correlated with increases in plasma estrogen concentration associated with each follicular phase. Estrus behavior is exhibited by 10% of queens on the first day of their follicular phase. The proportion of queens demonstrating estrus behavior then gradually increases until almost all queens show estrus behavior the day before the follicular phase ends (Fig. 33-2). Estrus behavior continues in many queens beyond the end of the follicular phase. Studies on days 1, 2, 3, and 4 after the end of the follicular phase revealed that approximately 60%, 40%, 20%, and 5% of the cats, respectively, continued to exhibit estrus behavior (Shille et al, 1979).

DURATION OF ESTRUS BEHAVIOR. *Average.* The average duration of estrus behavior in the queen is approximately 7 days. There is a wide range of duration, however, and healthy fertile queens may exhibit estrus for as little as 1 day to as long as 21 days. Queens experiencing coitus (whether or not they subsequently ovulate) are in estrus for approximately 8.5 days. Queens that do not have coital contact are in estrus for only 6 days on average (Shille et al, 1979).

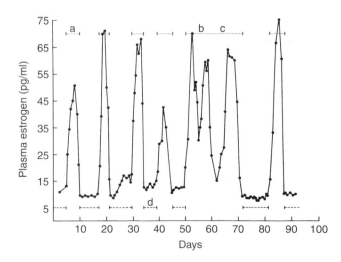

FIGURE 33-1. Schematic representation of the various estrogen secretion patterns that may occur in the cycle of the cat. Illustrated are the pronounced, rapid cyclic fluctuations in plasma estrogen concentration, representing ovarian follicle function. Also included are the periods of estrus (.....) that correlate with rises in plasma estrogen. The normal length of estrus is usually 2 to 10 days, averaging approximately 7 days (a). Note that some estrous periods overlap two or more follicular phases, often because estrogen concentrations fail to decline below 20 pg/ml (b), but not always (c). The interestrous period is also shown (- - -), lasting 3 to 15 days and averaging 8 days in duration (d).

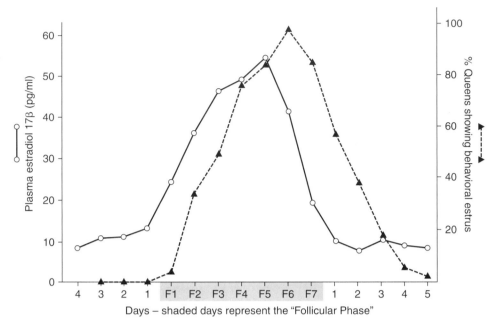

FIGURE 33-2. Schematic representation of the feline follicular phase (estrogen >20 pg/ml) versus the number of cats that have behavioral estrus on each day of the follicular phase.

Effect of coital contact on the duration of estrus. It has been hypothesized that the factors which initiate the ovulatory release of luteinizing hormone (LH) may also influence the centers that control sexual behavior. Vaginal stimulation is transmitted via a spinal afferent nervous pathway to the hypothalamus, where it is converted to a hormonal (gonadotropin-releasing hormone [GnRH]) signal. Release of GnRH following coitus may potentiate or extend sexual receptivity. Coital contact certainly does not immediately bring the queen out of estrus, nor does it shorten the period of receptivity, even if the coital contact induces ovulation.

Effect of personality on exhibition of estrus. Absence of behavioral estrus or extreme prolongation of estrus behavior has been and is observed during regularly recurring "normal" follicular phases in healthy cats. Failure to manifest estrus behavior at expected times, predicted by plasma hormone (estrogen) concentrations, has been seen in a few queens thought to be timid and at the lower end of the "social scale" (Shille et al, 1979). However, this personality trait is not always obvious in a queen with active follicular phases but no behavioral estrus. It is difficult to simply label these queens abnormal. Many queens failing to exhibit behavioral estrus during one season may appear normal in subsequent seasons.

Prolonged estrus. Prolonged estrus behavior is another trait occasionally seen in queens that may later be shown to be fertile and otherwise normal. In some cases, prolonged estrus is the result of overlapping waves of maturing follicles and persistent exposure to increased plasma estrogen concentrations (see Fig. 33-1). However, prolonged or continuous estrus behavior is also seen in cats experiencing distinct, repeated

follicular phases. These cats have estrogen concentrations indistinguishable from those observed in queens exhibiting the more typical, repeated sexual receptivity patterns. The reason for the lack of coordination between sexual behavior and plasma estrogen concentrations in a small percentage of queens remains, for the present, unexplained.

CLINICAL SIGNS OF ESTRUS. The queen in behavioral estrus looks to an owner like the proestrual cat. However, the rubbing, vocalizing, and rolling become more intense. These cats respond to stroking of the back and rubbing of the area at the base of the tail by lowering the forequarters with the elbows on the ground, raising the pelvis (lordosis), and deviating the tail to one side. The male is permitted to mount and breed. Behavioral estrus is described in greater detail in a subsequent section of this chapter (see Sexual Behavior in Estrus).

VAGINAL CYTOLOGY. *Interpretation.* Two major findings are observed in vaginal smears from queens in estrus. The first change is the background clearing, and the second is reapportionment of the percentage of each type of vaginal epithelial cell. Background clearing is defined as the absence of noncellular debris and eosinophilic or basophilic strands of mucus, allowing the vaginal epithelial cells to be easily visualized. This process is due, in part, to vaginal mucus being liquefied by estrogen. Clearing begins before the onset of the follicular phase in approximately 10% of queens, and one-third of the females studied had cytologic clearing prior to their showing any evidence of estrus behavior. During the follicular phase, at least 90% of the vaginal smears have clear backgrounds. This clearing of the vaginal smear continues in some queens after the follicular phase ends, with 20% of smears continuing to show clearing 5 days later (Shille et al, 1979). Vaginal clearing is easily recognized on the smear and is one of the most consistent alterations, other than blood hormone (estrogen) concentrations, that allow identification of an actively cycling queen.

Progressive changes are seen in the relative proportion of the types of vaginal epithelial cells during estrus (see Table 33-1). The anuclear superficial cells increase to 10% of the total on the first day of the follicular phase and continue to increase in number, reaching approximately 40% of the total from the 4th through 7th days, before slowly returning to less than 10% by the 12th to 13th day (5th to 6th day after the end of the follicular phase). Intermediate cells decrease in number, from approximately 40% to 50% of the total during the interestrous period to less than 10% during the 4th through 7th days of the follicular phase. Parabasal cells disappear during the follicular phase, returning to 5% to 10% of the total 5 days after the follicular phase has ended. The nucleated superficial cell maintains its 40% to 60% proportion of the vaginal epithelial cell population throughout the follicular phase (see Table 33-1) (Shille et al, 1979).

Clinical uses. Occasionally, the veterinarian is consulted regarding a queen that is failing to cycle. A number of these cats experience repeated follicular phases and appropriate fluctuations in plasma estrogen concentration. However, the shy queen or one housed with others and at the bottom of the "pecking order" may not display behavioral estrus. Vaginal smears obtained and reviewed once or twice weekly for 1 to 2 months, especially during February and March, reveal the cyclic nature of the queen's hormonal status.

One can teach owners how to obtain and make smears. They can then bring the air-dried slides to their veterinarian for staining and analysis. This becomes a simple, cost-effective method for studying an apparently healthy but noncycling queen. Vaginal cytology is not commonly used in feline practice, but recognition of subclinical cycles is one important use for this tool. Queens that are shipped for breeding can also be studied in this manner, especially if they fail to exhibit estrus behavior after being placed in a new environment.

Vaginal smears can be obtained after coital contact, following the after-reaction, to determine whether the male ejaculated and whether he is fertile. One can simply look for sperm. However, even when sperm are present, it is not possible to know whether or not the breeding induced an LH surge and thus ovulation.

The interestrous period

DEFINITION. Cats are polyestrous and have repeated phases of sexual receptivity (estrus) throughout the season of ovarian activity (see Fig. 33-1). The phases of sexual activity are associated with "waves" of follicular function separated by brief periods of sexual or reproductive inactivity. The ovaries are believed to be hormonally inactive during the periods between active follicular waves. These periods of inactivity are the "interestrous intervals" or "interestrous periods."

HORMONAL CHANGES AND DURATION OF THE INTERESTROUS PERIOD. *Effect of plasma estrogen concentration.* The interestrous period follows cessation of follicular function, which is characterized by an abrupt decline of plasma estrogen concentration to levels below 20 pg/ml. The estrogen concentration remains at the low, or basal, level for the duration of the interestrous period, which averages 8 days and ranges from 2 to 19 days (Shille and Sojka, 1995).

Effect of coital contact. The duration of the interestrous period is probably not affected by coital contact that fails to induce ovulation. Interestrous periods in queens experiencing coitus but not ovulation were shorter in duration than those in animals that had not experienced coitus (8 days versus 10 days, respectively).

Estrus spanning two or more follicular phases. Occasionally, queens appear to miss an interestrous interval (i.e., estrus activity spans two or more follicular phases despite typical cyclic follicular function; see Fig. 33-1). These queens do experience a hormonal interestrous period but not the behavioral interval one would expect. In some cats, the estrus behavior spanned interestrous intervals with typical basal plasma estrogen concentrations below 20 pg/ml. The estrogen surges during their follicular phases were not, as a rule, different from those seen in the average cat in behavioral interestrus. In other queens, however, cyclic estrogen fluctuations were observed in which the lowest estrogen concentrations remained above the 20 pg/ml plateau. In this latter situation, persistent estrus behavior, without an interestrous interval, is easier to comprehend because the queen is constantly under the influence of follicular estrogen secretion.

The interestrous period is much longer than the 8-day average if ovulation is induced (pseudopregnancy or pregnancy). The ovulation results in development of corpora lutea that secrete progesterone. Because sexual phases of progesterone dominance are referred to as "diestrus" phases, these are discussed in the subsequent section on diestrus.

BEHAVIOR. The interestrous period is characterized by a return to normal personality. Queens do not breed, do not attract males, and lose the extremely affectionate behavior patterns that typify estrus. The intense rubbing, rolling, and vocalizing disappear.

VAGINAL CYTOLOGY. During the interestrous period, nucleated superficial and intermediate vaginal epithelial cells again dominate the smears. The percentage of the various cell types remains static throughout this phase (see Table 33-1). The average numbers of each cell type, identified in one study during the interestrous interval, were parabasal cells, 2%; intermediate cells, 48%; superficial cells, 46%; and anuclear cells, 4% (Shille et al, 1979). Fluctuations in cell type were seen, but these were not typically dramatic and would not be confused with the changes consistent with estrus. Additionally, background debris is obvious on the vaginal smear of a queen in the interestrous period. Background debris interferes with the ability to visualize vaginal epithelial cells.

Diestrus

Diestrus is defined as a phase of progesterone dominance in the queen or bitch. The queen must have coital contact or similar vaginal stimulation to induce ovulation before corpora lutea develop and begin secreting progesterone. Within 24 to 48 hours of ovulation, functioning corpora lutea capable of secreting progesterone exist. Assuming that the cat has ovulated but is not pregnant, plasma estrogen concentrations are basal and plasma progesterone concentrations increase (ovulation and pregnancy are reviewed in separate sections in this chapter). Plasma progesterone concentrations greater than 1 to 2 ng/ml are associated with diestrus and are greater than 20 ng/ml within 14 to 18 days.

The ovaries contain several firm, tan to orange corpora lutea that remain functional for 35 to 37 days. Plasma progesterone concentrations decreasing to basal levels are consistent with cessation of luteal function. It may then take as long as 35 additional days for a queen to again exhibit estrus; the mechanism for the variable delay in cyclicity is not well understood. The uterus is largest in diestrus, because of the extreme thickening of the endometrium. The horns become turgid and twisted inside the serosa, forming irregular corkscrew bulges that may be palpable. Vagina, vestibule, and vulva are normal in appearance.

Anestrus

DEFINITION AND CLINICAL SIGNS. Anestrus is a period of clinical reproductive quiescence. Cats in anestrus do not attract males and do not display sexual behavior or exhibit evidence of active ovarian function. It is difficult to differentiate the queen in anestrus from one that has been ovariohysterectomized.

SEASONALITY AND DURATION. Anestrus typically begins in October and ends in late December. Anestrus has been described in some colonies and/or individual queens as beginning in midsummer (June through August) and lasting through January. Individual variability is common, although shortening day lengths plus the heat of summer are factors that may induce the onset of anestrus. Anestrus usually ends as the days begin to lengthen following the winter solstice.

It is possible to delay the onset of anestrus in cats by maintaining them in at least 10 hours of artificial light (equivalent to that provided by a 100-watt bulb in a 4- × 4-meter room); this regimen causes some queens to cycle throughout the year (Concannon and Lein, 1983). Some queens, however, still may enter anestrus during November and December, despite artificial light supplementation. The effect of the artificial light exposure experienced by pet cats living indoors has not been evaluated.

HORMONE CONCENTRATIONS AND VAGINAL CYTOLOGY. Hormonally, anestrus is similar to a prolonged interestrous interval. Plasma estrogen and progesterone concentrations remain at basal levels, and pituitary hormone concentrations undergo minor fluctuations. The vaginal cytology is consistent with an interestrous period. The exfoliated vaginal epithelial cells consist of less than 10% parabasal cells, 40% to 70% intermediate cells, and 30% to 40% nucleated superficial cells. Background debris is obvious.

PHYSIOLOGY OF OVULATION

Coital Induction of Ovulation

Vaginal stimulation by the penis of the tomcat is followed immediately by an increase in neural activity within areas of the hypothalamus that are known to contain large amounts of GnRH. Release of this GnRH is thought to cause the surge in serum LH that follows vaginal stimulation in induced ovulators, such as the cat. LH surges have been shown to occur within 15 minutes of copulation in cats (Concannon et al, 1980; Johnson and Gay, 1981).

The measured surges in serum LH have been correlated with the number of copulations. Maximal LH levels are attained 4 hours after the onset of 8 to 12 copulations. Serum LH concentrations return to basal levels 24 hours later. Peak serum LH concentrations were significantly lower when the queens were allowed to copulate only four times during a 4-hour period. Peak LH concentrations were even lower when only one copulation was allowed. Ovulation was associated with LH concentrations that were higher than when ovulation failed to occur (Concannon et al, 1980).

Each copulation does result in a release of LH, which may or may not be sufficient to cause ovulation. Fewer than 50% of queens in full estrus ovulate following a single breeding. This must be contrasted with the fact that most queens do ovulate following four or more copulations. Copulations may continue for several days, and major LH surges occur day after day. LH release becomes negligible following 2 to 4 hours of copulation in any 24-hour period. Ovulation occurs approximately 24 hours after the rapid release of LH (Concannon and Lein, 1983). Some queens may not release adequate LH concentrations to induce ovulation despite repeated matings with proven fertile tomcats. However, mating several days later during the same estrus, with the same male, may result in ovulation.

Adequate LH secretion, following vaginal stimulation, does not always result in ovulation. It is likely that a certain intrinsic maturity of the developing follicle is a necessary prerequisite for an ovulatory stimulus to be effective. If true, this is one explanation for the apparent variability noted in success of copulatory efforts and induction of ovulation. Some queens may be sexually receptive before follicle maturation has proceeded sufficiently to allow an ovulatory response to the LH surge. Alternatively, copulation and the LH surge may occur too late in a given cycle to result in ovulation. Finally, the apparent variability of the coitus-to-ovulation time interval, following a single series of breedings, could be the result of variations in the relationship of sexual responsiveness and follicle maturity.

Variability in Induction

The outcome of each feline estrous cycle usually (not always) depends on the queen's contact with a male. Four distinct possibilities are recognized (Fig. 33-3): first, an anovulatory cycle may occur in which no contact occurs with the male during estrus; second, an anovulatory cycle may occur in which coital contact with the male is insufficient (too few coital contacts or timing of breeding that is either too early or too late in the cycle); third, a pseudopregnancy cycle may occur as the result of a failure to fertilize ova following coitus in which the ovulatory stimulus is adequate; and fourth, ovulation and fertilization can occur with subsequent development of fetuses.

Induction of Ovulation Without Copulation

Spontaneous ovulation occasionally occurs without male contact or intromission. Stroking of the lower back or tail head may be sufficient stimulus to induce ovulation (Lofstedt, 1982). LH surges may accompany mating in cats when mounting occurs without intromission (Concannon et al, 1980). LH release and subsequent ovulation can also be induced by artificial stimulation of the vagina and/or cervix. This can be accomplished by probing the vagina with a cotton swab, such as when obtaining vaginal cytology smears.

When attempting to induce ovulation, the clinician should probe the vagina with a rod or cotton swab at least four to eight times, at 5- to 20-minute intervals. Each probing need last only 2 to 5 seconds. As with natural breedings, repeated stimulation does not induce ovulation in all queens. In some queens, repeat stimulation several days following an initial series of probes may succeed. The timing of artificial stimulation within an estrus may have an effect on the success of attempts at inducing ovulation. Successful stimulation of ovulation does not shorten an estrus period.

Ovulation can also be induced or enhanced medically. Human chorionic gonadotropin (hCG) can be administered at a dose of 250 IU intramuscularly on days 1 and 2 of estrus (Lein and Concannon, 1983).

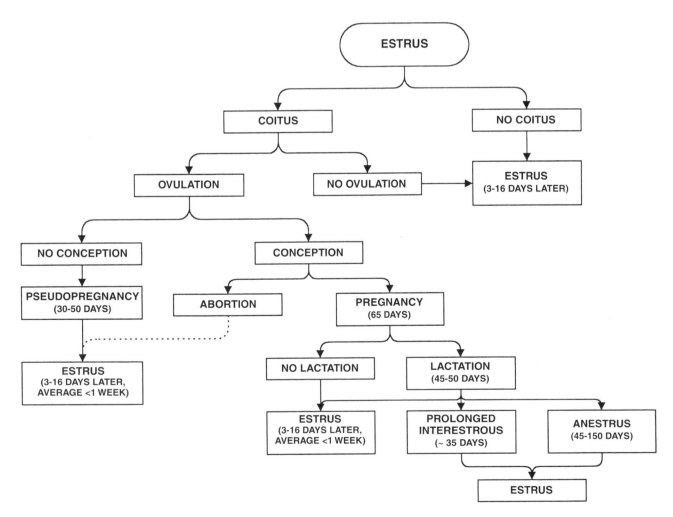

FIGURE 33-3. The potential courses of the reproductive cycle of the queen.

PSEUDOPREGNANCY

Definition

Pseudopregnancy is a physiologic alteration that usually occurs when a queen has been induced to ovulate but fails to become pregnant. Induction of ovulation results in development of corpora lutea that synthesize and secrete progesterone. The progesterone inhibits secretion of hypothalamic GnRH and, in turn, pituitary LH/FSH (follicle-stimulating hormone). The inherent lifespan of feline corpora lutea is approximately 35 days. Thus pseudopregnant queens do not exhibit ovarian cyclic activity for the time they are under the influence of progesterone plus the time required for a subsequent wave of follicle development. The typical duration of pseudopregnancy is 40 to 50 days.

Causes

Numerous natural and artificial causes induce ovulation without subsequent fertilization. These include use of an infertile male, a blockage inhibiting contact between sperm and eggs, artificial induction of ovulation (e.g., cotton swab, hCG), genital tract problems that are spermicidal, and myriad other potential explanations. Each cause has in common adequate "coital" contact to stimulate sufficient LH secretion at the appropriate time to induce ovulation. Regardless of the induction stimulus, the queen fails to become pregnant.

Physiology

In pregnancy or pseudopregnancy, ovulation is followed by formation of corpora lutea. Several carnivores, such as the dog, fox, and ferret, have luteal phases that are similar in duration, regardless of the presence or absence of pregnancy. The cat is one of several species that differ from other carnivores in that the luteal phase of the nonpregnant queen is only approximately one-half the duration of the normal gestation period. The cat thus appears to have a reproductive advantage over other carnivores in that the shorter, nonpregnant, luteal phase allows for a more rapid return to a potentially fertile state.

The cat has an additional reproductive advantage over the dog: in queens, the reestablishment of ovarian activity can begin as quickly as 7 to 10 days following pseudopregnancy, whereas in the average bitch at least 4.5 to 5 months elapse before ovarian activity can begin. It appears that a queen may undergo as many as four or five pseudopregnancies during the course of one polyestrous season.

Basal progesterone concentrations (<0.5 ng/ml) are associated with no functioning corpora lutea. Luteal activity in pseudopregnant cats begins approximately 4 days after the first day of copulation and approximately 1 to 2 days following ovulation. Luteal function

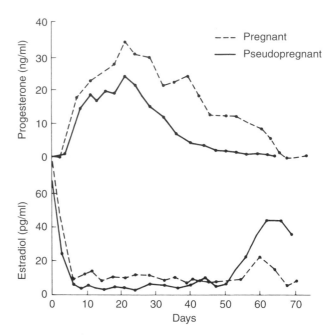

FIGURE 33-4. Average concentrations of progesterone and estradiol in pregnant and pseudopregnant queens. (From Christiansen IJ: Reproduction in the Dog and Cat. London, Bailliere Tindall, 1984.)

is usually defined as beginning when the plasma progesterone concentration increases above 1 ng/ml. Hormone synthesis and secretion in newly formed corpora lutea increase rapidly. Plasma progesterone concentrations are typically greater than 5 ng/ml on the third day of luteal function, and peak concentrations greater than 20 ng/ml are common by the 16th to 25th day. The progesterone concentrations then decline progressively, reaching relatively low levels by day 35 of luteal function. The mean duration of luteal activity in pseudopregnant cats was found to be 36.5 days, with a range of 30 to 50 days (Fig. 33-4; Concannon and Lein, 1983).

Behavior

The pseudopregnant cat usually ceases breeding behavior for 35 to 70 days, averaging 45 days (Concannon and Lein, 1983). The actual luteal phase lasts approximately 36 to 37 days, followed by a 7- to 10-day interestrous interval. Therefore the interval between two estrus periods is significantly prolonged in pseudopregnant cats as compared with the intervals that are not interrupted by ovulation and progesterone secretion. One might speculate that the gradual decline in plasma progesterone concentrations, which begins at about day 21 following coitus, suggests that corpus luteum function in the pseudopregnant cat is not terminated by the acute application of lytic factors but may have a lifespan predetermined at ovulation in the absence of gestational luteotrophic influences.

One important physiologic effect of progesterone in some species, such as the mare, sow, and ewe, is the

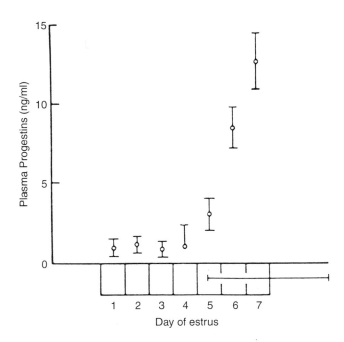

FIGURE 33-5. Schematic representation of behavioral estrus (horizontal scale) in the queen despite rising plasma progesterone concentrations induced by coital contact, ovulation, and development of corpora lutea. Note that estrus persists an average of 7 days, regardless of the progesterone secreted.

suppression of estrus. The queen and bitch are sexually receptive despite rising progesterone concentrations. As seen in Fig. 33-5, the cat maintains sexual receptivity in spite of rising progesterone concentrations for 3 days during the average estrus.

SEXUAL BEHAVIOR IN ESTRUS

The Queen

INITIAL SIGNS. The queen in estrus usually demonstrates obvious personality changes. As in proestrus, queens in estrus may be seen to show continuous rubbing of the head and neck against any convenient object. They also may tend to roll or rub their backs on the ground or floor. The queen vocalizes more frequently, often producing a moaning sound. She may urinate more frequently, be more restless, and show an increased desire to leave the home. Some females are much more affectionate toward their owners, but a few become aggressive. Some of these cats might be thought to be ill by an inexperienced pet owner. Owners may notice an increased number of male cats near their home.

When petted by a human or approached by a male cat, the queen in estrus stops rolling and rubbing. She crouches with her forequarters and elbows pressed to the ground and, by hyperextending her back, causes elevation of the pelvis and presentation of the perineal region (lordosis). She may deviate her tail to one side and "tread" with her back legs in response to human contact as well as to male cats.

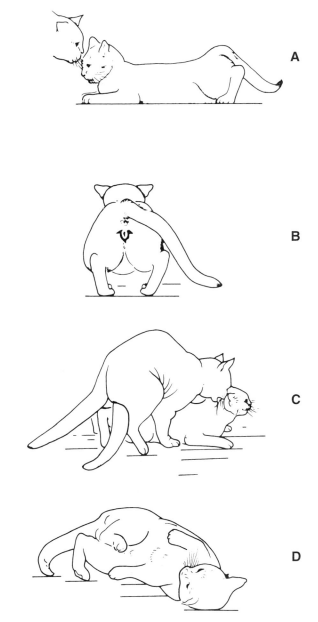

FIGURE 33-6. A and B, The typical posture adopted by the queen in estrus. Note the flexion of the limbs, lordosis, and deflection of the tail. C, Tomcat holds the queen during intromission. D, Postcoital rolling by the queen. (After Scott PP: In Hafez ESE (ed): Reproduction and Breeding Techniques for Laboratory Animals. Philadelphia, Lea & Febiger, 1970.)

DIFFERENTIATING "NORMAL" BEHAVIOR FROM "ESTRUS" BEHAVIOR. Many pet cats are quite affectionate. They enjoy human contact and commonly rub against their owners or objects in an attempt to elicit petting or to be held. Stroking along the back and rubbing at the base of the tail often results in raising of the pelvis and treading of the rear legs, even in ovariohysterectomized cats. Behavioral estrus can sometimes be recognized in normally affectionate queens only when sexual displays are out of character for that individual or when a male cat is present (Fig. 33-6). Some affectionate queens exhibit "friendly" behavior with much greater intensity and frequency when in estrus; thus their estrus periods are recognized (Voith, 1980).

BREEDING. *Female behavior.* Mating is initiated by the female. A point is reached during proestrus when the queen progresses into an "estrus posture." This lordosis posture (with or without other possible factors) is quickly recognized by the male. The queen in estrus allows the male to grasp her neck from the side (Table 33-2; see Fig. 33-6). Once held, most females elevate the pelvis, deviate the tail, and tread with the rear legs. If this behavior is not elicited, it still may occur following mounting, the alternating stepping movements of the male's hind feet, or the stroking of the female's thorax by the front feet of the male. Treading of the female's back feet may stimulate pelvic thrusting and intromission by the male, but lordosis and treading by the queen are not always seen (Voith, 1980).

Intromission. Intromission (penetration) follows several copulatory thrusts. Ejaculation occurs quickly after intromission is accomplished. Intromission is associated with the female emitting a characteristic yowl. The time from grasping the neck to intromission can vary from 30 seconds to 5 minutes, with intromission lasting only 1 to 4 seconds and rarely as long as 20 seconds (Concannon and Lein, 1983). In contrast to most species, penetration and ejaculation occur so quickly that observers are rarely able to determine whether normal copulation was completed. Recognition of copulation usually depends on seeing a typical display of an "after-reaction" by the queen.

Male behavior. If the mating sequence is disturbed, breeding may be interrupted for hours to days. A male spends considerable time establishing territory via urine spraying. If his territory is cleaned too thoroughly (especially with scented sprays) the male may ignore or even attack the estrus female until his territory has been reestablished. This territorial behavior mandates that females be brought to males for breeding. However, this concept must be tempered by the knowledge that change in environment may adversely affect the behavior or hormonal status of the female. Therefore it is recommended that a female be brought to a new surrounding several weeks early in order to allow her to adapt. Maintaining the male in the same general area as the female hastens the onset of estrus.

POSTCOITAL "AFTER-REACTION." During or immediately following intromission, the queen screams or yowls. She then attempts to break contact with the male by rolling underneath him and striking at him with her claws. Once free of the male, the queen lies on her side and vigorously rubs herself on the ground, rolling or thrashing from side to side (see Fig. 33-6). The intense rolling and rubbing action is interrupted by equally obsessive licking of the vaginal area. The after-reaction continues for 30 seconds to 9 minutes, during which time the queen actively repels any approach by the male.

"AFTER-REACTION" IN THE MALE. The male is surprisingly passive during the period of the queen's after-reaction. He usually remains several feet away from the queen and seems to ignore her. The experienced male is adept at avoiding any strike attempts by the queen, which are characteristic of after-reaction. He may either stand or sit, occasionally licking his penile area. Within minutes he may cautiously approach the queen, and if rejected, he may again just sit and wait. This behavior is repeated until he boldly approaches the queen and successfully grasps her neck (see Fig. 33-6). He may still be repelled at this point. Repeated breedings are common, improving the chance for induction of ovulation.

REPEAT BREEDINGS. As the after-reaction subsides, the queen may again solicit the attention of a male. She may reach out and touch the male with her paw or simply approach him. The more aggressive queen assumes a lordosis and treading posture (Voith, 1980). Subsequent mating may occur soon after completion of the after-reaction, with the interval between these two events lengthening with each coital contact. It has been reported that a queen may breed as many as 30 times in 24 hours and 36 times in 36 hours. The average number of breedings throughout an estrus has not been reported (Concannon and Lein, 1983).

ABNORMAL BREEDING BEHAVIOR. Extremely shy or intimidated queens may not demonstrate typical estrus behavior, and an estrus or "season" may be entirely missed, even by experienced owners. Therefore it is helpful for the queen to be kept in familiar, comfortable surroundings until estrus behavior is obvious. The queen is then traditionally brought to the tomcat for breeding. The queen that refuses breeding attempts by the male may be intimidated by new or strange surroundings. If this occurs, the queen should be placed in the breeding area by herself for several hours each

TABLE 33–2 DURATION AND CHARACTERISTICS OF THE PREMATING, MATING, AND POSTMATING PERIODS

Duration	Tomcat	Queen
Premating (10 sec-5 min)	Moves forward Sniffs female's genitalia Circulates Calls Moves forward	Lordosis posture Rolls Calls Treads hindlegs
Mating (1-3 min)	Neckbiting Mounts with forelegs Mounts with hindlegs Rakes with forelegs Treads with hindlegs Arching of the back	Crouches Treads with hindlegs
(5-10 sec)	Pelvic thrusting Erection Intromission Ejaculation Withdraws penis	Bends tail to one side Raises pelvis Copulation scream Turns on tomcat
Postmating (30 sec-10 min)	Licks penis Licks forepaws	Licks genitalia Rolls Licks forepaws Views tomcat Re-encourages tomcat

day before introducing the male. She can then become acclimated to the new environment but still be in the territory of the male, improving the likelihood of a positive response from both cats.

Use of an experienced tomcat is also helpful when breeding an inexperienced or shy queen. The experienced male is less likely to be easily repelled by a queen in estrus, improving the chances of breeding and minimizing the problem of a queen habitually rejecting contact with the male.

It has been suggested that one remedy for a queen that aggressively rejects a male is to stimulate the queen manually, induce a display of sexual behavior, and then hold her for the tom (Voith, 1980). This can be difficult to accomplish and sometimes requires a rather well-behaved male. The owner attempting this approach should not be surprised by an attack from either cat. It would be more prudent, perhaps, to use a second male if successful breeding is not apparent with one tomcat. Partner preferences are well-recognized, and the queen that repels one male may accept another (Voith, 1980).

ARTIFICIAL BREEDING

Estrus Induction

Artificial induction of estrus is rarely performed in clinical veterinary practices. This procedure can be used to synchronize estrous cycles among several queens. Estrus induction is also an important component of embryo transfer and in vivo fertilization protocols. It is used to stimulate ovarian activity in embryo donors and to achieve synchrony with embryo recipients. No regimen has equaled the pregnancy rate or embryo quality typical of natural estrus. The most successful protocol includes administration of 150 IU equine chorionic gonadotropin (eCG, IM) followed in no less than 80 hours and no more than 88 hours with 100 IU human chorionic gonadotropin (hCG, IM). The resulting pregnancy rate was 80% (Donoghue et al, 1992). An alternative protocol is administration of FSH, 2 mg intramuscularly once daily for 5 to 6 days, with the cat mated daily during the induced estrus (Shille and Sojka, 1995).

Artificial Insemination

Although artificial insemination is commonly performed in a variety of species, including dogs, it is rarely performed in clinical veterinary practices on cats. Even if semen is successfully collected from the male (which is rare), two commonly encountered problems include (1) inadequate penetration of intravaginally deposited sperm through the cervix; (2) inadequate induction of ovulation. After cats ovulated, intrauterine insemination under anesthesia with laparoscopy resulted in a 50% conception rate (Howard et al, 1992; see Semen Collection, Storage, and Preservation in this chapter). Semen was deposited into the cranial third of each

uterine horn using a 17-gauge catheter. These procedures may be employed by practitioners in the future but are currently reserved for research animals.

Embryo Transfer

Embryo transfer has been reported; however, like artificial insemination, this is not a procedure employed by private practitioners. Embryos can be collected via laparoscopy from donors 7 to 8 days after mating. A catheter is placed close to the uterotubular junction in each uterine horn. The embryos are then flushed caudally and collected into gridded tissue culture dishes via a catheter located at the uterine bifurcation. The embryos are then surgically transferred into a reproductive stage–matched recipient (Goodrow et al, 1988).

PREGNANCY

Gestation Length

Gestation length, defined as the interval from a fertile mating to parturition, lasts 56 to 69 days. In one colony of cats, the average gestation was 66 days (Lein and Concannon, 1983). The duration of pregnancy is more uniform (63 to 66 days) when timed to the first rise in serum progesterone concentration. Variation in the duration of coitus-to-parturition interval is likely explained by coitus failing to consistently induce ovulation.

Implantation and Fetal Development

After ovulation, eggs remain in the oviducts for 3 to 4 days. Fertilization is presumed to occur within the oviducts. The zygotes migrate into the uterus 4 to 5 days after fertilization. Blastocysts become localized and recognized as spherical enlargements within the uterus 13 to 14 days into gestation, perhaps later if the estrus is artificially induced (Thatcher et al, 1991). Trophoblastic attachment occurs near day 15 following coitus.

The *fetal stage* is recognized after development of species characteristics (at about 4 weeks). At that time fetuses have a crown-to-rump length of 2.4 cm. In the fifth week of pregnancy, eyes and ear pinnae are present and closed, the digits can be recognized to have claws, and the crown-to-rump length is 4.7 cm. Fine body hair without color is seen at 7 weeks, and full body hair with color patterning can be recognized by the eighth week of gestation.

Hormonal Characteristics

Progesterone concentrations during the initial 14 to 20 days of pregnancy are similar to those seen in pseudopregnant cats. Thereafter, plasma progesterone concentrations are increased in the pregnant queens (see Fig. 33-4; Concannon and Lein, 1983). The elevated plasma progesterone concentrations are a reflection of continuing function by corpora lutea. In addition, progesterone begins to be synthesized and secreted by the placenta after 30 days of gestation.

Plasma progesterone concentrations vary markedly among pregnant cats (5 to 50 ng/ml; Shille and Sojka, 1995). The corpora lutea produce progesterone for approximately 40 to 50 days, but the amounts produced after day 40 day are minimal. By gestation day 40 to 50, ovariectomy does not result in termination of pregnancy because placental progesterone maintains pregnancy. Before day 40, ovariectomy can terminate pregnancy in the cat. At the end of gestation, plasma estrogen (see Fig. 33-4) and prolactin concentrations rise.

Behavior

The relatively subtle increases in plasma concentrations of estrogen near the end of gestation can bring about changes in the queen's behavior. Estrus behavior and matings may occur prior to or following parturition. These matings are neither common nor fertile. Postpartum lactation tends to suppress normal estrous cycles, and pregnancies would be rare.

Pregnancy Diagnosis

FETAL AGE.   Accurate fetal age is best determined by serial assessment of plasma progesterone concentrations in the queen. Onset of pregnancy should be defined as the first day that plasma progesterone exceeds 2.5 ng/ml. Assuming that pregnancy is subsequently confirmed with ultrasonography or radiography, dating can be quite specific.

ABDOMINAL PALPATION.   Abdominal palpation remains the most commonly used tool for diagnosing pregnancy in cats. Palpation of discrete, firm spherical structures, representing developing fetuses, can be accomplished by day 17 of gestation. These isolated structures can usually be felt through day 25 of gestation, making this 7- to 8-day period the ideal time for pregnancy diagnosis via palpation. Less commonly, one may be able to palpate individual fetuses through day 35 day of gestation. An enlarged uterus should be palpable from day 25 of gestation through parturition. The queen, not being as difficult a challenge as many bitches, is usually easy to palpate.

ULTRASONOGRAPHY.   Abdominal ultrasonography is easily the most sensitive and reliable tool available for early pregnancy diagnosis. Developing fetuses can be visualized as early as 11 to 14 days into gestation, and the functioning hearts can be seen by day 22 to day 24 (Davidson et al, 1986). As with the bitch, it is not always possible to reliably count fetuses with ultrasonography, especially if the litter is four kittens or larger. Ultrasonography requires no anesthesia or sedation, takes only a few minutes after removing the ventral hair with a clipper, and is not harmful. Furthermore, the ultrasound measurement of fetal head and body diameter is a practical and accurate tool in the assessment of gestational age and is a potentially useful indicator of parturition date (Table 33-3; Beck et al, 1990).

RADIOLOGY.   Radiographic diagnosis of pregnancy in the cat depends on calcification of fetal skeletons. Radiographic diagnosis is possible after day 38 of gestation, but consistent results are seen after day 43. Uterine enlargement before fetal calcification is a nonspecific finding that might be recognized in cats with pyometra, hydrometra, or other causes for enlargement. It is recommended that owners bring cats to their veterinarian for radiographic pregnancy diagnosis 45 days after the first breeding to avoid an inconclusive study.

Return to Fertile Cycles

Following normal lactation and weaning, return to estrus takes 2 to 8 weeks, averaging 4 weeks. If kittens are removed from the queen at 3 days of age, estrus behavior may begin as soon as 6 to 8 days (Concannon and Lein, 1983). Abortion of developing kittens may be the result of, or may cause, a shortened luteal phase. Queens can begin to cycle within a week of aborting a litter.

TABLE 33–3   ULTRASOUND PREDICTION OF PARTURITION

Queen	HD (cm)	BD (cm)	Predicted Days Prepartum	Actual Days Prepartum	Predicted Minus Actual	Number of Kittens
1	0.6	—	46	36	10	5
2	0.8	—	41	40	1	4
3	1.3	—	29	29	0	7
4	1.6	1.8	22 (HD) 24 (BD)	22	0 (HD) 2 (BD)	4
5	1.6	2.0	22	21	1	3
6	1.6	2.2	22 (HD) 19 (BD)	21	1 (HD) –2 (BD)	3
7	2.1	—	9	9	0	4
8	2.4	—	2	4	–2	3

From Beck KA, et al: Ultrasound prediction of parturition in queens. Vet Radiol 31:32, 1990.
HD, Head diameter; BD, body diameter.

Care of the Queen

The pregnant queen should be fed a well-balanced diet consisting of canned and kibbled commercial cat foods. Such foods are easy to obtain and provide the necessary nutrients. The total caloric requirement during pregnancy usually increases 25% to 50%. During lactation, queens often eat twice the amount of food they consume when they are not pregnant. Breeding queens should be vaccinated, dewormed, and tested for feline leukemia virus (FeLV) prior to estrus. Vaccinating pregnant cats is not recommended.

Hemograms of pregnant cats (weeks 3 to 9 of gestation) demonstrate normocytic normochromic anemia with a 20% reduction in hematocrit or red blood cell count. Medications of any type are discouraged in pregnant cats. A list of drugs and potential problems associated with their administration to pregnant animals is available (see Chapter 20). When queening approaches, a warm, dry, secluded area with nesting material (e.g., shredded disposable baby diapers) should be provided.

PARTURITION

Endocrinology

Hormonal interrelationships are assumed to be similar during parturition in most species (see Chapter 20 on parturition in the bitch). One potential difference between the queen and the bitch is the source of progesterone during the final 2 weeks of gestation. Decreasing plasma progesterone concentrations, below some critical level, is an essential event in initiating parturition. The queen has placental progesterone during the final weeks of gestation. As progesterone concentrations decline, the rectal temperature usually decreases (<99° F), signifying that parturition has commenced and that obvious uterine contractions will begin within 12 to 36 hours.

Labor

STAGE I OF LABOR. The first stage of labor (uterine contractions and dilation of the cervix) may persist for 2 to 24 hours and be characterized by restlessness, frequent grooming, pacing, panting, vomiting, and vocalization. Neither uterine nor abdominal contractions can be seen, although small amounts of clear mucus may be seen at the vulva. Just before stage II labor (delivery of the newborn), nesting behavior, antagonism toward strangers or other cats, and the desire to find seclusion are intensified. The queen may be anorectic or inappetent, or she may eat normally throughout parturition. Toward the end of stage I labor, the cat may settle in the "nest" and purr loudly.

STAGES II AND III OF LABOR. Stage II labor is defined as delivery of the newborn(s). Stage III labor is the passage of the placenta. The process of the fetus entering the uterine body and then passing through cervix and vagina, is associated with strong visible uterine contractions. The entire birthing process of a litter is usually complete 2 to 6 hours after delivery of the first kitten, although it may take as long as 12 hours. Kittens may be delivered rapidly, within minutes of each other, or at 30- to 60-minute intervals. Breech and headfirst presentations are normal.

Nesting behavior can be obvious for 12 to 48 hours prior to queening. The decline in rectal temperature usually precedes delivery of kittens by at least 12 hours, but rectal temperature is a notoriously unreliable indicator of the onset of labor. The first kitten may follow a few obvious contractions or take as long as 30 to 60 minutes to be born. Expulsion of this first newborn may be accompanied by a good deal of loud vocalizing by the queen.

Between deliveries, the queen removes and eats any placental tissue, severs the cord, cleans kittens, and licks her vulvar area. Some queens nurse kittens while labor continues (milk may be expressed from the mammary glands 24 to 48 hours before queening).

Uncommonly, parturition may be interrupted and take as long as 1 to several days, in contrast to the more rapid sequence of events just described. Interruption in parturition may occur for a variety of reasons, such as some disturbing environmental factor that causes a queen to move her newborn(s) to a new location. After the birth of the first kitten(s), labor activity and contractions may cease for 12 to 24 hours. The queen may nurse her newborn, eat, rest, and act as if parturition were complete. The remaining kittens are usually delivered live and without difficulty when labor begins again. This phenomenon is not considered abnormal but must be differentiated from dystocia (Christiansen, 1984).

The fetal membranes are typically expelled (stage III labor) shortly after the delivery of each kitten, or two placentas may pass following the birth of two kittens. Many queens ingest the fetal membranes soon after they are passed. No evidence suggests that this material is beneficial or harmful to the queen, so placentas can be gently removed from the queening box.

Providing a Proper Environment

The queen usually has little difficulty during delivery (queening). Most cats instinctively search for a secluded location for delivery of their kittens. It is wise to provide the pregnant cat with a dry, quiet, warm area with nesting material (such as shredded baby diapers) 4 to 7 days before queening is expected to begin. The queen then has an opportunity to become familiar with her surroundings. A "queening box" or cage is used by many breeders. The chosen location should be free of other cats or excessive human activity. A queen recently moved to a new area or disturbed by her environment can delay the onset of parturition or interrupt queening between delivery of kittens in order to seek a more desirable location. She usually then moves her newborn kittens to the new area, or less commonly, she may neglect her kittens. A visual barrier, such as a sheet or towel, cardboard box, or the back of a closet, usually provides the seclusion needed by the queen during parturition (Voith, 1980).

A small number of queens may actually seek their owners, who should attempt to remain with the queen until the newborn kittens demand the attention of the queen. Once this occurs, the owner can usually leave without disturbing the mother cat.

PERIPARTURIENT AND POSTPARTUM PROBLEMS

Ectopic Pregnancy

Ova fertilized outside of the fallopian tubes or fertilized ova expelled from the ovarian bursa can result in an ectopic pregnancy. Ectopic pregnancy is defined as a fetus developing within the abdominal cavity, outside of the uterus. Such queens have been described as having no signs of illness or as having an abdominal mass, abdominal enlargement, and/or vague signs of illness. Abdominal ultrasonography is the best means of diagnosing this extremely rare condition. Radiographs are less likely to be diagnostic. Surgical removal of the fetus resolves the condition (Olson et al, 1986).

Prepartum Vaginal Hemorrhage

The pregnant cat with a bloody vaginal discharge must be monitored closely. Bleeding that occurs between the second and eighth week of gestation is abnormal. This discharge may represent the only clue that a queen may be resorbing or aborting a litter. Less common signs include nonspecific listlessness and/or anorexia. Little can be recommended for treating these queens, aside from keeping them indoors in a quiet location away from animals or children and offering them highly palatable food.

The queen with a hemorrhagic vaginal discharge occurring after the eighth week of gestation also requires close monitoring. At this point in gestation, delivered kittens have at least a 50% chance at survival. In this context, the queen is not aborting her litter; rather, she is delivering the kittens prematurely. Queens with a small amount of hemorrhagic discharge (a few drops per day) should be kept quiet, comfortable, and indoors. Queens with larger amounts of discharge are in greater danger of losing their litter. In either situation, the source of blood is likely to be separation of placental sites, the premature tearing away of the placenta from the endometrium. Excessive tearing seriously interrupts vital blood supply to the fetus. Therefore excessive bleeding (15 ml or greater) is a strong indication to intercede with a cesarean section.

Dystocia

DIAGNOSIS. A major component of managing dystocia is determining the health of the queen. Before any diagnostic or therapeutic measures are employed, a complete history and physical examination are imperative. Dystocia rarely occurs in the cat but should be suspected if strong nonproductive contractions persist beyond 60 minutes. Dystocia should also be suspected if a kitten is visible in the vaginal vault but cannot be delivered or if a large quantity of bloody vaginal discharge is seen during parturition. Dystocia may also be present if gestation is prolonged or if labor ceases. If a kitten is visible in the vaginal vault, the veterinarian may be able to remove it physically. Radiographs of the abdomen are extremely valuable in evaluation of possible dystocia. If fetuses are normally positioned and sized and the birth canal is anatomically normal, medical management can be attempted. Radiographic abnormalities suggest the need for a cesarean section.

FETAL DYSTOCIA. Fetal dystocias can be the result of abnormal positioning that creates too large a mass for the birth canal. If only one or two normal kittens are present, each may be too large for the pelvis of the queen. Fetal deformities may also result in dystocia. Any of these problems are best diagnosed with abdominal radiography and managed by cesarean section.

MATERNAL DYSTOCIA. *Causes.* Maternal dystocias may include a congenitally narrowed pelvis or an acquired problem, such as a previously fractured pelvis. Torsion of (1) the uterus, (2) a single uterine horn, or (3) a segment of one horn are potential causes of dystocia, as would be inguinal hernias or a prolapsed uterus. Uterine torsion, usually diagnosed during laparotomy, has been described in eight queens in the veterinary literature (Johnston, 1983). Again, these problems are best managed by cesarean section.

Uterine inertia (primary = no kittens delivered; secondary = a portion of the litter delivered) is another maternal cause of dystocia. If the clinician believes that uterine inertia is present, most commonly seen in older obese queens and rarely in queens with large litters, medical intervention may succeed (Laliberte, 1986).

Medical management. Usually 2 to 4 U of oxytocin are administered intravenously to induce uterine contractions. If this fails, oxytocin can be repeated 20 minutes later after administering a slow intravenous infusion of 1 to 2 ml 10% calcium gluconate. If this treatment also fails, it should be followed in 20 minutes by repeating oxytocin administration after giving 2 ml of 50% dextrose by slow IV infusion. Cesarean section should follow failure of this third attempt to induce parturition.

Instrumentation. The use of instrumentation or rectal and abdominal manipulation is discouraged. The queen is usually too small for procedures that can be successful in larger animals. Cesarean section is a straightforward, commonly used procedure that is less traumatic than excessive digital or instrument maneuvers. Heroic, nonsurgical procedures are usually reserved for a neonate that is visible or readily palpable within the vagina.

Kitten Mortality

Various problems can result in death of newborn kittens. Several kittens can be delivered within a short time span; if the queen fails to separate the kittens from their membranes they can become entangled (Fig. 33-7, *A*). Several kittens may share one umbilical cord, which also can result in entanglement. The entanglement can result in trauma, with strangulation of a limb (Fig. 33-7, *B*) or death of one or more kittens. This problem can be avoided with conscientious owner involvement.

Because neonatal mortality has numerous causes, a specific diagnosis cannot usually be made by viewing gross specimens. Specimens from abnormal vaginal discharges, stillborn kittens, mummified fetuses, weak kittens that die, or placental tissues should be carefully handled. Any specimen available should be submitted to a veterinary diagnostic laboratory for examination (e.g., cytology, necropsy, histology, and cultures) in the hope that a definitive diagnosis can be made and specific treatment, control, or preventive measures instituted. Because contagious agents may be the source of the problem, the queen and any remaining kittens should be strictly isolated from other cats and kittens. Pregnant queens and kittens certainly should be protected as completely as possible.

Postpartum Vaginal Hemorrhage

Small amounts of hemorrhagic (red to blackish) vaginal discharge are common following normal parturition or dystocia. The discharge usually persists for several days to as long as 3 weeks. Noticing the vaginal discharge depends, to some degree, on the cleanliness of the queen. If the queen and kittens are healthy, persistent hemorrhagic discharge should be monitored but need not be treated. If the amount of discharge seems excessive, the red blood cell count and hematocrit should be monitored. With a decline in these parameters, coagulation disorders must be considered. After ruling out a bleeding problem, the veterinarian may be forced to recommend an ovariohysterectomy. An alternative to surgery is prostaglandin therapy, as discussed in the section of this chapter on pyometra. Oxytocin injections, administered within 24 to 36 hours of completing parturition, may serve as prophylaxis in preventing postpartum hemorrhage.

Occasionally, the normal bloody postpartum vaginal discharge becomes mucopurulent in appearance. This may be a reflection of a uterine infection, which can be diagnosed via physical examination (fever, listlessness, dehydration), increased white blood cell count, or refusal of the queen to nurse the kittens. Therapeutic alternatives include administration of antibiotics, prostaglandin therapy, or ovariohysterectomy.

Subinvolution of Placental Sites

Prolonged postpartum vaginal bleeding (>3 weeks' duration) may be a result of subinvolution of placental sites (SIPS) within the endometrium. This condition is usually self-limiting, and therapy is not necessary. The diagnosis of SIPS is suggested by persistent vaginal bleeding beyond 3 weeks after parturition. Administration of antibiotics, ergot products, or prostaglandins is of no value. Treatment is necessary only if the queen becomes anemic or if metritis/pyometra develops. In the latter conditions, therapies to consider include transfusions and/or ovariohysterectomy.

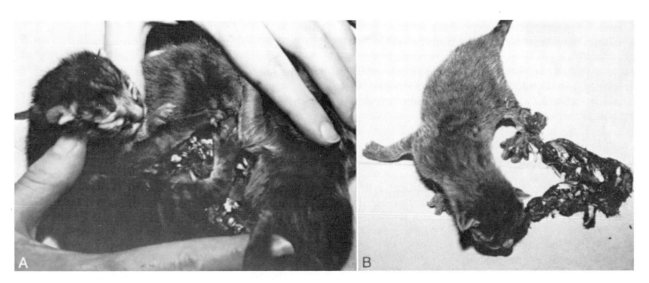

FIGURE 33-7. *A,* Kittens tied together by their entangled umbilical cords. *B,* Trauma to one leg of a kitten entangled within its umbilical cord. (Courtesy of Anthony Buffington, DVM.)

Retained Placenta

Retained placentas are usually described as causing fever, anorexia, depression, and absence of nursing instincts in the queen and bitch. However, the diagnosis of retained placenta remains extremely difficult. Owner observation and/or palpation of the queen's abdomen is subjective and quite unreliable in diagnosing this condition. Radiographs of the abdomen are also difficult to interpret following parturition because the uterus is invariably enlarged and often irregular in shape, potentially creating a false impression of a uterine mass. Queens that have been evaluated with abdominal ultrasonography rarely have retained placentas. A majority of those that have evidence of a retained placenta have remained healthy despite continued presence of potential foreign material within the uterus. Some queens pass the membranes naturally several days later. Others have subsequently been bred, queened healthy litters, and passed the placenta during the subsequent parturition. Therefore retained placenta is an uncommon cause for the queen to be ill postpartum and does not consistently result in metritis.

Acute Metritis

Acute metritis is seen 12 to 96 hours following parturition. Acute metritis involves infection secondary to disorders such as retained fetus, retained placenta, and injury from instruments and other trauma. The diagnosis is based on the presence of an off-color, foul-smelling vaginal discharge and uterine enlargement on abdominal palpation. The queen is typically depressed, listless, and anorectic. She usually ignores her kittens, and her rectal temperature may be normal, subnormal, or elevated. A complete blood count often reveals a left shift to immature neutrophils in association with a normal or elevated white blood cell count. Uncommonly, the total white blood cell count is low.

Therapy for this condition includes administration of IV fluids and antibiotics. Our experience with trimethoprimsulfa has been excellent. Ovariohysterectomy is the treatment of choice. Use of subcutaneously administered prostaglandins for 3 to 5 days has been extremely beneficial in treating cats whose owners did not wish to consider ovariohysterectomy.

Uterine Prolapse

Uterine prolapse may occur during parturition or in the following 48 hours. The condition has been described in numerous case reports and usually follows delivery of an entire litter. One empty uterine horn may prolapse while the other still contains fetuses, suggesting some obstruction preventing delivery of the remaining fetuses despite strong contractions.

Therapy consists of manual reduction and replacement of the uterus under general or epidural anesthesia if the uterus appears to be healthy and viable (Christiansen, 1984). Some cats may require laparotomy with both internal and external manipulation of the tissue to accomplish reduction. Ovariohysterectomy is recommended when extensive tissue damage is present.

Inadequate Care of Kittens

A queen that appears unwilling to nurse her kittens requires close attention. Some cats seem restless, stay with kittens for only brief periods, or even show aggressive behavior toward the newborns. Often, this unacceptable behavior is a result of environmental disturbances. Placing the queen and litter in a quiet, isolated area may prove beneficial. Light tranquilization of the queen also may improve her disposition (Christiansen, 1984). Admittedly, some queens do not tolerate kittens in any environment.

Maternal Care and Hand-Raising Orphan Kittens

The lactating queen may accept and nurse orphaned kittens that are similar in size to her own kittens. The greater the age and size differences between orphaned kittens and a queen's litter, the less likely she is to accept and nurse them. Use of a foster mother is ideal for raising orphan kittens. The queen usually remains with her kittens for 24 to 48 hours when parturition is complete and provides them with approximately 1 ml of milk per hour. The content of the milk changes during the nursing period (Table 33-4).

Kittens consume 5 to 7 ml of milk per feeding in the second week of life, weighing double their birth weight. Their eyes open by 8 to 10 days of age. After each feeding, the queen cleans and grooms the kittens, stimulating urination and defecation. The queen then consumes the urine and feces (Christiansen, 1984). At 3 weeks of age, kittens are more active and they learn to urinate and defecate some distance from their nest. Solid food should be supplemented by the fourth week of life and the kittens weaned between 5 and 8 weeks. Hand-raising kittens can be a difficult and time-consuming chore.

Hand-raised kittens should be kept together in a group. They must be kept warm with heating blankets or light bulbs to provide an ambient temperature of 75

TABLE 33–4   AVERAGE FAT, PROTEIN, AND LACTOSE CONTENT IN CAT MILK*

Content (Percent)	DAYS AFTER PARTURITION	
	1 to 10	11 to 60
Fat	3.7	3.3
Protein	6.5	8.7
Lactose	3.6	4.0

*After Hwini H, Montalta J: Z Versuchstierk 22:32, 1980.

TABLE 33–5 DOSAGE AND FREQUENCY OF MEALS FOR KITTENS*

Weeks Postpartum	Feed	Number of Meals/24 hr	Volume of Milk/Meal (ml)	Caloric Requirement	Expected Body Weight (g)
1	Milk mixture	9–12	1–7	40–80	100–200
2	Milk mixture	9	7–9	80–100	200–300
3	Milk mixture	9	10	112	300–360
4	Milk mixture	7	10	115	350–420
5	Introduce solids, reduce milk volume, increase solids	7	8–10	120	400–500
6	Milk in bowl, plus solids	6		125	450–600
7	Weaning from milk	3		130	500–700

*Adapted from Scott PP: Cats. *In* Hafez ESE (ed): Reproduction and Breeding Techniques for Laboratory Animals. Philadelphia, Lea & Febiger, 1970, p 192.

to 80° F. They can be fed with a stomach tube, from a bottle with a small nipple, or from a syringe with an adapter. Commercial milk replacements are available. Alternatively, one can formulate a diet using 20 g of skimmed milk powder, 90 ml of water, and 10 ml of olive oil (Christiansen, 1984). For the first few days, 80 μg of vitamin A should be added to the milk and 50 μg thereafter. The milk should be warmed to 98 to 99° F (37° C) before administration (Christiansen, 1984). Stomach tubes can be used quickly and safely, realizing that it is difficult to pass a tube into the trachea because of the kitten's sensitive laryngeal reflex. The tube length from mouth to stomach should be measured, further ensuring correct placement. If using a bottle, one should burn a hole in the nipple, 1 mm in diameter, with a hot needle to provide a smooth-edged opening of sufficient size (Voith, 1980).

The newborn kitten should be given hourly meals, each consisting of 1 ml of formula. Each day 0.5 ml should be added until a maximum of 10 ml is reached. By 4 to 5 weeks of age the kittens can be fed four to six times per day, and they can begin eating soft food and water from a dish (Table 33-5). After feeding, it is important to groom kittens with a warm, moist, soft towel to keep them clean and to stimulate urination and defecation.

Mammary Hyperplasia

DEFINITION AND CLINICAL DESCRIPTION. Massive enlargement of mammary glands can develop soon after (1) pregnancy, (2) pseudopregnancy, or (3) any time within a year of ovariohysterectomy. This condition appears to result from the rapid removal of progesterone from the system. The decreasing plasma progesterone is presumed to stimulate prolactin secretion from the pituitary, which in turn stimulates growth of mammary tissue. The glands are typically firm and easily distinguished from the abdominal wall. Growth can be so rapid that skin ulcers may develop in the most prominent areas. Infection of this tissue is catastrophic because it appears to quickly overwhelm the immune system, resulting in severe systemic septicemia/bacteremia.

TREATMENT. Treatment of mammary hyperplasia involves radical mastectomy or use of prolactin-suppressive drugs. Surgery may not be possible because the size of these glands and the amount of tissue lost if mastectomy is attempted prevent any ability to close the incision. Bromocriptine has been recommended at a dose of 0.25 mg, once daily, orally for 5 to 7 days. This drug, however, can cause vomiting, anorexia, and depression. Conservative measures include keeping the tissue clean, preventing nursing by other cats, and preventing self-mutilation (Elizabethan collar). Use of mibolerone or megestrol acetate has not been consistently helpful.

Mastitis and Eclampsia

These disorders are diagnosed and treated as described in Chapter 21.

SPONTANEOUS RESORPTION/EARLY PREGNANCY LOSS/ABORTION

Incidence

The incidence of abortion or resorption remains speculative in queens because ultrasonographically confirmed pregnancies are not common. Often, the diagnosis of pregnancy is made by the owner based on a queen's behavior or abdominal size. Less commonly, pregnancy is diagnosed by the owner or veterinarian via abdominal palpation. Such subjective methods of diagnosis can be quite misleading.

History and Signs

Various signs are associated with abortion or resorption. The queen may have a history of failing to have kittens despite normal matings or fail to deliver kittens in spite of a previous "positive" pregnancy diagnosis. Stronger evidence is recognition of a vaginal discharge (bloody or purulent) during gestation with or without fever, inappetence, anorexia, depression, vomiting, or diarrhea. Premature expulsion of fetuses cannot be disputed, but the queen may consume such evidence before it is seen. It is possible for a queen to remain clinically healthy despite resorbing fetuses or aborting a litter.

Causes

INFECTION. *Feline panleukopenia.* Panleukopenia virus is known to attack tissue with high mitotic activity such as an embryo or rapidly developing tissue within a fetus. The queen may have adequate neutralizing antibodies for self-protection but insufficient for the developing fetuses. Depending on the gestational age of the fetuses at the time of exposure, the result could be either infertility due to inapparent loss of embryos or abortion of mummified or macerated fetuses. Later exposure could cause blindness, hydrencephaly, and/or ataxia due to retinal, cerebral, and/or cerebellar degeneration, respectively. Definitive diagnosis in the cat with reproductive failure but without illness may be difficult, because even serologic testing is reliable only during the acute stage of viremia (Shille and Sojka, 1995).

Feline leukemia. Infection with the FeLV may result in unobserved early embryonal deaths, resorption of fetuses, or abortion of normal-appearing fetuses. In late pregnancy, fetuses may acquire lymphocyte-associated virus transplacentally, or neonates may be infected from the queen's saliva or milk. Kittens may fail to nurse, become dehydrated, and die within the first few weeks of life. The queen may develop pyometra as a result of her immunosuppressed condition. Management involves identification of all positive reactors on serologic testing and removal of those cats from the household. Because seronegative healthy carriers exist, it is prudent to recommend that testing be continued at 90-day intervals until no positive cats are identified on two consecutive tests. Vaccination of seronegative cats is recommended. Because the virus is relatively fragile in the environment, routine cleanliness interrupts spread of the disease.

Other infections. Various other infectious agents may interfere with pregnancy in queens. Feline viral rhinotracheitis may cause abortion, fetal mummification, and delivery of stillborn kittens. Queens with signs of upper respiratory tract disease have been observed to abort fetuses or deliver stillborn kittens (Colby, 1980a). FeLV virus has been incriminated as a cause of fetal resorption, abortion, fading kitten syndrome, and infertility (Colby, 1980a). Toxoplasmosis has been associated with abortions. Coliform bacteria, streptococci, staphylococci, and salmonellae are among the numerous bacteria associated with aborting queens (Christiansen, 1984).

FETAL DEFECTS. Numerous fetal disorders can result in death and kittens with congenital defects may be part of an otherwise normal litter. Less severe defects are seen in young kittens because the most severe problems result in the fetuses being resorbed or aborted earlier in gestation.

MATERNAL PROBLEMS/CYSTIC ENDOMETRIAL HYPERPLASIA. Poor nutrition, trauma, and abnormalities of the genital tract are among the maternal causes of pregnancy failure. These can be extremely difficult to recognize or diagnose. Cystic endometrial hyperplasia (CEH), endometritis, or endometrial infection should be suspected if the queen has a radiographically visible uterus. Better success in diagnosis is achieved with ultrasonography, which allows thickening of the uterine wall and/or fluid in the uterus to be visualized. Occasionally, one detects evidence of a retained or mummified fetus, extrauterine pregnancy, fetal remnants (skeleton), or fetal membranes. With any of these problems, the veterinarian can recommend an exploratory laparotomy in order to complete an evaluation.

At surgery one can perform a uterine biopsy or intrauterine culture and/or remove any abnormal tissue. The patency of the uterine horns and oviducts can also be assessed by holding off each horn at the uterine body and infusing saline into the horn. Saline should fill each horn homogeneously and leak through the oviducts into the surgical field. Remember that the uterotubular junction is tight (closed) in proestrus. The infusion procedure is quick and safe, using a small-gauge needle to pass into the uterine lumen.

Many of the disorders that can be diagnosed with the above procedures are not easily treated. Infection should be treated chronically (2 to 4 months) with the appropriate antibiotic. CEH has no proven therapy, although induction of prolonged anestrus may allow complete uterine involution and resolution of the condition. Because progestagens may worsen the problem, androgens such as mibolerone are recommended. Oviductal or uterine aplasia, causing lack of patency, cannot be treated, and ovariohysterectomy should be recommended.

ENVIRONMENTAL STRESS. Many of the causes for pregnancy failure can be the result of "stress." Environmental stress can be caused by shipping a queen by air or land, moving a cat away from a familiar location, adding new pets to the queen's environment, poor nutrition, dirty surroundings, parasites, infectious diseases, and numerous other factors. All are stresses that may terminate pregnancy (Voith, 1980).

ENDOCRINE DISORDERS—HYPOLUTEOIDISM. *Definition.* Among the endocrine problems that could account for premature termination of pregnancy is luteal phase inadequacy (hypoluteoidism). This condition is defined as inadequate secretion of progesterone for maintenance of pregnancy. As in the dog, this condition has not been confirmed to be a true clinical entity. However, its diagnosis and suggested therapy are commonplace. Because luteal phase inadequacy was first described in women as a potential cause of infertility and abortion, a large amount of information has accumulated, supporting the notion that this syndrome, if it exists, is complex and heterogeneous.

Physiology. Luteal phase inadequacy is characterized by incomplete or delayed secretory transformation of the endometrium due to the inadequate secretion of progesterone from corpora lutea. This renders the endometrium a poor substrate for implantation of the blastocyst, which would likely be considered an infertile cycle by most owners (Taubert, 1984). Later in gestation, progesterone deficiency (due to insufficient synthesis from corpora lutea or the placentae) would cause resorption/abortion, either of which may go unrecognized or be considered a non-fertile cycle. Various causes for subnormal progesterone concentrations during pregnancy have been described in addition to simple primary ovarian dysfunction: delayed onset of luteinization, inadequate stimulation by LH, interference with function of corpora lutea by intermittent moderate hyperprolactinemia, hyper-androgenemia, or improper follicular maturation due to a relative deficiency of FSH in the early follicular phase (Di Zerega and Hodgen, 1981). The investigations into this complex disorder have involved primarily women, not animals.

Diagnosis. Demonstration of abnormally low circulating diestrual progesterone concentrations (<1.0 ng/ml) is critical to the diagnosis of this condition. However, demonstration of concurrent pregnancy is also needed to rule out the occurrence of natural (normal) shortening of luteal phase duration, recognized in any pseudopregnant queen. Therefore diagnosis of pregnancy early in gestation via abdominal ultrasonography is vital. Ultrasonography can be performed as early as 2 weeks following breeding and repeated every 4 to 7 days. With each recheck, the plasma progesterone concentration should be assayed (using in-house ELISA kit or via a laboratory). If the queen is demonstrated to be pregnant but with prematurely decreasing or low plasma progesterone concentrations, she should resorb or abort her litter. Once this has been demonstrated, it is reasonable to consider progesterone supplementation during a sub-sequent pregnancy.

Treatment. Therapy consists of medroxyprog-esterone acetate, 10 mg orally per week, starting 1 week before previous abortions were identified and continuing until 1 week before anticipated parturition (Christiansen, 1984). Alternatively, 1 to 2 mg/kg of repositol progesterone intramuscularly, weekly, can also be used (Christiansen, 1984). Therapy is under-taken rarely, because an inadequate luteal phase is an uncommon cause of either infertility, resorption, or abortion in queens. Progesterone administration, as a treatment for hypoluteoidism, may increase the chances for development of pyometra (Colby, 1980a; Christiansen, 1984) or result in masculinization of the external genitalia of female kittens (Johnston, 1983).

Therapy

For the majority of the conditions described in this section, prevention is the easiest and most successful therapy. Cats used in breeding should be kept current on vaccinations, and good husbandry practices are essential. Breeding cats should be tested and treated for intestinal parasites, periodically checked for FeLV, and guarded against unnecessary exposure to cats that are ill or untested. Pregnant cats should not be vaccinated, and all other medications should be used with the realization that there is always potential for harm to the fetus.

CYSTIC ENDOMETRIAL HYPERPLASIA/PYOMETRA

Pathophysiology

The pathophysiology of cystic endometrial hyperplasia (CEH) appears to be similar in cats and dogs (a detailed discussion is available in Chapter 23). The endometrium becomes abnormally thickened with fluid-filled cystic structures, accounting for the term *cystic endometrial hyperplasia*. If uncontaminated, the fluid is clear and is present primarily within cystic structures in the uterine mucosa. This same fluid, if free in the uterus, represents an excellent medium for bacterial growth. Bacterial contamination of the fluid leads to breakdown of the cystic structures, dissemination of the infection, and development of pyometra. Bacteria are most likely derived from vaginal flora that ascends into the uterus via the cervix. Like dogs, normal and healthy cats commonly have bacteria within their vaginal tracts (Table 33-6; Clemetson and Ward, 1990).

The most common bacterium isolated in pyometra is *Escherichia coli,* although numerous other bacteria have been isolated (Davidson et al, 1992). The cystic structures occur, in part, as a result of progesterone's effect on the endometrium. The susceptibility to bacteria appears increased when the queen is under the influence of both progesterone and estrogen. Estrogens may dilate the cervix, allowing the initial contamination of uterine contents. Pyometra or metritis may also develop secondary to such problems as a retained fetus, retained fetal membranes, trauma during parturition, or instrumentation used in relieving dystocia. Pyometra has also been reported in queens with an extrauterine pregnancy (Vasseur and Feldman, 1982) and in a cat with uterus masculinus (Schulman and Levine, 1989).

Signalment, History, and Physical Examination

HISTORY. The CEH/pyometra complex can be diagnosed at any age. It is interesting to note that the disorder has been described as being prevalent in queens over 5 years of age that have never had kittens (Lein and Concannon, 1983), as well as being most common in queens that have had one or more litters (Colby, 1980a). In our review of queens with pyometra, the past history of previous litters has not appeared to influence susceptibility. CEH is typically a subclinical condition or results in prolonged anestrus until bacterial infection occurs. The signs that are seen with pyometra (Table 33-7) include copious vaginal dis-charge, anorexia or inappetence, depression, listless-ness, weight loss, unkempt appearance, polyuria and polydipsia, occasional vomiting, and/or diarrhea. Only the cats with open-cervix pyometra have an obvious watery or thick and viscous vaginal discharge. The discharge is often creamy and light tan–pink to dark brown in color. Some of these cats have relatively mild signs of inappetence or depression. In more advanced

TABLE 33–6 BACTERIAL ISOLATES FROM THE REPRODUCTIVE TRACTS OF THREE GROUPS OF CATS

Bacteria Isolated	NUMBER OF ISOLATES		
	Group 1* (n = 13)	Group 2† (n = 10)	Group 3‡ (n = 30)
Vaginal Aerobes			
Staphylococcus (coagulase negative)	7(54)§	7(70)	10(33)
S aureus	0(0)	1(10)	0(0)
S intermedius	0(0)	1(10)	0(0)
Streptococcus canis	9(69)	8(80)	6(20)
Str uberis	0(0)	0(0)	4(13)
Str agalactiae	0(0)	0(0)	2(7)
Str dysgalactiae	0(0)	0(0)	1(3)
Str faecalis	1(8)	0(0)	0(0)
Str mitis	1(8)	0(0)	1(3)
Streptococcus (unidentified)	1(8)	0(0)	8(10)
Aerococcus sp	2(15)	0(0)	1(3)
Micrococcus sp	0(0)	1(10)	0(0)
Bacillus sp	1(8)	0(0)	0(0)
Corynebacterium sp (nonhemolytic)	5(38)	3(30)	7(23)
Actinomyces pyogenes	0(0)	0(0)	4(13)
Gardnerella sp-like	1(8)	0(0)	0(0)
Escherichia coli	6(46)	2(20)	20(66)
Klebsiella ozaenae	0(0)	0(0)	2(7)
Flavobacterium sp	1(0)	0(0)	2(7)
CDC IIJ	1(8)	1(10)	3(10)
Moraxella sp	2(15)	2(20)	3(10)
Acinetobacter sp	2(15)	1(10)	5(16)
Pasteurella haemolytica	0(0)	1(10)	1(3)
P multocida	2(15)	0(0)	0(0)
Pseudomonas sp	0(0)	0(0)	1(3)
Haemophilus paracuniculus	0(0)	0(0)	4(13)
Haemophilus sp	2(15)	0(0)	0(0)
Haemophilus sp-like (unidentified)	0(0)	2(20)	8(26)
Simonsiella sp	0(0)	0(0)	1(3)
Vaginal Anaerobes			
Bacteroides fragilis	ND	ND	1(3)
B oralis	ND	ND	1(3)
B asaccharolyticus	ND	ND	1(3)
Peptococcus sp	ND	ND	2(7)
Uterine Flora			
Lactobacillus sp (anaerobe)	ND	ND	1(3)
Acinetobacter sp	ND	ND	1(3)
E coli	ND	ND	1(3)

From Clemetson LL, Ward ACS: Bacterial flora of the vagina and uterus of healthy cats. JAVMA 196:902, 1990.
*Multiparous adult cats (≥3 years old) that had been in a cat-breeding colony for at least 2 years.
†5–7-month-old kittens born in that colony.
‡6–16-month-old, privately owned and nonspayed cats (Group 3).
§The percentage of cats within each group infected with a bacterial isolate is enclosed in parentheses. *ND*, Not determined.

disease, abdominal enlargement is described (Lawler et al, 1991; Potter et al, 1991).

PHYSICAL EXAMINATION. Physical examination usually reveals the vaginal discharge in a mildly depressed, dehydrated animal with a normal or increased rectal temperature and a palpably enlarged

TABLE 33–7 CLINICAL SIGNS OF PYOMETRA IN 21 CATS

Copious vaginal discharge	21/21	100%
Palpable uterus	21/21	100%
Fever	5/21	24%
Anorexia	5/21	24%
Lethargy	5/21	24%
Weight loss	3/21	14%
Unkempt appearance	2/21	9%
Polydipsia/polyuria	2/21	9%

uterus. Severe toxemia can be associated with marked illness and subnormal temperatures. Cats with closed-cervix pyometra have no vaginal discharge but they may have significant uterine distention causing abdominal enlargement and severe illness.

Diagnosis

CYSTIC ENDOMETRIAL HYPERPLASIA. Cats with CEH are usually normal on physical examination. Occasionally, the uterus can be palpated. Blood and urine tests are normal. Visualizing the uterus radiographically in a nonpregnant queen supports the diagnosis of CEH, although radiographs are often negative. Ultrasonography of the abdomen has been a sensitive and reliable tool for recognizing a nonpregnant, enlarged uterus due to a thickened endometrium, with or without intraluminal fluid. The diagnosis can be confirmed only by laparotomy and histologic evaluation of a uterine biopsy.

PYOMETRA. Queens with pyometra do not pose the difficult diagnostic challenge one associates with CEH. A queen with an abnormal vaginal discharge should be assumed to have pyometra, and further evaluation is undertaken to substantiate the diagnosis. The diagnosis is supported by finding uterine enlargement radiographically. Ultrasonography readily distinguishes between pregnancy and pyometra 21 days after the last breeding date. Many, but not all, cats with pyometra have an increase in white blood cell count (mean of 35,000 cells/mm^3) and/or a shift to more immature neutrophils on the white blood cell differential (Davidson et al, 1992). If the cat is or was recently in diestrus, if she recently queened a litter, or if no other explanation for a vaginal discharge is obvious (proestrus, vaginal foreign body or mass, vaginitis, trauma), therapy for pyometra should begin.

Before and during treatment for pyometra, various other parameters should be monitored. In the extremely ill queen, abnormalities in rectal temperature, blood urea nitrogen, urine output, and serum sodium/potassium concentrations are among the factors that can contribute to the animal's illness. Correcting secondary problems, as well as the primary abnormalities, improves the success of any mode of therapy.

Treatment

SUPPORTIVE CARE—ANTIBIOTICS AND INTRAVENOUS FLUIDS. The incidence of bacteremia in bitches with pyometra approaches 10% to 15%. It is presumed that a similar percentage of queens with pyometra also have bacteremia. Therefore all such cats should receive antibiotics. *E. coli* is the most prevalent bacterium in the pyometra complex. Either trimethoprim/sulfadiazine (Tribribrissin, Burroughs Wellcome Co., Research Triangle Park, NC) or amoxicillin trihydrate/clavulanate potassium (Clavamox, Beecham Inc, Bristol, TN) is the initial antibiotic of choice. A culture and sensitivity test on material obtained from the anterior vaginal vault could assist in determining the efficacy of any antibiotic, but such procedures are not commonly employed in cats. Antibiotics used as the sole form of therapy are rarely effective. The hydration status of any cat suspected of having pyometra should be carefully assessed and appropriate therapy used.

SURGERY. *Ovariohysterectomy (OVH).* Hysterectomy has traditionally provided consistent and successful results. OVH remains the treatment of choice. Surgery permanently eliminates the site of infection, and most cats quickly recover.

Surgical drainage of the uterus. Draining and lavaging the uterus via laparotomy and uterotomy has been reported (Vasseur and Feldman, 1982). The procedure involves packing off the uterus and aspirating all purulent uterine contents after making a small longitudinal incision in the ventral uterine surface. The uterus can then be thoroughly lavaged with a balanced electrolyte solution. One fenestrated feeding tube should be placed in each uterine horn with an end passed through the cervix and out the vagina to allow postsurgical lavage (Fig. 33-8). This protocol does involve major surgery on an infected organ involving a debilitated cat. Although successful in a limited number of cats, the procedure is not recommended.

PROSTAGLANDIN THERAPY. *Criteria for therapy.* Various medical therapies have been proposed for use in the management of pyometra, but none has gained the acceptance or success of prostaglandins. Our experience with prostaglandin $F_{2\alpha}$ ($PGF_{2\alpha}$) in cats with postpartum metritis and in those with open-cervix pyometra has been excellent. Treatment with $PGF_{2\alpha}$ has been reserved for queens that are 6 years of age or younger with no evidence of retained fetal tissue (abdominal ultrasonography is extremely valuable) and are owned by individuals who would prefer to avoid OVH in order to preserve the reproductive capability of the cat. Using these criteria, we have treated 32 queens with open-cervix pyometra and 8 queens with open draining postpartum endometritis. None of these cats was thought to be in critical condition.

Initial protocol and immediate response. Queens should be treated with 0.1 mg/kg of dinoprost tromethamine (Lutalyse, The Upjohn Co., Kalamazoo, MI) SC twice daily for 5 days. We have not had experience with the more potent synthetic analogues. The $PGF_{2\alpha}$ had one major effect on the reproductive tract: contraction of the myometrium resulting in progressive expulsion of uterine contents over a period of days. Most but not all of the queens with open-cervix pyometra have had plasma progesterone concentrations suggestive of active luteal function (>1.0 ng/ml). The $PGF_{2\alpha}$ did not appear to consistently inhibit synthesis of progesterone or cause lysis of corpora lutea. The ability of $PGF_{2\alpha}$ to dilate the cervix could not be assessed.

Prostaglandin's ability to cause contraction of the uterus was not often obvious in the bitch. However, in the queen we often noted a dramatic increase in the amount of vaginal discharge present soon after $PGF_{2\alpha}$ administration, reflecting an obvious effect of the drug on the myometrium.

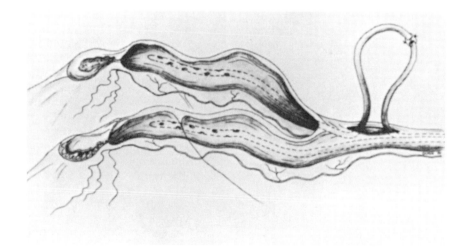

FIGURE 33-8. Schematic drawing showing the placement of intrauterine tubes when treating pyometra surgically. (From Vasseur PB, Feldman EC: Pyometra associated with extrauterine pregnancy in a cat. JAAHA 18:870, 1982.)

Concurrent antibiotic therapy is recommended. Each treated queen should be closely monitored with complete physical examinations at least twice daily, although they do not need to be hospitalized during the entire period. Treated cats should be hospitalized during the day for observation following prostaglandin administration. If the cat develops worsening fever, abdominal pain, or other worrisome problems, white blood cell count and abdominal ultrasonography should be reevaluated. Although neither systemic infection nor peritonitis has developed in any of our treated cats, either is possible. If signs worsen and/or peritonitis is suspected, the owner can be apprised of the situation and OVH with or without abdominal lavage should be recommended. To date, surgery has not been necessary in any cat we have medically managed with prostaglandins.

Side effects. Many of the side effects caused by $PGF_{2\alpha}$ in cats are similar to those described in the bitch (Nelson et al, 1982; Davidson et al, 1992; see Chapter 23). Within 30 to 120 seconds, the queen may begin vocalizing and panting; become restless; exhibit intense grooming behavior; have tenesmus, salivation, diarrhea, kneading, and mydriasis; and vomit, urinate, defecate, and/or exhibit a lordosis posture. The grooming is directed at the flanks and/or vulva. Additional side effects have included tail flagging and tearing at newspapers in the cage (Table 33-8).

The side effects usually persist for 2 to 20 minutes. In virtually every treated queen, the reactions to $PGF_{2\alpha}$ therapy have been less obvious following each successive injection. By the fifth day, the side effects, if any, are minimal and short-lived.

Long-term follow-up. Queens that have received $PGF_{2\alpha}$ should be rechecked 1 and 2 weeks following the last injection. A clear, serous vaginal discharge 7 days after completion of treatment strongly suggests that the pyometra has been successfully managed, and no further injections are usually required. The clear discharge is present transiently (2 to 10 days). The white blood cell count is usually normal 7 days after treatment and certainly should be normal by day 14. Typically, cats are normal by day 14 posttreatment. One may need to consider a second 5-day series of injections if a sanguineous or mucopurulent vaginal

discharge, uterine enlargement, high white blood cell count, or fever has persisted through the 14-day recheck.

Breeding. Queens frequently return to estrus within 1 to 6 weeks of therapy. We have recommended that the queen be bred at that time to obtain a litter and reduce the likelihood of recurring infection.

Results. The results in treating 32 cats with open-cervix pyometra and 8 queens with postpartum endometritis have been excellent. All cats responded to $PGF_{2\alpha}$ therapy. At the time of discharge from the hospital all queens demonstrated improved appetite, normal rectal temperature, and diminished or no vaginal discharge. At the 14-day recheck all queens were clinically normal with no vaginal discharge or palpable uterine enlargement. Of the 40 queens, 39 had a normal estrous cycle after prostaglandin treatment. Estrus was observed 0.5 to 12 months after treatment, with an average 4-month delay. One queen had recurrence of purulent vaginal discharge 1 month after completing treatment, was treated a second time, and responded without complication.

Successful breedings were reported for 39 of the 40 queens, 2 weeks to 5 years after treatment. Of these, 37 queens produced live kittens. One queen had three litters of stillborn kittens, one queen was spayed 1 year after treatment because of recurrence of the pyometra (she never had kittens), and one queen was never bred despite normal estrous cycles. Of the 37 queens that delivered healthy kittens after treatment, 3 later redeveloped pyometra. One of these was spayed, but the other two were once again treated with prostaglandins, and each subsequently carried pregnancies to term and delivered normal kittens.

INFERTILITY

Evaluating the Problem

Infertility is a broad term that refers to any cause for a queen to fail in producing a litter. Infertility is not a diagnosis but rather a sign of a problem. Because of the wide variety of problems that can contribute to or cause infertility, a thorough understanding of an individual queen is quite helpful. The questionnaire used in evaluating a bitch with infertility can easily be adapted for use in cats (see Chapter 24). A few of the questions should be altered to ascertain whether the breeding queen has the expected postcopulatory yowl and displays a typical postcoital afterreaction and to determine the number of times per day breeding takes place, the number of days bred during an estrus, and so forth.

Infertility: Breeding Queen with a Normal Polyestrous Cycle (Fig. 33-9)

GENERAL HEALTH OF THE QUEEN. In order to eliminate an unnecessary evaluation of the reproductive system,

TABLE 33–8 PHYSICAL REACTIONS TO SUBCUTANEOUS PROSTAGLANDIN $F_{2\alpha}$ OBSERVED IN 21 CATS TREATED FOR PYOMETRA

Vocalization	13/21	62%
Panting	8/21	38%
Restlessness	7/21	33%
Grooming	5/21	24%
Tenesmus	5/21	24%
Salivation	5/21	24%
Diarrhea	4/21	19%
Kneading	4/21	19%
Mydriasis	3/21	14%
Emesis	2/21	9%
Urination	2/21	9%
Lordosis	2/21	9%

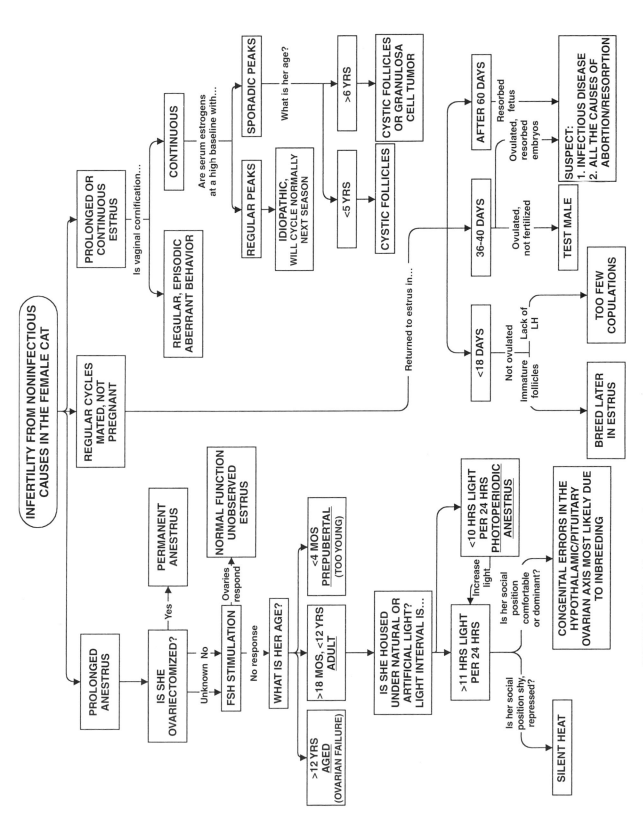

FIGURE 33-9. Algorithm for evaluating an apparently infertile queen that does not have an infection.

obvious problems should first be identified. The queen with liver, renal, or other major organ disturbances may specifically be infertile because of that problem. The veterinary clinician should obtain a complete history and perform a thorough physical examination. Any abnormalities identified should be investigated. In addition, most infertility evaluations should include a review of complete blood count (CBC), serum chemistry profile, urinalysis, FeLV status, and, if the cat is quite thin, a serum T_4 concentration. Titers for feline infectious peritonitis (FIP) and toxoplasmosis can be considered. Any cardiac problem suspected should be evaluated with thoracic radiography, electrocardiography, and, when possible, ultrasonography or echocardiography.

An ultrasonographic evaluation of the abdomen is strongly recommended. Among its attributes, ultrasonography is an excellent tool for examining the uterus, uterine contents (if any), and the ovaries (e.g., tumor, cysts). In addition, this tool allows evaluation of remaining abdominal structures. Radiographs are not as useful but should be completed following a 12- to 24-hour fast and one or two enemas. This preparation should allow visualization of the kidneys, liver, gastrointestinal tract, urinary bladder, and spine for obvious abnormalities. Unexpected visualization of the uterus, fetal structures, or unidentified masses may provide a diagnosis.

THE MALE. The fertility of the male cat is not evaluated as easily as that of his canine counterpart. However, any time that an apparently healthy queen fails to conceive, the soundness of the male should be questioned. If the male has not sired a litter within a 6- to 12-month period, he remains a potential cause of the infertility. Use of a proven sire should be recommended before beginning sophisticated studies in an apparently normal queen.

REVIEW OF BREEDING MANAGEMENT PRACTICES. Food, housing, parasite control, vaccination procedures, FeLV testing, and isolation of cats before they are added to a colony should be considered in the assessment of infertility cases. Cats should be fed high-quality commercial cat foods. This becomes more important when more than one queen from a household or colony is suspected of being infertile.

The owner should be carefully questioned on breeding management. As discussed earlier in this chapter, a queen bred only once each day (or once total) during estrus has a much lower incidence of ovulation induction than a queen bred four to eight times every other day. A queen bred too early or too late in estrus also may have a decreased chance of ovulating. The owner should be made aware that the queen and tom should be allowed to breed at least four times, every day or every other day, as long as the queen is in estrus. This ensures the greatest chance of successfully inducing ovulation and conception.

The owner should also report what is observed during breeding. Is the male allowed to mount, is there a postcoital yowl by the queen, and does she exhibit an after-reaction? If the yowl and after-reaction are not observed, it is likely that breeding never occurred. In this situation, another male should be used. If the problem persists, the queen should be evaluated for refusing to allow breeding. If the owners never observe breeding, they cannot provide the answers to these extremely important questions. The differential diagnosis is entirely different for queens that refuse to breed versus those that apparently fail to conceive (see Fig. 33-9).

INTERESTROUS INTERVALS. The owner and veterinarian should review breeding dates. This gives the veterinarian an opportunity to assess an owner's record system and observation skills. The average queen allows breeding for an average of 7 consecutive days (range is 4 to 9 days). If a sufficient number of breedings took place to induce ovulation, the nonpregnant queen should become pseudopregnant, and the interestrous interval should persist for 35 to 70 days. If pseudopregnancy is induced, the queen either is failing to conceive or is resorbing or aborting fetuses, or the male is sterile. The presence of pseudopregnancy can be confirmed with a plasma progesterone concentration obtained 1 to 3 weeks after breeding ceases. If pseudopregnancy is not induced, it must be determined whether breeding did occur and whether there were sufficient breedings at the correct time (see Fig. 33-9).

IMPLANTATION FAILURE; RESORPTION; ABORTION. See discussions on Cystic Endometrial Hyperplasia or Abortion/Resorption in this chapter.

Failure to Cycle

PREVIOUS OVARIOHYSTERECTOMY. If a queen displays no estrous activity whatsoever, the veterinarian should check to see whether she has previously undergone an OVH. Usually, checking for a "spay" incision is all that is needed (see Fig. 33-9).

GENERAL HEALTH. The cat's general health must be thoroughly evaluated. This usually involves a good history, complete physical examination, and a routine blood and urine data base. Estrous cycles can be interrupted or can cease in an animal under the stress of a poor diet, compromising illness, overcrowding, exposure to extremes in temperature, or inadequate exposure to light. The stress of a show circuit and traveling can also influence the estrous cycle. Drug therapy, especially progestagens and glucocorticoids, can interrupt estrous activity via negative feedback to the pituitary. A variety of ovarian and uterine neoplasias have been recognized. Ovarian granulosa–theca cell tumors and ovarian dysgerminomas are the most common neoplasias (Loar, 1989). These could result in prolonged anestrus, CEH, or prolonged estrus (Herron, 1986).

SILENT HEAT. Perhaps the best example of silent heat is the cat housed with a number of other cats. If a cat is low on the "pecking order" or if overcrowding exists, its cycles may be completely undetectable, or "silent," to humans and apparently to other cats. This is a difficult syndrome to recognize, although several simple diagnostic methods can be used (see Fig. 33-9). The easiest method is to teach an owner how to obtain vaginal smears from the cat and to do this procedure once or twice weekly from January through March. The slides can be air-dried and brought to the veterinarian for staining and review. Follicular phases are reflected as an increase in the percentage of superficial cells present. Alternatively, once- or twice-weekly plasma samples can be assayed for estrogen concentration. If either study suggests normal follicular function, the cat should be completely isolated and maintained on 14 hours of light and 10 hours of darkness. Usually, her estrous activity is more apparent on this regimen and removal from the other cats. Another approach is to attempt to induce estrus medically (see below).

PREMATURE OVARIAN FAILURE. The functional longevity of the ovaries in queens is not known, although many queens do not continue estrous cycle activity beyond 11 to 13 years of age. Queens beyond 8 years of age are not usually used in breeding programs. The ovaries, abnormally, may cease functioning earlier. This results in a permanent condition interpreted as prolonged anestrus by the owner. Premature ovarian failure is suspected when all other differentials are excluded from the list of potential diagnoses and induction procedures fail. It is a difficult diagnosis, however, to confirm. The clinician may assay LH and FSH concentrations in the plasma. Persistent elevation of these hormones is consistent with nonfunctioning ovaries (see Fig. 33-9).

DISORDERS OF SEXUAL DEVELOPMENT. Phenotypically normal females may not have functional ovaries secondary to chromosomal abnormalities. Several such cats have been reported (Nicholas et al, 1980; Johnston et al, 1983). Karyotyping can be performed at the University of California and other institutions to recognize these disorders, which are described in detail in Chapter 24. Another option is to perform exploratory surgery to examine the reproductive tract and to biopsy or remove any abnormal tissue. The veterinarian can also attempt to induce estrus medically to rule out any likelihood of a disorder in sexual development.

INDUCTION OF ESTRUS. *Indications.* Once the veterinarian is certain that no anatomic defect, organic illness, or medication explains the failure to cycle, an attempt can be made to induce a cycle medically. This procedure can be used in queens that have never cycled, queens with prolonged acquired anestrus, or queens with highly irregular cycles. Because the queen is an induced ovulator, one must rely on the male to induce ovulation once estrus is induced, or an attempt can be made to induce ovulation medically.

Exposure to correct amounts of light. Before administration of hormones, altering light exposure should be tried. The queen should be exposed to 8 to 10 hours of light and 14 to 16 hours of dark for 1 week, followed by 12 to 14 hours of light and 10 to 12 hours of dark for as long as 4 to 8 weeks. This protocol can be used repeatedly to induce estrus (Hurni, 1981).

Housing with cycling queens. The queen in anestrus can also be housed with several queens that have normal estrous cycles in an attempt to induce estrus. This has been reported to be successful, especially when working with a family pet that may have been isolated from other cats for a prolonged period of time (Christiansen, 1984).

Use of hormones to induce estrus. See the discussion under Artificial Breeding on page 1027.

Prolonged Interestrous Intervals

PSEUDOPREGNANCY. A queen that enters estrus every 30 to 60 days may be ovulating and experiencing repeated pseudopregnancies. This has been observed in queens that have never been bred. Ovulation in some queens can be induced by petting, by obtaining vaginal cytology smears, or by less obvious factors. These queens are typically healthy and are fertile if bred. The diagnosis of pseudopregnancy can be confirmed by demonstrating an elevation in the plasma progesterone concentration 1 to 3 weeks after estrus. See the discussion on page 1024.

REVIEW OF MANAGEMENT. Queens must receive adequate food, housing, light, and general care if they are to cycle normally. Owner observation is valuable to ensure that some cycles are not missed. A general health examination and laboratory evaluation are also worthwhile, because an underlying illness may interrupt cyclic ovarian activity.

Cystic Follicles

DIAGNOSIS. Cystic follicles could result in either prolonged estrus behavior or a prolonged interestrous interval. Although difficult to diagnose, functioning follicles create persistent estrus via production of estrogen, which can be assayed. The most reliable and easiest method of diagnosing cystic follicles is abdominal ultrasonography. Cystic structures are usually easily identified and remain relatively static in size and shape. If the plasma estrogen concentration is persistently increased (>20 pg/ml), the diagnosis is further supported (see Fig. 33-9).

PROLONGED SEXUAL RECEPTIVITY—NYMPHOMANIA. Normal queens may exhibit prolonged sexual receptivity despite having normal waves of follicular function. In other words, their estrus behavior overlaps interestrous intervals, and persistent estrus results (Colby, 1980b). In most cats, this is considered a normal phenomenon, not requiring treatment. The ideal therapy, if any, is to induce ovulation via breeding to a normal or vasectomized tomcat. Artificial vaginal stimulation could also be used to induce ovulation and cause an end to persistent behavioral estrus.

Follicular cysts often produce signs of persistent estrus. A persistent follicle becomes a persistent source of estrogen. Any queen under a constant influence of estrogen displays continuous estrus behavior. The diagnosis is made by demonstrating increased plasma estrogen concentrations for more than 3 weeks without evidence of normal cyclicity in a queen with a cystic structure associated with one ovary on abdominal ultrasonography.

Persistent estrus in cats older than 5 years is consistent with the presence of granulosa cell tumors. This is the most common ovarian neoplasm in cats. Such tumors are more likely to be malignant in cats than in other species (McEntee, 1990).

TREATMENT. Treatment may consist of attempts at breeding to ovulate the cyst. The veterinarian can attempt to induce rupture of the follicle(s) by administering 250 IU of hCG IM once daily for 2 days (see discussion below). The recommended treatment is surgical removal of the cyst, with or without the associated ovary. Usually surgeons have not been able to remove the cyst without the ovary. These cats remain fertile with one ovary.

Failure to Permit Breeding

Review the appropriate sections in Chapters 24 and 25 on failure to permit breeding in the bitch. A similar group of differential diagnoses exist in the queen, including management problems, behavior disorders, vaginal or vulvar defects, and miscellaneous obstructions. Vulvar and vaginal atresias have been diagnosed in our practices. Vaginal strictures are rare but must be considered in a queen that fails to permit breeding.

ESTRUS IN OVARIOHYSTERECTOMIZED CATS

Cats that have been spayed but subsequently attract males may or may not have ovarian remnants as a result of incomplete surgery. Increased plasma estrogen concentrations and cornification of exfoliated vaginal cells suggest presence of an ovarian remnant or estrogen excess due to an adrenocortical problem. It has been suggested that oral administration of prednisolone (2.2 mg/kg, once daily, for 5 days) results in permanent disappearance of signs of estrus within 3 to 5 days (Shille and Sojka, 1995).

Ovarian remnant can be confirmed by luteinizing follicles with one injection of either hCG (250 IU, IM) or GnRH (25 µg, IM) and then documenting an increase in luteal progesterone. If the plasma progesterone concentration increases above 2.5 ng/ml 5 to 7 days after the stimulus, exploratory surgery to identify and remove the remnant tissue is warranted. It is recommended that surgery be performed during an estrus, because during the estrus phase, vascularized ovarian tissue is easier to identify (Shille and Sojka, 1995).

PREVENTION OF ESTROUS CYCLES; CONTRACEPTION

Surgical Contraception

OVH is the method of choice for permanently sterilizing female cats. This common procedure is safe, inexpensive, and successful. No strong evidence exists that OVH has any harmful effects on cats. Ovariectomy alone is not recommended, because the uterus would remain as a potential site of infection. Oviductal ligation or hysterectomy is rarely acceptable to an owner of a cat that will continue to cycle, display estrus, and attract males.

Laparoscopic sterilization can be accomplished in the queen. The uterine horns or the uterotubal junctions can be occluded by electrocoagulation or the use of plastic clips. Using either technique, the veterinarian must be certain that bilateral occlusion of the reproductive tract has been complete. Laparoscopic sterilization can be quick and safe, can be performed on young, prepubertal queens, and could potentially be a practical method for mass sterilization (Wildt and Lawler, 1985). However, queens would continue to cycle, breed, and attract males. Thus the disadvantages of continued ovarian activity must be realized.

Chemical Contraception

PROGESTAGENS. *General approach.* The use of progestagens is fully discussed in Chapter 22. In the queen, progestagen therapy should begin during true anestrus (i.e., the period of sexual inactivity usually seen during October, November, and December). This approach should minimize any risk of inducing uterine disorders. If given to the postpartum queen, therapy may need to be initiated soon after parturition to avoid the first postpartum estrus. Prolonged administration of any progestagen may result in CEH, pyometra, or mammary hyperplasia. Because this form of therapy is not benign (see below), it is not recommended for valuable future-breeding queens.

Megestrol acetate in prevention of estrous cycling. Megestrol acetate represents a relatively benign progestagen used in estrus prevention. There are few side effects (see below), and conception rates after withdrawal of this drug are excellent. Because megestrol acetate is metabolized by the liver, its use is discouraged in cats with liver dysfunction (Henik et al, 1985). Estrus prevention involves administration of 2.5 mg/day for 8 weeks or 2.5 mg/week for up to 18 months (Christiansen, 1984). A rest period of 2 or 3 months is recommended following each treatment period. If the cat is to be bred, she should breed on the second estrus following cessation of the therapy (Christiansen, 1984).

If the queen is entering estrus, megestrol acetate can still be used. Megestrol acetate, 5 mg daily for 3 days, followed by 2.5 to 5.0 mg/week for 10 weeks, is one recommended schedule. The queen should be isolated from males for the first few days of treatment. Rapid remission of estrus behavioral signs can be expected. Vocalization, rolling, awkward body contortions, and seeking males disappeared in 41% of cats after 3 days of treatment; 47% of the queens were in anestrus on day 5, and 90% were in anestrus by the end of the first week (Christiansen, 1984).

Side effects of megestrol acetate. Progestational compounds have numerous potential side effects in cats (Romantowski, 1989). These include possible increased friendliness toward humans, lethargy, depression, increased appetite, weight gain, polydipsia, and polyuria (Henik et al, 1985). Long-term oral megestrol acetate therapy can cause epidermal atrophy in cats (Henik et al, 1985), and cutaneous xanthomatosis was reported in one cat (Kwochka and Short, 1984). Some cats receiving megestrol acetate have had mammary hyperplasia (Chen and Bellenger, 1987; Shille and Sojka, 1995).

An association exists between excess progesterone and stimulation of growth hormone secretion with resultant signs of acromegaly and insulin resistance in dogs and cats (Eigenmann, 1985). Some megestrol-treated cats have developed diabetes mellitus that is usually transient, resolving with discontinuation of the drug. Some cats, however, develop a permanent diabetic state. Cats treated with common doses of megestrol acetate have been shown to have marked adrenocortical suppression without clinical signs of glucocorticoid insufficiency (Chastain et al, 1981). These cats should be considered to have hypoadrenocorticism and should receive glucocorticoid therapy if they develop any serious stress (illness, trauma, surgery).

Use of megestrol acetate in the United States. The labeling of megestrol acetate in veterinary medicine is solely for use in dogs. However, it is commonly used in cats for a variety of conditions, and this use is recognized in various veterinary publications.

ANDROGENS. Mibolerone (Cheque, The Upjohn Co., Kalamazoo, MI) is an androgenicanabolic steroid that has not received FDA approval for use in cats but does prevent estrous cycles in a large percentage of queens. A dose of 50 µg/day should be given, starting at least 30 days before the expected onset of estrus. As long as treatment continues, ovarian activity is suppressed without apparent effect on any subsequent estrus or on mating, conception, litter size, or parturition (Christiansen, 1984). If a queen is in proestrus or estrus, mibolerone should be withheld. This medication often causes enlargement of the clitoris and thickening of the cervical dermis. Mibolerone is considered contraindicated for cats because of reports of hepatotoxicity and thyrotoxicosis (Shille and Sojka, 1995).

MISMATING; PREVENTION OF IMPLANTATION

Mismating is not a common problem for veterinarians to treat in cats. As with the bitch, attempts can be made to determine whether mating actually occurred through history, vaginal smears (attempting to determine the stage of estrus and/or the presence of sperm), or physical findings such as scratches, bites, or hair loss on the back of the neck. Estrogens can be used as in the bitch, but they are not recommended. Megestrol acetate in a single oral dose of 2.0 mg during estrus has been reported to prevent implantation. Prostaglandins can be used to terminate pregnancy after 30 to 35 days of gestation. The dose is similar to that used in the treatment of pyometra.

THE MALE (TOM)

ANATOMY AND PHYSIOLOGY

Penis

The feline penis is ventral to the scrotum, is directed backwards, and is within a free prepuce. The cranial two-thirds of the penis has on its surface 100 to 200 cornified papillae. These papillae are 0.75 to 1 mm in length and are directed toward the base of the penis. They are fully developed at sexual maturity (approximately 9 months of age), and their rasping effect may have importance in mating by increasing the stimulus for ovulation (Christiansen, 1984).

Testicles

Androgen concentrations in the testicular vein exceed that assayed in the peripheral blood by as much as 70-fold. Administration of exogenous testosterone may suppress release of hypothalamic GnRH and pituitary LH, interrupting testosterone synthesis by Leydig cells. Consequently, cells undergoing spermatogenesis are deprived of essential testosterone despite exogenous administration. Sterility may result.

The testicles are usually in the scrotum at birth. At the time of the first vaccination and veterinary examination (6 to 8 weeks of age), they are usually easily palpable. Leydig cells mature by 5 months of age, and spermatozoa may be present in the tubules shortly thereafter. Congenital testicular hypoplasia may be the result of fetal or neonatal panleukopenia (Lein and Concannon, 1983), as well as chromosomal abnormalities, especially in tortoise shell–colored tomcats.

EXAMINATION

Scrotum, Testes, Prepuce, and Penis

EXAMINATION. The examination of a tomcat is similar to that of a male dog. The testes should be spherical, smooth, firm, bilaterally symmetrical in size and shape, and nonpainful. The head of the epididymis points dorsocranially, and the body of the epididymis is on the dorsolateral aspect of each testis, with the vas deferens returning along the medial border.

ORCHITIS. Problems encountered include traumatic injuries, resulting in orchitis. Orchitis can be treated with antibiotics and use of moist, warm compresses to maintain cleanliness. Orchitis can also occur secondary to various viruses or bacteria.

CRYPTORCHIDISM. Cryptorchidism, unilateral and bilateral, is not seen frequently (<2% of cats; Millis et al, 1992) but may be an inherited trait. Castration is usually recommended. Testicular tumors are rare.

PENIS AND PREPUCE. Few problems are encountered that involve the penis and prepuce. The major disorders are trauma and urethral obstruction. Urethral obstruction is quite common, and some degree of penile trauma is caused by the obstructive process, the male licking the penis, and the veterinarian relieving the blockage. Usually, gentle handling and time are needed to treat this trauma.

Unsuccessful matings without intromission, in spite of mounting and pelvic thrusting, may be caused by an accumulation of hair around the base of the glans penis. This is easily removed by sliding the ring of hair over the glans after retracting the sheath.

Semen Collection, Storage, and Preservation

MANUAL COLLECTION. It has been estimated that 20% of tomcats can be trained to ejaculate into an artificial vagina (Shille and Sojka, 1995). The artificial vagina consists of a 1-ml rubber pipette bulb with the end cut off, fitted onto a small test tube. This apparatus can be placed in a water jacket consisting of a 60-ml plastic bottle filled with warm (52° C) water. The rolled end of the bulb is stretched over the rim of the plastic bottle. When the tomcat mounts a teaser queen and an erection develops, the lubricated artificial vagina is slipped onto the penis and the ejaculate is collected within a brief time (seconds). Normal volume of semen is approximately 0.2 to 0.8 ml.

ELECTROEJACULATION. Under total anesthesia, a Teflon rectal probe has been used to ejaculate tomcats. The probe is 10 mm × 12 cm and has three longitudinal stainless steel electrodes, 5 cm in length apiece. Stimuli of 1 to 8 V and 5 to 250 mA are applied (Christiansen, 1984). In one report, each electroejaculation consisted of a series of 60 stimuli. Each series used a sinusoidal waveform at a frequency of 30 Hz. The first 40 stimuli were given at 2.0 V, 20 to 30 mA, and these were followed immediately with 20 stimuli at 3.0 V, 30 to 40 mA. There was an interval of approximately 2 seconds between stimuli of each series. The lubricated probe was inserted into the rectum to a depth of 6 cm and directed ventrally (Pineda et al, 1984).

SEMEN ANALYSIS. The ejaculate obtained with an artificial vagina usually has 0.15 to 13.0×10^6 total sperm, a volume of 0.02 to 0.12 ml, and motility in 60% to 95% of the sperm. An aliquot of 0.005 ml can be used for evaluation. Fewer than 10% morphologically abnormal sperm are usually detected. The ejaculate obtained with electroejaculation is similar except that the volume is usually greater (0.05 to 0.14 ml; Pineda et al, 1984). Electroejaculation can be performed once weekly, whereas ejaculate can be collected from a tomcat using an artificial vagina several times a week. Semen evaluation is completed as described for the male dog (see Chapter 32).

SEMEN ANALYSIS AFTER NATURAL BREEDING. Immediately following natural breeding, a moistened cotton swab can be inserted into the vaginal vault, as is done when obtaining vaginal cytology. The cotton is rolled along a slide, which can then be checked for sperm.

SEMEN STORAGE. Successful overnight storage has been accomplished by extending feline semen immediately after collection in TEST buffer with 20% yolk and keeping it at 4° C. For cryopreservation, 5% glycerol was added to the extended semen and the suspension placed into straws or pellets for liquid nitrogen storage (Dooley et al, 1983; 1986; Howard et al, 1986; Pope et al, 1991).

ARTIFICIAL INSEMINATION. See page 1027.

INFERTILITY

Only limited information is available on infertility in tomcats. The differential diagnosis is similar to that seen in male dogs. Intersex conditions do exist, especially with the so-called Calico. A diagnosis is not often made, but a cat placed in a new or unfamiliar environment may show decreased sexual drive for 1 to 2 months. An aggressive or dominant queen can discourage an inexperienced male, as can restricted movement due to continual housing in a cage (Christiansen, 1984). As with any animal, nutrition, exercise, environment, presence of parasites or illnesses, heat or cold, show circuits, and a variety of other stresses may affect libido and fertility.

The role of the tomcat in venereal spread of infectious disease is not known. It is wise to ascertain that the male has no obvious infectious diseases and that he is adequately vaccinated. In-house healthy cats should be used for breeding, or a quarantine period of at least 2 weeks should follow every contact outside the cattery.

REFERENCES

Banks DR: Physiology and endocrinology of the feline estrous cycle. *In* Morrow DE (ed): Current Therapy in Theriogenology. Philadelphia, WB Saunders Co, 1986, p 795.

Beck KA, et al: Ultrasound prediction of parturition in queens. Vet Radiol 31:32, 1990.

Chastain CB, et al: Adrenocortical suppression in cats given megestrol acetate. Am J Vet Res 42:2029, 1981.

Chen JC, Bellenger CR: Obese appearance, mammary development and retardation of hair growth following megestrol acetate administration to cats. J Small Anim Pract 28:1161, 1987.

Christiansen IJ: Reproduction in the Dog and Cat. London, Bailliere Tindall, 1984.

Clemetson LL, Ward ACS: Bacterial flora of the vagina and uterus of healthy cats. JAVMA 196:902, 1990.

Colby ED: Infertility and disease problems. *In* Morrow DE (ed): Current Therapy in Theriogenology. Philadelphia, WB Saunders Co, 1980a, p 869.

Colby ED: The estrous cycle and pregnancy. *In* Morrow DE (ed): Current Therapy in Theriogenology. Philadelphia, WB Saunders Co, 1980b, p 832.

Concannon PW, et al: Reflex LH release in estrous cats following single and multiple copulations. Biol Reprod 23:111, 1980.

Concannon PW, Lein DH: Feline reproduction. *In* Kirk RW (ed): Current Veterinary Therapy VIII. Philadelphia, WB Saunders Co, 1983, p 932.

Davidson AP, et al: Pregnancy diagnosis with ultrasound in the domestic cat. Vet Radiol 27:109, 1986.

Davidson AP, et al: Treatment of pyometra in cats, using prostaglandin F_{2alpha}: 21 cases (1982–1990). JAVMA 200:825, 1992.

Di Zerega GS, Hodgen GD: Luteal phase dysfunction: A sequel to aberrant folliculogenesis. Fertil Steril 35:489, 1981.

Donoghue AM, et al: Influence of gonadotropin treatment interval on follicular maturation, in vitro fertilization, circulating steroid concentrations, and subsequent luteal function in the domestic cat. Biol Reprod 46:972, 1992.

Dooley MP, et al: An electroejaculator for the collection of semen from the domestic cat. Theriogenology 20:297, 1983.

Dooley MP, et al: Effect of method of collection on seminal characteristics of the domestic cat. Am J Vet Res 47:286, 1986.

Eigenmann JE: Growth hormone and insulin-like growth factor in the dog: Clinical and experimental investigations. Domest Anim Endocrinol 2:1, 1985.

Goodrow KL, et al: A comparison of embryo recovery, embryo quality, estradiol-17 beta and P4 profiles in domestic cats (Felis catus) at natural and induced oestrus. J Reprod Fertil 82:553, 1988.

Henik RA, et al: Progesterone therapy in cats. Compend Cont Educ 7:132, 1985.

Herron MA: Infertility from noninfectious causes. *In* Morrow DA (ed): Current Therapy in Theriogenology. Philadelphia, WB Saunders Co, 1986, p 829.

Howard JG, et al: Semen collection, analysis and cryopreservation in non-domestic animals. *In* Morrow DE (ed): Current Therapy in Theriogenology. Philadelphia, WB Saunders Co, 1986, p 1047.

Howard JG, et al: The effect of preovulatory anaesthesia on ovulation in laparoscopically inseminated domestic cats. J Reprod Fertil 96:175, 1992.

Hurni H: Day length and breeding in the domestic cat. Lab Anim 15:229, 1981.

Johnson LM, Gay VL: Luteinizing hormone in the cat. II. Mating-induced secretion. Endocrinology 109:247, 1981.

Johnston SD: Management of pregnancy disorders in the bitch and queen. *In* Kirk RW (ed): Current Veterinary Therapy VIII. Philadelphia, WB Saunders Co, 1983, p 952.

Johnston SD, et al: X-Chromosome monosomy (37, XO) in a Burmese cat with gonadal dysgenesis. JAVMA 182:986, 1983.

Kwochka KW, Short BG: Cutaneous xanthomatosis and diabetes mellitus following long-term therapy with megestrol acetate in a cat. Compend Cont Educ 6:185, 1984.

Laliberte L: Pregnancy, obstetrics, and postpartum management of the queen. *In* Morrow DE (ed): Current Therapy in Theriogenology. Philadelphia, WB Saunders Co, 1986, p 812.

Lawler DF, et al: Histopathologic features, environmental factors and serum estrogen, progesterone and prolactin values associated with ovarian phase and inflammatory uterine disease in cats. Am J Vet Res 52:1747, 1991.

Lein DH, Concannon PW: Infertility and fertility treatments and management in the queen and tomcat. *In* Kirk RW (ed): Current Veterinary Therapy VIII. Philadelphia, WB Saunders Co, 1983, p 936.

Loar AS: Tumors of the genital system and mammary glands. *In* Ettinger SJ (ed): Textbook of Veterinary Internal Medicine. Philadelphia, WB Saunders Co, 1989, p 1814.

Lofstedt RM: The estrous cycle of the domestic cat. Compend Cont Educ 4:52, 1982.

McEntee K: Reproductive Pathology of Domestic Animals. New York, Academic Press, 1990.

Millis DL, et al: Cryptorchidism and monorchism in cats: 25 cases (1980–1989). JAVMA 200:1128, 1992.

Nelson RW, et al: Treatment of canine pyometra and endometritis with prostaglandin F_2 alpha. JAVMA 181:899, 1982.

Nicholas FW, et al: An XXY male Burmese cat. J Hered 71:52, 1980.

Olson PN, et al: A need for sterilization, contraceptives and abortifacients: Abandoned and unwanted pets. Part II. Contraceptives. Compend Cont Educ 98:173, 1986.

Pineda MH, et al: Long-term study on the effects of electroejaculation on seminal characteristics of the domestic cat. Am J Vet Res 45:1038, 1984.

Pope CE, et al: Semen storage in the domestic felid: A comparison of cryopreservation methods and storage temperatures [abstract]. Biol Reprod 44:117, 1991.

Potter K, et al: Clinical and pathologic features of endometrial hyperplasia, pyometra, and endometritis in cats: 79 cases (1980–1985). JAVMA 198:1427, 1991.

Romantowski J: Use of megestrol acetate in cats. JAVMA 194:700, 1989.

Schulman J, Levine SH: Pyometra involving uterus masculinus in a cat. JAVMA 194:690, 1989.

Shille VM, et al: Follicular function in the domestic cat as determined by estradiol-17□ concentrations in plasma: Relation to estrous behavior and cornification of exfoliated vaginal epithelium. Biol Reprod 21:953, 1979.

Shille VM, Sojka NJ: Feline reproduction. *In* Ettinger SJ, Feldman EC (eds): Textbook of Veterinary Internal Medicine. Philadelphia, WB Saunders Co, 1995, p 1690.

Taubert HD: Luteal phase inadequacy: A quest for new insights. *In* Taubert HD, Kuhl H (eds): The Inadequate Luteal Phase. Lancaster, England, MTP Press Ltd, 1984, p 1.

Thatcher MJD, et al: Characterization of feline conceptus proteins during pregnancy. Biol Reprod 44:108, 1991.

Vasseur PB, Feldman EC: Pyometra associated with extrauterine pregnancy in a cat. JAAHA 18:870, 1982.

Voith VL: Female reproductive behavior. *In* Morrow DE (ed): Current Therapy in Theriogenology. Philadelphia, WB Saunders Co, 1980, p 839.

Wildt DE, Lawler DF: Laparoscopic sterilization of the bitch and queen by uterine horn occlusion. Am J Vet Res 46:864, 1985.

INDEX*